DISORDERS OF THE SHOULDER

Diagnosis and Management

DISORDERS OF THE SHOULDER

Diagnosis and Management

Edited by

Joseph P. Iannotti, M.D., Ph.D.
Professor of Orthopaedic Surgery
Chief, Shoulder and Elbow Service
Penn Musculoskeletal Institute
University of Pennsylvania Health System
Philadelphia, Pennsylvania

Gerald R. Williams, Jr., M.D.
Associate Professor of Orthopaedic Surgery
Shoulder and Elbow Service
Penn Musculoskeletal Institute
University of Pennsylvania Health System
Philadelphia, Pennsylvania

Illustrations by Jennifer Smith, AMI

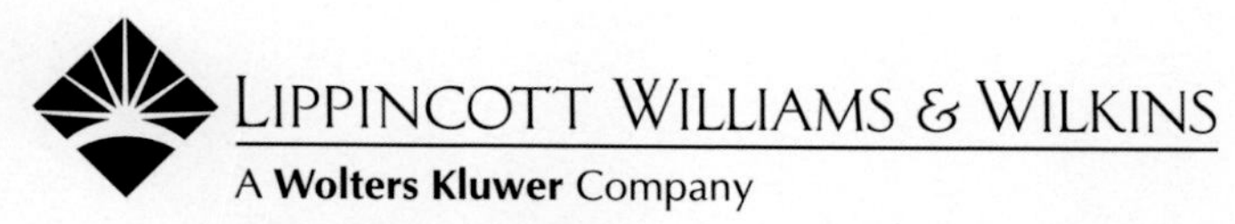

Acquisitions Editor: Danette Knopp
Developmental Editor: Juleann Dob
Manufacturing Manager: Timothy Reynolds
Production Manager: Jodi Borgenicht
Production Editor: Karen G. Edmonson
Cover Designer: Patricia Gast
Indexer: Pamela Edwards
Compositor: Maryland Composition Inc.
Printer: Imago

Printed and bound in Singapore

9 8 7 6 5 4 3 2 1

Library of Congress Cataloging-in-Publication Data

Disorders of the shoulder : diagnosis and management / edited by Joseph P. Iannotti and Gerald R. Williams, Jr ; illustrations by Jennifer Smith.
p. cm.
Includes bibliographical references and index.
ISBN 0-7817-1320-X
1. Shoulder—Surgery. 2. Shoulder—Diseases. I. Iannotti, Joseph P. II. Williams, Gerald R., 1958– .
[DNLM: 1. Shoulder—surgery. 2. Shoulder Joint—surgery. 3. Joint Diseases—surgery. 4. Joint Diseases—diagnosis. WE 810D612 1999]
RD557.5.D56 1999
617.5′72–dc21
DNLM/DLC
for Library of Congress 98-37040
CIP

To our wives Robin Williams and Cindy Iannotti.
We thank them for their support and patience without which we would have not been able or willing to start or complete this work;

To our children Alexis and Mark Williams and Matthew Iannotti.
To our parents for their unending encouragement and support.
We are truly fortunate to have such warm and loving families; and

To our mentors and teachers for their support, knowledge, and friendship.

Contents

Part VII. Sternoclavicular Joint

Part VIII. Neuromuscular Disorders and the Scapulothoracic Articulation

Part IX. Arthroscopy and Imaging

Part X. Neoplasms

Part XI. Infection

Part XII. Rehabilitation

Part XIII. Outcome Measurement

Part XIV. Pain Management

Contributing Authors

Julian S. Arroyo, M.D.
Lakewood Orthopaedic Surgeons
5605 100th Street Southwest
Tacoma, Washington 98499

Louis U. Bigliani, M.D.
Professor and Chairman of Orthopaedic Surgery
Department of Orthopaedic Surgery
Columbia University, College of Physicians and Surgeons
Chief, The Shoulder Service
Columbia-Presbyterian Medical Center
161 Fort Washington Avenue, Room 245
New York, New York 10032

Randip Bindra, M.D.
Consultant Orthopaedic Surgeon
Department of Orthopaedic Surgery
Gwynedd Hospitals NHS Trust
Bangor, United Kingdom LL572PW

Mark K. Bowen, M.D.
Assistant Professor
Northwestern University
Attending Orthopaedic Surgeon
Northwestern Memorial Hospital
211 East Chicago Avenue, #1336
Chicago, Illinois 60611

Anthony R. Brown, M.D.
Associate Clinical Professor of Anesthesiology
Department of Anesthesiology
Director, Orthopaedic and Regional Anesthesia
Columbia-Presbyterian Medical Center
630 West 168th Street
New York, New York 10032

Wayne Z. Burkhead, Jr., M.D.
W.B. Carrell Memorial Clinic
2909 Lemmon Avenue
Dallas, Texas 75204

Win Chang, M.D.
Attending Physician
Department of Orthopaedic Surgery
Putnam Hospital Center
Stoneleigh Avenue
Carmel, New York 10512

Anthony J. Checroun, M.D.
Shoulder Fellow
Shoulder Service
New York University Hospital for Joint Diseases
301 East 17th Street
New York, New York 10003

Robert H. Cofield, M.D.
Professor
Mayo Medical School
Department of Orthopaedics
The Mayo Clinic and Mayo Foundation
200 First Street, Southwest
Rochester, Minnesota 55905

Brian J. Cole, M.D.
Department of Orthopaedics
Rush-Presbyterian-St. Luke's Medical Center
Chicago, Illinois 60612

David N. Collins, M.D.
Clinical Assistant Professor
Department of Orthopaedic Surgery
University of Arkansas for Medical Sciences
4301 West Markham
Little Rock, Arkansas 72205

Frank A. Cordasco, M.D.
Assistant Clinical Professor
Department of Orthopaedic Surgery
Columbia University College of Physicians and Surgeons
St. Luke's-Roosevelt Hospital Center
Columbia-Presbyterian Medical Center
343-345 West 58th Street
New York, New York 10019

Frances Cuomo, M.D.
Assistant Professor
Department of Orthopaedic Surgery
New York University
Chief, Shoulder Service
New York University Hospital for Joint Diseases
301 East 17th Street
New York, New York 10003

Donald F. D'Alessandro, M.D.
Chief
Sports Medicine and Shoulder Service
Carolinas Medical Center
Associate, Miller Orthopaedic Clinic
1001 Blythe Boulevard, Suite 200
Charlotte, North Carolina 28203

Jeffrey J. Eckardt, M.D.
Professor
Department of Orthopaedic Surgery
UCLA Medical Center
Box 956902, 10833 Le Conte Avenue
Los Angeles, California 90095-6902

John L. Esterhai, Jr., M.D.
Associate Professor
Department of Orthopaedic Surgery
Hospital of the University of Pennsylvania
3400 Spruce Street
Philadelphia, Pennsylvania 19104

John M. Fenlin, Jr., M.D.
Clinical Professor
Department of Orthopaedic Surgery
Jefferson Medical College
Walnut Street
Philadelphia, Pennsylvania 19107

F. Michael Ferrante, M.D.
Associate Professor
Department of Anesthesia and Medicine
University of Pennsylvania School of Medicine
Director, Pain Medicine Center
Hospital of the University of Pennsylvania
3400 Spruce Street
Philadelphia, Pennsylvania 19104

Evan L. Flatow, M.D.
Professor of Orthopaedics
Chief of the Shoulder Service
Mount Sinai Medical Center
5 East 98th Street
New York, New York 10029

Barbara Frieman, M.D.
Clinical Associate Professor
Department of Orthopaedic Surgery
Jefferson Medical College
Walnut Street
Philadelphia, Pennsylvania 19107

Christian Gerber, M.D.
Professor and Chairman
Department of Orthopaedics
University of Zürich
Balgrist
Forchstrasse 340
8008 Zürich, Switzerland

Thomas P. Goss, M.D.
Professor of Orthopaedic Surgery
Department of Orthopaedic Surgery
University of Massachusetts Medical School
55 Lake Avenue North
Worcester, Massachusetts 01655

Sean M. Griggs, M.D.
Park Plaza Hand and Upper Extremity Center
1200 Binz Street, Suite 1200
Houston, Texas 77004

Dan Guttmann, M.D.
Resident, Orthopaedic Surgery
Department of Orthopaedic Surgery
Albert Einstein Medical Center
5501 Old York Road WCB/4
Philadelphia, Pennsylvania 19141

Shawn P. Hennigan, M.D.
Chief Resident, Department of Orthopaedic Surgery
Rush-Presbyterian-St. Luke's Medical Center,
1725 W. Harrison Street, Suite 1063
Chicago, Illinois 60612

G. Brian Holloway, M.D.
Knoxville Orthopaedic Clinic
1128 Weisgarber Road
Knoxville, Tennessee 37909

Joseph P. Iannotti, M.D., Ph.D.
Professor of Orthopaedic Surgery
Department of Orthopaedic Surgery
Chief, Shoulder and Elbow Service
Penn Musculoskeletal Institute
University of Pennsylvania Health System
One Cupp Pavilion, 39th and Market Streets
Philadelphia, Pennsylvania 19104

Christopher Jobe, M.D.
Professor
Department of Orthopaedic Surgery
Loma Linda University School of Medicine
11234 Anderson Street
Loma Linda, California 92350

Jesse B. Jupiter, M.D.
Chief of Hand Surgery Service
Massachusetts General Hospital
15 Parkman Street, ACC 527
Boston, Massachusetts 02114

Martin Kelley, M.S.
Musculoskeletal Team Leader
Department of Occupational and Physical Therapy
University of Pennsylvania Medical Center
3400 Spruce Street
Philadelphia, Pennsylvania 19104

John J. Klimkiewicz, M.D.
Department of Orthopaedic Surgery
Penn Musculoskeletal Institute
Presbyterian Medical Center
One Cupp Pavilion
39th and Market Streets
Philadelphia, Pennsylvania 19104

J. Bruce Kneeland, M.D.
Associate Professor of Radiology
Department of Radiology
Hospital of the University of Pennsylvania
3400 Spruce Street
Philadelphia, Pennsylvania 19104

Scott H. Kozin, M.D.
Assistant Professor
Department of Orthopaedic Surgery
Temple University Hospital
9331 Old Bustleson Avenue
Philadelphia, Pennsylvania 19115

John E. Kuhn, M.D.
Assistant Professor
Section of Orthopaedic Surgery
The University of Michigan Shoulder Group
24 Frank Lloyd Wright Drive
Ann Arbor, Michigan 48106-0363

Mark D. Lazarus, M.D.
Clinical Assistant Professor
Department of Orthopaedic Surgery
Temple University School of Medicine
Attending-Director of Shoulder and Elbow Surgery
Albert Einstein Medical Center
5501 Old York Road, WCB/4
Philadelphia, Pennsylvania 19141

Brian G. Leggin
Senior III Physical Therapist
Penn Therapy and Fitness
University of Pennsylvania Medical Center
3624 Market Street
Philadelphia, Pennsylvania 19104

Leslie S. Matthews, M.D.
Department of Orthopaedic Surgery
The Union Memorial Hospital
3333 North Calvert Street
Suite 400, Baltimore, Maryland 21218

Patrick J. McMahon, M.D.
Assistant Professor
Department of Orthopaedic Surgery
University of California Irvine
101 City Drive
Orange, California 92668

Tom R. Norris, M.D.
Department of Orthopaedic Surgery
California-Pacific Medical Center
2351 Clay Street, Suite 510
San Francisco, California 94115-1931

Gordon W. Nuber, M.D.
Associate Professor
Department of Orthopaedic Surgery
Northwestern University Medical School
211 East Chicago Avenue #1336
Chicago, Illinois 60611

Peter J. O'Rourke, M.D.
W.B. Carrell Memorial Clinic
2909 Lemmon Avenue
Dallas, Texas 75204

Lucas J. Pavlovich, Jr., M.D.
Department of Orthopaedic Surgery
The Union Memorial Hospital
3333 N. Calvert Street
Baltimore, Maryland 21218

Matthew D. Pepe, M.D.
Clinical Instructor
Department of Orthopaedic Surgery
University of Pennsylvania School of Medicine
Chief Resident
Hospital of the University of Pennsylvania
3400 Spruce Street
Philadelphia, Pennsylvania 19104

Matthew L. Ramsey, M.D.
Assistant Professor
Department of Orthopaedic Surgery
Shoulder and Elbow Service
Penn Musculoskeletal Institute
University of Pennsylvania Health System
One Cupp Pavilion
39th and Market Streets
Philadelphia, Pennsylvania 19104

Robin R. Richards, M.D.
Professor
Department of Surgery
Head, Division of Orthopaedic Surgery
St. Michael's Hospital
30 Bond Street
Toronto, Ontario, Canada

David Ring, M.D.
Resident
Department of Orthopaedics
Harvard University School of Medicine
Department of Orthopaedic Surgery
Massachusetts General Hospital
15 Parkman Street
Boston, Massachusetts 02114

Charles A. Rockwood, Jr., M.D.
Professor and Chairman Emeritus
Department of Orthopaedics
University of Texas Health Science Center at San Antonio
7703 Floyd Curl Drive, San Antonio, Texas 78284-7774

Anthony A. Romeo, M.D.
Assistant Professor
Department of Orthopaedic Surgery
Rush Medical College
Rush-Presbyterian/St. Lukes Medical Center
1725 West Harrison Street, Suite 1063
Chicago, Illinois 60612-3828

Thomas Schenk, M.D.
Fellow, Shoulder and Elbow Service
Department of Orthopaedic Surgery
Hospital of the University of Pennsylvania
3400 Spruce Street
Philadelphia, Pennsylvania 19104

Jerry S. Sher, M.D.
Clinical Assistant Professor
Department of Orthopaedics and Rehabilitation
University of Miami School of Medicine
Shoulder and Knee Institute of Florida
250 63rd Street, Morris Tower, 9-A
Miami Beach, Florida 33141

John G. Skedros, M.D.
Department of Orthopaedic Surgery
Ogden Clinic
4650 South Harrison Boulevard
Ogden, Utah 84403

John W. Sperling, M.D.
Resident, Orthopaedic Surgery
Department of Orthopaedics
Mayo Clinic and Mayo Foundation
200 First Street, Southwest
Rochester, Minnesota 55905

Virak Tan, M.D.
Instructor in Orthopaedics
Department of Orthopaedic Surgery
University Pennsylvania School of Medicine
3400 Spruce Street
Philadelphia, Pennsylvania 19104

James E. Tibone, M.D.
Professor
Department of Orthopaedics
University of Southern California
1510 San Pablo, #322
Los Angeles, California 90033

Jon J.P. Warner, M.D.
Chief, Shoulder Service
Department of Orthopaedics
Massachusetts General Hospital
275 Cambridge Street
Boston, Massachusetts 02114

Gerald R. Williams, Jr., M.D.
Associate Professor of Orthopaedic Surgery
Shoulder and Elbow Service
Department of Orthopaedic Surgery
Penn Musculoskeletal Institute
University of Pennsylvania Health System
One Cupp Pavilion, 39th and Market Streets
Philadelphia, Pennsylvania 19104

Phillip Wirganowicz, M.D.
Assistant Professor
Department of Orthopaedic Surgery
Hospital of the University of Pennsylvania
3400 Spruce Street
2 Silverstein Pavilion
Philadelphia, Pennsylvania 19104

Michael A. Wirth, M.D.
Chief, Shoulder Service
Augie Murphy Veterans Hospital
Associate Professor
Department of Orthopaedics
The University of Texas Health Science Center at San Antonio
7703 Floyd Curl Drive
San Antonio, Texas 78284-7774

Ken Yamaguchi, M.D.
Assistant Professor
Department of Orthopaedic Surgery
Washington University School of Medicine
Chief, Shoulder and Elbow Service
Barnes Jewish Hospital
One Barnes-Jewish Hospital Plaza, Suite 11300, West Pavilion
St. Louis, Missouri 63110

Joshua M. Zimmerman, M.D.
W.B. Carrell Memorial Clinic
2909 Lemmon Avenue
Dallas, Texas 75204

Joseph D. Zuckerman, M.D.
Chief, Shoulder and Elbow Service
Chairman, Department of Orthopaedic Surgery
New York University Hospital for Joint Diseases
301 East 17th Street
New York, New York 10003

Preface

The field of shoulder surgery is a relatively young discipline. As recently as 1975, subspecialty training in shoulder surgery was available only through loosely organized mentoring programs with a small number of individual surgeons who developed special interest and experience in the management of shoulder disorders. Very few textbooks on shoulder surgery existed, and the number of peer-reviewed articles in the orthopaedic literature dealing with shoulder disorders was relatively small.

Interest in the shoulder has increased dramatically over the past 25 years. The number of organized post-graduate fellowships offering subspecialty training in shoulder surgery has grown exponentially. Orthopaedic residency programs are also providing greater diversity of experience in treating shoulder pathology than ever before. Continuing medical education courses devoted to shoulder disorders are becoming increasingly popular and are often oversubscribed. Moreover, the amount of peer-reviewed literature dealing with the shoulder has increased so dramatically, that there is now a subspecialty journal devoted exclusively to shoulder and elbow research, both basic science and clinical. The end result of this explosion of information is an increase in the number of orthopaedic surgeons who are well trained in shoulder surgery. Most importantly, our patients have enjoyed the benefits of improved quality-of-life and function as a result of our better understanding of their shoulder conditions.

The current expansion of the subspecialty of shoulder surgery would not have been possible without the tireless efforts of a few pioneering surgeons in the United States and abroad. We owe a great deal of gratitude to these dedicated individuals who strove to advance the understanding of shoulder disorders through their teaching and writing. This textbook was written in the spirit of education that these dedicated scientists and clinicians fostered.

Our goal in compiling this text is to bring to a single comprehensive source the most current information available with regard to not only the basic concepts of diagnosis and management of common shoulder disorders, but also the more complex and controversial issues in adult shoulder reconstruction. We have attempted to assemble a group of authors with varied backgrounds and perspectives who share the common characteristics of excellence in their field and dedication to the art of teaching. Wherever possible, the format of the chapters has been standardized for the sake of uniformity. The bibliographies are intended to be complete reference sources for the initiated reader, but not so exhaustive as to be unmanageable. A unique feature of this text is the inclusion of treatment algorithms within each clinical chapter. We have found the systematic approach to the diagnosis and management of shoulder disorders to be rewarding and hope that the inclusion of these treatment algorithms is useful.

The CD-ROM which accompanies this text is in many ways complimentary to, rather than exclusive from, the traditional printed version. In addition to a complete electronic duplication of the printed text and figures, the CD-ROM contains modules dedicated to regional anatomy, clinical case examples, surgical footage of common procedures, and full text versions of selected references.

We believe that many of the concepts in this book will be valid for many years to come, but understand and hope that others will change in future years through continued research and clinical observations. The reader is encouraged to utilize the textbook to lay a foundation of knowledge that should be modified and updated through the continued advances of our understanding of the shoulder.

Joseph P. Iannotti, M.D., Ph.D.
Gerald R. Williams, Jr., M.D.

Acknowledgments

We acknowledge the work, dedication, and efforts of Danette Knopp and Julie Dob at Lippincott Williams & Wilkins. Their dedication to this textbook has resulted in what we believe to be a high quality, state-of-the-art publication. We sincerely thank them for all of their hard work. This textbook was also published and expanded in a CD-ROM at Lippincott Williams & Wilkins. We acknowledge the expertise and efforts of the staff in production of the CD-ROM. We would also like to acknowledge the contribution of Jennifer Smith whose artistic interpretation of many crude sketches enhanced this textbook greatly. This book would not have been possible without the work and expertise of the contributing authors. We acknowledge and thank them for their extraordinary efforts.

PART I

Rotator Cuff Diseases and Tendon Rupture

Disorders of the Shoulder: Diagnosis and Management,
edited by Joseph P. Iannotti and Gerald R. Williams, Jr.
Lippincott Williams & Wilkins, Philadelphia © 1999.

CHAPTER 1

Anatomy, Biomechanics, and Pathophysiology of Rotator Cuff Disease

Jerry S. Sher

The rotator cuff remains an area of active interest and research. Increasing information on the anatomy, pathogenesis, etiology, and natural history has improved our understanding of disorders surrounding this structure. Yet, although the function of the cuff and its contribution to maintaining dynamic stability of the glenohumeral joint has been well established, its role in pathologic conditions and its relation to symptomatology is not yet entirely clear. Moreover, despite the level of interest, numerous questions about the origin of rotator cuff tears remain unanswered. Multiple theories including vascular and impingement mechanisms have been implicated, but reports are often conflicting. Consideration of rotator cuff lesions as a result of solely intrinsic or extrinsic factors may be an oversimplification of the disease process. More likely, the heterogeneity of the disorder is a reflection of its multifactorial etiology which, in part, explains the difference in views concerning the origin of these tendon tears. Finally, the natural course of patients with rotator cuff disease can demonstrate considerable variability despite seemingly similar lesions. Its presence in asymptomatic persons raises further questions about diagnosis and treatment as well as causes of symptoms and dysfunction. Through continued investigative efforts, the origin, anatomy, function, and natural history of the rotator cuff and related disorders will be further unfolded.

J. S. Sher: Department of Orthopaedics and Rehabilitation, University of Miami School of Medicine and Shoulder and Knee Institute of Florida, Miami Beach, Florida 33140.

ROTATOR CUFF AND RELATED ANATOMY

Normal

The shoulder comprises a complex of four articulations that, under normal conditions, move in synchrony, affording smooth unhindered motion of the arm. An intricate relation exists between the osseous elements and the surrounding muscles and ligaments. In an attempt to better understand the anatomic arrangement of these structures, an organizational approach to the anatomy of the shoulder has been described.[36] The tissues were grouped into four separate and contiguous layers and demonstrate an alternation between muscular and fibrous elements. Layer 1, the most superficial level, includes the deltoid and pectoralis major muscles. Layer 2 is a continuous fascial layer that extends circumferentially from anterior to posterior and incorporates the clavipectoral and posterior scapular fascia. Layer 3, again a muscular layer, includes the rotator cuff, and layer 4, the deepest level, comprises the fibrous capsular elements. This classification can contribute to a better understanding of the shoulder's complex anatomy and safeguard against deviation from internervous planes during surgical procedures (Fig. 1).

The four muscles that compose the rotator cuff take their origin from the body of the scapula and envelope the humeral head as they insert along the tuberosities of the proximal humerus. The musculotendinous cuff is firmly adherent to the underlying glenohumeral capsule and provides circumferential reinforcement except at the rotator interval and axillary recess. The *rotator interval* is a triangular area

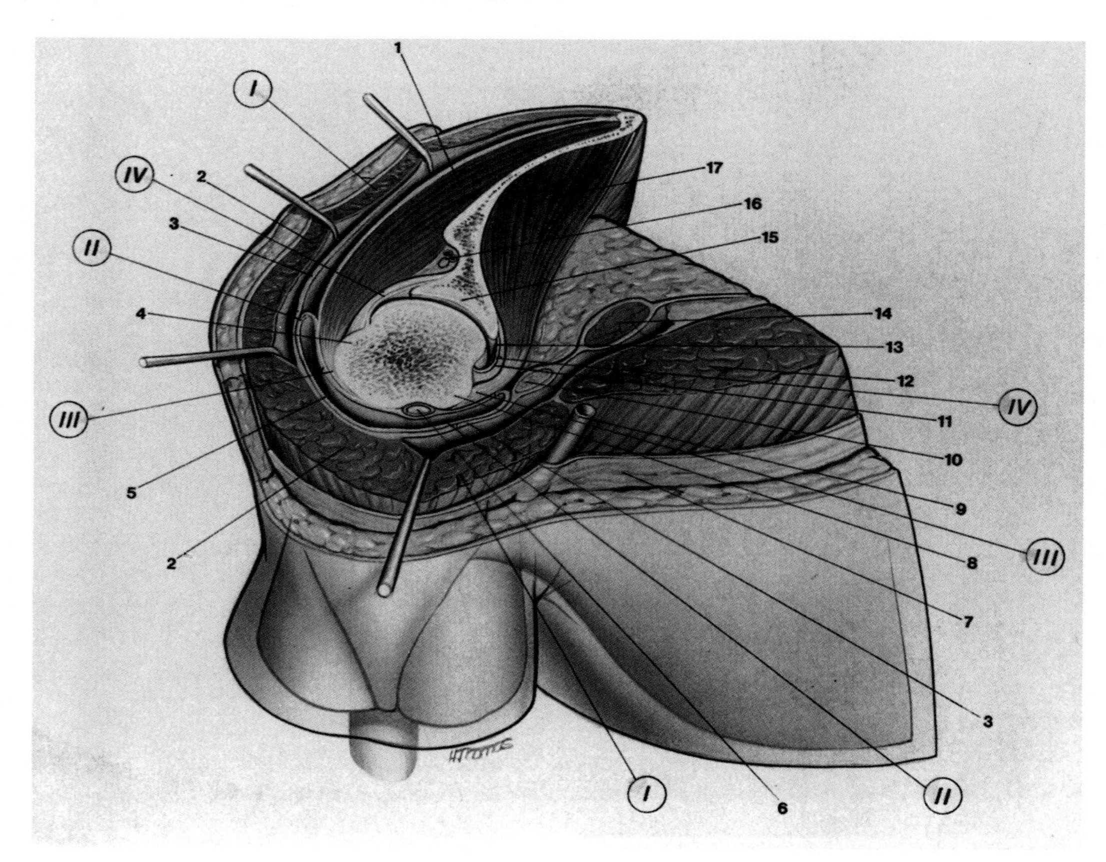

FIG. 1. Supporting layers of the glenohumeral joint: **Layer I**: Deltoid (*2*) and pectoralis major muscles (*12*); **Layer II**: clavipectoral fascia (*3*), conjoined tendon (*10*), coracoacromial ligament, posterior scapular fascia (*3*), and superficial bursal tissue (*5*); **Layer III**: Deep layer of subdeltoid bursa, rotator cuff (*1,17*); **Layer IV**: Glenohumeral joint capsule (*11*), synovium (*13*), coracohumeral ligament. (From ref. 36, with permission.)

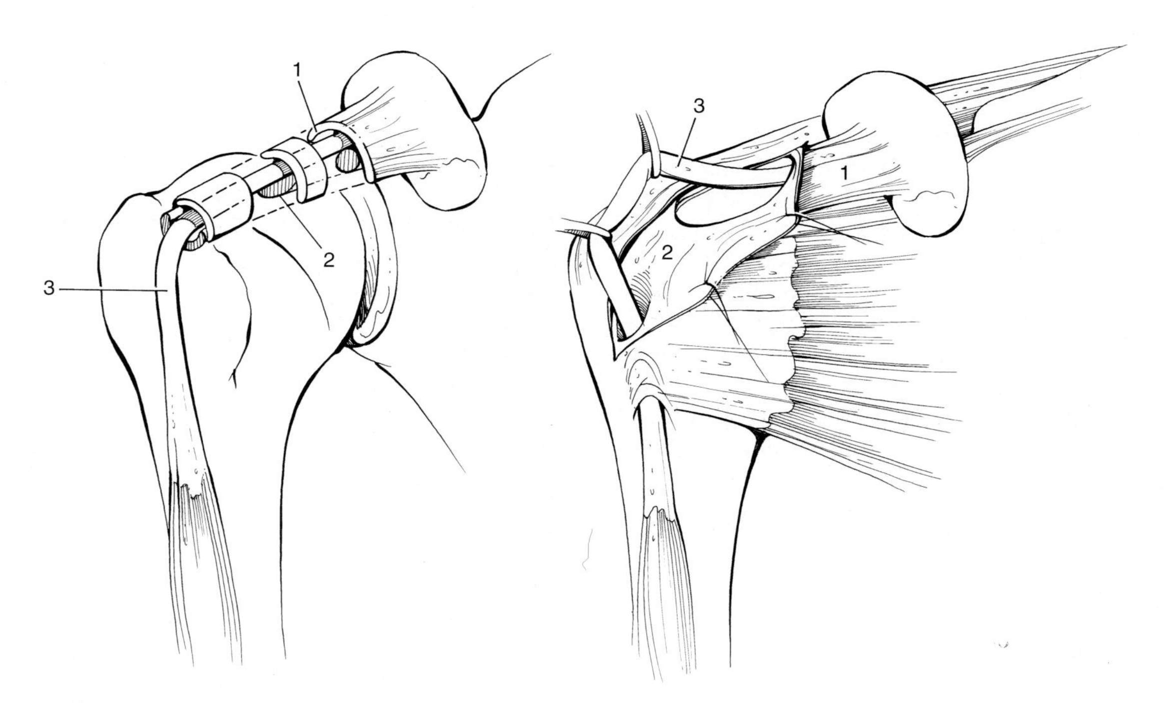

FIG. 2. Anatomy of the rotator interval. Coracohumeral ligament (1); superior glenohumoral ligament (2); bicepss tendon (3). (From Ref. 191, with permission.)

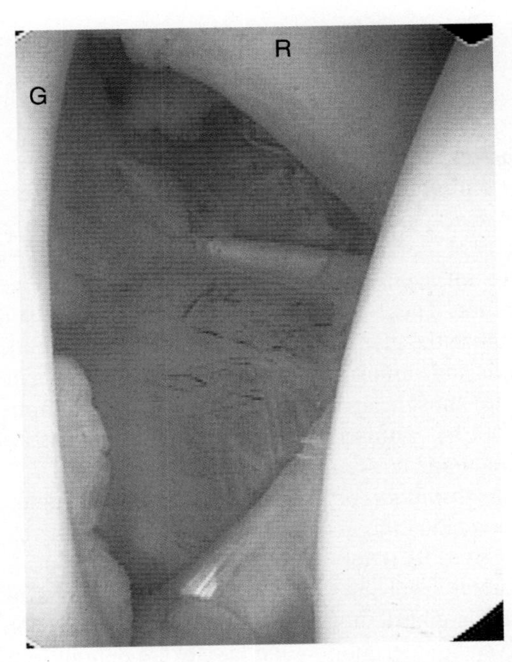

FIG. 3. Region of rotator interval as viewed arthroscopically. Safe portal of entry lies between the biceps tendon (R), upper border of subscapularis tendon (SSc), and glenoid rim (G).

that is made up of fibrous elements and bordered by the upper margin of the subscapularis tendon and anterior aspect of the supraspinatus. Within the interval lie the coracohumeral ligament, the biceps tendon, and the superior glenohumeral ligament. The coracohumeral ligament is seen superficially, whereas the superior glenohumeral ligament reflects around the biceps tendon and serves as an internal pulley at the floor of this space.[191] The coracohumeral and superior glenohumeral ligaments take origin from the lateral base of the coracoid and superior labrum, respectively[66,128] (Fig. 2). In one report, through gross anatomic study, variability was observed at the insertion of the coracohumeral ligament. Seventy-four percent of specimens demonstrated a predominant insertion into the rotator interval; in the remainder, the principal attachment was to the supraspinatus tendon.[128] Multiple functions have been attributed to the coracohumeral ligament, and most notably, they include limitation of external rotation in the adducted arm and restraint against inferior translation.[10,70,72,141,142,143] By serving as a "safe" portal for arthroscopic entry, the rotator interval affords passage into the glenohumeral joint without violation of the rotator cuff tendons. The intraarticular boundaries of this space can be easily visualized arthroscopically and are marked by the glenoid rim, the upper subscapularis tendon, and the intraarticular portion of the biceps tendon (Fig. 3). The *axillary recess*, which also lacks muscular or tendinous coverage by the rotator cuff, demonstrates capsular redundancy at the inferior aspect of the joint. This tissue laxity affords normal arm abduction, whereby patulousness or contracture can mediate joint instability or restriction of motion.

Anteriorly, the *subscapularis* muscle takes its origin along the costal surface of the scapula and inserts onto the lesser tuberosity of the humerus[114] (Fig. 4). It has a dual innervation from both the upper and lower subscapular nerves that arise from the posterior cord of the brachial plexus. The upper subscapular nerve innervates a greater portion of the muscle. Although commonly considered to be an internal ro-

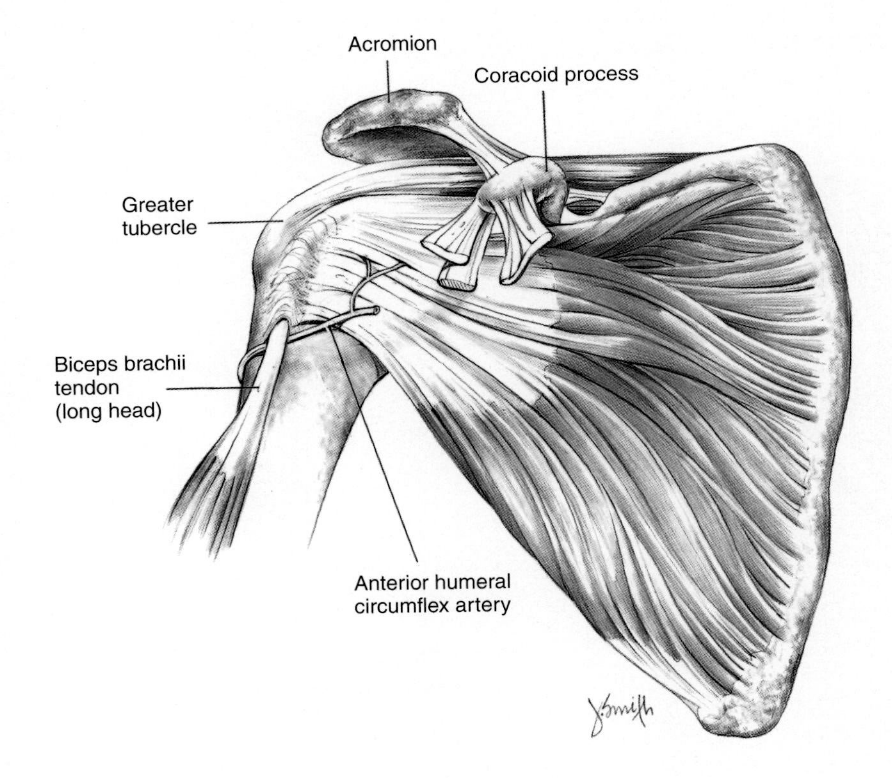

FIG. 4. Anatomical course of the subscapularis muscle.

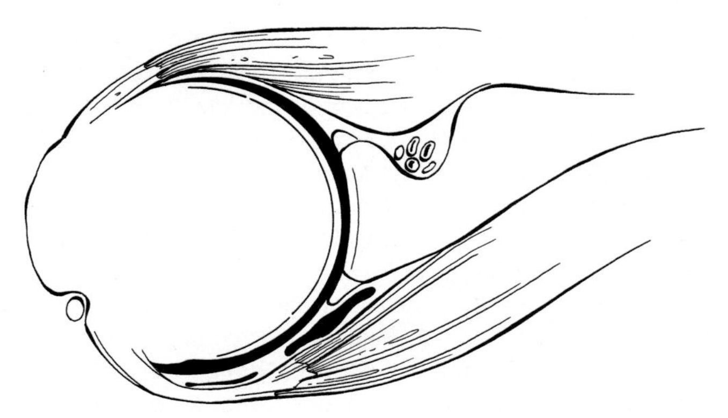

FIG. 5. The subscapularis bursa. Note its subcoracoid location between the glenoid neck and subscapularis muscle belly.

tator of the shoulder, its contribution to arm abduction and humeral head depression have also been emphasized.[81,139,140,171] The subscapularis bursa lies between the subscapularis tendon and neck of the scapula. It is found just inferior to the coracoid process and protects the tendon as it courses along the scapular neck and coracoid.[114] The bursa communicates with the glenohumeral joint capsule and can harbor intraarticular loose bodies (Fig. 5). Zlatkin and colleagues[204] described three areas of capsular insertion along the anterior glenoid neck. A type I capsule is inserted adjacent to the anterior glenoid labrum, whereas types II and III are inserted progressively more medial on the scapular neck. This categorization likely reflects the variation in morphology and size of the subscapular bursa, which can be readily identified on coronal magnetic resonance images (MRIs). While a predisposition to anterior glenohumeral instability in patients with a medial capsular insertion has been suggested, no controlled studies elucidating this issue have yet been conducted.

The *infraspinatus* and *teres minor* muscles make up the posterior portion of the rotator cuff. The infraspinatus is triangular and is often inseparable from the teres minor. They take origin from the infraspinatus fossa and dorsolateral border of the scapula, respectively, and insert onto the greater tuberosity of the humerus.[114] The suprascapular nerve innervates the infraspinatus, and the axillary nerve supplies the teres minor. These muscles externally rotate the humerus and stabilize the glenohumeral joint in concert with the subscapularis and supraspinatus muscles. The infraspinatus has a pennate muscle architecture with a central raphe that should not be confused with the intermuscular interval between it and the teres minor.

The *supraspinatus* originates from the suprascapular fossa and inserts along the greater tuberosity of the humerus (Fig. 6). It receives its innervation from the suprascapular nerve, which arises from the upper trunk of the brachial plexus. This muscle contributes to glenohumeral compression during active shoulder motion and assists the deltoid in effecting humeral abduction.[34,35,78] The supraspinatus is situated between the humeral articular surface and the acromial arch where it is protected by a synovial cavity on either side. The subacromial and subdeltoid bursae are found superficial to the tendon and separate it from the deltoid muscle. The bursa varies in size and extends laterally from the subacromial space to the proximal humeral metaphysis (Fig. 7).

The *suprascapular nerve* arises from the upper trunk of the brachial plexus and courses through the suprascapular notch just medial to the base of the coracoid process. It supplies the supraspinatus muscle before passing through the spinoglenoid notch where it finally provides neural innervation to the infraspinatus (Fig. 8). Warner and associates[193]

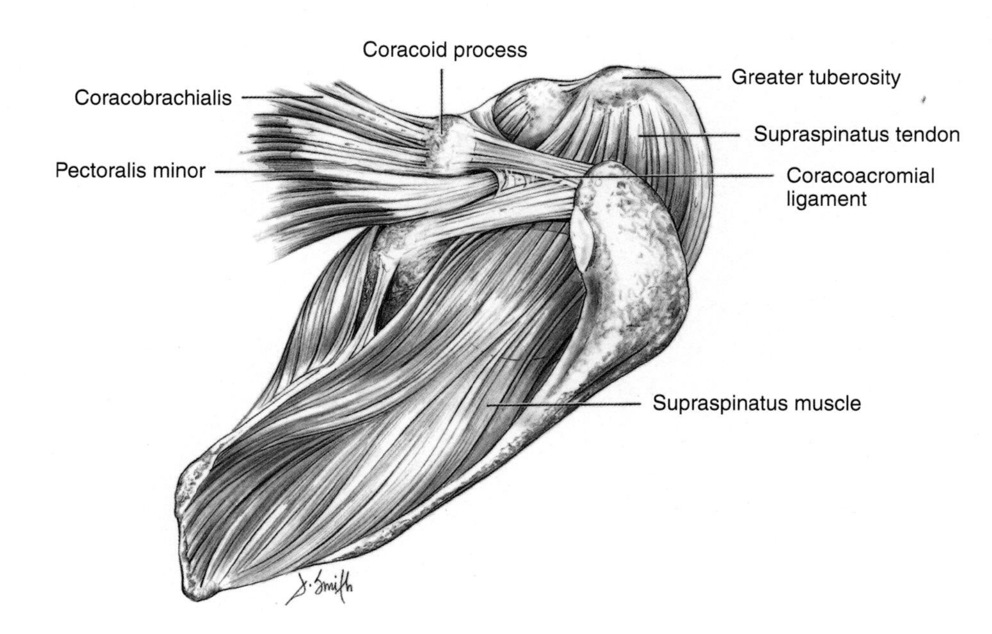

FIG. 6. The coracoacromial arch. Note the Y configuration of the coracoacromial ligament.

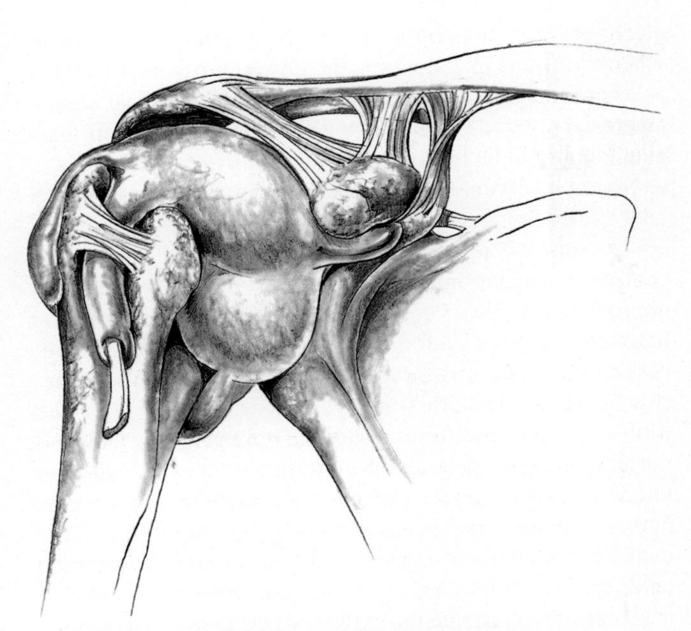

FIG. 7. The subacromial and subdeltoid bursae.

have highlighted the path and variational anatomy of the suprascapular nerve as it enters the posterior aspect of the shoulder. Eighty-four percent of 31 specimens revealed one or two branches of the nerve to the supraspinatus muscle. In 84% of specimens, the first branch originated either under the transverse scapular ligament or 1 mm distal to it. In 3%, the first motor branch originated proximal to the ligament and passed superficial to it. The infraspinatus muscle revealed three to four branches in approximately one-half of the specimens. Bigliani and coworkers[13] measured the distance of the nerve from fixed scapular landmarks and observed that it lay an average of 1.8 cm (range 1.4 to 2.5 cm) from the midposterior glenoid rim to the base of the scapular spine. The distance of the nerve from the supraglenoid tubercle to the base of the scapular spine measured an average of 2.5 cm (range 1.9 to 3.2 cm). These observations emphasize the caution required for surgical management of shoulder disorders such as mobilization of a torn and retracted rotator cuff, arthroscopic portal placement, transglenoid drilling, and neurolysis of an entrapped suprascapular nerve.

Superficial to the subacromial and subdeltoid bursae lies

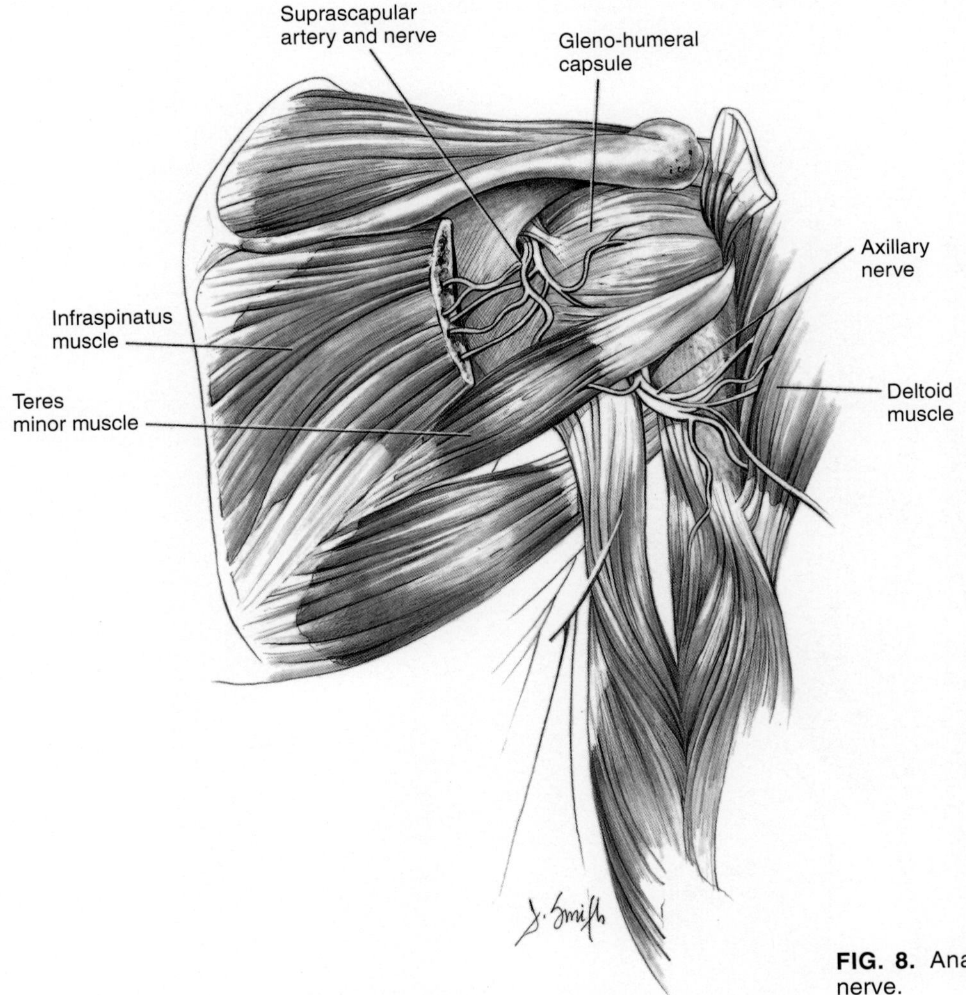

FIG. 8. Anatomic course of the suprascapular nerve.

the *deltoid* muscle. It is composed of three heads (anterior, middle, and posterior) that vary in structure and function. The muscle has an extensive origin, arising from the distal one-third of the clavicle, the acromion, and the lateral one-third of the scapular spine. It converges distally to insert on the deltoid tuberosity of the middiaphysis of the humerus (Fig. 9). Its broad origin, which is derived from the mobile scapula and clavicle, affords the deltoid a mechanical advantage by allowing the muscle to maintain its resting length at various arm positions. Furthermore, the bipennate structure of the large middle head contributes to abduction strength through contraction of its fibers at an angle to the line of pull, which also serves to maintain muscle fiber resting length and improve efficiency. In contrast, muscles with a parallel fiber arrangement, such as the anterior and posterior deltoid, by virtue of their structural configuration, result in considerably decreased strength during contraction.[39]

Differences in activity of the three portions of the deltoid relative to arm position have been observed through electromyographic analysis. The anterior and middle heads remain active at all angles of abduction and in multiple planes (coronal, scapular, and parasagittal), whereas the posterior deltoid, also an important shoulder extensor, contributes to elevation when the arm is above 110 degrees.[173] Moreover, when the arm is in abduction, the posterior deltoid functions as a secondary external rotator, for which its clinical importance is increased in patients with massive rotator cuff tears extending into the infraspinatus and teres minor tendons.

Neural innervation is afforded by the *axillary nerve* which takes a circuitous path before entering the deltoid muscle. It arises from the posterior cord of the brachial plexus and courses across the inferolateral border of the subscapularis approximately 3 to 5 mm medial to the musculotendinous junction.[98] It passes inferior to the glenohumeral axillary recess and exits the quadrangular space, along with the posterior humeral circumflex artery, where it divides into two trunks. The posterior trunk splits and innervates the teres minor and posterior deltoid before terminating as the superior lateral cutaneous nerve. The anterior trunk winds around the humerus and innervates the remaining deltoid muscle. It becomes subfascial and intramuscular at a point between the anterior and middle heads[24] (Fig. 10). Burkhead and colleagues[24] observed that the axillary nerve can occupy a position as close as 3.1 cm from the lateral tip of the acromion and that in 20% of specimens it was less than the generally accepted 5–cm distance.[1]

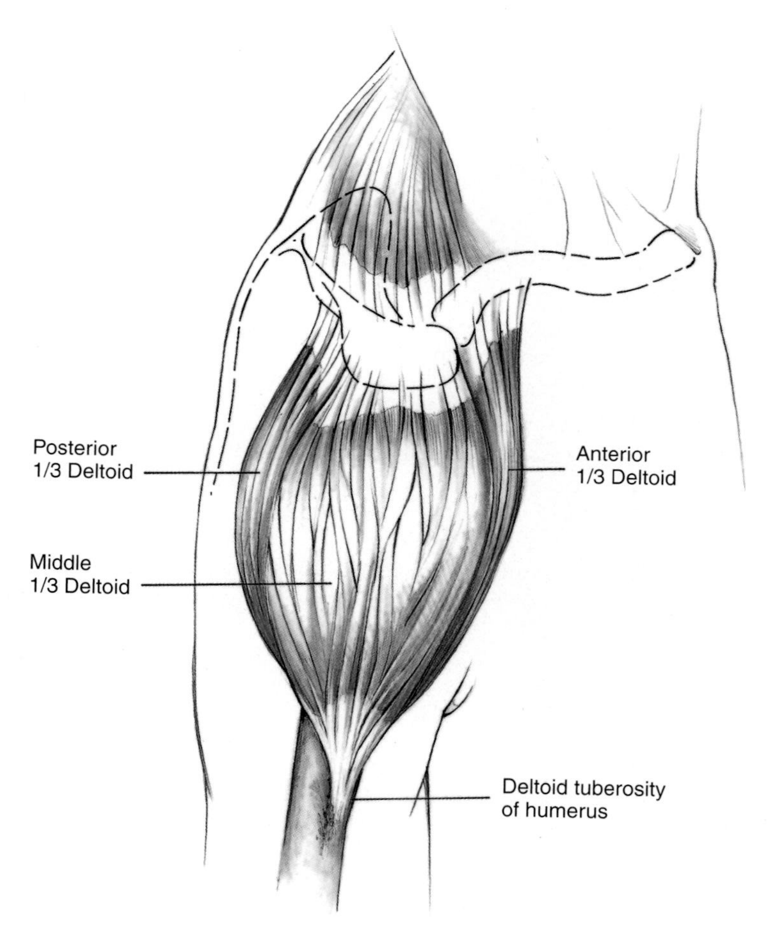

FIG. 9. The deltoid muscle.

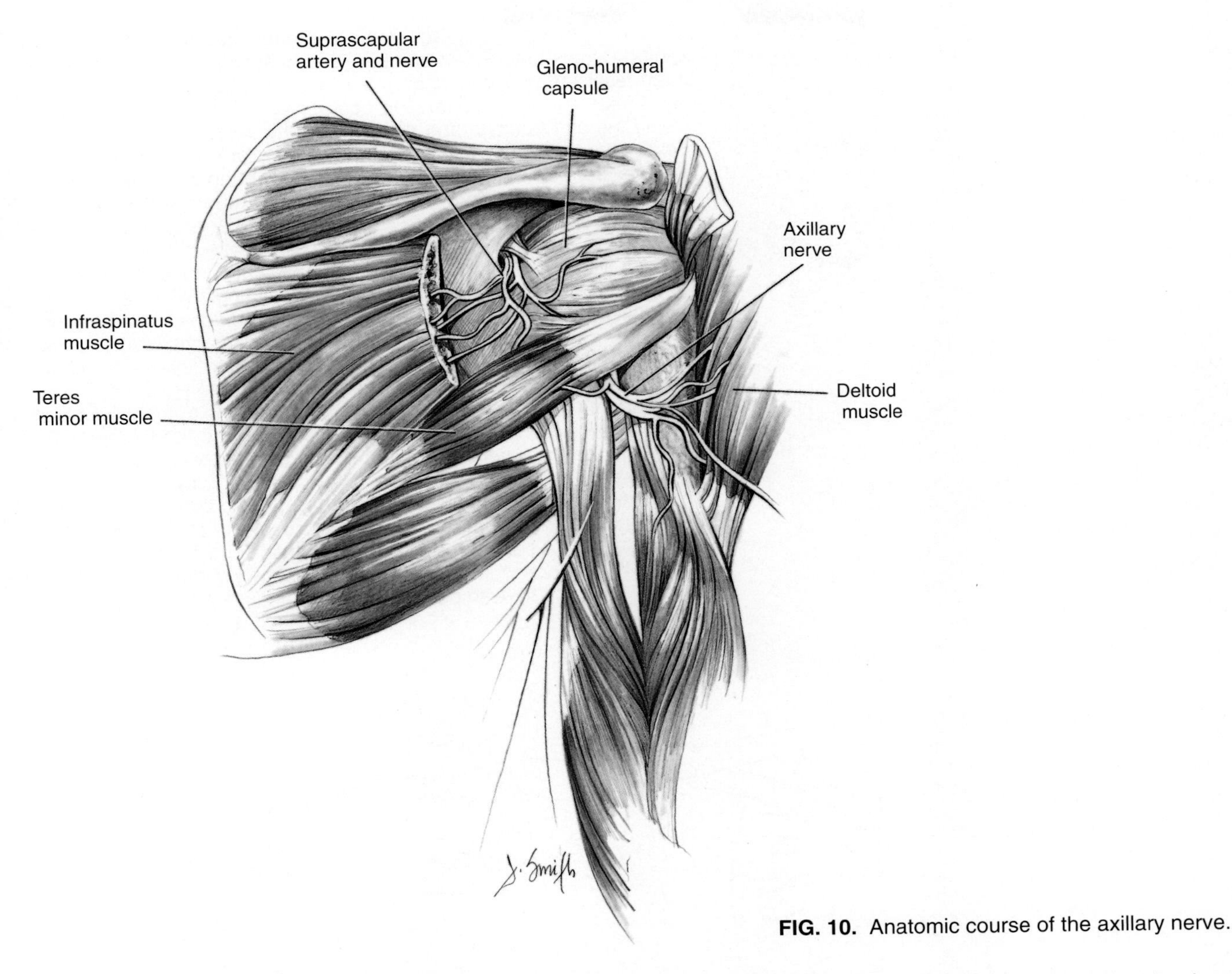

FIG. 10. Anatomic course of the axillary nerve.

The rotator cuff acts as a functional unit maintaining the humeral center within the glenoid during active arm elevation. These muscles are often considered as four distinct separate musculotendinous units that directly overlie the joint capsule and insert onto the proximal humerus. Clark and Harryman[30] performed gross anatomic and histologic studies in cadaveric specimens to better define the relation between the rotator cuff tendons and their underlying capsular elements. The fibers of the rotator cuff tendons interdigitate and fuse, forming a common insertion on the tuberosities of the humerus. Fibers from both the subscapularis and infraspinatus interdigitate with respective fibers of the supraspinatus. Microscopically, the rotator cuff complex is stratified into five distinct layers that also receive reinforcement from the coracohumeral ligament and is contiguous with the glenohumeral capsule (Fig. 11). This structural architecture may enhance the rotator cuff's resistance to failure with repeated loads, for tension generated in any single musculoskeletal unit could be expected to result in a distribution of forces over an expanded area.[30] Moreover, in circumstances under which the rotator cuff does fail, the network of interdigitating fibers contributes to the tissue's structural integrity, affording retention of sutures during operative repair.

Multiple vessels contribute to the vascularity of the rotator cuff. The anterior and posterior humeral circumflex arteries both supply the superior, as well as the anterior and posterior portions of the cuff, respectively. The suprascapular artery also supplies the superior cuff, and in the majority of persons the acromial branch of the thoracoacromial artery will nourish the supraspinatus. Additional contributions may include branches of the subscapular and the suprahumeral branches of the axillary artery. Osseous vessels emanating from the tuberosities of the proximal humerus have also been included in the vascular makeup of the rotator cuff[27,57,104,116,158] (Fig. 12).

Abnormal

Tears of the rotator cuff typically involve the supraspinatus tendon and, to a variable degree, they will often include the posterior cuff. The subscapularis tendon, although less

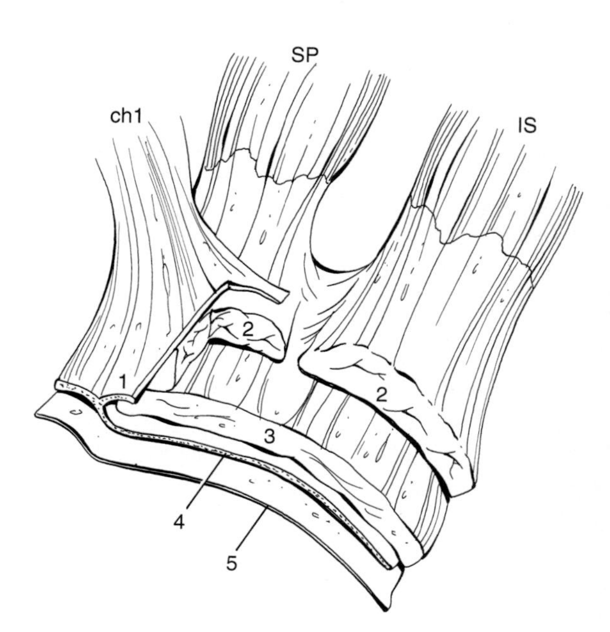

FIG. 11. Schematic diagram of the supraspinatus and infraspinatus tendinous insertions. Five discrete layers are identified. The orientation of the fascicles in the numbered layers are indicated by the lines on their upper surfaces. *Layer 1* is composed of superficial fibers that overlie the cuff tendons and extend from the coracoid process to the greater tuberosity. These fibers form an extension of the coracohumeral ligament (*chl*). *Layers 2* and *3* contain the fibers of the supraspinatus (*SP*) and the infraspinatus (*IS*) tendons. The fibers in layer 2 are oriented parallel to the axes of the supraspinatus and infraspinatus tendons. The fibers of layer 3 are smaller and are obliquely oriented with respect to the fibers of layer 2. Within layer 3, the fibers of the supraspinatus tendon fan out and intermingle with the fibers of the adjacent infraspinatus and subscapularis tendons. This intermingling between the infraspinatus and supraspinatus creates the variation in alignment of the fibers observed in layer 3. In *layer 4*, the fibers make up the deep extension of the coracohumeral ligament. These fibers branch off the main body of the ligament at the anterior border of supraspinatus tendon and then course between the tendon and capsule as far as the junction between the infraspinatus and supraspinatus. *Layer 5* is the true joint capsule of the shoulder, which forms a continuous fibrous cylinder extending from the glenoid labrum to the neck of the humerus. The synovial lining of the capsule is in direct contact with the articular surface of the humeral head. The orientation of the fibers within the capsule is quite variable and not identified in this diagram. (From ref. 30, with permission.)

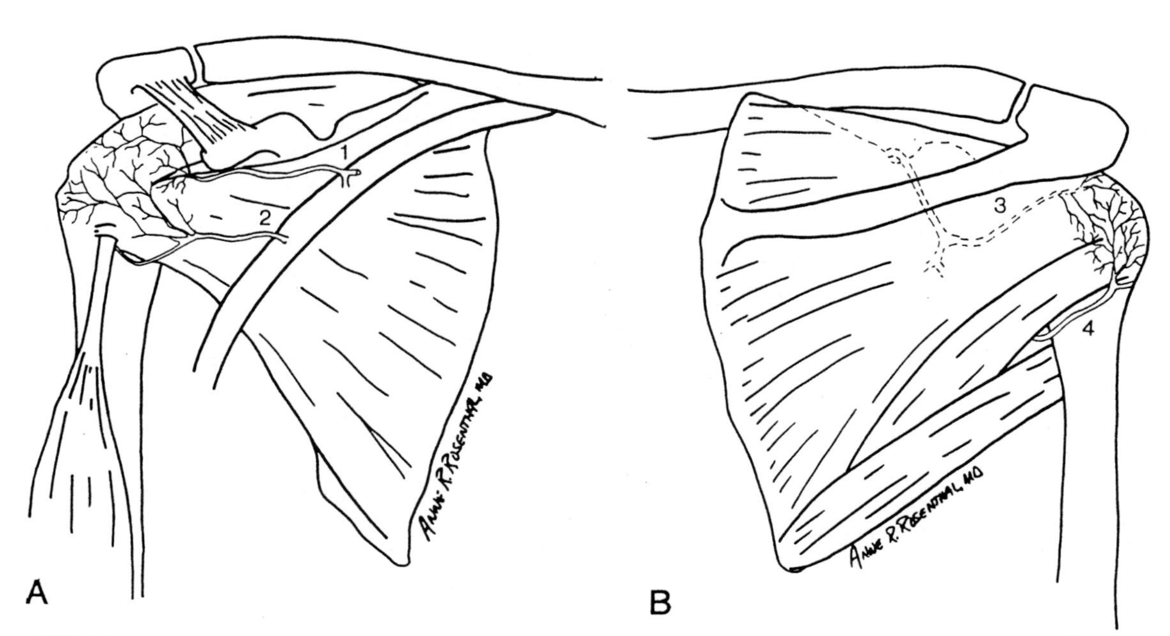

FIG. 12. Vascular supply to the rotator cuff. 1 = suprahumeral branch; 2 = anterior humeral circumflex artery; 3 = suprascapular artery; 4 = posterior humeral circumflex artery. (From ref. 27, with permission.)

frequently involved, may be easily overlooked if not considered during diagnostic evaluation.

The torn rotator cuff can demonstrate variably shaped defects that should be taken into consideration during surgical reconstruction. A vertical tear, in line with the course of the tendon, can often be repaired with a side-to-side closure. Horizontal tears run transverse to the normal course of the tendon and will demonstrate variability in size and extent of retraction. Typically, closure of such defects requires a transosseous repair to the greater tuberosity. Complex tears that contain both horizontal and vertical components also occur and may require a combination of the aforementioned techniques.

Tears involving the rotator interval, although less common, have also been described.[96,191] Surgical exploration of this interval in 116 patients with supposed isolated tears of the supraspinatus tendon, revealed occult lesions of the coracohumeral ligament, superior glenohumeral ligament, and upper border of the subscapularis in 19 cases. Treatment consisted of a rotator cuff repair and reconstruction of the rotator interval complex.[191] Although these lesions can be difficult to diagnose, their association with pain or dysfunction and the optimal method for their treatment remain undetermined.

Unfortunately, a universally accepted classification scheme for rotator cuff disease does not exist, making studies evaluating the results of surgical treatment difficult to compare. However, important parameters to consider when describing rotator cuff lesions include the duration, depth, and size of a tear, as well as the condition of the muscle and the tendon. Tears may be acute which typically present with the sudden onset of pain and dysfunction after a traumatic event. Chronic tears are present for longer than 3 months and may be associated with a variable degree of weakness and discomfort. Some patients may have a previously documented chronic rotator cuff tear and develop an acute extension of the lesion after a traumatic insult. The depth of a tear will differentiate partial from full-thickness lesions. Moreover, partial-thickness tears can be present on either the articular or bursal surface, or they may be intrasubstance. The thickness of the lesion may also vary until it extends through the entire tendon, at which point the subacromial space communicates with the glenohumeral joint. Gradation of partial-thickness lesions has been described; however, difficulty lies in the definition and accurate assessment of such lesions. For example, fraying of the tendon observed during an operation may be considered as a partial tear by some surgeons and not by others. Moreover, the incidence of such lesions in relation to symptoms and the results of treatment are not easily determined because of variability in imaging capabilities, interpretation, and lack of uniformity in classification.

Full-thickness tears may be described as small (less than 2 cm in diameter), medium (2 to 4 cm), large (4 to 5 cm) or massive (more than 5 cm). Additionally, a torn rotator cuff may be retracted, deficient, attenuated, or friable at the time of surgical assessment. The muscle can be best assessed with the aid of quality MRI scans on which cross-sectional area, degree of fatty infiltration and alterations in overall muscle signal intensity can be determined. A recent MRI investigation looked into the correlation of supraspinatus muscle atrophy in association with rotator cuff tears and residual function using electromyographic (EMG) analysis. As the supraspinatus became more atrophic, the EMG function of the muscle decreased.[118] Although these observations suggest a decrease in function in conjunction with MRI-evident supraspinatus atrophy, the influence of these findings on outcome after surgical repair of the rotator cuff will require further study.

Glenohumeral abnormalities have also been associated with tears of the rotator cuff. A prospective series of 100 patients with full-thickness tears, who underwent a diagnostic arthroscopy, revealed glenohumeral abnormalities in 74% overall. Common observations included lesions of the anterior labrum in 62%, intraarticular biceps tendon tears in 16%, and articular cartilage abnormalities in 28%.[113] Clearly, such lesions are being detected with increased frequency with the more widespread application of arthroscopic techniques. However, the relevance of these findings in association with full-thickness rotator cuff tears and the effect of their treatment on the overall outcome remains undetermined. Although the role of arthroscopic surgery in the evaluation and treatment of rotator cuff tears continues to be a subject of debate, it can offer prognostic and therapeutic benefits in selected cases.

THE CORACOACROMIAL ARCH

The coracoacromial arch marks the superior boundary of the subacromial space. It comprises the coracoid process, the coracoacromial ligament, and the acromion (see Fig. 7). Neer[121,123] described the role of this structure in the development of impingement syndrome and noted changes in the osseous and soft-tissue morphology in patients affected with this disorder.

The shape of the acromion exhibits variability among individuals. In an anatomic study of 140 cadaveric shoulders, Bigliani and Morrison[14] identified three predominant acromial forms when assessed in the sagittal plane (Fig. 13). A type I acromion had a flat undersurface and was present in 17% of cases. A type II acromion revealed a curved undersurface and was found in 43% of specimens. A hooked acromion, or type III, although present in 39% of cases, was found in 70% of shoulders with observed tears of the rotator cuff. A follow-up clinical study, using supraspinatus outlet radiographs to assess acromial morphology and arthrograms to determine rotator cuff integrity, affirmed the association between a "hooked" acromion and the presence of rotator cuff tears in patients presenting with various shoulder complaints.[115]

Despite the potential value of correlating specific acromial forms with lesions of the rotator cuff, other investigators have been unable to demonstrate comparable findings

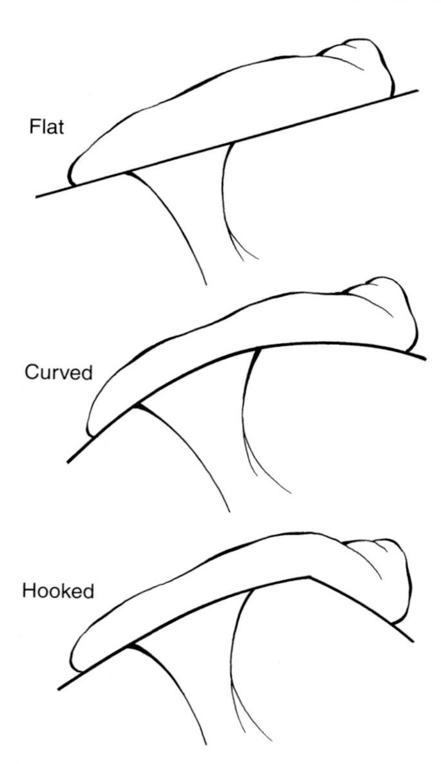

FIG. 13. Acromion morphology: **type I**, flat; **type II**, curved; **type III**, hooked. (Adapted with permission from ref. 14.)

and have questioned the reliability of radiographic acromial morphology assessment in the sagittal plane.[8,9,49,63,84,205] Moreover, even though a flat acromion could be readily detected by most clinicians, confusion has arisen with regard to discernment of the curved (type II) and hooked (type III) patterns. Jacobson and colleagues[84] studied 126 supraspinatus outlet radiographs in an attempt to determine the reliability of detecting acromion morphology. Inter- and intraobserver reliability coefficients of 0.516 and 0.888 were demonstrated, respectively. The data suggest that observers were each consistent in using a given set of classification criteria, but that these criteria differed among examiners. Furthermore, they also reflect the qualitative component of acromion morphology assessment and the potential difficulties in comparison of published studies. Some of the observed differences may best be explained by the potential for acromion architecture to exist as a continuum, ranging from a flat to a hooked configuration, with varying degrees of curvature within the extremes.

In an effort to objectively quantitate and standardize the classification of acromion morphology, Toivonen and coworkers[188] devised the measurement of an "acromial angle." This angle was formed between two lines drawn along the undersurface of the anterior third and posterior two-thirds of the acromion (Fig. 14). The authors reported reproducible methods and demonstrated a significant association between increasing acromial angle and rotator cuff tears. The types I, II, and III acromion had acromial angles of 0 to

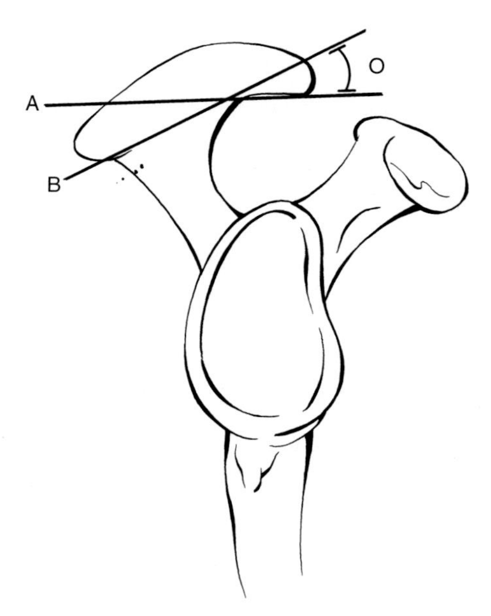

FIG. 14. Depiction of acromial angle. (From ref. 188, with permission.)

12, 13 to 27, and greater than 27 degrees, respectively. Moreover, their findings were consistent with those of Bigliani and Morrison[14] in that 89% of type III acromions were associated with tears of the rotator cuff.

Kitay and associates[93] called into question the use of supraspinatus outlet radiographs alone in evaluating acromial morphologic condition. Analysis of anteroposterior, axillary, 30-degree caudal tilt and supraspinatus outlet views in 23 surgically treated patients with impingement syndrome revealed the greatest interobserver reliability for the 30-degree caudal tilt view (0.84; Fig. 15). The caudal tilt x-ray

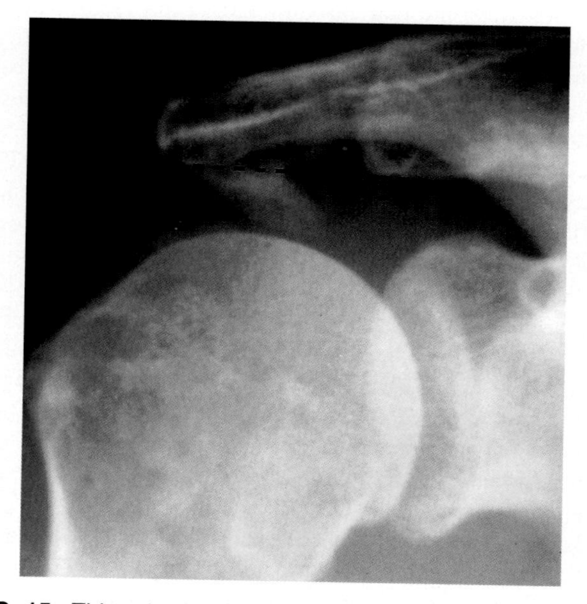

FIG. 15. Thirty-degree caudal tilt radiograph depicting anterior inferior projection of an acromial spur. The *solid line* designates the anterior cortical margin of the distal clavicle.

film reflected the acromial spur in its combined anterior and inferior projections, whereas the outlet view provided information on the inferior projection of the spur. The combined use of these two radiographs was believed to be the best predictor of intraoperative acromial spur size.

Whereas, acromial spurs have been identified by many as an acquired ossification of the coracoacromial ligament insertion, the distinction between native acromion morphology and developmental subacromial osseous excrescences has not always been clear. [25,29,136,144] Furthermore, the effect of age on acromial morphologic condition has not been sufficiently studied, leaving many questions unanswered about the potential for developmental alterations in acromial shape. Nicholson and coworkers[133] attempted to address this issue by quantifying osseous dimensions of the acromion and evaluating the relation between morphologic condition and age. Analysis of 420 scapulae in different age groups revealed no trends toward the alteration of acromial morphology. Although age did correlate with an increase in frequency of anterior acromial spur formation, it did not significantly change the dimensions of the acromion or alter morphology when assessed using supraspinatus outlet radiographs. The data suggest that the acromion's morphologic condition functions both independently and in association with age-related degenerative processes in the development of rotator cuff disease.

Other factors have also been implicated as potential contributors to subacromial impingement and rotator cuff disease. Neer and Poppen[124,127] suggested that both the slope of the acromion and acromioclavicular joint spurs can compromise the integrity of the rotator cuff through impingement mechanisms. Aoki and coworkers[4,5] measured acromial slope and found a decreased angle in patients with impingement syndrome when compared with normal controls. Qualitatively, this parameter refers to the pitch of the acromion in the sagittal plane. A more horizontal acromion would have a lower pitch and a corresponding low angle (Fig. 16). This lower pitch can result in a reduced area of the supraspinatus outlet, thereby creating the potential for rotator cuff compromise.[205]

Zuckerman and colleagues[205] studied the spatial anatomy of the coracoacromial arch and supraspinatus outlet as they relate to full-thickness tears of the rotator cuff. In an anatomic investigation of 140 shoulders, they demonstrated a significant association between rotator cuff tears and measured parameters, including a reduced supraspinatus outlet area, lower acromial tilt, and larger anterior projection of the acromion. These findings support the contention that elements other than sagittal plane acromial morphology can be important factors leading to disorders of the rotator cuff. Their work was further supported by Edelson and Taitz[44] who, in an anatomic study of 200 scapulas, observed that acromial slope, length, and height were most closely associated with osseous degenerative changes of the coracoacromial arch. Although such factors have also been implicated in the pathogenesis of rotator cuff disease, standard acromioplasty may not adequately address these elements and may explain failed surgical treatment in specific cases.

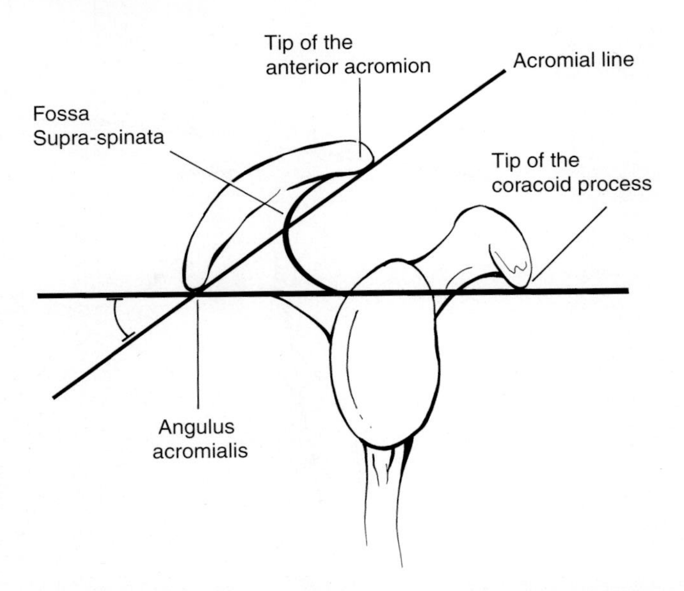

FIG. 16. Acromial slope (tilt). This angle reflects the pitch of the acromion and is formed by a line across the posterior acromion and coracoid tip and along the undersurface of the acromion. (From ref. 4, with permission.)

Attention to acromial morphology in other planes has also become an area of increasing interest. Banas and colleagues[8] described the "lateral acromion angle" after retrospectively reviewing 100 shoulder MRI scans in symptomatic patients. This angle is formed by a line along the undersurface of the acromion, as viewed in the coronal plane, and a second line joining the most superior and inferior margins of the glenoid (Fig. 17). As the lateral acromion angle decreased, a statistically significant increase in rotator cuff disease was observed. This parameter was felt to be an independent predictor of rotator cuff disease and further highlights the importance of acromial morphology assessment in multiple planes.

Moreover, inability to appreciate the variability in acromial shapes may make standard portal placement for arthroscopic procedures difficult and potentially hazardous. In a recent study, the posterior lip of the acromion was observed to project inferiorly, overlying the midpoint of the glenohumeral joint, in 16% of specimens.[45] Use of the posterior acromion as a sole reference for placement of the arthroscopic cannula may thus result in a portal that is potentially too low compromising of both the axillary nerve and arthroscopic visualization.

Recent interest has been focused on the structure and function of coracoacromial ligament. While commonly described as having an inverted "Y" configuration, other morphologic types have been noted.[75,165] Holt and Allibone[75] performed an anatomic and histologic analysis of the coracoacromial ligament in 50 shoulders and noted variable forms among individuals. They observed three predominant variants and described them as "quadrangular, Y-shaped or

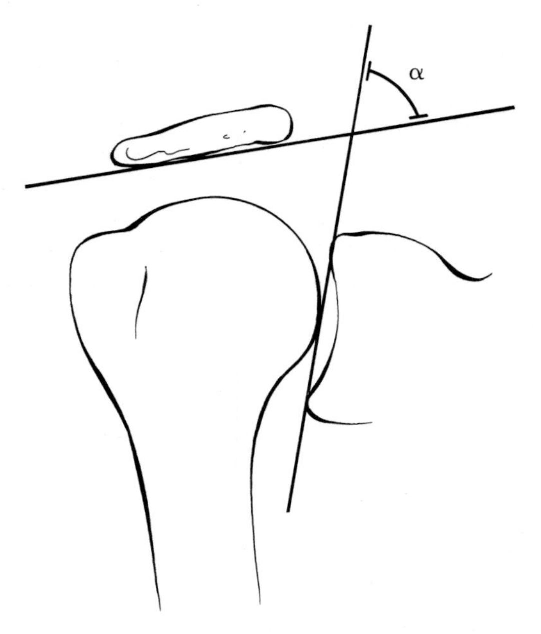

FIG. 17. Lateral acromion angle: This angle is formed by the intersection of a line along the undersurface of the acromion in the coronal plane and a second line connecting the superior and inferior margins of the glenoid. (From ref. 8, with permission.)

broad-banded" (Fig. 18). The quadrangular and Y forms demonstrated a frequency of 48 and 42%, respectively. In the Y type, the two limbs take origin from the medial and lateral aspects of the coracoid. As they project superolaterally to insert onto the undersurface of the acromion, the bands fuse and form the anterior soft-tissue boundary of the coracoacromial arch (see Fig. 6).

Mechanical forces about the coracoacromial arch, while not fully understood, have also been linked to the development of rotator cuff disease.[53,73,119,176] Biomechanical and geometric testing of the coracoacromial ligament has demonstrated that the lateral band was both shorter in length and smaller in cross-sectional area in shoulders with rotator cuff tears. Although histologically there were no structural differences in the ligament between normally formed shoulders and those with rotator cuff tears, there was evidence of decreased mechanical properties in the latter. The reduction in mechanical integrity of the ligament was thought to reflect the multiple directional loads imposed on this structure in shoulders with rotator cuff tears.[176] One additional investigation employing scanning electron micrographs in eight cadaveric shoulders demonstrated that observed degenerative changes of the rotator cuff were characteristic of alterations resulting from frictional and rubbing mechanisms. Observations support the contention that degenerative changes al-

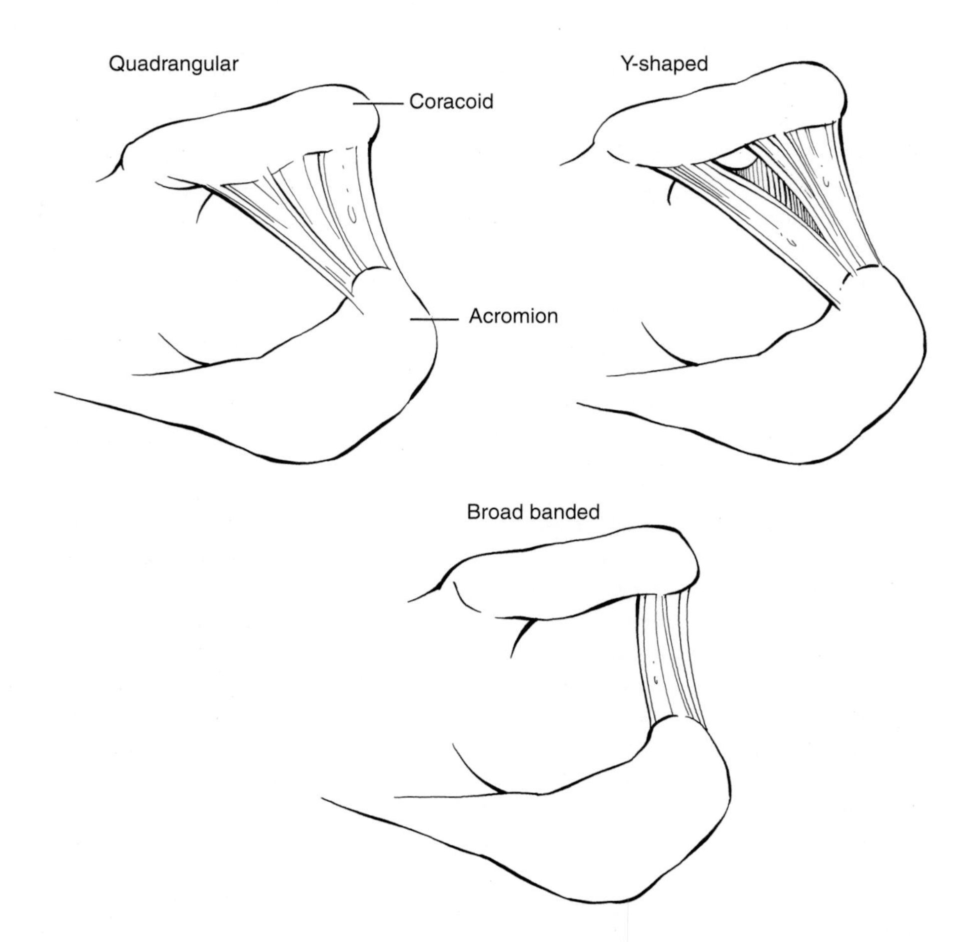

FIG. 18. Anatomic variants of the coracoacromial ligament. (From ref. 75, with permission.)

ready present in the cuff, irrespective of etiology, can be aggravated by proposed frictional or abrading type forces.[73] Additional reports have suggested that increases in measured subacromial pressures in patients with impingement syndrome may mediate the development and progression of rotator cuff disorders.[85,174,200]

In contrast with its implicated role in the pathogenesis of impingement syndrome, the coracoacromial ligament has been shown to function as a dynamic brace that lends support to the acromion and coracoid during loads imposed by the surrounding musculature. Putz and colleagues[152] used strain gauges to measure distortion of the coracoid and acromion after resection of the coracoacromial ligament in eight cadavers. With applied loads, significantly more distortion of the acromion was observed. Soslowski and associates[179] have noted that the coracoacromial arch acts as a buffer against superior translations when the humeral head is not centered in the glenoid. This may occur during normal obligate translation of the joint with humeral rotation and also in patients with glenohumeral instability. Furthermore, its role as a secondary restraint to anterosuperior migration of the humeral head in patients with large rotator cuff deficiencies has also been emphasized.[7,50,64,179,196] Salter and coworkers[165] have suggested that the coracoacromial ligament provides mechanical support to the acromioclavicular joint. Gross and microscopic anatomic evaluation revealed that fibers at its insertion under the anterior acromion were contiguous with the inferior acromioclavicular joint capsule.

Although such studies have provided quantitative analysis of the coracoacromial arch in relation to shoulder function, additional investigations are needed to further clarify subacromial stresses and contact areas in multiple planes of motion and in different pathologic states. Increased understanding of these issues may enhance our ability to effectively evaluate and treat patients with rotator cuff disease.

ROTATOR CUFF FUNCTION

Under normal conditions, the rotator cuff plays an important role in providing dynamic stability to the glenohumeral joint. The osseous architecture consists of an apparently flat glenoid and a larger, convex humeral head. Early studies have suggested that the radius of curvature of the glenoid closely approximates that of the humeral head (*conformity*), and that the differences observed represent a mismatch in the surface areas of the two articular surfaces (*constraint*).[76,162,164,167] Saha[162,164] emphasized the surface area mismatch and demonstrated that approximately 25% to 30% of the humeral head articulates with the glenoid at any given glenohumeral angle. He further described three different types of articulations that were based on the relation between the glenoid and humeral radii of curvature. Types A, B, and C exhibited a glenoid radius that was larger, equal, and smaller than that of the humeral head, respectively. However, conflicting data have fueled debate over conformity of the glenohumeral joint. More recently, Iannotti and coworkers[80] used both anatomic specimens and MRI to measure the dimensions of the glenohumeral articulation in 140 shoulders. They noted an elliptical contour of humeral head at the peripheral margins, whereas the central portion of the humerus was spherical and revealed a radius of curvature slightly less than that of the glenoid in the coronal plane (2.3 ±0.2 mm). Soslowski and colleagues[178] used stereophotogrammetry in cadavers to evaluate the three-dimensional geometry of the shoulder. This technique affords assessment of joint topography and takes into account the contribution of articular cartilage to joint conformity. Their observations affirmed the relative congruency of the glenohumeral joint, in that the radii of the glenoid and humeral articular surfaces were within 2 mm in 88% of cases. Differences in articular cartilage thickness were also noted. It was thickest at the glenoid periphery and central portion of the humeral head. Conversely, the thinner areas of cartilage were observed at the periphery of the humeral head and central portion of the glenoid. Even though plain radiographs depict the subchondral architecture and typically display a flat-appearing glenoid, differences in cartilage thickness across the joint, as determined through newer techniques, may help explain some of the disparate conclusions in the literature.

Obligate humeral translation, which occurs at the extremes of glenohumeral rotation, becomes more difficult to explain in light of conformity of the glenohumeral articulation.[70,77,201] Absolute conformity would suggest ball and socket kinematics, which would not account for this translatory motion. Howell and colleagues[77] radiographically studied glenohumeral patterns of motion in the horizontal plane and noted posterior humeral excursion when the arm was in maximum external rotation and extension (see chapter 8). Harryman and associates[70] noted similar findings in a biomechanical study using cadaveric shoulders. They demonstrated obligate posterior and anterior humeral translation when the arm was positioned in extension and flexion, respectively. Humeral excursion is thought to occur when the glenohumeral capsule becomes asymmetrically tight, such as at the extremes of motion. Yet, coupled translation with humeral rotation might also be considered in the context of the humeral head's shape. Translation occurring at the extremes of motion would correspond to articular contact at the peripheral and more elliptical portion of the humerus, thereby affording the potential for translatory motion. Moreover, a slight mismatch in joint conformity and, more importantly, the reversible deformation of the articular cartilage, may help further explain observed patterns of translational motion in light of the nearly conforming articulating surfaces.[70,80,178] Humeral translation has also been suggested to occur at the midranges of motion, either through pathologic asymmetric tensioning of the capsule, or by a dysfunctional rotator cuff. Additional in vivo investigations will be needed to further define and clarify this issue.

The wide arc of movement evident at the glenohumeral joint is largely due to its minimally constrained architecture. Moreover, a delicate balance between motion and stability exists such that increases in one parameter may occur at the expense of the other. The surrounding soft tissues, which include the rotator cuff as well as the glenoid labrum and glenohumeral ligaments, provide much of the added stability required for smooth unhindered motion of the shoulder. The labrum increases the depth and load bearing area of the glenoid, whereas the glenohumeral ligaments and capsule act as "check reins" limiting rotation at the extremes of motion. Dynamic stability is achieved predominantly through the coordinated and synchronous action of the rotator cuff (see chapter 17).

The rotator cuff comprises a group of muscles that are considerably smaller in size and cross-sectional area when compared with the more superficial structures, such as the deltoid, pectoralis major, latissimus dorsi, and trapezius. In addition, because they lie deep in the shoulder and in close proximity to the center of rotation of the glenohumeral joint, these muscles are collectively unable to generate the same degree of torque as the larger and more superficial structures. In part, the relatively shorter lever arm, or distance of the muscle from the center of rotation, accounts for observable differences in generated force. Consequently, given its anatomic architecture, maintenance of a stable glenohumeral fulcrum during active arm motion is one function that is both important and well-suited to the rotator cuff (Fig. 19).

A normal functioning rotator cuff achieves dynamic stability through multiple mechanisms. It acts through direct joint compression as well as through asymmetric contraction

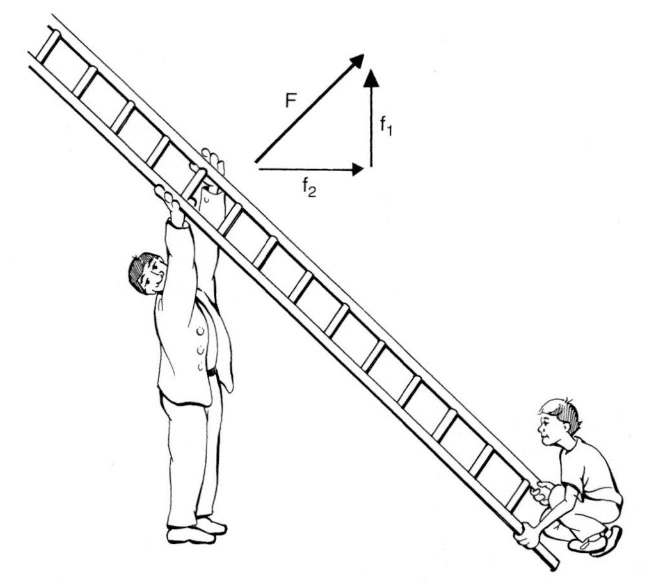

FIG. 19. The shoulder muscles can be grouped as either primary movers or primary stabilizers. This situation is somewhat analagous to that of a large man and a small boy teaming up to lift a ladder. Typically, the stronger one will lift or move the ladder, while the weaker one will hold it from sliding or lifting off the ground (stabilizer). There is a point at which the force generated by the stronger one can overpower the resistance of the weaker one and stability is lost. (From ref. 135, with permission.)

and "steering" of the humeral head into the glenoid during active motion.[11,101,135,146,163,199,202] Compression is achieved through the perpendicular vector of pull by the humeral head into the glenoid that serves to minimize tendencies toward joint subluxation.[101,135] Study of rotator cuff function in athletes who throw and in pathologic states has increased our understanding of dynamic stability under normal conditions. Warner and colleagues[194] noted a relative weakness of the humeral internal rotators in patients with anterior instability, resulting in a dynamic muscular imbalance. Glousman and associates[61] demonstrated similar findings using dynamic EMG in throwing athletes. Their observations revealed a decrease in muscle activity of the internal rotators and serratus anterior in persons with anterior instability. Other reports have noted the importance of the posterior cuff muscles in reducing strain of the inferior glenohumeral ligament with the arm in the cocked position. The infraspinatus and teres minor have been suggested to pull the humerus posteriorly when the arm is externally rotated and, thereby, minimize the potential for anterior subluxation.[25,146] However, EMG studies in both normal volunteers and throwers with anterior instability have not been able to validate these conclusions.[61,95] Despite a few inconsistencies in the literature, which may be related to differences in electrodiagnostic methods, the functional importance of the rotator cuff in maintaining dynamic glenohumeral stability should be realized. Moreover, although these data suggest a role for selective strengthening of affected muscles in an attempt to restore normal dynamic balance, a cause-and-effect relation between observed muscular inactivity and instability has not been established.

Alternative mechanisms through which the rotator cuff may function include action as a direct barrier to humeral head translation in the midranges of motion. Furthermore, the cuff may have a potential role in "dynamization" of the glenohumeral ligaments. The contiguous or intimate association between the rotator cuff and underlying capsule could permit asymmetric tensioning of the ligaments in the midranges at which they have been generally considered to remain lax. Through coordinated muscular contractions, the ligaments can be tensed affording further resistance to humeral translation (see chapter 8). Although this concept has gained more recent attention, the relation between the active and passive restraints of the shoulder remains poorly understood and will require further research to determine its contribution to glenohumeral stability.

Multiple forces pass across the shoulder during active motion to achieve a desired arm position. Force couples in various planes exist that can be defined as the action of two opposing muscle groups required to achieve a given movement. Inman and associates[81] initially described force couples involving the glenohumeral joint. They noted that the deltoid muscle acts to pull the humeral head in a cephalad direction, while the subscapularis, infraspinatus, and teres minor act as a functional unit counteracting the deltoid and effecting depression of the humeral head. Other biomechanical studies have highlighted the role of the infraspinatus and subscapularis in maintenance of normal glenohumeral kinematics.[21,170] In one cadaveric investigation, the isolated absence of an applied supraspinatus force appeared to have no appreciable difference on humeral head migration when measured radiographically in the anteroposterior plane. Absence of force generated by the infraspinatus, teres minor, and subscapularis, on the other hand, resulted in an increase in superior humeral translation because the deltoid was unopposed.[170] Burkhart[21] expanded on the importance of force couples in preserving normal kinematics in patients with rotator cuff tears. He noted that balanced forces in both the coronal and transverse planes afforded normal glenohumeral motion patterns as long as anterior and posterior portions of the cuff were preserved beyond a critical threshold (Fig. 20). The location, as opposed to size of the tendon tear, was suggested to be a more significant determinant in resultant glenohumeral kinematics.

The force couples across the shoulder remain integral to maintaining normal function, especially when placed in a perspective of the minimally constrained design of the glenohumeral joint. Although the importance of the rotator cuff in generating these force couples can be readily appreciated, its contribution in pathologic states and its relation to symptomatology remain uncertain and will require elucidation through further study.

The relative contribution of the rotator cuff to strength in arm abduction continues to remain an area of debate. Howell and coworkers[78] noted that, after selective blockade of the suprascapular and axillary nerves in normal volunteers, the supraspinatus and deltoid muscles contribute equally to measured torque in abduction. These findings are comparable with other reports on selective blocking of the axillary nerve in which it was noted that approximately 60% of the strength in abduction was attributable to the deltoid muscle.[34,35] Compromise of rotator cuff or deltoid function in such individuals could be expected to result in a progressive loss of muscle force with arm elevation and in early fatigability. The infraspinatus has also been implicated as a contributor to arm elevation. Otis and associates[140] reported decreases in abduction and external rotation torque of up to 45% and 75%, respectively, after selective paralysis of the infraspinatus muscle. These findings contrast with one EMG study that demonstrated silent electrical activity in the infraspinatus when it was elevated to 120 degrees.[151] In an effort to clarify the collective role of the infraspinatus, teres minor, and subscapularis, Sharkey and coworkers,[171] in a biomechanical cadaveric investigation, evaluated the contribution of these muscles to force in abduction. Because the tendons of the subscapularis and infraspinatus insert both above and below the humeral center of rotation, it is conceivable that portions of these muscles may act as arm abductors as well as humeral head depressors. Their data suggested that the combined contractions of these muscles contribute to arm abduction and that the magnitude of their contribution was similar to that of the supraspinatus. Otis and colleagues[139] provided further indirect evidence of the functional relation of the rotator cuff and deltoid to humeral elevation. By calculation of changes in moment arms and measurement of muscular excursion in cadaveric specimens, they demonstrated that both the infraspinatus and subscapularis contribute to abduction. Changes in rotation further affected the capacity of either muscle to augment elevation in the scapular plane. Internal and external rotation enhanced the ability of the upper portions of the infraspinatus and subscapularis, respectively, to abduct the arm. The data help partly explain how a supraspinatus defect may not necessarily limit functional abduction of the arm.

The complex interaction of the rotator cuff and surrounding muscles is largely responsible for the shoulder's considerable range of motion and the preservation of glenohumeral joint stability. Although debate continues over a few functions of the rotator cuff, the preponderance of data support its role as a dynamic stabilizer, providing humeral depression,

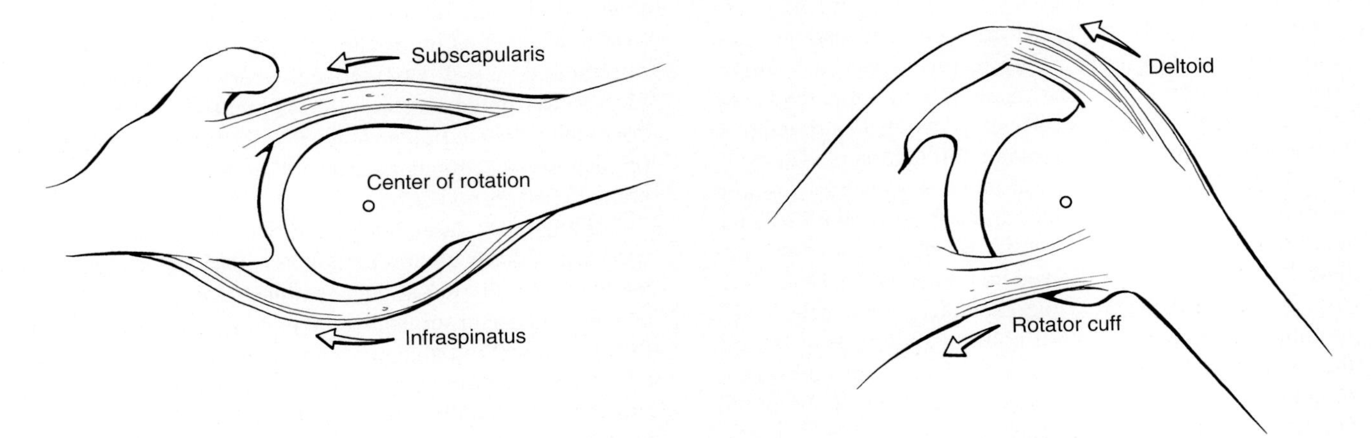

FIG. 20. Force couples of the shoulder. **Left:** The transverse plane force couple balances the opposing forces of the anterior and posterior cuff. **Right:** The coronal plane force couple consists of the deltoid counterpoised against the inferior portion of the rotator cuff. (From ref. 21, with permission.)

abduction, and joint compression. Its role in "dynamization" or tensioning of the glenohumeral ligaments in the midranges of motion remains unclear and will require validation with further study. Furthermore, the rotator cuff has an integral part in maintaining force couples in multiple planes, whereby its absence could potentially result in abnormal kinematics, an unstable fulcrum, and abnormal humeral head excursion. Through more sophisticated in vivo imaging and measuring applications, these muscle interactions may be unfolded and further increase our understanding of the pathomechanics underlying glenohumeral joint instability.

PATHOGENESIS

Controversy continues to exist concerning the pathogenesis of rotator cuff disease. The heterogeneity of the disorder, as well as the notion that rotator cuff disease may not actually represent a continuum of the same process, but rather, is a compilation of independent disorders, may partly explain the differing viewpoints on its origin. Two contrasting pathogenetic mechanisms have been extensively described and include vascular, or intrinsic, causes and impingement, or extrinsic, factors. Although other etiologies have also been reported that include trauma, congenital or developmental factors, and instability, they will be discussed in a subsequent section.

Vascular Factors

The relation between the microvascular blood supply of the rotator cuff and tendon degeneration remains a subject of debate. Conflicting reports describing the vascularity of the supraspinatus tendon exist; however, in many investigations, the methods employed were limited. Moreover, although vascular-mediated mechanisms have been suggested as an important factor in the genesis of rotator cuff disease, studies have been unable to sufficiently attribute hypovascularity as a direct cause for observed tears of the rotator cuff.

Mayer[108] initially dismissed the view that tendons were avascular and showed that they receive a vascular supply from three sources: muscular, osseous, and direct tendinous sites. Codman[31,32] subsequently proposed that a critical portion existed within the distal rotator cuff tendon predisposing it to degeneration and calcification. He suggested a vascular or ischemic mechanism, which in association with trauma, leads to tearing of the rotator cuff. McMaster[111] further supported this concept and showed that when normal musculotendinous specimens were placed under mechanical loads, the muscle became the initial point of failure. However, if the tendon was compromised secondary to an interrupted blood supply and repeated stress, it then became the initial site of failure while the integrity of the muscle was preserved.

Several investigators have observed a decrease in vascularity of the rotator cuff tendon. Notably, Lindblom[100] performed histologic analysis of 12 cadaveric shoulders and demonstrated a region of hypovascularity of the rotator cuff tendon near its insertion to the greater tuberosity. Rothman and Parke[158] also confirmed a region of relative hypovascularity within the distal rotator cuff tendon after arterial latex injection into 72 cadaveric shoulders. They noted consistent vascular patterns, which were independent of age, in their specimens; however, they felt that their methods were not sufficiently accurate to reflect age-related changes. Brooks and colleagues[17] performed postmortem quantitative histologic evaluations of the rotator cuff that showed a decrease in vessel number, size, and percentage of tendon occupied by vessels in both the distal supraspinatus and infraspinatus tendons. Because the hypovascular zone was not isolated to just the supraspinatus tendon, the authors concluded that other factors must be important in the pathogenesis of rotator cuff disease. This was further confirmed by the difference in observed frequency of tears of the supraspinatus and infraspinatus tendons.

In contrast, other reports failed to show similar decreases in vascularity of the rotator cuff tendon. Moseley and Goldie[116] performed microinjection studies on 72 cadaver shoulders and demonstrated a "watershed" area or zone of anastomoses between osseous and tendinous vessels supplying the rotator cuff tendon. They termed this region the "critical zone," which was 1 cm proximal to the rotator cuff insertion and was previously noted by Codman[31,32] to be the frequent site of rotator cuff tendon failure. Their findings were also independent of age.

Rathbun and Macnab[153] used both microangiographic and histologic techniques to evaluate the tendon vascularity of the rotator cuff in cadavers. They showed adequate vascularity when injections were performed on the abducted arm, but in the adducted arm the vessels were "wrung out" and no longer perfused. They hypothesized that the critical zone was subject to a transient hypovascularity that was mediated by position of the arm.

More recently, a vascular study in 18 anatomic specimens revealed differential vascularity between the bursal and articular surfaces of the rotator cuff. The bursal surface was observed to be well vascularized, whereas the articular surface demonstrated a sparse arteriolar pattern.[104] The authors concluded that deficient tendon vascularity differentially predisposed the articular surface of the rotator cuff to degenerative changes and failure.

Intraoperative laser Doppler flowtometry has also been used to assess rotator cuff tendon vascularity in symptomatic patients. One investigation was aimed at clarifying the discrepancy between surgical findings of increased vascularity in patients with impingement syndrome and previous cadaveric reports demonstrating a hypovascular zone within the supraspinatus tendon. The patients with tendinitis and intact tendons always demonstrated increased vascularity in the area of greatest mechanical impingement, or the critical zone. Increased vascularity was also observed at the tendon margins of those patients with partial-thickness tears. Patients with complete tendon tears had variable degrees of vascularity at the tendon edges. The authors concluded that impingement generates a hypervascular response that results in the resorption of injured tendon fibers by neovascular tissue and mediates the progression of rotator cuff disease.[182] These findings also corroborate an earlier cadaveric investigation in which an increase in the number of blood vessels was observed in areas of degenerative tendon. These vessels invaded degenerative tendons through ingrowth of granulation tissue from both the bursal and synovial joint surfaces; this was never observed in normal tendons. Interestingly, in normal tendons, the number of arterioles was noted to decrease with age.[197]

Despite the findings of earlier microinjection studies, many of the conclusions are limited by the inherent shortcomings of the methods used. Lack of small-vessel perfusion in a cadaveric specimen may not satisfactorily reflect vascular characteristics in vivo. Moreover, microinjection studies that do not use histologic techniques may not afford adequate assessment of tissue vascularity, for capillary networks cannot be identified. In addition, postmortem investigations lack the clinical correlation necessary to attribute specific findings to clinical symptoms. With further study, use of in vivo methods, and employment of microscopic tissue evaluation, some of the limitations of earlier reports can be overcome and may permit a more detailed assessment of tendon vascularity in relation to clinical findings.

Impingement

Even though multiple studies have reported satisfactory and reproducible results for subacromial decompression in patients with impingement syndrome, they have been unable to sufficiently address the etiology of impingement lesions.[2,48,68,71,121,156,180,185] The question of whether rotator cuff abnormalities result from mechanical impingement by the overlying coracoacromial arch or whether a pathologic cuff gives rise to secondary changes within the acromion and coracoacromial ligament remain unanswered.

Neer[121,123] initially popularized the concept of impingement syndrome, noting that the rotator cuff was potentially subject to repeated mechanical insult by the coracoacromial arch during elevation of the arm. His observations highlighted the anterior functional arc of shoulder motion, with resultant impingement of the rotator cuff by proliferative spurs and excrescences extending from the anterior third of the acromion and coracoacromial ligament. This was in contrast with impingement by the lateral acromion, as had been generally accepted.[6,175] He subsequently described three stages of the impingement syndrome that exist as a continuum, ultimately leading to tears of the rotator cuff. Stage I, characterized by subacromial edema and hemorrhage, was typical in symptomatic patients younger than 25 years of age. Stage II included fibrosis and tendinitis and was more common in persons 25 to 40 years old. With continued progression, stage III, or rotator cuff failure, would result and was characterized by partial or complete tendon tears typically in persons older than 40 years of age. He attributed 95% of all rotator cuff lesions to primary mechanical impingement.

Few biomechanical investigations have validated Neer's observations implicating the anterior acromion as a source of impingement.[25,51,106,120] Burns and Whipple[25] studied the anatomic sites of tendon compression against the coracoacromial arch. In the neutral arm position, the supraspinatus and intertubercular portion of the biceps tendon lies inferolateral to the coracoacromial ligament and anterior to the acromion. Arm elevation in the scapular plane resulted in contact of the supraspinatus and greater tuberosity with the junction of the anterior tuberosity with the junction of the anterior acromion and coracoacromial ligament. Biceps tendon impingement, on the other hand, occurred predominantly against the lateral free edge of the coracoacromial ligament. Macnab[106] also demonstrated that the supraspinatus insertion was damaged by the compression effect of the humeral head with repeated shoulder motions. Flatow and colleagues,[51] using stereophotogrammetry to evaluate subacromial contact areas with arm elevation, noted a progressive decrease in the acromiohumeral interval with scapular plane abduction. The humerus and acromion were at their closest proximity between elevations of 60 and 120 degrees. Moreover, contact and proximity were observed to begin at the anterolateral aspect of the acromion at zero degrees elevation and shift medially with progressive arm elevation. Only the anterior aspect of the acromion demonstrated the potential for subacromial contact. Additionally, acromiohumeral distances were decreased in shoulders with a hooked acromion morphology. In a subsequent investigation, Bigliani and colleagues[12] studied the effect of anterior acromioplasty on subacromial contact in seven cadaveric specimens. Their data suggested that flattening of the anterior third of the acromion was required to eliminate impingement. Although inherent limitations in a cadaveric model exist, they did note that flattening of just the anterior ridge of the acromion, rather than the anterior third, was insufficient to eliminate impingement in 50% of specimens.

Acromion morphology, or shape, has been further implicated in the etiology of impingement syndrome and rotator cuff disease. In a cadaveric study evaluating 140 anatomic specimens, Bigliani and Morrison[14] identified three predominant acromial forms. The acromion undersurface was categorized as flat (type I), curved (type II), or hooked (type III; see Fig. 13). Interestingly, 70% of observed rotator cuff tears were associated with hooked anterior acromions. Subsequently, Morrison and Bigliani[115] have verified these observations in a clinical setting in patients with various shoulder complaints.

Although a strong association between degenerative subacromial hypertrophic spur formation and full-thickness tears of the rotator cuff exists, a causal relation remains difficult to prove.[14,32,54,112,115,121,123,136,138,144,156] Biomechanical models have improved our understanding of humeral motion as it may relate to impingement syndrome; however, they are unable to sufficiently correlate findings with clinical symptoms. Furthermore, the role of scapulothoracic motion in altering subacromial contact requires further study. Because such movement is complex, multiplanar, variable, and difficult to reproduce in a laboratory setting, its potential contribution to rotator cuff impingement should be recognized.

The contribution of the coracoacromial ligament alone in the impingement syndrome has been investigated. It has been suggested that thickening of this ligament may predispose some patients to shoulder impingement. Uhtoff and coworkers[189] performed histologic analysis of the coracoacromial ligament in 17 patients with painful arc syndrome. Although they observed diffuse degenerative changes within the ligament, excessive proliferation of fibrous tissue could not be identified. Impingement in these patients was thought to occur as a result of expansion of the volume of the rotator cuff tendon or bursa, rather than the ligament itself. They highlighted the concept that any process that causes a decrease in the volume of the supraspinatus outlet can result in impingement syndrome. The coracoacromial ligament was believed to be one component of an unyielding tunnel that becomes too restrictive for its expanded contents.

Others have noted that coracoacromial ligament division alone may be sufficient for adequate decompression of the subacromial space in selected patients.[89,195] One report highlighted sectioning of the ligament in a subgroup of persons with clinical findings of impingement syndrome despite an absence of degenerative spur formation and the presence of a flat-appearing acromion.[89] Although satisfactory results were reported for most patients, the role of coracoacromial ligament division alone in such patients has not been sufficiently studied. Furthermore, although this structure has been implicated in the pathogenesis of rotator cuff disease, recent emphasis has focused on its important functional role as a secondary passive restraint to anterosuperior migration of the humeral head in cuff-deficient patients.[50,64,196] Questions on the benefits of limited subacromial decompression remain unanswered and continue to be an area of active investigation.

Proponents of intrinsic pathogenic mechanisms support the contention that subacromial spurs represent secondary changes occurring as a result of existing tears of the rotator cuff.[144] Conversely, others have suggested that observed lesions of the rotator cuff occur because of mechanical insult by inferiorly projecting subacromial bony excrescences.[121,123] The formation of such spurs has been suggested to occur as a result of repeated tension exerted on the coracoacromial ligament.[69,136] Despite controversy over the initial lesion, subacromial spurs appear to have a role in the development and progression of commonly observed rotator cuff tears. One histologic evaluation of bursal side rotator cuff tears in surgical specimens revealed variable thickness tears of the supraspinatus corresponding with areas of impingement of the overlying acromion and coracoacromial ligaments. Also observed were avascular regions of the proximal edge of the torn tendon. The combination of findings led the authors to conclude that multiple etiologies, including both intrinsic and extrinsic causes, were responsible for the observed abnormalities.[54] The pathogenesis question will likely remain unanswered until controlled studies are conducted. Retrospective clinical and cadaveric investigations remain limited in their ability to sufficiently address this issue. In search of an appropriate animal model, Soslowski and coworkers[177] have validated use of the rat in preliminary studies. However, further investigation will be necessary to determine its overall utility to the study of rotator cuff disease.

Alternative sources of impingement have been implicated in the development of rotator cuff disease. Distally pointing acromioclavicular osteophytes, the coracoid process, and the posterosuperior aspect of the glenoid can contribute to shoulder pain and rotator cuff lesions in certain patients.[38,43,58,59,65,86,94,102,121,123,124,127,145,147,169,183,187,190,192] Petersson and Gentz[147] studied the relation between distally pointing acromioclavicular osteophytes and ruptures of the supraspinatus tendon. By using radiographic analysis in patients with arthrographically confirmed rotator cuff tears and anatomic dissections in cadaveric subjects, they were able to demonstrate a strong association between ruptures of the supraspinatus tendon and periarticular osteophytes. Although acromial excrescences were also observed, their frequency in subjects with rotator cuff ruptures was less than that of acromioclavicular bone spurs. Seeger and coworkers[169] reviewed MRI scans in 107 patients with painful shoulders. Bony and soft-tissue abnormalities clinically described in impingement syndrome were evident in 53 persons. In these cases, the supraspinatus was noted to be compressed by either osseous spurs, hypertrophic capsular tissue of the acromioclavicular joint, or a low-lying acromion.

Whereas, abnormalities of the acromioclavicular joint have been associated with rotator cuff disorders, acromioclavicular joint arthrosis has also been observed in 65% of asymptomatic persons with and without tears of the rotator cuff.[172] These findings suggest that acromioclavicular joint abnormalities on imaging studies alone may not be a reliable predictor of disease in the absence of correlative symptomatology. Moreover, treatment of such periarticular abnormalities based on imaging studies alone, such as excision of small inferior acromioclavicular osteophytes during subacromial decompression, may convert a painless condition to a symptomatic joint in certain patients. However, patients with clinical evidence of the impingement syndrome and symptomatic arthritis of the acromioclavicular joint have been treated successfully with combined subacromial decompression and distal clavicle resection.[105]

Impingement of the rotator cuff between the humeral head and coracoid process can also occur with certain arm positions in some patients.[43,58,59,65,94,145] Gerber and coworkers[58] recognized the subcoracoid space (region between the tip of the coracoid process and humeral head or lesser tuberosity) as a source of shoulder pain and reported on idiopathic, iatrogenic, and traumatic causes of abnormalities affecting either the coracoid, glenoid, or humeral head. In all types, anterior shoulder pain was reproduced with either internal rotation of the arm in 90 degrees of abduction or adduction with the shoulder flexed to 90 degrees. Computed tomography scans of 47 shoulders in normal volunteers highlighted dimensional parameters of the subcoracoid space and suggested variational anatomic features that may predispose certain individuals to coracoid impingement. The subcoracoid space was confirmed as not being a free space, but rather a region just sufficient to accommodate gliding of the soft tissues between the coracoid process and humeral head. The distance between the coracoid and humerus decreased with the arm in forward flexion and internal rotation, especially in those persons with a coracoid projecting far laterally and close to the scapular neck. Moreover, the soft tissues in the space became folded with the arm in this position. Alterations in the coracohumeral relation (e.g., osteotomy or fracture) as studied in cadaveric controls highlighted the potential for impingement with the arm in a flexed and internally rotated position.[59] Although this entity remains an uncommon form of impingement and often a difficult diagnosis, satisfactory results have been reported with surgical treatment in selected patients.[43,58]

More recently, arthroscopic evaluations of throwing athletes who have the painful arc syndrome have demonstrated impingement of the deep surface of the rotator cuff against the posterosuperior glenoid rim with the arm in 90 to 150 degrees of abduction and maximal external rotation.[38,86,102,187,190,192] It has been suggested that abduction and external rotation of the arm can entrap a portion of the supraspinatus tendon between the humeral head and glenoid in susceptible persons. Increased glenohumeral external rotation, decreased humeral retroversion, scapulothoracic dysfunction, and poor throwing technique, all have been implicated in the development of this disorder. Associated findings, included partial-thickness tearing of the undersurface of the supraspinatus tendon, degenerative lesions of the posterosuperior glenoid labrum, and osteochondral impression fractures of the humeral head. Patients will typically complain of posterior shoulder pain that is elicited by overhead activity. Although these observations help emphasize alternative sources of shoulder impingement, further study is needed to better define this entity, its pathomechanics, and optimal treatment.

The impingement syndrome, as described by Neer, typically represents a specific diagnosis with characteristic findings. Clinical observation has suggested an overdiagnosis of this entity, which may partly explain why some patients do not improve with previously described and accepted treatment methods. Moreover, even if some patients may present with usual findings of impingement syndrome, alternative sources of pain should be considered. Ellman and colleagues[47] retrospectively reviewed 18 patients whose clinical findings were typical of impingement syndrome that had remained refractory to conservative management. Intraoperatively, they had coexisting degenerative changes of the glenohumeral joint that were evident arthroscopically, but had not been apparent radiographically. Because such findings can alter prognosis and treatment, increased suspicion, along with careful examination and both axillary and true scapular anteroposterior radiographs, may aid in preoperative detection of these lesions. Kessel and Watson[90] studied 97 patients with rotator cuff impingement lesions. Abnormalities in different regions of the rotator cuff were reported, and the potential for variability in presenting symptoms was highlighted. Hidden rotator interval lesions and traumatic tears within the rotator interval have also been associated with anterosuperior shoulder pain.[96,191] Despite the underlying etiology, the heterogeneity of rotator cuff disease, impingement syndrome, and other abnormalities that can mimic impingement disorders should be thoroughly considered to avoid potential pitfalls in diagnosis and treatment.

ETIOLOGY

Multiple etiologic factors have been associated with the development of rotator cuff disease (Table 1). They include tendon degeneration, trauma, glenohumeral instability, scapulothoracic dysfunction, and congenital abnormalities.

In early anatomic investigations, Codman[32] had suggested that degenerative processes, in association with trauma, were responsible for the genesis of rotator cuff tears. He noted that tendinous defects within the supraspinatus were commonly found 1 cm medial to its insertion on the greater tuberosity. The frequency of his findings increased with age. Subsequently, other anatomic investigations provided further evidence of degenerative changes about the shoulder with advancing age.[31,32,37,40,41,62,67,91,138,197]

Senescent changes of the rotator cuff likely occur in a manner similar to that of other joints in the body.[28,40,112] Through anatomic studies, DePalma[40,41] detailed these changes in the glenohumeral joint and rotator cuff. Observations included tearing of the cuff tendon and synovium, which became more pronounced with each successive decade of life. Moreover, DePalma and others[40,41,67,91,123,144] noted that partial-thickness tears typically begin to occur between 40 and 60 years of age and are also more frequent in older persons. Brewer[16] studied the rotator cuff in autopsy specimens and observed age-related changes, including a loss of cellularity, disorganization, and fragmentation that led to dissolution of the cuff in older subjects. It is difficult to determine whether degenerative processes are directly responsible for observed lesions, or whether they predispose the rotator cuff to tearing through alternative mechanisms. Additionally, although cadaveric age-related rotator cuff findings suggest that partial-thickness lesions develop into full-thickness tears, sufficient data in support of this concept are lacking.

More recently, Ozaki and coworkers[144] looked at the relation between anatomic changes of the acromion undersurface and pathologic findings within the rotator cuff. Histologic and radiographic evaluation demonstrated an association between bursal-side partial rotator cuff tears and abnormalities of the acromion undersurface. Changes on the acromion correlated with the severity of the bursal tear, and the prevalence increased with advancing age. Interestingly, shoulders that demonstrated joint surface partial tears revealed an intact acromion undersurface. Their data further support the contention that rotator cuff tears represent a degenerative age-related process and that acromial abnormalities reflect secondary changes resulting from a bursal surface cuff tear. Whether precarious tendon vascularity or mechanical insult by the overlying coracoacromial arch also mediate this process remains undetermined; however, it seems conceivable that both factors play a contributing role.

TABLE 1. *Etiologic factors in rotator cuff syndromes*

Traumatic factors
Rotator cuff
Acute high-velocity trauma (acute partial- or full-thickness tears)
Repetitive low-velocity microtrauma (overuse, athletic, or work-related syndromes)
Supraspinatus outlet
Acromioclavicular separation
Coracoid nonunion or malunion
Greater tuberosity malunion
Acromial malunion or nonunion
Degenerative factors
Proliferative and degenerative changes of the acromion, coracoacromial ligament, acromioclavicular joint, or greater tuberosity
Intrinsic degenerative changes of the rotator cuff
Dystrophic calcification
Developmental factors
Os acromiale
Coracoid malformation
Type II or type III acromial morphology
Low-lying acromioscapular angle
Capsuloligamentous factors
Instability
Traumatic, unidirectional
Atraumatic, multidirectional
Capsular contracture
Tight posterior capsule
Scapulothoracic neuromuscular dysfunction
Chronic cervical spondylosis
Serratus anterior palsy (long thoracic nerve injury)
Trapezius nerve palsy (spinal accessory nerve injury)
Scapulofascial muscular dystrophy
Scapulohumeral neuromuscular dysfunction
Entrapment syndromes
Axillary nerve
Suprascapular nerve
Inflammatory disease
Calcific tendinitis or bursitis
Rheumatoid arthritis
Crystal-induced arthropathy
Iatrogenic or acquired disorders
Hardware placement
Foreign materials
Inferior placement of the humeral prosthesis
Corticosteroid-induced tendonopathy

(From Iannotti JP, ed. Rotator cuff disorders: evaluation and treatment. American Academy of Orthopaedic Surgeons Monograph Series. Park Ridge, IL: American Academy of Orthopaedic Surgeons; 1991:2, with permission.)

Tearing of the rotator cuff may also result from differences in the mechanical properties of the bursal and articular surfaces of the tendon. Nakajima and coworkers[119] performed histologic and biomechanical analyses of the rotator cuff tendon in 20 autopsy specimens. The bursal layer demonstrated distinct tendon bundles that were more resistant to applied tensile loads. In contrast, tendon fibers of the articular surface were thinner, variable in their architectural arrangement, and more susceptible to tearing under tension. Fukuda and colleagues[53] histologically studied intra-tendinous tears of the rotator cuff in surgical specimens and implicated shear between the bursal and joint layers in the pathogenesis of observed lesions. Although such investigations provide further insight into potential underlying causes of rotator cuff tears, it is unlikely that one mechanism can explain the different types of tendon abnormalities. Additional study will be required to help define the etiology of the disparate lesions observed.

Traumatic insults to the shoulder can result in tearing of the rotator cuff tendon. Neviaser and coworkers[132] reported on a series of 30 patients who had a concurrent rupture of the rotator cuff with an anterior dislocation of the glenohumeral joint. All patients were older than 40 years of age and were unable to sufficiently elevate the arm in the postinjury period. The supraspinatus was torn in most of the patients, with variable degrees of infraspinatus involvement. All patients with recurrent anterior instability had disruption of the subscapularis tendon. These individuals were satisfactorily treated with primary repair of the tendon without reconstruction of the capsulolabral complex. Similar findings were noted in other reports that also included disruption of the infraspinatus and teres minor tendons in a patient with recurrent posterior dislocations.[83,130,131,154]

Overall, ruptures of the rotator cuff can occur in 14% to 63% of patients after an acute anterior or inferior dislocation.[74,107,148,154,186] The incidence increases in older persons and has been reported in 63% of patients older than 50 years of age.[154] Presumption that the rotator cuff tear is a result of the dislocation is based on negative patient accounts of shoulder pain or dysfunction before occurrence of the traumatic event.[130,131] However, it is conceivable that a tear may have been present before the injury and was extended or exacerbated after the dislocation. This may parallel patients who demonstrate acute extensions of a chronic, preexisting rotator cuff tear in the absence of instability. Although the chronicity of a potential preexisting rotator cuff lesion is sometimes difficult to determine, its influence on the prognosis and treatment should be considered. In such instances, surgical reconstruction of the rotator cuff may be more challenging than anticipated owing to the chronic component of the injury.

Fractures of the greater tuberosity, with or without a glenohumeral dislocation, can also result in tears of the rotator cuff. Neer[122] reported that a displaced greater tuberosity fracture results in an obligate longitudinal cuff tear at the region of the rotator interval. Posterior dislocations can result in a fracture of the lesser tuberosity, with disruption of the subscapularis. Interestingly, recurrent instability after fracture dislocations of the greater tuberosity is rare and is reported to range from 1% to 4%.[110,159,161]

Other forms of traumatic rotator cuff lesions include small partial-thickness tears of the supraspinatus or subscapularis in young, repetitive overhead athletes. Sports such as tennis, swimming, and baseball may predispose certain persons to rotator cuff tears through repeated mechanical stresses. One proposed mechanism suggests that fatigue of the scapular stabilizers results from repeated throwing, causing the humeral head and rotator cuff to abut against the acromion during arm elevation. The scapula is thought to "lag" behind the humerus, becoming unable to abduct sufficiently. Patients with neural impairments causing weakness of the trapezius or serratus anterior muscles can also develop secondary impingement through similar mechanisms. Loss of the suspensory mechanism of the scapula, such as in traumatic disruption of the acromioclavicular and coracoclavicular ligaments, may result in comparable rotator cuff abnormalities. In such cases, rotator cuff impingement occurs secondary to abnormal functional mechanics of the scapula.

Jobe and associates[87,88] popularized the concept of secondary mechanical impingement in throwing athletes. They noted that rotator cuff lesions are the end result of a continuum that progresses from instability, subluxation, impingement, and tension overload of the cuff, with resultant tearing. Repeated mechanical stresses cause failure of the glenohumeral static restraints and place increased demands on the dynamic stabilizers. The rotator cuff eventually fatigues, resulting in abnormal translation of the humeral head and secondary impingement. If left untreated, the impingement can progress and cause tearing of the cuff. The ability to distinguish between primary and secondary impingement, as described by Neer and Jobe, respectively, is paramount to effectively treating patients affected with these disorders. Although satisfactory results have been reported for subacromial decompression in patients with primary impingement, the same does not hold true for individuals with the secondary type.[2,48,56,60,68,71,149,168,180,184,185] Rather, treatment in this group requires attention to the underlying instability.

An association between an unfused acromial epiphysis or, "os acromiale," and tears of the rotator cuff has also been described.[117,125,134] The acromion has three centers of ossification that typically unite with the scapular spine by age 12 and with each other by age 15 to 18[52,129] (Fig. 21). These three centers are designated as the preacromion, mesoacromion, and metaacromion. The prevalence of os acromiale has been reported to range from 1% to 15%, with a 62% frequency of bilateral involvement.[46,66,99,133] Abnormal motion at the synostosis or synchondrosis is thought to decrease the capacity of the subacromial space and contribute to mechanical insult of the underlying rotator cuff.

An os acromiale can be identified on an axillary radiograph and should not be mistaken for a fracture of the acromion. Failure to recognize this entity can potentially compromise the results of treatment. Consensus on the optimal management is lacking and has ranged from conservative treatment to excision versus internal fixation and bone grafting.[22,79,117,134,181] Norris and associates[134] evaluated a group of 29 patients with os acromiale and suggested bone grafting in patients in whom the os was considered to be unstable. Standard acromioplasty was believed to be satisfactory in patients with a stable synostosis. Arthroscopic subacromial decompression alone has been reported to yield poor results in some patients, for symptoms were noted to recur within 1 year of surgery.[79] Whereas smaller fragments may be amenable to excision in symptomatic patients, no controlled studies exist comparing excision with internal fixation and bone grafting for meso os acromiale. Because the acromion serves as the origin for the deltoid, potential compromise of this important muscle should be considered during surgical management of affected patients.

The finding of an os acromiale may be incidental and not necessarily correlate with a patient's symptoms. Normal shoulder function has been noted in patients with an os acromiale.[22,99] Burkhart[22] reported on a high-performance tennis player who had competed without pain or dysfunction for 15 years before evaluation. Furthermore, clinical experience has demonstrated that many patients who present with shoulder pain and have an os acromiale had been asymptomatic

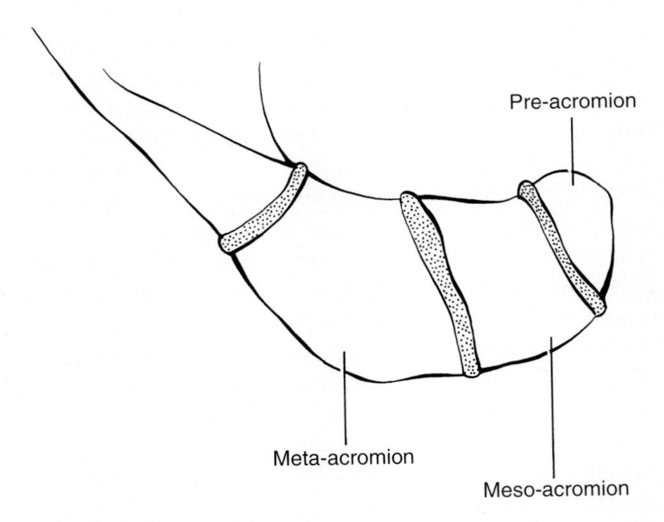

FIG. 21. Three ossification centers of the acromion. (From ref. 99, with permission.)

for many years before clinical presentation. Often, a traumatic event has been presumed to precipitate symptoms surrounding the os acromiale. If the prevalence of this anomaly is estimated at 1% to 15% of the general population, then it seems likely that many individuals with an os acromiale never develop symptoms given the frequency of cases seen in a clinical shoulder practice.

Other coracoacromial arch abnormalities associated with the development of rotator cuff disease include congenital subacromial stenosis. A narrow subacromial space, recently described after review of radiographs in a clinical setting, may predispose certain patients to impingement lesions of the rotator cuff.[20] Such findings likely parallel previous anatomic studies that linked rotator cuff disease to coracoacromial arch dimensional parameters resulting in a narrowed outlet.[44,205] The literature is sparse relative to this entity, and further investigation is required to better define, detect, and treat such patients.

It is apparent that rotator cuff disease represents a heterogeneous disorder that is likely of multifactorial etiology. Vascular factors, impingement syndrome, degenerative processes, and developmental influences, all appear to contribute, in some combination, to the formation and progression of rotator cuff lesions. Recognition of such processes will lead to an increased ability to effectively diagnose and treat patients who present with symptoms related to the rotator cuff.

NATURAL HISTORY

The rotator cuff is subject to substantial forces because it maintains the humeral head within the shallow glenoid. It is situated in a potentially tight subacromial space and undergoes senescent structural changes commonly observed in other joints of the body.[28,40,112] When the cuff fails, spontaneous healing of the torn tendon is not expected to occur, and multiple factors may be responsible. Its fibers are under tension and typically retract on tearing. In full-thickness lesions, only bursal tissue may bridge the area of tendon loss. Histologic evaluation of partial tears in surgical specimens has also demonstrated patterns of incomplete healing. Observations included neovascular tissue at the distal margin of the defect and relative avascularity of the proximal stump. Although the potential for a reparative process was felt to exist, there was no evidence of closure of the defect in any of the specimens. The findings were suggestive of a futile attempt at healing.[54] Other investigators have noted that resorption of tendon fibers by neovascular tissue can occur.[182,197] This may potentially weaken surrounding intact fibers placed under increased loads as a result of a tear. Because the torn cuff is bathed in synovial fluid, factors responsible for normal healing and formation of fibrin clots may be disrupted. Moreover, tearing may further impair the blood supply to a relatively dysvascular tendon.

The prevalence of rotator cuff tears in the general population can be extrapolated from both cadaveric and MRI studies. The frequency of complete and partial rotator cuff tears ranges from 5% to 39% and 13% to 3%, respectively.[32,55,67,91,92,123,144,147,172,197] Although anatomic studies have reported an increase in pathologic findings about the cuff with advancing age, they are limited by an inability to sufficiently correlate findings with symptomatology. Given the prevalence of rotator cuff tears in cadaveric studies alone, it remains unclear whether observed findings could be considered part of the normal-aging process.

More recently, a prospective investigation was conducted to determine the prevalence of rotator cuff tears in an entirely asymptomatic population by using shoulder MRI scans in 96 normal volunteers. Overall, complete and partial-thickness tears were found in 14% and 20% of individuals, respectively. In persons older than 60 years of age, the prevalence of complete and partial tears was 28% and 26%, respectively[172] (Fig. 22). The results provided in vivo evidence that asymptomatic individuals with rotator cuff tears can exhibit normal shoulder function. Moreover, they emphasized the dangers of basing operative decisions on MRI scans alone. The high prevalence of cuff tears in an asymptomatic population and their direct correlation with age support the contention that some rotator cuff tears occur as part of a normal age-related process. However, the natural history of these findings remains unknown; they may potentially represent an early phase of a pathologic process in which symptoms have not yet developed. Longitudinal follow-up studies in such persons can further help determine the natural course of these lesions.

The question of why some patients with rotator cuff tears develop symptoms, and others do not, has not been sufficiently addressed in the literature. Both prior reports and clinical observation affirm that many patients with cuff tears may not demonstrate significant pain or dysfunction.[15,18,109,160,166] Clearly, some individuals with symptomatic tears respond well to conservative treatment despite the persistence of a tendon defect. Other authors have documented good functional results, in the short term, in patients who had undergone debridement, rather than repair of a torn rotator cuff. Furthermore, satisfactory pain relief was predictably achieved despite lack of closure of the tendon tear.[19,97,137,155,157,206] As such lesions do not typically heal, it would seem conceivable that factors other than the tendon defect itself must contribute to the generation of symptoms. Fukuda and associates[53] suggested that subacromial bursal inflammation, as evidenced in surgical histologic specimens of partial-thickness rotator cuff tears, mediates symptoms in affected patients. They noted that the degree of inflammation likely correlates with the patient's level of symptoms. Others have suggested additional sources of shoulder pain that potentially include synovitis, intraarticular pathology, and mechanical factors.[23,47,121,123]

Alterations in normal glenohumeral kinematics have also been considered in the development of symptoms, but equally important, may be individual differences in scapular mechanics, compensatory action of surrounding muscles,

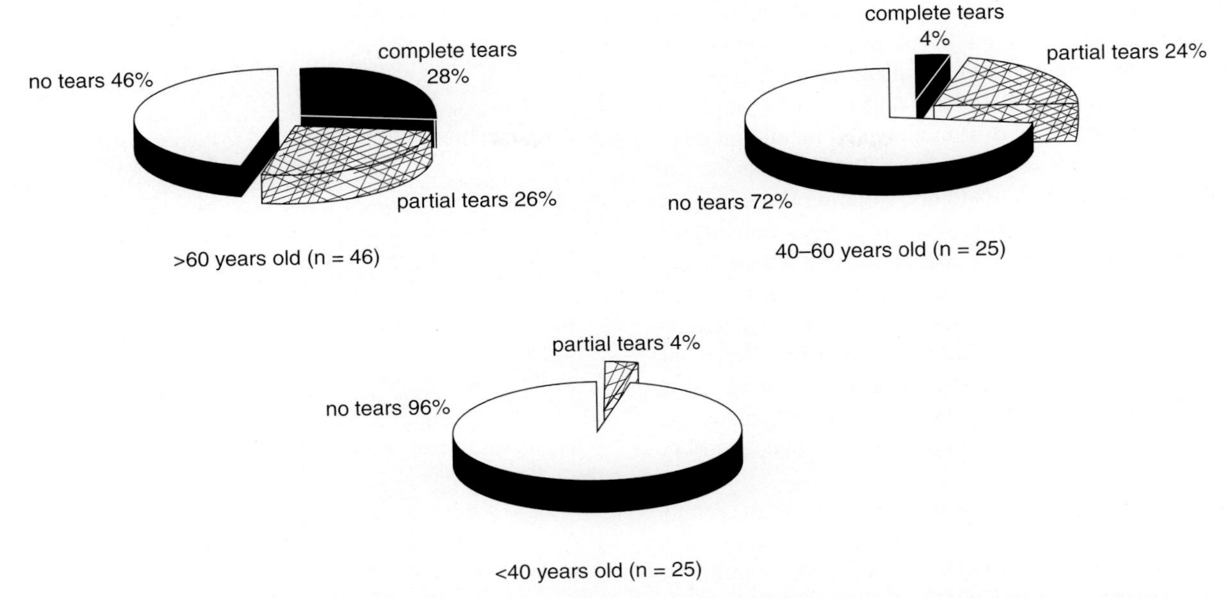

FIG. 22. Prevalence of MRI-evident rotator cuff tears in (**left**) asymptomatic volunteers older than 60 years of age, (**right**) those 40 to 60 years, and (**bottom**) those younger than 40 years. (Adapted with permission from ref. 172.)

and variable tolerances to pain. Multiple studies have shown abnormal superior migration of the humeral head during active arm elevation in shoulders with rotator cuff tears and the impingement syndrome.[21,42,103,150,170,203] In normal shoulders, on the other hand, the geometric center of the humeral head remains centered on the glenoid during active arm elevation.[3,150,170] Abnormal glenohumeral patterns of motion have thus been suggested to play a role in mediating pain. Burkhart[21] emphasized the concept of an anatomically deficient, but biomechanically intact, rotator cuff. Fluoroscopy was used to assess kinematics of the glenohumeral joint in patients with massive tears of the rotator cuff. Normal patterns were demonstrated, provided sufficient anterior and posterior cuff were present to preserve the normal transverse plane force couple. Location, rather than size of the tear was felt to have a more important role in preserving normal glenohumeral motion. Another biomechanical study evaluating glenohumeral motion in artificially created tendon defects highlighted the potential for normal kinematics, provided only a portion of the cuff was violated. Lesions of the supraspinatus did not alter normal motion patterns, whereas defects involving both the supra- and infraspinatus demonstrated an increase in humeral cephalad migration.[103]

A recent investigation attempted to address the relation between glenohumeral kinematics and symptoms in patients with rotator cuff tears. Computer-enhanced radiographic measurements were obtained during arm elevation in patients with known tears of the rotator cuff. An asymptomatic and symptomatic population were studied, which revealed progressive superior humeral head translation in both groups when compared with normal controls.[203] These data demonstrate that loss of glenohumeral kinematics, as measured in the coronal plane, does not correlate with the presence of symptoms. More likely, symptoms are the result of multiple factors that may not necessarily be independent of one another.

The fate of the many types of cuff lesions cannot always be predicted. It is difficult to conclude that all rotator cuff lesions fall within a continuum progressing from tendinitis to full-thickness tears, because conclusive evidence supporting this concept is lacking. Rather, it seems more plausible that the types of pathology observed reflect the multifactorial etiology and pathogenetic mechanisms so far identified. Moreover, we cannot definitively determine that partial tears heal, for evidence to the contrary exists.[54] The significance of bursal and joint surface partial lesions in relation to symptoms and their pathogenesis also remains uncertain.

The natural history of patients with symptomatic full-thickness rotator cuff tears is variable. Moreover, our ability to reliably predict a given patient's course is limited and may partly reflect insufficient knowledge about its pathogenesis. Clinical experience has demonstrated that patients with similar-appearing lesions may have differences in symptoms, function, and response to treatment. Cofield[33] noted that conservative management of patients with chronic painful rotator cuff tears will likely result in a successful outcome less than 50% of the time. Others have noted similar findings after nonoperative treatment and reported gradual deterioration of shoulder function with time in some patients.[82,166,198] Neer and coworkers[126] estimated that cuff tear arthropathy will develop in 4% of patients with complete rotator cuff tears. If the tear was not sufficiently large or became sealed off by bursal tissue, then development of cuff-related arthropathy was less likely. The surgical recommendations for patients with symptomatic complete tears are generally individualized and based on the duration of symptoms, severity of pain, degree of dysfunction, and functional goals. Although, satisfactory results can usually be achieved with surgical treatment in many patients, isolating those individuals likely to achieve similar outcomes with nonsurgical management continues to be a challenge. The heterogeneity, lack of uniform classification, nonuniformity in treatment strategies, and existence of similar lesions in normal asymptomatic persons make it difficult to predict the likely outcome of these patients. The use of appropriate animal models and execution of large longitudinal follow-up studies can help further identify prognostic criteria for rotator cuff lesions.

Given the evidence to date, it seems likely that the rotator cuff has some degree of reserve that affords functional use of the arm in cases of limited tendon deficiencies. Moreover, location rather than size of a tear may be more important in the development of symptoms; however, this issue requires elucidation with further study. Factors such as synovitis, subacromial bursitis, and intraarticular abnormalities may contribute to pain and dysfunction, but further basic science and clinical research can help define and isolate specific causes of pain in affected patients. Enhancement of our ability to identify individuals with cuff lesions prone to progression and dysfunction will afford the development of optimal treatment approaches individualized to a given patient's clinical findings.

REFERENCES

1. Abbott LC, Saunders JBM, Hagey H, Jones EW. Surgical approaches to the shoulder joint. *J Bone Joint Surg [Am]* 1949;31:235–244.
2. Altchek DW, Warren RF, Wickiewicz TL, Skyhar MJ, Ortiz G, Schwartz E. Arthroscopic acromioplasty. *J Bone Joint Surg [Am]* 1990;72:1198–1207.
3. An KN, Brown AO, Korinek S, Tanaka S, Morrey BF. Three-dimensional kinematics of glenohumeral elevation. *J Orthop Res* 1991;9:143–149.
4. Aoki M, Ishii S, Usui M. Clinical application for measuring the slope of the acromion. In: Post M, Morrey B, Hawkins R, eds. *Surgery of the shoulder*. St Louis: Mosby–Year Book; 1990:200–203.
5. Aoki M, Ishii S, Usui M. The slope of the acromion and rotator cuff impingement. *Orthop Trans* 1986;10:228.
6. Armstrong JR. Excision of the acromion in the treatment of the supraspinatus syndrome. Report of ninety-five excisions. *J Bone Joint Surg [Br]* 1949;31:436–442.
7. Arntz CT, Matsen FA, Jackins S. Surgical management of complex irreparable rotator cuff deficiency. *J Arthroplasty* 1991;6:363–370.
8. Banas MP, Miller RJ, Totterman S. Relationship between the lateral acromion angle and rotator cuff disease. *J Shoulder Elbow Surg* 1995;4:454–461.
9. Barthel T, Gohlke F, Loehr J, Eulert J, Gandorfer A. The reliability of the supraspinatus outlet view in assessing acromial morphology. Presented at the Fifth International Conference on Surgery of the Shoulder; Paris, France, July 12–15, 1992. *J Shoulder Elbow Surg* 1993;2:S18.
10. Basmajian JV, Bazant FJ. Factors preventing downward dislocation of the adducted shoulder joint in an electromyographic and morphological study. *J Bone Joint Surg [Am]* 1986;41:1182–1186.
11. Bechtol CO. Biomechanics of the shoulder. *Clin Orthop* 1980;146:37–41.
12. Bigliani LU, Colman WW, Kelkar R, et al. The effect of anterior acromioplasty on rotator cuff contact: an experimental and computer simulation. Presented at the American Shoulder and Elbow Surgeons, eleventh open meeting, Orlando, FL, February 19, 1995.
13. Bigliani LU, Dalsey RM; McCann PD, April EW. An anatomical study of the suprascapular nerve. *Arthroscopy* 1990;6:301–305.
14. Bigliani LU, Morrison DS, April EW. The morphology of the acromion and rotator cuff impingement. *Orthop Trans* 1986;10:288.
15. Bokor DJ, Hawkins RJ, Huckell GH, Angelo RL, Schickendantz MS. Results of nonoperative management of full-thickness tears of the rotator cuff. *Clin Orthop* 199;294:103–110.
16. Brewer BJ. Aging of the rotator cuff. *Am J Sports Med* 1979;7:102–110.
17. Brooks CH, Revell WJ, Heatley FW. A quantitative histological study of the vascularity of the rotator cuff tendon. *J Bone Joint Surg* 1992;74-B:151–153.
18. Brown JT. Early assessment of supraspinatus tears: procaine infiltration as a guide to treatment. *J Bone Joint Surg [Br]* 1949;31:423.
19. Burkhart SS. Arthroscopic debridement and decompression for selected rotator cuff tears. *Orthop Clin North Am* 1993;24:111–123.
20. Burkhart SS. Congenital subacromial stenosis. *Arthroscopy* 1995;11:63–68.
21. Burkhart SS. Flouroscopic comparison of kinematic patterns in massive rotator cuff tears. A suspension bridge model. *Clin Orthop* 1992;284:144–152.
22. Burkhart SS. Os acromiale in a professional tennis player. *Am J Sports Med* 1992;20:483–484.
23. Burkhart SS. Reconciling the paradox of rotator cuff repair versus debridement: a unified biomechanical rationale for the treatment of rotator cuff tears. *Arthroscopy* 1994;10:4–19.
24. Burkhead WZ, Scheinberg RR, Box G. Surgical anatomy of the axillary nerve. *J Shoulder Elbow Surg* 1992;1:31–36.
25. Burns WC, Whipple TL. Anatomic relationships in the shoulder impingement syndrome. *Clin Orthop* 1993;294:96–102.
26. Cain PR, Mutschler TA, Fu FH, Lee SK. Anterior stability of the glenohumeral joint. *Am J Sports Med* 1987;15:144–148.
27. Chansky HA, Iannotti JP. The vascularity of the rotator cuff. *Clin Sports Med* 1991;10:807–822.
28. Chard MD, Cawston TE, Riley GP, Gresham GA, Hazleman BL. Rotator cuff degeneration and lateral epicondylitis: a comparative histological study. *Ann Rheum Dis* 1994;53:30–34.
29. Ciullo JV, Guise ER. Histopathologic findings in clinical coracoacromial arch impingement (abstr). *Orthop Trans* 1986;10:228.
30. Clark JM, Harryman DT. Tendons, ligaments, and capsule of the rotator cuff. *J Bone Joint Surg [Am]* 1992;74:713–725.
31. Codman EA. Rupture of the supraspinatus tendon. *Clin Orthop* 1990;254:3–26.
32. Codman EA, Akerson TB. The pathology associated with rupture of the supraspinatus tendon. *Ann Surg* 1931;93:348–359.
33. Cofield RH. Rotator cuff disease of the shoulder. *J Bone Joint Surg [Am]* 1985;67:974–979.
34. Colachis SC, Strohm BR. Effect of suprascapular and axillary nerve blocks on muscle force in upper extremity. *Arch Phys Med Rehabil* 1971;52:22–29.
35. Colachis SC, Strohm BR, Brechner VL. Effects of axillary nerve block on muscle force in the upper extremity. *Arch Phys Med Rehabil* 1969;50:647–654.
36. Cooper DE, O'Brien SJ, Warren RF. Supporting layers of the glenohumeral joint. An antomic study. *Clin Orthop* 1993;289:144–155.
37. Cotton RE, Rideout DF. Tears of the humeral rotator cuff. A radiological and pathological necropsy survey. *J Bone Joint Surg [Br]* 1964;46:314–328.
38. Davidson PA, Elattrache NS, Jobe CM, Jobe FW. Rotator cuff and posterior–superior glenoid labrum injury associated with increased glenohumeral motion: a new site of impingement. *J Shoulder Elbow Surg* 1995;4:384–390.
39. DePalma AF. Biomechanics of the shoulder. In: DePalma AF, ed. *Surgery of the shoulder*, 3rd ed. Philadelphia; JB Lippincott Co; 1983.
40. DePalma AF. In: DePalma AF, ed. *Surgery of the shoulder*, 3rd ed. Philadelphia; JB Lippincott Co; 1983:211–241.
41. DePalma AF, Callery G, Bennett GA. Variational anatomy and de-

generative lesions of the shoulder joint. Instructional Course Lectures, American Academy of Orthopaedic Surgeons 1949;6:255–281.

42. Deutsch A, Altchek DW, Schwartz E, Otis JC, Warren RF. Radiologic measurement of superior displacement of the humeral head in impingement syndrome. *J Shoulder Elbow Surg* 1996;5:186–193.
43. Dines DM, Warren RF, Inglis AE, Pavlov H. The coracoid impingement syndrome. *J Bone Joint Surg [Br]* 1990;72:314–316.
44. Edelson JG, Taitz C. Anatomy of the coraco-acromial arch: relation to degeneration of the acromion. *J Bone Joint Surg [Br]* 1992;74:589–594.
45. Edelson JG, Taitz C. Bony anatomy of coracoacromial arch: implications for arthroscopic portal placement in the shoulder. *Arthroscopy* 1993;9:201–208.
46. Edelson JG, Zuckerman J, Hershkovitz I. Os acromiale: anatomy and surgical implications. *J Bone Joint Surg [Br]* 1993;75:551–555.
47. Ellman H, Harris E, Kay SP. Early degenerative joint disease simulating impingement syndrome: arthroscopic findings. *Arthroscopy* 1912;8:482–487.
48. Ellman H, Kay SP. Arthroscopic subacromial decompression for chronic impingement. Two to five year results. *J Bone Joint Surg [Br]* 1991;73:395–398.
49. Farley TE, Neumann CH, Steinbach LS, Peterson SA. The coracoacromial arch: MR evaluation and correlation with rotator cuff pathology. *Skeletal Radiol* 1994;23:641–645.
50. Flatow EL, Connor PM, Levine WN, Arroyo JS, Pollock RG, Bigliani LU. Coracoacromial arch reconstruction for anterosuperior instability. Presented at American Shoulder and Elbow Surgeons 13th Open Meeting, San Francisco, February 1997.
51. Flatow EL, Soslowski LJ, Ticker JB, et al. Excursion of the rotator cuff under the acromion. Patterns of subacromial contact. *Am J Sports Med* 1994;22:779–788.
52. Folliasson A. Un cas d'os acromial. *Rev Orthop* 1933;20:533–538.
53. Fukuda H, Hamada K, Nakajima T, Tomonaga A. Pathology and pathogenesis of the intratendinous tearing of the rotator cuff viewed from en bloc histologic sections. *Clin Orthop* 1994;304:60–67.
54. Fukuda H, Hamada K, Yamanaka K. Pathology and pathogenesis of bursal-side rotator cuff tears viewed from en bloc histologic sections. *Clin Orthop* 1990;254:75–80.
55. Fukuda H, Mikasa M, Ogawa K, Yamanaka K, Hamada K. The partial thickness tear of the rotator cuff. *Orthop Trans* 1983;7:137.
56. Gartsman GM. Arthroscopic acromioplasty for lesions of the rotator cuff. *J Bone Joint Surg [Am]* 1990;72:169–180.
57. Gerber C, Schneeberger AG, Vinh TS. The arterial vascularization of the humeral head: an anatomical study. *J Bone Joint Surg [Am]* 1990;72:1486–1494.
58. Gerber C, Terrier F, Ganz R. The role of the coracoid process in the chronic impingement syndrome. *J Bone Joint Surg [Br]* 1985;67:703–708.
59. Gerber C, Terrier F, Zehnder R, Ganz R. The subcoracoid space. An anatomic study. *Clin Orthop* 1987;215:132–138.
60. Glousman RE. Instability versus impingement syndrome in the throwing athlete. *Orthop Clin North Am* 1993;24:89–99.
61. Glousman RE, Jobe F, Tibone J, Moynes D, Antonelli D, Perry J. Dynamic electromyographic analysis of the throwing shoulder with glenohumeral instability. *J Bone Joint Surg [Am]* 1988;70:220–226.
62. Godsil RD, Linscheid RL. Intratendinous defects of the rotator cuff. *Clin Orthop* 1970;69:181–188.
63. Gohlke F, Barthel T, Gandorfer A. The influence of variations of the coracoacromial arch on the development of rotator cuff tears. *Arch Orthop Trauma Surg* 1993;113:28–32.
64. Gohlke F, Daum P, Eulert J. The stabilizing function of the capsule of the glenohumeral joint and the corresponding role of the coracoacromial arch (abstr). *J Shoulder Elbow Surg* 1994;2:S22.
65. Goldthwait JE. An anatomic and mechanical study of the shoulder joint. Explaining many of the cases of painful shoulder, many of the recurrent dislocations and many of the cases of brachial neuralgias or neuritis. *Am J Orthop Surg* 1909;6:579.
66. Grant JCB. *An atlas of anatomy*, 6th ed. Baltimore: Williams & Wilkins; 1972:26, 40.
67. Grant JCB, Smith CG. Rupture of the supraspinatus tendon. *Anat Rec* 1948;100:666.
68. Ha'eri GB, Wiley AM. Advancement of the supraspinatus muscle in the repair of ruptures of the rotator cuff. *J Bone Joint Surg [Am]* 1981;63:232–238.
69. Harris JE, Blackney M. The anatomy and function of the coracoacromial ligament (abstr). *J Shoulder Elbow Surg* 1993;2:S6.
70. Harryman DT, Sidles JA, Clark JM, McQuade KJ, Gibb TD, Matsen FA. Translation of the humeral head on the glenoid with passive glenohumeral motion. *J Bone Joint Surg [Am]* 1990;72:1334–1343.
71. Hawkins RJ, Brock RM, Abrams JS, Hobeika P. Acromioplasty for impingement with an intact rotator cuff. *J Bone Joint Surg [Br]* 1988;70:795–797.
72. Helmig P, Sojberg JO, Kjaersgaard-Anderson P, et al. Distal humeral migration as a component of multidirectional shoulder instability: an anatomical study in autopsy specimens. *Clin Orthop* 1990;252:139–143.
73. Hijioka A, Suzuki K, Nakamura T, et al. Degenerative change and rotator cuff tears. An anatomical study in 160 shoulders and 80 cadavers. *Arch Orthop Trauma Surg* 1993;112:61–64.
74. Hintermann B, Gachter A. Arthroscopic findings after shoulder dislocation. *Am J Sports Med* 1995;23:545–551.
75. Holt EM, Allibone RO. Anatomic variants of the coracoacromial ligament. *J Shoulder Elbow Surg* 1995;4:370–375.
76. Howell SM, Galinat BJ. The glenoid–labral socket. A constrained articular surface. *Clin Orthop* 1989;243:122–125.
77. Howell SM, Galinat BJ, Renzi AJ, Marone PJ. Normal and abnormal mechanics of the glenohumeral joint in the horizontal plane. *J Bone Joint Surg [Am]* 1988;70:227–232.
78. Howell SM, Imobersteg AM, Seger DH, Marone PJ. Clarification of the role of the supraspinatus muscle in shoulder function. *J Bone Joint Surg [Am]* 1986;68:398–404.
79. Hutchinson MR, Veenstra MA. Arthroscopic decompression of shoulder impingement secondary to os acromiale. *Arthroscopy* 1993;9:28–32.
80. Iannotti JP, Gabriel JP, Schneck SL, Evans BG, Misra S. The normal glenohumeral relationships. An anatomical study of one hundred and forty shoulders. *J Bone Joint Surg [Am]* 1992;74:491–500.
81. Inman VT, Saunders JB, Abbott LC. Observations on the function of the shoulder joint. *J Bone Joint Surg* 1944;26:1–30.
82. Itoi E, Tabata S. Conservative treatment of rotator cuff tears. *Clin Orthop* 1992;275:165–173.
83. Itoi E, Tabata S. Rotator cuff tears in anterior dislocation of the shoulder. *Int Orthop* 1993;17:64.
84. Jacobson SR, Speer KP, Moor JT, et al. Reliability of radiographic assessment of acromial morpholgy. *J Shoulder Elbow Surg* 1995;4:449–453.
85. Jalovaara P, Lanotto V. Local pressures in the subacromial space at different positions of the humerus. *Acta Orthop Scand Suppl* 1992;247:23–24.
86. Jobe CM, Sidles J.Evidence for a superior glenoid impingement upon the rotator cuff (abstr). *J Shoulder Elbow Surg* 1993;2:S19.
87. Jobe FW, Kvitne RS. Shoulder pain in the overhand or throwing athlete: the relationship of anterior instability and rotator cuff impingement. *Orthop Rev* 1989;18:963.
88. Jobe FW, Pink M. Classification and treatment of shoulder dysfunction in the overhead athlete. *J Orthop Sports Phys Ther* 1993;18:427–432.
89. Johansson JE, Barrington TW. Coracoacromial ligament division. *Am J Sports Med* 1984;12:138–141.
90. Kessel L, Watson M. The painful arc syndrome. Clinical classification as a guide to management. *J Bone Joint Surg [Br]* 1977;59:166–172.
91. Keyes EL. Anatomical observations on senile changes in the shoulder. *J Bone Joint Surg [Am]* 1935;17:953–960.
92. Keyes EL. Observations on rupture of the supraspinatus tendon: based upon a study of 73 cadavers. *Ann Surg* 1933;97:849–856.
93. Kitay GS, Iannotti JP, Williams GR, Haygood T, Kneeland BJ, Berlin J. Roentgenographic assessment of acromial morphologic condition in rotator cuff impingement syndrome. *J Shoulder Elbow Surg* 1995;4:441–448.
94. Ko JY, Shih CH, Chen WJ, Yamamoto R. Coracoid impingement syndrome caused by a ganglion from the subscapularis tendon. A case report. *J Bone Joint Surg [Am]* 1994;76:1709–1711.
95. Kronberg M, Brostrom LA, Nemeth G. Differences in shoulder muscle activity between patients with generalized joint laxity and normal controls. *Clin Orthop* 1991;269:181–192.
96. LeHuec JC, Schaeverbeke T, Moinard M, et al. Traumatic tear of the rotator interval. *J Shoulder Elbow Surg* 1996;5:41–46.
97. Levy HJ, Gardner RD, Lemak LJ. Arthroscopic subacromial decom-

pression in the treatment of full thickness rotator cuff tears. *Arthroscopy* 1991;7:8–13.
98. Levy HJ, Uribe JW, Delaney LG. Arthroscopic assisted rotator cuff repair: preliminary results. *Arthroscopy* 1990;6:55–60.
99. Liberson F. Os acromiale: a contested anomaly. *J Bone Joint Surg* 1937;683–689.
100. Lindblom K. On the pathogenesis of ruptures of the tendon aponeurosis of the shoulder joint. *Acta Radiol* 1939;20:563–577.
101. Lippitt S, Matsen F. Mechanisms of glenohumeral joint stability. *Clin Orthop* 1993;291:20–28.
102. Liu SH, Boynton E. Posterior superior impingement of the rotator cuff on the glenoid rim as a cause of shoulder pain in the overhead athlete. *Arthroscopy* 1993;9:697–699.
103. Loehr JF, Helmig P, Sojberg JO, Jung A. Shoulder instability caused by rotator cuff lesions. An in vitro study. *Clin Orthop* 1994;304: 84–90.
104. Lohr JF, Uhthoff HK. The microvascular pattern of the supraspinatus tendon. *Clin Orthop* 1990;254:35–38.
105. Lozman PR, Hechtman KS, Uribe JW. Combined arthroscopic management of impingement syndrome and acromioclavicular joint arthritis. *J South Orthop Assoc* 1995;4:177–181.
106. Macnab I. Rotator cuff tendinitis. *Ann R Coll Surg Engl* 1973;53: 271–287.
107. Mallon WJ, Bassett FH, Goldner RD. Luxatio erecta: the inferior glenohumeral dislocation. *J Orthop Trauma* 1990;4:19–24.
108. Mayer L. The physiologic method of tendon transplantation. *Surg Gynacol Obstet* 1915;22:182.
109. McLaughlin HL. Repair of major cuff ruptures. *Surg Clin North Am* 1963;43:1535.
110. McLaughlin HL, MacLellan DI. Recurrent anterior dislocation of the shoulder: II. A comparative study. *J Trauma* 1967;7:191–201.
111. McMaster P. Tendon and muscle ruptures. *J Bone Joint Surg* 1933;15: 705.
112. Meyer AW. The minuter anatomy of attrition lesions. *J Bone Joint Surg [Am]* 1931;13:341–360.
113. Miller C, Savoie FH. Glenohumeral abnormalities associated with full-thickness tears of the rotator cuff. *Orthop Rev* 1994;23:159–164.
114. Moore KL. *Clinically oriented anatomy*, 2nd ed. Baltimore: Williams & Wilkins; 1985:626–793.
115. Morrison DS, Bigliani LU. The clinical significance of variations in acromial morphology. *Orthop Trans* 1987;11:234.
116. Moseley HF, Goldie IG. The arterial pattern of the rotator cuff of the shoulder. *J Bone Joint Surg [Br]* 1963;45:780–789.
117. Mudge MK, Wood VE, Frykman GK. Rotator cuff tears associated with os acromiale. *J Bone Joint Surg [Am]* 1984;66:427–429.
118. Nakagaki K, Ozaki J, Tomita Y, Tamai S. Function of supraspinatus muscle with torn cuff evaluated by magnetic resonance imaging. *Clin Orthop* 1995;318:144–151.
119. Nakajima T, Rokuuma N, Hamada K, Tomatsu T, Fukuda H. Histologic and biomechanical characteristics of the supraspinatus tendon: reference to rotator cuff tearing. *J Shoulder Elbow Surg* 1994;3: 79–87.
120. Nasca RJ, Salter EG, Weil CE. Contact areas of the subacromial joint. In: Bateman JE, Welsh RP, eds. *Surgery of the shoulder*. New York: Marcel Decker; 1984:134–139.
121. Neer CS. Anterior acromioplasty for the chronic impingement syndrome. A preliminary report. *J Bone Joint Surg [Am]* 1972;54:41–50.
122. Neer CS. Displaced proximal humeral fractures. Part I. Classification and Evaluation. *J Bone Joint Surg [Am]* 1970;52:1077–1089.
123. Neer CS. Impingement lesions. *Clin Orthop* 1983;173:70–77.
124. Neer CS. Cuff tears, biceps lesions and impingement. In: Neer CS. *Shoulder reconstruction*. Philadelphia: WB Saunders; 1990;44–48.
125. Neer CS. Rotator cuff tears associated with os acromiale. *J Bone Joint Surg [Am]* 1984;66:1320–1321.
126. Neer CS, Craig EV, Fukuda H. Cuff-tear arthropathy. *J Bone Joint Surg [Am]* 1983;65:1232–1244.
127. Neer CS, Poppen NK. Supraspinatus outlet (abstr). *Orthop Trans* 1987;11:234.
128. Neer CS, Satterlee CC, Dalsey RM, Flatow E. The anatomy and potential effects of contracture of the coracohumeral ligament. *Clin Orthop* 1992;280:182–185.
129. Neumann W. Uber das "Os Acromiale". *Fortschr Geb Rontgenstr* 1918;25:180–191.
130. Neviaser RJ, Neviaser TJ. Recurrent instability of the shoulder after age 40. *J Shoulder Elbow Surg* 1995;4:416–418.
131. Neviaser RJ, Neviaser TJ, Neviaser JS. Anterior dislocation of the shoulder and rotator cuff rupture. *Clin Orthop* 1993;291:103–106.
132. Neviaser RJ, Neviaser TJ, Neviaser JS. Concurrent rupture of the rotator cuff and anterior dislocation of the shoulder in the older patient. *J Bone Joint Surg [Am]* 1988;70:1308–1311.
133. Nicholson GP, Goodman DA, Flatow EL, Bigliani LU. The acromion: morphologic condition and age related changes. A study of 420 scapulas. *J Shoulder Elbow Surg* 1996;5:1–11.
134. Norris TR, Fischer J, Bigliani L, et al. The unfused acromial epihysis and its relationship to impingement syndrome. *Orthop Trans* 1983;7: 505–506.
135. O'Driscoll SW. Atraumatic instability: pathology and pathogenesis. In: Matsen FA, Fu FH, Hawkins RJ, eds. *The shoulder: a balance of mobility and stability*. Rosemont: American Academy of Orthopaedic Surgeons; 1993:305–316.
136. Ogata S, Uhthoff HK. Acromial enthesopathy and rotator cuff tear. A radiologic and histologic postmortem investigation of the coracoacromial arch. *Clin Orthop* 1990;254:39–48.
137. Ogilvie-Harris DJ, Demaziere A. Arthroscopic debridement versus open repair for rotator cuff tears: a prospective cohort study. *J Bone Joint Surg [Br]* 1993;75:416–420.
138. Olsson O. Degenerative changes of the shoulder joint and their connection with shoulder pain. *Acta Chir Scand* 1953;181:1–130.
139. Otis JC, Jiang CC, Wickiewicz TL, Peterson MG, Warren RF, Santer TJ. Changes of the moment arms of the rotator cuff and deltoid muscles with abduction and rotation. *J Bone Joint Surg [Am]* 1994;76: 667–676.
140. Otis JC, Jiang CC, Wickiewicz TL, Warren RF. Contribution of the infraspinatus muscle to shoulder abduction and external rotation torques. In: Torzilli PA, Friedman MH, eds. *1989 Biomechanics symposium*. New York: The American Society for Mechanical Engineers; 1987.
141. Oveson J, Nielson S. Anterior and posterior shoulder instability: a cadaver study. *Acta Orthop Scand* 1986;57:324–327.
142. Oveson J, Nielson S. Posterior instability of the shoulder. A cadaver study. *Acta Orthop Scand* 1986;57:436–439.
143. Oveson J, Nielson S. Stability of the shoulder joint: cadaver study of stabilizing structures. *Acta Orthop Scand* 1985;56:149–151.
144. Ozaki J, Fujimoto S, Nakagawa Y, Masuhara K, Tamai S. Tears of the rotator cuff of the shoulder associated with pathologic changes in the acromion. *J Bone Joint Surg [Am]* 1988;70:1224–1230.
145. Patte D. The subcoracoid impingement. *Clin Orthop* 1990;254:55–59.
146. Perry J. Anatomy and biomechanics of the shoulder in throwing, swimming, gymnastics, and tennis. *Clin Sports Med* 1983;2:247–270.
147. Petersson CJ, Gentz CF. Ruptures of the supraspinatus tendon. The significance of distally pointing acromioclavicular osteophytes. *Clin Orthop* 1983;174:143–148.
148. Pettersson G. Rupture of the tendon aponeurosis of the shoulder joint in anterior–inferior dislocation. A study on the origin and occurrence of the ruptures. *Acta Chir Scand* 1942;77(suppl):1–187.
149. Pieper HG, Quack G, Krahl H. Impingement of the rotator cuff in athletes caused by instability of the shoulder joint. *Knee Surg Sports Traumatol Arthrosc* 1993;1:97–99.
150. Poppen NK, Walker PS. Normal and abnormal motion of the shoulder. *J Bone Joint Surg* 1976;58A:195–201.
151. Poppen NK, Walker PS. Forces at the glenohumeral joint in abduction. *Clin Orthop* 1978;135:165–170
152. Putz R, Liebermann J, Reichelt A. Funktion des Ligamnetum coracoacromiale. *Acta Anat* 1988;131:140–145
153. Rathbun JB, Macnab I. The microvascular pattern of the rotator cuff. *J Bone Joint Surg [Br]* 1970;52:540–553.
154. Ribbans WJ, Mitchell R, Taylor GJ. Computerized arthrotomography of primary anterior dislocation of the shoulder. *J Bone Joint Surg [Br]* 1990;72:181–185.
155. Rockwood CA, Burkhead WZ. Management of patients with massive rotator cuff defects by acromioplasty and rotator cuff debridement. *Orthop Trans* 1988;12:190–191.
156. Rockwood CA, Lyons FR. Shoulder impingement syndrome: diagnosis, radiographic evaluation, and treatment with a modified Neer acromioplasty. *J Bone Joint Surg [Am]* 1993;75:409–424.
157. Rockwood CA, Williams GR, Burkhead WZ. Debridement of degenerative irreparable lesions of the rotator cuff. *J Bone Joint Surg [Am]* 1995;77:857–866.
158. Rothman RH, Parke WW. The vascular anatomy of the rotator cuff. *Clin Orthop* 1965;41:176–186.

159. Rowe CR. Prognosis in dislocations of the shoulder. *J Bone Joint Surg [Am]* 1956;38:957–977.
160. Rowe CR. Ruptures of the rotator cuff: selection of cases for conservative treatment. *Surg Clin North Am* 1963;43:1531.
161. Rowe CR, Pierce DS, Clark JG. Voluntary dislocation of the shoulder. A preliminary report on a clinical, electromyographic, and psychiatric study of 26 patients. *J Bone Joint Surg [Am]* 1973;55:445–460.
162. Saha AK. Dynamic stability of the glenohumeral joint. *Acta Orthop Scand* 1971;42:491–505.
163. Saha AK. Mechanics of elevation of the glenohumeral joint. *Acta Orthop Scand* 1973;44:668–678.
164. Saha AK. *Theory of shoulder mechanism: descriptive and applied.* Springfield, IL: Charles C Thomas; 1961.
165. Salter EG, Nasca RJ, Shelley BS. Anatomical observations on the acromioclavicular joint and supporting ligaments. *Am J Sports Med* 1987;15:199–206.
166. Samilson RL, Binder WF. Symptomatic full thickness tears of the rotator cuff. *Orthop Clin North Am* 1975;6:449–466.
167. Sarrafian SK. Gross and functional anatomy of the shoulder. *Clin Orthop* 1083;173:11–19.
168. Schneider T, Straus JM, Fink B, Jerosch J, Menke W, Ruther W. Influence of joint stability on the results of arthroscopic subacromial decompression. *Acta Orthop Belg* 1996;62:94–99.
169. Seeger LL, Gold RH, Bassett LW, Ellman H. Shoulder impingement syndrome: MR findings in 53 shoulders. *AJR: Am J Roentgenol* 1988; 150:343–347.
170. Sharkey NA, Marder RA. The rotator cuff opposes superior translation of the humeral head. *Am J Sports Med* 1995;23:270–275.
171. Sharkey NA, Marder RA, Hanson PB. The entire rotator cuff contributes to elevation of the arm. *J Orthop Res* 1994;12:699–708.
172. Sher JS, Uribe JW, Posada A, Murphy BJ, Zlatkin MB. Abnormal findings on magnetic resonance images of asymptomatic shoulders. *J Bone Joint Surg [Am]* 1995;77:10–15.
173. Shevlin MG, Lucci JA. Electromyographic study of the function of some muscles crossing the glenohumeral joint. *Arch Phys Med Rehabil* 1969;50:264–270.
174. Sigholm G, Styf J, Korner L, Hereberts P. Pressure recordings in the subacromial bursa. *J Orthop Res* 1988;6:123–128.
175. Smith-Peterson MN, Aufranc OE, Larson CB. Useful surgical procedures for rheumatoid arthritis involving joints of the upper extremity. *Arch Surg* 1943;46:764–770.
176. Soslowski LJ, An CH, Johnston SP, et al. Geometric and mechanical properties of the coracoacromial ligament and their relationship to rotator cuff disease. *Clin Orthop* 1994;304:10–17.
177. Soslowski LJ, Carpenter JE, DeBano CM, Banerji I, Moalli MR. Development and use of an animal model for investigations on rotator cuff disease. *J Shoulder Elbow Surg* 1996;5:383–392.
178. Soslowski LJ, Flatow EL, Bigliani LU, Mow VC. Articular geometry of the glenohumeral joint. *Clin Orthop* 1992;285:182–190.
179. Soslowski LJ, Flatow EL, Bigliani LU, Mow VC. Stabilization of the glenohumeral joint by articular contact and by contact in the subacromial space. In: Matsen FA, Fu FH, Hawkins RJ, eds. *The shoulder: a balance of mobility and stability*. Rosemont, IL: American Academy of Orthopaedic Surgeons; 1993:107–124.
180. Speer KP, Lohnes J, Garrett WE. Arthroscopic subacromial decompression; results in advanced impingement syndrome. *Arthroscopy* 1991;7:291–296.
181. Sterling JC, Meyers MC, Chesshir W, Calvo RD. Os acromiale in a baseball catcher. *Med Sci Sports Med Exerc* 1995;27:795–799.
182. Swiontowski MF, Iannotti JP, Boulas HJ, et al. Intraoperative assessment of rotator cuff vascularity using laser doppler flowtometry. In: Post M, Morrey BF, Hawkins RJ, eds. *Surgery of the shoulder.* St Louis: Mosby–Year Book; 1990:208–212.
183. Taylor GM, Tooke M. Degeneration of the acromioclavicular joint as a cause of shoulder pain. *J Bone Joint Surg [Br]* 1977;59:507.
184. Tibone JE, Elrod B, Jobe FW, et al. Surgical treatment of tears of the rotator cuff in athletes. *J Bone Joint Surg [Am]* 1986;68:887–891.
185. Tibone JE, Jobe FW, Kerlan RK, et al. Shoulder impingement syndrome in athletes treated by anterior acromioplasty. *Clin Orthop* 1985; 198:134–140.
186. Tijmes J, Loyd HM, Tullos HS. Arthrography in acute shoulder dislocations. *South Med J* 1979;72:564–567.
187. Tirman PF, Bost FW, Garvin GJ, et al. Posterosuperior glenoid impingement of the shoulder: findings at MR imaging and MR arthrography with arthroscopic correlation. *Radiology* 1994;193:431–436.
188. Toivonen DA, Tuite MJ, Orwin JF. Acromial structure and tears of the rotator cuff. *J Shoulder Elbow Surg* 1995;4:376–383.
189. Uhthoff K, Hammond DI, Sarkar K, Hooper GJ, Papoff WJ. The role of the coracoacromial ligament in the impingement syndrome. A clinical, radiological and histological study. *Int Orthop* 1988;12:97–104.
190. Walch G, Boileau P, Noel E, et al. Impingement of the deep surface of the supraspinatus tendon on the posterosuperior glenoid rim: an arthroscopic study. *J Shoulder Elbow Surg* 1992;1:238–245.
191. Walch G, Laurent NJ, Levigne C, Renaud E. Tears of the supraspinatus tendon associated with "hidden" lesions of the rotator interval. *J Shoulder Elbow Surg* 1994;3:353–360.
192. Walch G, Liotard JP, Noel E. Postero-superior impingement: another shoulder impingement. *J Orthop Surg* 1992;6:78–81.
193. Warner JJP, Krushell RJ, Masquelet A, Gerber C. Anatomy and relationships of the suprascapular nerve: anatomical constraints to mobilization of the supraspinatus and infraspinatus muscles in the management of massive rotator cuff tears. *J Bone Joint Surg [Am]* 1912;74: 36–45.
194. Warner JJP, Micheli LJ, Arslanian LE, Kennedy J, Kennedy R. Patterns of flexibility, laxity, and strength in normal shoulders and shoulders with instability and impingement. *Am J Sports Med* 1990;18: 366–375.
195. Watson M. Major ruptures of the rotator cuff. The results of surgical repair in 89 patients. *J Bone Joint Surg [Br]* 1985;67:618–624.
196. Wiley AM. Superior humeral dislocation. A complication following decompression and debridement for rotator cuff tears. *Clin Orthop* 1991;263:136–141.
197. Wilson CL, Duff GL. Pathologic study of degeneration and rupture of the supraspinatus tendon. *Arch Surg* 1943;47:121–135.
198. Wolfgang GL. Surgical repairs of tears of the rotator cuff of the shoulder. Factors influencing the result. *J Bone Joint Surg [Am]* 1974;56: 14–26.
199. Wuelker N, Plitz W, Roetman B, Wirth CJ. Function of the supraspinatus muscle. Abduction of the humerus studied in cadavers. *Acta Orthop Scand* 1994;65:442–446.
200. Wuelker N, Roetman B, Roessig S. Coracoacromial pressure recordings in a cadaveric model. *J Shoulder Elbow Surg* 1995;4:62–67.
201. Wuelker N, Schmotzer H, Thren K, Korell M. Translation of the glenohumeral joint with simulated active elevation. *Clin Orthop* 1994; 309:193–200.
202. Wulker N, Rossig S, Korell M, Thren K. Dynamic stability of the glenohumeral joint. A biomechanical study. *Sportverletz Sportschaden* 1995;9:1–8.
203. Yamaguchi K, Sher JS, Andersen WK, et al. Glenohumeral motion in patients with rotator cuff tears: a comparison of asymptomatic, symptomatic, and normal shoulders. Presented at American Shoulder and Elbow Surgeons 13th Open Meeting, San Francisco, Feb. 16, 1997.
204. Zlatkin MB, Bjorkengren AG, Gylys-Morin V, Resnick D, Sartoris DJ. Cross-sectional imaging of the capsular mechanism of the lenohumeral joint. *AJR: Am J Roentgenol* 1988;150:151–158.
205. Zuckerman JD, Kummer FJ, Cuomo F, Simon J, Rosenblum S, Katz NJ. The influence of coracoacromial arch anatomy on rotator cuff tears. *J Shoulder Elbow Surg* 1992;1:4–13.
206. Zvijac JE, Levy HJ, Lemak LJ. Arthroscopic subacromial decompression in the treatment of full thickness rotator cuff tears: a 3- to 6-year follow-up. *Arthroscopy* 1994;10:518–523.

Disorders of the Shoulder: Diagnosis and Management,
edited by Joseph P. Iannotti and Gerald R. Williams, Jr.
Lippincott Williams & Wilkins, Philadelphia © 1999.

CHAPTER 2

Management of Rotator Cuff Disease: Intact and Repairable Cuff

Julian S. Arroyo and Evan L. Flatow

INTRODUCTION

In the 19th century the etiology of chronic shoulder pain was poorly understood, and most cases were lumped together and vaguely ascribed to "periarthritis."[56] In a series of papers beginning in 1904, Codman shifted attention away from the glenohumeral joint and toward the subdeltoid bursa and its contents, especially the supraspinatus tendon.[32–45] In 1911 he reported his first repair, performed in 1909, of a full-thickness supraspinatus tear.[39] Although scattered reports of procedures that included repair of the tendons of the short rotators have been identified in the older literature,[25,146] Codman's reports and lectures eloquently presented the clinical and pathologic findings of rotator cuff injuries, and influenced a generation of orthopedic surgeons on the importance of these disorders. The field was further advanced by McLaughlin, who published a series of practical reports on the treatment of rotator cuff tears over a 30-year period.[111–114]

J. S. Arroyo: Lakewood Orthopaedic Surgeons, Tacoma, Washington 98499.

E. L. Flatow: The Shoulder Service, Mount Sinai Medical Center, New York, New York 10029.

Codman emphasized the role of trauma in causing rotator cuff tears, and disputed Meyer's theory of attrition.[43,116] Other authors recognized that the acromion could pinch underlying structures, advocating complete or lateral acromionectomy[6,85,181] for a variety of painful conditions, usually when the cuff was intact. Neer's report in 1972 described the impingement syndrome and its role in rotator cuff disease.[124] He identified the anteroinferior acromion as the principal area of pathology, and advocated anterior acromioplasty to enlarge the subacromial space and decompress the rotator cuff.[124,125] Neer argued that total acromionectomy was unnecessary, and in fact, was deleterious to shoulder function.[128] He thus advocated a reshaping (without removal) of the anteroinferior acromion, preservation of the deltoid, and mobilization and repair of the tendons. These principles led to a revolution in rotator cuff surgery. The results of rotator cuff repairs had been unpredictable and often disappointing before 1970, with unsatisfactory results reported in as many as 26% to 46% of patients.[20,39,43,44,52,80,93,186] More recent experience, using techniques that follow the principles established by Neer, have documented predictably satisfactory results for pain relief and function.[1,9,13,46,48,49,60,67,91,119,125–127,135,143,148,152,153]

The advent of arthroscopy has had a dramatic effect on the evaluation and treatment of rotator cuff pathology.[26,61,62,63]

The combination of the arthroscope's ability to routinely visualize the glenohumeral joint as well as the undersurface of the rotator cuff tendon and the information gained from the widespread use of magnetic resonance imaging (MRI) has uncovered a bewildering array of "lesions." Although occasionally diagnostic accuracy has been improved, it has been hard to quantify the clinical value of the new information. More clear has been the therapeutic value of arthroscopic techniques.[76,189] Arthroscopic anterior acromioplasty, arthroscopic rotator cuff repair, and arthroscopic-assisted "mini-open" repair are new tools available to the orthopedic surgeon for the care of rotator cuff disorders.

The anatomy, biomechanics, pathoetiology, and classification of rotator cuff tears are discussed in Chapter 1, so these areas will be mentioned only when necessary to place surgical principles in context. This chapter will focus on the reparable (or intact) cuff tendon. The management of irreparable tears will be discussed in Chapter 3, as will biceps lesions in Chap. 6, complications of cuff repairs in Chap. 4, and arthritis with cuff deficiency in Chap. 21.

EVALUATION

Clinical History

Patients with rotator cuff problems will typically complain of pain or weakness or both. Many patients cannot recall an injury, and in others, symptoms may have begun after a trivial trauma (e.g., catching their balance by holding onto a railing). However, more severe injuries may play a role, especially when a cuff tear occurs in association with a dislocation in an older patient. The pain is usually described as anterior, either in the front of the shoulder or down the anterior humeral region, often as far as the elbow. Pain in the back of the shoulder or trapezius, or that which radiates down past the elbow into the hands is more consistent with a cervical radiculopathy, although there are exceptions. Pain from rotator cuff pathology is usually increased with use of the arm, particularly for overhead activities, and is often most severe at night, frequently interrupting sleep.

Because splinting from pain may simulate weakness, lack of strength does not always indicate a large tear unless a subacromial anesthetic injection has been given first. Furthermore, patients with massive tears may still have remarkably good motion and function. However, it is more common for patients with large or massive tears to report weakness and fatigue with overhead use, and difficulty in raising their arm. If the onset of weakness is sudden after an injury, especially one causing a glenohumeral dislocation, then not only a rotator cuff injury needs to be suspected, but also a neurologic injury (most commonly suprascapular or axillary nerve) should be ruled out.

Physical Examination

Visual inspection for shoulder symmetry will often reveal atrophy of the supraspinatus or infraspinatus in the presence of long-standing cuff tears. Asymmetry of the biceps muscle belly may be a clue to a partial recession or dislocation of the tendon of the long head of the biceps.[126] A complete rupture, not infrequently, is seen with large cuff tears.

Range of motion of the shoulder should be performed actively and passively and compared with the asymptomatic side.[2] It is surprisingly infrequent for patients with rotator cuff tears to have decreased passive range of motion, although this can occur. More commonly, there is a limitation of active range of motion caused either by weakness or pain (Fig. 1). Subacromial injections with 1% lidocaine (Xylo-

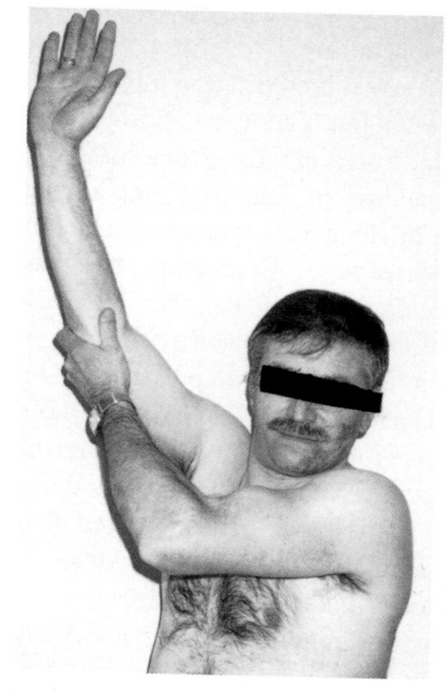

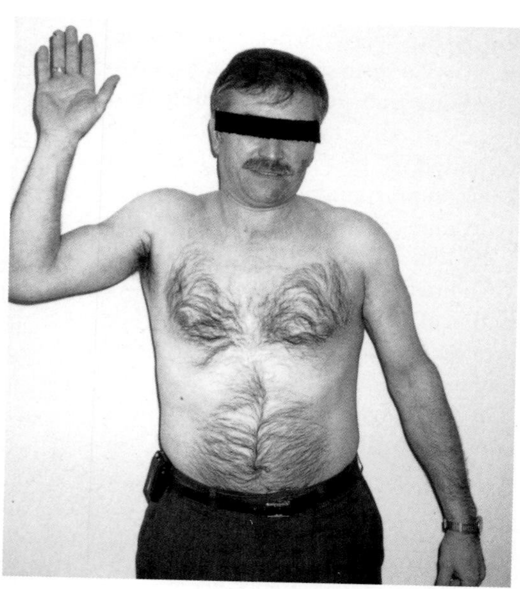

FIG. 1. (A) This patient with a massive cuff tear, has full passive elevation when assisted with the other arm. **(B)** Active elevation, however, is severely impaired.

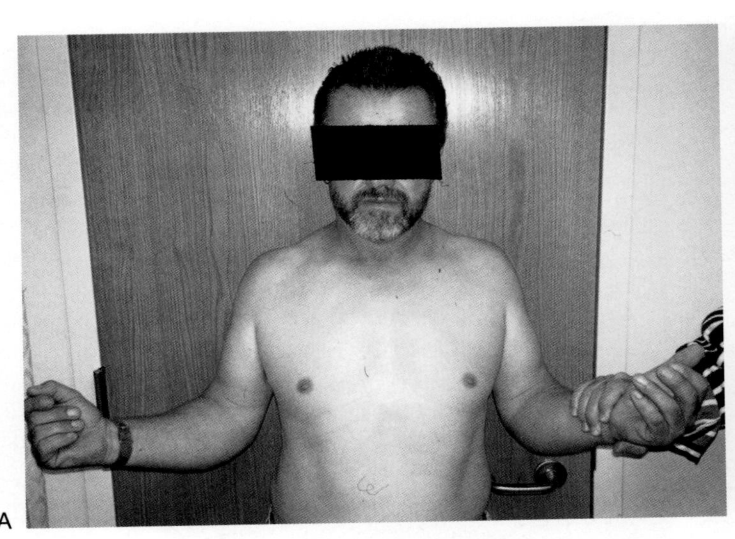
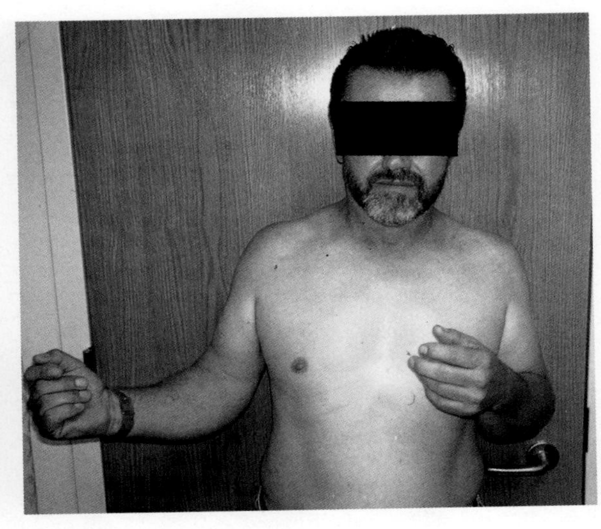
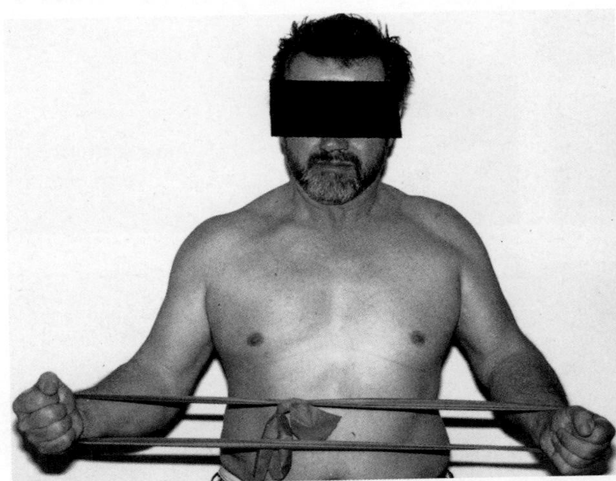
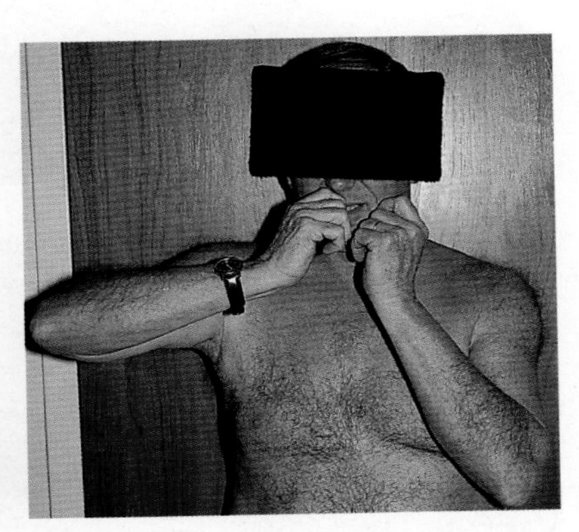

FIG. 2. (A) This patient with a massive tear involving the posterior cuff can be passively externally rotated. **(B)** When the arm is let go it "falls off" into internal rotation, demonstrating severe weakness. **(C)** One year after rotator cuff repair he has regained active external rotation, although his strength is not full. **(D)** Signe de clairon: Right arm must be elevated higher than left to reach mouth since active external rotation is impaired.

caine) can be used to help distinguish between the two. If there is limited range of motion, but no difference between active and passive, then adhesive capsulitis or arthritis should be suspected.

Strength of the shoulder should be examined in elevation, abduction, external rotation, and internal rotation. For large or massive tears, strength may be reduced when compared with the contralateral side. Weakness of external rotation is a common finding, particularly when the infraspinatus is involved in the tear. Patients with large or massive tears involving the infraspinatus will often be unable to maintain their arm in external rotation: If the patient sits with the arm at the side and the elbow bent 90 degrees the arm may be fully externally rotated passively, but once the arm is let go it will "fall off" into internal rotation[13] (Fig. 2A–C). The similar inability to actively externally rotate the abducted arm has been termed the "signe de clairon," since it puts the arm in the position used to blow a bugle[77] (see Fig. 2D)

Weakness of terminal internal rotation indicates involvement of the subscapularis. Internal rotation strength can be evaluated with the "lift-off" test[78] (Fig. 3A–C). Patients are asked to reach up their backs and then lift their hand away from their trunk. The test is considered positive when they cannot do so. Another method to test the strength of the subscapularis is to have the patient place their hands on their abdomen, internally rotate their shoulders, bringing their elbows in front of their torso, and then push their hands into their abdomen (see Fig. 3D). When the subscapularis is deficient the patient's elbow will fall back behind the coronal plane of the body because they cannot maintain terminal internal rotation. Hertel and coworkers[94] have quantified these findings by describing external rotation and internal rotation "lag signs," that measure the difference between passive and active terminal rotation.

Provocative tests are used to elicit symptoms of impingement by maneuvering the biceps and rotator cuff under the

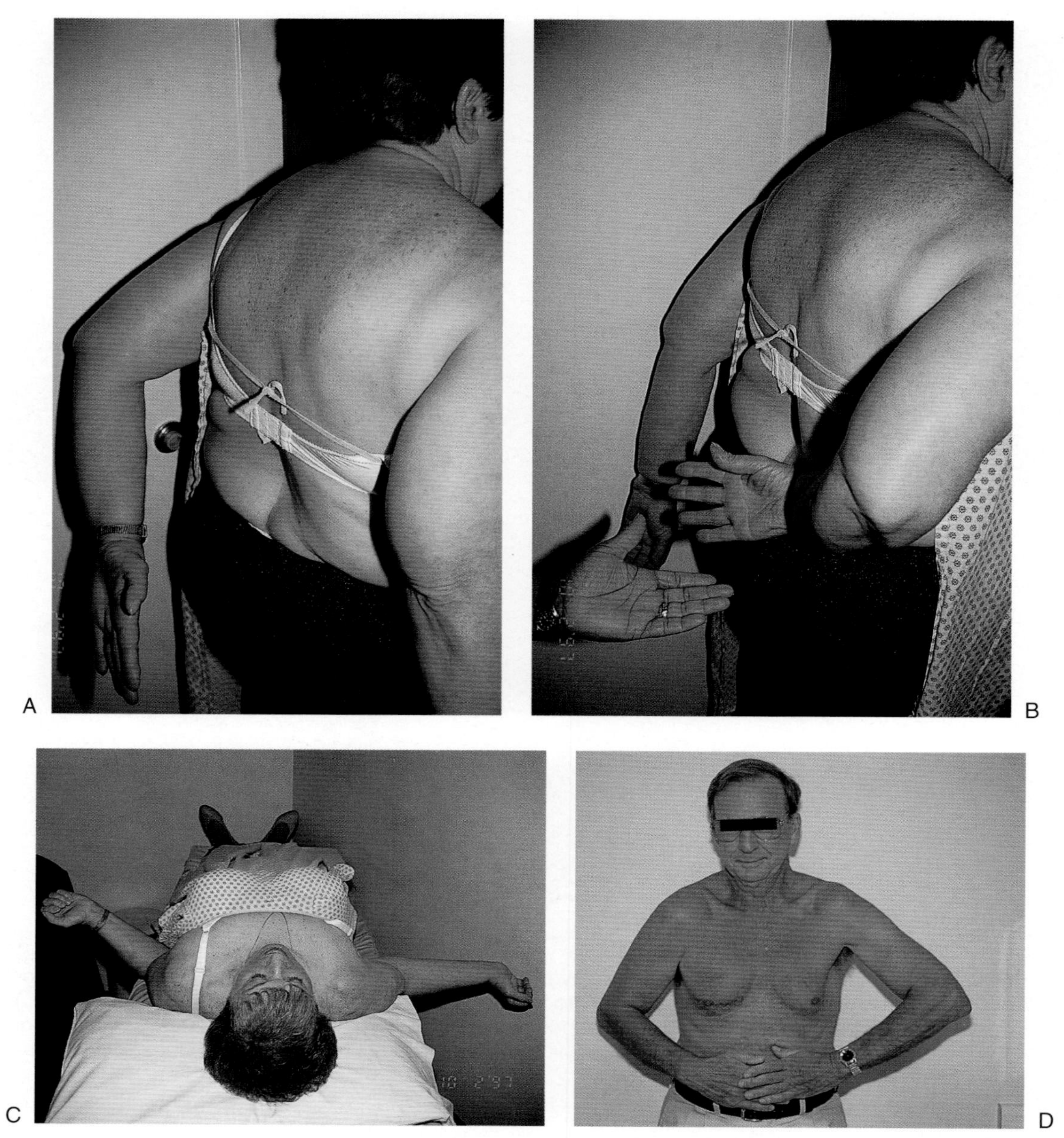

FIG. 3. **(A)** The lift-off test is used to evaluate the integrity of the subscapularis tendon.[78] Although originally it was described as asking the patient to lift their hand off the small of their back, it can be more sensitive if the examiner holds the hand to maximally internal rotate the arm and then lets go. This patient is able to maintain maximal internal rotation with her left shoulder. **(B)** Her right shoulder, which has an isolated subscapularis tear, has an internal rotation lag because she cannot maintain maximal internal rotation. **(C)** Her right shoulder has increased external rotation, another finding in subscapularis ruptures. **(D)** Abdominal compression test: the right elbow falls back when the patient tries to compress his abdomen.

coracoacromial arch. The Neer impingement test entails elevation with the arm internally rotated,[125] whereas Hawkin's test for impingement is elevation to 90 degrees, adduction across the chest, and internal rotation[88] (Fig. 4). Both of these tests bring the biceps, rotator cuff, and greater tuberosity directly under the coracoacromial arch. However, these maneuvers may also cause pain in other shoulder conditions such as stiffness, calcium deposits, and arthritis. In patients with classic impingement syndrome, pain will not only be produced by these impingement maneuvers, but should be nearly completely eliminated following a subacromial injection of 10 mL of 1% lidocaine.

The acromioclavicular (AC) joint is often a source of impingement and pain; it should be inspected for prominence and palpated for tenderness. Maneuvers to elicit signs of impingement can also exacerbate pain from the AC joint. When there is uncertainty about the source of shoulder pain, serial injections, first into the subacromial space followed by an in-

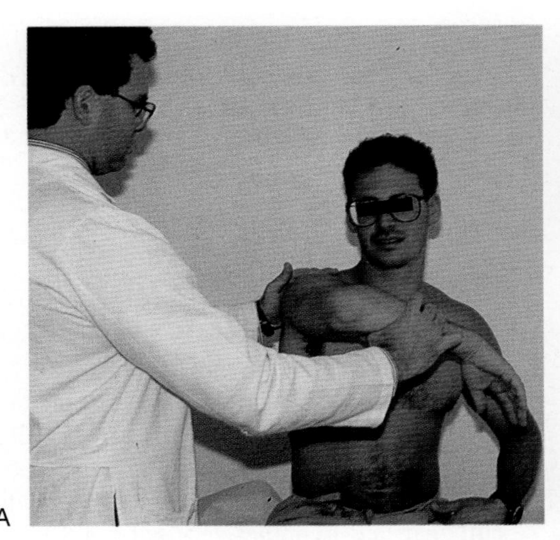

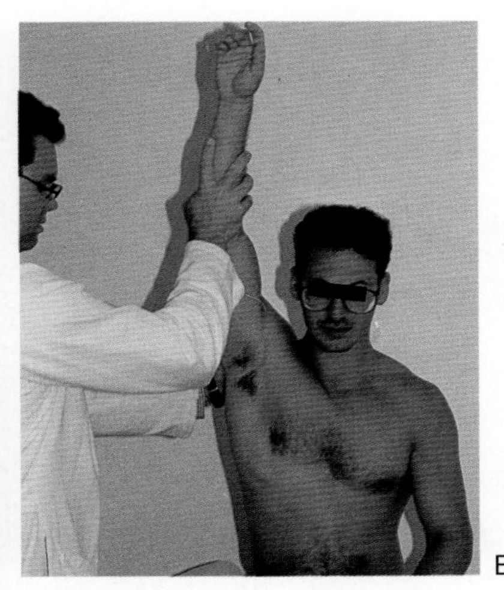

FIG. 4. (A) Hawkins impingement sign. **(B)** Neer impingement sign.

jection into the AC joint can be performed and patient responses recorded. It is not uncommon for patients to have prominent, arthritic AC joints that are asymptomatic. Resection of the distal clavicle should be performed only when the AC joint itself is tender and painful. Finally, instability testing should be performed in those patients, especially throwing athletes, in whom the relative contributions of instability and rotator cuff pathology are uncertain.

IMAGING

Radiographs

Plain radiographs are used to determine the bony morphology of the acromion and to evaluate the position of the humeral head relative to the glenoid fossa and acromion. Plain radiographs are also important to rule out other sources of shoulder pain such as calcific tendinitis, glenohumeral osteoarthritis, or destructive bone lesions. Patients with rotator cuff pathology are evaluated with five views of the shoulder. Anteroposterior (AP) views in the plane of the scapula in neutral, internal, and external rotation are obtained to visualize the glenohumeral joint and greater and lesser tuberosities, and to bring small calcium deposits into relief. The AP view may also reveal an excrescence or cysts on the greater tuberosity, suggestive of rotator cuff disease. The acromiohumeral interval can also be assessed on the AP views and, if reduced, may be an indication of a torn or nonfunctioning rotator cuff.[148,184]

On the axillary view, the glenohumeral joint and tuberosities can be inspected. The acromion is usually well visualized on the axillary view and can be evaluated for the presence of an os acromiale, or unfused anterior acromial epiphysis. The axillary view is also useful to look for subtle joint space narrowing (seen in early arthritis).

Finally, a supraspinatus outlet view will show the subacromial space and the coracoacromial arch. To obtain this view, a lateral x-ray film of the scapula is obtained while the x-ray beam is angled downward 10 degrees.[15,126,129] The supraspinatus outlet view will reveal any spurs encroaching on the subacromial space from the AC joint or anteroinferior acromion (Fig. 5). It is also the view used to determine the acromial morphology (Fig. 6).

Tendon Imaging

Arthrograms are extremely accurate for the detection of full-thickness rotator cuff tears, but are invasive procedures that do not give accurate information on tear size or the condition of the rotator cuff muscles. Also, partial-thickness tears are unreliably assessed.

High-resolution real-time ultrasound has also been used to

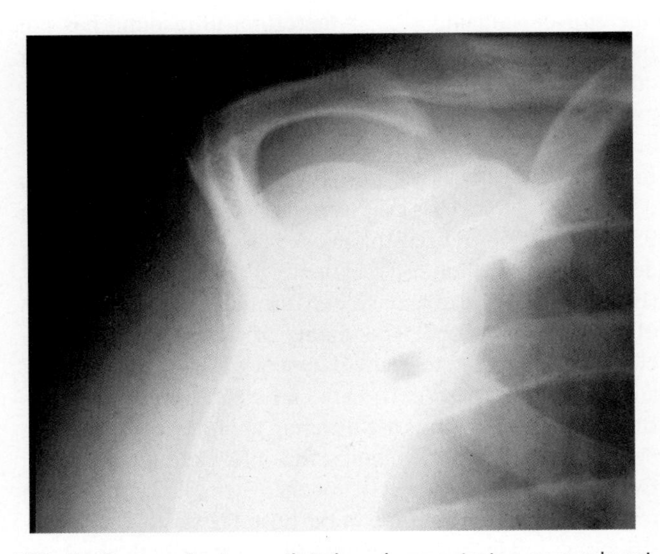

FIG. 5. Supraspinatus outlet view demonstrates a prominent anterior acromion in a 31-year-old former college outfielder. This can be a clue that despite the patient's young age, extrinsic impingement may be involved.

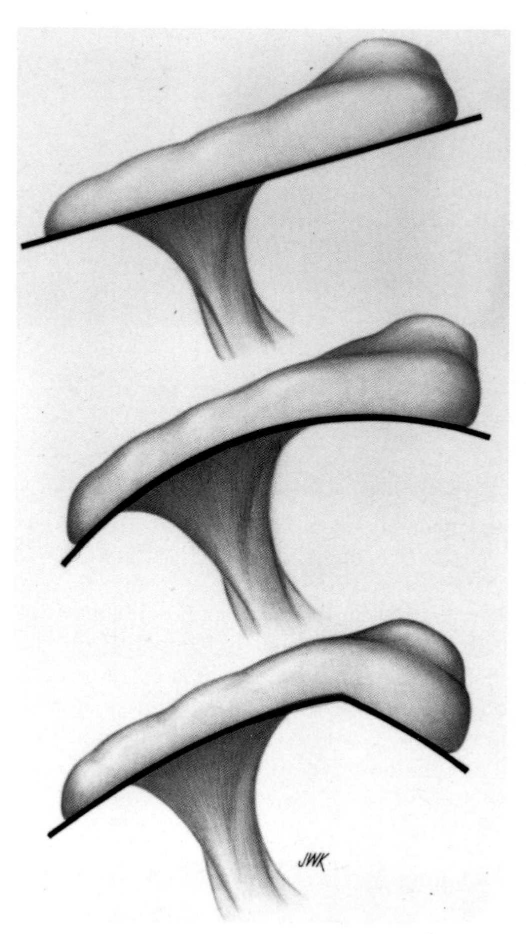

FIG. 6. Acromion morphology as described by Bigliani et al.[15]: *type I* flat, *type II* curved, and *type III* hooked.

evaluate the integrity of the rotator cuff.[30,108,118] Accuracy is operator-dependant;[95,108,118] therefore, ultrasound has not become a commonly employed method to assess the rotator cuff. However, it retains the advantages of being quick, inexpensive, safe, and tolerated by claustrophobics.

Magnetic resonance imaging (MRI) has become the cuff-imaging study of choice in many centers. The accuracy in detecting full thickness cuff tears has been reported between 93% and 100%. Partial-thickness tears are less accurately detected and are more dependent on the technique used[21] (Fig. 7). The main advantage of MRI, however, is the wealth of information gained. The quality of the rotator cuff muscles, the size of the tear, involvement of the biceps tendon, and partial-thickness cuff tears can clearly be determined. Because many surgeons use different approaches, depending on tear size and muscle quality, this information is of value. Even when the approach will not change, many patients wish realistic projections of time in the hospital, postoperative restrictions, and length of rehabilitation to prepare themselves. Finally, some patients base their decision whether to undergo an operation at all on what functional gains can reliably be expected, and an MRI scan of cuff muscle atrophy can help the surgeon give an accurate prognosis. The main disadvantage of MRI, its cost, has been greatly reduced owing to wider availability, competition, and the effects of changes in health care reimbursement.

NONOPERATIVE TREATMENT

Rotator cuff pathology is a common cause of shoulder pain, with a reported incidence of rotator cuff tears ranging from 5% to 40%, with an increased incidence in older patients.[54,82 02,106,125,147,167,187] Clearly not all patients with rotator cuff tears are disabled by this condition. McLaughlin noted approximately 25% of cadavers studied had a rotator cuff tear and hypothesized that not all of these had been symptomatic in life,[112] as has been shown in more recent MRI studies of asymptomatic patients.[164] The aim of nonoperative treatment, then, is to help a patient with symptomatic rotator cuff disease become aymptomatic.

A review of the literature suggests that nonoperative treatment of rotator cuff tears is successful in 33% to 92% of cases,[18,23,90,99,174,175,187] with most studies reporting a satisfactory result in approximately 50% of patients. Boker and coworkers[18] reported on 53 patients with documented rotator cuff tears undergoing nonoperative treatment at an average follow-up of longer than 7 years. Seventy-five percent of patients had satisfactory pain relief, particularly those presenting after an acute injury. Patients with long-standing pain (over 6 months) did not respond well to nonoperative therapy. Wirth and coworkers[187] reported on 60 patients with documented rotator cuff tears, and at a minimum of 2

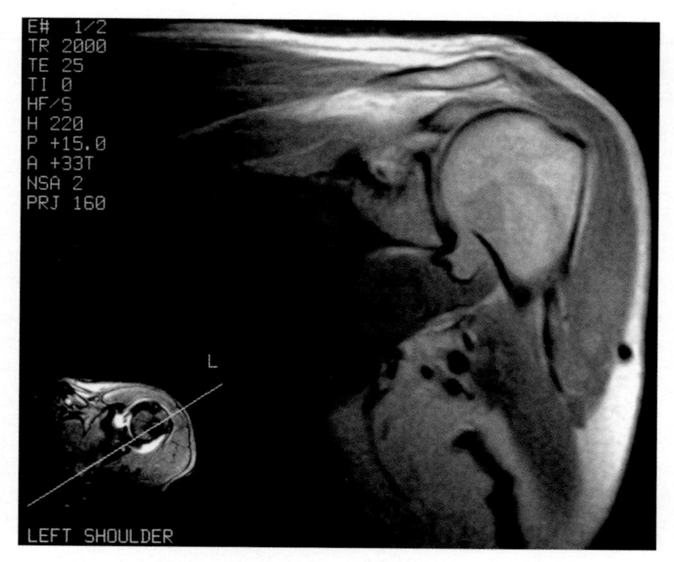

FIG. 7. T1 weighted MRI of a left shoulder with a large full-thickness rotator cuff tear. The supraspinatus tendon is retracted to the middle of the humeral head.

years follow-up, only 62% of patients had a satisfactory result. Furthermore, only 4% of the patients were rated as excellent.

Authors' Preferred Treatment

Our own approach would be to recommend nonoperative treatment for patients with rotator cuff disease who present with pain without dramatic or progressive weakness. Treatment would be instituted after a history, physical examination, and plain radiographs. Unless there was diagnostic confusion, we would not image the cuff initially, but rather consider an MRI later if this approach had failed, once surgery was being considered. Patients with weakness, especially if the onset was sudden after an injury, are imaged more expeditiously.

Patients are taught a home exercise program, and sent to physical therapy for supervision and education.[99,122] Also instituted is a course of oral nonsteroidal antiinflammatory drugs, heat application, and modification of activities to eliminate offending motions. Initial exercises aim at eliminating any subtle stiffness (especially posterior capsular tightness, which can exacerbate impingement) and strengthening the rotator cuff and parascapular muscles. The patient's progress is monitored after 4 to 6 weeks. If adequate progress has not been made, a subacromial injection may be considered, especially if pain is limiting the patient's ability to perform exercises. We prefer a mixture of 3 mL of lidocaine (1%), 3 mL of bupivicaine (0.25%), and a depot corticosteroid (usually 8 mg of dexamethasone acetate in 1 mL). This can be very helpful,[16] even though pathologic studies have shown that true inflammation is rarely present in degenerative rotator cuff disease.[177] This injection is occasionally repeated after a few months, but repeated injections are not used.

For patients with pain as their chief complaint, this type of program is continued for 4 to 6 months before an MRI is obtained and surgical options are discussed. When weakness is prominent or progressive, this process is accelerated. A common presentation is that of sudden loss of strength after a relatively trivial injury. Because splinting from pain (e.g., from hemorhagic bursitis) can simulate weakness, we would generally start with a therapy program. However, if there has not been dramatic improvement after a few weeks, an MRI is obtained. If a cuff tear is found of sufficient size to explain the weakness, timely repair is considered,[9] for it is likely that this is an acute tear, or at least an acute extension of a prior small tear. If the tear size seems inconsistent with the physical findings, other etiologies of weakness, especially a nerve injury, should be considered. Occasionally an older patient will present with dramatic weakness after a dislocation, and both a cuff tear and a brachial plexopathy will be present, and their relative contributions to the patient's weakness may be unclear. However, because waiting for the nerve lesion to resolve would likely allow irreservible atrophy of the cuff muscles to develop, it seems prudent to recommend early cuff repair in most of these patients.

SURGICAL MANAGEMENT

Surgical Indications

The presence of a rotator cuff tear is not necessarily an indication for surgery. As previously mentioned, MRI and cadaver studies have shown asymptomatic patients to have cuff tears.[164] The indications for surgical repair of rotator cuff tears are, therefore, the presence of pain or functional deficits that interfere with activities and have not responded to conservative measures. Most surgeons would continue nonoperative treatment for at least 3 to 4 months before considering repair; when weakness is prominent or progressive, more timely repair may be considered. Bassett and Cofield reported that in patients who have an acute injury and a full-thickness rotator cuff tear, repair within the first 3 weeks resulted in the best surgical outcome.[9] Specific indications are discussed in the following according to pathology (see Algorithm).

Surgical Approaches

There are three basic approaches to the rotator cuff: arthroscopic, arthroscopic-assisted (miniopen), and open.

Arthroscopic Approach

Arthroscopy may be performed in either the lateral or beach chair position. We prefer the beach chair position because it allows scalene anesthesia (awake patients do not tolerate the lateral position well), provides a standard anatomic orientation (same as open cases), facilitates conversion to an open procedure, and avoids the risks of fixed traction.[168] The torso is angled approximately 60 degrees from the horizontal plane[151,189] (Fig. 8). A head rest that allows access to the superior and posterior aspects of the shoulder is used. The arm is draped free, allowing shoulder rotation, extension, and elevation. Two small towels are placed under the scapula to elevate the shoulder off the table.

On our service all rotator cuff procedures are performed under regional interscalene anesthesia, because this avoids the morbidity of general anesthesia, allows improved relaxation, and facilitates outpatient surgery.[22,149] There is a misperception among some surgeons that patients are loath to undergo a scalene block. Although it is true that patients often express unease with being awake during surgery, they generally become highly accepting when reassured that they will be as sedated as they wish, especially if it is added that the other option is to have a tube down their throat and be connected to a respirator. Before beginning the arthroscopy, 10 mL of 0.25% bupivicaine with epinephrine is injected into the subacromial space. This distends the subacromial space, provides hemostasis, and improves postoperative pain

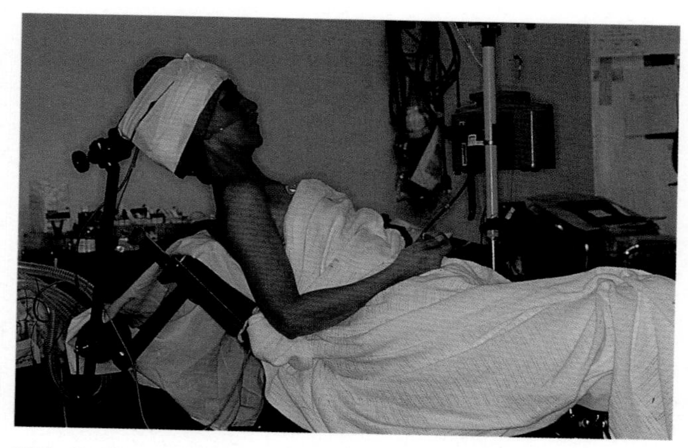

FIG. 8. Beach chair position with the torso angled approximately 60 degrees from the horizontal plane.

control. Epinephrine is added to the irrigation fluid (saline) to a concentration of 1:300,000 for hemostasis, except in the rare instance of a medical contraindication such as a cardiac arrythmia. The glenohumeral joint is accessed through a posterior portal located in the posterior "soft spot," the location of which which may vary from patient to patient but typically is 2 cm inferior and 2 cm medial to the posterolateral corner of the acromion. Care must be taken not to go below the teres minor into the quadrangular space, which transmits the axillary nerve and posterior humeral circumflex artery. The glenohumeral joint is inspected, with particular attention to the long head of the biceps tendon, rotator cuff, and glenoid labrum. The insertion of the rotator cuff is best visualized with the arm abducted 90 degrees and externally rotated (Fig. 9). If a working portal is needed it is placed anteriorly 1 cm lateral to the coracoid and brought in at the rotator cuff interval (between the biceps tendon and the subscapularis) under direct visualization from within the joint.

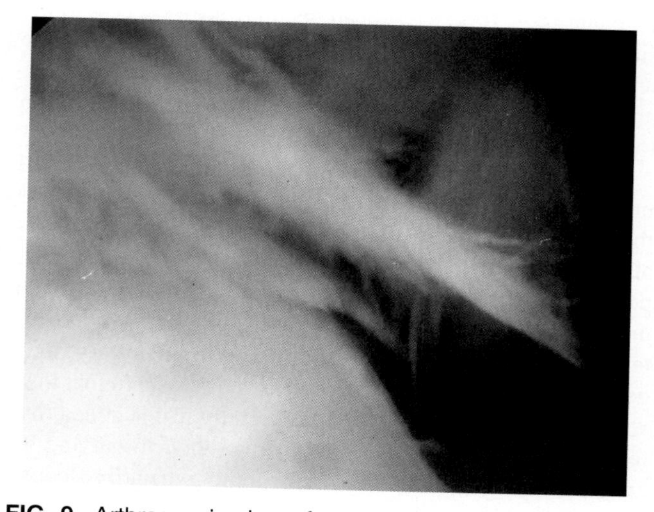

FIG. 9. Arthroscopic view of a partial-thickness rotator cuff tear on the undersurface of the supraspinatus tendon. This tear involves less than 50% of the tendon and will be treated with debridement followed by an anterior acromioplasty.

This is a dangerous portal in that if it is placed medial to the coracoid the brachial plexus or brachial artery could be injured, and if it is placed inferior to the coracoid, the axillary or musculocutaneous nerves may be injured.

Once the glenohumeral joint arthroscopy is completed, the posterior portal may be redirected into the subacromial space. A lateral or anterolateral portal is then created for instrumentation. An arthroscopic bursectomy, anterior acromioplasty, and coracoacromial ligament resection may then be performed as needed. If there is a full-thickness tear, the cuff may be mobilized with traction sutures. The most commonly used techniques of tendon repair involve using the anterior, lateral, and posterior portals to place suture anchors in the tuberosity, pass the sutures through the cuff tendon edge, and tie down the knots arthroscopically.

Mini-open Approach

In an arthroscopic-assisted approach the initial procedure is the same as with an arthroscopic repair, usually including an arthroscopic subacromial decompression. Then a small incision is used to directly repair the tear through a deltoid split without detachment. This approach is especially useful for small and medium cuff tears. Although some authors have made quite large skin incisions, and still called it a "mini-open" approach, if only a deltoid split is used, most surgeons have kept the incision small and in the skin creases. We have preferred a "portal-extension" approach in which the anterolateral portal is extended to a length of 3 cm, anterior to posterior[151,189] (Fig. 10). Flaps are elevated, and the deltoid is split in the direction of its fibers to just posterior to the anterolateral corner of the acromion. The deltoid split should be no longer than 3 or 4 cm and should incorporate the small defect from the arthroscopic portal. None of the deltoid is detached from the acromion. A stay suture is then placed in the deltoid to prevent propagation of the split and possible damage to the axillary nerve. By maneuvering the arm, the entire extent of the tear can be seen. This approach provides good exposure of the supraspinatus and infraspinatus tendons, but access to the subscapularis and teres minor is difficult.

Standard Superior Approach

Many skin incisions can be used to gain access to the rotator cuff, but in our experience the most versatile and cosmetic incision is one extending from the middle of the acromion anteriorly to approximately 2 cm lateral to the coracoid in the lines of Langer (Fig. 11). This incision can be moved medially if access to the AC joint is necessary or laterally if a large tear is anticipated and the AC joint does not need to be addressed. We use this approach for all large and massive tears.

Following the skin incision, subcutaneous flaps are raised. A 3- to 5-cm deltoid split is then made from the anterolateral corner of the acromion in the direction of the muscle fibers

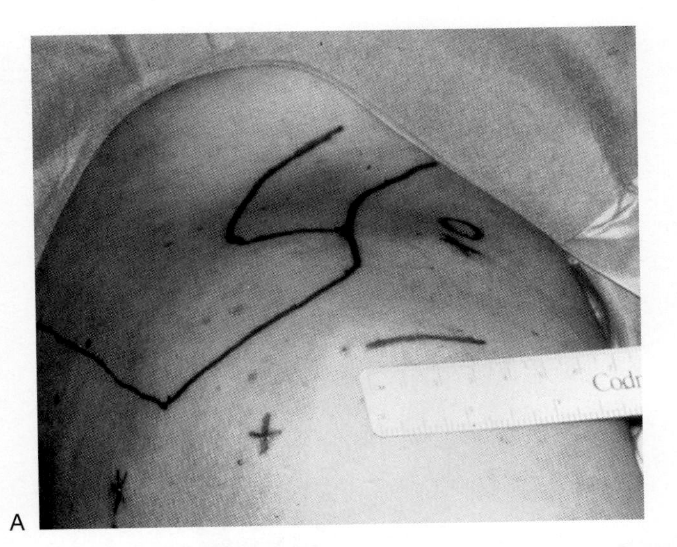

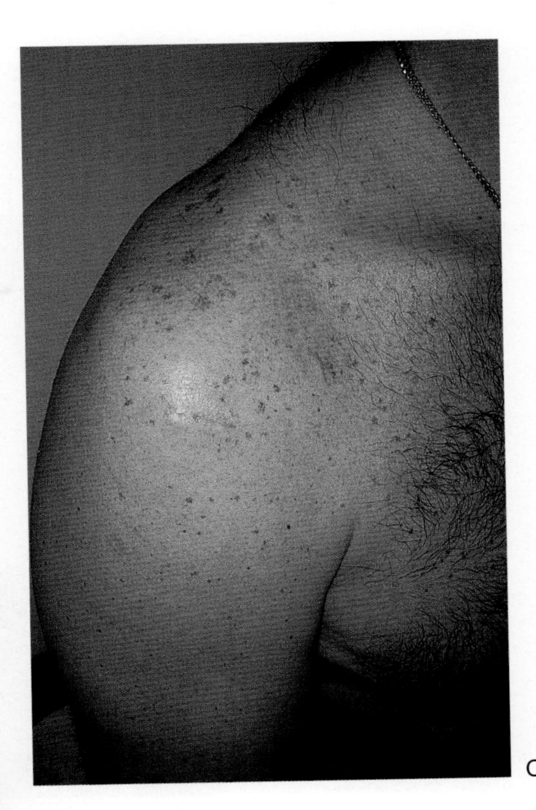

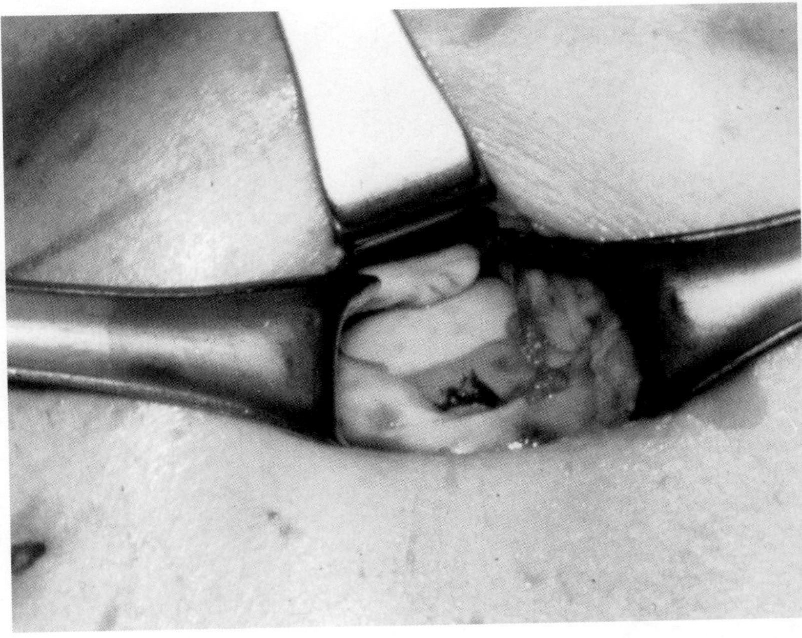

FIG. 10. In the portal-extension approach, the anterolateral arthroscopic portal is extended to a total length of 3 cm in Langer's lines. This approach gives excellent visualization of small rotator cuff tears. **(A)** Before arthroscopy the skin incision is marked, for extravasation of arthroscopy fluid will make Langer's lines difficult to detect. **(B)** View of an isolated supraspinatus tendon tear from the portal-extension approach. **(C)** Typical "portal extension" miniopen incision seen at 3 months after surgery.

using needle tip electrocautery. A stay suture is placed at the end of the split to avoid extension of the split and possible damage to the axillary nerve, which generally lies 5 to 6 cm from the tip of the lateral acromion. If the posterior portion of the cuff is thought to be intact, then the split can be placed along the anterolateral raphe of the deltoid. However, by curving the split more posteriorly, greater exposure of the back of the cuff is possible.[13] The incision is then taken up over the anterosuperior edge of the acromion to the front of the AC joint, essentially along the line at which the acromioplasty will be performed (Fig. 12). The deltoid is then elevated subperiosteally with electrocautery. The coracoacromial ligament is taken down with the deltoid as one thick flap. The split is deepened through the deltoid until the subacromial bursa is encountered.

Following a subacromial decompression and mobilization and repair of the rotator cuff, the deltoid is repaired. A perfect repair of the deltoid is as important as the rotator cuff repair itself. A heavy no. 2 nonabsorbable suture is used to reattach the deltoid back to the anterior acromion. An anatomic repair can be achieved by passing one suture through the AC joint capsule and then two sutures through the bone of the acromion. A Mason–Allen suture[79] technique (Fig. 13) is used to hold the deltoid fibers securely. The deltoid split is closed in a side-to-side fashion with simple buried knots.

Surgery for Subacromial Impingement, Cuff Intact

Subacromial impingement results from irritating contact between the rotator cuff and biceps tendon and the coracoacromial arch. The various causes of this syndrome, as

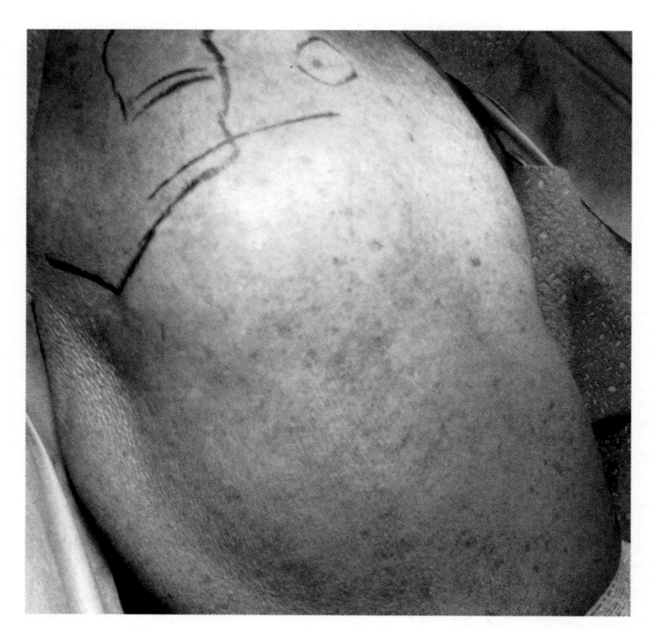

FIG. 11. Skin incision in Langer's lines at the superoanterior aspect of the shoulder extending from the lateral aspect of the anterior third of the acromion inferiorly to the lateral aspect of the coracoid.

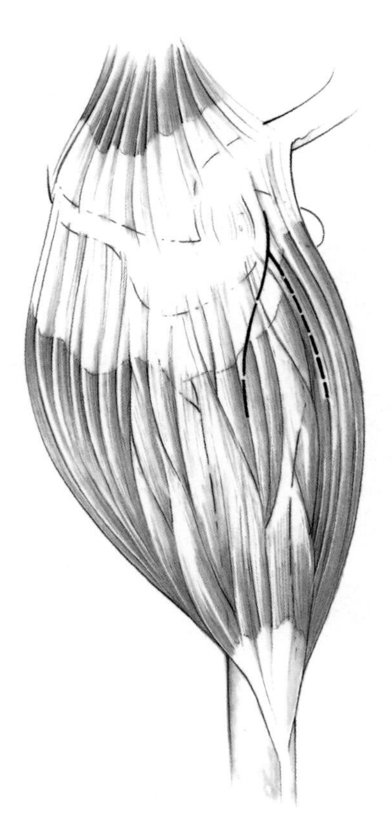

FIG. 12. The posterior curve of the deltoid incision allows the exposure to be centered over the greater tuberosity for better access to the cuff. The dotted line demonstrates the less desirable anterior exposure provided by the older and more anterior type of deltoid incision. (From ref. 13, with permission.)

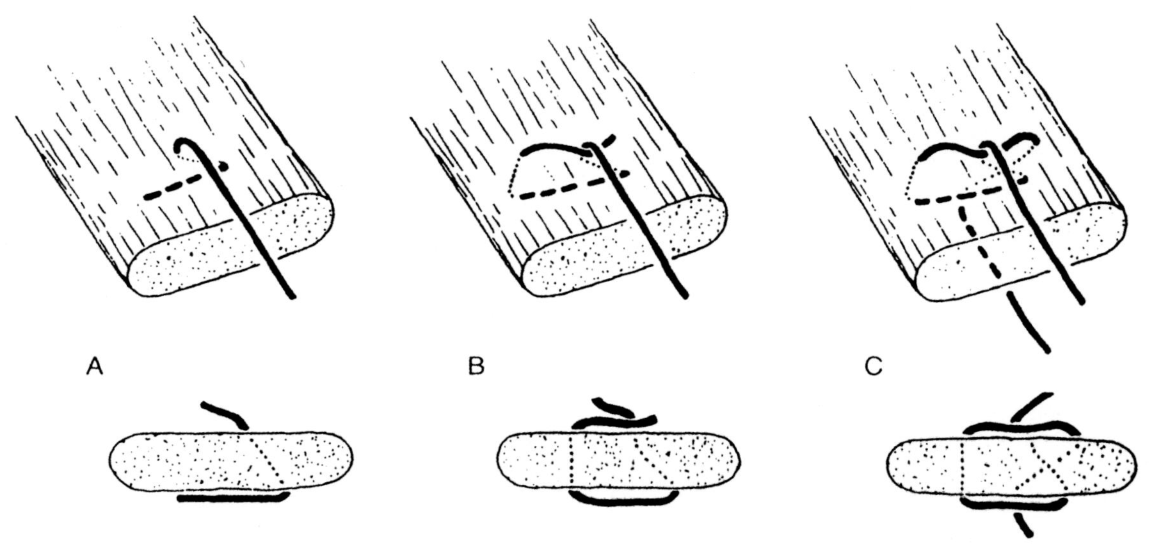

FIG. 13. Schematic illustration of the Mason–Allen stitch used in rotator cuff repair. **(A)** The stitch is passed obliquely from the superior tendon surface to the inferior tendon surface. **(B)** The suture is then passed directly through the tendon from the inferior surface to the superior surface. **(C)** Finally, the suture is passed in front of the stitch placed in panel A, and brought obliquely through the tendon such that it passes just behind the transverse suture lines present on the inferior tendon surface. This illustration assumes that the suture is now going to be passed through the bone. If the suture has already been passed through a bone tunnel, the steps are inverted (the suture first enters through the inferior surface of the tendon). (From ref. 79, with permission.)

well as the pathomechanics involved, are reviewed in chapter 1. Whether or not impingement is thought to be primary or secondary in a particular patient, if a prominent anterior acromion is felt to be contributing to pain and tendon injury at the time that surgery is considered, then an acromioplasty is considered. Open acromioplasty[124] has been an effective procedure, with long-term satisfactory results ranging from 80% to 90% in most series.[84,89,125,152]

In 1985 Ellman introduced the technique of arthroscopic subacromial decompression.[57] His preliminary findings were that the results of arthroscopic subacromial decompressions are comparable with open decompressions. In a follow-up study,[58] he demonstrated an 88% satisfactory outcome for arthroscopic subacromial decompression. Similarly, in a prospective, randomized study, Sachs and associates[160] found that patients having an arthroscopic acromioplasty did better in the first 3 months following surgery than did patients undergoing an open procedure. After 3 months the two groups were equal. Long-term follow-up showed no difference between the two procedures, with an overall success rate of 90%. These findings are consistent with other reports in the literature.[3,62,63,75,144,158,159,171]

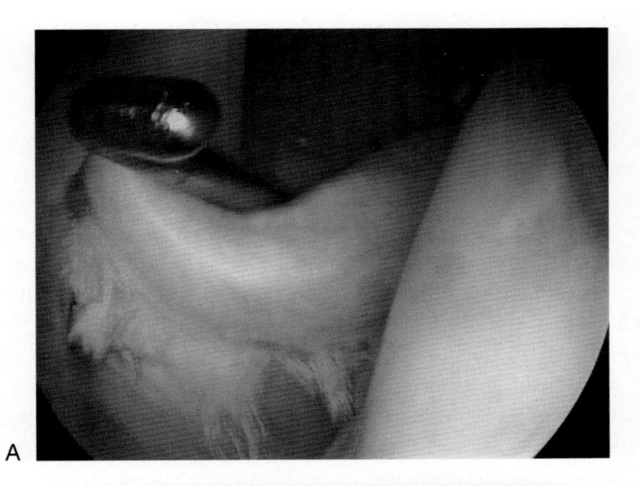

A

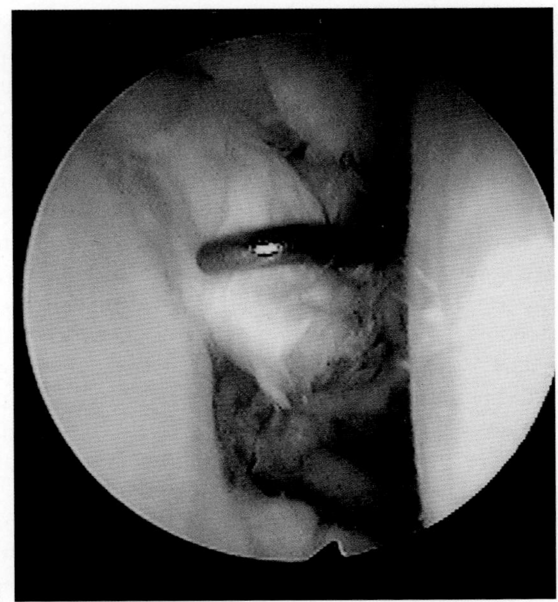

B

FIG. 14. (A) Partial biceps tear seen on glenohumeral arthroscopy as the biceps is pulled down into the joint. This will be debrided. **(B)** Proximal stump of a torn biceps tendon. This will be resected back to the base.

Authors' Preferred Treatment

We prefer to perform routine decompressions arthroscopically. The procedure begins with glenohumeral joint inspection. Any inflamed synovium should be debrided and glenohumeral pathology addressed as indicated.[51] (Fig. 14) Attention is then focused on the undersurface of the rotator cuff, evaluating for any irritation or tears. Once the glenohumeral joint has been examined, the subacromial space is entered with the arthroscope. Typically a thick bursitis is encountered, and this is removed with a 5.5-mm full-radius gator. Once there is good visualization of the subacromial space, the undersurface of the acromion and coracoacromial (CA) ligament are inspected. Although there may be a synovitic or inflamed appearance to the ligament, the usual finding is hypertrophy of the ligament, with a degenerative, attritional lesion of the anteroinferior acromion, including frayed fibers hanging down (Fig. 15). In young, athletic patients there may be no bone abnormalities, but just scarring of the bursa and thickening of the coracoacromial ligament.[8] In these patients, a soft-tissue decompression with debridement without release of the ligament, combined with renewed rehabilitation to treat any subtle underlying instability, may be helpful.

In older patients with a more degenerative profile, the ligament is removed and an acromioplasty performed. The CA

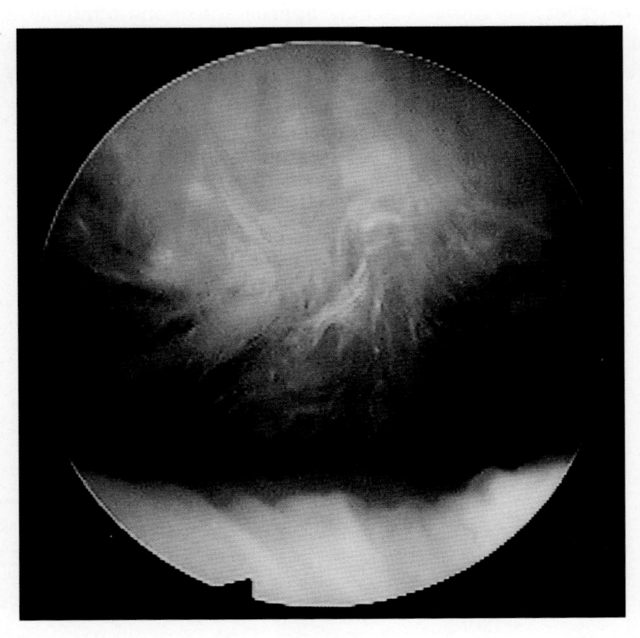

FIG. 15. Attritional lesion of the anteroinferior acromion at the insertion of the coracoacromial ligament.

ligament is sequentially removed from the undersurface of the acromion using electrocautery and then freed at its margins laterally and medially. Once the ligament has been released from the anterior acromion, a full-radius gator will remove it, or it can be removed in one piece with a grasper. Frequently, the acromial branch of the thoracoacromial artery will be encountered, and the surgeon must be prepaired with electrocautery to cauterize the vessel and prevent a "red-out." The undersurface of the acromion, and frequently a spur, are now exposed with the ligament resection. It is important to visualize the entire acromion, from the AC joint to the lateral margin to perform an adequate acromioplasty. We routinely use the electrocautery to expose the anterolateral and lateral aspect of the acromion to better appreciate the acromial morphology and spur size. Newer bipolar cautery devices have made acromial exposure easier.

To perform the bony acromioplasty a 6.0-mm–tapered burr is used. The thickness and morphology of the acromion as well as the size of any bone spur will dictate the amount of bone removed in an individual patient. A popular technique for determining the amount of bone removal is the "cutting-block" technique.[29] (Fig. 16). In this method the burr is brought in from the posterior portal, applied to the posterior acromion, and then advanced to plane down the anterior acromion, thereby flattening the entire acromion. This approach aims to convert the acromion to a type I after Bigliani and Morrison.[15] However, this may remove an excessive amount of bone if the burr is brought into the subacromial space at an acute angle to the posterior surface of the acromion. In the past, the coracoacromial arch has been often thought of as a purely harmful structure, causing impingement and good for little else. Indeed, in 1984, Rockwood advocated the routine removal of the CA ligament at the time of any shoulder operation.[155] This encouraged, in past years, a "more is better" approach to bone removal at acromioplasty. However, in a study in our laboratory, we found contact by the acromion on the underlying rotator cuff and humerus in normal shoulders.[70] We and others believe that the arch has a passive, stabilizing function.[68,103,121,137,180,185] In a later study simulating different amounts of bone removal at acromioplasty, smoothing the anterior third of the acromial undersurface removed all focused contact on the supraspinatus insertion, which we termed impingement; therefore, total flattening of the acromion was not only unnecessary to relieve impingement, but destroyed much of the broad contact, termed "buffering," which was likely important for stability.[66]

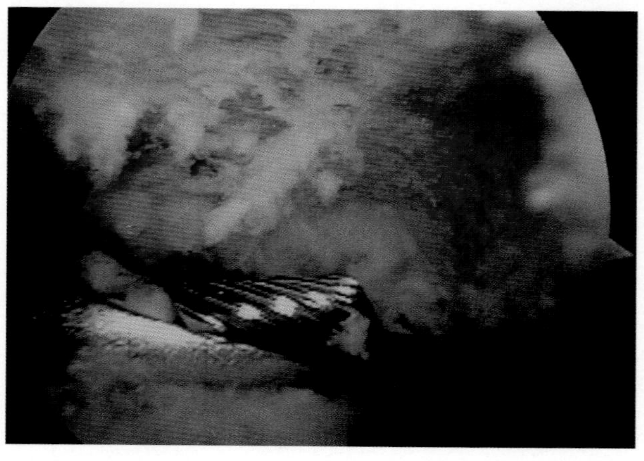

FIG. 16. Cutting block technique for arthroscopic acromioplasty.

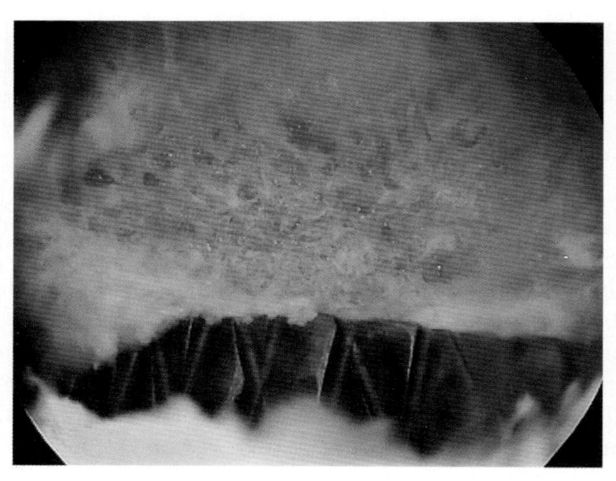

FIG. 17. An instrument of known size, such as a burr or rasp as seen here, may be used to estimate the amount of bone resection. The rasp may also be used to smooth and contour the acromion.

In addition to removing excessive bone, the arthroscopic cutting block technique may risk injuring the deltoid origin, especially in curved acromions in which a line drawn up against the posterior acromial undersurface essentially transects the anterior acromion. Indeed, some surgeons who purport to use this technique will depart from it when they notice a thin, curved acromion (J Rogerson, personal communication, 1997). We prefer to aim for opening up the subacromial space by resculpting the anteroinferior acromion so that it curves gently away from the underlying humerus and cuff. The amount of bone removal may be estimated from the preoperative outlet view and measured intraoperatively by comparison with the known diameter of an instument (Fig. 17). The transition to the posterior acromion is then smoothed. All debris is removed, and the bursal space is irrigated. After decompression, the instruments are removed and portals are closed with absorbable suture. The patient is placed in a removable sling for 1 to 2 days for initial comfort. Postoperative motion exercises are generally started immediately, and progressed as tolerated.

The major advantage of arthroscopic over open decompression is that deltoid detachment is avoided.[2] Use of the arthroscope also allows inspection of the glenohumeral joint, as well as the undersurface of the rotator cuff, and any pathology encountered can then be addressed. Finally, arthroscopic decompressions are less invasive and can be performed more easily on an outpatient basis.

Surgery for Partial-Thickness Rotator Cuff Tears

The literature remains unclear and somewhat confusing on the treatment of partial-thickness rotator cuff tears. Recommendations range from conservative therapy to open rotator cuff debridement and repair. Prior to arthroscopic surgery, excision and repair of significant partial cuff tears seemed logical and added little morbidity to an open procedure.[73,127] However, after the advent of arthroscopic acromioplasty, but before techniques of arthroscopic tendon repair had been developed, simple debridement with or without decompression became more widely used for partial tears and even many full-thickness tears.[59,63] Later, as data accumulated indicating that not all of these patients did well,[115,182] primary excision of the damaged part of the tendon with tendon repair came back into vogue, especially because this now involved only additional arthroscopic steps or at most a miniopen incision, rather than conversion to a full open procedure.[64] Currently, recommendations for the operative management of partial tears vary between investigators. Essentially, there are three surgical options: debridement alone, decompression and debridement, and excision of damaged tendon with primary repair (usually along with decompression). Let us examine each of these in turn.

Andrews reported good success with debridement,[4] but his population was young and athletic. It is likely that overuse and tensile failure were involved, rather than any acromial abnormalities. Snyder and coworkers[170] reported their results on arthroscopic cuff debridement with or without subacromial decompression. They had 85% satisfactory results, with similar results between those patients having a decompression and those not having a decompression. However, patients were not randomized for decompression, but were selected on clinical criteria, likely correctly identifying patients in whom impingement was prominent. Arroyo and coworkers noted that young, overhead athletes frequently develop subacromial scarring and bursitis owing to overuse and instability, and that soft-tissue cleanout of the subacromial space may be helpful.[8] Altchek and Carson studied 50 throwing athletes with anterior shoulder pain, which was refractory to nonoperative treatment,[2] and found that most had fraying of the articular surface of the cuff. Debridement of this area, combined with debridement of bursitis and coracoacromial ligament hypertrophy when noted, was associated with favorable results in 80% of cases.[2]

The role of internal impingement, in which the cuff undersurface abuts the glenoid rim in abduction and external rotation,[100,101,178] also adds complexity to decision making. This mechanism, as well as other causes of cuff failure, is discussed in chapter 9. When deep-surface cuff partial tears are associated with internal impingement, most surgeons have employed simple debridement;[64] however, little data are available on the effectiveness of this approach. In some cases, anterior subluxation has been thought to play a role, and capsulorraphy recommended.[101] Indeed, one author has suggested that derotational humeral osteotomy be considered.[178] In any event, this group of younger patients, who are often involved in throwing sports, is a different group from that of older patients with degenerative tendon failure.

In such older patients, simple debridement has been far less satisfactory. Ogilivie Harris and coworkers treated 57 partial tears with arthroscopic debridement alone, and found that only half achieved satisfactory results.[139] In this group, acromioplasty appears to improve results.[21,59,75,140,189] Arthroscopic decompression has also been effective. Gartsman noted that 33 of 40 patients (83%) with partial-thickness tears had major improvements in their shoulders at an average of 29 months after arthroscopic acromioplasty.[75] However, not all patients do well with this approach. Altchek and coworkers noted that the results of debridement and decompression of partial tears were not as favorable as those from decompression in shoulders with intact cuffs.[3] But which subgroups of partial tears need more than decompression?

Weber felt that degree of tendon involvement was important.[182] He reported inferior results in patients undergoing debridement and decompression of partial cuff tears that involved more than half the tendon's thickness, as compared with a miniopen approach in which the damaged tendon was excised and healthy tissue repaired side-to-side.[182] Interestingly, his recommendations are the same as those of Neer[127] (done open), although less aggressive than Fukuda and coworkers, who performed excision of damaged tissue on most partial tears[73] and achieved a 92% success rate. Further

Algorithm for surgical decision making

Pathology		Treatment
Subacromial bursitis/tendonitis	⇒	Arthroscopic subacromial bursectomy
. . . if prominent/worn coracoacromial ligament	⇒	. . . arthroscopic coracoacromial ligament excision
. . . if prominent acromion, bone spur, <50% thickness partial rotator cuff tear	⇒	. . . arthroscopic acromioplasty, cuff debridement
. . . if >50% thickness partial rotator cuff tear, small or medium full-thickness rotator cuff tear	⇒	. . . arthroscopically-assisted ("miniopen") rotator cuff repair
Large or massive rotator cuff tear		Open acromioplasty, rotator cuff repair, coracoacromial ligament preservation

study is needed to make definitive recommendations for treatment.

Authors' Preferred Treatment

We treat minor degrees of tendon injury in a young, athletic patient with rehabilitation. If that fails, arthroscopy is considered. This population will often have subtle degrees of instability, but if cuff and bursal findings are dominant clinically, and if clear signs of instability, especially anteroinferior labral detachment, are not found, then initially, we would not likely perform a capsulorraphy. We would debride the partial tear and any labral fraying, and then inspect the bursa. If there is bursitis and coracoacromial ligament hypertrophy, then we would debride those areas, performing in effect a soft-tissue subacromial decompression (Table 1).

For older patients with degenerative partial cuff tears who fail nonoperative treatment, we will perform a shoulder arthroscopy to determine the depth and size of the tear. If the tear is less than 50% in thickness then we will perform an arthroscopic cuff debridement followed by an anterior acromioplasty with CA ligament excision (Fig. 18). The retracted edge of the "rim-rent" can be bulky, and may cause the tendon to buckle and jam in the subacromial space. Debridement includes trimming this edge to decrease its bulk. A colored absorbable (in case a piece breaks off) suture is passed through the partial tear with a spinal needle to aid in identifying the corresponding bursal surface of the tendon later. This will help to avoid missing a full-thickness perforation and to find cases in which the tendon is thinned from both sides. If the tear involves more than 50% of the tendon's thickness in an active patient, we will perform the arthroscopic anterior acromioplasty and proceed to a portal-extending mini-open rotator cuff debridement, with elliptical excision of the degenerative tendon, followed by a side-to-side or tendon-to-bone repair. For patients with partial tears of less than 50%, their rehabilitation is the same as patients undergoing arthroscopic anterior acromioplasty for chronic

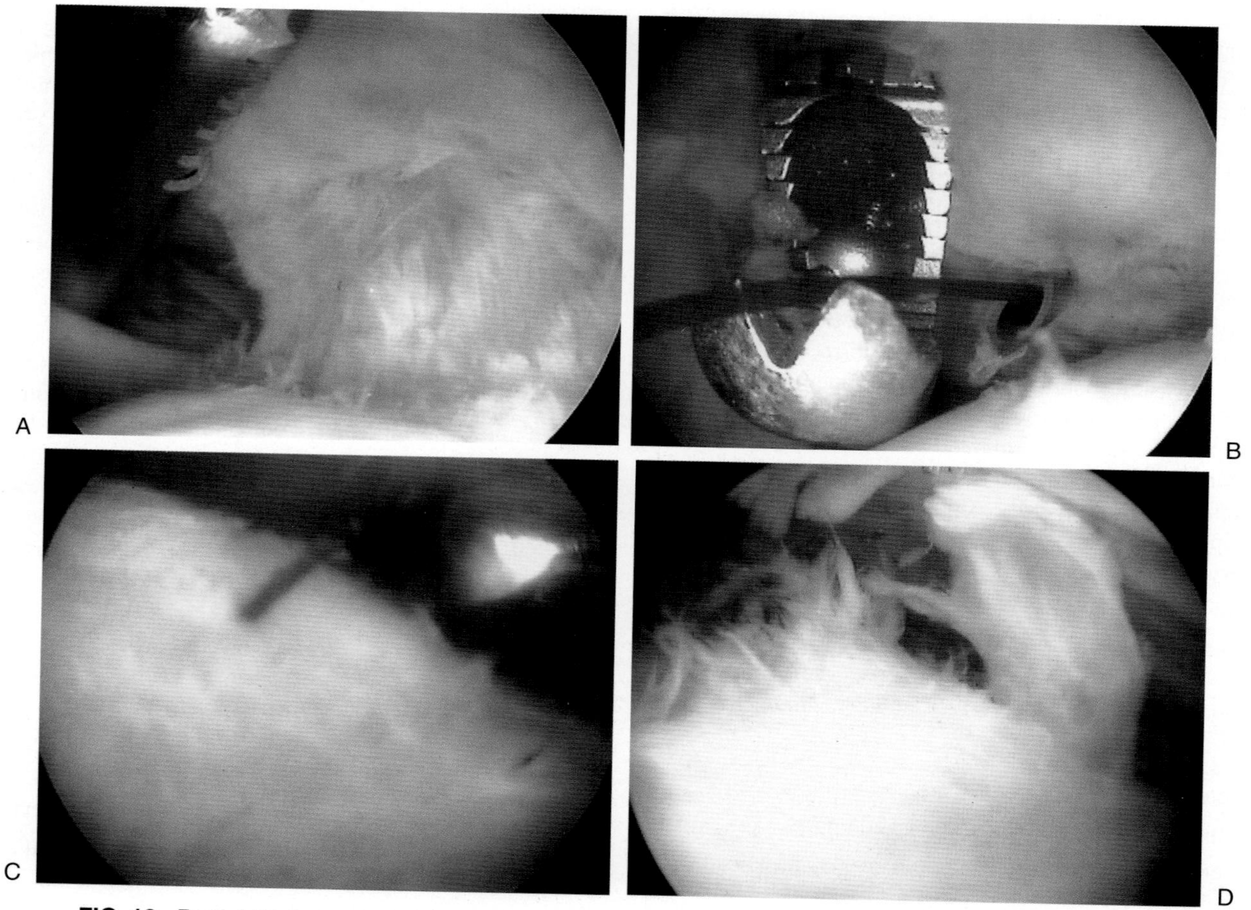

FIG. 18. Partial-thickness tears of the rotator cuff can be treated with debridement if the tear is less than 50% of the thickness of the tendon. **(A)** Arthroscopic view from the posterior glenohumeral portal of an articular-sided partial-thickness tear of the supraspinatus. **(B)** An absorbable suture is placed through the tendon with a spinal needle to allow bursal-sided inspection. **(C)** Subacromial view of the bursal side of the tendon showing that the tear does not extend to the bursal surface. **(D)** Subacromial view of a different patient who has a partial bursal-sided tear.

impingement. Those with tears of more than 50%, and who have a miniopen procedure, receive the same rehabilitation as patients with a small full-thickness tear.

Full-Thickness Rotator Cuff Tears

History

Codman performed his first cuff repair in 1909,[39] and in 1934 he noted that 20 of 31 patients followed after repair of full-thickness rotator cuff tears obtained a good result.[43] Four years later Outland and Shepherd published a series of 12 rotator cuff repairs; satisfactory results were obtained in 67%.[141] McLaughlin, using a transacromial approach, reported 94% pain relief and 100% return to manual labor in 32 patients after cuff repair.[111] In the 1950s and 1960s overall satisfactory results after cuff tendon repair were seen in 77% of Mosely's cases,[123] 74% of Godsil and Linscheid's cases,[80] 60% of Heikel's cases,[93] and 66% of Debeyre et al.'s cases.[52]

In 1972, Neer advocated routine anterior acromioplasty at the time of rotator cuff repair.[124] Of 20 patients with full-thickness tears treated by acromioplasty and repair, 19 (95%) achieved satisfactory results (patient satisfied, no significant pain, less than 20 degrees of limitation of elevation and at least 75% of normal strength). In this and in other writings,[124,126–128] Neer argued for certain principles in rotator cuff surgery:

1. Reshaping rather than removing the acromion, avoiding procedures that damage the deltoid origin
2. Restoring motion
3. Releasing, mobilizing, and repairing the torn tendons
4. Surgeon-directed individualized rehabilitation

Although most modern surgeons have employed an approach similar to Neer's, there have been exceptions. Repair of the tendons without acromioplasty has been advocated,[138,166] as has acromioplasty without tendon repair.[157] Some have even continued to advocate acromionectomy.[20] Nevertheless, decompression and repair remains the most common treatment for full-thickness tears requiring surgery. With recent advancements in arthroscopy, many authors are advocating arthroscopic repair of rotator cuff tears. Preliminary results appear to be promising and equal to those for miniopen repairs.[76,169,176] Arthroscopic repair follows the same principles as those for open repairs, including subacromial decompression, cuff mobilization, and repair of the tendon back to the tuberosity (Fig. 19). Technically, this can be very challenging and time-consuming, particularly on the upslope of the learning curve.

Principles and Technique

Approach

Although stiffness is surprisingly infrequent in shoulders with large cuff tears, it can occur.[127] Even if superior structures may be released during an open repair, the inferior capsule and axillary recess are difficult to reach through an open anterosuperior approach. Consequently, stiff shoulders are gently manipulated at the beginning of the procedure.

A variety of surgical approaches for cuff repair has been reported.[109] Norwood has described a posterior approach,[138] whereas Leffert has preferred an anterior, deltopectoral exposure,[104] also advocated by Gerber for subscapularis ruptures.[78] Most authors, however, have employed an anterosuperior approach through a split or takedown of the proximal deltoid.[109] In an attempt to visualize large tears with retraction, takedown of the anterior or lateral deltoid origin has been used, as have acromion-splitting approaches. However, Codman,[43] after trying various techniques, came to prefer a deltoid split combined with rotation of the head beneath the split to expose the involved area of the cuff. Diamond, in 1964, described an extensile approach for acromionectomy in which a deltoid split was taken up over the acromion, which was then exposed subperiosteally.[55] Neviaser employed a split taken into the AC joint with superiosteal reflection of the flaps to expose the tear, made easier because the distal clavicle was routinely resected.[135] However, exposure of a retracted posterior tear may be difficult with an anterior split, occasionally even requiring a supplemental posterior incision.[127] For this reason Bigliani has shifted the split posteriorly by beginning it at the anterolateral corner of the acromion; this affords excellent posterior exposure[13,50] (see Fig.12).

Athroscopic approaches generally involve three bursal portals: anterior, lateral, and posterior. Whereas a decom-

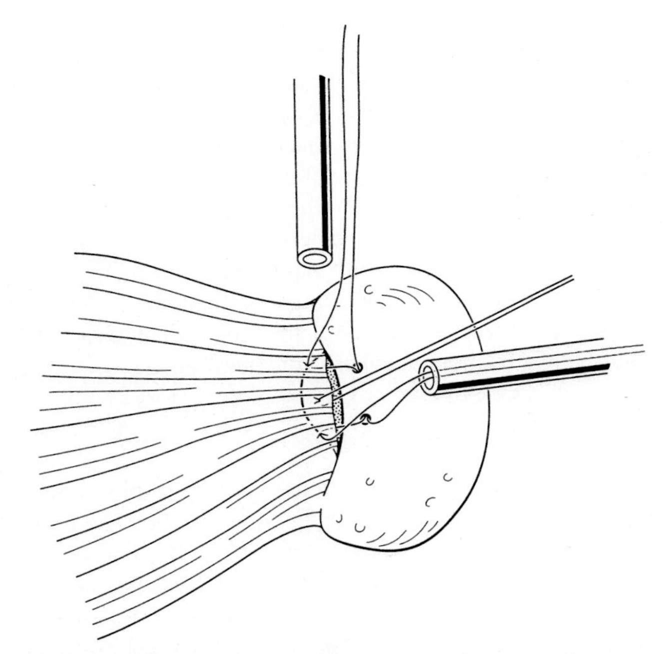

FIG. 19. Most arthroscopic techniques rely on passing a suture anchor in the greater tuberosity, passing sutures through the tendon edge and tying the knots arthroscopically. (From ref. 76, with permission.)

pression and, if indicated, a distal clavicle resection involve visualizing the anteroinferior and anteromedial acromion, the cuff tear and tuberosity are generally quite lateral to the acromion, and the lateral portal must not be placed too high. Mini-open approaches are considered to be those that employ only a split of the deltoid, without any takedown of the origin. The actual skin incision may range from a 3-cm portal extension in the skin creases[151] to a fairly large longitudinal incision.[145]

Decompression

Traditionally, decompression at the time of cuff repair has consisted of anterior acromioplasty, resection of the coracoacromial ligament, and if needed, resection of downward-projecting acromioclavicular osteophytes.[124] It has become increasingly appreciated that the coracoacromial arch has a normal buffering role in passively resisting superior humeral translation,[66,68,70,103,121,137,180,185] especially when the dynamic stabilizing function of the cuff muscles has been lost. Wiley reported that anterosuperior subluxation could result from decompression without repair of massive cuff tears,[185] but we have noticed this also after decompression and repair when the repair fails or the muscles, although reattached, are too atrophied to generate the force necessary to center the head. Indeed, Watson, noting that his cases of cuff repair did better when the coracoacromial ligament was incised, rather than resected, conjectured that coracoacromial ligament "removal may allow the strong deltoid muscle to pull the humeral head proximally," stretching and potentially damaging the cuff repair.[180]

Preservation of the coracoacromial arch for stability has been employed at the time of arthroplasty for cases of end-stage rheumatoid arthritis and cuff-tear arthropathy;[7,150] however, the prosthetic humeral component to some extent spaces the tuberosity (which, if bare, may also be trimmed) away from the acromion, so that decompression is not required. In 1991 the senior one of us (ELF) began to preserve the coracoacromial ligament when repairing massive tears, and reported on the initial experience a few years later.[71] This has not appeared to result in postoperative impingement or inadequate pain relief. Whether this should be used for all tears or only large ones, and if the latter, what size cutoff there should be, remain unanswered questions.

Tendon Mobilization and Repair

The aim of tendon mobilization is not only to allow repair, but to free the cuff muscle–tendon units so they can glide, and to prevent postoperative stiffness.[126,127] It is unfortunate that the cuff literature has emphasized concepts such as "coverage of the head," as if cuff repair were a plastic surgery procedure. No hand surgeon would sew a graft into an old, scarred flexor tendon laceration and say that he or she had "covered" the proximal interphalangeal joint. The goal should be to restore the cuff's dynamic function as best possible. Therefore, the tendons must be not only repaired, but also must be freed from adhesions to surrounding structures so that the muscle–tendon unit can glide and function. Also, passive shoulder motion may be normal, despite extensive cuff scarring, because the capsule is detached from the humerus along with the cuff tendons, so motion occurs "through the tear." If the tendons (and the attached capsule) are repaired without being adequately released, a stiff shoulder may result, and stretching exercises will improve motion only by pulling out the repair.

Arthroscopic techniques have progressed to the point where experts report that the same tendon releases traditionally performed open may be accomplished arthroscopically.[72,76] A possible exception may be chronic subscapularis tears, which may have extraarticular adhesions (especially including the axillary nerve).

Repair is performed with the arm at the side. Performing the repair with the arm in abduction and then placing the patient in an airplane splint will usually lead to pullout of the repair when the brace is discontinued.[133] However, protection of a repair of a large tear (performed with the arm at the side) with a brace was employed by Neer,[127] and has been more recently advocated by Gerber (C. Gerber personal communication, 1993). Recently developed braces are more comfortable than earlier models, are less likely to rotate into extension, and allow for more intermediate positions rather than wide abduction and external rotation. The proper role of postoperative bracing remains in dispute.

Traditionally, many surgeons preferred repairing the tendon to a trough in bone.[113] Many techniques have been reported in which the tendon edge is pulled into a deep cancellous trough with mattress sutures. Several factors have contributed to a trend away from cancellous troughs. First, use of mattress sutures often allows some mobility of the free edge of the tendon, or at least some discontinuity between the repair and the tuberosity. We have preferred simple or Mason–Allen sutures that hold the tendon edge flat against the tuberosity and present a smooth surface. Second, concern for the holding power of sutures in osseous tunnels, and especially for the pullout strength of suture anchors, has prompted a desire to preserve the cortical bone at the articular–tuberosity junction. Finally, doubts have been raised as to whether, in fact, cancellous bone is a better healing bed for tendon than cortical bone—a recent study in sheep found no difference in repair strength.[172] Most surgeons freshen the bone at the articular–tuberosity junction, to remove nonhealing bursal tissue and scar, but do not necessarily expose the cancellous bone.

Numerous suture techniques have been described. An influential study recently suggested that modified Mason–Allen sutures provided the best holding power in a weak tendon while minimizing strangulation.[79] However, simple sutures elongate least under load, and thus gap less in a strong tendon. The most accepted arthoscopic techniques involve placing suture anchors, threading the sutures through the edge of the torn tendon, and then arthroscopically tying knots to effect the repair. Alternatively, a transfixing implant such as a tack or staple may be used, or a suture anchor with attached suture may be threaded directly through the tendon edge. Attempts to place transosseous tunnels have been made,[69] but the risk of injury to the circumflex branch of the axillary nerve has kept most surgeons to suture-anchor techniques. These approaches are still in rapid evolution, but do appear to reproduce the steps of the open repair well.

Deltoid Repair

In open surgery the deltoid must be securely repaired; indeed, some of the worst complications in cuff surgery involve damage to or detachment of the deltoid. The deltoid may be repaired back to bone, to a cuff of soft-tissue, or both. Some surgeons detach a portion of the deltoid with a sliver of acromial bone, so that it can be repaired bone-to-bone.

The major advantage of arthroscopic repair is believed to be the preservation of the deltoid origin. However, Rockwood has suggested that subperiosteal elevation of the deltoid, as is performed with arthroscopic acromioplasty, may detach a large proportion of the Sharpey fibers of the deltoid origin, causing substantial weakening.[156] Indeed, with the advent of miniopen cuff repair, surgeons have been able to examine the deltoid after an arthroscopic acromioplasty, and many have noted (anecdotally) occasional thin areas or even frank detachment of the anterior fibers.

Rehabilitation

Passive motion begun early after repair is used by most rotator cuff surgeons, and active motion is generally deferred until tendon healing can be expected. The limits of motion must be based on the surgeon's impressions of the security of the repair and the quality of the tissues. These factors are highly variable. Stiffness is unusual after repair of massive tears, because most of the capsule was off with the tendon and both are often thin and insubstantial. Pulling out of the repair is the more likely complication, so slow, gradual, passive motion is generally the core of the postoperative program. Conversely, patients with small tears, with thick, robust tendon (and attached capsule), not infrequently may become stiff after repair, whereas repair dehiscence is far less frequent than after repair of massive tears.[86] For these patients, a more aggressive mobilization program is used. In any event, the program must be directed by the surgeon who performed the repair, and progress must be closely monitored.

Results

The long term results of rotator cuff repair have been evaluated. Wolfgang[188] in 1974 reported on 65 full-thickness rotator cuff repairs that were first evaluated at 9.8 months, and then at 8.2 years postoperatively. In addition to cuff repair, 55% of the shoulders in this series underwent lateral acromionectomy. Sixty-nine percent of the shoulders in this series demonstrated good to excellent results at 9.8 months; 46 of these patients were again evaluated at an average of 8.2 years postoperatively, and 74% of these had good to excellent results at that time. Petersson[147] in a different study in 1981, also demonstrated that the results of rotator cuff repair do not deteriorate over time. Of 66 original surgical patients in the study, 43 shoulders were available for reexamination at an average of 14 years after the original procedure. These results were compared with the results obtained in these same patients only 6 months after their original procedures. A good result was judged to be a shoulder with more than 150 degrees of elevation, as well as being devoid of pain. At 6 months postoperatively, 63% of the shoulders were rated as good, and at 14 years postoperatively, 58% were judged to be good results.

Samilson and Binder[161] in 1975 evaluated the results obtained in 33 shoulders with full-thickness tears undergoing surgical repair. The coracoacromial ligament was excised in all cases, and an anterior acromioplasty was performed in 21% of the shoulders in addition to the tendon repair. After average follow-up of 23 months, 84% of these shoulders were rated as good or excellent results; 76% of the patients returned to work and 70% of the shoulders demonstrated increased strength in external rotation postoperatively.

By 1985, the techniques of rotator cuff repair became more standardized for surgeon acceptance of the importance of physical therapy, anterior acromioplasty, and the preservation of the deltoid muscle origin. Hawkins and coworkers[91] reviewed 100 consecutive rotator cuff repairs at a mean of 4.2 years postoperatively. Repair of the tendon and anterior acromioplasty were employed in all surgical procedures. Postoperately, 86% of these 100 patients had no or slight pain. The average active abduction postoperatively was 125 degrees (compared to 81 degrees preoperatively). Of the patients in Hawkins' series, 78% could use their affected arm above the shoulder level either normally, or with minimal compromise postoperatively, compared with 16% of patients being able to do this preoperatively. Postoperative strength in external rotation of the shoulder was considered to be normal in 42%, compared with 22% of shoulders preoperatively. All but 6 of the patients (94%) considered themselves to be improved after rotator cuff surgery. Although a statistically significant improvement in strength of the shoulder was demonstrated postoperatively, the authors of this study were of the opinion that the improvement in function was primarily related to relief of pain.

Ellman and coworkers[60] reviewed 50 rotator cuff repairs after an average follow-up duration of 3.5 years. A full-thickness tear was present in 49 of the shoulders (98%). Anterior acromioplasty was performed in 48 of the shoulders (96%), and in 20 of these same 48 shoulders, distal clavicle excision was also performed. These authors rated their results according to the criteria of Neer.[124] They obtained a satisfactory result in 84% of the shoulders when pain, function, and strength of forward flexion were evaluated. Forty-nine of the patients (98%) were satisfied with their result.

A large series of rotator cuff repairs was reviewed by Neer and coworkers[127] in 1988. These authors analyzed 245 shoulders with tears of the cuff necessitating repair, and 243 of these (99%) also underwent anterior acromioplasty. Follow-up averaged 5.5 years and results were graded as "excellent" (essentially normal shoulder), "satisfactory" (no significant pain, active elevation above horizontal, and patient pleased with result) or "unsatisfactory." Excellent or satisfactory results were obtained in 92% and excellent results were obtained in 78% of these shoulders.

Recently, Cofield and coworkers[48] examined 81 shoulders following rotator cuff repair an average of 7.5 years following surgery. Anterior acromioplasty and repair of the tendon defect were performed on all of the shoulders at surgery. Ninety-three percent obtained satisfactory pain relief and 94% of the patients were of the opinion that they were much better after surgery; 83% returned to work. Overall, 65% had excellent results and 79% had either excellent or satisfactory results.

Cofield[46] reviewed many different series of rotator cuff repairs, and averaged the results as described by the various authors. Overall, pain relief occurred in 87% of shoulders, and patient satisfaction averaged 77%.

Factors appearing to influence the outcome of rotator cuff repair appear to be the size of the tear, patient age, and preoperative function. Hattrup evaluated patient age relative to outcome following rotator cuff repair.[87] He was able to show that patients older than the age of 65 years tended to have poorer results as well as larger cuff tears. Cofield and coworkers found that tear size is the single most important factor influencing long-term results.[48] Pollock and coworkers[148] also found that cuff tear size directly correlated with final outcome. Satisfactory results were obtained in 95% of small, 94% of medium, 88% of large, and 84% of massive tears. Others have also found that results for surgical repair of massive tears are inferior to those for smaller tears.[14,48,50,53,81,83,86,91,126,133,143] Harryman and coworkers suggested a reason why larger tears did less well: the repair was less likely to remain intact.[86]

Many techniques have been described for the management of massive rotator cuff tears, including debridement,[5,91,115,120,157,190] partial repair,[24] mobilization and repair of cuff tissue,[13,46,50,52,60,91,111,113,124,126,127] tendon transfer,[27,47,77,97,126,131,134] implantation of fascia,[11] allografts,[132] and the placement of synthetic material.[142] Mobilization and transposition of existing rotator cuff tissue has generally yielded better results than implantation of fascia, allografts, synthetic material,[13,46,50,67] or cuff debridement.[5,91,115,120,185,190]

Ellman and coworkers[60] were able to show a correlation between a poor result and preoperative strength and active range of motion. If patients had grade 3/5 strength or less or were unable to abduct their shoulder beyond 100 degrees, there was an increased risk of a poor result. When patients have an unsatisfactory result, it is usually associated with poor function and not pain relief. This is supported by Bigliani[13] and Hawkins[91] who found that there was good pain relief for repairs of massive tears, but functional improvement was less predictable.

Finally, the final outcome of rotator cuff repair may not necessarily be directly related to complete healing of the tendon. Calvert and coworkers[28] demonstrated good function, pain relief, and satisfaction despite having a documented dye leak at follow-up shoulder arthrography. Packer and coworkers had similar findings[143] and suggest a "water-tight closure" of a cuff defect is not necessary. Likewise, Harryman and coworkers[86] found up to 50% of their cuff repairs had a postoperative defect. This did not adversely influence patient satisfaction or pain relief, but it did affect shoulder strength. Indeed, in their study the most important factor affecting strength and function at follow-up was a maintained tendon repair. This, combined with the poor results reported for decompression without repair of cuff tears,[115] has led to an increased emphasis on the technical adequacy of tendon repair, including the use of stronger sutures, tendon or bone augmentation, and postoperative bracing.[79,173]

A particularly careful and well-documented study[98] found 88% good or excellent results after cuff repair, and good correlation between patient satisfaction and objective measures such as the Constant score.[96,97] Increased preoperative tear size, poorer tissue quality, increased difficulty of tendon mobilization, and the presence of a rupture of the tendon of the long head of the biceps, together, adversely affected outcome. We are currently undertaking a study, funded by the Orthopaedic Research and Education Foundation, of the outcome of cuff repair, looking at costs, quality of life, ASES evaluation scheme, Constant score, AAOS DASH form, and SF-36 assessment; early results show consistent gains in most domains in the first year after repair (unpublished data).

The results of arthroscopic acromioplasty with a miniopen rotator cuff repair are good. Levy and coworkers reported 80% satisfactory result.[105] Of their patients 96% were satisfied with the procedure. We have recently reported our experience with miniopen rotator cuff repairs following an arthroscopic acromioplasty.[151] All 30 of our patients had an excellent result at an average of 25 months follow-up. All the tears in this study group were either small or medium.

Entirely arthroscopic repair is still in evolution, but early results have been promising.[76,183] Weber compared 39 entirely arthroscopic repairs with 101 arthroscopic-assisted miniopen repairs: he found lower early morbidity, but also a higher complication rate, including 3 loose anchors (8%), in the arthroscopic group.[183] After 6 weeks, the outcomes were identical. Three recent series contained 137 patients followed for at least 1 year after arthroscopic cuff repair:[117,163,176] overall, 88% achieved good or excellent results.

Authors' Preferred Treatment

For small and medium cuff tears we perform an arthroscopic anterior acromioplasty and a portal-extending mini-open repair of the rotator cuff (see Fig. 10). We employ a 3-cm skin incision in the skin creases centered over the anterolateral portal. Subcutaneous flaps are elevated, and a 3-cm deltoid split is made in the direction of its fibers created from just behind the anterolateral corner of the acromion distally. If the split is brought too anteriorly, the anterior deltoid may be inadvertently pulled off the anterior acromion with retraction, especially if the anterior deltoid origin has been weakened during the acromioplasty (as discussed earlier). The tendon mobilization and repair is as described in the following for large tears. With practice and effort, it is remarkable how large a tear may be repaired through a mini-open approach. We generally limit this technique, however, to supraspinatus tears, for several reasons. First, the releases for large, retracted tears seem more reliably and more rapidly performed open. Second, preservation and repair of the coracoacromial ligament is easier through an open approach. Finally, as the tear comes to involve multiple tendons, the tissue is usually thinner and of poorer quality, and the postoperative regimen (limits of rehabilitation, delay in active use, restrictions on sports and occupation) is dominated by concern for the tendon repair, rather than protection of the deltoid repair.

After the tendon repair, the deltoid split is repaired side-to-side. A buried no. 0 permanent braided suture is used to anchor the repair at the acromial edge, and then no. 0 absorbable sutures are used for the rest of the split. The incision is repaired in a layered fashion, and the skin is closed with a 4-0 absorbable subcuticular stitch.

For tears that involve the subscapularis or infraspinatus in addition to the supraspinatus, an open procedure is performed. A 6- to 7-cm skin incision is made in the direction of the skin creases, centered over the anterolateral corner of the acromion (see Fig. 11). A 3- to 5-cm deltoid split is made from the anterolateral corner of the acromion distally in the direction of the delotid fibers. For massive tears with posterior retraction, the split is slanted posteriorly for exposure. The incision is then taken up over the anterior acromion to the anterior aspect of the acromioclavicular joint, traveling 2 to 3 mm posterior to the anterior edge of the acromion. This keeps a thick, rindlike flap of tissue with the anterior deltoid, allowing secure repair to the acromion with transosseous sutures. The incision is then continued around the anterior edge of the acromion to continue underneath the anteroinferior acromion, so that the entire coracoacromial ligament is subperiosteally elevated and stays as one flap with the anterior deltoid (Fig. 20).

Once the coracoacromial ligament is detached, there is excellent exposure of the anterior acromion and any spurs that may have developed (see Fig. 12). An acromioplasty is then performed. A wide osteotome is used to remove the anteroinferior aspect of the acromion from the AC joint to the lateral edge of the acromion. The amount of bone removal depends on the thickness of the acromion, the degree of anteroinferior acromial prominence, and the size of any spurs. The emphasis should be on contouring a smooth undersurface of the acromion. Rongeurs, rasps, and a burr are used to obtain a perfectly smooth surface. The wedge of bone excised should, however, consist of the full width of the acromion from the medial to the lateral border. If the AC joint is tender preoperatively, a distal clavicle excision will be performed. This is performed from the undersurface using either a rongeur or a burr. The superior and posterior AC ligaments are left intact for distal clavicle stability. If the AC joint is not tender preoperatively, then the AC joint is left undisturbed, even if it is arthritic. If it is felt that inferior AC osteophytes are contributing to impingement, then they are removed, and the undersurface of the AC joint is smoothed. Some surgeons have found a high incidence of late AC pain after such undersurface trimmings, and have suggested that perhaps it is better to either leave the joint unviolated or to completely resect the distal clavicle (M. Gross, personal communication, 1997; F. Savoie, personal communication, 1997). However, this has not been our experience.

Once the acromioplasty is performed, the rotator cuff is more easily visualized. Mobilization of the rotator cuff is the first step in repairing the tendon. Any heaped-up portion of the bursa that lies over the defect or the tendon edges is removed for exposure as well as to free the rotator cuff from bursal adhesions. Stay sutures are placed in the retracted rotator cuff tendon, beginning anteriorly and working posteriorly. These can be used for traction while mobilizing the tendon. Clamps (which might crush the tissue) are not employed. To mobilize the tendon, all adhesions are freed, beginning on the bursal side, bluntly separating the tendons from the undersurface of the acromion and deltoid. After complete bursal surface release and exposure, the posterior tissues are assessed to determine the full extent of the cuff tear. Usually a portion of the posterior cuff remains attached to the humeral head.

Releases are performed systematically. First the tendon edges are freshened to remove nonsticking bursal tissue and to stimulate healing, and to remove a tapered edge to yield a thick edge that will hold sutures. This generally means removing 1 to 2 mm of tissue; resection of tendon edges to bleeding tissue is not advocated, as despite a white, nonbleeding appearance, the edges of cuff tears are, in fact, usually well-vascularized. The plane between the cuff tendons and the overlying acromion and deltoid is bluntly developed. The retracted tendons are often scarred to the coracoid base, with fixed shortening of the coracohumeral ligament.[130] This ligament is divided (Fig. 21), and the coracoid base is freed anteriorly, laterally, and posteriorly, but not medially (to avoid injury to the suprascapular nerve).

As the tendons retract, the capsule may shorten until the tendons are tenodesed to the glenoid rim. To release them, the capsule is divided external to the labrum. Care must be taken to avoid going more than 1 cm medial to the glenoid rim, lest injury to the suprascapular nerve ensue. The use of

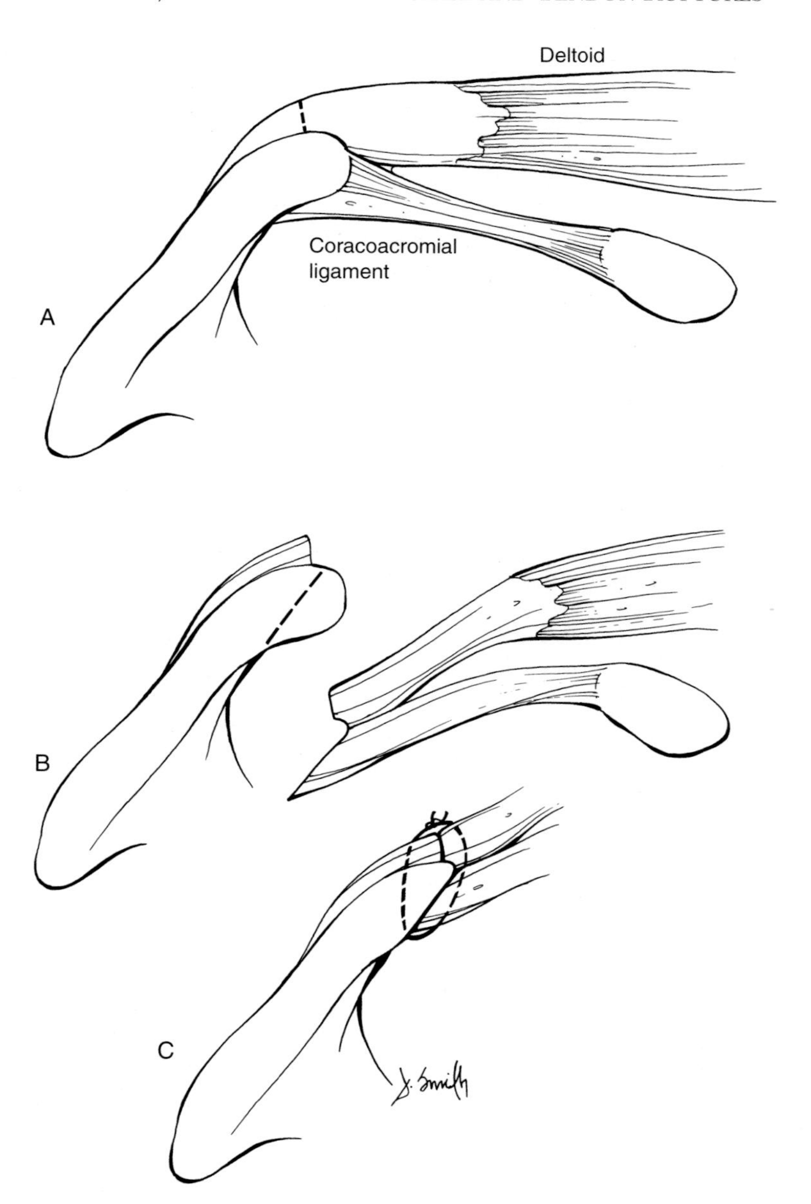

FIG. 20. (A) An incision is made just behind the anterior acromion. **(B)** This is then skived under the acromion to elevate the deltoid and coracoacromial ligament as one flap. The *dotted line* shows the amount of the acromioplasty. **(C)** The coracoacromial ligament is repaired with transosseous sutures.

a distracting device, designed by Gerber (see Chap. 3), to sublux the humeral head inferiorly, can be extremely helpful in performing these releases.

The tendons commonly retract variable amounts. A frequent pattern is that the supraspinatus is retracted medially, whereas the subscapularis is out to length. In such a situation the anterior margin of the supraspinatus, being medially retracted, is scarred to the medial aspect of the subscapularis. To realign it an "interval release (slide)"[13] may be helpful. The interval between the supraspinatus and subscapularis is divided to the coracoid base (Fig. 22). If there is differential retraction between the supraspinatus and infraspintus posteriorly, it can also be useful to free the interval between these two tendons (Fig. 23). Not only do interval releases allow realignment of retracted tendons, but they function as "relaxing incisions"[179] so that the tendons, scarred into a circle with the attached capsule at the glenoid rim, may be brought out over the larger-diameter humeral head (much as the collar of a turtleneck shirt must be stretched to pull it over one's head).

Next the articular surface of the tendon is mobilized. Usually, when the tendon is retracted, the capsule shortens, so that the tendon is essentially tenodesed to the glenoid rim. This may be released by incising the capsule external to the labrum (Fig. 24). Care must be taken to avoid injury to the suprascapular nerve at the base of the scapular spine or to the biceps tendon origin. Once the undersurface is freed, the excursions of the tendons are assessed.

If the biceps tendon is intact and gliding in its groove, it is preserved. It is often enlarged and may have minor degrees of fraying. If a significant portion of the biceps tendon is damaged, or if it is subluxed out of its groove (usually in as-

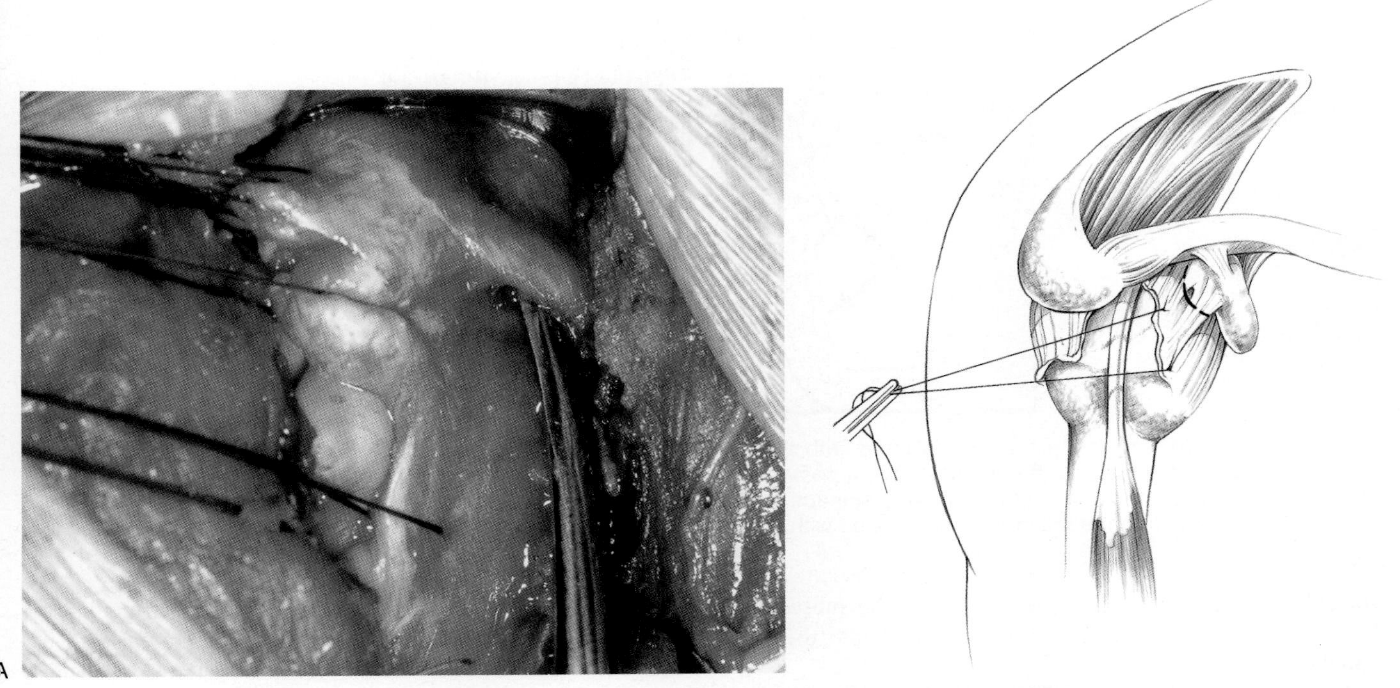

FIG. 21. (A) The coracohumeral ligament (*at end of instrument*) is contracted, tethering the retracted tear edge to the coracoid. **(B)** This ligament must be divided (*dotted line*) and the coracoid base freed to mobilize the tendon. (From ref. 130, with permission.)

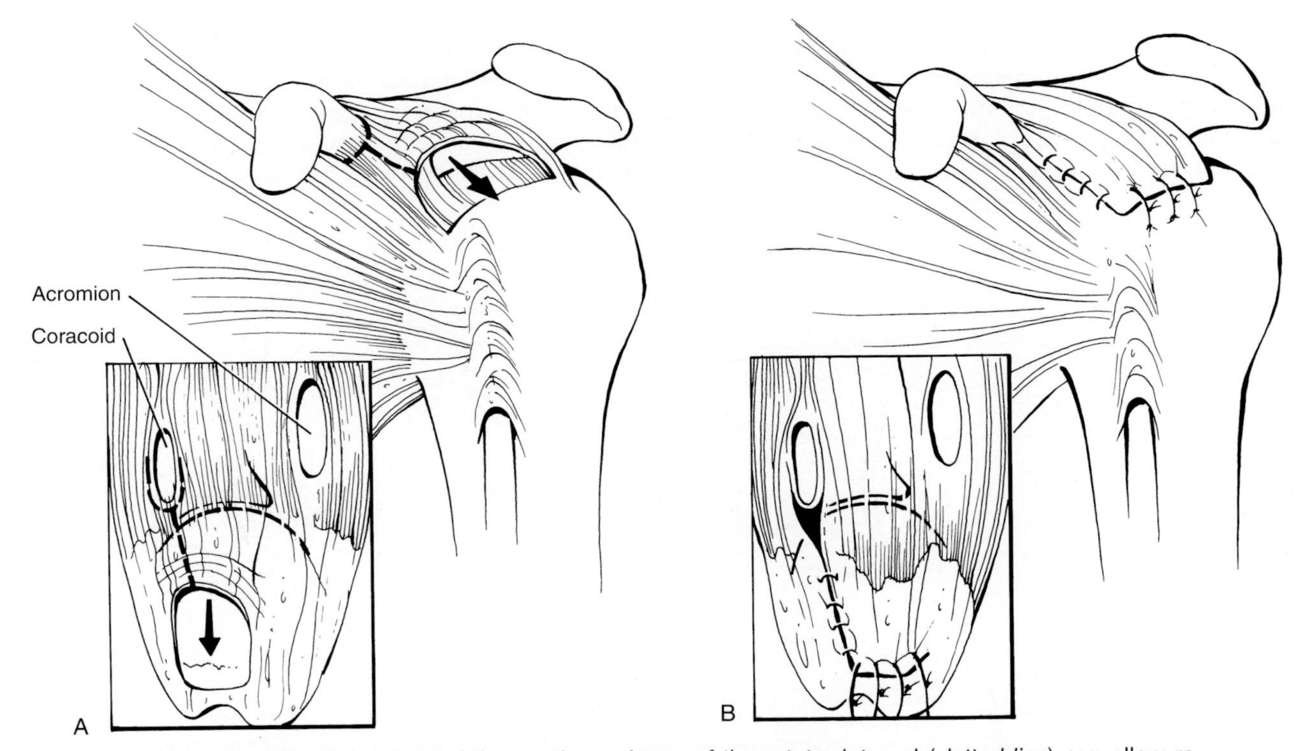

FIG. 22. (A) If there is differential retraction, release of the rotator interval (*dotted line*) can allow realignment of the supraspinatus tendon (*arrow*). **(B)** After the tendon is repaired to the bone, the interval is sutured. (Redrawn from ref. 31, with permission.)

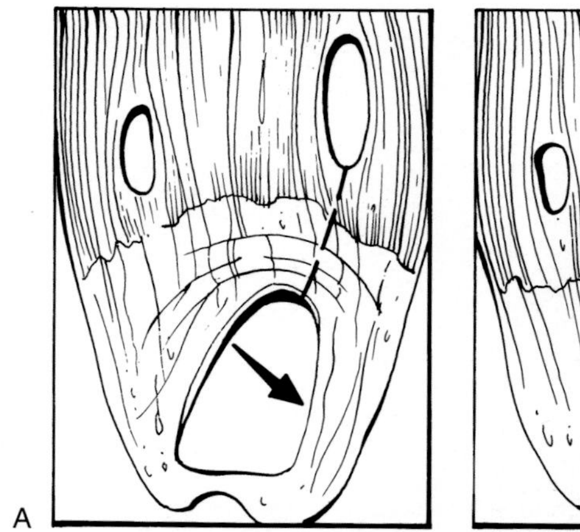

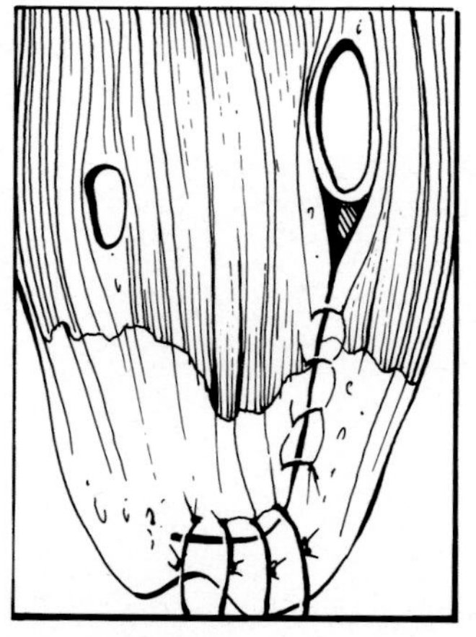

FIG. 23. (A) If the tear is retracted with the greatest differential retraction between the posterior supraspinatus and the infraspinatus, a posterior interval release (*dotted line*) is performed, separating these two tendons so that the supraspinaus tendon may be mobilized (*arrows*). **(B)** After the tendon is repaired to bone the interval is repaired with sutures. (Redrawn from ref. 31, with permission.)

sociation with a tear or the upper portion of the subscapularis), it is either tenodesed of incorporated into the repair.[27,127]

Intact muscles are generally not rerouted, and tendon transfers for cuff repair are described in Chapter 3. By using the techniques of tissue mobilization described in the foregoing, tendon repair may be achieved in all but a few rare situations. These repairs may sometimes be imperfect, reattaching an atrophied muscle by thin, poor-quality tendon tissue. However, reattachment gives the muscle–tendon units a better chance for functional recovery than leaving them disinserted. If there is significant loss of cuff tissue and full repair is not possible, the anterior and posterior cuff are mobilized cephalad as much as is possible to gain a better fulcrum for head depression.[24]

The greater tuberosity is prepared for tendon repair by freshening or scarifying the anatomic neck area with a rongeur or curette. Sharp excrescences are removed. A deep trough is not used, for it requires more tendon mobilization and has not been shown to be necessary to promote tendon-to-bone healing. Reusable curved awls (Link America, Denville, N.J.) are used to create transosseous tunnels and pass heavy nonabsorbable no. 2 sutures. The tendon is then repaired to the greater tuberosity, with the arm at the side in a neutral position. A combination of simple and Mason–Allen stitches are used at the tendon edge.

We still prefer transosseous sutures over metallic suture anchors in cuff surgery because of the variable strength of the tuberosity bone in these often elderly cuff-disease patients (unlike the uniformly hard bone of the anterior glenoid

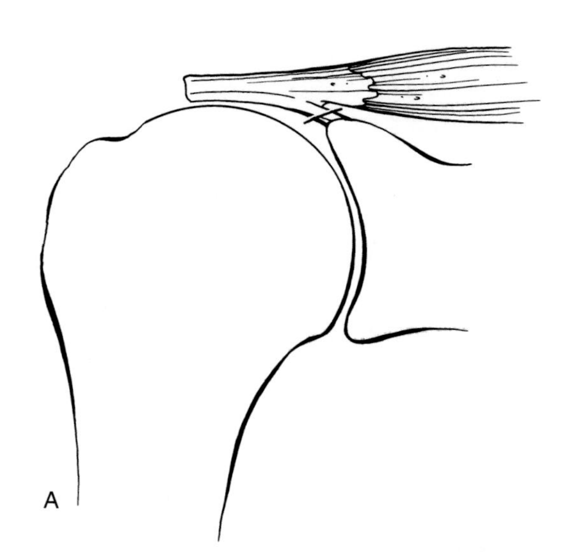

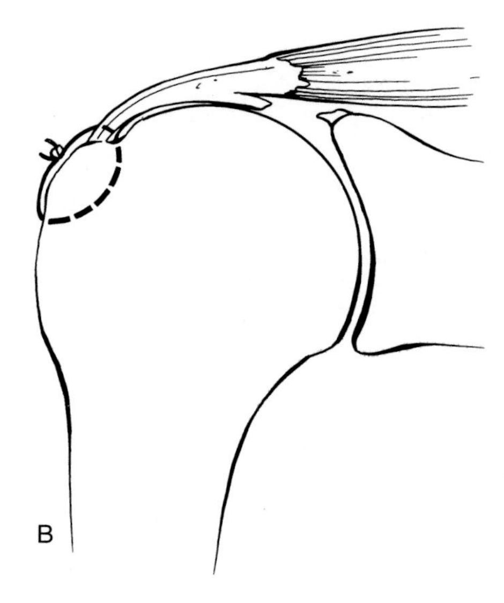

FIG. 24. (A) If the retracted tendon is tethered to the glenoid rim by a shortened, fibrotic capsule, the capsule should be incised (*dotted line*). **(B)** This allows mobilization and repair of the tendon.

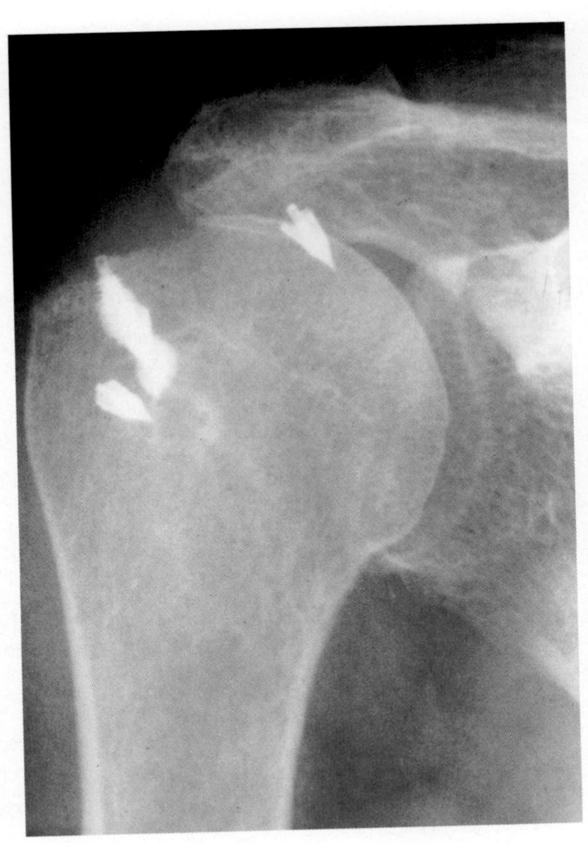

FIG. 25. This metal anchor has pulled out of the soft bone of the tuberosity. Because it is attached to sutures on the cuff edge it has stayed adjacent to the articular surface.

in instability patients). Also, the attached sutures tend to hold loose anchors in the superior joint, where articular damage may result (Fig. 25). However, technical improvements, including plastic anchors, resorbable anchors, and better fixation techniques, may make implants more attractive in the future.

If there is a large or massive tear, the coracoacromial ligament is repaired together with the anterior deltoid flap to the anterior acromion. This provides a buttress that may provide restraint from superior migration or anterosuperior instability of the humeral head. The deltoid is meticulously repaired as outlined in the section on surgical approaches.

Depending on the quality of tissue and repair, postoperative rehabilitation is tailored to the security of the repair and the quality of the tissues. Braces that hold the arm in wide abduction and external rotation are not used. However, occasionally, the posterior cuff is repaired with some tension, and a brace to hold the arm in slight abduction and neutral rotation may be used; this avoids the sling position of internal rotation across the body. Passive motion is still begun immediately, with the therapist or a trained family member raising the arm in the scapular plane above the brace.

A physician-directed rehabilitation program is always begun on the first postoperative day. For very massive tears with poor tissue, only pendulum and passive elevation in the scapular plane by the surgeon, the therapist, or a trained family member are used for the first 6 weeks. Pulley elevation is not used owing to the significant active cuff recruitment that results.[110] Elevation is allowed to a level determined at the time of repair, usually between 120 and 140 degrees. Assistive exercises are begun at 6 weeks, but active elevation and light resistive exercises are not allowed until 3 months after repair of these massive tears. Patients after repair of medium and large tears with good tissue begin an assistive program immediately, and active exercises (progressing slowly to light resistive) are added between 6 and 8 weeks postoperatively.

When using these principles for rotator cuff repair, Cofield, in a review of the literature, found an average of 85% of patients had satisfactory results with reports up to 100%.[46] We have recently reviewed our experience on The Shoulder Service at New York Orthopaedic Hospital for rotator cuff repairs in 486 patients and found 96% had satisfactory pain relief and 80% had substantial functional improvement.[148]

REFERENCES

1. Adamson GJ, Tibone JE. Ten-year assessment of primary rotator cuff repairs. *J Shoulder Elbow Surg* 1993;2:57–63.
2. Altchek DW, Carson EW. Arthroscopic acromioplasty: current status. *Orthop Clin North Am* 1997;28:157–168.
3. Altchek DW, Warren RF, Wickiewicz TL. Arthroscopic acromioplasty. Technique and results. *J Bone Joint Surg [Am]* 1990;72: 1198–1207.
4. Andrews JR, Broussard TS, Carson WG. Arthroscopy of the shoulder in the management of partial tears of the rotator cuff: a preliminary report. *Arthroscopy* 1985;1:117–122.
5. Apoils A, Augereau B. Anterosuperior arthrolysis of the shoulder for rotator cuff degeneration lesions. In: Post M, Morrey BF, Hawkins RJ. eds. *Surgery of the shoulder*. St Louis: Mosby-Year Book, 1990: 257–260.
6. Armstrong JR. Excision of the acromion in treatment of the supraspinatus syndrome. *J Bone Joint Surg [Br]* 1949;31:436–442.
7. Arntz CT, Jackins S, Matsen FA III. Prosthetic replacement of the shoulder for the treatment of defects in the rotator cuff and the surface of the glenohumeral joint. *J Bone Joint Surg [Am]* 1993;75:485–491.
8. Arroyo JS, Hershon SJ, Bigliani LU. Special considerations in the athletic throwing shoulder. *Orthop Clin North Am* 1997; 28:69–78.
9. Bassett RW, Cofield RH. Acute tears of the rotator cuff. The timing of surgical repairs. *Clin Orthop* 1983;175:18–24.
10. Bateman JE. The diagnosis and treatment of ruptures of the rotator cuff. *Surg Clin North Am* 1963;43:1523–1530.
11. Bayne O, Bateman JE. Long-term results of surgical repair of full-thickness rotator cuff tears. In: Bateman JE, Walsh RP, eds. *Surgery of the shoulder*. Philadelphia: BC Decker, 1984:166–171.
12. Bigliani EL, Flatow EL, Codd TP. History, physical examination, and diagnostic modalities. In: McGinty JB, Caspari RB, Jackson RW, Poehling GG, eds. *Operative arthroscopy*, 2nd ed. Philadelphia: Lippincott–Raven, 1996:635–646.
13. Bigliani LU, Cordasco FA, McIlveen SJ, Musso ES. Operative treatment of massive rotator cuff tears: long-term results. *J Shoulder Elbow Surg* 1992;1:120–130.
14. Bigliani LU, Cordasco FA, McIlveen SJ, Musso ES. Operative treatment of failed repairs of the rotator cuff. *J Bone Joint Surg [Am]* 1992; 74:1505–1515.
15. Bigliani LU, Morrison DS, April EW. The morphology of the acromion and its relationship to rotator cuff tears. *Orthop Trans* 1986; 10:228.

16. Blair B, Rokito AS, Cuomo F, Jarolem K, Zuckerman JD. Efficacy of injections of corticosteroids for subacromial impingement syndrome. *J Bone Joint Surg [Am]* 1996;78:1685–1689.
17. Blevins FT, Djurasovic M, Flatow EL, Vogel KG. Biology of the rotator cuff tendon. *Orthop Clin North Am* 1997;28:1–16.
18. Boker DJ, Hawkins RJ, Huckell GH, et al. Results of nonoperative management of full-thickness tears of the rotator cuff. *Clin Orthop* 1993;294:103–110.
19. Bosley RC. Total acromionectomy. A twenty-year review. *J Bone Joint Surg [Am]* 1991;73:961–968.
20. Bosworth DM. An analysis of twenty-eight consecutive cases of incapacitating shoulder lesions, radically explored and repaired. *J Bone Joint Surg* 1940;22:369–392.
21. Braezeale NM, Craig EV. Partial-thickness rotator cuff tears: pathogenesis and treatment. *Orthop Clin North Am* 1997;28:145–156.
22. Brown AR, Weiss R, Greenberg CP, Flatow EL, Bigliani LU. Interscalene block for shoulder arthroscopy: comparison with general anaesthesia. *Arthroscopy* 1993;9:295–300.
23. Brown JT. Early assessment of supraspinatus tears. Procain infiltration as a guide to treatment. *J Bone Joint Surg [Br]* 1949;31:423–425.
24. Burkhart SS. Partial repair of massive rotator cuff tears: the evolution of a concept. *Orthop Clin North Am* 1997;28:125–132.
25. Burkhead WZ Jr, Habermeyer P. The rotator cuff: a historical review of our understanding. In: Burkhead WZ Jr, ed. *Rotator cuff disorders*. Baltimore: Williams & Wilkins, 1996:3–44.
26. Burns TP, Turba JE. Arthroscopic treatment of shoulder impingement in athletes. *Am J Sports Med* 1992;20:13–16.
27. Bush LF. The torn shoulder capsule. *J Bone Joint Surg [Am]* 1975;57: 256–259.
28. Calvert P, Packer N, Stoker D, et al. Arthrography of the shoulder after operative repair of the torn rotator cuff. *J Bone Joint Surg [Br]* 1986;68:147–150.
29. Caspari RB, Thal R. A technique for arthroscopic subacromial decompression. *Arthroscopy* 1992;8:23–30.
30. Cervilla V, Schwetzer ME, Ho C, et al. Medial dislocations of biceps tendon dislocation: appearance at MR imaging. *Radiology* 1001;180: 523–526.
31. Codd TP, Flatow EL. Anterior acromioplasty, tendon mobilization, and direct repair of massive rotator cuff tears. In: Burkhead WZ Jr, ed. *Rotator cuff disorders*. Baltimore: Williams & Wilkins, 1996: 323–334.
32. Codman EA. Some points on the diagnosis and treatment of certain neglected minor surgical lesions. *Boston Med Surg J* 1904;150: 371–374.
33. Codman EA. On stiff and painful shoulders. The anatomy of the subdeltoid or subacromial bursa and its clinical importance. Subdeltoid bursitis. *Boston Med Surg J* 1906;154:613–620.
34. Codman EA. Bursitis subacromialis, or peri-arthritis of the shoulder-joint (subdeltoid bursitis). *Boston Med Surg J* 1908;159:533–537.
35. Codman EA. Bursitis subacromialis, or peri-arthritis of the shoulder-joint (subdeltoid bursitis). *Boston Med Surg J* 1908;159:576–582.
36. Codman EA. Bursitis subacromialis, or peri-arthritis of the shoulder-joint (subdeltoid bursitis). *Boston Med Surg J* 1908;159:615–616.
37. Codman EA. Bursitis subacromialis, or peri-arthritis of the shoulder-joint (subdeltoid bursitis). *Boston Med Surg J* 1908;159:723–726.
38. Codman EA. Bursitis subacromialis, or peri-arthritis of the shoulder-joint (subdeltoid bursitis). *Boston Med Surg J* 1908;159:756–759.
39. Codman EA. Complete rupture of the supraspinatus tendon. Operative treatment with report of two successful cases. *Boston Med Surg J* 1911;164:708–710.
40. Codman EA. Abduction of the shoulder. An interesting observation in connection with subacromial bursitis and rupture of the tendon of the supraspinatus. *Boston Med Surg J* 1912;166:890–891.
41. Codman EA. Obscure lesions of the shoulder; rupture of the supraspinatus tendon. *Boston Med Surg J* 1927;196:381–387.
42. Codman EA. The pathology associated with rupture of the supraspinatus tendon. *Ann Surg* 1931;93:348–359.
43. Codman EA. *The shoulder: rupture of the supraspinatus tendon and other lesions in or about the subacromial bursa*. Boston: Thomas Todd, 1934.
44. Codman EA. Rupture of the supraspinatus—1834 to 1934. *J Bone Joint Surg* 1937;19:643–652.
45. Codman EA, Akerson TB. The pathology associated with rupture of the supraspinatus tendon. *Ann Surg* 1911;93:354–359.
46. Cofield RH. Rotator cuff disease of the shoulder. *J Bone Joint Surg [Am]* 1985;67:974–979.
47. Cofield RH. Subscapular muscle transposition for repair of chronic rotator cuff tears. *Surg Gynecol Obstet* 1982;154:667–672.
48. Cofield RH, Hoffmeyer P, Lanzar WH. Surgical repair of chronic rotator cuff tears. *Orthop Trans* 1990;14:251–252.
49. Constant CR. Shoulder function after rotator cuff tears by operative and nonoperative means. In: Post M, Morrey BF, eds. *Surgery of the shoulder*. St Louis: Mosby-Year Book, 1990:231–233.
50. Cordasco FA, Bigliani LU. Large and massive tears: technique of open repair. *Orthop Clin North Am* 1997;28:179–194.
51. Cordasco FA, Steinmann S, Flatow EL, Bigliani LU. Arthroscopic treatment of glenoid labral tears. *Am J Sports Med* 1993;21:425–430.
52. Debeyre J, Patte D, Elmelik E. Repairs of rupture of the rotator cuff of the shoulder: with a note on advancement of the supraspinatus muscle. *J Bone Joint Surg [Br]* 1965;47:36–42.
53. DeOrio JK, Cofield RH. Results of a second attempt at surgical repair of a failed initial rotator cuff repair. *J Bone Joint Surg [Am]* 1984;66: 563–567.
54. Depalma AF. *Surgery of the shoulder*, 3rd ed. Philadelphia: JB Lippincott, 1983:221–225.
55. Diamond B. *The obstructing acromion: underlying diseases, clinical development, and surgery*. Springfield, IL: Charles C Thomas, 1964: 131–136.
56. Duplay S. De la peri-arthrite scapulo-humerale et de raideurs de l'epaule qui en sont la consequence. *Arch Gen Med* 1872;20:513–542.
57. Ellman H. Arthroscopic subacromial decompression. *Orthop Trans* 1985;9:49.
58. Ellman H. Arthroscopic subacromial decompression: analysis of one- to three-year results. *Arthroscopy* 1987;3:173–181.
59. Ellman H. Diagnosis and treatment of incomplete rotator cuff tears. *Clin Orthop Rel Res* 1990;254:64–74.
60. Ellman H, Hanker G, Bayer M. Repair of the rotator cuff. End-result study of factors influencing reconstruction. *J Bone Joint Surg [Am]* 1986;68:1136–1144.
61. Ellman H, Kay SP. Arthroscopic subacromial decompression for chronic impingement. Two- to five-year results. *J Bone Joint Surg [Br]* 1991;73:395–398.
62. Esch JC. Arthroscopic subacromial decompression and postoperative management. *Orthop Clin North Am* 1991;24:161.
63. Esch JC, Ozerkis LR, Helgager JA, Kane N, Lilliott N. Arthroscopic subacromial decompression: results according to the degree of rotator cuff tear. *Athroscopy* 1988;4:241–249.
64. Flatow EL, Altchek DW, Gartsman GM, et al. Commentary. *Orthop Clin North Am* 1997;28:277–294.
65. Flatow EL, Bigliani LU. Complications of rotator cuff repair. *Complications Orthop* 1992;8:298–303.
66. Flatow EL, Coleman WW, Kelkar R, et al. The effect of anterior acromioplasty on rotator cuff contact: an experimental and computer simulation. *J Shoulder Elbow Surg* 1995;4:S53–S54.
67. Flatow EL, Fischer RA, Bigliani LU. Results of surgery. In: Ianotti JP, ed. *Rotator cuff disorders: evaluation and treatment.* Park Ridge, IL: American Academy of Orthopaedic Surgeons, 1991:53–63.
68. Flatow EL, Kelkar R, Raimondo RA, et al. Active and passive restraints against superior humeral translation: the contributions of the rotator cuff, the biceps tendon, and the coracoacromial arch. *J Shoulder Elbow Surg* 1996;5:S111.
69. Flatow EL, Rodosky MW, Compito CA, et al. Arthroscopic rotator cuff repair with suture to bone technique: a cadaver study. *Arthroscopy* 1994;10:353–354.
70. Flatow EL, Soslowsky LJ, Ticker JB, et al. Excursion of the rotator cuff under the acromion. Patterns of subacromial contact. *Am J Sports Med* 1994;22:779–788.
71. Flatow EL, Weinstein DM, Duralde XA, Compito CA, Pollock RG, Bigliani LU. Coracoacromial ligament preservation in rotator cuff surgery. *J Shoulder Elbow Surg* 1994;3:73.
72. Fleega BA. Arthroscopic operative reconstruction of full-thickness rotator cuff ruptures in athletes using a new giant needle technique. *J Shoulder Elbow Surg* 1996;5:S47.
73. Fukuda H, Craig EV, Yamanaka K. Surgical treatment of incomplete thickness tears of the rotator cuff: long-term follow-up. *Orthop Trans* 1987;11:237.
74. Fukuda H, Hamada K, Nakajima T, Tomonaga A. Pathology and

pathogenesis of the intratendinous tearing of the rotator cuff viewed from en bloc histologic sections. *Clin Orthop* 1994;304:60–67.

75. Gartsman GM. Arthoscopic acromioplasty for lesions of the rotator cuff. *J Bone Joint Surg [Am]* 1990;72:169–180.
76. Gartsman GM, Hammerman SM. Full-thickness tears: arthroscopic repair. *Orthop Clin North Am* 1997;28:83–98.
77. Gerber C, Hersche O. Tendon transfers for the treatment of irreparable rotator cuff defects. *Orthop Clin North Am* 1997;28:195–204.
78. Gerber C, Hersche O, Farron A. Isolated rupture of the subscapularis tendon: results of operative repair. *J Bone Joint Surg [Am]* 1996;78: 1015–1023.
79. Gerber C, Schneeberger AG, Beck M, Schlegel U. Mechanical strength of repairs of the rotator cuff. *J Bone Joint Surg [Br]* 1994;76: 371–380.
80. Godsil RD, Linscheid RL. Intratendinous defects of the rotator cuff. *Clin Orthop* 1970;69:181–188.
81. Gore DR, Murray MP, Sepic SB, et al. Shoulder muscle strength and range of motion following surgical repair of full-thickness rotator cuff tears. *J Bone Joint Surg [Am]* 1996;68:266–272.
82. Grant JCB, Smith GC. Age incidence of rupture of the supraspinatus tendon. *Anat Rec* 1948;100:666.
83. Gupta R, Leggin BG, Iannotti JP. Results of surgical repair of full-thickness tears of the rotator cuff. *Orthop Clin North Am* 1997;28: 241–250.
84. Ha'eri GB, Wiley AM. Shoulder impingement syndrome: results of operative release. *Clin Orthop* 1982;168:128.
85. Hammond G. Complete acromionectomy in the treatment of chronic tendinitis of the shoulder. *J Bone Joint Surg [Am]* 1962;44:494–504.
86. Harryman DT, Mack LA, Wang KY, Jackins SE, Richardson ML, Matsen FA III. Repairs of the rotator cuff: correlation of functional results with integrity of the cuff. *J Bone Joint Surg [Am]* 1991;73: 982–989.
87. Hattrup SJ. Rotator cuff repair: relevance of patient age. *J Shoulder Elbow Surg* 1995;4:95–100.
88. Hawkins RJ, Abrams JS. Impingement syndrome in the absence of rotator cuff tear (stages 1 and 2). *Orthop Clin North Am* 1987;18: 373–382.
89. Hawkins RJ, Brock RM, Abrams JS, et al. Acromioplasty for impingement with an intact rotator cuff. *J Bone Joint Surg [Br]* 1988;70: 795.
90. Hawkins RJ, Dunlop R. Nonoperative treatment of rotator cuff tears. *Clin Orthop* 1995;178–188.
91. Hawkins RJ, Misamore GW, Hobeika PE. Surgery for full-thickness rotator-cuff tears. *J Bone Joint Surg [Am]* 1985;67:1349–1355.
92. Hawkins RJ, Mohtadi N. Rotator cuff problems in athletes. In: De Lee JC, Drez D Jr, eds. *Orthopedic sports medicine: principles and practice*. Philadelphia: WB Saunders, 1994:623–656.
93. Heikel HVA. Rupture of the rotator cuff of the shoulder. Experiences of surgical treatment. *Acta Orthop Scand* 1968;39:499–502.
94. Hertel R, Ballmer F, Lombert SM, Gerber C. Lag signs in the diagnosis of rotator cuff rupture. *J Shoulder Elbow Surg* 1996;5:307–313.
95. Hodler J, Fretz CJ, Terrier D, et al. Rotator cuff tears: correlation of sonographic and surgical findings. *Radiology* 1988;169:791–794.
96. Iannotti JP. Postoperative outcome assessment of the shoulder following rotator cuff repair. In: Vastamaki M, Jalovaara P, eds. *Surgery of the shoulder*. Amsterdam: Elsevier, 1995:353–362.
97. Iannotti JP. Full-thickness rotator cuff tears: factors affecting surgical outcome. *J Am Acad Orthop Surg* 1994;2:87–95.
98. Iannotti JP, Bernot MP, Kuhlman JR, Kelley MJ, Williams GR. Postoperative assessment of shoulder function: a prospective study of full-thickness rotator cuff tears. *J Shoulder Elbow Surg* 1996;5:449–457.
99. Itoi E, Tabata S. Conservative treatment of rotator cuff tears. *Clin Orthop* 1992;275:165–173.
100. Jobe, CM. Posterior superior glenoid impingement: expanded spectrum. *Arthroscopy* 1995;11:530–536.
101. Jobe CM. Superior glenoid impingement. *Orthop Clin North Am* 1997;28:137–144.
102. Keyes EL. Observations on ruptures of the supraspinatus tendon based upon a study of seventy-three cadavers. *Ann Surg* 1933;97:849.
103. Lazarus MD, Yung S-W, Sidles JA, Harryman DT. Anterosuperior humeral displacement: limitation by the coracoacromial arch. American Academy of Orthopaedic Surgeons, 62nd Annual Meeting, Orlando, Florida, February, 1995.
104. Leffert RD, Rowe CR. Tendon ruptures. In: Rowe CR, ed. *The shoulder*. New York: Churchill-Livingstone, 1988:131–154.
105. Levy HJ, Gardner RD, Lemak LJ. Arthroscopic subacromial decompression in the treatment of full-thickness rotator cuff tears. *Arthroscopy* 1991;7:8–13.
106. Lindblom K. On pathogensis of ruptures of the tendon aponeurosis of the shoulder joint. *Acta Radiol* 1939;20:563–577.
107. Liu SH, Baker CL. Arthroscopically assisted rotator cuff repair: correlation of functional results with integrity of the cuff. *Arthroscopy* 1994;10:54–60.
108. Mack LA, Matsen FR, Kilcoyne JF, et al. Ultrasound evaluation of the rotator cuff. *Radiology* 1985;157:205–209.
109. Matsen FA III, Arntz CT. Rotator cuff tendon failure. In: Rockwood CA Jr, Matsen FA III, eds. *The shoulder*. Philadelphia: WB Saunders, 1990:647–677.
110. McCann PD, Wooten ME, Kadaba MP, Bigliani LU. A kinematic and elecromyographic study of shoulder rehabilitation exercises. *Clin Orthop* 1993;288:179–188.
111. McLaughlin HL. Lesions of the musculotendinous cuff of the shoulder: 1. The exposure and treatment of tears with retraction. *J Bone Joint Surg* 1944;26:31–51.
112. McLaughlin HL. Ruptures of the rotator cuff. *J Bone Joint Surg [Am]* 1962;44:979–983.
113. McLaughlin HL. Repair of major cuff ruptures. *Surg Clin North Am* 1963;43:1535–1540.
114. McLaughlin HL, Asherman EG. Lesions of the musculotendinous cuff of the shoulder, IV: some observations based upon the results of surgical repair. *J Bone Joint Surg [Am]* 1951;33:76–86.
115. Melillo AS, Savoie FH 3d, Field LD. Massive rotator cuff tears: Debridement versus repair. *Orthop Clin North Am* 1997;28:117–124.
116. Meyer AW. Further observations upon use-destruction in joints. *J Bone Joint Surg* 1922;4:491–511.
117. Mileski RA, Snyder SJ, Karzel RP. Results of arthroscopic cuff repair. *Arthroscopy* 1997;13:399.
118. Miniaci A, Salonen D. Rotator cuff evaluation: imaging and diagnosis. *Orthop Clin North Am* 1997;28:43–58.
119. Misamore GW, Ziegler DW, Rushton JL 2nd. Repair of the rotator cuff. A comparison of results in two populations of patients. *J Bone Joint Surg [Am]* 1995;77:1335–1339.
120. Montgomery TJ, Yerger B, Savoie FH 3d. A comparison of arthroscopic debridement with open surgical repair for full-thickness tears of the rotator cuff. *J Shoulder Elbow Surg* 1994;3:70–78.
121. Moorman CT III, Deng XH, Warren RF, Torzilli PA, Wickiewicz TL. The coracoacromial ligament: is it the appendix of the shoulder? *J Shoulder Elbow Surg* 1996;5:S9.
122. Morrison DS, Frogameni AD, Woodworth P. Non-operative treatment of subacromial impingement syndrome. *J Bone Joint Surg [Am]* 1997; 79:732–737.
123. Moseley HF. Ruptures of the rotator cuff. *Br J Surg* 1951;38:340.
124. Neer CS 2d. Anterior acromioplasty for the chronic impingement syndrome in the shoulder: a preliminary report. *J Bone Joint Surg [Am]* 1972;54:41–50.
125. Neer CS 2d. Impingement lesions. *Clin Orthop* 1983;173:70–77.
126. Neer CS 2d. *Shoulder reconstruction*. Philadelphia: WB Saunders, 1990:41–142
127. Neer CS 2D, Flatow EL, Lech O. Tears of the rotator cuff. long term results of anterior acromioplasty and repair. *Orthop Trans* 1988;12: 735.
128. Neer CS 2D, Marberry TA. On the disadvantages of radical acromionectomy. *J Bone Joint Surg [Am]* 1981;63:416–419.
129. Neer CS II, Poppen NK. Supraspinatus outlet. *Orthop Trans* 1987;11: 234.
130. Neer CS II, Satterlee CC, Dalsey RM, Flatow EL. The anatomy and potential effects of contracture of the coracohumeral ligament. *Clin Orthop* 1992;280:13–16.
131. Neviaser JS.: Ruptures of the rotator cuff of the shoulder: new concepts in the diagnosis and operative treatment of chronic ruptures. *Arch Surg* 1971;102:483–485.
132. Neviaser JS, Neviaser RJ, NEviaser TJ. The repair of chronic massive ruptures of the rotator cuff. *J Bone Joint Surg [Am]* 1978;60:681–684.
133. Neviaser RJ, Neviaser TJ. Reoperation for failed rotator cuff repair: analysis of fifty cases. *J Shoulder Elbow Surg* 1992;1:283–286.
134. Neviaser RJ, Neviaser TJ. Transfer of the subscapularis and teres mi-

nor for massive defects of rotator cuff. In: Bayley JL, Kessel L, eds. *Shoulder surgery*. New York: Springer, 1982:60–63.
135. Neviaser TJ, Neviaser RJ, Neviaser JS. The four-in-one arthroplasty for the painful arc syndrome. *Clin Orthop* 1982;163:107–112.
136. Nicholson GP, Goodman DA, Flatow EL, Bigliani LU. The acromion: morphologic condition and age-related changes. A study of 420 scapulas. *J Shoulder Elbow Surg* 1996;5:1–11.
137. Nirschl RP. Rotator cuff tendinitis: basic concept of pathoetiology. In: Barr JS Jr, ed. *Instructional course lecture*. Park Ridge, IL: American Academy of Orthopaedic Surgeons, 1989:447–462.
138. Norwood LA, Barrack R, Jacobson KE. Clinical presentation of complete tears of the rotator cuff. *J Bone Joint Surg [Am]* 1989;71: 499–505.
139. Ogilvie-Harris DJ. Arthroscopic surgery of the shoulder: a general appraisal. *J Bone Joint Surg [Am]* 1986;68:201–207.
140. Olsewski JM, Depew AD. Arthroscopic subacromial decompression and rotator cuff debridement for stage II and stage III impingement. *Arthroscopy* 1994;10:61–68.
141. Outland TA, Shepherd WF. Tears of the supraspinatus tendon. Resume of twelve operated cases. *Ann Surg* 1938;107:116–121.
142. Ozaki J, Fujuimoto S, Masuhara K, et al. Reconstruction of chronic massive rotator cuff tears with synthetic materials. *Clin Orthop* 1986; 202:173–183.
143. Packer NP, Calvert PT, Bayley JIL, Kessel L. Operative treatment of chronic ruptures of the rotator cuff of the shoulder. *J Bone Joint Surg [Br]* 1983;65:171–175.
144. Paulos IF, Franklin JL. Arthroscopic subacromial decompression development and application: a five year experience. *Am J Sports Med* 1990;18:235–244.
145. Paulos LE, Kody MH. Arthroscopically enhanced "miniapproach" to rotator cuff repair. *Am J Sports Med* 1993;21:113–120.
146. Perthes G. Uber operationen bei habitueller schulterluxation. *Dtsch Z Chir* 1906;85:199–227.
147. Petersson CJ. Ruptures of the supraspinatus tendon: cadaver dissection. *Acta Orthop Scand* 1984;55:52.
148. Pollock RG, Black AD, Self EB, Flatow EL, Bigliani LU. Surgical management of rotator cuff disease. *J Shoulder Elbow Surg* 1996;5: S37.
149. Pollock RG, Brown AR, Flatow EL, Bigliani LU. Regional anesthesia for shoulder arthroscopy: the interscalene block. *Contemp Orthop* 1993;26:452–457.
150. Pollock RG, Deliz ED, McIlveen SJ, Flatow EL, Bigliani LU. Prosthetic replacement in rotator cuff-deficient shoulders. *J Shoulder Elbow Surg* 1992;1:173–186.
151. Pollock RG, Flatow EL. Full-thickness tears: mini-open repair. *Orthop Clin North Am* 1997;28:169–178.
152. Post M, Cohen J. Impingement syndrome: a review of the late stage II and early stage III lesions. *Clin Orthop* 1986;207:126.
153. Post M, Silver R, Singh M. Rotator cuff tear. Diagnosis and treatment. *Clin Orthop* 1983;173:78–92.
154. Rathbun JB, Macnab I. The microvascular pattern of the rotator cuff. *J Bone Joint Surg [Br]* 1970;52:540–553.
155. Rockwood CA Jr. Subluxations and dislocations about the shoulder. In: Rockwood CA Jr, Green DP, eds. *Fractures in adults*, 2nd ed. vol 1. Philadelphia: JB Lippincott, 1984:795.
156. Rockwood CA Jr, Lyons FR. Shoulder impingement syndrome: diagnosis, radiographic evaluation, and treatment with a modified Neer acromioplasty. *J Bone Joint Surg [Am]* 1993;75:409–424.
157. Rockwood CA Jr, Williams GR Jr, Burkhead WZ Jr. Debridement of degenerative, irreparable lesions of the rotator cuff. *J Bone Joint Surg [Am]* 1995;77:857–866.
158. Roye RP, Grana WA, Yates CK. Arthroscopic subacromial decompression: two- to seven-year follow-up. *Arthroscopy* 1995;11: 301–306.
159. Ryu RK. Arthroscopic subacromial decompression: a clinical review. *Arthroscopy* 1992;8:141–147.
160. Sachs RA, Stone ML, Devine S. Open vs. arthroscopic acromioplasty: a prospective, randomized study. *Arthroscopy* 1994;10:248–254.
161. Samilson RL, Binder WF. Symptomatic full-thickness tears of the rotator cuff: an analysis of 292 shoulders in 276 patients. *Orthop Clin North Am* 1975;6:449–466.
162. Seeger LL, Gold RH, Bassett LW, Ellman H. Shoulder impingement syndrome: MR findings in 53 shoulders. *AJR Am J Roentgenol* 1988; 150:343–347.
163. Shea KP, Jennings JE, Stahl EJ, Stoller SM, King WD. Arthroscopic rotator cuff repair using a transhumeral suture technique: a prospective 1 year follow-up. *Arthroscopy* 1997;13:399–400.
164. Sher JS, Uribe JW, Posada A, Murphy BJ, Zlatkin MB. Abnormal findings on magnetic resonance images of asymptomatic shoulders. *J Bone Joint Surg [Am]* 1995;77:10–15.
165. Shuman WP, Kilcoyne RF, Matsen FA, et al. Double-contrast computed tomography of the glenoid labrum. *AJR Am J Roentgenol* 1983; 141:5584–5812.
166. Siekanowicz AJ, Nirschl RP. Open repair of full thickness rotator cuff tears with preservation of the acromion and coracoacromial ligament. *Orthop Trans* 1996;20:401.
167. Skinner HA. Anatomical considerations relative to rupture of the supraspinatus tendon. *J Bone Joint Surg* 1937;19:137.
168. Skyhar MJ, Altchek DW, Warren RF, et al. Shoulder arthroscopy with the patient in the beach-chair position. *Arthroscopy* 1988;4:256–259.
169. Snyder SJ. Arthroscopic evaluation and treatment of the rotator cuff. In: *Shoulder arthroscopy*. New York: McGraw-Hill, 1994:133–178.
170. Snyder SJ, Pachelli AF, Del Pizzo W, Friedman MJ, Ferkel RD, Pattee G. Partial thickness rotator cuff tears: results of arthroscopic treatment. *Arthroscopy* 1991;7:1–7.
171. Speer KP, Lohnes J, Garrett WE. Arthroscopic subacromial decompression: results in advanced impingement syndrome. *Arthroscopy* 1991;7:291.
172. St Pierre P, Olson EJ, Elliott JJ, O'Hair KC, McKinney LA, Ryan J. Tendon-healing to cortical bone compared with healing to a cancellous trough. A biomechanical and histological evaluation in goats. *J Bone Joint Surg [Am]* 1995;77:1858–1866.
173. Sward L, Hughes JS, Amis A, Wallace WA. The strength of surgical repairs of the rotator cuff. A biomechanical study on cadavers. *J Bone Joint Surg [Br]* 1992;74:585–588.
174. Tabata S, Kida H, Takahara M, et al. A comparative study of nonsurgical treatment and surgical treatment of complete tears of the rotator cuff. In: Tagishi S, ed. *The shoulder*. Tokyo: Professional Postgraduate Services, 1987:241.
175. Takagishi N. Conservative treatment of ruptures of the rotator cuff. *J Jpn Orthop Assoc* 1978;52:781–787.
176. Tauro JC, Campolattaro R. Arthroscopic rotator cuff repair: 2 to 3 year follow-up. *Arthroscopy* 1997;13:398.
177. Uhthoff HK, Sano H. Pathology of failure of the rotator cuff tendon. *Orthop Clin North Am* 1997;28:31–42.
178. Walch G, Boileau P, Noel E, Donell ST. Impingement of the deep surface of the supraspinatus tendon on the posterosuperior glenoid rim: an arthroscopic study. *J Shoulder Elbow Surg* 1992;1:238–245.
179. Warren RF. Surgical considerations of rotator cuff tears in athletes. In: Jackson DW, ed. *Shoulder surgery in the athlete*. Rockville, MD: Aspen, 1985:73–82.
180. Watson M. Major ruptures of the rotator cuff. The results of surgical repair in 89 patients. *J Bone Joint Surg [Br]* 1985;67:618–624.
181. Watson-Jones R. *Fractures and joint injuries*, 5th ed. vol 2. London: Churchill Livingstone, 1976:524–527.
182. Weber SC. Arthroscopic debridement and acromioplasty versus mini-open repair in the management of significant partial-thickness tears of the rotator cuff. *Orthop Clin North Am* 1997;28:79–82.
183. Weber SC. All arthroscopic verus mini open repair in the management of complete tears of the rotator cuff. *Arthroscopy* 1997;13:368.
184. Weiner DS, Macnab I. Superior migration of the humeral head. *J Bone Joint Surg [Br]* 1979;52:524–527.
185. Wiley AM. Superior humeral dislocation: a complication following decompression and debridement for rotator cuff tears. *Clin Orthop* 1991;263:135–141.
186. Wilson PD. Complete rupture of the supraspinatus tendon. *JAMA* 1931;96:433–438.
187. Wirth MA, Basamania C, Rockwood CA Jr. Nonoperative management of full-thickness tears of the rotator cuff. *Orthop Clin North Am* 1997:28:59–68.
188. Wolfgang GL. Surgical repair of tears of the rotator cuff of the shoulder: factors influencing the result. *J Bone Joint Surg [Am]* 1974;56: 14–26.
189. Yamaguchi K, Flatow EL. Arthroscopic evaluation and treatment of the rotator cuff. *Orthop Clin North Am* 1995;26:643–659.
190. Zvijac JE, Levy HJ, Lemak LJ. Arthroscopic subacromial decompression in the treatment of full-thickness rotator cuff tears. A 3- to 6-year follow-up. *Arthroscopy* 1994;10:518–523.

Disorders of the Shoulder: Diagnosis and Management,
edited by Joseph P. Iannotti and Gerald R. Williams, Jr.
Lippincott Williams & Wilkins, Philadelphia © 1999.

CHAPTER 3

Massive Rotator Cuff Tears

Christian Gerber

The rotator cuff undergoes progressive degenerative changes during aging. This natural process results in weakening and in a remarkable prevalence of structural failure of the cuff's tendons with increasing age.[38,98,115,119,131,151] Necropsy studies on cadavers with a known or unknown prior history of shoulder pain, as well as imaging studies in asymptomatic individuals, document that not only the prevalence of tears, but also their size increase with age.[20,38,119]

The high prevalence of what are often small rotator cuff tendon tears in elderly patients who are beyond the age of retirement is frequently not associated with relevant dysfunction despite the undeniable structural lesion. Conversely, younger asymptomatic persons have structurally intact rotator cuff tendons. The large or "massive" tears are not observed in asymptomatic patients of working age: One ultrasound study[98] did not document any complete full-thickness tear in those younger than 50 years, and another magnetic resonance imaging (MRI) study documented an incidence of only 4% for full-thickness rotator cuff tears in asymptomatic persons younger than the age of 60 years.[131] Tears involving two or more tendons are associated with weakness and may be associated with incapacitating, chronic pain and severe functional impairment that is resistant to conservative treatment.[26,31,34,117,136,143] Unfortunately, not all these patients are amenable to successful surgical treatment and there is a need to distinguish between cases in whom surgical treatment will be truly beneficial and those for whom nonsurgical treatment, including possibly skillful neglect, would be a better treatment option.

To be successful, conservative or surgical treatment must improve the disability of the patient, which consists of pain, dysfunction, very rarely, deformity, or some combination thereof. Pain and dysfunction can be treated only indirectly by addressing the diseased anatomic structures presumably responsible for the actual disability. Whereas we have become very successful in identifying structural pathology, our knowledge concerning the precise role of the structural lesion responsible for the disability of the patient is often less reliably defined. In addition, there is uncertainty in predicting the reparability of a given structural abnormality by a given surgeon. Moreover, after repair, the functional outcome and satisfaction of the patient may not correlate with the structural result. Decision making, therefore, remains difficult, and a personal approach, as presented here, is admittedly based not only on established facts, but also heavily on personal experience.

ETIOLOGICAL FACTORS FOR ROTATOR CUFF TEARS

As early as 1931 Codman and Akerson[29] considered the following as the potential causes for rotator cuff tears:

- Trauma
- Defects after calcification
- Attritional lesions
- Necrosis (or another intrinsic pathological process)

These are still the most discussed hypotheses for the etiology of this condition, except for calcific deposits, which are

C. Gerber: Department of Orthopaedics, University of Zürich, 8008 Zürich, Switzerland.

no longer considered a relevant cause and thus will be discussed relative to their particular role in massive tears.

The rotator cuff of a young person can withstand very high forces[123], and trauma must be of extraordinary magnitude to cause a massive rupture of a healthy, young cuff. I have observed only one single case, in a 19-year-old patient involved in a car crash (Fig. 1), in whom the entire cuff was avulsed from the lesser and the greater tuberosity. The entire proximal humerus was denuded and the entire "hoodlike" cuff was interposed into the joint space. The axillary nerve was ruptured. The rotator cuff could be repaired, the axillary nerve was left alone. Interestingly enough, the humeral head went on to develop complete avascular necrosis. In the presence of complete deltoid wasting, avascular necrosis, and a poorly functioning cuff, the shoulder was fused.

Trauma is very *rarely the sole etiologic factor*, it very frequently precipitates the development of *symptoms* of rotator cuff deficiency. Asymptomatic partial or complete full-thickness rotator cuff tears may be traumatically enlarged by minor or major trauma, and this enlargement may transform a well-functioning, almost asymptomatic shoulder into a completely dysfunctional arm that is incompatible with manual work. Preexisting cuff pathology is an important consideration in "acute" rotator cuff tears and may significantly affect treatment plans in any patient older than 40 years. Traumatic shoulder dislocation sustained at an age older than 40 is a typical injury that may lead to rupture of a previously weak, but continent, or a previously ruptured rotator cuff.[70] In such a situation, a conventional, true (central beam parallel to the joint line) anteroposterior x-ray film of the shoulder, taken with the arm in neutral rotation, is the mandatory minimal diagnostic imaging modality. It serves to verify whether there is already static superior subluxation of the humeral head, with an acromiohumeral distance of less then 7 mm.[35,90,141,146] If this is true, a massive rotator cuff tear must have been present before the current injury, and the possibilities of successful repair are severely compromised: indeed, repair may be impossible (Fig. 2). If the acromiohumeral distance is more than 7 mm and a rotator cuff tear is proved, it can be assumed that the traumatic event has caused or enlarged a mechanically compensated rupture of the rotator cuff and repair may be achieved. Relevant trauma may injure not only the rotator cuff, but also other structures, such as the axillary nerve, and thereby dramatically worsen the prognosis.[65]

Most tears develop progressively. *Impingement* of the bursa and the tendinous units against the undersurface of the acromion[4,13,14,95,57,105,110] or against the posterosuperior glenoid rim[88,139] are often thought to be the most important reasons for development of large rotator cuff tears. *Subacromial* impingement has been considered to be of particular relevance, and the changes observed at the undersurface of the acromion have prompted Neer to recommend routine subacromial decompression for symptomatic cuff disease.[105] Convinced that "95% of the rotator cuff tears are caused by subacromial impingement,"[106] he advocated acromioplasty not only to relieve pain, but also because he believed that this would mostly eliminate the single most important etiologic factor for the development of tears of the rotator cuff.

This attritional hypothesis[59,95,96,105,106] and others has always remained in conflict with the concept that rotator cuff tearing was a result of age-related, *degenerative changes* in the rotator cuff.[20,29,28,38,86,88,115,138,149] Despite the common belief that impingement is responsible for vitually all rotator cuff tears, very few experimental studies have substantiated this hypothesis. A recent study from our laboratory has attempted to clarify this aspect.[129] In a rat model, we took one or two platelike autogenous bone grafts from the scapular spine of the rat. The undersurface of the anterior acromion was then modified by passing a suture through the acromion, or by fixing one or two plates to the undersurface of the acromion, such that an iatrogenic, controlled impingement of the infraspinatus tendon was created. Whereas rats with a sham operation or treated with only a suture did not show any evidence of infraspinatus tendon degeneration (Fig. 3A), the animals treated with one or with two plates showed distinct lesions of the tendon. All lesions were on the bursal side, showed clear-cut attritional changes, without any abnormalities on the articular side of the tendon (see Fig. 3B). The bursal side tears were deeper and larger if two plates were used than when one plate was used, and the tears increased in depth and width with increasing duration of the iatrogenic impingement. Our experimental data, therefore, support the concept that the most commonly seen changes, such as undersurface tears and intratendinous lamination, cannot be attributed to primary attrition under the acromion, and that the commonly observed attritional changes are explained better as a consequence of a rotator cuff dysfunction than as its cause. These experimental results also support clinical studies which have indicated that impingement is not the primary cause, but rather, it is a consequence of rotator cuff dysfunction.[86,115] The experimental results of Soslowsky et al. also suggest that attrition alone is probably not the cause of those tears that are most commonly seen.[132] Also, degenerative changes are a well-established fact, caused by the particular vascularity of the cuff.[21,102,121,127] These changes are better able to explain the failures of repair than does the impingement concept, because impingement is usually relieved with acromioplasty; hence, recurrent tears should be less frequent than observed clinically.[47,51,67,90,121]

Degenerative changes of the tendon tissue, atrophy of the greater tuberosity,[35,54,58] have been in focus for many years. Chronic rotator cuff tendon tears, however, are also associated with severe degenerative changes of the rotator cuff *muscles*.[59] Whether atrophy and fatty degeneration are caused by the absence of tensile stimuli owing to the tendinous rupture,[15] or whether they are caused by high subacromial[11] or intramuscular pressures compromising the vascularization of the cuff during strenuous use,[77,78] or by yet other unknown mechanisms, is not yet well established. We have recently been able to document that the structural changes in the cuff muscles are associated with profound changes in their mechanical behavior, characterized by in-

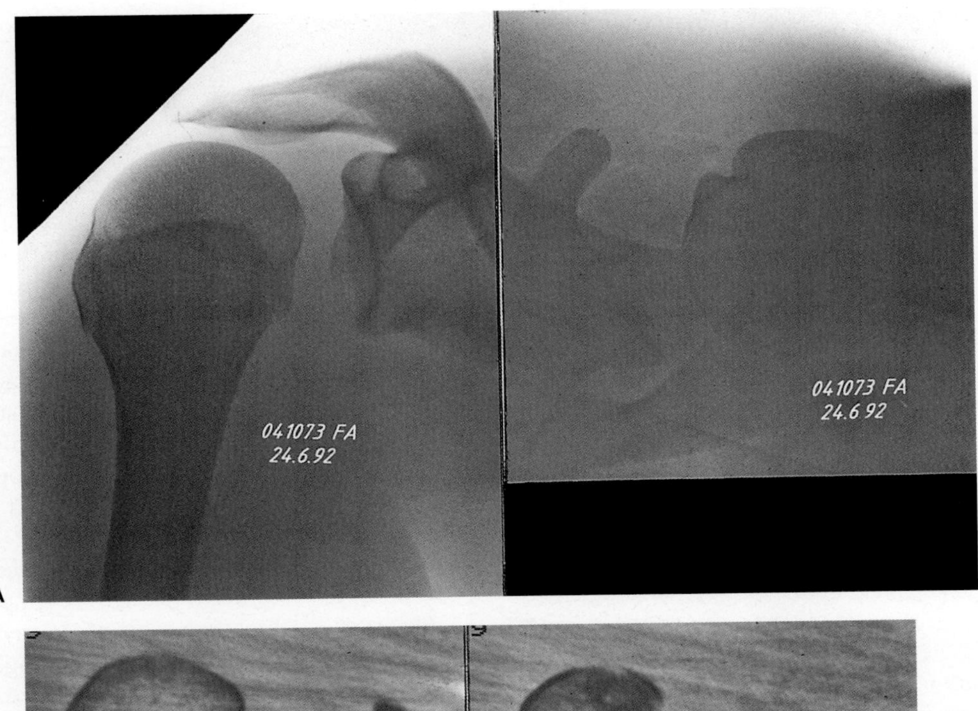

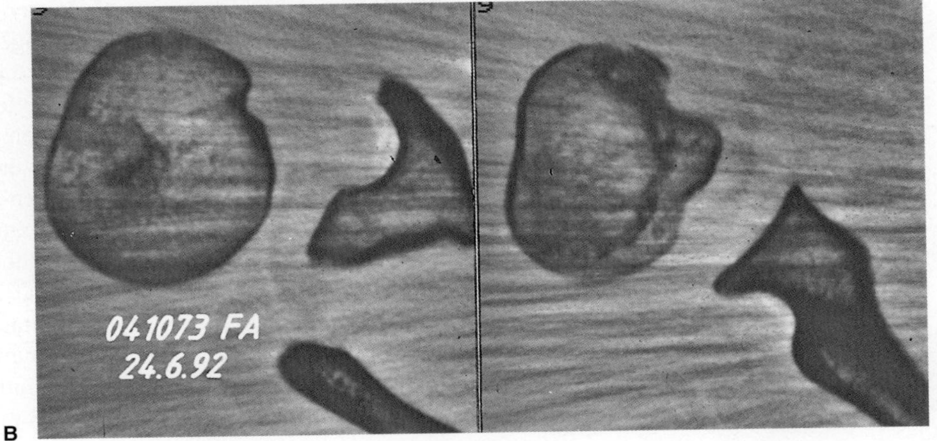

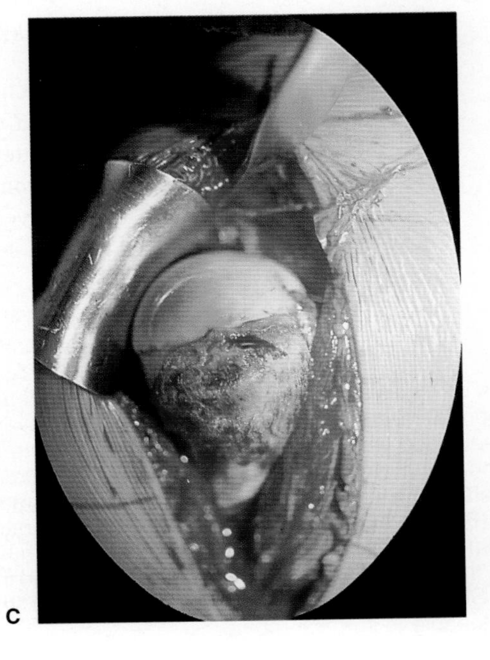

FIG. 1. A severe motor vehicle accident with apparent "shoulder dislocation." **(A)** After "reduction" under anesthesia, there is a large joint line on the conventional x-ray films, as well as on **(B)** the CT scans. The CT scan shows interposed soft tissue. Operative revision through a deltopectoral approach revealed **(C)** complete stripping of the entire cuff from the humeral insertion and interposition of the entire hood (including the biceps tendon) between humeral head and glenoid.

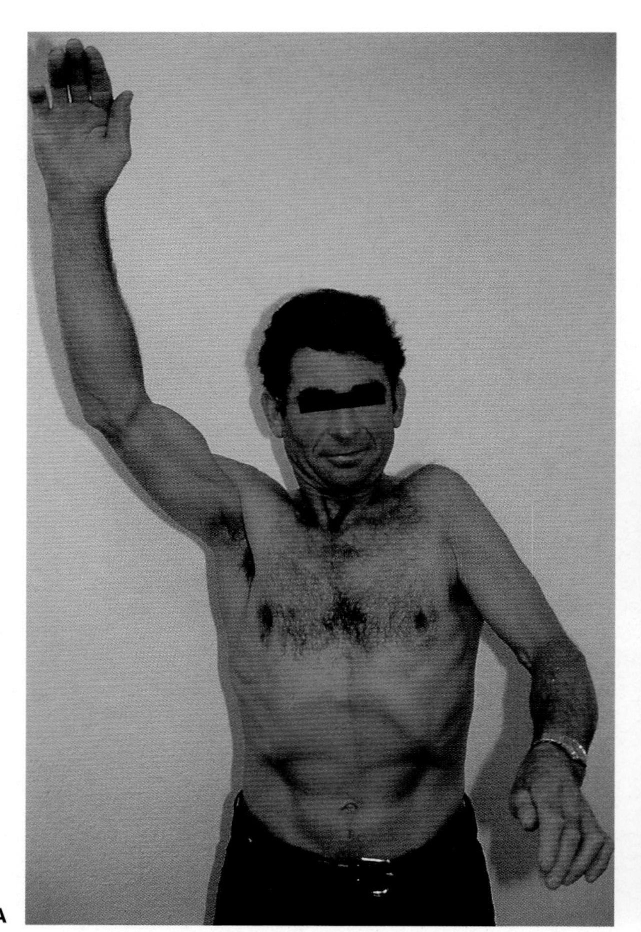

A

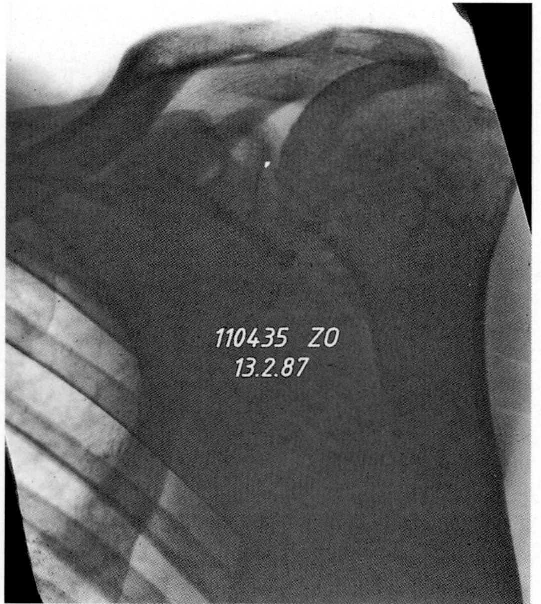

C

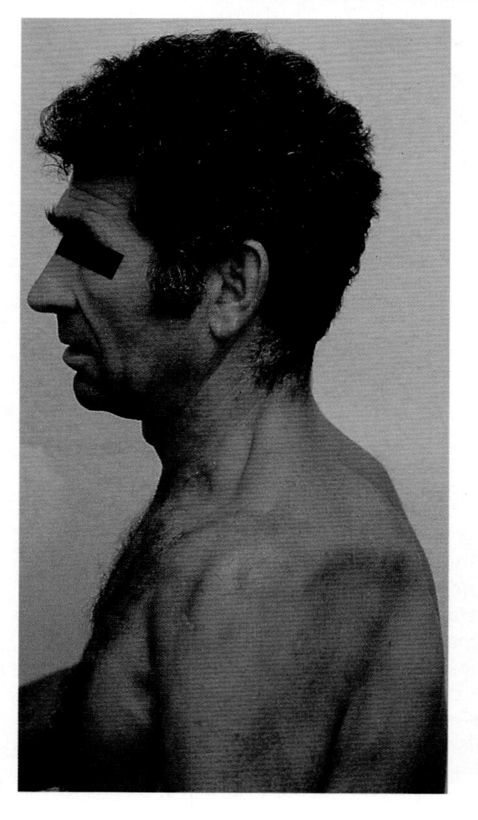

B

FIG. 2. A 52-two-year old mason: He had an anterior shoulder stabilization 20 years ago and was without any relevant problems until 2 weeks ago when he sustained a traumatic anterior shoulder dislocation. At examination he showed **(A)** a pain-free "pseudoparalysis," with elevation to 30 degrees and abduction to 30 degrees. **(B)** Conventional x-ray films show an obliterated acromiohumeral space, with a statically cranially displaced humeral head. Clinically, there is **(C)** severe wasting of the supra- and infraspinatus muscles. Such tears are not to be considered acute tears and will not be amenable to surgical repair.

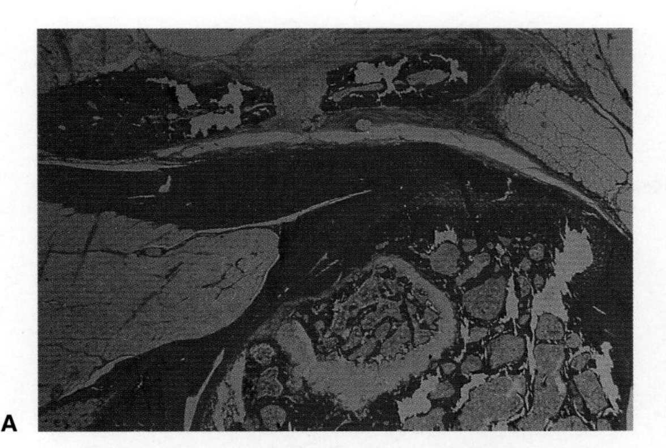

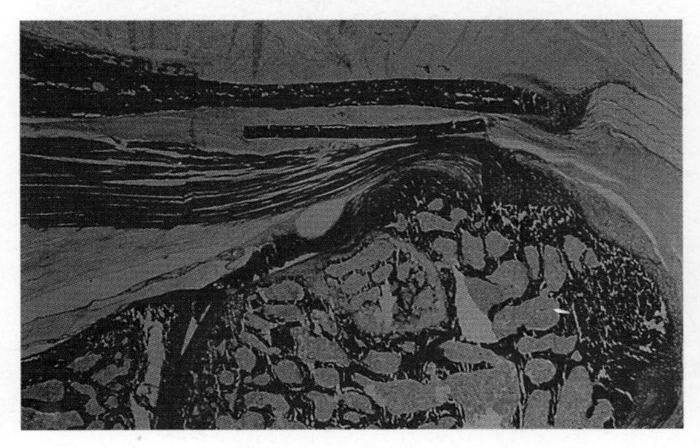

FIG. 3. Histological section through the frontal plane of a normal shoulder of a rat: The infraspinatus tendon (as opposed to the supraspinatus in the human) passes freely underneath the acromion. **(A)** The muscuotendinous unit is intact, as shown by a frontal histologic section through a normal rat shoulder. After fixation of a thin bone plate underneath the acromion **(B)** there are marked attritional changes on the bursal side of the infraspinatus tendon, but there is no change on the articular side of the joint. This experimental impingement study of Schneeberger et al.[129] could not reproduce the most frequent type of tear seen in the human, which does involve the articular side of the joint.

creased passive tension during tensile loading, thus creating a pathologic stress–strain behavior that compromises the stability and healing of tendon-to-bone repairs.[71]

These observations are of utmost importance for our personally preferred treatment concepts: Because we do not believe that impingement on the undersurface of the acromion is a primary reason for rotator cuff tears, an acromioplasty is not considered to be a mandatory part of the surgical treatment and most frequently is not carried out. The degenerative nature of the pathology is heavily weighed in our decision-making process: Watson[145] has documented that the mechanical properties of the tendinous stumps of the rotator cuff are often poor in the clinical situation. In our own sheep experiments,[55] we have observed that a ruptured tendon undergoes

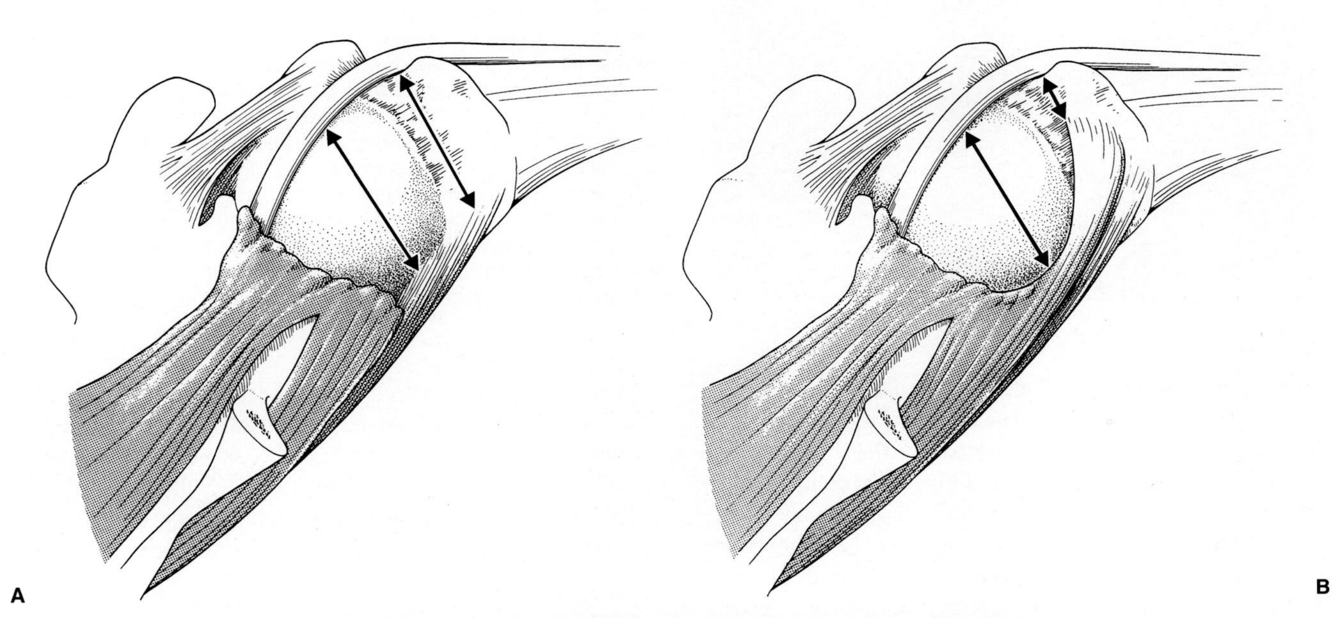

FIG. 4. If the rotator cuff size is measured in centimeters, this should be done by measuring the distance of disinsertion of the cuff tendons from their insertion at the greater and lesser tuberosity. This will also document **(A)** that two tendons are torn. If the size of the tear is measured on top of the head, a relatively small tear **(B)** can be mistaken for a massive tear owing to buttonholing of the proximal humerus through the defect.

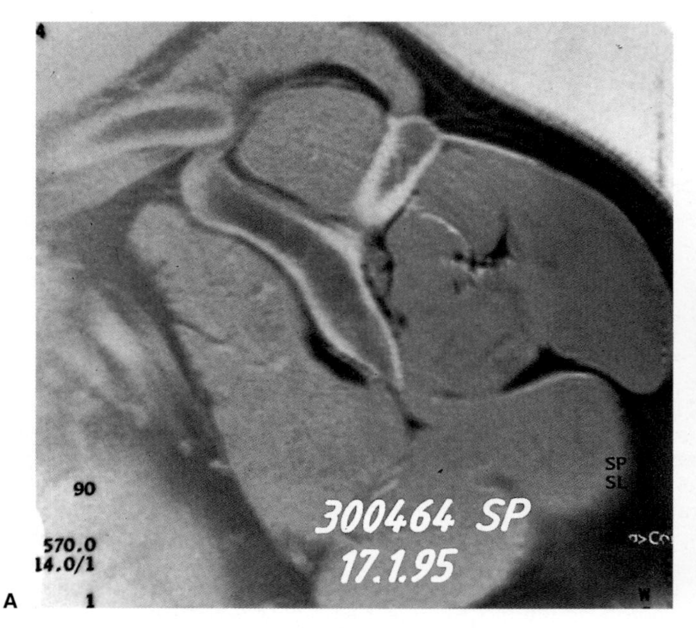

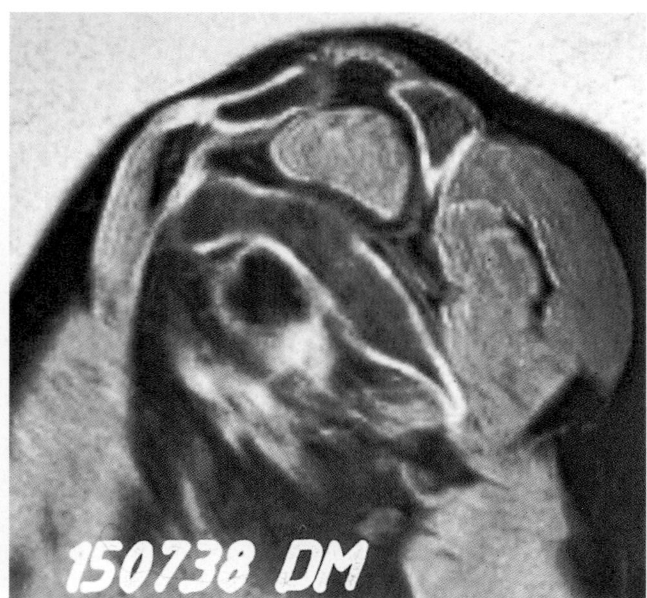

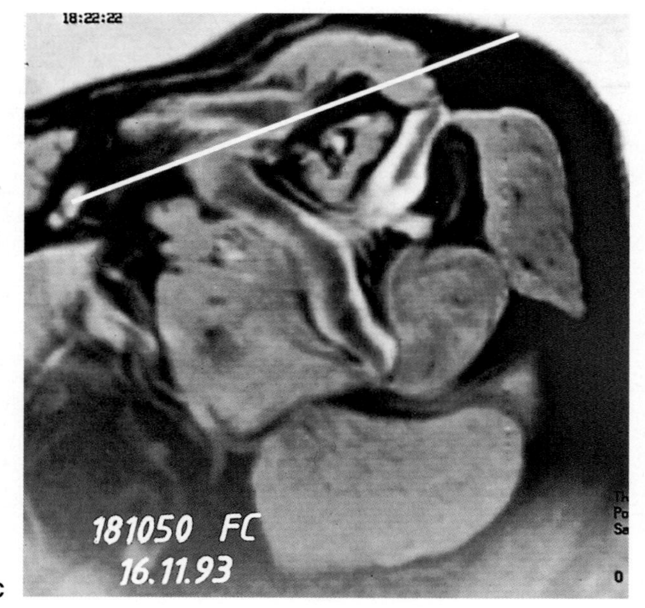

FIG. 5. Magnetic resonance images parallel to the glenoid plane through the base of the coracoid. **(A)** The subscapularis, supraspinatus, infraspinatus, and teres minor (the two latter muscle bellies can sometimes not be distinguished with certainty on MRI) are homogeneous, convex, and voluminous in a normal rotator cuff. **(B)** In an isolated tear of the subscapularis, the subscapularis muscle has virtually disappeared, the subscapularis fossa is filled with fat, scar, and some minimal remaining muscle tissue, whereas the supra- and infraspinatus exhibit normal signals and are of normal volume. **(C)** In a massive posterolateral tear, the subscapularis is normal, but the supraspinatus shows fatty infiltration and atrophy. If a line is drawn (a,b) from the top of the scapular spine to the highest point of the coracoid, this tangent line goes through the supraspinatus muscle in the absence of atrophy. In severe atrophy this tangent sign is positive and indicates atrophy of the supraspinatus in its body. The infraspinatus is virtually replaced by fat, whereas the teres minor is hypertrophic.

a myxoid degeneration, becomes hard and brittle, and at first sight it appears strong but, unable to resist pullout of a suture on repetitive loading. Histologically, the degenerative changes are of variable degree and may be accompanied by reparative processes coming especially from the bursa. Because of the poor mechanical properties of the degenerated tendon, the cuff edges are resected generously until good, solid tendon material, without any myxoid changes, can be safely grasped with strong sutures. To deal with the mechanical changes of the muscle, the arm is protected in an abduction splint, even though the advantage of this aftercare is not scientifically established. Because the muscle is the only strength-generating organ and because preliminary data suggest that the muscular changes are irreversible, we try to repair the rotator cuff tears before the advent of severe muscular changes in patients who need a strong shoulder, and if such changes have been established, musculotendinous transfers are used to dynamically augment repairs.[56]

DEFINITION OF "MASSIVE" ROTATOR CUFF TEARS

There is no agreement on the definition of a *massive* rotator cuff tear, but in North America, Cofield's [31] definition of such as a tear that is larger than 5 cm in maximal diameter, is generally used. The diameter of the tear is not the only and

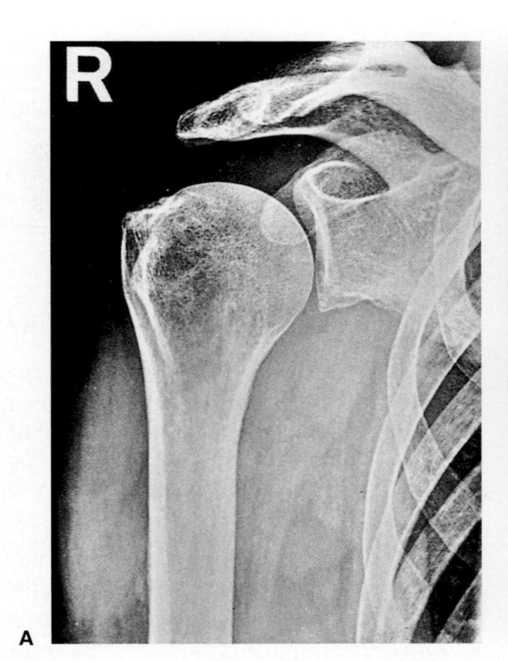

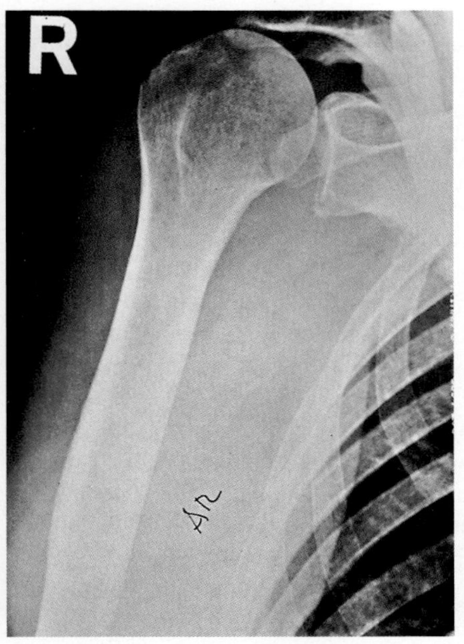

FIG. 6. True anteroposterior radiograph of the right shoulder of a 64-year-old woman, who has sustained a fall and developed a pseudoparalysis. Because she had already previously suffered from chronic shoulder pain, **(A)** a conservative treatment program was started. At 7 months, the patient continues to be unable to lift her arm, the head has migrated cranially, the acromiohumeral distance is 1 mm. **(B)** Chances to repair the cuff tear successfully at this point are virtually nil. Note that cranial migration after trauma to a shoulder with a prior cuff problem can occur very rapidly.

possibly not the best indication of the size, because there is a wide variation in the height and size of the patient, and most reports rarely state whether the size of the tear has been measured before or after resection of nonviable edges of the tendinous stump. In addition, if the humerus is pushed cranially, the diameter of the tear increases, and it decreases if the head is pulled distally (Fig. 4). The most appropriate variable to define the size of a tear is the amount of tendinous disinsertion.[117,118] Therefore, we define rotator cuff tears as massive, *if they involve a disinsertion of at least two complete tendons.* Most of these tears involve the supra- and the infraspinatus, but anterosuperior tears involving the supraspinatus and subscapularis exist in surprising frequency.[51,113,117] Most massive and all irreparable tears have a high degree of chronic degenerative changes and are, thereby, associated with two phenomena that are of crucial importance in defining the type of massive tear:

1. There are the previously discussed fatty degeneration and atrophy that may render repair of doubtful value (Fig. 5).
2. There is progressive cranial migration of the humeral head: Normally the humeral head is centered within the glenoid, and this fact is most readily represented by an acromiohumeral distance of 7 mm or more, as measured on an anteroposterior x-ray film with the arm in neutral rotation. An acromiohumeral distance of less than 7 mm is pathologic and indicates static proximal humeral migration (Fig. 6). If the head has migrated proximally, repair is very unlikely to be successful.[40,90,141,146]

Massive rotator cuff tears may or may not be reparable. We have defined tears as *irreparable*, if at least two tendons are disinserted and, if despite all attempts at mobilization—including release of the coracohumeral ligament, differential slide (release between supraspinatus and infraspinatus to the level of the glenoid, release between supraspinatus and subscapularis to the base of the coracoid), and circumferential capsulotomy—the tendinous stump cannot be brought into a bony trough between the cartilage of the humeral head and the tuberosity with the arm abducted to less than 60 degrees.[56] Such irreparable tears may merit specific considerations.

Massive or irreparable, massive rotator cuff tears are exceedingly rare in the asymptomatic working population,[131,98,119] and contrary to small tears, they do not represent a variant of normal in persons younger than 70 years. In most surgical series, they represent only a relatively small proportion of the observed tears. In Neer's series of 340 rotator cuff tears operated on over a 13-year period, 145 were classified as massive; Bigliani[12] reported on 61 cases treated in a referral center over a 6-year period. Of the 50 cases reported on by Ellman, only 9 (18%) were massive; in Hawkins' series,[69] 27% were massive tears. The definition used was not identical in all studies and the results may not be fully comparable, but the review of the literature shows that even experienced surgeons operate rather rarely on these lesions.

NATURAL HISTORY OF MASSIVE ROTATOR CUFF TEARS

The natural history of rotator cuff tears has not been studied in great detail. Most of our information stems from retrospective studies and may be somewhat biased. Gazielly[46,47] reported that 82% of his patients were satisfied with conservative management of massive rotator cuff tears. Of the 23 patients who were still of working age, 35% had already received a disability pension or had to be retrained at 18 months follow-up. Wallace has reported the fate of 37 workmen with confirmed rotator cuff tears, who were observed for 5 years. At follow-up, 54% were no longer professionally active and 81% had still moderate to intense pain. In Hawkins' series, 42% of the patients were dissatisfied at 3.8 years; and the series of Bokor,[17] which reports 74% satisfactory results at 7.6 years, is severely biased, for all patients who were operated on during the study period were excluded from the follow-up. The studies of Takagishi and of Noël[112,136] unequivocally document that the natural history of a large rotator cuff tear is much less favorable than that for small tears. If the results of arthroscopic cuff debridement for massive rotator cuff tears are taken into consideration,[41,155] the functional prognosis of nonrepaired, massive rotator cuff tears is not favorable. Although pain seems to remain a manageable problem in mid- to long-term, function deteriorates and is not compatible with manual labor. These data clearly suggest that the spontaneous outcome of the massive rotator cuff tear in young individuals who wish or need to use their arms with the elbow away from their side is not satisfactory, whereas it may be satisfactory for elderly patients who suffer solely from pain and have very little functional demands on their arms.

Diagnostic Considerations

It is not the purpose of this chapter to review the methods of diagnosis of rotator cuff tears. Suffice to say that the diagnosis of massive rotator cuff tears must prove the simultaneous, complete rupture of at least two tendons and, because the supraspinatus is torn in every massive tear, it has to focus on the diagnosis of infraspinatus (teres minor) and subscapularis tears. The assessment includes clinical evaluation and imaging studies. An important external rotation lag sign[72] and severe weakness for external rotation with the arm adducted document infraspinatus failure; weakness for external rotation with the arm in abduction suggests teres minor failure; weakness in abduction points to supraspinatus insufficiency;[72,79] and an abnormal lift-off or belly press test[50] proves subscapularis deficiency. A rupture of the tendon of the long head of the biceps may be diagnosed with the bulging biceps; however, this clinical finding may often be missing in elderly patients. Our preference is first for thorough analysis of conventional x-ray films,[18,35,58] then imaging with MRI or arthro-MRI[42,57,103,131] because this is the modality that most precisely allows one to assess the size of the rupture and the degree of atrophy and retraction of the musculature. Computed tomography (CT) scans are an alternative, especially if the interest is focused on fatty degeneration of the muscle.[59,61] Ultrasonographic evaluation is a less costly alternative.[97] If rupture of more than two complete tendons and significant atrophy of at least two muscle bellies are documented, the diagnosis of a massive tear is established.

TABLE 1. *Physiological cross-sectional areas for rotator cuff muscles (in % of total cuff)*

Muscle	Bassett[9]	Keating[82]	Herzberg[73a]
Subscapularis	46	52	51
Supraspinatus	16	15	16
Infraspinatus	38	33	33

PATHOMECHANICAL CONSIDERATIONS

The role of the rotator cuff muscles and of the deltoid have been studied clinically and experimentally in great detail.[22,33,57,73,76,82,91] The force potential of each of the rotator cuff muscles can be determined on the basis of their physiologic cross-sectional areas (PCSA).[73,82] The leverage can be determined from the length of a perpendicular line drawn from its line of action to the center of the joint's rotation.[9,10,19] Each muscle's force potential multiplied by its leverage determines its functional contribution (Tables 1 and 2). The supraspinatus muscle is relatively weak, and its relative contribution decreases with increasing abduction. The amplitude during simple plane abduction is less than half the amplitude available and is small compared with the tendon excursion of the deltoid;[49] hence, the cuff muscles act mostly as stabilizers during simple scapular plane abduction. Yet they have much larger amplitudes, necessary for more complex movements (Table 3). Clinical[23,124] and experimental data show that the shoulder may remain well compensated even though there is a structural lesion in the rotator cuff tendons. Extension posteriorly may favor cranial migration,[140,141] and extension anteriorly may favor loss of elevation and possibly allow anterosuperior subluxation.[23,48,113] That small tears may be associated with poor function and larger tears with relatively good function is certainly relative to the balance of the forces,[23,24,25] but still remains a puzzling theoretical problem and an irritating clinical fact.

TREATMENT OF MASSIVE ROTATOR CUFF TEARS

The Search for the Most Appropriate Treatment

If a patient with a documented tear involving at least two complete tendons is symptomatic enough to ask for treatment, it is the level of functional demands that determines the hierarchy of the preferred treatment options.

TABLE 2. *Rotational potential of rotator cuff (percentage)*

Muscle	Bassett[9] arm 90 abd + 90 er[a]	Keating[82] arm at side[a]
Subscapularis	42 (2.8 cm)	52 (2.3 cm)
Supraspinatus	13 (2.1 cm)	14 (2.0 cm)
Infraspinatus + teres minor	45 (3.1 cm)	32 (2.2 cm)

[a] Numbers in parentheses are average movement of the arms.

TABLE 3. *Tendon excursion and amplitude of the rotator cuff muscles*

Muscle	Amplitude of the rotator cuff muscles (cm)[9]	Tendon excursion during scapular plane abduction (cm)[73]
Subscapularis	7.3	0.4
Supraspinatus	6.7	3.8
Infraspinatus	8.6	3.5
Deltoid		6.5

Low Functional Demands

Functional demand heavily depends on age, gender, occupation, and handedness. It is considered low if a patient uses his or her arm almost exclusively with the elbow at the side and if he or she can easily compensate for the dysfunction with the opposite arm. The regular use of the arm at shoulder level or higher that cannot be compensated for by the opposite arm, or the presence of a symptomatic bilateral cuff tear, implies high demands on cuff function.

Even in low functional demand situations there are different scenarios:

If a patient with low functional demands has had an asymtomatic, strong shoulder and sustains a trauma with a pseudoparalysis, we inject 10 mL of 1% lidocaine into the subacromial (per definition also intraarticularly) space, with all precautions to avoid iatrogenic infection. If, with local anesthesia, the patient can hold his or her arm at 90 degrees of abduction, we will continue with conservative management, for the chances for functional recovery are still reasonably favorable.[22] If the pseudoparalysis persists, despite subacromial injection of local anesthetic,[22] we favor immediate surgical repair if there is not enormous wasting in the supraspinatus and infraspinatus fossa and if conventional x-ray films show an acromiohumeral distance of 7 mm or more. The recovery of active elevation seems to depend on the length of time during which the inability to lift the arm has been present.[10]

If a patient with low functional demands and a massive rotator cuff tear has gradually developed a pseudoparalysis with tolerable pain, wasting is pronounced, and the acromiohumeral distance is less than 7 mm, we feel that skillful neglect, with occasional intermittent physical therapy is generally the most advisable form of treatment. In the rare instances when a patient exhibits a mixture of pain and a desire to have some forward elevation, we have been using a constrained prosthesis.[62] This has not been used in patients with higher functional demands or in younger patients.

If a patient with low functional demands has a massive cuff tear with significant pain, there is usually no need for rapid surgical intervention because there is no proof that pain can be surgically managed any better in the early rather than in the late course of the disease. Conservative treatment, which may include one-time subacromial (intraarticular) injection of steroids, is the first step. Self-administered home programs of stretching are added. If this treatment fails, arthroscopic evaluation is considered. If the long head of the biceps is still present, a biceps tenotomy is performed, followed by a bursectomy and minimal trimming of the edges of the rotator cuff. Whereas we routinely debride inflamed parabursal tissues, we do not routinely perform an acromioplasty. If the patient has pain radiating into the neck and is tender over the acromioclavicular joint, a resection of the acromioclavicular joint, with debridement of inferior surface spurs, is added.

High Functional Demands

Laborers and persons who need or wish to use their affected arm higher than shoulder level are considered to have high demands on their shoulder.

If a young patient with high functional demands has had an asymptomatic, strong shoulder and sustains a trauma with a relevant rotator cuff tear, we advocate surgical repair as soon as the shoulder has free passive mobility. Because irreversible atrophy will develop, a shoulder with a large rotator cuff tear is unlikely to be compatible with heavy work[143] and because the functional results of repairs of traumatic rotator cuff tears are better if surgery is performed within 6 weeks of injury,[10] we prefer to proceed with surgery as soon as convenient, and all our experimental and clinical data suggest that an attempt at conservative treatment in this particular group of patients is unwise.[50,51,55,71] Primary repair is almost invariably possible in these circumstances. Should primary repair be impossible, we would proceed with partial repair to obtain coverage of the equator and augment this repair with the most appropriate musculotendinous transfer.

If a young patient with high functional demands and a massive rotator cuff tear has gradually developed a pseudoparalysis with tolerable pain, a careful analysis of the extent of the structural damage is mandatory. A complete drop or external rotation lag sign,[72] with a passive external rotation lag of 30 degrees or more is a definitive sign for a complete, probably irrecoverable, absence of infraspinatus (and supraspinatus) function. Because a severe functional deficit of the infraspinatus caused by a rotator cuff tear is basically never observed without rupture of the supraspinatus, a severe external rotation lag sign[72] defines a massive rotator cuff tear and implies important weakness in abduction: If the biceps is intact and the result of lift-off test[50,53,64] is negative, we proceed with direct repair if the acromiohumeral distance is 7 mm or more and if, on an MRI scan, the musculature seems still adequate. In the more likely situation of significant fatty degeneration and atrophy, we will proceed with an attempt at repair, followed by latissimus dorsi transfer.[48,56] If the acromiohumeral distance is less than 5 mm, an attempt at direct repair is worthless. Under these conditions, we will consider equatorial (partial) repair plus latissimus dorsi transfer for restoration of external rotation, but without the hope of regaining significant overhead strength. Whereas constrained prostheses are currently not considered for young patients with high functional demands and severe disability, arthrodesis remains an option, and it should be remembered that fusion is compatible with manual labor in many professions.

If, in addition to supraspinatus and infraspinatus deficiency, there is also a subscapularis lesion identified by a positive lift-off test, arthro-CT or MRI is mandatory to determine the state of the subscapularis.

- If the subscapularis is torn and shows fatty degeneration or atrophy, functional restoration using direct repair is extremely likely to fail and would be carried out only under very special circumstances involving an unusually motivated patient.
- If the biceps is still intact, the subscapularis is partially torn, but of good volume and signal quality, repair of the subscapularis, including an attempt at repair of the supra- and infraspinatus muscles plus transfer of the latissimus dorsi, are considered. The role of combined transfers (latissimus dorsi for external rotator function and pectoralis major transfer for augmentation of internal rotator function) is not yet established.
- Pseudoparalytic shoulders with global tears and static proximal migration of the humeral head in which pain and functional improvement is looked for at all cost, may lead us to consider hemiarthroplasty,[43,148] constrained total shoulder (but exclusively with the goal to be able to lift the arm and not to use it to do heavy work) or shoulder fusion.
- In the situation with chronic pseudoparalysis and absence of pain, an acromiohumeral distance of less then 7 mm, and severe atrophy of at least two complete muscles, the chances of functional restoration using any reconstructive procedures are minimal. Fortunately this situation is exceedingly rare in very young, manual laborers. Although such a procedure is extremely rarely performed, we continue to feel that for the exceptional, young patient with very high functional demands and complete destruction of the cuff, shoulder fusion should remain a consideration.

If the true demands of a person are safely established and agreed on, the likelihood of achieving the treatment goals with the different modalities of treatment outlined in the following are discussed with the patient, and the decision to proceed with a treatment plan is reached.

Conservative Management

Nonoperative treatment has received more and more attention and has now repeatedly been reported to be successful in a large proportion of patients.[26,36,124,130] Whereas it appears that subacromial injection of triamcinolone is (at least at short-term follow-up) beneficial for incomplete rotator cuff tears,[16] we do not know of any study that has established the superiority of one conservative program over another or over the natural history of the disease. Older studies of Kessel,[83] Patte,[117] and others suggest that posterolateral rotator cuff tears are better tolerated and can be treated by subacromial injection of steroids and different types of physiotherapy. Treatment of anterosuperior lesions involving supra- and subscapularis appear to yield less favorable results, and those tears that are centered over the supraspinatus, and possibly involve the long head of the biceps, often appear to be resistant to conservative management. It is known, however, that shoulder stiffness is often associated with pain and that stiff shoulders do not do well postoperatively. Therefore, it is our practice to rehabilitate all patients with reduced passive range of motion until their external and internal rotation with the arm at the side is normal and pain-free at the extremes of motion. It is not unusual to observe the disappearance of the pain when passive mobility is regained; accordingly, treatment decisions should be taken after restoration of free passive joint motion. If passive mobility is restored in a patient with a large rotator cuff tear who needs or wishes to use his or her arm overhead, we try to determine whether a direct repair is possible or whether other forms of reconstructive surgical treatment are in order. If this is the case, we proceed with surgical reconstruction as soon as the patient is ready and willing to undergo the operation and following rehabilitation. If the tear (very severe atrophy, acromiohumeral distance less than 5 mm) is beyond repair, we continue conservative management, or we plan biceps tenotomy or subacromial decompression. If the patient puts very low functional demands on his or her shoulders and specifically does not need to use the arm above the head level, we proceed with subacromial (which in these patients also means intraarticular) injection of steroids, followed by a self-administered home program of nonaggressive stretching exercises. Formal supervised physical therapy is rarely prescribed, the use of nonsteroidal antiinflammatory drugs is exceptional.

Surgical Options and Their Results

If the natural history of a massive rotator cuff disease is considered to be too unfavorable for a certain individual, the various surgical options must be considered relative to their invasiveness and potential benefit,[8,68] because it is clearly the desire to offer the patient the least invasive procedure to reach his or her treatment goals.

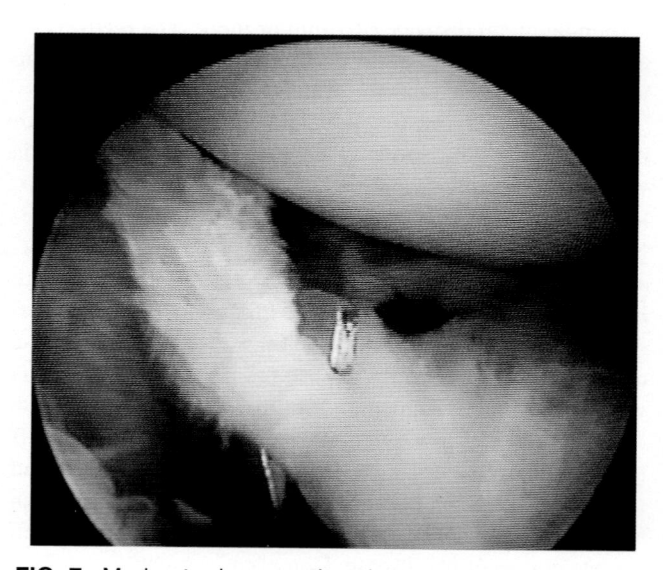

FIG. 7. Moderate degenerative changes of a biceps tendon in the presence of a massive rotator cuff tear in the nondominant shoulder of an elderly woman. The biceps is tenotomized at its origin.

Arthroscopic Treatments

Biceps Tenotomy

In recent years, simple tenotomy of the biceps has become an often discussed procedure in Europe (Fig. 7). Historically, it has been observed that the spontaneous rupture of the tendon of the long head of the biceps can lead to sudden, almost complete relief of pain and to a substantial improvement of function. This observation has prompted Walch and coworkers to consider that the long head of the biceps could be the major source of pain in patients with chronic massive rotator cuff tears and that its surgical division might reproduce the analgesic result of a spontaneous rupture.

Biomechanically the role of the biceps tendon is debated. It probably does not play a major role as a head depressor in the healthy shoulder. If the tendon is dislocated out of its groove, however, it acts similarly to the short head of the biceps, and its contraction will cause an upward thrust of the humeral head. Therefore, tenotomy of a dislocated biceps abolishes a force that is creating possibly painful impingement. Arthroscopic tenotomy of the tendon of the long head of the biceps in massive rotator cuff tears has been reported by Walch in a series of 86 rotator cuff tears treated. A tenotomy without any additional procedure was performed in 54 patients, an acromioplasty was associated in another 32 patients. The distal stump was left to retraction and was never tenodesed. At an average follow-up of 48 months, the results were excellent in 9%, satisfactory in 43%, fair in 36%, and poor in 11%. The relative constant score rose from 62% of an age- and sex-matched normal shoulder to 83% of an age- and sex-matched shoulder: 85% of the patients were very satisfied and only 2.4% were dissatisfied. Although the overall results became less favorable with increasing size of the rupture, the relative constant score remained at a level of 77% for ruptures involving all three tendons. Acromioplasty did not significantly affect the results, and the patients with additional acromioplasty did not fare better than those without acromioplasty. The author observed that the acromiohumeral distance decreased by 4 years after surgery, but this cranial migration of the humeral head was not compared with the natural history and may statistically still be within the natural evolution of the disease. Although these results of biceps tenotomy are not yet confirmed by multiple authors, the results reported by Walch, as well as the much smaller experience in our center, are favorable in a short- to midterm follow-up. We have observed slightly less complete pain relief after biceps tenotomy alone, but in patients who have an irreparable lesion and suffer from significant pain, biceps tenotomy may be a very valuable, minimally invasive, palliative procedure that requires minimal rehabilitation (Fig. 8). Although it is considered unwise by some authors, this procedure indeed either accelerates the natural history, which is very often characterized by a relatively pain-free shoulder as soon as the humeral head has migrated far enough proximally to have reached a stable situation under the acromion, or it treats a mechanically unfavorable situation (dislocated biceps acting as a head raiser) and, therefore, is a logical, minimally invasive procedure. Personal long-term to midterm results clearly document that this procedure can not be generally condemned. There are patients with massive rotator cuff tears who have received very significant benefit from biceps tenotomy, but the detailed role of this procedure remains to be established in larger series of patients.

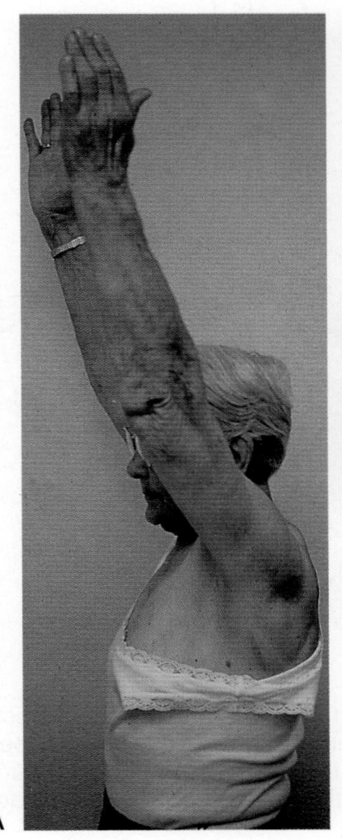

A

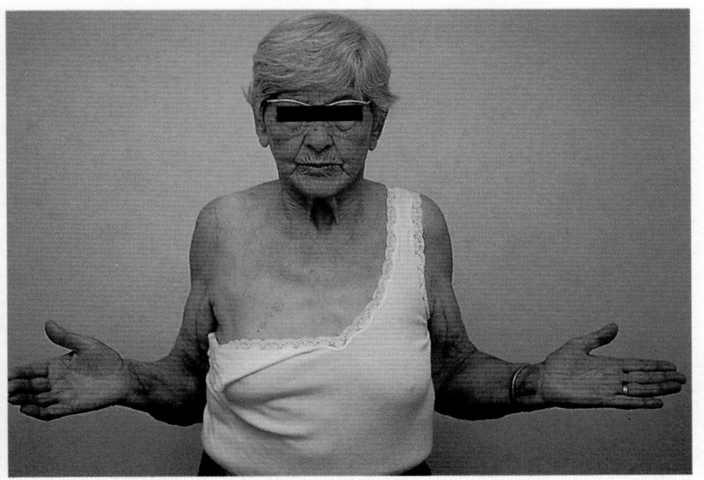

B

FIG. 8. (A,B) An 85-year-old woman with a painful, massive rotator cuff tear treated by biceps tenotomy: Three years after surgery she has sufficient active mobility with moderate weakness, but is pain-free and considers the result as excellent for her needs. The retraction of the lateral head of the biceps is usually not visible at this age.

Subacromial Decompression and Debridement

Open subacromial decompression has been used for many years to provide freedom from pain in shoulders in which repair of rotator cuff tears could not be achieved. Apoil has reported on the concept of the "antero-superior arthrolysis" as early as in 1977.[3] This operation (Fig. 9) consisted of a resection of the coracoacromial ligament, a resection of the hypertrophic edges of the ruptured cuff and a resection of the tendon of the long head of the biceps, a resection of the acromioclavicular joint, and the use of an abduction brace for 6 weeks. Although the results were favorable on short-term follow-up and

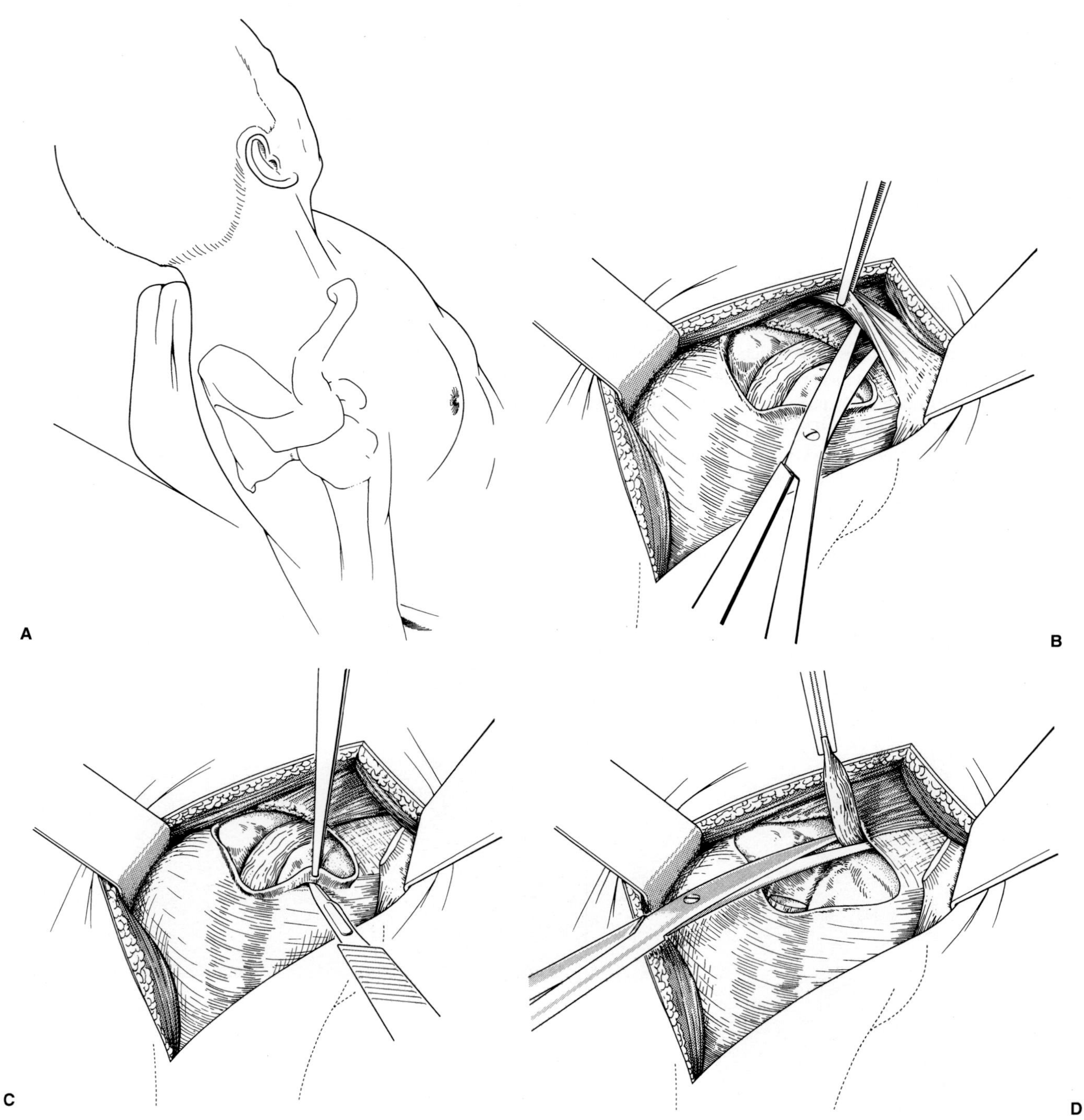

FIG. 9. Rotator cuff debridement according to Apoil and Dautry: After **(A)** a deltoid splitting approach, the operation consisted of **(B)** a resection of the coracoacromial ligament, **(C)** a resection of the hypertrophic edges of the ruptured cuff, and **(D)** a resection of the tendon of the long head of the biceps and a resection of the lateral end of the clavicle. Aftercare was performed with the use of an abduction brace for 6 weeks.

remained satisfactory for small tears even at longer follow-up, the long-term results for tears of more than 3 cm were so unsatisfactory that the authors abandoned the procedure for these large tears.[2,3,5,6] Conversely, Rockwood et al.[125,126] reported very satisfactory long-term results with anterior acromioplasty and cuff debridement in large tears mainly performed in elderly patients suffering from pain. These authors were often able to restore the mobility that had been lost owing to pain.

Currently, subacromial decompression is an arthroscopic procedure. Also, anterior acromioplasty, as well as the resection of the bursa and the hypertrophic edges of the cuff, can be performed easily and the adjunct of a resection of the acromioclavicular joint is possible without undue technical problems. The pain relief of subacromial decompression for full-thickness rotator cuff tears is satisfactory, but not more. The larger the tear, the less favorable the results. Proof that subacromial decompression is better than the natural history, treatment with subacromial infiltration, or than biceps tenotomy is lacking. There is proof, however, that subacromial decompression is less effective than open repair of rotator cuff tears. All studies that have compared arthroscopic subacromial decompression with open repair of full-thickness tears have documented the superiority of the repair approach,[41,44,45,63,100,155] and most importantly, the results of subacromial decompression deteriorate with time.[2,6,40,41,45,155] Therefore, it is believed that subacromial decompression is a procedure that should be reserved for either elderly persons with low functional demands or for tears that are unquestionably beyond repair (severe atrophy on MRI, acromiohumeral distance of less than 5 mm). We feel that subacromial decompression has a very limited role in the treatment of massive cuff tears, that it can often be replaced by subacromial injection or biceps tenotomy, and that it is occasionally detrimental; if the anterosuperior arch is compromised, anterosuperior dynamic subluxation, with severe functional disturbance may iatrogenically be caused (Fig. 10).

Open Surgical Management

Although some authors continue to perform rotator cuff debridement using open surgical techniques,[125] we think that this is a procedure that we prefer to perform arthroscopically, with no known substantial disadvantages, but with the advantage of a much smaller chance of violating the origin of the deltoid.[87] Open surgery, therefore, focuses on reconstruction.

Direct Cuff Repair

Direct cuff repair is the procedure of choice if repair is feasible and if the patient needs a strong, functional arm.

The patient is in a semi-sitting position except if a latissimus dorsi transfer is planned. Under these circustances the patient is positioned in the lateral decubitus position. An anterosuperior approach is selected, unless there is a major tear of the subscapularis. In the presence of retracted subscapularis tears we prefer a deltopectoral approach. In the superolateral approach we elevate the lateral deltoid with an osteotome. The anterior deltoid and the coracoacromial ligament are left undisturbed. The lateral 1 cm of the clavicle is resected if the acromioclavicular joint is symptomatic:[120] acromionectomy[4,66,109] has never been considered. A classic anterior acromioplasty[105,106,108] is not routinely added, and it is never performed in anterosuperior tears. We have not seen any negative effect from no longer routinely performing acromioplasty and concur with Watson that acromioplasty may not be mandatory for the postoperative improvement of the patient's symptoms.[145] The musculotendinous units are then mobilized as far as possible. A circumferential capsulotomy[154] is performed between capsule and labrum, the coracohumeral ligament is released, and the individual musculotendinous units are sharply separated from each other to permit an optimal ex-

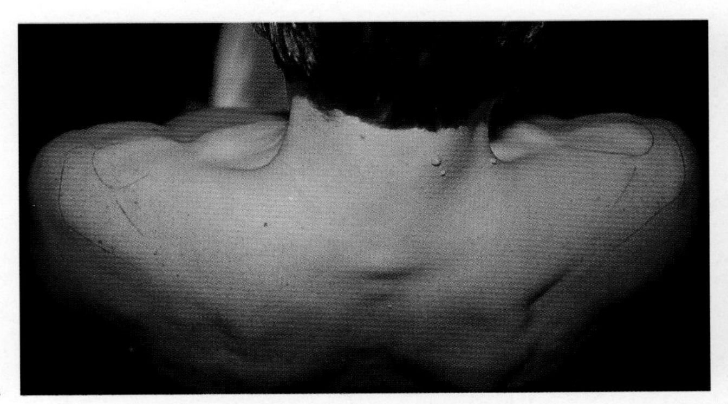

A

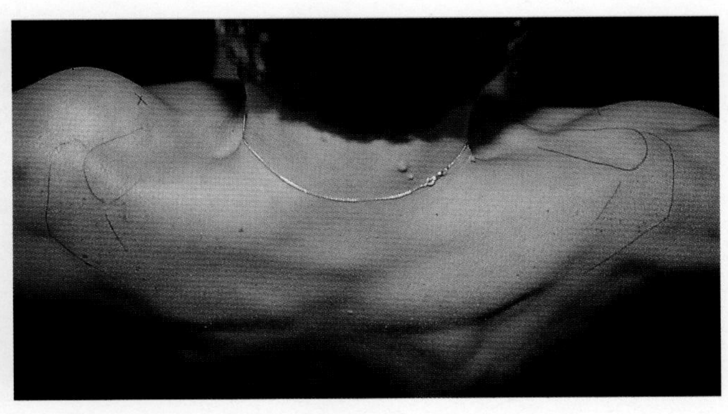

B

FIG. 10. Dynamic anterosuperior subluxation indicates major injury to supraspinatus and subscapularis, which is very difficult to correct surgically. The clinical diagnosis is made if **(A)** the patient has a normal contour of both shoulders at rest and **(B)** subluxates his shoulder anterosuperiorly while resisting abduction. The condition of anterosuperior subluxation can be precipitated by open or arthroscopic subacromial decompression, with release of the coracoacromial ligament. If anterosuperior subluxation becomes static (is also present at rest, as seen clinically or radiologically), successful restoration of overhead elevation by direct surgical repair is exceptional, and subacromial decompression is detrimental.

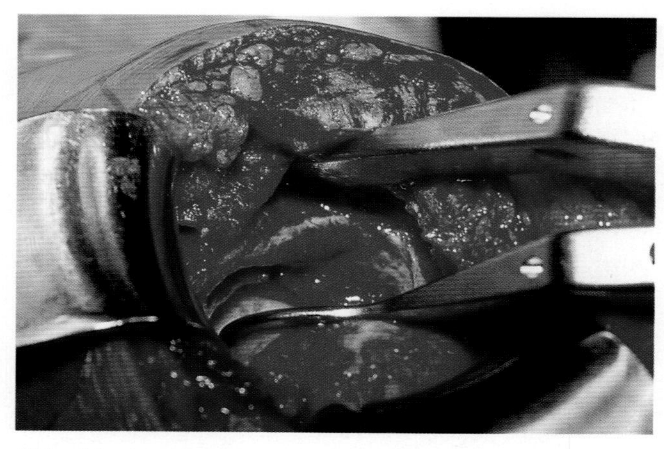

FIG. 11. A subacromial spreader (Sulzer Medica, Winterthur, Switzerland) is in place with its ring on the humeral head and its straight branch on the acromion and distracts the subacromial space. This greatly facilitates identification and mobilization of a retracted rotator cuff tendon.

cursion of each unit. Instruments are not used more than 2 cm medial to the glenoid to avoid injury to the suprascapular nerve.[144] Despite extensive mobilization, we can confirm that iatrogenic lesions of the suprascapular nerve are very rare.[152] The mobilization of the cuff is greatly facilitated by a subacromial spreader that distracts the subacromial space and permits one to work easily on the retracted cuff (Fig. 11). The cuff is mobilized to allow repair to a bony trough with the arm abducted to no more than 30 to 45 degrees. The repair should have a high initial fixation strength, allow minimal gap formation, and maintain mechanical stability until healing has occurred. Repair techniques of direct rotator cuff repair have been discussed on multiple occasions.[7,47,54,55,90,134] After extensive analysis of different methods in vitro,[54] we have concluded the following:

1. Suture failure is likely to occur after repairs of the rotator cuff tendons if sutures thinner than no. 2 or 3 are used.
2. Monofilament sutures (Maxon, PDSII) are very elastic and allow gapping during physiologic tensile loading.
3. Standard tendon-grasping techniques are weak. A modified Mason Allen tendon stitch (Fig. 12) improves suture pullout strength by a factor of at least 2.[54] For cyclic loading this modified tendon-grasping technique is by far superior to any other grasping technique studied.
4. The bone of the greater tuberosity is always osteoporotic in chronic rotator cuff tears, and it becomes the weakest link in the chain. Sutures may pull through the bone and repairs may, therefore, fail. Augmentation of the cortical bone with a buttonlike plate, which does not cut the sutures, augments the strength of the repair significantly.
5. Suture anchors that are reliable in good quality bone do not provide sufficient holding power for sutures in the osteoporotic greater tuberosity (Fig. 13).
6. The use of a no. 3 polyester suture, with the Mason–Allen tendon-grasping technique and a cortical bone augmentation device, improves the mechanical strength of a rotator cuff repair by a factor of at least 2.

The results of the in vitro study have been confirmed in a more recent in vivo experiment in sheep,[55] in which these modified repair techniques demonstrated their superiority in vivo. Because we believe that the repaired cuff is vascularized from the bony trough, which is never deep, but is merely a bony surface cleaned from fibrous tissue, we do not routinely close the bursa to enhance vascularization,[137] but often resect it to provide better visualization.

Care after Operative Repair

There is relatively little disagreement over the techniques of repair, but there is major disagreement concerning aftercare. Many surgeons feel that there is no need and no benefit to abduction splints. They are considered cumbersome for the patient without proof of efficacy in any study. We are not aware of a randomized trial comparing patients with compa-

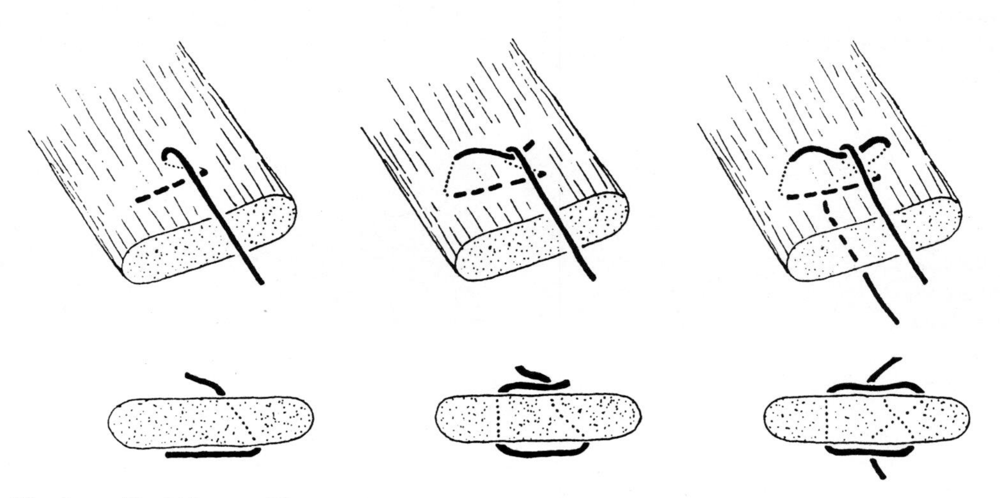

FIG. 12. A modified Mason–Allen tendon-grasping technique increases the pullout strength of the suture by a factor greater than 2 when compared with a simple stitch or with a mattress-type suture.

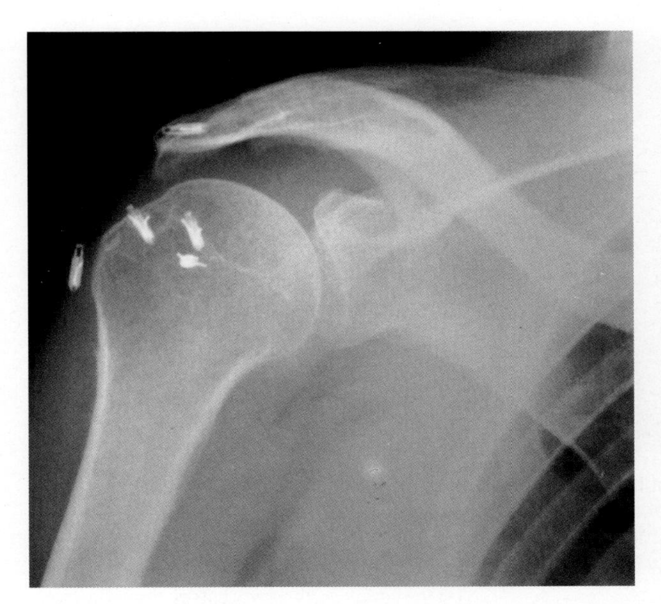

FIG. 13. Suture anchors do not have sufficient holding power and may pull loose in the weak, osteoporotic greater tuberosity that is typical for chronic rotator cuff tears .

rable tears who would have been treated with or without an abduction splint. Indirect evidence coming from clinical and experimental experience, however, has led us to routinely use an abduction splint in about 30 to 45 degrees (Fig. 14) of abduction on all large or massive tears. The following facts have led to this conviction:

- The in vivo experiments with rotator cuff repairs in the sheep have shown[51] that almost any repair technique will fail unless the animal is protected from weight bearing. Standard techniques failed by pulling of the suture out of the tendon or through the bone; modified techniques failed by failure of the (no. 3) sutures. The most important information gained from these animal experiments was that any repair will fail unless it is protected from undue, uncontrolled strain.
- We have intraoperatively measured passive tension of the rotator cuff musculotendinous units in the normal human shoulder, in partial tears, and in massive rotator cuff tears.[71] In stepwise elongation from 10 to 20 mm, passive tension increased by a factor of 2.2 ± 0.4 in chronic rotator cuff tears, but only by a factor of 1.3 in normal or partially torn musculotendinous units. Mean tension in 60 degrees of abduction was 14.25 ± 3.4 N in the four long-standing ruptures and 10 N in the control case. If the arm was adducted, tension rose to 25 N in the control case, whereas mean tension increased to 59.25 ± 12.7 N in long-standing rupture of the supraspinatus muscle. These findings demonstrate that passive tension in the supraspinatus is increased after long-standing rupture of its tendon. They also indicate that active force generation by these muscles will be compromised after surgery, and that the high strain imposed by repair may expose the musculotendinous unit to further damage.

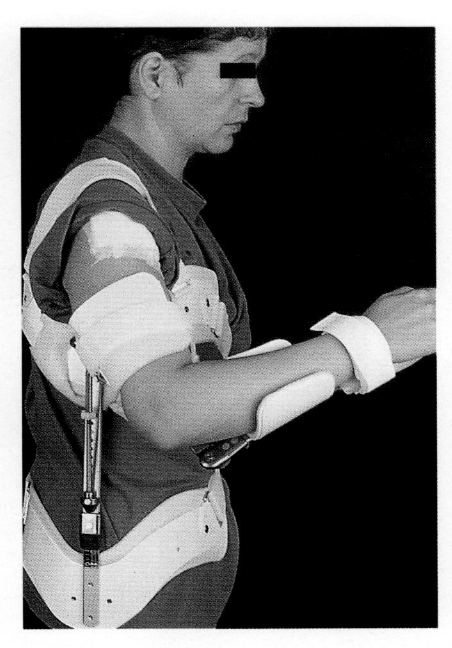

FIG. 14. Adjustable abduction splints are routinely used to protect repairs of massive cuff ruptures. They are mounted according to the tension observed intraoperatively and are used for 6 to 8 weeks. For passive range of motion exercises the arm is elevated from the splint; for hydrotherapy in the pool, the splint is removed. After 4 weeks abduction may be slightly lowered.

Therefore, we strongly believe that the postoperative use of abduction splints (see Fig. 14) is justified. The arm is brought into roughly 30 to 45 degrees of abduction, a position without relevant tension on the repaired musculotendinous unit. From this position, passive exercises are carried out daily, therapy in the pool is possible as long as adduction is prevented, and the splint is discontinued after 6 weeks. Physical therapy is usually continued for 3 months, unrestricted work can be resumed after 9 months.

Direct repair has yielded good to excellent clinical results in many studies addressing this problem.[1,10,11,12,27,28,31,32,34,37,40,47,51,63,67,75,84,89,93,94,99,100,108,116,121,128,141,145] The drawbacks of most studies that report their excellent results is that there is no detailed analysis of the failures and, more importantly, there is insufficient information concerning the selection of the patients.

We have recently reviewed[51] the results of a series of 38 consecutive massive rotator cuff tears treated by direct repair using modern techniques, such as modified Mason-Allen stitches, no. 3 braided polyester suture, and cortical bone augmentation devices. There were 15 cases that involved the supraspinatus and subscapularis muscles who were treated with a deltopectoral approach (Fig. 15) and 23 cases that involved either the supraspinatus and infraspinatus, or the supra-, infraspinatus, and subscapularis tendons who were treated by a superolateral approach.

Of these 38 cases, all had a tear of at least two complete tendons, but an acromiohumeral distance of at least 6 mm.

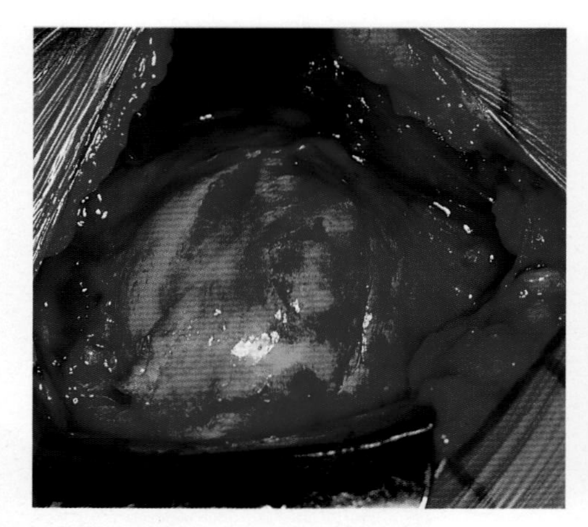

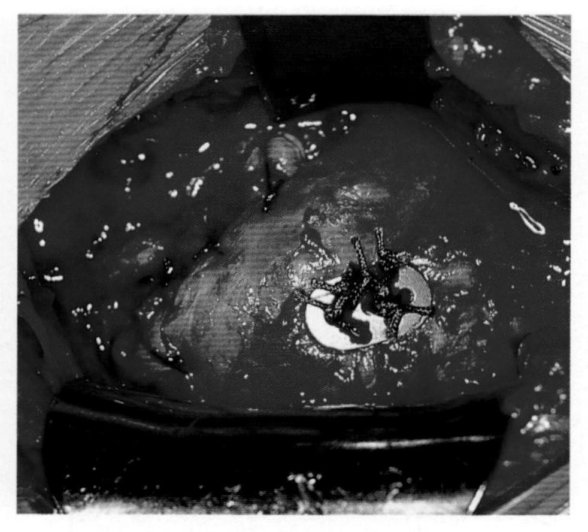

FIG. 15. (A) A massive rotator cuff tear involving the subscapularis and the supraspinatus approached through the deltopectoral interval. **(B)** Direct repair is achieved by transosseous sutures using the Mason–Allen tendon grasping technique, and fixation of the no. 3 suture to the soft bone, which is augmented with a cortical bone augmentation device to prevent cutting of the sutures through the bone. (Stratec/Synthes, Paoli, USA)

Statically, subluxated humeral heads had never before been considered for direct repair. Direct repair of these lesions improved the constant score of these shoulders[34] from 39 points preoperatively to 78 points at an average follow-up of 24.7 months, corresponding to an increase of 40% of the function, as measured on an age- and sex-adjusted functional score. The rerupture rate was 34%, which was lower than in other reported series,[47,67] but obviously still (too) high. As opposed to other series, however, all documented reruptures were smaller than the original tear, so that the retears actually represented partial repairs of massive cuff tears.[25] The clinical overall outcome in this consecutive series was most satisfactory, and we can confirm that primary repair is an excellent means of treatment for those massive tears that are amenable to direct repair (Fig. 16).

There are numerous patients with large rotator cuff tears who either are not or are seldom selected for surgical treatment. As opposed to other authors, we have not been as successful as they have in repairing cuffs of patients who could not be protected postoperatively (e.g., because they were wheelchair-bound[11,27]), or in patients with severe destruction of the cuff with subacromial nearthrosis and destruction of the humeral head.[92,107] In addition, our experience has shown that the following preoperative findings should be a caution to one before proceeding with surgery:

- Glenohumeral joint stiffness (limited passive external and internal rotation, tested with the arm in adduction)
- Long-standing pseudoparalysis without significant pain (see Fig. 2A)
- Severe atrophy of the supra- or infraspinatus muscle (see Figs. 2C and 5C)
- Injury, detachment, or paralysis of the deltoid muscle (Fig. 17)
- Anterosuperior subluxation (see Fig. 10)
- An acromiohumeral distance of less than 5 mm measured on an anteroposterior x-ray film, with the arm in neutral rotation (static superior subluxation, particularly negative if associated with anterior subluxation; see Fig. 2B)

Glenohumeral joint stiffness can usually be treated by physiotherapy and possibly surgical release so that direct repair may become possible. Severe anterior and even more so anterosuperior static subluxation associated with pseudoparalysis are currently not amenable to treatment by reconstructive procedures, and if surgery becomes mandatory, nonconstrained arthroplasty for pain relief and fusion, or possibly constrained arthroplasty,[62] are the only options. There is, however, a rather large group of patients who either have subjectively handicapping weakness, but no pseudoparalysis, in whom the humeral head may or may not have migrated cranially, or patients who have a relatively recent nonrecovering pseudoparalysis, but with an acromiohumeral distance of at least 5 mm. For this patient group, we feel that new and relevant advances have been made in palliative musculotendinous transfer surgery.

Musculotendinous Transfer Surgery

Most authors have come to agree that there are defects of the musculotendinous units of the rotator cuff that are not technically reparable because of the size of the structural defect, or who have accepted that structural healing does not reliably occur after technically successful repair of massive tears.[47,51,67,121] The defects that are beyond successful repair are probably indeed more frequent than previously believed, and alternatives to direct repair should probably be considered for more defects than is now current practice.[52]

Tendon "transfers" have been introduced into the treatment of massive or irreparable rotator cuff tears in the form of advancement of local musculotendinous units,[37] local transposition (rotational flaps) of musculotendinous units of the rotator cuff,[30,111] as well as by the use of the overlying deltoid muscle.[3,135] Attempts at reconstruction of massive defects with the use of the trapezius muscle[60,152] have also been performed, but reliable results have not been easily reproducible; hence, this indication remains controversial.

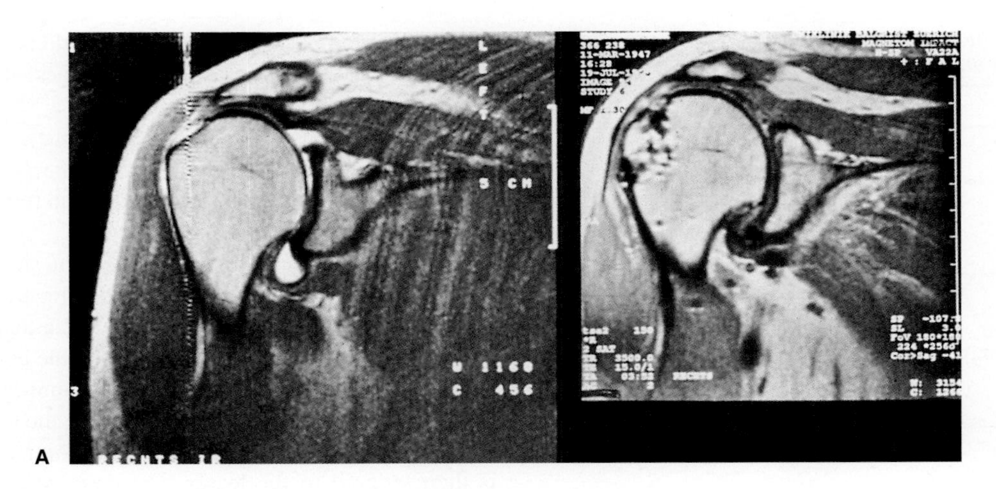

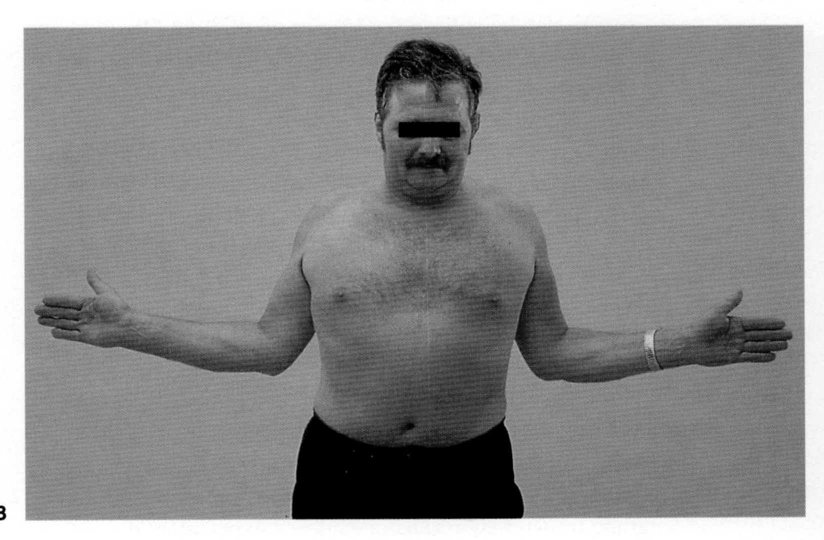

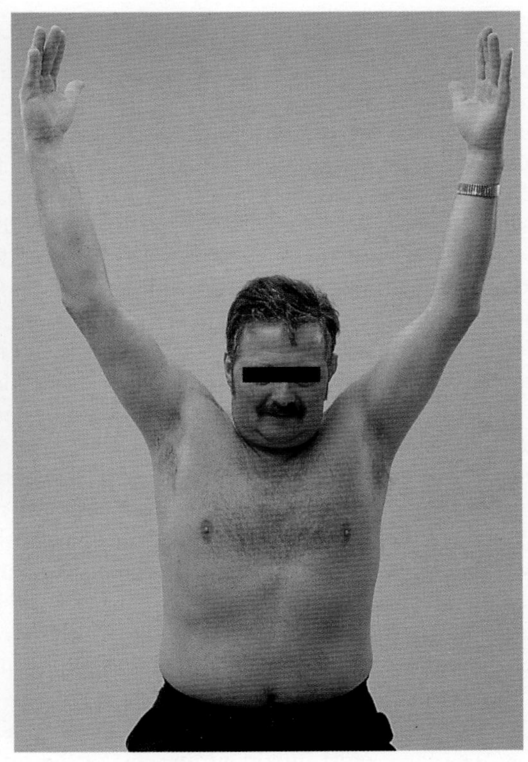

FIG. 16. Direct repair of a massive tear of the rotator cuff: 26 months after surgery, **(A)** the formerly ruptured cuff is in continuity. The patient is pain-free, and **(B,C)** function is excellent.

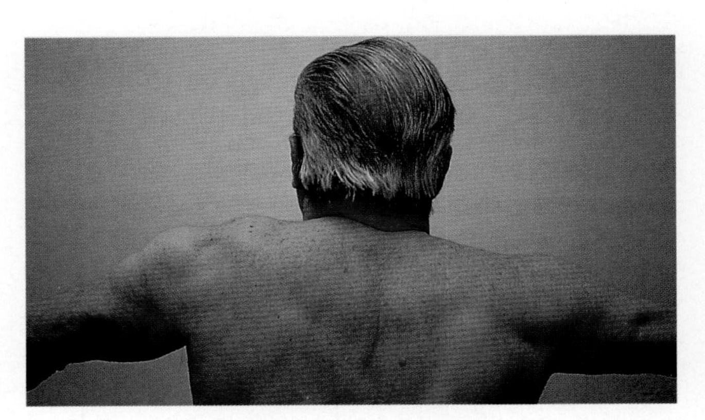

FIG. 17. Weakness after repair of the left rotator cuff: The deltoid is detached from its acromial origin. This condition results in weakness and often pain and must be prevented at all cost because it is very difficult to correct surgically.

Early in our experience, we had observed that tendinous tears are associated with so much muscular atrophy and degeneration that even a successful "watertight" repair is of limited functional value.[56] The contractile elements of the musculotendinous unit remain nonfunctional, and the fibrotic or degenerated muscle does not generate strength through a reasonable amplitude of motion, despite a successful tendon-to-bone repair. Transfer of musculotendinous units, therefore, appeared to be a logical solution that had certainly proved its value in surgery of the hand or the foot, and it was felt that it should be a consideration in any rotator cuff tear that is beyond repair.

The most frequent massive tear comprises the supra- and the infraspinatus tendons and if the defect is not reparable, the problem is the substitution of the function of the infra- and the supraspinatus. In analogy to a palliative procedure

TABLE 4. *Amplitude and relative strength of rotator cuff muscles and their potential substitutes*

Muscle	A (cm)	RS (%)
Subscapularis	7.3	14.5
Supraspinatus	6.7	5.1
Infraspinatus	8.6	9.6
Trapezius acr.	10.1	3.5
Pectoral minor	13.1	2.1
Pectoral major clavicle	14.5	2.2
Sternum	18.8	5.4
Trapezius, acromion	10.1	3.5
Deltoid (50% III [Fick])	9.0[a]	3.5[a]
Latissimus dorsi	33.9	5.8
Teres major	14.9	4.3

[a] Data from Ref. 73a.

for neurologic loss of infra- and supraspinatus function in obstetric plexus palsy.[74] The possibility of transfer of the musculotendinous unit of the latissimus dorsi to the posterolateral humeral head was studied anatomically and biomechanically and was then introduced as a salvage procedure to compensate for irreparable posterolateral rotator cuff defects.[48,56]

Basis of Musculotendinous Transfers about the Shoulder. To properly apply the methods of musculotendinous transfers, some basic concepts need to be reemphasized. Brand,[19] Herzberg,[73] and others have shown that two types of muscles have to be distinguished if tendon transfer surgery is considered: One group consists of short, strong muscles, with a short amplitude, the other group consists of relatively long muscles, with a large amplitude, that are less able to develop tension. The anatomic and physiologic basis for musculotendinous transfers about the shoulder had been established by Shiino[132] in the early part of the century, and they were recently refined by Herzberg.[73] These data can be of use to define which transferred muscle is most likely to optimally compensate for the absence of each of the individual muscles of the rotator cuff.

Transfers for Substitution of Individual Rotator Cuff Muscles. The three most important muscles of the rotator cuff have remarkably similar amplitudes (see Table 3), and they account for about 30% of the total strength generated by the muscles about the shoulder, with the subscapularis being by far the strongest (see Tables 1,2, and 4).

Subscapularis. The subscapularis is an intrinsic (going from scapula to the humerus) internal rotator and head depressor. It pulls the head posteriorly and, with its tendinous insertion situated high on the humeral head, it internally rotates and abducts the humerus. In Herzberg's experiments,[73] isolated contraction of the subscapularis compromised abduction, whereas its contraction, simultaneously with contraction of the infraspinatus, greatly facilitated abduction. It appears, therefore, that the subscapularis acts in synergy with the infraspinatus for abduction and elevation of the arm. This is a very important finding that should be borne in mind whenever reconstruction of only one of these muscles can be achieved.

For substitution of the subscapularis, the acromial part of the trapezius, the pectoralis minor, or the pectoralis major have been proposed. Their amplitudes and relative strengths are summarized in Table 4.

Although too weak and of somewhat short amplitude, thereby requiring optimal length adjustment, the trapezius has been tried as a substitute for the subscapularis. Its tendon is released from the acromion leaving some bone on the tendon (Fig. 18A). The musculotendinous unit is elevated and mobilized, the lateral clavicle is resected, the tendon brought through the enlarged acromioclavicular joint, and the tendon is then secured to the lesser tuberosity. Alternatively, the acromion can be split in the frontal plane,[37] and the transfer can be passed underneath the split (see Fig. 18B). The pull of the transferred muscle is backward, but unfortunately upward, and it is not active as an internal rotator. Nonetheless, Goutallier et al.[20] have reported early results of trapezius transfer for compensation of subscapularis deficiency in 25 cases: They have obtained good to excellent pain relief and functionally acceptable results in cases where they replaced the subscapularis as well as the supraspinatus with their transfer. The authors feel that this transfer probably prevents superior migration of the head, but that it does not recenter a cranially migrated head.

We have not had experience with trapezius transfer, because the muscle does not optimally fulfill the criteria for a muscle to be transferred to replace the function of the subscapularis. Further reports of clinical results are still awaited, and the transfer should be considered experimental.

The pectoralis major can be released from the humeral shaft and be transferred to the greater tuberosity. It is much better suited in terms of strength and amplitude to replace the subscapularis, but it is coming from anterior to the chest; therefore, it does not pull the humeral head backward. Nonetheless, Wirth and Rockwood[149] have reported good to excellent success with pectoralis major transfer for irreparable subscapularis lesions. Resch (personal communication) has suggested that, especially in cases with associated anterior shoulder instability, the tendon can be mobilized and then be brought laterally underneath the conjoined tendon, without any danger to the plexus, to be reinserted at the lesser tuberosity. If this can indeed be realized without loosening gliding properties for the transfer and with rerouting the tendon to come from more posteriorly, the transfer should mechanically be substantially better. The early results of Resch are no better than those of Wirth and Rockwood, but the population in whom it was used may be slightly different, and it will be most interesting to see the long-term results.

Our personal experience comprises 15 cases of transfer of the *entire* pectoralis major to the greater tuberosity. The del-

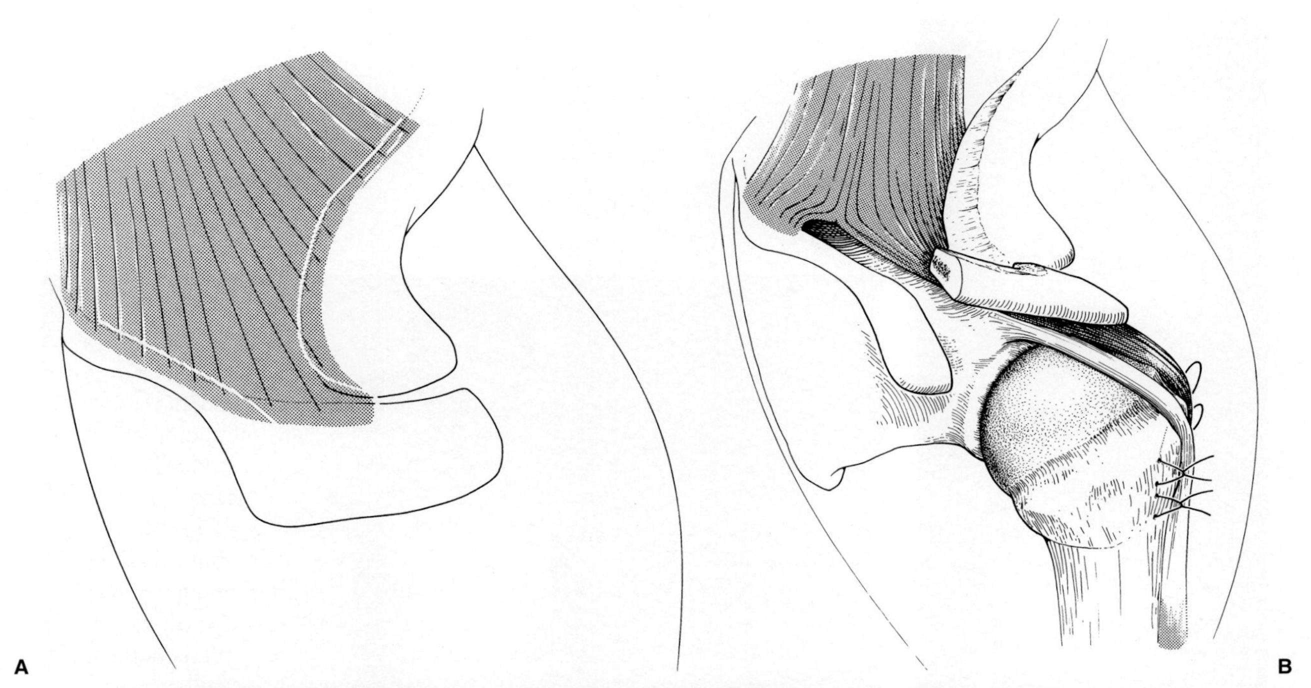

FIG. 18. Technique of trapezius transfer for substitution of subscapularis deficiency.[60] **(A)** The trapezius is elevated with a piece of the underlying acromion. **(B)** After elevation of the musculotendinous unit, it is either passed through the enlarged acromioclavicular joint or through the split acromion and reinserted at the lesser tuberosity. If a frontal split of the acromion has been used, this is closed with simple transosseous sutures.[37]

topectoral interval is extended 4 cm distally, the entire tendon is released from the humerus, and the musculotendinous unit is mobilized and pulled proximally to be reinserted on the greater tuberosity. Follow-up for the entire series is too short to allow definitive conclusions, but our results are encouraging. Elevation is usually restored, internal rotation is weak at the end of the amplitude, sufficient to reach behind the body. The transfer is rarely necessary, as most subscapularis tears can be repaired. Our encouraging results have prompted us to use the transfer for augmentation of a tenuous subscapularis repair, and the results are truly good if the lowermost part of the subscapularis could be repaired directly together with the anteroinferior capsule and the superior two-thirds of the subscapularis could be substituted for with the transfer (Fig. 19). We are surprised how often others have found the subscapularis to be irreparable and think that every attempt at repair should be carried out because no muscle can really replace the subscapularis. In our hands the transfer was first used for only isolated subscapularis tears and has alleviated pain and improved function substantially. In time we have also used it for the treatment of combined tears, and it also seems to be of value for massive tears. However, in cases with static anterior subluxation of the humeral head, the transfer does not appear to recenter the humeral head.

There is still no optimal transfer to replace the subscapularis, because restoring an optimal vector with a muscle of sufficient strength and amplitude appears as yet impossible. Pectoralis major transfer is currently the most reasonable for palliation. Future research is oriented toward transfer of the latissimus dorsi to the lesser tuberosity and rerouting the pectoralis major underneath the conjoined tendon.

Supraspinatus. The supraspinatus alone is almost never torn and retracted to a degree that it cannot be repaired. On a shoulder model, isolated contraction of the supraspinatus leads to an anterolateral elevation of 50 to 60 degrees and to an external rotation of about 20 degrees. Herzberg has shown[15] that it is much more efficient if it is activated simultaneously with the lateral deltoid. The supraspinatus has an optimal vector for abduction, and is relatively strong and short.

Although not really a transfer, but rather a slide of the muscle, the supraspinatus advancement designed by Debeyre et al.[37] merits review (Fig. 20). Indeed, release of the muscle bellies of the supra- and infraspinatus allows lateralization of the respective tendons far beyond that possible without release and without injury to the neurovascular bundle.[144] The concept is to release the muscle belly from the supraspinatus fossa without injury to the suprascapular neurovascular bundle and to advance the musculotendinous unit laterally, thereby rotating it around its neurovascular pedicle (see Fig. 20). Without being very widely used, the technique has stood the test of time for

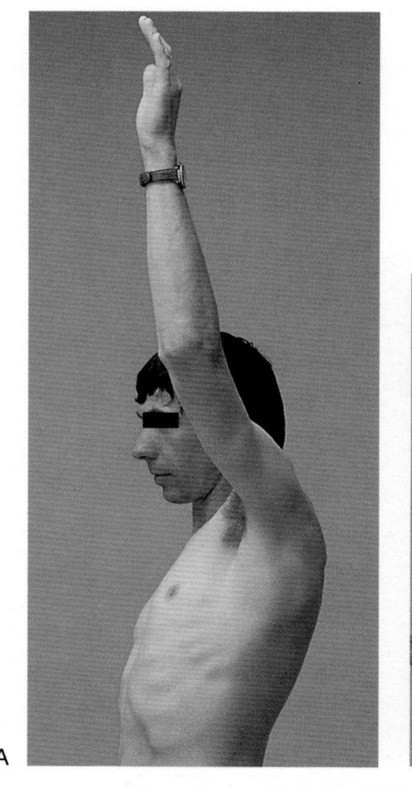

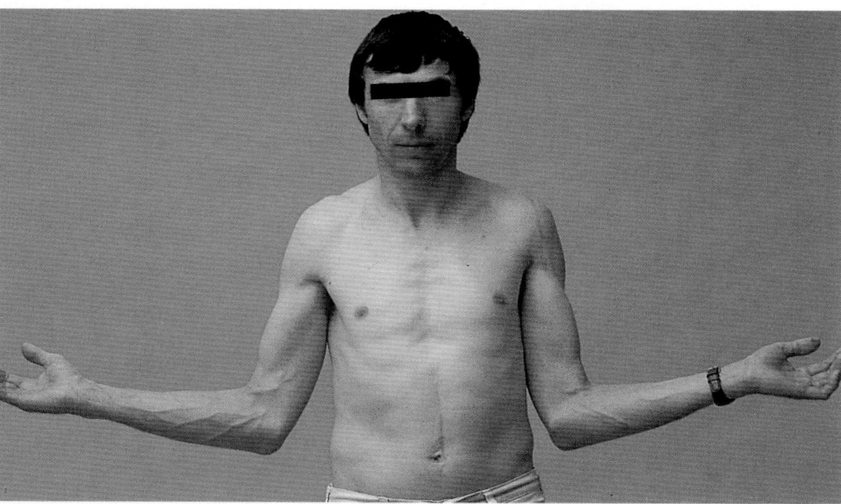

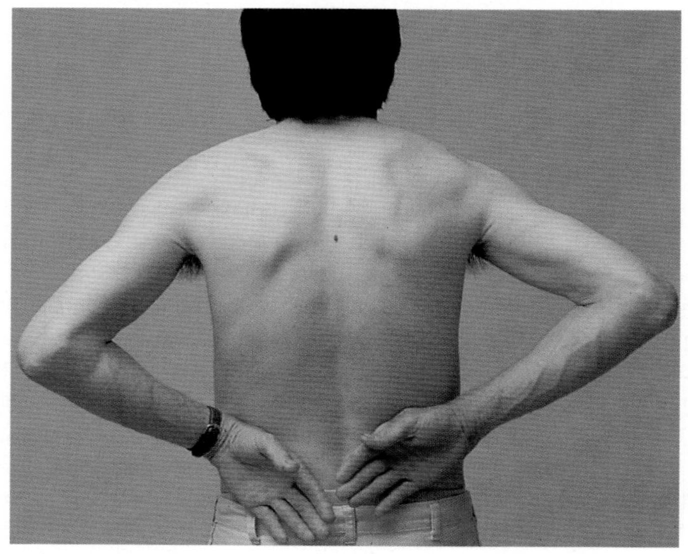

FIG. 19. Clinical result of a pectoralis major transfer for irreparable subscapularis tear: The lowermost fourth of the subscapularis was repaired directly, the superior aspect of the retracted subscapularis was not repaired, the entire pectoralis major was transferred to the greater tuberosity. **(A)** Elevation is pain-free and symmetrical, **(B)** external rotation is restored, and **(C)** internal rotation is diminished by three vertebral levels, but is functional.

Debeyre and his pupils, who continue to use supraspinatus advancement and have adopted the same concept for the infraspinatus,[117,118,121] with highly satisfactory results.

Another much better-known form of advancement is the subscapularis transfer proposed by Cofield.[30] A rotational flap is created by using the superior two-thirds of the subscapularis to cover the defect caused by rupture of the supraspinatus. We feel that the subscapularis is of crucial importance and is often already tenuous in very large tears; thus, we have often hesitated to use it under these circumstances. This rotational flap, which yields good results in moderate-sized tears,[30] has not been as successful in the treatment of massive tears.[81]

In terms of true musculotendinous transfers there are two major proposals for substitution of supraspinatus function: a transfer of the trapezius[152] and the transfer of the lateral deltoid, as independently described by Takagishi[135] and Apoil and Augereau.[2] Table 3 indicates that both muscles are well suited in terms of amplitude and strength.

The trapezius can be transferred with a technique that is analogous to the technique of transfer in subscapularis deficiencies. Instead of insertion into the lesser tuberosity, the ten-

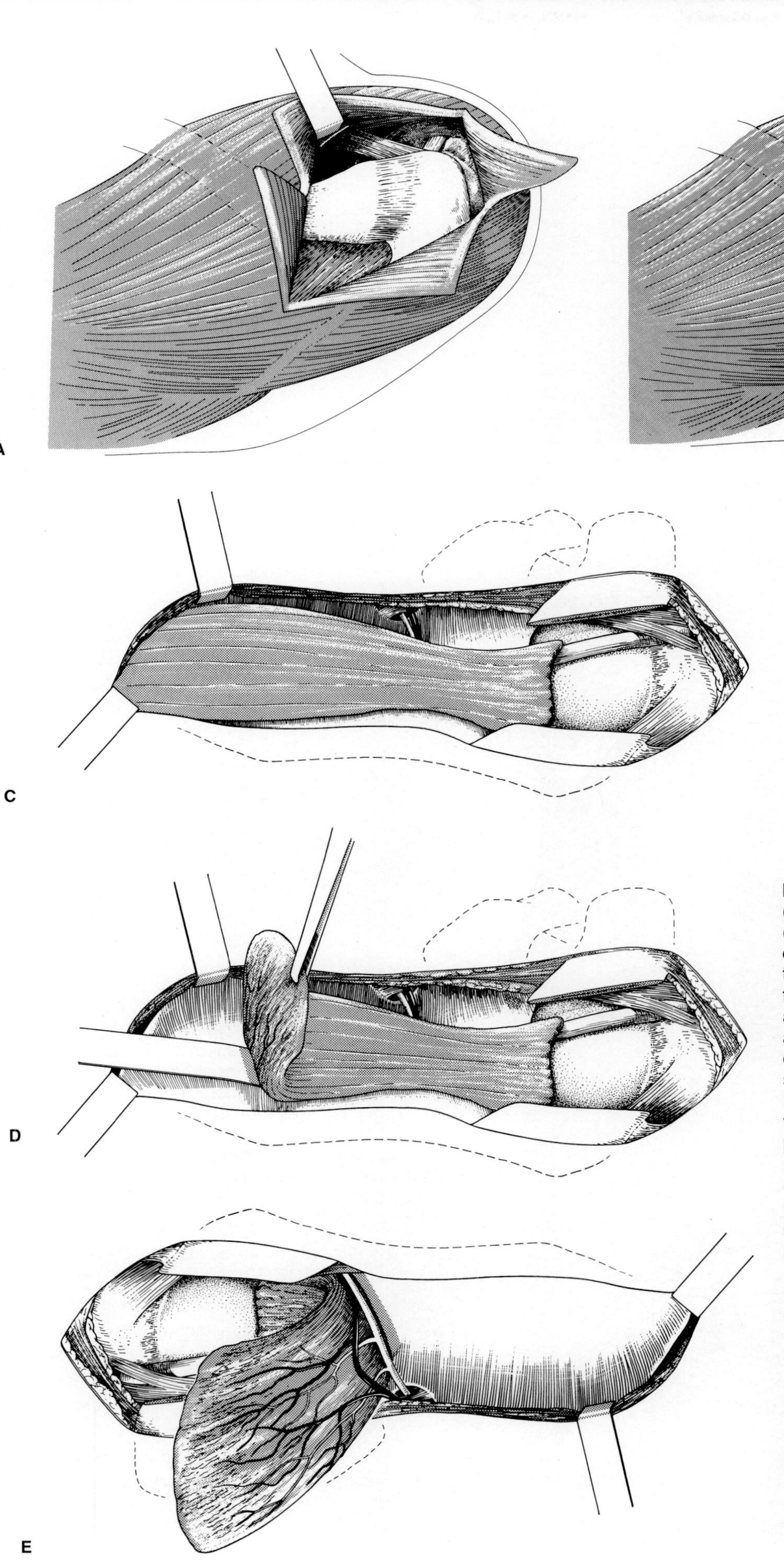

FIG. 20. Supraspinatus advancement (Debeyre) and infraspinatus advancement (Goutallier) for massive posterosuperior cuff tears. The operation is performed with the patient in the sitting position. **(A)** A frontal incision over the acromion with an anteroposterior extension is made, the acromioclavicular joint and the coracoacromial ligament are generously resected (Grande liberation antérieure of Patte). **(B)** The retracted supraspinatus tendon is identified. If mobilization is not possible, **(C)** the trapezius is divided more medially and the entire supraspinatus is exposed. **(D)** The supraspinatus is released from its fossa starting laterally until **(E)** the neurovascular pedicle is fully exposed. If the infraspinatus is also retracted medially, **(F)** a second incision is made over the infraspinatus fossa (Goutallier). **(G)** The infraspinatus is released from the infraspinatus fossa. **(H)** The insertion of the rhomboids at the medial border of the scapula is then also released. **(I)** Both musculotendinous units are then advanced and the tendon stumps are sutured to a bony trough at the greater tuberosity. **(J)** The rhomboids are then sutured to the infraspinatus hoping to augment the dynamic effect of the musculotendinous unit and protect the infraspinatus from sliding too laterally.

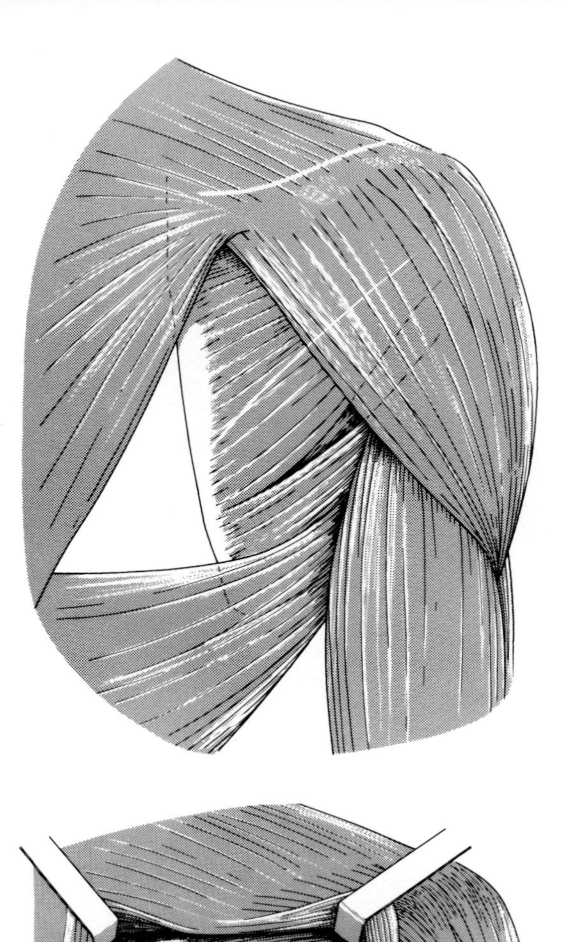

F

FIG. 20. *Continued*

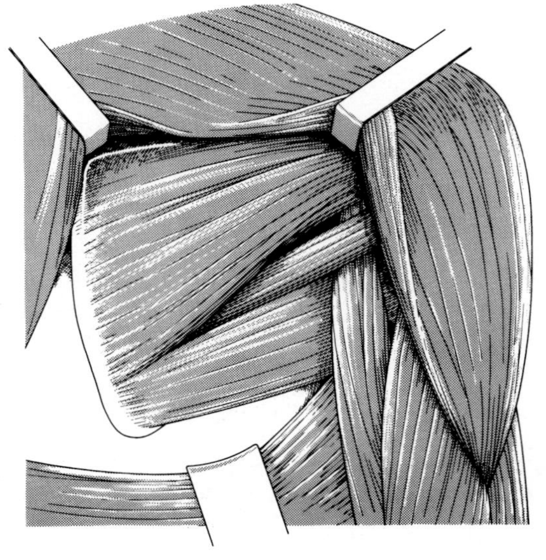

G

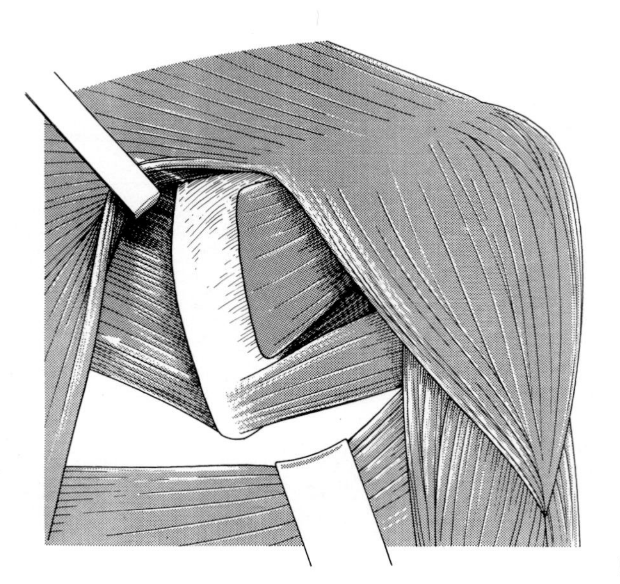

H

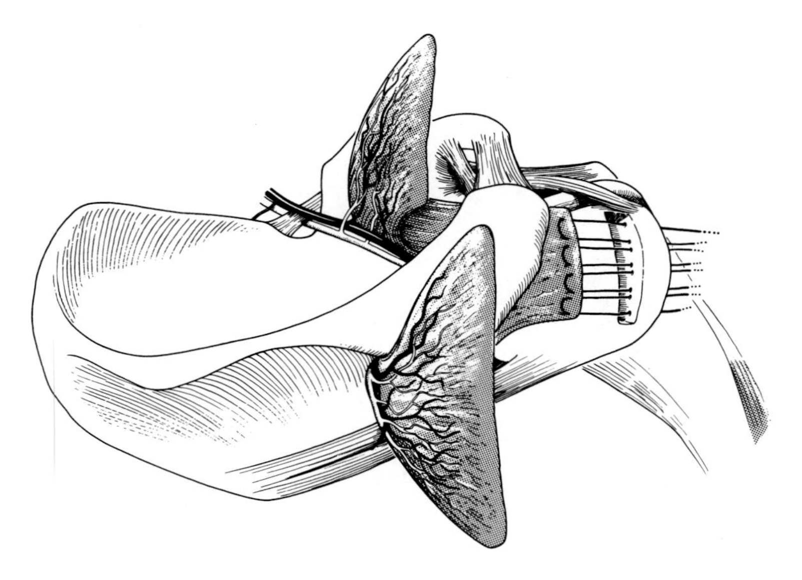

I

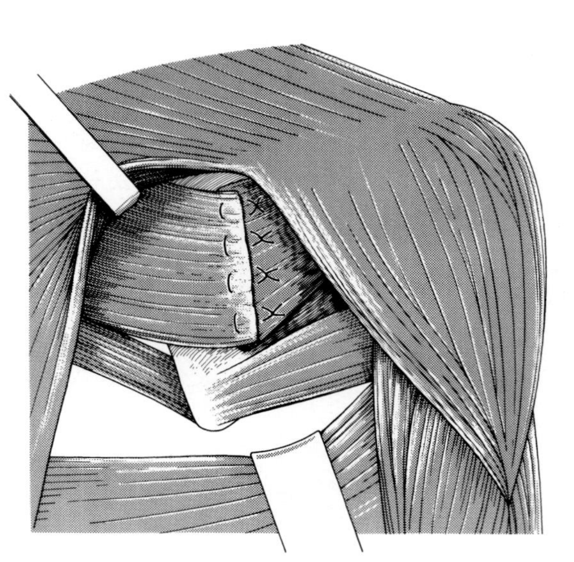

J

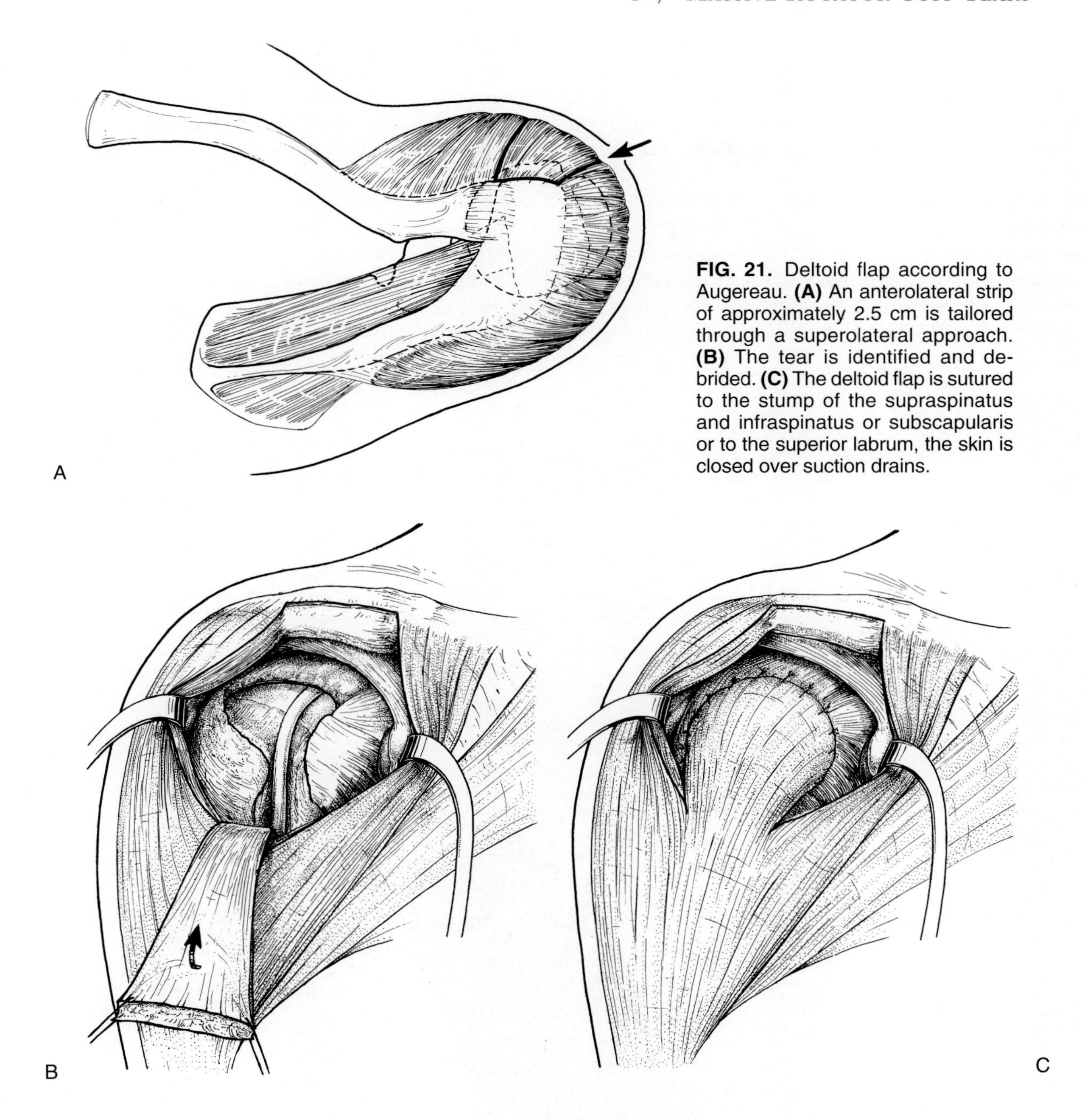

FIG. 21. Deltoid flap according to Augereau. **(A)** An anterolateral strip of approximately 2.5 cm is tailored through a superolateral approach. **(B)** The tear is identified and debrided. **(C)** The deltoid flap is sutured to the stump of the supraspinatus and infraspinatus or subscapularis or to the superior labrum, the skin is closed over suction drains.

don is implanted into the greater tuberosity. Yamanaka and Mikasa[152] used an acromion-split technique, rather than a resection of the lateral clavicle. The orientation of the transfer is not optimal; it pulls the head superiorly and it does not really act as an external rotator. The clinical results of this procedure are somewhat controversial; the recent report of Yamanaka and Mikasa[152] dealt with only seven cases and there are some good results, but there are almost no excellent results. We have elected to not use this procedure for this indication until there are results available from further investigators.

The deltoid flap was originally described by Takagishi.[135] It was then independently developed by Augereau, who has also performed this surgery on a very large series of cases and popularized the transfer. With this procedure, approximately a 2.5-cm–wide strip of the anterolateral deltoid is released from the acromion (Fig. 21), mobilized without injury to the axillary nerve, and then sutured to the supraspinatus stump or the superior aspect of the glenoid, thereby providing coverage of the humeral head and a dynamic abductor. This flap can be tailored to cover defects of the supraspinatus or to extend somewhat anteriorly to also cover defects of the superior aspect of the subscapularis, or it may be extended posteriorly to cover defects of the superior portion of the infraspinatus. Augereau has obtained excellent results in the treatment of massive tears with this technique. Gazielly[46] has recently summarized his own results in 20 cases. Whereas 5 cases had an excellent result, there were also 5 who had a poor result, and the overall results were definitely less favorable than the results reported by Bigliani[12] for primary repair. Another study by Dierickx et al.[39] also reported

20 cases with satisfactory results, but these results were no better than those of cuff debridement. A most recent prospective trial has yielded very satisfactory pain relief, high patient satisfaction, but essentially no gain in strength.[85] Accordingly, it must be concluded that deltoid flap has not proved its superiority over any other alternative.

It is important to recognize that it is extremely difficult to analyze the material currently presented, especially because it appears that this flap is often used for moderate- to large-sized tears. In our own experience, we have used this transfer only for truly irreparable tears involving more than two complete tendons. The results for this indication were good in terms of pain relief, but they were no better than cuff debridement or attempts at direct repair in terms of regaining function. The hesitation to compromise the deltoid by this surgery is waning, but it may remain a serious consideration in patients for whom the deltoid flap leads to an unsatisfactory result. We personally had to revise three cases of failed deltoid flaps, who had been sent for further treatment. All three cases were very painful and had an additional irreparable cuff tear. Although treatment of pain was possible, satisfactory function could not be regained in any of the three patients, and we remain reluctant to use the deltoid flap for irreparable tears.

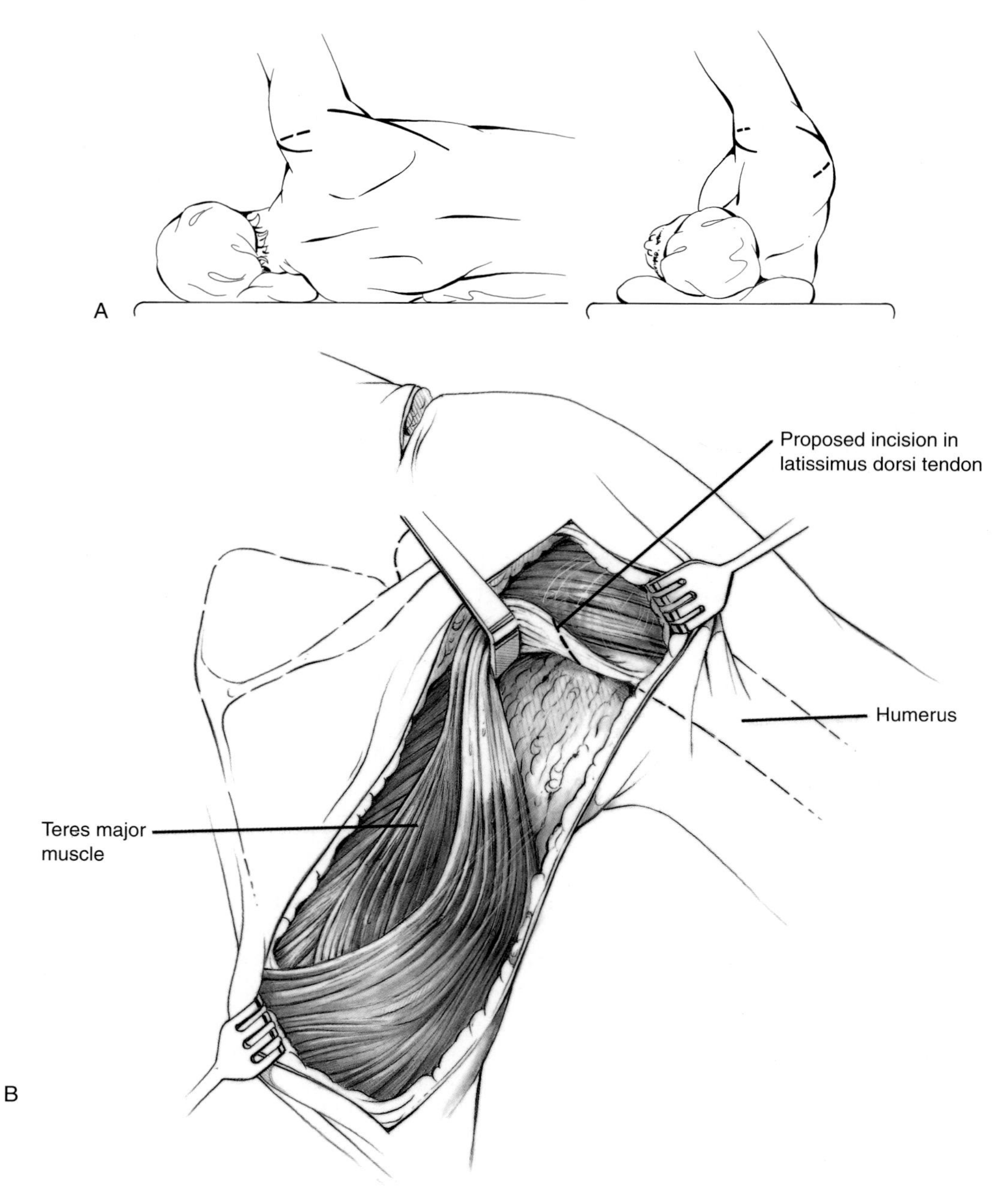

FIG. 22. Technique of latissimus dorsi transfer. **(A)** The patient is in a lateral decubitus position. After an attempt at conventional repair of the cuff through a superolateral approach, **(B)** an incision in the posterior axillary line is made, the latissimus is exposed and its tendon released from its insertion at the humerus. (*continued*)

Infraspinatus. The infraspinatus is almost never torn without a concomitant, large tear of the supraspinatus. The infraspinatus is an external rotator and at the end of its amplitude it is an elevator of the shoulder.

Advancement of the infraspinatus, as described in the foregoing, is a possibility with which we have no experience. It is used by Goutallier et al.[121] and has given satisfactory results for these authors.

In the light of musculotendinous transfer, Table 4 indicates that Herzberg[15] has shown that the *latissimus dorsi* is a relatively strong muscle, with an extremely large amplitude, which makes it better suited for transfer than the teres major.

The technique of the tendon transfer has been described in detail,[48,56] and only the most important elements are reviewed herein (Fig. 22): The patient is in a lateral decubitus position with the trunk elevated. A superolateral approach is

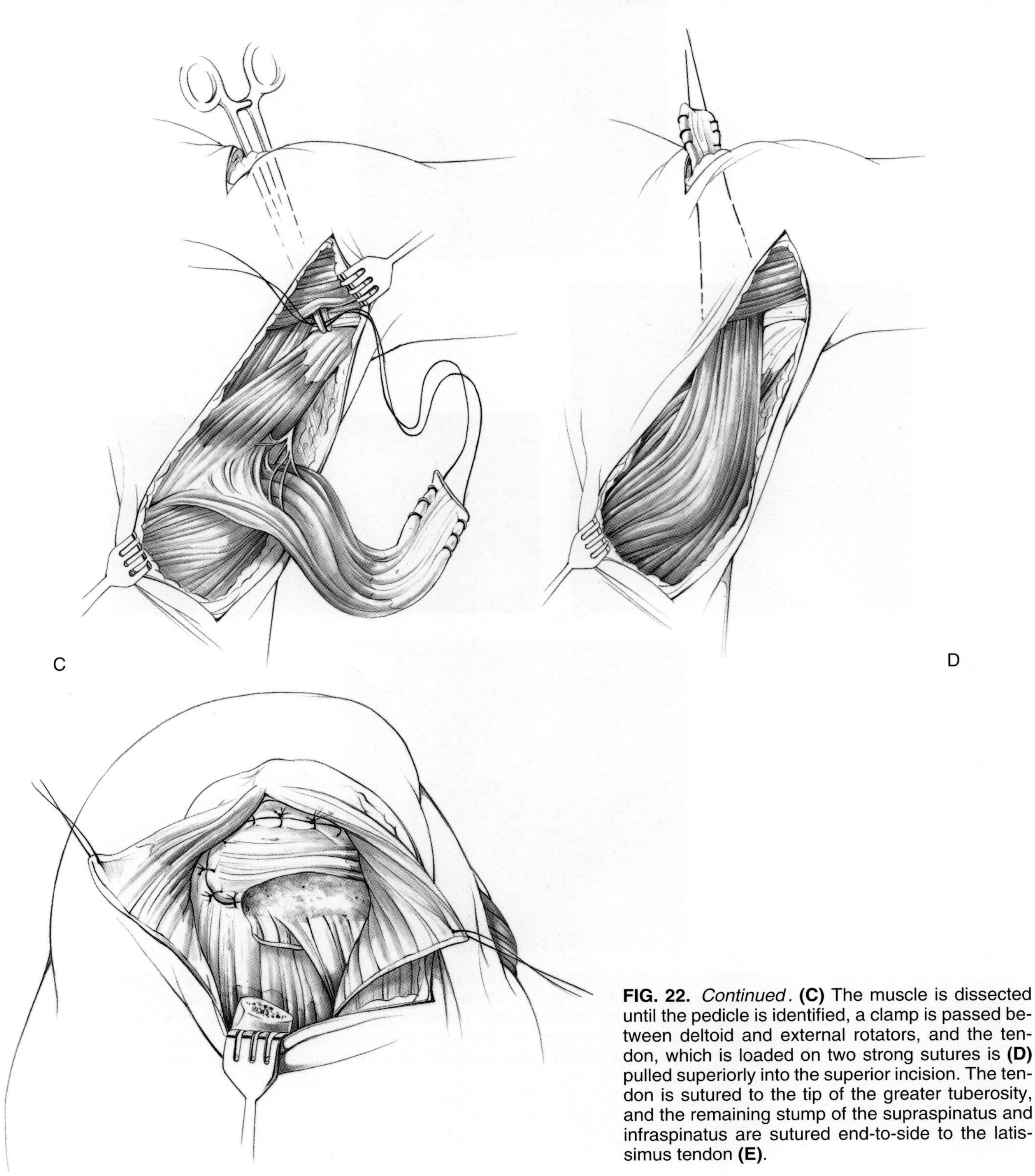

FIG. 22. *Continued*. **(C)** The muscle is dissected until the pedicle is identified, a clamp is passed between deltoid and external rotators, and the tendon, which is loaded on two strong sutures is **(D)** pulled superiorly into the superior incision. The tendon is sutured to the tip of the greater tuberosity, and the remaining stump of the supraspinatus and infraspinatus are sutured end-to-side to the latissimus tendon **(E)**.

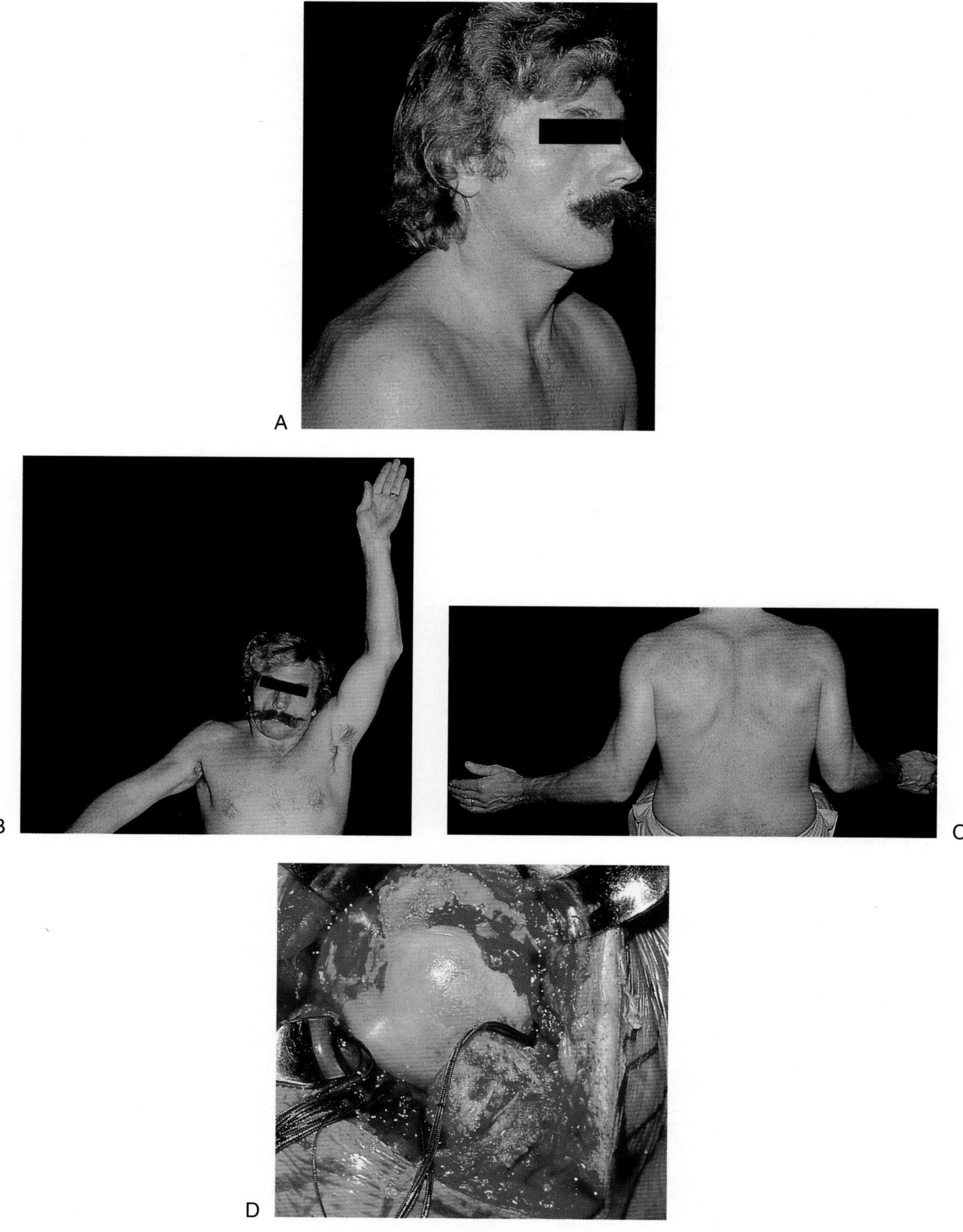

FIG. 23. (A) A young patient with a massive tear and severe atrophy of supra- and infraspinatus. **(B and C)**. He has a pseudoparalysis for scapular plane abduction and for external rotation. **(H)** Intraoperatively the supra- and infraspinatus tears are not reparable, and a latissimus dorsi transfer is performed. **(F)**: At 2 years postoperatively the patient has recovered elevation and external rotation and is pain-free. At 10 years he still has normal elevation of his right arm (but a painful left arm), restored external rotation, and is working as a truck driver **(G and H).**

used for the attempt at a conventional repair. If direct repair is impossible, a posterior approach along the posterior axillary line is performed to identify the latissimus dorsi. The tendon is released from the humeral shaft, and the muscle is mobilized until the neurovascular pedicle can be identified. The tendon is then brought into the superolateral approach by pulling it upward between the deltoid and the teres minor. It is then inserted at the very top of the humeral head–greater tuberosity transition zone. The end of the tendon is sutured to the subscapularis tendon, and it comes to lie exactly at the insertion of the supraspinatus. Herzberg[15] has studied the mechanical effect of transfer of the tendon to different sites at the humeral head, and has determined that the tip of the greater tuberosity or the region of the supraspinatus insertion is optimal.

Of all cases operated on, we have recently reviewed the first consecutive 16 after a minimal follow-up of 5 years, and the 13 surviving patients were reviewed after a minimal follow-up of 10 years (Fig. 23). All had chronic irreparable, massive rotator cuff tears. At 65 months after latissimus dorsi transfer, as originally described, pain relief was excellent or good in 94% of the shoulders at rest, and in 75% on exertion. Pain-free active flexion increased, postoperatively, by 40 degrees from 83 degrees. Active external rotation was restored for the adducted arm, and the transfer successfully served as an external rotation tenodesis for the elevated arm. The average ultimate function of the shoulders was assessed by the constant score and calculated to be 73% of an age- and gender-matched normal shoulder. The 12 shoulders with a functionally intact subscapularis scored an average of 83%, but those without an intact subscapularis scored only 54%. The latissimus dorsi transfer, therefore, yielded durably good to excellent subjective and objective results in chronically painful dysfunctional shoulders with irreparable tears of the rotator cuff if the subscapularis was intact. However, it was of no benefit in the presence of massive cuff tears with subscapularis insufficiency.

After 10 years of experience, we know that the results obtained at 3 and 5 years are maintained at 10 years, provided that the subscapularis does not fail. The best indications for latissimus dorsi transfer are patients who can still elevate their arm, but by internally rotating it. They are very weak in elevation and abduction and have complete

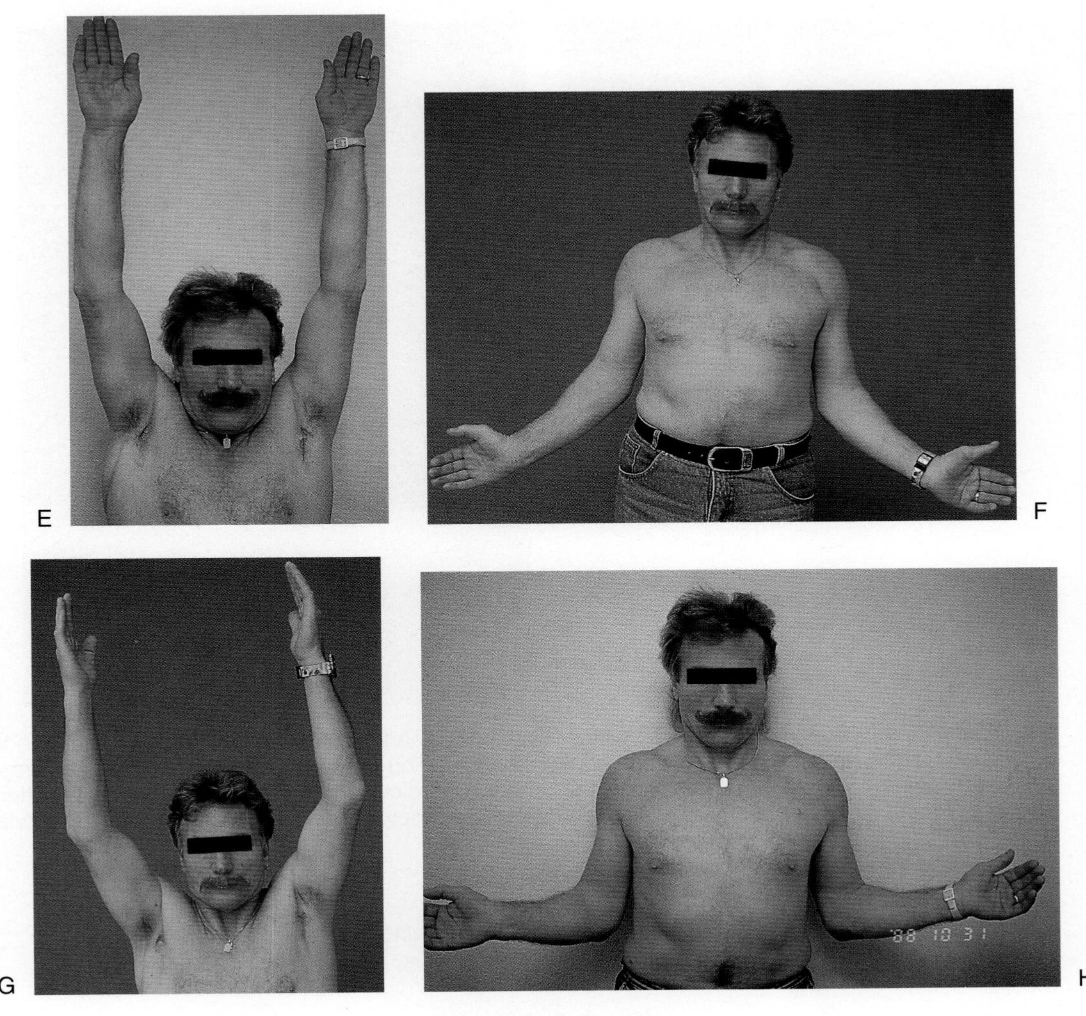

FIG. 23. *Continued*

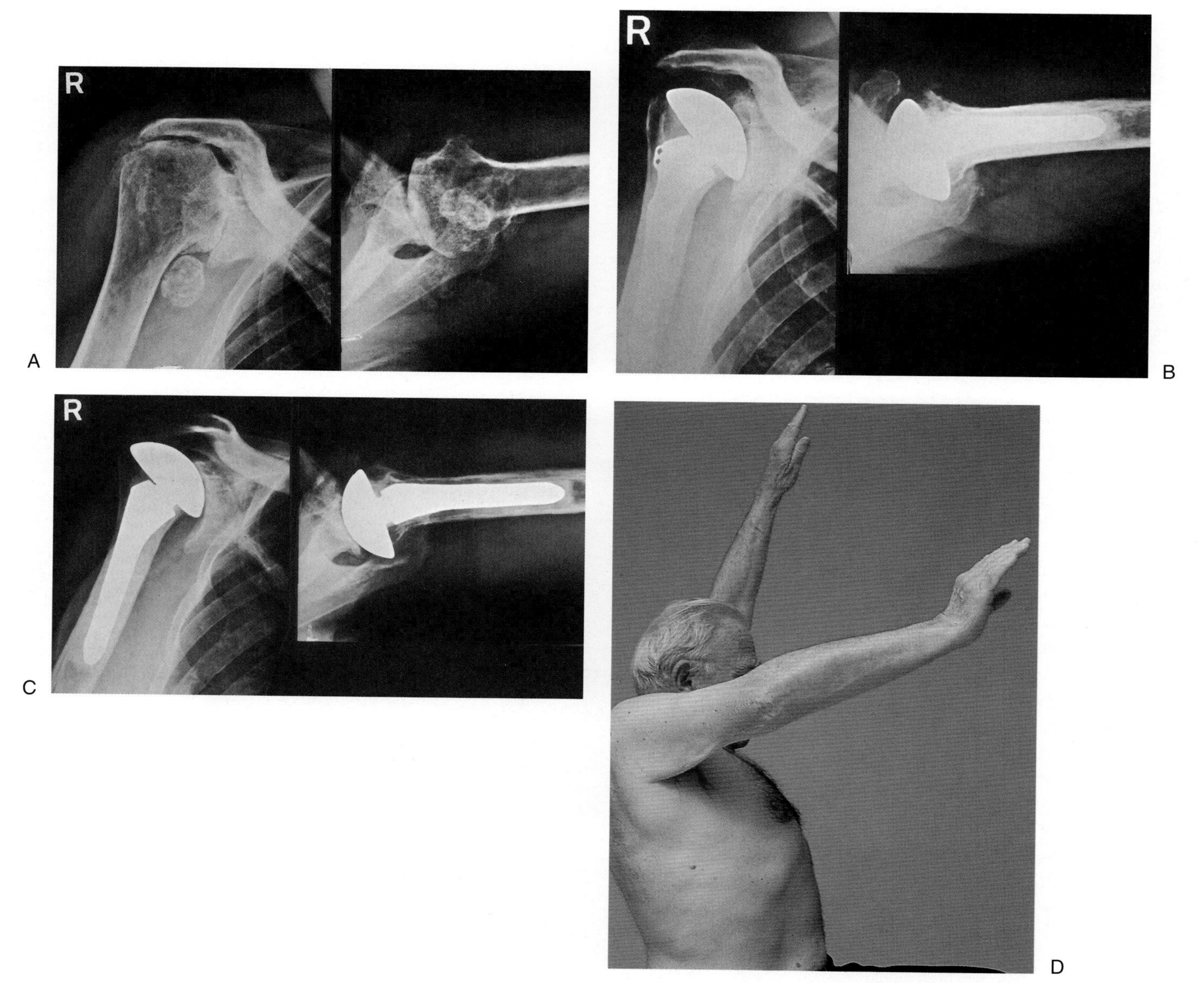

FIG. 24. (A) A massive rotator cuff tear, with advanced osteoarthrosis. The humerus is centered in the anteroposterior direction. **(B)** An exact anatomic reconstruction of the proximal humerus is performed with use of an anatomic prosthesis (Anatomica®; Sulzer Medica, Winterthur, Switzerland). **(C)** After 1 year the glenoid shows remodeling and wear. **(D)** Anterior elevation preoperatively is painful. (*continued*)

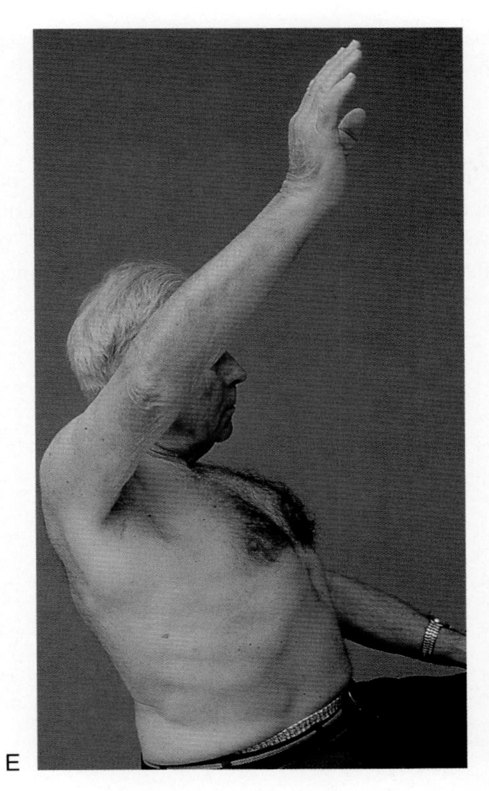

FIG. 24. *(Continued).* **(E)** At 1 year, it is pain-free.

loss of functional external rotation. It is this functional loss of external rotation (inability to reach forward with the hand, inability to stabilize the arm in space; e.g., in front of the mouth) that is consistently improved by this technique, provided the contraindications are respected. Conversely, patients with positive lift-off test results are definitely not candidates for transfer. In cases of deltoid deficiency, the transfer is also less successful.

In cases of complete pseudoparalysis, the results are also less predictable. We have recovered full anterior elevation in some patients and could not reduce the pseudoparalysis in others. We currently perform the procedure in patients who are suffering from their deficit in active external rotation and flexion and in abduction, and we can be sure to relieve pain and restore functional external rotation with the arm at the side, but we are uncertain whether we will restore strong overhead motion. The latissimus dorsi is clearly superior to any treatment alternatives that we have used for this very well-defined small segment of patients.

Although transfer surgery is currently considered only in irreparable tears, we believe that transfer surgery should always be considered if functional restoration is mandatory and muscular atrophy or degeneration is present. In our current practice, latissimus dorsi for certain posterolateral cuff lesions and pectoralis major for subscapularis lesions are best established and are also used more and more frequently as an augmentation procedure if the primary repair is critical. Other transfers, such as deltoid muscle flaps, have their clear indication for other authors. This field of reconstructive surgery of the cuff is young, and few authors have accepted the challenge of trying to restore function with a treatment concept that is not well established. The presently reported results justify us in continued evaluation of the currently available procedures and the study of further alternatives.

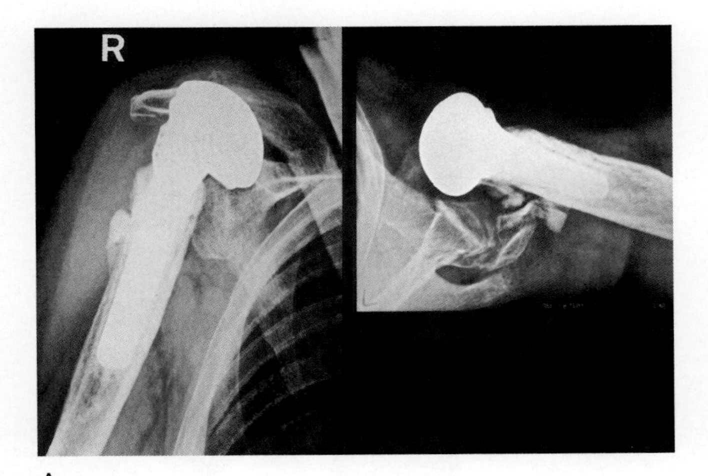

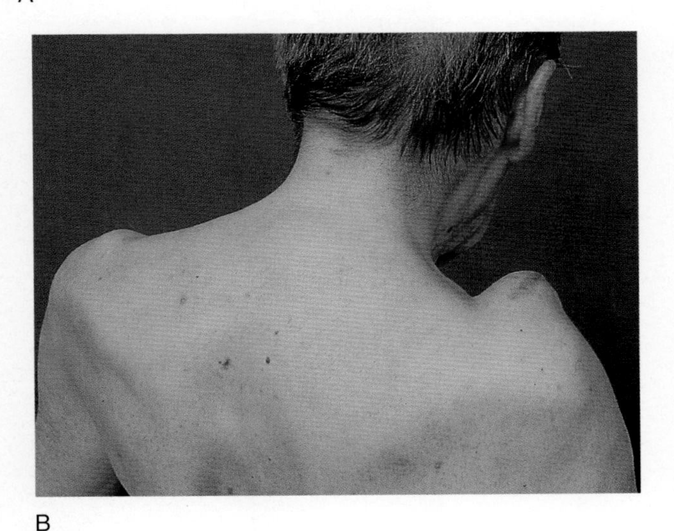

FIG. 25. Hemiarthroplasty after anterior acromioplasty. **(A)** The prosthesis is dislocated anterosuperiorly, is painful, and **(B)** is almost piercing the skin. Hemiarthoplasty is not used in the presence of anterosuperior subluxation of the humeral head.

Arthroplasty

Massive rotator cuff tears may be associated with moderate to severe osteoarthrosis[119] or with true rotator cuff tear arthropathy.[107] Prior surgery, including anterior acromioplasty with coracoacromial ligament resection, may complicate the situation. Nonconstrained (hemi-) arthroplasty has become a more and more frequently used and established form of treatment. Despite its poor reputation, constrained arthroplasty may need to be reconsidered for certain specific indications and, therefore, will be briefly discussed.

Nonconstrained Hemiarthroplasty

Nonconstrained arthroplasty is being used for patients with irreparable rotator cuff tears and so-called eccentric superiorly migrated arthrosis. Two recent reports[43,148] present the results after 3 to 4 years using usually a slightly oversized

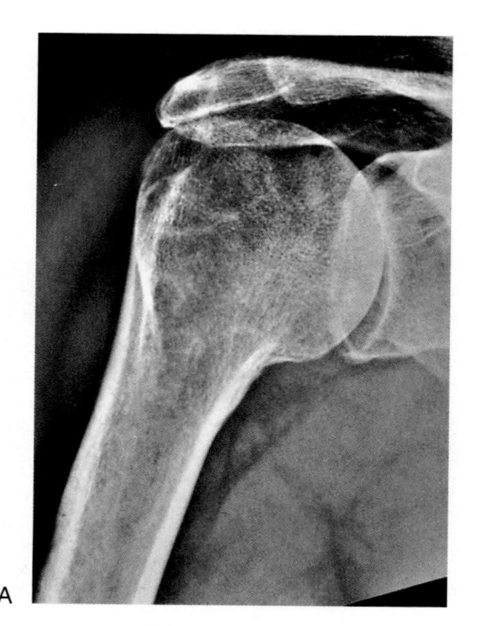

A

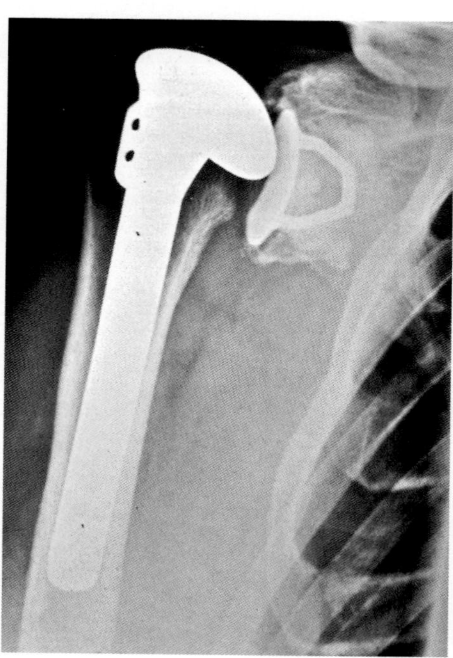

B

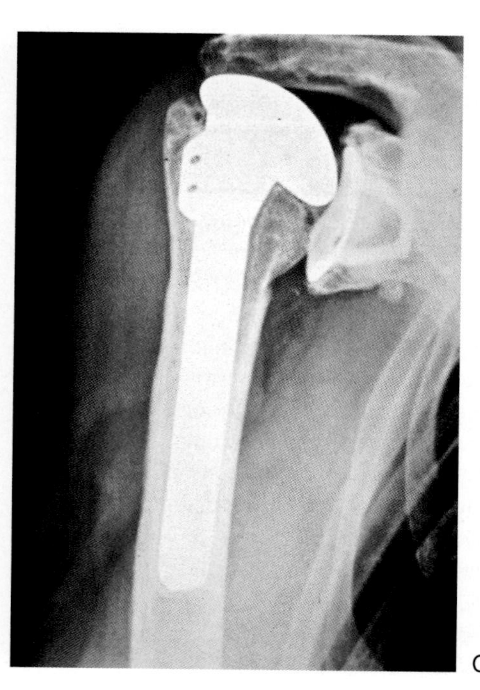

C

FIG. 26. (A) A massive rotator cuff tear with superiorly migrated arthrosis. At surgery **(B)**, the glenoid cartilage was worn and a glenoid component was implanted, despite the irreparable rotator cuff tear. Eight years later, the patient is pain-free, with an elevation of 90 degrees. **(C)** Although the noncemented shaft shows signs of loosening, there is no evidence of progressive radiological loosening of the glenoid component.

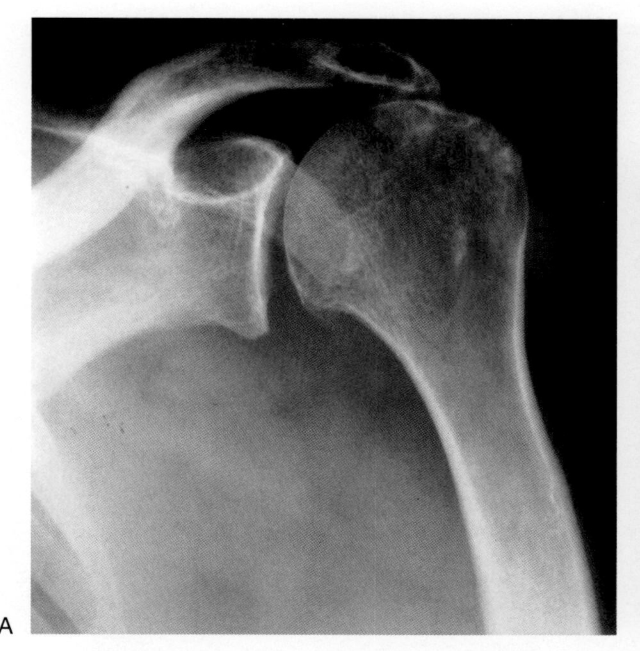

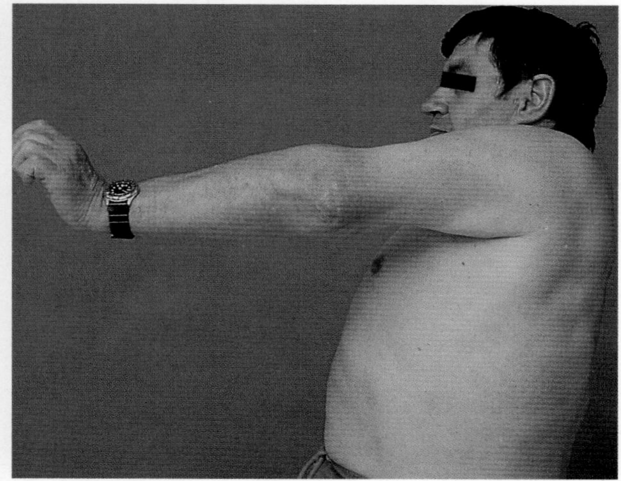

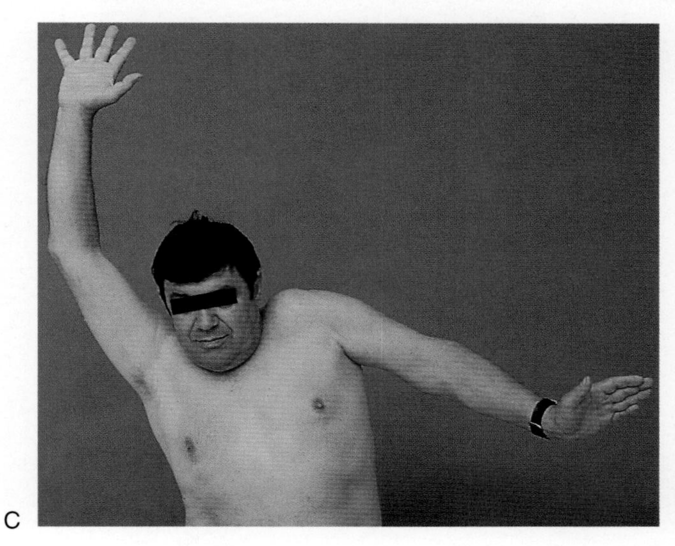

FIG. 27. (A) Static anterosuperior subluxation in an irreparable cuff tear. **(B)** Elevation is 60 and **(C)** abduction is 45 degrees.

head. In one series only 63% had satisfactory results,[43] and in the other series only 12 of 21 patients became pain-free. It was concluded that hemiarthroplasty is a reasonable alternative for the treatment of this condition, but that prior surgery involving attempts at cuff repair and rotator cuff tear arthropathy are significant risk factors.[43]

We use hemiarthroplasty in superiorly migrated arthrosis and rotator cuff tear only if there is no anteroposterior instability and if the head is well centered in the glenoid in the horizontal plane (Fig. 24). We do not use hemiarthroplasty in cases with lack of anteroposterior stability or after acromioplasty, including coracoacromial ligament resection, because untreatable anterosuperior subluxation or dislocation is a very real complication that almost cannot be dealt with because prosthetic replacement also compromises later arthrodesis (Fig. 25). It has been our experience that obtaining freedom from pain requires a very long time, and the patient is often well only after about 1 year. In fact, it is almost usual to see the patient somewhat dissatisfied at 3 and 6 months, and it should be remembered that there is no point in revising hemiarthoplasties for pain at this point. Chances are that patients will become better, in terms of pain, by themselves.

For the use of nonconstrained arthroplasty for massive rotator cuff tears, we conceptually differ from many authors in two specific points:

1. We do not oversize the head, with the understanding that, indeed, there are many patients with massive cuff tears and a nonarthritic, spherical humeral head who have excellent function and never need any operation. These patients invariably have humeral heads of physiologic size, and we think that our chances to improve function by using an unphysiologic implant are minimal (see Fig. 24).

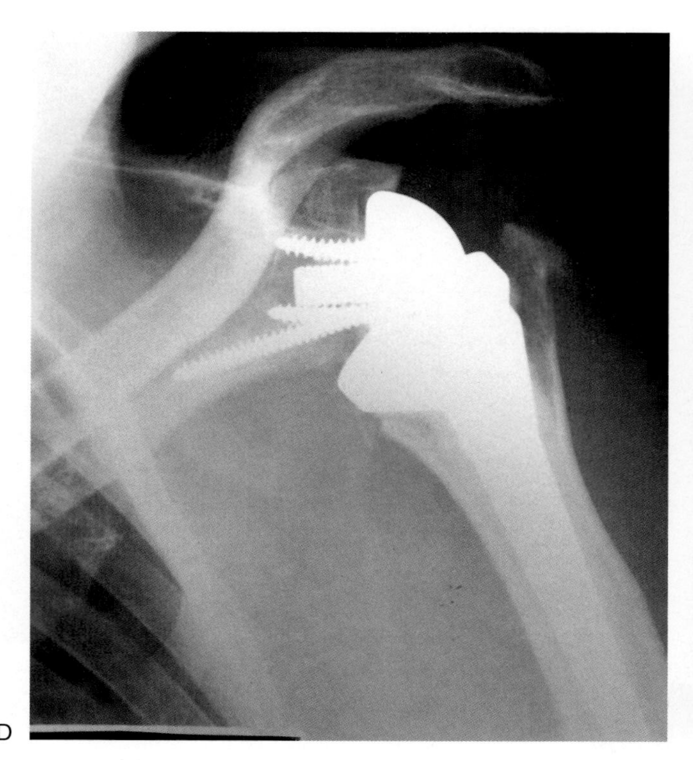
D

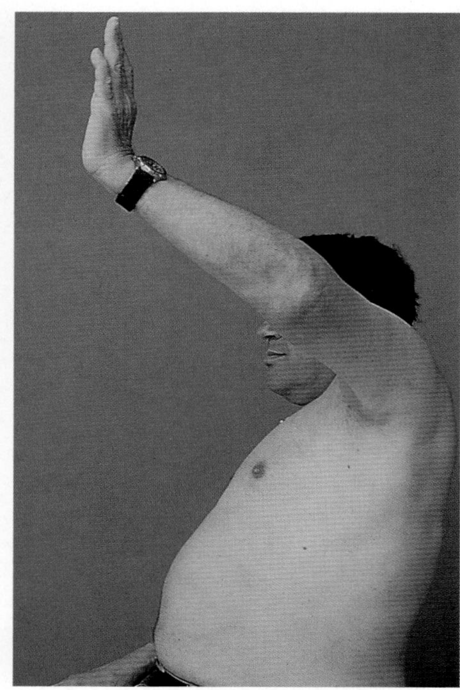
E

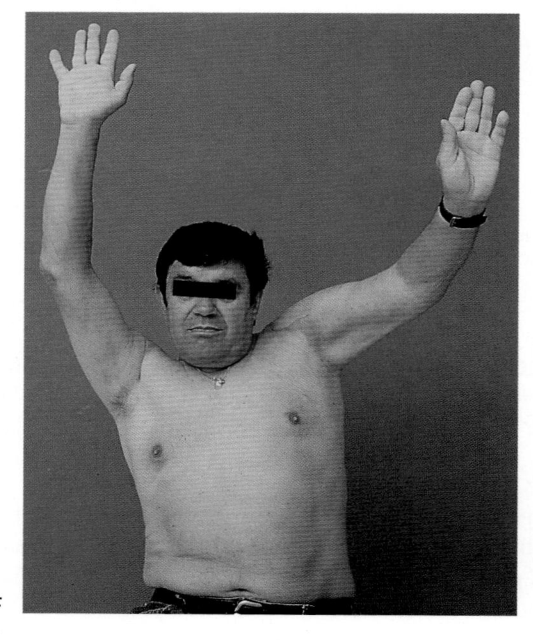
F

FIG. 27. (*Continued*). **(D)** A constrained prosthesis, according to Grammont, is implanted. Already 6 weeks after surgery **(E)**, elevation is 90 and abduction is 95 degrees **(F)**. This implant is only used exceptionally and in relatively old patients with very low functional demands; long-term follow-up is not yet available.

2. Sometimes the glenoid is worn, and passive rotational movements of the arm are painful. Despite the knowledge that rim loading can lead to earlier loosening of a glenoid component, we doubt that the very general agreement that irreparable rotator cuff tear is a formal contraindication against a glenoid component is justified. If the head is centered in the anteroposterior direction, and the glenoid can be implanted in a high position, loosening may occur no earlier than in other shoulders (Fig. 26) and be associated with freedom from pain, which is better than the pain relief reported in the two aforementioned series of hemiarthroplasties.[43,148].

Constrained Shoulder Arthroplasty

Constrained shoulder arthroplasty has again become en vogue in Europe through the work of Grammont,[62] who designed a prosthesis with a convex glenoid and a concave humerus. The glenoid component has its center of rotation in the scapular neck so that a relevant proportion of the stress during motion of the shoulder is applied almost perpendicularly to the noncemented glenoid component. Long-term results of 68 cases are currently being assessed by Molé and Favard (Molé personal communication 1997), and it appears that these results are much better than expected, provided the prosthesis was used in elderly patients with low functional demands.

We do use this prosthesis extremely rarely in elderly patients, with anterosuperior subluxation (Fig. 27) of the humeral head and an intact deltoid, who have relatively low functional demands, but feel very handicapped by their complete pseudoparalysis. Early subjective results are excellent, objective early functional results are good for elevation and abduction, active external rotation is never restored, and we have already had to revise one glenoid component which, however, had been inserted as a revision after a cemented glenoid component. We consider the prosthesis to be an experimental implant.

Other Surgical Alternatives

We have not had experience with freeze-dried cuffs[110] and have only seen cases with synthetic cuffs that need to be revised.[104] Currently, neither of these possibilities seems to be sufficiently promising to continue its use. Shoulder arthrodesis is not discussed in this chapter, but remains an invaluable option in cases of failed cuff with infection, in cases with concomitant cuff disease and nerve injury, and in cases of ir-

Acromiohumeral distance > 7 mm
- *Tear usually reparable*
- *Indications for transfer exceptional*

Antero-superior tear (Lift-off positive, supraspinatus torn but repairable)	"Isolated" irreparable supraspinatus (exceptional!!)	Postero-superior tears (lift-off negative infra and supra torn); usually recent cases
■ Supraspinatus repair + repair lower part subscapularis + pectoralis major transfer (possibly as augmentation of subscapularis repair)	■ Shift of infraspinatus if weak: (possibly) deltoid flap	■ Repair; if quality of supraspinatus and infraspinatus poor. ■ Latissimus dorsi transfer

Acromiohumeral distance < 7, > 5 mm (infraspinatus torn)

Lift-off positive Subscapularis torn		Lift-off negative Subscapularis intact
No fatty degeneration, reparable (elevation often >90°) Subscapularis tendon repair, tenodesis biceps repair, postero-lateral + latissimus dorsi transfer	Fatty degeneration, irreparable (elevation often <90°) - Conservative treatment - Constrained prosthesis in elderly patients - Biceps tenotomy in young painful shoulders	Repair of supraspinatus and infraspinatus If fatty degeneration of infrapinatus is ≥ grade 3 (Goutallier), → Latissimus dorsi transfer

Acromiohumeral distance < 5 mm
- *repair impossible!*

Subscapularis torn (elevation usually <90°)	Subscapularis intact	
	Functional demand ↑	Functional demand ↓
- Conservative Treatment - Biceps tenotomy - Constrained prosthesis for elderly patients - Unconstrained hemiarthroplasty for young patients with cuff tear arthropathy	Latissimus dorsi transfer	- Conservative treatment - Biceps tenotomy

Acromiohumeral distance on an AP radiograph taken without muscular contraction in neutral rotation.

reparable rotator cuff tears with a relevant deltoid injury. We feel that, especially for young persons, shoulder arthrodesis is probably underutilized.

THE FAILED CUFF

There are numerous reasons for failure of repairs of the cuff[80] or persistent pain after rotator cuff surgery.[147] This problem is beyond the scope of this chapter. However, in our opinion, failure is more frequently caused by errors in indication than by errors in surgical execution of a procedure. The surgeon tends to overestimate the potential of repair and is reluctant to accept that there are rotator cuff pathologies that are beyond repair despite all our advancements in the management of this disease. In addition, it is our feeling that the failure to protect the cuff repairs postoperatively is one of the most frequent reasons for recurrent tears, and this concept of aftercare without any immobilization should be revisited.

We think that substantial improvements have been made in the assessment, the surgical treatment, and in the aftercare of the patient with a massive rotator cuff tear. The daily practice, however, teaches that we still have a long way to go before we can reliably predict our results and achieve our goals in all patients.

REFERENCES

1. Adamson GJ, Tibone JE. Ten-year assessment of primary rotator cuff repairs. *J Shoulder Elbow Surg* 1993;2:57–63.
2. Apoil A, Augereau B. Reparation par lambeau déltoidien des grandes pertes de substance de la coiffe des rotateurs. *Chirurgie* 1985;111: 287–290,
3. Apoil A, Dautry P, Moinet P, Koechlin P. Le syndrome dit "de rupture de la coiffe des rotateurs de l'épaule.". A propos de 70 observations. *Rev Chir Orthop* 1977;63(suppl 2):145–149.
4. Armstrong JR. Excision of the acromion in treatment of the supraspinatus syndrome. *J Bone Joint Surg [Br]* 1949;31:436–442.
5. Augereau B Apoil A. La réparation des grandes ruptures de la coiffe des rotateurs de l'épaule. *Rev Chir Orthop* 1988;74(suppl 2):59–62.
6. Augereau B, Koechlin, Moinet PH, Apoil A, Bonnet JC, Doursounian L. L'arthrolyse antéro-supérieure de l'épaule pour lésions trophiques de la coiffe des rotateurs sur tête centrée. *Rev Chir Orthop* 1988;74: 292–296.
7. Barber FA, Cawley P, Prudich JF. Suture anchor failure strength—an in vivo study. *Arthroscopy* 1993;9:647–652.
8. Bartolozzi A, Andreychik D, Ahmad S. Determinants of outcome in the treatment of rotator cuff disease. *Clin Orthop* 1994;90–97.
9. Bassett RW, Browne AO, Morrey B, An KN. Glenohumeral muscle force and moment mechanics in a position of shoulder instability. *J Biomech* 1990;23:405–415.
10. Bassett RW, Cofield RH. Acute tears of the rotator cuff. *Clin Orthop* 1998;175:18–24.
11. Bayley JC, Cochran TP, Sledge CB. The weight-bearing shoulder. The impingement syndrome in paraplegics. *J Bone Joint Surg [Am]* 1987;69:676–678.
12. Bigliani LU, McIlveen SJ, Cordasco F, Musso E. Operative repair of massive rotator cuff tears: long term results. *J Shoulder Elbow Surg* 1992;1:120–130.
13. Bigliani LU, Morrison DS, April EW. The morphology of the acromion and its relationship to rotator cuff tears. *Orthop Trans* 1996; 10:216,
14. Bigliani LU, Ticker JB, Flatow EL, Soslowsky L, Mow VC. The relationship of acromial architecture to rotator cuff disease. *Clin Sports Med* 1991;10:823.
15. Bjorkenheim J-M. Structure and function of the rabbit's supraspinatus muscle after resection of its tendon. *Acta Orthop Scand* 1989;60: 461–463.
16. Blair B, Rokito AS, Cuomo F, Jarolem K, Zuckerman JD. Efficacy of injections of corticosteroid for subacromial impingement syndrome. *J Bone Joint Surg [Am]* 1996;78:1685–1689.
17. Bokor DJ, Hawkins RJ, Huckell GH, Angelo RL, Schickendantz MS. Results of nonoperative management of full-thickness tears of the rotator cuff. *Clin Orthop* 1993;294:103–110.
18. Bonnin M. La radiographie simple dans les ruptures de coiffe. In: Walch G, Noël E, Liotard J-P, eds. *Journées Lyonnaises de l'epaule 1.2.3.avril 1993.* Lyon: Clinique de Chirurgie Orthopédique Centre Hospitalier Lyon Sud; 1993:14–19.
19. Brand PW, Beach RB, Thompson DE. Relative tension and potential excursion of muscles in the forearm and hand. *J Hand Surg* 1997;6: 209–219.
20. Brewer BJ. Aging of the rotator cuff. *Am J Sports Med* 1997;7: 102–110.
21. Brooks CH, Revell WJ, Heatley FW. A quantitative histological study of the vascularity of the rotator cuff tendon. *J Bone Joint Surg [Br]* 1992;74:151–153.
22. Brown JT. Early assessment of supraspinatus tears. Procaine infiltration as a guide to treatment. *J Bone Joint Surg [Br]* 1949;31:423–425.
23. Burkhart SS. Arthroscopic debridement and decompression for selected rotator cuff tears: clinical results, pathomechanics and patient selection based on biomechanical parameters. *Orthop Clin North Am* 1993;24:111–123.
24. Burkhart SS. Arthroscopic treatment of massive rotator cuff tears: clinical results and biomechanical rationale. *Clin Orthop* 1997;267: 45–56.
25. Burkhart SS, Nottage WM, Ogilvie-Harris DJ, Kohn HS, Pachelli A. Partial repair of irreparable rotator cuff tears. *Arthroscopy* 1994;10: 363–370.
26. Caroit M, Rouaud JP, Texier T. Le devenir des ruptures de la coiffe des rotateurs de l'épaule non opérées. *Rev Chir Orthop* 1988;74: 325–326.
27. Cochran TP, Bayley JC. The weight bearing shoulder: the shoulder in paraplegics (abstr). 53rd Annual Meeting of the AAOS, 1986.
28. Codman EA, *The shoulder.* Brooklyn: G Miller & Co; 1934.
29. Codman EA, Akerson IB. The pathology associated with rupture of the supraspinatus tendon. *Ann Surg* 1931;93:348–359.
30. Cofield RH. Subscapular muscle transposition for repair of chronic rotator cuff tears. *Surg Gynecol Obstet* 1982;154:667–672.
31. Cofield RH. Rotator cuff disease of the shoulder. *J Bone Joint Surg [Am]* 1985;67:974–979.
32. Cofield RH, Hoffmeyer P, Lanzer WL. Surgical repair of chronic rotator cuff tears (abstr). 6th Open Meeting of the American Shoulder and Elbow Surgeons, 1990.
33. Colachis SC, Strohm BR, Brechner VL. Effect of suprascapular and axillary nerve blocks on muscle force in upper extremity. *Arch Phys Med Rehabil* 1969;50;nov,647-654.
34. Constant CR, Murley AHG. A clinical method of functional assessment of the shoulder. *Clin Orthop* 1987;214:160–163.
35. Cotty P, Proust F, Bertrand P, et al. Rupture de la coiffe des rotateurs. Quantification des signes indirects en radiologie standard et manoeuvre de Leclercq. *J Radiol* 69:1988;633–638.
36. Dalton SE. The conservative management of rotator cuff disorders. *Br J Rheumatol* 1994;33:663–667.
37. Debeyre J, Patte D, Elmelik E. Repair of ruptures of the rotator cuff of the shoulder. *J Bone Joint Surg [Br]* 1965;47:36–42.
38. Depalma AF. *Surgery of the shoulder.* Philadelphia: JB Lippincott Co; 1983.
39. Dierickx C, Vanhoof H. Massive rotator cuff tears treated by a deltoid muscular inlay flap. *Acta Orthop Belg* 1994;60:94–100.
40. Ellman H, Hanker G, Bayer M. Repair of the rotator cuff. End-result study of factors influencing reconstruction. *J Bone Joint Surg [Am]* 1986;68:1136–1144.
41. Ellman H, Kay SP, Wirth M. Arthroscopic treatment of full-thickness rotator cuff tears: 2–7 year follow-up study. *Arthroscopy* 1993;9: 195–200.
42. Erickson SJ, Fitzgerald SW, Quinn SF, Carrera GF, Black KP, Lawson TL. Long bicipital tendon of the shoulder: normal anatomy and pathologic findings on MR imaging. *AJR. Am J Roentgenol* 1992;158: 1091–1096.

43. Field LD, Dines DM, Zabinski SJ, Warren RF. Hemiarthoplasty of the shoulder for rotator cuff arthropathy. *J Shoulder Elbow Surg* 1997;6: 18–23.
44. Gartsman GM. Arthroscopic acromioplasty for ruptures of the rotator cuff. *J Bone Joint Surg* 1990;72:169–180.
45. Gartsman GM. Massive, irreparable tears of the rotator cuff. results of operative debridement and subacromial decompression. *J Bone Joint Surg [Am]* 1997;79:715–721.
46. Gazielly DF. Deltoid muscle flap transfer for massive defects of the rotator cuff. In: Burkhead WZJ, ed. *Rotator cuff disorders*. Baltimore: Wiliams & Wilkins; 1996:356–367.
47. Gazielly DF, Gleyze P, Montagnon C. Functional and anatomical results after rotator cuff repair. *Clin Orthop* 1994;304:43–53.
48. Gerber C. Latissimus dorsi transfer for the treatment of irreparable tears of the rotator cuff. *Clin Orthop* 1992;275:152–160.
49. Gerber C. Massive rotator cuff tears. In: Kenwright J, Duparc J, Fulford P, eds. *European instructional course lectures*. London: British Editorial Society of Bone and Joint Surgery; 1997:85–89.
50. Gerber C, Farron A, Hersche O. Isolated ruptures of the subscapularis tendon. Results of operative repair. *J Bone Joint Surg [Am]* 1996;78: 1015–1023.
51. Gerber C, Fuchs B. The structural and clinical results of direct repair of massive rotator cuff tears. Presented at the14th meeting of the American Shoulder and Elbow Surgeons, New Orleans, 22.03.98.
52. Gerber C, Hersche O. Tendon transfers for the treatment of irreparable rotator cuff defects. *Orthop Clin North Am* 1997;28:195–203.
53. Gerber C, Krushell RJ. Isolated rupture of the tendon of the subscapularis muscle. Clinical features in 16 cases. *J Bone Joint Surg [Br]* 1991;73:389–394.
54. Gerber C, Schneeberger AG, Beck M, Schlegel U. Mechanical strength of repairs of the rotator cuff. *J Bone Joint Surg [Br]* 1994;76: 371–380.
55. Gerber C, Schneeberger AG, Nyffeler R. Experimental rotator cuff repair. An in-vivo study on 47 sheep. 1997 In press.
56. Gerber C, Vinh TS, Hertel R, Hess CW. Latissimus dorsi transfer for the treatment of massive tears of the rotator cuff; a preliminary report. *Clin Orthop* 1988;232:51–61.
57. Glousman RE, Sigman SA, Vanderwilde RS, Friedman SG, Flannigan BD,Raper PL. Abnormal MRI scans of the shoulder in asymptomatic patients (abstr). Closed Meeting of the ASES, October 20, Amelia Island, 1996:58.
58. Goupille P, Anger C, Cotty P, Fouquet B, Soutif D, Valat JP. Value of standard radiographies in the diagnosis of rotator cuff rupture. *Rev Rhum Ed Fr* 1993;60:440–444.
59. Goutallier D, Bernageau J, Patte D. L'évaluation par le scanner de la trophicité des muscles des coiffes des rotateurs ayant une rupture tendineuse. *Rev Chir Orthop* 1989;75:126–127.
60. Goutallier D, Lavau L, Postel JM. The trapezius flap in nonreinsertable tears of the subscapularis. In: Vastamäki M, Jalovaara P, eds. *Surgery of the shoulder*. Amsterdam: Elsevier; 1995:79–83.
61. Goutallier D, Postel J-M, Bernageau J, Lavau, Voisin M-C. Fatty muscle degeneration in cuff ruptures. *Clin Orthop* 1994;304:78–83.
62. Grammont PM, Baulot E. Delta shoulder prosthesis for rotator cuff rupture. *Orthopedics* 1993;16:65–68.
63. Grana WA, Teague B, King M, Reeves RB. An analysis of rotator cuff repair. *Am J Sports Med* 1994;22:585–588.
64. Greis PE, Kuhn JE, Schultheis J, Hintermeister R, Hawkins RJ. Validation of the lift-off test and analysis of subscapularis activity during maximal internal rotation. *Am J Sports Med* 1996;24:589–593.
65. Groh GI, Rockwood CA. The terrible triad: anterior dislocation of the shoulder associated with rupture of the rotator cuff and injury to the brachial plexus. *J Shoulder Elbow Surg* 1995;4:51–53.
66. Hammond G. Complete acromionectomy in the treatment of chronic tendinitis of the shoulder. *J Bone Joint Surg [Am]* 53:173–180.
67. Harryman DT, Mack LA, Wang KY, Jackins SE, Richardson ML, Matsen FA. Repairs of the rotator cuff. Correlation of functional results with integrity of the cuff. *J Bone Joint Surg [Am]* 1991;73: 982–989.
68. Hattrup SJ. Rotator cuff repair: relevance of patient age. *J Shoulder Elbow Surg* 1995;4:95–100.
69. Hawkins RH, Dunlop R. Nonoperative treatment of rotator cuff tears. *Clin Orthop* 1995;321:178–188.
70. Hawkins RJ, Bell RH, Hawkins RH, Koppert GJ. Anterior dislocation in the older patient. *Clin Orthop* 1986;206:192–195.
71. Hersche O, Gerber C. Passive tension in the musculotendinous unit of the supraspinatus after long standing rupture of its tendon. A preliminary report. *J Shoulder Elbow Surg* 1998;(In press).
72. Hertel R, Ballmer FT, Lambert SM, Gerber C. Lag signs in the diagnosis of rotator cuff rupture. *J Shoulder Elbow Surg* 1996;5:307–313.
73. Herzberg G. Anatomical bases of musculotendinous transfers about the shoulder. *J Shoulder Elbow Surg* 1998;(In press).
74. Hoffer MM, Wickenden R, Roper B. Brachial plexus birth injuries. Results of tendon transfer of the rotator cuff. *J Bone Joint Surg [Am]* 1997;60:691–695.
75. Iannotti JP, Bernot MP, Juhlman JR, Kelley MJ, Williams GR. Postoperative assessment of shoulder function: a prospective study of full thickness rotator cuff tears. *J Shoulder Elbow Surg* 1996;5:449–457.
76. Itoi E, Minagawa H, Sato T, Tabata S. Isokinetic strength after tears of the supraspinatus tendon. *J Bone Joint Surg [Br]* 1997;79:77–82.
77. Jarvholm U, Palmerud G, Styf J, Herberts P. Intramuscular pressure in the supraspinatus muscle. *J Orthop Res* 1988;6:230–238.
78. Jarvholm U, Styf J, Suurkula M, Herberts P. Intramuscular pressure and muscle blood flow in supraspinatus. *Eur J Appl Physiol* 1988;58: 219–224.
79. Jobe FW, Jobe CM. Painful athletic injuries of the shoulder. *Clin Orthop* 1983;173:117–124.
80. Karas EH, Iannotti JP. Failed repair of the rotator cuff. Evaluation and treatment of complications. *J Bone Joint Surg [Am]* 1997;79: 784–793.
81. Karas SE, Giaghello TL. Subscapularis transfer for reconstruction of massive tears of the rotator cuff. *J Bone Joint Surg [Am]* 1996;78: 239–245.
82. Keating JF, Waterworth P, Shaw-Dunn J, Crossan J. The relative strength of the rotator cuff muscles. *J Bone Joint Surg [Br]* 1993;75: 137–140.
83. Kessel L, Watson M. The painful arc syndrome. Clinical classification as a guide to management. *J Bone Joint Surg [Br]* 1997;59:166–172.
84. Kirschenbaum D, Coyle MP Jr, Leddy JP, Katsaros P, Tan F Jr, Cody RP. Shoulder strength with rotator cuff tears. Pre- and postoperative analysis. *Clin Orthop* 1993;288:174–178.
85. Lehuec JC, Liquois F, Schaeverbecke T, Zipoli B, Chauveaux D, Le Rebeller A. Results of a series of deltoid flaps for the treatment of massive rotator cuff tears with an average follow up of 3.5 years. *Rev Chir Orthop* 1997;82:22–28.
86. Lindblom J, Palmer F. Rupture of the tendon aponeurosis of the shoulder joint: the so-called supraspinatus rupture. *Acta Chir Scand* 1939; T1–82:133.
87. Lindh M, Norlin R. Arthroscopic subacromial decompression versus open acromioplasty. A two-year follow-up study. *Clin Orthop* 1993; 290:174–176.
88. Macnab I. Degenerative changes in the rotator cuff of the shoulder. A pathological and clinical study. *Jeff Orthop J* 1974;3:7–20.
89. Mallet J, Rouleau Y. A propos du traitement chirurgical des ruptures de la coiffe tendineuse de l'épaule. *Ann Orthop l'Ouest* 1969;1:27–31.
90. Mansat P, Cofield RH, Kersten TE, Rowland CM. Complications of rotator cuff repair. *Orthop Clin North Am* 1997;28:205–213.
91. Markhede G, Monastyrski J, Stener B. Shoulder function after deltoid muscle removal. *Acta Orthop Scand* 1985;56:242–244.
92. McCarty DJ, Swanson AB, Ehrhart RH. Hemorrhagic rupture of the shoulder. *J Rheumatol* 1994;21:1134–1137.
93. McLaughlin HL. Lesions of the musculotendinous cuff of the shoulder. I. The exposure and treatment of tears with retraction. *J Bone Joint Surg [Am]* 1944;26:31–49.
94. McLaughlin HL. Rupture of the rotator cuff. *J Bone Joint Surg [Am]* 1962;44:979–983.
95. Meyer AW. Further observations upon use—destruction in joints. *J Bone Joint Surg* 1922;4:491–511.
96. Meyer AW. Chronic functional lesions of the shoulder. *Arch Surg* 1937;35:646–674.
97. Middleton WD. Ultrasonography of rotator cuff pathology. *Top Magn Reson Imaging* 1994;6:133–138.
98. Milgrom C, Schaffler M, Gilbert S, Van Holsbeeck M. Rotator-cuff changes in asymptomatic adults. The effect of age, hand dominance and gender. *J Bone Joint Surg [Br]* 1995;77:296–298.
99. Misamore GW, Hobeika PE. Surgery for full-thickness rotator cuff tears. *J Bone Joint Surg [Am]* 1985;67:1349–1355.
100. Montgomery TJ, Yerger B, Savoie FH. Management of rotator cuff tears: a comparison of arthroscopic debridement and surgical repair. *J Shoulder Elbow Surg* 1994;3:71–78.

101. Morrison DS, Bigliani LU. The clinical significance of variations in acromial morphology. *Orthop Trans* 1987;11:234.
102. Moseley HF, Goldie I. The arterial pattern of the rotator cuff of the shoulder. *J Bone Joint Surg [Br]* 1963;45:780–789.
103. Nakagaki K, Ozaki J, Tomita Y, Tamai S. Alterations in the supraspinatus muscle belly with rotator cuff tearing: evaluation with magnetic resonance imaging. *J Shoulder Elbow Surg* 1994;3:88–93.
104. Nasca RJ. The use of freeze-dried allografts in the management of global rotator cuff tears. *Clin Orthop* 1988;228:218–226.
105. Neer CS. Anterior acromioplasty for the chronic impingement syndrome in the shoulder. A preliminary report. *J Bone Joint Surg [Am]* 1972;54:41–50.
106. Neer CS. Impingement lesions. *Clin Orthop* 1981;173:70–77.
107. Neer CS, Craig EV, Fukuda H. Cuff tear arthropathy. *J Bone Joint Surg [Am]* 1982;65:1232–1244.
108. Neer CS, Flatow EL, Lech O. Tears of the rotator cuff. Long term results of anterior acromioplasty and repair. *Orthop Trans* 1988;12:735.
109. Neer CS, Marberry TA. On the disadvantages of radical acromionectomy. *J Bone Joint Surg [Am]* 1981;63:416–419.
110. Neviaser JS, Neviaser RJ, Neviaser TJ. The repair of chronic massive ruptures of the rotator cuff of the shoulder by use of a freeze-dried rotator cuff. *J Bone Joint Surg [Am]* 1978;60:681–684.
111. Neviaser RJ, Neviaser TJ. Transfer of subscapularis and teres minor for massive defects of the rotator cuff. In: Bayley IL, Kessel L, eds. *Shoulder surgery*. Berlin: Springer; 1982:60—63.
112. Noel E. Les ruptures de la coiffe des rotateurs avec tête humérale centrée. Résultats du traitement conservateur. A propos de 171 épaules. *J Lyonnaises l'Epaule* 1993;283–297.
113. Nové-Josserand L, Gerber C, Walch G. Lesions of the anterosuperior rotator cuff. In: Warner JJP, Iannotti JP, Gerber P, eds. *Complex and revision problems in shoulder surgery*. Philadelphia: Lippincott-Raven; 1997:165–176.
114. Otis JC, Jiang CC, Wickiewicz TL, Peterson MGE, Warren RF, Santner TJ. Changes in the moment arms of the rotator cuff and deltoid muscles with abduction and rotation. *J Bone Joint Surg [Am]* 1996;76:667–676.
115. Ozaki J, Fujimoto S, Nakagawa Y, Masuhara K, Tamai S. Tears of the rotator cuff of the shoulder associated with pathological changes in the acromion. A study in cadavera. *J Bone Joint Surg [Am]* 1988;70:1224–1230.
116. Patte D, Debeyre J. Réparation chirurgicale des ruptures de la coiffe. *Ann Orthop l'Ouest* 1969;1:19–25.
117. Patte D, Debeyre J. Essai comparatif de deux séries de ruptures de coiffe opérées et non opérées. *Rev Chir Orthop* 1988;74:327–328.
118. Patte D, Goutallier D, Monpierre H, Debeyre J. Etude des lésions étendues. *Rev Chir Orthop* 1988;74:314–318.
119. Petersson CJ. Degeneration of the gleno-humeral joint. An anatomical study. *Acta Orthop Scand* 1983;54:277–283.
120. Petersson CJ, Gentz CF. Ruptures of the supraspinatus tendon—the significance of distally pointing acromioclavicular osteophytes. *Clin Orthop* 1983;174:143–148.
121. Postel JM, Goutallier D, Lavau L, Bernageau J. Anatomical results of rotator cuff repairs: study of 57 cases controlled by arthrography. *J Shoulder Elbow Surg* 1994;3:S20.
122. Rathbun JB, Macnab I. The microvascular pattern of the rotator cuff. *J Bone Joint Surg [Br]* 1970;52:540—553.
123. Reeves B. Experiments on the tensile strength of the anterior capsular structures of the shoulder in man. *J Bone Joint Surg [Br]* 1968;50:858–865.
124. Rockwood CA, Basmania C, Wirth MA. Nonoperative treatment of full-thickness rotator cuff tears (abstr). Closed Meeting of the ASES, October 20, Amelia Island, 1996:57.
125. Rockwood CA, Burkhead WZ. Management of patients with massive rotator cuff defects by acromioplasty and rotator cuff debridement. *Orthop Trans* 1988;12:190–191.
126. Rockwood CAJ, Williams GR, Burkhead WZ. Debridement of degenerative, irreparable lesions of the rotator cuff. *J Bone Joint Surg [Am]* 1995;77:857–866.
127. Rothman RH, Parke WW. The vascular anatomy of the rotator cuff. *Clin Orthop* 1965;41:176–186.
128. Samilson RL. Rotator cuff tears, management and end results of over 400 cases. *J Bone Joint Surg [Br]* 1980;62:277.
129. Schneeberger AG, Nyffeler R, Gerber C. Structural changes caused by experimental subacromial impingement in the rat. *J Shoulder Elbow Surg* 1997;(In press).
130. Seltzer DG, Kechele P, Basamania C, Rockwood CA. Conservative management of rotator cuff tears. In: Burkhead WZ, ed. *Rotator cuff disorders*. Baltimore: Williams & Wilkins; 1996:258–267.
131. Sher JS, Uribe JW, Posada A, Murphy BJ, Zlatkin MB. Abnormal findings on magnetic resonance images of asymptomatic shoulders. *J Bone Joint Surg [Am]* 1995;77:10–15.
132. Shiino K. Ueber die Bewegungen im Schultergelenk und die Arbeitsleistung der Schultermuskeln. *Arch Anat Physol Abtlg Anat* 1913; Suppl 1:89.
133. Soslowsky LJ, Carpenter JE, Flanagan MS, Thomopoulos S, Yian BS. Effect of overuse coupled with intrinsic or extrinsic modifications on rotator cuff tendons (abstr). Closed Meeting of the ASES, October 18, Amelia Island, 1996:26.
134. Sward L, Hughes JS, Amis A, Wallace WA. The strength of surgical repairs of the rotator cuff. A biomechanical study on cadavers. *J Bone Joint Surg* 1992;74:585–588.
135. Takagishi N. The new operation for the massive rotator cuff rupture. *J Jpn Orthop Assoc* 1978;52:775–80.
136. Takagishi N. Conservative treatment of the ruptures of the rotator cuff. *J Jpn Orthop Assoc* 1978;52:781–787.
137. Uhthoff HK, Sarkar K. Surgical repair of rotator cuff ruptures. The importance of the subacromial bursa. *J Bone Joint Surg [Br]* 1991;73:399–401.
138. Uhthoff HK, Sarkar K. The pathogenesis of rotator cuff disease with special reference to changes at the tendon insertion. In: Vastamäki M, Jalovaara P, eds. *Surgery of the shoulder*. Amsterdam: Elsevier; 1995:59–63.
139. Walch G, Liotard JP, Boileau P, Noel E. Le conflit glénoidien postéro-supérieur: un autre conflit de l'épaule. *Rev Chir Orthop* 1991;77:571–574.
140. Walch G, Madonia G, Pozzi I, Riand N, Levigne C. Arthroscopic tenotomy of the long head of the biceps in rotator cuff ruptures. In: Gazielly DF, Gleyze P, Thomas T, eds. *The cuff*. Paris: Elsevier; 1997:350–355.
141. Walch G, Marechal E, Maupas J, Liotard JP. Traitement des ruptures de la coiffe des rotateurs. Facteurs de pronostic. *Rev Chir Orthop* 1992;78:379–388.
143. Wallace WA, Wiley AM. The long term results of conservative management of full thickness tears of the rotator cuff. *J Bone Joint Surg [Br]* 1986;68:162.
144. Warner JJP, Krushell RJ, Masquelet AC, Gerber C. Anatomy and relationships of the suprascapular nerve: anatomical constraints to mobilization of the supraspinatus and infaspinatus muscles in the management of massive rotator cuff tears. *J Bone Joint Surg [Am]* 1992;74:36–45.
145. Watson M. Major ruptures of the rotator cuff. The results of surgical repair in 89 patients. *J Bone Joint Surg [Br]* 1985;67:618–624.
146. Weiner DS, Macnab I. Superior migration of the humeral head. A radiological aid in the diagnosis of tears of the rotator cuff. *J Bone Joint Surg [Br]* 1970;52:524–527.
147. Williams GR. Painful shoulder after surgery for rotator cuff disease. *J Am Acad Orthop Surg* 1997;5:97–108.
148. Williams GR, Rockwood CA. Hemiarthroplasty in rotator cuff deficient shoulders. *J Shoulder Elbow Surg* 1996;5:362–367.
149. Wirth MA, Rockwood CA. Operative treatment of irreparable rupture of the subscapularis. *J Bone Joint Surg [Am]* 1997;79:722–731.
150. Wilson CL, Duff GL. Pathologic study of degeneration and rupture of the supraspinatus tendon. *Arch Surg* 1943;47:121–135.
151. Yamanaka K, Matsumoto T. The joint side tear of the rotator cuff. *Clin Orthop* 1994;304:66–73.
152. Yamanaka K, Mikasa M. Trapezius transfer. In: Burkhead WZJ, ed. *Rotator cuff disorders*. Baltimore: Williams & Wilkins, 1996:374–379.
153. Zanotti RM, Carpenter JE, Blasier RB, Greenfield MLV, Adler RS, Bromberg MB. The low incidence of suprascapular nerve injury after primary repair of massive rotator cuff tears. *J Shoulder Elbow Surg* 1997;6:258–264.
154. Zuckerman JD, Leblanc J-M, Choueka J, Kummer F. The effect of arm position and capsular release on rotator cuff repair. *J Bone Joint Surg [Br]* 1997;73:402–405.
155. Zvijac JE, Levy HJ, Lemak LJ. Arthroscopic subacromial decompression in the treatment of full thickness rotator cuff tears: a 3- to 6-year follow-up. *Arthroscopy* 1994;10:518–523.

Disorders of the Shoulder: Diagnosis and Management,
edited by Joseph P. Iannotti and Gerald R. Williams, Jr.
Lippincott Williams & Wilkins, Philadelphia © 1999.

CHAPTER 4

Complications of Rotator Cuff Surgery

Gerald R. Williams, Jr.

INTRODUCTION

The term "rotator cuff surgery" is extremely broad and could potentially encompass a variety of surgical procedures. For the purposes of this chapter, *rotator cuff surgery* is defined as arthroscopic or open decompression of the subacromial space with or without rotator cuff repair. There are several causes of continued pain following rotator cuff surgery that are both intrinsic and extrinsic to the shoulder girdle (Table 1).[186] However, not all of these causes are a direct result of the surgical procedure. The complications discussed in this chapter, although not all-inclusive, are directly or indirectly related to subacromial decompression and rotator cuff repair. These complications include acromial stress fracture, persistent subacromial impingement, heterotopic ossification, frozen shoulder, infection, suprascapular nerve injury, axillary nerve injury, deltoid detachment, recurrent rotator cuff tear, and anterosuperior humeral head subluxation.

In general, subacromial decompression and rotator cuff repair are safe procedures, with a low incidence of complications. Mansat and colleagues[113] reviewed the results of 40 reported series of rotator cuff repairs. This represented 2,948 shoulders that were operated on from 1982 to 1985. The incidence of complications in these 2,948 shoulders after operation was 10.5% Table 2 indicates the type and frequency of complications encountered.

According to Mansat and colleagues,[113] complications following rotator cuff repair may be underreported or underappreciated. These authors reported a personal series of 116 rotator cuff repairs.[113] Their combined medical and surgical complication rate was 38% (44 shoulders). If the medical complications are subtracted, the remaining complication rate was 33% (38 shoulders). A major surgical complication that affected the final outcome occurred 23 times in 19 shoulders (16%). These 23 major surgical complications

G. R. Williams, Jr.: Shoulder and Elbow Service, Department of Orthopaedic Surgery, University of Pennsylvania School of Medicine, and Penn Musculoskeletal Institute, Presbyterian Hospital, Philadelphia, Pennsylvania 19104.

TABLE 1. *Causes of persistent shoulder pain after rotator cuff surgery*

Extrinsic shoulder pathology
Brachial plexopathy
Cervical radiculopathy
Long-thoracic neuropathy
Neoplasm
Reflex sympathetic dystrophy
Spinal-accessory neuropathy
Suprascapular neuropathy
Thoracic outlet syndrome
Intrinsic shoulder pathology
Intraarticular
Adhesive capsulitis
Articular cartilage defect
Bicipital tendinitis
Instability
Labral tears
Osteoarthritis
Extraarticular
Acromioclavicular arthropathy
Deltoid insufficiency
Rotator cuff defect
Subacromial impingement

From ref. 186, with permission.

comprised failure of tendon healing (17), frozen shoulder (3), deep infection (2), and anterosuperior humeral head dislocation (1). Mansat and colleagues[113] defined failure of tendon healing clinically as an inability to actively flex more than 120 degrees in the absence of stiffness. It is possible that the rate of rerupture or failure of tendon healing would have been higher if postoperative rotator cuff imaging had been employed.

Most studies report the results of the procedure, but do not specifically discuss the incidence of surgical complications. When complications of rotator cuff surgery are reported, they typically take the form of case reports or a series of patients with a given complication who were treated by a particular surgeon over a certain time peroid. There is often no knowledge of the number of patients who were treated successfully during the same period and, therefore, no knowledge of the true incidence of a particular complication. To a certain extent, each complication has its own incidence and etiologic factors. These will be discussed in the following section individually.

TABLE 2. *Incidence of postsurgical complications following rotator cuff surgery**

Complication	No. of shoulders (%)
Failed tendon repair	182 (6.2)
Nerve injury	33 (1.1)
Infection	31 (1.1)
Deltoid avulsion	16 (0.5)
Frozen shoulder	16 (0.5)
Suture granuloma	14 (0.5)
Wound hematoma	11 (0.4)
Dislocation	3 (0.1)
Reflex dystrophy	2 (0.1)
Greater tuberosity fracture	1
Acromion fracture	1
Total	310 (10.5)

* Complications reported in 40 series of patients undergoing surgical repairs for rotator cuff tears.[12–28,31–42] The series were published between 1982 and 1995; they included 2948 operated shoulders.

From ref. 113, with permission.

ETIOLOGY AND PREVENTION

Acromial Stress Fracture

Although fracture of the acromion could theoretically occur following either open or arthroscopic acromioplasty, it has only been reported following arthroscopic subacromial decompression.[117,147] The overall incidence is unknown. However, Paulos and colleagues[147] reported 1 case in 80 subacromial decompressions, not all of which included bone resection as part of the decompression. Etiologic risk factors that have been identified include osteopenia and overzealous bone resection.[117] The technique of arthroscopic acromioplasty is difficult to master and has a steep learning curve.[1,3,34,46–499,57,105,147] In addition, because arthroscopic surgery involves operating in three dimensions while visualizing in two dimensions, intraoperative appreciation of the amount of bone resection may be difficult, even for experienced surgeons.

The risk of acromial stress fracture following arthroscopic acromioplasty can be minimized by maintaining as much of the thickness of the acromion as possible while still removing the subacromial spur. There is no predetermined amount of bone to resect in all patients with subacromial impingement. In fact, it is likely that the amount of bone to be removed will vary depending on the size of the spur as well as the size of the acromion (i.e., patient). Furthermore, recent studies[13,53,96] have suggested that, acromial spur and size being equal, the amount of bone resection required to relieve abnormal subacromial contact may be small. There is probably an optimal range of bone resection that will both relieve impingement and minimize the risk of postoperative acromial fracture. Bone resections on either side of that range (i.e., too much or too little) may produce a higher percentage of poor results because of either acromial stress fracture or persistent impingement.

Preoperative radiographic assessment of acromial morphology should be used to provide an estimate of the amount of bone to be removed intraoperatively. The supraspinatus outlet view has been advocated by many authors as the best view to evaluate subacromial spurring.[122,126,127,132] Other authors have recommended a standing anteroposterior (AP) view with 30-degree–caudal tilt to determine anterior prominence of the acromion.[37,157] It is important to remember that the acromial spur occurs in more than one plane. For an anterior acromial spur to produce purely an inferior prominence, it would have to make a right angle with the anterior acromion. Likewise, straight anterior extension of the acromion is probably not clinically relevant, because the humeral head and rotator cuff could never make contact with it. Therefore, the best estimate of acromial spur size is actually the hypotenuse of the right triangle defined by the anterior and inferior extensions of the acromion (Fig. 1).[102] Use of both the outlet and 30-degree–caudal tilt views is recommended to provide the most preoperative information about spur size and acromial thickness.

Although many specific surgical techniques have been described to perform arthroscopic anterior acromioplasty, they differ primarily by which portal is used to perform acromial resection.[1,3,34,46,49,57,162] Acromioplasty may be performed by using a midlateral or anterolateral portal for visualization and a straight posterior portal for acromial resection, or by using a posterior or posterolateral portal for visualization and an anterolateral or midlateral portal for acromial resection. Overzealous bone resection can result from either technique. However, the mechanism is different depending on which operative portal is used.

Techniques that use a posterior portal for acromial resection key off the posterior third of the acromion as a template. The arthroscopic burr is introduced into the posterior portal parallel to the undersurface of the posterior acromion, which is used as a cutting block to progressively flatten the acromion from posterior to anterior.[34,163] If the posterior acromion and the arthroscopic burr are convergent, rather than parallel, it is possible to remove more of the anterior acromion than anticipated, which could weaken it and lead to postoperative stress fracture (Fig. 2). This complication can be minimized by recognizing the convergence of the posterior acromion and arthroscopic burr and adjusting the angle of resection accordingly, or by replacing the instrument through a different, more parallel posterior portal.

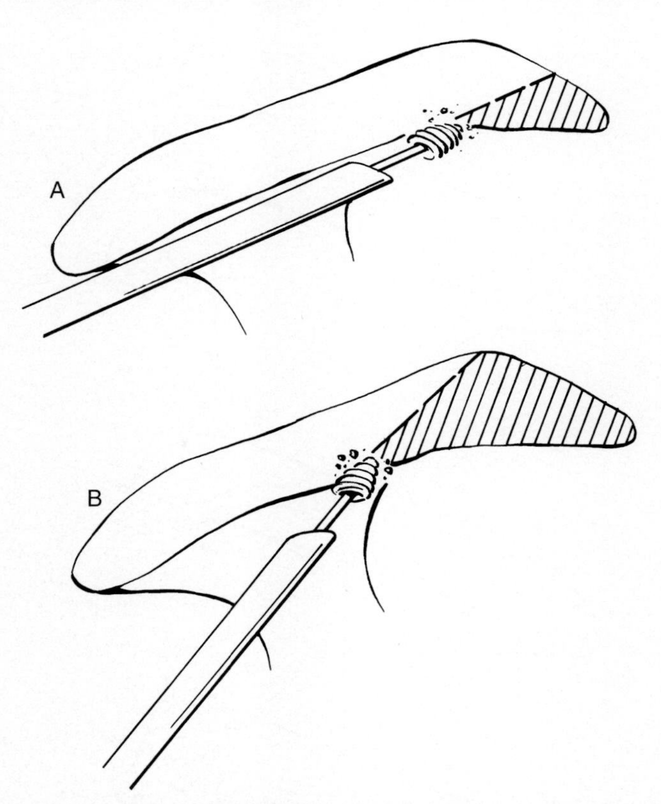

FIG. 2. Arthroscopic acromioplasty techniques that use a posterior portal for bone resection use the undersurface of the posterior third of the acromion as a template. **(A)** If the arthroscopic burr enters the subacromial space parallel to the undersurface of the posterior acromion, the anterior acromial resection produces a flat residual acromion with maximal thickness. **(B)** If the plane of the burr and the acromion are convergent, the additional bone removed leaves a thinner anterior acromion that may be prone to stress fracture.

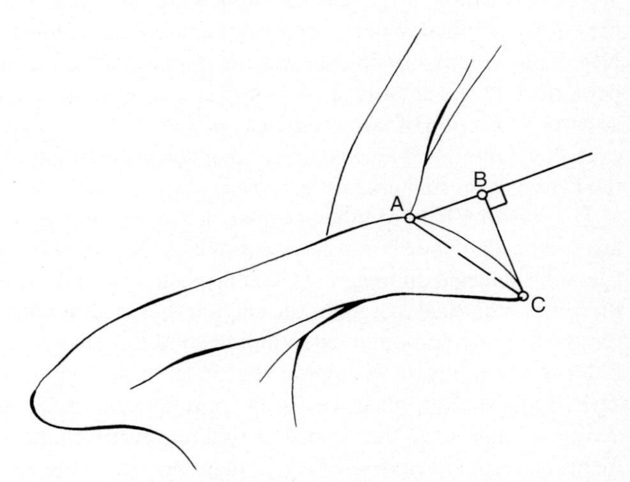

FIG. 1. The best estimate of acromial spur size is the hypoteneuse (*AC*) of the right triangle formed by three points: *A*, the point on the acromion that intersects an imaginary line drawn laterally from the anterior cortical border of the clavicle; *C*, the most inferior point on the anterior edge of the acromion; and *B*, the point on a line drawn parallel to the dorsal surface of the acromion through point *A* that intersects a perpendicular line drawn from point *C* to the first line.

Acromial resection through a midlateral or anterolateral portal requires that the arthroscopic burr sweep from anterior to posterior. It is important to remember that the amount of bone resected, or the depth of penetration of the burr, should be greatest at the anterior acromial margin and progressively tapered to zero at the posterior border of the acromioclavicular joint. Failure to remember this technical point may result in more resection of bone slightly posterior to the anterior edge, rather than on the anterior acromial edge. This will result in a thinner, C-shaped acromion that may be prone to stress fracture (Fig. 3). Care should also be taken to preserve at least 50% of the thickness of the anterior acromion. This can be accomplished by performing the acromioplasty in two stages. First, a full-thickness resection of a small portion of the anterior acromion, determined by extending a line laterally from the anterior cortical margin of the clavicle, is performed. This is followed by beveling the remaining acromion from anterior to posterior. The known thickness of

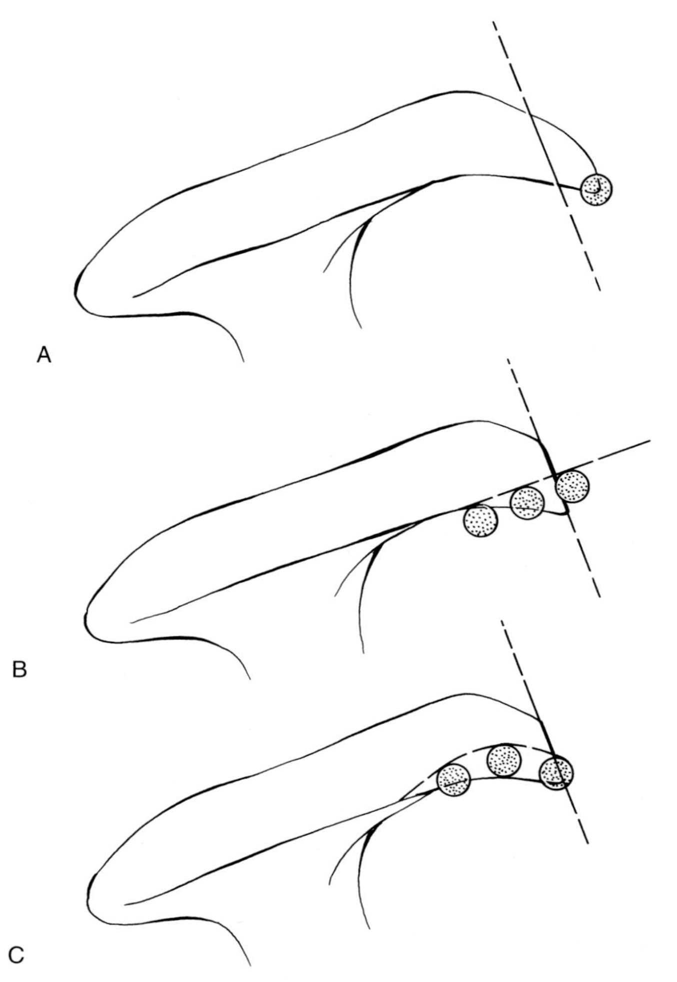

FIG. 3. Arthroscopic techniques that use an anterolateral portal for bone resection may also result in inappropriate bone resection. **(A)** The first step of the acromioplasty involves full-thickness resection of a small portion of the anterior acromion. **(B)** The remaining acromion is then beveled from anterior to posterior to produce a flat undersurface. If care is not taken to ensure that maximum bone resection occurs at the anterior acromial edge, a thinner C-shaped acromion may result. **(C)** The resultant acromion may be prone to stress fracture.

the arthroscopic burr is used to measure the thickness of the residual anterior acromion so that approximately 50% remains following the acromioplasty (see Fig. 3).

Persistent Subacromial Impingement

Persistent impingement following rotator cuff surgery is the result of inadequate supraspinatus outlet decompression. It has been reported to occur because of residual anterior acromial spurring,[55,84,142,158] inferiorly projecting acromioclavicular osteophytes,[126] and persistence or regrowth of the coracoacromial ligament.[126,142,158] Persistent subacromial impingement has been reported in 18% to 79% of patients with failed acromioplasty.[55,84,142,158,186] However, the actual incidence of inadequate supraspinatus outlet decompression or persistent impingement following acromioplasty is unknown.

The optimal amount of acromial resection to relieve painful subacromial contact has been debated for as long as supraspinatus outlet narrowing has been recognized as a pathologic condition. Sir Reginald Watson-Jones is credited with the first acromial excision for "supraspinatus tendon lesions."[5,184] His technique involved resection of the acromion beginning from a point "⅓ in. to the outer side of the acromioclavicular joint" and extending laterally. The most medial portion of the acromion as well as the acromioclavicular joint were preserved.[184] Although Watson-Jones stated that, in some cases, he had excised the entire acromion, including its clavicular articulating surface, it was Armstrong[5] who first emphasized that the residual medial acromion could be responsible for persistent symptoms. Therefore, he recommended that the entire acromion be excised in cases of chronic "supraspinatus syndrome."[5] Although radical and lateral acromionectomy have been advocated by some authors,[21,43,76,77,118,123,171] they remove more bone than is necessary to relieve subacromial impingement and have been associated with significant complications.[130]

Neer's dissatisfaction with the results of radical and lateral acrominectomy prompted him to investigate the role of the anterior acromion in the pathophysiology of impingement syndrome.[126,127] In his observation of 100 cadaver scapulae, Neer noted a "characteristic ridge of proliferative spurs and excrescences" on the undersurface of the anterior acromion.[127] In all cases, the posterior third of the acromion was spared of spurs and bony irregularities. Therefore, Neer recommended removal of a wedge of bone consisting of the anterior edge and lateral portion of the undersurface of the anterior acromion. It is clear from reviewing the text and figures of the original manuscripts that the intended purpose of Neer's anterior acromioplasty was not only to flatten the undersurface of the anterior acromion, but also to remove any anterior projection of the acromial spur (Fig. 4).[126–128] However, Neer cautioned against removal or shortening of any of the native or normal anterior acromion.[126]

The junction between the "normal" acromion and the anterior acromial spur is not always obvious. Rockwood and Lyons[157] selected an imaginary line projected laterally from the anterior cortical margin of the clavicle and recommended removal of any acromion extending beyond this line, in addition to beveling or flattening the undersurface (Fig. 5). They suggested an open, two-step technique in which the acromion anterior to the clavicle is first removed and the remaining acromial undersurface is then beveled. However, the same end result can be obtained using a single osteotomy.[128] In most instances, to make the undersurface of the anterior acromion parallel to the undersurface of the posterior third of the acromion, some portion of the anterior acromion (i.e., spur) will be resected. The boundary of this resection may not always coincide with the anterior cortical margin of the clavicle, but it is usually close. Therefore, the

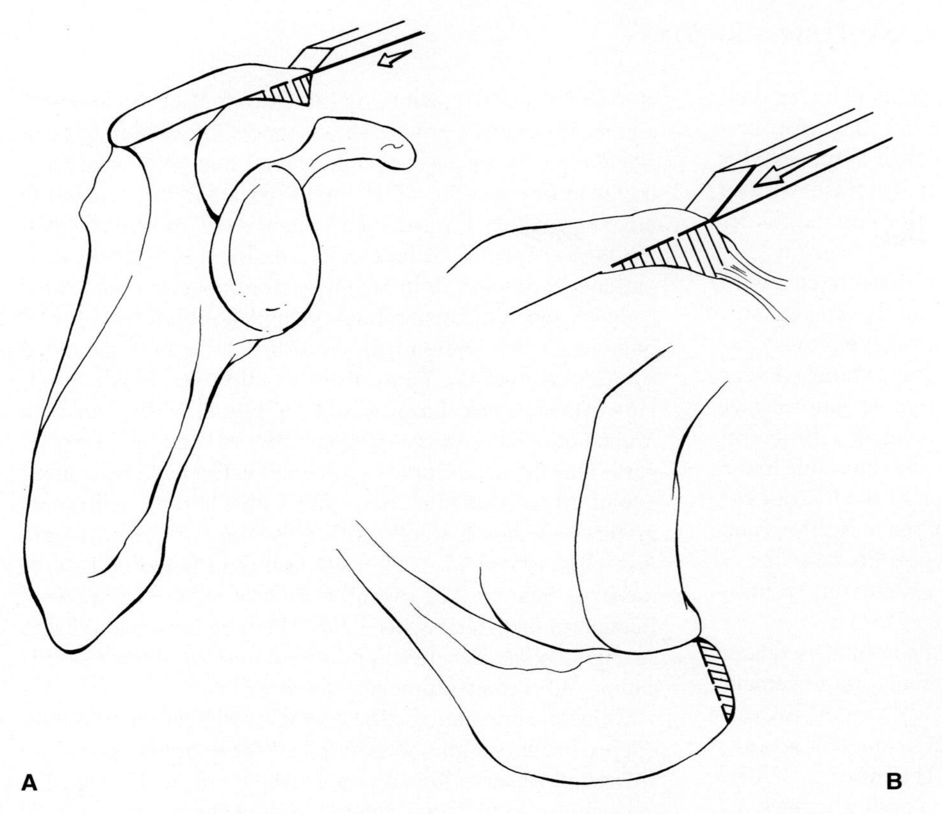

FIG. 4. Neer recommended anterior acromioplasty for refractory impingement syndrome. **(A,B)** The original figures depicted removal of the anterior acromial spur with an osteotome. They also demonstrated excision of enough of the anterior acromial edge (i.e., shortening the anteroposterior dimension) to remove the spur. Neer, however, cautioned against shortening the native acromion.[126]

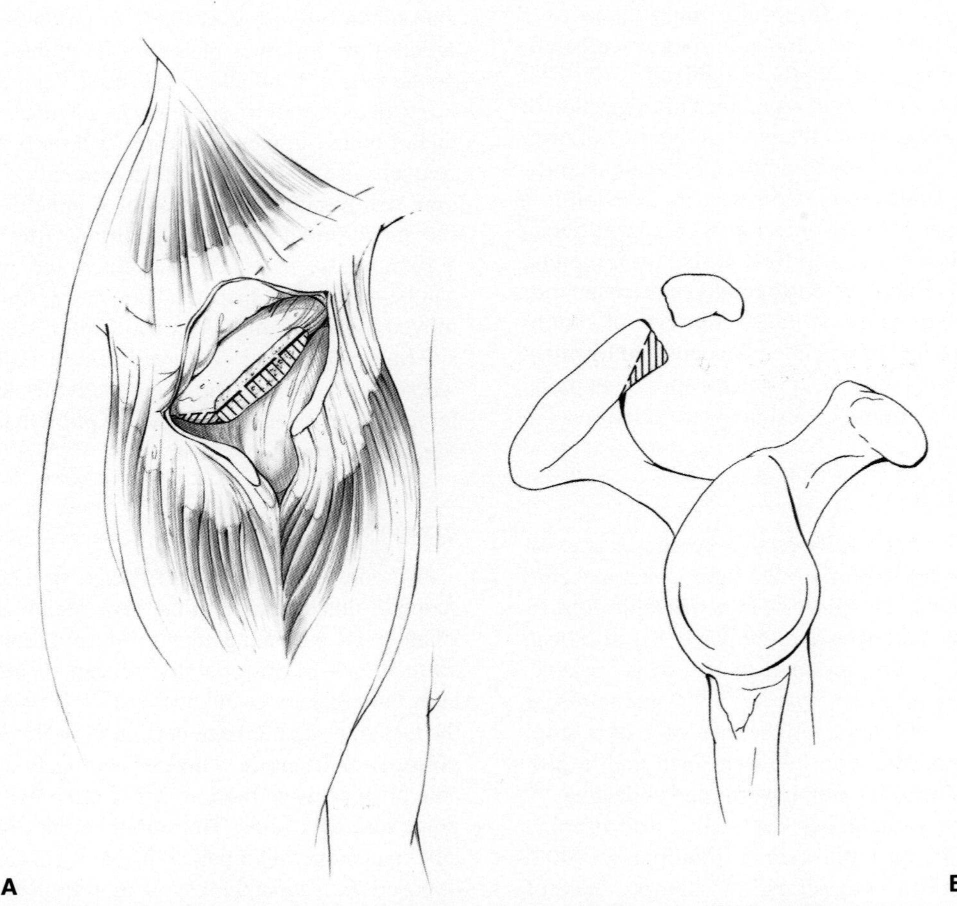

FIG. 5. (A,B) The two-step open acromioplasty technique recommended by Rockwood and Lyons[157] involves a full-thickness resection of the anterior acromion in line with the anterior cortical margin of the clavicle, followed by beveling the remaining acromial undersurface.

likelihood of persistent impingement related to residual acromial spurring can frequently be minimized by resecting enough of the undersurface and anterior edge of the anterior acromion to produce a flat inferior acromial surface, with an anterior edge that approximates the anterior cortical border of the clavicle.[128,157]

Inferiorly projecting osteophytes associated with acromioclavicular arthritis may also cause persistent impingement.[126] This can be avoided by identifying these patients preoperatively and addressing the acromioclavicular joint at the time of the original subacromial decompression. The acromioclavicular joint can be managed with lateral clavicle excision, if there are also symptoms referrable to the acromioclavicular joint, or with resection of the inferior osteophytes alone. A detailed discussion of the indications and techniques of lateral clavicle excision is beyond the scope of this chapter. The reader is referred to the chapter on acromioclavicular joint abnormalities (see Chap. 27).

Persistence or regrowth of the coracoacromial ligament has been reported to be a cause of continued impingement following subacromial decompression.[126,142,158] However, most often, the persistent coracoacromial ligament is accompanied by a persistent acromial spur.[158] Therefore, it is difficult to know the independent contribution of this ligament to continued symptoms. In addition, its importance as a humeral head containment mechanism in rotator cuff-deficient shoulders is being increasingly recognized.[54,106,120,185] In patients with an intact or small reparable cuff, resection of a portion of the coracoacromial ligament at the time of original acromioplasty is not likely to produce clinically significant anterosuperior subluxation. However, its excision in a patient with an irreparable cuff defect or with a large defect that is difficult to repair and, therefore, at risk for rerupture, may increase the likelihood of postoperative anterosuperior subluxation.[185] In these patients, the relative risk of continued impingement from a persistent coracoacromial ligament must be balanced with the risk of anterosuperior humeral subluxation when performing the original cuff repair.

Heterotopic Ossification

Heterotopic ossification involving the shoulder is unusual and is most often related to burns, brain injury, or spinal cord injury.[2,149,161,176] However, heterotopic ossification following both arthroscopic and open acromioplasty has also been reported.[5,11,12,77,105,188] The reported incidence is variable, with a range of 3.2% to 30%.[5,11,12,77,105,188] Although Berg and Ciullo[11] noted no difference in the incidence of postoperative heterotopic ossification between open and arthroscopic methods of bone resection, Lazarus and colleagues[105] noted a much higher incidence following arthroscopic acromioplasty compared with open acromioplasty—30% compared with 10%. In both series,[11,105] the presence of postoperative heterotopic ossification was associated with a worse result.

The etiology of heterotopic ossification following acromioplasty is probably multifactorial. Neer[128] cautioned against the use of a power burr or handheld rasp during open acromioplasty because it could spread morseled bone fragments throughout the subacromial space and could result in bone formation. Lazarus and colleagues[105] postulated that the high incidence of heterotopic ossification seen in their patients following arthroscopic acromioplasty could have been the result of subacromial or subdeltoid implantation of bone fragments created with the arthroscopic burr and aided by the arthroscopic pump used to improve visualization. However, because Lazarus and colleagues[105] did not take immediate postoperative radiographs, an alternative explanation for the heterotopic ossification could have been inadequate bone resection. Berg and Ciullo[11] obtained radiographs less than 8 weeks after either open or arthroscopic acromioplasty in 17 of their 40 cases and noted no heterotopic ossification. The overall incidence of heterotopic ossification in their series was 3.2%. These authors also noted a strong association between postoperative heterotopic ossification and chronic pulmonary disease.[11]

Complete prevention of heterotopic ossification following open or arthroscopic acromioplasty may not be possible. However, observation of some simple surgical principles may minimize the occurrence of this postoperative complication. An osteotome is likely to produce fewer bone fragments than a power burr or a handheld rasp.[128] When a power burr or handheld rasp is used, frequent irrigation with large quantities of irrigant may help reduce the number of retained bone fragments. During arthroscopic acromioplasty, frequent use of the suction attachment on the arthroscopic burr will minimize the amount of bone debris deposited in the subacromial space. In addition, after the arthroscopic acromioplasty has been completed, the subacromial space can be thoroughly inspected and any visible bone debris removed by suctioning. Berg and Ciullo[11] recommended considering prophylactic indomethacin or radiation in patients with a history of ankylosing spondylitis, hypertrophic pulmonary osteoarthropathy, chronic pulmonary disease, smoking, or hypertrophic arthritis.

Frozen Shoulder

A complete discussion of frozen shoulder is beyond the scope of this chapter and the interested reader is referred to Chapter 15, on management of the stiff shoulder. The overall incidence of postoperative frozen shoulder following rotator cuff surgery is unknown. This is primarily because of the lack of a standardized definition of frozen shoulder in the postoperative setting. There is obviously a range of acceptable postoperative motion that is often used to evaluate and grade surgical results. The amount of motion loss required to label a postoperative patient as having a frozen shoulder, as opposed to acceptable loss of motion, has not been consistently defined. The likelihood of encountering frozen shoulder following rotator cuff surgery, however, is much greater in patients who exhibit significant contracture preoperatively.[128] Patients with other medical conditions that are known to be associated with frozen shoulder, such as diabetes mellitus and hypothyroidism,[22,124,135,138,141,181] are also at increased risk of developing postoperative stiffness following rotator cuff surgery.

Shoulder stiffness following rotator cuff surgery is often the result of combined capsular and extracapsular factors. Capsular fibrosis may be localized or generalized. Generalized capsular contracture following surgery for rotator cuff disease is uncommon unless there was an element of generalized adhesive capsulitis preoperatively, prolonged postoperative immobilization, or a predisposing factor for the development of frozen shoulder such as diabetes mellitus, hypothyroidism, or subclinical glenohumeral arthritis. Conversely, localized capsular contracture, especially involving the posterior capsule, is common in subacromial impingement syndrome and rotator cuff disease.[114–116] If it is not addressed through stretching exercises preoperatively or through capsular release intraoperatively, posterior capsular contracture may persist following rotator cuff surgery and contribute to continued pain and dysfunction.

Extracapsular contracture following acromioplasty alone or in combination with cuff repair may result from postoperative adhesion formation between the raw cancellous undersurface of the acromion and the rotator cuff.[121,128] These subacromial adhesions can interfere with normal shoulder motion and function. In addition, reattachment and successful healing of the supraspinatus tendon, particularly if the rotator interval accompanies it, to an excessively medial position on the humeral head may lead to permanent loss of motion and, therefore, is a potential source of extracapsular contracture.

One of the most important principles to follow to prevent or minimize the occurrence of postoperative frozen shoulder is to avoid performing rotator cuff surgery on stiff shoulders.[114,127,128,157] Preoperative capsular contractures should be addressed with capsular stretching exercises before performing rotator cuff surgery. With recalcitrant stiffness, consideration should even be given to closed manipulation or arthroscopic capsular release[150,181] and continued physiotherapy before performing rotator cuff surgery.

Infection

Data relative to infection following rotator cuff surgery are sparse. However, the incidence of infection following arthroscopy has been reported to be approximately 0.4%.[6,15,170] Risk factors include patient age, coexistent medical problems such as diabetes mellitus, and technical issues related to instrument sterilization and operative time. It is likely that the incidence and associated risk factors of infection following rotator cuff surgery are similar to arthroscopic surgery. Postoperative infection following rotator cuff surgery is difficult to manage and often is associated with rotator cuff repair failure, permanent loss of motion or function, and a compromised result. Therefore, the most prudent treatment is prevention.[40,164]

The efficacy of prophylactic antibiotics in the prevention of postoperative infection following rotator cuff surgery has not been as extensively studied as in joint replacement surgery. However, at least for rotator cuff repair, some of the relevant issues are the same. Even if permanent implants, such as suture anchors, are not used, nonabsorbable sutures are commonly employed. These sutures are typically braided, which provides an increased surface area for potential bacterial adherence. Although widespread use of prophylactic antibiotics may be associated with the emergence of resistant bacterial strains, the potential cost of treatment and permanent sequelae associated with an infection following rotator cuff repair provide a strong argument for the use of prophylactic antibiotics. The most common organism is reported to be *Staphylococcus aureus*.[70] Therefore, the most common prophylactic agents utilized are the first-generation cephalosporins such as cefazolin.[164]

In addition to the use of prophylactic antibiotics, adherence to some simple surgical principles may also reduce the incidence of postsurgical infections. There are several techniques available for rotator cuff repair and subacromial decompression; some are more complicated than others and require a different level of surgical experience. The amount of time the surgical wound is open and, therefore, the infection risk should be minimized. In addition, operating room traffic should be minimized and, if arthroscopic equipment is sterilized by soaking in 2% glutaraldehyde, soaking time should be at least 20 minutes and the solution should be warm.[164]

Suprascapular Nerve Injury

The course of the suprascapular nerve after it leaves the superior trunk of the brachial plexus makes it vulnerable to potential direct and indirect injury during rotator cuff repair.[18,145,183] The nerve reaches the dorsal surface of the scapula by passing through the scapular notch, beneath the transverse scapular ligament. It innervates the supraspinatus muscle, then continues around the spinoglenoid notch to enter the infraspinatus fossa, where it innervates the infraspinatus muscle.[18,145,183] At the superior aspect of the glenoid, the branches of the suprascapular nerve that supply the supraspinatus are approximately 3 cm medial to the origin of the long head of the biceps; at the midportion of the glenoid, the branches to the infraspinatus are approximately 2 cm medial to the posterior glenoid rim.[183]

During mobilization and lateral advancement of retracted rotator cuff tears, the capsule may be incised to relieve its tenodesis effect on the overlying rotator cuff musculotendinous unit. Direct injury to the branches of the suprascapular nerve can be avoided by limiting the amount of medial dissection that occurs through the capsulotomy in the interval between the rotator cuff muscles and the scapula. In addition, the suprascapular nerve is tethered proximally at the scapular notch.[183] Therefore, indirect injury to the nerve may occur through traction on the free, retracted edge of the supraspinatus and infraspinatus tendons. According to Warner and colleagues,[183] safe lateral advancement of either the supraspinatus or infraspinatus tendon is limited by the neurovascular bundle to 1 cm. This safe zone can be increased to 3 cm if the muscle belly is also released from the underlying fossa and allowed to advance laterally with the tendon.[141,183]

Extrapolation of Warner and colleagues data,[183] which were obtained in cadavers without retracted cuff tears, to the clinical situation is difficult. Lateral mobilization of more than 1 cm may be possible when a retracted supraspinatus or infraspinatus musculotendinous unit is restored to its original, premorbid length. Conversely, it is probably not possible to restore a chronically retracted musculotendinous unit to its premorbid length without placing more tension on the neurovascular bundle than was present in the premorbid state. Therefore, the concept of limiting the amount of lateral advancement of chronic, retracted rotator cuff tears during repair is valid, even if the safe limit for advancement is unknown.

Suprascapular nerve injury following rotator cuff repair has been sparsely reported.[67,190] Zanotti and coworkers[190] reported on ten patients who underwent acromioplasty and rotator cuff repair, without muscular advancement,[41] for massive tears. All patients had postoperative electromyography; one of ten (10%) patients had suprascapular nerve injury. Goutallier and colleagues[67] reported electromyographically proved postoperative suprascapular nerve injury in 7 of 24 (29%) patients undergoing repair with muscular advancement for large and massive defects. In 1 patient, the suprascapular nerve was abnormal on preoperative electromyography. Two of the remaining 6 patients with positive postoperative electromyography did not have preoperative studies for comparison. Although the rate of suprascapular nerve injury following rotator cuff repair appears to be low,[67,190] postoperative electromyography, even in patients with continued weakness, is rarely reported. Consequently, the true incidence of iatrogenic suprascapular nerve injury during rotator cuff repair may be higher than reported.

Axillary Nerve Injury

The axillary nerve reaches the posterior aspect of the shoulder by passing through the quadrangular space with the posterior humeral circumflex artery. After giving off a cutaneous branch and a motor branch to the teres minor, the axillary nerve courses from posterior to anterior on the deep surface of the deltoid, which it innervates.[23,29,30,45,88,103,108,111] The distance from the lateral edge of the acromion to the axillary nerve is thought to be 5 cm.[88,111] However, Burkhead and associates[29] have demonstrated that this distance is subject to significant individual variation and is dependent on the size of the arm (i.e., patient). In one cadaver specimen, the axillary nerve was 3.5 cm from the edge of the acromion. Burkhead and associates[29] also reported that the distance between the lateral acromial margin and the axillary nerve could decrease by as much as 30% with abduction of the humerus.

During the superior, deltoid-splitting approach commonly used for rotator cuff repair, the axillary nerve can be injured by either direct laceration or by traction during overzealous retraction of the deltoid.[23,29,71,126–128] When this occurs, the entire deltoid anterior to the point of injury is dennervated, which uniformly produces significant disability[71]. Axillary nerve injury during rotator cuff repair is easily avoided by limiting the distal extent of the deltoid split. Even in small persons, a deltoid split of 3 cm or less should avoid axillary nerve injury.[29] If more distal exposure is necessary, palpation of the deep surface of the deltoid will allow identification of the axillary nerve, which can then be protected (Fig. 6). Neer recommended placement of a suture at the apex of the deltoid split to prevent distal propagation and axillary nerve injury during retraction of the deltoid for rotator cuff repair.[29,126–128]

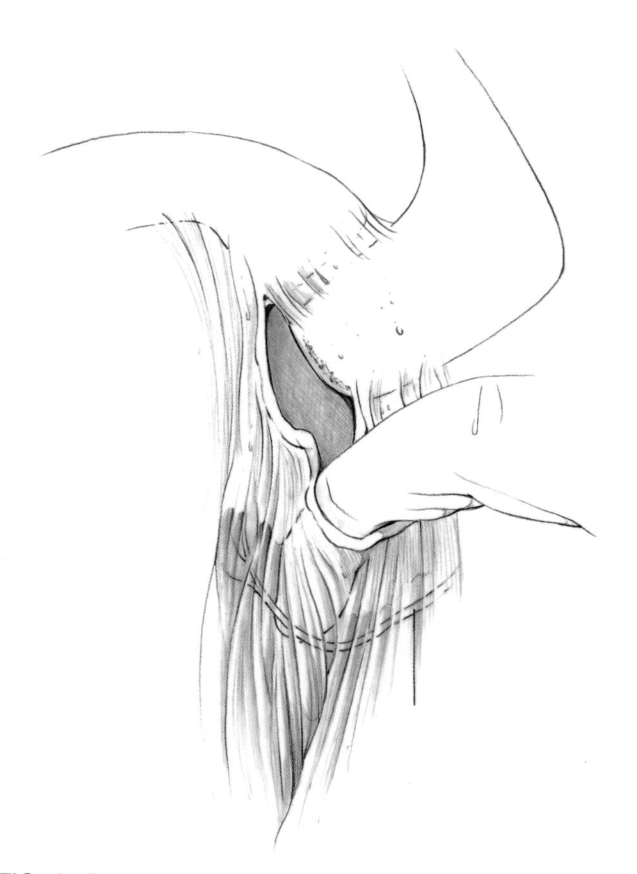

FIG. 6. Digital palpation of the deep surface of the deltoid can be used to identify the axillary nerve so that the deltoid split does not extend distal enough to cause injury to the nerve.

Deltoid Detachment

Detachment of the deltoid origin is a potentially devastating complication of rotator cuff surgery.[14,42,71,130,139,167,186] Because the deltoid origin encompasses the entire acromial surface, detachment of the deltoid origin could theoretically occur following either open or arthroscopic rotator cuff surgery.[104] However, it has been reported only following open acromioplasty.[14,42,71,130,139,167] Postoperative deltoid detachment may be the result of poor intraoperative management of the deltoid, poor tissue quality, overzealous acromial excision, postoperative infection, and inappropriate postoperative physiotherapy.[71,130,133,167] Poor prognostic factors associated with deltoid detachment include lateral acromionectomy, involvement of the middle deltoid, and a recurrent or persistent massive rotator cuff defect.[14,130,167]

The risk of postoperative deltoid detachment following open rotator cuff surgery can be minimized by observing several surgical principles. The fibers of the middle or lateral deltoid are oriented perpendicular to the lateral edge of the acromion, whereas the anterior deltoid fibers arise obliquely from the anterior acromion (Fig. 7). Therefore, deltoid-splitting approaches that either spare the deltoid origin completely or spare the middle deltoid origin by exploiting the interval between the perpendicularly oriented middle deltoid fibers and the obliquely oriented anterior deltoid fibers theoretically may be associated with fewer deltoid detachments and less retraction when detachment of the deltoid does occur.[56,114,119,169] However, repair of large or massive rotator cuff defects that extend into the infraspinatus and teres minor may require more extensive exposure than is possible with these conservative, deltoid-sparing approaches.[16]

Intraoperative management of the deltoid is an important factor in preventing postoperative deltoid detachment. The manner in which the deltoid origin is reflected from the acromion may have a direct influence on the quality of the deltoid repair. When the deltoid split is extended proximally to reflect the anterior deltoid, the incision should be placed at the anterior acromial edge or on the most anterior portion of the dorsal surface of the acromion to ensure a strong distal musculotendinous cuff of tissue for reattachment.[157] It is safest to err on making the incision too proximal, rather than too distal. As long as the distal musculotendinous cuff is adequate, it can always be repaired to bone. I attempt to avoid detachment of the middle deltoid, if possible. However, if more posterior exposure is required, and any of the middle deltoid origin is reflected, it should be detached in a fashion similar to the anterior deltoid origin. Following cuff repair, all portions of the deltoid origin that were reflected are repaired securely. The deep deltoid fascia, which has a tendency to retract distally after detachment, should be identified and incorporated into the repair. Tendon-to-tendon repair is possible if adequate soft-tissue exists proximally and distally. When the tendon quality is deficient proximally, the deltoid is repaired to the bone of the acromion.

One of the most difficult situations to salvage is deltoid detachment in the setting of prior lateral or radical acromionectomy.[14,130,157,168] Although good results have been reported following radical acromionectomy,[21,43,75–77,184] when the postoperative complication of deltoid detachment occurs it can be extremely disabling and irretrievable.[14,130,167] In addition, complete excision of the acromion is not required to relieve impingement.[53,127] Therefore, it should be avoided.

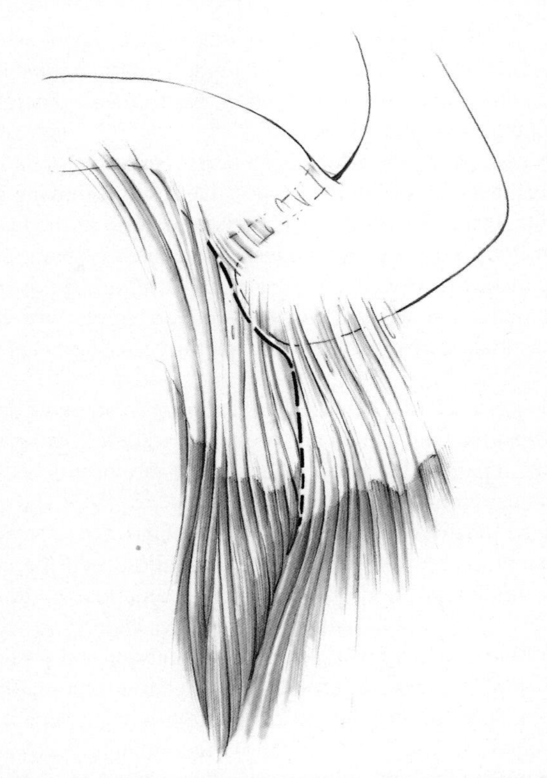

FIG. 7. The anterior deltoid fibers arise obliquely from the anterior acromion, and the middle deltoid fibers arise perpendicularly from the lateral acromion. Incisions that exploit this interval may be less likely to result in postoperative deltoid detachment and retraction.

The deltoid, as with any repaired tendon, should be protected. The length and manner of protection depends on the procedure performed and the quality of the repair. Acromioplasty, even if it is performed arthroscopically or through a conservative deltoid split, theoretically weakens the deltoid attachment.[104] Therefore, even with these relative deltoid-sparing techniques, some period of activity restriction may be justified. Following arthroscopic acromioplasty, I allow activities of daily living immediately, but restrict lifting to the weight of the arm for 2 weeks. Following open acromioplasty, the deltoid repair is protected by allowing only pendulum and passive exercises for 2 weeks.

Recurrent Rotator Cuff Tear

Persistent or recurrent rotator cuff defects following rotator cuff repair have been reported to occur in 20% to 65% of cases.[59,78,110] Associated risk factors include advanced age, large tear size, chronicity, poor tendon quality, poor bone quality, inappropriate rehabilitation, inadequate subacromial decompression, and smoking.[17,32,42,59,78,110,133] Controversy exists concerning the effect that a persistent or recurrent rotator cuff defect has on the postoperative result following rotator cuff repair. This controversy arises because of the lack of controlled, prospective, standardized, objective data; especially those for strength and function.[89] In addition, postoperative subjective and functional results are rarely correlated with anatomic results (i.e., postoperative rotator cuff status).[59,78,110]

The presence of a persistent or recurrent rotator cuff defect is compatible with a good postoperative result following rotator cuff repair.[19,31,110] Pain relief presumably occurs because of adequate subacromial decompression.[24–26,146,160] The quality of the functional result, however, depends on the size of the persistent defect, the integrity of the deltoid and the coracoacromial arch, and the functional demands of the patient.[49,78,127,160,185] Patients with persistent defects in whom the deltoid is intact and the remaining anterior and posterior rotator cuff muscles are sufficient to maintain a fulcrum for the humeral head during deltoid contraction will be capable of overhead function.[24–27,127,160] They are more likely, however, to complain of fatigue with overhead activities and limitation of activities requiring vigorous or sustained overhead strength than patients with an intact cuff repair.[59,78] Therefore, the goal of rotator cuff repair is long-term restoration of a functional, healed musculotendinous unit. This goal may not always be attainable in primary rotator cuff repair. However, the incidence of persistent or recurrent postoperative rotator cuff defects can be minimized through a combination of optimal preoperative patient selection, sound surgical technique, and appropriate postoperative protection and rehabilitation.

Selection of the appropriate patient for primary rotator cuff repair is a complex process that is influenced by many factors. A complete discussion of this topic is beyond the scope of this chapter and the interested reader is referred to Chapter 2 on primary cuff repair. Certain preoperative factors may have a considerable effect on the likehood of obtaining long-term tendon-to-bone healing and deserve emphasis. It is likely that the biologic potential for healing is greater in newly torn tendons than it is in tendons that have been torn for some time.[8] In addition, muscular atrophy may not be completely reversible and is thought to have a negative effect on outcome following rotator cuff repair.[66] Furthermore, tendon retraction that has been allowed to become chronic may prevent the surgeon from obtaining an adequate tendon-to-bone repair. Therefore, in patients with an acute or acute-on-chronic rotator cuff tear associated with retraction, early repair is more likely to result in long-term tendon-to-bone healing than late repair. This potential advantage, however, must be considered in the context of other preoperative patient selection criteria such as age, physical demand, and motivation before the recommendation of early surgical repair can be made.

The surgical technique of rotator cuff repair is discussed extensively in Chapter 2 on primary rotator cuff repair. The surgical principles that are most likely to affect the incidence of postoperative recurrent or persistent rotator cuff defects, which will be emphasized in this chapter, are tendon mobilization and tendon-to-bone repair techniques. The principle of tendon mobilization refers to the process of releasing various adhesions to a retracted rotator cuff tendon so that the tendon edge can be advanced and repaired to the humerus without excessive tension. It is, without question, the most difficult and most important component of rotator cuff repair to learn and master. The superficial surface of the retracted tendon must be released from overlying structures such as the subacromial or subdeltoid bursa, acromion, scapular spine, and the trapezius and deltoid muscles. The deep surface of the retracted tendon must also be released from the tenodesis effect of the underlying capsule.[192] Finally, rotator interval contractures and adhesions between the retracted musculotendinous unit and the intact portions of the rotator cuff must be released.[16,127–129] Even after these releases have been performed, intramuscular scarring may prevent adequate lateral mobilization of the tendon for repair. Management of the irreparable rotator cuff tear is discussed in Chapter 3.

The process of reattaching the torn tendon to bone presents the surgeon with several choices that may affect tendon-to-bone healing and, ultimately, postoperative outcome. Tendon-grasping suturing techniques, such as the Mason–Allen technique, provide better initial pullout strength, and presumably a more durable repair, than simple or mattress sutures.[64,165] Although extensive debridement of the retracted tendon edge may not be necessary, excision of necrotic, fibrinous material to produce a healthy tendon edge strong enough to hold sutures seems advisable. The rates of tendon healing to normal cortical versus cancellous bone have been equal in a goat model.[174] Consequently, complete removal of the cortical surface of the humeral attachment site during rotator cuff repair is probably neither desirable nor necessary. However, the cortical bone of the proximal humerus in the region of a chronic rotator cuff tear is probably not normal. Therefore, abrasion of the proposed humeral attachment site to expose a bleeding bone surface may enhance tendon healing.[72]

The popularity of suture-anchoring devices for reattachment of tendon to bone during rotator cuff repair is increasing rapidly.[28,33,58,148,172] Creation of bone tunnels and passage of sutures through them are tedious procedures that can add to the operative time and frustration level of rotator cuff repair. Suture anchors clearly offer the potential advantages of decreased operative time and frustration. One major disadvantage of suture anchors, however, is cost. Even if this disadvantage is disregarded, in certain patient populations, suture anchors may not be the best choice of anchoring technique. The bone of the proximal humerus in patients with a chronic rotator cuff tear, regardless of age, develops osteoporosis.[94] If this effect is combined with the age-related osteoporosis seen in postmenopausal women and elderly men, suture anchors may not provide adequate pullout strength.[165] Under these circumstances, passage of sutures through bone tunnels and tying of these sutures over a lateral bone bridge that has been augmented with a thin plate or button provides superior strength.[64,165] Suture anchors are an attractive alternative in young, active patients with relatively acute rotator cuff tears. However, more data and follow-up are necessary before anchors can be advocated in all patients undergoing rotator cuff repair.

Postoperative rehabilitation and protection of the repair may also help prevent postoperative recurrent or persistent rotator cuff defects. The importance of early passive mobilization of the shoulder following cuff repair is well known.[92,101,128,129,131,157] However, extreme extension, adduction, and internal rotation should be avoided in the early postoperative period because of the effect of these arm positions on rotator cuff tension.[192] In addition, active range of motion and strengthening exercises should not be instituted until 6 or 8 weeks postoperatively.[92,101,128,129,131,157] Weights and isokinetic strengthening machines should be used judiciously. The use of weights in the early postoperative setting has been associated with tendon repair failure.[139]

Immobilization of the arm following rotator cuff repair has limited usefulness and may be detrimental. However, protection of tendon repairs is a well-known principle that is routinely employed in virtually every other instance of tendon repair or reconstruction that comes to mind. Supporting the postoperative arm following rotator cuff repair in a sling, which places the shoulder in adduction, internal rotation, and (potentially) extension, is counterintuitive. Immobilizing the repaired superior and posterior rotator cuff in this position, which places the tendon under tension,[192] is analogous to immobilizing a repaired digital flexor tendon with the finger in extension. An orthosis, such as a commercially available abduction pillow or brace, which places the arm in a small amount of abduction and, more importantly, prevents internal rotation seems logical. This orthosis is meant to protect a tendon that was repaired with adequate length to reach the humeral attachment site with the arm at the side without excessive tension. It is not possible, in a live patient who is not paralyzed, to repair any tendon without tension. Therefore, the use of an abduction pillow or orthosis, at least in large or massive tears, will allow the repaired tendon to heal under a minimum of tension.

Anterosuperior Humeral Head Subluxation

Normal function of the rotator cuff and coracoacromial arch maintains the geometric center of the humeral head within 2 mm of the center of the glenoid during overhead elevation.[53,95,97,98,151,173] Although the greater tuberosity may come in contact with the coracoacromial ligament and anterior acromion at more than 60 degrees of elevation,[53] the major restraint to anterosuperior translation in the normal shoulder is the compression of the humeral head into the glenoid fossa provided by the contraction of the rotator cuff.[95,109,178] The coracoacromial arch assumes a more important role as a passive restraint to anterosuperior subluxation in the presence of a rotator cuff tear.[54,185]

Small rotator cuff tears allow the remaining anterior and posterior rotator cuff muscles to compensate for the loss of function that accompanies the tear. In these "compensated" rotator cuff tears, the intact rotator cuff tendons continue to provide the primary restraint to anterosuperior subluxation. The coracoacromial arch, as in the normal shoulder, plays a secondary, but probably more important, role as a passive restraint. Rotator cuff tears that are too large cannot be adequately compensated by the intact rotator cuff muscles that remain. In these relatively "uncompensated" rotator cuff tears, the humeral head subluxates proximally, and the coracoacromial arch is the only remaining restraint to continued anterosuperior subluxation. Incompetence of the coracoacromial arch from prior acromioplasty, particularly if the coracoacromial ligament has been excised, combined with a poorly compensated or uncompensated persistent or recurrent rotator cuff defect may result in severe compromise of overhead shoulder function.[185]

Although the incidence of this complication following rotator cuff repair is unknown, when it occurs, it has a devastating effect on function that often is not salvageable.[13,50,54,185] In an effort to prevent the occurrence of this complication, Flatow and colleagues[51] have recommended repair of the coracoacromial ligament following acromioplasty and cuff repair in selected rotator cuff tears. In addition to coracoacromial ligament repair, preservation of as much acromion as possible, while smoothing the undersurface, may also help maintain the stabilizing effect of the coracoacromial arch. This is particularly true of the anterior length of the acromion, because repair of the coracoacromial ligament may be more difficult, and the loss of the acromial fulcrum effect more pronounced, with significant shortening of the anterior acromion.[24,26,27,126,127]

Preservation of the coracoacromial arch during surgery for rotator cuff tears is an important concept. The problem with clinical application of this concept is one of patient selection. Clearly, repair of the coracoacromial ligament in all patients undergoing rotator cuff repair is not necessary. Acromioplasty combined with partial excision of the coracoacromial ligament has been reported with good results.[16,78,86,127,129,137,140,157,160] In addition, persistence of the coracoacromial ligament has been reported to be a cause of failure in some patients, with continued pain following rotator cuff surgery.[81,126,142,158,186] However, loss of the coracoacromial arch in patients with severe decrease in the acromiohumeral interval preoperatively and a failed cuff repair will often result in worse postoperative function than preoperative.

Indications for coracoacromial ligament preservation or repair during rotator cuff surgery continue to evolve. Coracoacromial ligament repair should be considered during open rotator cuff repair when there is decrease in the

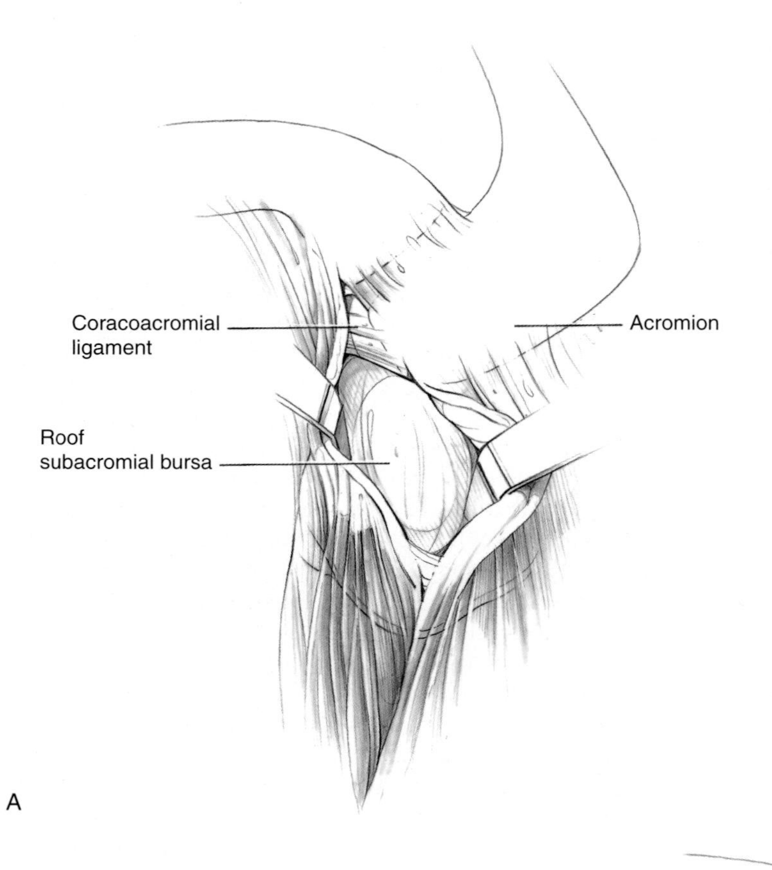

FIG. 8. (A) The coracoacromial ligament may be preserved during repair of selected rotator cuff tears by reflecting the anterior deltoid in one layer, leaving the roof of the subacromial bursa (i.e., the superficial layer of the bursa) and coracoacromial ligament attached to the acromion. **(B)** The roof of the bursa is then incised in line with the deltoid split and the acromial attachment of the anterior portion of the bursal roof and the coracoacromial ligament are released from the anterior acromion. **(C)** The superior edge of the bursal roof and the acromial attachment of the coracoacromial ligament are sutured to the deep surface of the anterior deltoid fascia.

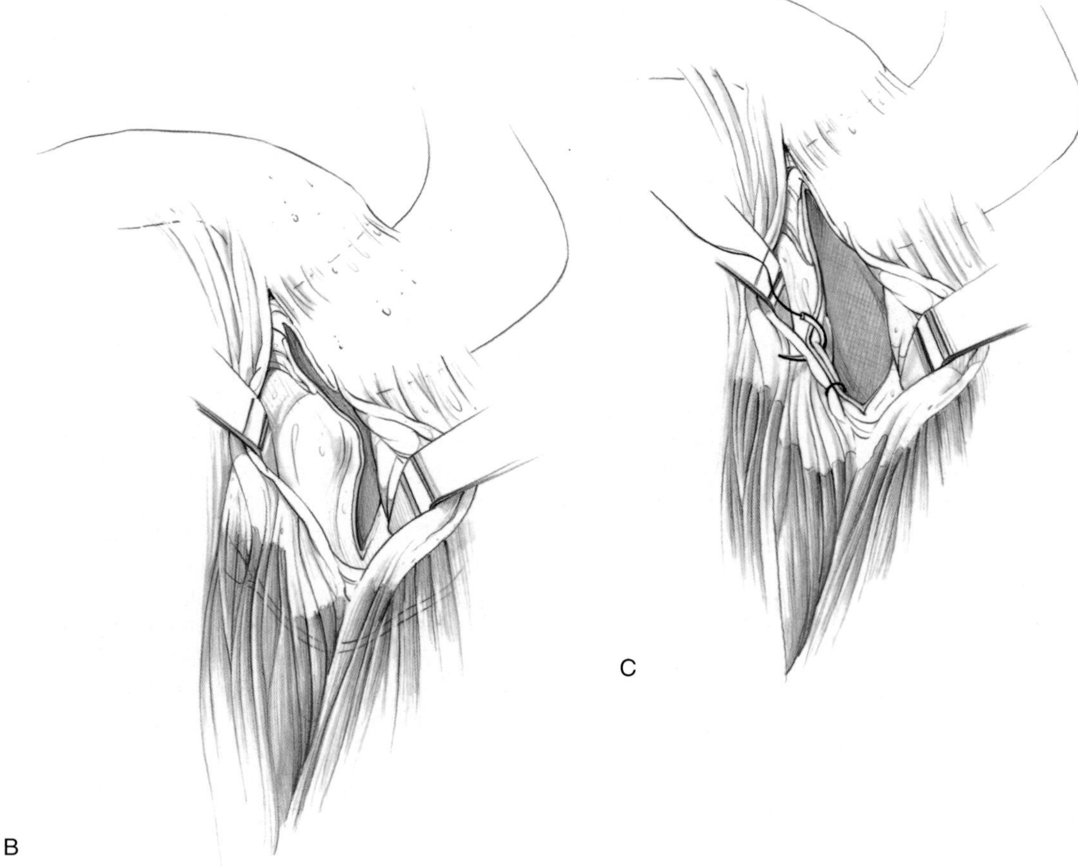

acromiohumeral interval preoperatively. This will likely involve many patients in whom the rotator cuff tear involves two tendons (i.e., supraspinatus and infraspinatus) and all patients with three-tendon involvement. Even if the rotator cuff defect is reparable, the rate of recurrence or persistence of the defect postoperatively in two- and three-tendon tears (45% to 65%) is high enough to justify consideration of coracoacromial ligament preservation or repair.[32,59,78] Patients with marginal overhead function and complete obliteration of the acromiohumeral interval preoperatively present the most risk for postoperative deterioration of function following subacromial decompression and attempted rotator cuff repair. If surgical treatment is elected in these unfortunate patients, it is sometimes helpful to attempt to ascertain preoperatively, with magnetic resonance imaging (MRI), ultrasound, or computed tomographic (CT) arthrography, whether the cuff defect is reparable. If it is likely not reparable, a more conservative deltoid-sparing or arthroscopic decompression can be considered. However, if there is any question on the reparability of the defect, the decision should be made intraoperatively.

Even if we assume that a surgical candidate who is dependent on the coracoacromial arch as a passive restraint to anterosuperior translation has been identified, the actual technique for coracoacromial ligament repair or preservation may vary.[51] If the decision to perform an isolated decompression without repair has been made preoperatively, an arthroscopic acromioplasty is a reasonable option. Arthroscopic removal of any portion of the anterior acromion, including its undersurface, is difficult, if not impossible, without detachment of some portion of the coracoacromial ligament. It is often possible to preserve the most medial acromial attachment of the ligament. Even if the entire acromial attachment of the ligament is released, it will likely grow back to the acromion postoperatively as long as the anteroposterior length of the acromion is preserved.

The coracoacromial ligament can be released and repaired in one of two ways during open subacromial decompresion. First, the deltoid insertion, roof of the subacromial bursa, and the acromial attachment of the coracoacromial ligament can all be released in a single layer. The ligament and bursa are reattached along with the deltoid at the completion of the procedure. Alternatively, the interval between the roof of the subacromial bursa and the deltoid can be developed and the deltoid can be released from the anterior acromion in a single layer. This will expose the underlying roof of the subacromial bursa and coracoacromial ligament, which can then be released from the acromial margin under direct vision. This technique offers the potential advantage of maximizing coracoacromial ligament length by allowing detachment of the ligament from the undersurface of the acromion, rather than from its anterior edge. The bursal roof and ligament are then immediately sewn to the deep deltoid fascia. This ensures that the ligament and bursa will be reattached with the deltoid and also provides a layer of reinforcement to the deltoid repair (Fig.8).

EVALUATION

The evaluation of patients with continued pain and dysfunction following rotator cuff surgery requires a thorough knowledge of the potential postsurgical complications. The most important diagnostic components are history and physical examination. In addition to obtaining a history from the patient, the surgical report(s) and medical records surrounding any prior rotator cuff surgery should be reviewed when possible. Potential adjunctive tests include magnetic resonance imaging, ultrasonography, arthrography, computed tomography, electrodiagnostic testing, and scintigraphy. The history, physical findings, and usefulness of various adjunctive diagnostic tests vary according to the complication(s) present.

Acromial Stress Fracture

Although acromial stress fractures following arthroscopic acromioplasty probably occur within the first 2 to 3 postoperative months, there is often a delay in diagnosis because of a low index of suspicion. The patient will often report a sudden, marked increase in pain associated with swelling. If an inciting event is recalled, it is usually minor. There is marked point tenderness over the dorsal aspect of the acromion, which corresponds to the area of fracture. This typically occurs at the junction of the anterior and middle thirds of the acromion in line with the posterior border of the clavicle and acromioclavicular joint. A relative stress riser exists in the transitional zone between the anterior third of the acromion, which has been partially resected, and the normal middle or posterior acromion. The diagnosis is confirmed with routine radiography (Fig. 9). Adequate visualization of the fracture is often not possible without an axillary view, supraspinatus outlet view, or an anteroposterior view with 30-degree–caudal tilt.[37,132,157]

Persistent Subacromial Impingement

The diagnosis of persistent subacromial impingement following rotator cuff surgery is made when physical findings associated with subacromial impingement are present, those findings improve sustantially with subacromial injection of a local anesthetic (i.e., positive impingement test), and there is radiographic evidence of continued supraspinatus outlet narrowing.[37,114,127,132,157] Patients may complain of continued night pain and difficulty in overhead use of the arm, with little or no postoperative improvement. The impingement and impingement reinforcement (i.e., Hawkins) signs are painful and may be associated with subacromial crepitus.[82,83,85,127] Passive motion should be checked carefully to determine the presence or absence of capsular contracture. Contracture involving the posterior capsule, as evidenced by decreased passive internal rotation and adduction with the arm at 90 degrees of elevation in the scapular plane, is commonly associated with impingement syndrome and may contribute to continued subacromial impingement following rotator cuff

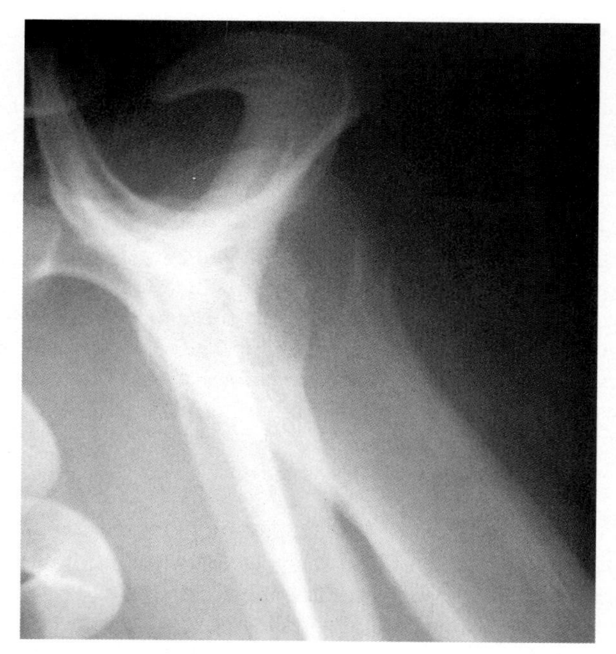

FIG. 9. A postoperative acromial stress fracture was suspected in this patient who had undergone arthroscopic acromioplasty approximately 6 weeks earlier. She presented with marked increase in pain and tenderness over the dorsum of the acromion. Radiographs confirmed the diagnosis.

surgery.[114,186] Supraspinatus outlet and 30-degree–caudal tilt radiographs[37,157] should demonstrate continued evidence of supraspinatus outlet narrowing (Fig. 10).

Continued pain and physical findings suggestive of persistent subacromial impingement may occasionally be present in patients whose postoperative radiographs show little or no evidence of continued anatomic narrowing of the supraspinatus outlet. Persistence or regrowth of the coracoacromial ligament as the cause for continued subacromial impingement is a diagnosis of exclusion that should be made cautiously, especially in patients with potential secondary gain.[81] The importance of a diagnostic subacromial injection with lidocaine as a confirmatory test in all patients with suspected continued subacromial impingement following rotator cuff surgery cannot be overemphasized.

Heterotopic Ossification

Patients who develop heterotopic ossification following rotator cuff surgery may or may not notice an initial period of postoperative pain relief. However, within 3 to 6 months, persistent pain will be apparent. Usually, the heterotopic ossification occurs within the subacromial space or deltoid attachment site and is not associated with significant decrease in passive motion (Fig. 11).[11,105] Rarely, severe periarticular heterotopic ossification may occur and is associated with significant loss of passive glenohumeral motion (Fig. 12). In patients in whom the ossification is subacromial and not associated with motion loss, the impingement sign, impingement reinforcement sign, and the impingement test may be positive.[82,83,85,127] Severe periarticular ossification will present with a picture resembling a frozen shoulder. In addition to severe restriction of passive glenohumeral motion, these patients may also present with erythema and warmth, suggestive of an infection. It is important to consider the possibility of postoperative heterotopic ossification in all patients with continued pain, with or without motion loss. Obviously, heterotopic ossification is a radiographic diagnosis. It is helpful to supplement standard anteroposterior and axillary

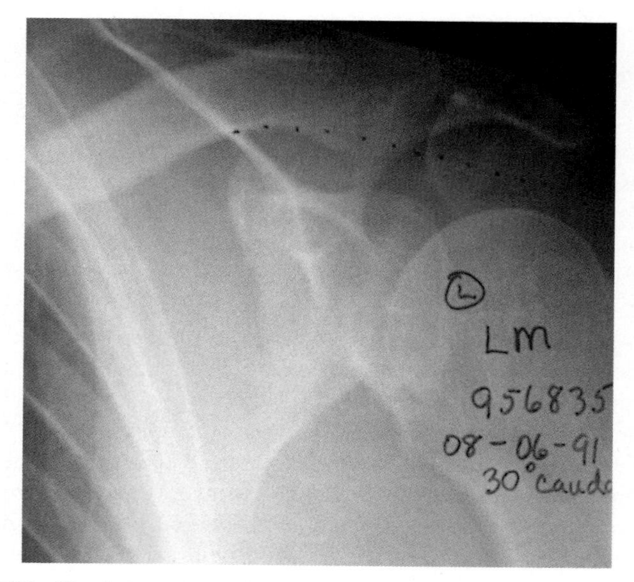

FIG. 10. A standing anteroposterior radiograph with 30-degree–caudal tilt in a patient with persistent pain following previous arthroscopic acromioplasty. Note the persistence of an anterior acromial spur.

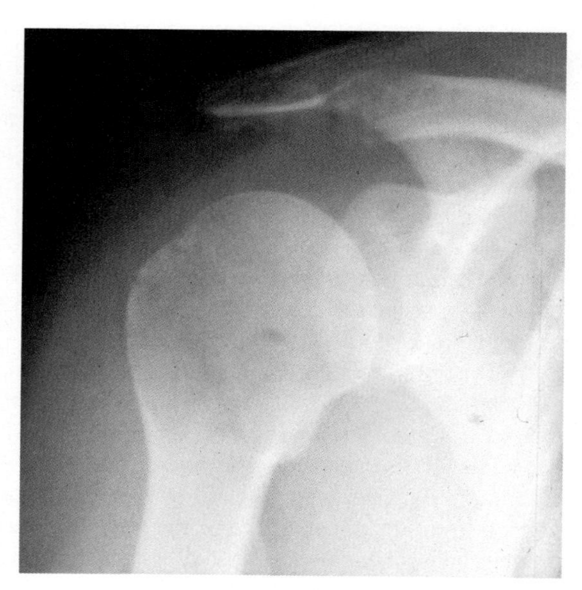

FIG. 11. A standing anteroposterior with 30-degree–caudal tilt radiograph in a patient with persistent pain following arthroscopic acromioplasty. This heterotopic ossification is located within the subacromial space and is not associated with passive motion loss.

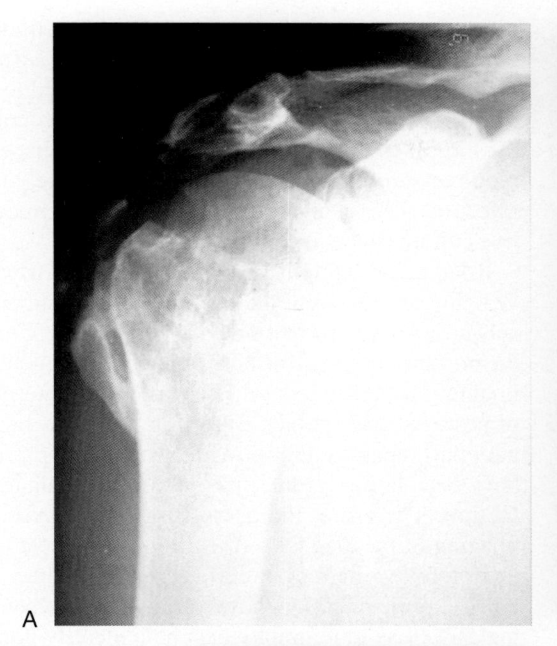

A

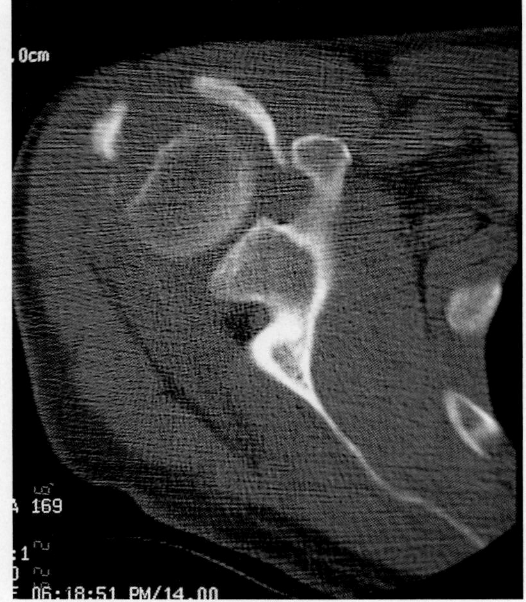

C

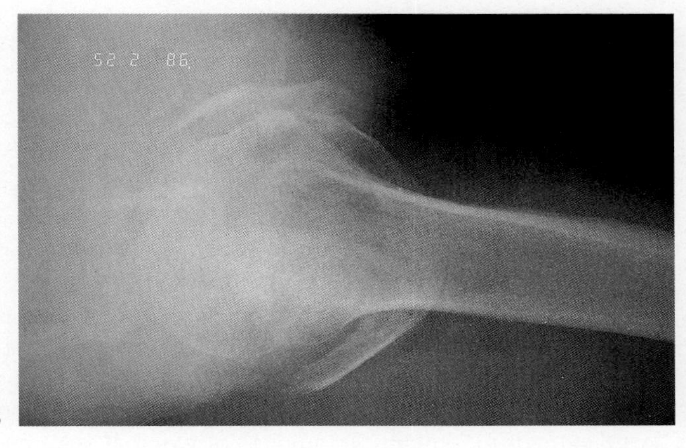

B

FIG. 12. **(A)** Anteroposterior and **(B)** axillary radiographs of a patient with severe glenohumeral motion loss associated with extensive subacromial and pericapsular heterotopic ossification following repair of a supraspinatus tendon rupture. **(C)** Computed tomography reveals anterior and posterior extension of the heterotopic bone.

views with supraspinatus outlet[132] and 30-degree—caudal tilt views[37,157] to fully inspect the subacromial space for heterotopic ossification.

Frozen Shoulder

In patients with a suspected frozen shoulder following rotator cuff surgery, it is important to elicit the history of any predisposing risk factors. These associated risk factors include diabetes mellitus, hypothyroidism, glenohumeral arthritis, and prolonged postoperative immobilization. The hallmark of frozen shoulder is symmetrical decrease in both passive and active glenohumeral motion.[135,138,141,181,186] Therefore, active as well as passive motion in all planes are measured and compared with those of the opposite, normal extremity. It is useful to perform motion testing in the upright as well as the supine position. When gravity is eliminated in the supine position, some patients are better able to relax during passive motion testing.

The effect of any capsular contracture on passive glenohumeral motion depends on which portion of the capsule is affected. If the contracture is localized to the rotator interval, there will be decreased passive external rotation with the arm at the side and relative sparing of elevation and rotational motion with the arm at 90 degrees of elevation in the scapular plane.[80] Isolated posterior capsular contracture will result in decreased terminal elevation and decreased internal rotation and adduction with the arm at 90 degrees of elevation in the scapular plane.[114] Generalized capsular contracture produces passive motion loss in all planes.

Occasionally, it can be difficult to determine whether decreased passive motion is the result of voluntary guarding or soft-tissue contracture. This is particularly true in those patients with secondary gain whose subjective complaints of pain are out of proportion to what would be expected based on their objective findings. The only way to know for sure whether there is significant soft-tissue contracture is by examination under anesthesia. However, a reasonable approximation can be obtained during examination of the awake patient by practical application of some simple anatomic observations. If, in the supine position with the arm at the side, there is passive external rotation that is equal to or approximates the opposite, normal side, there is no significant contracture of the superior capsuloligamentous structures. The presence of a rotational arc of motion that equals or approximates the opposite side with the arm at 90 degrees of elevation in the scapular plane indicates relative lack of inferior capsular contracture. If the arm cannot be passively elevated beyond 90 degrees under these circumstances, the cause is likely to be voluntary guarding, rather than contracture.

Radiographic findings in patients with frozen shoulder are normal. However, routine radiographs should be obtained to exclude glenohumeral arthritis or other concomitant osseous abnormalities, such as pericapsular heterotopic ossification. Magnetic resonance imaging and other adjunctive tests are superfluous in the diagnosis of frozen shoulder. However, if pain persists after motion has been regained, magnetic resonance imaging may be indicated.

Infection

The physical findings that accompany postoperative infection following rotator cuff surgery can be very subtle. Consequently, to make a timely diagnosis, a high index of suspicion must be maintained. Following arthroscopic rotator cuff surgery, infection is usually manifested by a low-grade fever, erythema around one or more of the portal sites, and prolonged drainage from one or more of the portal sites. Patients will often notice progressively increasing pain and a change in the nature of the drainage from thin, serous fluid to thick, yellow exudate. In the early postoperative period, a single white blood cell count may not be helpful because of the hydrocortisone (Cortisol)-induced increase in the peripheral white cell count commonly seen following the stress of surgery. The diagnosis is confirmed by a positive culture from the portal site or from a subacromial aspirate. An initial negative culture does not exclude infection, particularly if prophylactic antibiotics were administered at the time of surgery. Therefore, the surgeon must remain vigilant.

Patients who develop postoperative infection following open rotator cuff surgery may present with obvious signs of infection, including dehiscence of the wound, surrounding erythema, thick drainage, generalized malaise, fever, and leukocytosis. However, the presentation may be as subtle as increased pain, swelling, and erythema. Any patient who presents to their first postoperative visit (7 to 10 days) following open rotator cuff surgery with an erythematous wound and what appears to be a localized hematoma under the wound must be suspected of having a deltoid detachment, deep wound infection, or both.

There are several differences between postoperative wound infection and hematoma that may aid in making the correct diagnosis. First, a hematoma is most often present immediately after surgery. If the surgeon or patient noticed the localized swelling around the wound within the first 24 to 48 hours following surgery, it is more likely to represent hematoma than infection. Conversely, if the wound was benign-appearing and then suddenly developed swelling and erythema, infection should be more strongly suspected. Second, a hematoma should not be accompanied by erythema. Third, a 7- to 10-day-old hematoma should contain organizing clot. If the wound is aspirated and contains either liquid blood or serosanquinous fluid, it is more likely to represent infection. The diagnosis of infection is confirmed by a positive culture of the aspirate.

Routine radiographs may be obtained and usually will reveal soft-tissue swelling. The presence of subcutaneous or subacromial air at 7 to 10 days postoperatively may indicate the presence of a gas-forming organism. Magnetic resonance imaging, if performed, will be difficult to interpret because of postoperative artifact. Even if deltoid detachment and rotator cuff repair failure were identified, their presence would have been known at the time of surgical drainage of the infection. Therefore, the usefulness of magnetic resonance imaging in the diagnosis of early or acute postoperative infection following rotator cuff surgery is limited. In a potentially chronic infection, however, magnetic resonance imaging as well as scintigraphy may help identify potential areas of osteomyelitis.

Suprascapular Nerve Injury

The presence of significant external rotation weakness with the arm at the side and with the arm at 90 degrees of elevation in the scapular plane should suggest the possibility of either a recurrent rotator cuff tear or a suprascapular nerve injury. The cause of the external rotation weakness is more likely to be suprascapular nerve injury than recurrent rotator cuff tear if (a) prior records reveal that the cuff was intact at the time of surgery; (b) the size of the rotator cuff defect documented on preoperative studies or operative reports was not large enough to explain the amount of external rotation weakness present. In all patients with suspected suprascapular nerve palsy, the possibility of superimposed cervical radiculopathy should also be entertained. Under these circumstances, electrodiagnostic testing is indicated. If the suprascapular nerve is found to be normal, magnetic resonance imaging is ordered to investigate the possibility of recurrent or persistent rotator cuff tear.

Axillary Nerve Injury

Atrophy of the deltoid following rotator cuff surgery may be the result of disuse secondary to pain, detachment of the deltoid repair, or axillary nerve injury. These three causes can usually be disinguished on the basis of physical findings. Disuse atrophy affects all portions of the deltoid equally. The other muscles of the shoulder girdle may also appear atrophic, and there is no palpable defect at the deltoid origin. Deltoid detachment produces a palpable defect at the anterior acromion. However, there typically is intact deltoid origin medial to the acromion that can be seen to contract normally. Axillary nerve injury produces a characteristic pattern of deltoid atrophy because this nerve innervates the deltoid muscle from posterior to anterior.[23,29,30,45,88,103,108,111] All portions of the deltoid muscle anterior to the site of injury will be atrophic. In some cases, the previously placed skin incision will suggest an axillary nerve injury (Fig. 13). Although the axillary nerve does supply a sensory branch to the lateral aspect of the arm, it typically arises proximal to the most frequent zone of surgical injury. In addition, the cutaneous distributions of the axillary nerve and other surrounding cutaneous nerves overlap substantially. Therefore, sensory testing is unreliable.[20]

The suspected diagnosis of axillary nerve injury is confirmed by electromyography. The examining electromyographer should be made aware that the diagnosis of axillary nerve injury is being entertained. All three portions of the deltoid muscle should be tested so that a false-negative study report is not produced by isolated testing of the intact portion of the deltoid. Experienced electromyographers may be able to provide an opinion on the type of nerve injury present (i.e., whether the nerve is likely to be in continuity). Electromyography can also be used to follow the progress of regeneration of the nerve.

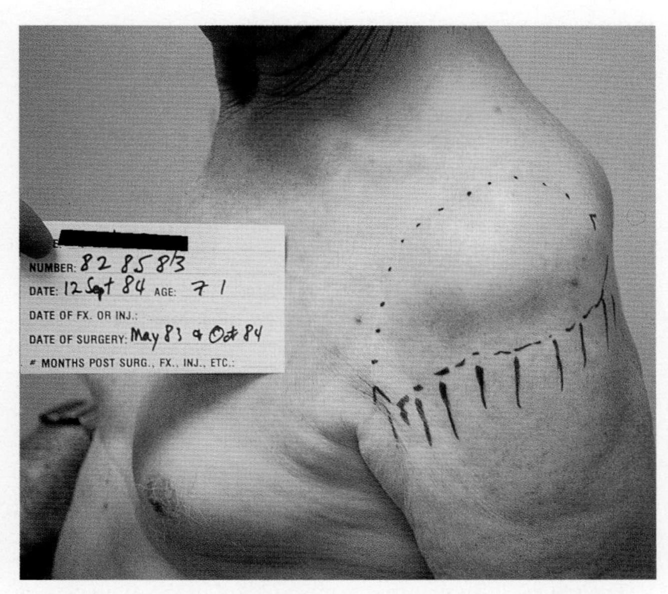

FIG. 14. Postoperative deltoid detachment is characterized by distal retraction of the detached deltoid, which can easily be seen as a mass or prominence in the anterior or lateral arm. Middle deltoid detachments exhibit more severe retraction. (Courtesy of C. A. Rockwood, Jr., M.D.; from ref. 186.)

Deltoid Detachment

Failure of the deltoid repair following open rotator cuff surgery obviously occurs in the early postoperative period. However, there is often a long delay in diagnosis. In one reported series, the average duration of symptoms before surgical treatment of the deltoid detachment was 17 months.[168] The presentation is variable and depends on the size of the deltoid defect, the portion of the deltoid affected, the status of the coracoacromial arch, the amount of acromion remaining, and the status of the rotator cuff. Acute cases are characterized by the sudden onset of increased pain and localized swelling over the anterior acromion. All patients who present with sudden onset of localized swelling over the anterior acromion within 7 to 10 days of open rotator cuff surgery should be suspected of having a deltoid detachment, deep wound infection, or both.

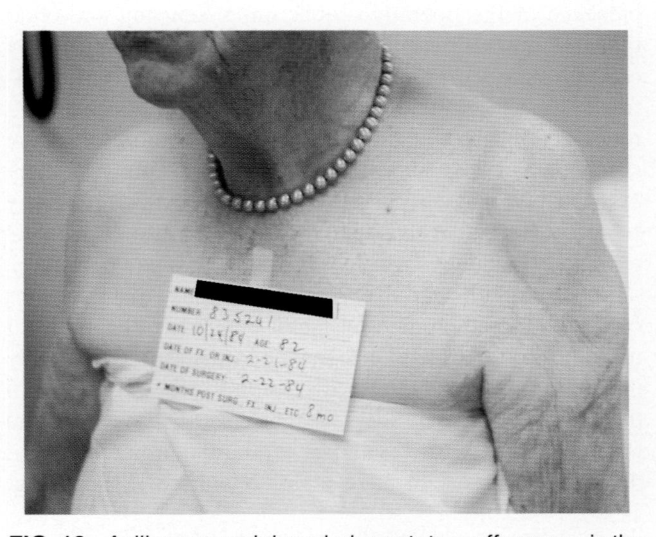

FIG. 13. Axillary nerve injury during rotator cuff surgery is the result of direct incision of the nerve or traction neuropathy. This patient exhibited denervation of the deltoid anterior to this surgical incision that extends far below the projected course of the axillary nerve. (Courtesy of C. A. Rockwood, Jr. M.D.)

In all cases of postoperative deltoid detachment, there is a visible and palpable defect present at the site of this detachment and the detached deltoid is retracted distally (Fig. 14). Because the fibers of the middle deltoid attach to the acromion perpendicular to their line of action, postoperative detachment of the middle deltoid results in a greater degree of distal retraction than detachment of the anterior deltoid. If the rotator cuff is intact and there is no capsular contracture, overhead elevation is often preserved in all but the largest deltoid detachments. Patients with concomitant recurrent or persistent rotator cuff defects, particularly if the coracoacromial arch is deficient from coracoacromial ligament excision or overzealous acromial excision, may present with severely compromised overhead function.[14,42,71,133,168,185]

Radiographic evaluation should include routine anteroposterior and axillary views, in addition to supraspinatus outlet and 30-degree–caudal tilt projections to assess the amount of acromion remaining.[37,132,157] Magnetic resonance imaging will demonstrate the deltoid detachment, but is more useful in evaluating any concomitant persistent or recurrent rotator cuff defect. If a deep wound infection is suspected in addition to deltoid detachment, aspiration of the subacromial space will provide material for culture.

Recurrent Rotator Cuff Tear

The incidence of recurrent or persistent rotator cuff tears is highest in older patients with chronic and retracted tears and tears that involve two or three tendons.[78] Therefore, the index of suspicion for a recurrent rotator cuff tear as the cause for continued pain and disability following its repair should be highest in these patients. Physical findings in patients with recurrent or persistent rotator cuff tears are variable and dependent on the size of the defect, the location of the defect (i.e., which tendons are affected), and the integrity of the coracoacromial arch. The most important initial step in physical examination is to exclude the presence of significant soft-tissue contracture. It is difficult, if not impossible, to determine the presence and clinical relevance of recurrent rotator cuff tears in a stiff shoulder. Once significant soft-tissue contracture has been excluded or corrected, the physical findings associated with the recurrent rotator cuff defect will become more apparent.

The physical finding that is most useful in the diagnosis of recurrent rotator cuff tears is weakness during isolated muscle testing. The reliability of strength testing may be limited by pain and, under these circumstances, improved through the use of subacromial lidocaine. The rotator cuff and other shoulder girdle muscles function largely as a coordinated unit, and complete isolation of individual musculotendinous units is difficult. However, muscle testing in certain arm positions may provide information about specific regions of the cuff.

Abduction strength with the arm elevated to 90 degrees in the scapular plane, the elbow extended, and the humerus internally rotated (i.e., the Jobe test) is thought to be largely a supraspinatus function.[87,91–93] Therefore, weakness of abduction in this position may be indicative of a persistent or recurrent defect of the supraspinatus tendon. Tension in the posterior capsule and rotator cuff is a function of arm position. The superior portions of the capsule and cuff are relatively taut with the arm at the side, whereas the inferior portions of the posterior capsule and cuff are relatively taut with the arm elevated to 90 degrees. Therefore, a potential recurrent or persistent defect involving the supraspinatus and upper portion of infraspinatus (i.e., the superior portion of the posterior cuff) is characterized by external rotation weakness with the arm at the side that is improved when the arm is abducted to 90 degrees in the scapular plane. Conversely, a recurrent defect that extends into the lower portion of infraspinatus or teres minor (i.e., the lower portion of the posterior cuff) produces external rotation weakness with the arm at the side and with the arm at 90 degrees of abduction in the scapular plane. External rotation lag signs, or the inability of the patient to actively maintain maximum passive external rotation, with the arm at the side and with the arm at 90 degrees in the scapular plane, also indicate recurrent defects involving the posterosuperior and posteroinferior rotator cuff, respectively.[87]

Recurrent defects involving the subscapularis tendon are accompanied by weakness of terminal internal rotation. This is best demonstrated by the "lift-off" sign.[63] A positive lift-off sign is characterized by inability of the patient to lift the dorsum of the hand away from the small of the back (Fig. 15). The examiner must prevent the patient from substituting shoulder or elbow extension for humeral internal rotation during testing to avoid false-negative results. The internal rotation lag sign, or the inability of the patient to maintain the dorsum of the hand away from the small of the back after it has been passively placed in this position of maximum internal rotation by an examiner, is also a sensitive test for subscapularis insufficiency (see Fig. 15).[87]

The lift-off test and the internal rotation lag sign require full passive internal rotation. Therefore, they are less useful in patients with internal rotation loss resulting from posterior capsular contracture. Under these circumstances, the abdominal compression test, which requires less internal rotation than the lift-off test or the internal rotation lag sign to perform, may be useful in documenting subscapularis insufficiency. Patients with normal subscapularis function are able to internally rotate the humerus to bring the flexed elbow anterior to the plane of the body while simultaneously maintaining the palm of the hand compressed against the abdomen (Fig. 16). Inability of the patient to maintain the flexed elbow anterior to or in the plane of the body with the palm of the hand compressed against the abdomen, once the arm has been passively placed in this position, is analogous to the internal rotation lag sign and is also indicative of subscapularis insufficiency. The effect of scapular protraction on the performance of the abdominal compression test is difficult to control. Therefore, the abdominal compression test may be less specific for subscapularis insufficiency than the lift-off test or the internal rotation lag sign.[69,175]

The presence of a recurrent or persistent rotator cuff defect can be verified with ultrasonagraphy, arthrography, or magnetic resonance imaging.[19,31,32,39,59,72,78,112,143,189] The presence of postoperative subacromial scarring and other types of postsurgical artifact makes interpretation of any type of rotator cuff imaging in the postoperative setting difficult. Therefore, the diagnostic criteria for a full-thickness rotator cuff defect in the postoperative shoulder are more stringent than in the shoulder that has had no surgery for any of these three modalities. Although all three modalities may be useful, we prefer magnetic resonance imaging. Magnetic resonance imaging is noninvasive and provides information on recurrent cuff tear size, rotator cuff muscle atrophy, biceps tendon pathology, and labral pathology. The clinical relevance of minor tendon signal abnormalities, particularly in the postoperative setting is uncertain. However, even in the postoperative shoulder, the presence of a well-defined tendon gap that is traversed by synovial fluid is a reliable indicator of a persistent or recurrent rotator cuff defect (Fig. 17).[72,143]

Anterosuperior Humeral Head Subluxation

Anterosuperior humeral head subluxation occurs when a massive recurrent rotator cuff defect exists in conjunction

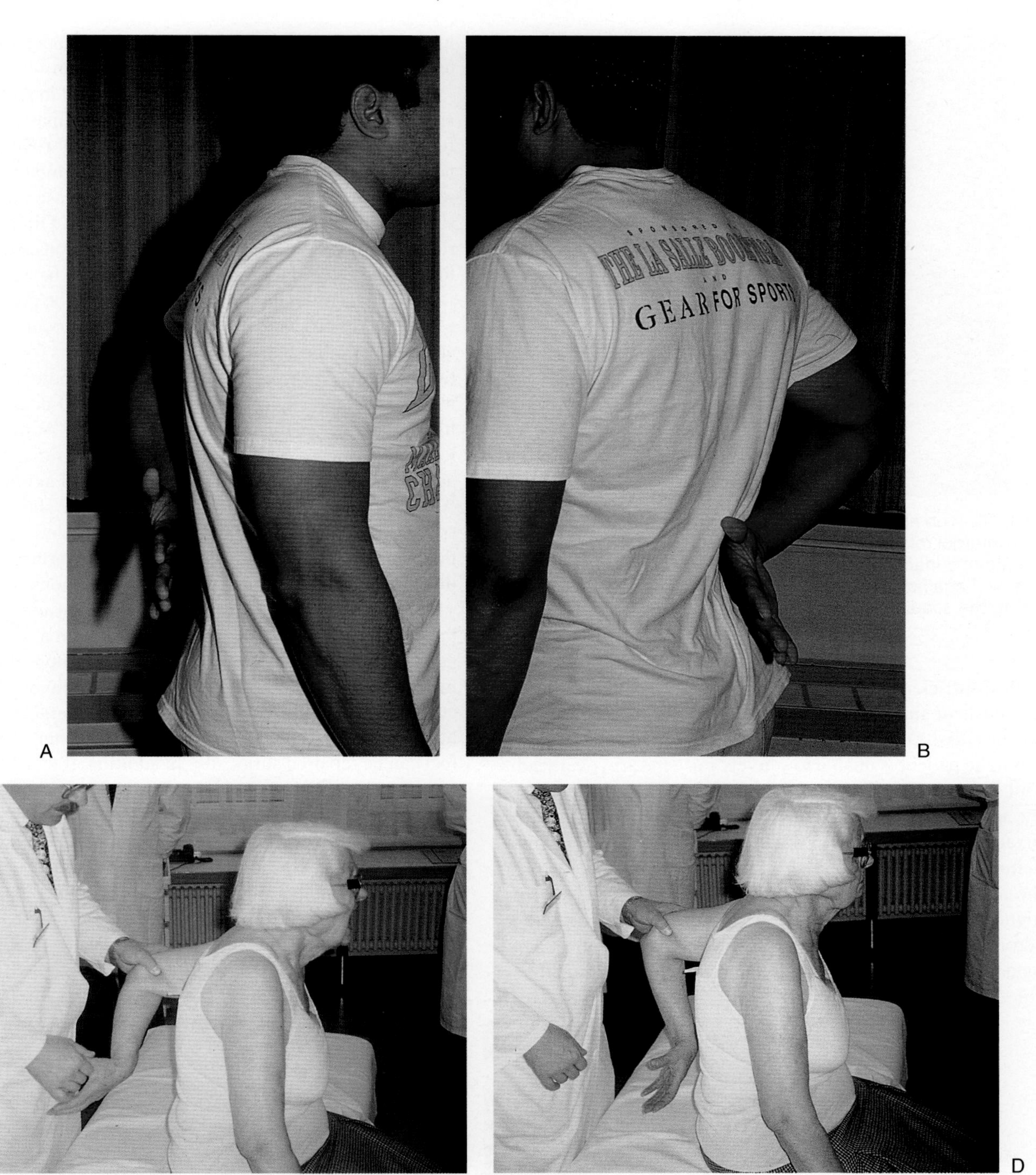

FIG. 15. (A) The patient has normal subscapularis function and is able to actively hold the dorsum of the hand away from the lumbar spine. **(B)** However, his contralateral shoulder has a chronic subscapularis rupture that prevents him from placing the affected hand in a similar position. The internal rotation lag sign also indicates subscapularis insufficiency. It is performed by **(C)** passively placing the patient's hand behind the back with the humerus maximally internally rotated. **(D)** This patient cannot actively maintain this position that was achieved passively because of subscapularis insufficiency. (**C** and **D**, courtesy of C. Gerber, M.D.)

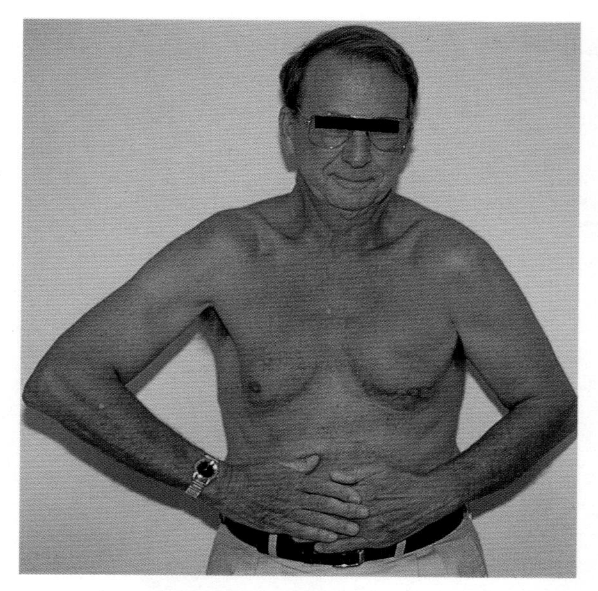

FIG. 16. The abdominal compression test requires less passive internal rotation to perform. A positive test is indicated by a pateint's inability to maintain the palm of the hand compressed against the abdomen while bringing the elbow anterior to the scapular plane.

with insufficiency of the coracoacromial arch.[54,106,185] The diagnosis of anterosuperior subluxation of the humeral head can usually be made purely on the basis of clinical examination. The patient is unable to actively raise the arm overhead. Full passive elevation, however, is usually possible unless the anterosuperior subluxation is chronic and fixed. The subluxation may not be obvious with the arm at the side and the deltoid relaxed. However, when the patient attempts to raise the arm, the humeral head can be seen to rise out of the glenoid into the subcutaneous tissues anterior to the acromion. Often, anterosuperior subluxation is accompanied by deltoid insufficiency.[185] Therefore, the deltoid should be inspected closely for a defect indicative of detachment of its origin or atrophy associated with denervation.

The size of the recurrent rotator cuff defect in patients with anterosuperior humeral head subluxation is massive. Therefore, patients will often demonstrate external rotation weakness with the arm at the side and with the arm at 90 degrees of elevation in the scapular plane. In addition, some degree of subscapularis involvement is usually present. Often, the inferior fibers of the subscapularis are present. Consequently, the lift-off and abdominal compression tests may be negative, but weak, and the internal rotation lag sign may be present.[63,87]

Radiographic evaluation is helpful for documenting the anterosuperior humeral subluxation as well as for evaluating the remaining coracoacromial arch. Useful radiographic projections include anteroposterior, axillary, 30-degree–caudal tilt, and supraspinatus outlet views.[37,132,157] Acromial bone loss, indicative of coracoacromial arch insufficiency, is best appreciated on the 30-degree–caudal tilt and axillary views. Anteroposterior and axillary radiographs should be inspected for signs of humeral head collapse and humeral articular incongruities indicative of cuff tear arthropathy, for this may have an influence on treatment options.

Magnetic resonance imaging is not necessary to confirm the diagnosis of anterosuperior subluxation or a recurrent rotator cuff defect. However, it may provide important information for treatment and prognosis. If the involved rotator cuff muscles exhibit atrophy and fatty degeneration, they are not likely to be functional, even if the persistent tendon defect can be repaired surgically. In addition, if tendon transfer techniques are being entertained as treatment options, it is important to know which muscles are still intact. For instance, functional results following latissimus dorsi transfer for irreparable posterior cuff insufficiency are better in the presence of an intact subscapularis.[61,62] Subscapularis insufficiency suspected on physical examination can be confirmed and quantitated by magnetic resonance imaging. This knowledge may facilitate treatment decision making.

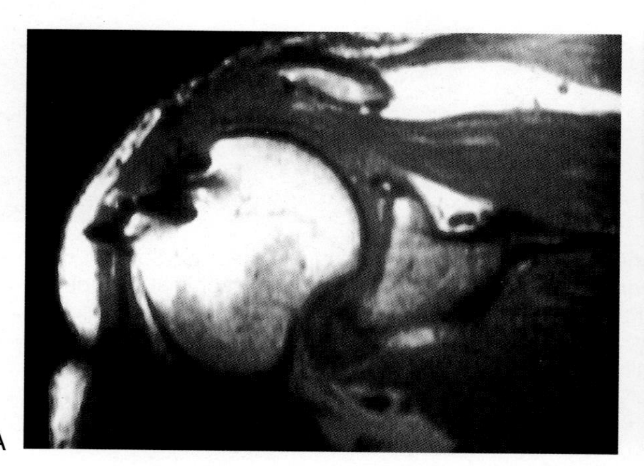

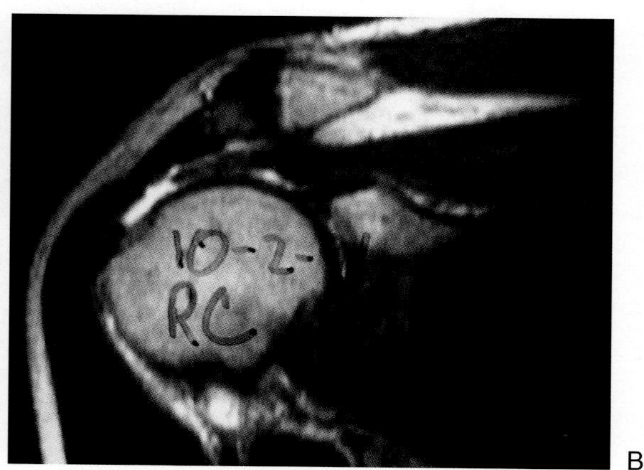

FIG. 17. Magnetic resonance imaging criteria for the diagnosis of a recurrent full-thickness defect must be stringent to avoid false-positive results secondary to postsurgical artifact. **(A)** Subtle signal intensity abnormalities may represent scarring, rather than a recurrent defect. **(B)** A well-defined tendon gap filled with synovial fluid that communicates with the subacromial space, however, is a reliable sign of a persistent or recurrent rotator cuff tear.

TREATMENT AND RESULTS

The treatment options for patients with complications following rotator cuff surgery are dependent on the complication present. Furthermore, multiple complications may coexist in the same patient and, therefore, require combined treatment strategies. In general, the results following treatment of complications of rotator cuff surgery are inferior to the results that would have been obtained after uncomplicated primary rotator cuff surgery. However, if patients are selected carefully, the symptoms associated with their complications can often be improved.

Acromial Stress Fracture

Nonoperative management of patients with acromial stress fracture following arthroscopic acromioplasty is usually unsuccessful. Patients frequently develop painful nonunion as the result of micromotion from deltoid contraction. Available surgical treatment options include excision or open reduction, internal fixation, and bone grafting.[117] The anterior fragment, which consists of the partially resected anterior third of the acromion, is thin and irregular. Therefore, adequate internal fixation is often difficult or impossible. Open excision requires detachment of the deltoid. After the thin anterior fragment has been carefully excised, the remaining deltotrapezius aponeurosis may be tenuous and prone to postoperative dehiscence, thereby leading to failure of the deltoid repair. Arthroscopic excision, which also leaves a thin layer of deltotrapezius aponeurosis, is theoretically less likely to lead to dehiscence of the deltoid because it does not require deltoid detachment through the thin fascia at the nonunion or fracture site.

If the diagnosis is made shortly after the fracture occurs, arthroscopic excision is delayed for 6 to 12 weeks. Although healing of the fracture or spontaneous resolution of pain is unlikely, this delay allows the aponeurosis within which the fracture has occurred to recover from the hemorrhage and edema of the acute injury. The resultant toughened fibrous tissue surrounding the fracture site is theoretically less likely to fail after the nonunited anterior fragment has been removed. It is important to maintain full passive motion during this period so that the patient is not prone to permanent stiffness following arthroscopic excision of the nonunited fragment.

Arthroscopic excision of the fragment is accomplished by placing the arthroscope into the subacromial space through either a posterior or posterolateral portal. An anterolateral portal is established slightly posterior to an imaginary line drawn straight laterally from the anterior cortical border of the clavicle (Fig. 18). The soft tissue on the undersurface of the acromion is removed and any remaining coracoacromial ligament is incised to allow visualization of the borders of the anterior fragment. The fragment is then removed using an arthroscopic burr that sweeps from the anterior lip of the nonunited fragment to the nonunion site. The resection starts laterally and proceeds medially. As the resection proceeds, a progressively thinner fragment results. Eventually, all that remains is the dorsal cortex of the fragment and the adherent deltotrapezial fascia. This cortical shell is carefully "peeled" away from its fascial envelope, leaving an intact sleeve of deltotrapezius aponeurosis in continuity with the remaining acromion and the anterior deltoid (see Fig. 18).

Postoperatively, the thin deltotrapezius aponeurosis is protected. Active elevation of the arm is discouraged for 4 to 6 weeks. Pendulum, supine passive flexion, and passive external rotation exercises are begun on the first postoperative day. An overhead pulley is added at 4 weeks. Full active elevation is instituted 4 to 6 weeks postoperatively. Subsequent rehabilitation exercises for the rotator cuff and scapular rotators are not significantly different from those used following primary rotator cuff surgery. Therefore, the interested reader is referred to Chapter 35.

Results following treatment of postoperative acromial stress fractures are sparsely reported and inconsistent.[117] Excision of the anterior acromion shortens its anteroposterior dimension, thereby compromising the deltoid lever arm.[130] This may result in weakness of elevation and fatigue during overhead activity. Pain relief is reportedly inconsistent.[117] However, if the deltoid remains attached to the residual acromion an excellent result is possible.

Persistent Subacromial Impingement

Persistent supraspinatus outlet narrowing from residual acromial spurs, a persistent coracoacromial ligament, or downward projecting acromioclavicular osteophytes is managed by repeat subacromial decompression.[55,84,143,158] This can be accomplished through either open or arthroscopic techniques. The surgical techniques and postoperative rehabilitation for revision acromioplasty, coracoacromial ligament release or excision, and excision of inferior acromioclavicular osteophytes are not significantly different from the analogous procedures in a nonoperated shoulder that has not had surgery. These techniques have been adequately described elsewhere in this book. The interested reader is referred to Chapters 2 and 35 on primary cuff repair and rehabilitation.

The reported results of repeat subacromial decompression in patients with persistent subacromial impingement following previous rotator cuff surgery are inferior to the results reported following primary subacromial decompression.[55,84,142,158,186] Satisfactory results have been reported in 10% to 75% of patients undergoing revision subacromial decompression.[55,84,142,158] Potential etiologic factors responsible for these inferior results include a high percentage of workman's compensation patients and other patients with secondary gain factors,[81] subacromial scarring related to multiple surgeries, unrealistic patient expectations, and unrecognized concomitant pathology. The importance of strict patient selection on the basis of continued radiographic supraspinatus outlet narrowing and positive subacromial injection tests cannot be overemphasized.

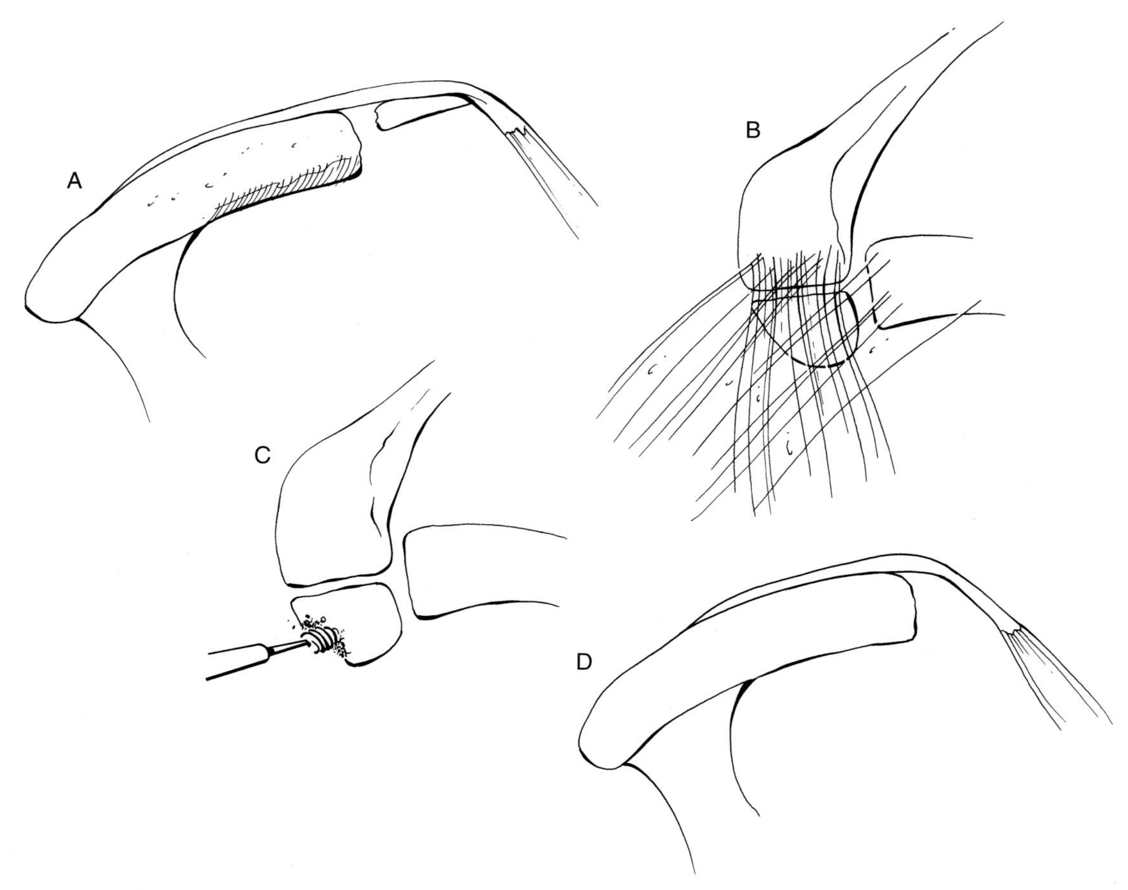

FIG. 18. **(A)** The ununited anterior acromial fragment lies within the anterior deltoid aponeurosis and **(B)** extends to the middle third of the acromion at a level corresponding to the posterior portion of the acromioclavicular joint. **(C)** Arthroscopic excision begins at the anterior edge of the anterior fragment and extends posteriorly toward the nonunion or fracture site. **(D)** Complete excision leaves the deltotrapezius aponeurosis on the dorsal surface of the acromion in continuity with the anterior and middle deltoid.

Heterotopic Ossification

The treatment of heterotopic ossification following rotator cuff surgery is dependent on the type and severity of ossification present. Ossification within the subacromial space which is not associated with loss of glenohumeral motion may be managed by open or arthroscopic debridement of the subacromial space. Open debridement requires deltoid detachment. However, it may be associated with a lower incidence of recurrent ossification and allow a more thorough excision than arthroscopic debridement.[105] Whichever method of surgical debridement is chosen, indomethacin (25 mg three times per day) is prescribed for 6 weeks postoperatively to prevent recurrent ossification.[11]

More aggressive heterotopic ossification involving the pericapsular soft tissue is often associated with significant loss of glenohumeral motion. Recurrence following excision is less likely if the excision is delayed until active ossification has ceased and the heterotopic bone has been allowed to mature. The optimum time for excision is difficult to determine because experience with aggressive postoperative heterotopic ossification about the shoulder is limited. An arbitrary delay of 1 year before excision of heterotopic bone should allow adequate maturation of the heterotopic bone and may decrease the likelihood of recurrence.

The extensive nature of this pericapsular ossification requires open excision. The surgical approach is dependent on the location of the largest amount of bone. Usually this is anterior; therefore, the initial approach is deltopectoral. If possible, anterior and inferior pericapsular ectopic bone is excised through a subscapularis splitting incision. If this is not possible, the subscapularis is incised 1 to 2 cm medial to its insertion and reflected medially to expose the heterotopic bone. Heterotopic ossification that involves the superior capsule and supraspinatus can then be excised by sharply dissecting the interval between the supraspinatus and the superior capsule. Significant posterior heterotopic bone may require a second, posterior incision for adequate exposure. Again, excision is preferred through muscle-splitting approaches, rather than muscle-detaching approaches, when possible. Single low-dose radiation or indomethacin is given postoperatively for 6 weeks to prevent recurrence.[11]

Frozen Shoulder

Frozen shoulder that develops subsequent to rotator cuff surgery is often the result of both intraarticular and extraarticular contractures.[121,150,181,182] Dense adhesions between the undersurface of the acromion and the rotator cuff in addition to capsular contracture contribute to the refractory nature of postoperative frozen shoulder.[121,182] As long as the patient demonstrates continued progress, nonsurgical joint mobilization techniques are pursued for 3 to 6 months. Judicious use of intraarticular corticosteroids, particularly in the early postoperative period, may provide pain relief, which facilitates compliance with physiotherapy. However, if the stiffness occurs following a rotator cuff repair, the merits of intraarticular corticosteroids in the early postoperative period must be balanced against the possibility of interference with tendon healing.

Closed manipulation without capsular release is most often unsuccessful in the refractory postoperative stiff shoulder, but should be attempted. Arthroscopic release is an excellent technique for management of the postoperative frozen shoulder that has been recalcitrant to nonsurgical treatment and unresponsive to closed manipulation.[79,182] However, arthroscopic capsular release in patients with stiffness following rotator cuff surgery must often be combined with resection of subacromial adhesions.[182] I prefer to place the arthroscope into the subacromial space before placing it into the glenohumeral joint. This is performed through a posterolateral portal (Fig. 19). After the posterolateral skin incision is made, the sheath for the arthroscope, with the blunt obturator in place, is inserted into the subacromial space. An attempt is then made to pass the sheath and obturator over the greater tuberosity and into the subdeltoid bursa. If this cannot be accomplished without substantial force, the obturator is removed from the sheath and the arthroscope is inserted. An anterolateral portal is established through which an arthroscopic resector is placed (see Fig. 19). The adhesions

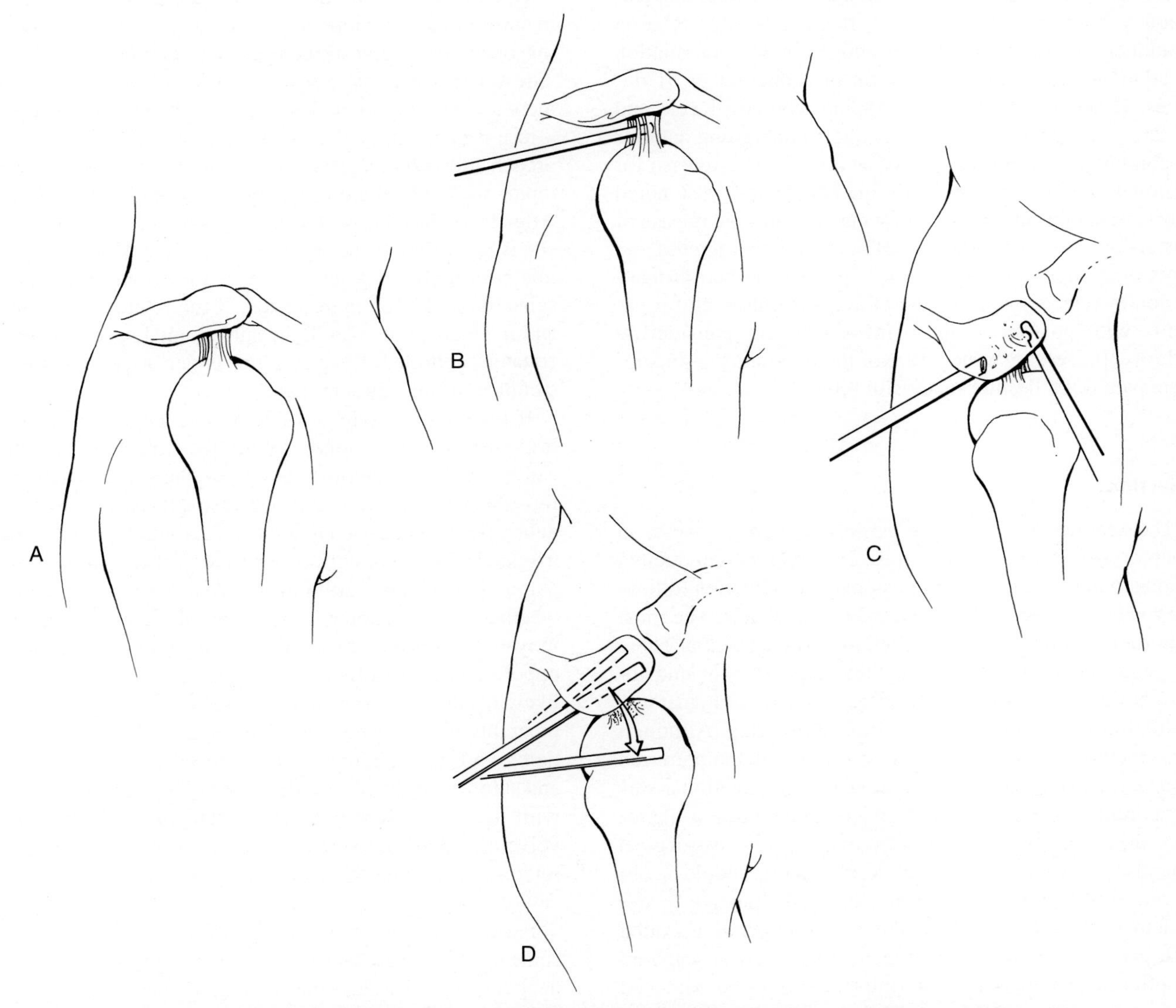

FIG. 19. Frozen shoulder following previous rotator cuff surgery is often characterized by dense adhesions between the undersurface of the acromion and the superficial surface of the rotator cuff **(A)**. A blunt obturator placed into the subacromial space is prevented from moving over the humeral head into the subdeltoid bursa by these dense adhesions **(B)**. After these adhesions have been resected and the subacromial space has been re-established **(C)**, the blunt obturator can easily be passed from the subacromial space to the subdeltoid bursa and back again **(D)**.

between the rotator cuff and the acromion are then resected. Electrocautery is used not only for hemostasis, but also for additional release of adhesions. Resection and release of adhesions is continued until the blunt obturator for the arthroscopic sheath can be passed freely from the subacromial space, over the greater tuberosity, into the subdeltoid bursa, and back into the subacromial space (see Fig. 19).

The arthroscope is then inserted into the glenohumeral joint through a standard posterior portal. Release of the anterior and posterior capsule is performed as necessary. The technique for arthroscopic anterior and posterior capsular release in the postoperative shoulder is not substantially different from the technique in the nonoperated shoulder.[10,79,166,181,182,191] The interested reader is referred to Chapter 15 on diagnosis and management of the stiff shoulder. Open release is reserved for patients who have failed arthroscopic release.

Return of motion following arthroscopic release for postoperative stiffness is usually excellent.[10,182] Warner and colleagues[182] reported mean gains in flexion, external rotation in adduction, external rotation in abduction, internal rotation in adduction, and internal rotation in abduction of 51 degrees, 31 degrees, 40 degrees, six spinous process levels, and 41 degrees, respectively, in 11 patients undergoing anterior or combined anterior and posterior arthroscopic release for postoperative stiffness. Beaufils and colleagues[10] also noted substantial gains in motion following arthroscopic release of postoperatively stiff shoulders. However, the pain relief and functional improvement was not as good as in their primary or nonoperated shoulders. Therefore, it is important for patients with postoperative stiffness who are considering arthroscopic release to be aware of the possibility of incomplete pain relief despite successful return of motion.

Infection

The treatment of shoulder sepsis is extensively covered in Chapter 34 on shoulder infections. However, certain factors unique to the management of postoperative infection following rotator cuff surgery deserve added emphasis. The most important of those factors is a high index of suspicion. There is a tendency to treat patients with postoperative wound abnormalities, such as mild erythema, drainage, or hematoma formation expectantly or with oral antibiotics. Although these methods may occasionally be successful, the preferred management of a deep, postoperative wound infection is surgical drainage. The sooner a deep wound infection is identified, the sooner it can be treated. Therefore, postsurgical wounds that exhibit any signs of deep infection should be observed closely for deterioration. Surgical drainage or debridement should be considered in any postoperative wound with persistent drainage or erythema. The modest potential benefits of prolonged oral antibiotics should be balanced against the possibility for a delay in diagnosis of a deep wound infection.

Early infection (i.e., within 4 weeks of surgery) following arthroscopic acromioplasty may be adequately managed by arthroscopic irrigation and debridement. If glenohumeral diagnostic arthroscopy was performed in addition to the initial arthroscopic acromioplasty, the glenohumeral joint as well as the subacromial space should probably be irrigated and debrided. I prefer to obtain as clean a subacromial space as possible before I enter the glenohumeral joint with the arthroscope. The subacromial space is often loculated and each of these loculations may contain infected debris. Therefore, an arthroscopic resector with frequent suction is used to break up these loculated pockets of infection. Once the subacromial space has been adequately debrided and irrigated, the arthroscope is inserted into the glenohumeral joint, and the joint cavity is irrigated with large quantities (3 to 6 L) of irrigant. It is helpful to establish a formal outflow portal with a large-bore (8-mm) cannula to facilitate flow of the irrigant through the joint.

Open irrigation and debridement are probably preferable in cases of early postoperative deep wound infection following open acromioplasty or open acromioplasty and rotator cuff repair. The relative advantages of arthroscopic management are less important, because the patient has already had a recent open surgical procedure. In addition, an open approach allows direct inspection of the deltoid and rotator cuff repair sites, which are often compromised by the infection. After the skin incision has been opened, the deltoid repair site is identified. If the repair is secure, the deltoid is split in line with its fibers at the site of the previous split, and the subacromial region is inspected. If the rotator cuff is intact and the loculations within the subacromial space can be adequately debrided, the procedure is performed without detachment of the deltoid repair.

If the deltoid repair has failed or if the subacromial debridement is compromised by limited exposure, the deltoid can be retracted anteriorly to expose the subacromial space for adequate irrigation and debridement. After all necrotic debris has been excised and the subacromial space has been irrigated, the rotator cuff is inspected. If there was a prior repair and the repair is still intact, a decision must be made on whether or not the potentially colonized suture material is removed. Removal of all suture material may provide the best opportunity for resolution of the infection. However, it will likely result in a chronically retracted tendon that may not be reparable after the infection has cleared. Therefore, in patients who are not immunocompromised, the repaired tendon and sutures are left in situ. Because the sutures communicate with the joint, there is the potential for intraarticular involvement of the infection. Therefore, a small incision in the rotator interval can be made to permit irrigation of the joint cavity.

Failure of the previous rotator cuff repair usually indicates some degree of necrosis of the tendon edge as a result of the deep infection. Because the suture material is no longer providing any function, it is debrided. Any suture-anchoring devices that are accessible may also be debrided. Whether the torn tendon is rerepaired depends on the condition of the remaining tendon and the size of the tendon defect. If the tendon is necrotic and the defect is small (i.e., one tendon), it may be best to leave it unrepaired until the infection has cleared (i.e., 6 weeks). The patient can then be reassesed for possible repair if necessary. Conversely, if the defect is large, particularly if preoperative overhead function had been compromised, consideration should be given to immediate rerepair at the time of the initial debridement. Regardless of whether or not the rotator cuff is repaired, the deltoid should be reattached. The soft tissues at the anterior edge of the acromion are often quite friable and are not ideal for suture placement. Under these circumstances, the deltoid is repaired to the bone of the acromion.

Antibiotics are withheld until intraoperative cultures have been obtained. Broad-spectrum coverage for skin organisms such as *Staphylococcus aureus* is then given. This is most often vancomycin or a first-generation cephalosporin such as cefazolin. The antibiotics are changed appropriately when the cultures return. The duration of antibiotic coverage is empiric and must be individualized. However, treatment generally includes 1 to 3 weeks of intravenous treatment followed by 1 to 3 weeks of oral treatment.

The additive trauma of the first surgery, the infection, and the second surgery predisposes to the development of stiffness. Therefore, passive mobilization is started immediately postoperatively in all cases. In patients who required deltoid or rotator cuff rerepair, an abduction brace or pillow is used to protect the repair for 3 weeks. These patients remove their arm from the pillow or brace only to perform their passive exercises. Active motion and strengthening are begun 6 weeks postoperatively.

Patients with an intact rotator cuff and deltoid at the time of the debridement use only a sling postoperatively. If the primary rotator cuff surgery did not include a cuff repair, active exercises and strengthening are begun as soon as symptoms allow. If the primary operation did include a rotator cuff repair, only passive exercises are performed for the first 6 weeks. Thereafter, active motion and strengthening exercises are added.

Late or chronic infection following rotator cuff surgery requires more aggressive treatment than early infection. It is often related to retained foreign bodies, such as nonabsorbable suture or suture-anchoring devices.[177] Complete eradication of the infection requires removal of all foreign bodies and radical debridement of all necrotic debris. If there are large quantities of necrotic material and the adequacy of debridement cannot be determined at the time of the initial debridement, repeat debridement may be necessary. Any rotator cuff defect identified at the time of debridement should be left unrepaired. It is only repaired if the infection has been successfully cleared. Intraoperative cultures should be sent not only for routine aerobes and anaerobes, but also for fungus, tuberculosis, and atypical mycobacteria. Intravenous antibiotics are continued for 6 weeks after debridement.

Reports on outcome following treatment of postoperative shoulder infections are lacking. All patients, regardless of rotator cuff or deltoid status, seem to have more pain with activity than their counterparts who have not been infected. The pain is usually not disabling, nor severe enough to require analgesics. Strength and overhead function, however, are directly related to rotator cuff and deltoid integrity. Most patients with an intact deltoid and rotator cuff have good overhead function. Even patients with an intact deltoid and a small unrepaired rotator cuff defect function overhead, albeit with some degree of fatigue. Postoperative wound infection following rotator cuff surgery undoubtedly has a negative effect on overall outcome. However, the results are not nearly as poor as those reported for spontaneous septic arthritis of the shoulder in adults.[60,99,100]

Suprascapular Nerve Injury

Suprascapular nerve injury following rotator cuff surgery is the result of aggressive lateral mobilization of a chronically retracted cuff tear.[183] The nerve presumably has been stretched over the lateral margin of the suprascapular notch, or it has been injured directly by surgical dissection too far medial to the glenoid rim. These rotator cuff tears are typically large or massive and are also at significant risk for recurrent tearing or incomplete healing following primary repair.[59,78] In addition, the functional results following primary repair of these large defects are not as favorable as results following repair of smaller, less retracted defects, regardless of the status of the suprascapular nerve.[86,89] Therefore, the added effect of the nerve injury may be difficult to quantitate.

The treatment of suprascapular neuropathy depends on the degree of functional impairment, the age and activity level of the patient, and the status of the supra- and infraspinatus muscle bellies. Treatment options include observation and activity modification, nerve exploration and decompression, and tendon transfer. Most patients with low overhead demands and many patients with high overhead demands will be willing to modify their activity and accept the limitations related to suprascapular nerve injury. In addition, these suprascapular nerve injuries are usually incomplete neuropraxias. Therefore, activity modification should be combined with external rotation strengthening exercises to obtain the most function possible from the remaining posterior rotator cuff muscles (i.e., the unaffected portions of the supra- and infraspinatus as well as the teres minor).

It is unusual for a young, active patient to present with suprascapular nerve injury following rotator cuff surgery. Suprascapular neuropathy in a young patient who has undergone subacromial decompression without cuff repair probably represents a failure in diagnosis, rather than a complication of the surgery and should be treated as a primary suprascapular neuropathy. In the rare instance of a young, active patient presenting with suprascapular neuropathy following mobilization and repair of a chronic, retracted rotator cuff tear, exploration and possible decompression of the nerve is considered only if there is significant functional impairment, there has been no electromyographic or clinical improvement in 6 months, the cuff repair is intact, and the supra- and infraspinatus muscle bellies have not undergone significant fatty degeneration.[66] Decompression of the nerve is performed at the suprascapular notch and should include enlargement of the lateral margin of the notch, in addition to division of the transverse scapular ligament.[4,155,156,179]

Tendon transfers are reserved for patients who either have failed decompression of the nerve or were not candidates for nerve decompression based on the foregoing criteria. It is very unlikely that a patient will have enough functional impairment related to the suprascapular neuropathy with an intact cuff repair to require tendon transfer to augment posterior rotator cuff function. If this rare circumstance is encountered, consideration is given to the tendon transfer techniques for irreparable posterior rotator cuff insufficiency described in Chapter 3 on management of the irreparable rotator cuff tear.

Axillary Nerve Injury

Axillary nerve injury during rotator cuff surgery results from extension of the deltoid split too far distally. This almost never occurs during isolated acromioplasty because of the limited exposure necessary. However, the added visualization necessary to repair large and massive rotator cuff tears occasionally results in distal extension of the deltoid split, either by overzealous retraction or direct incision. Treatment of the axillary nerve injury depends on the status of the cuff repair, the status of the coracoacromial arch, and the degree of functional impairment. The nerve injury typically occurs at the level of the mid- or anterior acromion. In this location, the caliber of the nerve and the proximity of the terminal branches to the anterior deltoid often preclude neurolysis, nerve repair, or nerve grafting. Therefore, available treatment options include activity modification and rehabilitation, muscle transfers, and arthrodesis. Most patients with an intact cuff repair will be able to use their arm at or near shoulder height and, therefore, are willing to pursue nonoperative management.

Management of axillary nerve injury in association with a failed cuff repair is dependent on the size and reparability of the recurrent rotator cuff defect and the status of the coracoacromial arch. If the recurrent rotator cuff defect is small and reparable, consideration is given to bipolar latissimus transfer to restore anterior deltoid function.[90] This is not performed, however, until after the revision cuff repair has been performed and the subsequent final result has been evaluated. Often the location of the axillary nerve injury spares enough of the middle deltoid that the patient may be willing to live with the axillary nerve injury if the repeat cuff repair has been successful.

Axillary nerve injury in the presence of a large or massive recurrent rotator cuff defect, particularly when the coracoacromial arch is deficient, is a very difficult problem, with no good solution. This is discussed further under the following sections on recurrent rotator cuff defects and anterosuperior humeral head subluxation. When the functional deficits of axillary nerve injury are added to the deficits associated with a recurrent massive cuff defect, the shoulder is nearly flail. The likelihood of restoring permanent rotator cuff function, coracoacromial arch integrity, and deltoid function is very low. Therefore, the choice for these patients is usually between acceptance of the deficits or arthrodesis. Patients considering arthrodesis should understand clearly that they will lose all rotational motion of the shoulder. Often, even the most disabled patients are able to use humeral rotation with the arm at the side. Loss of this only remaining function may not be worth the potential pain relief and improved stability afforded by an arthrodesis.

Deltoid Detachment

Detachment of the deltoid repair following open acromioplasty or acromioplasty and rotator cuff repair is best managed by prompt reattachment if the affected portion of the deltoid is functionally significant. Small (1- to 1.5-cm) detachments may not be symptomatic or clinicaly relevant. Larger deltoid detachments should be repaired as soon as they are recognized. If they are diagnosed early (within 4 to 6 weeks) the detached deltoid can be reattached easily. Reattachment to the bone of the acromion in addition to the deltotrapezius fascia is recommended. Any reparable recurrent rotator cuff defect identified at the time of deltoid repair is also rerepaired.

Unfortunately, most postoperative deltoid detachments go unrecognized for a long period.[71,167] This makes mobilization and reattachment of the chronically retracted deltoid difficult. This is particularly true when the detachment involves any significant portion of the middle deltoid.[167] After making a skin incision and undermining full-thickness skin flaps, an attempt is made to identify the intact portions of the deltoid at the margins of the detachment. This can sometimes be difficult, because thin scar tissue often occupies the void between the remaining intact portions of the deltoid. It can be helpful to identify the anterolateral corner of the residual acromion and incise the scar tissue attaching there in line with the perceived direction of the deltoid. Digital palpation with the index finger on the deep surface and the thumb on the superficial surface of the deltoid may identify the thicker area of the intact portions of the deltoid (Fig. 20).

Once the intact anterior and middle portions of the deltoid have been identified, the remaining scar tissue between the intact portions of the deltoid can be released from the acromion. The split at the anterolateral corner is then extended to the level of the axillary nerve, which is easily palpable on the deep surface of the deltoid fibers (see Fig. 20). The thickened fibrous edge of the retracted anterior deltoid can usually be palpated and distinguished from the adjacent scar within the anterior soft-tissue flap. This thin adjacent scar tissue is then excised up to the fibrous edge of the retracted anterior deltoid (see Fig. 20). The distance between the lateral edge of the intact anterior deltoid origin and the anterolateral corner of the acromion is measured. An equivalent distance is then measured along the fibrous edge of the anterior deltoid. A suture is placed at that point in the retracted deltoid origin (see Fig. 20). This point will eventually be reattached at the anterolateral corner of the residual acromion.

The fibrous thickened edge of the retracted middle deltoid origin is next identified in a similar fashion (see Fig. 20). The thin scar tissue that was attached to the acromion at the site of the middle deltoid detachment can usually be distinguished from the thickened middle deltoid origin and is excised. The detached and retracted middle deltoid is then mobilized proximally. This requires circumferential release of the detached portion of the middle deltoid. The location of the axillary nerve should always be remembered to avoid inadvertent injury. After the superficial and deep surfaces of the retracted portion of the middle deltoid have been completely dissected, the muscle is mobilized proximally to the lateral edge of the acromion. In a fashion similar to the anterior deltoid, the distance from the intact portion of the middle deltoid to the anterolateral acromion is measured. An equivalent distance along the fibrous edge of the retracted middle deltoid is measured and a suture is placed. This portion of the middle deltoid will be reattached to the residual anterior acromion, adjacent to the analogous portion of the anterior deltoid (Fig. 20).

The portions of the acromion that will receive the detached portions of the middle and anterior deltoid are freshened. The anterior and middle portions of the deltoid are then sutured to the acromion through drill holes using interupted, heavy, nonabsorbable sutures. Care is taken to ensure that the previously marked portions of the anterior and middle deltoid are reattached at the anterolateral corner of the acromion, adjacent to one another. The split in the deltoid is next repaired with interupted nonabsorbable sutures (see Fig. 20).

All deltoid detachments do not have the same configuration. In addition, acromial deficiency from overzealous acromion excision can make deltoid reattachment impossible. Therefore, relaxing incisions and transpositional flaps from the intact portion of the deltoid may be required to close the deltoid defect.[167] As the complexity of the required reconstructive procedures escalates, the expected results deteriorate.

Postoperatively, all patients undergoing deltoid reattachment or deltoid reconstruction are placed in an abduction orthosis for 3 to 6 weeks. This affords protection of the deltoid repair or reconstruction. Passive supine elevation and passive external rotation exercises are instituted within the first postoperative week. The patient removes the arm from the orthosis to perform these passive exercises three to five times each day, but wears the orthosis full-time otherwise. Active and active-assisted motion is allowed 4 to 6 weeks postoperatively. Strengthening exercises are added 6 to 8 weeks postoperatively.

Reported results following reattachment of the deltoid are sparse and, generally, poor.[14,133,167] This is especially true when these results are compared with the results of primary, uncomplicated rotator cuff repair. Sher and colleagues reported 67% unsatisfactory results in 24 patients who underwent deltoid repair or reconstruction for postoperative deltoid detachment.[167] However, patients with no or small residual rotator cuff defects, early recognition and treatment, no middle deltoid involvement, and no acromial insufficiency had a better prognosis.[167] Early recognition and treatment of the detachment is perhaps the strongest positive influence. In Sher and colleagues' series, patients whose detachment was treated within 2 and 12 months of the initial surgery had 62% and 88% satisfactory results, respectively.

Recurrent Rotator Cuff Tear

The treatment principles surrounding revision rotator cuff repair are the same as those surrounding primary rotator cuff repair. However, the chronicity of the rotator cuff tear inherent in revision surgery and the presence of other mitigating factors such as deltoid insufficiency, coracoacromial arch insufficiency, and subacromial scarring make revision rotator cuff repair much more challenging than primary cuff repair. Deltoid insufficiency and coracoacromial arch insufficiency are covered elsewhere in this chapter. Therefore, this section will cover only the management of recurrent rotator cuff defects.

Treatment options for recurrent or persistent rotator cuff defects are the same as for primary defects and include rehabilitation and activity modification, revision repair, debridement or partial repair, tendon substitution with allograft or prosthetic material, tendon advancement, local tendon transposition, and distant tendon transfer.[7,16,24,25,35,42,61,73,74,125,136,144,152,159,180] The specific treatment indicated is dependent on patient age, activity, motivation, tear size, the degree of impairment, and tissue quality. It is important to remember that significant stiffness should be corrected before considering revision rotator cuff surgery. This is particularly true in large recurrent defects. Lack of both active and passive elevation may be the result of capsular contracture, rather than residual cuff insufficiency. Correction of stiffness by arthroscopic capsular release may allow a patient with irreparable rotator cuff insufficiency to tolerate the residual cuff insufficiency and avoid a complicated reconstructive procedure.

Rehabilitation of the remaining portions of the rotator cuff, deltoid, and scapular stabilizers is a very reasonable initial treatment for most patients with a recurrent defect. Exceptions to this general rule are patients who had repair of an acute, large tear and patients who sustained an early rerupture with marked change in symptomatology. This is particularly true if the rerupture coincided with an easily identifi-

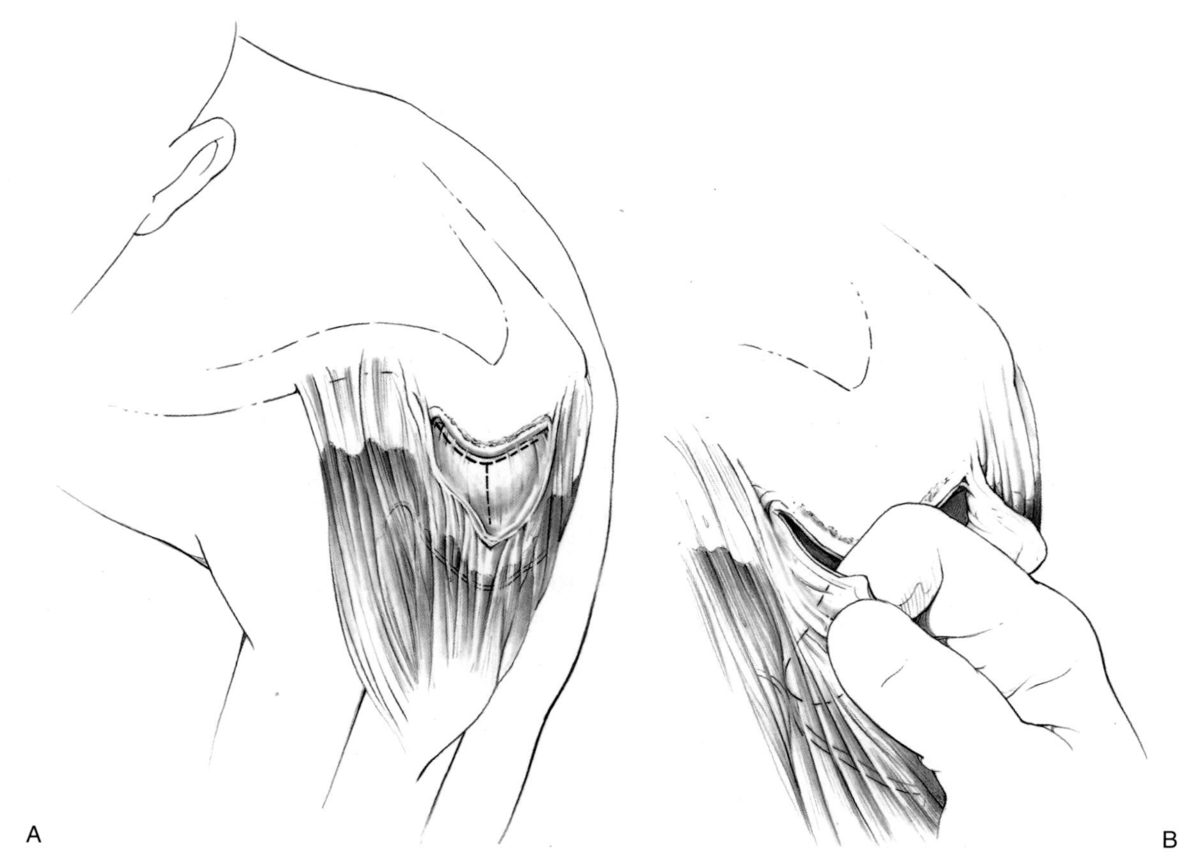

FIG. 20. When attempting to reattach the deltoid which has come detached following previous rotator cuff surgery, it can be difficult to identify the junction between the retracted deltoid edge and the thin scar tissue which has filled the gap between the acromion and the retracted deltoid **(A)**. (continued)

able event and if the original repair was thought to be of good quality. When rehabilitation is indicated, the methods are not substantially different from those employed in primary ruptures that are treated nonoperatively. The interested reader is referred to Chapter 35 on rehabilitation.

Revision rotator cuff repair is indicated in patients who have failed nonoperative management or who fit the criteria for early revision repair as outlined earlier. The specific surgical principles employed during revision rotator cuff repair are no different from those employed in primary repair as outlined in Chapter 2. The general surgical philosophy is to repair the rotator cuff tendon-to-bone securely enough to allow early passive motion and to facilitate tendon-to-bone healing. If the entire recurrent defect is not reparable, reattachment of some portion of the tendon to bone will likely result in improved function.[25] If no portion of the tendon can be repaired, a decision must be made on tendon reconstruction or transfer. If the patient had intact overhead function preoperatively, I prefer to ignore the defect and preserve the anterior and posterior rotator cuff force couple that remains by not transposing any of the intact anterior and posterior rotator cuff superiorly to close the defect.[24,27,35,134,137] In addition, any remaining portion of the coracoacromial ligament is preserved or repaired. The remaining rotator cuff is rehabilitated along with the deltoid and scapular rotators. If the patient is unhappy with their shoulder or their overhead function is not adequate after rehabilitation, tendon transfer is considered. Latissimus dorsi transfer has been described for irreparable posterior cuff insufficiency.[61,65] Currently, pectoralis major transfer is the most popular technique for anterior cuff insufficiency.[187] These techniques are outlined in Chapter 3 on management of the irreparable rotator cuff tear.

Most authors report disappointing results with revision rotator cuff repair.[17,42] Deorio and Cofield reported on 27 patients who underwent revision rotator cuff repair.[42] Seven patients (26%) required a third operative procedure before the completion of the study; of the remaining 20 patients, there were no excellent results and only 9 (42%) good results. Bigliani and colleagues reported only 52% satisfactory results in 31 patients undergoing revision rotator cuff repair.[17] Neviaser and colleagues reported more encouraging results in 50 patients who underwent revision rotator cuff repair.[133] They noted no correlation of the result with number of prior surgeries, size of the recurrent defect, or status of the long head of the biceps. A satisfactory outcome was most de-

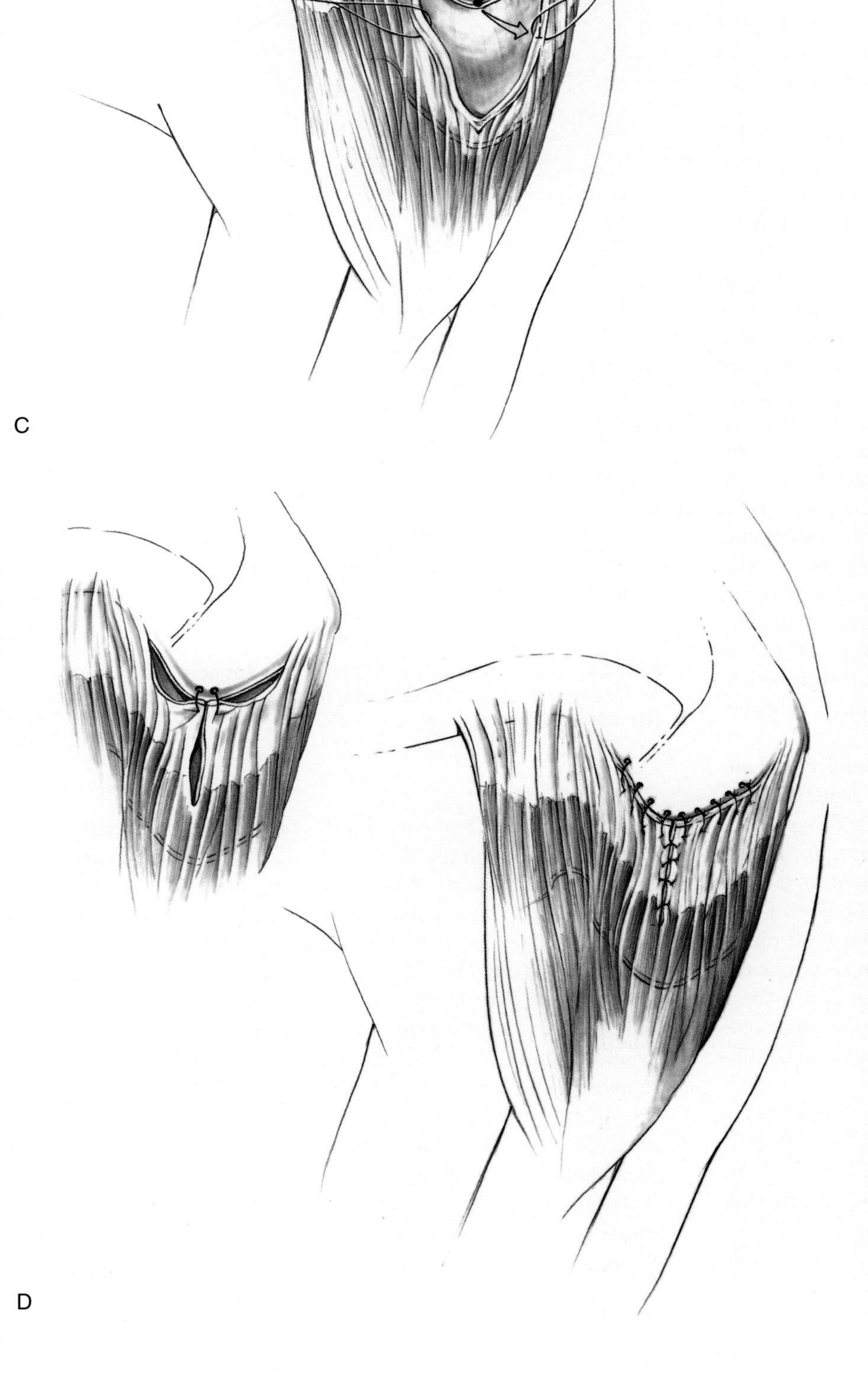

FIG. 20. *(Continued)* The antero-lateral corner of the acromion is identified and the soft-tissue attaching to it is incised in line with the perceived direction of the deltoid fibers for a distance of 3-3.5 centimeters. In addition, the soft-tissue along the anterior and lateral margins is incised for a short distance anterior and posterior to the anterolateral corner **(A)**. This creates an anterior flap, which contains the retracted anterior deltoid and the attached scar tissue, and a posterior flap, which contains the retracted middle deltoid and attached scar tissue. Digital palpation of the two flaps allows identification of the interface between the thicker retracted deltoid edge and the thinner scar tissue. The intact portions of the anterior and middle detoid origins can also be palpated. The scar tissue is excised up to the intact deltoid origins and up to the retracted deltoid edge. The split at the anterolateral corner is continued distally to the level of the axillary nerve, which is protected **(B)**. The respective distances from the intact portions of the middle and anterior deltoid to the anterolateral corner of the acromion are measured. Marking sutures are placed within the fibrous, retracted edges of the anterior and middle deltoids at points which correspond to the previous measured distances **(C)**. These two sutures are then passed through drill holes in the anterolateral corner so that they come to rest adjacent to one another. The remaining portions of the detached anterior and middle deltoid are also reattached to the acromion through drill holes **(D)**.

pendent on an adequate subacromial decompression, repair of the cuff with tendon-to-bone sutures, avoidance of weights in the early postoperative period, and an intact and functioning deltoid.[133]

Anterosuperior Humeral Head Subluxation

Surgical treatment options in patients with anterosuperior subluxation following prior rotator cuff repair should be considered salvage procedures. These patients are some of the most unhappy patients one will encounter with shoulder problems. Their pain and disability is often intolerable, even with significant activity modifications and analgesics.[50,185] Surgical options fall under two general categories: (a) motion preserving and (b) motion sacrificing. Motion-preserving procedures include various combinations of tendon transfers and coracoacromial arch reconstructions as well as constrained joint replacement.[50,61,68,185,187] Motion-sacrificing procedures include arthrodesis.[36]

Surgical management of anterosuperior humeral head subluxation without constrained arthroplasty or arthrodesis requires that both the rotator cuff and coracoacromial arch insufficiencies be addressed. These rotator cuff defects are usually not reparable. Therefore, one is left with partial repair, tendon transfer, or a combination of partial repair and tendon transfer as the best available options to improve rotator cuff function. The goal is to restore some semblance of a balanced anteroposterior rotator cuff force couple, even if the entire humeral head is not covered. Usually these patients have some portion of the subscapularis preserved or reparable. Therefore, latissimus dorsi transfer to augment or replace the posterior rotator cuff mechanism is most frequently indicated.[61] If irreparable posterior rotator cuff insufficiency is combined with irreparable subscapularis insufficiency, then reestablishment of a balanced force couple is probably not possible.

Theoretically, the coracoacromial arch could be reconstructed using soft tissue, bone, or prosthetic material. Currently described techniques employ either bone grafts or soft-tissue coracoacromial ligament reconstructions (Fig. 21).[50,185] Experience with either of these methods is preliminary and not extensive. Therefore, it is difficult to know which is the most reliable method. The goal with either method of coracoacromial arch reconstruction is to span the defect between the coracoid and the acromion to provide a static restraint which, when combined with appropriate tendon transfers, will prevent anterosuperior humeral head subluxation.

There has been renewed interest, especially in Europe, in constrained implants for the management of the cuff-deficient shoulder with anterosuperior subluxation.[9,68] Constrained implants in the shoulder have been plagued by high loosening and mechanical failure rates in the past.[38,44,107,153,154] Although constrained implants can reestablish a ful-

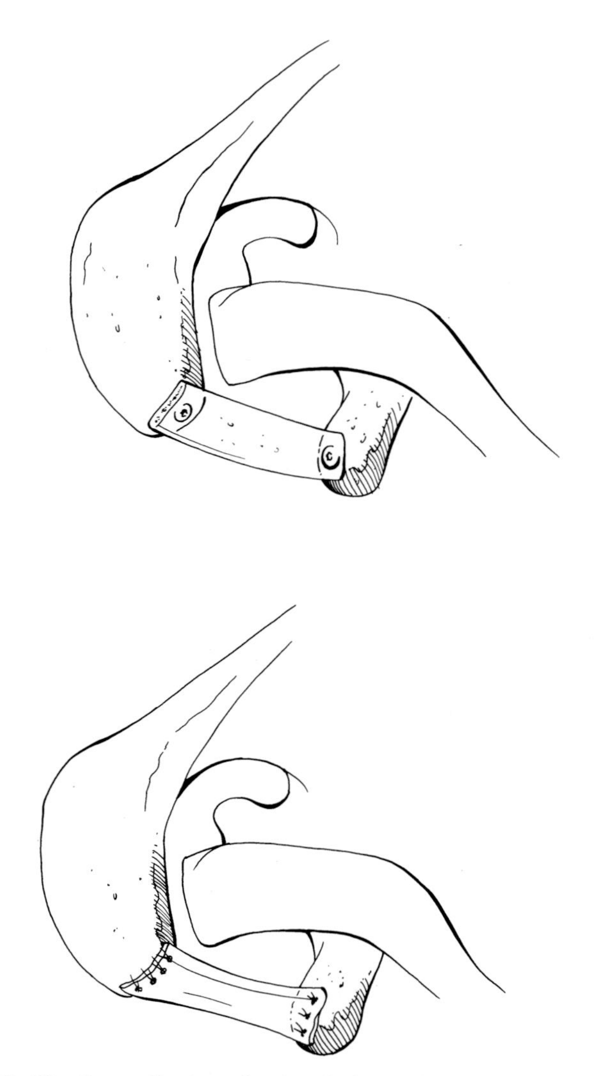

FIG. 21. Currently described techniques for coracoacromial arch reconstruction include bone grafting **(A)** and soft-tissue **(B)** interposition.

crum between the humerus and the scapula and potentially improve function in the short term, significant stress is imparted to the implants as well as to the implant–bone-anchoring points. The use of constrained implants in the United States should be considered investigational at this time.

Arthrodesis may be the only realistic surgical option in some patients with anterosuperior subluxation of the humeral head. A successful arthrodesis will improve stability and strength. However, the trade-off is complete loss of glenohumeral rotation. In many instances, patients with anterosuperior subluxation will be content to use their involved extremity as a helping hand with the arm at the side. Loss of glenohumeral rotation may actually represent a decrease in function in some patients. Therefore, glenohumeral arthrodesis is reserved for patients with severe pain who are willing to sacrifice glenohumeral rotation.

CONCLUSIONS AND TREATMENT ALGORITHM

Rotator cuff surgery is generally safe and efficacious. However, when complications occur, they are frequently accompanied by recurrent symptoms that may be worse than the original preoperative symptoms that prompted the patient to seek medical care in the first place. Reported results of surgical treatment of many of these complications are inconsistent. Surgical treatment of complications of rotator cuff surgery is demanding and requires both a motivated patient and a knowledgeable surgeon. It is impossible to establish rigid patient selection criteria and treatment protocols for all types of complications of rotator cuff surgery. However, adoption of a systematic approach that is based on known anatomic observations and well-established surgical principles affords the best opportunity for a successful outcome. One algorithmic approach to the management of patients with complications following rotator cuff surgery is depicted in Fig. 22.

Several principles used to develop this algorithm deserve emphasis. The first principle is that the presence of significant stiffness interferes with the interpretation of the significance of any other complications that accompany the stiffness, such as a recurrent rotator cuff tear. Frequently, patients with documented recurrent rotator cuff defects will present with inability to achieve elevation of their arm more than 90 degrees, either actively or passively. If these patients present, before their primary rotator cuff repair, with intact active overhead elevation, restoration of normal or near normal passive elevation will likely be accompanied by significant gains in active elevation. The patient may be satisfied with their shoulder function after a simple arthroscopic capsular release and be willing to forego more complicated sur-

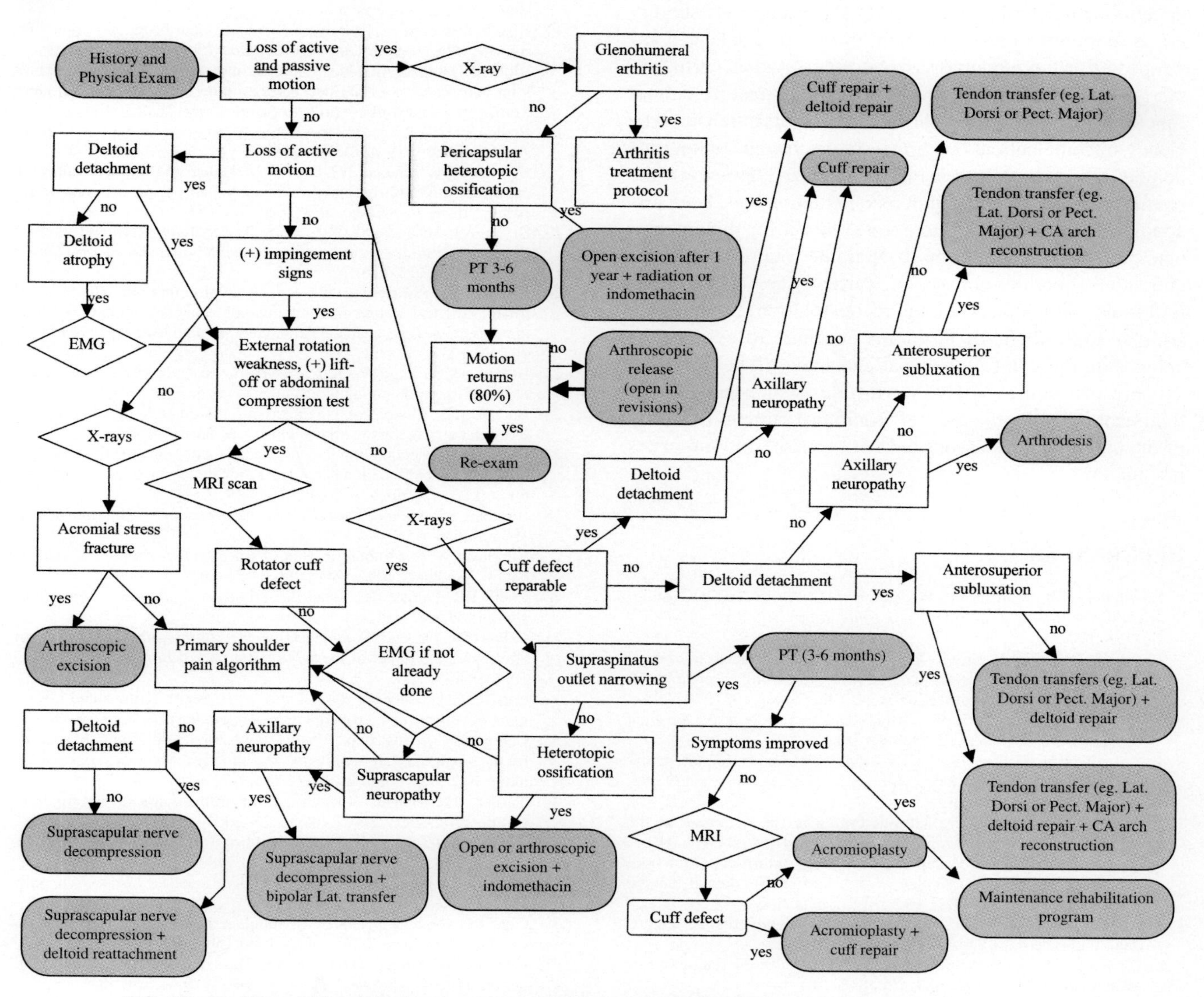

FIG. 22. Treatment algorithm for the management of complications following rotator cuff surgery.

gical procedures, particulary if their recurrent rotator cuff defect is irreparable.

Loss of active elevation in the presence of normal or near-normal passive motion may indicate deltoid insufficiency, rotator cuff insufficiency, or both. Furthermore, the presence of pain and voluntary guarding can make the interpretation of several physical findings difficult. This is particularly true for strength assessment of various portions of the rotator cuff. Subacromial lidocaine may improve the reliability of strength and functional assessments of the rotator cuff and is frequently used in the diagnosis of patients with continued pain and dysfunction following rotator cuff surgery.

Ultimately, the final outcome in patients who have undergone multiple operations for rotator cuff disease and complications related to their primary surgery is affected by many factors. If we assume that the original diagnosis was accurate, the goals of revision surgical intervention in most patients with complications of primary rotator cuff surgery are to reestablish passive motion; to restore a balanced anteroposterior force couple by rotator cuff repair, partial repair, or muscle transfer; and to preserve or restore deltoid function. The importance of coracoacromial arch insufficiency in some patients with massive recurrent rotator cuff defects is becoming increasingly recognized. However, the results of coracoacromial arch reconstruction have been disappointing. There is still no good solution for the unfortunate patient with a recurrent irreparable rotator cuff defect and anterosuperior subluxation, particularly when the deltoid is also deficient. Although reconstructive techniques to address these difficult problems continue to evolve, the choices for these unfortunate patients may still be limited to salvage procedures such as arthrodesis or nonoperative treatment. Clearly, the most efficacious treatment for many of the complications associated with rotator cuff surgery is prevention.

REFERENCES

1. Altchek DW, Warren RF, Wickiewicz TL. Arthroscopic acromioplasty: techniques and results. *J Bone Joint Surg [Am]* 1990;72: 1198–1207.
2. An HS, Ebraheim N, Kim K, Jackson WT, Kane JT. Heterotopic ossification and pseudoarthrosis in the shoulder following encephalitis. A case report and review of the literature. *Clin Orthop* 1987;291–298.
3. Andrews JR, Schemmel SP. Arthroscopic acromioplasty. *Surgical rounds for the orthopaedics* 1989:45–50.
4. Antoniadis G, Richter HP, Rath S, Braun V, Moese G. Suprascapular nerve entrapment: experience with 28 cases. *J Neurosurg* 1996;85: 1020–1025.
5. Armstrong JR. Excision of the acromion in the treatment of the supraspinatus syndrome. *J Bone Joint Surg [Br]* 1949;31:436–442.
6. Armstrong R, Bolding F. Septic arthritis after arthroscopy: the contributing roles of intra-articular steroids and environmental factors. *Am J Infect Control* 1994;22:16.
7. Augereau B. [Reconstruction of massive rotator cuff rupture using a deltoid muscle flap]. *Orthopade* 1991;20:315–319.
8. Bassett R, Cofield R. Acute tears of the rotator cuff: the timing of surgical repair. *Clin Orthop* 1983;175:18–24.
9. Baulot E, Chabernaud D, Grammont PM. [Results of Grammont's inverted prosthesis in omarthritis associated with major cuff destruction. Apropos of 16 cases]. *Acta Orthop Belg* 1995;61:112–119.
10. Beaufils P, Prevot N, Boyer T, et al. [Gleno-humeral arthroscopic arthrolysis for shoulder stiffness. Apropos of 26 cases. Societe Francaise d'Arthroscopie]. *Rev Chir Orthop* 1996;82:608–614.
11. Berg E, Ciullo JV. Heterotopic ossification after acromioplasty and distal clavicle resection. *J Shoulder Elbow Surg* 1995;4:188–193.
12. Berg EE, Ciullo JV, Oglesby JW. Failure of arthroscopic decompression by subacromial heterotropic ossification causing recurrent impingement. *Arthroscopy* 1994;10:158–160.
13. Bigliani L, Colman W, Kelkar R, et al. The effect of anterior acromioplasty on rotator cuff contact: an experimental and computer simulation. Presented at American Shoulder and Elbow Surgeons 11th open meeting. Orlando. FL, 1995.
14. Bigliani L, Dordasco F, McIlveen S, Musso E. Operative treatment of failed repairs of the rotator cuff. *J Bone Joint Surg [Am]* 1992;74: 1505–1515.
15. Bigliani L, EL, F, Deliz E. Complications of shoulder arthroscopy. *Orthop Rev* 1991;20:743.
16. Bigliani LU, Cordasco FA, McIlveen SJ, Musso ES. Operative repair of massive rotator cuff tears: long term results. *J Shoulder Elbow Surg* 1992;1:120–130.
17. Bigliani LU, Cordasco FA, McIlveen SJ. Operative management of failed rotator cuff repairs. *Orthop Trans* 1988;12:1974.
18. Bigliani LU, Dalsey RM, McCann PD, April EW. An anatomical study of the suprascapular nerve. *Arthroscopy* 1990;6:301–305.
19. Blauth W, Gartner J. Post operative results of arthrography following suturing of ruptured rotator cuff. *Orthopede* 1991;20:262–265.
20. Blom S, Dahlback LO. Nerve injuries in dislocations of the shoulder joint and fractures of the neck of the humerus. A clinical and electromyographical study. *Acta Chir Scand* 1970;136:461–466.
21. Bosley RC. Total acromionectomy. A twenty year review. *J Bone Joint Surg [Am]* 1991;73:961–968.
22. Bowman CA, Jeffcoate WJ, Pattrick M, Doherty M. Bilateral adhesive capsulitis, oligoarthritis and proximal myopathy as presentation of hypothyroidism. *Br J Rheumatol* 1988;27:62–64.
23. Bryan WJ, Schauder K, Tullos HS. The axillary nerve and its relationship to common sports medicine shoulder procedures. *Am J Sports Med* 1986;14:113–116.
24. Burkhart S. Arthroscopic debridement and decompression for selected rotator cuff tears: clinical results, pathomechanics and patient selection based on biomechanical parameters. *Orthop Clin North Am* 1993; 24:111–123.
25. Burkhart S, Nottage W, Ogilvie-Harris D, Kohn H, Pachelli A. Partial repair of irreparable rotator cuff tears. *Arthroscopy* 1994;10:363–370.
26. Burkhart SS. Fluoroscopic comparison of kinematic patterns in massive rotator cuff tears. *Clin Orthop* 1992;285:144–152.
27. Burkhart SS. Reconciling the paradox of rotator cuff repair versus debridement: a unified biomechanical rationale for the treatment of rotator cuff tears. *Arthroscopy* 1994;10:4–19.
28. Burkhart SS. Shoulder arthroscopy. New concepts. *Clin Sports Med* 1996;15:635–653.
29. Burkhead W, Scheinberg R, Box G. Surgical anatomy of the axillary nerve. *J Shoulder Elbow Surg* 1992;1:31–36.
30. Cahill BR, Palmer RE. Quadrilateral space syndrome. *J Hand Surg [Am]* 1983;8:65–69.
31. Calvert PT, Packer NP, Stoker DJ, et al. Arthrography of the shoulder after operative repair of the torn rotator cuff. *J Bone Joint Surg [Br]* 1986;68:147–150.
32. Cammerer U, Habermeyer P, Plenk A, Huber R. [Ultrasound assessment of reconstructed rotator cuffs]. *Unfallchirurg* 1992;95:608–612.
33. Caniggia M, Maniscalco P, Pagliantini L, Bocchi L. Titanium anchors for the repair of rotator cuff tears: preliminary report of a surgical technique. *J Orthop Trauma* 1995;9:312–317.
34. Caspari RB, Thal R. A technique for arthroscopic subacromial decompression. *Arthroscopy* 1992;8:23–30.
35. Cofield RH. Subscapularis muscle transposition for repair of chronic rotator cuff tears. *Surg Gynecol Obstet* 1982;154:667–671.
36. Cofield RH, Briggs BT. Glenohumeral arthrodesis. *J Bone Joint Surg [Am]* 1979;61:668–677.
37. Cone RO, Resnick D, Danzig L. Shoulder impingement syndrome: radiographic evaluation. *Radiology* 1984;150:29–33.
38. Coughlin MJ, Morris JM, West WF. The semiconstrained total shoulder arthroplasty. *J Bone Joint Surg [Am]* 1979;61:574–581.
39. Crass JR, Craig EV, Feinberg SB. Sonography of the post operative rotator cuff tear. *Am J Radiol* 1986;146:561–564.
40. D'Angelo G, Ogilvie-Harris D. Septic arthritis following arthroscopy,

with cost/benefit analysis of antibiotic prophylaxis. *J Arthrosc* 1988; 4:10.
41. Debeyre J, Patte D, Elmelik E. Repair of ruptures of the rotator cuff of the shoulder. *J Bone Joint Surg [Br]* 1965;47:36–42.
42. DeOrio JK, Cofield RH. Results of a second attempt at surgical repair of a failed initial rotator cuff repair. *J Bone Joint Surg [Am]* 1984;66: 563–567.
43. Diamond B. *The obstructing acromion*. Springfield, IL: Charles C Thomas, 1964.
44. Driessnack RP, Ferlic DC, Wiedel JD. Dissociation of the glenoid component in the Macnab/English total shoulder arthroplasty. *J Arthroplasty* 1990;5:15–18.
45. Duval MJ, Parker AW, Drez D Jr, Hinton MA. The anterior humeral circumflex vessels and the axillary nerve. An anatomic study. *Orthop Rev* 1993;22:1023–1026.
46. Ellman H. Arthroscopic subacromial decompression: analysis of one to three year results. *Arthroscopy* 1987;3:173–181.
47. Ellman H, Kay S. Arthroscopic subacromial decompression for chronic impingement: two- to five-year results. *J Bone Joint Surg [Br]* 1991;73:395–398.
48. Esch J. Arthroscopic subacromial decompression and postoperative management. *Orthop Clin North Am* 1993;24:161–171.
49. Esch J, Ozerkis L, Helgager J, Kane N, Lilliott N. Arthroscopic subacromial decompression: results according to the degree of rotator cuff tear. *Arthroscopy* 1988;4:241–249.
50. Flatow E, Connor P, Levine W, Arroyo J, Pollock R, Bigliani L. Coracoacromial arch reconstruction for anterosuperior subluxation after failed rotator cuff surgery. *J Shoulder Elbow Surg* 1997;6:228.
51. Flatow E, Weinstein D, Duralde X, Compito C, Pollock R, Bigliani L. Coracoacromial ligament preservation in rotator cuff surgery. *J Shoulder Elbow Surg* 1994;3:S73.
52. Flatow EL. Tendon-healing in goats [letter]. *J Bone Joint Surg [Am]* 1996;78:1785–1786.
53. Flatow EL, Soslowsky LJ, Ticker JB, et al. Excursion of the rotator cuff under the acromion. Patterns of subacromial contact. *Am J Sports Med* 1994;22:779–788.
54. Flatow EL, Wang VM, Kelkar R, et al. The coracoacromial ligament passively restrains anterosuperior humeral subluxation in the rotator cuff deficient shoulder. *Trans Orthop Res Soc* 1996;21:229.
55. Flugstad D, Matsen FA, Larry I, Jackins SE. Failed acromioplasty: etiology and prevention. *Orthop Trans* 1986;10:229.
56. Frieman B, Fenlin J. Anterior acromioplasty: effect of litigation and workers' compensation. *J Shoulder Elbow Surg* 1995;4:175–181.
57. Gartsman GM. Arthroscopic acromioplasty for lesions of the rotator cuff. *J Bone Joint Surg [Am]* 1990;72:169–180.
58. Gartsman GM, Hammerman SM. Full-thickness tears: arthroscopic repair. *Orthop Clin North Am* 1997;28:83–98.
59. Gazielly D, Gleyze P, Montagnon C. Functional and antomical results after rotator cuff repair. *Clin Orthop* 1994;304:43–53.
60. Gelberman RH, Menon J, Austerlitz MS, Weisman MH. Pyogenic arthritis of the shoulder in adults. *J Bone Joint Surg [Am]* 1980;62: 550–553.
61. Gerber C. Latissimus dorsi transfer for the treatment of irreparable tears of the rotator cuff. *Clin Orthop* 1993;275:152–160.
62. Gerber C, Hersche O. Tendon transfers for the treatment of irreparable rotator cuff defects. *Orthop Clin North Am* 1997;28:195–203.
63. Gerber C, Hersche O, Farron A. Isolated rupture of the subscapularis tendon. *J Bone Joint Surg [Am]* 1996;78:1015–1023.
64. Gerber C, Shneeberger A, Beck M, Schlegel U. Mechanical strength of repairs of the rotator cuff. *J Bone Joint Surg [Br]* 1994;76:371–380.
65. Gerber C, Vinh TS, Hertel R, Hess C. Latissimus dorsi transfer for the treatment of massive tears of the rotator cuff. *Clin Orthop* 1988;232: 51–61.
66. Goutallier D, Postel JM, Bernageau J, Lavau L, Voisin MC. Fatty infiltration of disrupted rotator cuff muscles. *Rev Rhum Engl Ed* 1995; 62:415–22.
67. Goutallier D, Postel JM, Boudon R, Lavau L, Bernageau J. [A study of the neurologic risk in tendino-muscular advancement of supraspinatus and infra-spinatus in the repair of large rotator cuff rupture]. *Rev Chir Orthop* 1996;82:299–305.
68. Grammont PM, Baulot E. Delta shoulder prosthesis for rotator cuff rupture. *Orthopedics* 1993;16:65–68.
69. Greis PE, Kuhn JE, Schultheis J, Hintermeister R, Hawkins R. Validation of the lift-off test and analysis of subscapularis activity during maximal internal rotation. *Am J Sports Med* 1996;24:589–593.
70. Gristina A, Kammire G, Voytek A, Webb L. Sepsis of the shoulder: molecular mechanisms and pathogenesis. In: Rockwood C, Matsen F, eds. *The shoulder*. Philadelphia: WB Saunders, 1990:920–939.
71. Groh G, Simoni M, Rolla P, Rockwood C. Loss of the deltoid after shoulder operations: an operative disaster. *J Shoulder Elbow Surg* 1994;3:243–253.
72. Gusmer PB, Potter HG, Donovan WD, SJ, OB. MR imaging of the shoulder after rotator cuff repair. *AJR Am J Roentgenol* 1997;168: 559–563.
73. Ha'Eri G, Wiley A. "Supraspinatus slide" for rotator cuff repair. *Int Orthop* 1980;4:231–234.
74. Ha'eri GB, Wiley AM. Advancement of the superspinatus muscle in the repair of ruptures of the rotator cuff. *J Bone Joint Surg [Am]* 1981; 63:232–238.
75. Hammond G. Complete acromionectomy in the treatment of tendinitis of the shoulder. *J Bone Joint Surg [Am]* 1961;43:1260.
76. Hammond G. Complete acromionectomy in the treatment of chronic tendinitis of the shoulder. *J Bone Joint Surg [Am]* 1962;44:494–504.
77. Hammond G. Complete acromionectomy in the treatment of chronic tendinitis of the shoulder. A follow-up of ninety operations on eighty-seven patients. *J Bone Joint Surg [Am]* 1971;53:173–180.
78. Harryman DT, Mack LA, Wang KY, Jackins SE, Richardson ML, Matsen FA. Repairs of the rotator cuff: correlation of functional results with integrity of the cuff. *J Bone Joint Surg [Am]* 1991;73: 982–989.
79. Harryman DT 2nd, Matsen FA 3rd, Sidles JA. Arthroscopic management of refractory shoulder stiffness. *Arthroscopy* 1997;13:133–147.
80. Harryman DT, Sidles JA, Harris SL, Matsen FA. The role of the rotator interval capsule in passive motion and stability of the shoulder. *J Bone Joint Surg [Am]* 1992;74:53–66.
81. Hawkins R, Chris T, Bokor D, Kiefer G. Failed anterior acromioplasty: a review of 51 cases. *Clin Orthop* 1989;243:106–111.
82. Hawkins RJ, Abrams JS. Impingement syndrome in the absence of rotator cuff tear (stages 1 and 2). *Orthop Clin North Am* 1987;18: 373–382.
83. Hawkins RJ, Brock RM, Abrams JS, Hobeika P. Acromioplasty for impingement with an intact rotator cuff. *J Bone Joint Surg [Br]* 1988; 70:795–797.
84. Hawkins RJ, Chris AD, Kiefer G. Failed acromioplasty. *Orthop Trans* 1986;10:229.
85. Hawkins RJ, Hobeika P. Physical examination of the shoulder. *Orthopedics* 1983;6:1270–1278.
86. Hawkins RJ, Misamore GW, Hobeika PE. Surgery for full thickness rotator cuff tears. *J Bone Joint Surg [Am]* 1985;67:1349–1355.
87. Hertel R, Ballmer FT, Lombert SM, Gerber C. Lag signs in the diagnosis of rotator cuff rupture. *J Shoulder Elbow Surg* 1996;5:307–313.
88. Hollinshead WH. *Anatomy for surgeons—the back and limbs*. Philadelphia: Harper & Row, 1982.
89. Iannotti JP, Bernot MP, Kuhlman JR, Kelley MJ, Williams GR. Postoperative assessment of shoulder function: a prospective study of full-thickness rotator cuff tears. *J Shoulder Elbow Surg* 1996;5:449–457.
90. Itoh Y, Sasaki T, Ishiguro T, Uchinishi K, Yabe Y, Fukuda H. Transfer of the latissimus dorsi to replace a paralyzed anterior deltoid. *J Bone Joint Surg [Br]* 1987;69:647–657.
91. Jobe FW, Bradley JP, Pink M. Impingement syndrome in overhead athletes. *Surgical rounds for orthopaedics* 1990:19–24, 39–41.
92. Jobe FW, Moynes DR. Deliniation of diagnostic criteria and a rehabilitation program for rotator cuff injuries. *Am J Sports Med* 1982;10: 336–339.
93. Jobe FW, Pink M. Classification and treatment of shoulder dysfunction in the overhead athlete. *J Orthop Sports Phys Ther* 1993;18: 427–432.
94. Kannus P, Leppala J, Lehto M, et al. A rotator cuff rupture produces permanent osteoporosis in the affected extremity, but not in those with whom shoulder function has returned to normal. *J Bone Miner Res* 1995;10:1263–1271.
95. Karduna AR, Williams GR, Williams JL, Iannotti JP. Kinematics of the glenohumeral joint: influences of muscle forces, ligamentous constraints, and articular geometry. *J Orthop Res* 1996;14:986–993.
96. Kelkar R, Colman WW, Ateshian GA, et al. Three-dimentional topography of the acromion: a quantitative study and simulation of surgical alterations. *Am Soc Mech Eng* 1995;31:149.
97. Kelkar R, Newton PM, Armengol J, et al. Glenohumeral kinematics. *J Shoulder Elbow Surg* 1993;2:S28.

98. Kelkar R, Newton PM, Armengol J, et al. Three-dimensional kinematics of the glenohumeral joint during abduction in the scapular plane. *Trans Orthop Res Soc* 1993;18:136.
99. Kelly PJ. Bacterial arthritis in the adult. *Orthop Clin North Am* 1975; 6:973–981.
100. Kelly PJ, Martin WJ, Coventry MB. Bacterial (suppurative) arthritis in the adult. *J Bone Joint Surg [Am]* 1970;52:1595–1602.
101. Kibler WB, Chandler TJ, Pace BK. Principles of rehabilitation after chronic tendon injuries. *Clin Sports Med* 1992;11:661–671.
102. Kitay G, Iannotti J, Williams G, Haygood T, Kneeland B, Berlin J. Roentgenographic assessment of acromial morphologic condition in rotator cuff impingement syndrome. *J Shoulder Elbow Surg* 1995;4: 441–448.
103. Kulkarni RR, Nandedkar AN, Mysorekar VR. Position of the axillary nerve in the deltoid muscle. *Anat Rec* 1992;232:316–317.
104. Kumar VP, Satku K, Liu J, Shen Y. The anatomy of the anterior origin of the deltoid. *J Bone Joint Surg [Br]* 1997;79:680–683.
105. Lazarus M, Chansky H, Misra S, Williams G, Iannotti J. Comparison of open and arthroscopic subacromial decompression. *J Shoulder Elbow Surg* 1994;3:1–11.
106. Lazarus M, Yung S, Sidles J, Harryman D. Anterosuperior humeral displacement: limitation by the coracoacromial arch. Presented at American Shoulder and Elbow Surgeons 11th open meeting. Orlando, FL, 1995.
107. Lettin AWF, Copeland SA, Scales JT. The Stanmore total shoulder replacement. *J Bone Joint Surg [Br]* 1982;64:47–51.
108. Linker CS, Helms CA, Fritz RC. Quadrilateral space syndrome: findings at MR imaging. *Radiology* 1993;188:675–676.
109. Lippitt SB, Vanderhooft JE, Harris SL, Sidles JA, Harryman DT, Matsen FA. Glenohumeral stability from concavity-compression: a quantitative analysis. *J Shoulder Elbow Surg* 1993;2:27–35.
110. Liu SH, Baker CL. Arthroscopically assisted rotator cuff repair: correlation of functional results with integrity of the cuff. *Arthroscopy* 1994;10:54–60.
111. Loomer R, Graham B. Anatomy of the axillary nerve and its relation to inferior capsular shift. *Clin Orthop* 1989;100–105.
112. Mack L, Nyberg D, Matsen F, Kilcoyne R, Harvey D. Sonography of the postoperative shoulder. *Am J Radiol* 1988;150:1089–1093.
113. Mansat P, Cofield RH, Kersten TE, Rowland CM. Complications of rotator cuff repair. *Orthop Clin North Am* 1997;28:205–213.
114. Matsen F, Artnz C. Subacromial impingement. In: Rockwood C, Matsen F, eds. *The shoulder*. Philadelphia: WB Saunders, 1990:623–648.
115. Matsen FA, Kirby RM. Office evaluation and management of shoulder pain. *Orthop Clin North Am* 1982;13:453–475.
116. Matsen FA, Lippitt SB, Sidles JA. *Practical evaluation and management of the shoulder*. Phildephia: WB Saunders, 1994.
117. Matthews L, Burkhead W, Gordon S, Racanelli J, Ruland L. Acromial fracture: a complication of arthroscopic subacromial decompression. *J Shoulder Elbow Surg* 1994;3:256–261.
118. McLaughlin HL. Lesions of the musculotendinous cuff of the shoulder I. The exposure and treatment of tears with retraction. *J Bone Joint Surg [Am]* 1944;26:31–51.
119. McShane R, Leinberry C, Fenlin J. Conservative open anterior acromioplasty. *Clin Orthop* 1987;223:127–144.
120. Moorman C, Deng X, Warren R, Torzilli P, Wickiewicz T. The coracoacromial ligament: is it the appendix of the shoulder? Presented at American Shoulder and Elbow Surgeons 11 open meeting. Orlando, FL, 1995.
121. Mormino MA, Gross RM, McCarthy JA. Captured shoulder: a complication of rotator cuff surgery. *Arthroscopy* 1996;12:457–461.
122. Morrison DS, Bigliani LU. The clinical significance of variations in acromial morphology. *Orthop Trans* 1987;11:234.
123. Moseley HF. *Shoulder lesions*. Edinburgh: E & S Livingstone, 1969.
124. Murnaghan JP. Adhesive capsulitis of the shoulder: current concepts and treatment. *Orthopedics* 1988;11:153–158.
125. Nasca RJ. The use of freeze-dried allografts in the management of global rotator cuff tears. *Clin Orthop* 1988;228:218–226.
126. Neer CS. Impingement lesions. *Clin Orthop* 1983;173:71–77.
127. Neer CS II. Anterior acromioplasty for the chronic impingement syndrome in the shoulder: a preliminary report. *J Bone Joint Surg [Am]* 1972;54:41–50.
128. Neer CS II. *Shoulder reconstruction*. Philadelphia: WB Saunders, 1990.
129. Neer CS II, Flatow EL, Lech O. Tears of the rotator cuff: long term results of anterior acromioplasty and repair. *Orthop Trans* 1988;12:673.
130. Neer CS II, Marberry TA. On the disadvantages of radical acromionectomy. *J Bone Joint Surg [Am]* 1981;63:416–419.
131. Neer CS II, McCann PD, Macfarlane EA, Padilla N. Earlier passive motion following shoulder arthroplasty and rotator cuff repair. A prospective study. *Orthop Trans* 1987;2:231.
132. Neer CS II, Poppen NK. Supraspinatus outlet. *Orthop Trans* 1987;11: 234.
133. Nevaiser R, Nevaiser T. Reoperation for failed rotator cuff repair: analysis of fifty cases. *J Shoulder Elbow Surg* 1992;1:283–286.
134. Neviaser JS. Ruptures of the rotator cuff of the shoulder. *Arch Surg* 1971;102:483–485.
135. Neviaser JS. Adhesive capsulitis and the stiff and painful shoulder. *Orthop Clin North Am* 1980;11:327–331.
136. Neviaser JS, Neviaser RJ, Neviaser TJ. The repair of chronic massive ruptures of the rotator cuff of the shoulder by use of a freeze-dried rotator cuff. *J Bone Joint Surg [Am]* 1978;60:681–684.
137. Neviaser RJ. Ruptures of the rotator cuff. *Orthop Clin North Am* 1987; 18:387–394.
138. Neviaser RJ, Neviaser TJ. The frozen shoulder. Diagnosis and management. *Clin Orthop* 1987;59–64.
139. Neviaser RJ, Neviaser TJ. Re-operation for failed rotator cuff repair: analysis of 50 cases. *J Shoulder Elbow Surgery* 1992;1:283–286.
140. Neviaser T, Neviaser R, Neviaser J. The four-in-one arthroplasty for painful arc syndrome. *Clin Orthop* 1982;163:108–112.
141. Neviaser TJ. Adhesive capsulitis. *Orthop Clin North Am* 1987;18: 439–443.
142. Ogilvie-Harris D, Wiley A, Sattarian J. Failed acromioplasty for impingement syndrome. *J Bone Joint Surg [Br]* 1990;72:1070–1072.
143. Owen R, Iannotti J, Kneeland J, Dalinka M, Deren J, Oleaga L. Shoulder after surgery: MR imaging with surgical validation. *Radiology* 1993;186:443–447.
144. Ozaki J, Fujimoto S, Masuhara K, et al. Reconstruction of massive rotator cuff tears with synthetic materials. *Clin Orthop* 1986;202: 173–183.
145. Ozer Y, Grossman JA, Gilbert A. Anatomic observations on the suprascapular nerve. *Hand Clin* 1995;11:539–544.
146. Packer NP, Calvert PT, Bayley JIL, et al. Operative treatment of chronic ruptures of the rotator cuff of the shoulder. *J Bone Joint Surg [Br]* 1983;65:171–175.
147. Paulos L, Franklin J. Arthroscopic shoulder decompression development and application: a five year experience. *Am J Sports Med* 1990; 18:235–244.
148. Peterson CA 2nd, Altchek DW. Arthroscopic treatment of rotator cuff disorders. *Clin Sports Med* 1996;15:715–736.
149. Peterson SL, Mani MM, Crawford CM, Neff JR, Hiebert JM. Postburn heterotopic ossification: insights for management decision making. *J Trauma* 1989;29:365–369.
150. Pollock RG, Duralde XA, Flatow EL, Bigliani LU. The use of arthroscopy in the treatment of resistant frozen shoulder. *Clin Orthop* 1994;30–36.
151. Poppen NK, Walker PS. Normal and abnormal motion of the shoulder. *J Bone Joint Surg [Am]* 1976;58:195–201.
152. Post M. Rotator cuff repair with carbon filament. *Clin Orthop* 1985; 196:154–158.
153. Post M. Constrained arthroplasty of the shoulder. *Orthop Clin North Am* 1987;18:455–462.
154. Post M, Jablon M. Constrained total shoulder arthroplasty. *Clin Orthop* 1983;109–116.
155. Post M, Mayer J. Suprascapular nerve entrapment. Diagnosis and treatment. *Clin Orthop* 1987;126–136.
156. Rask MR. Suprascapular nerve entrapment: a report of two cases treated with suprascapular notch resection. *Clin Orthop* 1977;123:73.
157. Rockwood C, Lyons F. Shoulder impingement syndrome: diagnosis, radiographic evaluation, and treatment with a modified Neer acromioplasty. *J Bone Joint Surg [Am]* 1993;75:409–424.
158. Rockwood CA, Williams GR. The shoulder impingement syndrome; management of surgical treatment failures. *Orthop Trans* 1992;16: 739.
159. Rockwood CA, Williams GR, Burkhead WZ. Debridement of irreparable degenerative lesions of the rotator cuff. *Orthop Trans* 1992; 16:740.
160. Rockwood CA Jr, Williams GR Jr, Burkhead WZ Jr. Debridement of degenerative, irreparable lesions of the rotator cuff. *J Bone Joint Surg [Am]* 1995;77:857–866.
161. Rothmeier J, Schreiber H, Froscher W. [Myositis ossificans circum-

scripta following unusual brain injury]. *Fortschr Med* 1990;108: 415–416.
162. Roye R, Grana W, Yates K. Arthroscopic subacromial decompression: two- to seven-year follow-up. *Arthroscopy* 1995;11:301–306.
163. Sampson TG, Nisbet JK, Glick JM. Precision acromioplasty in arthroscopic subacromial decompression of the shoulder. *Arthroscopy* 1991; 7:301–307.
164. Sawyer J, Esterhai J. Shoulder Infections. In: Warner J, Iannotti J, Gerber C, eds. *Complex and revision problems in shoulder surgery.* Philadelphia: Lippincott–Raven Publishers, 1997:385–398.
165. Schneeberger AG, Beck M, Gerber C. [In-vitro stability of rotator cuff repair techniques]. *Orthopade* 1995;24:268–274.
166. Segmuller HE, Taylor DE, Hogan CS, Saies AD, Hayes MG. Arthroscopic treatment of adhesive capsulitis. *J Shoulder Elbow Surg* 1995; 4:403–408.
167. Sher J, Iannotti J, Warner J, Groff Y, Williams G. Surgical treatment of postoperative deltoid origin disruption. *Clin Orthop* 1997;343: 93–98.
168. Sher J, Warner J, Groff Y, Williams G, Iannotti J. Treatment of postoperative deltoid origin disruption. Presented at Anerican Shoulder and Elbow Surgeons 12th open meeting. Atlanta, GA, 1996.
169. Skoff HD. Conservative open acromioplasty. *J Bone Joint Surg [Br]* 1995;77:933–936.
170. Small N. Complications in arthroscopic: the knee and other joints. *J Arthrosc* 1986;2:253.
171. Smith-Petersen MN, Aufranc OE, Larson CB. Useful surgical procedures for rheumatoid arthritis involving joints of the upper extremety. *Arch Surg* 1943;46:764–770.
172. Snyder SJ. Technique of arthroscopic rotator cuff repair using implantable 4-mm Revo suture anchors, suture shuttle relays, and no. 2 nonabsorbable mattress sutures. *Orthop Clin North Am* 1997;28: 267–275.
173. Soslowsky LJ, Flatow EL, Bigliani LU, Pawluk RJ, Ateshian GA, Mow VC. Quantitation of in situ contact areas at the glenohumeral joint: a biomechanical study. *J Orthop Res* 1992;10:524–534.
174. St Pierre P, Olson EJ, et al. Tendon-healing to cortical bone compared with healing to a cancellous trough. A biomechanical and histological evaluation in goats. *J Bone Joint Surg [Am]* 1995;77A:1858–1866.
175. Stefko JM, Jobe FW, VanderWilde RS, Carden E, Pink M. Electromyographic and nerve block analysis of the subscapularis liftoff test. *J Shoulder Elbow Surg* 1997;6:347–355.
176. Stover SL, Hataway CJ, Zeiger HE. Heterotopic ossification in spinal cord-injured patients. *Arch Phys Med Rehabil* 1975;56:199–204.
177. Ticker JB, Lippe RJ, Barkin DE, Carroll MP. Infected suture anchors in the shoulder. *Arthroscopy* 1996;12:613–615.
178. Vanderhooft E, Lippitt S, Harris S, Sidles J, Harryman DT II, Matsen FA III. Glenohumeral stability from concavity-compression: a quantitative analysis. *Orthop Trans* 1992;16:774.
179. Vastamaki M, Goransson H. Suprascapular nerve entrapment. *Clin Orthop* 1993;135–143.
180. Visuri T, Kiviluoto O, Eskelin M. Carbon fiber for repair of the rotator cuff: a 4-year follow-up of 14 cases. *Acta Orthop Scand* 1991;62: 356–359.
181. Warner JJ, Allen A, Marks PH, Wong P. Arthroscopic release for chronic, refractory adhesive capsulitis of the shoulder. *J Bone Joint Surg [Am]* 1996;78:1808–1816.
182. Warner JJ, Allen AA, Marks PH, Wong P. Arthroscopic release of postoperative capsular contracture of the shoulder. *J Bone Joint Surg [Am]* 1997;79:1151–1158.
183. Warner JJP, Krushell RJ, Masquelet A, Gerber C. Anatomy and relationships of the suprascapular nerve: anatomical constraints to mobilization of the supraspinatus and infraspinatus muscles in the management of massive rotator-cuff tears. *J Bone Joint Surg [Am]* 1992;74: 36–45.
184. Watson-Jones R. *Fractures and joint injuries*. Edinburgh: E & S Livingstone, 1943.
185. Wiley AM. Superior humeral dislocation. A complication following decompression and debridement for rotator cuff tears. *Clin Orthop* 1991;135–141.
186. Williams G. Painful shoulder after surgery for rotator cuff disease. *J Am Acad Orthop Surg* 1997;5:97–108.
187. Wirth MA, Rockwood CA Jr. Operative treatment of irreparable rupture of the subscapularis. *J Bone Joint Surg [Am]* 1997;79:722–731.
188. Wolfgang GL. Surgical repair of tears of the rotator cuff of the shoulder. *J Bone Joint Surg [Am]* 1974;56:14–26.
189. Wuelker N, Melzer C, Wirth C. Shoulder surgery for rotator cuff tears: ultrasonographic 3-year followup of 97 cases. *Acta Orthop Scand* 1991;62:142–147.
190. Zanotti RM, Carpenter JE, Blasier RB, Greenfield ML, Adler RS, Bromberg MB. The low incidence of suprascapular nerve injury after primary repair of massive rotator cuff tears. *J Shoulder Elbow Surg* 1997;6:258–264.
191. Zanotti RM, Kuhn JE. Arthroscopic capsular release for the stiff shoulder. Description of technique and anatomic considerations. *Am J Sports Med* 1997;25:294–298.
192. Zuckerman JD, LeBlanc J-M, Choueka J, Kummer F. The effect of aRm position and capsular release on rotator cuff repair: a biomechanical study. *J Bone Joint Surg [Br]* 1991;73B:402–405.

Disorders of the Shoulder: Diagnosis and Management,
edited by Joseph P. Iannotti and Gerald R. Williams, Jr.
Lippincott Williams & Wilkins, Philadelphia © 1999.

CHAPTER 5

Calcifying Tendinitis

Shawn P. Hennigan and Anthony A. Romeo

PATHOPHYSIOLOGY

Introduction

Calcifying tendinitis of the rotator cuff, a disease of unknown etiology, is characterized by multifocal, cell-mediated calcium deposition in viable tissue. These deposits normally undergo spontaneous resorption followed by subsequent healing of the tendon. The clinical presentation is variable; patients may have little or no symptoms during the formative phase, or they may have acute symptoms during the resorptive phase.

Definition and Classification

Calcifying tendinitis of the rotator cuff tendons differs from dystrophic calcification or other rotator cuff tendonopathies in several ways. First, calcifying tendinitis occurs in vascularized, viable soft tissue, whereas tendonopathies tend to occur in dysvascular, nonviable soft tissues. Next, calcifying tendinitis is a disease that proceeds toward resolution. Degenerative tendonopathies tend to worsen over time. It is unusual to see other signs of degenerative changes in calcifying tendinitis, whereas they are commonplace in dystrophic calcification and tendonopathies. Another difference between calcifying tendinitis and dystrophic calcification is in the radiographic location and appearance of the calcification. In dystrophic calcification, the calcifying deposits tend to occur at the insertion site of the tendon into the bone and are commonly stippled in appearance. In calcifying tendinitis, the calcification tends to occur 1 to 2 cm proximal to the insertion site of the tendon, and within the midsubstance of the tendon (Fig. 1).

Duplay first recognized the subacromial bursa as a source of shoulder pain in 1871.[27] He coined the term "scapulohumeral periarthritis." In 1907, Painter described subacromial calcium deposits, and felt that these deposits were the primary source of pathology.[96] There were later descriptions by Bergemann and Steida in 1908, who also believed that the subacromial bursa was the primary site of pathology.[10] In fact, this was the opinion of many authors at the beginning of this century. Codman, in 1909, was one of the first to demonstrate that the calcium deposits were located in the tendons of the rotator cuff, and not in the subacromial bursa.[21] In 1912, Wrede is credited with the first histologic description of the disease of calcifying tendinitis. He identified the presence of chondrocytes among tenocytes within the tendon.[141] The intratendinous location of the calcified deposits was later confirmed by other authors, such as Schaer in 1936,[119]

S. P. Hennigan and A. A. Romeo: Department of Orthopaedic Surgery, Rush–Presbyterian–St. Luke's Medical Center, Chicago, Illinois 60612.

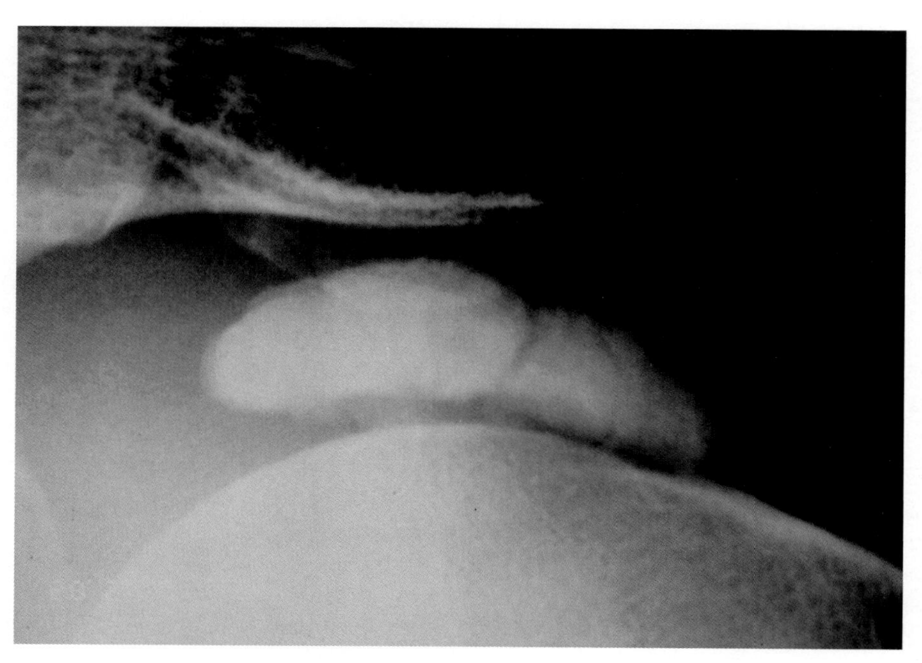

FIG. 1. The typical location of the calcific mass is within the midsubstance of the tendon, not at its insertion site. Calcifying tendinitis most commonly affects the supraspinatus tendon. (Courtesy of Docteur Gilles Walch.)

Sandstrom in 1938,[116] as well as McLaughlin in 1946.[76] These authors all believed that calcifying tendinitis was the result of a degenerative process. Bateman observed that calcium deposits occurred close to the site of tendon attachment that is now known as the "critical zone," an area that may have diminished vascularity. He thought that "abnormal aging of collagen fibers initiated the calcification mechanism."[8] This belief persisted despite the observation in 1937 by Sandstrom and Wahlgren that calcification occurs in viable, not in necrotic tissue.[117] Moseley, in 1963, stated that "at operation, I have noted that the tendon was well vascularized around the area of deposit and therefore disagree with the idea that the calcium salts were precipitated in an area of previous disease with resultant ischemia."[87]

DeSeze and Welfling in 1970 coined the term "tendinites calcifiantes," denoting an evolutionary process of calcifying tendinitis tending toward spontaneous healing.[25] This differs in many ways from degenerative tendinopathy and now appears to be the description of choice for calcifying tendinitis. Uhthoff, in 1975, elucidated the pathogenesis of calcification, correlating histological findings with clinical symptoms.[128]

Codman, in his classic text, pointed out that disease in the supraspinatus tendon tended to appear in a specific area of the tendon about "half inch proximal to the insertion degenerative of the tendon." He called this area the "critical portion."[21] This area was later renamed by Moseley and Goldie as the "critical zone."[88] Multiple studies of vascularity of the rotator cuff tendon by microangiographic techniques have been performed. The critical zone is a watershed area within the supraspinatus tendon, with its blood supply coming from the proximal muscular portion of the supraspinatus as well as from the osseotendinous junction. This may account for a relative decrease in perfusion. This was supported by studies performed by Rothman and Parke.[113] However, Moseley and Goldie thought that this area had a rich anastomosis.[88]

Rathbun and Macnab, in 1970, performed cadaveric studies to study the vascularity of the supraspinatus tendon.[106] They found that the perfusion to the critical zone in the supraspinatus tendon was largely dependent on the arm position. The critical zone was subject to a "wring-out" phenomenon, from pressure on the tendon exerted by the humeral head with the humerus in the adducted position.

Terminology

The terminology surrounding calcifying tendinitis has also evolved along with a better understanding of the pathogenesis. In 1907, Painter first used the term calcifying bursitis.[96] This was later used by Bergemann and Steida in 1908,[10] and again by Steida in 1908.[126] In 1937, Sandstrom coined the term "peritendinitis calcarea."[117] The first appearance of the term calcifying tendinitis appeared in the North American literature in 1952 by Plenk.[103] DeSeze and Welfling coined the term "Tendinite Calcifiante" in 1970.[25] In 1979, Dieppe referred to this condition as calcified peritendinitis.[26] The term *tendinitis* is preferred over tendinosis because of the acute nature of symptoms and the tendency toward complete resolution. *Tendinosis* is more appropriately used for conditions of a degenerative nature in which symptoms are chronic and tend toward a gradual deterioration over time.

Classification

There are many classification schemes created for calcifying tendinitis of the rotator cuff, some based on clinical presentation and others based on radiologic findings. DePalma divided calcifying tendinitis into three categories based on the presenting symptoms: acute, subacute, and chronic.[24] Bosworth classified calcifying tendinitis by the radiographic size of the deposits.[15]

Patte and Goutallier described two forms of calcifying tendinitis: localized and diffuse. Localized deposits were discrete, dense, and homogeneous in density, and they had a tendency to heal spontaneously. In contrast, the diffuse form tended to appear "fluffy" on radiograph, was heterogenous in density, and tended to heal more slowly. Patients with the diffuse type were believed to have a higher likelihood of clinical symptoms.[97]

Uhthoff and Sarkar proposed that calcifying tendinitis is a dynamic disease that progresses through a complete cycle in most patients. Calcifying tendinitis has two distinct pathologic phases: the formative phase, and the resorptive phase. Contained within these two phases are three distinct stages of calcification: the precalcifying stage, the calcifying stage, and postcalcifying stage[135] (Fig. 2).

Other causes of calcification about the shoulder are numerous, including arteriosclerosis of brachial and axillary vessels, calcified soft-tissue or bony neoplasms, patients with chronic renal failure, heterotopic ossification following acromioplasty and distal clavicle resection, subdeltoid calcifying bursitis in rheumatoid arthritis, chronic acromioclavicular separation with calcification of the coracoclavicular ligament, as well as in diabetes.[1,2,9,11,26,39,44,56,73,74,84,102,119] Other distinct causes of calcification about the shoulder include the "Milwaukee" shoulder. This is characterized by massive calcifications in association with a complete rotator cuff tear, severe glenohumeral arthritis, acromioclavicular arthritis, or some combination thereof. Dystrophic calcifications are seen at the torn ends of the rotator cuff tendon after a complete tear.

Pathogenesis

Considerable controversy still exists over the etiology of calcifying tendinitis. Codman initially proposed that calcifying tendinitis is a degenerative process of the rotator cuff tendon. He believed that the fibers of the tendon degenerate, become necrotic, then develop dystrophic calcification.[21] Other authors accepted this concept. In 1946, McLaughlin pointed out that the earliest lesion in rotator cuff tendon calcification is a focal hyalinization of fibers that eventually become fibrillated, detached from the tendon, and wound up into rice-like bodies that undergo calcification.[68] This theory was further supported by an experimental study performed

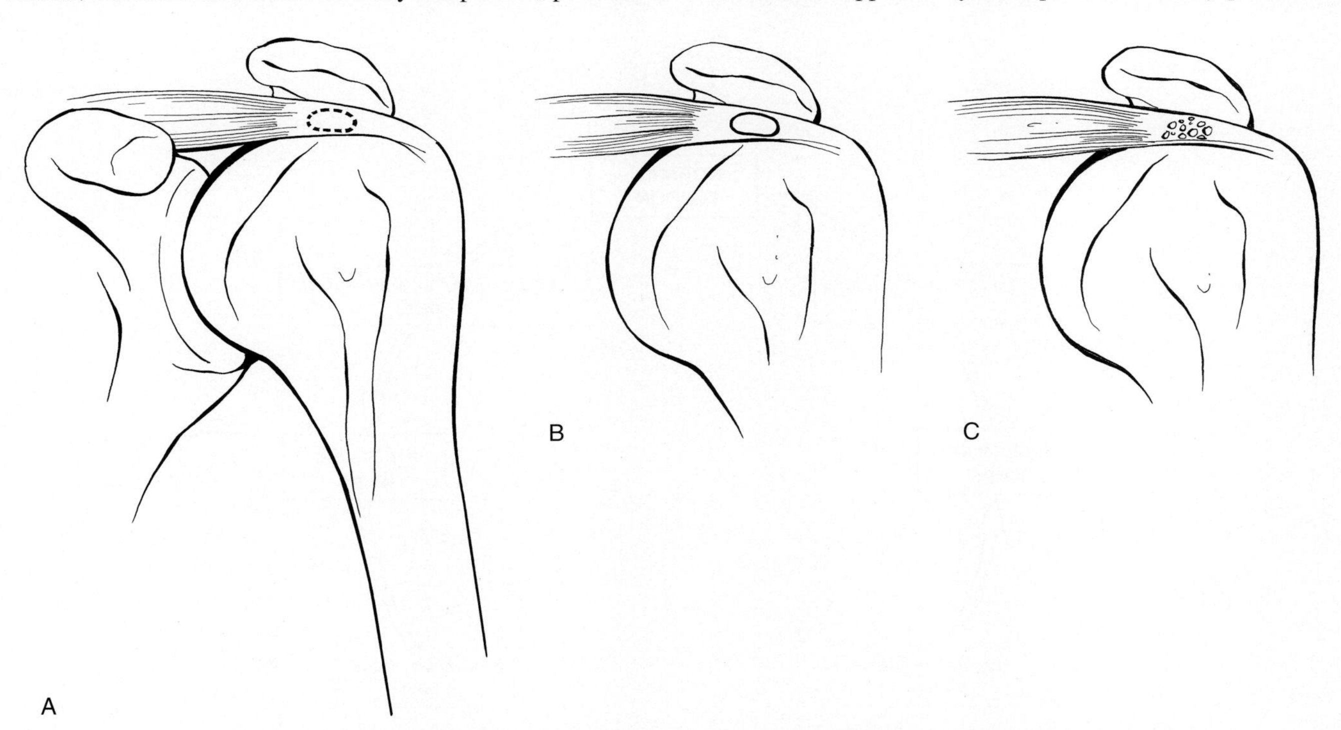

FIG. 2. The calcification of the rotator cuff tendon progresses through three distinct stages: **(A)** The precalcific stage demonstrates a metaplasia of the tenocytes into chondrocytes. Degenerative changes of the tendon are absent. The signal for this metaplasia is unknown. **(B)** The calcifying stage begins with the formative phase, with small foci of calcium deposits that can coalesce into a large homogeneous deposit. The absence of a vascular response distinguishes this calcification process from endochondral ossification. **(C)** The postcalcific stage begins with resorption of the calcific deposit and ends with reconstitution of the normal tendon.

by Macnab. He was able to show that interruption of the vascular supply to the Achilles tendon in rabbits can produce the hyalinization of the tendon fibers, followed by calcification.[68] Brewer has shown that as the supraspinatus tendon ages, its vascularity diminishes. By about the fourth or fifth decade, many fascicles in the tendon have thinned and fibrillated. The natural senescence of rotator cuff tendons with decreased vascularity is suggested as a contributing factor to the pathogenesis of calcifying tendinitis.[17]

In contrast, Uhthoff and Sarkar have pointed out that there are various aspects of calcifying tendinitis that are not consistent with a degenerative process.[128,131] In calcifying tendinitis, the calcification occurs in apparently viable tissue. Degenerative calcification occurs in nonviable or poorly vascularized tissue. The peak incidence of calcifying tendinitis is in the fourth and fifth decade in most studies. The incidence of calcifying tendinitis is rare in the sixth decade. Calcifying tendinitis has not been reported in patients who were older than the age of 71. This would include autopsy findings on patients older than 71, including those with a previous history of calcifying tendinitis. These well-documented characteristics of calcifying tendinitis support the concept that this distinct clinical entity is a reparative process progressing through a predictable disease cycle.

Uhthoff and Sarkar have divided the typical cycle of calcifying tendinitis into three distinct stages: precalcific, calcifying, and postcalcific. The precalcific stage is marked histologically by metaplasia of the tenocytes into chondrocytes. This is accompanied by increased proteoglycan formation. The cause for the initiation of this process is unknown. Codman suggested that hypoxia may play a role in initiating this process,[21] but other catalysts may include microtrauma, disuse, hormonal factors, or dietary factors. The formative phase marks the beginning of the calcification, the hallmark of which is calcium deposition, primarily into matrix vesicles within the chondrocytes. Histologic examinations reveal that, during the formative phase, the surrounding tissue is relatively avascular and is marked by the absence of vessels. This process of calcification is distinctly different from endochondral bone formation, which is marked by the presence of blood vessels at the time of calcification. Generally, the foci of calcium deposits coalesce to form large deposits until a very dense homogeneous and typically well-delineated calcium deposit is formed. Clinical symptoms are often absent. However, when clinical symptoms accompany the formative stage, the findings are typically similar to patients with mild to moderate subacromial impingement.[71] The lack of hyperalgesia, and the ability to use the shoulder for many activities may not lead to medical evaluation and confirmation of the diagnosis. Intermittent worsening of the symp-

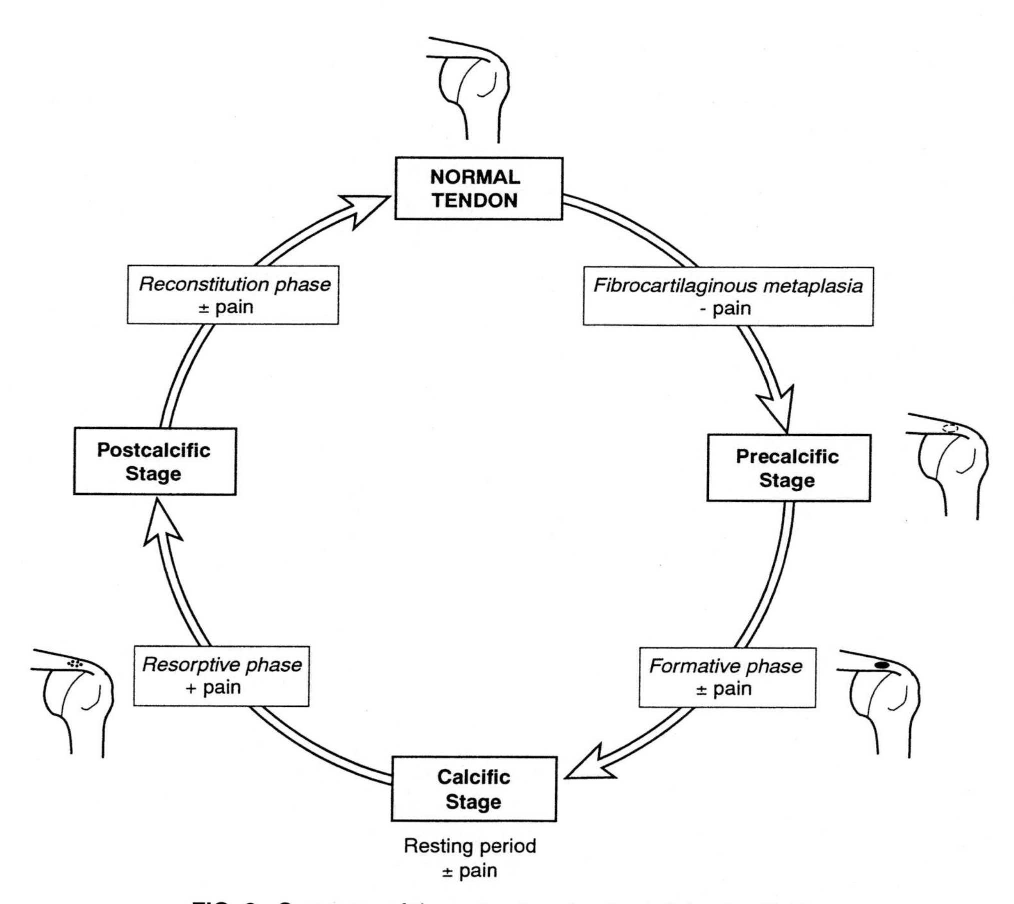

FIG. 3. Summary of the natural cycle of calcifying tendinitis.

toms, including diffuse pain, difficulty with overhead activities, and rest pain, defines the clinical picture of "chronic" calcifying tendinitis. At this stage, plain radiographs for the evaluation of nonspecific shoulder pain may detect a calcific deposit within the rotator cuff tendon, most typically the supraspinatus tendon.[37] During the formative phase, the calcium deposit exists primarily as a chalky deposit that is well demarcated within the tendon. The duration of the formative phase is variable, and it may last for many years.

The proliferation of blood vessels at the periphery of the calcium deposit heralds the phase of resorption. With the vascularization process, cellular infiltration occurs with macrophages, mononuclear giant cells, and fibroblasts initially seen at the periphery of the calcific deposit. These cells mediate an aggressive inflammatory process, releasing various cellular mediators and enzymes that break up the calcium deposit and phagocytose the calcium. With the vascular and cellular infiltration comes an obligate increase in the intratendinous pressure, largely as a result of the edema, which causes the classic acute hyperalgesia of calcifying tendinitis. The pressure may be so great that the deposit ruptures into the subacromial bursa, or into the area external to the subacromial bursa in the subacromial space. Roentgenographically, the calcium deposit now appears poorly delineated and fluffy. Concomitant with the inflammatory response, fibroblasts lay down collagen in the cavity left behind by the resolving calcium deposit. As the collagen matures and the resorptive process proceeds to conclusion, the fibers line themselves along the axis of the tendon, allowing return of the tendon structure, and eventual tendon function.

The postcalcific stage is marked by fibroblasts laying down collagen, primarily type III, which later remodels into type I collagen. This final stage completes the natural cycle of calcifying tendinitis. There is speculation, but no firm evidence, that the healed tendon may be more susceptible to degenerative tearing over time (Fig. 3).

Incidence

The incidence of calcifying tendinitis varies with diagnostic techniques, the patient population being studied, and the geographic location. At a recent meeting, North American shoulder surgeons reported an overall decrease in incidence of calcifying tendinitis.[135] In fact, Neer commented that surgical treatment of calcifying tendinitis was one of the most common procedures performed at his teaching hospital when he was a resident.[91] However, surgical treatment and the diagnosis of this disorder has become less common owing to factors that are not understood. The reported incidence of calcifying tendinitis seen by European and Japanese surgeons has not significantly changed during the same time period.

Bosworth reported a 2.7% incidence of calcifying tendinitis among 6,061 asymptomatic office workers.[14] In a report from France, Welfling reported an incidence of 7.5% of the disorder among 200 asymptomatic shoulders. However, in 925 symptomatic shoulders, there was a 6.8% incidence.[138] Ruttimann reported a 20% incidence in 100 asymptomatic shoulders.[115] Regional variation suggests that hereditary and dietary factors may play a role in the predisposition toward calcifying tendinitis.

Most authors report the highest incidence of calcifying tendinitis occurs between the ages of 40 and 50 years. Thirty-six percent of the patients in the study by DePalma and Kruper[24] fell into this age category, as did 42% of the patients in a report by Uhthoff and Sarkar.[130] Welfling, on the other hand, reported the highest incidence between the ages of 31 and 40 years. No patient was older than the age of 71 years.[138] Nutton reported a case of a 3-year-old child with acute calcific supraspinatus tendinitis.[94] Recently, Hsu et al., reporting on their patient population from Taiwan,[50] reported that 69% of the patients in their study were older than 60 years of age, the first report to suggest that calcifying tendinitis may have a distinct clinical variant in an Asian population, with its onset in an older-aged group.[50] Furthermore, the significant incidence of associated rotator cuff tears in Hsu's study is in distinct contrast with other studies of calcifying tendinitis.

The calcifying deposits are most commonly located in the supraspinatus tendon. Plenk reported an 82% incidence in the supraspinatus tendon.[103] In Bosworth's report, the supraspinatus was involved in 51% of his patients, the infraspinatus in 44.5% (Fig. 4), the teres minor in 23.3%, and the subscapularis in 3% (Fig. 5).[14] DePalma and Kruper reported that the supraspinatus was involved in 74% of their cases.[24] Hsu et al. reported a similar 70.7% involvement of the supraspinatus, with 26.8% involving the infraspinatus.[50]

There is still some controversy over the role of the subacromial bursa in calcifying tendinitis. It is commonly be-

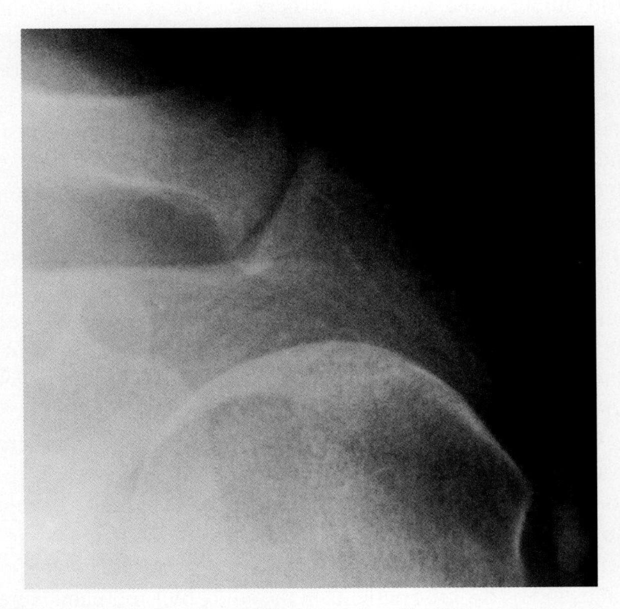

FIG. 4. Calcifying tendinitis involving the infraspinatus tendon, which occurs in approximately one-third of patients with calcifying tendinitis. (Courtesy of Docteur Gilles Walch.)

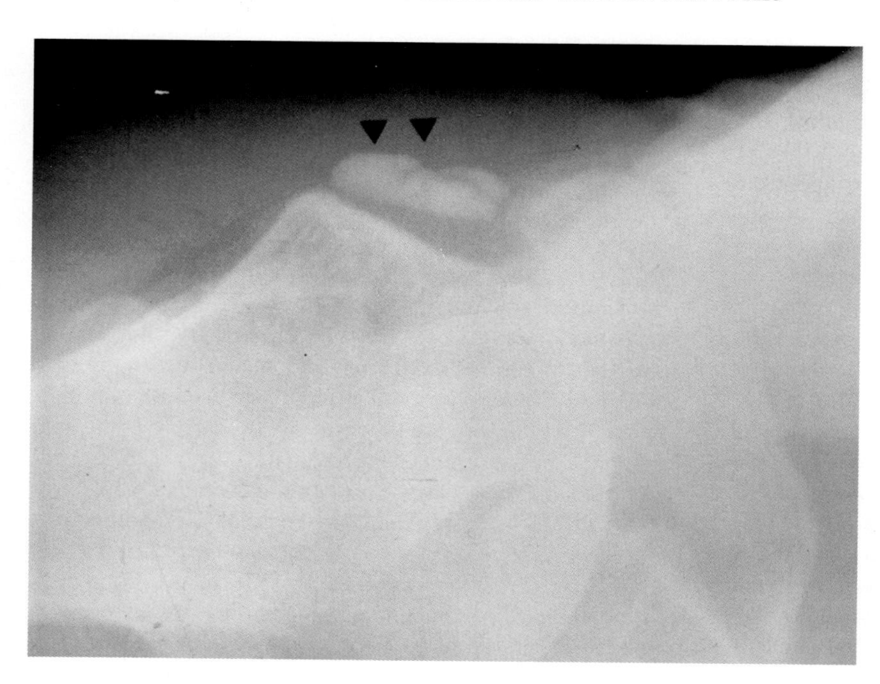

FIG. 5. Calcifying tendinitis involving the subscapularis tendon: Because the deposit is superimposed on the humerus with an anteroposterior radiograph, this rare situation can be easily missed if an axillary lateral radiograph is not obtained. (Courtesy of Docteur Gilles Walch.)

lieved, however, that the subacromial bursa is not a factor in the chronic phase of this disorder. This belief is supported by Carnett, who noted that bursitis forms a minor and infrequent feature of chronic calcifying tendinitis.[19] Ischii et al. noted bursal reactions in subacromial bursal specimens removed at the time of surgery from 63 patients, 6 of whom had calcifying tendinitis. Their findings clearly showed that the strongest bursal reaction was present with a rotator cuff tendon tear, and was weakest in calcifying tendinitis.[52] Pedersen and Key looked at the pathology of calcareous tendinitis and subdeltoid bursitis, and found at surgery the bursa was thin and translucent, light pink, and without evidence of acute inflammation. They did note some free calcium material in several instances. However, in each of these cases, there was also roentgenographic evidence of rupture of the calcium deposit into the bursa. As they stated "unless there was free material in the wall of the bursa, this was not the site of gross inflammatory change."[99] Sarkar and Uhthoff stated that "it has been known for a long time that calcification of rotator cuff tendons occurs primarily in the tendon substance and not in the bursa."[118] Thus, it appears the bursa may become involved secondarily from either impingement, with subsequent inflammation of the bursa, or from rupture of the calcifying deposit into the bursa, with secondary inflammation.

In the gender of the patients, most authors agree that there is a higher incidence among females than males. Uhthoff reported a 57% incidence of female involvement,[130] while Bosworth reported a 76.7% incidence.[14] Welfling[138] reported 62% of his patients with calcifying tendinitis were female, and 64% of the patients in the study by Lippmann were female.[64] DePalma and Kruper also reported that 60.3% of their patients were female.[24] However, Hsu and his collaborators reported only a 26% incidence of female patients, again drawing attention to the distinct difference in their Asian patient population and possibly the clinical condition they have reported.[50]

Calcifying tendinitis may be related to certain occupations or activities. DePalma and Kruper reported 41% of their patients were housewives, and 27% were executives and sales persons.[24] Uhthoff and Sarkar reported that 43% of their patients were housewives, and 44% were clerical workers.[130] It appears that heavy laborers suffer less from calcifying tendinitis than do sedentary workers or workers who primarily perform nonstrenuous tasks with their elbow at their side. There does not appear to be a direct relation between trauma and calcifying tendinitis.

The incidence of bilateral involvement increases with the length of follow-up. Welfling reported an incidence of 24.3% of bilateral calcifying tendinitis of the shoulder.[138] DePalma and Kruper reported a 13% incidence of bilateral calcifying tendinitis,[24] and Uhthoff and Sarkar reported a 17% incidence.[130]

In some instances, calcifying tendinitis appears to be part of a systemic disease.[102] This is supported by the incidence of calcifications occurring at other sites, most notably around the hip. No other study has suggested a similar incidence of hip involvement. Welfling reported that 62.5% of his patients with calcifying tendinitis of the shoulder had simultaneous calcifications around the hip, whereas in the control group, only 4% had calcifications about the hip.[138] Gschwend was unable to prove an association with diabetes or gout.[43] However, other authors feel that there is an increase in the incidence of calcifications in many areas of the body in patients with diabetes, including the shoulder region.[56,73] Abnormalities in calcium or phosphate metabolism have not been reported as part of the clinical syndrome of calcifying tendinitis, although they are clearly evident with other conditions leading to soft-tissue calcifications, such as renal osteodystrophy.[2] There have also been attempts to correlate HLA-A1 presence with calcifying tendinitis, although the role for HLA testing in diagnosis or management of patients is unclear.[123]

Clinical Presentation

The clinical presentation is highly variable. An understanding of the pathogenesis of calcifying tendinitis allows the clinician to make proper diagnostic as well as management decisions. The formative phase of calcification is frequently subclinical or even asymptomatic. It is often discovered serendipitously. As Baer observed during surgery, large deposits may lead to an impingement syndrome.[5] In contrast, the resorptive phase, which occurs later in the cycle of calcifying tendinitis, is commonly characterized by acute symptoms. The pain seen at this stage is related to the increase in intratendinous pressure from the vascular proliferation, influx in inflammatory cells, edema, and swelling. As tendon volume increases, the unyielding dimensions of the subacromial space may add additional pressure to the involved tendon, leading to evidence of secondary impingement.[128]

Bursitis has been suggested as a source of pain. However, during surgery, bursal reaction is minimal and is localized to a focal area with hyperemia. It is usually not severe enough to cause a bursal thickening. The rupture of the calcific material into the bursa may cause a crystalline-type bursitis. However, DeSeze and Welfling reported 12 patients who had rupture of the calcified deposit into the bursa, only 8 of whom showed symptoms.[25]

Many authors have stressed the typical subclinical nature of the formative phase. Codman noted that the "usual history is not acute pain in the beginning."[21] Gschwend observed that the calcification is often asymptomatic at the beginning, but its disappearance is marked with acute pain.[43] Wilson stated that many patients know about the calcium deposit for months to years before an acute attack.[139] Rowe broke down the clinical course of patients with calcifying tendinitis into the silent phase, the impingement phase, and the acute phase.[114] Pinals and Short,[102] Booth,[13] Simon,[124] Re and Karzel,[107] and Bosworth[15] provided similar descriptions.

Most authors discuss two primary clinical phases—acute and chronic—with some variation. The subacute or chronic phases are characterized by mild symptoms, whereas the acute phase has more severe symptoms.[31,36,138] DePalma and Kruper divided the clinical presentation of patients into three groups, based on the duration of symptoms. The acute cases had severe shoulder pain for less than 4 weeks duration, the subacute cases had more mild symptoms lasting anywhere between 1 and 6 months, and the chronic cases were those in which patients have had mild symptoms present for more than 6 months.[24] Jones observed that the onset of pain in patients with calcification of the supraspinatus tendon was very sudden and severe and usually not precipitated by injury. He stated that "there is inability to rest or sleep and sometimes patients have become mentally strange after several days of such pain."[54] He was most likely describing the presentation of hyperalgesia related to the resorption phase of calcifying tendinitis. Lapidus coined the term "dormant" deposits with which patients may be without symptoms, except for occasional aches and pains. He suggested that rupture of the tendinous tissue into the floor of the bursa, with extrusion of the calcifying material, was the cause of the developing acute symptoms.[61] Moseley described calcifying tendinitis in terms of four distinct phases: a silent phase, a mechanical phase, followed by rupture of the calcified material into the subbursal space, and finally intrabursal rupture of the calcific deposit.[86] Lippmann describes a phase of increment and a phase of disruption. The phase of increment correlates with very mild symptomatology. Radiographic appearance is discrete and homogeneous in density. The phase of disruption, however, is marked by severe pain and a radiographic appearance that is heterogeneous and fluffy.[64] As implied from these various clinical classification schemes, the pathologic stages of calcifying tendinitis correlate with the clinical presentation, with mild symptoms common with the formative stage, but severe symptoms being typical of the onset of the resorptive phase.

The intensity of the pain may be very severe with the acute clinical phase. Initially, rupture of the calcified deposit into the bursa was presumed to be the etiology of these symptoms. However, DeSeze and Welfling documented acute symptoms in only 8 of 12 patients who had roentgenographic evidence of rupture of the calcium deposit into the bursa. They postulated that the acute symptoms appear to be related to the increase in intratendinous pressure caused by vascular proliferation, inflammatory cell accumulation, and edema. Their explanation is supported by the common intraoperative observation that the calcium deposit literally spurts from the tendon when the tendon is incised during the acute clinical phase.[25]

Calcifying tendinitis should be understood as a continuum, not two distinct subgroups of a disease. Uhthoff and Sarkar stress that "the calcifying deposit must first be formed and thereafter be removed before the tendon is reconstituted." In their experience, the process of formation is usually without symptoms. Serendipitous roentgenographic discovery is common. However, during the stage of resorption, symptoms are usually severe, corresponding to the acute phase in other classification schemes. Once the resorptive phase has resolved, the tendon reconstitutes its fiberous architecture in this self-healing condition, completing the cycle of calcifying tendinitis.[130]

The duration of symptoms correlates with their acuity. The more acute the symptoms, the shorter the duration of symptoms. Simon reported a definite relation between the intensity of symptoms and duration. The acute symptoms last up to 2 weeks; subacute 3 to 8 weeks; and chronic more than 3 months.[124] DePalma stated that the acute symptoms last less than 1 month, subacute between 1 and 6 months and chronic longer than 6 months.[24] Booth stated that "acute calcifying tendinitis is a self-limited process with a natural history of 6 to 14 days."[13] According to Carnett, the chronic cases "ran a self-limiting course and irrespective of treatment, the patient made a complete recovery at varying periods from a few months up to 3 years."[19] Codman believed that few cases were exceedingly acute, and that most cases of calcifying tendinitis ran a subacute course over months to years.[21] In Howorth's series, the duration of symptoms in his patients with calcifying tendinitis was 2 days to 20 years with an average of 2 years. Only 24 patients out of a consecutive series of 100 patients had symptoms of less than 1 month's duration. Nearly all of the others came in because of intermittent exacerbations of pain.[49] Pendergrass and Hodes made the observation that acute symptoms subside in less than 2 weeks, even in the absence of treatment.[100] The importance of the relation between the acuity of symptoms and their resolution becomes paramount when discussing intervention and the "success" of treatment because it appears that most patients presenting with acute hyperalgesia will improve even without treatment.

The location of pain is typically referred to the insertion of the deltoid in over half of the patients. This referral pattern, common with supraspinatus tendinopathy, reflects the frequent involvement of the supraspinatus tendon with calcifying tendinitis. Less commonly, the pain radiates toward the neck. Most patients give a history of difficulty with overhead tasks, inability to sleep on the affected shoulder, or increasing pain during the night that often prevents sleep. Other complaints may include shoulder stiffness, less strength with the arm away from their side, or mechanical complaints, such as "snapping" or "catching" of the shoulder.

Physical Examination

Physical examination characteristics are dependent on the phase of presentation. With the subacute or chronic phase, examination findings often mimic subacromial impingement, with mild decreases in range of motion and a "positive" impingement sign.[71] Kessel and Watson describe the "painful arc of motion," with symptoms of pain elicited with motion of the arm between 70 and 110 degrees of elevation. The painful arc most commonly relates to subacromial pathology.[59] Patients may have a sensation of painful catching caused by a localized impingement of the calcified mass on the coracoacromial arch. The chronic phase of calcifying tendinitis may also present with supraspinatus and infraspinatus atrophy.

During the acute phase, pain is frequently intense, with patients often stating that they have never felt more severe pain. The severe pain leads to guarding against any motion, for they fear the examination may worsen their symptoms. Even if they allow motion, the glenohumeral motion and even the scapulothoracic motion may be severely limited by muscular spasm. Strength testing is prohibited by the pain. Provocative tests, such as the impingement sign, are impossible because of the loss of motion. This "pseudoadhesive capsulitis" is distinguished from idiopathic frozen shoulder by the severity of the pain, by the acute and rapid onset of the pain, and by the radiographic findings. The severity of the pain and the shoulder examination findings may also be confused with acute brachial plexitis (Parsonage-Turner syndrome), but is distinguished by the lack of pure neurologic findings and sparing of the elbow, wrist, and hand function.

Imaging Studies for Calcifying Tendinitis

The calcium deposits are localized to an area within a tendon that is approximately 1 to 2 cm from its insertion site on the tuberosity of the humerus.[21] The pattern of the deposit may be characteristic for the stage of calcifying tendinitis; therefore, a full understanding of the pathogenesis is essential to proper radiologic interpretation.

When a diagnosis of calcifying tendinitis is suspected, radiographs of the shoulder are mandatory. Radiographs can make or confirm the diagnosis, suggest the pathologic phase, and permit radiographic follow-up. Calcifying tendinitis can be suggested by the clinical features discussed, including the age of the patient, the pattern of symptoms, and examination findings. Furthermore, in patients presenting with findings suggestive of subacromial abnormality, a careful review of the radiographs is important. Harbin pointed out that a diagnosis of bursitis was frequently made in cases of calcifying tendinitis because of the failure to recognize the calcification on roentgenograms.[45]

Although many radiographic views of the shoulder may be helpful for specific conditions, routine radiographs must include a true anteroposterior view of the shoulder and an axillary lateral one.[72] Other views are directed by the history and the findings on clinical examination. Although many cases of calcifying tendinitis will be detected with a true anteroposterior view of the glenohumeral joint, additional anteroposterior films, with the shoulder in internal as well as external rotation, are recommended to see the tuberosities and the tendon insertions in multiple profiles. Anteroposterior radiographs with the humerus in neutral rotation show the greater tuberosity in profile, thereby bringing any calcium deposits within the supraspinatus tendon into view. Calcifications within the subscapularis tendon are detected with an anteroposterior view of the humerus in external rotation. With the humerus in internal rotation, precise localization of calcium deposits in both the infraspinatus and teres minor can be made based on their relative location on the greater tuberosity. If calcification is present in the middle one-third of the greater tuberosity, the infraspinatus tendon is likely involved. If the distal one-third of the greater tuberosity is involved, the teres minor is involved. These calcifications are frequently missed on standard anteroposterior radiographs owing to superimposition of the calcification over the proximal humerus (Fig. 6). In addition, calcifications within the long head of the

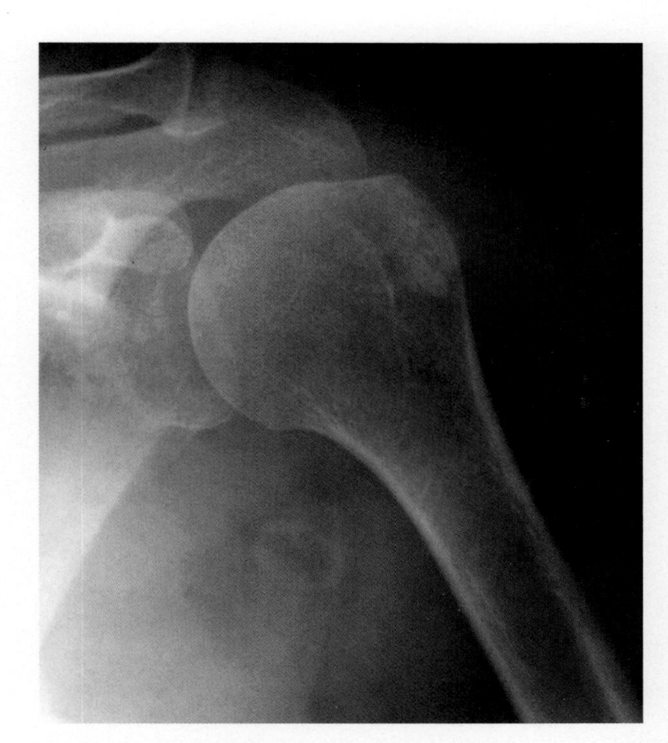

FIG. 6. Calcifying tendinitis involving the infraspinatus or teres minor can be readily seen on an anteroposterior radiograph of the shoulder with the humerus held in internal rotation.

biceps are frequently seen adjacent to the upper portion of the glenoid, and the position of these deposits are unchanged by external or internal rotation of the humerus. Calcifications in the region of the lower portion of the glenoid may represent involvement of the short head of the biceps or the triceps. Rupture of the calcium into the subacromial bursa may give a "skullcap appearance."[124] A supraspinatus outlet view is helpful in determining whether a deposit is in the supraspinatus or infraspinatus and whether it is encroaching on the coracoacromial arch (Fig. 7).

In 1934, Codman reported the presence of a pyramidal shadow in the region of the subacromial bursa just above the tip of the greater tuberosity and stated that this represented calcification within the region of the subacromial bursa. However, on exploration during surgery, he noted no bursal involvement. The calcium deposit was completely contained within the tendon of the rotator cuff.[21]

Bosworth believed that routine use of fluoroscopy was more accurate than routine roentgenographic examination, with concern that radiographs commonly missed calcifications that were superimposed over the humeral head or the acromion.[15] He claimed that "regardless of whether or not roentgenograms are taken, fluoroscopy should never be omitted as an essential part of the exam." He also pointed out that many calcified deposits are "discovered accidentally," with nothing being done about it. Howorth also felt that fluoroscopy may be useful to localize the calcium deposition.[49] Fluoroscopy may help with visualization of the calcific deposit, but its value over routine radiographs in determining treatment is unknown. He felt that his technique was a more sensitive way to detect the calcifications than even surgical exploration.[46]

Bosworth reported a classification scheme based on the size of the calcium deposit. Small deposits, up to 0.5 mm in diameter, were of little or no clinical significance; medium-sized deposits, 0.5 to 1.5 mm in diameter, were of moderate clinical significance; and the larger deposits, of more than 1.5 mm in diameter, were most likely to cause clinical symptoms.[15] Patte and Goutallier described a classification scheme that divided the radiographic appearance of calcifying tendinitis into a localized form and a diffuse form. The localized form was characterized by round or oval, homogeneously dense calcifications that were close to the bursal wall. These tended to heal spontaneously. The diffuse form was thought to be situated deeper than the localized form, close to the bony insertion of the tendons. The density was heterogeneous, and these were considered to cause more pain and to take longer to resolve.[97] Most authors feel that the classifications by both Bosworth and by Patte and Goutallier are not of much clinical value.

The French Society of Arthroscopy has classified rotator cuff calcifications into four categories (Fig. 8).[83] Type A is a homogeneous calcification, with well-defined limits, and represents approximately 20% of the patients presenting in a large multicenter review. Type B is heterogeneous calcification that is fragmented, but with well-defined limits and was seen in 45% of their patients. Type C calcification is a heterogeneous calcification, with poorly defined limits, sometimes with a punctate appearance; 30% of their patients present with this finding on radiographs. Type D calcification is

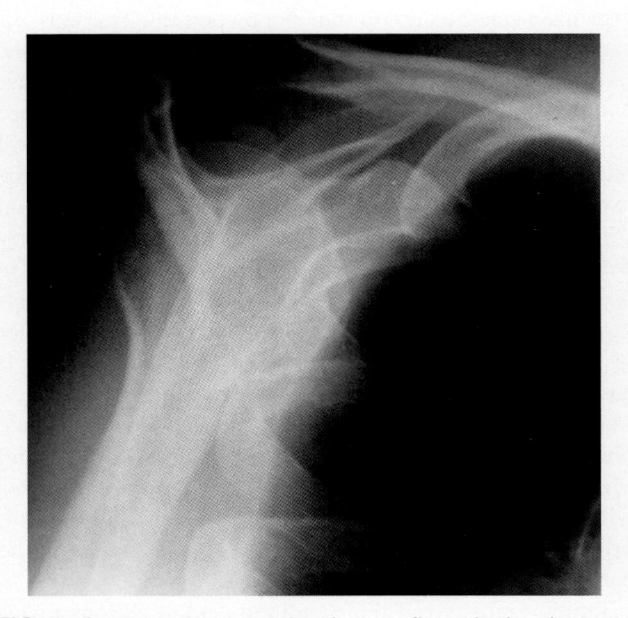

FIG. 7. A supraspinatus outlet view confirms the involvement of the supraspinatus tendon. Localizing the calcific deposit is essential for successful needling or surgical decompression of the lesion.

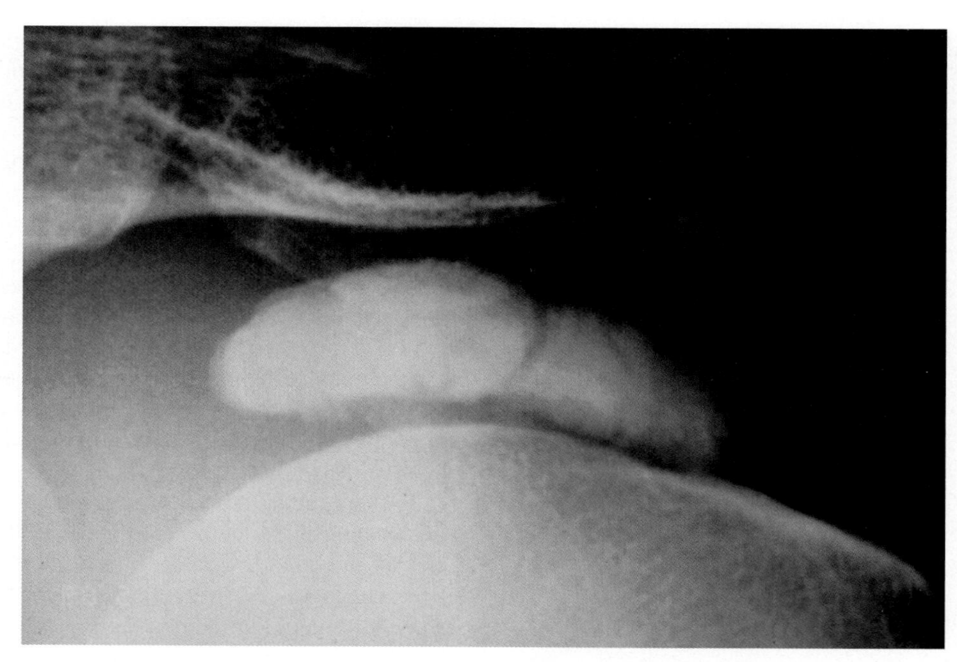

FIG. 8. The French Society of Arthroscopy has classified rotator cuff calcifications into four categories: *type A*: homogeneous, well-defined limits; *type B*: heterogeneous, fragmented, well-defined limits; *type C*: heterogeneous, poorly defined limits; *type D*: dystrophic pattern. A type B calcification is seen in approximately 45% of the patients in their multicenter evaluation. Fifty percent of patients with this pattern will have a pasty consistency to the calcific material at the time of surgery. (Courtesy of Docteur Gilles Walch.)

a dystrophic pattern at the insertion of the rotator cuff. This pattern clearly represents a degenerative process and should not be confused with calcifying tendinitis (Fig. 9). With Type A and B, the calcifications, at surgery, have a pasty consistency 50% of the time. Type C is diffuse, and a well-organized calcific deposit may not be present. This classification has relevance to the stage of calcifying tendinitis, the radiographic appearance, and implications for intervention.

Other authors have attempted to correlate the appearance of the calcified deposit on roentgenogram with the clinical phase of calcifying tendinitis. DePalma and Kruper describe two radiologic types. Type I was amorphous, "fluffy" and ""fleecy" in appearance, and heterogeneous, with a poorly defined periphery. This pattern was usually encountered in acute phases. Occasionally, they noted a contiguous overlying crescentlike streak that they believed represented rupture of the calcified deposit into the subacromial bursa. Type II had a well-defined outline and was homogeneous in density. This appearance was common in the subacute or chronic phase of calcifying tendinitis.[24] DeSeze and Welfling[25] and McKendry[75] were also able to correlate clinical symptoms with the radiographic appearance of the calcium deposit. Friedman could not find a correlation between the size of the particles and the severity of symptoms.[31]

Pulich emphasized that tendinous calcifications differ from capsular or bursal calcifications because the calcific deposit of calcifying tendinitis is contained within the tendons of the rotator cuff and remains confined to the points of insertion of the tendon. Bursal or capsular calcifications eventually conform to the cavity within which they are contained.[105]

Uhthoff and Sarkar do not believe that all cases end with rupture of the calcified deposit into the subacromial bursa.[131] When this did not occur in their patients, symptoms tended to be more prolonged and recurring. Furthermore, they demonstrated a strong correlation between the clinical symptoms, radiographic appearance, and intraoperative findings in 41 patients undergoing surgery for calcifying tendinitis.[75] Of the 41 patients, 31 had chronic or subacute symptoms, and 10 had acute symptoms. Twenty-four of 31 patients with chronic symptoms had roentgenograms consistent with the formative phase of calcifying tendinitis. Intraoperatively, the calcified deposit appeared chalklike in 29 of the 31 patients. Of the 10 patients with acute symptoms, 8 had x-rays films consistent with the resorptive phase; 9 patients also had a toothpastelike consistency of the calcified deposit.

Other radiographic concerns include coexisting conditions. Some authors have raised the question of concomitant presence of a rotator cuff tear with calcifying tendinitis. Although McLaughlin and Asherman stated that the presence of calcifying tendinitis is strong evidence against a rotator cuff tear,[78] other authors, including Hsu and his colleagues, believe that one should commonly consider the possibility of coexisting calcifying tendinitis and rotator cuff tear.[50] However, their study contrasts with many of the tenets concerning calcifying tendinitis that are confirmed in previous stud-

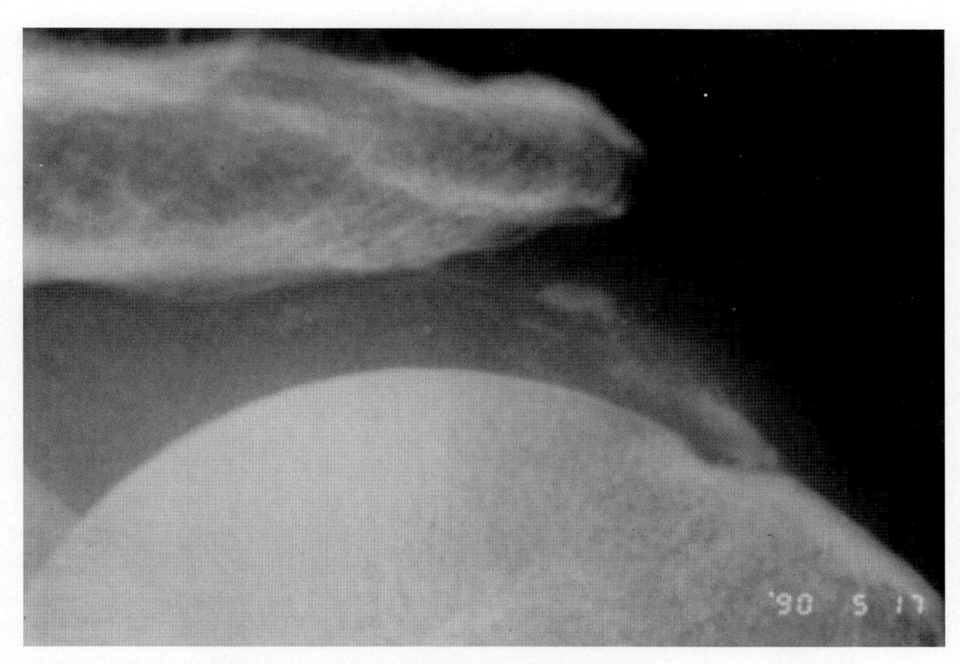

FIG. 9. Type D calcification with a dystrophic pattern typical of degenerative process, but not calcifying tendinitis. (Courtesy of Docteur Gilles Walch.)

ies, and suggests that the report by Hsu et al. is discussing a subset of calcifying tendinitis, a completely different condition, or a variation of calcifying tendinitis unique to his Taiwanese patient population. Also, many patients were older than the age of 60, at which an increased incidence of rotator cuff tears would be expected in a control population without calcifying tendinitis. However, others have suggested an increased incidence of rotator cuff tears with calcifying tendinitis. Kernwein observed that, in patients older than the age of 40 years with calcifying tendinitis, there was a 90% probability that an arthrogram would reveal rotator cuff tear.[58] This report has not been supported by others.[37] Wolfgang observed that 23% of the patients that had a rotator cuff tendon repair also had calcifying tendinitis.[140]

Jim et al. looked at the coexistence of calcifying tendinitis and rotator cuff tendon tears prospectively in their Taiwanese patient population. In 81 patients with calcifying tendinitis, an arthrogram was performed to look for concomitant rotator cuff tear. Twenty-two arthrograms were positive. Small amounts of calcifications were statistically more likely to be associated with rotator cuff tear in this population. They concluded that calcifying tendinitis with rotator cuff tendon tear is not uncommon, especially in older patients.[53]

Confounding this issue, Loew correlated the presence of calcifying tendinitis with subacromial impingement findings. They looked at 75 patients with calcifying tendinitis, and prospectively performed roentgenographic studies as well as magnetic resonance imaging (MRI) of these patients to identify additional findings of subacromial impingement. They found degenerative tendon changes in 11% of the 75 patients, and a type III acromion in 16% of these patients. Their conclusion was that there was little correlation between calcifying tendinitis and additional findings of subacromial impingement.[67]

The role of computed tomography (CT) and MRI in calcifying tendinitis is still unclear. Computerized tomography may help localize the calcific deposit, but is unlikely to add additional information that will influence treatment. On MRI, the T1-weighted images show calcifications as decreased signal intensity, whereas T2-weighted images may show perifocal increased uptake around the deposit, largely from edema during the resorptive phase.[48,51] A cautious interpretation of the MRI findings is important because the decreased signal intensity, combined with the relatively thin dimensions of the cuff lateral to the calcific deposit, may be interpreted as a large rotator cuff tear. This false MRI interpretation, when combined with a limited physical examination secondary to pain, may lead to a more aggressive surgical approach than is indicated by the true pathology. Re and Karzel stated that routine use of CT and MRI are probably unnecessary if adequate roentgenograms are obtained.[107] However, if evaluation of coexisting pathology is the intent, MRI is the most effective specialized radiographic study.[48,51] An arthrogram will also provide additional information on the integrity of the rotator cuff.

Ultrasound has also been used for evaluation of calcific deposits. Hartig and Huth demonstrated that ultrasonography was more sensitive than plain radiographs for detecting calcific deposits in the rotator cuff tendons.[47] In 217 cases of calcifying tendinitis, ultrasound detected 100% of the lesions, while plain radiographs demonstrated 90%. Ultrasound has the added benefit of not exposing the patient to unnecessary radiation. Unfortunately, ultrasonography is highly dependent on technicians and radiologists with significant experience in evaluating shoulder conditions.

Natural History

Calcifying tendinitis proceeds through a cycle of calcification, resorption, then tendon reconstitution in most cases (see Fig. 3). The self-healing nature of calcifying tendinitis has been emphasized. Carnett pointed out the "tendency for the hyperacute pain to ease up after a few days or within two weeks." He also stated that "in many chronic cases, the condition ran a self-limiting course and irrespective of treatment, the patient made complete recovery at varying periods from a few months up to 3 years."[19] Unfortunately, not all cases of calcifying tendinitis resolve expediently and without sequelae.

Codman questioned the ability of the involved rotator cuff tendon to completely heal and reconstitute its normal integrity. He stated that "although it is the rule that cases of calcified deposits recover with no known sequelae, I am more and more inclined to think that they must result in some atrophy of the tendon, whether they are absorbed naturally or are removed."[21]

Howorth noted that the calcareous deposits often change in size and density over a period of month or years, but may in fact change over a few days. He also noted that calcium deposits within the tendons commonly persist for many years unless there is spontaneous or surgical drainage. Rupture of the deposit into the subacromial bursa results not only in a change in the location and density of the calcified material, but also usually is followed by immediate relief of symptoms and absorption of the calcified material.[49]

McLaughlin, in 1946, reported that 90 patients who had calcified deposits discovered incidentally by roentgenograms returned at a later date with pain, presumably owing to irritation by the calcified deposit. Acutely painful lesions frequently had a portion of the calcified deposit in contact with the bursal floor and occasionally within the subacromial bursa itself. He suggested that if the lesion was left untreated it could produce constant mild pain for as long as 15 years. However, these calcified deposits were rarely found in unselected cadavers older than 66 years, which indicated that "most if not all deposits are limited by some spontaneous mechanism prior to the sixth decade."[76]

Lippmann observed that the phase of interval symptoms abides by no time schedule, and has been observed to persist for as long as 12 years. He noted that a close inverse relation between the severity of pain and its duration exists, but rarely does the painful absorption of calcium persist for longer than 3 weeks.[64] Moseley outlined a detailed natural history of calcified deposits in the rotator cuff. He described an initial "silent phase," which was characterized by minimal clinical signs and symptoms. The "mechanical phase" was characterized by impingement-type symptoms. These patients tended to have a painful arc of motion. The "subbursal rupture" phase is a result of partial evacuation of the calcified deposit. As such, symptoms in this phase of the disease tend to recur. The final phase, which he called "intrabursal rupture," is characterized by complete drainage of the calcified deposit under the floor of the bursa and secondarily into the bursa. Clinical symptoms were most severe with this phase, corresponding to resorption of the calcific deposit. He believed that the calcified deposit had to be completely eliminated before the patient was free of symptoms.[86]

Lapidus and Guidotti reported on "a number of cases of spontaneous recovery in the patients who came under observation days following the onset of the acute symptoms." They also noted complete disappearance of the deposit radiographically in those same patients.[62] Ghormley observed that although the tendency for complete resolution was the rule, some cases would go on to "heterotopic ossification."[36] This concept has not been supported by others.

Uhthoff and Sarkar have conclusively demonstrated that calcifying tendinitis is an active, cell-mediated process that tends to progress toward spontaneous resolution, including tendon reconstitution. The roentgenographic appearance, the clinical symptomatology, as well as the histologic and gross appearance can be reasonably predicted by knowing any one of the aforementioned features and by understanding the cyclic nature of this disorder.

Other authors have suggested that because the success of intervention is high and rapidly resolves the clinical symptoms, patients should not have to wait for the expected resolution of their condition. Codman felt that if he personally developed calcifying tendinitis, he would rather have surgical treatment than wait for the condition to resolve on its own.

Harbin also suggested that "conservative treatment in the acute cases seems to be unwise." He recommended that "since the operative treatment is so simple, offers so little danger, and promises complete relief in practically 90% of the cases, one should have little hesitancy in urging it in all cases in which the condition has persisted over a period of months without relief by the more conservative measures."[45]

Harmon reported that the natural course of calcifying tendinitis could be favorably influenced by treatment properly applied relative to the time in the cycle of the disease. He too recommended removal of large to medium-sized deposits within the rotator cuff tendons. This was based on his observations that few quiescent or mildly symptomatic deposits disappear spontaneously. However, in the acute and hyperacute deposits, these tended to disappear in 7 to 14 days with conservative treatment.[46] DePalma and Kruper believed that the natural history of calcifying tendinitis could usually be favorably altered by the treatment chosen. They reported on the results of a long-term follow-up study of shoulder joints treated for calcifying tendinitis, surgically as well as conservatively. They observed that 84% of the patients treated conservatively had favorable short-term results. However, long-term results revealed only 61% were favorable. In contrast, surgical management produced 96% favorable results. They noted that the convalescence period was longer when the calcifying tendinitis was treated surgically.[24]

Most recently, Kempf noted that although the natural evolution of this calcifying tendinitis is favorable, the cyclic natural history described by Uhthoff may in fact be blocked at any stage of the disease. Even though many studies have demonstrated that conservative treatment of these deposits can be successful in most of these patients, a study by Noel and Brantus encourages a cautious posture for prognosis because only 50% of their 124 cases treated without surgery demonstrated favorable results.[57]

TREATMENT

The treatment of calcifying tendinitis has tended to vary according to the expertise and experience of the treating physician. There have been a variety of treatment methods proposed, all of which have had some success in the treatment of calcifying tendinitis. An understanding of the pathophysiology of calcifying tendinitis is essential when determining the correct intervention. Uhthoff's explanation of the three pathophysiologic stages of calcifying tendinitis create a framework in which to establish an appropriate treatment algorithm.[135]

Determining the correct stage of calcifying tendinitis includes a careful history, physical examination, and appropriate plain radiographs. Acute calcifying tendinitis is severely painful, with patients splinting their upper extremity against any movement. Narcotic medications may be required to control pain and allow sleep at night. Patients often demand intervention because of the severity of their symptoms and the effect on their daily activities, even if they understand that their condition may actually be resolving. Because acute symptoms are associated with the resorption phase, which is frequently measured in days or weeks, treatment at this stage is likely to be associated with a favorable result, even though the treatment may have had no direct effect on the natural history of the patient's condition. With chronic symptoms secondary to calcifying tendinitis, intermittent worsening of symptoms may lead to patient dissatisfaction. The goal of intervention should be to establish a treatment plan that can accelerate the natural history of this condition or encourage the resolution of symptoms without significant risk to the patient.

Nonoperative Treatment

Virtually all patients with calcifying tendinitis are successfully treated with nonoperative management. Gschwend and colleagues estimate that more than 90% of patients are adequately treated with conservative management.[43] Litchman reported that he was able to treat 99 of 100 patients with calcifying tendinitis without surgical intervention.[65] Treatment options include analgesics, nonsteroidal antiinflammatory medications, physical therapy, infiltrations, needling or barbatoge with or without aspiration, extracorporial lithotripsy, and antiinflammatory radiotherapy.[6,16,39,43,46,66,69,89,98,100,101,112]

On initial presentation, patient complaints are most commonly related to pain. Nonsteroidal antiinflammatory medications are often prescribed. Their efficacy for the treatment of chronic or acute calcifying tendinitis and their effect on the natural history is unknown. During the acute hyperalgesia of the resorption phase, narcotic medication may be indicated for the relief of severe pain that interferes with sleep and daily activities.

Many authors recommend physical therapy for the treatment of patients with calcifying tendinitis, especially those patients presenting with mild pain and chronic symptoms.[14,30,36,43,64,76,87] The primary focus of physiotherapy is to reestablish normal shoulder motion. Some authors have suggested that therapy is necessary to prevent an idiopathic frozen shoulder. However, there is no evidence to confirm that calcifying tendinitis leads to a generalized contracture of the glenohumeral joint capsule, which is the hallmark of a frozen shoulder.[72] Restriction in motion is more likely to be secondary to pain, muscular spasm, and an increased volume of the rotator cuff within the confines of the coracoacromial space. Because the coracoacromial arch is congruent with the normal rotator cuff tendon and proximal humerus, a change in the volume of the rotator cuff tendon from a calcific deposit or the combined effects of the deposit and factors involved in the resorptive phase is likely to lead to mechanical irritation. This mechanical irritation will lead to decreased volitional movement of the shoulder to avoid discomfort. The primary focus of therapy is mobilization, avoiding the stiffness that accompanies inactivity and pain so that once the calcifying tendinitis has improved, there is no long-term restriction on shoulder motion. Exercises initially include pendulum exercise and gentle passive range of motion. As the symptoms improve, stretching of the shoulder can be accomplished with passive to active motion, including forward elevation, external rotation, internal rotation, and horizontal adduction.

Physical modalities, such as ultrasonography, infrared heat, and iontophoresis, have been used to treat calcifying tendinitis.[42] However, there is no evidence that any of these physical modalities have a beneficial effect on the resolution of the calcifying tendinitis, either in the acute or chronic clinical phase. Griffin and Karselis have observed that ultrasonography was unable to mobilize the calcium crystals or to stimulate the resorption of the calcium deposit.[42] However, ultrasonography did provide short-term pain relief.

Needling or Puncture Aspiration

Some form of needling of the calcific deposit has been commonly recommended for the treatment of calcifying tendinitis. The methods of needling or puncture aspiration have been varied and include the placement of a needle within the calcific deposit to decompress the pressure at the site of the calcifying tendinitis, an injection of a local anesthetic alone, an injection of a local anesthetic with needling of the deposit, followed by a cortisone injection, and injection of cortisone alone in the subacromial space, and a needle aspiration–irrigation to decompress and remove the calcifying tendinitis deposit. Each method has a proponent with some data to support its use. Much of the confusion arises from the treatment of calcifying tendinitis during the resorption stage. Because the acute symptoms are commonly associated with an expedient resolution of the condition, any treatment at this time is likely to be "successful." In fact, the treatment goal during the acute hyperalgesic clinical phase, corresponding to the stage of resorption, should be primarily directed toward improving patient comfort, with a secondary goal of avoiding any intervention that may inhibit the tendon restoration. Because each method may be effective, the single best treatment must also take into account the cost to the patient both in terms of potential risks as well as the costs related to the expense of the procedure.

Several authors have recommended needling or barbotage of the calcific deposit (Fig. 10). In Codman's treatise on rotator cuff disorders,[21] he refers to Flint's 1913 publication describing aspiration of the calcific deposit. After reading Flint's publication, Codman tried the aspiration and felt at the time of the aspiration he actually punctured the deposit, which allowed the contents to leak into the bursa and relieve the patient's pain. He stated this was not Flint's exact plan, but was his achievement nonetheless. Barbotage can be accomplished either with a blind approach, as described by DePalma and Kruper,[24] or may be done with a more sophisticated measure of localizing the lesion using either fluoroscopic control or ultrasound.

Patterson and Darrach recommended needling of the calcification in conjunction with an injection of local anesthetic in the subacromial space.[98] Friedman demonstrated the ability to achieve pain relief in 85% of patients treated with this method.[31] However, in 11 out of 70 shoulders, the method failed to relieve the acute pain. Furthermore, Friedman noted that the amount of actual calcium removed did not appear to be important to the outcome of the needling of the calcified deposit. He concluded that piercing the calcium deposit was essential, whether or not the calcium was removed by aspiration or irrigation.

In DePalma and Kruper's report, a 1% solution of a local anesthetic was used to anesthetize the area of the subacromial space.[24] After needling the deposit and attempting to remove as much of the calcific mass as possible, multiple punctures were then placed with the 18-gauge needle into the rotator cuff tendon. It was suggested that this would cause an active hyperemia, enhancing dissolution and absorption of remaining calcific material. After completion of the needling, 10 mL of hydrocortisone was injected at the site of needling. One hundred fifty-four shoulders were evaluated for calcifying tendinitis, 86 of these treated by conservative methods. Ninety-four of the shoulders were reevaluated at follow-up, with 41 of the shoulders being treated by multiple puncture of the deposit. Only 23 of the 41 shoulders treated conservatively were reexamined, with 13 having a good result, 5 having a fair result, and 5 having a poor result. In other patients contacted by questionnaire, 18 shoulders in total, 12 were rated as good, 4 fair, and 2 poor. It was their opinion that conservative management provides satisfactory short-term results in most cases.

Key recommended needling in acute cases when a single large deposit is seen on radiographs.[60] After needling and aspirating the deposit, multiple punctures were performed. He suggested needling under local anesthesia for patients who would best be treated by operative removal, but did not want to undergo an operation. Key felt that it was not a reliable

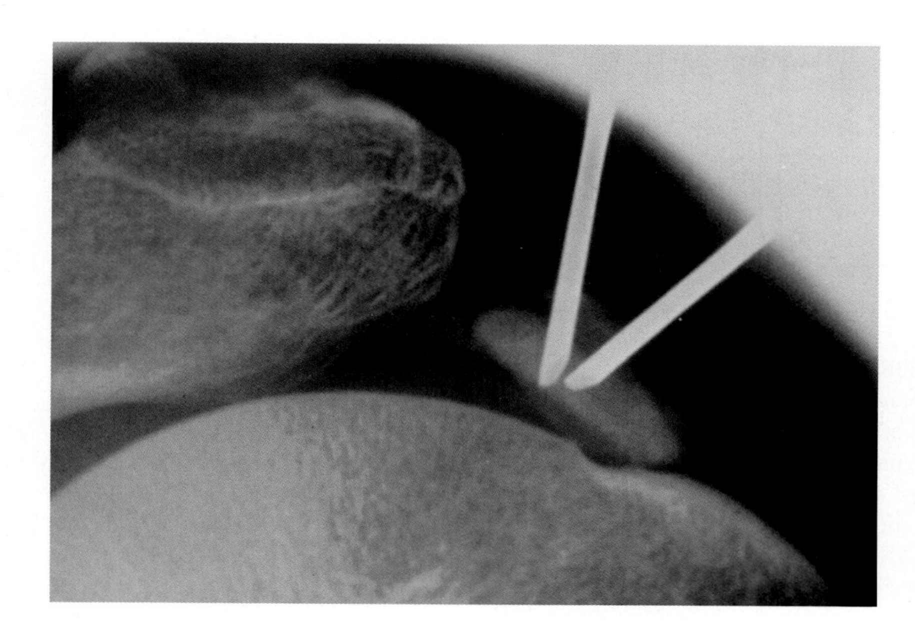

FIG. 10. Needling of the calcific deposit decompresses the lesion, decreases the pressure in the tendon, an subsequently alleviates the symptoms of calcifying tendinitis. Needling can be performed "blind" in the office, or by using specialized techniques, such as fluoroscopy, to accurately localize the deposit. A second needle can be inserted into the area of the deposit for additional decompression or lavage. (Courtesy of Docteur Gilles Walch.)

form of treatment, and he recommended surgery for those patients who did not respond to physical therapy and physical modalities.

Lapidus presented 16 cases of patients presenting with acute symptoms.[61] He found that treatment by infiltration with a local anesthetic and injection of saline into the calcified deposit caused relief of symptoms and disappearance of calcification soon afterward and, therefore, injection therapy was beneficial. It was clear that his treatment occurred at the time of resorption and it was likely that resolution of the calcium would occur without the injection. Moutounet and his colleagues discussed the radiological localization of the calcific deposit with subsequent needling.[89] After needling the deposit, corticosteroid was injected into the area of the deposit. They concluded that direct puncture of the calcification shortens the natural history of both acute or chronic calcifying tendinitis and accelerates resorption in 50% of the cases. With the addition of a small amount of cortisone, pain was relieved, and 80% good and very good results were achieved.

Clement also described a method of needling of the calcific deposit.[20] After spraying the skin with ethyl chloride, a no. 22 needle containing lidocaine and methylprednisolone was used to inject the solution into the subacromial space. Once the local anesthetic had become effective, the calcific deposit was needled repeatedly. Clement recommended 15 to 20 times. This was done without any type of radiologic localization of the calcific deposit. Clement mentioned that the acute pain subsided within 24 hours. Within a few days, the patients were referred to the therapist for ultrasonic treatment. He concluded that the pain was relieved with needling and injection and that the absorption of calcium was improved with ultrasonic treatments. There was no control group to evaluate whether the ultrasonic treatment had any effect in addition to the needling. In his series, there were no recurrences.

Farin et al. described a more sophisticated technique using ultrasonic-guided needling and aspiration, as well as lavage of the calcific deposits.[26] The technique of ultrasonographic localization was described, and two case reports were provided. The goal was direct needling of the deposit, followed by aspiration and lavage to remove as much of the calcific material as possible (Fig. 11). Within a few days of the treatment, both patients had a substantial reduction in their discomfort and were started on physical therapy programs. Bradley et al. reported 11 cases with radiographically evident calcific deposits. By using an ultrasound guidance technique, the deposit was needled and aspirated. Six of 11 patients had "relief" on the same day, 4 additional patients were pain-free after 2 weeks, and the remaining patient, who had no change in symptoms, had a supraspinatus tear seen on the ultrasonographic examination.[16]

Although needling of the deposit with adjunctive use of a local anesthetic is widely accepted, the addition of corticosteroid to the local treatment has been controversial. Harmon, discussing the treatment for calcific rotator cuff tendinitis in 609 shoulders, performed 263 needlings after local injection of hydrocortisone meticorten anesthetic drugs.[46] A total quantity of 20 to 40 mL suspension with one-half 1% lidocaine and one-half hydrocortisone, 25 mg (or prednisolone 25 or 50 mg/10 mL). This was blindly injected into multiple sites just proximal to the greater tuberosity, which was determined by the patient examination and radiographs. The results were considered excellent by this method alone, with the disappearance in 14 days or less after the last injection. However, approximately 54% of this group required two or more injections to alleviate the symptoms. Furthermore, there was no difference in those shoulders that were injected and needled with lidocaine alone or with the lidocaine and corticosteroid suspension. Subjectively, there did appear to be decreased muscle spasm and periarticular stiffening with the corticosteroid suspension.

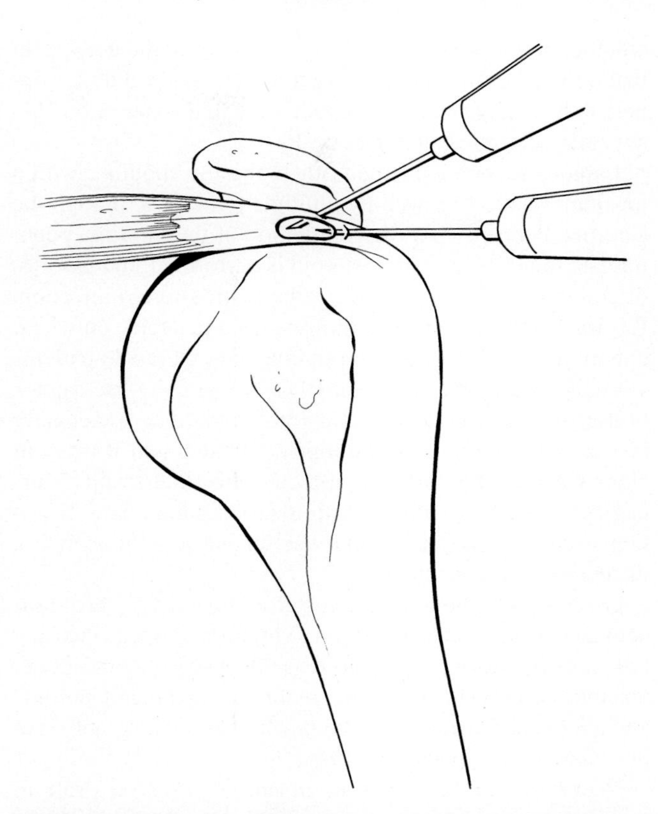

FIG. 11. Needling and lavage can be effective if the deposit is localized. Sophisticated imaging techniques, such as fluoroscopy or ultrasound, permit accurate localization and direct penetration of the calcific deposit.

Friedman noted that patients who had corticosteroid injected at the time of the calcium needling appeared to have less pain after the anesthetic effect of procaine (Novocaine) had worn off.[31] However, he emphasized the decompression of the calcific deposit was far more important than the local affect of hydrocortisone. Those deposits that had been definitely pierced or aspirated had results that were similar whether or not corticosteroid had been used. It did not appear that corticosteroids had any negative effect, nor did they appear to have any effect on the reduction in the size or the disappearance of the calcium deposit.

Lapidus recommended anesthetizing the shoulder with a local anesthetic followed by multiple punctures through the calcified deposit.[61] At the completion of the multiple puncture, an injection of corticosteroid is performed. In his series of 248 cases, 83 patients received a corticosteroid injection. It is unclear as to what criteria were used to decide on which patient received a corticosteroid injection. Of the 83 patients who did receive the injection, 19 (23%) actually had aspiration of the calcific deposit. Lapidus stated that "practically all" of our patients were promptly relieved, and it was unclear whether the cortisone affected the final result. Murnaghan treated 27 patients with local anesthetic and 24 patients with corticosteroid and was unable to demonstrate a difference in the results.[90]

Gschwend found that corticosteroid injections were short acting, and their effect was on symptoms alone.[43] Mosley felt that steroids injected into tense deposits may cause extensive necrosis and, therefore, recommended that if steroids and a local anesthetic are to be injected, it must be only into the subacromial space and bursa.[87]

Neer believes that cortisone injections do have a role in the treatment of patients with calcifying tendinitis.[91] When patients had pain and stiffness that could not be effectively treated with physiotherapy, he recommended a limited number of local steroid injections to reduce inflammation and resume exercises. When the resorptive phase had begun and pain was severe, he recommended an injection of lidocaine followed by needling, and then completed with an injection of corticosteroids. In those deposits that had occurred during the formative stage, again, injections, including cortisone injections, were recommended. Neer noted that when he was a resident, the most frequent shoulder operation in his hospital was excision of calcium. However, he believes that treatment using parenteral nonsteroidal antiinflammatory medications and corticosteroids has reduced the surgical excision of calcium to a rare procedure.

Other authors have expressed concern over the injection of corticosteroid and the disruption of the normal tendon-healing process, or tendon reconstitution. Lippman believed that corticosteroids could inhibit the resorptive phase and possibly return the calcifying tendinitis back to its static or resting phase.[64] Uhthoff has also stated that there is no indication for an injection of cortisone when treating the acute clinical or resorptive phase of calcifying tendinitis.[134]

In conclusion, an injection of corticosteroids is primarily effective as a long-acting pain reliever, possibly because of the resolution of the associated inflammatory process of the resorptive phase. Cortisone does not appear to have any benefit on the resolution of the calcific deposit. However, despite theoretical concerns, there is no evidence that an injection of corticosteroids into the subacromial space following needling of the calcific deposit has any adverse effects.

Radiotherapy

Radiation or x-ray therapy has been advocated for the treatment of calcifying tendinitis of the shoulder.[6,95,100,103] Treatments have varied from a single large dose of radiation to small doses on a repetitive basis. Improvement in symptoms has been reported in 70% to 100% of patients. Radiotherapy was initially proposed in Europe and later used in the United States. Plenk evaluated the effect of radiation therapy in 21 patients, with an additional 17 patients as a control group.[103] In the control group, the patients were set up exactly as the study group; only a lead shutter was placed in front of the x-ray tube housing to prevent any radiation of the shoulder. Remarkably, a definite improvement or complete relief of pain within 6 weeks after therapy was discovered in 15 of the treated patients and 15 of the control patients. It was Plenk's opinion that "calcifying tendinitis of the shoulder is essentially a self-limiting disease." He argued that there was no benefit from radiation therapy, and stressed the importance of understanding the natural history of calcifying tendinitis.

Recently, Ollagnier and coworkers reported on a group of 44 patients receiving what they termed "antiinflammatory radiotherapy."[95] All patients were treated with a dose of radiotherapy ranging from 600 to 1,200 R, divided between five and nine sessions. With a mean follow-up of longer than 2 years, 68% of the patients were satisfied or very satisfied with the treatment. However, when the treatment was broken down into the various stages of calcifying tendinitis, it was clear that patients presenting with the formative stage of calcifying tendinitis had equivocal results, with 6 out of the 14 patients not a part of the satisfied group. In those patients in the resorption phase or demonstrating heterogeneous pattern to the calcific deposit, 6 out of the 8 were in the satisfied group. The author speculated that antiinflammatory radiation therapy was effective and that it is "at least as efficient as needle aspiration or lithotripsy."

Baird reported on 18 cases of calcifying tendinitis:[6] 9 patients were in the acute phase, 5 patients in the subacute phase, and 4 patients in the chronic phase. He suggested that only one exposure was required to relieve the pain completely and restore normal function for patients in the acute phase and some patients in the subacute phase. No serious adverse effects were noted. Given the cost, potential risks to the patient, and the lack of evidence demonstrating its effectiveness, it would appear that radiation therapy for calcifying tendinitis is primarily of historical importance.

Extracorporeal Shockwave Treatment

Dahmen initially reported on the efficacy of extracorporeal shockwave therapy using low-pulse energy.[23] There was no investigation into the changes of the calcific deposit after the shockwave application, but clinically there was a significant improvement in shoulder pain.

Loew studied 20 patients who were treated with a lithotripter in two sessions of 2,000 pulses each.[66] Twelve weeks following the treatment, 15 of the 20 patients had a marked reduction of symptoms, with a 30% improvement overall. Fourteen patients had a transient subcutaneous hematoma. Magnetic resonance imaging failed to demonstrate any damage to the tendon or the bone. These patients demonstrated chronic calcifying tendinitis, with a history of symptoms for longer than 12 months and radiologically proven calcification of the rotator cuff measuring greater than 10 mm in the anteroposterior roentgenogram, consistent with the formative stage. The calcific deposits were of homogeneous consistency and would correspond to the type A classification by the French Society of Arthroscopy. No patients had rotator cuff tears. Radiographic studies 6 weeks following the extracorporeal shockwave therapy demonstrated 11 of the 20 patients had a change in their radiographic architecture. At 12 weeks, 12 patients demonstrated radiographic changes, with 7 showing a complete resolution of the calcium deposit.

Rompe evaluated the treatment of extracorporeal shockwave therapy in the treatment of 46 patients with calcific deposits of the supraspinatus tendon. Inclusion criteria included persistent shoulder pain, in combination with the calcific deposit of the supraspinatus, that had been present for more than 12 months and had failed conservative therapy for at least 6 months. The deposits were sharply outlined and densely structured, with a minimum diameter of 10 mm. This technique uses an electromagnetic shockwave generator in a mobile fluoroscopy unit. A regional anesthetic agent was necessary to complete the procedure. At 6 weeks, partial resorption of the calcium deposit was noticed in 43% of the patients, with complete resorption in 10%. By 24 weeks there was a 48% partial resorption and a 15% complete disintegration. Again, based on the results, Rompe noted that extracorporeal shockwave therapy was more effective than injections or needle irrigation for the treatment of calcifying tendinitis in the formative stage. However, the results of shockwave therapy remain inferior to surgical debridement.

Surgical Treatment

Codman wrote: "My personal opinion is that surgical removal of the deposit is practically free from danger, sure to relieve the severe symptoms at once, and, in fact, that it generally will relieve all really troublesome symptoms within a few weeks."[21] He further opined "it would be rational to thrust a large aspirating needle into the deposit under guidance of the fluoroscope, but I would prefer to be operated upon were I the patient." He suggested the operation could be performed with a local anesthetic despite an open approach to the supraspinatus tendon. Bosworth concurred, stating that the most dependable way of eliminating the symptoms and the disease of calcifying tendinitis is by open surgery.[14]

Lippman reviewed his results of 100 consecutive cases treated with surgical decompression of the calcific deposit.[64] His conclusion was that patients with calcifying tendinitis treated surgically can expect return of normal function to the shoulder. McLaughlin discussed the operative decompression and removal in over 200 cases.[77] Surgical treatment was believed to be necessary in less than 10% of all cases of calcifying tendinitis. In most of the surgical cases, he believed the severity of the patient's symptoms and their request for treatment of their pain led to surgical management. He concluded that surgical treatment produced the most certain and permanent results.

Gschwend recommended surgical treatment when there was a progression of symptoms, interference with activities of daily living, and a failure of conservative management.[43] Such treatment was correlated with a good or an excellent result in more than 90% of patients. Neer states that surgical indications should include the failure of conservative treatment, as well as multiple hard, gritty deposits with long-standing symptoms.[91] Despite a practice dedicated entirely to the treatment of shoulder problems, he was performing the procedure only once or twice a year. He also was keenly aware that the recovery period for long-standing lesions is longer than one might expect from relatively minimal open surgery and removal of the calcifying deposit, suggesting residual tendonopathy despite removal of the calcific lesion.

McKendry et al. reported on the surgical treatment of 57 patients with calcifying tendinitis.[75] Surgery was performed after an average follow-up of 2.8 years after the onset of symptoms. Sixty percent of patients were pain-free postoperatively at 6 weeks, although 30% had continuing pain beyond 12 weeks. Preoperative factors predicting a longer convalescence could not be identified. They emphasized that a fluffy appearance to the calcium deposit is associated with the resorptive phase; therefore, a trial of conservative treatment was recommended.

In summary, many investigators have shown that surgical management is effective for the treatment of calcifying tendinitis. Surgery is primarily indicated for the treatment of symptomatic patients with calcifying tendinitis in the formative stage, which is confirmed on radiographs demonstrating a relatively homogeneous calcific deposit. Patients who have acute severe symptoms or patients with evidence of heterogeneous calcification are likely to be in the resorptive phase and, therefore, continued conservative management would be recommended. Patients treated surgically during the resorptive phase are likely to have favorable results because the natural history is that most of these patients will go on to resolve their calcifying tendinitis, no matter what treatment is performed.

Surgical Technique

Open Approach

Traditionally, an open surgical technique through a split in the deltoid muscle has been demonstrated to be effective in visualizing and removing the calcific deposit. Codman recommended a local anesthetic, exposure through a split in the deltoid muscle, and removal of the calcific deposit.[21]

McLaughlin felt that local anesthetic and treatment in the office was an "invitation to catastrophe." Others have suggested a general anesthetic, with the patient in a sitting position and support for the head.[60] The incision begins over the margin of the acromion and extends downward for approximately 4 cm. The deltoid fibers are split and the calcium deposit is readily apparent if it is in the supraspinatus, the most common location (Fig. 12). The site of the deltoid split may need to be modified, depending on the exact location of the deposit. The deposit is incised in line with the fibers of the rotator cuff tendon, and the contents are allowed to escape or are removed with a curette. Postoperative immobilization is unnecessary.

Howorth reported on the surgical treatment of 23 shoulders and 22 patients over a 6-year period.[49] Relief of pain and improved motion was noted in all cases. Eighteen patients were reevaluated at an average of 19 months after their surgery. Only 5 of 18 patients demonstrated excellent results, with no pain, weakness, disability, or limitation of motion; 10 patients demonstrated good results, and 3 patients demonstrated fair results. Analysis of his study group suggests that 4 out of the 5 patients with excellent results were in the resorptive phase, whereas the 10 patients with good results were in the formative phase. Two of the 3 patients with fair results were also in the formative stage. The other patient had been initially treated for severe shoulder stiffness. Howorth concluded that operative removal of the calcific deposit was the surest and most rapid method of relief.

Friedman treated 20 shoulders in 15 patients with surgical removal.[31] Most of his patients had acute pain a few days to 2 weeks before the surgery. Twelve of the shoulders had deposits measuring over 2 cm, with 5 of the shoulders having deposits measuring more than 3 cm. Eleven of the 20 shoulders had been treated initially with infiltration and needling that had failed to relieve the acute symptoms. A deltoid split was used to approach the deposit. The deposit was either decompressed by incising the center and allowing the material to escape under pressure, or curetted if the deposit was dry and gritty. In most patients, acute pain was relieved within 1 or 2 days after surgery. Friedman noted that there is a select group of patients who seem to take an extended period of time to recover from a limited surgical approach. In 1 patient, severe stiffness developed, with range of motion returning after 4 months.

Harmon performed a direct surgical excision of the calcific deposit in 104 shoulders, which represented 17% of his patient population with calcifying tendinitis.[46] His indications for surgery included two different classes of patients: (a) Those who had failed repeated needlings and injections, and (b) those with fulminating hyperacute symptoms. He considered the latter group a surgical emergency and, after surgical decompression, relief was instantaneous. He recommended nonsurgical treatment in any case of calcific deposits in the subscapularis tendon, for none of his patients presented with acute symptoms, and all were recovering following a simple needling procedure. The outpatient procedure was performed using a local anesthetic and a split through the upper deltoid. Full active motion was attained in 80% of his patients within 3 to 5 days. It was unclear how many patients represented the second class or those with "fulminating hyperacute symptoms." Because these patients are in the resorptive phase of the calcifying tendinitis, it is likely that nonsurgical treatment would also have demonstrated good results.

Moseley recommended operative treatment for patients with mechanical symptoms in addition to pain, or when conservative treatment fails and the patient continues to demonstrated a "stiff and painful" shoulder.[87] He reported 304 cases treated with an open operative approach and direct exploration and removal of the deposit. In his opinion, the "few

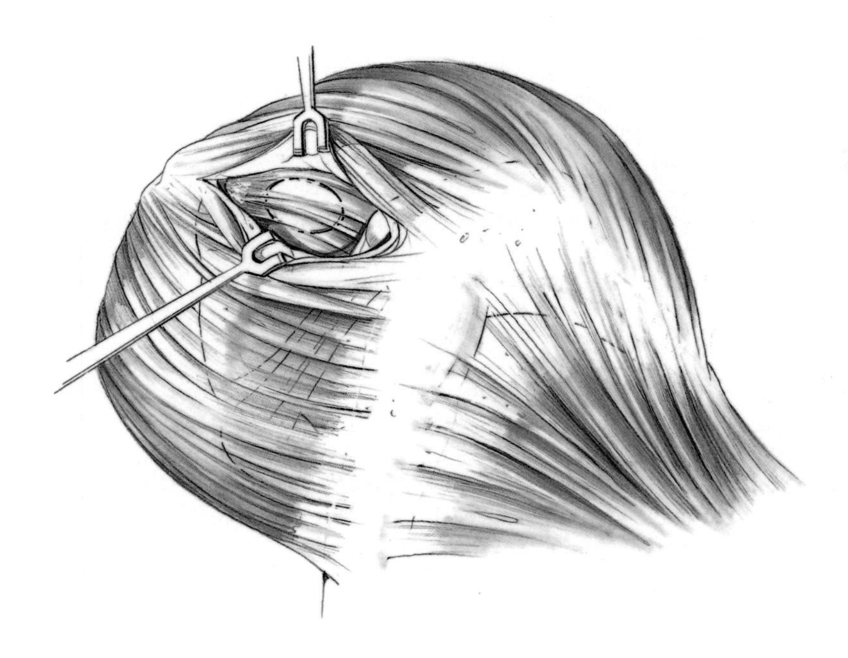

FIG. 12. The approach to the calcific deposit is dependent on its location. For deposits in the supraspinatus tendon, the most common location, a small skin incision in Langer's lines is followed by a split of the deltoid at the anterolateral deltoid raphe. After incising the underlying bursa, the deposit is seen within the substance of the tendon. Incision of the tendon is performed in line with the fibers of the tendon, then the calcific material is completely removed. At the completion of the procedure, all layers are closed "side-to-side" permitting an accelerated rehabilitation program.

recurrences" are due to remaining calcific deposit after the procedure. Ghormley also stated that it was essential that all of the calcified material be removed and the tendon be left intact. He reported three case reports, all with successful results.[36]

Litchman et al. analyzed 100 consecutive cases of calcific tendinitis treated with an open surgical approach over a 10-year period.[65] They stated that these 100 cases represented less that 1% of the patients seen for calcifying tendinitis, which suggests that 1,000 patients a year presented to their practice with evidence of calcifying tendinitis. The patients were divided into four clinical categories: acute (12%), acute–recurrent (13%), chronic (45%), and chronic with acute exacerbation (30%). These authors concluded that the patients presenting with chronic or chronic with acute exacerbation symptoms benefitted the most from the surgical approach. The surgical procedure is performed under a general anesthesia with the arm draped free for rotation during the procedure. The deltoid muscle is split and the deposit identified. Serial vertical incisions in the rotator cuff tendon may be necessary to identify the deposit in chronic cases. The calcareous material is removed and an elliptical portion of the tendon is excised, followed by curettage. The tendon defect is then closed with an absorbable suture. In the review of the 100 cases, patients generally regained normal function of the shoulder. The duration of convalescence following the surgery to full recovery was directly related to the degree of chronic disability before the surgery. The average patient returned to full activities after 4 weeks, but in patients who demonstrated severe restrictions of glenohumeral motion, the time to full recovery was "often doubled or tripled."

Vebostad reported on the surgical treatment of 43 shoulders with calcifying tendinitis treated over a 13-year period.[136] He divided the groups into three different types of operations: group A was simple excision of the calcific deposit; group B was excision of the deposit combined with partial resection of the acromion; and group C was a partial resection of the acromion alone. There were no specific indications for deciding whether the partial acromion resection should be performed when an identifiable calcific deposit was present; when the deposit could not be easily identified, patients were treated with a partial resection of the acromion alone (group C). Of 43 operations, 34 were considered to be "successful." On average, at 2.4 months following the surgery the pain had been relieved. Patients in the group that had undergone resection of the calcium alone had a much shorter period of recovery. There was no difference in the final results in all three groups. Vebostad recommended a simple removal of the deposit as the preferred procedure. However, in patients who have substantial increase in pain in the middle range of abduction or when the deposit could not be localized, an acromioplasty was beneficial.

Uhthoff should be credited with much of our current understanding of the cell-mediated, nondegenerative characteristics of calcifying tendinitis.[128,131] Armed with an understanding of the basic pathophysiology underlying this disorder, he sought a better understanding of the surgical indications and pathologic findings for this disorder. In a report authored by McKendry et al., 57 patients with calcifying tendinitis were treated with an open procedure by 11 different orthopedic surgeons.[75] All patients were treated with a simple curettage of the calcified material, with removal of a small segment of the adjacent tendon. Surgery was performed an average of 2.8 years after the onset of symptoms. By 6 weeks, 61% of patients were pain-free, but 30% continued to have pain beyond 12 weeks. They concluded that patients with a radiographic fluffy appearance of the deposit associated with acute pain were in a self-healing stage of the disease, and nonoperative treatment is recommended. Patients with long-standing symptoms unresponsive to conservative measures with a radiographic homogeneous appearance of the deposit are appropriately treated with curettage of the calcified material.[134]

Despite the relative success of open decompression of the calcific deposit, some patients failed surgical treatment, with continued symptoms of pain and stiffness. Clinical findings suggested pathology localized to the relation between the affected tendon and the coracoacromial arch; therefore, some authors have investigated the efficacy of an open anterior acromioplasty in the treatment of calcifying tendinitis. Postel reviewed a group of 31 shoulders, with the diagnosis of calcifying tendinitis, that were treated by an acromioplasty alone, without excision of the calcification.[104] The mean duration of symptoms before the operation was 4.6 years. In 14 cases, lavage and needling was attempted, followed by an injection of cortisone, but relief of pain was incomplete. Normal mobility was noted in 15 patients, but the remainder of the patients had significant limitations in arm elevation. Preoperatively, the calcification in 13 cases was heterogeneous, corresponding to the resorptive phase. Eight cases demonstrated a dense homogeneous calcification, and 6 cases had multiple, small, and dense calcifications. Four cases had a history of calcifying tendinitis, but the calcification had resorbed despite their persistent symptoms. Sixteen cases demonstrated a type II acromion.[12] Acromioplasty was performed using an open technique in 24 cases, with an arthroscopic technique used in 7 cases. Adding to the complexity of the evaluation, the acromioclavicular joint was also resected in 13 cases. The results were better in the group for whom the acromioclavicular joint was resected, with no failures and 70% excellent and very good results. Only 40% excellent and good results were achieved in the group with a simple acromioplasty. Improvements in range of motion and decrease in pain were noted in most patients. The authors proposed that when a superficial homogeneous deposit is noted, incision and curettage is effective. However, when there is intratendinous heterogeneous calcification, an acromioplasty should be strongly considered. The authors suggested that the acromioplasty permits reduction in the inflammation of the rotator cuff tendon. It is possible that there are other effects from the acromioplasty in addition to alleviating the mechanical aspects, such as decreasing the pressure within the tendon, thereby facilitating the resorptive process, and the natural cycle of calcifying tendinitis by improving blood flow to the rotator cuff tendon.

Gazielly et al. evaluated the results of open acromioplasty combined with excision of the calcium deposit in 39 patients who had at least a 1-year history of shoulder calcification.[34] All patients underwent an anterior acromioplasty, as well as an excision of the calcification and suturing of the curetted tendon. Follow-up averaged over 2 years. Seventy-four percent of the patients had calcification in the supraspinatus, 20% in the infraspinatus, and 6% in the subscapularis. Intraoperative findings of the calcification demonstrated 74% of patients with a solid or chalklike consistency, 18% with a fluid consistency, and the remaining 8% with mixed consistency. The functional rating for the operative shoulder corresponded to 98% of the contralateral shoulder function compared with 63% preoperatively. Radiographic follow-up demonstrated that the main calcium deposit had been fully eliminated in 98% of the shoulders. Eighty-two percent of patients felt that they had recovered from their condition, whereas the remaining 18% judged that their condition was much improved or improved. It was the opinion of the authors that the clinical results were dependent on the total excision of the calcification, as well as the suturing of the edges of the tendon, which could only be done through an open approach. The authors then went on to look at their own personal series of having treated more than 100 calcifications by arthroscopic surgery over a 6-year period. From a comparison of their personal series, it was their opinion that arthroscopic excision is difficult, the learning curve for the surgical skills is steep, and the postoperative morbidity from an open procedure is not significantly different from the arthroscopic technique.

Arthroscopic Approach

Arthroscopic treatment of calcifying tendinitis has several potential advantages. The deltoid split to approach the calcific deposit can now be performed through a small arthroscopic portal. Furthermore, as some authors have suggested, an acromioplasty can also be performed arthroscopically, minimizing the iatrogenic risk of deltoid detachment following open acromioplasty. Ark et al. reported on the results of the arthroscopic treatment of chronic calcific tendinitis in 23 patients at an average of 26 months after the procedure.[4] Indications for surgery were persistent shoulder pain, in the presence of calcific tendinitis despite at least 1 year of conservative treatment. Conservative treatment included physical therapy (8 patients), nonsteroidal antiinflammatory medications (16 patients), and steroid injections (14 patients). All patients continued to have pain at night. The calcium deposit was localized to the supraspinatus tendon in 20 patients, the infraspinatus tendon in 2 patients, and the subscapularis in 1 patient. Nineteen patients demonstrated a dense calcific deposit consistent with formative phase, whereas 4 patients demonstrated a fluffy deposit. The arthroscopic procedure was performed in the beach chair or the sitting position. The authors noted that hypertrophic bursitis was often noted on arthroscopic examination of the subacromial space, and a partial bursectomy was necessary. Other authors have demonstrated that the bursal reaction is primarily a localized reaction to the specific area of pathology.[52] Ark reported the release of the coracoacromial ligament in 9 of their patients for hypertrophy or localized inflammation. In 3 patients that demonstrated a prominence to the anterior acromion, an arthroscopic acromioplasty was also performed. A needle was used to identify and, if possible, release the calcific deposit (Fig. 13). Needling was followed by a small longitudinal incision within the cuff in line with its fibers (Fig. 14). If necessary, up to three incisions were made to completely expose the deposit. Finally, a small curette was used to further liberate the calcific deposit (Fig. 15). Any contents from the deposit and "inflamed tissue" were debrided. Bupivacaine without cortisone, was injected at the completion of the procedure.

At follow-up at an average of 26 months after the procedure, 11 patients (50%) had full relief of pain, and an additional 9 patients (41%) were satisfied with the results, although they had occasional episodes of discomfort. Two patients had persistent pain and after a second arthroscopic procedure were relieved following 5 months of recuperation. The authors felt that these patients had undergone an inadequate removal of the calcium deposit during the primary procedure.[4]

Follow-up radiographic studies performed in this patient group demonstrated 1 patient with an intact large calcium deposit, 12 patients with partial removal of the deposit, and

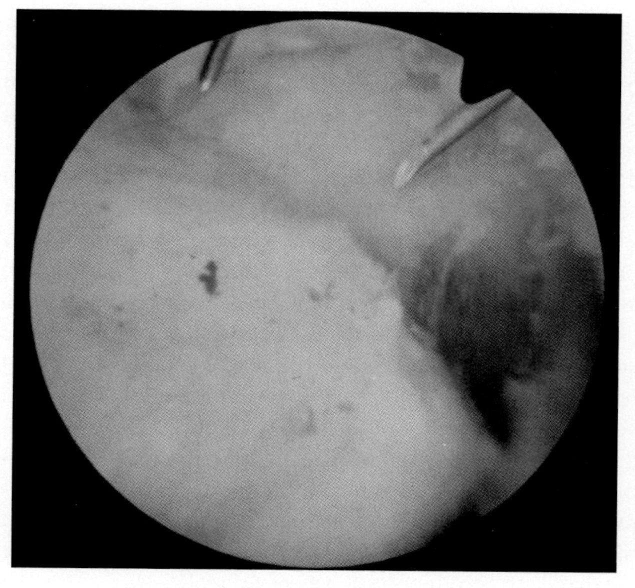

FIG. 13. Arthroscopic treatment of calcifying tendinitis offers the ability to localize and decompress the deposit with minimal injury to the surrounding healthy tissues. Once the deposit is localized, puncturing the deposit will release the calcific contents. (Courtesy of Docteur Gilles Walch.)

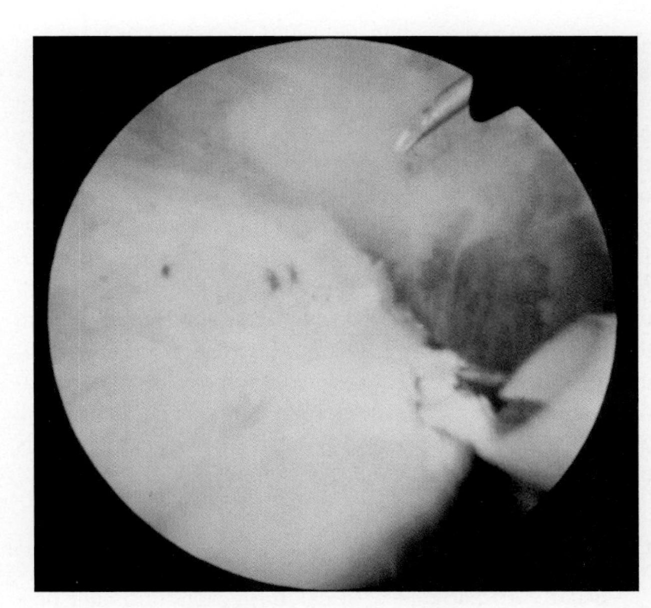

FIG. 14. A small longitudinal incision in line with the fibers of the tendon can be performed with an 18-gauge needle or a knife. The release of the calcific material is dramatic when the contents are under pressure. (Courtesy of Docteur Gilles Walch.)

9 patients with complete removal of the calcium. Twelve of 14 patients in whom there was persistent calcium still had significant relief of their pain. The authors, therefore, concluded that complete excision of the calcific deposit during the arthroscopic procedure was not essential for a good outcome.

In fact, a report by Barchilon and Gazielly specifically looked at the amount of calcium deposit removed at the time of shoulder arthroscopy and its relation to overall results.[7] Over a 4-year period, 78 patients with chronic calcifying tendinitis were treated with arthroscopic evaluation and removal of the calcific deposit. From preoperative plain radiographs, the average area of the deposit was 2.1 cm^2. Overall, an average of 74% of the calcific deposit was removed. Removal of deposits from the infraspinatus was less effective than removing deposits from the more common location in the supraspinatus (86%). They also found no correlation between the amount of calcium remaining after surgery and the final result. Kempf et al. also favored isolated excision of the calcific deposit, emphasizing that calcifying tendinitis occurs in an otherwise globally healthy tendon.[57]

However, as noted before, not all patients respond to decompression of the deposit alone, whether it is performed with needling, an open procedure, or an arthroscopic procedure. The poor results have led some surgeons to consider the role of an acromioplasty in the treatment of calcific tendinitis. Ellman and Kay reported satisfactory results in 15 of 16 patients who were treated with a debridement or removal of the calcific deposit followed by an arthroscopic subacromial decompression.[28]

Synder and Eppley also described satisfactory results using arthroscopic techniques for decompression of the deposit in 13 of 13 patients, but also suggest that arthroscopic evidence of impingement or hypertrophy of the coracoacromial ligament indicates the need to include an arthroscopic acromioplasty.[125] Re and Karzel support this recommendation, suggesting that arthroscopic treatment includes decompression of the deposit, with an arthroscopic acromioplasty indicated only in those patients with clinical or arthroscopic evidence of impingement.[107]

Molé et al., in the French Society of Arthroscopy, organized a multicenter study to evaluate the results of arthroscopic treatment of chronic calcifying tendinitis.[83] This retrospective review did not randomize patient treatment, but instead looked at the results of treatment by the individual members of the society. One hundred twelve patients were included in the analysis. The surgeons used a variety of treatment options, including excision of the calcific deposit, excision of the deposit with acromioplasty, and acromioplasty without treatment of the calcific deposit. There was no statistically significant difference in the final results using these different treatments. Functional results were evaluated using the constant score.[35] Excellent results were achieved in 61% of patients, very good results in 24%, good results in 7%, and fair results in 5%. Eight patients had poor results. Acromioplasty did not provide any additional improvement in the final results. However, the authors recommended that an acromioplasty be performed when the calcification could not be found, which occurred in 12% of their patients. The most important factor for a successful result appeared to be the ability to remove the deposit. Poor prognostic factors included the preoperative limitation of passive mobility, the

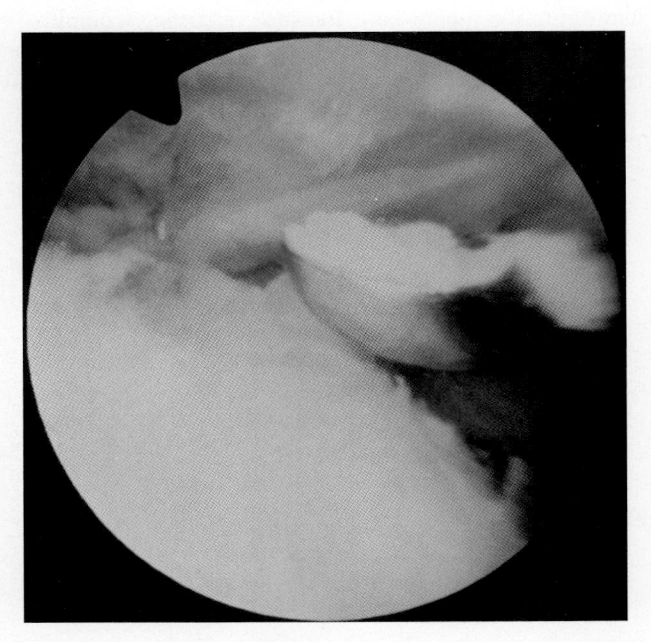

FIG. 15. A currette can be used to remove any remaining calcific material from the deposit site. (Courtesy of Docteur Gilles Walch.)

existence of calcific deposits of the lesser tuberosity, and the existence of a rare complete or significant intertendinous tear of the rotator cuff tendon that was found in 4% of the cases.

Gleyze and colleagues also concluded that isolated excision of the calcification is the appropriate treatment, with little evidence for the routine performance of an acromioplasty.[37] However, using the French Society of Arthroscopy classification of radiographic findings in calcifying tendinitis, an acromioplasty is recommended with or without excision of the remaining calcific deposit in patients with type C calcification (heterogeneous) and a lack of clinical evidence of acute pain. This is true for supraspinatus calcific deposits alone. This pattern, radiographically, may be part of the resorptive process; however, the lack of hyperalgesic pain and the presence of chronic symptoms suggest the resorptive process has paused or has failed. In this study, symptoms were present for more than 1 year. It is suggested by Kempf that these tendons have been unable to complete the typical calcifying tendinitis cycle and, therefore, the patient is left with a pathologic supraspinatus tendon.[57] Consequently, an acromioplasty may remove the mechanical irritation from the overlying acromion, or decrease the intratendinous pressure, allowing increased blood flow and possibly stimulating the completion of the resorption cycle with improved tendon healing. The physiologic effects of an acromioplasty for chronic calcifying tendinitis are unknown.

AUTHORS' RECOMMENDED TREATMENT

The treatment of calcifying tendinitis is based on a thorough understanding of its cycle, the clinical presentation, and the radiographic findings. All three aspects are crucial to avoid treatment that is not only less successful but possibly harmful to the rotator cuff. Because calcifying tendinitis is generally a transient phenomenon, any treatment that is potentially harmful or may disrupt normal tissues around the shoulder must be clearly indicated before it can be recommended.

With these principles in mind, patients presenting with acute pain representing the resorptive phase of calcifying tendinitis are most appropriately treated with nonsurgical measures. Patients with calcifying tendinitis in the formative phase are best treated initially with nonoperative measures. If the condition fails to resolve, surgical treatment is effective in alleviating the patient's symptoms and allowing a return of shoulder function. The most difficult decision is with those patients for whom there appears to have been the initiation of the resorptive process, and yet, symptoms and radiographic findings persist. Despite the same epidemiologic attributes, the various manifestations of calcifying tendinitis must be managed with unique strategies (Fig. 16).

Conservative Treatment

Virtually all patients with calcifying tendinitis are best treated nonoperatively. When patients present with the acute symptoms of the resorptive phase of this disorder, intervention is dictated by the patient's severity of symptoms. In this phase, patients often present with severe pain and an inability to move their shoulder. Palpation may lead to tears. Many patients are desperate for relief from the pain that interferes with every aspect of their life, including sleep. Explaining to the patient the transient nature of their severe pain is not reassuring at this time. Although nonsteroidal antiinflammatory medications and even narcotics are helpful, their benefit is minimal, and usually it does not allow patients to sleep comfortably. Physical therapy and gentle motion exercises are likely to aggravate the symptoms; therefore they are not initially indicated.

The primary goal of treatment is pain relief, and the most effective method to accomplish this task is needling of the deposit. The deposit is carefully evaluated using plain radio-

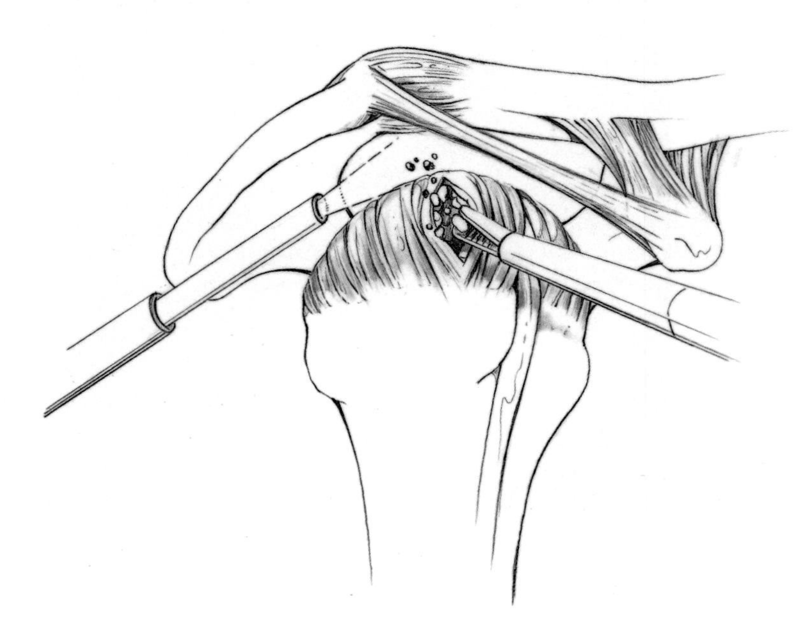

FIG. 16. Arthroscopic approach to a calcific deposit within the tendon of the supraspinatus. The arthrosope is in the posterior portal, with the working instruments in the lateral portal. An anterior portal is created for outflow. A basket forceps or small curette placed in the lateral portal can be used to remove the calcific material.

graphy. Bilobular or multilobular involvement should be noted. The anteroposterior views of the shoulder, including rotation views, will allow the deposit to be localized. Fortunately, most deposits are in the supraspinatus, which is easily approached without concern for injuring neurovascular structures. Deposits in the infraspinatus will often demonstrate an area of localized soft-tissue prominence and tenderness on the lateral side of the shoulder. With the arm at the patient's side, lesions in the supraspinatus are referenced from the anterolateral corner of the acromion, which is usually in close proximity to the deposit. Furthermore, palpation of the bicipital groove provides an additional reference point on physical examination. Palpation directly over the deposit is accompanied by a severe worsening of the pain. If necessary, the arm can be placed into a slight amount of extension to move the site of the deposit from under the acromion. Once this site is localized, then 20 to 30 mL of lidocaine is used to anesthetize the skin at a site that will allow directed needle penetration. Most commonly, this is at the anterolateral edge of the acromion. A local anesthetic is used to anesthetize the skin, then the needle is directed toward the deposit in the rotator cuff tendon. A small amount of local anesthetic is injected as the needle progresses towards the deposit, anesthetizing the entire path. Slowly progressing the tip of the needle may allow the physician to sense the resistance or roughness of the calcific material. Aspiration is attempted at this time, although this is difficult and often unsuccessful. A repeated needling or puncturing of the area containing the deposit is performed approximately five to ten times. At the completion of the procedure a corticosteroid injection accompanied with a long-acting anesthetic is placed into the subacromial space, not the tendon. The use of cortisone has not been associated with any adverse effects specific to the treatment of calcifying tendinitis. Patients are instructed to rest their shoulder for 1 to 2 days and then to gradually work on regaining their range of motion. Furthermore, they are provided with a prescription for either a nonsteroidal antiinflammatory medication or mild narcotic. Application of ice to the site of pain may also help alleviate their symptoms. Frequently, pain relief is dramatic, and the symptoms quickly dissipate. Although physical therapy may be necessary for patients who demonstrate shoulder stiffness, this is frequently not prescribed, for patients will return with close to a full range of motion and decreased pain within a few weeks, sometimes as quickly as a few days.

If the first attempt has been unsuccessful in alleviating symptoms, a second needling is performed. If a partial response was achieved, a second "blind" needling using the technique described is attempted in the office. However, if their was no response to the first needling, the second needling procedure is performed in the radiology suite with the assistance of fluoroscopy to accurately locate the deposit. Again, after anesthetizing the skin and soft tissue along the path to the deposit, the deposit is directly needled, followed by an injection of a solution of anesthetic and cortisone into the subacromial space. In our experience, this treatment plan has been successful in resolving pain rapidly with generally a full return of shoulder function. Surgical intervention has been unnecessary for the treatment of acute symptoms associated with the normal resorptive phase of calcifying tendinitis.

Treatment during the formative stage, or resting stage, is based on the duration and severity of the symptoms, as well as the examination findings. Initial conservative measures include nonsteroidal antiinflammatory medications for pain relief. There is no evidence that these medications accelerate the disappearance of the calcium or positively affect the completion of the calcifying tendinitis cycle. When pain is under control, a daily program of stretching exercises will help maintain the mobility of the shoulder. Physical modalities, such as ice or heat, may be beneficial. Other physical modalities provided under the supervision of a therapist, such as ultrasound or diathermy, may have some short-term benefit by relieving pain, but again, these have not been proved effective in the resolution of this condition. The cost of these physical modalities is substantial and, therefore, the authors cannot recommend their use until some benefit is proved other than short-term pain relief.

Corticosteroid injections are recommended if the symptoms persist despite oral medications and therapy. Corticosteroids may be used initially in those patients with an intolerance or allergy to nonsteroidal antiinflammatory medications. There is no evidence that a corticosteroid injection will facilitate the resolution of the calcifying tendinitis cycle. Uhthoff has recommended against their routine use owing to the theoretical concern that the effect of corticosteroids may actually interrupt or delay the resorptive phase.[134] However, this concern has not been validated in a well-controlled study, and we have noted marked improvement in symptoms with one or two injections in those patients who have had symptomatic calcifying tendinitis for less than 6 months.

"Blind" needling of the calcific deposit during the formative stage is not recommended. These dense homogeneous deposits do not permit an easy release of the calcific material. Dual needling and lavage may be beneficial. To be successful, this technique requires fluoroscopic isolation and may also involve a regional or general anesthetic agent to relax the patient, permit the dual needling of the calcific deposit, followed by lavage. The goal of needling and lavage should be removal of as much of the deposit as possible. Following the procedure, a brief period of rest is recommended, along with nonsteroidal antiinflammatory medications or a mild narcotic for pain relief. Physical therapy is directed toward reestablishing normal shoulder motion, then progressing to recovery of shoulder function. Patients should be forewarned that even successful recovery from this procedure is extended, often lasting 3 to 6 months.

Patients who have had chronic symptoms for more than 6 months with radiographic evidence of calcifying tendinitis meet the appropriate criteria for surgical intervention. Imaging of the rotator cuff tendon is also recommended if surgical intervention is contemplated. Although we have rarely seen evidence of true tendonopathy, such as a significant partial-thickness or full-thickness tearing of the rotator cuff, others have reported an incidence of approximately 4% in this patient population.[83] Furthermore, two studies from the same institution in Taiwan suggest a significantly higher incidence of rotator cuff tearing in older patients and in patients with Asian heritage presenting with long-standing calcifying tendinitis in the formative phase.[50,53] Knowledge of a significant tendonopathy will enable better preoperative planning for the patient and the surgeon.

We prefer an arthroscopic approach to the surgical treatment of calcifying tendinitis. Arthroscopy permits localization of the deposit, removal of the contents of the deposit, while minimizing injury to the unaffected tissues. In our opinion, an acromioplasty is rarely necessary. However, an acromioplasty may be indicated when significant clinical or arthroscopic findings of impingement are present. Furthermore, an acromioplasty appears to be beneficial when the calcific deposit can not be localized owing to a poorly circumscribed lesion, usually seen as a type C calcification pattern on preoperative radiographs. Although arthroscopic techniques are preferred, open procedures performed through a split in the deltoid tendon without detaching the anterior acromion attachment of the deltoid origin, are equally effective for localization of the deposit and removal of the contents. Both surgical procedures are performed on an outpatient basis, and patients are started on an early range of motion program. Postoperative corticosteroid injections have not been indicated.

Open Surgical Technique

Exposure of the involved rotator cuff tendon depends on its location. Most rotator cuff calcifications will be within the substance of the supraspinatus tendon. This tendon is readily approachable through a split in the deltoid muscle centered at the anterolateral edge of the acromion. Regional anesthesia, general anesthesia, or a combination of the two techniques can be used for the surgical procedure. A long-acting local anesthetic is injected at the surgical site. The use of local anesthesia alone has been described, but is not recommended. An incision is made in Langer's lines from the lateral corner of the acromion towards the coracoid process. The deltoid raphe is identified perpendicular to this skin incision. Dissection is carried through the anterolateral deltoid raphe, beginning at the acromion and progressing inferiorly. The fibers are split and separated by self-retaining retractors. Three centimeters of exposure provides a generous approach to the supraspinatus tendon without risk of injuring the innervation of the anterior deltoid. The patient is positioned in the beach chair position for the surgical procedure.

Once the split in the deltoid tendon is made, the overlying bursa is incised to expose the rotator cuff tendon. A partial bursectomy is performed to have adequate visualization of the rotator cuff tendon. When locating the deposit, the most significant intraoperative landmark is the biceps tendon. In general, a supraspinatus calcific deposit will be approximately 1 cm posterior to the biceps tendon and approximately 1.5 cm from the attachment site of the supraspinatus tendon on the greater tuberosity. Once the site of the calcific deposit is identified, either by direct visualization, palpation, or estimation from the preoperative radiographs and intraarticular landmarks, an incision is made at the site of the calcific deposit in line with the fibers of the rotator cuff tendon. The calcium is exposed, irrigated, and then debrided with a curette to remove as much of the calcific deposit as possible. Although it is not necessary to completely remove all of the calcium, it does appear to be beneficial to remove as much of the contents as possible to decrease the intratendinous pressure, the thickness of the tendon, and risk for an acute inflammatory reaction to remaining calcific debris. If a significant amount of the tendon appears to be involved, side-to-side repair of the tendon edges with absorbable sutures can be performed, but the benefit is unclear. At the completion of the removal of the calcific deposit, the subacromial space is irrigated thoroughly. The deltoid is closed with a side-to-side repair using absorbable sutures. The skin is closed with a running subcuticular closure supported with small adhesive strips. Patients are allowed range of motion as tolerated. Sutures are removed within 5 to 7 days. If the patient has difficulty regaining range of motion, a supervised therapy program may be initiated. Recurrence of the calcific deposit does not occur, although some of the deposit may persist after surgery. Patients may exhibit a prolonged course of recovery taking 3 to 6 months to regain their motion, strength, and function.

Arthroscopic Technique

Preoperative assessment with radiographs including an anteroposterior view of the humerus in neutral rotation, external rotation, and internal rotation is essential to predict the site of the calcific deposit. Anesthesia can be delivered through a regional interscalene block, a general anesthetic agent, or a combination of the two. We prefer a beach chair position, but a lateral decubitus position with a gentle amount of traction on the arm is also effective. In the lateral position, the arm is placed at approximately 20 degrees of abduction with slight forward flexion. Approximately 10 lb (4.5 kg) of traction are used for smaller patients, 15 lb (6.8 kg) for larger patients. A posterior portal is established and the glenohumeral joint is evaluated. The anterior portal is established with an inside-out technique. The arthroscope is placed above the subscapularis tendon and below the biceps tendon directly against the anterior capsule of the glenohumeral joint. A Wissinger rod is then placed through the cannula for the arthroscope and bluntly directed out of the capsule through the deltoid, becoming prominent underneath the anterior skin of the shoulder. An anterior incision is then made directly over the site of the Wissinger rod prominence and the Wissinger rod is advanced out of the shoulder anteriorly. A second disposable cannula with a water dam is then slid over the top of the Wissinger rod and advanced into the shoulder joint. Once the cannula is allowed to advance within the center of the glenohumeral joint, the Wissinger rod is slowly removed to separate out the scope cannula posteriorly from the disposable cannula anteriorly. As soon as the two cannula separate, they are then pushed past one another to ensure that they stay within the glenohumeral joint. The arthroscope is then placed back into its cannula. To maximize visualization of the glenohumeral joint, the outflow is connected to the disposable cannula anteriorly.

The glenohumeral joint inspection is carried out in a systematic fashion. In general, inspection of the biceps and superior labrum begins the examination and then the arthroscope is used to visualize various points of interest, including the rotator cuff tendon at its insertion site, the biceps tendon, and the anterior ligaments. Partial-thickness and full-thickness rotator cuff tears have been seen with calcifying tendinitis and can be evaluated with standard arthroscopic techniques.

After a completion of the glenohumeral joint inspection, which takes no longer than 5 min, the calcific deposit is marked with a suture. Marking the deposit is possible if the area of involvement can be identified from the glenohumeral joint. An 18-gauge spinal needle is passed through the skin, into the area of the deposit, then into the glenohumeral joint while the arthroscope is maintained in the glenohumeral joint. A stiff synthetic suture is then passed through the needle into the glenohumeral joint. A grasper is used to put the suture out the anterior portal. After marking the location of the deposit, the arthroscopic equipment is then advanced into the subacromial space. Marking the deposit is particularly helpful when the lesion involves the subscapularis or infraspinatus, as these areas are more difficult to visualize in the subacromial space. This technique is also used to mark partial- or small full-thickness rotator cuff tears for later inspection from the subacromial space.

Once the subacromial space has been established and is acceptable, which often includes removing some of the bursa, the examination of the subacromial space also proceeds in a systematic fashion. In addition to evaluating the coracoacromial ligament and undersurface of the acromion, careful inspection of the rotator cuff tendon is necessary. Once the site of the calcific deposit is located, it is generally necessary to establish a third lateral portal for a direct approach to the calcific deposit. This portal is 2 cm below the lateral edge of the acromion at the anterior one-third of the acromion when the lesion is located in the supraspinatus. An 18-gauge needle can be advanced through the skin and deltoid to ensure that a direct approach to the calcific deposit is possible. The lateral portal becomes the working portal for incision and removal of the calcific deposit. A second disposable cannula is beneficial to help maintain the pressure within the subacromial space and minimize the amount of trauma to the deltoid with the exchange of instruments. Once the calcific deposit has been clearly visualized, a no. 11 blade on a long-handled knife, an arthroscopic blade, or an 18-gauge needle can be advanced through the lateral portal. The supraspinatus tendon is incised in line with its fibers to expose the calcific material. Visualization is maintained using an arthroscopic pump. Once the calcific deposit has been incised and some of the material removed, a curette can be advanced through the lateral portal to debride the remaining contents of the deposit (Fig. 17). An arthroscopic power shaver is not recommended because inadvertent removal of some of the normal tendon is likely. A hooded shaver may be beneficial without risking injury to the remaining intact tendon. The shoulder should be irrigated thoroughly and exchange of fluid should be rapid to maximize removal of the calcific material. The skin is closed with an interrupted suture closure of the portals. Patients are allowed range of motion as tolerated. Sutures are removed within 5 to 7 days. If the patient has difficulty regaining range of motion, a supervised therapy program may be initiated. Recurrence of the calcific deposit does not occur, although some of the deposit may persist after surgery. Despite the minimally invasive arthroscopic technique, a prolonged course of recovery that takes 3 to 6 months to regain motion, strength, and function is not uncommon, similar to the results of an open surgical procedure.

If the calcific deposit is indistinct or can not be localized, an arthroscopic acromioplasty is advised. The benefit of the acromioplasty appears to be related to the decompression or widening of the subacromial space, decreasing the mechanical irritation of the rotator cuff tendon. There may also be underlying physiologic changes, such as decreased tendon pressure and improved blood flow, that may allow tendon healing or simply the resolution of pain. The need for an acromioplasty may be predicted from the preoperative radiographs. An inhomogeneous, poorly circumscribed lesion associated with chronic symptoms suggests a stop in the normal cycle of calcifying tendinitis. The calcific material is within the tendon fibers, but not readily accessible; therefore, it cannot be directly addressed with surgical removal. In our opinion, a well-performed arthroscopic acromioplasty in this setting has distinct clinical advantages over a traditional open acromioplasty.

SUMMARY

The key to successful treatment of calcifying tendinitis is a complete understanding of the pathophysiology of this disease. Calcifying tendinitis tends to follow a characteristic disease cycle in most patients. The cycle includes the formation of the calcific deposit, the resorption of the deposit, then tendon restoration. Some patients demonstrate findings that suggest an aborted cycle, with chronic symptoms and radiographic evidence of persistent calcific material or incomplete resorption. However, clinical characteristics and cadaveric studies suggest that resorption of the deposit always occurs, even though the resorption may occur over many years.

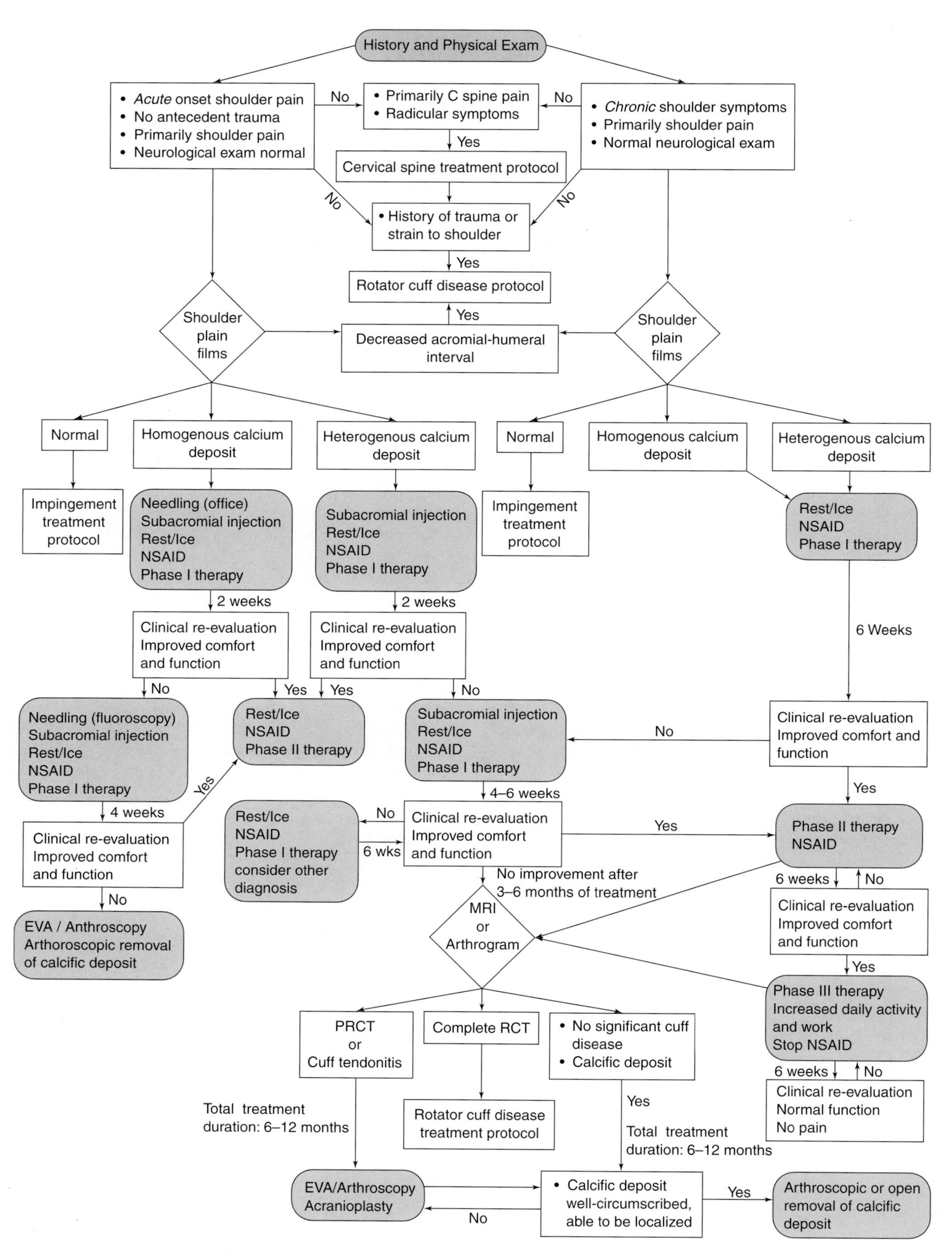

FIG. 17. Algorithm for evaluation and treatment of calcifying tendinitis.

Calcifying tendinitis is a condition of unknown etiology, although it is understood that the calcium deposition is a cell-mediated process that occurs in nondegenerative rotator cuff tendons. The epidemiology of this disease is the same despite various physiologic, clinical, and radiographic stages. Understanding the pathology, then combining this understanding with the presenting clinical and radiographic features enables one to formulate successful treatment strategies.

Treatment options are numerous, but the most successful strategies have included decompression of the calcific deposit. During the acute hyperalgesic stage, consistent with the resorptive phase, pain relief is the primary goal. This can be rapidly accomplished by needling the calcific deposit without interrupting the natural resolution of the resorptive phase. Chronic symptoms are more difficult to treat, and they may require direct surgical intervention. The primary goal of surgery is the decompression and removal of the calcific material without causing undo harm to tissues not involved in the disease process. Arthroscopic decompression and removal of the deposit offers an accurate and effective approach for this condition. When symptoms persist despite the absence of a homogeneous, well-circumscribed lesion, an acromioplasty is beneficial in the treatment of the persistent tendonopathy, although the postoperative recovery is longer than expected. In the future, a better understanding of the etiology and the cellular signals that trigger the resorptive process may permit better medical management of this condition.

REFERENCES

1. Anderson HC. Calcific diseases. *Arch Pathol Lab Med* 1983;107: 341–348.
2. Andresen J, Nielsen HE. Juxta-articular erosions and calcifications in patients with chronic renal failure. *Acta Radiol Diagn (Stockh)* 1981; 22:709–713.
3. Archer RS, Bayley JI, Archer CW, Ali SY. Cell and matrix changes associated with pathological calcification of the human rotator cuff tendons. *J Anat* 1993;182(pt 1):1–11.
4. Ark JW, Flock TJ, Flatow EL, Bigliani LU. Arthroscopic treatment of calcific tendinitis of the shoulder. *Arthroscopy* 1992;8:183–188.
5. Baer WS. The operative treatment of subdeltoid bursitis. *Johns Hopkins Hosp Bull* 1907;18:282–284.
6. Baird LW. Roentgen irradiation of calcareous deposits about the shoulder. *Radiology* 1941;37:316–324.
7. Barchilon V, Gazielly DF. Radiographic study of the amount of calcium deposit removed by shoulder arthroscopy. In: Gazielly DF, Gleyze P, Thomas T, eds. *The cuff.* Elsevier, Paris 1994 1997: 176–180,
8. Bateman JE. *The shoulder and neck.* Philadelphia: WB Saunders, 1978.
9. Berg EE, Cuillo JV. Heterotopic ossification after acromioplasty and distal clavicle resection. *J Shoulder Elbow Surg* 1995;4:188–194.
10. Bergemann D, Steida A. Uber die mit kalkablagerungen einhergehende entzundung der schulterschleimbeutel. *Munch Med Wochenschr* 1908;52:2699–2702.
11. Berger LS, Ziter FM Jr. Calcifications with enlarged subdeltoid bursae in rheumatoid arthritis. *Br J Radiol* 1972;45:530–531.
12. Bigliani LU, Morrison DS, April EW. The morphology of the acromion and its relationship to rotator cuff tears. *Orthop Trans* 1986; 10:228.
13. Booth RE Jr, Marvel JP Jr. Differential diagnosis of shoulder pain. *Orthop Clin North Am* 1975;6:353–379.
14. Bosworth BM. Calcium deposits in the shoulder and subacromial bursitis: a survey of 12,122 shoulders. *JAMA* 1941;116:2477–2482.
15. Bosworth BM. Examination of the shoulder for calcium deposits. *J Bone Joint Surg* 1941;23:567–577.
16. Bradley M, Bhamra MS, Robson MJ. Ultrasound guided aspiration of symptomatic supraspinatus calcific deposits. *Br J Radiol* 1995;68: 716–719.
17. Brewer BJ. Aging of the rotator cuff. *Am J Sports Med* 1979;7: 102–110.
18. Brickner WM. Shoulder disability: stiff and painful shoulder. *Am J Surg* 1912;26:196–204.
19. Carnett JB. The calcareous deposits of so-called calcifying subacromial bursitis. *Surg Gynecol Obstet* 1925;41:404–421.
20. Clement BL. Shoulder bursitis with calcification. *Am J Orthop* 1966; 8:160–161.
21. Codman EA. Rupture tendon of the supraspinatus tendon and other lesions in or about the subacromial bursa. In: *The shoulder.* Boston: Thomas Todd 1984:178–215.
22. Crass, JR. Current concepts in the radiographic evaluation of the rotator cuff. *CRC Crit Rev Diagn Imaging* 1988;28:23–73.
23. Dahmen GP, Meiss L, Nam V, Cruodis B. Extracorparale, stossweilentherapie in knochennaher. Weisheibereich an der schulner. *Extra Orthop* 1992;15:25–17.
24. DePalma AF, Kruper JS. Long-term study of shoulder joints afflicted with and treated for calcific tendinitis. *Clin Orthop* 1961;20:61–72.
25. DeSeze S, Welfling J. Tendinites calcifiantes. *Rhematologie* 1970;2: 5–14.
26. Dieppe P. Crystal deposition disease and the soft tissues. *Clin Rheum Dis* 1979;5:807–822.
27. Duplay S. De la periarthrite scapulohumerale et des raideurs de l epaule qui en sont la consequence. *Arch Gen Med* 1872;513:542.
28. Ellman HK. Arthroscopic treatment of calcific tendinitis. *Orthop Trans* 1989;13:240.
29. Farin PU, Jaroma H, Soimakallio S. Rotator cuff calcifications: treatment with US-guided technique. *Radiology* 1995;195:841–843.
30. Faure G, Daculsi G. Calcified tendinitis: a review. *Ann Rheum Dis* 1983;42(suppl):49–53.
31. Friedman MS. Calcified tendinitis of the shoulder. *Ann J Surg* 1957; 94:56–61.
32. Gartner J, Heyer. [Calcific tendinitis of the shoulder. A review]. *Orthopade* 1995;24:284–302 [in German].
33. Gartner J, Simons B. Analysis of calcific deposits in calcifying tendinitis. *Clin Orthop* 1990;254:111–120.
34. Gazielly DF, Bruyere G, Gleyze P, Thomas T. Open acromioplasty with excision of calcium deposits and tendon suture. In: Gazielly DF, Gleyze P, Thomas T, eds. *The cuff.* Elsevier, Paris 1997:172–175.
35. Gerber C. Integrated scoring systems for the functional assessment of the shoulder. *The shoulder: a balance of mobility and stability.* Rosemont: American Academy of Orthopaedic Surgeons, 1992:545–559
36. Ghormley JW. Calcareous tendinitis. *Surg Clin North Am* 1961;4: 1721–1728.
37. Gleyze P, Montes P, Thomas T, Gazielly DF. Compared results of the different treatments in calcifying tendinitis of the rotator cuff. A multicenter study of 149 shoulders. In: Gazielly DF, Gleyze P, Thomas T, eds. *The cuff.* Elsevier, Paris 1997:181–184.
38. Goldman AB. Calcific tendinitis of the long head of the biceps brachii distal to the glenohumeral joint: plain film radiographic findings. *AJR Am J Roentgenol* 1989;153:1011–1016.
39. Goodman CR. Ultrasonic therapy for chronic acromioclavicular separation with calcific deposits. *N Y State J Med* 1972;72:2884–2886.
40. Goutallier D, DuParc F. Surgical treatment of calcifying tendinitis by decompression without removal of a deposit—a four year follow-up. The Rotator Cuff of the Shoulder. An International Symposium. Ottawa, Canada, May 20–22, 1993.
41. Gravanis MB, Gaffney EF. Idiopathic calcifying tenosynovitis. Histopathologic features and possible pathogenesis. *Am J Surg Pathol* 1983;7:357–361.
42. Griffin EJ, Karselis TC. Physical agents for physical therapists. *Ultrasonic energy*, 2nd ed. Springfield, IL: Charles C Thomas, 1982.
43. Gschwend N, Patte D, Zippel J. Therapy of calcific tendinitis of the shoulder. *German Arch Orthop Unfallchir* 1972;73:120–135.
44. Halverson PB, McCarty DJ, Cheung HS, Ryan LM. Milwaukee shoulder syndrome. *Ann Rheum Dis* 1984;43:734–741.
45. Harbin M. Deposition of calcium salts in tendon of supraspinatus muscle. *Arch Surg* 1929;18:1491–1512.

46. Harmon HP. Methods and results in the treatment of 2,580 painful shoulders with special reference to calcific tendinitis and the frozen shoulder. *Ann J Surg* 1958;95:527–544.
47. Hartig A, Huth F. Neue aspekte zur morphologie und therapie der tendinosis calcarea der schultergelenke. *Arthroskopie* 1995;8: 117–122.
48. Herzog RJ. Magnetic resonance imaging of the shoulder. *J Bone Joint Surg [Am]* 1997;79:934–953.
49. Howorth NB. Calcification of the tendon cuff of the shoulder. *Surg Gynecol Obstet* 1945;80:337–345.
50. Hsu HC, Wu JJ, Jim YF, Chang CY, Lo WH, Yang DJ. Calcific tendinitis in rotator cuff tearing: a clinical and radiographic study. *J Shoulder Elbow Surg* 1994;3:159–164.
51. Ianotti JP, Zlatkin MB, Esterhai JL, Kressel HY, Dalinka MK, Spindler KP. Magnetic resonance imaging of the shoulder: sensitivity, specificity and predictive value. *J Bone Joint Surg [Am]* 1991;73: 17–29.
52. Ishii H, Brunet JA, Welsh RP, Uhthoff HK. Bursal reactions in rotator cuff tearing, the impingement syndrome, and calcifying tendinitis. *J Shoulder Elbow Surg* 1997;6:131–136.
53. Jim YF, Hsu HC, Chang CY, Wu JJ, Chang T. Coexistence of calcific tendinitis and rotator cuff tear: an arthrographic study. *Skeletal Radiol* 1993;22:183–185.
54. Jones GB: Calcification of the supraspinatus. *J Bone Joint Surg [Br]* 1949;31:433–435.
55. Jozsa L, Baliut BJ, Reffy A. Calcifying tendinopathy. *Arch Orthop Trauma* 1980;97:305–307.
56. Kaklamanis P, Rigas A, Giannatos J, Matsas S, Economou P. Calcification of the shoulders in diabetes mellitus [letter]. *N Engl J Med* 1975;293:1266–1267.
57. Kempf JF, Bonnomet F, Nerisson D, Gastaud F, Lacaze F, Geraud H. Arthroscopic isolated excision of the rotator cuff calcium deposits. In: Gazielly DF, Gleyze P, Thomas T, eds. *The cuff.* Elsevier, Paris 1997: 164–168
58. Kernwein GA. Roentgenographic diagnosis of shoulder dysfunction. *JAMA* 1965;194:1081–1085.
59. Kessel L, Watson M. The painful arc syndrome. *J Bone Joint Surg [Br]* 1977;59:166–172.
60. Key LA. Calcium deposits in the vicinity of the shoulder and other joints. *Ann Surg* 1949;129:737–753.
61. Lapidus PW. Infiltration therapy of acute tendinitis with calcification. *Surg Gynecol Obstet* 1943;76:715–725.
62. Lapidus PW, Guidotti FP. Common shoulder lesions—report of 493 cases. Calcific tendinitis, tendinitis of the long head of the biceps frozen shoulder, fractures and dislocations. *Bull Hosp Joint Dis* 1968; 29:293–306.
63. Lenggenhager K. [On the origin and therapy of degeneration and calcification of the supraspinal tendon.] *Langenbecks Arch Chir* 1966; 315:310–322 [in German].
64. Lippmann RK. Observations concerning the calcific cuff deposits. *Clin Orthop* 1961;20:49–60.
65. Litchman HM, Silver CM, Simon SD, Eshragi A. The surgical management of calcific tendinitis of the shoulder. *Int Surg* 1968;50: 474–482.
66. Loew M, Jurgowski W, Mau HC, Thomsen M. Treatment of calcifying tendinitis of rotator cuff by extracorporeal shock waves: a preliminary report. *J Shoulder Elbow Surg* 1995;4:101–106.
67. Loew M, Sabo D, Wehrle M, Mau H. Relationship between calcifying tendinitis and subacromial impingement: a prospective radiography and magnetic resonance imaging study. *J Shoulder Elbow Surg* 1996; 5:314–319.
68. MacNab I. Rotator cuff tendinitis. *Ann R Coll Surg* 1973;53:271–287.
69. Marchetti PG, Angeletti P, Jacchia GE. [Treatment of calcified periarthritis of the shoulder by use of two way lavage.] . *Minerva Orthop* 1971;22:399 [in Italian].
70. Marecek V, Peleska L, Urbanek K. [Surgical management of calcareous subacromial bursitis.] *Acta Chir Orthop Traumatol Czech* 1967; 34:343–346 [in Czech].
71. Matsen FA III, Arntz CT. Subacromial impingement. In: Rockwood CA Jr, Matsen FA III, eds. *The shoulder*. Philadelphia: WB Saunders, 1990:623–646.
72. Matsen FA III, Lippitt SB, Sidles JA, Harryman D II. Synthesis: practice guidelines. *Practical evaluation in management of the shoulder.* Philadelphia: WB Saunders, 1994:221–230.
73. Mavrikakis ME, Drimis S, Kontoyannis DA, Rasidakis A, Moulopoulou ES, Kontoyannis S. Calcific shoulder periarthritis (tendinitis) in adult onset diabetes mellitus: a controlled study. *Ann Rheum Dis* 1989;48:211–214.
74. McCarty DJ, Halverson PB, Carrera GF, et al. "Milwaukee shoulder": association of microspheroids containing hydroxyapatite crystals, active collagenase, and neutral proteas with rotator cuff defects. I. Clinical aspects. *Arthritis Rheum* 1981;24:464–473.
75. McKendry RJ, Uhthoff HK, Sarkar K, St. George-Hyslop P. Calcifying tendinitis of the shoulder: prognostic value of clinical, histologic and radiologic features in 57 surgically treated cases. *J Rheumatol* 1982;9:75–80.
76. McLaughlin HL. Lesions of the musculotendinous cuff of the shoulder. III. Observations on the pathology, course and treatment of calcific deposits. *Ann Surg* 1946;124:354–362.
77. McLaughlin HL. Selection of calcium deposits for operation—the technique and result of operation. *Surg Clin North Am* 1963;43: 1501–1504.
78. McLaughlin, HL, Asherman, EG. Lesions of the musculotendinous cuff of the shoulder. *J Bone Joint Surg [Am]* 1951;33:76–86.
79. Michiels VI, Menke W, Apel R, Benner A. [Calcarious tendinitis—special forms of the upper extremities. Clinical aspects and differential diagnosis.] *Fortschr Med* 1991;109:273–276 [in German]
80. Milone FP, Copeland MM. Calcific tendinitis of the shoulder joint. *AJR Am J Roentgenol* 1996;85:901–913.
81. Molé D, Gonzalez M, Roche O, Scarlat M. Introduction to calcifying tendinitis. In: Gazielly DF, Gleyze P, Thomas T, eds. *The cuff.* Elsevier, Paris 1997:141–143.
82. Molé D. Calcifying tendinitis. In: Gazielly DF, Gleyze P, Thomas T, eds. *The cuff.* 1997:185.
83. Molé D, Kempf JF, Gleyze P, Rio B, Bonnomet F, Walch G. Results of arthroscopic treatment of tendinitis of the rotator cuff of the shoulder. Second part: calcified lesions of the rotator cuff. *Rev Chir Orthop* 1993;79:532–541.
84. Mortier G, Vandevelde L. The pathogenesis of periarticular calcifications of the shoulder. *J Belge Rhumatol Med Phys* 1965;20:89–93 [in French].
85. Moschkowitz E. Histopathology of calcification of the spinatous tendons associated with subacromial bursitis. *Ann J Med Sci* 1915;149: 351–361.
86. Moseley HF. The natural history and clinical syndromes produced by calcified deposits in the rotator cuff. *Surg Clin North Am* 1963;43: 1489–1494.
87. Moseley HF. The results of nonoperative and operative treatment of calcified deposits. *Surg Clin North Am* 1963;43:1505–1506.
88. Moseley HF, Goldie I. The arterial pattern of the rotator cuff of the shoulder. *J Bone Joint Surg* [Br] 1963;45:780–789.
89. Moutounet J, Chevrot A, Wybier M, Godefroy D. [X-ray guided puncture-aspiration of refractory calcifications of the shoulder.] *Ann Radiol (Paris)* 1992;35:157–159 [in French].
90. Murnaghan GF, McIntosh D. Hydrocortisone in painful shoulder. Controlled trial. *Lancet* 1955;25:798–800.
91. Neer CS II. Less frequent procedures. *Shoulder reconstruction.* In: Neer CS II, ed. Philadelphia: WB Saunders, 1990:427–433.
92. Noel E, Brantus JF. Les tendinopathies calcifiantes de la coiffe rotateurs: traitement medical. A propos de 124 epaules. *J Lyonnaises Epaule.* 1993;547:199–213.
93. Noel E, Carrillon Y, Gaillard T, Bouvier M. Needle aspiration irrigation in calcifying tendinitis of the rotator cuff. Gazielly DF, Gleyze P, Thomas T, eds. *The cuff.* Elsevier, Paris 1997:152–158.
94. Nutton RW, Stothard J: Acute calcific supraspinatus tendinitis in a 3 year old child. *J Bone Joint Surg [Br]* 1987;69:148.
95. Ollagnier E, Bruyere G, Gazielly DF, Thomas T. Medical treatment of calcifying tendinitis of the rotator cuff. Results of a series of 47 cases of calcifying tendinitis. In: Gazielly DF, Gleyze P, Thomas T, eds. *The cuff.* Elsevier, Paris 1997:147–151.
96. Painter CF. Subdeltoid bursitis. *Boston Med Surg J* 1907;156: 345–349.
97. Patte D, Goutallier D. Calcifications. *Rev Chir Orthop* 1988;74: 277–278.
98. Patterson RL, Darrach W. Treatment of acute bursitis by needle irrigation. *J Bone Joint Surg* 1937;19:993–1002.
99. Pedersen HE, Key JA. Pathology of calcareous tendinitis and subdeltoid bursitis. *Arch Surg* 1951;62:50–63.

100. Pendergrass EP, Hodes PJ. Roentgen irradiation in treatment of inflammations. *AJR Am J Roentgenol* 1941;45:74–106.
101. Pfister J, Gerber H. Treatment of calcific humero-scapular periarthropathy using needle irrigation of the shoulder. Retrospective study. *Z Orthop* 1994;132:300–305.
102. Pinals RS, Short CL. Calcific periarthritis involving multiple sites. *Arthritis Rheum* 1966;9:566–574.
103. Plenk HP. Calcifying tendinitis of the shoulder. *Radiology* 1952;59: 384–389.
104. Postel JM, Goutallier D, Lambotte JC, Duparc F. Treatment of chronic calcifying or postcalcifying shoulder tendinitis by acromioplasty without excision of the calcification. In: Gazielly DF, Gleyze P, Thomas T, eds.*The cuff.* Elsevier, Paris 1997:159–163.
105. Pulich JJ. Calcific tendinitis of the shoulder joint and its roentgen manifestations. *J Am Osteopath Assoc* 1976;75:987–993.
106. Rathbun JB, Macnab J. The microvascular pattern of the rotator cuff. *J Bone Joint Surg [Br]* 1970;52B:540–553.
107. Re LP, Karzel RP. Management of rotator cuff calcifications. *Orthop Clin North Am* 1993;24:125–132.
108. Remberger K, Faust H, Keyl W.[Calcific tendinitis. Clinical aspects, morphology, pathogenesis and differential diagnosis.] *Pathologe* 1985;6:196–203 [in German].
109. Resch H, Povacz P, Seykora P. Excision of calcium deposit and acromiolpasty? In: Gazielly DF, Gleyze P, Thomas T, eds. *The cuff.* Elsevier, Paris 1997:169–171.
110. Riley GP, Harrall RL, Constant CR, Chard MD, Cawston TE, Hazleman BL. Glyocosaminoglycans of human rotator cuff tendons: changes with age and in chronic rotator cuff tendinitis. *Ann Rheum Dis* 1994;53:367–376.
111. Riley GP, Harrall RL, Constant CR, Chard MD, Cawston TE, Hazleman BL. Tendon degeneration and chronic shoulder pain: changes in the collagen composition of the human rotator cuff tendons in rotator cuff tendinitis. *Ann Rheum Dis* 1994;53:359–366.
112. Rompe JD, Rumler F, Hopf C, Nafe B, Heine J. Extracorporal shock wave therapy for calcifying tendinitis of the shoulder. *Clin Orthop* 1995;321:196–201.
113. Rothman RH, Parke WW. The vascular anatomy of the rotator cuff. *Clin Orthop* 1965;41:176–186.
114. Rowe CR. Calcific tendinitis. *Instr Course Lect* 1985;34:196–198, 1985.
115. Ruttiman G. Uber die Haufigkeit rontgenologischer Veranderungen bei Patienten mit typischer Periarthritis humeroscapularis und Schultergesunden. Inaugural Dissertation, Zurich, 1959.
116. Sandstrom C. Peritendinitis calcarea: common disease of middle life: its diagnosis, pathology and treatment. *AJR Am J Roengenol* 1938;40: 1–21.
117. Sandstrom C, Wahlgren F. Bietrag zur Kenntnis der Peritendinitis calcarea (sog. bursitis calculosa) speziell vom pathologisch histologischen Gesichspunkt. *Acta Radiol Stockh* 1937;18:263–296.
118. Sarkar K, Uhthoff HK. Ultrastructural localization of calcium and calcifying tendinitis. *Arch Pathol Lab Med* 1978;102:266–269.
119. Schaer H. Die Periarthritis humeroscapularis. *Ergebn Chir Orthop* 1936;29:211–309.
120. Scutellari PN, Orzincolo C, Mazzilli MP, Ghedini M, Bonari RL, Stabellini R. [The shoulder and basic calcium phosphate microcrystal deposit disease.] *Radiol Med (Torino)* 1986;72:724–728 [in Italian].
121. Seifiert G. Morphologic and biochemical aspects of experimental extraosseous tissue calcification. *Clin Orthop* 1970;69:146.
122. Selye H. The experimental production of calcific deposits in the rotator cuff. *Surg Clin North Am* 1963;43:1483–1488.
123. Sengar DP, McKendry RJ, Uhthoff HK. Increased frequency of HLA-A1 in calcifying tendinitis. *Tissue Antigens* 1987;29:173–174.
124. Simon WH. Soft tissue disorders of the shoulder. Frozen shoulder, calcific tendinitis, and bicipital tendinitis [review]. *Orthop Clin North Am* 1975;6:521–539.
125. Snyder SJ, Eppley RA. Arthroscopic removal of subacromial calcification. Presented at the 10th Annual Meeting of the Arthroscopy Association of North America, April, 1991.
126. Steida A. Zur Pathologie der Schultergelenkschleimbeutel. *Arch Klin Chir* 1908;85:910–924.
127. Toriyama K, Fukuda H, Hamada K, Noguchi T. Calcifying tendinitis of the infraspinatus tendon stimulating a bone tumor. *J Shoulder Elbow Surg* 1994;3:165–168.
128. Uhthoff HK. Calcifying tendinitis, an active cell-mediated calcification. *Virchows Arch A Pathol Anat Histopathol* 1975;366:51–58.
129. Uhthoff HK, Sarkar K. Calcifying tendinitis. *Baillieres Clin Rhumatol* 1989;3:567–581.
130. Uhthoff HK, Sarkar K. Classification and definition of tendinopathies [review]. *Clin Sports Med* 1991;10:707–720.
131. Uhthoff HK, Sarkar K, Maynard JA. Calcifying tendinitis. A new concept of its pathogenesis. *Clin Orthop* 1976;118:164–168.
132. Uhthoff HK, Sarkar K. An algorithm for shoulder pain caused by soft-tissue disorders. *Clin Orthop* 1990;254:121–127.
133. Uhthoff HK. Anatomopathology of calcifying tendinitis of the cuff. In: Gazielly DF, Gleyze P, Thomas T, eds. *The cuff.* 1997:144–146.
134. Uhthoff HK, Sarkar K. Calcifying tendinitis. In: Rockwood CA, Matsen FA, eds. *The shoulder.* Philadelphia: WB Saunders, 1990, 774–790.
135. Uhthoff HK, Loehr JW. Calcific tendinopathy of the rotator cuff. *J Am Acad Orthop Surg* 1997;5:183–191.
136. Vebostad A. Calcific tendinitis in the shoulder region. A review of 43 operated shoulders. *Acta Orthop Scand* 1997;46:205–210.
137. Vigario GD, Keats TE. Localization of calcific deposits in the shoulder. *AJR Am J Roetgenol* 1970;108:806–811.
138. Welfling J, Kahn MF, Desroy M, Paolaggi JB, DeSeze S. [Calcifications of the shoulder. II. The disease of multiple tendinous calcifications.] *Rev Rheum* 1965;32:325–334 [in French].
139. Wilson CL. Lesions of the supraspinatus tendon. Degeneration, rupture and calcification. *Arch Surg* 1943;46:307–325.
140. Wolfgang GL. Surgical repairs of the rotator cuff of the shoulder. *J Bone Joint Surg [Am]* 1974;56:14–26.
141. Wrede L. Uber kalkablagerungen in der Umgebung des Schultergelenkes und ihre bezielhungen zur periarthritis Humeroscapularis. *Langenbecks Arch Klin Chir* 1912;99:259–272.

Disorders of the Shoulder: Diagnosis and Management,
edited by Joseph P. Iannotti and Gerald R. Williams, Jr.
Lippincott Williams & Wilkins, Philadelphia © 1999.

CHAPTER 6

Disorders of the Biceps Tendon

Ken Yamaguchi and Randip Bindra

INTRODUCTION

The clinical significance of the long head of the biceps tendon to shoulder function has been a subject of controversy for some time. Opinions on the contribution of the intraarticular biceps tendon have varied across an entire spectrum, with proponents suggesting a vestigial function that is analogous to an appendix of the shoulder, to those who believe it can play a critical role in shoulder stability. Historically, there have been wide shifts in surgical treatment of the long head of the biceps tendon. In the 1940s, the biceps tendon was seen as a major source of shoulder pain, and tenodesis was favored as a primary procedure.[25,38,65] As the focus shifted to the rotator cuff, tenodesis of the long head of the biceps became less popular. Later, concerns about a possible secondary role of the long head of the biceps tendon led to recommendations for preservation whenever possible.[58,69,87] More recently, previously accepted theories on the functional role of the biceps in head depression have undergone reexamination in the context of an increased awareness about the symptomatic significance of a retained, chronically inflamed tendon.[9,73,83,102]

With the accumulation of research and clinical experience specific to the long head of the biceps tendon, it is becoming increasingly accepted that pathology in this structure can have significant symptomatic consequences that will require

K. Yamaguchi: Department of Orthopaedic Surgery, Washington University School of Medicine, St. Louis, Missouri, 63110.
R. Bindra: Department of Orthopaedic Surgery, Gwynedd Hospitals, Penrhosgarnedd, Bangor, UK LL572PW.

directed treatment plans. As with most controversial treatment issues, the proper strategy will ultimately reflect a balance of previously recognized concerns about functional deficits and persistent symptoms. The purpose of this chapter is to review the anatomic, functional, and clinical information about the long head of the biceps tendon that is required to formulate logical treatment plans.

ANATOMY

The long head of the biceps tendon arises from the posterosuperior labrum and the supraglenoid tubercle. The site of origin of the long head is variable. Habermeyer et al. described the long head origin in most cases (50%) as being completely labral. Attachment to the supraglenoid tubercle alone was less common (20%), the tendon more commonly (30%) arising from both origins, sometimes appearing bifurcated.[22,41] Another study of the origin of the tendon of the long head of the biceps in 105 cadaveric shoulders showed that 40% to 60% arose from the supraglenoid tubercle and surrounding labrum.[97] The remainder of the origins were from labrum alone. The labral attachment has been further described as being in four types: type I, the labral attachment is entirely posterior (22%); type II, most of the labral contribution is posterior, with some anterior component (33%); type III, equal contributions from both the anterior and posterior labrums (37%); and type IV, most of the contribution are anterior (8%)[97] (Fig. 1). Additionally, the orientation of the tendon attachment to the superior glenoid tubercle was dependent on the type of labral attachment. In those biceps tendons with a mostly posterior labral attachment, the superior glenoid tubercle origin was more likely to be posterior at a 1-o'clock position for a left glenoid. In those situations with an anterior labral attachment, the glenoid tubercle origin was more likely to be slightly anterior at an 11-o'clock orientation for a left glenoid.

The tendon is encased within the synovial sheath of the glenohumeral joint (Fig. 2). It traverses obliquely within the shoulder joint arching anteriorly over the head of the humerus and exits the shoulder joint beneath the transverse humeral ligament along the intertubercular sulcus, also referred to as the bicipital groove (Fig. 3). Open only at the glenohumeral cavity medially, the synovial sheath ends as a blind pouch at the end of the bicipital groove. The long head

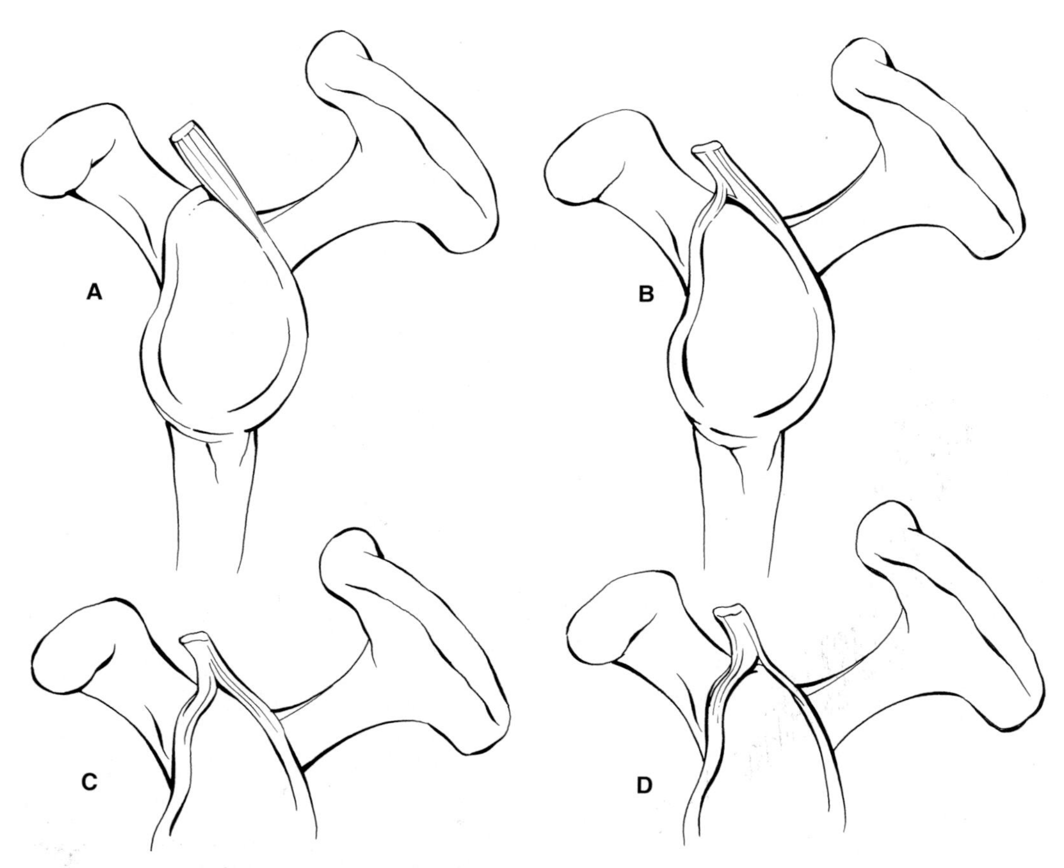

FIG. 1. Schematic drawings of the variations in the biceps origin. **(A)** *Type I.* The labral attachment is almost entirely posterior. This is seen 22% of the time. **(B)** *Type II.* Most of the labral contribution is posterior with a small amount of anterior contribution. This is seen 33% of the time. **(C)** *Type III.* There are equal contributions from both the anterior and posterior labrums and this is seen 37% of the time. **(D)** *Type IV.* Most of the labral contribution is anterior with only a small posterior contribution; this is seen 8% of the time.

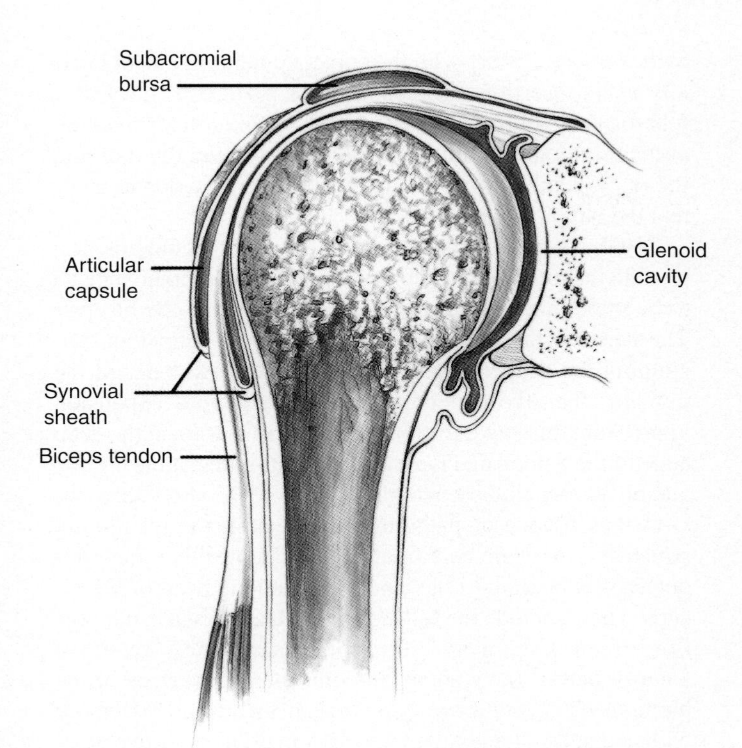

FIG. 2. A schematic of a sagittal section taken through the glenohumeral joint. The biceps tendon is covered by reflection of the synovial sheath that maintains a tendon as an extra synovial structure despite its intraarticular location. The synovial sheath ends as a blind path distally outside of the bicipital groove.

of the biceps tendon is thus intraarticular, but extrasynovial (see Fig. 2). In 50 cadaveric dissections, Habermeyer and coauthors found the mean length of the tendon to be 9.2 cm.[40,41] The tendon was widest at its origin (mean 8.5 by 2.8 mm), and progressively narrowed down to form the muscle belly (mean 4.5 by 2.8 mm). At the level of the insertion of the deltoid, the tendon evolves into an elongated muscle belly joined medially by the short head. The two bellies lie closely approximated, but are separable until about 7 cm from the elbow joint.

The ascending branch of the anterior humeral circumflex artery runs adjacent to the tendon and is the main arterial supply to the long head in the bicipital groove. Labral branches of the suprascapular artery may also contribute to the blood supply of the long head of the biceps tendon at its origin.[85] The musculocutaneous nerve (C5-7) constitutes the motor innervation to the muscle.

RESTRAINTS OF THE LONG HEAD OF THE BICEPS TENDON

Although the greater and lesser tuberosities help to contain the tendon within the bicipital groove, retention of the long head of the biceps is provided mainly by the surrounding soft tissues.

The bicipital groove is hourglass shaped, being narrowest and deepest in its midportion. With a mean width of 9.6 mm and depth of 2.2 mm it is wide and shallow at its entrance. The mean measurements at the midportion are 6.2 mm wide and 5.0 mm deep. The tunnel flattens out at its exit, 7.3 mm wide and 2.4 mm deep.[40,41] The medial wall angle varies widely among individuals, with reported mean values from 56 degrees to 64 degrees.[50] Although the humeral head size is larger in men, there is no significant difference between the two sexes in the relative size of the groove.[3] In some cases, a supratubercular ridge extends forward and downward from the region of the articular cartilage to the upper and dorsal portion of the lesser tuberosity. First described by Meyer, it is estimated to occur in 17.5% of humerii.[63,64] The significance of the supratubercular ridge is unclear; but according to Meyer, it diminishes the efficacy of the tuberosity as a trochlea, and when present can predispose to dislocation of the long head of the biceps tendon out of the groove.

Laterally, the long head of the biceps tendon runs in the rotator interval. This triangular space between the supraspinatus and the subscapularis tendons is devoid of rotator cuff and is bridged by fibrous tissue. The transverse humeral ligament bridging the bicipital groove forms the lat-

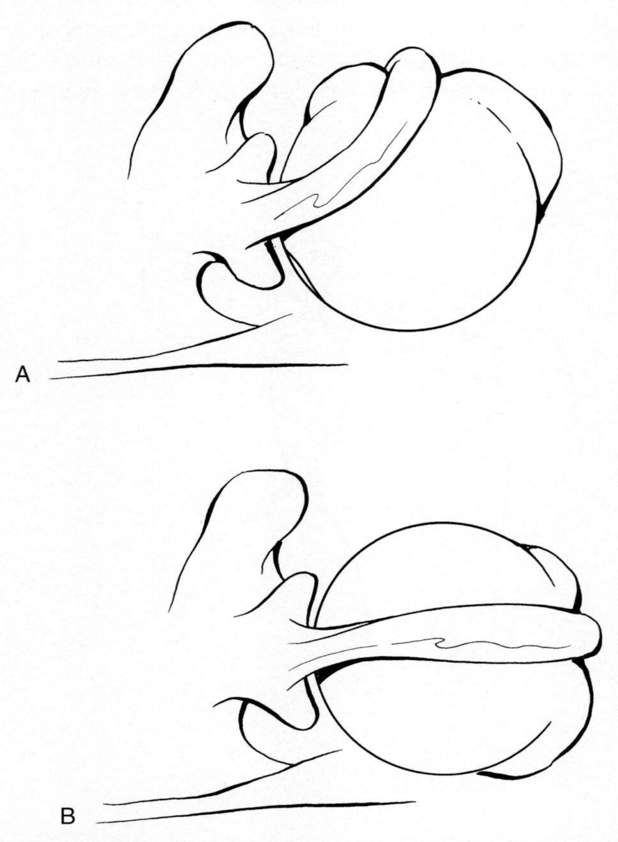

FIG. 3. (A,B) A schematic of an axial view of the glenohumeral joint showing the relative position of the biceps tendon from internal to external rotation. In internal or neutral rotation, the biceps maintains an oblique course across the joint starting from an anterior location. It is only in external rotation that the biceps tendon courses over the apex of the humeral head.

eral apex of the triangle. The coracoid process, with the origin of the coracohumeral ligament medially, constitutes the base. The coracohumeral ligament has a broad origin extending from the base of the coracoid process along the lateral border of the coracoid for about 18 mm[46] and forms the roof of the space. Located in the floor are the long head of the biceps and the superior glenohumeral ligaments (Fig. 4).[19,20,36,40]

Most authors agree that the transverse humeral ligament bridging the bicipital groove, does not play an important role in retaining the biceps tendon.[1,40,63,64,81] The ligament is often weak or absent and is present lower down in the bicipital groove. Rather, the coracohumeral ligament is believed to be more important. It consists of two bands; the superior band blends into the adjacent tendinous edge of the supraspinatus and inserts into the greater tuberosity.[19,20,29,40] The inferior band blends with the superior border of the subscapularis and inserts into the lesser tuberosity and the transverse humeral ligament. The superior glenohumeral ligament is also important for biceps tendon retention within the groove. It has two narrow osseous attachments medially. One attachment is from the apex of the labrum, shared with the biceps tendon, and the other is from the base of the coracoid process.[96] Whereas it is distinct from the coracohumeral ligament at its medial attachment to the superior labrum and the neck of the scapula, the superior glenohumeral ligament blends imperceptibly with the coracohumeral ligament laterally at its insertion into the superior surface of the lesser tuberosity.[20] Thus, in the lateral part of the rotator interval, at the proximal portion of the bicipital groove, the roof and the floor blend to form a sling for the biceps tendon as it enters the bicipital groove.

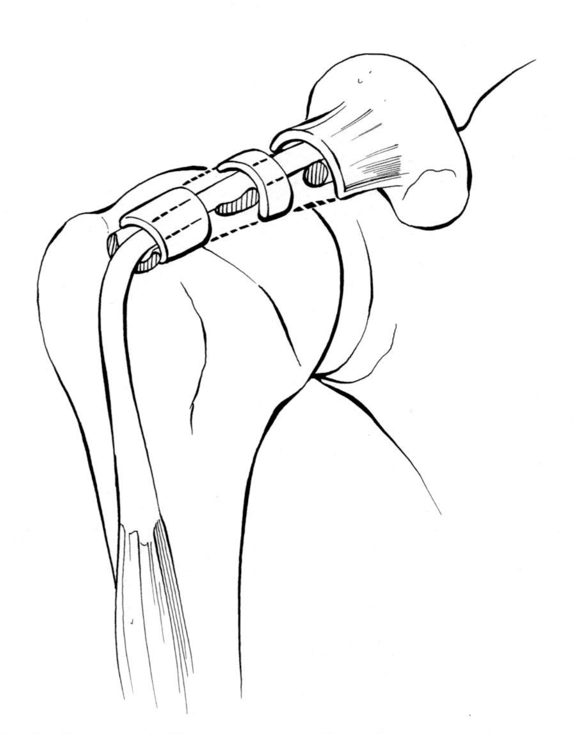

FIG. 4. A schematic representation of the relations of the coracohumeral ligament and superior glenohumeral ligament to the long head of the biceps tendon. The long head of the biceps tendon is stabilized in the bicipital groove by the coracohumeral ligament (*black*) which forms the roof and the superior glenohumeral ligament (*hatched*), which forms the floor.

Distal to the summits of the greater and lesser tuberosities, it is the insertion of the pectoralis major tendon that appears to be important in retention of the long head of the biceps.[1] The sternocostal portion of the pectoralis major tendon, constituting the deeper lamina, inserts more proximally in the humerus than the clavicular portion. A fibrous expansion arises from this head, forming a falciform margin at the deep edge of the tendon and is attached to both sides of the groove and blends proximally with the capsule of the shoulder joint.

In the absence of pathologic changes in the restraining structures, there are certain anatomic features that may predispose dislocation of the tendon of the long head of the biceps. These include the following: (a) The intraarticular portion of the tendon may lie more eccentrically over the anterior half of the sloping, smooth, rounded surface of the humeral head, favoring its medial dislocation; (b) a more widened and flattened tendon origin may occur at the superior glenoid; (c) a shallow medial wall of the groove may be present. This would not provide as substantial a restraint to medial subluxation of the tendon because the tendon of the long head of the biceps makes an abrupt turn from a horizontal direction to a vertical course at the intertubercular sulcus. The lesser tuberosity acts as the trochlea for the tendon at this point. (d) The supracondylar ridge, when present, diminishes the prominence of the lesser tuberosity, decreasing its efficacy as a trochlea.[38,64]

FUNCTIONAL ANATOMY OF THE LONG HEAD

Perhaps no aspect of the long head of the biceps tendon has raised as much controversy as its function at the shoulder. The biceps extends from the scapula to the bones of the forearm and thus has potential function at both the shoulder and elbow. Elbow function includes both flexion and supination. The actions of the proximal tendon around the shoulder have been incompletely defined. Although the long head of the biceps has been postulated to have several roles or functions about the shoulder, definitive experimental proof has been sparse and contradictory, leaving its exact role controversial.

More complete characterization of the functional role of the long head of the biceps can be clinically important in determining indications for tenodesis. Some reports have suggested a weak humeral head depressor role that increases in relative importance in the presence of rotator cuff tears. Other studies have suggested that the long head of the biceps works solely in relation to the elbow, with no significant shoulder-related activity. Neer warned against thoughtless tenodesis of the long head of the biceps because it destroys its function as a head depressor and may precipitate or escalate an impingement problem.[69] Leffert and Rowe offered the observation that increased size of the tendon with chronic rotator cuff rupture represented an increased function that compensated for the loss of the rotator cuff, and they strongly discouraged tenodesis.[58] However, this phenomenon has been seen only with large rotator cuff tears in which the tendon was exposed to constant impingement and more plausibly reflected a chronic inflammatory response. Additionally, the more physiologic response of increased muscle mass, as opposed to increased tendon size, has not been noted. Aside from clinical observations, there have been several approaches employed to study the potential function of the biceps tendon. These include comparative anatomy observations, cadaveric biomechanical studies, and dynamic electromyographic (EMG) analysis.

Comparative Anatomy

The asymmetrical size of the greater and lesser tuberosities and the angular orientation of the bicipital groove are exclusive to the human shoulder and represent an evolutionary adaptation to the vertical posture. The presence of two heads is unique to primates. In certain quadrupeds, such as the horse, which does not have a deltoid muscle, this head is large and functions to elevate the extremity in conjunction with a comparatively large supraspinatus.[52] In quadrupeds, the biceps passes over the center of the spherical humeral head in the bicipital groove, which is located between two symmetrical tuberosities and oriented perpendicular to the glenoid. Because the scapula and glenoid face are oriented toward the forward plane, the biceps tendon in quadruped animals contributes to flexion of the shoulder.

In adaptation to an upright posture, the anteroposterior diameter of the chest wall has decreased progressively, and the scapula has rotated dorsally over the flattened chest wall.[50] To allow the articular surface of the humerus, which previously faced dorsally, to continue facing the scapula, the humeral shaft has undergone torsion. This has resulted in a displacement of the bicipital groove medially and ventrally to form an angle of 30 to 40 degrees with the plane of the scapula (Fig. 5). This developmental change in the tendon orientation to the glenoid has resulted in a significant decrease in effectiveness of the biceps as an arm elevator, which can only be partially restored with full external rotation of the arm. There has been a compensatory developmental adaptation by the deltoid muscle, which becomes a much more effective elevator in primates secondary to its more distal insertion, increased muscle mass, and adaptations of the acromion to increase the leverage of the muscle.[51]

Hitchcock and Bechtol studied the anatomy of the bicipital tuberosity in 100 dry human specimens and compared

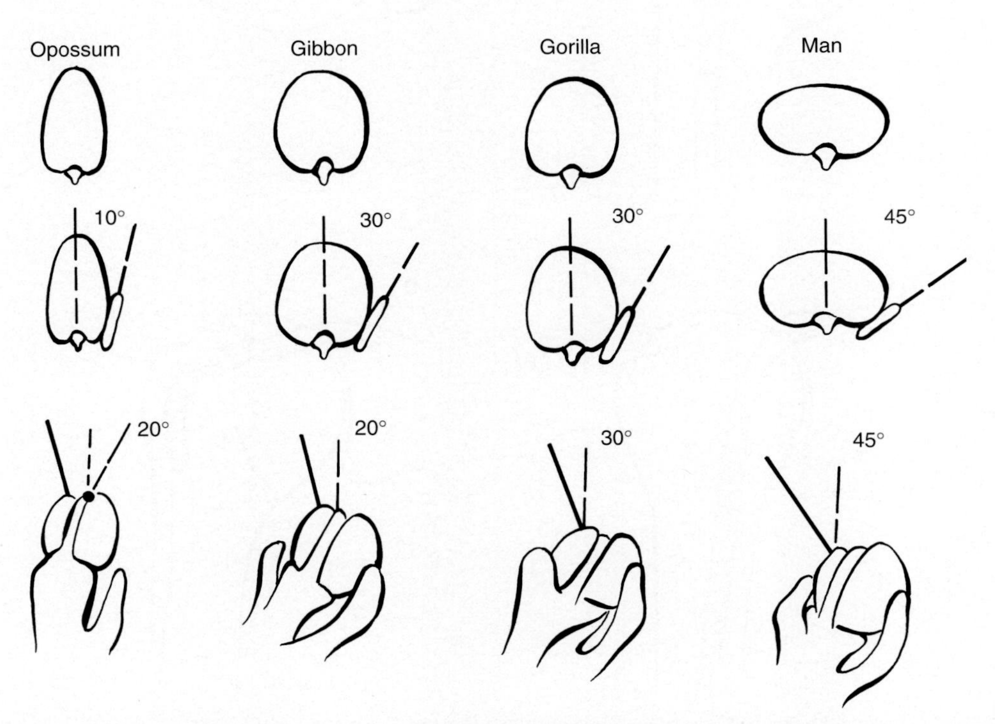

FIG. 5. A schematic showing progressive change in positioning of the scapula and bicipital groove from the quadruped to the biped. As an adaptation for upright posture, the anteroposterior dimension of the chest wall has decreased progressively. This has resulted in secondary humeral torsion and a displacement of the bicipital groove medially and ventrally in relation to the scapula. Whereas the bicipital groove follows a straight course over the top of the humeral head in the quadruped (opossum), in humans it now resides against the lesser tuberosity over the anterior portion of the head. This has resulted in a significant decrease in effectiveness of the biceps to act as an arm elevator.

them with primate humerii from the Chicago Natural History Museum.[50] The human specimens demonstrated a wide variation in the depth of the bicipital groove. This was expressed as the angle of the medial wall, a smaller angle representing a shallow wide groove. Although most human specimens demonstrated a medial wall angle of 60 to 75 degrees, values of 45 degrees or less were observed in 20% of specimens. Except the orangutan (a primate with greater predisposition to tree climbing), which presented values similar to humans, other apes demonstrated deep bicipital grooves, with consistent medial wall angles of 90 degrees in all specimens. The shallow bicipital groove in humans was postulated to be important for the development of instability and subsequent inflammation of the long head of the biceps.[50] The considerable variability of the biceps groove was considered to reflect a developmental loss of function in elevation for the biceps muscle. These authors also noted the relative ventral orientation of the long head of the biceps in relation to other mammals. Additionally, they emphasized that humans will habitually hold their humerus in the forward plane and internal rotation, increasing the poor anatomic arrangement for the biceps to act in abduction. They concluded that an operation to fix the tendon in the bicipital groove, while removing a portion of the tendon above the groove, can relieve the symptoms caused by biceps tendon pathology and does not materially weaken the shoulder.[50]

Anatomic and Biomechanical Studies

Lippmann surgically observed, in patients under local anesthesia, that the long head of the biceps is a passive structure, sliding in its groove with movements of the shoulder[61] (Fig. 6). No motion was seen to be transmitted to the humeral head by contractions of the long head of the biceps during active elbow flexion. He believed the biceps played a minimal active role in producing motion at the shoulder joint. Rather,

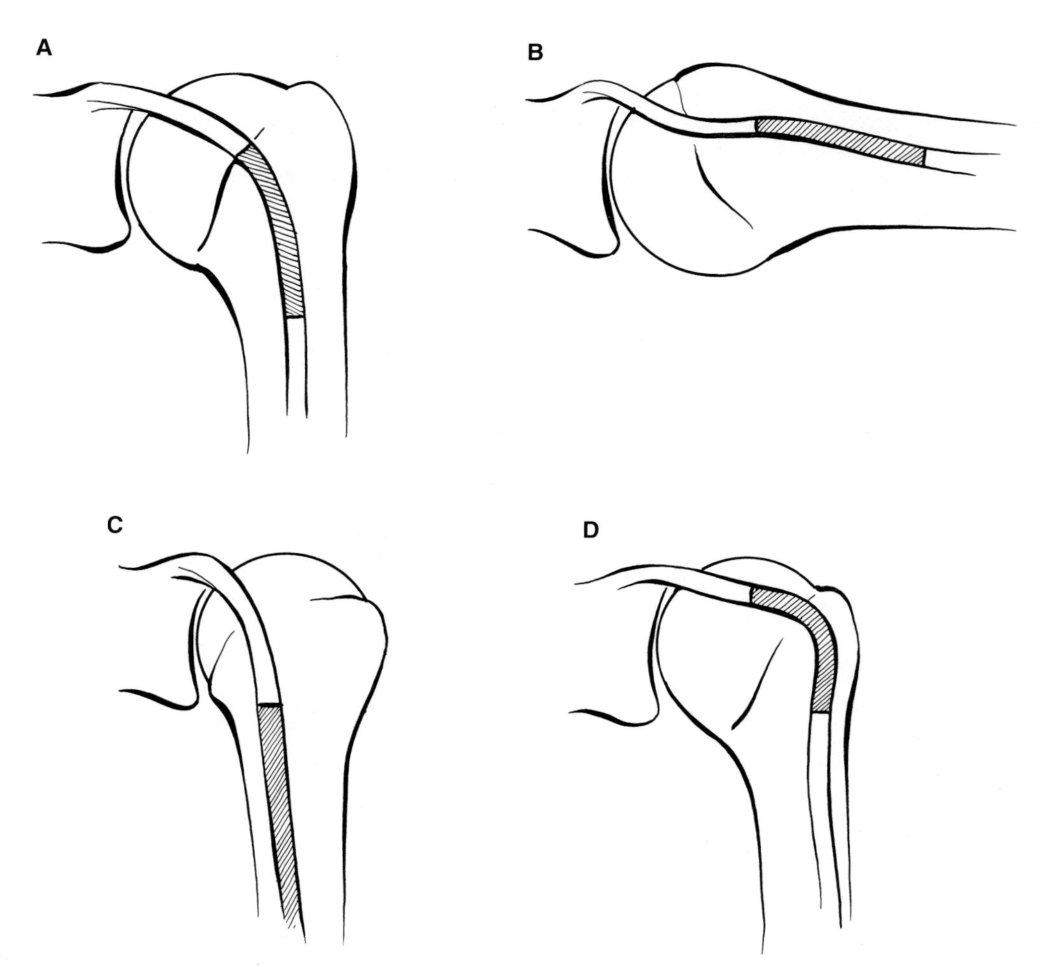

FIG. 6. Schematic of the relation of the biceps tendon to the humerus with glenohumeral motion. As described by Lippmann, with direct surgical observation, the biceps tendon played a passive role during humeral motion. The biceps tendon slid freely between the sheath and the joint proper as the shoulder was moved. Varying amounts of the tendon were intraarticular, depending on shoulder position. A maximum of intraarticular tendon was seen with external rotation and adduction. A minimal amount of intraarticular tendon was present during elevation: **(A)** neutral rotation; **(B)** elevation; **(C)** internal rotation; **(D)** external rotation.

the humeral head was believed to passively move on the biceps tendon. This passive motion of the biceps tendon within the intertubercular groove is necessary for normal motion.[47] Biceps tendon adhesion within the bicipital groove, either after injury, immobilization, inflammation, or incorporation of the tendon during tuberosity repairs, potentially limits the maximal recovery of motion. The shorter the intraarticular tendon length during adhesion, the greater the motion restriction. This was particularly evident if the adhesion occurred in internal rotation and adduction.

In contrast, by electrically stimulating the biceps muscle during shoulder arthroscopy in five patients, Andrews et al. observed that the tendon became taut and raised its origin at the superior labrum off the glenoid.[6] They also observed compression of the humeral head into the glenoid. These authors suggest that such compressive forces afford stress protection to the humerus during the act of throwing. They also suggested that sudden forceful transmission of contraction of the biceps on the superior labrum may be one mechanism for the development of superior labral anterior and posterior (SLAP) lesions.

Studies using simulated muscle contractions in freely hanging cadaveric specimens have been difficult to interpret because of difficulties in reproducing physiologic tension of the muscles around the shoulder. Extrapolation of the findings of these studies to the clinical situation have been difficult. Kumar et al., in a cadaveric study of 15 dependent shoulder specimens, radiographically measured changes to the acromiohumeral interval when applying tension to the short and long heads of the biceps before and after division of the long head of the biceps.[57] There was no attempt to recreate contributions from the rotator cuff. An average decrease in the acromiohumeral interval by 15.5 mm was observed when the short head was tensed in the absence of an intact long head of the biceps. The authors suggested that a function of the long head of the biceps was to stabilize the humeral head on the glenoid during powerful elbow flexion and forearm supination by the biceps brachii. In this study, all recordings were performed with the arm by the side and the contribution of the biceps tendon in motion at the shoulder was not examined.

Flatow et al. studied possible restraints against superior humeral translation in a cadaveric model in which the long head of the biceps and rotator cuff muscle activity was simulated with a cable system.[32] Superior migration of the humeral head with abduction of the shoulder was then studied in the cuff-intact situation and with simulated tears of various size. Force along the biceps tendon restrained superior migration of the humeral head most significantly in the presence of a large rotator cuff defect.

Itoi et al., in two separate cadaveric studies, looked at the stabilizing function of the long head of the biceps.[52] In the first study, nine cadaveric specimens were tested in a hanging arm position in which the biceps was spring-loaded to simulate contractions. In this model, with the biceps in the hanging arm position, anterior and posterior displacement was significantly decreased by loading the long head of the biceps. Additionally, inferior displacement and external rotation were significantly decreased by long head loading. Interestingly, long head loading in this model produced small amounts of superior displacement of the shoulder. Similar to the study by Kumar et al., no attempt was made to re-create the actions of the rotator cuff. In the second study, biceps function was studied in simulated stable and unstable shoulders. Again, anterior displacement of the head was significantly decreased by both the long head and short head loading when the arm was in 60 to 90 degrees of external rotation. It was concluded that the long head of the biceps and short head of the biceps had functions similar to the anterior stabilizers of the glenohumeral joint when the arm is in abduction and external rotation, and that the stabilizing increases as shoulder stability decreases.

A functional role for the long head of the biceps in anterior stability was also shown in a study by Rodosky et al.[88] In this study, performed in seven fresh-frozen cadaveric shoulders, the biceps was tested in the context of simulated rotator cuff contractions by use of pneumonic cylinders. In this dynamic model, simulated contractions of the biceps muscle contributed to anterior stability of the glenohumeral joint by increasing the shoulder's resistance to torsional forces. This was particularly apparent in the vulnerable abducted and externally rotated position.

Pagnani, in a study of ten cadaveric shoulders, also tested the effect of simulated contraction of the long head of the biceps on glenohumeral translation.[78] In the presence of a joint reactive force of 22 N, a 50 N anterior, posterior, superior, and inferior force was partly resisted by contraction of the long head of the biceps. This was more pronounced at middle and lower elevation angles. The reduction in anterior translation was 10.4 mm. There was only a 1.2-mm reduction in superior translation.

Interpretation of these cadaveric studies has been difficult because of an inability to reproduce the dynamic interplay and bulk effect of surrounding musculature. However, one in vivo analysis of the role of the long head of the biceps has been performed by Warner et al.[99] In this study, performed in seven patients, with isolated loss of the proximal tendon of the long head of the biceps, superior migration of the instant center of rotation of the humeral head was measured at 0, 45, 90, and 120 degrees of humeral abduction in the scapular plane. A significant increase in the superior translation was measured in comparison with the contralateral uninvolved side. The amount of the superior translation, however, was small, and the authors concluded that it may be more important in conditions where the subacromial space was more narrow, such as in patients with a type II or type III acromion.

Electromyographic Analysis Studies

Interpretation of cadaveric studies of the long head of the biceps muscle requires relevant EMG analysis to predict the quality of applied loads. A consistent, but potentially inaccurate, assumption with all of these studies has been the inclusion of significant biceps muscle activity associated with shoulder motion. Multiple studies have attempted to evaluate biceps muscle function during shoulder motion through the use of EMG analysis. Electromyographic analysis has a significant advantage over cadaveric studies by allowing an in vivo observation of potential long head of the biceps function.

With the use of EMG data gathering, some studies have suggested a biceps role in shoulder stabilization. Ting et al., in a study of five patients with unilateral rotator cuff tears, showed increased biceps activity on the ipsilateral side in comparison with contralateral controls.[95] Additionally, Jobe et al., in a study of baseball pitchers with symptoms consistent with instability, showed increased biceps activity in comparison with stable controls.[54]

In a similar study, Basmajian and Latif noted activity in the long head of the biceps on shoulder abduction only with an externally rotated and supinated forearm.[7] They concluded that the primary action of the biceps was at the elbow for flexion of the supinated forearm, the activity in the tendon diminishing with forearm pronation. The biceps tendon was also active with forearm supination with the elbow flexed or supination against resistance. The actions of the long and short heads of the biceps were similar, but the long head was generally more active. Similar findings were reported by Habermeyer et al. when they studied 12 shoulders in healthy subjects.[41] These authors observed EMG activity in the biceps with shoulder abduction from 90 to 166 degrees, peaking at 132 degrees. On flexion of the shoulder, EMG activity was recorded in the biceps from 0 to 164 degrees, peaking at 84 degrees. Lesser activity was recorded with other shoulder movements, with no activity observed in internal rotation.

In contrast, several EMG studies have shown that the biceps is active only during elbow motion. Furlani, in 30 healthy shoulders, showed that the biceps was completely inactive with abduction and elbow extension.[34] Only 1 subject showed slight activity in abduction with elbow flexion. When the shoulder was abducted against a significant load, only 3 of the 30 subjects showed some activity, and 2 of these subjects were considered tense. Pauly et al., in a study of 18 volunteers, showed no significant biceps activity with shoulder abduction or rotation in any subject.[79] Gowan et al. in an EMG study of the shoulder during pitching, showed the biceps acting primarily in late cocking.[39] Moderate activity in the biceps was noted with elbow flexion in the cocking phase, reaching an intensity of about 34% of a maximal manual muscle test. With the elbow position relatively stable during the acceleration phase, the intensity of biceps action diminished to less than 25%. Peak activity in the biceps tendon was recorded during the follow-through phase, the muscle contracting to decelerate the rapidly extending elbow. Given their findings, they concluded that the biceps acts in concert with the brachialis and triceps to control the elbow, with no significant effect at the shoulder, during the throwing action.

As the biceps muscle traverses two joints, interpretation of previous EMG studies has been difficult because no attempt was made to control for elbow-related actions. Yamaguchi et al., in a study of 44 shoulders, including 14 with rotator cuff tears, showed no significant shoulder-related activity of the biceps muscle when elbow function was controlled with the use of a brace (Fig. 7).[102] Biceps levels remained relatively flat throughout various shoulder motions and were insignificant compared with supraspinatus levels, which increased in a motion-specific fashion. Brachioradialis controls were similarly minimal, and they mirrored biceps activity patterns, suggesting that any biceps activity was either background or elbow-related. No significant increase was seen in patients with rotator cuff tears. In contrast, supraspinatus activity levels showed significant increase in the presence of rotator cuff tears. The results of this study were further substantiated by Levy et al., in a study of ten shoulders controlled for elbow motion.[59] In this study, fast and slow motions, as well as loaded and unloaded shoulder motions, were tested for the presence or absence of biceps activity. As previously reported by Yamaguchi, no significant electroactivity was identified in the long head of the biceps in response to isolated shoulder motion when elbow and forearm position were controlled. The authors of both of these studies concluded that any function attributed to the long head of the biceps was not likely to be active. Rather, the long head of the biceps had either a passive role or an active role dependent on an association with elbow and forearm activity.[53]

Summary of Functional Anatomy

The exact function of the long head of the biceps tendon in shoulder function still remains incompletely characterized. Whereas the comparative anatomy analysis and EMG observations would suggest a minimal role for the biceps tendon, the biomechanical data would suggest otherwise. The latest EMG data with controlled elbow motion would suggest that very little coordinated biceps activity occurs specific to the shoulder joint.[59,102] The previously used loads on the biceps tendon for cadaveric analysis may have been misleading. Even in complex activities, such as pitching, the axial muscle contractions noted in the biceps muscle have been about 30% to 40% of those attainable.[39] Given vector analysis of the pull of the biceps, a head depression role would be unlikely to occur in most ranges of motion short of full external rotation. This does not preclude a role in anterior instability that appears to be better supported by both the EMG and biomechanical analysis.[52,54,88] In the context of anterior instability, the biceps plays a significant role in dynamic cadaveric models and in vivo during which an increase EMG response was seen in unstable pitchers versus those without stability symptoms.[52,54,88]

The absence of supportive evidence on a coordinated ac-

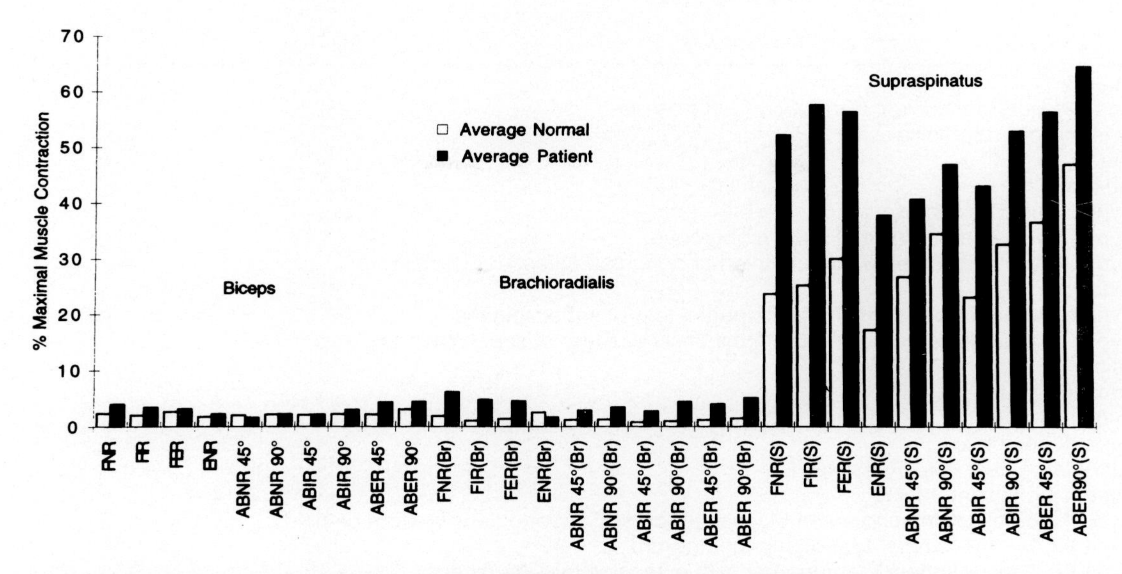

FIG. 7. Column graph showing the combined electromyographic activity from the biceps, brachioradialis, and supraspinatus in normal control subjects and patients with rotator cuff tears. When elbow activity was controlled, minimal biceps and brachioradialis activity was achieved, which was shown for both normal and rotator cuff tear patients. In contrast, significant amounts of supraspinatus activity were seen, and the amounts increased when a rotator cuff tear was present. The results suggest a lack of biceps activity coordinated with shoulder motion. y-axis = EMG activity as a percent of maximal muscle contraction: *x*-axis, various types of active shoulder motion.

tive role of the biceps does not preclude a significant passive role or active role secondary to elbow activity. It is possible that resting tension on the biceps may be helpful in both anterior and superior instability. Additionally, proprioceptive roles for the biceps tendon remain to be studied.

PATHOPHYSIOLOGY

Shoulder pain arising solely from the long head of the biceps can be quite severe, causing marked loss of shoulder motion. Disorders of the biceps tendon may arise from inflammatory changes in and around the tendon or may develop as a consequence of a significant injury or repeated microtrauma. These two major group of pathological processes (i.e., inflammatory and traumatic) are a result of the location of the tendon and its unique anatomic structure.[15,69,71,73,75,86] Although the eventual clinical presentation of these afflictions of the long head of the biceps tendon is shoulder pain, they affect different patient populations with dissimilar pathogeneses. In this section, we will discuss the various disorders of the long head of the biceps tendon by classifying them into inflammatory, unstable, or traumatic, on the basis of the original initiating event (Table 1). It must be stressed that the distinction is not always clear; the degenerated and inflamed tendon is more prone to trauma and, conversely, repeated trauma may result in changes in the tendon indistinguishable from those of inflammation. Nevertheless, this classification can help with the organization of the pathogenesis of these disorders and formulation of protocols for appropriate management.

Inflammatory Lesions of the Biceps Tendon

Biceps Tendinitis Concurrent with Rotator Cuff Tendinitis

Tendinitis of the long head of the biceps was described by Neer to be secondary to impingement syndrome for most of the cases encountered in clinical practice.[69] Because the sheath of the biceps tendon is an extension of the synovial lining of the glenohumeral joint and intimately related to the rotator cuff, any inflammatory process affecting one of the structures can also eventually affect the others.[14,40,71–75] The terms subacromial bursitis, rotator cuff tendinitis, and impingement syndrome have been used to describe the inflammatory changes occurring in the subacromial space as a result of the impingement syndrome. This and other forms of bursitis, such as rheumatoid arthritis, gout, and other crystal arthropathies, and infections, usually involve intraarticular synovitis.

In addition to a secondary involvement of the surrounding synovitis, the long head of the biceps tendon is susceptible to the same mechanical abutment seen with impingement of the rotator cuff tendons.[15,69,75] Whether primary or secondary causes of impingement exist, the long head of the biceps occupies an anterior location within the impingement zone that predisposes its involvement with rotator cuff disease. Besides these compressive forces, the biceps tendon is further subjected to a medial displacing force across the lesser tuberosity as it moves in the groove.[81,90]

The mechanical effects on the rotator cuff and long head of the biceps tendon appear to be age-related and tend to oc-

TABLE 1. *Classification of biceps tendon disorders*

- I. Inflammatory
  1. Biceps tendinitis concurrent with rotator cuff disease
  2. Primary bicipital tendinitis
- II. Instability
  1. Subluxation
     - Type I: superior subluxation
     - Type II: unstable at proximal portion of groove
     - Type III: subluxation following malunion or nonunion of lesser tuberosity
  2. Dislocation
     - Type I: extraarticular, combined with partial tear of subscapularis
     - Type II: intraarticular, combined with full-thickness tear of subscapularis
- III. Traumatic
  1. Traumatic rupture
     - Type I: partial
     - Type II: complete
  2. Superior labral tear (SLAP lesion)
     - Type I: significant fraying
     - Type II: complete detachment of biceps tendon and superior labrum from glenoid
     - Type III: "bucket-handle" tear of superior labrum
     - Type IV: Central superior labrum tear with extension into the biceps

cur together. Petersson performed 151 shoulder dissections in 76 cadavera.[80] No degenerative changes were observed before the age of 60. The long head of the biceps demonstrated fraying and flattening in 12 shoulders, and was ruptured in 6. Four shoulders demonstrated dislocation of the tendon out of its groove. The number of shoulders with degenerative changes in the biceps tendon seemed to increase with increasing age, involving 5 of 6 cases over the age of 90.

Neviaser performed a prospective arthroscopic evaluation of the biceps tendon in 153 patients requiring surgery for chronic rotator cuff disease.[76] Synovial biopsies as well as direct examination of the intertubercular groove portion of the biceps tendon were performed in all cases: 17% of the biceps tendons were completely normal; 24% in cases of no rotator cuff tear; 15% in cases with partial tear; and 10% in those with full-thickness rotator cuff tears. Marked inflammatory changes, without gross degeneration of the tendon, were seen in 64%; 56% in those with no tears; 64% with partial tears; and 74% with full tears. Thirteen percent had fibrosis of the biceps tendon. Thus, there appeared to be a strong association of coexistent biceps tendon disease with rotator cuff disease. This association increased with increasing severity of the rotator cuff disease.

Synovitis of the biceps tendon, likened to deQuervain's stenosing tenosynovitis, is generally found in the segment within the bicipital groove, under the transverse humeral ligament (Fig. 8).[73] Surgical exploration can reveal the synovial sheath of the tendon as hemorrhagic and bulging slightly above and below the transverse humeral ligament. At incision of the outer layer of the synovial sheath, an effusion can escape into the wound. Not present normally between the two layers of the synovial sheath around the tendon, this fluid represents the inflammatory exudate. The contained segment of the tendon will appear dull, swollen, and discolored, but is still mobile in the groove. These findings correspond to the acute painful stage of the disease.[61] In later cases, the sheath appears thickened, fibrotic, and less vascular. The tendon is roughened and lies in a bed of hemorrhagic adhesions. The inflamed tendon can appear reddened, but initially normal in size. In later stages, the tendon may appear atrophic or hypertrophic. The atrophic tendon is thin and frayed and represents a prerupture stage. In the hypertrophic type, inflammatory changes within the tendon result in an enlarged appearance.

Microscopically, the inflammatory changes in the tendon have been well documented. There is a pronounced round cell infiltration of the tendon, degeneration of the tendon fibers, and edema.[61,76] The hypertrophied tendon, as seen in relation to large cuff tears, most plausibly represents a chronic inflammatory response from continuing impingement of the tendon.[102] Eventually, the tendon can become firmly bound down in the groove with adhesions or spontaneously rupture. This can be associated with resolution of the symptoms of tendinitis. Rupture of the intraarticular portion of the tendon has been reported in 3% of anatomic dissections.[61] These changes appear age-related, with more pronounced changes occurring in patients past middle life.[25] When spontaneous rupture is seen, it is often accompanied with an instant and gratifying relief of the long-standing shoulder pain. Perhaps no other clinical observation is more supportive of the significant role biceps tendinitis can contribute toward shoulder pain.

Primary Bicipital Tendinitis

The term *primary bicipital tendinitis* has been reserved for isolated inflammation of the long head of the biceps tendon in the intertubercular groove, without any evidence of associated shoulder pathology. Most authors believe that primary tendinitis of the biceps tendon is uncommon and must be diagnosed only after exclusion of rotator cuff pathology or subacromial impingement.[26,69]

Tendinitis may also commence as a result of direct or indirect trauma, unusual or increased activity, an underlying inflammatory disease, a result of trauma, or secondary to instability of the tendon.[83] Often no specific factor is identifiable, constituting the idiopathic group that, in some series, accounts for 43% of cases.[23] Whatever the inciting factor, the pathologic changes are restricted to the intertubercular groove and are indistinguishable from secondary tendinitis. However, primary tendinitis almost surely also exists as a separate entity. This bicipital tenosynovitis has been likened to that seen in deQuervain's tenosynovitis.[23,25,61,65,83] The thickening of synovitis of the tendon occurs under the transverse humeral ligament in the bicipital groove. The intraarticular portion of the tendon has been reported to always be normal.

The etiology of biceps tendonitis can be multifactorial. DePalma described anomalies of the bicipital groove, together with repeated trauma, as a major factor in younger persons.[25] Degenerative changes were described to be the more common factor in older persons. Rathbun and Macnab, in a microvascular injection study of the shoulder, showed a critical zone in the long head of the biceps tendon similar to that seen in the supraspinatus.[84] This critical zone of avascularity, however, was primarily in the intracapsular portion of the tendon.

Long Head of the Biceps Tendon Instability

The spectrum of instability of the biceps tendon varies from subluxation, that is excessive mobility of the tendon within the groove, to dislocation or complete displacement of the tendon out of its groove in the humerus.

We have used the term *primary instability* to include all the spectrum of biceps instabilities, from subluxation, to frank dislocation. The biceps tendon passes at an angle of 30 to 40 degrees from its origin to the groove in the humerus, where it descends vertically. The tendon is relatively fixed from the point of its entrance into the bicipital groove, and it swings from one angle to another as the arm is rotated. When the arm is cocked to abduction and external rotation, the forces tend to displace the tendon medially, compressing it against the medial edge of the bicipital groove. In internal rotation, the tendon is thrust against the lateral margin of the groove, moving through an arc of more than 90 degrees in the process.[77] If the groove is shallow, the tendon may force its way over the greater or lesser tuberosity. If the groove is narrow and tight, the constant pressure on the tendon may lead to tendinitis.

Luxation of the long head of the biceps tendon is most

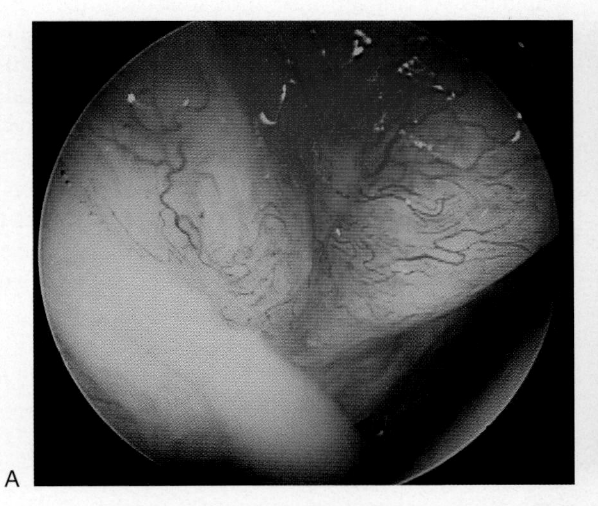

A

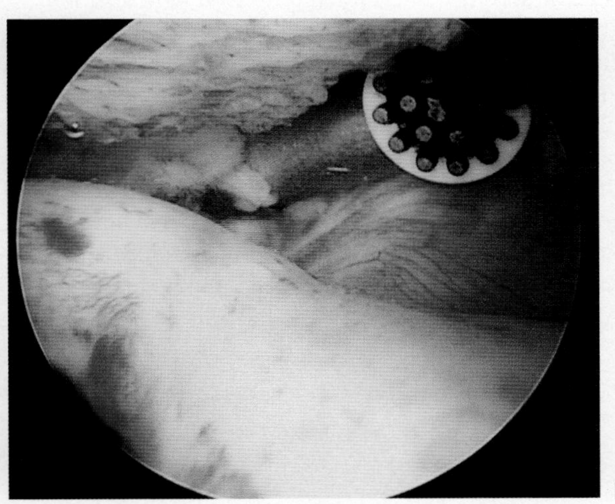

B

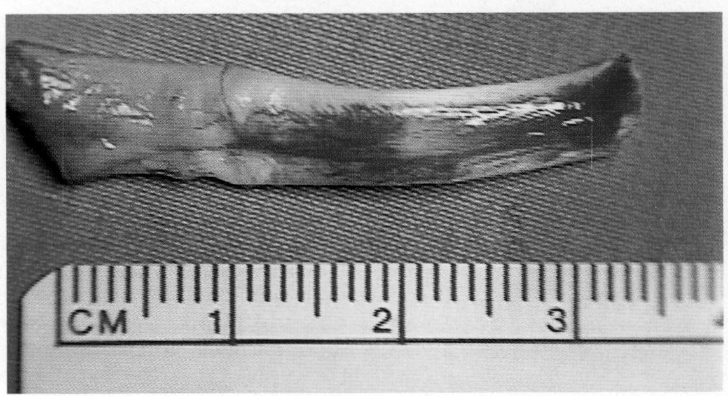

C

FIG. 8. Intraoperative photos showing the marked synovitis that could be seen on the under surface of the rotator cuff with chronic rotator cuff tendinitis: **(A)** Synovitis on the under surface of the rotator cuff is encircling the biceps tendon during its intraarticular path. **(B)** Involvement of synovitis at the biceps origin. **(C)** Removed tendon obtained from a patient who had failed a previous decompression for chronic rotator cuff tendinitis. Following this revision procedure, in which this tendon was removed, the patient had a resolution of symptoms.

commonly secondary to loss of the soft-tissue restraints with degenerative rotator cuff tears.[14,40,81,98] It is generally agreed that the main restraint to medial dislocation of the tendon of the long head of the biceps is the integrity of the rotator interval, which can be disrupted with rotator cuff tears that involve either the superior aspect of the subscapularis or the anterior portion of the supraspinatus tendon.[14,19,20,40,46] Displacement of the biceps tendon out of its groove, in association with tears of the rotator cuff, has been reported with incidences as high as 20%.[90] The tendon lies medial to the lesser tuberosity, over the subscapularis, covered by a sling of the subscapularis tendon. In a cadaveric study of 153 shoulders, Petersson found two patterns of medial dislocation of the long head of the biceps tendon: the dislocated tendon sliding over the subscapularis, and a dislocated tendon sliding beneath a deep tear of the subscapularis.[81] The latter pattern occurred in four of the five cases in Petersson's series. In patients with full-thickness tears of the supraspinatus tendon with rupture of the coracohumeral ligament, the tendon can displace medially over the subscapularis tendon. In the presence of a partial tear of the subscapularis tendon involving its deep surface, however, the tendon can sublux medially deep to the subscapularis muscle. At external inspection, the subscapularis tendon can appear intact, and a dislocated tendon may be missed if the region is not carefully examined at surgery.[98]

Contrary to common perceptions about subluxation, the biceps tendon does not intermittently reduce with arm motion. Rather, these luxations appear to be fixed. Subluxation has been classified by Habermeyer and Walch into three types (Fig. 9).[40]

Type I, a superior subluxation, comes as a consequence of a loss of the coracohumeral ligament and rotator interval sling. The subscapularis tendon is intact, preventing an otherwise true dislocation. There is often a partial lesion of the supraspinatus lesion. In Type II subluxation, the biceps tendon is unstable at the entrance to the bony groove. In this situation, the tendon slips over the medial rim of the lesser tuberosity, short of complete dislocation. The pathologic lesion here is a detachment of the superior-most fibers of the subscapularis tendon. Type III subluxations follow a malunion or nonunion lesser tuberosity. In this situation, a fracture of the lesser tuberosity without healing or any malunited fracture compromises the medial bony restraint to the long head of the biceps tendon, allowing subluxation. Symptoms are more prominent in internal rotation. Each of these types of subluxation are associated with tendinitis and capsular synovitis in the area of the rotator interval. Chronic cases of this tendonitis can lead to attrition and later rupture of the long head of the biceps tendon.

A frank dislocation rupture of the long head of the biceps is nearly always associated with a tear of the subscapular tendon. Thus, observation of a completely dislocated biceps tendon either on preoperative imaging, such as magnetic resonance imaging (MRI) or ultrasonography, or during direct observation arthroscopically, should alert the treating physician to the possibility of a concurrent full-thickness rupture of the subscapularis tendon. Habermeyer and Walch have classified these types of dislocations into type I and type II lesions.[40] Type I lesions are extraarticular dislocations combined with a partial tear of the subscapularis tendon. In this situation, the long head of the biceps tendon is completely dislocated over the lesser tuberosity. There is a rupture of the common attachment of the superior glenohumeral ligament and coracohumeral ligament. Superficial and lateral fibers of the subscapularis tendon are also torn, releasing the soft-tissue restraints to the tendon. However, deep fibers of the subscapularis tendon remain intact, preventing intraarticular displacement. The lesion essentially corresponds to a more advanced evolution of a type II subluxation. In type II dislocations of the biceps tendon, there is an intraarticular dislocation of the long head of the biceps tendon. This occurs in conjunction with a complete full-thickness tear of the subscapularis. This type of dislocation is associated with an extensive tearing of the tendinous portion of the subscapularis tendon and approximately half of these result from a traumatic incident.

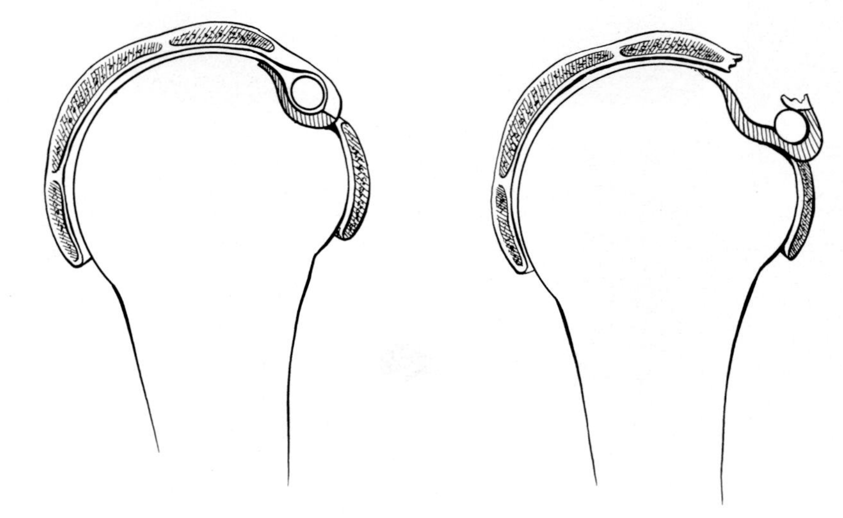

FIG. 9. Schematic showing the anatomic basis of biceps subluxations. Subluxation can occur as a consequence of the loss of the coracohumeral ligament (*hatched*) and superior glenohumeral ligament sling (*black*). An intact subscapularis acts to prevent an otherwise complete dislocation. In type I lesions there is only a superior luxation from a loss of the interval sling. In type II subluxations, the biceps tendon is more unstable distally secondary to a tear of the superior-most fibers of the subscapularis tendon.

Traumatic Lesions of the Biceps Tendon

Traumatic Rupture of the Long Head of the Biceps Tendon

Traumatic rupture of a normal long head of the biceps tendon is extremely uncommon. When ruptures of the long head of the biceps tendon are seen following trauma, they are generally in the context of a previously degenerated tendon. Often the trauma can be relatively minor in these circumstances and is usually preceded by history consistent with rotator cuff tendinitis. However, isolated ruptures of the long head of the biceps can occur in the absence of previous history of subacromial impingement.[25,64,65,83,89] These can be seen in the context of significant trauma involving either a powerful supination force, powerful deceleration of the forearm during pitching, or fall on an outstretched arm as in SLAP lesions.[6,91–93] Type IV SLAP lesions, which include an extension of the labral tear into the intratendinous substance of the biceps, are an example of primary partial ruptures of the biceps tendon from trauma.

When partial tearing of the biceps tendon occurs, often significant pain and dysfunction are associated with the lesion. A higher suspicion of a partial-thickness traumatic tear of the biceps tendon again should be considered in the context of previous tendinitis or bicipital-like pain. In contrast, full-thickness traumatic ruptures of the biceps tendon are generally less consequential from a symptomatic point of view.[16,40,100] In these cases, the patient may have experienced significant pain in the upper and anterior brachium. This is often associated with bruising down the biceps muscle. After a period of discomfort, the pain generally subsides and the patients are generally without significant consequence to the shoulder function.

Tears of the Superior Labrum at the Origin of the Biceps Tendon

Even though tendinitis of the biceps tendon has long been recognized as a cause of shoulder pain, a symptomatic tear of the superior labrum at the origin of the biceps tendon has only recently been established as a pathologic entity. First described in athletes by Andrews et al., the lesion has been further characterized and classified by Snyder et al., who are also responsible for attaching the acronym SLAP to these findings.[6,91–93] Although both reports included patients with tears of the superior labrum at the origin of the biceps tendon, diagnosed arthroscopically, the patient populations seem to differ. Andrews et al. retrospectively identified 73 throwing athletes (51 baseball players) with no history of a single episode of significant trauma and a mean age of 23 years.[6] In Snyder's series, the 27 patients with superior labral lesions represented about 4% of the total arthroscopic procedures performed over a 4-year period.[93] With a mean age of 37.5 years, the most common mechanism of injury (48%) was compression injury resulting from a fall on the outstretched hand. The remainder seemed to arise from traction injuries, either as a sudden pull on the arm (22%) or repetitive traction with overhead throwing activities (8%). The mechanism was unclear in the remaining 22% with no history of these activities.[93]

Both of these populations, although different in presentation, most likely represent a spectrum of the same pathology, one arising from the repetitive trauma of overhead activities, the latter from a single traumatic episode.

It is postulated that a fall on the outstretched hand with the shoulder abducted and in slight forward flexion provides a proximal subluxing force, resulting in direct compression at the superior labrum and biceps origin. An additional traction force may be provided by the reflex contraction of the biceps during the fall. Starting posteriorly on the superior aspect of the labrum, the tear extends anteriorly, ending near the middle glenoid notch. The tear may involve and extend along the long head of the biceps tendon. Repeated transmitted force through the origin of the long head of the biceps may account for the detachment of the labrum in throwing athletes.[6] The maximum traction probably occurs as a consequence of the burst of activity in the biceps during the deceleration of the follow-through phase of the throwing act.[4]

Although it would appear that the production of symptoms in superior labral lesions may be a consequence of repeated displacements of the unstable labral–tendinous complex, some authors believe that superior labral lesions are symptomatic by leading to anterosuperior microinstability of the glenohumeral articulation.[30]

Traumatic disruption of the superior labrum can occur to varying extents and has been classified into four types, based on the labral injury and the stability of the labrum–biceps complex found at arthroscopy (Fig. 10).[92]

Type I: This lesion represents the mildest of the spectrum. The superior labrum appears degenerated and frayed. The attachment of the labrum and long head of the biceps tendon are preserved and stable when probed. The long head of the biceps has a normal appearance.

Type II: The frayed superior labrum and the attached tendon of the long head of the biceps are stripped off the underlying glenoid in association with avulsion of the superior glenohumeral ligament complex. The superior labrum arches away from the glenoid and can be lifted off with a probe. The peripheral detachment of the labrum seen in type II lesions differentiates these from the normal loose attachment of the superior labrum in its central portion.

Type III: In type III lesions, the superior labrum develops a tear, with a stable labrum–biceps complex, similar to the bucket-handle tear of the knee meniscus. The origin of the long head of the biceps and the superior glenohumeral ligament complex retain their attachment to the glenoid, differentiating it from a type II lesion. The torn labrum devoid of any peripheral attachment can be displaced into the glenohumeral joint.

Type IV: The central tear includes a portion of the biceps tendon. The biceps tendon is thus split longitudinally into an intact peripheral portion and a central portion displaced

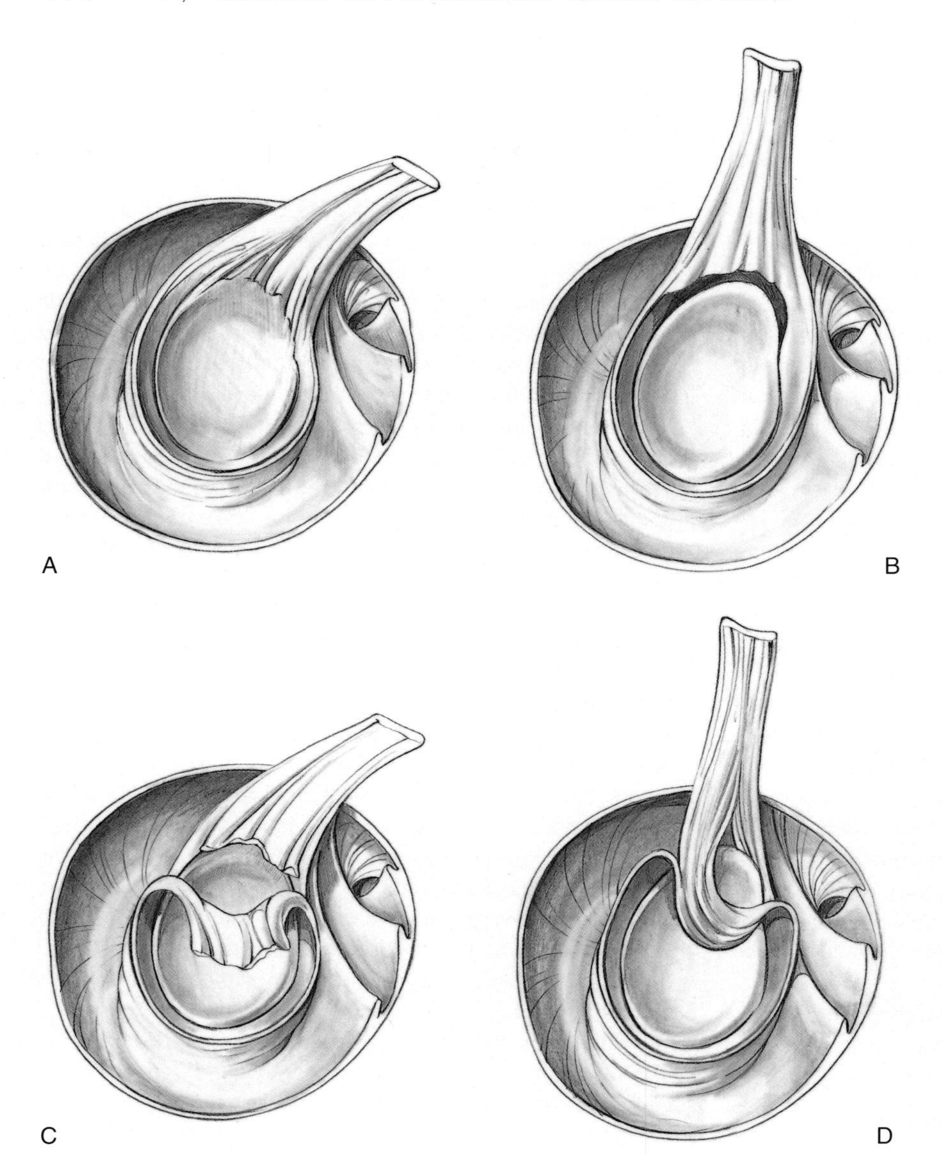

FIG. 10. Schematic of the four types of SLAP lesions: **(A)** Type I is a significant fraying or degeneration of the superior labrum. **(B)** Type II SLAP lesions are characterized by detachment of the superior labrum and biceps tendon from the glenoid rim. **(C)** Type III SLAP lesions are seen as a bucket-handle tearing of the superior labrum. The remaining labral tissue maintains the biceps as anchored to the glenoid rim. **(D)** Type IV SLAP lesions consist of an extension of the bucket-handle labral tear into the substance of the biceps tendon.

into the joint with the attached bucket-handle tear of the labrum.

Type II and type III lesions were the most common in Snyder's series, accounting for 41% and 33% of the cases, respectively. Although type IV lesions were observed in 15%, type I lesions were the least common, accounting for 11% of the series.

CLINICAL EVALUATION

History

As with all other orthopedic conditions, an accurate and directed history and physical examination is a basic and essential part of the clinical evaluation. This is particularly true in biceps tendon disorders, for imaging studies are often nondiagnostic.

Patients with biceps tendinitis or pain from subluxation always have pain at the bicipital groove.[14,40,71,72] This pain, however, can be difficult to distinguish from anterior subdeltoid pain from impingement syndrome or rotator cuff tendinitis. In most persons, the bicipital groove can be felt as a distinct entity between the greater and lesser tuberosities when the arm is placed in neutral rotation. The pain felt in this location should migrate laterally with external rotation of the arm. Often, this pain radiates down anteriorly to the biceps muscle belly. This is different from the pain of rotator cuff tendinitis that generally radiates to the deltoid insertion. Generally, the patient experiences the pain with activities, particularly repetitive overhead types seen in sports. Resting pain is seen later in the disease progression and can be a significant component of night pain. When involved with calcific tendinitis, the pain can be of such intensity that it may mimic a septic shoulder.

In bicipital tendinitis, it is almost always accompanied by rotator cuff inflammatory symptoms.[69] The patient will complain of pain in the anterior aspect of the arm, particularly with extension and internal rotation. Impingement signs, such as those described by Neer and Hawkins, are generally positive.[70,71] We have found the lift-off sign, as described by Gerber, to be helpful not only for detecting subscapularis tears, but also as a sensitive test for eliciting impingement-type pain in patients with bicipital tendinitis.[37] Additionally, those patients with rotator cuff tendinitis with more severe symptoms and signs, including restriction of shoulder motion, are those more likely to have a component of bicipital tendinitis. Whether they are in association with tendinitis or full-thickness tears of the cuff, inflammation of the biceps tendon can be a major source of additional discomfort. A significant pain that can sometimes accompany inflammation of the long head of the biceps has led some authors to believe it to be a possible etiology in the development of frozen shoulder. DePalma reported a 40% incidence of frozen shoulder in bicipital tendinitis, particularly in the 45- to 55-year-old age group.[25] Modern interpretation of those findings is that the intraarticular synovitis associated with frozen shoulder preceded the bicipital involvement. When long-standing, the pain from the long head of the biceps tendon can spontaneously resolve, following a full thickness rupture (Fig. 11). This dramatic relief of symptoms has been termed rupture salvatrice or saving rupture. The rupture of the degenerated long head of the biceps is sometimes accompanied by bruising down the front of the arm, along the biceps muscle belly, in the presence of a lump on the anterior lateral aspect of the arm. When impingement-like pain is persistent following a rupture, further evaluation of the rotator cuff is warranted.

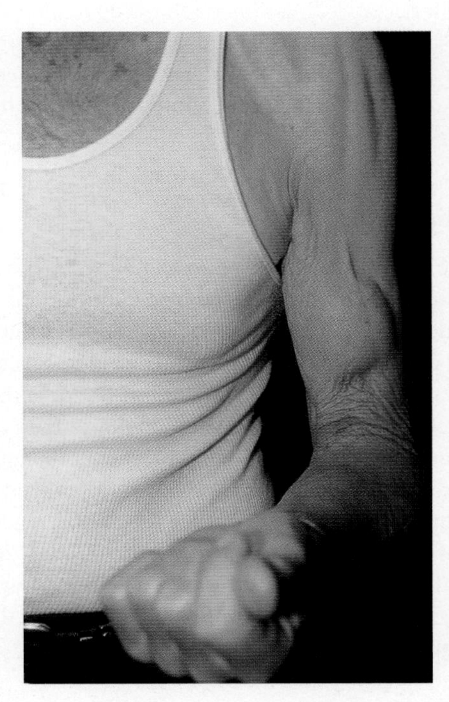

FIG. 11. This is a 68-year-old patient, with a long history of pain in the shoulder. The patient experienced a spontaneous resolution of the pain following a full-thickness rupture of the long head of the biceps tendon. The rupture of the long head of the biceps tendon is noted by a shortening of the lateral biceps muscle seen as a lump on the anterior lateral aspect of the arm.

Instability of the biceps tendon, in the form of subluxation, is extremely difficult to assess nonsurgically. Patients who develop this condition are more likely to be young, overhead athletes.[77] They can often notice a painful snapping or clicking sensation in the shoulder, especially with overhead positions going from internal to external rotation. It is unclear why these symptoms occur, for the tendon is generally fixed in a luxated location. As subluxation generally occurs in the presence of partial- or full-thickness surrounding rotator cuff defects, the symptoms are concurrent with those usually found with rotator cuff disease.

Frank dislocations of the long head of the biceps tendon are seen in the dominant shoulder of middle-aged men.[80,81] The cause of this location is traumatic in most cases. As with subluxation of the biceps, motion of the shoulder will aggravate the pain, especially in those of forced internal–external rotation, as seen with throwing. Recurrent dislocation of the tendon of the groove can often be accompanied by a snapping sensation, sometimes causing a sudden reflex dropping of the arm. The symptoms are similar to those seen in recurrent subluxation or dislocation of the glenohumeral joint.

Lesions of the superior labrum (SLAP) are similarly difficult to assess from history alone. These lesions are generally seen in younger patients who are extremely active in overhead activities. The most common cause, however, is a fall on the outstretched arm in which the proposed mechanism is a pinching of the humeral head against the superior labrum.[93] A history of snapping or popping can also accompany these types of disorders.[24,93,84]

Physical Examination

The most common finding on physical examination for disorders of the long head of the biceps tendon is point tenderness over the intertubercular sulcus. This is most easily distinguished with the arm in 10 degrees of internal rotation, when the biceps groove generally faces anteriorly and can be palpated approximately 7-cm distal to the acromion. In this position, the lesser and greater tuberosities can generally be palpated to locate the bicipital groove. The pain at the bicipital groove can be distinguished from the anterior shoulder pain, commonly associated with rotator cuff disorders, by externally rotating the arm. Pain specific to the biceps tendon should move laterally with external rotation in the arm in contrast to subcoracoid pain.[36] Unless there is complete disruption of the transverse humeral ligament and luxation of the biceps tendon out of the groove, the long head of the biceps tendon can not be directly palpated. When dislocated, the biceps tendon can be rolled under the fingers of the examiner, and this can exacerbate the tenderness.[25] Actual palpation of the tendon, however, is generally rare, and symptoms emanating from the bicipital groove are difficult to distinguish between tendinitis and instability.

Several specific physical examination tests have been described to isolate the biceps tendon as a source of pathology. These tests help localize the tenderness to the biceps tendon, but they are not specific for any particular pathology. They include the following:

1. Speed's test or bicipital resistance test: The patient attempts to flex the arm with the forearm supinated and the elbow at approximately 30 degrees of flexion. A positive test is indicated by pain in the region of the bicipital groove.[38,71]
2. Yergason's test: Resisted supination of the forearm, with the elbow flexed 90 degrees and the arm at the side, can cause pain, specifically at the bicipital groove.[104]
3. Biceps instability test: In this test, dislocation of the tendon is elicited as a palpable and sometimes audible clicking as the biceps tendon is forcibly subluxated or dislocated. This is performed by placing the arm in full abduction and external rotation. The arm is then slowly brought down to the side in the plane of the scapula in progressive internal rotation.[1]
4. Shoulder compression test: This is performed with the patient supine, the shoulder abducted to 90 degrees, and the elbow flexed to 90 degrees. The compression force is applied to the humerus, which when rotated, can sometimes elicit either pain or snapping of labrum. The test is analogous to the McMurray's compression test for meniscal tears in the knees.[93]
5. Modified biceps tension test: This test, designed to test superior labral lesions, is performed by holding the shoulder in 90 degree abduction and the forearm supinated. Pain is seen on application of a downward-directed force applied to the distal forearm.[84]
6. Lift-off examination: Because instability of the biceps is so often associated with a loss of integrity of the subscapularis tendon, the lift-off test is an essential portion of the biceps evaluation. The lift-off test, as described by Gerber, is performed by placing the arm just short of maximal internal rotation and extension. The patient is then asked to actively lift the back of the hand off the belt line or buttock, depending on the amount of internal rotation achievable. The modified lift-off test is performed by placing the arm in maximal internal rotation, with the back of the hand posterior to the belt line or the buttock. A positive result is seen when the patient cannot keep the hand in this position, and it falls to the buttock or belt line. The hallmark of a positive test is a significant difference between active and passive maximal internal rotation and extension.[36] Positive examination results are highly suggestive of subscapularis tears. Additionally, as noted by Gerber, pain during this test serves as a sensitive indicator of impingement. Placement of the humeral head in internal rotation and extension positions the posterior rotator cuff under stretch and up against the acromial arch.

Once these tests are performed, an essential part of the clinical evaluation for disorders of the long head of the biceps is the use of differential injections. Initially, a subacromial injection should be performed with lidocaine. The injection of a local anesthetic into a subacromial space is generally very effective for temporarily alleviating symptoms associated with rotator cuff tendinitis.[9,18,55] In the absence of a full-thickness tear, pain from the biceps tendon should remain persistent. Because the long head of the biceps occupies an intraarticular location, the use of a subacromial injection should not have a direct and immediate effect on pain associated with the tendon. In those cases with persistent pain, despite a subacromial injection, an intraarticular injection of lidocaine is then administered.[9,14] Resolution of symptoms, particularly at the biceps groove or with any of the specific biceps examinations following an intraarticular injection, is relatively accurate for biceps tendon pathology.[9,72] When symptoms are not improved with an intraarticular injection, two clinical scenarios should be considered: (a) Marked inflammation within the intertubercular portion of the biceps tendon is preventing the infiltration of a local anesthetic in this location, or (b) an alternative etiology for anterior shoulder pain exists.

When a significant concern for biceps tendon pathology exists despite a negative intraarticular test, a direct injection of the biceps tendon sheath within the bicipital groove can be attempted. When done in a blind fashion, this injection can be difficult because direct injection of the tendon should be avoided.[55] Accuracy of this injection can be improved significantly by performing it under ultrasound guidance. An injection of a local anesthetic should reliably relieve pain specific to the long head of the biceps tendon.

Diagnostic Imaging

Despite significant progress in shoulder diagnostic techniques, such as MRI or high-resolution ultrasound, imaging for disorders of the biceps tendon and superior labrum has remained difficult and nonspecific. The value of plain films, MRI, ultrasonography, or arthrography has come more from the characterization of associated pathology, such as rotator cuff disease. Although the long head of the biceps tendon and superior labrum can at times be well visualized by some of these methods, any finding must be strictly placed in the context of a history and physical examination. Conversely, the lack of positive findings does not rule out, or even deem less likely, the presence of significant long head of the biceps tendon pathology.

Plain Films

The imaging of a painful shoulder begins with plain films. In our institution a standard shoulder series of plain radiographs includes, anteroposterior view with the humerus in internal rotation, posterior oblique true anteroposterior view of the shoulder in external rotation, supraspinatus outlet view, and axillary lateral. Plain radiography of the shoulder may demonstrate radiographic changes of an associated long-standing rotator cuff disease, with sclerosis of the greater tuberosity, anterior acromial spurs, and decrease in the subacromial space.[43] When a disorder of the long head of the biceps is suspected, specific additional views can be a useful adjunct.

Although the tuberosities are visible on anteroposterior and axillary views, special views to visualize the bicipital groove have been described. The groove view described by Cone permits measurement of the depth and width of the groove as well as the slope of the medial wall and may demonstrate degenerative changes in half the patients with tendinitis.[2–4] This study is obtained with the patient supine and the arm in external rotation. The x-ray beam is directed cephalad and 15 degrees medial to the long axis of the humerus toward the film cassette, which rests on the superior aspect of the shoulder.

Arthrography

Arthrography can be a valuable adjunctive tool in the evaluation of biceps-related shoulder pain. The accuracy in the diagnosis of rotator cuff disease has been well established when leakage of dye injected into the shoulder joint is seen in the subacromial space.[2] The ability to visualize the tendon sheath by arthrography has extended its indications to evaluation of the long head of the biceps tendon. There are two openings normally present in the shoulder capsule: the first being the subscapularis bursa, and the second, the biceps tendon synovial sheath. Preliminary scout films are obtained, anteroposterior views in internal and external rotation and abduction of the shoulder, axillary view, and a bicipital groove view. In obtaining anteroposterior views, the tube is tilted approximately 15 to 20 degrees caudad to allow visualization of the subacromial space, without posterior overlap by the acromion.[87] Normally the entire shoulder should fill from the glenoid to the anatomic neck without any irregularities. When the biceps tendon sheath and tendon outline is easily visualized without any narrowing or vacuolization, significant inflammation is unlikely (Fig. 12).[70] Loss of the sharp delineation of the long head tendon may suggest the presence of associated synovitis. The main drawback of arthrography is that filling of the sheath of the biceps tendon is unreliable, and it may be absent in up to 31% of arthrograms, especially in the presence of full-thickness cuff tears.[66,67] The absence of filling of a normal tendon, hence, may be difficult to differentiate from rupture. Although vacuolization of the sheath with narrowing of the contrast may be noted in some cases, often there may be no difference in the pattern of filling of the tendon sheath in tendinitis compared with normal tendons.[3,4] Because of this, arthrography of the shoulder can be of limited value in the diagnosis of bicipital tendinitis without atrophy, fraying, or subluxation of the tendon.[4] Arthrography can be useful for demonstration of the bony configuration of the bicipital groove and sensitive for the detection of subluxation of the biceps tendon medially out of the groove.[71] The sensitivity for detection of subluxation or dislocation of the tendon can be enhanced with computed tomographic (CT) arthrography.[40] Although useful at times, arthrography has become less popular in the age of MRI and ultrasonography

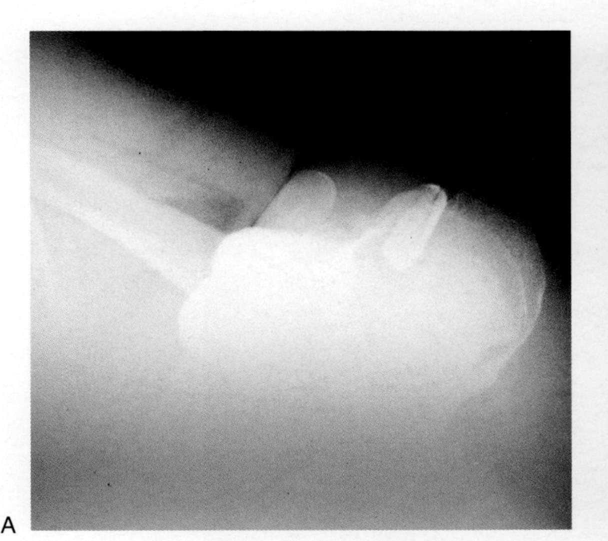
A

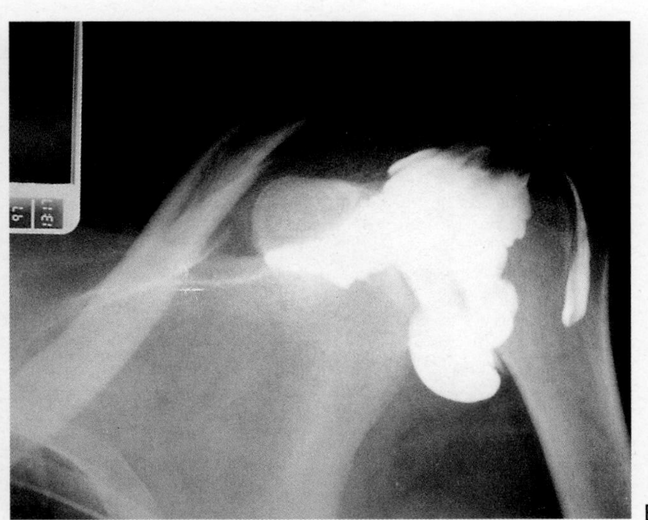
B

FIG. 12. Arthrogram of the glenohumeral joint showing the relation of the biceps tendon. **(A)** Contrast dye is normally seen down the biceps tendon sheath, and a tendon outline can generally be visualized. In absence of any significant narrowing or vacuolization, this generally indicates that inflammation is unlikely. **(B)** Dye in the bicipital groove can also be seen on the biceps view.

because it is an invasive procedure with potential side effects, such as exacerbation of shoulder pain, and complications, such as allergic reaction to the contrast medium, and infection.[42]

Ultrasonography

In the late 1980s, with improving technology and expertise, ultrasonography became increasingly applied for the diagnosis of shoulder pathologies. Ultrasonography has the advantage of correlating, in a dynamic fashion, abnormal findings with clinical sites of tenderness.[5,60,66,67] The test is noninvasive, relatively inexpensive, and offers the opportunity for bilateral examinations at the same sitting. The tendon can be best imaged by transverse scanning at the bicipital groove.[66,67] The normal tendon appears as an echogenic ellipse within the groove (Fig. 13). Proximal to the groove, the tendon is visible lying against the humeral head, covered by the supraspinatus posterosuperiorly, and by the subscapularis anteroinferiorly. On longitudinal imaging, the tendon appears as a narrow band of tissue between the humerus and the deltoid, differentiated from the latter by its greater echogenicity. Absence of the biceps tendon in its sheath indicates rupture, or dislocation, out of the groove. Ultrasound can detect effusions within the sheath of the biceps and can also detect other abnormalities in the groove, such as osteo-

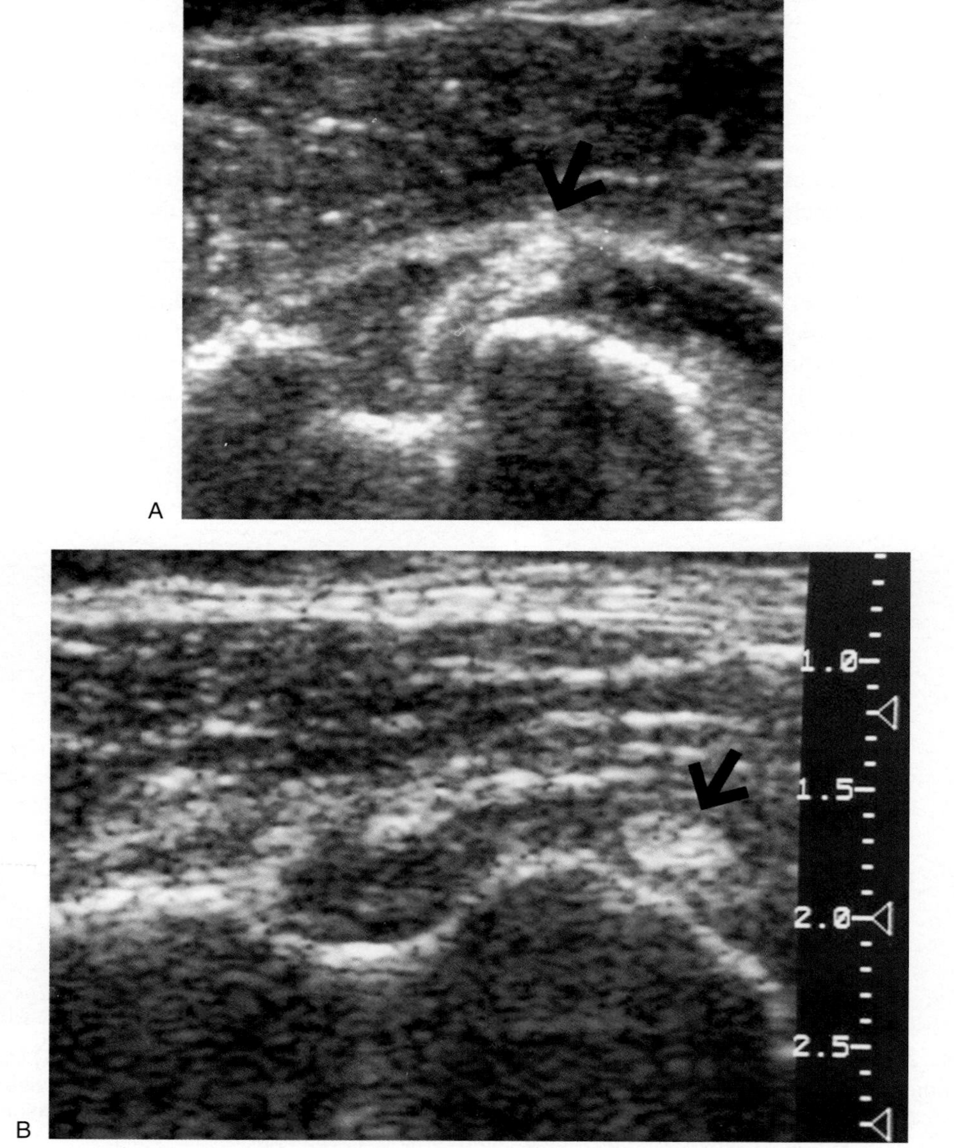

FIG. 13. (A,B) Ultrasound views of the biceps tendon and its relation to the intertubercular groove.

cartilaginous loose bodies. In a prospective study of 80 patients, Middleton et al. compared the value of sonography and arthrography for the detection of lesions at the bicipital groove and distally in the biceps tendon.[66] In 20% of cases, who had negative arthrograms for biceps lesions, effusions of the sheath of the biceps tendon were demonstrated by ultrasonography. Most of these patients had other associated pathology in the shoulder.

In our experience, ultrasonography has been extraordinarily accurate in defining not only the presence of associated rotator cuff defects, but also in precise characterization of the morphology.[103] Subtle partial-thickness or full-thickness defects in the anterior edge of the supraspinatus or superior edge of the subscapularis, as seen with tendon instability, can be visualized with surprising accuracy. These improvements have followed recent technologic gains in the resolution of the scanners and refinements in technique gained with increasing clinical experience.

There are some limitations to ultrasonography. The test is highly dependent on the technical expertise of the radiologist, and currently is not widely available. Additionally, the viewing area is constrained by the bony anatomy. Because the acromial process can not be penetrated, medial pathology at the joint line, such as labral defects, are not well visualized. Given these disadvantages it is anticipated that ultrasonography will become increasingly popular secondary to significant advantages in cost-effectiveness, patient tolerance, bilateral information, and associated accuracy.

Magnetic Resonance Imaging

Magnetic resonance imaging provides high-resolution soft-tissue imaging in a noninvasive fashion and has the advantage of a multiplanar study of the shoulder.[49] In addition, the morphology of the bicipital groove can be studied, and bony osteophytes or other abnormalities can be detected.[17] Images in the axial plane and in the coronal oblique and sagittal oblique planes (with reference to the plane of the subscapularis) are used for a routine shoulder study. In axial images, the biceps tendon can be identified on T1-weighted images as a round, low-signal intensity structure contained in the bicipital groove. The tendon of the subscapularis muscle can be visualized sweeping anterior from the tendon to its insertion on the lesser tuberosity. In the coronal oblique sections, the tendon is seen as a linear structure between the greater and lesser tuberosities. Sagittal oblique sections can demonstrate segments of the tendon within the groove. In bicipital tendinitis, an effusion may be noted in the tendon sheath, with or without, a corresponding effusion in the shoulder joint. A thickening of the tendon may be observed in some patients with hypertrophic tendinitis. An empty groove in the axial section suggests rupture or dislocation of the tendon. A medially dislocated tendon should be considered in these patients. It is important to follow the tendon on serial axial sections to avoid mistaking osteophytes in the groove for the tendon. As a high incidence of abnormalities or disruption of the subscapularis tendon is reported in association with luxation of the biceps tendon, special attention should be given to it. Because the long head of the biceps tendon is not visualized in continuity, it is easy to miss subluxations or even dislocations of the tendon between slices.

Use of MRI has not proved useful in the diagnosis of superior labral lesions, with reports of a positive scan in only about a third of cases.[30] Magnetic resonance arthrography, employing the intraarticular injection of gadolinium, has been reported to provide better definition of labral lesions than conventional MRI, but the accuracy has not been sufficient to make definitive diagnosis.[31]

The value of MRI appears to be more for defining associated shoulder pathology, such as partial- or full-thickness rotator cuff tears.[49] However, it is an expensive, and sometimes poorly tolerated test, and is generally not recommended as the procedure of choice for imaging the long head of the biceps tendon or superior labrum.

TREATMENT

Nonoperative

Nonoperative treatment of long head of the biceps tendinitis has generally been directed toward treatment of the rotator cuff. A failure to improve, or a deterioration, in symptoms is more often seen in those patients with a component of biceps tendinitis. Biceps tendinitis is typically more resistant to treatment and does not respond to subacromial steroid injections.[14,71–73] Consequently, direct tendon sheath injections have been suggested when subacromial ones have failed. DePalma, in a series of 18 cases treated for isolated bicipital tenosynovitis, reported improvement in 10 when given a series of hydrocortisone injections into the tendon directly under the transverse ligament.[25] More modern concerns for atrophic tendon changes from the steroid have led to recommendations for sheath injections in preference to intratendinous ones.[55] A 74% favorable and excellent result has been reported with this approach.[55] Technical difficulties associated with blind injection of biceps tendon sheath have led to recommendations for intraarticular injections as an alternative method.

Very little information is available about the nonoperative treatment of SLAP lesions or long head of the biceps instability. Because tendon instability almost invariably follows the development of major rotator cuff pathology, treatment is again directed primarily along those guidelines. With instability of the biceps, nonoperative measures are less likely to be successful and earlier operative intervention or prolonged activity restriction is required.

Spontaneous or traumatic ruptures of the long head of the biceps tendon do not require operative intervention.[14,16,40] Although, associated with a cosmetic defect, the long-term functional and symptomatic sequelae are minimal. Mariani et al. compared 26 patients who underwent early tenodesis of a rupture of the long head of the biceps with 30 patients who had nonsurgical treatment.[62] Residual pain was infrequent for both groups. On biomechanical testing the nonsurgical group lost 21% of supination strength versus 8% for the surgical group. There was no significant difference in elbow flexion. The nonsurgical patients returned to work earlier. Similar results were reported by Warren, who showed no loss of elbow flexion strength and only 10% supination loss.[100]

Authors' Preferred Treatment

Long Head of the Biceps Tendinitis

Nonoperative treatment is primarily directed at the accompanying rotator cuff tendinitis. This includes rest, local modalities, such as ice, nonsteroidal antiinflammatory medication, physical therapy, and local steroid injections.[68,82] When patients present with acute or significantly painful shoulders, initial treatment is directed toward inflammation control instead of strengthening. Starting physical therapy at this time may cause exacerbation of symptoms. Rather, a short period of rest or reduction of activities is recommended.

Nonsteroidal oral medication given at antiinflammatory doses is used in conjunction with local measures such as ice. Many patients who present for orthopedic consultation have some history of nonsteroidal use. However, dosages and compliance are often insufficient for anything more than an analgesic effect. To achieve maximal antiinflammatory benefit, such medication should be taken in a sustained fashion and at antiinflammatory doses.

Subacromial injections are given only in the context of severe night pain or a failure to improve with 6 weeks of treatment. Physical therapy is instituted only after some initial improvement in symptoms. It is directed toward range of motion stretching and rotator cuff strengthening. There is no attempt made to specifically strengthen the biceps muscle. If there are strong signs or suspicions of biceps-related pain, then an intraarticular injection of steroids is considered. Theoretically, to achieve maximum benefit, the steroid should be injected only into the tendon sheath and intratendinous injection avoided. Because this is technically difficult to achieve on a consistent basis, we prefer to inject the solution into the shoulder joint cavity, thereby addressing the intraarticular and extraarticular portions of the tendon.

We generally prefer to perform intraarticular injections from a superior approach, analogous to the superior arthroscopic portal, as described by Neviaser.[74] A spinal needle is required. The entry site is in the supraclavicular region. The needle is inserted 1-cm medial to the medial border of the acromion, just posterior to the clavicle and anterior to the scapular spine. A soft spot can be reliably palpated there. The needle is advanced, aiming 30 degrees anteriorly and 30 degrees laterally. To assist in orientation, the arm is placed 30 degrees of coronal plane abduction, and the needle is directed down the long axis of the arm. On contact with the humeral head, the needle is withdrawn by a few millimiters, and a solution of local anesthetic and water-soluble steroid suspension is injected. Immediate and temporary relief of symptoms is diagnostic and it is hoped, therapeutic.

The patient is monitored at 6-week intervals throughout the nonoperative treatment period (Fig. 14). At each of these follow-up consultations, a reevaluation of progress is coordinated with indications for further workup or treatment changes. When significant improvements are made, a gradual tapering of nonsteroidal medication and progression of activities and physical therapy is attempted. When there are no significant changes, depending on the severity and nature of the symptoms, further observation, without treatment changes, is reasonable. The deterioration of symptoms or a continuation of severe symptoms should alert the treating physician that further workup, or treatment modification, may be indicated. Treatment modification should include differential injections, including intraarticular, as described in the foregoing. Further workup may include imaging for rotator cuff tears and biceps tendon subluxation. Ultrasound, MRI, and CT arthrography are examples of modalities that may provide information about both the rotator cuff and long head of the biceps tendon. If a strong suspicion remains for biceps-related pain despite a negative intraarticular injection, a bicipital groove injection is considered. In our institution, this injection can be performed with high accuracy with the use of ultrasonic guidance. In the absence of any major findings with these studies, nonoperative treatment, including repeat injections (maximum of three) is continued for a minimum of 6 months if the injections are positive (patient experiences some relief of symptoms). In the absence of copathology, such as rotator cuff tears or tendon instability, a high percentage of patients (more than 80%) are expected to experience satisfactory improvement. A negative finding for both imaging studies and injections should alert the treating physician to alternative causes of anterior shoulder pain, including instability, adhesive capsulitis, glenohumeral arthritis, acromioclavicular arthrosis, coracoid impingement syndrome, neurogenic causes, and medical conditions.

Instability of the long head of the biceps and SLAP lesions are generally considered operative indications in those rare circumstances when a strong preoperative diagnosis is available and there is longer than 3 months of pain. Nonoperative treatment for these disorders is limited to rest and intraarticular injections.

Surgical Treatment

As a reflection on the remaining controversies about the functional and symptomatic significance of the long head of the biceps tendon, multiple and often contradictory treatment strategies and indications have been recommended. Options for surgical treatment include benign neglect, with treatment of associated pathology only (i.e., rotator cuff or labral defects); inspection and synovectomy; repair of partial tears; or tenodesis in the intertubercular groove. Currently, concerns

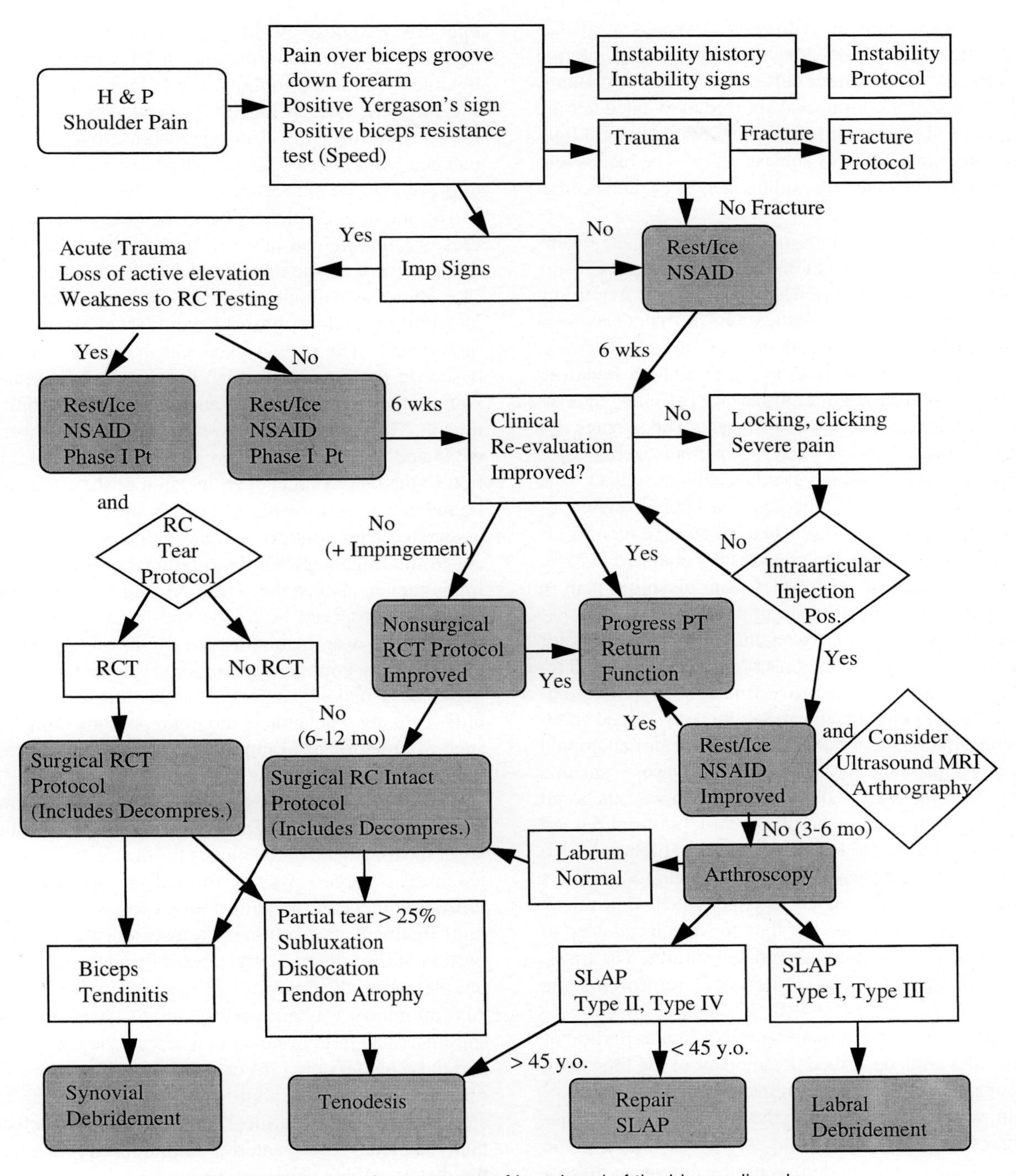

FIG. 14. Algorithm for treatment of long head of the biceps disorders.

about functional deficits created by loss of the long head of the biceps tendon have led to a prevailing operative strategy for avoidance of tenodesis whenever possible.

Treatment for Biceps Tendinitis Associated with Rotator Cuff Disease

Surgery for rotator cuff disorders accounts for most of the cases in which biceps pathology is encountered. Neer recommended routine inspection of the long head of the biceps and intertubercular groove as part of the surgical procedure for impingement syndrome.[69] Neviaser noted pathologic changes in the biceps tendon in all patients with preoperative arthrography.[70] These included vacuolization within the sheath, partial or complete obstruction of dye flow, or subluxation of the tendon. Operative examination of the biceps tendon in the groove at surgery always confirmed these findings of tenosynovitis.[71] Given this experience, they recommended inclusion of biceps tenodesis with excision of the intraarticular segment as part of the surgical procedure for the treatment of impingement syndrome.[73] Walch et al. described the presence of hidden lesions of the rotator interval in 19 of 116 cases with rotator cuff tears.[98] In these patients, exploration of the rotator interval showed associated tearing of the superior glenohumeral ligament, coracohumeral ligament, and superior portion of subscapularis. The biceps tendon was ruptured in 2 patients, subluxated in 14, and normal in 5.

Although the high association of long head of the biceps tendon pathology has not been disputed, indications for surgical treatment have been varied and inconsistent. According to Crenshaw and Kilgore, the indications for tenodesis were pain present for an average of about 5 months, bicipital tenderness, and restriction of motion.[23] The authors reviewed 89 patients who had undergone surgery for bicipital tenosynovitis, with a minimum followup of 1 year. The average age at the time of surgery was 52 years. All patients were treated with bicipital tenodesis using various techniques; most were treated as described by Hitchcock (see later discision).[50] Maximum improvement was reached at about 12 months after surgery, with excellent and good results obtained in 87%. Pain relief was dramatic with relief from disabling pain in 80% by the end of the month, and in 95% by 3 months.

Other early reports similarly recommended tenodesis for shoulder pain unresponsive to conservative measures and regardless of the extent of operative findings. Lippmann observed a relief of symptoms in patients who developed spontaneous adhesion of the tendon in its groove and attempted to surgically reproduce the same in acute cases.[61] In this technique, the long head of the biceps tendon was anchored in its groove with several nonabsorbable sutures passed through drill holes in the lesser tuberosity. Hitchcock also described fixation of the tendon in the bicipital groove.[50] His technique, however, created an osteoperiosteal flap raised from the floor of the groove. The tendon was placed deep to this flap and secured with nonabsorbable sutures. The transverse humeral ligament was sutured over reinforcing the repair.

With concerns over the remaining intraarticular portion of the tendon, DePalma described detachment of the long head of the biceps from its origin and removal from the groove.[25] The origin was then transferred to the coracoid process adjacent to the conjoined tendon of the coracobrachialis and the short head of the biceps tendon. With the extensive dissection involved and development of tenderness over the coracoid in some patients, he later discontinued this treatment and recommended fixation of the tendon in the roughened groove by a staple. An alternative and popular technique for the long head of the biceps tenodesis after release of the intraarticular origin, as described by Froimson and termed the keyhole technique, involved placement of a rolled or knotted biceps tendon into a keyhole-shaped through which had been drilled in the bicipital groove (Fig. 15).[33]

Neer highlighted the importance of mechanical impingement from the anterior acromial arch as the primary cause of anterior shoulder pain.[69] In a series of 50 shoulders, with preoperative diagnosis of biceps tenosynovitis, only 30% had significant biceps abnormalities and favorable results were obtained with acromioplasty alone. In this series, tenodesis was rarely performed, and biceps-related symptoms were reliably resolved from decompression alone. Neer recommended avoidance of biceps tenodesis, whenever possible, to prevent a loss of head depressor effect.[69]

The importance of treating associated rotator cuff disorders was highlighted in several other series. In a retrospective review of 20 shoulders in 18 patients who underwent biceps tenodesis without subacromial decompression, Dines et al. reported good results in 14 shoulders at a mean follow-up of 3 years.[26] The patients were categorized into two groups based on findings at surgery: those with inflammatory lesions in the bicipital groove, and those with instability of the tendon. Most of the patients were young, with an average age of 33 and 35 years in the two groups, respectively. In addition to the biceps procedure, incision of the coracoacromial ligament was performed in 14 of 20 cases. Poor results were associated with younger age and failure to release the coracoacromial ligament. Of the 6 failures, 4 were attributed to impingement against the acromion, and glenohumeral instability was observed in 2. The authors recommend careful preoperative examination for the exclusion of glenohumeral instability in younger patients and suggest that acromioplasty be a major component of the surgical procedure in older patients. The authors did not report any complications, such as superior head migration, arising from tenodesis of the long head.

Becker and Cofield reported the long-term follow-up of 54 shoulders at an average of 13 years after surgical tenodesis of the long head of the biceps for the treatment of chronic tendinitis.[8] Surgery was performed through a limited deltopectoral incision. As part of the exposure, the coracoacromial ligament was routinely transected, the intraarticular portion of the long head was removed and the remainder was tenodesed at the bicipital groove or to the short head. Acromioplasty was not performed. At latest follow-up, 22 shoulders had mild or no pain, whereas, the other 22 continued to be moderately (16) or severely (10) painful. Twenty-nine patients needed additional treatment in the form of steroid injections or surgical procedures (8%), including rotator cuff tear repairs, anterior acromioplasty, or excision of the distal clavicle. They advised against bicipital tenodesis without decompression as the primary surgical procedure because of deteriorating long-term results. In their opinion tenodesis is indicated if, during a surgical procedure directed primarily at the rotator cuff, degenerative changes are encountered in the biceps tendon, or if the tendon is unstable or displaced from its groove.

In contrast to the Becker and Cofield, tenodesis of the long head of the biceps has been reported to have good results even when not performed in conjunction with a decompression of the coracoacromial arch. Post and Benca showed 94% excellent results in a series of 13 patients with primary bicipital tendinitis.[83] Berlemann and Bayley reported im-

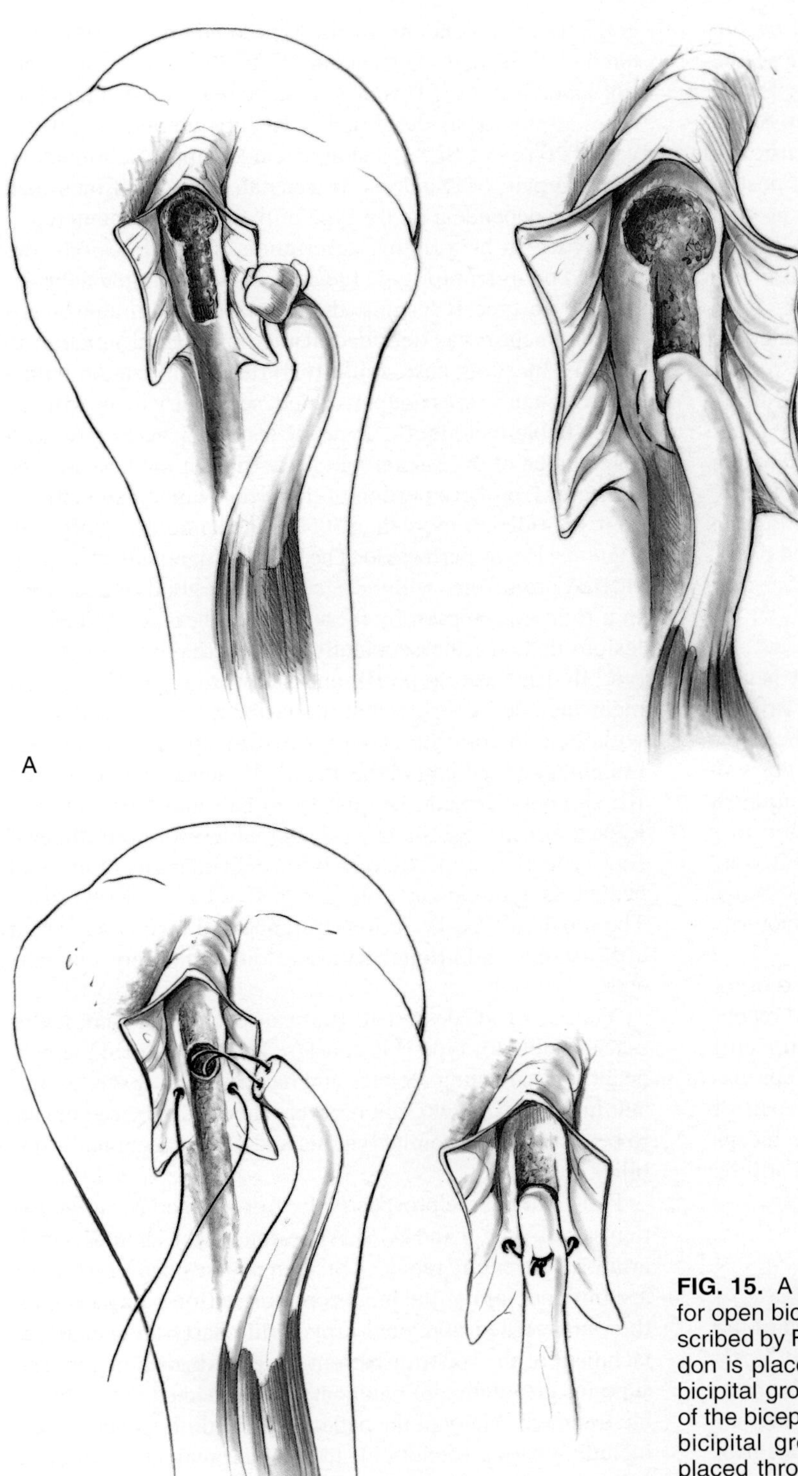

FIG. 15. A schematic representation of two popular techniques for open biceps tenodesis. **(A)** In the keyhole technique, as described by Froimson, the knotted proximal end of the biceps tendon is placed into a keyhole slot that had been drilled into the bicipital groove. **(B)** In the Post technique, the proximal portion of the biceps tendon is inserted into a round hole drilled into the bicipital groove. A tendon-grasping stitch, which had been placed through the proximal end of the tendon, is brought into the hole and out through two drill holes. The tendon is then sutured into itself.

proved results of biceps tenodesis with long-term follow-up.[9] Of interest, 8 of the 15 cases in this series had persistent pain following decompression. Six of the 8 then had complete resolution of the symptoms following biceps tenodesis.

Although the long-term results as reported by Becker and Cofield would suggest a relatively poor outcome for an isolated biceps tenodesis, no studies have shown adverse results when performed in conjunction with a decompression of the coracoacromial arch. Neviaser and coauthors reported their experience with 89 patients who underwent routine biceps tenodesis as part of the procedure for subacromial decompression.[73] They operated on 89 patients, the average age being 42 years, and evaluated the results at 2 to 8 years. Patient results were based on pain relief and range of motion. All but 1 patient reported no pain (86%) or pain with unaccustomed exertion (13%). Adhesive capsulitis was diagnosed postoperatively in 1 patient, who continued to have pain at night and intermittently during the day. The authors did not report any functional loss secondary to tenodesis of the biceps tendon.

Despite the excellent results reported for biceps tenodesis performed in conjunction with acromioplasty, the routine employment of this procedure is unsupported.[69,87] Multiple studies in which biceps tenodesis was generally avoided during treatment of the rotator cuff have shown good results with decompression and cuff repair alone.[10–13,21,27,28,35,45,48,56,94] It is unclear, however, how many of the failures may have been secondary to persistent biceps-related pain.

Treatment of Biceps Instability

Similar to biceps tendinitis, rotator cuff pathology is generally coexistent with tendon instability. Contrary to surgical treatment of tendinitis, tenodesis has historically been the procedure of choice. O'Donoghue performed tenodesis of the biceps tendon in the groove, using the technique of Hitchcock, as a treatment for unstable biceps tendon in a young population involved in athletic pursuits.[77] Fifty-six operations were performed in 53 patients, with an age range of 15 to 35. Seventy-seven percent could throw satisfactorily and resumed sports.

More recently, biceps instability, seen in the context of rotator interval lesions, has been treated with attempted reconstruction of the coracohumeral ligament and rotator cuff tear.[98] In a series of 14 shoulders with subluxated biceps tendons, an attempt at reinsertion of the tendon and repair of torn structures resulted in secondary rupture of the biceps tendon in 25%. When rupture is not seen, there can still be concerns with autotenodesis with this operative strategy.

Treatment of Long Head of the Biceps Ruptures

Spontaneous or traumatic ruptures of the long head of the biceps do not generally require surgical intervention.[16] Although little information is available about surgical treatment of long head ruptures, one study showed a 21% supination and 8% elbow flexion strength deficit.[63] Pronation, grip, and elbow extension strength were normal. When comparing operative versus nonoperative patient groups in 27 patients, residual pain was uncommon for both, and the nonsurgically treated patients returned to work faster.

Treatment of Superior Labral Disorders

Since the initial description of superior labral lesions, associated with the biceps origin by Snyder, treatment has generally been dependent on the type of pathology encountered.[24,91] Seen, at most, about 5% to 6% of the time, superior labral lesions (SLAP lesion) have been divided into four types as previously described.[92] Treatment options for these various types of SLAP lesions include simple debridement, suture repair, or tenodesis. In general, the type of treatment has been dependent on the type of pathology encountered.

Snyder, in his original description of SLAP lesions, described treatment for type I lesions as being simple debridement.[92] In type II lesions, the superior labrum and biceps tendon anchor was debrided at the bone labral junction to obtain a bleeding base. Initially, further stabilization with a screw or suture was not performed, secondary to an absence of available techniques. Type III lesions were treated with an excision of the bucket-handle portion of the tear. In type IV lesions, the torn portion of the biceps tendon and labrum were debrided. If more than 50% of the tendon was torn then a tenodesis was performed. The short-term results were considered promising, with 88% considered good or excellent. In a follow-up report, by these same authors, of 140 SLAP lesions treated arthroscopically, 21% were type I, 55% were type II, 10% were type III, and 5% were type IV.[93] Treatment included debridement alone for type I; debridement with glenoid abrasion alone for half of the type II, and debridement with repair in the other half; debridement for type III; and debridement for type IV in half and repair in half. Repeat arthroscopy in 18 of the shoulders showed three of five type II lesions treated with debridement alone had healed, in comparison with four of five treated with repair. The repaired type IV lesions all appeared healed on repeat arthroscopy. Additional data and outcome were unavailable.

Yoneda et al. described the use of an arthroscopically placed staple for type II lesions.[105] They performed the procedure in ten young athletes and had a good or excellent result in eight. The two failures were thought to be secondary to persistent subacromial bursitis and multidirectional instability.

Field and Savoie prospectively treated 20 consecutive patients, with type II and IV SLAP lesions of the shoulder, with arthroscopic suture repair.[30] Sixteen patients had a history of a significant injury, the most common reason being a fall on the outstretched abducted arm. Arthroscopy revealed detachment of the superior labrum–biceps tendon anchor. The superior glenohumeral ligament was connected to the unstable fragment. Many of the patients had additional pathology, including partial rotator cuff tears (eight patients), impingement syndrome (five patients), and acromioclavicular arthritis (three patients), which were addressed at the same time. All patients underwent arthroscopic debridement and reattachment of lesion using transglenoid sutures. At an average follow-up of 21 months, the authors report excellent results in 80% and good results in 20%. Although the scores for motion, strength, and stability were improved after surgery, the increase in the pain and function scores was statistically significant.

Arthroscopy

Authors' Preferred Treatment

In the treatment of biceps tendon pathology, the initial modality is generally arthroscopic. Arthroscopy provides a valuable tool to accurately visualize both intraarticular and intertubercular biceps pathology as well as any associated disorders such as rotator cuff tears. As we perform arthroscopy in the beach chair position, open approaches can be easily conducted during the same sitting. Beach chair arthroscopy is performed on a standard operating table. The patient is positioned as far laterally on the table as possible using a universal joint head holder and lateral pad to secure the patient safely. Arthroscopy is then initially performed in the glenohumeral joint through the standard posterior portal. The rotator interval is easily identified within a triangle demarcated by the biceps tendon superiorly, the subscapularis inferiorly and the glenoid medially (Fig. 16). An anterior portal is established in an outside-in fashion by first placing a spinal needle just lateral to the coracoid tip. Needle placement is verified intraarticularly with arthroscopic visualization. A 6.5-mm cannula is then placed with a sharp plastic trocar from outside to in. A standard diagnostic arthroscopy is performed with the arm under slight in-line traction. The articular surfaces of both the humerus and glenoid are thoroughly evaluated. The anterior glenoid labrum is visualized from the midportion of the glenoid to the inferior, observing for labral fraying or detachment, which may suggest instability. Glenohumeral ligaments, particularly the inferior glenohumeral ligament, are then inspected. The scope is then brought to the rotator interval, the superior subscapularis muscle, and the tendon. From this position, the 30-degree scope is pointed laterally out toward the intersection of the biceps tendon and subscapularis (Fig. 17). In this fashion, the entire portion of the superior subscapularis is inspected. The scope is then brought posterior to the biceps tendon to visualize the supra, infra, and teres minor insertions. The scope is then brought out over the top of the humeral head to inspect the bare area for any Hill Sachs type impression fractures. Following this, the scope is then brought up through the posterior aspect glenoid inspecting for any posterior labral defects or any posterior superior inflammation suggestive of internal impingement. The biceps tendon is then inspected at length from its superior labral attachment laterally to the bicipital groove. Under normal conditions, the entrance of the biceps tendon into the groove distally can be easily visualized. The probe is then placed anteriorly under the anterosuperior labrum and the origin of the biceps examined for any detachment suggestive of a superior labral lesion (Fig. 18). The probe is then placed over the top of the biceps tendon to pull the tendon further into the joint to inspect the portion normally within the intraarticular groove (Fig. 19). The humeral head is brought from a position of external rotation into internal rotation to observe whether the biceps tendon is subluxated from the bicipital groove.

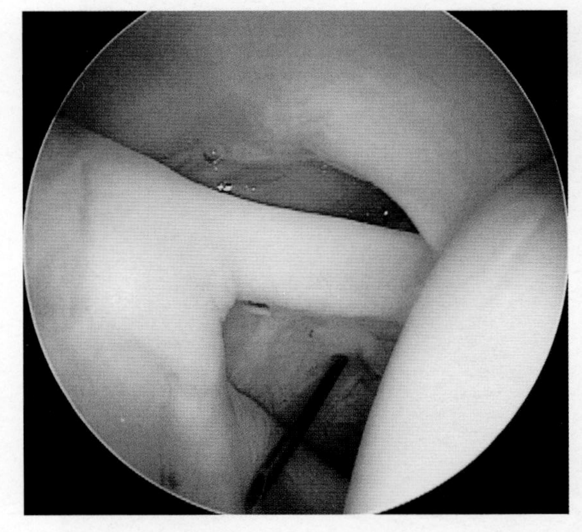

FIG. 16. An arthroscopic view showing the rotator interval. A needle is placed just lateral to the coracoid under arthroscopic visualization to verify the location of the anterior portal.

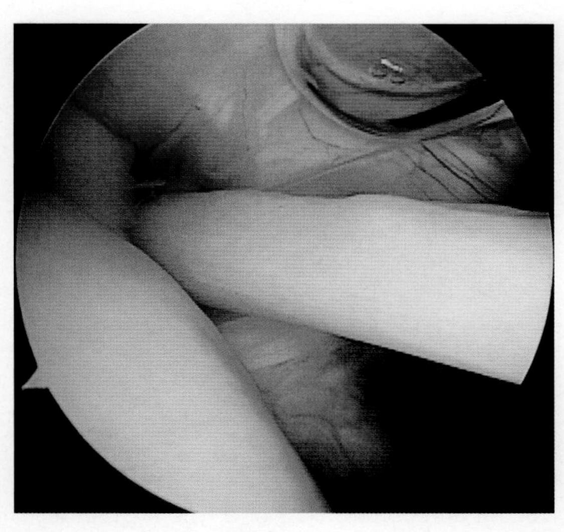

FIG. 17. Arthroscopic view of the entrance to the bicipital groove. The intersection of the subscapularis and supraspinatus with the biceps tendon can be seen at the proximal portion of the bicipital groove. Pathology in this location may indicate a disruption of the rotator interval sling.

Treatment of Bicipital Tendinitis

We determine appropriate surgical treatment for the long head of the biceps tendon according to observations made during surgery. We feel that the biceps tendon can be a significant source of shoulder pain if not specifically addressed during a surgical procedure. This is partly based on multiple observations of patients who had spontaneous resolution of shoulder pain with rupture of the long head. Additionally, as previously described in other studies, we have seen patients, who have failed subacromial decompressions for chronic ro-

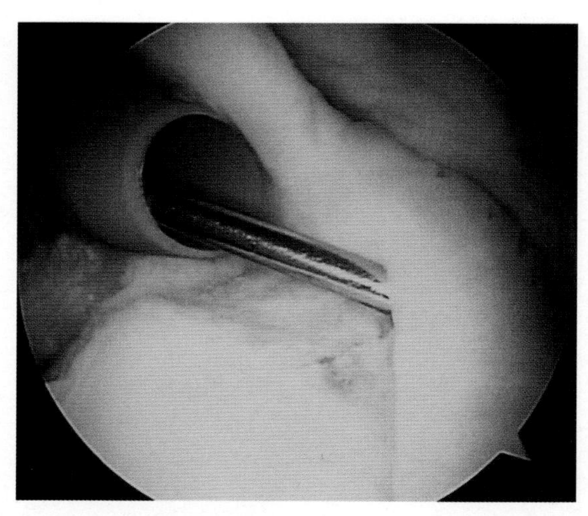

FIG. 18. An arthroscopic view of a type II SLAP lesion. A probe is placed under the anterior superior labrum to detect any detachment of the biceps origin. The probe is placed in from the anterior portal. Notice that easy access for abrasion of the glenoid rim can be achieved from this same portal.

tator cuff tendinitis or rotator cuff tears, who later can achieve satisfactory pain relief from a revision surgery in which a biceps tenodesis is performed. However, we do not feel routine biceps tenodesis is indicated. Given the symptomatic concerns of a significant biceps tendon disorder, we also do not feel a policy of avoidance of tenodesis whenever possible is appropriate. Rather, avoidance of tenodesis is employed whenever it is felt that the inflammatory changes to the biceps tendon are reversible. In general, the criteria for a biceps tendon with reversible changes include less than 25% partial tearing from a normal-width tendon, a normally located tendon within the bicipital groove, and normal tendon size, regardless of associated synovitis. Those surgical observations that are consistent with a biceps tendon with irreversible changes include partial-thickness tearing or fraying of the tendon for more than 25% of the normal width of the tendon, any luxation of the biceps tendon from the bicipital groove, any disruption of the associated bony or ligamentous anatomy of the bicipital groove that would make autotenodesis likely, and any significant reduction or atrophy in the size of the tendon that is more than 25% of the normal ten-

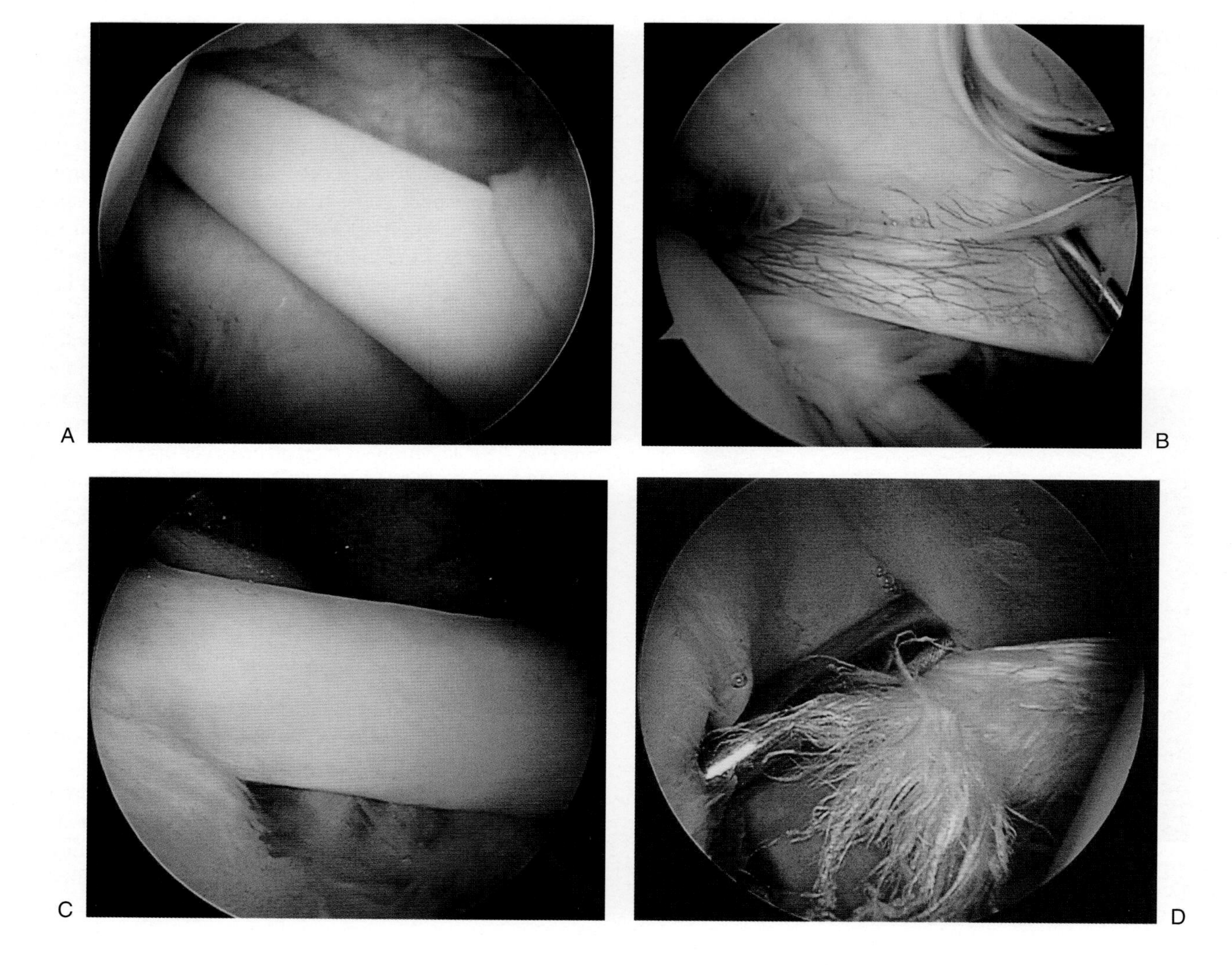

don's width (Fig. 20). Relative indications for biceps tenodesis also include any biceps pathology in the context of a failed acromioplasty, or any significant biceps pathology in the context of a SLAP lesion.

Inflammation of the biceps tendon, or involvement of the biceps tendon within the marked inflammation seen with rotator cuff disease, is treated in the standard fashion for rotator cuff disease alone. It is generally anticipated that adequate treatment of a rotator cuff tendinitis will resolve concurrent bicipital tendinitis. Generally, a florid subscapular synovitis is present, descending from the rotator interval to encompass the anterosuperior and posterosuperior labrum and bicipital groove portion of the biceps tendon (see Fig. 8). We have found a wide dispersion cautery device, such as the multifilament bipolar device (Arthrocare), quite useful in ablating the synovitis. The cautery device is used to vaporize the red, inflamed tissues on the undersurface of the rotator cuff without any penetration through the capsule to the cuff itself. No attempt is made to debride the inflamed synovian overlying the bicipital groove portion of the long head of the biceps.

When a biceps tenodesis is indicated, based on the foregoing criteria, an arthroscopic-assisted approach is generally employed. In this technique, the biceps tendon is first tagged with a no. 2 PDS suture. This is accomplished by placing a spinal needle anterolaterally through the rotator interval. Under arthroscopic guidance, the needle is placed through the substance of the tendon near the bicipital groove entrance (Fig. 21). A no. 2 PDS suture is then threaded through the 18-gauge spinal needle into the joint. A suture grasper is inserted, and the suture is brought out through the anterior portal. In this fashion, the suture prevents any excursion of the long head of the biceps tendon down the arm. Once the biceps tendon is secured with the suture, the origin is released with either electrocautery or an arthroscopic scissor. Generally, after release of the origin, the excursion of the tendon is only 1 to 2 cm. The stay suture is only a preventive measure, for the biceps tendon is wider at the base and generally will not travel down the bicipital groove unless atrophic changes are present.

Securing the tendon in the bicipital groove is achieved by one of two approaches. If a miniopen repair is being performed, then tenodesis is accomplished through the miniopen deltoid splitting approach. The arm is externally rotated at the side to bring the bicipital groove out laterally underneath the deltoid split. The transverse humeral ligament is then divided in line with the groove. The biceps tendon is then delivered out through the deltoid split with the PDS suture in place (Fig. 22). The floor of the groove is roughened with a curette and a single suture anchor placed into the groove. The length of the tendon in the tenodesis is determined by the stay suture that was placed close to the insertion of the biceps tendon in the groove. A tendon grasping stitch is run through the biceps and then back to the suture anchor, to secure it in place. The transverse humeral ligament is then sutured on top of the secured tendon. The excess intraarticular portion of the tendon is excised.

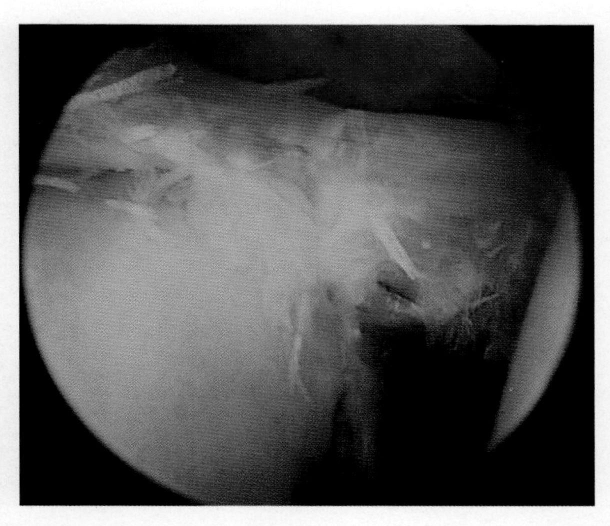

FIG. 20. Arthroscopic view of a biceps tendon with more than 25% fraying in the width of the tendon. In this situation significant, chronic, or posttraumatic changes have occurred that make healing of the tendon less likely and concerns about persistent pain more significant. This is considered an indication for tenodesis.

When a deltoid split is not being performed for the rotator cuff, then an alternative inferior axillary approach is employed, as described for shoulder instability procedures.[101] A 4-cm incision is placed in the axilla, centered on the inferior border of the pectoralis major tendon. Most of the incision should be in the axilla, when the arm is at the side. This incision, made along this line is quite cosmetic and for the most part not visible. Subcutaneous dissection is then taken to the deltoid pectoral interval, and this is then followed to the bicipital groove. The inferior portion of the transverse humeral ligament is then divided in line with the bicipital groove. The tendon is visualized and drawn out of the groove using a curved clamp. It is then secured within the groove us-

FIG. 19. Inspection of the biceps tendon must include the intertubercular groove portion. This is inspected by placing a probe over the top of the biceps tendon and drawing the intertubercular groove portion into the joint: **(A)** A normal-appearing biceps tendon. **(B)** When the intertubercular groove portion is drawn into the joint with a probe, a marked amount of synovitis is recognized. **(C)** Again, the biceps tendon appears to be normal in the intraarticular portion. **(D)** When a probe is used to draw in the intertubercular groove portion a significant partial tear is detected.

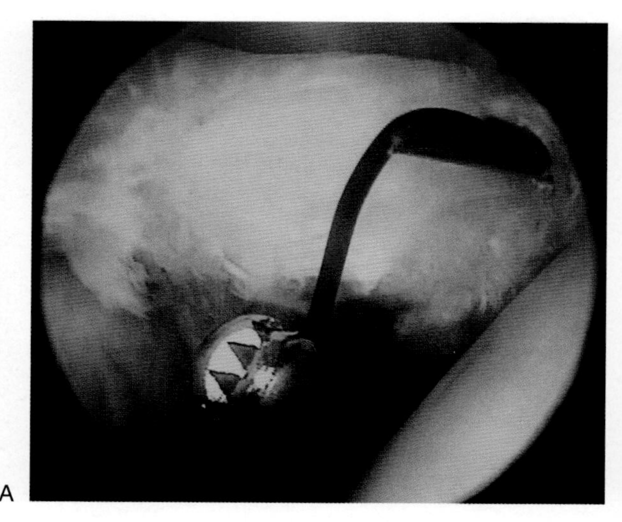

A

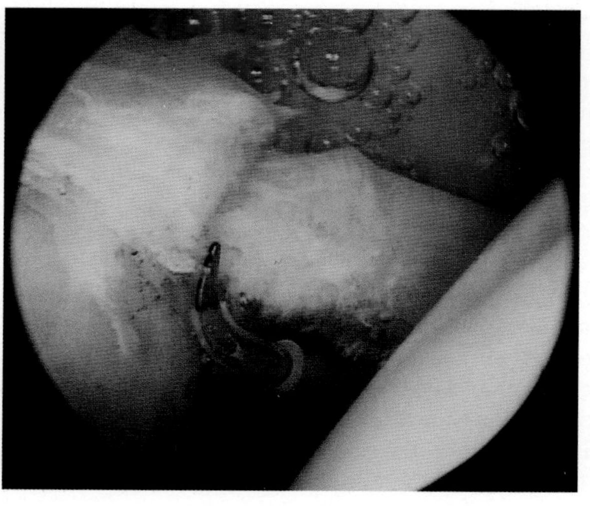

B

FIG. 21. Arthroscopic views from a biceps tenodesis: **(A)** A spinal needle is used to insert a no. 2 PDS suture into the biceps tendon near its entrance to the bicipital groove. This suture is then grasped and brought out through the anterior portal. **(B)** The origin is then released with an electrocautery device.

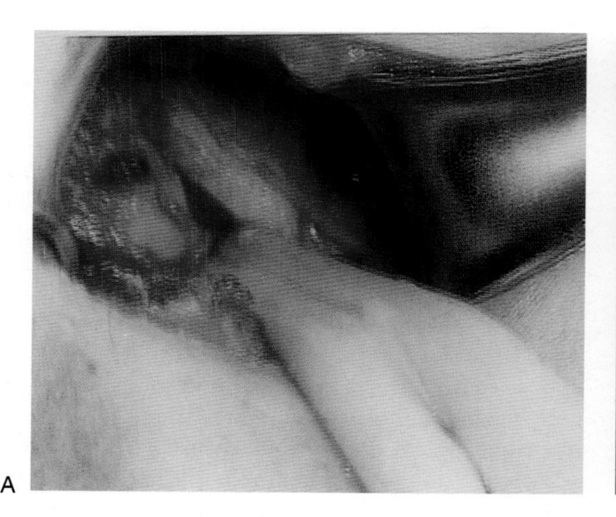

A

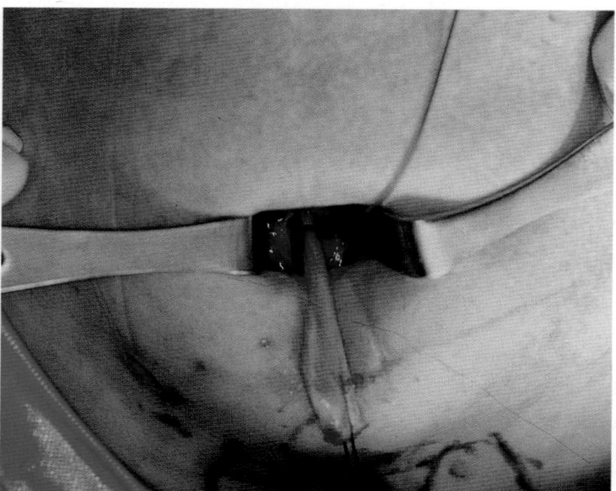

B

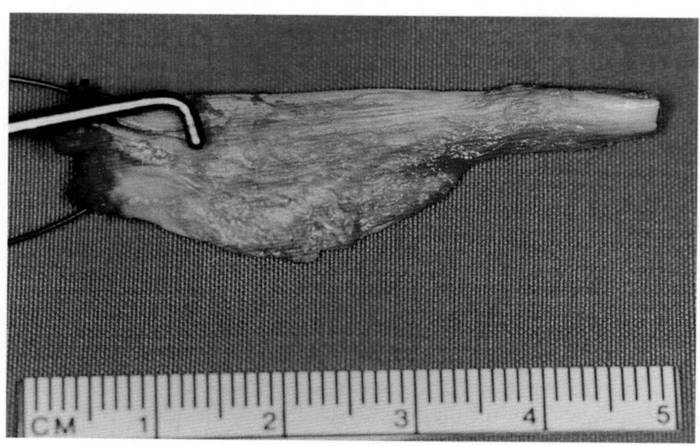

C

FIG. 22. Intraoperative photo of an arthroscopically assisted biceps tenodesis done through a miniopen deltoid-splitting approach. The biceps tendon is brought out through a deltoid split. **(A)** By externally rotating the arm, the bicipital groove is positioned underneath the deltoid split. A longitudinal incision is then made through the transverse humeral ligament to draw the tendon into the wound. **(B)** A close-up view showing the longitudinal split in the transverse humeral ligament. **(C)** The removed intraarticular portion of the biceps tendon showing the significant degenerative changes.

ing a single suture anchor. The appropriate tendon length is once again estimated by the PDS suture placed during the arthroscopic portion of the procedure.

Treatment of SLAP Lesions

Treatment of superior labral lesions of the biceps origin is generally according to those as described by Snyder et al.[92,93] Type I lesions, seen as significant fraying about the superior labrum, are debrided with a shaver placed through the anterior portal. Type II lesions, in which the biceps origin and superior labrum are detached from the bony base of the glenoid, are treated, depending on the instability of the lesion and the age of the patient. Many type II lesions, as described by Snyder et al., are relatively stable and can be treated by debridement and bony abrasion alone. When the labral detachment is significant and it can easily be pulled off of the superior glenoid, either repair or tenodesis should be considered. Tenodesis, in our practice, is preferred for those patients generally older than the age of 45. Younger patients and those with an increased propensity toward overhead activities are treated with repair. Repair is performed through a combination of the standard anterior and posterior portals as well as the superior Neviaser portal (Fig. 23). The location of the Neviaser portal is established under direct arthroscopic visualization by placing a spinal needle through the soft spot approximately 1 to 2 cm medial to the medial border of the acromion and posterior to the clavicle. It is directed anteri-

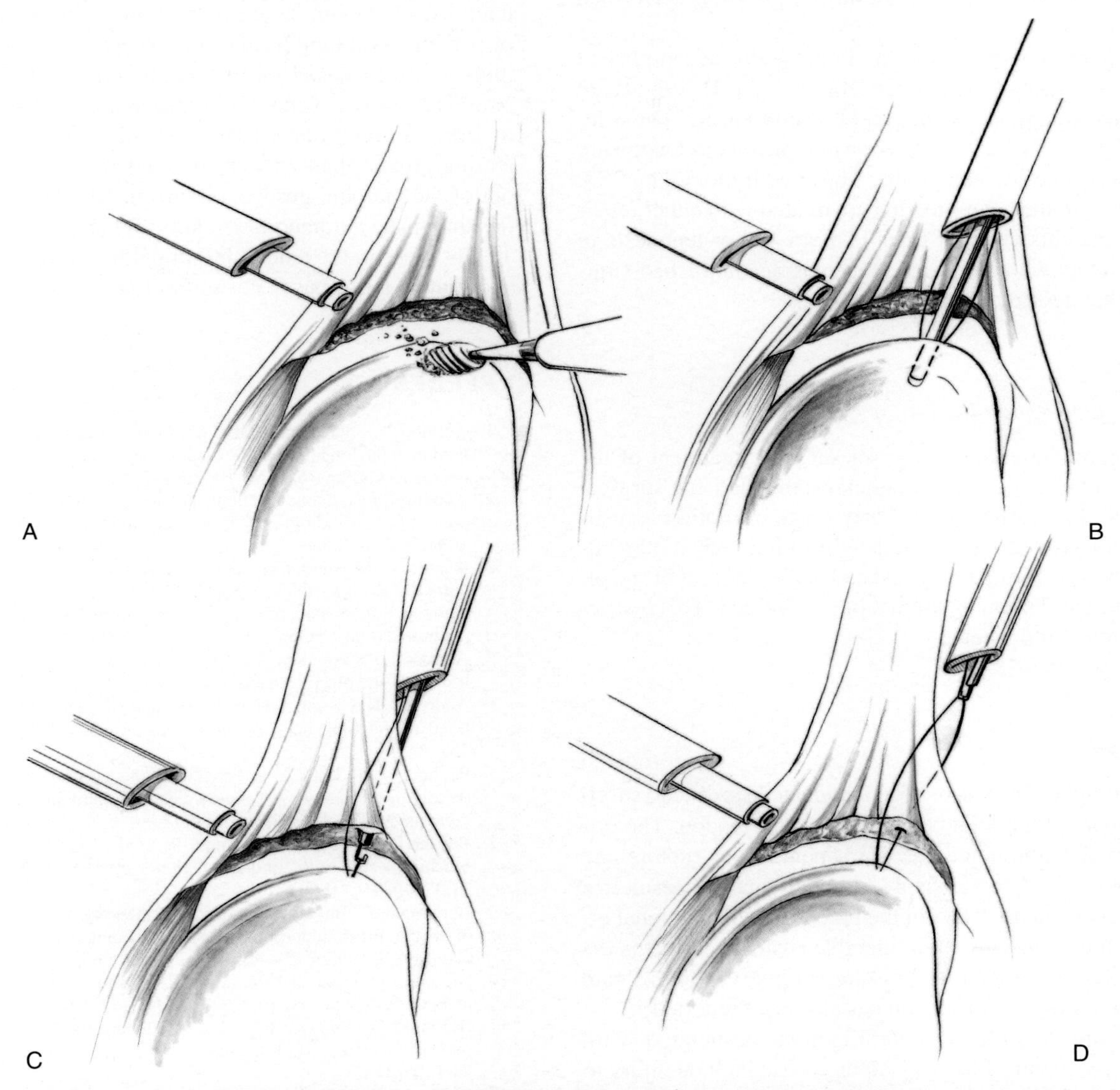

FIG. 23. Schematic representation of an arthroscopic repair of a type II SLAP lesion. **(A)** The superior glenoid rim is debrided with a round burr from the anterior portal. **(B)** A suture anchor is then placed into the superior glenoid rim from the superior portal. Both of the free ends of the suture are brought out through the superior portal. **(C)** An arthroscopic suture grasper (Innovasive Devices, Inc.) is used to simultaneously grasp one of the free ends of the suture and bring it through the superior glenoid labrum. This is then drawn out through the superior portal. **(D)** An arthroscopic knot is then brought down from the superior portal using an arthroscopic knot pusher.

orly 30 degrees and laterally 30 degrees. The entrance site into the glenohumeral joint is generally just behind the biceps tendon origin. The spinal needle is then generally directed right through the labrum, close to the biceps origin. Bone debridement is generally performed through the anterior portal, with visualization from posterior. Following this, a suture anchor is brought in through the superior portal, determined by spinal needle orientation, and then placed in the superior glenoid near the approximate location of the biceps origin. One limb of the attached suture is brought out the superior portal. The other limb of the suture from the suture anchor is then grasped by a suture grasper that simultaneously inserts it through the labrum. This is then brought out through the superior portal. The free ends of the sutures from the suture anchor are tied with arthroscopic knots performed from superiorly.

Treatment of type III lesions is generally accomplished with debridement of the flapped labrum. Type IV lesions are treated dependent on the amount of biceps tearing. Those lesions with less than 25% extension into the biceps tendon are treated with debridement alone. Those with more than 25% extension into the biceps tendon are treated with either repair in those patients younger than 45 years old or tenodesis in those patients who are older. Repair is accomplished similarly to that described for type II lesions.

Postoperative Rehabilitation

Postoperative rehabilitation for surgical treatment of the biceps tendon follows guidelines established for surgical treatment of the rotator cuff. Early range of motion is instituted in a passive to active-assisted fashion. When a biceps tenodesis is performed, any resisted active motion of the elbow, either in flexion or supination, is avoided. This restriction remains for 6 weeks.

Complications

Few complications have been recognized specific to surgical treatment of the long head of the biceps tendon. The primary complication noted has been spontaneous rupture and shortening of the lateral biceps. Although this may result in a significant cosmetic defect in the brachium, its functional effects are minimal. Thus an intolerable cosmetic defect is the primary indication for revision surgical intervention. A rare case of heterotopic ossification has also been reported.[44]

There are theoretical complications associated with arthroscopic repair of SLAP lesions. These include injury to the suprascapular nerve, which resides 1.6 cm medial to the superior glenoid labrum. Additionally, hardware such as suture anchors placed in this location may fail or loosen, resulting in intraarticular hardware. These complications have not yet been reported, but are a concern with the increasing popularity of these procedures.

SUMMARY

Without a clear understanding of the functional role for the long head of the biceps tendon, treatment recommendations have been subject to controversy. An objective review of the available information would suggest that some humeral head stability may be imparted through the tendon. However, the magnitude of this function is likely to be small and possibly insignificant. In contrast, the symptomatic significance of the long head of the biceps is less controversial. It clearly can be an important source of shoulder pain that may remain persistent when not specifically addressed with either nonoperative or operative treatment. When present, persistent pain from the long head of the biceps is likely to have more negative functional consequences than loss of the tendon itself. Given these concerns, evaluation and treatment of patients with long head of the biceps disorders should be individualized based on the likelihood that biceps-related pain will resolve. Tenodesis is recommended in the context of irreversible structural changes, such as atrophy, partial tearing greater than 25% of the tendon width, any luxation out of the bicipital groove, or surrounding bony abnormalities that make autotenodesis likely. When structural changes are not present, the tendon inflammation is likely to resolve, and routine tenodesis is not supported.

REFERENCES

1. Abbott LC, Saunders JB DEC M. Acute traumatic dislocation of the tendon of the long head of the biceps brachii. A report of six cases with operative findings. *Surgery* 1939;6:817–840.
2. Ahovuo J, Paavolainen P, Slätis P. The diagnostic value of arthrography and plain radiography in rotator cuff tears. *Acta Orthop Scand* 1984;55:220–223.
3. Ahovuo J. Radiographic anatomy of the intertubercular groove of the humerus. *Europ J Radiol* 1985;5:83–86.
4. Ahovuo J, Paavolainen P, Slätis P. Radiographic diagnosis of biceps tendinitis. *Acta Orthop Scand* 1985;56:75–78.
5. Ahovuo J, Paavolainen P, Slätis P. Diagnostic value of sonography in lesions of the biceps tendon. *Clin Orthop* 1986;202:184–188.
6. Andrews JR, Carson WG Jr, McLeod WD. Glenoid labrum tears related to the long head of the biceps. *Am J Sports Med* 1985;13: 337–341.
7. Basmajian JV, Latif A. Integrated actions and functions of the chief flexors of the elbow. A detailed electromyographic analysis. *J Bone Joint Surg [Am]* 1957;39:1106–1118.
8. Becker DA, Cofield RH. Tenodesis of the long head of the biceps brachii for chronic bicipital tendinitis. *J Bone Joint Surg [Am]* 1989; 71:376–381.
9. Berlemann U, Bayley I. Tenodesis of the long head of biceps brachii in the painful shoulder: improving results in the long term. *J Shoulder Elbow Surg* 1995;4:429–435.
10. Bigliani LU, Kimmel J, McCann PD, Wolfe I. Repair of rotator cuff tears in tennis players. *Am J Sports Med* 1992;20:112–117.
11. Bigliani LU, Cordasco FA, McIlveen SJ, Musso ES. Operative treatment of failed repairs of the rotator cuff. *J Bone Joint Surg [Am]* 1992; 74:1505–1515.
12. Bigliani LU, D'Alessandro DF, Duralde XA, McIlveen SJ. Anterior acromioplasty for subacromial impingement in patients younger than 40 years of age. *Clin Orthop* 1989;246:111–116.
13. Björkenheim J-M, Paavolainen P, Ahovuo J, Slätis P. Surgical repair of the rotator cuff and surrounding tissues. Factors influencing the results. *Clin Orthop* 1988;236:148–153.
14. Burkhead WZ Jr. The biceps tendon. In: Rockwood CA, Matsen FA III, eds. *The shoulder*. Philadelphia: WB Saunders, 1990:791–836.

15. Burns WC II, Whipple TL. Anatomic relationships in the shoulder impingement syndrome. *Clin Orthop* 1993;294:96–102.
16. Carroll RE, Hamilton LR. Rupture of biceps brachii. A conservative method of treatment. *J Bone Joint Surg [Am]* 1967;49:1016.
17. Chan TW, Dalinka MK, Kneeland JB, Chervrot A. Biceps tendon dislocation: evaluation with MR imaging. *Radiology* 1991;179:649–652.
18. Clark D, Ricker JH, MacCollum MS. The efficacy of local steroid injection in the treatment of stenosing tenovaginitis. *Plastic Reconstr Surg* 1973;Feb:179–180.
19. Clark J, Sidles JA, Matsen FA. The relationship of the glenohumeral joint capsule to the rotator cuff. *Clin Orthop* 1990;254:29–34.
20. Clark JM, Harryman DT II. Tendons, ligaments, and capsule of the rotator cuff. Gross and microscopic anatomy. *J Bone Joint Surg [Am]* 1992;74:713–725.
21. Cofield RH. Tears of rotator cuff. *Instr Course Lect.* 1981;30: 258–273.
22. Cooper DE, Arncozky SP, O'Brien SJ, Warren RF, DiCarlo E, Allen AA. Anatomy, histology, and vascularity of the glenoid labrum. An anatomical study. *J Bone Joint Surg [Am]* 1992;74:46–52.
23. Crenshaw AH, Kilgore WE. Surgical treatment of bicipital tenosynovitis. *J Bone Joint Surg [Am]* 1966;48:1496–1502.
24. Curtis A, Snyder SJ. Evaluation and treatment of biceps tendon pathology. *Orthop Clin North Am* 1993;24:33–43.
25. DePalma AF, Callery GE. Bicipital tenosynovitis. *Clin Orthop* 1954; 3:69–85.
26. Dines D, Warren RF, Inglis AE. Surgical treatment of lesions of the long head of the biceps. *Clin Orthop* 1982;164:165–171.
27. Ellman H, Hanker G, Bayer M. Repair of the rotator cuff. End-result study of factors influencing reconstruction. *J Bone Joint Surg [Am]* 1986;68:1136–1144.
28. Essman JA, Bell RH, Askew M. Full-thickness rotator cuff tear. An analysis of results. *Clin Orthop* 1991;265:170–177.
29. Ferrari DA. Capsular ligaments of the shoulder. Anatomical and functional study of the anterior superior capsule. *Am J Sports Med* 1990; 18:20–24.
30. Field LD, Savoie FH III. Arthroscopic suture repair of superior labral detachment lesions of the shoulder. *Am J Sports Med* 1993;21: 783–790.
31. Flannigan B, Kursonoghi-Brahme S, Snyder SJ, et al. MR arthrography of the shoulder: comparison with conventional MR imaging. *AJR Am J Roentgenol* 1990;155:829.
32. Flatow EL, Raimondo RA, Kelkar R, et al. Active and passive restraints against superior humeral translation. The contributions of the rotator cuff, the biceps tendon and the coracoacromial arch. Presented at the annual meeting of the American Society of Shoulder and Elbow Surgeons. 1996.
33. Froimson AI, Oh I. Keyhole tenodesis of biceps origin at the shoulder. *Clin Orthop* 1975;112:245–249.
34. Furlani J. Electromyographic study of the m. biceps brachii in movements at the glenohumeral joint. *Acta Anat* 1976;96:270–284.
35. Gazielly DF, Gleyze P, Montagnon C. Functional and anatomical results after rotator cuff repair. *Clin Orthop* 1994;304:43–53.
36. Gerber C, Terrier F, Ganz R. The role of the coracoid process in the chronic impingement syndrome. *J Bone Joint Surg [Br]* 1985;67: 703–708.
37. Gerber C, Krushell RJ. Isolated rupture of the tendon of the subscapularis muscle. Clinical features in 16 cases. *J Bone Joint Surg [Br]* 1991;73:389–394.
38. Gilcreest EL. Dislocation and elongation of the long head of the biceps brachii. An analysis of six cases. *Ann Surg* 1936;104:118–138.
39. Gowan ID, Jobe FW, Tibone JE, Perry J, Moynes DR. A comparative electromyographic analysis of the shoulder during pitching. Professional versus amateur pitchers. *Am J Sports Med* 1987;15:586–590.
40. Habermeyer P, Walch G. The biceps tendon and rotator cuff disease. In: Burkhead WZ Jr, ed. *Rotator cuff disorders.* Baltimore: Williams & Wilkins 1996:142—159.
41. Habermeyer P, Kaiser E, Knappe M, Kreusser T, Wiedemann E. Zur funktionellen anatomie und biomechanik der langen bizepssehne. *Unfallchirurg* 1987;90:319–329.
42. Hall FM, Rosenthal DI, Goldberg RP, Wyshak G. Morbidity from shoulder arthrography: etiology, incidence and prevention. *AJR Am J Roentgenol* 1981;136:59–62.
43. Hamada K, Fukuda H, Mikasa M, Kobayashi Y. Roentgenographic findings in massive rotator cuff tears. A long-term observation. *Clin Orthop* 1990;254:92–96.
44. Harris AI, Bush-Joseph CA, Bach BR Jr. Massive heterotopic ossification after biceps tendon rupture and tenodesis. *Clin Orthop* 1990; 255:284–288.
45. Harryman DT, Mack LA, Wang KY, Jackins SE, Richardson ML, Matsen FA. Repairs of the rotator cuff. Correlation of functional results with integrity of the cuff. *J Bone Joint Surg [Am]* 1991;73: 982–989.
46. Harryman DT, Sidles JA, Harris SL, Matsen FA III. The role of the rotator interval capsule in passive motion and stability of the shoulder. *J Bone Joint Surg [Am]* 1992;74:53–66.
47. Harryman DT, Basta J, Sidles JA. Is biceps glide essential to glenohumeral motion? Presented at Annual Open Meeting, ASES, San Francisco, 1997.
48. Hawkins RJ, Misamore GW, Hobeika PE. Surgery for full-thickness rotator-cuff tears. *J Bone Joint Surg [Am]* 1985;67:1349–1355.
49. Herzog RJ. Magnetic resonance imaging of the shoulder. *J Bone Joint Surg [Am]* 1997;79:934–953.
50. Hitchcock HH, Bechtol CO. Painful shoulder. Observations on the role of the tendon of the long head of the biceps brachii in its causation. *J Bone Joint Surg [Am]* 1948;30:263–273.
51. Inman VT, Saunders JB DEC M, Abbott LC. Observations on the function of the shoulder joint. *J Bone Joint Surg* 1944;26:1–30.
52. Itoi E, Kuechle DK, Newman SR, Morrey BF, An K-N. Stabilising function of the biceps in stable and unstable shoulders. *J Bone Joint Surg [Br]* 1993;75:546–550.
53. Itoi E, Motzkin NE, Morrey BF, An KN. Stabilizing function of the long head of the biceps in the hanging arm position. *J Shoulder Elbow Surg* 1994;3:135–142.
54. Jobe FW, Moynes DR, Tibone JE, Perry J. An EMG analysis of the shoulder in pitching. A second report. *Am J Sports Med* 1984;12: 218–220.
55. Kennedy JC, Willis RB. The effects of local steroid injections on tendons: a biomechanical and microscopic correlative study. *Am J Sports Med* 1976;4:11–21.
56. Kumar K, Kapahtia NK. Surgery for full-thickness rotator-cuff tears [letter]. *J Bone Joint Surg [Am]* 1986;68:634.
57. Kumar VP, Satku K, Balasubramaniam P. The role of the long head of the biceps brachii in the stabilization of the head of the humerus. *Clin Orthop* 1989;244:172–175.
58. Leffert RD, Rowe CR. Tendon rupture. In: Rowe CR, ed. *The shoulder.* New York: Churchill Livingstone, 1988:131–163.
59. Levy AS, Kelly B, Lintner S, Speer KP. The function of the long head of the biceps at the shoulder; An EMG analysis. *Clin Orthop* (in press).
60. Lind T, Reimann I, Larsen JK, Karstrup S. Sonography in soft-tissue trauma of the shoulder. *Acta Orthop Scand* 1989;60:49–53.
61. Lippmann RK. Bicipital tenosynovitis. *NY State J Med* 1944;Oct: 2235–2241.
62. Mariani EM, Cofield RH, Askew LJ, Li G, Chao EYS. Rupture of the tendon of the long head of the biceps brachii. Surgical versus nonsurgical treatment. *Clin Orthop* 1988;228:233–239.
63. Meyer AW. Unrecognized occupational destruction of the tendon of the long head of the biceps brachii. *Arch Surg* 1921;2:130–144.
64. Meyer AW. Spontaneous dislocation and destruction of tendon of long head of biceps brachii. Fifty-nine instances. *Arch Surg* 1928;17: 493–506.
65. Michele AA. Bicipital tenosynovitis. *Clin Orthop* 1960;18:261–267.
66. Middleton WD, Reinus WR, Totty WG, Melson GL, Murphy WA. US of the biceps tendon apparatus. *Radiology* 1985;157:211–215.
67. Middleton WD, Reinus WR, Totty WG, Melson GL, Murphy WA. Ultrasonographic evaluation of the rotator cuff and biceps tendon. *J Bone Joint Surg [Am]* 1986;68:440–450.
68. Morrison DS, Frogameni AD, Woodworth P. Non-operative treatment of subacromial impingement syndrome. *J Bone Joint Surg [Am]* 1997; 79:732–737.
69. Neer CS II. Anterior acromioplasty for the chronic impingement syndrome in the shoulder. A preliminary report. *J Bone Joint Surg [Am]* 1972;54:41–50.
70. Neviaser TJ. Arthrography of the shoulder. *Orthop Clin North Am* 1980;11:205–217.
71. Neviaser RJ. Lesions of the biceps and tendinitis of the shoulder. *Orthop Clin North Am* 1980;11:343–348.
72. Neviaser TJ, Neviaser RJ. Lesions of long head of biceps. *Instr Course Lect* 1981;30:250–257.
73. Neviaser TJ, Neviaser RJ, Neviaser JS, Neviaser JS. The four-in-one

arthroplasty for the painful arc syndrome. *Clin Orthop* 1982;163:107–112.
74. Neviaser TJ. Arthroscopy of the shoulder. *Orthop Clin North Am* 1987;18:361–372.
75. Neviaser TJ. The role of the biceps tendon in the impingement syndrome. *Orthop Clin North Am* 1987;18:383–386.
76. Neviaser TJ. The incidence of pathological changes of the long head of the biceps tendon. (Personal communication.)
77. O'Donoghue DH. Subluxing biceps tendon in the athlete. *Clin Orthop* 1982;164:26–29.
78. Pagnani MJ, Deng XH, Warren RF, Torzilli PA, O'Brien SJ. Role of the long head of the biceps brachii in glenohumeral stability: a biomechanical study in cadavera. *J Shoulder Elbow Surg* 1996;5:255–262.
79. Pauly JE, Rushing JL, Scheving LE. An electromyographic study of some muscles crossing the elbow joint. *Anat Rec* 1967;159:47–54.
80. Petersson CJ. Degeneration of the gleno-humeral joint. An anatomical study. *Acta Orthop Scand* 1983;54:277–283.
81. Petersson CJ. Spontaneous medial dislocation of the tendon of the long biceps brachii. An anatomic study of prevalence and pathomechanics. *Clin Orthop* 1986;211:224–227.
82. Petri M, Dobrow R, Neiman R, Whiting-O'Keefe Q, Seaman WE. Randomized, double-blind, placebo-controlled study of the treatment of the painful shoulder. *Arthritis Rheum* 1987;30:1040–1045.
83. Post M, Benca P. Primary tendinitis of the long head of the biceps. *Clin Orthop* 1989;246:117–125.
84. Rames RD, Karzel RP. Injuries to the glenoid labrum including SLAP lesions. *Orthop Clin North Am* 1993;24:45–53.
85. Rathbun JB, Macnab I. The microvascular pattern of the rotator cuff. *J Bone Joint Surg [Br]* 1970;52:540–553.
86. Refior HJ, Sowa D. Long tendon of the biceps brachii: sites of predilection for degenerative lesions. *J Shoulder Elbow Surg* 1995;4:436–440.
87. Rockwood CA, Lyons FR. Shoulder impingement syndrome: diagnosis, radiographic evaluation, and treatment with a modified Neer acromioplasty. *J Bone Joint Surg [Am]* 1993;75:409–424.
88. Rodosky MW, Harner CD, Fu FH. The role of the long head of the biceps muscle and superior glenoid labrum in anterior stability of the shoulder. *Am J Sports Med* 1994;22:121–130.
89. Schrager VL. Tenosynovitis of the long head of the biceps humeri. *Surg Gynecol Obstet* 1938;66:785–790.
90. Slatis P, Aalto K. Medial dislocation of the tendon of the long head of the biceps brachii. *Acta Orthop Scand* 1979;50:73.
91. Snyder SJ, Karzel RP, Del Pizzo W, Ferkel RD, Friedman MJ. SLAP lesions of the shoulder (Lesions of the superior labrum both anterior and posterior). *Orthop Trans* 1990;14:257–258.
92. Snyder SJ, Karzel RP, Del Pizzo W, Ferkel RD, Friedman MJ. SLAP lesions of the shoulder. *Arthroscopy* 1990;6:274–279.
93. Snyder SJ, Banas MP, Karzel RP. An analysis of 140 injuries to the superior glenoid labrum. *J Shoulder Elbow Surg* 1995;4:243–248.
94. Tibone JE, Elrod B, Jobe FW, et al. Surgical treatment of tears of the rotator cuff in athletes. *J Bone Joint Surg [Am]* 1986;68:887–891.
95. Ting A, Jobe FW, Barto P, Ling P, Moynes D. An EMG analysis of the lateral biceps in shoulders with rotator cuff tears. Presented at American Shoulder and Elbow Surg. Open Meeting, San Francisco. *Orthop Trans* 1987;11:237.
96. Turkel SJ, Panio MW, Marshall JL, Girgis FG. Stabilizing mechanisms preventing anterior dislocation of the glenohumeral joint. *J Bone Joint Surg [Am]* 1981;63:1208–1217.
97. Vangsness CT, Jorgenson SS, Watson T, Johnson DL. The origin of the long head of the biceps from the scapula and glenoid labrum. An anatomical study of 100 shoulders. *J Bone Joint Surg [Am]* 1994;76:951–954.
98. Walch G, Nove-Josserand L, Levigne C, Renaud E. Tears of the supraspinatus tendon associated with hidden lesions of the rotator interval. *J Shoulder Elbow Surg* 1994;3:353–360.
99. Warner JJP, McMahon PJ. The role of the long head of the biceps brachii in superior stability of the glenohumeral joint. *J Bone Joint Surg [Am]* 1995;77:366–372.
100. Warren RF. Lesions of the long head of the biceps tendon. *Instr Course Lect* 1985;34:204–209.
101. Yamaguchi K, Flatow EL. Management of multidirectional instability. *Clin Sports Med* 1995;14:885–902.
102. Yamaguchi K, Riew KD, Galatz LM, Syme JA, Neviaser RJ. Biceps activity during shoulder motion: an electromyographic analysis. *Clin Orthop* 1997;336:122–129.
103. Yamaguchi K, Hasan SA, Teefey SA, Middleton WD, Wright RW. High resolution ultrasonography for the detection of rotator cuff tears: a retrospective analysis of 90 consecutive scans compared to operative findings. Presented AAOS annual meeting 1998.
104. Yergason RM. Supination sign. *J Bone Joint Surg* 1931;13:160.
105. Yoneda M, Kirooka A, Saito S, Yamamoto T, Ochi T, Shino K. Arthroscopic stapling for detached superior glenoid labrum. *J Bone Joint Surg [Br]* 1991;73:746–750.

Disorders of the Shoulder: Diagnosis and Management,
edited by Joseph P. Iannotti and Gerald R. Williams, Jr.
Lippincott Williams & Wilkins, Philadelphia © 1999.

CHAPTER 7

Traumatic Muscle Ruptures

Donald F. D'Alessandro

INTRODUCTION

Traumatic muscle ruptures involving the shoulder girdle are relatively uncommon. This brief chapter focuses on the isolated muscle ruptures that rarely do occur: namely, the pectoralis major, deltoid, coracobrachialis, and triceps. Excluding the rotator cuff and biceps, which are discussed in other sections of this text, the pectoralis major and triceps tendons are the most prone to avulsion, whereas traumatic injuries to the deltoid and coracobrachialis are rare.

Muscle injuries may vary in severity from minor strains to complete disruption of muscle fibers. These injuries involve different locations within the musculotendinous unit, including the site of origin, within the muscle belly itself, at the musculotendinous junction, and complete tendinous avulsion from bone. Clinical factors, such as mechanism of injury, rate of loading, and the specific anatomic features of a given muscle determine the site of injury.[51,87] It has been shown experimentally that normal tendons are the strongest link of the muscle–tendon–bone construct.[51] Direct trauma to a contracted muscle generally causes disruption of fibers within the muscle belly.[28,50,80] Indirect trauma from which the affected extremity is subjected to an overwhelming force against a maximally contracted muscle usually results in distal tendon avulsion from the bony insertion.[17]

Although traumatic ruptures of the shoulder musculature are uncommon, the physician's heightened awareness and understanding of the pathomechanics, combined with a careful clinical evaluation and judicious use of imaging studies, will lead to prompt diagnosis and optimal management.

PECTORALIS MAJOR RUPTURES

Surgical Anatomy and Biomechanics

The pectoralis major is a thick triangular muscle, with a broad origin including the medial clavicle, anterior surface of the sternum, the costal cartilages down to the sixth rib, and the aponeurosis of the external oblique muscle of the abdomen.[30] The muscle converges laterally to form two distinct heads: the smaller clavicular head and the larger sternocostal head (Fig. 1). The architecture of the tendinous insertion consists of two lamina that cross over the long head

D.F. D'Alessandro: Miller Orthopaedic Clinic and Carolinas Medical Center, Charlotte, North Carolina 28203.

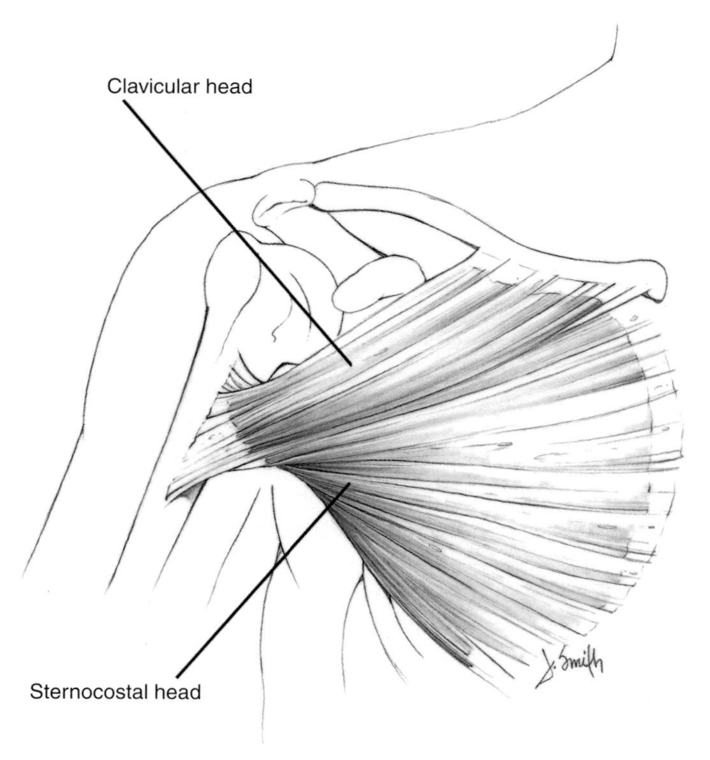

FIG. 1. Anatomy of the pectoralis major: The triangular muscle converges to form two distinct segments: the smaller clavicular head and the larger sternocostal head. The sternocostal portion spirals on itself to insert proximally and underneath the clavicular portion of the muscle.

of the biceps and is inserted on the lateral edge of the bicipital groove. The upper clavicular head constitutes the anterior lamina, whereas the lower and deeper fibers of the sternocostal head form the posterior lamina. The sternocostal head spirals on itself approximately 180 degrees, inserting proximally underneath the clavicular portion. This rolled edge creates the anterior axillary fold. Kretzler and Richardson found that the actual pectoralis tendon was about 1 cm long on its anterior surface and 2.5 cm long on its posterior surface.[38]

The function of the pectoralis major depends on the arm's relative position to the chest at the time of contraction. For example, the muscle functions to flex the humerus if it is extended behind the plane of the body; whereas the pectoralis major's lower fibers will extend the shoulder when the contraction is initiated with the arm in a flexed position. The pectoralis is also a powerful adductor and internal rotator of the humerus.[48] Weight lifting, and particularly the bench press, is a commonly reported mechanism of injury for pectoralis major rupture. Wolfe et al.[89] examined muscle fiber lengths at various points along the muscle, both at rest and during a simulated bench press maneuver in a cadaveric model. They demonstrated that the short inferior fibers of the muscle lengthened disproportionately during the final 30 degrees of humeral extension when compared with the superior fibers of the sternal head. Therefore, these inferior fibers are theoretically placed at a mechanical disadvantage in the eccentric phase of the lift, predisposing them to injury.[89]

The pectoralis major is innervated by the lateral and medial pectoral nerves, which principally serve the clavicular and sternocostal heads, respectively. These nerves course from a superior to inferior direction and enter the muscle along its posterior surface. The muscle's innervation is not in jeopardy during mobilization of the tendon for surgical repair.

Incidence and Pathophysiology

Rupture of the pectoralis major muscle is relatively uncommon, first reported in 1822 by Patissier.[61] Since that time approximately 86 cases have been reported, but only half have been confirmed by exploration for surgical repair.[11] McEntire and associates published a literature review of pectoralis major ruptures in 1972 and added 11 new cases to the 45 already in the literature.[50] However, only 22 of these 56 cases were confirmed surgically. Two large series of new cases have more recently been reported. Kretzler, in 1989, reported 19 new cases of which 16 were repaired.[38] Wolfe et al., in 1992, published on 14 new cases with 7 being managed with surgery.[89]

Most of these injuries occur in men during the third or fourth decade.[35] To date, not a single case of a pectoralis major rupture has been reported in a woman.

The mechanism of injury usually described involves an overwhelming extension force applied to a maximally contracted pectoralis muscle, resulting in a complete tendinous avulsion from bone. The single most common mechanism causing pectoralis rupture has been the bench press exercise, comprising 31 cases in the literature.[6,32,35,38,42,66,83,89,90] Other sports activities, such as boxing, football, ice hockey, sail boarding, skiing, water skiing, and wrestling, all have been associated with cases of pectoralis rupture. The mechanism of injury involves either an indirect sudden force applied to the upper extremity or, in a small number of cases, a direct blow to the contracted muscle. Reaching out to break a fall or grabbing a railing to prevent a fall are two commonly described mechanisms.

Pectoralis major ruptures may be complete or partial. Partial injuries are treated nonsurgically and, consequently, the pathoanatomy of these lesions has not been documented. Partial injuries of the musculotendinous unit may occur in the muscle belly, at the musculotendinous junction, or at the tendinous insertion site. Partial tendinous disruption at the bony insertion site most often involves a complete rupture of the sternal portion of the muscle, while the smaller clavicular part remains intact. Palpation of the intact clavicular head may be interpreted as an incomplete injury not requiring surgical intervention. However, the sternal portion constitutes approximately two-thirds of the muscle mass and its repair is warranted in active individuals. This pattern of disruption is consistent with the common mechanism of injury involving the terminal eccentric part of the bench press where the lower muscle fibers of the pectoralis are stretched disproportionately. Complete rupture of both the sternal and clavicular head is less common, but has been reported.[42,45,50,60,83,89]

A survey of the recent literature shows that most reported cases involving the pectoralis major are distal disruptions at the insertion site and musculotendinous junction, rather than proximal ruptures of the muscle belly. Proximal muscle belly ruptures occasionally do occur and tend to result from a direct blow to the contracted muscle.[34,50] Interestingly, there are only two cases in the literature in whom a bone fragment from the humerus was avulsed at the time of injury.[58,84] In one case the bone fragment was small and inconsequential. In the other, a large fragment of humeral cortex was reinserted with screws and spiked washers.[84]

Evaluation

The principal clue to the diagnosis of a pectoralis major rupture is the patient's history of an acute traumatic event associated with burning pain and a tearing sensation of the upper arm and chest. Most often the mechanism of injury described by the patient involves an overpowering extension force on the extremity. An audible pop is not usually appreciated.

The specific physical findings depend on the exact site and extent of muscle rupture. The more common distal ruptures will have swelling and ecchymosis of the lateral chest and upper arm region. The muscle retracts medially and superiorly, although the absence of the anterior axillary fold may not be immediately obvious in the acute setting. With complete avulsion of the sternal head, one may still be able to palpate the thin, tendinous clavicular insertion. Zeman describes one patient who, at surgery, had a complete avulsion at the musculotendinous junction, but a persistent overlying fascia layer had clinically masqueraded as a segment of intact tendon.[90] Weakness of adduction and internal rotation with a medial muscle bulge that is accentuated with resistance can usually be appreciated.

Conversely, proximal or medial muscle injury causes ecchymosis and swelling on the anterior part of the chest wall. The muscle belly retracts toward the axillary fold and a visible and palpable medial defect is seen. Again, these injuries are often a result of a direct blow or crush injury. A useful clinical test involves having the patient firmly press his hands together in front of his chest to allow for simultaneous inspection and palpation of the involved and uninvolved pectoralis muscles.

In the chronic setting, the diagnosis is very straightforward. The patient will complain of fatigue, ache, and weakness to strenuous internal rotation and adduction activities. Weight lifters and body builders, in particular, will complain of the gross asymmetry compared with the uninvolved side. Weakness on manual muscle testing of adduction and internal rotation can usually be appreciated. Isokinetic testing has been used to quantify and document this weakness.[38,43,69,72,89]

Occasionally, associated injuries will present with pectoralis major ruptures. Injuries to the anterior deltoid, rotator cuff, latissimus dorsi, and brachial plexus have all been seen.[34,50] Interestingly, pectoralis major disruption has only been reported in combination with an anterior traumatic dislocation of the shoulder in one case.[3] The mechanism for these two anterior shoulder injuries is similar, albeit with traumatic instability usually occurring at greater degrees of abduction and external rotation. It is important to consider this differential diagnosis when assessing football players who have been injured while tackling with their arm in an abducted and extended position.

Radiographic evaluation of the shoulder and chest is usually negative, except in the rare case of an avulsion of a small bone fragment.[58,84] The subtle finding of a loss of the normal pectoralis major shadow has been described.[48,60,90] The use of magnetic resonance imaging (MRI) in the early diagnosis has been mentioned in only one case report.[53] The potential benefit of MRI in the acute setting would be to specifically identify the extent and site of muscle injury when the clinical diagnosis is unclear because of swelling and pain (Fig. 2). In most cases, an MRI is unnecessary, as subsequent examination within 7 to 10 days after the acute event will usually clarify the diagnosis. This brief delay in diagnosis has no influence on decision making or the ultimate result.

Treatment

The treatment of pectoralis major muscle ruptures is determined by the specific location and degree of injury. Tears from the origin or within the muscle belly, whether a mild strain, partial tear or complete disruption, are not amenable to surgical intervention and respond satisfactorily to conser-

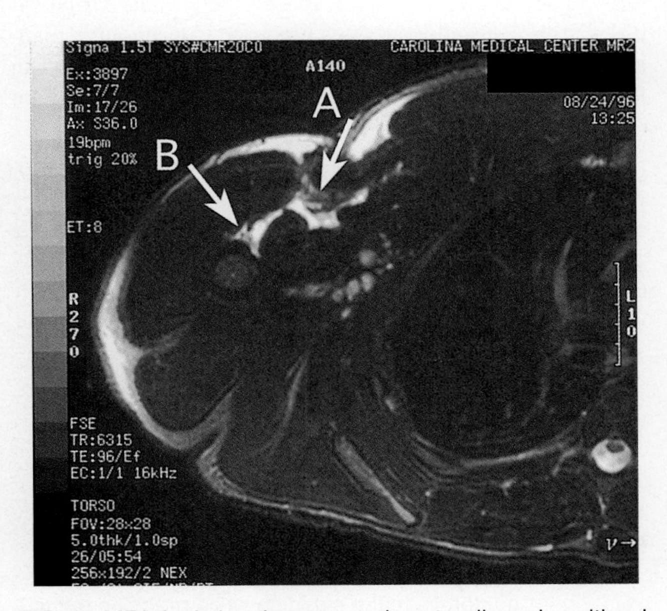

FIG. 2. MRI depicting the retracted pectoralis major with adjacent hematoma (*A*) and the tract leading from the humeral insertion underneath the deltoid (*B*).

vative treatment.[11,28] There are several case reports in the literature of wrestlers who sustained medial pectoral injuries and successfully returned to competition. Injuries at the musculotendinous junction are usually of partial severity, and conservative management will yield acceptable function despite the residual cosmetic defect.[50,69,78] Magnetic resonance imaging may help the surgeon decide on operative versus nonoperative management by providing information on the exact location of a distal injury and the degree of muscle involvement.[15,53] Distal tendinous avulsion may be complete involving both heads of the pectoralis major or partial, for which just the larger inferior sternal portion is detached. Most authors would recommend surgical repair of these injuries, particularly in athletes and laborers who require optimal function and prefer upper body muscular symmetry (Fig. 3).[6,8,19,32,38,42,43,46,48,50,60,90] This recommendation is based on subjective complaints of weakness interfering with recreational or occupational function and cosmetic deformity. Isokinetic testing has demonstrated 25% to 50% muscle deficits in adduction and internal rotation in both preoperative patients and in those treated nonoperatively.[38,43,69,72,89]

The literature is divided in the recommendations for treatment of chronic ruptures. A few authors have suggested nonoperative treatment for the chronic tear, based on satisfactory functional recovery in a few cases while avoiding the potential difficulties of late repair.[48,69] The more recent literature tends to favor late repair of complete disruptions, with satisfactory results achieved with surgery done up to 5 years after rupture.[6,38,42,43,72,89]

Nonoperative Treatment

Nonoperative treatment is recommended for medial ruptures of the pectoralis origin, muscle belly, and partial injuries at the musculotendinous junction. Conservative management is also appropriate for complete distal ruptures in lower-demand individuals, particularly if the nondominant extremity is involved. Initial treatment includes immobilization in a sling and icing to control pain and to allow stabilization of the hematoma. Gentle active and passive range of motion exercises are begun at 7 to 10 days postinjury. In the partial distal injury, care is taken to avoid humeral extension and abduction to protect the vulnerable inferior fibers of the sternal portion of the muscle. Resisted exercises are begun at 6 weeks. Isokinetic exercises for horizontal adduction can assist in the rehabilitation to develop strength and endurance. Depending on the severity of the initial injury and the specific occupational or athletic demands, patients may return to unrestricted activity at between 8 and 12 weeks.

Surgical Management

The goal of surgical intervention is to achieve optimal functional recovery in high-demand individuals requiring full strength. Surgery is best suited for complete tendinous avulsion of both the clavicular and sternal heads or complete disruption at the musculotendinous junction. Serious consideration for surgical repair should be given for partial tendinous avulsions in active athletes or heavy laborers in whom the sternal head has been completely avulsed, but the smaller clavicular head remains. Surgery is not indicated for proximal tears of the muscle origin or muscle belly.

Anatomic repair is accomplished using heavy nonabsorbable suture placed in Bunnell fashion in the distal tendon passed through drill holes lateral to the biceps tendon at the humeral insertion site.[38,89] Other technical options reported include using pullout wires,[50] a barbed staple,[20] and most recently, suture anchors.[53] Disruptions within the distal tendon itself occur rarely, but should also be secured directly to bone.

Repair of musculotendinous junction tears is more difficult because of the inability to obtain secure suture fixation in the torn muscle. For this reason, most partial tears are probably best managed nonoperatively. Very large defects or complete musculotendinous junction disruptions are accom-

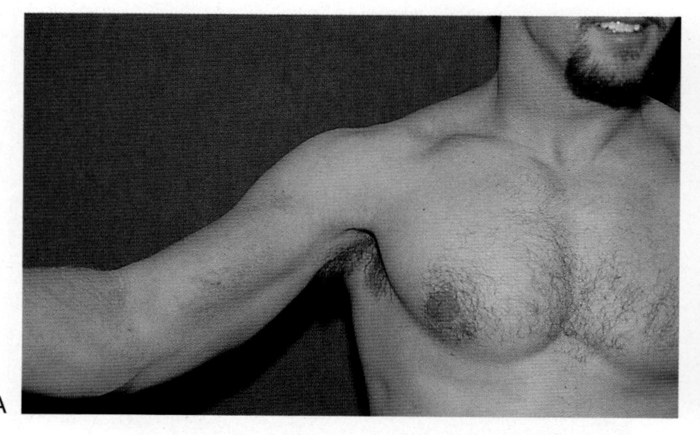
A

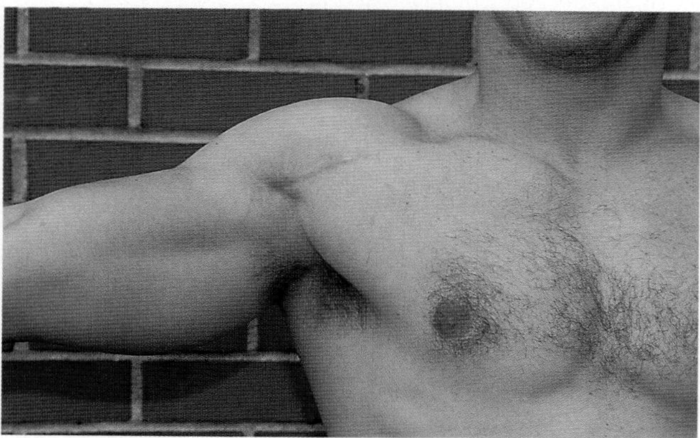
B

FIG. 3. (A) Preoperative photograph of a professional football player who had sustained a complete pectoralis major avulsion while reaching out to make a tackle. Note the web appearance of the anterior axilla. **(B)** Postoperative photograph showing restoration of the anterior axillary fold after a pectoralis major repair.

plished with standard suturing techniques. Less vigorous postoperative rehabilitation is recommended in this setting.

Late primary repair for chronic ruptures can be accomplished, even up to 5 years after the initial injury, although surgical dissection through scar and mobilization of the chronically retracted muscle is more difficult.[6,38,42,43,72,89]

Postoperative management is relatively aggressive. The arm is immobilized for 1 to 2 weeks and then gradually weaned out of the sling by 4 weeks after surgery. Progressive active exercises and gentle use out of the sling are begun at 2 weeks postoperatively. Passive stretching is avoided. Resisted exercise begins at 6 weeks. Isokinetic machines can offer an objective assessment of strength and endurance and are used at 8 to 10 weeks in anticipation of return to full activities by 3 to 4 months after surgery. The postoperative rehabilitation program must be less aggressive in those cases of musculotendinous junction repair.

Results

Although there are 85 cases presented in the literature, the results of treatment, whether nonoperative or surgical, are generally described anecdotally. There are very few large series in the literature that offer objective criteria with which we can critically analyze results. In 1970 Park and Espiniella reviewed 30 cases of pectoralis major ruptures. The results in those patients treated with surgical repair were 80% excellent and 10% good. These results were superior to the 17% excellent and 58% good outcomes in patients treated nonoperatively.[60] McEntire et al., in 1972, presented 11 new cases and combined the results with the 45 cases that were already in the literature. They identified a similar trend favoring surgical management. In those patients for whom outcomes could be determined by the data available, surgical treatment yielded 77% excellent and 11% good results. By comparison, results in those patients who received conservative treatment or no formal treatment at all were 29% excellent and 54% good.[50]

Zeman et al., in 1979, reported on nine athletes with ruptures of the pectoralis major. Four cases were treated surgically and all had excellent results. The five patients managed nonoperatively had residual weakness, with two weight lifters and one professional boxer dissatisfied with their ability to perform at return to athletic competition.[90]

Kretzler and Richardson in 1989 repaired 16 distal avulsions, and 81% achieved full return of range of motion, strength, and normal contour. Two patients were repaired 5 years after injury and, although they had a satisfactory clinical result, both patients have persistent weakness in horizontal adduction of 16% and 20%, respectively, by Cybex evaluation.[38]

Wolfe et al., in 1992, evaluated 14 sports-related ruptures, 7 treated surgically and 7 conservatively. Cybex testing demonstrated marked strength and work deficits in those patients treated conservatively, compared with normal strength in the repaired group.[89]

Surgical repair of chronic pectoralis ruptures is technically feasible, even up to 5 years after injury. Acceptable results can be obtained, albeit somewhat inferior in recovery of strength compared with those repaired immediately.[6,32,38,42,43,72,89] Jones in 1988 reviewed the literature and concluded that ruptures repaired within 7 days had 57% excellent and 30% good results, but those patients with delayed repair had no excellent and 60% good results.[32] Although delayed primary repair of chronic ruptures is possible, patients should be told that a satisfactory outcome is probable, but there is a likelihood of mild persistent weakness and cosmetic asymmetry.

Complications

Complications from surgical intervention are infrequent. One patient was slightly limited in abduction postoperatively,[38] and another had postoperative fourth and fifth digit paresthesias of unknown cause.[89] Interestingly, there have been several early reports of complications from pectoralis major rupture related to the associated hematoma in patients treated nonoperatively. Sepsis from an infected hematoma caused the death of one patient and precipitated the death of a second with pneumonia.[56,61] Additionally, a pseudocyst had formed from a hematoma.[70] Finally, myositis ossificans was reported to develop in a patient 4 months after rupture.[66] Rerupture after surgical repair has not been documented.

Author's Preferred Treatment

Conservative treatment is indicated for all proximal injuries involving the pectoralis major origin and muscle belly. Partial injuries at the musculotendinous junction can be similarly managed nonoperatively. One may wish to consider operative intervention if a large defect at the musculotendinous junction occurs in a high-demand individual or body builder who requires symmetry and optimal strength. An MRI can be helpful in this setting to determine the exact location and extent of the defect when the clinical evaluation is obscured by swelling and hematoma.

Acute surgical repair is recommended not only for complete avulsion, but also for partial distal injuries that involve the entire sternal head of the pectoralis major and leave the clavicular head intact. I prefer approximating the tendon to a bony trough by sutures passed through cortical bone tunnels. The humeral cortex in young, active individuals is fairly thick and the bone holes should be drilled in a convergent orientation. Suture passage can be facilitated using a contoured loop of a 24-gauge wire. Sutures passed in mattress fashion through these tunnels maximize the tendon-to-bone contact (Fig. 4). Suture anchor fixation is another option, but cinching the tendon firmly down to the bone may be difficult and to date there is only one case in the literature advocating this technique.[53]

Postoperative rehabilitation is fairly aggressive, with early

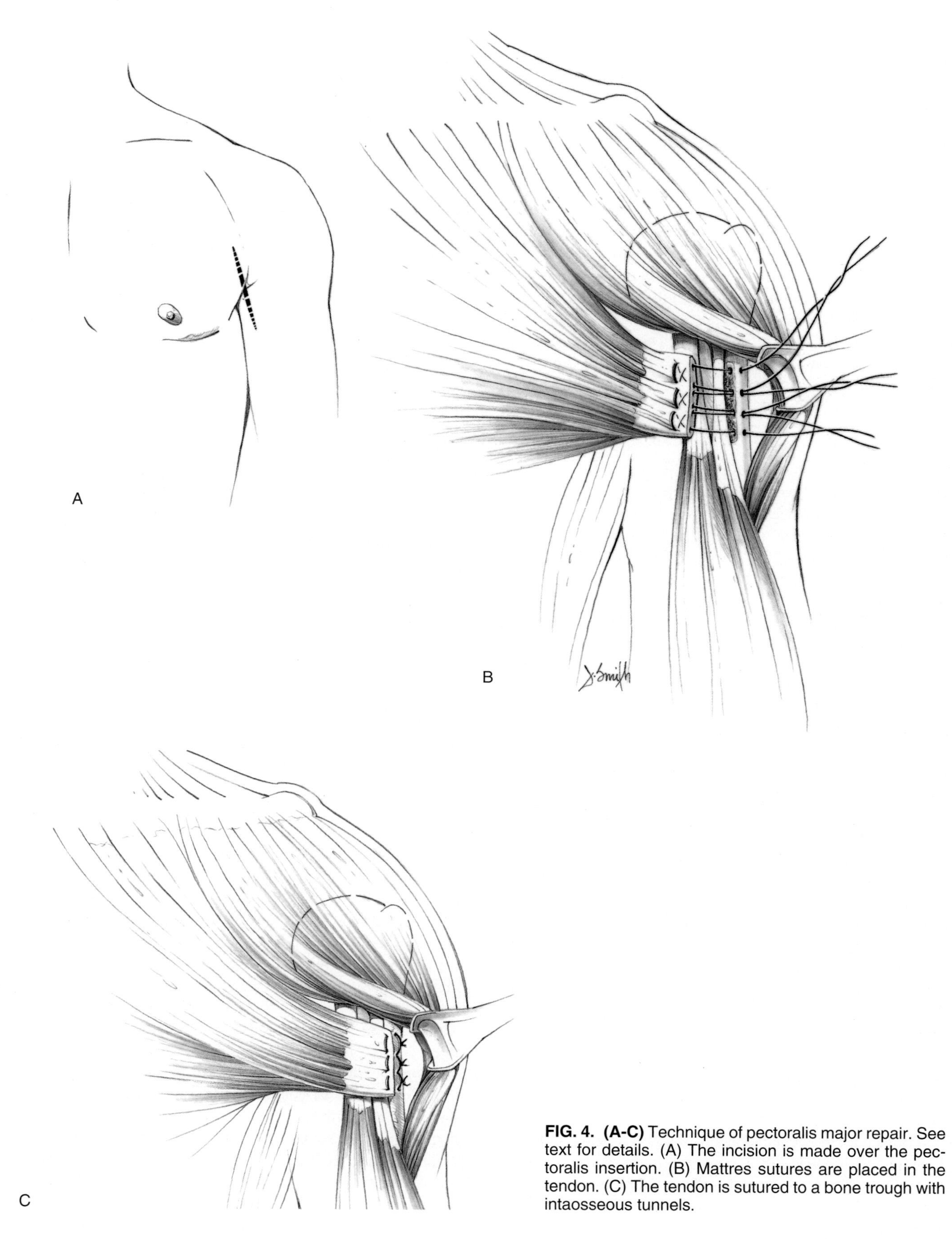

FIG. 4. (A-C) Technique of pectoralis major repair. See text for details. (A) The incision is made over the pectoralis insertion. (B) Mattres sutures are placed in the tendon. (C) The tendon is sutured to a bone trough with intaosseous tunnels.

mobilization and return to unrestricted activity by 3 to 4 months after repair.

DELTOID RUPTURES

Surgical Anatomy and Biomechanics

The deltoid is the largest muscle of the shoulder girdle and its integrity is critical to shoulder function. It consists of three major parts, with the anterior deltoid taking origin from the anterior and superior surfaces of the outer third of the clavicle and anterior acromion, the middle deltoid from the lateral margin of the acromion, and the posterior deltoid from almost the entire scapular spine (Fig. 5).[30] The fibers converge from this wide origin to insert into the deltoid tuberosity on the lateral humeral shaft. Anterior and posterior fibers are essentially unipennate, meaning they run parallel to each other. The more powerful middle part is multipennate, with an internal structure consisting of tendinous septae serving as both origin and insertion sites for its relatively short and multiply oriented muscle fibers.[30] The axillary nerve innervates the muscle after exiting the quadrangular space posteriorly and courses along its undersurface from posterior to anterior.

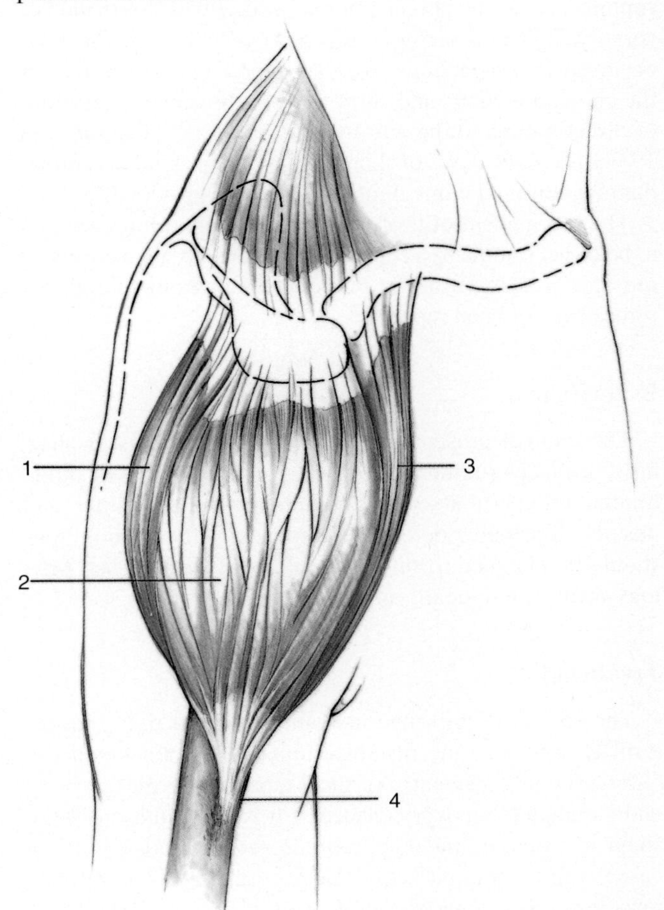

FIG. 5. Anatomy of the deltoid muscle. 1) posterior 1/3 deltoid; 2) middle 1/3 deltoid; 3) anterior 1/3 deltoid; 4) deltoid tuberosity of humerus.

The most important function of the deltoid is forward elevation in the scapular plane. The anterior and middle deltoid contribute to this motion. All three components of the muscle, but particularly the middle third, abduct the humerus, whereas the posterior deltoid extends the humerus.

Incidence and Pathophysiology

Traumatic rupture of the deltoid is rare. Deltoid detachment as a complication of cuff tear arthropathy or previous shoulder surgery is addressed in Chapter 4. There are only five reported cases in the literature from which we can draw information concerning the etiology and management of this injury. Deltoid disruption appears to be a result of a sudden force applied to the muscle, sometimes associated with a concomitant direct blow. The first case was described by Clemens in 1913 and occurred while the patient was carrying a heavy rail.[14] Gilcreest and Albi reported two cases in 1939; one was sustained in an automobile accident and the other occurred with an overhead lifting accident.[26] McEntire et al. published a case of a deltoid rupture associated with a pectoralis major tear.[50] Caughey and Welsh, in review on this subject, described a chronic deltoid detachment in a 62-year-old guide who sustained the injury when a snowmobile rolled over him.[11] Finally, Davis in 1919 reported a case not of traumatic etiology, but of a deltoid origin detachment caused by osteomyelitis of the distal clavicle.[18]

In a general orthopaedic practice, minor strains of the deltoid are not uncommon and are often related to participation in athletic activity, particularly throwing sports. Contusions from direct blows may be associated with a subcutaneous hematoma, but usually do not involve significant muscle fiber disruption. Complete traumatic disruption as evidenced by the foregoing literature accounts is extremely rare and is caused by an abrupt external force applied either directly or indirectly to the contracted deltoid muscle.

Evaluation

Physical examination findings are dependent on the site of rupture and extent of muscle involvement. The clinical presentation is also determined by whether the injury is acute or chronic.

A mild strain or direct contusion will be manifest by local tenderness, mild swelling, and decreased active range of motion secondary to pain. The degree of weakness in either forward flexion or abduction will reflect the exact location and magnitude of the injury.

Acute complete deltoid rupture may occur in the context of a severe traumatic event to the upper extremity or in conjunction with a multiple trauma case. Rupture from the acromial origin can involve an isolated anterior, middle, or posterior head of the deltoid. Acute swelling may mask the proximal muscle defect. Resisted deltoid contraction will accentuate the distal muscle retraction and reveal the asymmetrical deltoid contour and muscle defect. Passive range of motion may be only slightly limited because of pain. Weakness in forward elevation, abduction, or extension reflects injury to the anterior, middle, and posterior heads, respectively. If significant weakness is present, but no defect is appreciated, the possibility of axillary nerve injury must be entertained, particularly if there is a history of concomitant shoulder dislocation. Serial examinations, MRI, or electromyography may be helpful if the diagnosis is uncertain.

Treatment

Deltoid strains and contusions are treated nonoperatively, with early icing and passive range of motion exercises to avoid stiffness. After resolution of the acute injury phase, heat, electrical stimulation, and graduated stretching and strengthening exercises are instituted. Full recovery is anticipated within 4 to 6 weeks of injury.

There is limited published information with which to base recommendations for treatment of acute traumatic ruptures. Disruptions involving an entire segment of the deltoid, particularly the anterior or middle portions, will significantly alter shoulder function and should be surgically repaired back to the acromion. An MRI may help quantify the extent of deltoid origin involved. Prompt surgical repair is necessary to achieve an optimal result. A midsubstance muscle tear is certainly more difficult to repair securely, raising the question of whether repair should be attempted for these injuries. If severe soft-tissue and muscle injury of the shoulder girdle presents in association with a closed head injury, one may wish to consider prophylactic use of indomethacin (Indocin) to avoid heterotopic ossification.

Postoperatively the deltoid repair should be protected in an abduction pillow or splint for 4 to 6 weeks. Passive range of motion in forward elevation, and internal and external rotation from the abduction pillow or brace should begin immediately. Humeral extension or internal rotation with the arm behind the back must be avoided for 6 weeks. Progressive active exercises are started at 6 weeks postoperatively.

Complications

A miss or a delay in diagnosis of an acute deltoid rupture will significantly compromise the surgeon's ability to restore normal shoulder function. Discussion on complications of deltoid detachment more commonly pertain to dehiscence of the deltoid repair following shoulder surgery and are considered in Chapter 4 of this text.

CORACOBRACHIALIS AND SHORT HEAD OF BICEPS RUPTURES

Surgical Anatomy and Biomechanics

The coracobrachialis muscle originates underneath and medial to the short head of the biceps on the coracoid process with a fleshy, tendinous attachment. It inserts on the anterior medial surface of the middle of the humerus.[30] The short head of the biceps takes origin from the lateral tip of the coracoid. The muscle belly of the short head fuses distally with the larger long head, ultimately inserting by a singular stout tendon across the elbow into the radial tuberosity.

The musculocutaneous nerve penetrates the coracobrachialis muscle and runs between the biceps and brachialis muscles, before emerging distally as the lateral antebrachial cutaneous nerve.[30] The innervation of the coracobrachialis is supplied by both a small direct branch from the lateral cord and the musculocutaneous nerve. The main nerve enters the coracobrachialis between 3.1 and 8.2 cm from the tip of the coracoid. Small nerve twigs may enter the muscle as close as 1.7 cm from the coracoid.[23] The coracobrachialis is a flexor and adductor of the arm. The short head of the biceps contributes to arm adduction, but is principally an elbow flexor.

Incidence and Pathophysiology

Rupture of the coracobrachialis muscle and short head of the biceps is extremely rare. Two case reports of coracobrachialis rupture exist in the literature. Gilcreest and Albi, in 1939, described a case of coracobrachialis muscle belly rupture caused by direct trauma, which was confirmed at surgery.[26] The second case recorded by Tobin et al., in 1941, occurred in a parachutist who sustained a complete tear of the coracobrachialis and short head of the biceps as a result of direct trauma to the arm by his static line.[80] Gilcreest, in 1934, listed two cases of short head of biceps tendon rupture, but no additional clinical information was provided.[25]

The mechanism of this unusual injury, therefore, appears to be direct trauma to a contracted muscle. Avulsion of these muscles' origin from the coracoid as a result of indirect forces has not been reported.

Evaluation

The clinical presentation of a coracobrachialis or short head of biceps rupture is presumed to be a history of direct trauma to the arm associated with tenderness, swelling, and possibly a palpable defect in the muscle belly. Radiographs should be obtained to rule out a coracoid fracture. An MRI may be useful in identifying this unusual injury.

Treatment

The paucity of information available on this injury makes it difficult to give any firm recommendations for treatment. Gilcreest performed early surgical repair of the muscle belly and a complete recovery ensued.[26] It is not unreasonable to suggest exploration and appropriate surgical repair in those cases of direct trauma to the anterior arm when a significant muscle defect is appreciated by examination or MRI evaluation. Clinical factors, such as arm dominance and the patient's physical demands, should also play a role in the choice of treatment.

TRICEPS TENDON AVULSION

Surgical Anatomy and Biomechanics

The triceps muscle occupies the entire posterior aspect of the arm and comprises three distinct heads. The long head takes origin from the infraglenoid tubercle of the scapula and courses downward anterior to the teres minor and posterior to the teres major muscles. It serves as the medial border of the quadrangular space through which the axillary nerve and posterior humeral circumflex vessels emerge. The lateral head arises from the posterior surface of the humerus above the radial groove. The long and lateral heads converge distally to create the V-shaped triceps contour that can be appreciated superficially on the back of the arm. The medial head has a broad origin along the entire posterior surface of the humerus below the radial groove, and it fuses with the deep surface of the combined long and lateral heads. Ultimately, the entire muscle then transitions to form the substantial triceps tendon that inserts into the olecranon. Some of the superficial fibers of the tendon proceed over the surface of the olecranon and extend into the fascia of the forearm.[30]

The radial nerve innervates the triceps brachia, giving off multiple small branches to all three heads as it spirals downward along the posterior aspect of the arm. Although the nerve is at risk with posterior approaches to the humerus, it is not in jeopardy during the distal exposure associated with repair of a triceps avulsion.

The triceps muscle is essentially the sole extensor of the elbow, assisted only by the small anconeus muscle. The integrity of the triceps function is necessary to perform many activities of daily living, such as getting out of a chair and pushing objects away from the body.

Incidence and Pathophysiology

Since Partridge documented the first case of triceps tendon avulsion in 1868, approximately 50 cases have been reported in the American and European literature.[10] Anzel et al. reviewed a Mayo Clinic series of 1,014 tendon injuries and found only 8 cases of triceps tendon injury, 4 of which were from a direct laceration.[2,55] The three largest series include Levy (16 cases), Pantazopoulos (7 cases) and Tarsney (7 cases). Most of the remaining cases in the literature are presented as individual case reports.

Bach et al.[5] cumulated the cases of triceps tendon avulsion in the English literature up to 1987, and their study produced interesting epidemiologic data. The mean age at the time of injury was 26 years, ranging from 7 to 72. Males constituted 71% (29 of 41) of the patients. There was no correlation with the patient's dominant side.[5]

The mechanism of injury for triceps tendon avulsion is a fall on an outstretched arm in most cases. The pathomechanics have been described as "a deceleration stress, superimposed upon a contracting triceps muscle with or without a concomitant blow to the posterior aspect of the elbow."[21] An abrupt, forceful, eccentric contraction of the triceps causes most triceps avulsions. Less frequently, a concomitant direct blow to the posterior aspect of the triceps at its insertion has been described in the mechanism of injury.[1,7,16,21,62,74,77] There are two case reports of triceps avulsion that occurred during participation in athletics that illustrate this latter mechanism. One was a football player who was kicked on the posterior aspect of his outstretched arm and the other a skier whose ski struck his arm while he was falling. Recently, four cases of triceps tendon avulsion injury have been reported in body builders and power lifters during the act of weight lifting, specifically the bench press or military press exercises.[5,10,29,33] The occurrence of this injury in body builders raises a question of the potential role of anabolic steroids in this injury.[5,29] Although steroid use was denied in these cases, this issue has been considered for predisposition to pectoralis major and distal biceps ruptures. The deleterious effects of either local steroid injections on tendon[36,82] or systemic anabolic steroid use on the strength of tendons and ligaments,[31,37,52] have been well-documented. A recent case report illustrates this point. A body builder who had received a series of six steroid injections for olecranon bursitis sustained an intrasubstance rupture of the triceps tendon while bench pressing.[76] In addition, he had a 5-year history of systemic anabolic steroid use. Individuals who use anabolic steroids are at risk for tendon ruptures because their abnormal muscular strength is applied to tendons that are stiffer and absorb less energy to failure.[52]

The literature contains a number of systemically compromised patients in whom triceps tendon rupture has occurred spontaneously or as a result of trivial trauma. Medical conditions reported in association with tendon ruptures include renal osteodystrophy and secondary hyperparathyroidism,[12,22,44,47,49,57,64,65,73,81] chronic acidosis,[57] Marfan's syndrome,[71] and steroid treatment for lupus erythematosus.[81,88] The pathophysiology is not well understood, but calcification within the tendon from the chronic hypercalcemia of secondary hyperparathyroidism has been implicated.[65]

The site of triceps muscle injury may be at the muscle belly, musculotendinous junction, or the osseous tendon insertion. The vast majority of authors have described tendoosseous avulsions usually associated with a small fleck of bone.[21,55,77] Ruptures of the musculotendinous junction[24,29,54] and muscle belly tears[4,54,62] are unusual, having been noted in only a few cases. Although complete disruption is the rule, incomplete or partial tears do occur occasionally.[10,21,77] It is important to differentiate a partial tear from a complete rupture because surgical repair is necessary for the complete injury, whereas partial lesions are treated nonoperatively.[16,55]

Triceps tendon avulsions are sometimes associated with other upper extremity injuries, resulting from the fall on the outstretched arm. Levy et al.[40,41] documented 16 patients with radial head fractures associated with triceps rupture.

Lee[39] described a case of triceps rupture occurring in conjunction with a wrist fracture.

In the adolescent population, triceps avulsions involve complete separation of the olecranon epiphysis.[63,68] The secondary ossification center of the olecranon appears in the area of the triceps insertion at about 9 years of age. The physis fuses in an anterior to posterior direction at about 14 years of age.[9,75] The triceps expansion extends beyond the epiphysis, attaching to the surface of the metaphysis.[68] The injury sustained when the physis is incompletely fused produces a Salter-Harris type II fracture.[27]

Evaluation

The diagnosis of a complete triceps tendon avulsion is not difficult. The patient will relate a history of falling on the outstretched arm causing acute pain, a tearing sensation, and subsequent swelling and ecchymosis of the arm. The patient's complaint and physical findings will depend on whether the triceps is partially or completely torn. With a complete disruption, an indentation of the posterior contour of the arm can be seen, particularly as swelling subsides. A defect in the triceps mechanism is usually palpable. If a partial injury has occurred, tenderness is usually localized to the musculotendinous junction, and a discrete defect may not be appreciated. A complete tear results in the loss of extension against gravity, whereas an incomplete lesion is manifested by weakness, but the ability to actively extend the elbow is maintained.

In the acute setting, extension strength can be difficult to assess because of pain. In 1990, Viegas described a modification of the Thompson test[79] (traditionally used to identify complete ruptures of the Achilles tendon) for the assessment of a triceps injury.[85] The modified test can be performed either with the patient seated and the arm draped over the back of the chair, or with the patient in the prone position, letting the forearm hang over the table. In the normal extremity, squeezing the triceps muscle belly produces slight elbow extension, but no motion will occur if a complete rupture is present.[85] This test is helpful for distinguishing between partial and complete triceps injuries.

The presence of associated injuries must be considered, particularly when falling on an outstretched hand is the mechanism of injury. Radial head fractures have been most frequently associated with triceps avulsions,[40,41,77] and distal wrist injuries[39] have also been reported. The differential diagnosis of triceps weakness includes nontraumatic etiologies. A C-7 nerve root lesion will cause isolated triceps weakness. As noted previously, spontaneous ruptures or injuries resulting from trivial forces may be the result of chronic medical conditions, including renal osteodystrophy with secondary hyperparathyroidism, and long-term steroid use associated with systemic lupus erythematosus.

A plane lateral radiograph of the elbow will often confirm the diagnosis. A small avulsion fracture of the olecranon, called a "flake sign"[21,77] is estimated to be present in two-thirds of cases[29] and implies a complete rupture (Fig. 6). Additional studies, such as an MRI or ultrasound,[10] may be useful for defining the extent of partial lesions, but are usually not necessary in cases of complete rupture.

Treatment

Surgical repair is the recommended treatment for complete avulsions. As opposed to cases of pectoralis major or distal biceps tendon ruptures for which other muscles adequately compensate for the loss of these specific muscle functions, no compensatory muscle exists to substitute for triceps function. Even in those chronically ill patients who are suboptimal surgical candidates, triceps function is essential for transfers and the use of ambulatory aids. Operative repair is, therefore, necessary in this group as well.

The surgical technique universally proposed in the literature involves anatomic reattachment of the triceps tendon through drill holes in the olecranon, most commonly using a nonabsorbable suture. Primary repair can be accomplished, even with delays in diagnosis and treatment of up to 6 months. Several case reports involving 3-, 4.5-, and 6-month delays in surgical treatment have achieved excellent results.[5,74,77] Other authors have suggested augmentation of the repair when faced with poor quality tissue or in the set-

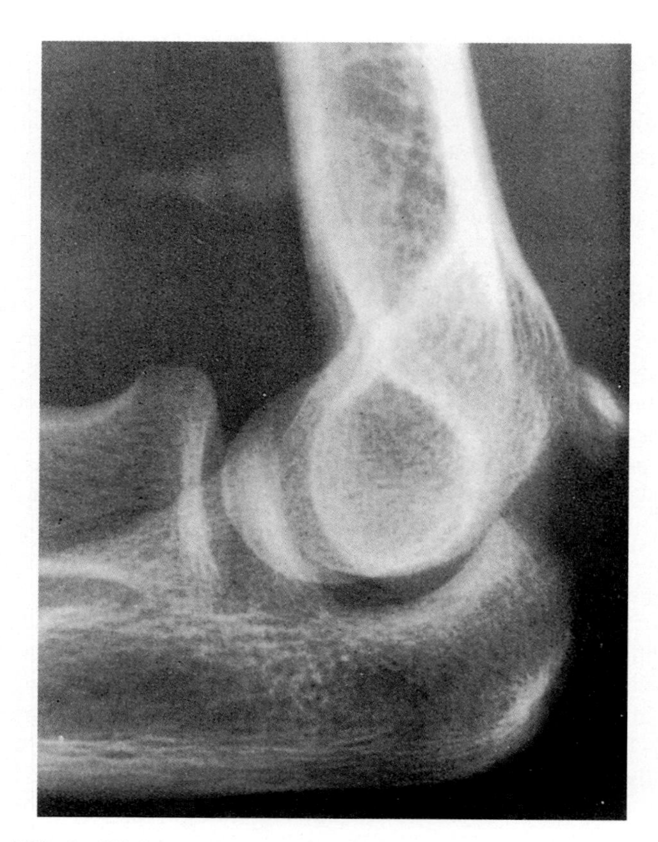

FIG. 6. "Flake sign": A small avulsion fracture of the olecranon, best seen on a lateral radiograph of the elbow, is pathognomonic of a complete triceps avulsion (From ref. 55, with permission.)

ting of a late repair.[13,21,55] Bennett described reinforcing the repair by reflecting a proximally based flap of the posterior forearm fascia and suturing it to the triceps.[7] Clayton and Thirupathi supplemented a triceps repair using an inverted tongue of triceps fascia in an elderly patient with chronic bursitis.[13] Carpentier et al. described Z-plasty lengthening of the triceps to avoid undue tension when repairing a chronic rupture.[10]

The results of operative repair are uniformly excellent in the literature. Authors usually have based their results on the patients' or physicians' subjective assessment. Range of motion is almost always reported as normal. Occasionally a loss of approximately 5 degrees of terminal extension has been seen, but this trivial loss of motion has not affected the functional outcome.[9,49,75] Cybex evaluation has provided objective confirmation of strength recovery in two case reports.[5,74]

Ulnar neuritis has been seen in conjunction with triceps injury in two cases. In both instances, a delay in surgical intervention resulted in the formation of scar tissue encompassing the ulnar nerve.[1,29] Anterior transposition of the nerve at the time of triceps repair has produced satisfactory results.

Nonoperative treatment is appropriate for a partial triceps injury. The rate of progression with range of motion and strengthening exercises following 2 to 3 weeks of immobilization is dependent on the degree of muscle involvement. With adequate rehabilitation, essentially full restoration of strength and function can be anticipated after a partial tear.[4,10,21]

Author's Preferred Treatment

Early anatomic repair through bone holes in the proximal ulna is strongly recommended for all patients with acute complete avulsions.

A posterior approach to the arm and elbow can be accomplished with the patient in the supine, lateral, or prone position. A tourniquet may be used to facilitate the dissection, particularly around the ulnar nerve. However, it must be deflated to permit maximal advancement of the triceps mechanism in the latter stages of the procedure. A posterior linear incision is used passing lateral to the olecranon and parallel to the lateral border of the ulna (Fig. 7A). The ulnar nerve must be identified and protected, but formal mobilization or transposition is not necessary. The small bone fleck often associated with triceps avulsion is excised. If a large fragment has been avulsed, which usually occurs in the adolescent population, repair is amenable to tension band technique or screw-and-washer fixation.

A nonabsorbable no. 5 suture is woven through the freshened tendon in Bunnell fashion. Criss-crossed bone tunnels in the olecranon, as described by Morrey, is an excellent method to secure the suture (see Fig. 7B).[55] Again, care must be taken not to tether or entrap the ulnar nerve, which lies immediately adjacent to the repair. The suture is tied with the tourniquet deflated and the arm extended. Placing the knot on the lateral side of the ulna will help avoid ulnar nerve irritation and local tenderness when the arm is resting on a hard surface (see Fig. 7C). After routine closure, the arm is splinted at 30 to 45 degrees of elbow flexion, depending on the quality of tissue and tension on the repair.

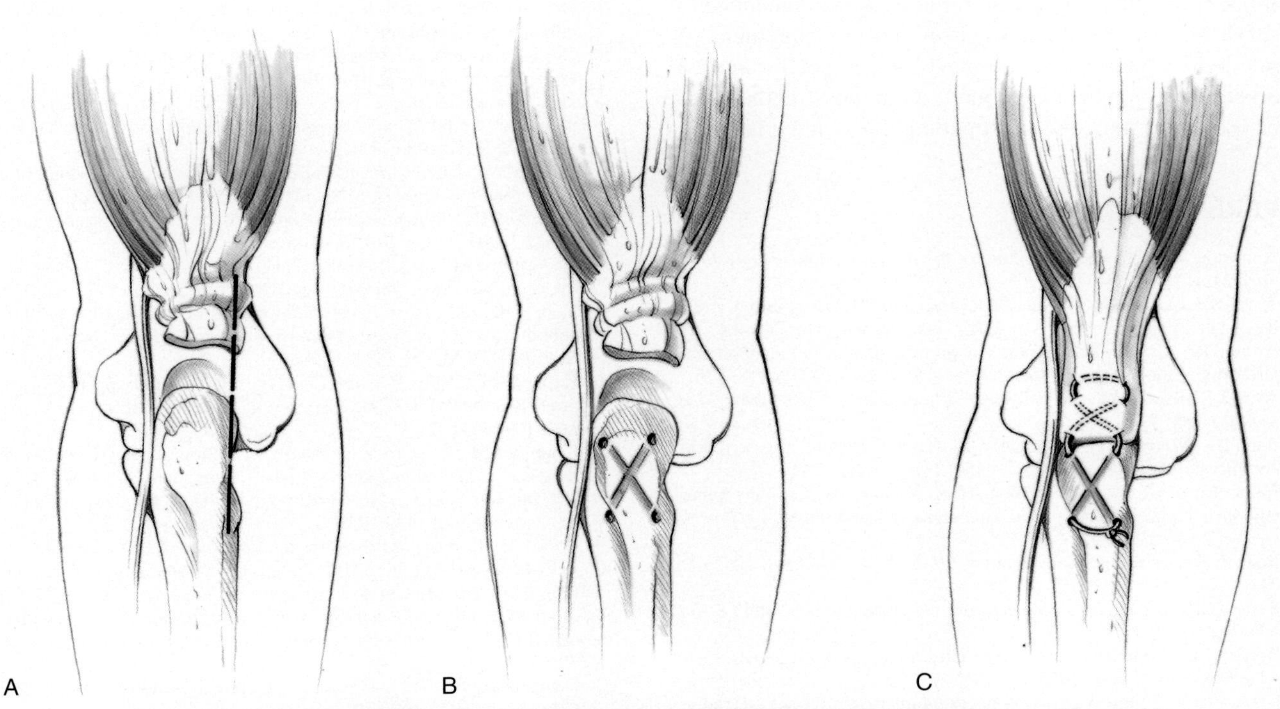

FIG. 7. (A-C) Surgical technique for repair of triceps tendon avulsion. See text for details. (Adapted from ref. 55, with permission.)

I would recommend immobilizing the arm in a posterior splint for approximately 2 to 3 weeks postoperatively. The duration of postoperative immobilization in the literature ranges from 10 days to 6 weeks, averaging 3 weeks.[5] Gentle active elbow flexion and passive extension are begun 2 to 3 weeks after surgery. Resisted exercises are initiated at 6 weeks. Return to full unrestricted activity occurs between 4 and 6 months after surgery and is determined by the quality of the tissue repaired and the patient's specific functional demands.

Complications

No significant complications, such as rerupture or ulnar nerve injury, have been reported with operative repair of triceps avulsions. Wire sutures did cause a bursa over the olecranon in one case and, therefore, should probably be avoided.[59] Not a single case of failed repair was found in the literature.

SUMMARY

Muscle ruptures about the shoulder girdle are relatively uncommon. Unrecognized or untreated rupture of the deltoid origin will severely affect shoulder function. It is difficult to predict the consequences of an isolated coracobrachialis or short head of biceps disruption. Complete pectoralis major rupture from its tendinous insertion will significantly impair strength in high-demand athletes and laborers. The triceps is the sole extender of the elbow, and therefore its integrity is essential for normal upper extremity function. In general, anatomic repair of acute tendon ruptures is recommended to preserve normal shoulder function. The management of muscle belly ruptures is determined by the specific muscle involved and the extent of injury. Awareness of these injuries is the first step toward proper diagnosis and treatment.

REFERENCES

1. Anderson KJ, LeCocq JF. Rupture of the triceps tendon. *J Bone Joint Surg [Am]* 1957;39:444–446.
2. Anzel SH, Covey KW, Weiner AD, Lipscomb PR. Disruption of muscles and tendons: an analysis of 1,014 cases. *Surgery* 1959;45:406.
3. Arciero RA, Cruser DL. Pectoralis major rupture with simultaneous anterior dislocation of the shoulder. *J Bone Joint Surg* 1997;6:318–320.
4. Aso K, Torisu T. Muscle belly tear of the triceps. *Am J Sports Med* 1984;12:485–487.
5. Bach BR, Warren RF, Wickiewicz TL. Triceps rupture. A case report and literature review. *Am J Sports Med* 1987;15:285–289.
6. Baratz M, ElAttrache N, Herndon JH. Rupture of the pectoralis major tendon: a report of 2 cases: an acute and a delayed repair. *Pittsburgh Orthop J* 1990;1:42.
7. Bennett BS. Triceps tendon ruptures. *J Bone Joint Surg [Am]* 1962;44:741.
8. Berson BL. Surgical repair of pectoralis major rupture in an athlete. *Am J Sports Med* 1979;7:348–351.
9. Brodeur AE, Silberstein MJ, Graviss ER. *Radiology of the pediatric elbow.* Boston: GK Hall, 1981.
10. Carpentier E, Tourne Y, Vernay A. Les traumatismes fermes du tendon du triceps brachial. *J Chir* 1992;129:99–102.
11. Caughey MA, Welsh P. Muscle ruptures affecting the shoulder girdle. In: Rockwood CA, Matsen FA, eds. *The shoulder.* 2nd vol. Philadelphia: WB Saunders, 1990:863–873.
12. Cirincione RJ, Baker BE. Tendon ruptures with secondary hyperparathyroidism. A case report. *J Bone Joint Surg [Am]* 1975;57:852.
13. Clayton ML, Thirupathi R. Rupture of the triceps tendon with olecranon bursitis. *Clin Orthop* 1984;184:183–185.
14. Clemens H. Traumatische hemie des m. deltoideus. *Dtsch Med Wochenschr* 1913;39:2197.
15. Curtis RJ. Injuries of the proximal humerus region. In: DeLee JC, Drez D, eds. *Orthopaedic sports medicine.* Philadelphia: WB Saunders, 1994:664–716.
16. D'Alessandro DF, Shields CL. Biceps rupture and triceps avulsion. In: Jobe FW, ed. *Operative techniques in upper extremity sports injuries.* St Louis: CV Mosby, 1996:506–517.
17. D'Alessandro DF, Shields CL, Tibone JE, Chandler R. Repair of distal biceps tendon ruptures in athletes. *Am J Sports Med* 1993;21:114–119.
18. Davis CB. Plastic repair of the deltoid muscle. *Surg Clin* 1919;3:287–289.
19. Delport HP, Piper MS. Pectoralis major rupture in athletes. *Arch Orthop Trauma Surg* 1982;100:135–137.
20. Egan TM, Hall H. Avulsion of the pectoralis major tendon in a weight lifter: repair using a barbed staple. *Can J Surg* 1987;30:434.
21. Farrar EL, Lippert FG. Avulsion of the triceps tendon. *Clin Orthop* 1981;161:242–246.
22. Fery A, Sommelet J, Schmitt D, Lipp B. Avulsion bilaterale simultanee des tendons quadricipital et rotulien et rupture du tendon tricipital chez un hemodialyse hyperparathyroidien. *Rev Chir Orthop* 1978;64:175.
23. Flatow EL, Bigliani LU, April EW. An anatomic study of the musculocutaneous nerve and its relationship to the coracoid process. *Clin Orthop* 1989;244:166–171.
24. Gilcreest EL. Rupture of muscle and tendons, particularly subcutaneous rupture of the biceps flexor cubiti. *JAMA* 1933;84:1819–1822.
25. Gilcreest EL. The common syndrome of rupture, dislocation and elongation of the long head of the biceps brachii; an analysis of 100 cases. *Surg Gynecol Obstet* 1934;58:322.
26. Gilcreest EL, Albi P. Unusual lesions of muscles and tendons of the shoulder girdle and upper arm. *Surg Gynecol Obstet* 1939;68:903.
27. Grantham SA, Kiernan HA. Displaced olecranon fractures in children. *J Trauma* 1975;15:197–204.
28. Heckman JD, Levine MI. Traumatic closed transection of the biceps brachii in the military parachutist. *J Bone Joint Surg [Am]* 1978;60:369–372.
29. Herrick RT, Herrick S. Ruptured triceps in a powerlifter presenting as cubital tunnel syndrome. *Am J Sports Med* 1987;15:514–516.
30. Hollinshead WH, ed. *Anatomy for surgery: the back and limbs.* 3rd ed. Philadelphia: Harper & Row, 1982.
31. Hunter MB, Shybut GT, Nuber G. The effect of anabolic steroid hormones on the mechanical properties of tendons and ligaments. *Trans Orthop Res Soc* 1986;11:240.
32. Jones MW, Matthews JP. Rupture of pectoralis major in weight lifters: a case report and review of the literature. *Injury* 1988;19:219.
33. Jorgensen U, Hinge K, Rye B. Rupture of the distal biceps brachii tendon. *J Trauma* 1986;26:1061–1062.
34. Kawashima M, Sato M, Torisu T, Himeno R, Iwabuchi A. Rupture of the pectoralis major: report of two cases. *Clin Orthop* 1975;109:115.
35. Kelley JD, ElAttrache N. Muscle ruptures of the shoulder girdle. In: Jobe FW, ed. *Operative techniques in upper extremity sports injuries.* St Louis: CV Mosby, 1996:360–372.
36. Kennedy JC, Willis RB. The effects of local steroid injections on tendons: a biomechanical and microscopic correlative study. *Am J Sports Med* 1976;4:11–21.
37. Kramhoft M, Solgaurd S. Spontaneous rupture of the extensor pollicis longus tendon after anabolic steroids. *J Hand Surg [Br]* 1986;11:87.
38. Kretzler HH, Richardson AB. Rupture of the pectoralis major muscle. *Am J Sports Med* 1989;17:453.
39. Lee MHL. Rupture of the triceps tendon. *Br Med J* 1960;2:197.
40. Levy M, Fishel RE, Stern GM. Triceps tendon avulsion with or without fracture of the radial head: a rare injury? *J Trauma* 1978;18:677–679.
41. Levy, M, Goldberg I, Meir I. Fracture of the head of the radius with tear or avulsion of the triceps tendon. *J Bone Joint Surg [Br]* 1982;64:70–72.
42. Lindenbaum BL. Delayed repair of a ruptured pectoralis major muscle. *Clin Orthop* 1975;109:120.
43. Liu J, Wu J, Chang S, Chou Y, Lo W. Avulsion of the pectoralis major tendon. *Am J Sports Med* 1992;20:366–368.

44. Lotem M, Bernheim J, Conforty B. Spontaneous ruptures of tendons—A complication of hemodialyzed patients treated for renal failure. *Nephron* 1978;21:201–208.
45. Mackenzie DB. Avulsion of the insertion of the pectoralis major muscle. *S Afr Med J* 1981;7:147.
46. Manjarris J, Gershuni DH, Miotoza J. Rupture of the pectoralis major tendon. *J Trauma* 1985;25:810–811.
47. Mankin HJ. Rickets, osteomalacia, and renal osteodystrophy. Parts I & II. *J Bone Joint Surg [Am]* 1974;56:101–128, 352–386.
48. Marmor L, Bechtol CO, Hall CB. Pectoralis major muscle function of sternal portion and mechanism of rupture of normal muscle: case reports. *J Bone Joint Surg [Am]* 1961;43:81–87.
49. Martin JR, Wilson CL, Mathews WH. Bilateral rupture of ligamenta patellae in case of disseminated lupus erythematosus. *Arthritis Rheum* 1958;6:548–552.
50. McEntire JE, Hess WE, Coleman S. Rupture of the pectoralis major muscle: a report of eleven injuries and review of fifty-six. *J Bone Joint Surg [Am]* 1972;54:1040.
51. McMaster PF. Tendon and muscle ruptures. Clinical and experimental studies and locations of subcutaneous ruptures. *J Bone Joint Surg* 1933; 15:705–722.
52. Miles JW, Grana WA, Egle D, Min K, Chitwood J. The effect of anabolic steroids on the biomechanical and histological properties of rat tendon. *J Bone Joint Surg [Am]* 1992;74:411–422.
53. Miller DM, Johnson DL, Fu FH, Thaete FL, Blanc RO. Rupture of the pectoralis major muscle in a collegiate football player: use of magnetic resonance imaging in early diagnosis. *Am J Sports Med* 1993;21: 475–477.
54. Montgomery AH. Two cases of muscle injury. *Surg Clin Chicago* 1920;4:871.
55. Morrey BF. Tendon injuries about the elbow. In: Morrey BF, ed. *The elbow and its disorders*. 2nd ed. Philadelphia: WB Saunders, 1993: 492–504.
56. Moulonguet G. Rupture spontanee du grand pectoral chez un vieillard: enorme hematome. *Mort Bull Mem Soc Anat Paris* 1924;94:24.
57. Murphy KJ, McPhee I. Tears of major tendons in chronic acidosis with elastosis. *J Bone Joint Surg [Am]* 1965;47:1253.
58. Orava S, Sorasto A., Aalto K, Kvist H. Total rupture of pectoralis major muscle in athletes. *Int J Sports Med* 1984;5:272–274.
59. Pantazopoulos T, Exarchou E, Stavrou Z, Hartofilakidis-Garofalidis G. Avulsion of the triceps tendon. *J Trauma* 1975;15:827.
60. Park JY, Espiniella JL. Rupture of pectoralis major muscle: a case report and review of the literature. *J Bone Joint Surg [Am]* 1970;52:577.
61. Patissier P. Traite des Maladies des Artisans. Paris: 1822:162–164.
62. Penhallow DP. Report of a case of ruptured triceps due to direct violence. *NY Med J* 1910;91:76.
63. Poland J, ed. *A practical treatise on traumatic separation of the epiphyses*. London: Smith, Elder & Company, 1898.
64. Preston ET. Avulsion of both quadriceps tendons in hyperparathyroidism. *JAMA* 1972;221:406–407.
65. Preston FS, Adicoff A. Hyperparathyroidism with avulsion at three major tendons. *N Engl J Med* 1961;266:968.
66. Purnell R. Rupture of the pectoralis major muscle: a complication. *Injury* 1988;19:284.
67. Ritchie AJ, Rocke LG. Spontaneous rupture of the triceps in the presence of a patella cubiti. *Arch Emerg Med* 1990;7:114–117.
68. Rockwood CA, Wilkins KE, King RE. *Fractures involving the proximal physis of the olecranon: fractures in children*. Philadelphia: JB Lippincott, 1991.
69. Roi GS, Respizzi S, Dworzak F. Partial rupture of the pectoralis major muscle in atheltes. *Int J Sports Med* 1990;11:85.
70. Ronchetti G. Rottura sottocutanea parziale del muscolo grand pettorale con formazione di pseudocistie ematica. *Minerva Chir* 1959;14: 22–28.
71. Schutt RC, Powell RL, Winter WG. Spontaneous ruptures of large tendons. American Academy of Orthopedic Surgeons Annual Meeting, New Orleans, January 25, 1982.
72. Scott BS, Wallace WA, Barton MAJ. Diagnosis and assessment of pectoralis major rupture by dynamometry. *J Bone Joint Surg [Br]* 1992;74: 111.
73. Searfoss R, Tripi J, Bowers W. Triceps brachii rupture: a case report. *J Trauma* 1976;16:244–246.
74. Sherman OH, Snyder SJ, Fox JM. Triceps tendon avulsion in a professional body builder. *Am J Sports Med* 1984;12:328–329.
75. Silberstein MJ, Brodeur AE, Graviss ER, Atchawee L. Some vagarities of the olecranon. *J Bone Joint Surg* 1981;63:722–725.
76. Stannard JP, Bucknell AL. Rupture of the triceps tendon associated with steroid injections. *Am J Sports Med* 1993;21:482–485.
77. Tarsney FF. Rupture and avulson of the triceps. *Clin Orthop* 1972;83: 177–183.
78. Tietjen R. Closed injuries of the pectoralis major muscle. *J Trauma* 1980;20:262.
79. Thompson TC. A test for rupture of the tendo achilles. *Acta Orthop Scand* 1962;32:461–465.
80. Tobin WJ, Cohen LJ, Vandover JT. Parachute injuries. *JAMA* 1941; 117:1318.
81. Twinning RH, Marcus WY, Garey JL. Tendon ruptures in systemic lupus erythematosus. *JAMA* 1964;187:120–124.
82. Unverferth JL, Olix ML. The effects of local steroid injections on tendon. *J Sports Med* 1973;1:31–37.
83. Urs ND, Jani DM. Surgical repair of the pectoralis major muscle: a case report. *J Trauma* 1976;16:749.
84. Verfaillie SM, Claes T. Bony avulsion of the pectoralis major muscle. *J Bone Joint Surg* 1996;5:327–329.
85. Viegas S. Avulsion of the triceps tendon. *Orthop Rev* 1990;19: 533–536.
86. Waugh RL, Hathcock TA, Elliott JL. Ruptures of muscle and tendons. *Surgery* 1949;25:370.
87. Welsh RP, Macnab I, Riley V. Biomechanical studies of rabbit tendon. *Clin Orthop* 1971;81:171–177.
88. Wener JA, Shein AJ. Simultaneous bilateral rupture of the patello tendon and quadriceps expansions in systemic lupus erythematosus. A case report. *J Bone Joint Surg [Am]* 1974;56:823.
89. Wolfe SW, Wickiewicz TL, Cavanaugh JT. Ruptures of the pectoralis major muscle: an anatomic and clinical analysis. *Am J Sports Med* 1992;20:587.
90. Zeman SC, Rosenfeld RT, Liscomb PR. Tears of the pectoralis major muscle. *Am J Sports Med* 1979;7:343.

PART II

Glenohumeral Instability

Disorders of the Shoulder: Diagnosis and Management,
edited by Joseph P. Iannotti and Gerald R. Williams, Jr.
Lippincott Williams & Wilkins, Philadelphia © 1999.

CHAPTER 8

Anatomy, Biomechanics, and Pathophysiology of Glenohumeral Instability

Brian J. Cole and Jon J.P. Warner

INTRODUCTION

The complexity of the shoulder joint is best appreciated from our understanding of how shoulder anatomy and biomechanics are intrinsically related to the pathophysiology of shoulder instability. A multidisciplinary collaboration between surgeons, biomechanical engineers, anatomists, biochemists, and several other basic scientists is responsible for recent advances in these areas. No longer is our understanding of shoulder instability based on anecdotal and qualitative clinical experiences documenting shoulder pathology. A plethora of gross and histologic cadaveric studies, radiographic studies, and biomechanical studies now provides a sound foundation to understand how a minimally constrained articulation can balance mobility and stability. Alterations in any of the anatomic or biomechanical factors requisite for shoulder stability provide the pathogenesis for clinical instability.

The purpose of this chapter is to review the current anatomic and biomechanic factors that control glenohumeral joint motion and stability. Because anatomy and biomechanics are two interdependent disciplines, they will be discussed together as each of the relevant structures is reviewed. A deeper understanding of this relation will provide substantive data critical to classify and appreciate the pathophysiology of glenohumeral instability. More importantly, the application of anatomic and biomechanic principles provides a rational approach to the treatment of glenohumeral instability for optimal functional restoration.

DEFINING THE PROBLEM

Laxity is asymptomatic, passive translation of the humeral head on the glenoid as determined by clinical examination and is unassociated with pain. Laxity is required for normal

B.J. Cole: Department of Orthopaedics, Rush-Presbyterian St. Luke's Medical Center, Chicago, Illinois 00612.
J.J.P. Warner: Harvard Shoulder Service, Harvard Medical School, Massachusetts General Hospital, Boston, Massachusetts 02114.

glenohumeral motion and may be affected by age,[45] gender, and congenital factors. In general, laxity changes with the position of the arm. At the extremes of rotation, the static restraints tighten and decrease laxity. Whether laxity is a risk factor for the development of clinical instability is a matter of debate.[127]

Instability is a pathologic condition that manifests as pain or discomfort in association with excessive translation of the humeral head on the glenoid fossa during active shoulder motion. Both clinical[35,45,54] and experimental studies[62,63,158,183,184,192] demonstrate a wide range of normal "play" in the glenohumeral joint; thus, it is the association with symptoms that clearly separates instability from excessive laxity. A spectrum of instability exists, representing increasing degrees of injury and dysfunction of the dynamic and static factors that function normally to contain the humeral head within the glenoid.

ANATOMIC AND BIOMECHANIC CONSIDERATIONS

Anatomic control of glenohumeral joint stability can be divided into static (e.g., ligaments and tendons) and dynamic (e.g., muscular contraction) factors (Table 1). The cooperative role that these factors play is complex, and no single factor is responsible for glenohumeral joint stability. Similarly, no single lesion is responsible for clinical instability (Table 2). Contemporary approaches to the treatment of glenohumeral joint instability are directed at restoring normal anatomy and biomechanics, as opposed to simply constraining motion, as has been historically described.[33,46]

Establishing criteria for "normal" and "pathologic" conditions of the glenohumeral joint is often difficult owing to the considerable individual variation in capsuloligamentous anatomy[42,47,123,125,183,184] and in inherent shoulder laxity.[45,62,63,98] Dynamic factors (i.e., rotator cuff and biceps) are affected by their level of conditioning and strength. Scapulothoracic motion[191] is a more subtle, but equally important, dynamic factor helping to maintain shoulder stability. To add to this complex equation, an interaction between static capsuloligamentous factors and dynamic muscular factors, mediated through proprioception, has been postulated.[18,31,95,98]

Anatomic and biomechanic dysfunction leading to glenohumeral instability results from varying levels of applied stress (i.e., a single traumatic event versus cumulative microtrauma), the relative risk of injury associated with an activity, the quality and integrity of the static stabilizers, and the strength and conditioning of the dynamic stabilizers. An individual's "susceptibility" for glenohumeral instability is dependent on these factors, each of which will be discussed in the following sections. The consequences of deficiency of any one component will be presented.

TABLE 1. *Factors maintaining joint stability*

Factors
Static factors
Articular components
Articular version
Glenoid labrum
Negative intraarticular pressure
Adhesion–cohesion
Capsule and ligament
Rotator cuff
Dynamic factors
Rotator cuff
Biceps brachii
Scapular rotators
Proprioception

Static Factors

Articular Version

Both arthrographic and roentgenographic studies have characterized the relation between the humeral head and the glenoid surface of the scapula. With the arm hanging at the side in an adducted position, the scapula faces 30 degrees anteriorly on the chest wall, tilts 3 degrees upward relative to the transverse plane and 20 degrees forward relative to the sagittal plane (Fig. 1).[123] As described by Saha,[155] in 75% of persons the average glenoid orientation is in 7 degrees of retroversion, with 25% persons having anteversion ranging from 2 to 10 degrees. Saha[155] and others[10] have observed that the glenoid has an average superior tilt of 5 degrees (Fig. 2). Scapular inclination may have a contributory role in controlling inferior stability.[184] However, the difficulty in interpreting these studies arises from a wide range of interindividual variability, the reproducibility of techniques used to measure these factors, and an unknown relative contribution to clinical instability.

Recently, the anatomy of the proximal humerus has been significantly clarified. Saha[155] was one of the first to radiographically show that the neck-shaft angle averages 130 to 140 degrees and retroversion averages 30 degrees relative to the transepicondylar axis of the distal humerus (see Fig. 2).

Walch and Boileau,[181] using a micron precision probe and a computer to render a three-dimensional image of 65 humeri, determined that the inclination of the articular surface varies between 114 and 147 degrees with an average value of 130 degrees. In this same study, the average humeral retroversion measured 17.9 degrees (range, −6.5 to 47.5 degrees).

Articular Conformity

The glenohumeral joint in the adult consists of the humeral head and glenoid surface of the scapula. Understanding the glenoid and humerus as separate, but interdependent, congruent structures is integral to appreciate how these two joint surfaces can maintain stability, yet provide for a relatively large range of motion. This congruent articulation provides the foundation for the rotator cuff to establish a concavity–compression effect as it dynamically com-

TABLE 2. *Normal and abnormal anatomy and biomechanics*

Stability factor	Pathoanatomy
Glenoid version	Congenital: abnormal version; dysplasia
	Fracture causing abnormal version
Humeral version	Congenital: abnormal version; dysplasia
	Fracture/surgery causing abnormal version
Articular congruity	Congenital: dysplasia
	Acquired: fracture, Bankart lesion, osteoarthritis
Labrum	Bankart lesion
	"Fraying" secondary to laxity
Capsuloligamentous	Traumatic tear, cumulative microtrauma with plastic deformation
	Congenital laxity
	Loss of proprioceptive feedback
Negative intraarticular pressure	Capsular tear
	"Rotator interval" defect
	Lax capsule
Rotator cuff deficiency	Traumatic tear, cumulative microtrauma
Biceps	SLAP lesion
	Tendon rupture
Scapulothoracic motion	Dyskinesis: fatigue and weakness of serratus
	Long thoracic nerve palsy

presses the convex humeral head into the matched concavity of the glenoid.[99] Furthermore, as an extension of the glenoid, the labrum functions to increase the depth and surface area of the glenohumeral articulation enhancing this effect.[71]

The glenoid surface is "pear-shaped," similar to an inverted comma, being approximately 20% narrower superiorly than inferiorly (Fig. 3). The average vertical and transverse dimensions are 35 and 25 mm, respectively. In contrast, the larger humeral head has vertical and transverse dimensions averaging 48 and 45 mm, respectively.[123] Approximating a sphere, the humeral head has a surface area that is three times that of the glenoid.[162] In any position of rotation there is a surface area mismatch such that only 25% to 30% of the humeral head is in contact with the glenoid surface.[154] In other words, the glenoid's relatively smaller surface area is insufficient to cover the humeral head. This emphasizes the importance of the soft tissues and muscles surrounding the joint in providing stability during shoulder function.

Walch and Boileau[180] determined that the humeral head is comparable to a sphere in 90% of the 160 humeri they examined, with the articular surface constituting about one-third of the sphere. The diameter of the head was variable with an average of 43.2 mm (range, 36.5 to 51.7 mm) with an articular cartilage thickness on average of 15.2 mm (range, 12 to 18 mm). They demonstrated that the spherical humeral head sits with a frontal plane medial offset of 6.9 mm on average (range, 2.9 to 10.6 mm) and a sagittal plane posterior offset of 2.6 mm (range, 0.8 to 6.1 mm). These parameters, however, may have more implications for shoulder arthroplasty design than for shoulder stability. Similarly, Iannotti et al.[75] reported that the humeral head approximates

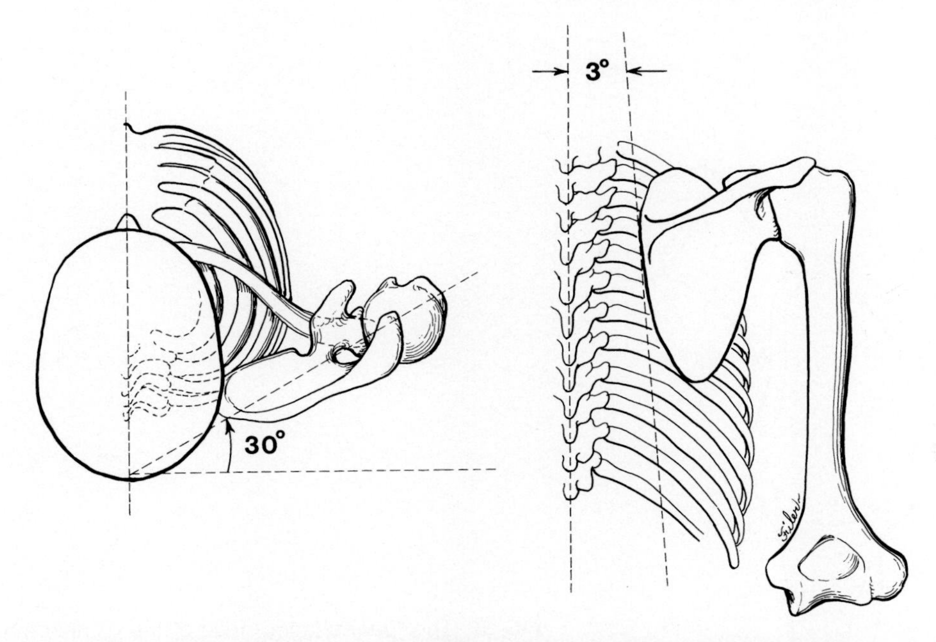

FIG. 1. Scapular orientation on chest wall. **(Left)** 30 degrees anterior; **(Right)** 3 degrees upward. (From Warner JJP. The gross anatomy of the joint surfaces, ligaments, labrum and capsule. In: Matsen FA III, Fu FH, Hawkins RJ, eds. *The shoulder: a balance of mobility and Stability.* Rosemont: American

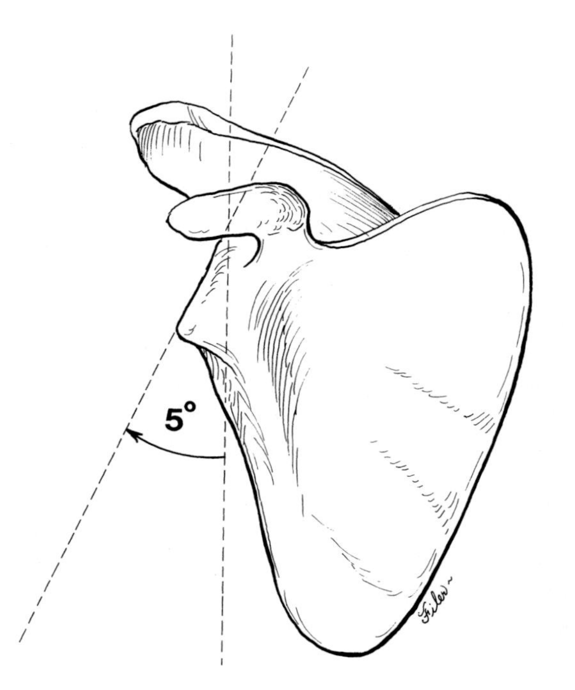

FIG. 2. (Left) Superior tilt of the glenoid (see text). (From Warner JJP. The gross anatomy of the joint surfaces, ligaments, labrum and capsule. In: Matsen FA III, Fu FH, Hawkins RJ, eds. *The shoulder: a balance of mobility and stability*. Rosemont: American Academy of Orthopaedic Surgeons, 1993: 9, with permission.) **(Center and right)** Glenoid and humeral version, and neck-shaft angle of proximal humerus (see text). (From Warner JJP, Caborn DNM. Overview of shoulder instability. *Crit Rev Phys Rehabil Med* 1992;4:145–198, with permission.)

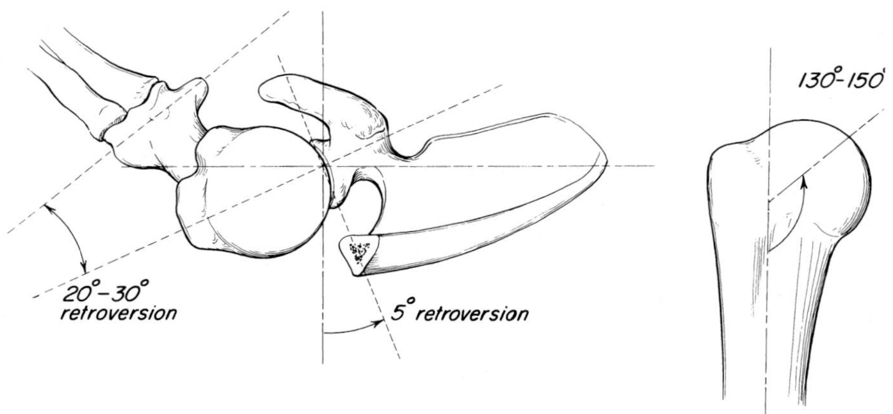

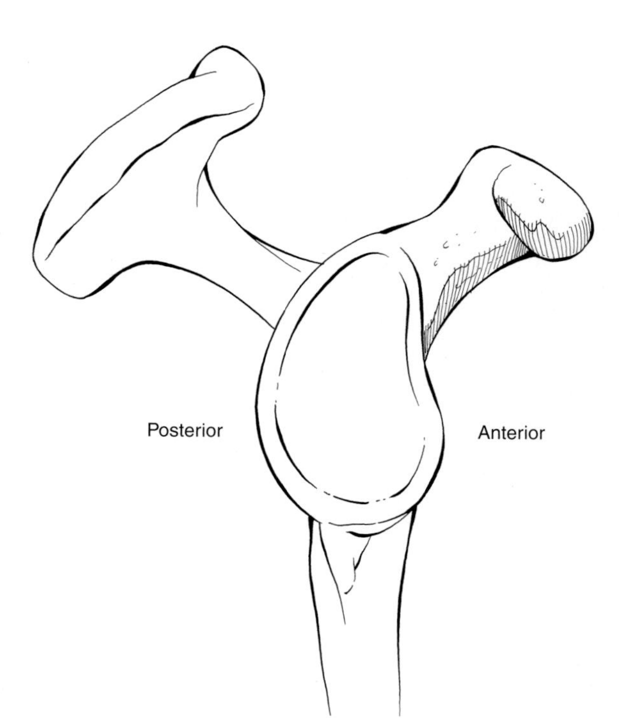

FIG. 3. The "pear-shaped" face of the glenoid that articulates with the humeral head. (From Boardman ND III, Fu FH. Shoulder biomechanics. In: McGinty JB, Caspari RB, Jackson RW, Poehling GG, eds. *Operative arthroscopy*. Philadelphia: Lippincott–Raven, 1996: 627, with permission.)

a sphere in the central articular areas and becomes slightly elliptical peripherally. Variations in these findings and their effect on the pathophysiology of shoulder instability is not clearly understood.

Conceptually, the glenohumeral joint has been compared to a "golfball sitting on a tee"[123] (Fig. 4). This analogy is based on historical beliefs sighting the relatively small area of the glenoid and its relative shallowness compared with the humeral head, allowing only a limited portion of the humeral head to contact the glenoid in any single shoulder position.[22,155,156] In fact, the articular surfaces of the humeral head and glenoid are almost perfectly matched with a congruence within 3 mm, with deviations from sphericity of less than 1%.[112,162] Additionally, the cartilage of the glenoid is thicker peripherally, and thus, plain radiographs tend to underestimate the relative concavity of the glenoid. This would imply that the glenohumeral joint would function similar to a ball-and-socket articulation as described by Kelkar et al.[87,88]

Although some coupled translation occurs at the extremes of glenohumeral rotation,[62,63,98] tracking of the geometric center of the cartilaginous articular surface with simulated muscle forces actually approximates ball-in-socket motion.[88] In the stable shoulder, external and internal rotation is associated with posterior and anterior humeral head translation, respectively. These relations may be altered in the unstable shoulder. McMahon et al.,[106] in an elegant model using a dynamic shoulder testing apparatus, measured muscle force values and tendon excursions across the glenohumeral joint during abduction in the scapular plane. They determined that humeral head translations on the glenoid were less than 2 mm under all testing conditions used and that the joint does behave kinematically as a "ball-and-socket" articulation during glenohumeral abduction. The importance of these findings is that articular incongruency is probably less of a predisposing factor for instability than is surface area mismatch, as seen in glenoid dysplasia or glenoid fracture.[6,90,97,149,151,166] Additionally, the integrity of the soft tissues influences coupled translation, and this may also be a greater predisposing factor to instability than is articular incongruency.[25,62,71,72]

Glenoid Labrum

The relative lack of depth and surface area of the bony glenoid is compensated by the fibrous labrum acting to maintain normal glenohumeral biomechanics. As determined by Cooper et al.,[38] the labrum is a fibrous ring attaching to the glenoid articular cartilage through a narrow fibrocartilaginous transition zone. Above the glenoid equator, the labrum is relatively more mobile. In contrast, below the equator, the labrum is more consistently tightly attached to the glenoid articular cartilage. The tendon fibers of the long head of the biceps brachii blend with the superior labrum, and the inferior glenohumeral ligament (IGHL) blends into the inferior labrum. Cooper et al.[38] examined the vascular supply of the labrum and found that the superior and anterosuperior parts of the labrum were less vascular than the posterosuperior and inferior portions. Blood supply was limited to the periphery.

The labrum contributes to stability of the glenohumeral joint through several mechanisms. It acts as an anchor point for the capsuloligamentous structures.[38,110,142] Howell and Galinat[71] have shown how the labrum enhances stability by

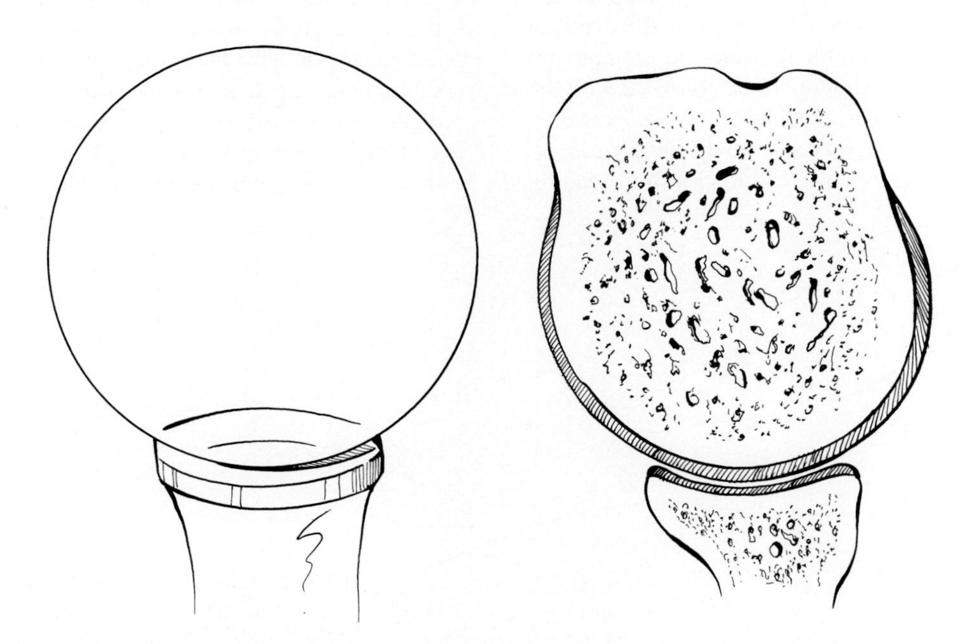

FIG. 4. Analogy of the glenohumeral joint to a golf ball and tee. (Boardman ND III, Fu FH. Shoulder biomechanics. In: McGinty JB, Caspari RB, Jackson RW, Poehling GG, eds. *Operative arthroscopy.* Philadelphia: Lippincott–Raven, 1996:627, with permission.)

deepening the concavity of the glenoid socket to an average of 9 and 5 mm in the superoinferior and anteroposterior planes, respectively (Fig. 5). Loss of the labrum decreases the depth of the socket by 50% in either direction. Functionally, this acts as a "chock-block" preventing the head from slipping over the edge of the glenoid. Lippitt et al.[99] demonstrated that resection of the labrum reduced resistance to translation by 20%, and it was especially effective in doing so in combination with joint compression in the midrange of glenohumeral motion. The labrum also acts to increase the surface area of contact, acting as a load-bearing structure similar to the function of the meniscus in the knee.[24,163] Unlike the meniscus, however, the labrum lacks the microscopic architecture to disperse hoop stress and, therefore, is unlikely to effectively bear load.

Vanderhooft et al.[178] and Bowen et al.[25] have shown that the labrum plays a significant stabilizing role during rotator cuff contraction, facilitating the concavity–compression mechanism as the humeral head is compressed into the glenoid. Recently, Lazarus et al.[94] have defined a *stability ratio*, as a measure of the effectiveness of concavity–compression in the stabilization of the glenohumeral joint, as the ratio between the maximum dislocating force that can be stabilized in a given direction and the load compressing the head into the glenoid. They determined that by creating a chondral–labral defect, an 80% reduction in the height of the glenoid occurred, with a concomitant reduction in the stability ratio of 65% for translation in the direction of the defect.

A Bankart lesion represents a lesion of the labrum corresponding to the detachment of the anchoring point of the IGHL and middle glenohumeral ligament (MGHL) from the glenoid rim.[9,149] A Bankart lesion disrupts the concavity–compression effect during rotator cuff contraction, eliminates the "chock-block" effect, and decreases the depth of the socket by 50% with detachment of the capsuloligamentous structures. This lesion should not be confused with the normal anatomic variants of a sublabral sulcus underneath a cordlike MGHL or a loosely attached labrum superiorly. Whether the Bankart lesion is the "essential lesion" leading to recurrent anterior instability, as suggested by several authors, is currently a topic of interest.[9,22,110] Isolated detachment of the labrum as a singular entity leading to recurrent instability was challenged early in the literature by Townley[174] and now recently by Speer et al.[164] and others.[80] Today, its role as a glenohumeral restraint remains in debate.

Recently, Pagnani et al.[133] have demonstrated the importance of the superior portion of the glenoid labrum. In a cadaver study, isolated lesions of the anterosuperior portion of the labrum did not have a significant effect on glenohumeral translation. However, complete lesions of the superior portion of the labrum associated with destabilization of the biceps insertion resulted in significant increases in anteroposterior and superoinferior glenohumeral translations in the lower and middle ranges of elevation. The implications of these findings are that destabilization of the glenoid insertions of the superior glenohumeral ligament (SGHL), MGHL, and biceps insertion may be associated with subtle increases in translation and may be related to the symptoms present in patients who have isolated lesions of the superior labrum.[133,161]

Negative Intraarticular Pressure

In normal shoulders, a relative vacuum exists as a result of high osmotic pressure in the interstitial tissues, causing water to be drawn out of the glenohumeral joint.[102] As the articular surfaces are pulled apart, a suction effect develops to resist further displacement. The magnitude of this negative pressure has been shown to be about −42 cm of water in the adducted and relaxed shoulder. This increases to −82 cm water during the application of a 25-N inferior force applied to the cadaver shoulder.[27] Negative intraarticular pressure becomes especially important when the rotator cuff is not contracting or when tension has not developed in the superior and coracohumeral ligaments during glenohumeral motion.

Pathologic conditions may include those that cause venting of the glenohumeral joint, leading to inferior subluxation, as has been shown experimentally by Warner et al.[185]

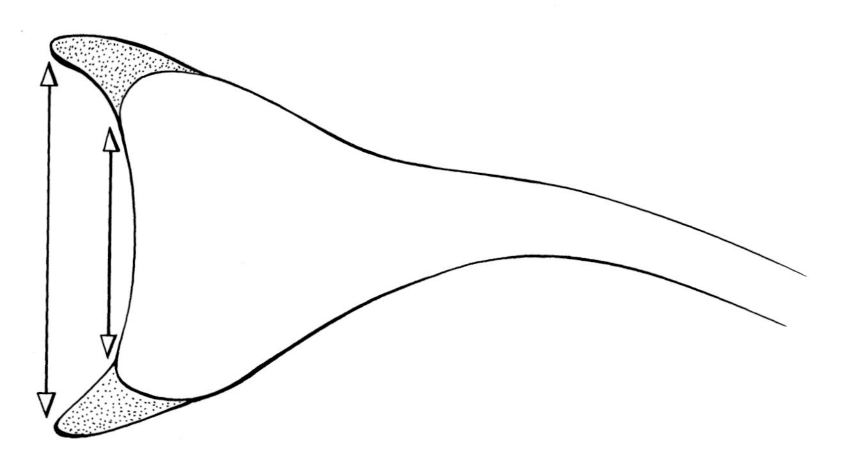

FIG. 5. Glenoid labrum increases the surface area and depth of the glenoid socket. (From Warner JJP, Caborn DNM. Overview of shoulder instability. *Crit Rev Phys Rehabil Med* 1992:4: 145–198, with permission.)

and others.[92] Wuelker et al.[196] observed that venting of the joint increased displacement significantly in the anterior, posterior, and inferior planes. Anterior translation also increased by 55%[56] after capsular venting. This restraint becomes negligible, however, when the muscles contract with shoulder abduction or when the IGHL or superior capsular structures are under tension.[27,185] In a study by Helmig et al.,[68] venting of the capsule led to significant increases in anteroposterior translation and external rotation. The implications of their findings were that evaluation of shoulder stability in biomechanical investigations should be performed before violation of the negative intraarticular pressure mechanism occurs, or at the very least, measures should be corrected for this factor.

Thus, as a static restraint, negative intraarticular pressure appears to be important in limiting translation of the humeral head. Habermeyer et al.[60] noted that the presence of a Bankart lesion somehow eliminated the intraarticular seal to atmospheric pressure. A traumatic capsular rupture or an enlarged rotator interval capsular defect, possibly present at birth, presumably could lead to excessive glenohumeral translation, predisposing to instability.[36] Recently, Hashimoto et al.[65] have indicated that dynamic changes in intraarticular pressure can help differentiate patients with adhesive capsulitis, partial- and full-thickness rotator cuff tears, and instability. Practically, from a clinical perspective, reestablishing negative intraarticular pressure remains a theoretical concern and plays no role in the treatment of shoulder instability.

Adhesion–Cohesion

The glenohumeral joint contains less than 1 mm of synovial fluid that provides articular nourishment through diffusion and lubrication through several mechanisms (e.g., hyrodynamic, boundary, weeping, or boosted). Viscous and intermolecular forces help to create this adhesion–cohesion effect. Functionally, this is a stabilizing mechanism that permits sliding motion between the two joint surfaces while simultaneously limiting them from being pulled apart.[102] This is analogous to two glass plates separated by a thin film of water that slide easily over one another, but are difficult to separate. Clinically, like negative intraarticular pressure, this factor probably plays a minor role in maintaining glenohumeral stability and only at very low load levels.

Capsuloligamentous Structures

Few structures in the shoulder have received as much attention by investigators as the capsule and ligaments surrounding the glenohumeral joint. Traditionally, the ligaments of the capsule were described as discreet thickenings constituting the "glenohumeral ligaments."[42,123,125,157] Clinical observations at the time of surgery[4,22,51,110,114,134,149,151,152] or by cadaver shoulder dissections[32,9,42,47,71,120,125,149,152,175] have enhanced our understanding of these structures from an anatomic perspective. To obtain a concise appreciation of these structures, anatomic investigations must minimally distort the ligamentous relationships (Fig. 6). With increasing sophistication, the biomechanical function,[56,124,126,129,148,184] material properties,[16,21,61,86,145,173] and the interrelation of the rotator cuff and capsule have been described.[29,73,103,120,148,183] Synthesizing the available data into a cohesive algorithm applicable to the clinical setting of glenohumeral instability is a formidable task for most.

In a classic anatomic study, DePalma[42] described the variability of the shoulder capsule, categorizing it into six basic types based on the pattern of the synovial recesses. Other anatomic studies have since confirmed and clarified the variable architecture of the glenohumeral ligaments.[47,110] Contemporary investigators suggest, as did DePalma,[42] that some anatomic findings correlate with the risk of developing shoulder instability.[108,184] The basis for the functional roles of the capsular structures lies in their anatomic arrangement throughout the capsule. A significant advance in our knowledge came from Turkel et al.,[175] who confirmed by anatomic radiographic studies that different portions of the capsuloligamentous complex provided static stability that depends on arm position and the direction of the load applied to the proximal humerus.

The glenohumeral ligaments function principally during rotation of the arm to reciprocally tighten and loosen, thus limiting translation and rotation in a load-sharing fashion.[186] In the midrange of rotation when these structures are relatively lax, stability is maintained primarily by the action of the rotator cuff and biceps through the concavity–compression effect across the glenohumeral joint.[63,99] The ligaments principally protect against instability when the joint is placed at the extremes of motion and become especially important when all other stabilizing mechanisms have been overwhelmed.[102]

Clinically, this becomes important during capsular reconstruction. Tensioning these structures in the midrange can potentially overtighten and constrain the joint, limiting rotation.[100,188] In the extreme case, this may lead to posterior humeral subluxation or arthritis.[13,17] The static role of each component of the capsuloligamentous structure is summarized in Table 3. In the sections that follow, each structure will be reviewed in terms of contemporary research describing the anatomy and biomechanics as well as a limited discussion on the relevant material properties.

Superior and Coracohumeral Ligaments

These structures are considered together because their anatomic courses are parallel and they constitute the reinforcing structures of the "rotator interval" region.[21,36,64,114,120,123,149] The rotator interval subtends a medially based triangular space, bordered superiorly by the anterior margin of the supraspinatus tendon, inferiorly by the superior border of the subscapularis tendon, medially by the base of the coracoid, and laterally by the long head of the bi-

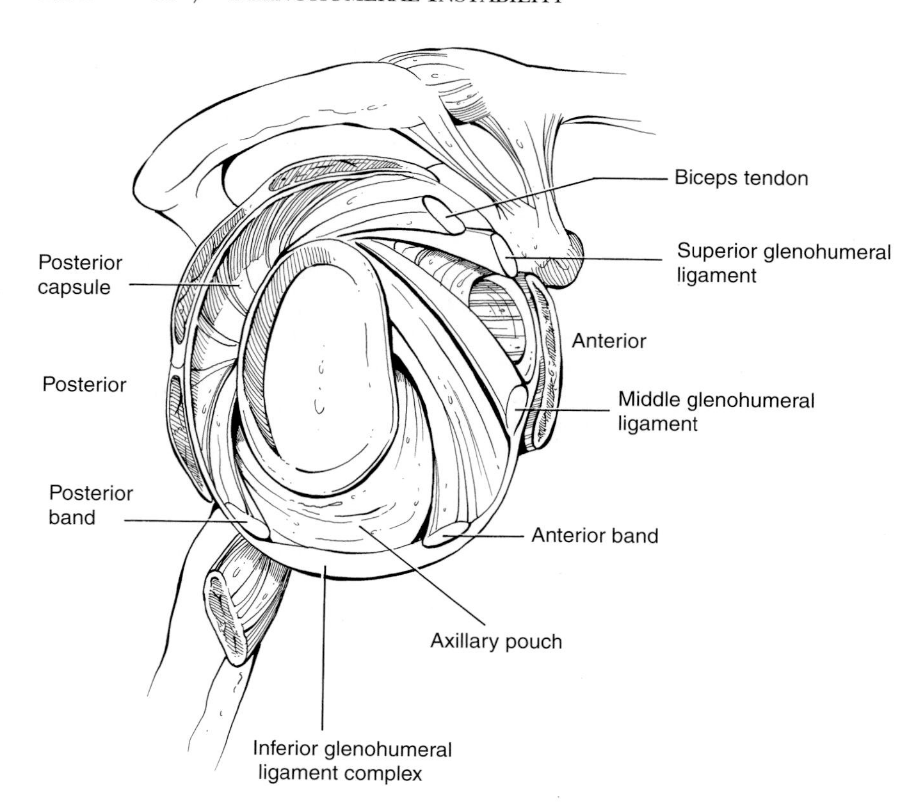

FIG. 6. Capsuloligamentous anatomy viewed from the side with the anterior *(S)* aspect to the right and the posterior aspect *(P)* to the left. The humeral head has been removed, leaving the glenoid. The superior (*SGHL*) and middle (*MGHL*) ligaments are labeled. The inferior glenohumeral ligament complex (*IGHLC*) consists of an anterior band (*AB*), posterior band (*PB*), and interposed axillary pouch (*AP*). The posterior capsule (*PC*) is the area above the posterior band (*PB*). The biceps (*B*) is also labeled. (From O'Brien SJ, et al. The anatomy and histology of the inferior glenohumeral ligament complex of the shoulder. *Am J Sports Med* 1990;18:449–456, with permission.)

ceps tendon and sulcus. The floor of the rotator interval is normally bridged by capsule. Occasionally, a complete opening within the tissue spanning the rotator interval is present and is described as a "rotator interval capsular defect" (Fig. 7).

The coracohumeral ligament (CHL) is a dense fibrous extraarticular structure originating on the lateral surface of the coracoid process as a broad (1 to 2 cm) and thin structure. It inserts into the greater and lesser tuberosities adjacent to the bicipital groove and becomes intermingled with the tendinous edges of the supraspinatus and subscapularis, respectively.[42,64] Cooper et al.[39] questioned the significance of the CHL, describing it as a capsular fold creating a "pup tent" of capsule within the rotator interval. Others argue that the CHL is a well-defined structure that prevents excessive inferior translation of the adducted humerus in either position of humeral rotation.[116,129]

The SGHL lies deep to the CHL and is variable in size and is present in over 90% of cases.[42,123,126,152,158,184] Usually quite diminutive, it originates from the superior glenoid tubercle just inferior to the biceps tendon and runs parallel to the CHL as it inserts into the superior aspect of the lesser tuberosity just medial to the bicipital groove.

Opinions vary on the specific functions of these two ligaments. Harryman et al.[64] characterized the relative biomechanical contribution of the rotator interval capsule to shoulder stability in cadaver specimens. A transverse incision in the rotator interval region including the capsule, CHL, and SGHL allowed statistically significant increases in humeral head translations in all planes tested. Imbrication of the rotator interval decreased inferior translation in adduction and posterior translation in flexion to less than the intact state. No attempt was made to isolate the role of specific capsular ligaments. Basmajian et al.,[10] using electromyographic and anatomic dissections, showed that the superior capsule and the CHL resisted downward displacement with the arm adducted, independent of load.

Patel et al.[135] recently described the CHL to consist of an anterior and posterior band originating at the coracoid and inserting into the lesser and greater tuberosities, respectively. During adduction and external rotation, the SGHL and anterior band of the CHL shortened from a maximally lengthened position. These changes were opposite those of the posterior band of the CHL that was maximally lengthened with adduction and internal rotation. Warner et al.[184] suggested that the SGHL resists inferior translation of the adducted shoulder and that the CHL is not important here. However, subsequent work by Boardman et al.[21] suggested that the CHL is the principal functional component of the capsule within the rotator interval.

Despite varying opinions in the literature (see Table 3), the current consensus is that these two structures constrain the humeral head on the glenoid, limit inferior translation and external rotation when the arm is adducted, and posterior translation when the shoulder is in a position of forward flexion, adduction, and internal rotation. There has been renewed interest in this portion of the shoulder capsule because openings within the rotator interval have been associated with recurrent anteroinferior and multidirectional instability.[48,64,119,149] As suggested by several of these studies, addressing this pathology may be important in preventing recurrence. Conversely, contracture or scarring of this portion of the shoulder capsule has been associated with adhesive capsulitis.[64,116]

Middle Glenohumeral Ligament

As described by DePalma[42] and others,[123,125,158,183,184] the MGHL has the greatest variation in size and presence of all the ligaments of the shoulder. It is absent or poorly defined in 40% of individuals.[47,125] It originates from the supraglenoid tubercle and anterosuperior labrum, often along with the SGHL, and inserts just anterior to the lesser tuberosity, blending with the posterior aspect of the subscapularis tendon. Its variable morphology usually takes one of two forms: (a) sheetlike and confluent with the anterior band of the IGHL or (b) cordlike, with a foraminal separation between it and the anterior band of the IGHL. Moseley and Overgaard[110] reported that the MGHL originated from the scapular neck and formed an anterior pouch accommodating the humeral head in some patients with recurrent anterior instability.

It is generally believed that the MGHL functions as a passive restraint to both anterior and posterior translation of the humeral head when the arm is abducted in the range from 60 to 90 degrees in external rotation and limits inferior translation when the arm is adducted at the side. Those who are "MGHL dominant" individuals with a cordlike MGHL may be more dependent on this structure to provide a protective role against anterior instability.[108,184] Clinically, the MGHL may be detached from the anterior glenoid and constitutes the leading edge of a Bankart lesion, which typically includes the anterior band of the IGHL. However, the sublabral hole should not be confused with a detached labrum, for generally the labrum is more mobile above the equator of the glenoid.

Inferior Glenohumeral Ligament Complex

Originally described by DePalma,[42] several descriptions of the IGHL exist in the literature ranging from a triangular-shaped structure coursing from the labrum to the humeral neck, to one with well-defined thickenings at its leading edge.[125,173,175] Typically, it originates from the anteroinferior labrum or inferior half of the neck of the glenoid adjacent to the labrum and inserts just inferior to the MGHL at the humeral neck. Our current understanding has advanced to the point at which we now consider this structure to be quite developed, with very specific functions attributed to its individual components. O'Brien et al.[125] have defined this structure, through arthroscopic, gross, and histologic evaluation, as the inferior glenohumeral ligament complex (IGHLC) consisting of three components. They described a discrete anterior and posterior band (ligament) with an interposed thinner axillary pouch (see Fig 6). The complex consists of three well-defined layers of collagen fibers extending from the glenoid to the humerus (inner and outer) and running circumferentially around the joint (middle). Ticker et al.[173] and Bigliani et al.[16] have recently challenged the presence of a discrete posterior band and found all regions of the IGHLC to be thicker near the glenoid than the humerus.

O'Brien et al.[125] suggested that the IGHLC functions as a hammock to support the humeral head as it undergoes reciprocal tightening–loosening with abduction or rotation as the orientation of the complex changes. In adduction, it forms a dependent fold, acting as a secondary restraint limiting large inferior translations.[125,184] In abduction, however, this complex moves underneath the humeral head, becoming taut, in

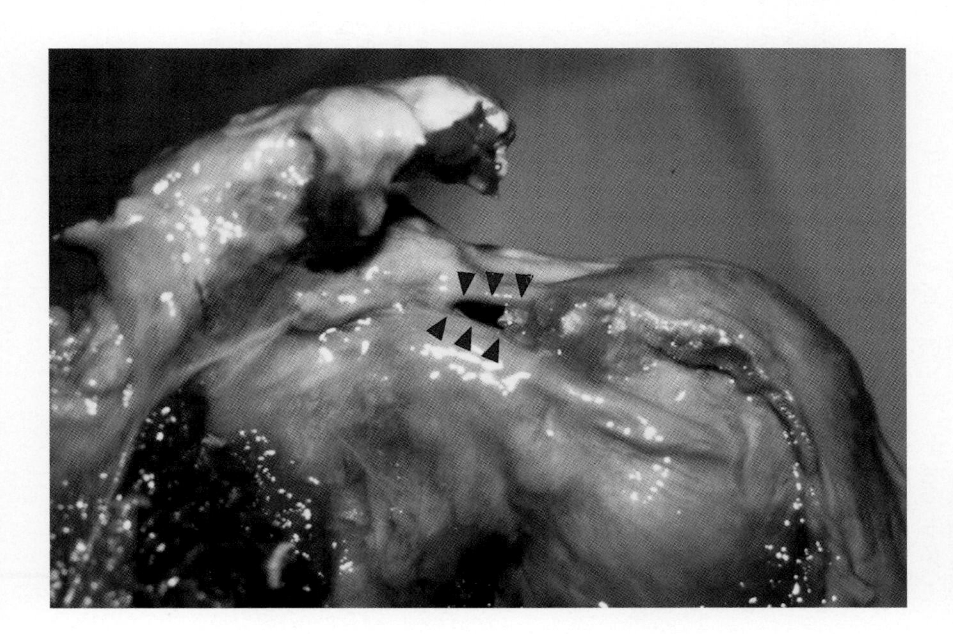

FIG. 7. Gross anatomic specimen of a left shoulder demonstrating the opening within the rotator interval situated between the supraspinatus and subscapularis muscle tendons.

TABLE 3. *Functions of the ligaments*

Author	SGHL	CHL	MGHL	IGHLC	Other
Turkel et al.[175]	Little role in anterior stability		Primary stabilizer for anterior stability at 45-degrees abduction; limits ER in mid-ABD	Primary stabilizer for anterior instability in ABD	Subscapularis is secondary stabilizer at 45-degrees ABD
Ovesen and Nielsen[128–130]	Secondary stabilizer to posterior instability	Secondary stabilizer to posterior instability; primary stabilizer against inferior instability in ABD	Important for anterior instability at 45-degree ABD	Posterior capsule plays role in anterior and posterior stability	
Schwartz et al.[158]; O'Brien etal.[124]	Little role in stability			1 degree and 2 degree stabilizers against anterior and posterior instability in ABD	
Basmajian and Bazant[10]	Primary restraint to inferior translation in ADD	Primary restraint to inferior translation in ADD			
Warren et al.[193]	Secondary restraint to posterior instability in ADD, flexed, IR				Posterior capsule is primary restraint to posterior translation
O'Connell et al.[126]	Primary restraint to ER in ADD		Secondary restraint to ER in ABD; primary restraint to anterior instability at 45-degree ABD		
Ferrari[47]	Primary restraint to ER in lower range of ABD		Important restraint to ER at 60 and 90 degrees ABD		
Helmig et al.[67]		Primary restraint to inferior instability			
Harryman et al.[62]		Primary restraint to ER			
Warner et al.[183]	Primary restraint to inferior translation in ADD	Minimal role in inferior stability	Secondary stabilizer for inferior translation in ADD	Primary stabilizer to inferior translation in ABD and secondary stabilizer in ADD	

ER, external rotation; ABD, abduction; ADD, adduction; IR, internal rotation.

the fashion of a hammock, effectively limiting inferior translation. As the arm is internally rotated, the complex moves posteriorly, and as the arm is externally rotated, the complex moves anteriorly, forming a barrier to posterior and anterior dislocation, respectively (Fig. 8). Horizontal flexion and extension in abduction will also tighten the posterior or anterior components, respectively, thereby limiting anteroposterior translation.[158] Recently, another biomechanical study by O'Brien et al.[124] verified that the primary anteroposterior stabilizer of the 90-degree abducted shoulder is the IGHL. The anterior band was the primary stabilizer in 30 degrees of horizontal extension and the posterior band at 30 degrees of horizontal flexion.

Injury to the IGHLC plays an integral role in the development of anterior instability. Surgical reconstruction directed at anatomic restoration of this part of the capsule has been advocated even in the earliest reports on the surgical management of shoulder instability.[9] Although all of the structures that define the shoulder capsule have at least a limited role, alterations of the IGHLC is believed by most to be a significant factor in the pathophysiology of anterior shoulder instability.

Posterior Capsule

This is the capsule extending from superior to the posterior band of the IGHLC to the intraarticular portion of the biceps tendon.[125] Other than the capsule found within the rotator interval, this is the thinnest region of the joint capsule.[36,125] There are no direct posterior ligamentous reinforcements. Its role is to limit posterior translation when the shoulder is forward-flexed, adducted, and internally rotated.[193] Clinically, this becomes relevant in patients who present with posterior instability.

Material Properties

Because instability is often associated with failure of the static constraints (e.g., the capsuloligamentous structures), recent investigations have focused on the individual material properties and the modes of failure. The shoulder capsule is quite redundant, having a surface area two times that of the humeral head.[123] Material properties of the capsule refer to the intrinsic mechanical characteristics of its composition, molecular structure, and ultrastructure. Presumably anatomic variability (e.g., the SGHL and MGHL) may have clinical implications. In other words, a more robust ligament (e.g., IGHL) is presumably more tolerant of strain or force and would be expected to play a more significant role in helping to maintain glenohumeral stability.

Similar to other joint capsules in the body, the shoulder capsule is composed primarily of type I collagen, with lesser amounts of types II and III. Reeves[145] determined that the average maximum tensile strength of the anteroinferior capsule measured in cadaver shoulders is 70 N (at least 20 kg), decreasing after age 50. Between the ages of 10 and 40, the anteroinferior labral insertion was the weakest portion of the

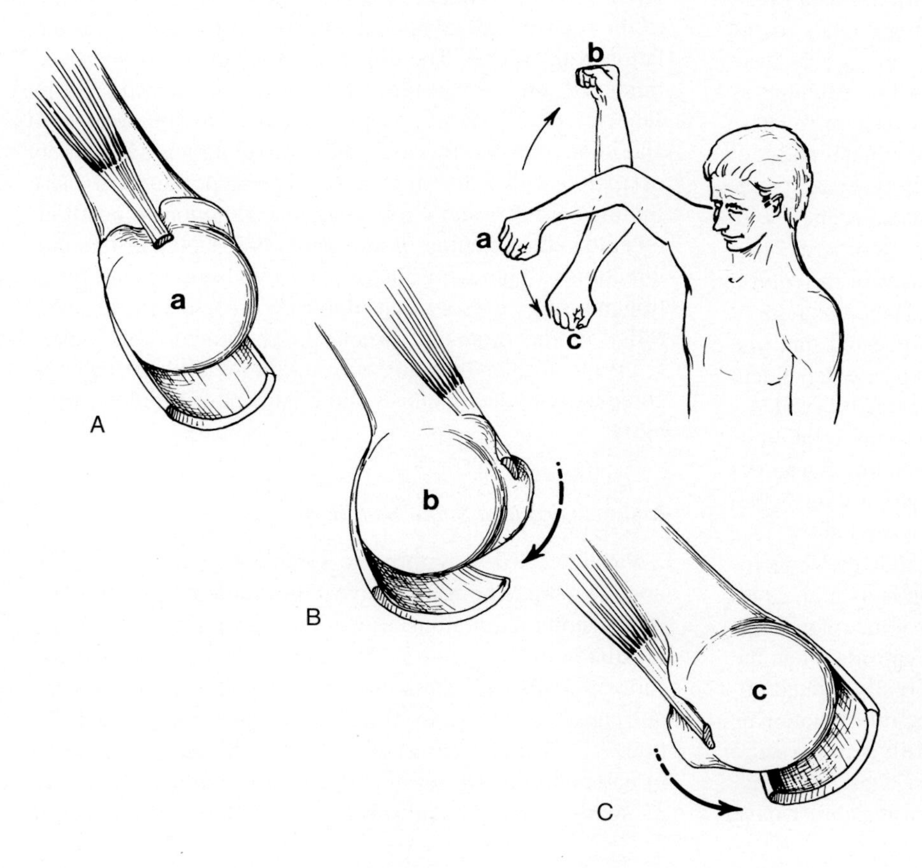

FIG. 8. The "hammock"-like anatomy of the inferior glenohumeral ligament complex allows for reciprocal tightening of its anterior and posterior portions when the arm moves from neutral rotation in **(a)** abduction to external **(b)** and internal **(c)** rotation. (From Warner JJP, Caborn DNM. Overview of shoulder instability. *Crit Rev Phys Rehabil Med* 1992;4:145–198, with permission).

whole complex, with more than two-thirds of the failures occurring there. Specimens in the fifth to seventh decades experienced capsular rupture and subscapularis tendon failure more frequently than failure at the labrum.[145] That the anteroinferior portion of the capsule fails first and capsular strength varies inversely with age has also been demonstrated by Kaltsas.[86] Recently, Hara et al.[61] evaluated the glenoid labrum and capsule and determined that the anteroinferior labrum close to the glenoid cartilage was weakest, rupturing with a mean force of 3.84 kg/5 mm.

The properties of the IGHL have been well described by Bigliani et al.[16] who used tensile testing to analyze strength and failure modes in humerus–IGHLC–glenoid specimens. The region of the anterior band had the greatest thickness (average 2.8 mm), progressively decreasing in the axillary pouch (average 2.3 mm) and posterior capsular regions (average 1.7 mm). In contrast to O'Brien et al.,[125] no discrete posterior band was identified, and the axillary pouch was not the thickest region. Additionally, there were no significant differences in the resting length or width of these areas.[16]

Stress at failure of the anterior axillary pouch (average 5.5 MPa) was substantially lower than that described for the knee ligaments (estimated at 35 to 80 MPa[198]), emphasizing the importance of other stabilizing mechanisms in protecting the IGHLC from structural failure. Similar inferior strength characteristics have been described for the SGHL and CHL.[21] The superior band and anterior axillary pouch exhibit significant strain rate-dependent viscoelastic behavior. These effects were explained by compositional data determining that a proteolglycan content gradient exists, being greatest anterosuperiorly and least posteroinferiorly. Mechanically, this property leads to viscoelastic stiffening as the collagen fibers are "uncrimped" during tension.[16] These investigators also determined that the predominant modes of failure were at the glenoid insertion, with slower strain rates as seen in the Bankart lesion, and in the midsubstance, with faster strain rates as seen with capsular laxity or stretching. This is explained by a nearly elastic behavior in the central region of the IGHL and principally viscoelastic behavior at the bony insertion.[16,173] These authors suggested that viscoelastic behavior during tension and strain rate-dependent properties of the IGHL support its role as a humeral head stabilizer in the position of abduction and external rotation as force is rapidly applied. Thus, functional adaptation may occur to stabilize the head during high-energy activities when other static or dynamic restraints are overwhelmed.

Morrey and Chao[109] have calculated that the anterior shear force in the position of apprehension is as high as 60 kg. To counteract these forces, contraction of the rotator cuff significantly reduces stress in the anterior capsule when the arm is in the maximally abducted and externally rotated position.[29] Thus, the dynamic restraints to stability function as a protective mechanism against structural failure of the static restraints. Although investigated to a lesser degree, the material properties of the restraints to posterior instability have been described. Weber and Caspari displaced the humeral head posteriorly in 90 degrees of flexion and full internal rotation, resulting in a horizontal split in the posterior capsule and posterior labral avulsion from the glenoid.[195] Because the results of these studies depend on a simulated mechanism of injury in the presence of an inactive rotator cuff, rigid interpretation and extrapolation to the pathoanatomy of instability is somewhat speculative.

Obligate Translations

A relatively new area of research interest is focused on understanding the relation between glenohumeral rotation and obligate translation caused by asymmetrical tightening–loosening of the capsuloligamentous structures. Howell and Galinat[72] used axillary radiographs of patients to measure anteroposterior excursion during glenohumeral rotation. Except for maximal extension with external rotation, the humeral head remained centered on the glenoid. In normal subjects, the extended and externally rotated position caused the humeral head to translate posteriorly. In patients with anterior instability, posterior excursion did not occur. Taken a step further, Harryman et al.[63] monitored loads and translations with a magnetic-tacking device in cadaver specimens. Anterior translation occurred with flexion beyond 55 degrees, and posterior translation occurred with extension beyond 35 degrees. Interestingly, these authors found that surgical tightening of the posterior capsule resulted in increased anterior translation with flexion that occurred earlier in the arc of motion compared with normal specimens. Tightening of the rotator interval also increased obligate anterior translation with flexion. The effects of Bankart repair and overtightened inferior capsular shifts were also investigated by Janevic et al.[80] These procedures shifted the humeral head and joint contact posteriorly during loading with abduction, extension, and external rotation. The importance of these findings are that static restraints may function in positions other than the extremes of rotation. It is conceivable that unidirectional tightness, primary (e.g., overhead athlete) or iatrogenic (e.g., anterior capsulorrhapy), could lead to instability in the opposite direction. These concepts, while requiring further investigation, add an additional layer of complexity to the diagnosis and treatment of shoulder instability.

Rotator Cuff as a Static Stabilizer

Passive tension within the rotator cuff musculotendinous structures appear to have some static role in preventing glenohumeral translation. The "posterior mechanism of dislocation" occurs in older patients who sustain supraspinatus and infraspinatus tendon tears, with or without capsular injury, in association with anterior dislocation.[41,145] Rupture of the subscapularis has also been noted in patients with recurrent dislocations who are older than 35 years of age.[117] The subscapularis statically limits anterior translation in lower ranges of abduction with similar limitations to posterior translation found from the infraspinatus and teres minor.[129,130] Recently, the contribution of passive bulk tissues and the deltoid to static inferior glenohumeral stability was investigated by Motzkin et al.[111] This study determined that in both humeral adduction and abduction, passive bulk tissues (i.e., all tissues superficial to the deltoid) and the deltoid did not provide significant stability to the shoulder joint. Thus, the rotator cuff appears to be one of the few dynamic restraints that has a concomitant passive role in preventing glenohumeral instability.

Dynamic Factors

Clinical experience suggests that static stabilizers by themselves may not be as important in enhancing glenohumeral stability as that provided by the dynamic stabilizers or the relation between them. Experimentally, specimens dissected free of the rotator cuff and long head of the biceps tend to demonstrate at least some degree of inferior subluxation.[92,129] Active contraction of these structures contributes to the dynamic stabilization of the glenohumeral joint through two mechanisms: (a) joint compression (e.g., concavity–compression) resulting from synergistic and coordinated rotator cuff activity and (b) ligament dynamization through direct attachments to the rotator cuff muscles. Augmenting these mechanisms are the long head of the biceps brachii, coordinated scapulothoracic rhythm, and proprioception providing feedback about extremity position and movement.

Joint Compression

Contraction of the rotator cuff and long head of the biceps brachii augments joint stability by enhancing the conforming fit and increasing the load needed to translate the humeral head through compression of the humeral head into the glenoid.[29,99,102] Lipitt et al.[99] quantified the magnitude of the tangential forces required to produce glenohumeral dislocation in the setting of applied joint-compressive loads of 50 and 100 N. Tangential forces were as high as 60% of the applied joint-compressive load. The stability of the joint was markedly reduced if a portion of the labrum was removed. Vahey et al.[177] introduced the concept of "scapulohumeral balance" to illustrate that glenoid geometry coupled with joint compression is a major stabilizing force. Bowen et al.[25] determined that a joint compression load of 111 N was sufficient to stabilize the glenohumeral joint in the face of a 50 N force, despite sectioning of three-fourths of the joint capsule. It has been suggested from the results of ligament cutting studies and direct quantification of the efficiencies of the dynamic stabilizers that joint compression is a more important stabilizer to translation than are static capsular constraints.[20,25]

Poppen and Walker[141] showed that the joint reaction force was a maximum of 0.89 times body weight directed into the face of the glenoid at 90 degrees of abduction using a simplified two-dimensional cadaveric model with digitized radiographs. Also, the subscapularis had a greater mechanical advantage at lower abduction angles (i.e., 60 degrees), whereas the deltoid had a greater advantage at higher abduction positions. McKernan et al.[103] have validated these findings and attributed them to the anterior location of the subscapularis tendon in lower ranges of elevation, making it a more effective stabilizer against a given translation. This effect is reduced as the shoulder is elevated and the line action of the subscapularis moves superior to the joint.

All portions of the rotator cuff are probably important in enhancing stability as was shown by Blasier et al.[19] In their biomechanical study, omission of tension in any one of the rotator cuff muscles led to a substantial reduction in anterior joint stability. Rotator cuff tears result from either single traumatic or cumulative microtraumatic (i.e., overuse injuries) events. Because of age-related attrition, a dislocation in individuals older than the age of 40 is not uncommonly associated with a rotator cuff tear.[86,117,145] Rotator cuff tears result in superior translation of the humeral head during scapular plane abduction, thereby demonstrating the importance of synchronous contraction of the entire cuff in maintaining containment of the humeral head in the glenoid.[141,192]

Increasing the joint compressive load appears to "center" the humeral head, reducing subsequent translation. In overhead athletes, for example, in whom the rotator cuff functions as an important decelerator to anterior translation, imbalanced muscle recruitment may play a role in those with more subtle forms of instability.[57,82] This has been validated by Warner et al.,[191] who demonstrated that patients with shoulder instability had altered rotator cuff strength patterns compared with normal controls. Asynchronous contraction of the rotator cuff, leading to voluntary instability, is an example in the extreme of the relative importance of the rotator cuff in enhancing dynamic stability of the glenohumeral joint.[150] Conversely, capsuloligamentous insufficiency could subject the rotator cuff to overuse, fatigue, and injury.

The importance of these findings is that rotator cuff-strengthening programs can improve the function of a weak or ineffective cuff by limiting translation of the humeral head on the glenoid during active shoulder motion.[28] Initial therapeutic approaches to shoulder instability, therefore, should emphasize strengthening, conditioning, and coordination of the rotator cuff as an integral part of the treatment program.

Ligament Dynamization

There appear to be direct connections between the rotator cuff tendons and the capsuloligamentous system.[32,47] Clark et al.[32] reported a complex anatomic relation between the tendons of the rotator cuff and the capsule adjacent to the humeral tuberosities. Conceptually, active shoulder motion may "dynamize" the capsule and ligaments, thereby becoming a significant stabilizing factor in the midranges of rotation at which the ligaments and capsule are relatively lax. Warner et al.,[183] in a dynamic shoulder model, were able to define and document the orientation and interrelation between the glenohumeral ligaments during simulated rotator cuff contraction. Although this study clearly elucidated the effect of shoulder rotation on the orientation of the undisturbed and intact capsuloligamentous system, the dynamic effects of rotator cuff contraction upon the ligaments remains unclear.

Pagnani et al.[132] suggested that because the biceps inserts into the relatively mobile superior labrum, it is conceivable that tension would be transmitted by the labrum to the SGHL and MGHL to dynamize these static structures and indirectly enhance stability. A similar relation may exist owing to the proximity of the triceps to the medial aspect of the axillary pouch of the IGHLC.[32,38] Anterosuperiorly, the subscapularis and supraspinatus interconnect with the CHL, providing an additional site for dynamic interaction between static and dynamic restraints.

Active rotation may also have the effect of altering capsular tension, potentially providing a protective mechanism against failure. For example, coupled posterior humeral head translation with active external rotation may actually reduce anterior ligamentous strain.[63,72] McKernan et al.[104] and others[29,147] have shown in cadaveric experiments that contraction of the posterior rotator cuff muscles (i.e., infraspinatus and teres minor) and biceps tendon reduced IGHL strain in the late cocking phase of throwing. These dynamic factors may provide relative protection of the IGHLC or other anterior structures as they contribute to anterior stability by dynamically increasing the resistance to torsional forces in the position of apprehension. Recently, however, the role of the infraspinatus, as determined by electromyographic (EMG) analysis in patients with recurrent anterior instability, was not believed to be a critical component in providing anterior stability.[73] Clinically, that a stabilizing relation may exist between the capsule and musculature about the shoulder signifies the importance in reestablishing length tension relations by either operative or nonoperative means in patients with shoulder instability.

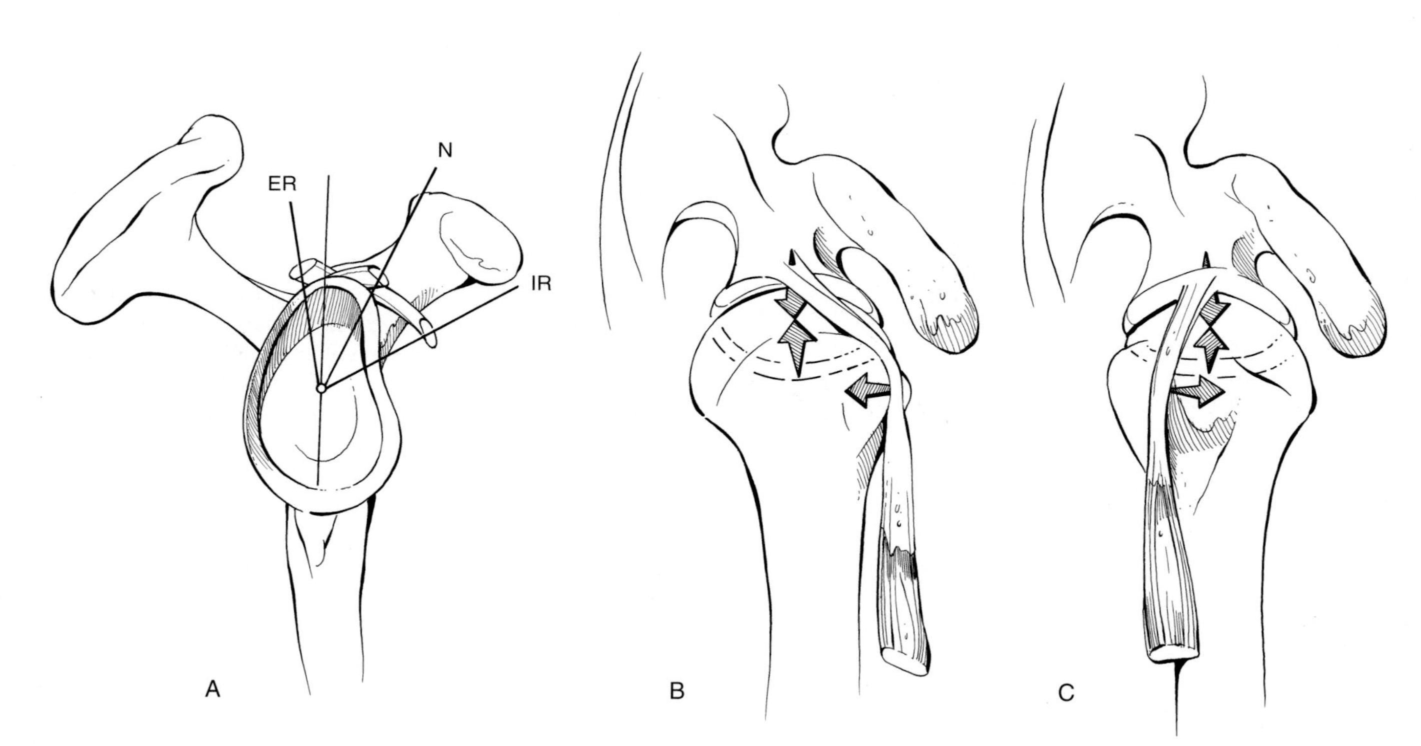

FIG. 9. Diagrammatic representation of forces created with simulated contraction of long head biceps brachii. **(A)** Rotation of humerus changes orientation of biceps tendon relative to the joint. In neutral rotation (*N*) tendon generally occupies a slightly anterior position. With internal rotation (*IR*) the tendon lies anterior to joint. In contrast, the tendon occupies a slightly posterior position with external rotation (*ER*). **(B)** With internal rotation of humerus, the biceps appears to generate joint compressive forces (*paired arrows*) and posteriorly directed force (*single arrow*), which restrain glenohumeral translation. **(C)** With external rotation of the humerus, anteriorly directed force (*single arrow*) appears to accompany joint compressive forces (*paired arrows*). (From ref. 132, with permission.)

Long Head of the Biceps Brachii

As the tendon of the long head of the biceps passes to its insertion in the supraglenoid tubercle, it occupies an intraarticular position. The relative importance as a dynamic stabilizer probably becomes significant when the rotator cuff or capsuloligamentous structures are overwhelmed. Several experimental studies have demonstrated the dynamic-stabilizing role of the long head of the biceps brachii for the glenohumeral joint.[3,57,76,78,132 147] Rodosky et al.[147] showed that, in the late cocking phase of throwing, contraction of the biceps tendon can significantly reduce anterior translation and increase torsional rigidity of the joint helping to resist external rotation. Additionally, strain in the IGHL was noted to increase after sectioning of the tendon.

Pagnani et al.[132] determined that the effect of the long head of the biceps is dependent on the shoulder position being greatest in middle and lower elevation angles. The biceps tended to stabilize the joint anteriorly when the arm was internally rotated and served as a posterior stabilizer when the humerus was externally rotated (Fig. 9). Superoinferior translation was also reduced with simulated contraction of the biceps, which was believed to help center the humeral head on the glenoid, thereby stabilizing the fulcrum and allowing more efficient arm elevation. Recently, Levy et al.[96] emphasized through dynamic EMG analysis that elimination of elbow flexion or supination resulted in complete inactivity of the biceps brachii. Thus, the role of biceps function at the shoulder is either due to a passive mechanism or depends on tension developing in association with elbow and forearm activity.

These concepts may help explain why the biceps tendon or superior labrum may demonstrate lesions in throwers[3,161] and why it is occasionally found to be hypertrophied in the rotator cuff-deficient patient.[101,169] Clinically, this suggests that nonoperative treatment of instability or rotator cuff deficiency should be directed at rehabilitation of the biceps brachii in addition to the rotator cuff muscles.

Scapular Rotators

Until recently, scapulothoracic motion has been relatively ignored as an important dynamic factor maintaining stability of the glenohumeral joint. The scapular rotators include the following muscles: trapezius, rhomboids, latissimus dorsi, serratus anterior, and levator scapulae. Codman[34] first introduced the concept of "scapulohumeral rhythm," which has now been recognized by others to be an important contributor to joint stability.[10,77,155,190] Even though somewhat variable, the normal scapulohumeral rhythm motion relation is two of glenohumeral rotation for every one of scapulothoracic rotation during scapular plane abduction.[140,141] Clinical and radiographic studies have documented abnormal scapulothoracic motion in patients with shoulder instability.[131,190] EMG analysis of the scapulothoracic musculature has demonstrated fatigue of the serratus anterior and trapezius with repetitive overhead activities, leading to poor scapulothoracic control.[57,122]

The scapular rotators function to provide a stable platform beneath the humeral head during shoulder motion (Fig. 10). These muscles allow the glenoid to adjust to changes in arm position. The scapular inclination angle is a significant factor preventing inferior translation of the adducted shoulder.[77] For example, the scapula normally rotates upward (i.e., protraction) in synchrony with arm elevation as the serratus anterior contracts. Thus, clinically, scapulothoracic weakness or dysfunction is associated with varying degrees of scapular winging, which is often found in patients with shoulder instability.[190] Warner et al.[190] have hypothesized that scapulothoracic dysfunction may be a cause of "nonoutlet" impingement, as the advancing greater tuberosity is unable to avoid impingement on the coracoacromial arch during forward flexion. Presently, however, it is unclear if scapulothoracic dysfunction is a cause or product of shoulder instability. Despite these unanswered questions, nonsurgical management of shoulder instability must include rehabilitation of the scapular rotators.

Proprioception

The perception of joint position and joint motion is termed *proprioception*. Proprioceptive interaction between ligaments and muscles may mediate a protective mechanism against capsular failure and instability.[18,31,89,95] Murakami et al.[113] described what were thought to be mechanorecepetors in the transition zone between the labrum and capsule in primates. Since then, others[81,179] have described similar findings in the capsule and ligaments of the glenohumeral joint. Mechanoreceptors are specialized nerve endings (e.g., pacinian corpuscles; Ruffini endings; and Golgi tendonlike endings) that transduce mechanical deformation into electric signals that transmit information about joint position and motion.[58,59]

Lephart et al.[95] and Warner et al.[189] have hypothesized that the capsuloligamentous structures may contribute to stability by providing an afferent feedback for reflex muscular contraction of the rotator cuff and biceps. It is plausible, as these authors discuss, that as these receptors respond to tension changes in the capsule during rotation, active stabilization may occur through reflex arcs from the capsule to the surrounding rotator cuff, allowing selective contraction of the rotator cuff and biceps muscles in response to changes in acceleration.

With use of a specialized proprioception testing device, Lephart et al.[95] evaluated subjects with and without traumatic anterior instability preoperatively and postoperatively after arthroscopic or open Bankart repairs. In normal shoulders, the threshold to detect passive motion (TTDPM) averaged 1.5 to 2.2. In those with instability, TTDPM was 2.8. These differences were statistically significant. Postoperatively, patients' TTDPM was that no different from normal. One criticism of this study was that the speeds at which patients were tested were much slower than the speeds that occur with overhead sports. Ito et al.[79] has stated that traumatic dislocation may, in fact, occur sooner than the response time of the rotator cuff stretch reflex. Thus, the relative impor-

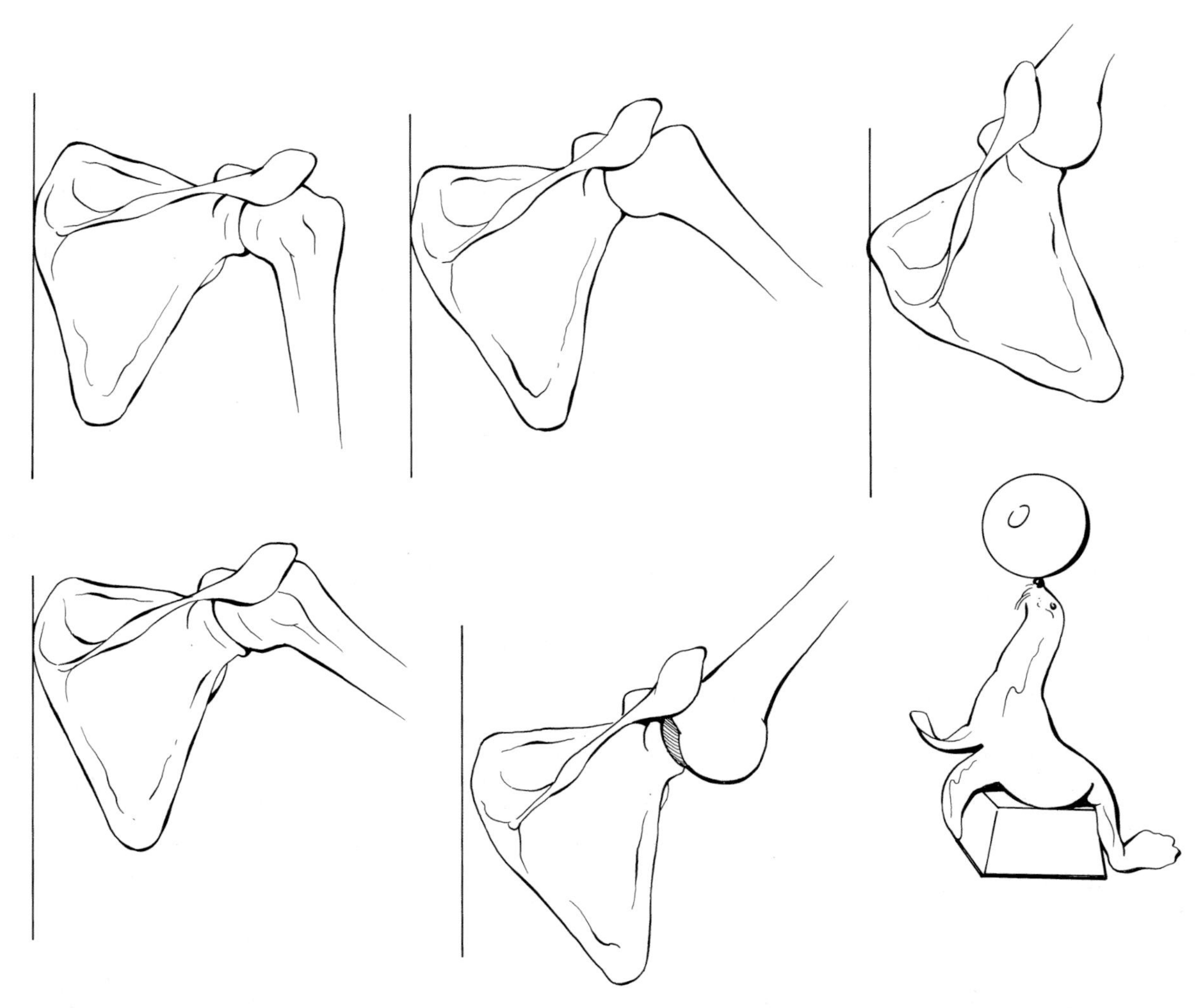

FIG. 10. (Top row) Normal scapulothoracic rotation positions the glenoid underneath the humeral head so that it acts as a stable platform. **(Bottom row)** Failure of proper scapulothoracic motion results in loss of the stable glenoid platform underneath the humeral head. This is analogous to a seal balancing a ball on its nose. (From Warner JJP, Caborn DNM. Overview of shoulder instability. *Crit Rev Phys Rehabil Med* 1992;4:145–198, with permission.)

tance of this proposed mechanism may be more significant in lower-energy situations when the rotator cuff or biceps has time to react to relative changes in capsular tension. Furthermore, it is postulated that proprioception may be a way to protect the capsuloligamentous structures from failure owing to repetitive microtrauma, leading to excessive translation or instability.[95,189]

PATHOANATOMY OF SHOULDER INSTABILITY

In addition to the "essential lesion" (i.e., labral detachment), recurrent instability has been attributed to several pathologic entities. As indicated in Table 2, each of the factors already discussed plays a role in the pathogenesis of shoulder instability. Several authors have cited attenuation of the capsule and capsular ligaments,[16,110,174,175] impression fracture of the humeral head (Hill-Sachs or reverse Hill-Sachs lesion),[37,70,105] attenuation of the subscapularis tendon,[43,167] and capsular rupture.[84,144,146] Recently, several authors have observed humeral avulsion of the glenohumeral ligaments as an additional cause of anterior instability.[7,168,197] A thorough history is important to ascertain the mechanism of injury. A single violent trauma will focus the injury on a specific anatomic region (e.g., Bankart lesion or capsular damage). On the other hand, repetitive microtrauma may cause more subtle capsular stretch, emphasizing the pathoanatomic continuum of capsular injury. Clinically, appreciation of the pathoanatomy of shoulder instability is important because surgical intervention is ultimately directed at anatomic and biomechanic restoration.

Bankart Lesion

The most common form of shoulder instability is recurrent anterior subluxation or dislocation resulting from trauma. Perthes[137] and Bankart[9] (e.g., Perthes–Bankart lesion) originally described the detachment of the capsulolabral complex from the glenoid rim and scapular neck as the "essential lesion" leading to recurrent anterior dislocation. This has been challenged by Speer et al.,[164] who found that simulation of the Bankart lesion in cadaveric cutting studies resulted in only minimal increases in anterior translation. Baker et al.[8] established a classification system based on arthroscopic findings of initial anterior shoulder dislocations. Sixty-two percent had evidence of a Bankart or equivalent lesion, with all of these patients demonstrating gross instability with examination under anesthesia. Thirteen percent were stable on examination and demonstrated no evidence of labral detachment. Recently, Taylor et al.[168] studied first-time patients with traumatic anterior shoulder dislocations and determined arthroscopically that 97% had evidence of isolated detachment of the capsuloligamentous complex from the glenoid rim and neck, without evidence of intracapsular injury. Others have noted a similarly high incidence of Bankart lesions at the time of surgery.[170]

Despite experimental and clinical evidence of increased anterior translation of the humeral head on the glenoid caused by a Bankart lesion, most patients present with recurrent anterior instability with additional pathology that may have developed or advanced over time. Additionally, plastic deformation or capsular injury in patients with first-time dislocations may not be appreciated by macroscopic evaluation because it may represent microscopic ultrastructural failure not visible to the naked eye. It is now believed that recurrent complete dislocation requires an additional pathoanatomic component (e.g., capsular plastic deformation or stretch).[9,16,149,164]

Recognition of this concept is clinically relevant. Isolated arthroscopic Bankart repair is technically challenging and has been associated with higher failure rates, possibly because of overapplication, poor patient selection, and minimal scar formation.[5,40,93,107,165,181] Conversely, open Bankart procedures that address "only" the labral detachment may create enough capsular scarring to prevent recurrence. Thus, the choice of operative procedure will depend on the patients history, examination under anesthesia, arthroscopic anatomy, and appreciation for capsular injury. These tenants become more complex in the patient with multidirectional instability in whom capsular laxity is the dominant pathology, and Bankart lesions are less frequently found.

Capsular Injury

Traumatic Intrasubstance Injury

Clinical observations indicate that capsular injury is commonly associated with traumatic anterior shoulder dislocation. Capsular injury resulting from traumatic anterior shoulder dislocation was recognized as early as the 13th century. Reeves demonstrated capsular rupture by arthrography in 55% of the anterior dislocations he treated.[144,146] Symenoides[167] observed that 15% of his patients treated for anterior dislocation had both labral detachment and anterior capsular ruptures. Johnson[84] observed that 54% of his patients at the time of arthroscopy for anterior dislocation had torn glenohumeral ligaments.

Experimentally, Bigliani et al.[16] measured the stress–strain data at failure of the IGHLC in bone–IGHL–bone preparations and concluded that before failure, significant plastic deformation (e.g., strain) occurred. The implications of these findings are that laxity of the IGHLC leading to instability is not only a congenital finding, but that it may be acquired through submaximal trauma (single or repetitive) without causing rupture or detachment. When the anterior shear force overcomes the capsular tensile strength or when the rotator cuff fatigues or cannot effectively contract (e.g., rotator cuff tears), the ligaments may fail on an ultrastructural level. Similarly, age-related attrition of the rotator cuff tissues is greater than in capsular tissues such that anterior dislocation commonly results in a rotator cuff tear, potentially leading to capsular injury in older patients.[145] Clinically, capsular injury leading to laxity and labral detachment can be found to coexist supporting concomitant capsulorraphy and Bankart repair in the surgical management of instability. Bigliani et al.[14] and Altchek et al.[2] have advocated addressing capsular pathology as part of the surgical treatment of recurrent anterior shoulder instability.

Humeral Avulsion

First described in 1942 by Nicola,[118] avulsion of the capsule from the humerus can occur with forceful hyperabduction. Disruption of the lateral capsule from the humeral neck is probably rare, but has been reported in two cases by Bach et al.[7] and in one case by Taylor et al.[168] in association with anterior dislocation. Wolf et al.[197] has termed this a "HAGL lesion" representing humeral avulsion of the glenohumeral ligament. Appreciation for this variant of capsular injury at the time of arthroscopy can be difficult. Humeral avulsion of the glenohumeral ligament should be repaired anatomically at the time of surgical reconstruction.

Repetitive Injury

The overhead athlete (e.g., pitchers, throwers, swimmers, volleyball, tennis, water polo players, and javelin throwers) represents a special category of patients with complaints relating to instability. These patients subject their shoulder to repetitive stresses that potentially lead to microtrauma not readily appreciated at the time of arthroscopy. Repetitive injury may be the cause of acquired laxity, as seen in gymnasts, and may present as multidirectional instability, rather than pure unidirectional instability. These patients are often confused as having isolated subacromial impingement and inappropriately treated as such.[50,172] It is now believed that "subtle glenohumeral instability" is the cause of subacromial impingement, and capsular laxity is the primary pathology that should be addressed.[171]

Capsular Laxity

Capsular laxity is a prerequisite to allow a large range of glenohumeral motion. The degree of laxity varies among individuals and attempts at correlating the extent and direction of laxity under anesthesia can be confusing, for the overlap between normal laxity and clinical instability is difficult to ascertain.[35,45,54,63,64,127,176,191] In the preadolescent shoulder joint, more than two-thirds may be asymptomatically subluxated on examination.[45] That asymptomatic subluxation or even dislocation may occur in the "normal" shoulder at the time of anesthesia was also appreciated by O'Driscoll and Evans[127] and Warner et al.[187] Thus, it is unclear if constitutional laxity is a risk factor for clinical instability of the shoulder joint. With a proper history of the mechanism and symptoms, correlation with drawer testing under anesthesia can be useful if one considers the effect of arm position on different portions of the capsule.

Humeral and Glenoid Bone Loss

Humeral Bone Loss

Articular abnormalities of the humeral head can disrupt the anatomic relation of the glenohumeral joint, predisposing to recurrent instability. A large Hill-Sachs or reverse Hill-Sachs impression fracture (Fig. 11) on the posterolateral or anterolateral margin of the humeral head, respectively, is created when the humeral head dislocates over the anterior or posterior glenoid rim.[30,136,149,153] This lesion is present in more than 80% of anterior dislocations and 25% of anterior subluxations.[30,136] Hill-Sachs lesions have been noted at the time of arthroscopy in patients with recurrent anterior instability up to 100% of the time.[30,121,168] The small Hill-Sachs lesions are not usually thought to be a major contributor to recurrent anterior instability.[30] The incidence with posterior instability is unknown.

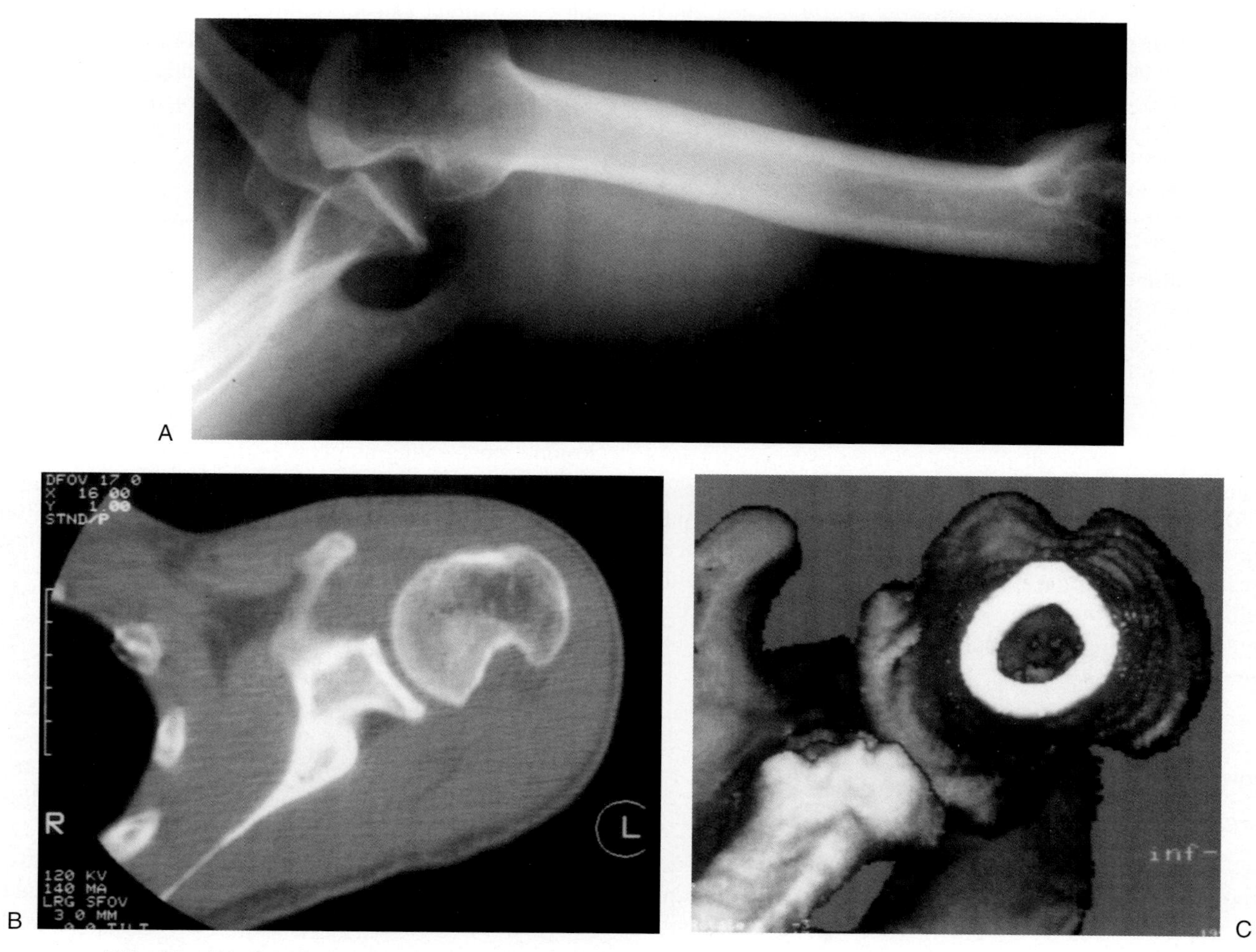

FIG. 11. (A) Anterior dislocation in a patient with a large Hill-Sachs lesion (more than 30% of the humeral head). **(B)** Computed tomographic scan in the same patient. **(C)** A three-dimensional CT reconstruction also shows a large Bankart lesion in addition to the large Hill-Sachs lesion.

The Hill-Sachs lesion is larger with dislocations of longer duration, recurrent dislocations, and inferior displacement of the humeral head.[49,69] In most instances this lesion is relatively small and plays little role in ongoing shoulder instability or its surgical management. Relatively small lesions may be prevented from coming into contact with the anterior glenoid rim simply by performing a more generous anterior capsulorrhaphy (Fig. 12). Caution is warranted by this practice because excessively tight anterior repairs may be associated with the development of late arthrosis.[13,17] However, when the Hill-Sachs lesion involves more than 30% of the humeral articular surface, it may contribute to recurrent anterior instability, even with capsular repair.[151,153]

The mechanism for this persistent instability is that with increasing external rotation, the lesion slips over the anterior glenoid (i.e., as in the original injury) and sits in an anteromedial position outside of the glenoid cavity. Surgical treatment of these defects involves filling the defect with allograft bone (Fig. 13),[55,83] muscle tendon transfer,[37,49,105] (e.g., infraspinatus or subscapularus) or humeral head replacement in older individuals. Alternatively, the lesion can be rotated out of contact with the glenoid with proximal humeral osteotomy.[194]

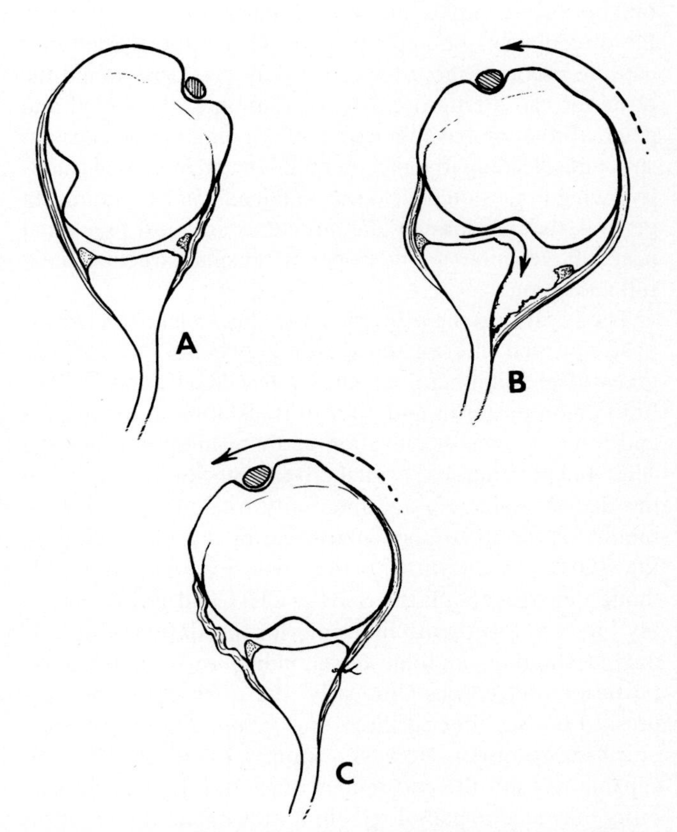

FIG. 12. Role of the Hill-Sachs lesion in anterior shoulder instability: **(A)** With the arm in internal rotation, the Hill-Sachs lesion is not in contact with the glenoid. **(B)** With external rotation, the humeral head translates anteriorly because of the incompetent anterior capsular mechanism. This allows the humeral head to dislocate through the Hill-Sachs lesion. **(C)** An adequate Bankart repair keeps the Hill-Sachs lesion contained on the glenoid, unless it is greater than 30% of the humeral articular surface. (From Warner JJP, Schulte KR, Imhoff AB. Current concepts in shoulder instability. In: *Advances in operative orthopaedics*, vol. 3. Mosby–Year Book, 1995;217–247, with permission.)

Glenoid Bone Loss

Bony lesions of the anterior or posterior glenoid rim have also been described and are believed by some to be important enough to be formally reconstructed during open capsulorrhaphy. These lesions are either due to an osseous Bankart or wear related to repeated instability. Pavlov et al.[136] described an osseous Bankart lesion of the anterior glenoid in 15% of patients with recurrent anterior dislocation and in approximately 50% of patients with recurrent anterior subluxation. Gerber[53] has advocated intraarticular iliac bone graft to formally reconstruct the glenoid cavity before capsular repair to restore normal anatomy of the glenoid. Steinman et al.[166] believes that compromise of 25% or more of the glenoid surface warrants bony reconstruction.

Defects smaller than 20% can be rendered extraarticular by repairing the capsule and labrum back to the edge of the intact glenoid. Larger fragments can be mobilized and fixed through traditional means.[23] Unlike the Hill-Sachs lesion, there are few data available to suggest which glenoid defects require repair, debridement, or neglect. The overall aim of any reconstructive procedure directed at larger defects is to deepen the socket and support the capsule.

Articular Version Abnormalities

Clinically, excessive glenoid retroversion is thought to be a contributing factor to posterior instability and may infrequently be due to a variant of glenoid dysplasia. In most cases, however, excessive version is acquired from eccentric articular surface wear. Some surgeons recommend glenoid osteotomy in addition to soft-tissue procedures.[26,91,159] Several other authors[91,143] have reported varying degrees of normal glenoid and humeral articular version, indicating that further study is needed to support a relation between the development of instability and bony alignment. Glenoid osteotomy and rotational humeral osteotomies, seemingly reasonable treatment options in the presence of articular version abnormalities, have been associated with the development of glenohumeral arthritis.[74,85] Currently, in North America, humeral rotational osteotomy or glenoid osteotomy is not generally practiced, perhaps reflecting the unclear relation between these factors and clinical instability.

PUTTING IT ALL TOGETHER

Successful management of shoulder instability requires a thorough knowledge of all factors responsible for stability in addition to those pathologic factors contributing to instabil-

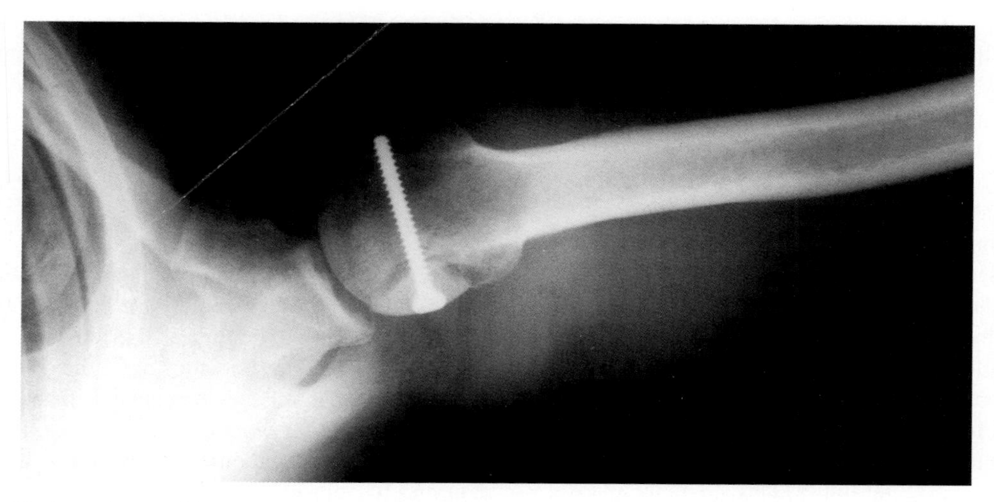

FIG. 13. This large Hill-Sachs defect was treated with a Bankart repair and osteochondral allograft reconstruction of the humeral head.

ity. Because the large spherical head of the humerus articulates with a relatively small and shallow glenoid, the glenohumeral joint requires several mechanisms to maintain stability while providing for a large range of motion. Static and dynamic stability is provided by the combined effects of the capsuloligamentous structures, and rotator cuff and biceps. In the midranges of rotation, most joint stability is through the dynamic action of the rotator cuff and biceps tendons through concavity–compression of the humeral head within the glenoid socket. The ligamentous structures function only at the extreme positions of rotation, preventing excessive rotation of the humeral head on the glenoid. Contraction of the muscles around the shoulder may act secondarily by protecting the relatively weak ligamentous structures from being overwhelmed from excessive tension. Because interpretations of the literature are often confusing, this section is an effort to synthesize the findings already discussed.

The labrum provides an attachment site for the glenohumeral ligaments and the tendon of the long head of the biceps. Its principal function is to increase the depth of the glenoid socket and to act as a chock block in preventing the head from rolling over the anterior edge of the glenoid. Recently, however, the role of the labrum in preventing translation or instability has been challenged. The Bankart lesion, by its anatomic definition, implies dysfunction of the IGHLC, and possibly the SGHL and MGHL. Thus, virtually all labral lesions, especially those below the glenoid equator, are thought to be associated with glenohumeral instability. However, plastic deformation, capsular rupture, abnormal laxity, periosteal stripping, or any combination of these lesions may also be associated with complete dislocation, with or without the Bankart lesion. Thus, one of the goals of reconstructive surgery for glenohumeral instability is to anatomically reconstruct both the labral and capsular deficiency independent of cause (e.g., genetic predisposition or extrinsic forces).

The role of the capsule and ligaments in preventing instability is quite complex and depends on shoulder position and the direction of the applied force. Generally, the anterior capsule becomes more important during extension and the posterior capsule during flexion. Extremes of internal and external rotation have the effect of winding up the capsular structures, leading to joint compression and increased stability owing to tension developing in the relevant structures. In general, the inferior capsular structures are most functional near full elevation and the superior capsular structures near full adduction.

The IGHLC is the primary static check against anterior, posterior, and inferior translation between 45 and 90 degrees of glenohumeral elevation. The SGHL and MGHL limit anteroposterior and inferior translation in the middle and lower ranges of elevation as the arm approaches the adducted position. Experimentally, posterior translation in the flexed, adducted, and internally rotated position may require disruption of the anterosuperior capsule (including the SGHL) in addition to the posterior structures. Although controversial, the SGHL, CHL, and IGHL probably function together to limit inferior translation of the adducted shoulder and act as secondary restraints against posterior translation. Clinically, these structures are addressed during either arthroscopic or open Bankart repair or capsulorrhaphy. However, simply overtightening the capsule to limit the end-ranges of motion to achieve stability may lead to pathologic limitation of shoulder motion and late arthrosis.

The rotator interval region between the subscapularis and supraspinatus may be associated with abnormal translation, especially inferior translation of the adducted arm and, possibly, anteroposterior translation. Contraction of the rotator cuff and long head of the biceps brachii affects both static and dynamic factors that enhance stability. Primarily, they act in concert to increase compression across the glenohumeral joint, increasing the loads required to translate the humeral head. These factors are especially important in the midranges of motion where the capsuloligamentous structures are more lax. The scapulothoracic stabilizers help accurately time and position the glenoid beneath the humeral head. Dysfunction in any of these stabilizers can lead to subsequent instability as residual stabilizing mechanisms become overwhelmed. Furthermore, proprioceptive mechanisms help to coordinate and time this system and can be restored after instability surgery.

Finally, the effects of abnormal articular surfaces, articular version, negative intraarticular pressure, and adhesion–cohesion, either in part or in combination, can lead to or worsen shoulder instability. By themselves, however, they may play only a small role in the pathogenesis of shoulder instability. Rarely is bone loss significant enough to warrant surgical correction. Unfortunately, clinical data are lacking for most of these factors, and an algorithmic approach to their treatment is currently evolving as experimental models improve.

CLASSIFICATION

The importance of a classification system for shoulder instability is best appreciated from observations of treatment failures resulting from improper matching of a surgical procedure with the appropriate pathology. Careful classification improves our ability to tailor individualized treatment programs for patients with glenohumeral instability. Although other classification systems exist for shoulder instability,[139] a system based on four factors is commonly employed: the degree of instability, the frequency of occurrence, direction, and etiology of the instability (Table 4).

The degree of instability is proportional to the level of injury to the capsulolabral structures. *Dislocation* is defined as complete separation of the articular surfaces, often requiring a reduction maneuver to restore joint alignment. *Subluxation* is symptomatic instability without complete dislocation of the articular surfaces. These patients may complain of only pain without an appreciation for actual instability.

Subtle degrees of instability may be due to microtrauma, which may occur from overuse, as seen with repetitive overhead throwing. As in those with subluxation, some of these patients present with pain, with no knowledge of underlying instability. Additionally, patients with multidirectional or posterior instability may have associated tendinitis and pain without a sense of actual shoulder instability.[52,152,160] The avid overhead athlete may also present with pain in the posterior aspect (e.g., internal impingement of the posterior rotator cuff on the posterosuperior glenoid) of the shoulder during the late cocking or early acceleration phase of throwing. Impingement, when present, is due to altered biomechanics and is a secondary phenomenon, rather than true mechanical impingement from the coracoacromial arch.[1,72,183] These can be difficult diagnostic and therapeutic problems.

The frequency of instability is described as acute or chronic. The temporal delineation between acute and chronic is not well defined in the literature, and those definitions that do exist may not have direct clinical relevance. However, for descriptive purposes, an *acute episode* of glenohumeral instability generally refers to the primary dislocation and is defined as one in which the patient is seen in the acute period (within several hours or even a few days) of the injury. These injuries may or may not need to be manually reduced, for occasionally they will reduce spontaneously. *Chronic instability* is in reference to either recurrent episodes of acute instability (AKA: recurrent instability) or dislocations that remain displaced for greater periods of time. The latter type may be more appropriately termed fixed or locked dislocations. Most commonly, this is seen in a missed or neglected posterior dislocation.[66]

The etiology of instability may be categorized as traumatic, atraumatic, microtraumatic, congenital, or neuromuscular. As our understanding of the pathophysiology of shoulder instability has evolved, we now recognize that simplifying etiology into atraumatic or traumatic is somewhat limiting. Thomas and Matsen[171] originally introduced the acronyms TUBS and AMBRI to help us think about the etiology and treatment of most patients who have shoulder instability. The TUBS variety of instability describes a patient with macrotraumatic unidirectional instability associated with a Bankart lesion that typically responds well to surgery. The AMBRI variety of instability describes a patient with atraumatic multidirectional instability that is bilateral and often responds to rehabilitation; rarely, this type of instability requires an inferior capsular shift.

Patients with this atraumatic instability may demonstrate the ability to voluntarily dislocate their shoulders. By se-

TABLE 4. *Shoulder instability classification*

I. Degree
  A. Dislocation
  B. Subluxation
  C. Subtle
II. Frequency
  A. Acute (primary)
  B. Chronic
    1. Recurrent
    2. Fixed
III. Etiology
  A. Traumatic (macrotrauma)
  B. Atraumatic
    1. Voluntary (muscular)
    2. Involuntary (positional)
  C. Acquired (microtrauma)
  D. Congenital
  E. Neuromuscular (Erb's palsy, cerebral palsy, seizures)
IV. Direction
  A. Unidirectional
    1. Anterior
    2. Posterior
    3. Inferior
  B. Bidirectional
    1. Anteroinferior
    2. Posteroinferior
  C. Multidirectional

lective muscle contraction and relaxation, these patients can position their shoulder resulting in subluxation or dislocation. Most commonly, this is seen in cases of posterior and multidirectional instability, but pure anterior instability can also be produced. Rowe et al.[150] have observed that voluntary subluxation can be associated with emotional and psychiatric disorders of secondary gain. In general, this category of voluntary instability has a high rate of recurrence after surgical stabilization if the underlying psychopathology is not addressed.[114,150] A subtype of voluntary instability includes those who have an unconscious behavioral tic leading to selective muscular contraction. This form of voluntary instability may respond best to biofeedback techniques.[11]

Alternatively, dislocation may occur voluntarily with underlying involuntary instability, as with activities or even during sleep owing to instability that is positional. Although patients can voluntarily reproduce disabling instability just by positioning their arm, they prefer not to do so. Most commonly, these patients may have involuntary posterior instability that can be demonstrated by positioning the arm into flexion, adduction, and internal rotation. These patients often adapt by avoiding positions of risk where the shoulder might dislocate.[160] This positional type of involuntary instability, unlike voluntary instability caused by psychiatric factors or a behavior muscular tic, may respond well to surgical stabilization.[15,51]

Neer[115] recognized acquired instability that results from repetitive microtrauma (overuse) to the glenohumeral joint. These patients often provide a history of being an avid overhead athlete (e.g., baseball, swimming, tennis, and such) as they subject their anterior and inferior capsuloligamentous structures to repetitive injury and stretch causing symptomatic instability. These patients are not uncommonly found to have a preexistent constitutional congenital hyperlaxity.[44,45,127] Conceivably, these patients excel at their sport because of this excessive laxity and may develop symptomatic instability through subsequent trauma. Finally, neurologic disorders can lead to instability including stroke, Erb's palsy, and seizures, which can cause both anterior or posterior instability. Thus, rather than a discrete etiology, there remains a spectrum of instability, with traumatic and atraumatic mechanisms occupying the extremes. This is reflected by the variety of findings observed at the time of surgery that may include any combination of a Bankart lesion, capsular laxity, or capsular rupture.

The direction of instability can be anterior, posterior, inferior, or any combination of these. Unidirectional instability occurs in only one of these directions. Multidirectional instability as in the AMBRI variety may demonstrate all three directions of instability in addition to generalized ligamentous laxity. The principal direction of instability in both the TUBS and AMBRI variety of instability is usually anterior. However, the presence of inferior instability is the hallmark of the diagnosis of multidirectional instability. To add to already confusing nomenclature, Pollock and Bigliani[138] and Bigliani et al.[14] have described patients with an intermediate degree of instability, who demonstrate an inferior component in addition to an anterior or posterior component as bidirectional (e.g., anteroinferior or posteroinferior). This type of instability is more common in overhead athletes who expose their anterior and inferior capsular restraints to repetitive microtrauma, leading to plastic deformation and stretch. An additional subtlety is that patients with posterior instability often exhibit smaller degrees of inferior and even anterior instability.

Recognition of global capsular laxity and instability in more than one direction that is due to either of the extremes of causation (e.g., traumatic or atraumatic) is critical for determining appropriate surgical management so as not to exacerbate the instability in the direction left unaddressed.[114] Often, it is the primary direction of instability that causes most of the patients symptoms and is, therefore, most commonly addressed surgically. However, procedures that treat anterior capsular laxity by Bankart repair or capsular plication may not adequately manage the associated components of inferior and or posterior instability. In the extreme, asymmetrical tightening during capsulorrhaphy can lead to a fixed subluxation in the opposite direction.[12,100] Thus, establishing the principal direction of the instability and acknowledging the lessor components by the time of surgical intervention is critical to obtain a successful outcome.

CONCLUSIONS

The aims of this chapter were to review the anatomy, biomechanics, and pathophysiology of shoulder instability. An understanding of what is "normal" provides a foundation for diagnosing and treating what is considered to be pathologic. Because current research endeavors have focused on the basic science of shoulder instability, we no longer have to rely on an anecdotal and qualitative account of the associated pathology noted at the time of treatment. We now have an organized and quantitative approach to the treatment of shoulder instability. Anatomic studies have provided abundant information on the macro- and ultrastructure of the static and dynamic restraints to stability. Experiments examining the biomechanics of shoulder instability have helped clarify the effects of articular version, the labrum, negative intraarticular pressure, the material properties and limits of function of the capsuloligamentous complex, and the dynamic interaction between static and dynamic restraints. There are still several unanswered questions. As technology is advancing, we must continue to evaluate how older and newer techniques correct anatomic and biomechanic abnormalities leading to glenohumeral instability. Newer forms of "heat therapy" and arthroscopic techniques are exciting means to perform less invasive surgery. However, meticulous analysis will be required to determine their value. Our current understanding of anatomy and biomechanics should greatly facilitate this goal.

REFERENCES

1. Altchek D, Dines D. Shoulder injuries in the throwing athlete. *J Am Acad Orthop Surg* 1995;3:159–165.
2. Altchek DW, Dines DM. The surgical treatment of anterior instability. Selective capsular repair. *Oper Tech Sports Med* 1993;1:285–292.
3. Andrews J, Carson W, McLeod W. Glenoid labrum tears related to the long head of the biceps. *Am J Sports Med* 1985;13:337–341.
4. Andrews J, Carson WJ, Ortega K. Arthroscopy of the shoulder: technique and normal anatomy. *Am J Sports Med* 1985;12:1–7.
5. Arciero R, Wheeler J, Ryan J, et al. Arthroscopic Bankart repair versus nonoperative treatment for acute, initial anterior shoulder dislocations. *Am J Sports Med* 1994;22:589–594.
6. Aston JJ, Gregory C. Dislocation of the shoulder with significant fracture of the glenoid. *J Bone Joint Surg [Am]* 1973;55:1531–1533.
7. Bach B, Warren R, Fronek J. Disruption of the lateral capsule of the shoulder: a cause of recurrent dislocation. *J Bone Joint Surg [Br]* 1988;70:274–276.
8. Baker C, Uribe J, Whitman C. Arthroscopic evaluation of acute initial anterior shoulder dislocations. *Am J Sports Med* 1990;18:25–28.
9. Bankart A. The pathology and treatment of recurrent dislocation of the shoulder-joint. *Br J Surg* 1938;26:23–29.
10. Basmajian J, Bazant F. Factors preventing downward dislocation of the adducted shoulder joint in an electromyographic and morphological study. *J Bone Joint Surg [Am]* 1959;41:1182–1186.
11. Beall MJ, Diefenbach G, Allen S. Electromyographic biofeedback in the treatment of voluntary posterior instability of the shoulder. *Am J Sports Med* 1987;15:175–178.
12. Bigliani L, Flatow E, Kelkar R, et al. Effect of anterior tightening on shoulder kinematics and contact. Presented at the Second World Congress of Biomechanics, Amsterdam, July 10–15, 1994:304.
13. Bigliani L, Flatow E, Kelkar R, et al. The effect of anterior capsular tightening on shoulder kinematics and contact. *J Shoulder Elbow Surg* 1994;3:S65.
14. Bigliani L, Kurzweil P, Schwartzbach C, et. al. Inferior capsular shift procedure for anterior–inferior shoulder instability in athletes. *Am J Sports Med* 1994;22:578–584.
15. Bigliani L, Pollock R, Endrizzi D, et al. Surgical repair of posterior instability of the shoulder: long-term results. *Orthop Trans* 1993;17: 75–76.
16. Bigliani L, Pollock R, Soslowsky L, et al. Tensile properties of the inferior glenohumeral ligament. *J Orthop Res* 1992;10:187–197.
17. Bigliani L, Weinstein D, Glasgow M, Pollock R, Flatow E. Glenohumeral arthroplasty for arthritis after instability surgery. *J Shoulder and Elbow Surg* 1995;4:87–94.
18. Blasier R, Carpenter J, Huston L. Shoulder proprioception: effect of joint laxity, joint position, and direction of motion. *Orthop Rev* 1994; 23:44–50.
19. Blasier R, Guldberg R, Rothman E. Anterior shoulder stability: contributions of rotator cuff forces and the capsular ligaments in a cadaver model. *J Shoulder Elbow Surg* 1992;1:140–150.
20. Blasier R, Soslowsky L, Malicky D, et al. Anterior glenohumeral stabilization efficiency in a biomechanical model combining ligamentous and muscular constraints. *J Shoulder Elbow Surg* 1994;3(suppl):S23.
21. Boardman DI, Debski R, Warner J, et al. Tensile properties of the superior glenohumeral and coracohumeral ligaments. *J Shoulder Elbow Surg* 1996;5:249–254.
22. Bost FC, Inman VT. The pathological changes in recurrent dislocation of the shoulder. A report of Bankart's operative procedure. *J Bone Joint Surg [Am]* 1942;24:595–613.
23. Boulris C, Horwitz D, Pollock R, Flatow E. Open reduction internal fixation of intra-articular glenoid fractures. *Orthop Trans* 1996;20:12.
24. Bowen M, Deng X, Hannafin J, Arnoczky S, Warren R, Warner J. An analysis of the patterns of glenohumeral joint contact and their relationship to the glenoid "bare area." *Trans Orthop Res Soc* 1992;17: 496.
25. Bowen M, Deng X, Warner J, Warren R, Torzilli P. The effect of joint compression on stability of the glenohumeral joint. *Trans Orthop Res Soc* 1992;38:289.
26. Brewer B, Wubben R, Carrera G. Excessive retroversion of the glenoid cavity: a cause of non-traumatic posterior instability of the shoulder. *J Bone Joint Surg [Am]* 1986;68:724–731.
27. Browne A, Hoffmeyer P, An K, et al. The influence of atmospheric pressure on shoulder stability. *Orthop Trans* 1990;14:259.
28. Burkhead WJ, Rockwood CJ. Treatment of instability of the shoulder with an exercise program. *J Bone Joint Surg [Am]* 1992;74:890–896.
29. Cain P, Mutschler T, Fu F, et al. Anterior stability of the glenohumeral joint: a dynamic model. *Am J Sports Med* 1987;15:144–148.
30. Calandra J, Baker C, Uribe J. The incidence of Hill-Sachs lesions in initial anterior shoulder dislocations. *Arthroscopy* 1989;5:254–257.
31. Carpenter J, Blasier R, Pellizzan G. The effect of muscular fatigue in shoulder propriocepition. *Trans Orthop Res Soc* 1993;39.
32. Clark J, Sidles J, Matsen F. The relationship of glenohumeral joint capsule to the rotator cuff. *Clin Orthop* 1990;254:29–34.
33. Clarke H. Habitual dislocation of the shoulder: the Putti–Platt operation. *J Bone Joint Surg* 1948;30:198–202.
34. Codman EA, ed. *The shoulder: rupture of the supraspinatus tendon and other lesions in or about the subacromial bursa.* Boston: Thomas Todd, 1934.
35. Cofield R, Irving J. Evaluation and classification of shoulder instability: reference to examination under anesthesia. *Clin Orthop* 1987;223: 32–42.
36. Cole B, Rodeo S, O'Brien S, et al. The developmental anatomy of the rotator interval capsule and the rotator interval defect. An anatomic and histologic analysis of fetal and adult cadaver specimens with clinical implications. American Orthopaedic Society for Sports Medicine Specialty Day, San Francisco, CA, 1997.
37. Conolly J. Humeral head defects associated with shoulder dislocation. The diagnostic and surgical significance. *Instr Course Lect* 1972;21: 42–52.
38. Cooper D, Arnoczky S, O'Brien S, et al. Anatomy, histology, and vascularity of the glenoid labrum: an anatomical study. *J Bone Joint Surg [Am]* 1992;74:46–52.
39. Cooper D, O'Brien S, Arnoczky S, Warren R. The structure and function of the coracohumeral ligament: an anatomic and microscopic study. *J Shoulder Elbow Surg* 1993;2:70–77.
40. Coughlin L, Rubinovich M, Johansson J, et al. Arthroscopic stable capsulorrhaphy for anterior shoulder instability. *Am J Sports Med* 1992;20:253–256.
41. Craig E. The posterior mechanism of acute anterior shoulder dislocations. *Clin Orthop* 1984;190:212–216.
42. Depalma A, Callery G, Bennet G. Part 1. Variational anatomy and degenerative lesions of the shoulder bone. In: Blount W, Banks S, eds. *American Academy of Orthopaedic Surgeons Instructional Course Lectures XVI.* Ann Arbor: JW Edwards, 949:225–281.
43. Depalma A, Cooke A, Prabhaker M. The role of the subscapularis in recurrent anterior dislocations of the shoulder. *Clin Orthop* 1967;54: 35–49.
44. Dowdy P, O'Driscoll S. Shoulder instability. An analysis of family history. *J Bone Joint Surg [Br]* 1993;75:728–784.
45. Emery R, Mullaji A. Glenohumeral joint instability in normal adolescents: incidence and significance. *J Bone Joint Surg [Br]* 1991;73: 406–408.
46. Ferlic D, Digiovine N. A long-term retrospective study of the modified Bristow procedure. *Am J Sports Med* 1988;16:469–474.
47. Ferrari D. Capsular ligaments of the shoulder: anatomical and functional study of the anterior–superior capsule. *Am J Sports Med* 1990; 18:20–24.
48. Field LD, Warren RF, O'Brien SJ, Altchek DW, Wickiewicz TL. Isolated closure of rotator interval defects for shoulder instability. *Am J Sports Med* 1995;23:557–563.
49. Flatow E, Miller S, Neer CI. Chronic anterior dislocation of the shoulder. *J Shoulder Elbow Surg* 1993;2:2–10.
50. Fly W, Tibone J, Glousman R. Arthroscopic subacromial decompression in athletes less than 40 years old. *Orthop Trans* 1990;14:250–251.
51. Fronek J, Warren R, Bowen M. Posterior subluxation of the glenohumeral joint. *J Bone Joint Surg [Am]* 1989;71:205–216.
52. Garth W, Allman F, Armstrong W. Occult anterior subluxation of the shoulder in noncontact sports. *Am J Sports Med* 1987; 15:579–585.
53. Gerber C. Chronic, locked anterior and posterior dislocations. In: Warner J, Iannotti J, Gerber C, eds. *Complex and revision problems in shoulder surgery.* Philadelphia: Lippincott–Raven, 1997:99–113.
54. Gerber C, Ganz R. Clinical assessment of instability of the shoulder: with special reference to anterior and posterior drawer tests. *J Bone Joint Surg [Br]* 1984;66:551–556.
55. Gerber C, Lambert S. Allograft reconstruction of segmental defects of the humeral head for the treatment of chronic locked posterior dislocation of the shoulder. *J Bone Joint Surg [Am]* 1996;78:376–382.

56. Gibb DT, Sidles JA, Harryman DT, McQuade KJ, Matsen FAI. The effect of capsular venting on glenohumeral laxity. *Clin Orthop* 1991; 268:120–127.
57. Glousman R, Jobe F, Tibone J, Moynes D, Antonelli D, Perry J. Dynamic electromyographic analysis of the throwing shoulder with glenohumeral instability. *J Bone Joint Surg [Am]* 1988;70:220–226.
58. Grigg P. Response of joint afferent neurons in cat medial articular nerve to active and passive movements of the knee. *Brain Res* 1976; 118:482–485.
59. Grigg P, Hoffman A. Calibrating joint capsule mechanoreceptors as in-vivo soft tissue load cells. *J Biomech Res* 1989;22:781–785.
60. Habermeyer P, Schuller U, Wiedermann E. The intra-articular pressure of the shoulder: an experimental study on the role of the glenoid labrum in stabilizing the joint. *Arthroscopy* 1992;8:166–172.
61. Hara H, Nobuyuki I, Iwasaki K. Strength of the glenoid labrum and adjacent shoulder capsule. *J Shoulder Elbow Surg* 1996;5:263–268.
62. Harryman DI, Sidles J, Clark J, et al. Translation of the humeral head on the glenoid with passive glenohumeral motion. *J Bone Joint Surg [Am]* 1990;72:1334–1343.
63. Harryman DI, Sidles J, Harris S, et al. Laxity of the normal glenohumeral joint: a quantitative in vivo assessment. *J Shoulder Elbow Surg* 1992;1:66–76.
64. Harryman DT, Sidles JA, Harris SL, Matsen FA. The role of the rotator interval capsule in passive motion and stability of the shoulder. *J Bone Joint Surg [Am]* 1992;74:53–66.
65. Hashimoto T, Suzuki K, Nobuhara K. Dynamic analysis of intraarticular pressure in the glenohumeral joint. *J Shoulder Elbow Surg* 1995; 4:209–218.
66. Hawkins R, Neer CI, Pianta R, et al. Locked posterior dislocation of the shoulder. *J Bone Joint Surg [Am]* 1987;69:9–18.
67. Helmig P, Sojberg J, Kjaersgaard-Andersen P, et al. Distal humeral migration as a component of multidirectional shoulder instability: An anatomical study in autopsy specimens. *Clin Orthop* 1990;252: 139–143.
68. Helmig P, Sojbjerg J, Sneppen O, Loehr J, Stgaard S, Suder P. Glenohumeral movement patterns after puncture of the joint capsule: an experimental study. *J Shoulder Elbow Surg* 1993;2:209–215.
69. Hermodsson I. Rontgenologische studern uber due traumatischen und habituellen schultergelenk-verrenhungen. Nach vorn un nach unten. *Acta Radiol Suppl* 1934;20:1–173.
70. Hill H, Sachs M. The grooved defect of the humeral head. A frequently unrecognized complication of dislocations of the shoulder joint. *Radiology* 1940;35:690–700.
71. Howell S, Galinat B. The glenoid–labral socket: a constrained articular surface. *Clin Orthop* 1989;243:122–125.
72. Howell S, Galinat B, Renzi A, Marone P. Normal and abnormal mechanics of the glenohumeral joint in the horizontal plane. *J Bone Joint Surg [Am]* 1988;70:227.
73. Howell S, Kraft T. The role of the supraspinatus and infraspinatus muscles in glenohumeral kinematics of anterior shoulder instability. *Clin Orthop* 1991;263:128–134.
74. Huber H. Incidence of recurrence and of osteoarthritis after rotational humeral osteotomy according to Weber. *J Bone Joint Surg [Br]* 1992; 74:7.
75. Iannotti J, Gabriel J, Schneck S, Evans B, Misra S. The normal glenohumeral relationships: an anatomical study of one hundred and forty shoulders. *J Bone Joint Surg [Am]* 1992;74:491–500.
76. Itoi E, Kuechle D, Newman S, Morrey B, An K-N. Stabilizing function of the biceps in stable and unstable shoulders. *J Bone Joint Surg [Br]* 1993;75:834–836.
77. Itoi E, Motzkin N, An K, Morrey B. Scapular inclination and inferior instability of the shoulder. *J Shoulder Elbow Surg* 1992;1:131–139.
78. Itoi E, Motzkin N, Newman S, Morrey B, An K-N. The stabilizing function of the long head of the biceps with the arm in the hanging position. *Orthop Trans* 1992–1993;16:775.
79. Itoi N, Eto M, Teshima K, Iwaski K. The mechanism of anterior shoulder dislocation. *Shoulder* Joint (Japan) 1991;15:200–204.
80. Janevic J, Craig E, Hsu K-C, et al. Biomechanics of repair of anterior instability. *Trans Orthop Res Soc* 1992;17:495.
81. Jerosch J, Clahsen H, Grosse-Hackmann A, et al. Effects of proprioceptive fibers in the capsule tissue in stabilizing the glenohumeral joint. *Orthop Trans* 1992;16:773.
82. Jobe F, Tibone J, Perry J, et al. An EMG analysis of the shoulder in throwing and pitching: a preliminary report. *Am J Sports Med.* 1983; 11:3–5.
83. Johnson D, Warner J. Osteochondritis dissecans of the humeral head: treatment with a matched osteochondral allograft. *J Shoulder Elbow Surg* 1997;6:160–163.
84. Johnson L. Techniques of anterior glenohumeral ligament repair. In: Johnson L, ed. *Arthroscopic surgery: principles and practice*. St Louis, MO: CV Mosby, 1986:1405–1420.
85. Johnston H, Hawkins R, Haddad R, Fowler P. A complication of posterior glenoid osteotomy for recurrent posterior shoulder instability. *Clin Orthop* 1984;187:147–149.
86. Kaltsas D. Comparative study of the properties of the shoulder joint capsule with those of other joint capsules. *Clin Orthop* 1983;173: 20–26.
87. Kelkar R, Flatow E, Bigliani L, Mow V. The effects of articular congruence and humeral head rotation on glenohumeral kinematics. *ASME Adv Bioeng* 1994;28:19–20.
88. Kelkar R, Newton P, Armengol J, et al. Three-dimensional kinematics of the glenohumeral joint during abduction in the scapular plane. *Trans Orthop Res Soc* 1993;18:136.
89. Kocher M, Lephart S, Warner J, Winge S, Fu F. Proprioception in patients with shoulder instability. *Trans Orthop Soc* 1993;39:312.
90. Kozlowski K, Scougall J. Congenital bilateral hypoplasia: a report of four cases. *Br J Radiol* 1987;60:705–706.
91. Kronberg M, Brostrom L. Humeral head retroversion in patients with unstable humeroscapular joints. *Clin Orthop* 1990;260:207–211.
92. Kumar V, Balasubramaniam P. The role of atmospheric pressure in stabilizing the shoulder. An experimental study. *J Bone Joint Surg [Br]* 1985;67:719–721.
93. Lane J, Sachs R, Riehl B. Arthroscopic staple capsulorrhaphy: a long-term follow-up. *Arthroscopy* 1993;9:190–194.
94. Lazarus M, Sidles J, Harryman DI, Matsen F. Effect of a chondral–labral defect on glenoid concavity and glenohumeral stability. *J Bone Joint Surg [Am]* 1996;78:94–102.
95. Lephart S, Warner J, Borsa P, et al. Proprioception of the shoulder joint in healthy, unstable, and surgically repaired shoulders. *J Shoulder Elbow Surg* 1994;3:371–380.
96. Levy A, Kelly B, Lintner S, Speer K. The function of the long head of the biceps at the shoulder: an EMG analysis. Presented at the American Orthopaedic Society for Sports Medicine. San Francisco, CA, 1997.
97. Lintner D, Sebastianelli W, Hanks G, et al. Glenoid dysplasia: a case report and review of the literature. *Clin Orthop* 1992;283:145–148.
98. Lippitt S, Harris S, Harryman DI, et al. In vivo quantification of the laxity of normal and unstable glenohumeral joints. *J Shoulder Elbow Surg* 1994;3:215–223.
99. Lippitt S, Vanderhooft J, Harris S, Sidles J, Harryman DI, Matsen FI. Glenohumeral stability from concavity–compression: a quantitative analysis. *J Shoulder Elbow Surg* 1993;2:27–35.
100. Lusardi D, Wirth M, Wurtz D, Rockwood CJ. Loss of external rotation following anterior capsulorrhaphy of the shoulder. *J Bone Joint Surg [Am]* 1993;75:1185–1192.
101. Matsen FI, Arntz C. Rotator cuff failure. In: Rockwood C, Matsen F, eds. *The shoulder*. Philadelphia: WB Saunders, 1990:647–665.
102. Matsen FI, Thomas S, Rockwood CJ. Anterior glenohumeral instability. In: Rockwood C, Matsen F, eds. *The shoulder*. Philadelphia: WB Saunders, 1990;526–622.
103. McKernan D, Mutschler T, Rudert M, et al. Significance of a partial and full Bankart lesion: a biomechanical comparison. *Trans Orthop Res Soc* 1989;14:231.
104. McKernan D, Mutschler T, Rudert M, et al. The characterization of rotator cuff muscle forces and their effect of glenohumeral joint stability: a biomechanical study. *Orthop Trans* 1990;14:237–238.
105. McLaughlin H. Posterior dislocation of the shoulder. *J Bone Joint Surg [Am]* 1952;34:584–590.
106. McMahon P, Debski R, Thompson W, Warner J, Fu F, Woo S. Shoulder muscle forces and tendon excursions during glenohumeral abduction in the scapular plane. *J Shoulder Elbow Surg* 1995;4:199–208.
107. Morgan C, Bodenstab A. Arthroscopic Bankart suture repair. Technique and early results. *Arthroscopy* 1987;3:111–122.
108. Morgan C, Rames R, Snyder S. Arthroscopic assessment of anatomic variations of the glenohumeral ligaments associated with recurrent anterior shoulder instability. Presented at the Annual Meeting of the American Shoulder and Elbow Surgeons. Washington, DC, 1993.
109. Morrey B, Chao E. Recurrent anterior dislocation of the shoulder. Clinical and anatomic considerations. In: Block J, Dumbleton J. eds. *Clinical biomechanics*. New York: Churchill Livingston, 1981:22–46.

110. Moseley H, Overgaard B. The anterior capsular mechanism in recurrent anterior dislocation of the shoulder: morphological and clinical studies with special reference to the glenoid labrum and the glenohumeral ligaments. *J Bone Joint Surg [Br]* 1962;44:913–927.
111. Motzkin N, Itoi E, Morrey B, An K-N. Contribution of passive bulk tissues and deltoid to static inferior glenohumeral stability. *J Shoulder Elbow Surg* 1994;3:313–319.
112. Mow V, Bigliani L, Flatow E, et al. Material properties of the inferior glenohumeral ligament and the glenohumeral articular cartilage. In: Matsen FI, Fu F, Hawkins R, eds. *The shoulder: a balance of mobility and stability*. Rosemont, IL: American Academy Orthopaedic Surgeons, 1993:29–67.
113. Murakami M, Kojima Y, Maeda T, et al. Sensory nerve endings in the shoulder joint capsule of the monkey as sensors of dynamic stabilizing system. *Trans Comb Mtg ORS USA, Japan, Canada* 1991:315.
114. Neer C, Foster C. Inferior capsular shift for involuntary inferior and multidirectional instability of the shoulder. *J Bone Joint Surg [Am]* 1980;62:897–908.
115. Neer CS I. *Shoulder reconstruction*. Philadelphia: WB Saunders, 1990.
116. Neer CS, Satterlee CC, Dalsey RM, Flatow EL. The anatomy and potential effects of contracture of the coracohumeral ligament. *Clin Orthop* 1992;280:182–185.
117. Neviaser R, Neviaser T, Neviaser J. Concurrent rupture of the rotator cuff and anterior dislocation of the shoulder in the older patient. *J Bone Joint Surg [Am]* 1988;70:1308–1311.
118. Nicola T. Anterior dislocation of the shoulder. The role of the articular capsule. *J Bone Joint Surg [Am]* 1942;24:614–616.
119. Nobuhara K. The rotator interval lesion. In: Wayne J, Burkhead Z, eds. *Rotator cuff disorders*. Baltimore: Williams & Wilkins, 1996:182–192.
120. Nobuhara K, Ikeda H. Rotator interval lesion. *Clin Orthop* 1987;223: 44–50.
121. Norlin R. Intraarticular pathology in acute, first-time anterior shoulder dislocation: An arthroscopic study. *Arthroscopy* 1993;9:546–549.
122. Nuber G, Jobe F, Perry J, et al. Fine wire electromyography analysis of muscles of the shoulder during swimming. *Am J Sports Med* 1986; 14:7–11.
123. O'Brien S, Arnoczky S, Warren R, et al. Developmental anatomy of the shoulder and anatomy of the glenohumeral joint. In: Rockwood CJ, Matsen FI, eds. *The shoulder*. Philadelphia: WB Saunders, 1990:1–33.
124. O'Brien S, Schwartz R, Warren R, Torzilli P. Capsular restraints to anterior–posterior motion of the abducted shoulder: a biomechanical study. *J Shoulder Elbow Surg* 1995;4:298–308.
125. O'Brien SJ, Neves MC, Arnoczky SP, et al. The anatomy and histology of the inferior glenohumeral ligament complex of the shoulder. *Am J Sports Med* 1990;18:449–456.
126. O'Connell P, Nuber G, Mileski R, et al. The contribution of the glenohumeral ligaments to anterior stability of the shoulder joint. *Am J Sports Med* 1990;18:579–584.
127. O'Driscoll S, Evans D. Contralateral shoulder instability following anterior repair: an epidemiological investigation. *J Bone Joint Surg [Br]* 1991;73:941–946.
128. Ovesen J, Nielsen S. Experimental distal subluxation in the glenohumeral joint. *Arch Orthop Trauma Surg* 1985;104:78–81.
129. Ovesen J, Nielsen S. Stability of the shoulder joint: cadaver study of stabilizing structures. *Acta Orthop Scand* 1985;56:149–151.
130. Ovesen J, Nielson S. Anterior and posterior instability of the shoulder: a cadaver study. *Acta Orthop Trauma Surg* 1986;57:324–327.
131. Ozaki J. Glenohumeral movements of the involuntary inferior and multidirectional instability. *Clin Orthop* 1989;238:107–111.
132. Pagnani M, Deng X-H, Warren R, Torzilli P, O'Brien S. Role of the long head of the biceps brachii in glenohumeral stability: a biomechanical study in cadavera. *J Shoulder Elbow Surg* 1996;5:255–262.
133. Pagnani M, Xiang-Hua D, Warren R, Torzilli P, Altchek D. Effect of lesions of the superior portion of the glenoid labrum on glenohumeral translation. *J Bone Joint Surg [Am]* 1995;77:1003–1010.
134. Pappas A, Goss T, Kleinman P. Symptomatic shoulder instability due to lesions of the glenoid labrum. *Am J Sports Med* 1983;11:279–288.
135. Patel PR, Imhoff AB, Debski RE, et al. Anatomy and biomechanics of the coracohumeral and superior glenohumeral ligaments. Presented at Specialty Day, American Shoulder and Elbow Surgeons, 12th Open Meeting, Academy of Orthopaedic Surgeons. Atlanta, GA, 1996.
136. Pavlov H, Warren R, Weiss C, et al. The roentgenographic evaluation of certain surgical conditions. *Clin Orthop* 1985;184:317–321.
137. Perthes G. Uber operation bei habitueller schulterluxation. *Dtsch Z Chir* 1906;85:199–227.
138. Pollock R, Bigliani L. Recurrent posterior shoulder instability: diagnosis and treatment. *Clin Orthop* 1993;291:85–96.
139. Pollock R, Flatow E. Classification and evaluation. In: Bigliani L, ed. *The unstable shoulder*. Rosemont: American Academy of Orthopaedic Surgeons, 1996:25–36.
140. Poppen N, Walker P. Normal and abnormal motion of the shoulder. *J Bone Joint Surg [Am]* 1976;58:195–201.
141. Poppen N, Walker P. Forces at the glenohumeral joint in abduction. *Clin Orthop* 1978;58:165–170.
142. Prodromos C, Ferry J, Schiller A, et al. Histological studies of the glenoid labrum from fetal life to old age. *J Bone Joint Surg [Am]* 1990;72:1344–1348.
143. Randelli M, Gambrioli P. Glenohumeral osteometry by computed tomography in normal and unstable shoulders. *Clin Orthop* 1986;208: 151–156.
144. Reeves B. Arthrography in acute dislocation of the shoulder. *J Bone Joint Surg [Br]* 1968;48:182.
145. Reeves B. Experiments on tensile strength of the anterior capsular structures of the shoulder in man. *J Bone Joint Surg [Br]* 1968;50: 858–865.
146. Reeves C. Acute anterior dislocation of the shoulder: clinical and experimental studies. *Ann R Coll Surg Engl* 1969;44:255–273.
147. Rodosky M, Harner C, Fu F. The role of the long head of the biceps muscle and superior glenoid labrum in anterior stability of the shoulder. *Am J Sports Med* 1994;22:121–130.
148. Rodosky M, Rudert M, Harner C, et al. Significance of a superior labral lesion of the shoulder. *Trans Orthop Res Soc* 1990;15:276.
149. Rowe C, Patel D, Southmayd W. The Bankart procedure: a long-term end-result study. *J Bone Joint Surg [Am]* 1978;60:1–16.
150. Rowe C, Pierce D, Clark J. Voluntary dislocation of the shoulder: a preliminary report on clinical, electromyographic, and psychiatric study of twenty-six patients. *J Bone Joint Surg [Am]* 1973;55:445–460.
151. Rowe C, Sakellarides H. Factors related to recurrences of anterior dislocations of the shoulder. *Clin Orthop* 1961;20:40–48.
152. Rowe C, Zarins B. Recurrent transient subluxation of the shoulder. *J Bone Joint Surg [Am]* 1981;63:159–168.
153. Rowe C, Zarins B, Ciullo J. Recurrent anterior dislocation of the shoulder after surgical repair. *J Bone Joint Surg [Am]* 1984;66: 159–168.
154. Saha A. *Theory of shoulder mechanism: descriptive and applied*. Springfield, IL: Charles C Thomas, 1961.
155. Saha A. Dynamic stability of the glenohumeral joint. *Acta Orthop Scand* 1971;42:491–505.
156. Saha A. Mechanics of elevation of the glenohumeral joint: its application in rehabilitation of flail shoulder in upper brachial plexus injuries and poliomyositis and in replacement of the upper humerus by prosthesis. *Acta Orthop Scand* 1973;44:668–678.
157. Sarrafin S. Gross and functional anatomy of the shoulder. *Clin Orthop* 1983;173:11–19.
158. Schwartz RE, O'Brien SJ, Torzilli PA, Warren RF. Capsular restraints to anterior and posterior motion of the shoulder. *Orthop Trans* 1988; 12:727.
159. Scott DJ. Humeral head retroversion in patients with unstable humeroscapular joints. *Clin Orthop* 1967;260:207–211.
160. Silliman J, Hawkins R. Classification and physical diagnosis of instability of the shoulder. *Clin Orthop* 1993;291:7–19.
161. Snyder S, Karzel R, DelPizzo W, et al. SLAP lesions of the shoulder. *Arthroscopy* 1990;6:274–279.
162. Soslowsky L, Flatow E, Bigliani L, et al. Articular geometry of the glenohumeral joint. *Clin Orthop* 1992;285:181–190.
163. Soslowsky L, Flatow E, Bigliani L, Pawluk R, Ateshian G, Mow V. Quantitation of in situ contact areas at the glenohumeral joint: a biomechanical study. *J Orthop Res* 1992;10:524–534.
164. Speer K, Deng X, Torzilli P, Altchek D, Warren R. A biomechanical evaluation of the Bankart lesion. *Trans Orthop Res Soc* 1993;39:315.
165. Speer K, Warren R, Pagnani M, Warner J. An arthroscopic technique for anterior stabilization of the shoulder with a bioresorbable tack. *J Bone Joint Surg [Am]* 1996;78:1801–1807.
166. Steinmann S, Bigliani L, McIlveen S. Glenoid fractures associated with recurrent anterior dislocation of the shoulder. Presented at the American Academy of Orthopaedic Surgeons 57th Annual Meeting. New Orleans, LA. Park Ridge: American Academy of Orthopaedic Surgeons, 1990.

167. Symeonides P. The significance of the subscapularis muscle in the pathogenesis of recurrent anterior dislocation of the shoulder. *J Bone Joint Surg [Br]* 1972;54:476–483.
168. Taylor D, Arciero R. Pathologic changes associated with shoulder dislocations. *Am J Sports Med* 1997;25:306–311.
169. Terry G, Hammon D, France P, Norwood L. The stabilizing function of passive shoulder restraints. *Am J Sports Med* 1991;19:26–34.
170. Thomas S, Matsen FI. An approach to the repair of avulsion of the glenohumeral ligaments in the management of traumatic anterior glenohumeral instability. *J Bone Joint Surg [Am]* 1989;71:506–513.
171. Tibone J. Glenohumeral instability in overhead athletes. In: Bigliani L, ed. *The unstable shoulder*. Rosemont, IL: American Academy of Orthopaedic Surgeons, 1996:91–98.
172. Tibone J, Jobe F, Kerlan R, et al. Shoulder impingement syndrome in athletes treated by anterior acromioplasty. *Clin Orthop* 1985;198: 134–140.
173. Ticker J, Bigliani L, Soslowsky L, Pawluk R, Flatow E, Mow V. Inferior glenohumeral ligament: geometric and strain-rate dependent properties. *J Shoulder Elbow Surg* 1996;5:269–279.
174. Townley C. The capsular mechanism in recurrent dislocation of the shoulder. *J Bone Joint Surg [Am]* 1950;32:370–380.
175. Turkel S, Panio M, Marshall J, Girgis F. Stabilizing mechanisms preventing anterior dislocation of the glenohumeral joint. *J Bone Joint Surg [Am]* 1981;63:1208–1217.
176. Uthoff H, Piscopo M. Anterior capsular redundancy of the shoulder: congenital or traumatic? An embryological study. *J Bone Joint Surg [Br]* 1985;67:363–366.
177. Vahey J, Lippitt S, Matsen FI. Scapulohumeral balance: the limits of angular stability provided by glenoid geometry. Presented at the Annual Meeting of the American Academy of Orthopaedic Surgeons. San Francisco, CA, 1993
178. Vanderhooft E, Lippitt S, Harris S, Sidles J, Harryman DI, Matsen FI. Glenohumeral stability from concavity-compression: a quantitative analysis. Presented at the 8th Annual Meeting of the American Shoulder and Elbow Surgeons. Washington, DC, 1993.
179. Vangsness CJ, Ennis M. Neural anatomy of human glenoid labrum and shoulder ligaments. Proceedings of the American Academy of Orthopaedic Surgeons 59th Annual Meeting. Washington, DC. Park Ridge: American Academy of Orthopaedic Surgeons, 1992.
180. Walch G, Boileau P. Morphological study of the humeral proximal epiphysis. *J Bone Joint Surg [Br]* 1992;74:14–20.
181. Walch G, Boileau P, Levigne C, Mandrino A, Neyret P, Donell S. Arthroscopic stabilization for recurrent anterior shoulder dislocation: result of 59 cases. *Arthroscopy* 1995;11:173–179.
182. Walch G, Boileau P, Noel E, Donell S. Impingement of the deep surface of the supraspinatus tendon on the posterosuperior glenoid rim: an arthroscopic study. *J Shoulder Elbow Surg* 1992;1: 238–245.
183. Warner J, Caborn D, Berger R. Dynamic capsuloligamentous anatomy of the glenohumeral joint. *J Shoulder Elbow Surg* 1993;2:115–133.
184. Warner J, Deng X, Warren R, et al. Static capsuloligamentous restraints to superior–inferior translation of the glenohumeral joint. *Am J Sports Med* 1992;20:675–685.
185. Warner J, Deng X, Warren R, et al. Superior–inferior translation in the intact and vented glenohumeral joint. *J Shoulder Elbow Surg* 1993;2: 99–125.
186. Warner J, Flatow E. Anatomy and biomechanics. In: Bigliani L, ed. *The unstable shoulder*. Rosement, IL: American Academy of Orthopaedic Surgeons, 1996:1–24.
187. Warner J, Janetta-Alpers C, Miller M. Correlation of glenohumeral laxity with arthroscopic ligament anatomy. *J Shoulder Elbow Surg* 1994;3(suppl):S32.
188. Warner J, Johnson D, Miller M, Caborn D. Technique for selecting capsular tightness in repair of anterior–inferior shoulder instability. *J Shoulder Elbow Surg* 1995;4:352-364.
189. Warner J, Lephart S, Fu F. Role of proprioception in pathoetiology of shoulder instability. *Clin Orthop* 1996;330:35–39.
190. Warner J, Micheli L, Arslanian L, et al. Scapulothoracic motion in normal shoulders and shoulders with glenohumeral instability and impingement syndrome: a study using Moire topographic analysis. *Clin Orthop* 1992;285:191–199.
191. Warner J, Micheli L, Arslanian L, Kennedy D, Kennedy R. Patterns of flexibility, laxity, and strength in normal shoulders and shoulders with instability and impingement. *Am J Sports Med* 1990;18: 366–325.
192. Warner J, Paletta G, Warren R. Biplaner roentgenographic evaluation of glenohumeral instability and rotator cuff tears. Presented at the Annual Meeting of the American Academy of Orthopaedic Surgeons. Anaheim, CA, 1991.
193. Warren R, Kornblatt I, Marchand R. Static factors affecting posterior shoulder stability. *Orthop Trans* 1984;8:89.
194. Weber B, Simpson L, Hardegger F, et al. Rotational humeral osteotomy for recurrent anterior dislocation of the shoulder associated with a large Hill-Sachs lesion. *J Bone Joint Surg [Am]* 1984;66: 1443–1450.
195. Weber S, Caspari R. A biochemical evaluation of the restraints to posterior shoulder dislocation. *Arthroscopy* 1989;5:115–121.
196. Weulker N, Brewe F, Sperveslage C. Passive glenohumeral joint stabilization: a biomechanical study. *J Shoulder Elbow Surg* 1994;3: 129–134.
197. Wolf E, Cheng J, Dickson K. Humeral avulsion of glenohumeral ligaments as a cause of anterior shoulder instability. *Arthroscopy* 1995; 11:600–607.
198. Woo S, Gomez M, Seguchi Y, Endo C, Akeson W. Measurement of mechanical properties of ligament substance from a bone-ligament-bone preparation. *J Orthop Res* 1983;1:22–29.

Disorders of the Shoulder: Diagnosis and Management,
edited by Joseph P. Iannotti and Gerald R. Williams, Jr.
Lippincott Williams & Wilkins, Philadelphia © 1999.

CHAPTER 9

Biomechanics and Pathologic Lesions in the Overhead Athlete

James E. Tibone and Patrick J. McMahon

INTRODUCTION

The goal in treating overhead athletes is not simply to eliminate pain, but also to enable return to play. Today knowledge of shoulder anatomy, pathoanatomy, and biomechanics has dramatically improved treatment of injuries in the overhead athlete. Return to play is possible after treatment of numerous, common shoulder maladies, such as acromioclacular joint arthritis[16] and glenohumeral joint instability.[54,8]

An enormous range of mobility is essential at the shoulder to enable the prehensile hand to be placed in all the positions required in everyday life. As a consequence, there is less bony stability at the shoulder than other diarthrodial joints, such that soft tissues that guide and limit motion when injured can cause significant loss of function. This is especially true when the physiologic limits of the tissues are exceeded or impaired. This situation is less common in the general population, but is a frequent finding in individuals who participate in competitive overhead athletics. When one considers that simple shoulder motion necessitates the coordinated actions at four separate articulations, it is apparent that the demands placed on the shoulder during rigorous athletics is appreciable.

In this chapter, the anatomy and biomechanics of the shoulder are described with reference to the overhead athlete. The stages of the throwing motion, including electromyographic (EMG) data are described for both the normal and the injured shoulder. Baseball pitching is used as an example, but both swimming and tennis will also be described.

J. E. Tibone: Kerlan–Jobe Orthopaedic Clinic and University of Southern California, Inglewood, California 90301.
P. J. McMahon: Department of Orthopaedic Surgery, University of California, Orange, California 92668.

Then, evaluation of the injured shoulder in the overhead athlete will be detailed. Lastly, the clinical conditions resulting from overhead athletics will be reviewed.

SURGICAL ANATOMY AND BIOMECHANICS: NORMAL AND PATHOLOGIC

Before the description of the shoulder anatomy relevant to the overhead athlete, some definitions of the terms are necessary. Even though the term shoulder is often used to refer to the glenohumeral joint, normal function of the shoulder requires the coordinated function of four articulations: the sternoclavicular, the acromioclavicular, the glenohumeral, and the scapulothoracic. Furthermore, the shoulder is composed of approximately 30 muscles and 3 bones (humerus, clavicle, and scapula) in addition to the upper thorax. In this chapter, shoulder motion refers to the complex interaction of all these structures.

The actions (either translations or rotations) between the humerus and the glenoid are described as follows. Small linear movements that take place between the articular surfaces of the humeral head and the glenoid are termed *translations*. When large, these translations are exhibited clinically as glenohumeral joint instability. Large angular rotations also occur between the humerus and the scapula. In normal shoulders, motion is composed of large angular rotations and small glenohumeral translations.[33,67] For clarity, we define the three possible translations as anteroposterior, superoinferior, and mediolateral. The three rotations are internal–external, adduction–abduction in the scapular plane, and adduction–abduction in the horizontal plane.

Overview of Anatomy Relevant to Throwing and Overhead Athletics

Glenohumeral Anatomy and Motion

Four muscles compose the rotator cuff: the supraspinatus, subscapularis, infraspinatus, and teres minor. The supraspinatus has its origin on the posterosuperior scapula, superior to the scapular spine. It passes under the acromion, through the supraspinatus outlet and inserts on the greater tuberosity. The supraspinatus is active during the entire arc of scapular plane abduction; paralysis of the suprascapular nerve results in an approximately 50% loss of abduction torque.[15]

The infraspinatus and the teres minor muscles originate on the posterior scapula, inferior to the scapular spine, and insert on the posterior aspect of the greater tuberosity. Their tendinous insertions are not separate from each other or the supraspinatus tendon. These muscles function together to externally rotate and extend the humerus. Both account for approximately 80% of external rotation strength in the adducted position.

The subscapularis muscle arises from the anterior scapula and is the only muscle to insert on the lesser tuberosity. The subscapularis is the sole anterior component of the rotator cuff and functions to internally rotate and flex the humerus. The tendinous insertion of the subscapularis is continuous with the anterior capsule; therefore, these two structures have been considered responsible for providing anterior glenohumeral stability.[79,81]

The deltoid is the largest of the glenohumeral muscles and covers the proximal humerus on a path from its tripennate origin at the clavicle, acromion, and scapular spine to its insertion midway down the humerus at the deltoid tubercle. The three sections of the deltoid have three separate functions. The anterior portion is primarily a forward flexor and abductor of the glenohumeral joint; the middle portion is an abductor; and the posterior portion extends the humerus. The deltoid is active throughout the entire arc of glenohumeral abduction; paralysis of the axillary nerve results in a 50% loss of abduction torque.[15] The deltoid muscle can fully abduct the glenohumeral joint with the supraspinatus muscle inactive.

The humeral head represents approximately one-third of a sphere, the diameter being approximately 45 mm. The glenoid, on the other hand, has a 35-mm–vertical diameter and a 25-mm–horizontal diameter.[80,13,18,35,43] Relative to the plane of the scapula, the fossa is angled superior and posterior approximately 5 degrees,[26,67] offering little bony support to inferior instability with the arm at the side.

The proximal humerus is generally separated anatomically into four parts: the articular surface, the greater tuberosity, the lesser tuberosity, and the diaphyseal shaft. Relative to the shaft, the humeral head is angulated medially 45 degrees to the long axis of the humeral shaft and retroverted 30 degrees relative to the transcondylar axis of the distal humerus.[38] Between the two tuberosities is the intertubercular groove, in which the tendon of the long head of the biceps brachii muscle lies. This tendon is held in place by the coracohumeral ligament and the transverse humeral ligament. During abduction of the glenohumeral joint, the proximal humerus slides on the tendon of the long head of the biceps brachii. If the tendon ruptures, translation of the humeral head is increased.[83]

Soslowsky and coworkers[78] used stereophotogrammetry to demonstrate that the radius of curvature of the humeral head and the glenoid are not statistically different. Additionally, they showed that both surfaces approximated the surface of a sphere. However, this point is controversial, and others believe the surfaces are not conforming and that the contact between them is variable.[9,35]

In the glenohumeral joint, three actions are possible: spinning, sliding, and rolling. Spinning occurs when the contact point on the glenoid remains the same while the humeral head contact point is changing. Sliding is pure translation of the humeral head on the articular surface of the glenoid. At the extremes of motion, and certainly in unstable joints, glenohumeral translations occur. In this circumstance, the contact point on the glenoid is moving, while that for the humerus remains the same. The third type of action, rolling, may also occur at the glenohumeral joint. Rolling is a combination of humeral head translation and spinning relative to the glenoid, and the contact point changes on both the glenoid and the humeral head.[55] All three motions may take place at the glenohumeral joint.[55]

Capsuloligamentous and Labral Anatomy

Although originally disputed, it is now agreed that the glenohumeral ligaments are consistently present, although some variations in the insertion sites have been described. The superior glenohumeral ligament (SGHL) arises near the origin of the long head of the biceps brachii. If the glenoid had the markings of a clock with the 12 o'clock position superiorly and the 3 o'clock anteriorly, the origin of the SGHL would correspond to the area from the 12 o'clock to the 2 o'-clock positions. The SGHL runs inferiorly and laterally to insert on the humerus, superior to the lesser tuberosity. The middle MGHL usually arises from the neck of the glenoid just inferior to the origin of the SGHL and inserts into the humerus just medial to the lesser tuberosity. The presence of the MGHL is the most variable.[20]

The inferior glenohumeral ligament (IGHL) is a complex structure. Most recently, the IGHL has been described as having an anterior and a posterior band, with an axillary pouch between the two bands.[60] With abduction and external rotation, the anterior band fans out, and the posterior band becomes cordlike. Likewise, with internal rotation the posterior band fans out, and the anterior band appears cordlike. The anterior band of the IGHL arises from various areas corresponding to the 2 o'clock to 4 o'clock positions on the glenoid. The insertion site of this ligament has two attachments, one to the glenoid labrum and the other directly to the anterior neck of the glenoid.[53] The latter attachment is larger and likely more important in resisting anterior translation of the humeral head. The posterior band originates at the 7 o'clock to 9 o'clock positions. With the arm at the side, both the anterior and posterior bands pass through a 90-degree arc and insert on the humerus.

The labrum surrounds the periphery of the glenoid and is a site of attachment of the capsuloligamentous structures. It is composed of dense fibrous connective tissue, with a small fibrocartilaginous transition zone at the anterior inferior attachment of the osseous glenoid rim.[56,17,53] Other investigators have suggested that the labrum may act as a load-bearing structure for the humeral head and serve to increase the surface area of the glenoid.[9,77] Howell and Galinat showed that the labrum deepened the glenoid socket by nearly 50%.[32] Lippett and coworkers have shown that removal of the labrum decreases the joint's stability to shear stress by 20%. In this way, the triangular cross section of the labrum allows it to act as a chock-block to help prevent subluxation.

Scapulothoracic Anatomy and Motion

The scapulothoracic muscles include the trapezius (upper, middle, and lower portions), levator scapulae, serratus anterior, pectoralis minor, and rhomboid muscles. They all act to position the scapula in the proper orientation on the thoracic cage for a given shoulder motion. Postural support is provided by the levator scapulae and the upper trapezius. The middle trapezius and rhomboids retract the scapula, whereas the serratus anterior protracts the scapula. Upward rotation of the scapula is accomplished with the trapezius and serratus anterior. The upper trapezius and levator scapulae can also elevate the scapula. These muscles position the scapula to provide maximum stability at the glenohumeral joint while maintaining a large range of motion.

Motion between the scapula and the thorax—the scapulothoracic articulation—is an integral part of normal shoulder function. Other than muscular attachments, the scapula is supported only by the acromioclavicular joint and the coracoacromial ligaments. The scapula is mobile in many directions because of this unique articulation. The relative motion between the scapulothoracic articulation and the glenohumeral joint, during abduction, is termed the scapulothoracic rhythm. For the first 30 degrees of abduction, glenohumeral motion is much greater than scapulothoracic motion, the ratio of motions being reported to range from 4:1 to 7:1.[22,67] Thereafter, both joints move approximately the same amount.[22,67] In summary, over the entire arc of abduction, the glenohumeral joint moves more than the scapulothoracic joint; however, the difference is large at the beginning of abduction and is minimal at the end.

In the resting position, the superior edge of the scapular spine is rotated anteriorly from the frontal plane a mean of 31 degrees.[49] With the initiation of abduction, the scapula can translate medially or laterally, or in rare instances, oscillate on the chest wall.[38] As the shoulder abducts, the scapula rotates not only in the plane of abduction, but also in a plane perpendicular to it. The superior edge of the scapula first rotates anteriorly about 6 degrees with the first 90 degrees of shoulder abduction. Beyond 90 degrees, 16 degrees of posterior scapular rotation occurs.[14]

Acromioclavicular and Sternoclavicular Anatomy and Motion

The sternoclavicular joint is stabilized by four ligaments and the intraarticular disk. The interclavicular ligament provides restraint to superior joint motion and is taut when the shoulder is at the side.[70] Anterior and posterior motion is prevented by the anterior and posterior capsular structures, the anterior being the stronger of the two.[5] Inferiorly, the joint is stabilized by the costoclavicular ligaments, which run obliquely and laterally from the first rib to the clavicle. The anterior structures resist superior motion, and the posterior structures resist downward motion of the medial clavicle.[5]

At the acromioclavicular joint, the clavicle is stabilized to superior motion by the coracoclavicular ligaments: the conoid and the trapazoid. The acromioclavicular capsule is the primary restraint to anterior and posterior motion, with the acromioclavicular ligament being a superior thickening of the capsule.

The clavicle moves with shoulder motion; the lateral edge rotates approximately 30 degrees superiorly in the coronal plane during shoulder abduction. The lateral edge also rotates anteriorly, approximately 10 degrees with the first 40 degrees of shoulder abduction. No additional anterior rotation of the lateral edge occurs until 130 degrees of shoulder abduction; then 15 degrees of anterior clavicle rotation occurs until the end of shoulder abduction.[38]

The large axial rotations initially reported by Inman[38] have been questioned. By placing pins in the clavicle and the acromion, Rockwood and Green[70] have shown that the clavicle rotates axially less than 10 degrees over the entire arc of shoulder abduction. This finding is supported by the clinical observation that fixing the clavicle to the scapula does not significantly limit shoulder motion.

Stages of the Pitching and Throwing Motion, Including Electromyographic Data

Overhead throwing is a total body activity. It is an elaborate, synchronous progression of body movements that starts in the legs and trunk, proceeds to the upper extremities, and concludes in the rapid propulsion of the ball. The effectiveness of a thrower is determined by various factors, including velocity, accuracy, spin production, and endurance. Synchrony of muscular contractions and neurologic control throughout the body are essential to produce an effective throwing motion. Effectiveness also necessitates repetitive performance at a level that maximally stresses the physiologic limits of the shoulder. A delicate balance exists between mobility and stability of the joints of the upper extremities while throwing, and maintenance of this fragile balance is paramount. Small aberrations in the mechanisms that control stability have a significant and cumulative effect on upper extremity function and increase the risk of crossing the fine line between maximal throwing effectiveness and injury.

Sporting activities that involve the overhead throwing mechanism include softball, tennis, and swimming; but the complex biomechanics of throwing has been most studied in baseball.[10,27,29,30,47,45,46,63] Although the mechanics of throwing seem to differ slightly between player positions, in essence, the motions are quite similar. Most throwing studies have concentrated on the pitcher, because the motion is more constant, the collection of EMG data is easier, and pitchers frequently injure their arms. From a virtual standstill, a professional pitcher will accelerate a 142-g baseball to a release velocity of more than 90 mph in just 50 msec. Tremendous tensile, compressive, and rotational forces must be created and dissipated in the shoulder. A detailed description of the throwing motion will help clarify how this is done.

The Normal Shoulder

The baseball pitch is divided into five stages (Fig. 1): stage I is the windup, stage II is the early cocking stage, stage III is the late cocking stage, stage IV is the short propulsive stage of acceleration, stage V is the early follow-through or deceleration stage, which can also be divided into early and late.

At stance, the pitcher stands facing the batter with the shoulders parallel to the rubber. The pivot foot (right for right-handers) is positioned on the rubber.

In the windup stage, the body mechanics are quite individual. In general, windup begins with the stride foot (left for right-handers) coiling backward, away from home plate, and the arms swinging overhead. At this time, the position of the fingers on the ball is finalized while screened by the glove. The pivot foot rotates on the rubber as weight is transferred to it. This stage ends with the ball leaving the glove hand and the body balanced on the pivot foot. The EMG activity of the shoulder girdle and upper extremities is low during the windup, which reflects a lack of critical events related to performance or to injury potential.

Cocking is divided into early and late stages. Early cocking starts with pivot leg extension that propels forward the stride leg, nondominant upper extremity, and trunk. The gluteus maximus of the pivot leg is important in providing this propulsion. Temporarily, the dominant upper extremity lags behind the rest of the body. The trapezius and the serratus anterior muscles form a force couple to upwardly rotate and protract the scapula. This scapula motion is essential to place the glenoid in a stable position for the abducting and rotating humeral head. If the scapula is not positioned correctly, impingement can occur.[21] The deltoid and supraspinatus muscles act in synergy to abduct the humerus. Saha[73] described the glenohumeral muscles as drivers and steerers. In this case, the deltoid is the driver of the motion, and the supraspinatus is the steerer that fine-tunes the position of the humeral head in the glenoid. The remainder of the rotator cuff muscles have less activity during this phase,[21] indicating the importance of the supraspinatus in functioning with the deltoid in humeral abduction during this stage. Early cocking is terminated as the stride foot contacts the ground.

Late cocking begins with rapid forward motion of the trunk.[27] The dominant shoulder rotates forward. Abduction of the humerus is maintained and external rotation increases from 46 to 170 degrees.[24] Muscle forces are needed to overcome the inertia and gravity that act on the shoulder in horizontal abduction, external rotation, and adduction. Static and dynamic restraints combine to stabilize against these forces. In this position, the primary static anterior stabilizer of the glenohumeral joint is the anterior band of the inferior glenohumeral ligament.[81] Although the supraspinatus and the deltoid activity diminish as the humerus ceases to abduct, the other rotator cuff muscles increase in activity to stabilize the humeral head.[21] The subscapularis acts as a barrier to anterior translation, together with the pectoralis major and the latissimus dorsi. These muscles act as a dynamic sling to augment the inferior glenohumeral ligament.[21] The posterior rotator cuff muscles are also quite active during late cocking as the infraspinatus and teres minor actively externally rotate the humerus. Their posterior placement also enables them to act as checkreins to anterior subluxation.

Although there is no further abduction of the shoulder during late cocking, the scapulothoracic muscles continue to be active to produce a stable platform for the humeral head and to enhance maximal humeral external rotation.[21] The middle portion of the trapezius, the rhomboids, and the levator scapulae are all key in providing scapular stabilization. The serratus anterior is also important in opposing retraction to stabilize the scapula. Sometimes symptoms of anterior instability of the glenohumeral joint are demonstrated during this stage, because of an imbalance of the scapula-stabilizing mechanisms.[47]

The acceleration stage begins with maximal shoulder external rotation and terminates with ball release. The humerus internally rotates approximately 100 degrees in one-half second.[24] The humeral internal rotation torque is 14,000 in.-lb, with an angular velocity of 6100 degrees/sec.[42,27,30] The acceleration of the arm is coincident with the deceleration of the rest of the body, producing efficient transfer of energy to the upper extremity and ball.[27] A large glenohumeral joint compressive force (860 N), which has a stabilizing effect, also occurs. Synchronous muscular contraction about the glenohumeral joint balances the requirements of stabilization and rapid motion. A stable scapula is needed, and all of the scapular muscles have high activity in providing this function.

Shoulder angular velocity during acceleration is transferred from the trunk, with augmentation by the latissimus dorsi and the pectoralis major. The latissimus dorsi has even higher activity than the pectoralis major,[21] and it is anatomically positioned to generate large torques.[4] These two muscles are important in actively contributing to ball velocity, evidenced by a clinical study that reported they are the only two muscles to have a positive correlation between peak torque in isokinetic testing and pitching velocity.[2] The subscapularis, especially the upper portion, also has very high

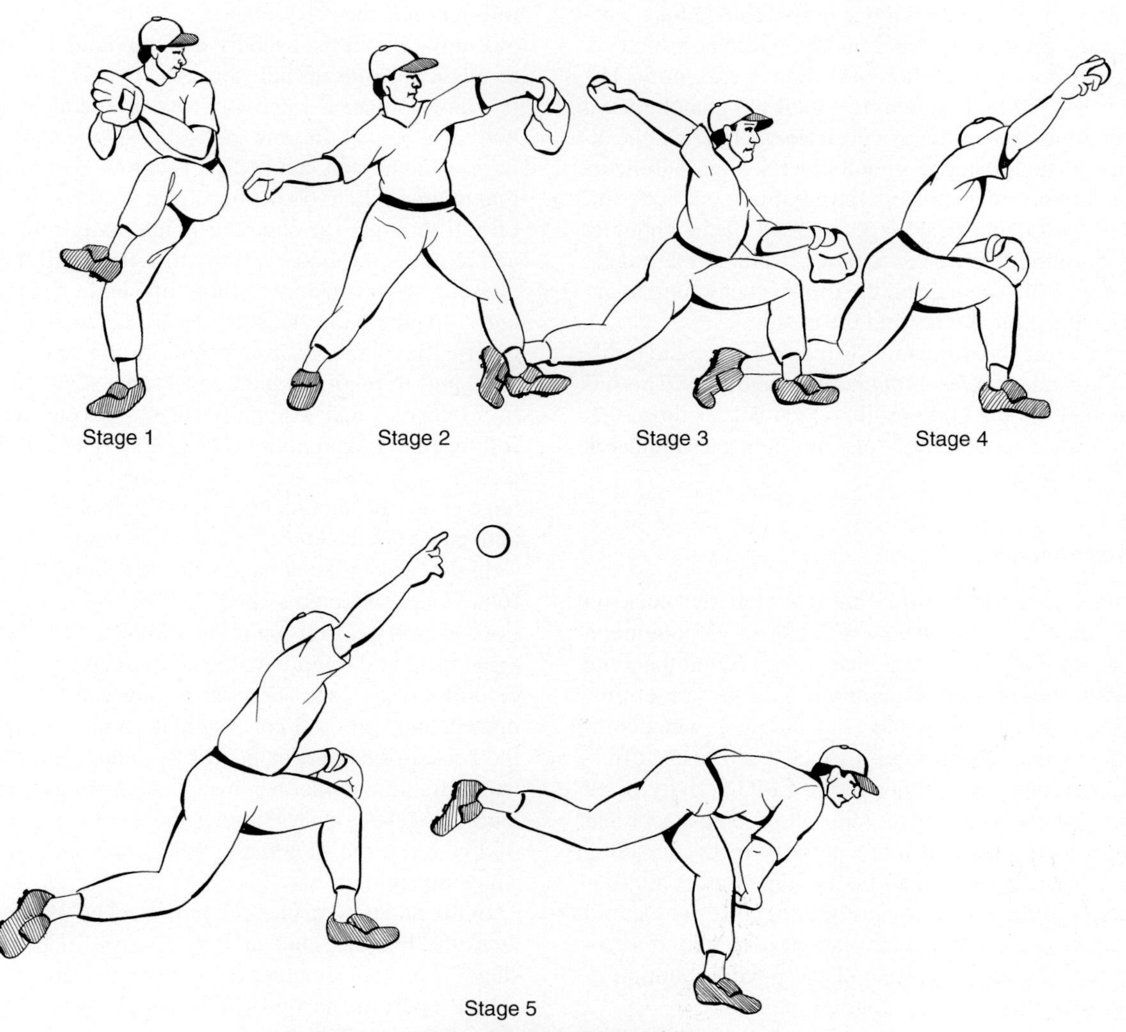

FIG. 1. The five phases of the baseball pitch.

activity during the acceleration stage and functions with the pectoralis major and latissimus dorsi.[21] Whereas the pectoralis major and the latissimus dorsi are the primary propellers of the arm, the subscapularis functions as a steering muscle to position the humeral head precisely in the glenoid. This coordinated function of the suscapularis with the latissimus dorsi has been observed in other overhead athletics as well.[66,65] The teres minor activity is also high, with the muscle acting as a checkrein to anterior instability. Athletes may note symptoms during this stage of throwing, the most typical problem being anterior instability.

Follow-through is after ball release and can also be divided into early and late stages. Initially the trunk and dominant lower extremity rotate forward. The shoulder continues to adduct and internally rotate to 30 degrees. Kinetic energy not transferred to the ball must be absorbed by the decelerating arm and body. Deceleration is estimated to be 500,000 degrees/sec^2 at the shoulder, with an external rotation torque of approximately 15,000 in.-lb at the humerus.[27,63] In general, deceleration of the upper extremity is accomplished by simultaneous contraction of opposing muscles around the shoulder.[21] The trapezius, serratus anterior, and rhomboids, all demonstrate high or very high activity. The deltoid is active, especially the posterior and middle portions, which are positioned to oppose the motion of the upper extremity. The teres minor has the highest activity of all the glenohumeral muscles, continuing to provide a posterior stabilizing checkrein. Injury to the posterior glenohumeral joint stabilizers will commonly become apparent during this stage. Late follow-through is a noncritical stage, with all of the shoulder muscles exhibiting decreasing activity.[21] All of the kinetic energy has been dissipated, and the trunk is beginning to extend, allowing the pitcher to field the position.

In summary, the throwing motion requires the rapid transmission of immense forces throughout the shoulder. This has been estimated to be 27,000 in.-lb, which is four times that in the leg during a soccer kick,[27] and this puts the shoulder at great risk for injury.

The Injured Shoulder

Alterations from these normal muscle activities occur in the injured shoulder. In athletes with anterior glenohumeral joint instability, Glousman and coworkers[29] found that elite pitchers with anterior joint instability had decreased serratus anterior EMG activity in all stages of the pitch when compared with normal. There were, in fact, significant differences between these two groups in the EMG activity of all the muscles tested, except the middle deltoid. The biceps and supraspinatus muscles had more activity in the unstable shoulders. This was thought to be a compensatory mechanism to help stabilize the humeral head against the glenoid fossa. In addition the infraspinatus showed increased activity during the late cocking phase of the pitching motion in those with instability.

Alterations from normal serratus anterior muscle activities are meaningful. Because of the rapidity of upper extremity motions, observation of scapula motion is nearly impossible during these overhead activities. But, during simple shoulder motions such as abduction, EMG activity in the serratus anterior muscle in the shoulder with anterior joint instability is diminished when compared, normal.[52] These findings indicate an abnormality in the coordinated rotation of the scapula on the thorax, termed *scapulothoracic rhythm*. Known primarily as a protractor that prevents winging of the scapula, the serratus anterior muscle is also important in the scapulothoracic rhythm during shoulder elevation.[3] Normal scapulothoracic rhythm has been extensively studied,[38,67,26,22,58] and these studies indicate the normal scapulothoracic rhythm has been altered, possibly resulting in a scapular lag.

Stages of Swimming Motion, Including Electromyographic Data

The swimming strokes can be divided into the pull-through and recovery phases.[69] In the freestyle stroke the pull-through phase is subdivided into hand entry, mid–pull-through, and end of pull-through (Fig. 2). During hand entry, the shoulder is internally rotated and abducted, and the body roll begins. In mid–pull-through the shoulder is at 90 degrees abduction and neutral rotation. Body roll reaches a maximum of 40 to 60 degrees from horizontal. With the end of pull-through, the shoulder is internally rotated and fully adducted as the body returns to horizontal. The recovery phase is subdivided into elbow lift, midrecovery, and hand entry. In elbow lift, the shoulder begins to abduct and rotate externally. The body roll begins in the opposite direction from pull-through. In midrecovery, the shoulder is abducted to 90 degrees and externally rotated beyond neutral. Body roll reaches a maximum of 40 to 60 degrees in the opposite direction. Breathing occurs by turning the head to the side. In hand entry, the shoulder is externally rotated and maximally abducted, and the body is returned to neutral roll.

In the backstroke at hand entry, the shoulder is externally rotated and abducted as body roll begins from neutral position. In mid–pull-through, the shoulder is abducted 90 degrees in neutral rotation with maximum body roll. At the end of pull-through, the shoulder is internally rotated and adducted, and body roll is horizontal. In the recovery phase of the backstroke, there is hand lift, rather than elbow lift. In hand lift, the shoulder begins with abduction and external rotation, and the body roll allows the arm to clear the water. In midrecovery, the shoulder is 90 degrees abducted and body roll is maximum.

In the butterfly stroke, the pull-through phase is the same as in the freestyle, but there is absence of body roll in all stages. To avoid shoulder flexion or extension, the hands are spread apart at the mid–pull-through stage. The recovery

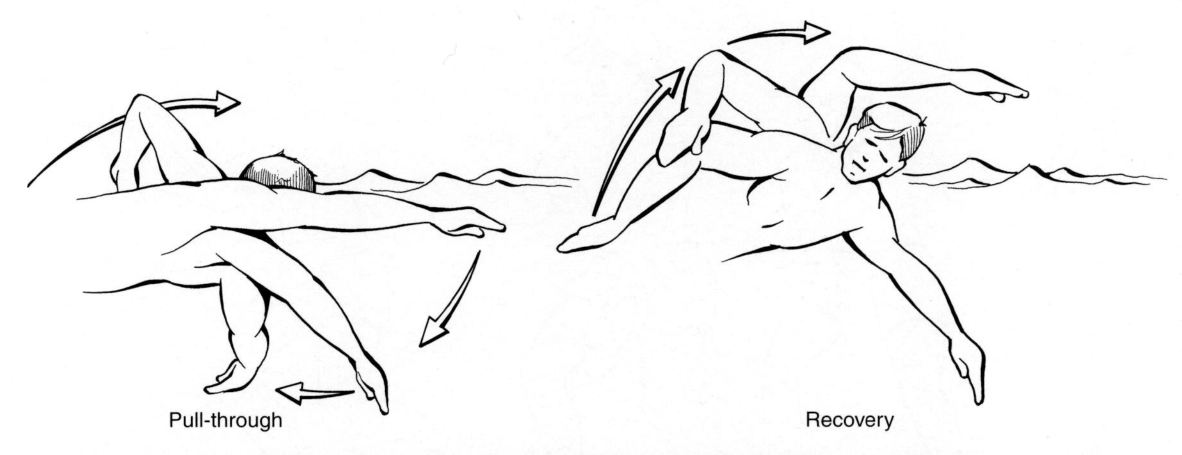

FIG. 2. The pull-through phase of the freestyle stroke can be subdivided into hand entry, mid–pull-through, and end of pull-through. The recovery phase can be subdivided into elbow lift, midrecovery, and hand entry.

phase is again similar to that in the freestyle, with an absence of body roll. Body lift allows both arms to clear the water. Shoulder flexion and extension do not occur.

The EMG indicates the rotator cuff is important during swimming.[66,65] The supraspinatus, infraspinatus, and middle deltoid activities are predominant in the recovery phase. They abduct and externally rotate the extremity in preparation for a new pull-through. This position, similar to the cocking phase of throwing, places the shoulder at risk for subacromial impingement.[31] The serratus anterior also has an important function during recovery. It allows the acromion to rotate clear of the abducting humerus and provides a stable glenoid base on which the humeral head can rotate. The serratus anterior works at nearly maximal levels to accomplish this. Significantly decreased EMG activity of the serratus anterior muscle was found in swimmers with shoulder pain. During the pulling stage of the freestyle stroke there was significantly less activity in the serratus anterior in subjects with a painful shoulder when compared with normal.[75] The serratus anterior demonstrates similar findings during the pull-through stage of the butterfly stoke in subjects with a painful shoulder.[64] If this muscle becomes fatigued during the course of a number of cycles, scapular rotation may not coincide with humeral abduction. As a result, impingement syndrome may occur.

The biceps brachii muscle exhibited erratic activity during all of the strokes and functioned primarily at the elbow, which is similar to its role in pitching. The latissimus dorsi and pectoralis major were propulsive muscles, with a resulting action similar to that of the acceleration phase of throwing.

In summary, particular attention must be paid to conditioning the rotator cuff and serratus anterior muscles in an effort to decrease the common problem of swimmer's shoulder impingement syndrome. Exercises must concentrate specifically on increasing the endurance of the serratus anterior muscle.

The Stages of Tennis Motion, Including Electromyographic Data

The tennis serve can be divided into the same stages of complex muscle activity as a baseball pitch. The deltoid muscle function is low during cocking compared with pitching because trunk rotation contributes to shoulder abduction. The acceleration and follow-through stages in the tennis serve demonstrate muscle patterns and activity that are similar to those observed in throwing a baseball. Because the motions for serving the tennis ball are similar to those for pitching, tennis players may benefit from the same conditioning program as that outlined for pitchers. Likewise, emphasis should be placed on rehabilitating the rotator cuff and serratus anterior muscles.

The ground strokes, both forehand and backhand, can be divided into three stages (Fig. 3). In stage I, racquet preparation begins with shoulder turn and ends with the initiation of weight transfer to the front foot. Stage II is acceleration and begins with weight transfer to the front foot accompanied by forward racquet movement and culminates at ball impact. Stage III is follow-through and begins at ball impact and ends with completion of the stroke. The forehand ground stroke reveals a relatively passive wind-up sequence. Trunk rotation provides some of the force for shoulder motion. In follow-through, there is a marked decrease in activity among the accelerating muscles and a concomitant increase in the external rotators responsible for deceleration. The backhand ground stroke is similar in concept, but opposite in muscle activity, to the forehand. Follow-through demonstrates deceleration with increased activity of the internal rotators.

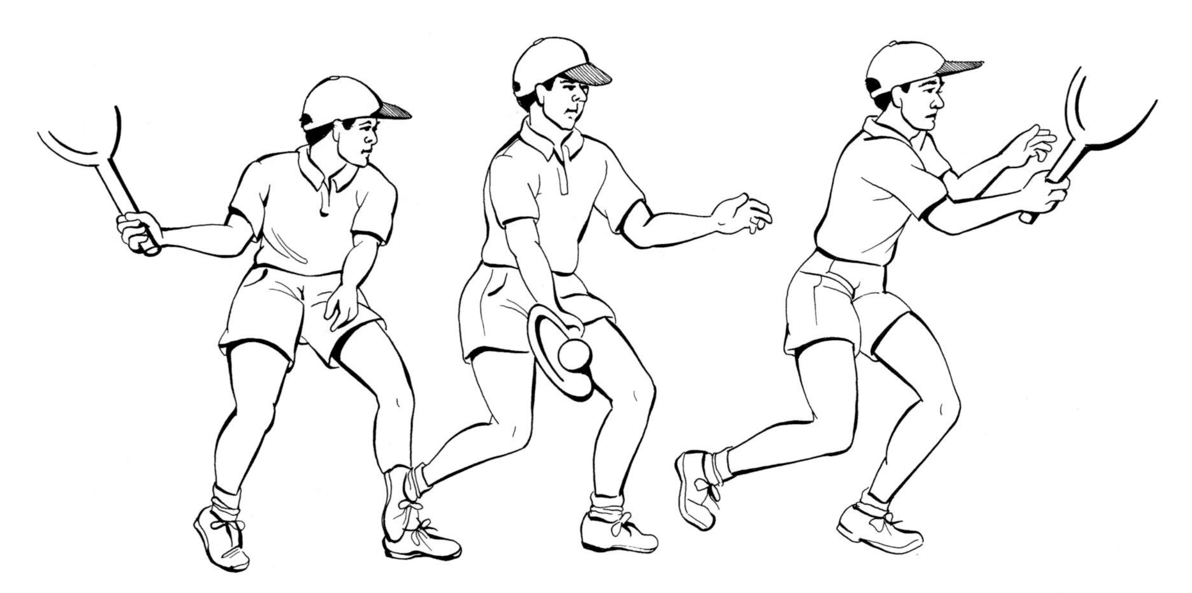

FIG. 3. The ground strokes of the tennis stroke, both forehand and backhand, can be divided into three stages: racquet preparation, acceleration, and follow through.

EVALUATION

Clinical

Clinical evaluation of the overhead athlete requires knowledge of normal mechanics of the sport and is best assessed on the field. The most important aspect of proper mechanics is that the motion is natural. This applies to all players, whether in baseball (when the ball is thrown from the outfield or the pitching mound), swimming, tennis, or any of the other activities that require an overhead motion. Baseball throwing is the best example. When an outfielder throws the ball, he or she first takes a step backward and then lands on the opposite forefoot with the knee slightly flexed. A pitcher should do the same. When the pitcher overthrows to get more speed on the ball, he tends to hyperextend the knee and land on the heel.[74] This places sudden, large forces on the shoulder during the cocking stage of throwing. Additionally, when the pitcher starts to fatigue, the elbow begins to drop and he increases the lordosis in his spine. A pitcher with back pain may later develop shoulder problems from poor mechanics. These signs are important in recognizing the thrower who is prone to injury. For a specific athlete, any deviation from the normal, natural motion is indicative of injury.

History

Injuries to the shoulder account for most injuries to adult baseball players.[1] Most of these injuries occur during the throwing motion. A professional baseball pitcher may play 30 to 40 games in a season. He or she may throw as many as 150 pitches in a game, many of these at high velocity.[63] Although amateur pitchers may not play as many games in a season, they still try to throw the ball as fast as possible while maintaining accuracy. It is not surprising that shoulder pain is a frequent complaint among baseball pitchers.

Clinical assessment of shoulder injuries in athletes should not focus attention on the shoulder joint entirely, because other disease processes may be overlooked. One must always be aware of other potential causes of shoulder pain when obtaining a history and physical examination from an injured player. Pain can be referred to the shoulder from the hand (e.g., carpal tunnel syndrome), or neck (e.g., radicular symptoms).

The history should be meticulous, including the patient's age and chief complaint. Loss of velocity, accuracy, and distance usually alert the thrower to injury more serious than usual aches and pains. The effect of the injury on the patient's activities of daily living may provide as many clues to the diagnosis as the effect of the injury on sports performance. Pain is a subjective symptom, but careful assessment can provide insight into disease pathology. The duration, anatomic location, and character of the pain should be specifically assessed. In addition, the presence of night pain and analgesic requirements should be considered. The temporal relation to sports activity and the postural relation to arm motion should be obtained from the patient with shoulder pain. For example, a pitcher who complains of anterior shoulder pain during the cocking stage of the throwing motion usually has anterior shoulder instability. The pitcher who has pain during the follow-through stage may have posterior shoulder instability. The onset of night pain, especially when lying on the affected side, may indicate a rotator cuff tear. Pain with overhead activities is possibly indicative of impingement syndrome.

Physical Examination

The physical examination of the shoulder consists of several phases, including visual inspection, palpation, range-of-motion testing, strength testing, neurovascular assessment, and general physical evaluation. Visual inspection includes examining the skin and the contour of the entire shoulder girdle. Special attention should be given to areas of swelling or muscle atrophy. Side-to-side differences should be recorded, with knowledge that there are some normal changes that occur in the throwing arm. For example, the musculature is usually hypertrophied and the scapula is often displaced slightly inferiorly in the throwing arm. Palpation should be performed from the neck to the fingers on all sides of the upper extremities. Motion of all four joints (sternoclavicular, acromioclavicular, scapulothoracic, and glenohumeral) is essential to normal shoulder kinematics. This can be assessed both actively and passively. Differences between active and passive motion can be the result of a deficiency, such as a rotator cuff tear. Motion should always be compared with the contralateral shoulder. Brown et al.[11] found that Major League pitchers have different ranges of motion between the shoulders. In the pitching arm, with the shoulder in abduction, there is 11 degrees less extension, 15 degrees less internal rotation, and 9 degrees more external rotation. Therefore, comparison with the contralateral arm should be done with this variance in mind.

In the load and shift test, the examiner applies a compressive load to the relaxed glenohumeral joint and an attempt is made to translate the humeral head. This test should be done in a number of shoulder positions and attempts made to translate the humeral head anterior, posterior, and inferior. It is important to compare the contralateral shoulder because, for example, many shoulders in asymptomatic athletes can be subluxated posteriorly (55%).[51] Simple translational testing can also be helpful. The patient should be in a supine position and the shoulder muscles relaxed. Then the humeral head is grasped and an attempt made to translate it anteriorly and posteriorly. As with the load and shift test it is best to compare with the contralateral shoulder and examine the translation several shoulder positions

Inferior laxity is then evaluated by applying an inferiorly directed load to the shoulder with the upper extremity at the side, the sulcus test. Once again, comparison with the contralateral shoulder and assessment of symptoms of pain or apprehension are important indicators of instability.[51]

Relocation Test

Diagnosis of shoulder injuries in the throwing athlete who is younger than 35 years old is often based on subtle findings. Sometimes there are symptoms related to a number of problems. For example an athlete may present with symptoms of impingement syndrome and anterior glenohumeral joint instability. Whereas the impingement signs are generally obvious, the instability is not. The most sensitive test we have found for occult anterior instability is the relocation test. With the patient supine and the muscles relaxed, the shoulder is placed into the position of apprehension by abducting to 90 degrees and then gently externally rotating the shoulder to the limit of motion (Fig. 4A). Usually the overhead athlete with subtle instability will not have apprehension that the joint will dislocate. Instead, this maneuver produces posterosuperior shoulder pain as the tuberosity or the rotator cuff impinges against the posterosuperior glenoid rim. A gentle anterior-directed force may be applied to the humeral head, and the signs become more obvious. The relocation test is performed by reproducing this position and applying a posteriorly directed force to the humeral head

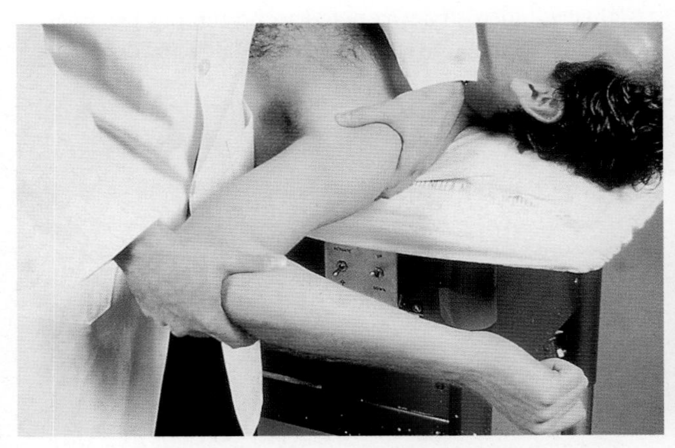

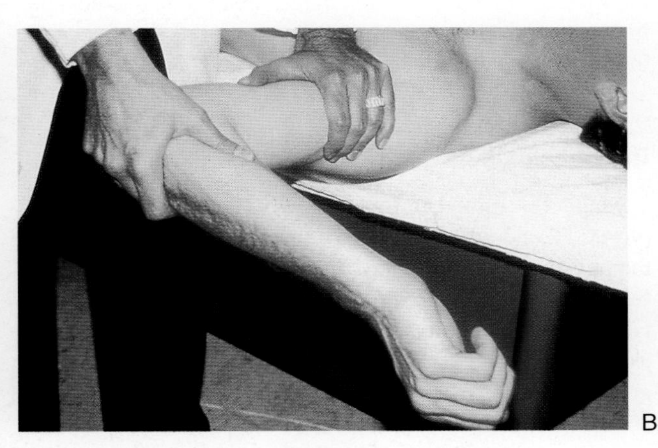

FIG. 4. (A) With the patient supine and the muscles relaxed, the shoulder is placed into the position of apprehension by abducting to 90 degrees and then gently externally rotating the shoulder to the limit of motion. The overhead athlete with subtle instability feels pain as the tuberosity or the rotator cuff impinges against the posterior superior glenoid rim. A gentle anterior directed force may be applied to the humeral head and the signs become more obvious. **(B)** The relocation test is performed by reproducing this position and applying a posteriorly directed force to the humeral head.

(see Fig. 4B) The posteriorly directed force likely keeps the joint located, so that in the athlete with anterior instability, the pain resolves. Continuous maximal external rotation is applied throughout the test, and usually, the shoulder can be externally rotated further with the posteriorly directed force being applied. The pain reproduced with this test is that of internal impingement.

Superior Labrum Anterior and Posterior Tests

O'Brien and coworkers[61] described a test for diagnosing superior labrum anterior and posterior (SLAP) lesions of the shoulder. The standing patient is asked to forward flex the affected arm to 90 degrees, with the elbow in full extension. The patient then adducts the arm 10 to 15 degrees medial to the saggital plane of the body and internally rotates so the thumb points downward. The examiner, standing behind the patient, applies a downward force to the arm and the patient resists the downward motion. With the arm in the same position, the forearm is then fully supinated and the maneuver is repeated. The test is considered positive if pain is elicited during the first step and is then reduced or eliminated with the second step. Sometimes there is a painful click inside the shoulder. This test will also be positive if the patient has acromioclavicular joint pathology, but the pain will be localized on top of the shoulder.

Another test for diagnosing SLAP lesions of the shoulder was described by Kibler[48] and reported to have sensitivity of 78% and specificity of 92%. The patient is examined either standing or sitting, with the hands on the hips, such that the thumbs are directed posteriorly. The examiner places one hand on top of the patient's acromion and the other hand behind the elbow. Force is then applied to the elbow, attempting to slide the humeral head anterior and superior. The patient is asked to resist this force. Pain localized to the front of the shoulder or a pop or click in this area is considered a positive test. If the test reproduces the symptoms that occur during the overhead athletic endeavor, the test is also positive.

Imaging Studies

Magnetic resonance imaging (MRI), computed tomography (CT), and other imaging studies can be used to reinforce the physical findings in the difficult case. It can also be helpful in a few special circumstances. If there is suspicion of rotator cuff abnormality, the MRI is useful in delineating the extent of injury. An MRI can also be used when the radiographs are not sufficient in identifying humeral and glenoid abnormalities. It is also helpful in the athlete with a strong suspicion of instability, but without a strong indication for surgery unless a specific labral lesion can be identified. The use of an intraarticular contrast agent is generally recommended. Iodine injection into the glenohumeral joint before CT, or gadolinium or saline injection into the glenohumeral joint before MRI, is helpful to outline the labrum. Routine use of these studies is not recommended or cost-effective in athletes with suspected instability.

Examination Under Anesthesia

The load and shift, translation, and sulcus tests can be performed under anesthesia to confirm the diagnosis of anterior instability. In our experience, valuable information can be gleaned from a variation of the simple translation testing done with the athlete under anesthesia. With the shoulder abducted and in neutral rotation the amount of anterior translation is assessed. With increasing external rotation of the shoulder, the amount of translation decreases and then becomes zero. At this point the position of the shoulder is noted. The test is then repeated with the contralateral shoulder. In the shoulder with instability, there is considerably more external rotation of the shoulder before anterior translation halts.

PATHOPHYSIOLOGY

Common Injuries

Internal Glenoid Impingement

Internal glenohumeral impingement is associated with anterior glenohumeral joint instability. The pitcher with internal impingement commonly complains of pain and decreased effectiveness. Pitch control is usually maintained, but velocity is diminished. Pain is located in the posterosuperior shoulder and is associated with throwing. After throwing is completed, the pain diminishes and then resolves after sufficient rest until throwing resumes.

Cadaveric studies indicate the rotator cuff can be pinched against the posterosuperior glenoid rim with the shoulder abducted to 90 degrees and then maximally externally rotated. With the glenohumeral joints fixed in this position, the greater tuberosity was noted to be forcing the rotator cuff against the glenoid rim[44] (Fig. 5). Walch and coworkers[82] re-

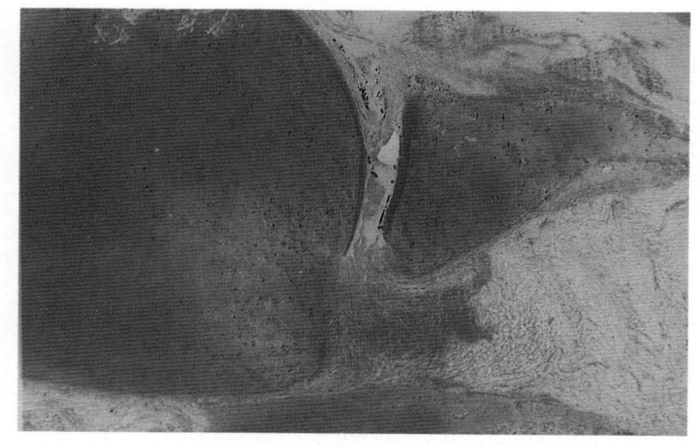

FIG. 5. Cadaveric section of the glenohumeral joint with the shoulder put into the apprehension position of abduction and maximal external rotation, the rotator cuff pinches against the posterior superior glenoid rim.

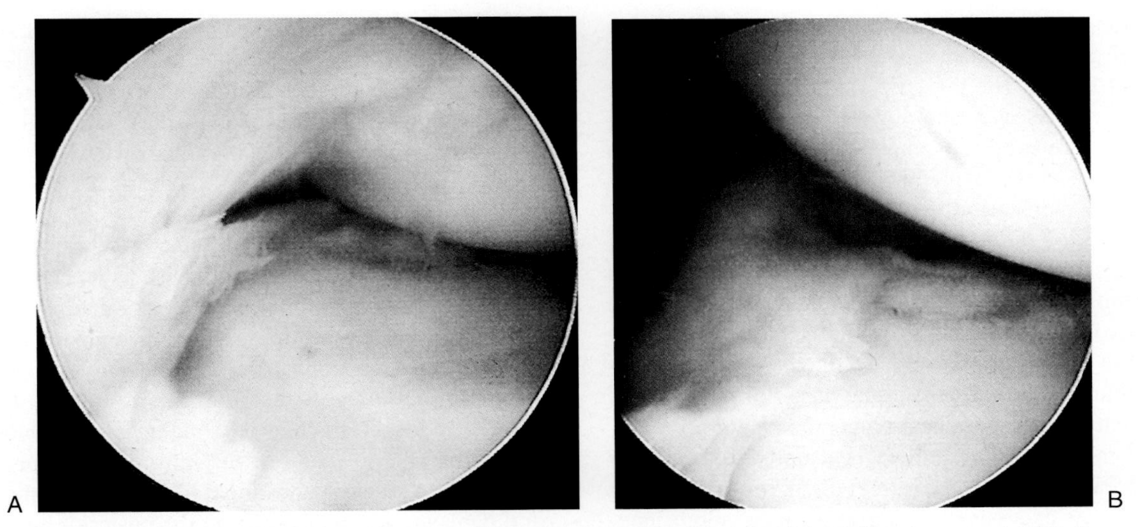

FIG. 6. (A) View of the relocation test from inside the joint demonstrating internal impingement. With the arthroscope in the posterior portal, the shoulder is put into the position of abduction and maximal external rotation. The rotator cuff pinches against the posterior superior glenoid rim. **(B)** With a posteriorly directed force applied to it, the humeral head returns to a normal position, and the greater tuberosity is posterior to the glenoid rim.

ported similar findings in an arthroscopic study. Davidson and coworkers[19] suggest that a subtle increase in anterior glenohumeral translation can cause internal impingement. Normally, both static and dynamic stabilizers act to prevent anterior instability, but in the apprehension position the normal distance from the rotator cuff to the posterosuperior rim of the glenoid is small so that little tolerance exists. Fatigue of the shoulder musculature from repetitive throwing may result in damage to the static stabilizers, such as stretching of the anterior band of the IGHL. During the throwing motion an increased humeral angulation may then occur. In the cocking or acceleration stage of throwing when the shoulder is in the apprehension position, this results in internal impingement. Increased anterior translation would then aggravate the internal impingement. As the humeral head translates anteriorly, with the shoulder in the apprehension position, more of the rotator cuff would contact the glenoid rim.

The shoulder relocation test, as described in the foregoing, is the best test for internal impingement. When necessary, arthroscopic evaluation of the glenohumeral joint reveals characteristic lesions. There is fraying of the supraspinatus tendon in a location slightly more posterior to that seen with classic impingement. Fraying of the posterosuperior glenoid rim is also seen. At arthroscopy the intraarticular effects of the relocation test can be directly visualized. With the arthroscope in the posterior portal, the shoulder is put into the apprehension position of abduction and maximal external rotation, the internal impingement can be seen as the rotator cuff abuts against the posterior superior glenoid rim (Fig. 6A). Then, with a posteriorly directed force applied to the humeral head, this is relieved (see Fig. 6B). This can also be visualized with MRI (Fig. 7).

In the normal glenohumeral joint, Howell and coworkers[33] described the humeral head translating 4 mm posteri-

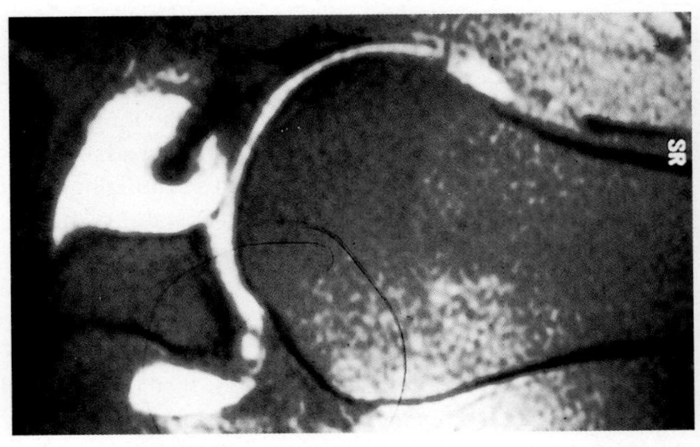

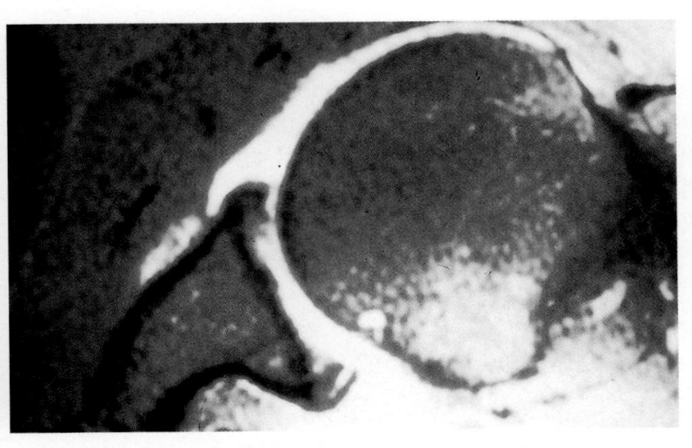

FIG. 7. (A) An MRI of a shoulder positioned in the apprehension position demonstrating internal glenoid impingement. **(B)** An MRI of a normal shoulder positioned in the apprehension position. The rotator cuff does not impinge on the posterior superior glenoid rim.

orly when the shoulder was abducted and externally rotated. This normal posterior translation helps to minimize abnormal contact of the rotator cuff on the posterosuperior glenoid. Individuals with anterior joint instability, by contrast did not demonstrate movement in the posterior direction and in some cases the humeral head translated anteriorly. This abnormal translation increases internal glenoid impingement. During the first part of the relocation test in the joint with instability, the anterior translation of the humeral head results in rotator cuff tendon compression between the greater tuberosity and the posterosuperior glenoid rim. The application of the posteriorly directed humeral force then relocates the humeral head to its normal posterior position and the rotator cuff tendon does not contact the glenoid rim.[19]

Because internal impingement is usually a secondary problem, treatment must be directed to the underlying causes, which are excessive humeral angulation, subtle anterior glenohumeral joint instability, and fatigue. Muscular development of the dynamic restraints and correction of problems with the throwing mechanics are indicated. Physical therapy aimed at strengthening and conditioning the shoulder muscles, including the rotator cuff, deltoid, and scapular muscles is instituted. It is important to include the scapular muscles in the rehabilitation efforts to restore the normal scapulothoracic rhythm. Both concentric and eccentric strengthening and conditioning exercises are included. Although posterior capsular stretching may also be beneficial, care is taken not to stretch the static restraints to anterior translation. Additionally, cardiovascular and general muscular conditioning is incorporated in the rehabilitation program to minimize fatigue. Generally there will be meaningful improvement in symptoms within 3 months, and throwing can resume with return to the prior level of competition after 6 months of treatment. Most overhead athletes (greater than 80%) can be successfully treated without surgery.

When anterior translation is markedly increased these efforts may prove to be insufficient to allow the thrower to return to pain-free activities. If the individual is intent on returning to overhead athletics, surgery is then indicated. In our experience, arthroscopic debridement of the rotator cuff and posterior superior glenoid fraying is unsuccessful if there is meaningful anterior joint instability. Only those individuals who would have responded successfully to the rehabilitation program have successful results with debridement alone. If there is meaningful anterior instability, operative repair of the anterior capsuloligamentous structures is required. Rehabilitation is then instituted, with expectation to return to the prior level of competition after 12 months.

Anterior Instability: Rotator Cuff Problems

Neer,[57] among others, described the impingement syndrome as compromise of the space between the humeral head and the coracoacromial arch. In the classic case, the coracoarcomial ligament and the anterior inferior aspect of the acromion are compressed against the bursal side of the rotator cuff during forward flexion of the shoulder. Classic impingement syndrome is unusual in overhead-throwing athletes. The overhead-throwing athletes generally represent a younger population than individuals with classic impingement syndrome resulting from anterior acromial spurs. In those younger than 35 years of age, the impingement syndrome is almost exclusively associated with anterior glenohumeral instability. Classically, these patients have positive impingement signs and will also demonstrate a positive relocation test. Under anesthesia, they have glenohumeral joint instability, but it is so subtle that it may go undetected. Arthroscopic findings, such as a classic Bankart lesion or a Hill-Sachs lesion, are unusual. Findings may include stretching of the anterior band of the inferior glenohumeral ligament, labral fraying, and minimal labral separation. Chondral damage, seen as a defect in the posterior humeral head articular cartilage, may also be present. Rotator cuff damage is usually on the articular surface of the supraspinatus tendon from internal impingement or overuse failure. Conservative care emphasizes strengthening and conditioning of the rotator cuff and scapular muscles. Return to sport should be gradual, with careful attention to symptoms. Initially after return to overhead throwing, if pain occurs it should be mild in intensity and resolve within a few hours of cessation of the activity. Within a short time, pain should be absent during the overhead throwing activity. If the pain persists, the duration or vigor of the activity must be diminished. Most individuals will improve with such a program. If after 6 months of rehabilitation, the symptoms continue, operative repair of the anterior capsuloligamentous structures is indicated. Isolated acromioplasty is not warranted and can lead to increased anterior instability.

Superior Labrum Anterior and Posterior Lesions

It has long been suggested that the long head of the biceps tendon has a role in preventing superior translation of the humeral head.[23,28] Experimental work has subsequently demonstrated that it stabilizes the humeral head on the glenoid in both the anterior to posterior direction[41,62] and the superior to inferior direction.[41,83,62] More recently, superior translation of the humeral head has been demonstrated in vivo in individuals after isolated rupture of the long head of the biceps.[83] Both the long head and the short head of the biceps contribute to anterior stability and this stabilizing effect is more significant when there is joint instability from a Bankart lesion.[40] In summary, the origin of the biceps is one of the structures that acts in synchrony to stabilize the humeral head on the glenoid.

Snyder and coworkers[76] described lesions of the biceps origin and the superior glenoid labrum, that they termed SLAP (superior labral anterior and posterior) lesions. They postulated that these lesions were the result of superior subluxation of the joint. There may be a history of minimal trauma in older individuals, for there appears to be a propensity for degenerative lesions of the labrum and biceps tendon in this location.[68] These authors report that there are five types of SLAP lesions (Fig. 8). A simple degenerative fraying of the superior labrum is a type I lesion. The peripheral edge of the labrum remains firmly attached to the glenoid and the biceps tendon attachment on the supraglenoid tubercle of the glenoid is intact. A type II lesion is most common. It is a tear of the superior labrum where the labrum with the biceps tendon attachment is avulsed from the glenoid (Fig. 9). Sometimes this lesion is similar to an anatomic variant because the labrum superiorly is meniscoid with a free edge.[17] Complete detachment of the labrum where bare bone is visible is abnormal. A bucket-handle tear of the labrum with preservation of the biceps anchor is a type III lesion (Fig. 10). In these cases the edge of the labrum is torn and can be displaced into the joint, whereas the peripheral portion of the labrum remains firmly attached to the glenoid. Additionally, the biceps tendon attachment is intact. When the biceps tendon is split with a portion remaining attached to the supraglenoid tubercle the lesion is a type IV. This lesion is similar to the type III lesion except that a portion of the biceps tendon attachment is also involved. A type V lesion is any combination of these. Iannotti and Wang[37] also described avulsion fracture of the supraglenoid tubercle as an early noninvasive finding that may help in the early diagnosis of the SLAP lesion.

Rokito and coworkers[72] have provided a simplified classification of the SLAP lesion that may better relate to treatment. Lesions are classified based on anatomic location and the probability of associated pathology. A type I lesion involves a tear of the labrum or the biceps tendon, or both. This is a mechanical lesion that does not result in instability. Type II lesions, which involve an avulsion of the anterior superior labrum and type III lesions, which involve an avulsion of the biceps tendon anchor complex, result in glenohumeral joint instability. Type I lesions should be debrided because there is no associated glenohumeral joint instability and type II and III lesions should be debrided of loose tissue and the involved labrum fixed to glenoid bone. Results correlated with the type of lesion. Eighty-eight percent of athletes with a type I lesion were able to successfully return to their sport, compared with 64% of athletes with a type II lesion and 92 treated for a type III lesion. Many individuals with a SLAP lesion, however, have recurrent glenohumeral joint instability, and this is often best treated with a concomitant anterior glenohumeral stabilization procedure. If there is minimal increase in joint translations, repair of the SLAP lesion alone is sufficient. But with meaningful symptoms of instability, the anterior glenohumeral stabilization procedure should also be performed.

Posterior Instability

Individuals with posterior instability of the glenohumeral joint can be divided into two distinct groups: those with traumatic posterior dislocation or subluxation, and those with posterior subluxation from repetitive microtrauma. The traumatic posterior instability is usually the result of a fall on the outstretched upper extremity with a normal shoulder. Athletes very rarely suffer a posterior shoulder dislocation. Recurrent posterior subluxation is more typical in overhead athletes and results from chronic, insidious microtrauma to the posterior capsule, which subsequently becomes attenuated. For example, if a pitcher overthrows, does not warm up properly, or has poor mechanics that lead to a limited follow-through, then the posterior capsule can be injured. Repeated, daily injuries during participation in practice and games lead to chronic subluxation. However, chronic subluxation can also result from a single traumatic episode that results in subluxation with repeated use in overhead athletics. A football quarterback who is tackled and falls on his outstretched hand may feel a pulling sensation in the posterior shoulder. There may or may not be appreciation of joint instability. When the acute pain has subsided, there may be posterior shoulder pain with throwing, and velocity may be diminished.

It is common for overhead athletes with recurrent, posterior subluxation to complain of pain during the offending sporting activity. Pain may be absent at other times, and specific complaints of joint instability are unusual. On physical examination there is no asymmetry of the shoulders and range of motion is normal, as is strength. The pain of subluxation is sometimes felt when the shoulder is placed in the position of 90 degrees of forward flexion, horizontally adducted across the body and internally rotated. Suspected posterior joint instability can be further evaluated by having the patient lie supine with the shoulder over the edge of the examination table, in the same position as described earlier, while a posterior force is applied to the shoulder. Although meaningful when positive, apprehension of posterior instability is rare. Accompanying symptoms of pain or apprehension are very important, for asymptomatic posterior subluxation present at physical examination may represent normal laxity and may not indicate pathologic instability. Anterior instability tests should also always be performed as described earlier in this chapter. It must be remembered that the athlete may be able to voluntarily subluxate the shoulder posteriorly, and this can be demonstrated by the patient on examination with the shoulder in the forward flexed and internally rotated position. These athletes are usually not psychologically disturbed and do not use their shoulders for secondary gain. They can be treated the same as the athlete who is unable to voluntarily subluxate the joint.

Rehabilitation of the shoulder muscles, including the rotator cuff and the scapular muscles is generally helpful in reducing symptoms of posterior instability. Strengthening of the infraspinatus, the teres minor, and the posterior deltoid muscles should be specifically addressed and biofeedback to rehabilitate the posterior shoulder muscles may have a place. When rehabilitation is maintained for at least 6 months, about 70% of individuals with posterior instability will improve symptomatically, and many athletes will be able to return to their sport.[34] When instability is recalcitrant to this re-

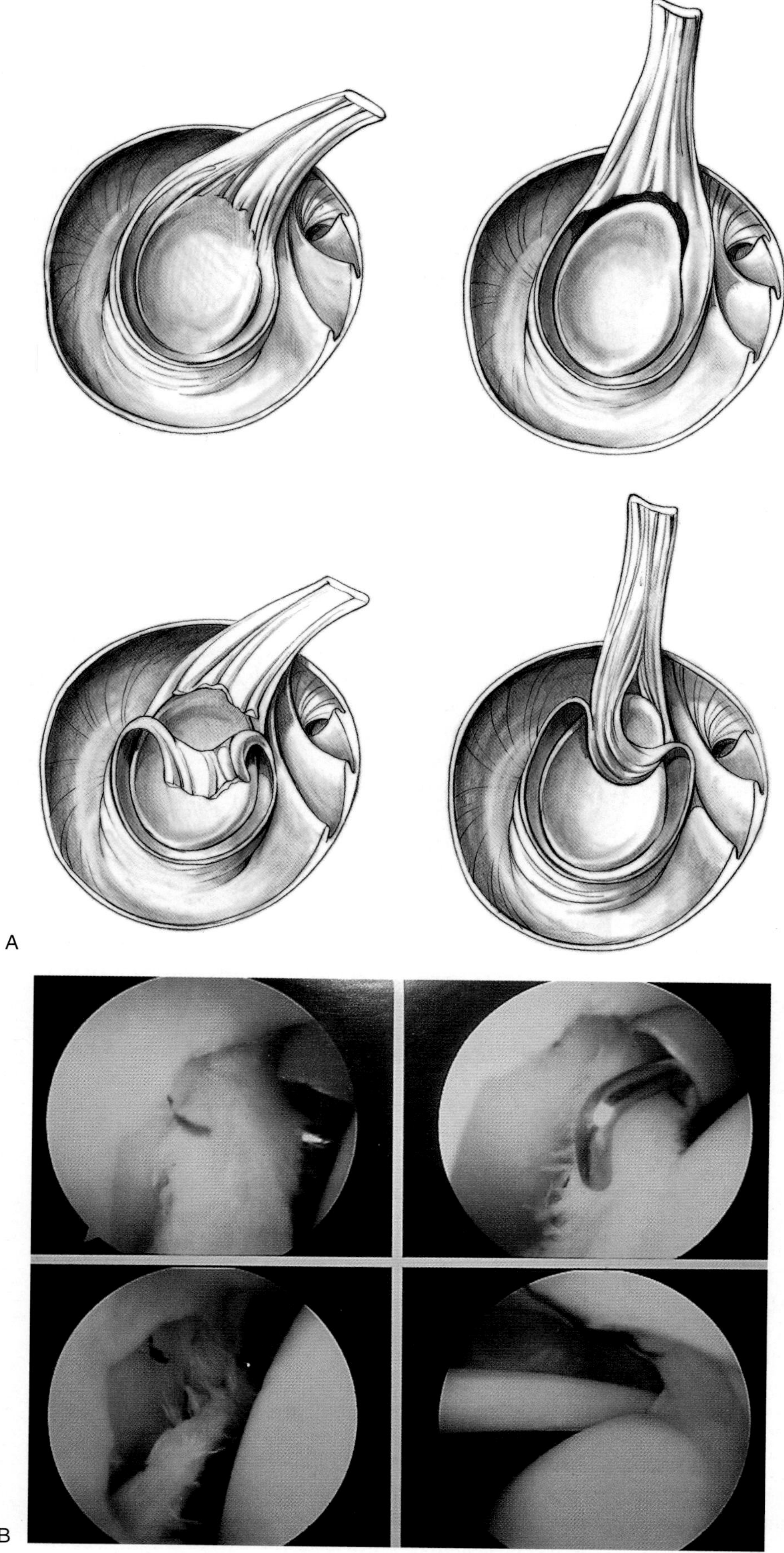

FIG. 8. (A) Line drawing of the SLAP lesion types. **(B)** Arthroscopic photograph of a type III SLAP lesion. (*continued*)

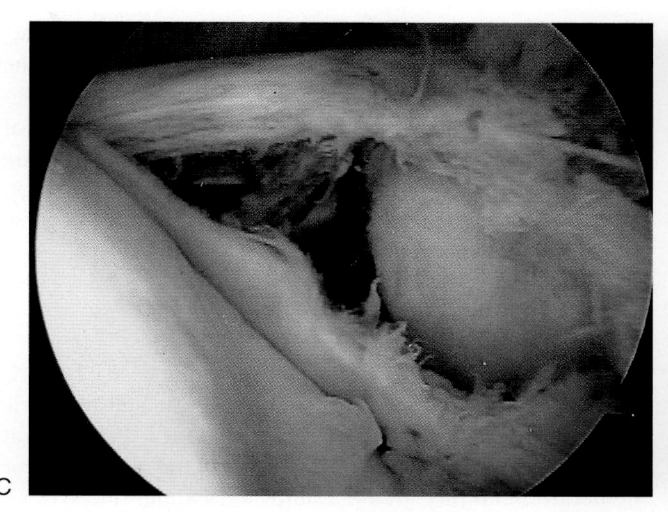

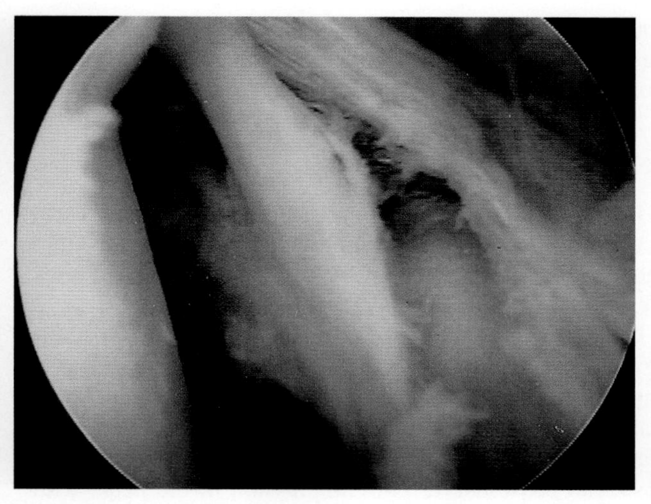

FIG. 8. *Continued.* **(C and D)** Athroscopic photograph of a type IV SLAP lesion. (B and C courtesy of JP Iannotti.)

habilitation program, we recommend a posterior capsulorrhaphy because the capsule is usually redundant. An osteochondral lesion (the reverse Hill-Sachs lesion) or a capsulolabral avulsion (the reverse Bankart lesion) is usually not seen. Generalized ligamentous laxity associated with posterior joint instability is a particular therapeutic problem best treated with an aggressive rehabilitation program; surgery is not recommended.

Bennett Lesion

The Bennett lesion is an ossification or calcification of the posterior inferior glenoid found in overhead athletes, most commonly baseball players. Generally, the thrower complains of pain while throwing and physical examination reveals tenderness in the posterior inferior glenoid region.

In 1941 Bennett[6] described a posteroinferior glenoid lesion, similar to an arthritic osteophyte, that he thought was the result of a traction injury of the long head of the triceps brachii. Pain accompanied the lesion. This was thought to be because of proximity to the axillary nerve and subsequent irritation. Radiographic analysis of the lesion necessitated direction of the x-ray beam 5-degrees cephalad, with the shoulder abducted and externally rotated. Initially, treatment of the Bennett lesion was resection from a posterior approach, but later Bennett stated that this was not necessary.[7] Ferrari and coworkers[25] used CT–arthography in seven elite pitchers to demonstrate that the Bennett lesion was extraarticular. Six had posterior labral tears. The Bennett lesion was described as a posteroinferior ossification associated with posterior labral injury.[25] Treatment included a period of rest followed by a rehabilitation program and treatment with

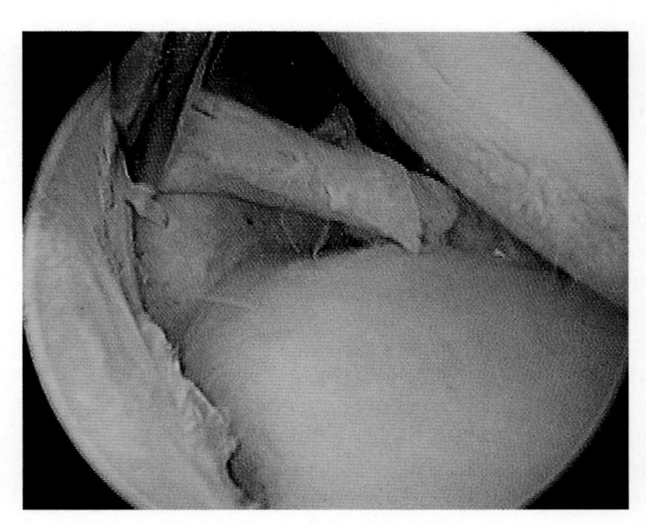

FIG. 9. Arthroscopic view from the posterior portal of a joint that demonstrates a type II SLAP lesion.

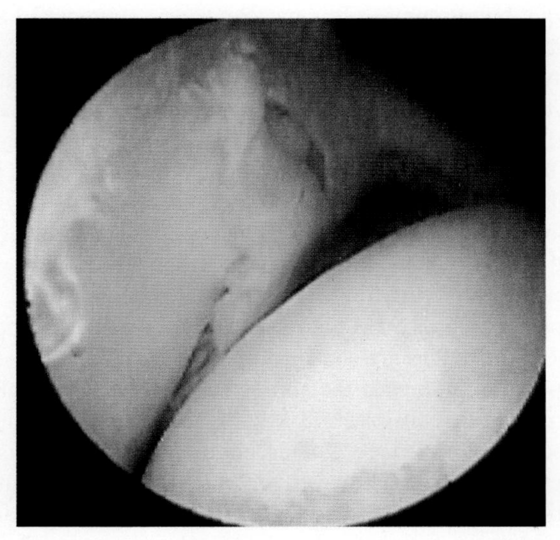

FIG. 10. Arthroscopic view from the posterior portal of a joint that demonstrates a type III SLAP lesion.

nonsteriodal antiinflammatory drugs for 3 to 4 months. If this failed, arthroscopic debridement of associated labral lesions may be indicated.

Neurologic Injury

Chronic neurologic injuries about the shoulder can present in overhead athletes of all ages. The neurologic examination should include complete sensory evaluation, testing of reflex arcs, observation for atrophy, and strength testing.

Cervical spine pain can be confused with shoulder pathology. These athletes may initially complain of shoulder pain, but neck pain is usually present on careful questioning. Physical examination and cervical spine radiographs enable correct localization of the pathology. A herniated nucleus pulposis can cause nerve root compression in the neck, with pain radiating down the arm in the distribution of the affected nerve.

Suprascapular Nerve Injury

The suprascapular nerve originates from the upper trunk of the brachial plexus to innervate the supraspinatus and infraspinatus muscles. Along its path, there are two areas of the scapula where it can be tethered and compressed: the suprascapular notch and the neck of the spine (spinoglenoid notch). Compression results in pain or weakness. Symptoms may preclude pitching more than one or two innings. In the chronic situation, the correct diagnosis can be elusive, because the disease has an insidious onset and vague symptoms. Muscle pain and diminished endurance are the important presenting symptoms. There is weakness of external rotation and sometimes of abduction, depending on the location of the compression. Either the infraspinatus is involved alone or both shoulder muscles are, depending on the location of the compression. Physical examination demonstrates muscle atrophy. The trapezius overlies the supraspinatus muscle, but atrophy of this muscle can be appreciated as a depression over the supraspinatus fossa of the shoulder. Atrophy of the infraspinatus is easy to appreciate as a depression over the lower half of the scapula. EMG can be used to confirm the diagnosis. Suprascapular nerve palsy can be confused with rotator cuff tears, which present with pain in a similar area and weakness of the same musculature. Surgical exploration and decompression of the nerve generally gives good results when the nerve is compressed at the suprascapular notch. In this case, the supraspinatus and infraspinatus muscles are both involved. However, if atrophy and EMG changes are confined to the infraspinatus muscle, the nerve is injured at the spinoglenoid notch. A ganglion cyst can be responsible, and MRI is helpful in determining its location.[36] When present, resection of the ganglion cyst is effective treatment. However, when the injury is a result of traction, nonsurgical treatment is recommended, because surgical decompression has not always been successful. The effects of chronic compression may not be reversible in either event. If the infraspinatus is not completely deinnervated, the authors have had good results with maximizing the residual muscle function with a daily exercise program. Because this muscle seldom contracts more than 30% to 40% of its maximum effort, the return to the prior level of pitching is sometimes possible. A meticulous history and physical examination for proper diagnosis early in the disease course yields the best chance for success.

Quadrilateral Space Syndrome

Bounded by the humerus, teres major, long head of the triceps brachii, and the inferior rotator cuff (the subscapularis anteriorly and the teres minor posteriorly) the quadrilateral space is crossed by the axillary nerve and the posterior humeral circumflex artery. Cahill and Palmer[12] described the etiology of pain in this location as compression of the axillary nerve by fibrous bands in the quadrilateral space. Symptoms occur when the athlete abducts and externally rotates the shoulder as in the cocking stage in throwing. There is tenderness over the teres minor muscle, and symptoms can be reproduced by placing the shoulder into this position. The neurologic examination is usually normal, as are EMG studies. Arteriography of the subclavian artery, which enables visualization of the posterior humeral circumflex artery as it passes through the quadrilateral space, is helpful in making the correct diagnosis. With the arm at the side, the artery is patent, but with abduction and external rotation of the shoulder the artery occludes. It is necessary to perform comparative studies of the contralateral shoulder. A test is positive only if the symptomatic side occludes and the normal side does not. In the athlete with this condition, a short period of rest and cortisone injections into the space are often helpful. If symptoms persist, operative decompression of the quadrilateral space is indicated. This can be performed through a posterior approach, inferior to the deltoid. The tendon of the teres minor can be incised to decompress the axillary nerve,[1] but in our experience, the long head of the triceps is often the offending structure. Results have been favorable.

Arterial and Venous Problems

Shoulder and arm pain in the overhead athlete does not often elicit a diagnosis of vascular injury, but misdiagnosis can result in disastrous outcomes, such as arterial thrombosis and embolization. Identifying vascular compression injuries is difficult in the overhead athlete, and these injuries are relatively uncommon. Unless vascular compromise is recognized as a possible source of pain, misdiagnosis is likely.

Early fatigue of the upper extremity in a well-conditioned athlete is a frequent initial complaint. In baseball pitchers, decreased endurance and measurable loss of pitch velocity after three innings are common findings. Forearm pain, throwing arm heaviness, and hand coldness are sometimes present. Loss of pitching control is not a symptom. Physical examination may reveal a diminished pulse or a loud bruit. Doppler ultrasonography and duplex scanning indicate that subclavian artery compression by the scalene muscles is the most likely etiology in symptomatic athletes.[50,59] When the shoulder is positioned in abduction and external rotation this finding is common in asymptomatic individuals as well as overhead athletes[71] and, therefore, is not specific. Physical examination findings must correlate. Sometimes symptoms are the result of subclavian artery aneurysm with thrombosis, and in these cases, embolization to the hand and severe ischemia may occur.[59] Compression of the axillary artery,[59] the posterior humeral circumflex artery,[39] the suprascapular artery, or the subscapular artery[50] can also result in localized symptoms. Treatment includes avoidance of all exacerbating activities until symptoms subside and a carefully supervised program of muscle strengthening for the entire shoulder girdle. Postural training may also be helpful, but this requires strengthening and conditioning of the trunk muscles. If conservative measures fail, the involved areas can be surgically decompressed with excellent results.[59]

SUMMARY

To successfully treat the overhead athlete: knowledge of (a) the biomechanics of the sport, (b) common findings in the history and physical examination, and (c) common shoulder pathology is necessary. Subtle anterior instability is a frequent entity in the overhead athlete. Examination while the patient is anesthetized and arthroscopy may be required to make the proper diagnosis. Internal impingement and SLAP lesions are associated with anterior instability and may lead to confusing symptoms and signs. Early diagnosis of the precise injury, shoulder rehabilitation, and appropriate surgical intervention optimize return to overhead athletics.

REFERENCES

1. Barnes DA, Tullos HS. An analysis of 100 symptomatic baseball players. *Am J Sports Med* 1978;6:63–67.
2. Bartlett LR, Storey MD, Simons BD. Measurement of upper extremity torque production and its relationship to throwing speed in the competitive athlete. *Am J Sports Med* 1989;17:89–91.
3. Basmajian J. The upper limb. In: *Muscles alive*. Baltimore: Williams & Wilkins, 1974:189–212.
4. Bassett R, Browne A, Morrey B, An K. Glenohumeral muscle force and moment mechanics in a position of shoulder instability. *J Biomech* 1990;23:405–415.
5. Bearn J. Direct observation of the function of the capsule of the sternoclavicular joint in clavicular support. *J Anat* 1967;101:159–170.
6. Bennett GE. Shoulder and elbow lesions of the professional baseball pitcher. *JAMA* 1941;117:510–514.
7. Bennett GE. Elbow and shoulder lesions of baseball players. *Am J Surg* 1959;98:484–492.
8. Bigliani LU, Kurzweil PR, Schwartzbach CC, Wolke IN, Flatow EL. Inferior capsular shift procedure for anterior–inferior shoulder instability in athletes. *Am J Sports Med* 1994;22:578–583.
9. Bowen MK, Deng XH, Hannafin JA, et al. An analysis of the patterns of glenohumeral joint contact and their relationship to the glenoid "bare area." *Trans Orthop Res Soc* 1992;17:496.
10. Bradley JP, Perry J, Jobe FW. The biomechanics of the throwing shoulder. *Pespect Orthop Surg* 1990;1:49–59.
11. Brown LP, Niehues SL, Harrah A, Yavorsky P, Hirshman HP. Upper extremity range of motion and isokinetic strength of the internal and external rotators in major league baseball players. *Am J Sports Med* 1988; 16:577–585.
12. Cahill BR, Palmer RE. Quadrilateral space syndrome. *J Hand Surg* 1983;8:65–69.
13. Clarke I, Gruen T, Hoy A, Hirschowitz D, Maki S, Amstutz H. Problems in glenohumeral surface replacements—real or imagined? *Eng Med* 1979;8:161–175.
14. Cleland FRS. Notes on raising the arm. *J Anat Physiol* 1884;18:275.
15. Colachis S, Strohm B. Effect of suprascapular and axillary nerve blocks on muscle force in upper extremity. *Arch Phys Med Rehabil* 1971;52: 22–29.
16. Cook FF, Tibone JE. The Mumford procedure in athletes: an objective analysis of function. *Am J Sports Med* 1988;16:97–100.
17. Cooper DE, Arnoczky SP, O'Brien SJ, et al. Anatomy, histology and vascularity of the glenoid labrum. *J Bone Joint Surg [Am]* 1992;74: 46–52.
18. Cyprien J, Vasey H, Burdet A, Bonvin J, Kritsikis N, Vuagnat P. Humeral retrotorsion and glenohumeral relationship in the normal shoulder and in recurrent anterior dislocation. *Clin Orthop Rel Res* 1983;175:8–17.
19. Davidson PA, Elattache NS, Jobe CM, Jobe FW. Rotator cuff and posterio-superior glenoid labrum injury associated with increased glenohumeral motion: a new site of impingement. *J Shoulder Elbow Surg* 1995;4:384–390.
20. DePalma AF, Callery G, Bennett GA. Variational anatomy and degenerative lesions of the shoulder joint. *Am Acad Orthop Surg Instr Course Lect Ser* 1949;6:225–281.
21. DiGiovine NM, Jobe FW, Pink M, Perry J. An electromyographic analysis of the upper extremity in pitching. *J Shoulder Elbow Surg* 1992;1: 15–25.
22. Doody SG, Freedman L, Waterland JC. Shoulder movements during abduction in the scapular plane. *Arch Phys Med Rehabil* 1970;51: 595–604.
23. Duchenne GB. *Physiology of motion*. Philadelphia: JB Lippincott, 1949.
24. Feltner M, Dapena J. Dynamics of the shoulder and elbow joints of the throwing arm during the baseball pitch. *Int J Sports Biomech* 1986;2: 235–259.
25. Ferrari JD, Ferrari DA, Coumas J, Pappas MM. Posterior ossification of the shoulder: the Bennett lesion: etiology, diagnosis and treatment. *Am J Sports Med* 1994;22:171–175.
26. Freedman L, Munro R. Abduction of the arm in the scapular plane: scapular and glenohumeral movements. *J Bone Joint Surg [Am]* 1966; 48:1503–1510.
27. Gainor B, Piotrowski G, Paul J, William A, Hagen R. The throw: biomechanics and acute injury. *Am J Sports Med* 1980;8:114–118.
28. Gilcreest EL. The common syndrome of rupture, dislocation and elongation of the long head of the biceps brachii: an analysis of one hundred cases. *Surg Gynecol Obstet* 1934;58:322–340.
29. Glousman R, Jobe F, Tibone D, Moynes D, Antonelli D, Perry J. Dynamic electromyographic analysis of the throwing shoulder with glenohumeral instability. *J Bone Joint Surg [Am]* 1988;70:220–226.
30. Gowan I, Jobe F, Tibone J, Perry J, Moynes D. A comparative electromygraphic analysis of the shoulder during pitching. *Am J Sports Med* 1987;15:586–590.
31. Hawkins RJ, Hobeika PE. Impingement syndrome in the athletic shoulder. *Clin Sports Med* 1983;2:391–405.
32. Howell S, Galinat B. The glenoid–labral socket. *Clin Orthop Rel Res* 1989;243:122–125.
33. Howell S, Galinat B, Renzi A, Marone P. Normal and abnormal mechanics of the glenohumeral joint in the horizontal plane. *J Bone Joint Surg [Am]* 1988;70:227–232.
34. Hurley JA, Anderson TE, Dear W, Andrish JT, Bergfeld JA, Weiker GG. Posterior shoulder instability: surgical vs. nonsurgical results with evaluation of glenoid version. *Am J Sports Med* 1992;20:396.
35. Iannotti JP, Gabriel JP, Schneck SL, Evans BG, Misra S. The normal glenohumeral relationships. An anatomical study of one hundred and forty shoulders. *J Bone Joint Surg [Am]* 1992;74:491–500.
36. Iannotti JP, Ramsey ML. Arthroscopic decompression of a ganglion cyst causing suprascapular nerve compression. *J Arthrosc Rel Res* 1996;12:739–745.
37. Iannotti JP, Wang ED. Avulsion fracture of the supraglenoid tubercle: a variation of the SLAP lesion. *J Shoulder Elbow Surg* 1992;1:26–30.

38. Inman V, Saunders M, Abbott L. Observations on the function of the shoulder joint. *J Bone Joint Surg* 1944;27:1–30.
39. Itoh T, Wakaro K, Takeda T, Murakami T. Circulatory disturbances in the throwing hand of baseball pitchers. *Am J Sports Med* 1987;15: 264–269.
40. Itoi E, Kuechle DK, Neuman SR, Morrrey B, An K-N. Stabilizing function of the biceps in stable and unstable shoulders. *J Bone Joint Surg [Br]* 1993;75:546–550.
41. Itoi E, Motzkin N, Morrey B, An K-N. Stabilizing function of the long head of the biceps in the hanging position. *J Shoulder Elbow Surg* 1994; 3:135–142.
42. Janda DH, Wojtys EM, Hankin FM, Benedict MA. Softball sliding injuries: a prospective study comparing standard and modified bases. *JAMA* 1988;259:1848–1850.
43. Jobe CM, Iannotti JP. Limits imposed on glenohumeral motion by joint geometry. *J Shoulder Elbow Surg* 1995;4:281–285.
44. Jobe CM, Sidles L. Evidence for a superior glenoid impingement upon the rotator cuff [abstr]. *J Shoulder Elbow Surg* 1993;2:S19.
45. Jobe F, Moynes D, Tibone J, Perry J. An EMG analysis of the shoulder in pitching: a second report. *Am J Sports Med* 1984;12:218–220.
46. Jobe F, Tibone J, Perry J, Moynes D. An EMG analysis of the shoulder in throwing and pitching: a preliminary report. *Am J Sports Med* 1983; 11:3–5.
47. Jobe FW, Bradley JP. Rotator cuff injuries in baseball: prevention and rehabilitation. *Sports Med* 1988;6:377–387.
48. Kibler WB. Specificity and sensitivity of the anterior slide test in throwing athletes with superior glenoid labral tears. *J Arthrosc Rel Res* 1995; 11:296–300.
49. Laumann U. Kinesiology of the shoulder. In: Kobel R, ed. *Shoulder replacement*. Berlin: Springer-Verlag, 1985:23.
50. McCarthy WJ, Yao JS, Schafer MF. Upper extremity arterial injury in athletes. *J Vasc Surg* 1989;9:317–326.
51. McFarland EG, Campbell G, McDowell J. Posterior shoulder laxity in asymptomatic athletes. *Am J Sports Med* 1996;24:468–471.
52. McMahon P, Jobe F, Pink M, Brault J, Perry J. Comparative electromyographic analysis of shoulder muscles during planar motions: anterior glenohumeral instability versus normal. *J Shoulder Elbow Surg* 1996;5:118–123.
53. McMahon PJ, Tibone JE, Dettling JR, Peatman TW, Lee TQ. Shoulder instability: a multidisciplinary study of the glenoid origin of the anterior band of the inferior glenohumeral ligament. In: *American shoulder and elbow surgeons*, San Francisco: 1997.
54. Montgomery WH, Jobe FW. Functional outcomes in athletes after anterior capsulolabral reconstruction. *Am J Sports Med* 1994;22:352–358.
55. Morrey B, An K-N. Biomechanics of the shoulder. In: Rockwood CJ, Matsen F, eds. *The shoulder*. Philadelphia: W B Saunders, 1990:216.
56. Moseley H, Overgaard B. The anterior capsular mechanism in recurrent anterior dislocation of the shoulder: morphological and clinical studies with special reference to the glenoid labrum and glenohumeral ligaments. *J Bone Joint Surg [Br]* 1962;44:913–927.
57. Neer CS. Anterior acromioplasty for the chronic impingement syndrome in the shoulder: a preliminary report. *J Bone Joint Surg [Am]* 1972;54:41–50.
58. Nobuhara K, Ikeda H. Rotator interval lesion. *Clin Orthop Rel Res* 1987;223:44–50.
59. Nuber GW, McCarthy WJ, Yao JST, Schafer MF, Sulker JR. Arterial abnormalities of the shoulder in athletes. *Am J Sports Med* 1990;18: 514–519.
60. O'Brien SJ, Arnoczsky SP, Warren RF, Rozbruch SR. Developmental anatomy of the shoulder and anatomy of the glenohumeral joint. In: Matsen F, Rockwood C, eds. *The shoulder*. Philadelphia: WB Saunders, 1990:1–33.
61. O'Brien SJ, Pagnani MJ, McGlynn SR, Fealy S, Wilson JB . A new and effective test for diagnosing labral tears and A. C. joint pathology. In: *American shoulder and elbow surgeons*, 19. Atlanta, GA: 1996.
62. Pagnani MJ, Deng X-H, Warren RF, Torzilli PA, O'Brien SJ. Role of the long head of the biceps brachii in glenohumeral stability: a biomechanical study in cadavera. *J Shoulder Elbow Surg* 1996;5:255–262.
63. Pappas AM, Zawak RM, Sullivan TJ. Biomechanics of baseball pitching: a preliminary report. *Am J Sports Med* 1985;13:216–222.
64. Pink M, Jobe FW, Perry J, Browne A, Scovazzo ML, Kerrigan J. The painful shoulder during the butterfly stroke. *Clin Orthop Rel Res* 1993; 288:60–72.
65. Pink M, Jobe FW, Perry J, Kerrigan J, Browne A, Scovazzo ML. The normal shoulder during the backstroke: an EMG and cinematogaphic analysis of twelve muscles. *Clin J Sports Med* 1992;2:6–12.
66. Pink M, Perry J, Jobe FW, Browne A, Scovazzo ML, Kerrigan J. The normal shoulder during freestyle swimming: an EMG and cinematographic analysis of twelve muscles. *Am J Sports Med* 1991;19: 569–575.
67. Poppen N, Walker P. Normal and abnormal motion of the shoulder. *J Bone Joint Surg [Am]* 1976;58:195–201.
68. Refior HJ, Sowa D. Long head of the biceps brachii: sites of predilection for degenerative changes. *J Shoulder Elbow Surg* 1995;4:436–440.
69. Richardson AB, Jobe FW, Collins HR. The shoulder in swimming. *Am J Sports Med* 1980;8:159–163.
70. Rockwood C, Green D. *Fractures in adults*. Philadelphia: JB Lippincott, 1984.
71. Rohrer MJ, Cardillo PA, Pappas AM, Phillips DA. Axillary artery compression and thrombosis in throwing athletes. *J Vasc Surg* 1990;11: 761–768.
72. Rokito SE, Reinhard GA, Elattrache NS, Jobe FW. 2 to 4 year clinical followup of superior glenoid labral lesions. (In Press).
Saha AK. Mechanics of elevation of the glenohumeral joint. *Acta Orthop Scand* 1973;44:668–678.
73. Sain J, Andrews JR. Proper pitching technique. In: Zarins B, Andrews JR, Carson WG, eds. *Injuries to the throwing arm*. Philadelphia: WB Saunders, 1985:31–37.
74. Scovazzo ML, Browne A, Pink M, Jobe FW, Kerrigan J. The painful shoulder during the freestyle stroke. *Am J Sports Med* 1991;19: 577–582.
75. Snyder SJ, Karzel RP, Pizzo WD, Ferkel RD, Friedman MJ. SLAP lesions of the shoulder. *J Arthrosc Rel Res* 1990;6:274–279.
76. Soslowsky L, Flatow E, Bigliani L, Pawluk R, Ateshian G, Mow V. Quantitation of in situ contact areas at the glenohumeral joint: a biomechanical study. *J Orthop Res* 1992;10:524–534.
77. Soslowsky LJ, Flatow EL, Bigliani LU, Mow VC. Articular geometry of the glenohumeral joint. *Clin Orthop Rel Res* 1992;285:181–190.
78. Terry G, Hammon D, France P, Norwood L. The stabilizing function of passive shoulder restraints. *Am J Sports Med* 1991;19:26–34.
79. Testut L. Traite d'anatomie humaine. In: Tome I, ed. *Osteologie, arthrologie, myologie*. Paris: Doin, 1921:504.
80. Turkel S, Panio M, Marshall J, Girgis F. Stabilizing mechanisms preventing anterior dislocation of the glenohumeral joint. *J Bone Joint Surg [Am]* 1981;63:1208–1217.
81. Walch G, Liotard JP, Boileau P, Noel E. In: Fifth International Conference on Surgery of the Shoulder, July 12–15, Paris, France: 1992.
82. Warner JP, McMahon PJ. The role of the long head of the biceps brachii in superior stability of the glenohumeral joint. *J Bone Joint Surg [Am]* 1995;77:366–372.

Disorders of the Shoulder: Diagnosis and Management,
edited by Joseph P. Iannotti and Gerald R. Williams, Jr.
Lippincott Williams & Wilkins, Philadelphia © 1999.

CHAPTER 10

Anterior and Anteroinferior Instability: Diagnosis and Management

Leslie S. Matthews and Lucas J. Pavlovich, Jr.

INTRODUCTION

An understanding of the pathomechanics and treatment of the unstable shoulder has evolved over the past 100 years. The current belief that multiple mechanisms and anatomic variations combine to create an unstable shoulder has evolved from the original theory of Perthes[64] and Bankart[6] that a single "essential lesion" creates instability. Etiologic theories continue to develop based on the advances in understanding of the disease process. The manifestations of instability will vary based on host factors and the magnitude of force required to create the injury. A traumatic force creating an initial dislocation is the most frequent cause of anterior instability. More subtle events may create a spectrum of instability, such as subluxations in patients with increased capsular laxity and microtrauma secondary to repetitive large forces (e.g., in overhead-throwing athletes or in swimmers). The diagnosis and management of anterior shoulder instability should be individualized based on etiology, various host factors, and associated pathology. This chapter presents an algorithmic approach to the treatment of anterior shoulder instability based on the natural history and pathology of the condition.

L. S. Matthews and L. J. Pavlovich, Jr.: Department of Orthopaedic Surgery, The Union Memorial Hospital, Baltimore, Maryland 21218.

EVALUATION

In most (more than 90%) cases, the diagnosis of shoulder instability is established by history and physical examination. Other modalities (such as radiographic imaging, examination under anesthesia, and diagnostic arthroscopy) can assist in establishing the diagnosis, confirming or defining pathology and, thereby, directing treatment.

In obtaining a history, it is important to acquire accurate information not only about the current incident (i.e., the injury mechanism and the magnitude or direction of causative forces), but also about previous incidents (i.e., the number and frequency of previous dislocations—if any—and the reduction method required). Because genetic factors may also play a role in shoulder instability,[17] it may be helpful to establish whether or not a family history of shoulder instability exists.

The clinician should distinguish between subluxation and dislocation events to help identify the severity of the event and determine prognosis. For the purposes of this chapter, *subluxation* is defined as a pathologic increase in glenohumeral translation without loss of articular contact between the humerus and glenoid; *dislocation* is the complete loss of contact between the articular surfaces. Primary shoulder dislocations that result from high-energy forces have an increased risk of associated injuries, such as neurovascular injuries, rotator cuff tears, and fractures.

Classification of Anterior Instability

Thomas and Matsen[83] have described the acronyms TUBS and AMBRI to classify most patients with instability. TUBS refers to patients with a *t*raumatic lesion, who have a *u*nidirectional component to their disease that frequently has a *B*ankart lesion and responds well to *s*urgery. AMBRI refers to patients who have an *a*traumatic etiology of their *m*ultidirectional disease that often has *b*ilateral shoulder findings and responds to *r*ehabilitation. As the understanding of the natural history, pathology, and treatment of shoulder instability has evolved, so has the classification scheme. Rockwood[67] described four patterns of instability: type I, traumatic subluxation without previous dislocation; type II, traumatic subluxation after a previous dislocation; type IIIA, voluntary subluxation in patients with psychiatric problems; type IIIB, voluntary subluxation in patients without psychiatric problems; type IV, atraumatic involuntary subluxation. The authors prefer to use an algorithmic approach (Fig. 1) to the classification of anterior instability based on etiology, direction, frequency, and volition.

Although trauma is the most commonly identified cause of anterior instability, more subtle factors may exist in patients with anterior subluxation and multidirectional instability. Patients who are classified as having multidirectional instability demonstrate a component of inferior instability. For a diagnosis of instability, patients must have symptoms that accompany increased translation, such as anterior or posterior shoulder pain or a feeling of apprehension. Multidirectional instability does not usually exist in all planes, but it commonly exists in two.

Acute Traumatic Anterior Dislocation

The most common mechanism of a traumatic initial dislocation is an anteriorly directed force applied to the posterior aspect of the externally rotated abducted arm, which levers the humeral head anterior in relation to the glenoid, as when the patient's arm is in the overhead position. The patient's age and the force required to create an initial dislocation are important factors in determining prognosis and associated injuries. Patients who are younger than 30 years old at the time of initial dislocation are more likely to suffer recurrent dislocation, whereas patients older than 50 years of age are more likely to suffer rotator cuff tears with the initial dislocation. In older patients, the inability to lift the arm over the head is more likely to be related to a rotator cuff tear than to an axillary nerve palsy. Neviaser et al.[57] noted an 85.7% incidence of rotator cuff tears and a 10.8% incidence of axillary nerve palsy in patients with initial traumatic shoulder dislocation occurring after age 40.

Anterior shoulder dislocation is diagnosed on the basis of the physical and radiographic examinations. The patient may present with an adducted and internally rotated arm and may be unable to externally rotate or fully abduct the arm. The humeral head may be palpated on the anterior aspect of the shoulder; whereas the posterior aspect may appear hollow.

Anterior Subluxation

In an anterior subluxation, it is often difficult to identify an initial traumatic event. Rowe and Zarins[71] described recurrent transient subluxation of the shoulder, causing a "dead arm syndrome," which is characterized by a sudden sharp or paralyzing pain in the affected arm when the shoulder is forcibly moved into a position of maximum external rotation in elevation or is subjected to a direct blow. This condition is most common in overhead-throwing athletes.

The shoulders of baseball pitchers are exposed to high-energy repetitive stresses that can exceed the rate of tissue repair.[36] This process can damage the static stabilizing structures and, in turn, place an increased amount of responsibility for glenohumeral stability on the dynamic stabilizers. As the static stabilizers become more attenuated and more stress is placed on the dynamic stabilizers, they may become fatigued. As the compensatory mechanism becomes overloaded, anterior subluxation may occur. As the humeral head subluxes anteriorly and contacts the coracoacromial arch, subacromial impingement occurs. With anterior subluxation, the tendinous portion of the supraspinatus and infraspinatus may impinge on the posterosuperior border of the glenoid rim, resulting in glenoid impingement as well. Swimmers, volleyball players, and other overhead-throwing athletes may experience similar symptoms.

Occult instability may also be present in nonthrowing athletes. For weight lifters,[22] anterior subluxation may be the primary etiologic factor of shoulder dysfunction and pain. Weight-lifting maneuvers that produce forced abduction, extension, and external rotation (such as military presses, flies, and latissimus pull-downs) may cause subluxation.

Multidirectional Instability

Patients with multidirectional instability have symptomatic instability in more than one plane of motion. Signs and symptoms are frequently subtle, and the condition in athletes is often mistaken for unidirectional instability. Standard treatments used for unidirectional instability often fail because they do not address the underlying pathology. The pathology of atraumatic multidirectional instability is related to a large, lax capsule. This laxity may extend anteriorly, inferiorly, and even posteriorly in these patients. Traumatic

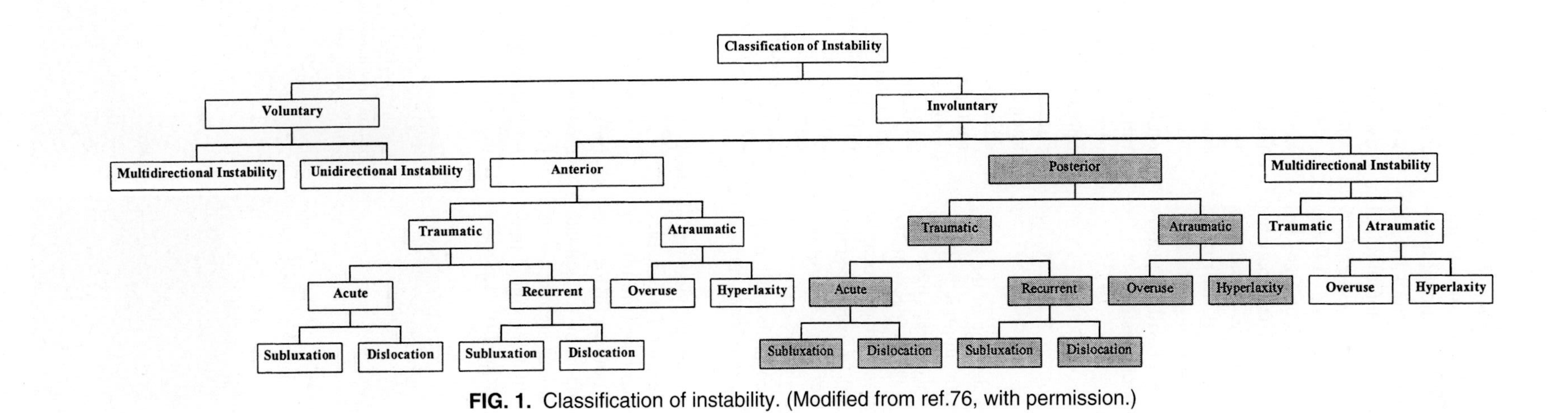

FIG. 1. Classification of instability. (Modified from ref.76, with permission.)

multidirectional instability may exhibit a labral detachment in association with capsular laxity.

Although diagnosis is frequently difficult, certain physical examination findings differentiate this condition from unidirectional instability. The patient with multidirectional instability exhibits inferior instability on examination of the affected shoulder,[55] as evidenced on downward longitudinal traction of the humerus, which may exhibit a sulcus sign. A 2-cm distance between the humeral head and inferior acromion or an asymmetrical difference in sulcus signs between the shoulders is considered positive. These patients may also have generalized ligamentous laxity. Swimmers and gymnasts with multidirectional instability will often demonstrate capsular laxity without other pathologic lesions, in contrast to athletes in contact sports who will frequently exhibit an associated Bankart or Hill–Sachs lesion.

Physical Examination

General Principles

It is important to obtain an overall evaluation of the musculoskeletal system through a systematic approach of inspection, palpation, range of motion analysis, strength testing, neurologic evaluation, shoulder stability assessment, and specialized testing. Range of motion and provocative testing of the cervical spine are required to exclude spinal disorders, which may present as shoulder pain. Neurologic manifestations of cervical disease may be assessed by range of motion testing. It is unlikely that a patient with a full, painless range of motion will have clinically significant cervical spine pathology.

Visual inspection before examination may provide valuable information. The skin should be inspected for evidence of collagen disorders, which can present as thinning or widening of surgical or traumatic scars. Shoulder dislocation may injure the axillary nerve, so it is important to evaluate for deltoid atrophy and weakness. The sulcus sign, a visible depression inferior to the lateral edge of the acromion, may occur in patients with multidirectional instability caused by inferior luxation of the humeral head. Winging of the scapula may be evident in patients with anterior subluxation or secondary impingement and pain.

Both active and passive range of motion should be recorded. Forward flexion, abduction, internal rotation, and external rotation should be tested. The clinician should note dyskinesia and whether or not accessory muscles are activated with range of motion testing.

The shoulder girdle should be palpated for local tenderness and muscle tone. Patients with anterior subluxation often have tenderness over the posterior capsule, whereas those who are compensating for multidirectional instability may be tender along the medial angle of the scapula. Patients with anterior instability caused by subluxation and secondary impingement may have tenderness over the greater tuberosity or biceps tendon. Crepitation occurring on range of motion testing should be noted. While the motion of the upper extremity is being assessed, it is important to examine strength in the pain-free range of motion, paying particular attention to external rotation, internal rotation, and abduction strength to rule out rotator cuff pathology. These results should be compared with the uninjured side.

Generalized ligamentous laxity is commonly associated with shoulder instability. This should be assessed by evaluating range of motion in several joints. The degree of thumb hyperabduction, with volar flexion of the wrist, as well as index finger, elbow, and knee hyperextension, should be noted. The tip of the thumb should not touch the volar aspect of the wrist and the index metacarpophalangeal angle should not exceed 90 degrees (Fig. 2).

Specific Tests

After the preliminary examination, specific tests for instability should be performed. The examination should be initiated on the unaffected shoulder first to obtain baseline data for each subsequent test. This approach also provides the patient with the opportunity to become comfortable with each maneuver. Two components are considered when assessing

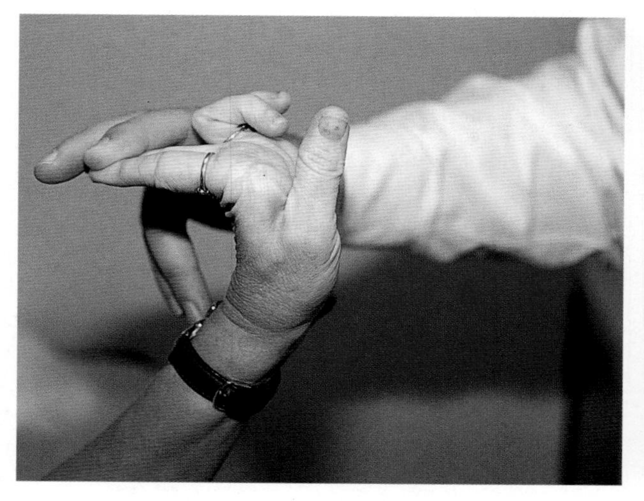
A

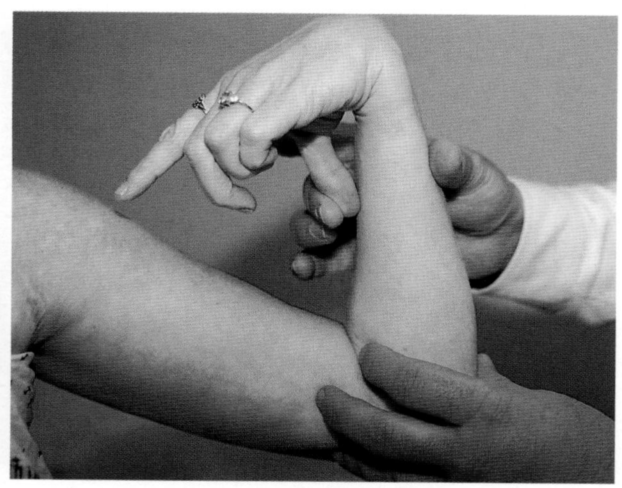
B

FIG. 2. Patient with ligamentous laxity and index metacarpophalangeal angle of 90 degrees.

the stability of the glenohumeral joint: (a) the amount of passive translation of the humeral head and glenoid fossa on stress testing, and (b) attempts to reproduce the symptoms of subluxation and apprehension by provocative testing of the shoulder in positions of compromise.

Sulcus Sign Test. The sulcus sign test establishes the presence of inferior laxity, which if symptomatic is necessary to establish the diagnosis of multidirectional instability. In a patient with gross instability, a depression may be seen inferior to the posterior aspect of the acromion when the arms of a sitting patient are positioned along the side of the body. However, it is usually necessary to apply a traction force along the longitudinal axis of the humerus by pulling the humerus in an inferior direction. The distance between the acromion and the humeral head is then observed and recorded in centimeters. A measurement of 2 cm or more or an asymmetrical sulcus sign is considered positive for inferior instability (Fig. 3).

Load and Shift Test. Glenohumeral translation should be evaluated in both the upright and supine positions. The load and shift test establishes whether clinically significant posteroanterior translation of the humeral head is possible and if this translation reproduces the patient's symptoms. The examiner stands behind the seated patient, with one hand on the affected shoulder. The other hand holds the proximal humerus, with the thumb on the posterior aspect of the humeral head and the index finger on the anterior aspect. The initial movement is to load the humeral head into the glenoid fossa, reducing the inherent subluxation. Then the examiner attempts to shift the humeral head in anterior and posterior directions while observing the area adjacent to the acromion for a sulcus sign. Translation should also be evaluated in the

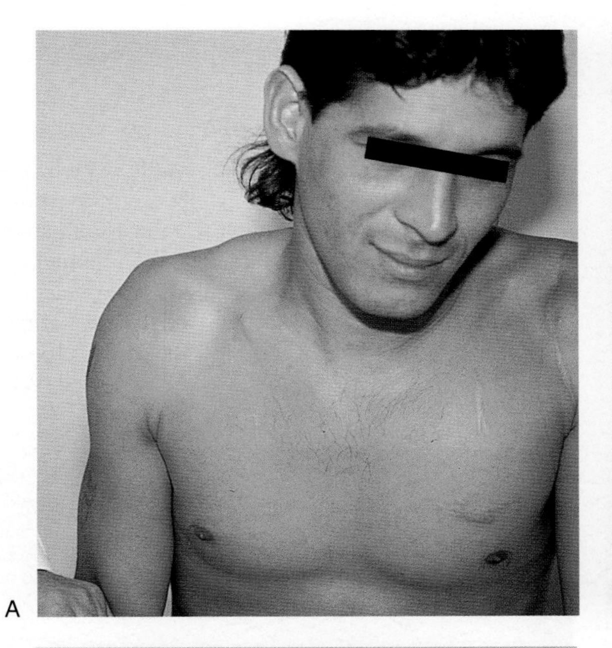
A

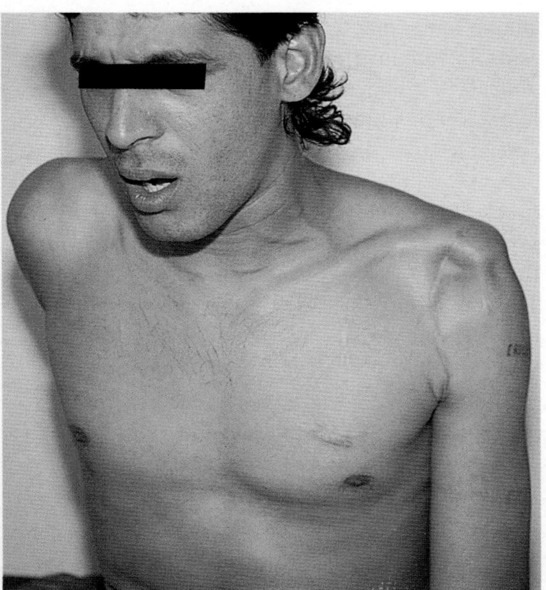
B

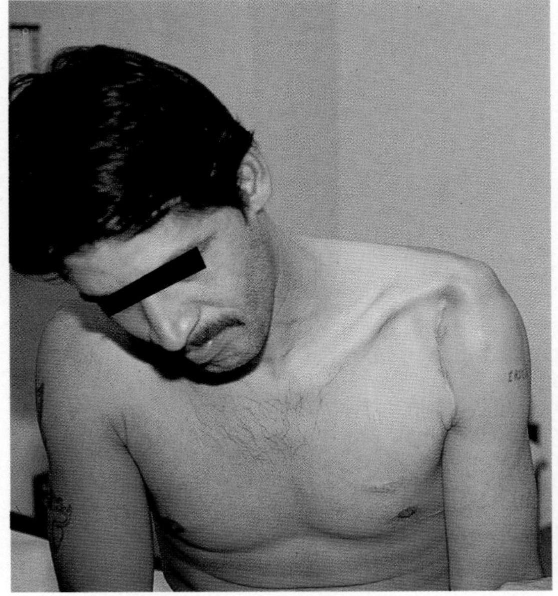
C

FIG. 3. (A) A 32-year-old man, with symptomatic asymmetrical positive sulcus sign on the left shoulder of 2 cm, after two failed anterior ligament reconstructions. **(B)** The sulcus sign is negative on the right shoulder. **(C)** One year after allograft reconstruction of the rotator interval and anterior capsule, the patient is asymptomatic and the sulcus sign is negative. (Courtesy of JP Iannotti MD, PhD.)

supine position. The examiner grasps the humerus in a position of 20 degrees abduction and forward flexion in neutral rotation. The humeral head is loaded and then posteriorly and anteriorly stressed while the examiner notes the amount of excursion.

Editors' Preferred Technique

Anterior Instability

Examination of the shoulder for instability using the load and shift technique is performed with the patient in the supine position. To test for anterior translation on the patient's right shoulder, the examiner positions the patient's arm in the plane of the scapula, at 45 to 60 degrees of abduction and neutral external rotation (Fig. 4). The examiner then places the left hand around the patient's arm at approximately the level of the deltoid insertion site with the thumb posterior and the remaining fingers anterior. The examiner's right arm controls arm position and provides an axial load to the humeral head to center it into the glenoid fossa. The examiner uses the left hand to provide an anterior or anteroinferior translation force to the humerus. When performed correctly, the scapula remains still and the amount of humeral head translation can be determined by both visual inspection and palpation. In almost all patients, there is some anterior or anteroinferior translation of the humeral head. As the examiner maintains an axial load to the humerus with the right arm, the patient's arm can be incrementally rotated into external rotation. With progressive external rotation of the humerus, the inferior glenohumeral ligament (IGHL) complex becomes taut (Fig. 5). With increased tension on the IGHL, there is decreasing anterior translation of the humeral head in the glenoid fossa.

Posterior Instability

To examine the patient's right shoulder, the arm is held in the plane of the scapula at 45 to 60 degrees of abduction and 45 to 60 degrees of external rotation. The examiner's hands are positioned in the same way as described for anterior translation testing, and an axial load is placed onto the humerus. The examiner's left hand is used to shift the head posteriorly. The examiner's right arm is used to incrementally internally rotate the patients arm. During internal rotation, the posteroinferior capsule becomes increasingly tight, which should result in decreased posterior translation of the humeral head.

Inferior Instability

The patient is examined in the seated position. The examiner first places a downward distraction force on the dependent humerus by applying traction at the distal humerus. The arm is in neutral rotation and the degree of humeral inferior translation (sulcus sign) is assessed in centimeters. The distraction force is then released, and the patient's arm is placed in maximum external rotation. The traction force is then reapplied and the sulcus sign is again measured. With exter-

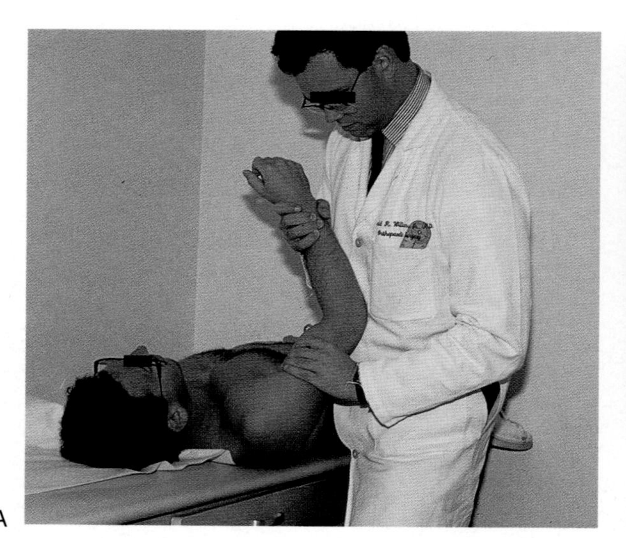

A

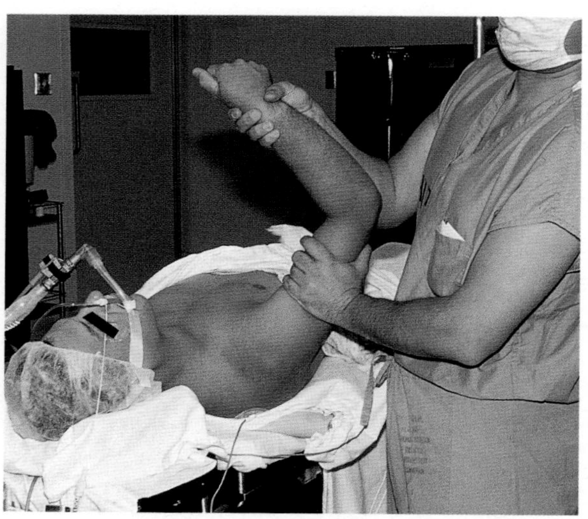

B

FIG. 4. Initial position for load and shift test for anterior instability testing of the shoulder. For a right shoulder examination, the examiner's left hand grasps the patient's upper arm with the fingers anterior. The examiner's right arm positions the patient's arm and controls its rotation. The arm is placed in the plane of the scapula, abducted 40 to 60 degrees, and maintained in zero degrees of rotation. The examiner's right arm places an axial load to the patient's arm through the humerus. The examiner's left hand then shifts the humeral head anteriorly, or anteroinferiorly over the glenoid rim. Grade 1 translation occurs if then the humeral head diameter rides over the anterior glenoid rim. Grade 2 translation occurs when the entire humeral head rides over the glenoid rim, but reduces when the dislocation force is released. Grade 3 translation occurs when the entire humeral head diameter translates over the glenoid rim and does not reduce when the dislocation force is released. This test can be performed in **(A)** the relaxed awake patient or **(B)** the anesthetized patient.

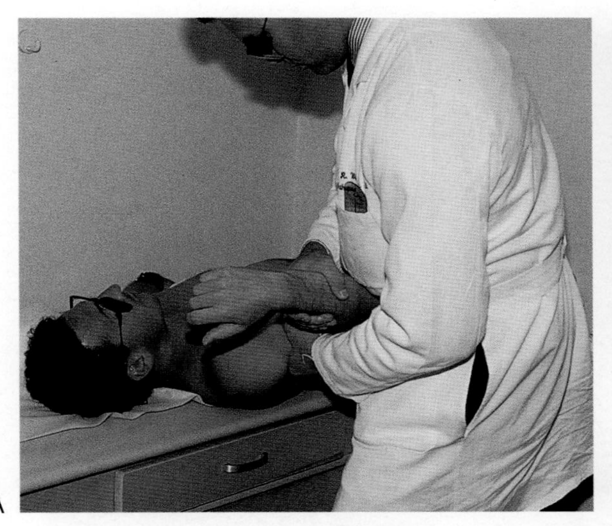

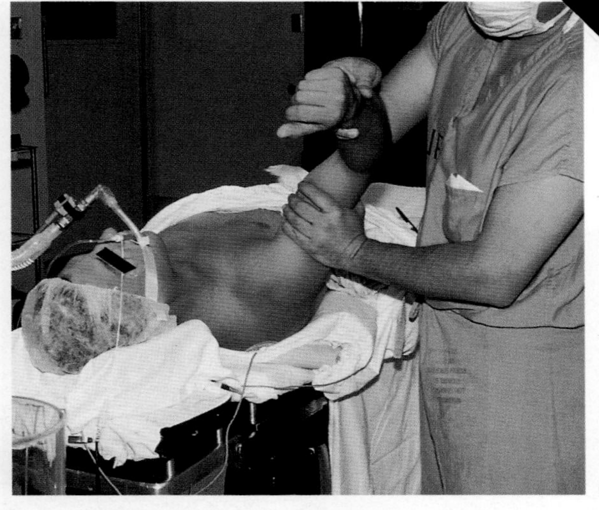

FIG. 5. The second position for the load and shift test for anterior stability is as described in Fig. 4 for the initial position, except that the arm is progressively externally rotated in 10- to 20-degree increments while the anterior dislocation force is alternatively applied and released. The examiner quantifies the degree of external rotation required to reduce the translation from grade 3 or 2 to grade 1. The examiner compares the normal and abnormal shoulders for this difference in translation with humeral rotation. The degree of rotation required to reduce the translation is an indicator of the functional laxity of the anterior inferior capsular ligaments. This examination is performed in **(A)** the relaxed awake patient or **(B)** the anesthesized patient.

nal rotation, the anterior and rotator interval capsule is tightened (Fig. 6). Tightening these tissues should decrease the amount of inferior translation of the humeral head.

The examiner evaluates differences between shoulders, assuming the opposite shoulder is normal. In the awake patient, this examination may be limited by muscular guarding, which is not an issue with the examination under anesthesia. The examination in the awake patient may illicit painful grating or apprehension that can reproduce the patient's symptoms. The symptoms in the awake patient can help in defining the diagnosis; these symptoms are, of course, absent in the anesthetized patient. Therefore, it is our practice to perform this examination in both the awake and anesthesized patient, for we believe that both examinations provide useful and complementary pieces of information.

Silliman and Hawkins[76] have provided a clinical grading system for this test. Grade I translation indicates that the humeral head can be felt to ride up on the face of the glenoid but cannot be moved over the glenoid rim. In grade II translation, the humeral head can be felt to glide over the glenoid rim, but it reduces spontaneously with release of pressure. This corresponds to clinical subluxation. Grade III exists

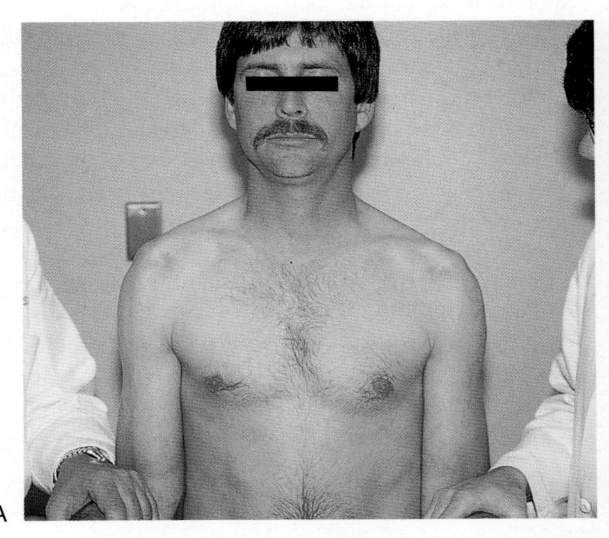

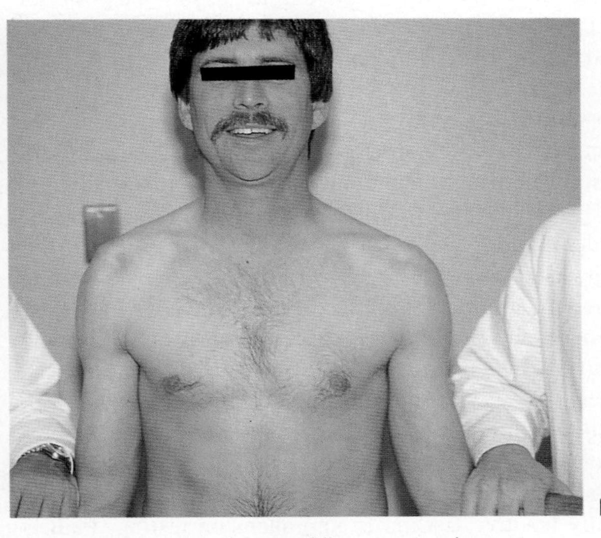

FIG. 6. The sulcus sign tests the functional integrity of the superior glenohumeral ligament and rotator interval capsule. These tissues are lax in neutral rotation and tighten with external rotation. **(A)** A mildly positive sulcus sign (1 cm) on the *right*, which **(B)** does not reduce with external rotation, whereas the minor translation on the *left* does reduce with external rotation.

ITY 257

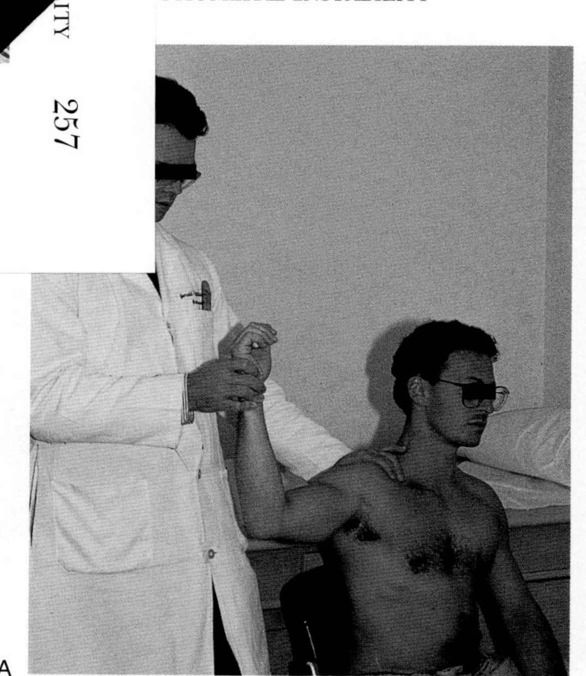

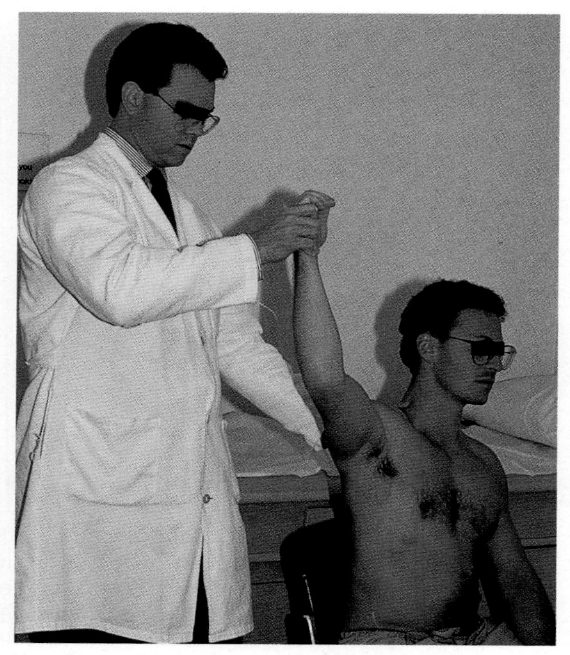

A B

FIG. 7. The apprehension test is performed by placing the arm in a position of abduction and external rotation in an attempt to produce a patient's feeling of subluxation or dislocation. The patient is tested in the seated position with the arm **(A)** at 90 degrees of abduction and **(B)** at 120 degrees of abduction. The higher degree of abduction places greater stress on the inferior capsular pouch.

when the head remains dislocated after release of pressure, corresponding to clinical dislocation.

Apprehension Test. The apprehension test places the shoulder in a provocative position of abduction and external rotation in an attempt to reproduce the patient's sensation of impending subluxation or dislocation (Fig. 7). This test should be performed in both the seated and supine positions. The examiner stands behind the seated patient, raises the patient's arm to 90 degrees of abduction, and begins to externally rotate the humerus. The hand of the examiner is placed over the humeral head with the thumb pushing the posterior aspect of the humeral head for extra leverage. Fingers are placed anteriorly to control any sudden instability that might occur. With increasing external rotation and controlled gentle forward pressure exerted against the humeral head, the patient may have an apprehensive feeling of impending instability. The patient communicates this apprehension verbally, by facial expression, or by protectively contracting the shoulder muscles.

This test is more easily performed in the supine position because the scapula is stabilized against the edge of the examining table, giving the examiner more control over the maneuver. The edge of the table acts as a fulcrum and the arm acts as a lever. As the humeral head is levered anteriorly, the amount of external rotation required to produce apprehension is noted.

Jobe et al.[32,34] have described pain in throwing athletes as the only positive finding in apprehension testing. Pain is suggestive of anterior subluxation, even in the absence of apprehension. Shoulder pain in this position must be differentiated from that secondary to impingement by performing a relocation test (discussion follows). However, Speer et al.[80] showed that pain was poorly correlated with instability and that apprehension was more specific to the diagnosis of instability. Pain with abduction and external rotation that is relieved by the relocation test may reflect internal glenoid impingement.

Relocation Test. The relocation test should be performed in conjunction with the apprehension test (Fig. 8). With the arm in the position that produces apprehension, a posteriorly directed stress is exerted on the proximal humerus. Both the apprehension and the pain should disappear with this maneuver. This test reduces the subluxation by pushing the humeral head posteriorly, thus relieving symptoms.

However, patients with rotator cuff involvement, but no instability, may have pain in the apprehension position and experience relief of pain with the relocation test. Such a patient may have a deep surface tear of the supraspinatus tendon, which is painful in the apprehension position because the tendon is trapped between the greater tuberosity and superior glenoid rim. The augmentation test, performed by pulling the humeral head forward while in the apprehension position, will increase the pain felt by rotator cuff patients, but will not augment pain in those with pure instability.

After a thorough physical examination, further diagnostic testing should be performed to clarify the nature and pattern of the instability.

Radiographic Evaluation

Initial plain film evaluation of the shoulder should include an anteroposterior (AP) view (Fig. 9), a true AP view of the

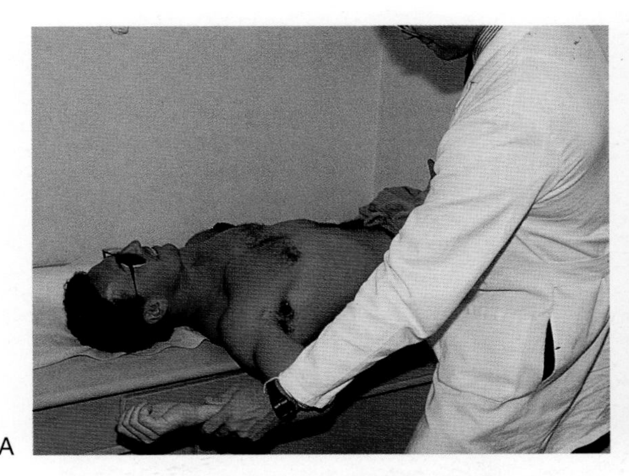
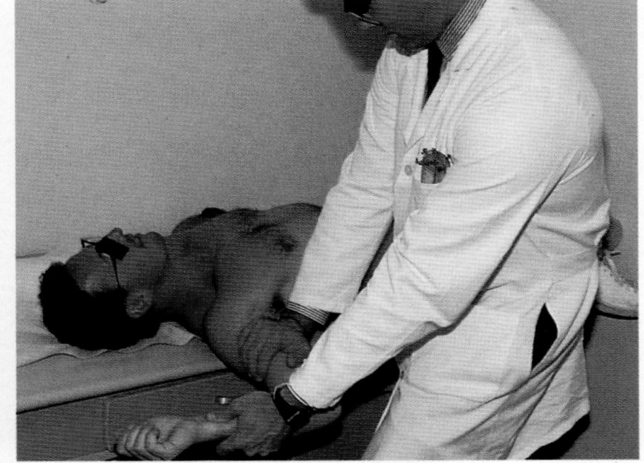
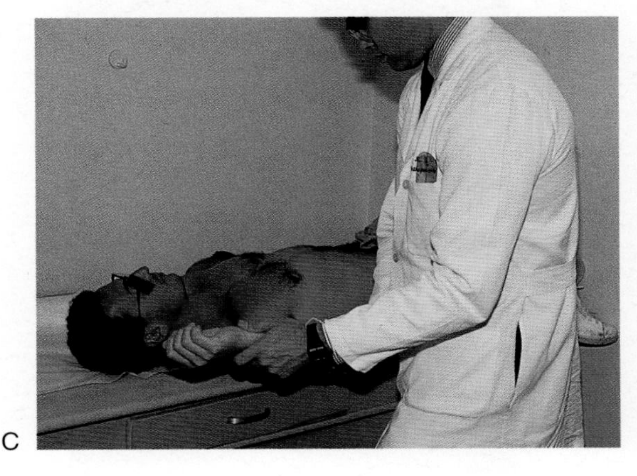

FIG. 8. Relocation test performed in the supine position: **(A)** The arm is first placed in a position of apprehension, 90 degrees of abduction, and maximum external rotation and extention posterior to the coronal plane of the body. **(B)** A posteriorly directed force is applied to the proximal humerus "relocating" the humeral head while the arm is in abduction and external rotation. Alternatively, **(C)** the arm can be kept in the same degree of abduction and external rotation and the arm brought into the coronal plane. A positive test is recorded if the symptoms of apprehension are eliminated.

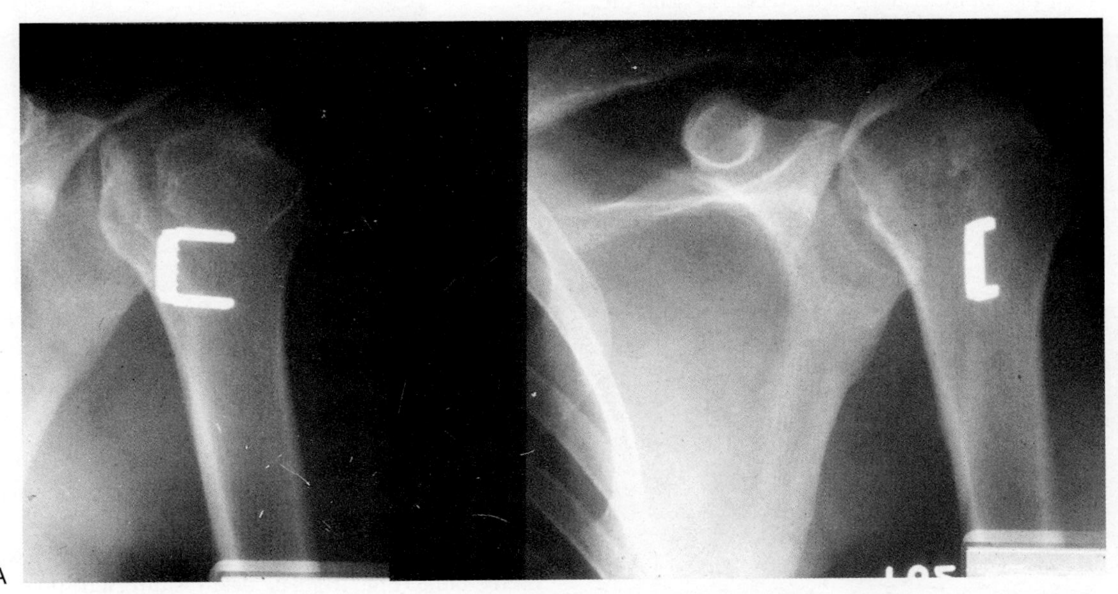

FIG. 9. (A,B) Initial radiographic series should include an AP view of the shoulder. This example shows the glenohumeral articulation to be overlapping (i.e., the x-ray beam is taken in the coronal plane of the body). This x-ray film was taken in both internal and external rotation, as shown by the position of the tuberosities and the metal staple used for a Magnussen-Stack procedure.

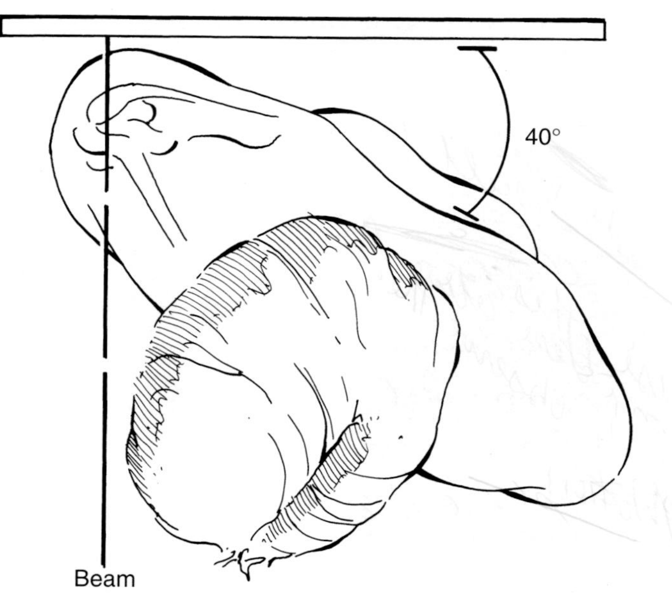

FIG. 10. Positioning for the Grashey view.

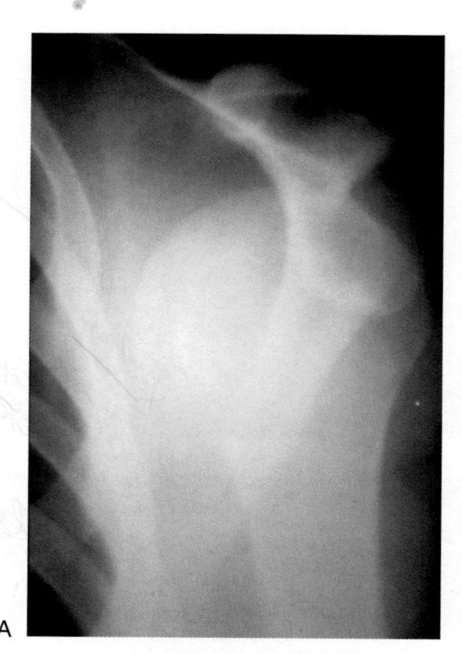

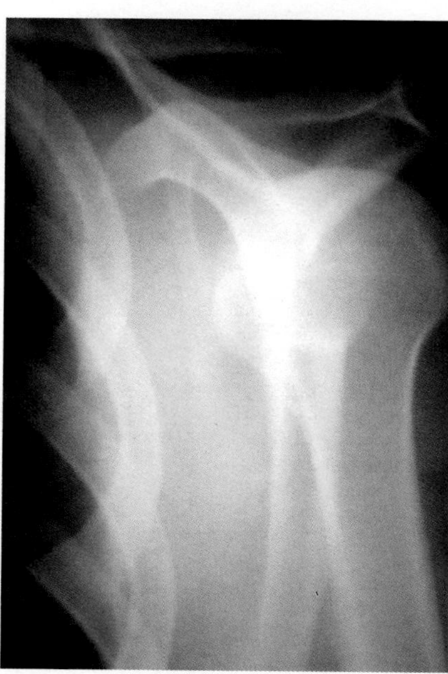

FIG. 12. Scapulolateral "Y" view showing **(A)** anterior dislocation and **(B)** reduction of glenohumeral joint.

glenoid (also called the Grashey projection; Figs. 10 and 11), a scapulolateral "Y" view (Fig. 12), and an axillary view (Fig. 13). Additionally, the West Point, Stryker notch, Didiee, and the Velpeau views are useful.

West Point View

To obtain a West Point axillary view, the patient is positioned prone with the shoulder abducted 90 degrees and the elbow bent and hanging off the edge of the table. The film cassette is positioned at the superior aspect of the shoulder (Fig. 14). The x-ray beam passes through the axilla at a 25-degree angle to the table top and is centered inferomedial to the acromioclavicular joint. This view provides the best evaluation of the anteroinferior glenoid rim, which is seen in tangent (Fig. 15).

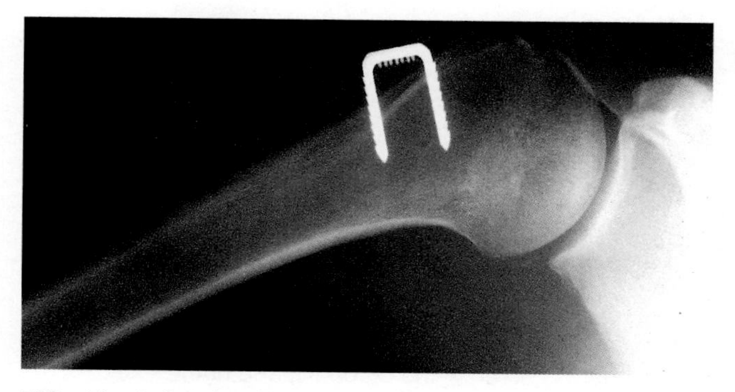

FIG. 11. A Grashey/AP view of the glenoid: The same patient is shown as in Fig. 9. The glenohumeral articulation is not overlapping and the glenoid is better visualized. With the arm in external rotation, the metal staple is seen in profile. This radiographic view is taken in the plane of the scapula.

Velpeau View

The Velpeau view is a modified axillary view that does not require arm abduction. With the arm in internal rotation at the side of the body (while wearing a sling), the standing patient leans backward 30 degrees over the cassette, which is on the table (Fig. 16). The beam is directed superoinferiorly through the shoulder.

Stryker Notch View

For the Stryker notch view, the patient is positioned supine, with the elbow elevated over the head and facing for-

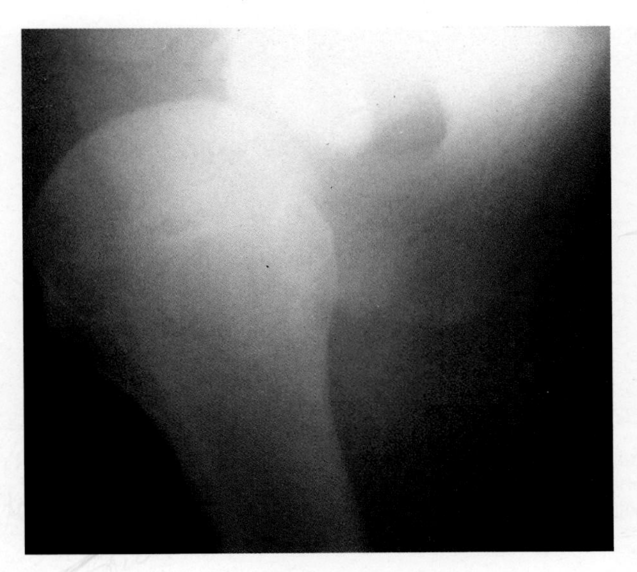

FIG. 13. Axillary view of the shoulder showing a bony Bankart lesion.

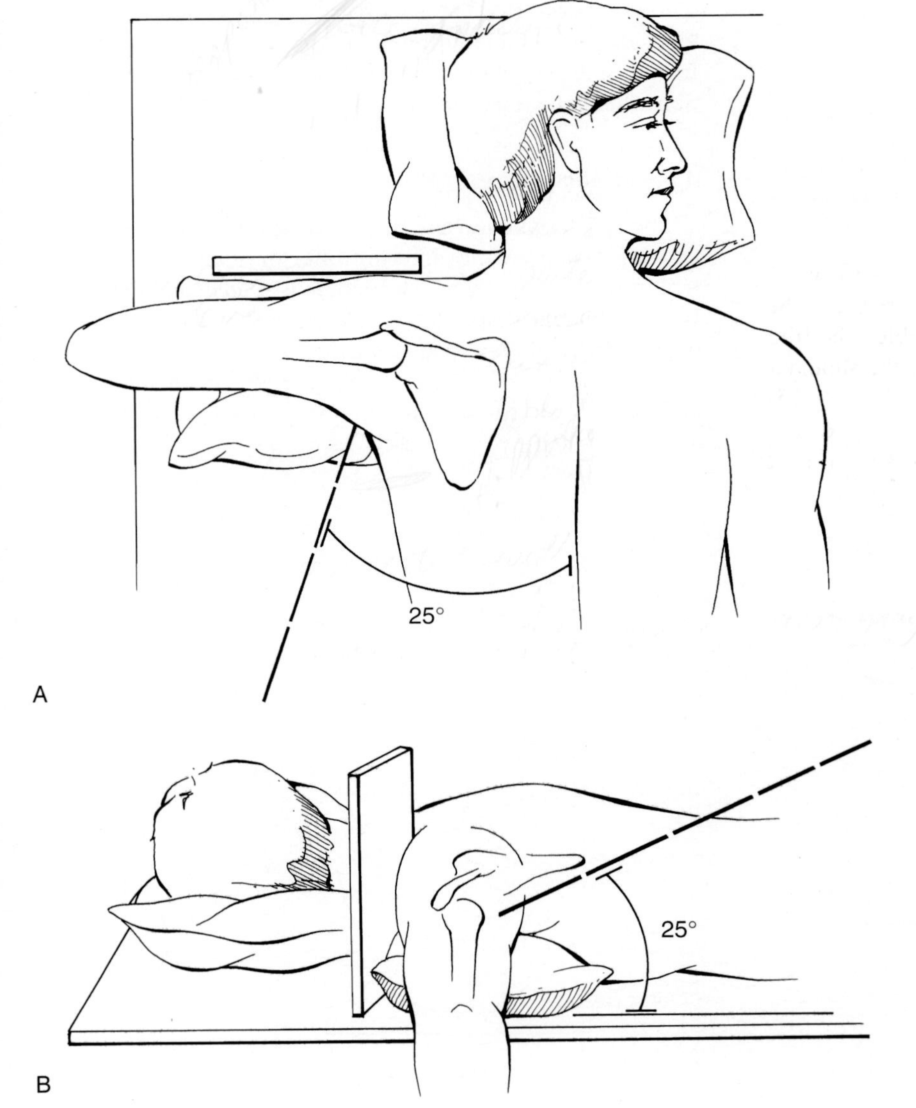

FIG. 14. Positioning for the West Point view.

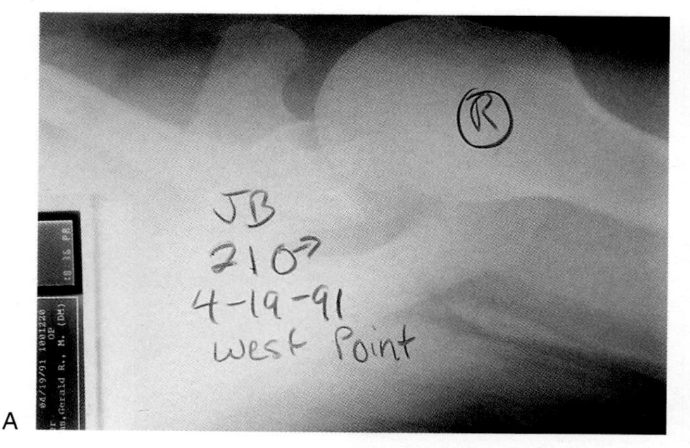

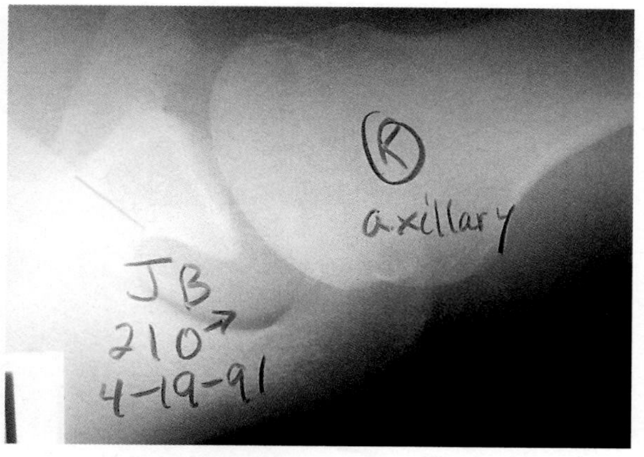

FIG. 15. **(A)** West Point axillary view showing the anterior and posterior glenoid rim. There is no abnormal glenoid bone identified, although it appears as if there is some anterior glenoid wear. **(B)** In this patient, the standard axillary view demonstrates a small glenoid rim fracture.

ward. The film cassette is placed under the shoulder, and the beam is directed cephalad at a 45-degree angle, centered on the axillary fold (Fig. 17). This view demonstrates the posterolateral humeral head to advantage and is useful for evaluating Hill–Sachs deformity (Fig. 18).

Didiee View

The Didiee view is obtained with the patient in the prone position, with the arm abducted and slightly flexed at the elbow; the dorsum of the hand is on the iliac crest. The film cassette is placed under the shoulder and the beam is directed from the lateral aspect toward the humeral head at a 45-degree angle (Fig. 19). These radiographic views allow assessment of glenohumeral alignment, as well as detection of fractures, degenerative changes, loose bodies, and calcification around the joint capsule.

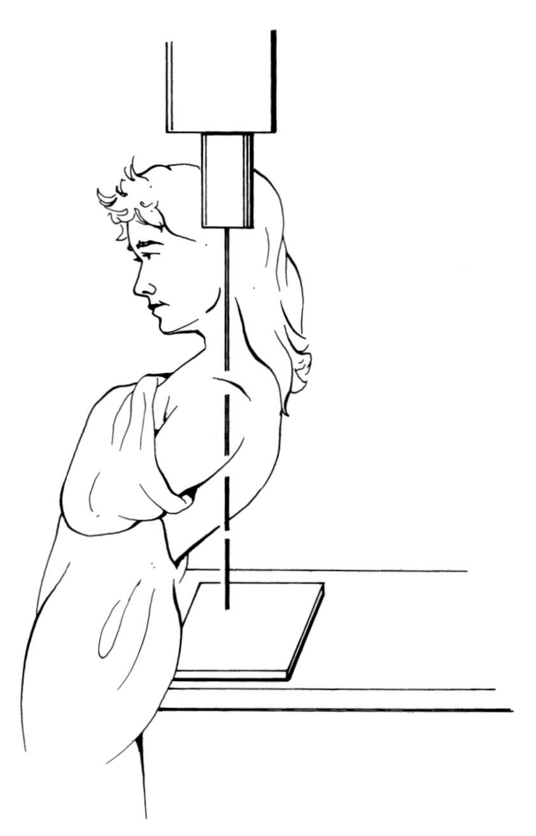

FIG. 16. Positioning for a Velpeau view.

Apical Oblique (Garth) View

The apical oblique view was described by Garth, et al.[18a] to best visualize the anterior inferior glenoid rim for fractures or calcification. The patient is seated, and the arm is on the patient's lap. The x-ray beam is directed angled 45 degrees to the thorax (plane of the scapula) and 45 degrees caudad. The beam is centered over the glenohumeral joint, and the cassette is placed posterior to the shoulder (Figs. 20 and 21).

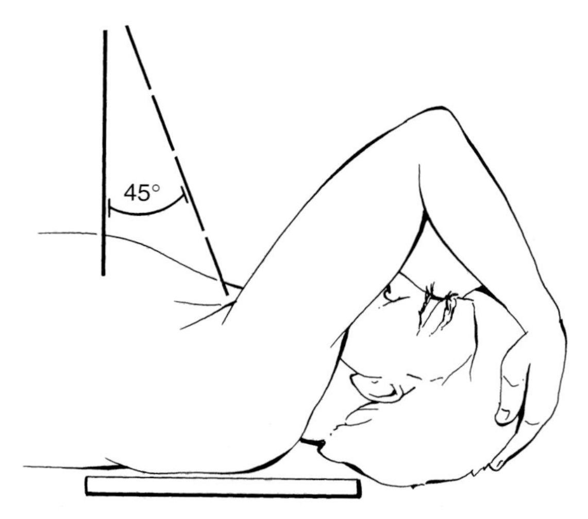

FIG. 17. Positioning for a Stryker notch view.

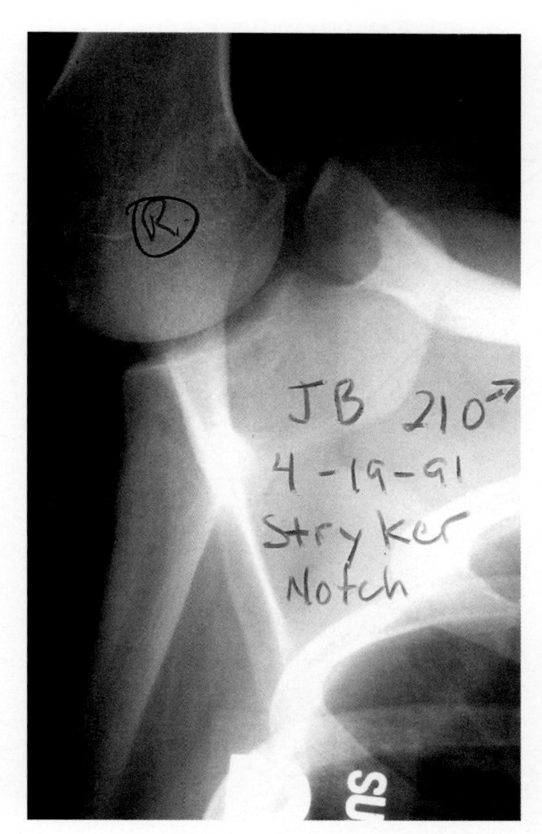

FIG. 18. Stryker notch view of the same patient in Fig. 15 shows a small wedge-shaped defect on the posterolateral humerus, which represents the Hill–Sachs lesion.

General Considerations

Anterior dislocations are usually accompanied by a degree of inferior displacement, making the injury apparent on the AP projection. Because of pain in the acute setting, the patient may be unable to abduct or rotate the shoulder, making the axillary, West Point, Stryker notch, and Didiee views difficult to obtain. The Velpeau and scapulolateral Y views are usually more comfortable for the patient because they do not require abduction. External rotation views are not recommended after reduction, because this position predisposes the patient to redislocation. (Algorithm 1 on p. 291).

The anterior, inferior, and medial displacement that occurs during anterior dislocation of the shoulder causes the posterolateral aspect of the superior humerus to impinge on the anteroinferior rim of the glenoid. This may result in an osteochondral compression fracture of the posterolateral humeral head, known as the Hill–Sachs lesion.[27] This fracture can occur as a sequela of the first or any subsequent dislocation episode. It is best seen on the AP view of the shoulder with internal rotation of the humeral head or on the Stryker notch view.[63,73]

Osteochondral glenoid lesions may also occur and are difficult to detect on prereduction films. A fracture of the glenoid rim, also called a bony Bankart lesion,[6,7] is best visualized on West Point or Didiee views[63] or on a Grashey view.[20]

The nonosseous Bankart lesion involves only the cartilaginous glenoid labrum; therefore, it cannot be evaluated by

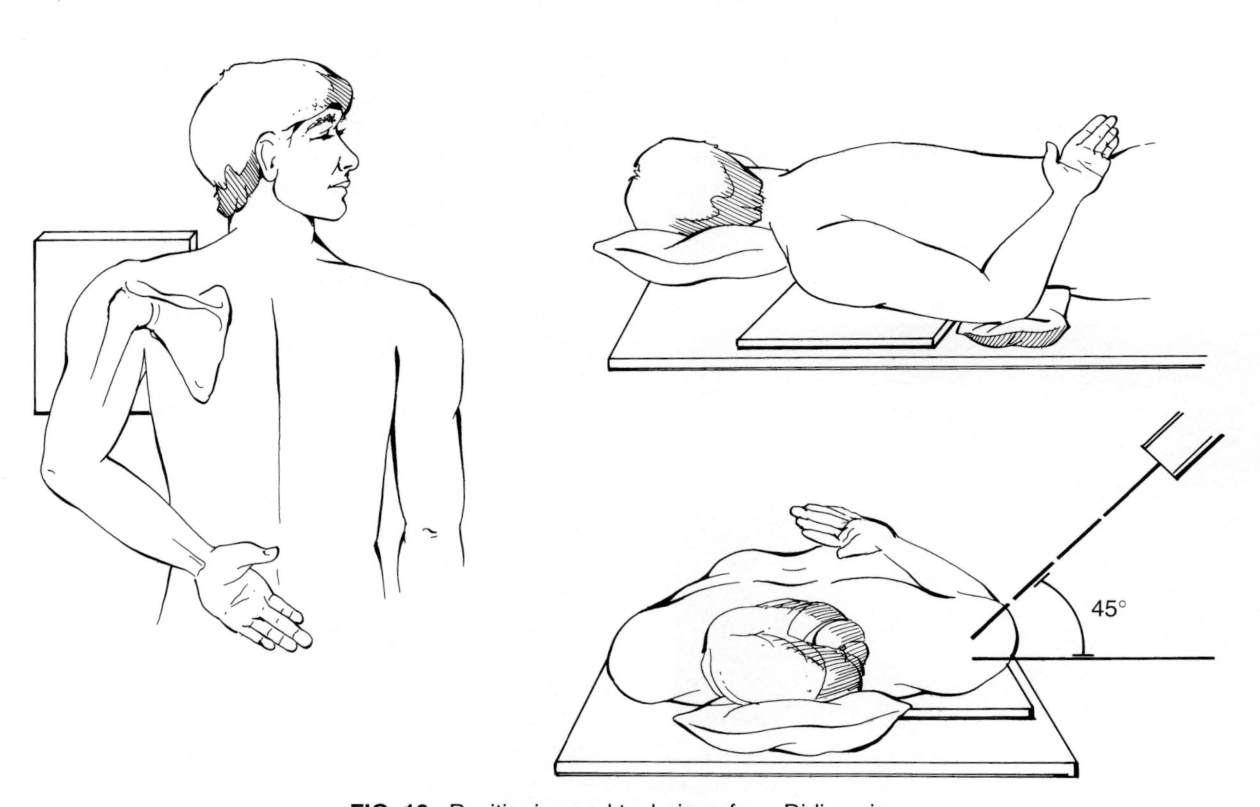

FIG. 19. Positioning and technique for a Didiee view.

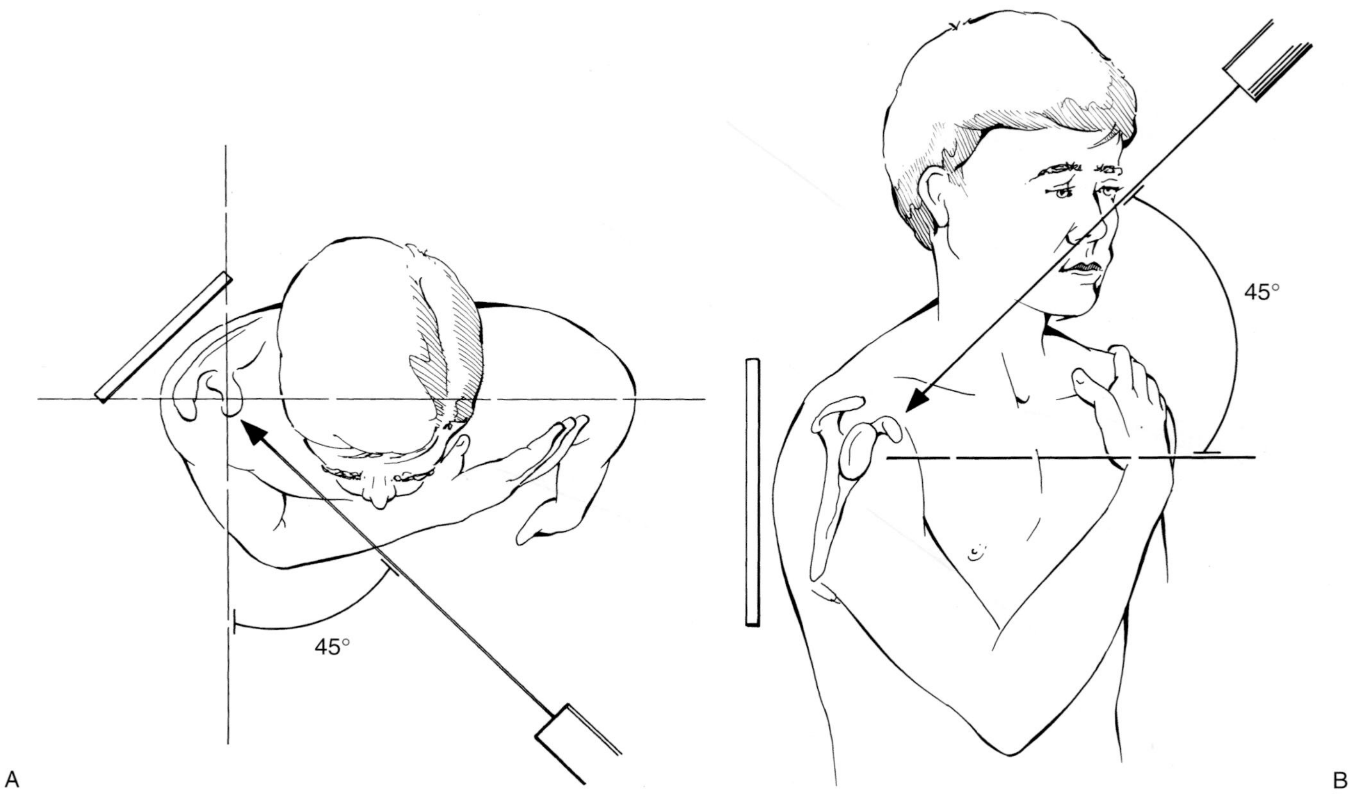

FIG. 20. (A,B) Positioning and technique for the apical oblique view (Garth) view

plain films. This lesion is best demonstrated by magnetic resonance imaging (MRI; Fig. 22), computed tomographic (CT) arthrography (Fig. 23), or arthroscopy (Fig. 24). In addition, a CT scan and MRI can visualize small bony lesions that may be difficult to see or quantify on plain films (Figs. 25 through 27). The advantages of MRI include lack of ionizing radiation and the ability to detect small changes in soft-tissue composition without relying on intravenous or intraarticular injection of contrast material. An MRI of the shoulder can demonstrate rotator cuff pathology, labral morphology, and osseous integrity.

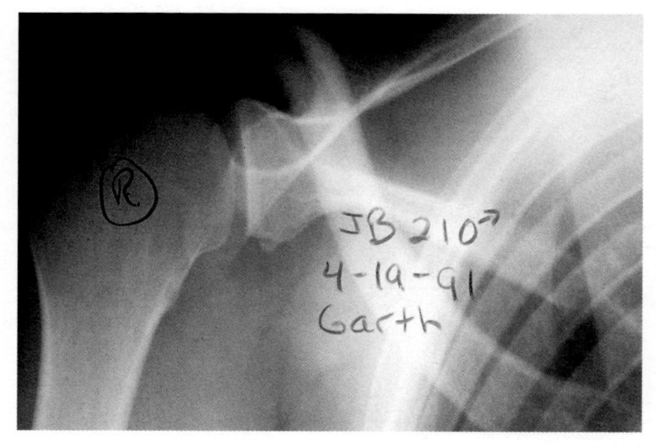

FIG. 21. An apical oblique view of the same patient in Figs. 15 and 18 demonstrates calcification of the anterior inferior glenoid rim associated with anterior glenohumeral instability.

Several investigators have studied labral morphology in normal patients. Although the posterior labrum maintains either a triangular or rounded shape, the appearance of the anterior labrum is variable. Neumann et al.[56] studied 30 asymptomatic volunteers and found cleaved, notched, or flat anterior labra in 30% and described absent portions of the anterior superior labrum in 6%. McCauley et al.[51] disagreed, finding labral clefts in only 4% of healthy subjects. Because of the variability in the appearance of normal glenoid labra, an MRI scan may overestimate the frequency of labral tears.

Complex labral tears are easier to detect. One can often see fragments that have migrated into the axillary pouch or labral cysts associated with labral tears. An MRI scan can also show capsular stripping from the glenoid, rotator cuff tears, muscle atrophy caused by suprascapular and axillary nerve injury, and osseous injuries such as Hill–Sachs lesions. Focal thinning of the articular cartilage of the glenoid may indicate areas of recurrent instability.

Use of MRI arthrography in the detection of labral and capsular pathology is controversial. Gusmer et al.[23] found noncontrast MRI to be 95% accurate in detecting labral tears. However, Flannigan et al.[18] believed that the presence of intraarticular contrast affords improved visualization of the labrum and rotator cuff and enhances the accuracy of MRI for

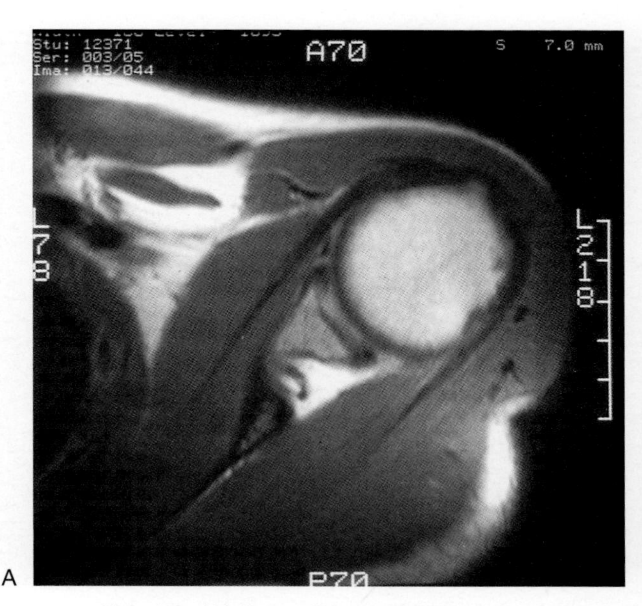

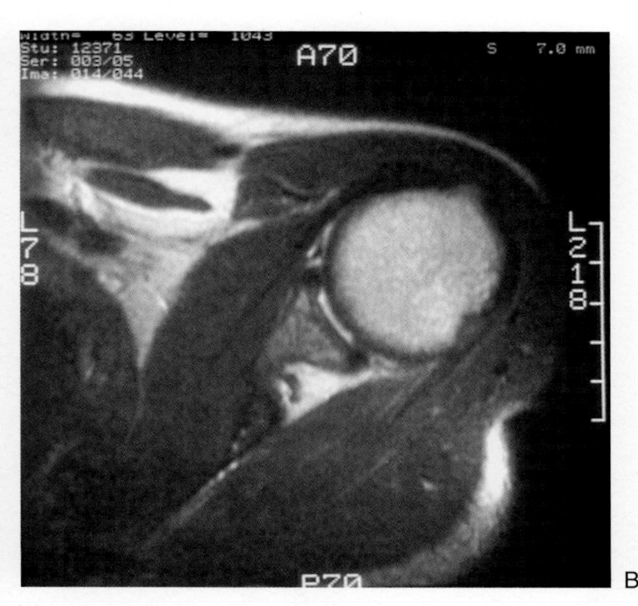

FIG. 22. **(A)** T-1 weighted and **(B)** T-2 weighted axial cuts demonstrating a small Hill–Sachs lesion on the posterosuperior humeral head and an anterior labrum tear that is best indicated by the high signal fluid between the labrum and the anterior glenoid rim.

the detection of labral and rotator cuff tears. Palmer and Caslowitz[61] evaluated MRI arthrography and found this method to have 92% sensitivity and 92% specificity for the detection of labral tears. One pitfall of MR arthrography is that the presence of intraarticular contrast may lift the superior labrum from the articular cartilage, simulating labral detachment.[46] Normal anatomic structures adjacent to the labrum, such as the glenohumeral ligaments and articular cartilage of the glenoid fossa, may be misinterpreted as labral tears.[46]

Use of CT arthrography can reliably define the osseous structures of the shoulder and assess both labral and capsular integrity. The disadvantages of this technique include exposure to ionizing radiation, an invasive procedure, and inability to assess partial-thickness tears of the rotator cuff, biceps tendon, or labrum.

Although imaging studies can provide useful anatomic information, they do not reflect a dynamic situation. Additional information can be obtained by fluoroscopic stress evaluation of the glenohumeral joint. In a study of 50 patients, Papilion and Shall[62] evaluated fluoroscopic examination of shoulder instability under general anesthesia. Translation was expressed as the percentage of displacement of

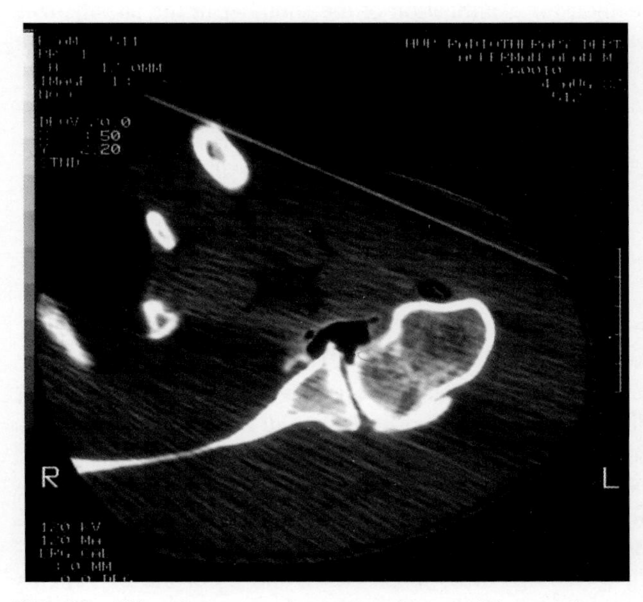

FIG. 23. CT arthrogram demonstrating avulsion of the anteroinferior capsule from the glenoid rim.

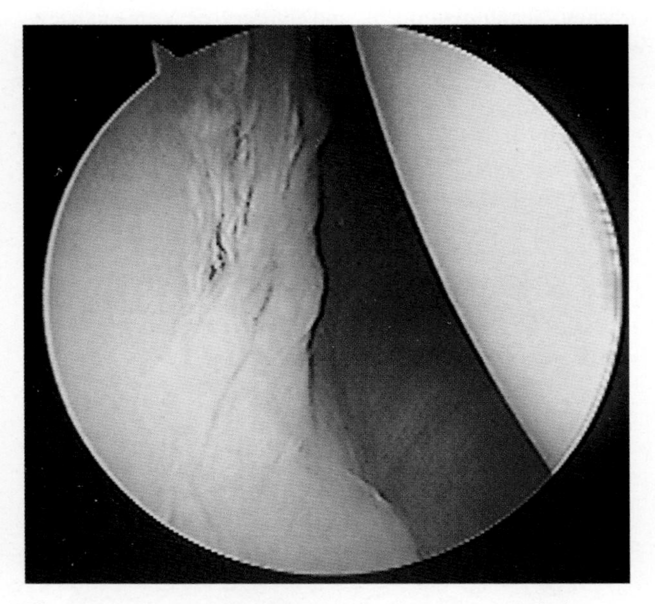

FIG. 24. Arthroscopic photograph of an anteroinferior capsular avulsion (Bankart lesion).

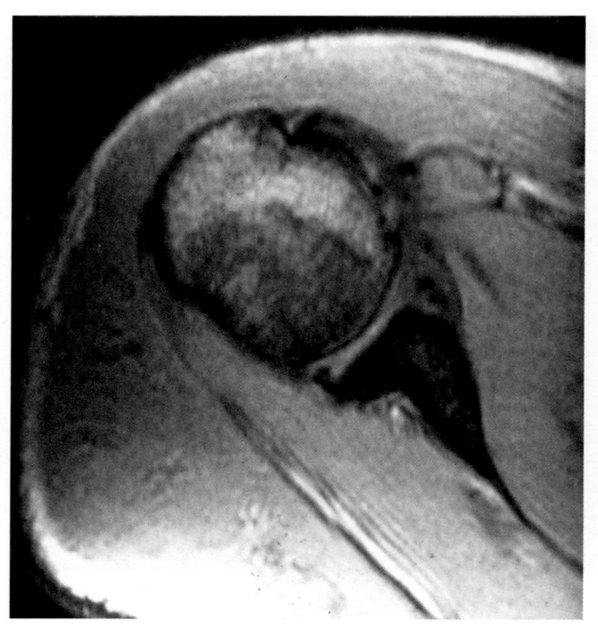

FIG. 25. MRI axial cut demonstrating a nondisplaced anterior glenoid fracture.

the humeral head relative to the glenoid. They found that up to 14% anterior translation and 37% posterior translation are "normal." A greater percentage of translation indicated instability. These criteria had an overall sensitivity of 93% and specificity of 100% for the diagnosis of the presence and direction of instability. It must be emphasized that an absolute degree of translation cannot be correlated with instability. The amount of translation can vary greatly among individuals, and the degree of translation must be correlated with the opposite normal shoulder when present.

We prefer to obtain a series of plain films that include AP, Grashey, scapulolateral Y, and axillary or Velpeau views. We use CT of the shoulder to evaluate the glenoid rim and volume of a Hill–Sachs deformity and use MRI only if there is a question of rotator cuff pathology.

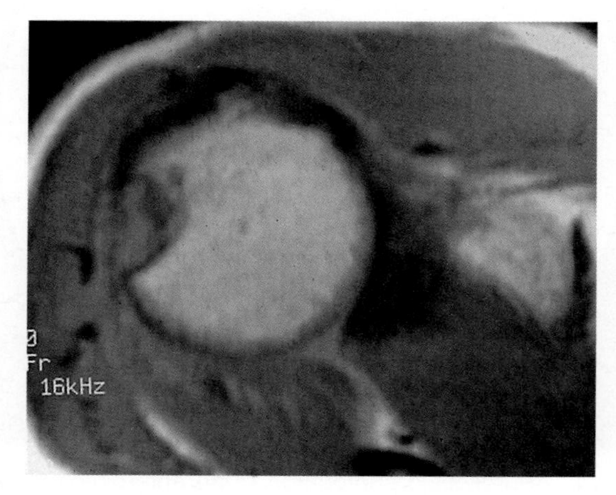

FIG. 26. MRI axial cut of a medium-sized Hill–Sachs lesion.

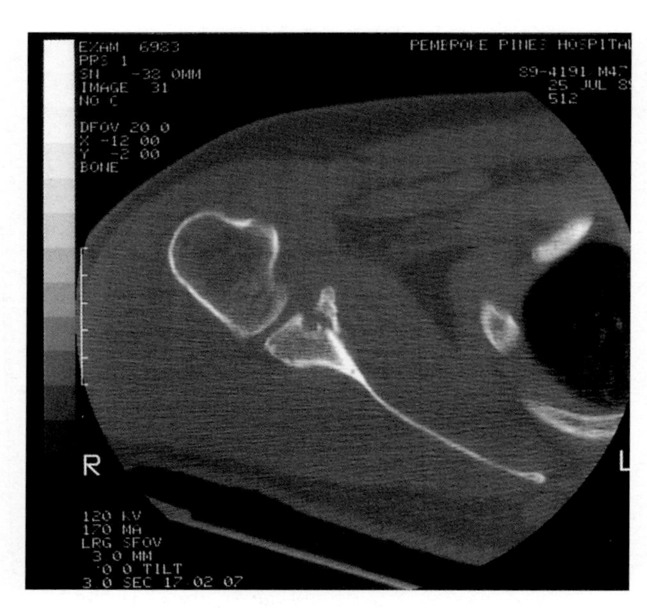

FIG. 27. CT scan of a anterior glenoid fracture.

Examination under Anesthesia

The numerous methods available for diagnosing shoulder instability may not provide enough information to proceed confidently to surgical treatment. Anesthesia is sometimes necessary to produce sufficient muscle relaxation and freedom from pain for an adequate examination. Under anesthesia, only a small amount of force is necessary to stress the ligaments of the joint capsule.

Simonet and Cofield[77] studied 55 patients thought to have shoulder instability. They compared the findings of the examination under anesthesia with the pathologic condition identified at surgery. They also described a systematic method for examination of the shoulder in the anesthetized patient and stated that both shoulders should be examined:

> On examination of the right shoulder, the right wrist of the patient is held by the right hand of the examiner. The left hand of the examiner is placed across the superolateral aspect of the shoulder, such that the palm of the hand is over the acromion and distal clavicle and the fourth and fifth fingers rest on the coracoid process. The thumb is positioned on the posterior aspect of the humeral head and the index and long fingers are placed on the anterior aspect of the humeral head. The right hand of the examiner positions the arm of the patient in various degrees of abduction and rotation. The left hand of the examiner applies pressure to the humeral head.

For the optimal determination of translation in the anterior direction, the arm is positioned in 80 degrees of external rotation and a load and shift test is performed. If the affected side demonstrates a higher grade of translation than does the unaffected side, the test for instability is positive.[76] In one study,[76] negative examinations correlated with negative surgical findings in 28 of 28 cases, and 25 of the 27 patients with positive findings on examination under anesthesia had pathology at surgery. Examination under anesthesia, when combined with diagnostic shoulder arthroscopy, can provide (in most cases) an accurate assessment of instability.

Diagnostic Arthroscopy

We routinely perform diagnostic arthroscopy on all patients before surgical repair of shoulder instability. It provides precise diagnosis of the type of instability and associated injuries. A systematic approach should be developed in examining a shoulder with suspected instability.[48]

Shoulder arthroscopy may be performed in the lateral decubitus or beach chair position. The beach chair position requires additional assistance for control of the arm. It does, however, provide more versatility in arthroscopic examination and allows easier positioning for conversion to an open procedure if desired. After systematic examination of the joint for other pathology, we examine the inferior recess for free bodies and the humeral head for the presence and size of a Hill–Sachs deformity. We evaluate for ease of movement of the arthroscope anteriorly through the glenohumeral joint and into the axillary pouch. A positive "drive-through" sign (described by Pagnani and Warren[60]) results from substantial laxity in the IGHL. A positive drive-through sign is considered present when, under distraction loading, the humeral head separates widely from the glenoid, facilitating easy passage (or "drive through") of the arthroscope from posterior to anterior. Finally, we direct our attention to the anterior labrum and capsule to confirm the diagnosis and direct the appropriate treatment.

If present, a Bankart lesion is usually obvious, and it confirms the diagnosis of anterior instability (Fig. 28). It is not uncommon, however, to find a detached labrum with scar filling the defect. These lesions are not always apparent with initial inspection of the labrum, but can be defined with careful probing.

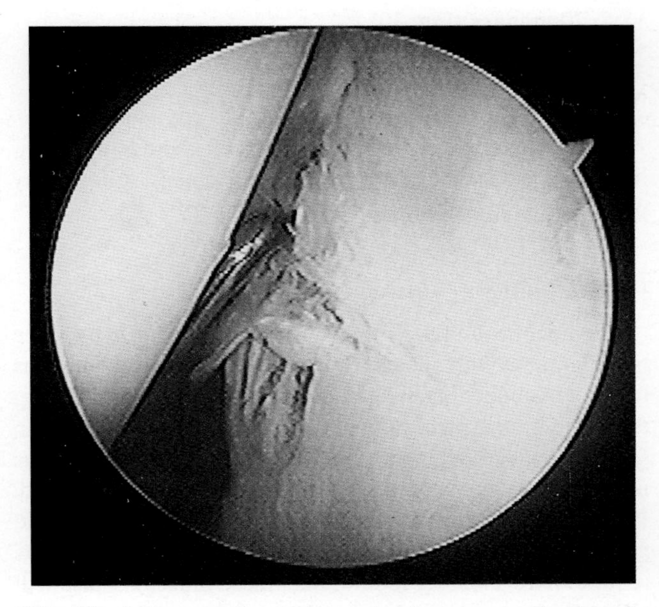

FIG. 28. Arthroscopic photograph of an acute Bankart lesion.

Hintermann and Gachter[28] performed a prospective arthroscopic study of 178 patients, each of whom had at least one episode of shoulder dislocation. Reporting the arthroscopically determined pathologic findings, they concluded that associated injuries were more common than expected and that there were significant differences between preoperative and postoperative diagnoses. The most frequent arthroscopic findings were anterior glenoid labral tears (85%), ventral capsule insufficiency (80%), Hill–Sachs lesions (67%), glenohumeral ligament insufficiency (55%), rotator cuff tears (20%), posterior glenoid labral tears (8%), and superior labral anterior to posterior lesions (SLAP lesions; 5%). They also noted that the labrum and anteroinferior glenoid rim showed abnormalities corresponding to different types of anterior instability. They concluded that preoperative shoulder arthroscopy increases the accuracy of diagnosis and has the potential to identify the optimal surgical procedure. Caspari[13] described other arthroscopic manifestations that occur in anterior shoulder subluxations and dislocations, including varying severity of labral pathology and anterior capsular injuries, which directed his surgical treatment.

MANAGEMENT

The goal of management of anterior shoulder instability is to return the patient as rapidly as possible to his or her preinjury level of activity. The first step toward this goal is adequate, prompt, and atraumatic reduction of an anteriorly dislocated shoulder. Decisions (often individualized) then need to be made for immobilization and rehabilitation (algorithm 2 on p. 292).

Once the diagnosis is made, the glenohumeral joint should be reduced as rapidly and gently as possible. If diagnosed in the field, a reduction maneuver may be attempted immediately before spasm of the shoulder muscles has occurred. A neurovascular examination should be performed before and after the reduction. When attempting such a reduction in the field without sedation, we prefer to place the patient's shoulder in a small amount of forward flexion and abduction and then slowly internally rotate the arm. If this does not achieve the desired results, the patient should be transported to an emergency room where reduction under sedation may be performed.

Many reduction maneuvers have been successfully performed with appropriate muscle relaxation. One technique is the traction and countertraction method described by Matsen et al. (Fig. 29).[47] In this method, the patient lies supine with a sheet passed around his or her thorax and around the assistant's waist. The assistant should be standing on the unaffected side of the patient to provide a countertraction force. The surgeon should be standing on the affected side of the patient with a second sheet looped around his or her waist and the patient's forearm. The surgeon leans back and applies steady, gradually increasing traction while grasping the

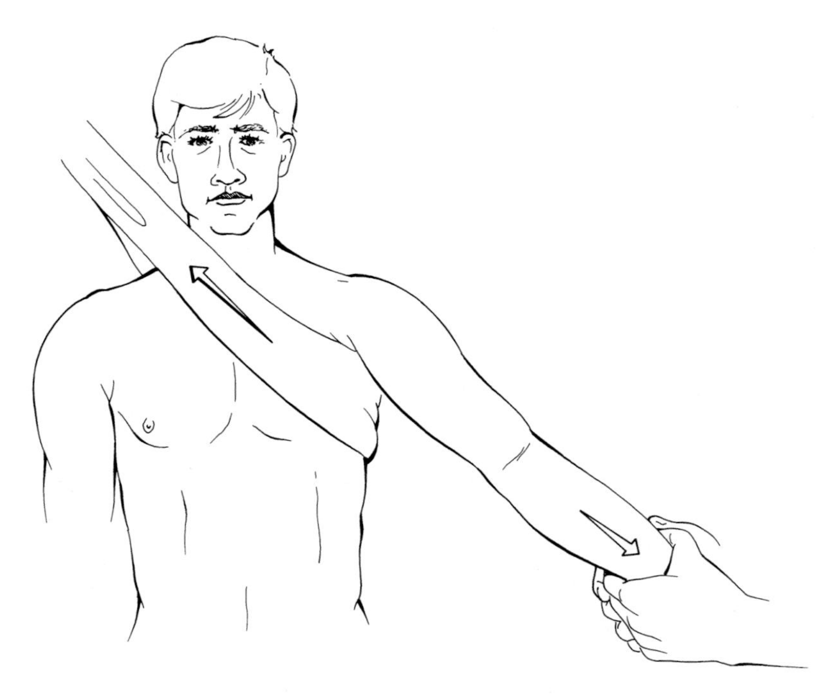

FIG. 29. Reduction technique using the traction–countertraction method.

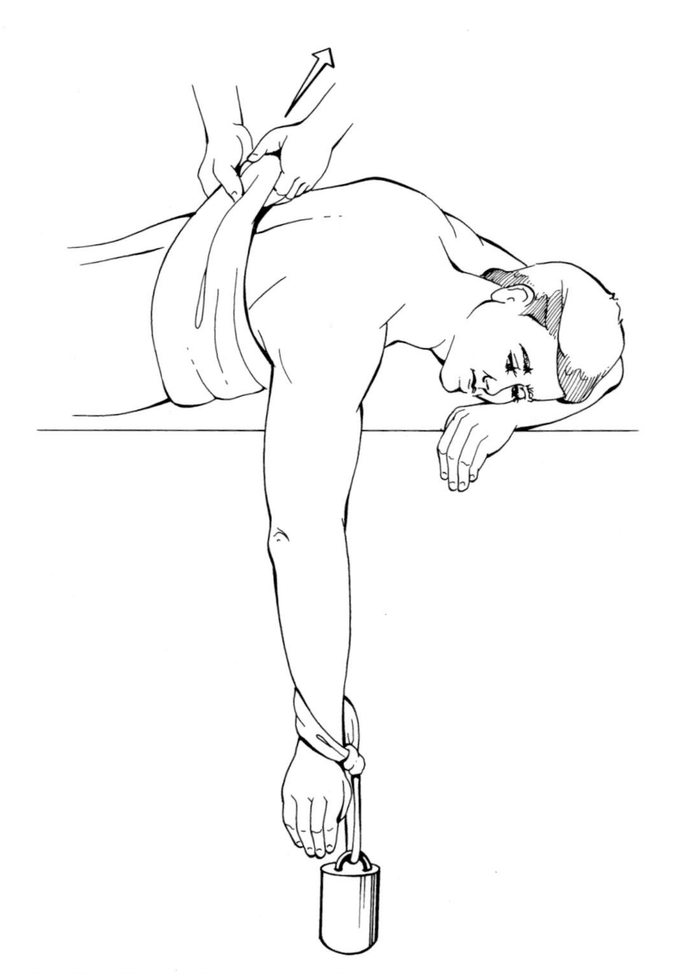

FIG. 30. Stimson's technique for closed reduction of dislocation.

forearm at the same time as the assistant provides countertraction around the patient's waist. The surgeon may be required to gently rotate the arm internally and externally or to attempt to apply gentle outward pressure to the humeral head with his or her hand in the axilla.

In Stimson's technique, the patient is placed in the prone position on the edge of the examining table, with the affected arm hanging over the side. If the weight of the arm is not sufficient to reduce the shoulder, gentle downward traction is applied with an appropriate weight (usually 5 lb or less) attached to the wrist. With this technique, reduction may take 15 to 20 minutes (Fig. 30).[47]

Nonoperative Treatment

Nonoperative management begins with shoulder immobilization (the duration of which is controversial), followed by physical therapy and (occasionally) bracing.

Immobilization

Shoulder instability in athletes has been managed by brace treatment, but with unclear results. The purpose of bracing is to prevent abduction and external rotation, thereby avoiding the position that places the patient at risk for dislocation. In sports such as basketball, baseball, and volleyball, this is nearly impossible because of the shoulder mobility required. Football players may have varying results based on the field position. Wide receivers, quarterbacks, and defensive backs require more shoulder motion than these braces usually will allow. However, braces have been used successfully for football linemen, hockey players, and wrestlers, where the motions of abduction and external rotation are not necessary for participation in the sport (Fig. 31). Restriction of motion is adjusted by a trainer to each individual athlete's needs to prevent subluxation and dislocation. Data available on the usefulness of these braces are largely anecdotal, and no biomechanical data exist, despite manufacturer's claims of success.

Controversy remains over the role of immobilization after first-time anterior shoulder dislocations and this treatment's ability to affect the rate of recurrence.

Hovelius et al.[30] prospectively followed 257 patients (all younger than 40 years) after first dislocation. Approximately half were treated with immobilization for 3 to 4 weeks; the others were treated with early range of motion. At the 2-year follow-up, recurrence rates were similar, with the highest recurrence rates seen in the younger patients, regardless of treatment. Yoneda et al.[89] reported the results of a more prolonged period of immobilization (5 weeks) and limited range of motion for an additional 6 weeks in a young, athletic population. At 13-years follow-up, 17.3% had had a recurrence; 13.5% of those required surgical repair. Kiviluoto et al.[35] showed a higher incidence of recurrence among patients younger than 30 years and, in this younger group, there was a higher incidence in those immobilized 1 week compared with those immobilized for 3 weeks. These authors recommended longer immobilization (3 weeks) for patients younger than 30 years old and shorter immobilization (1 week) for patients older than 30 years.

Rehabilitation

After an appropriate period of immobilization, a physical therapy program should be initiated for all patients with anterior instability, regardless of the underlying pathology.

Individualizing a rehabilitation program should take into account several factors, including knowledge of the patient's instability pattern and associated injury pathology. Patients with multidirectional instability should be encouraged to avoid activities that stress the shoulder in an inferior direction, and those who have had severe trauma causing dislocation should avoid prolonged time in positions at risk. Patients with subluxation may require less immobilization time before initiating a therapy program. It should be stressed that throughout the rehabilitation period, the patient should not be exercising in pain. If pain develops during a particular exercise, the patient should limit or modify the existing exercise level and avoid progressing to the next level until the pain resolves. Several studies support the usefulness of early rehabilitation programs in diminishing the rate of redislocation.[1,2] When using a strict rehabilitation protocol in a population of Naval midshipmen, Aronen et al.[2] reported a 75% success rate in preventing dislocation over a 3.5-year period. Arciero et al.[1] reported an 80% reduction rate in consistently treated West Point cadets after primary dislocation. However, Hovelius[29] reported that age at time of initial dislocation was more important than rehabilitation or length of immobilization.

Attempting to restore range of motion is the initial goal in any shoulder rehabilitation program. After an acute injury and appropriate initial immobilization, modalities should be performed to decrease the amount of pain. Ice, heat, ultrasound, and electrical stimulation treatments may improve pain and swelling. Oral nonsteroidal antiinflammatory medications may help decrease inflammation. Pendulum exercises are begun as soon as the immobilization is removed.

Isometric exercises are also initiated for resisted internal rotation and resisted adduction at this time. The position of abduction with external rotation is to be avoided. When the

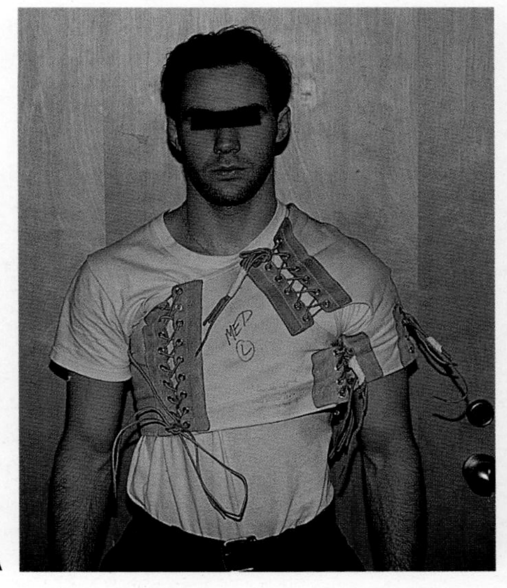

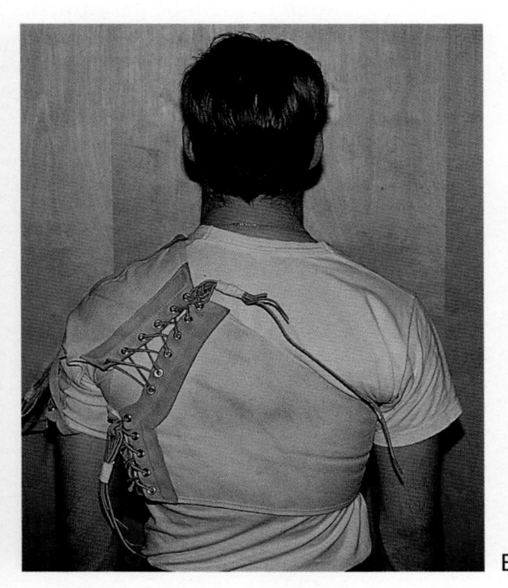

FIG. 31. Dennison-Duke brace worn to prevent shoulder dislocation in athletic competition.

patient can perform isometric exercises without pain, he or she may advance to isotonic exercises that strengthen the stabilizers. The scapular stabilizers are strengthened to provide a stable base for humerus rotation and maintain the glenoid in a position that has maximal congruency with the humeral head. Any change in position of the scapula will produce increased stress on the rotator cuff. In addition, many overhead athletes present with anterior tilt and lateral displacement of the scapula. This produces additional stress on the anterior structures of the shoulder. Moseley et al.[54] described a series of four scapular stabilizer exercises based on electromyographic findings to strengthen the scapula-stabilizing musculature. They recommended rowing, push-ups with maximal protraction (Fig. 32), scaption (which involves elevation of the humerus in the scapular plane with the humerus externally rotated) (Fig. 33A), and press-ups (which utilize the pectoralis minor) (Fig. 33B). Closed-chain exercises, such as push-ups, enhance joint stability by providing a compressive force across the joint and diminish tensile forces across the capsule. However, care must be taken to avoid abducting the shoulder, which places increased pressure on the anterior joint.

Muscle strengthening of the rotator cuff may help stabilize the humeral head by providing compression across the glenohumeral joint and preventing impingement. Initially, exercises for shoulder strengthening should occur in the scapular plane. This provides several advantages.[74] This position offers an optimal length–tension relation between the deltoid and rotator cuff muscles and minimizes the stress on the anterior and posterior capsule and rotator cuff.[16] The supraspinatus may be selectively strengthened in the scapular plane or by prone horizontal lifts with the shoulder slightly externally rotated. The subscapularis may be strengthened by side-lying internal rotation lifts against resistance. The isotonic program should be followed by an isokinetic strengthening program as pain allows.

Internal and external rotation exercises can be performed using Theraband tubing, whereas scaption strengthens the infraspinatus and deltoid. When strengthening the rotator cuff, it is important to include eccentric strength exercises because many throwing activities use the posterior rotator cuff to decelerate the arm during follow-through.[15] Before progressing to strengthening in an overhead position, apprehension must be eliminated. Muscular balance of the rotator cuff is important in restoring dynamic stability, and all muscular stabilizers must be taught to act synchronously.

Many overhead-throwing athletes present with excessive external rotation and a tightened posterior capsule.[11] Posterior tightness can lead to superior migration of the humeral head and anterior instability symptoms, with secondary impingement occurring as a result. When asymptomatic, such a patient should begin a stretching program to correct posterior capsular tightness. Gentle internal rotation stretches in 90 degrees of shoulder abduction is a more specific stretch for posterior capsular tightness than cross-body adduction stretches, which tend to stretch the scapular muscles.[21]

The biceps brachii should be strengthened to assist in anterior stabilization, and the deltoid should be able to provide abduction. The latissimus dorsi and pectoralis major should then be strengthened because they play an important role in deceleration of the shoulder in overhead activities.

Proprioception and neuromuscular control must also be emphasized in rehabilitation for shoulder instability (Fig. 34). Lephart et al.[40] recommended four exercises, emphasizing joint position and kinesthesia to accomplish this goal.

Once joint sensibility and dynamic muscular control is obtained, training for functionally specific activities may be initiated. Continued muscle strengthening as well as endurance training specific for each sport should be performed. Posterior capsular stretches should be continued. An interval training program should be initiated and continued until the patient is able to return to full function in the chosen activity.

Athletes require strong legs and trunk to provide torque to their arms. The legs and trunk are responsible for more than 50% of the kinetic energy consumed during throwing.[8,87] Therefore, any rehabilitation program involving the arm must include conditioning exercises for the legs, hips, abdominal muscles, and back muscles before the patient resumes over-

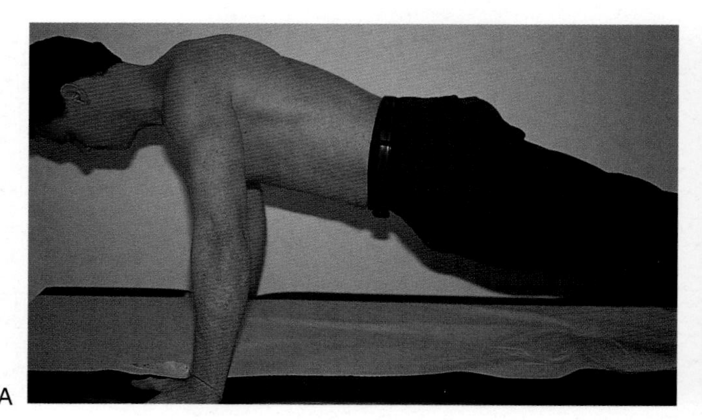
A

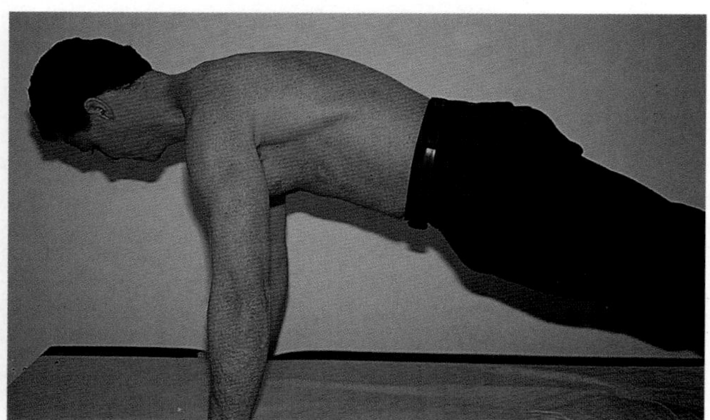
B

FIG. 32. Push-ups with a plus involves a normal push-up with maximum shoulder and scapular protraction with the elbows fully extended.

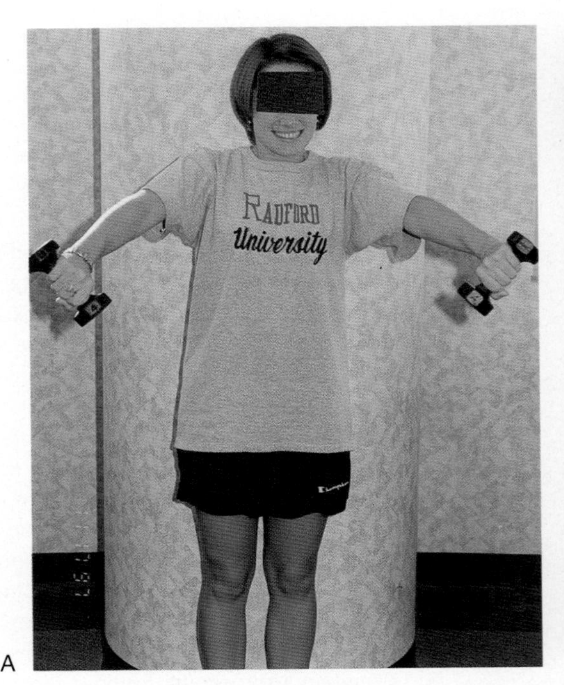

A

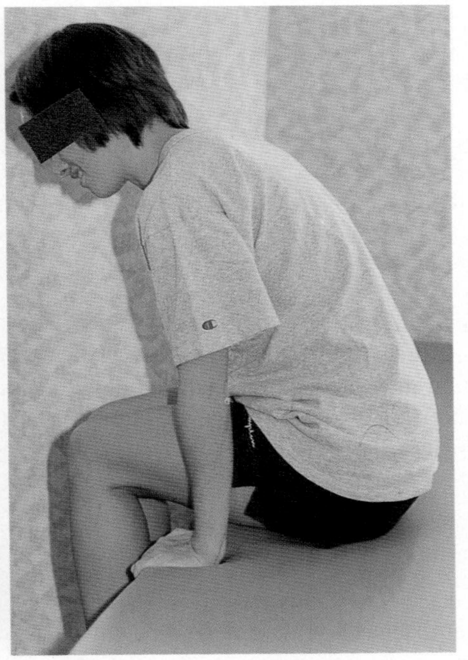
B

FIG. 33. Scapula-stabilizing exercises include **(A)** scaption, which involves elevation of the humerus in the scapular plane with the humerus in external rotation, and **(B)** press-up exercises.

head activities to diminish the amount of work required of the arms in reestablishing preinjury overhead performance.

Anterior Subluxation

These patients usually respond well to nonoperative treatments without the need of surgical treatment once the underlying pathology is determined. Rest, followed by oral nonsteroidal antiinflammatory medications and a supervised physical therapy program focusing on the rotator cuff and scapular stabilizers, will usually provide resolution of symptoms. When nonoperative treatment fails, surgery must correct capsular laxity and the associated labral pathology. Gross et al.[22] recommended technical modifications to elim-

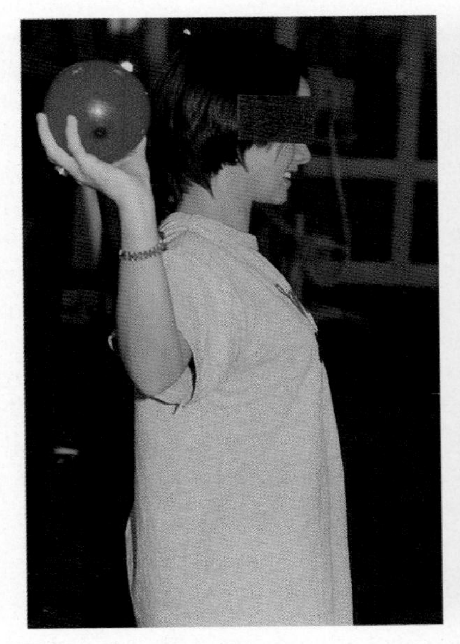

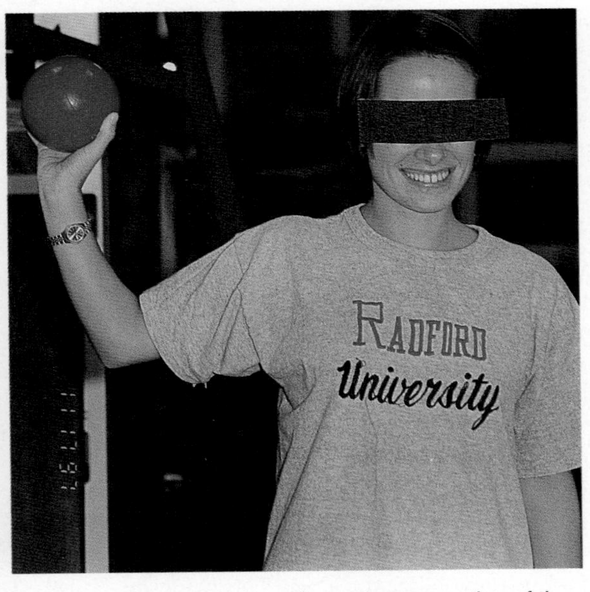

FIG. 34. Stretch-shortening exercise with a Plyoball uses the elastic and reactive properties of the muscle to generate maximum force production. These exercises serve as an excellent transition between traditional-strengthening exercises and throwing activities.

inate forces in the at-risk position, including positioning elbows anterior to or in the plane of the body during any maneuver.

Multidirectional Instability

Patients with multidirectional instability should be treated initially with a prolonged course of physical therapy, with the goal of strengthening the dynamic stabilizers and improving proprioception of the glenohumeral joint. For patients with trauma-induced multidirectional instability and other correctable pathology, surgery may be considered at an earlier time than for those with nontraumatic etiologies. Before initiating more aggressive treatment, the clinician must differentiate between patients who can voluntarily dislocate their shoulders and those whose dislocations are involuntary.

Surgical Intervention

Over the past decade, new concepts and techniques have evolved for the surgical management of anterior shoulder instability, including surgical treatment for first-time dislocators, arthroscopic intervention, and new open surgical procedures.

Role of Surgery for Patients with Initial Dislocations

Management of initial dislocations in young, active, athletic patients has become controversial. A high incidence of recurrence in young, active athletic patients has been previously reported.[29,77] Physical therapy alone has provided mixed results. Aronen and Regan[2] reported a 75% success rate among 20 midshipmen at the Naval Academy using a strict physical therapy regimen. Because these results have not been replicated by others, many clinicians believe that patients with initial dislocations would benefit from a more aggressive surgical approach, given the natural history and associated pathology. The high rate of redislocation that exists in patients younger than 30 years old reinforces the concept that such patients may have a different pathologic basis than those older than 40, who have a much lower redislocation rate. In a cadaveric study of 182 shoulders, Hertz[26] demonstrated a difference in pathology in the two age groups. He showed that identical movements producing dislocation caused different lesions. In the younger age group, there was either disruption of the labrum from the osseous margin of the scapula or splitting of the fibers near their bases. In the older age group, there were no lesions of the labrum, but ruptures of the joint capsule occurred. Increased forces were required to produce dislocations in the younger group. Hertz[26] believed that these data supported the explanation that the primary disruption of the labrum in younger patients was responsible for redislocation and that these lesions could not heal by immobilization alone. This work supported a previous cadaveric study by Reeves,[65] who showed decreased capsular tensile strength as individuals aged. This occurred while the strength of the glenoid labral attachment remained constant.

Baker et al.[4] reported arthroscopic results on the pathology of first-time dislocators younger than age 30. They examined 45 shoulders within 11 days of the initial dislocation and developed a classification system based on the pathology observed: group I, capsular tear with no labral lesion; group II, capsular tear with partial labral detachment; and group III, capsular tears with complete labral detachment. Group III patients were grossly unstable on examination under anesthesia, whereas group I patients were stable. Of the 45 patients in the study, only six (13%) had no labral lesion; 39 (87%) had Bankart lesions.

Military personnel have provided a large population for studying the results of treatment in young, active patients with first-time dislocations. Wheeler et al.[86] reported a 92% recurrence rate after initial anterior dislocation of the shoulder in West Point cadets. This occurred despite traditional nonoperative treatment programs, which included 3 weeks of immobilization and a physical therapy program that was poorly followed. Given these retrospective results, Wheeler et al. performed an arthroscopic Bankart repair in nine subsequent patients and noted labral detachment in all nine, but no interstitial damage in the IGHL. The recurrence rate for the nine was only 22%.

Arciero et al.[1] performed a prospective study using two treatment modalities for patients with first-time dislocations. One group of patients was treated nonoperatively with immobilization for 4 weeks and subsequent rehabilitation. The second group underwent diagnostic arthroscopy, arthroscopic Bankart repair, and the same rehabilitation program as the first group. Of the 15 patients in the nonoperative group, 80% developed recurrent instability. Of the 21 patients in the operative group (all with grade III Bankart lesions), only 14% developed recurrent instability. Arciero et al.[1] noted that after initial dislocation, one would not expect to see a degenerated or absent labrum, marked capsular attenuation, or a large Hill–Sachs lesion, which are commonly encountered in a patient with chronic instability. This led them to believe that acute dislocation provides the optimal situation for success with arthroscopic repair. Neither West Point study, however, addressed the treatment of patients with other than grade III lesions of the labrum. This is inconsistent with Baker's study, which showed that 18 of 45 patients had such lesions.[4]

Despite the promising results reported by Arciero et al.[1] for arthroscopic repair of first-time dislocations, we prefer to manage all patients with grade I and grade II lesions nonoperatively and to treat grade III lesions by diagnostic arthroscopy followed by open repair.

Indications for Arthroscopic Stabilization

The role of arthroscopy in the treatment of anterior shoulder instability has continued to evolve. Although there are no clearly defined indications for arthroscopic repair of anterior instability lesions, the ideal patient is a noncontact-sport athlete with anterior instability secondary to a traumatic injury, with a thick mobile Bankart lesion and little or no discernable capsular laxity.

Currently, the rate of recurrent instability after treatment with arthroscopic techniques exceeds the rate of recurrence reported with open surgical procedures (Table 1).[21] Nevertheless, arthroscopic repair has several theoretical advantages compared with open procedures, including minimizing surgical dissection, damage to surrounding tissues, and scarring. These factors may allow more rapid rehabilitation and improved range of motion. The arthroscope also allows improved visualization of the capsulolabral complex as well as other articular lesions[79] and is associated with less morbidity than open techniques. Theoretically, increased scarring associated with open surgery may contribute to postoperative loss of motion. Limited external rotation after anterior shoulder surgery may be caused by loss of normal elasticity of the shoulder or by overtightening of the anterior capsule and subscapularis. Unlike some open procedures, all arthroscopic methods address the pathology of the anterior capsulolabral complex. However, the technical manner by which the anterior capsulolabral complex is reattached to the glenoid rim and how much the anterior capsule is advanced also differs between arthroscopic and open procedures. One potential disadvantage of the arthroscopic approach is that it may not afford as precise a repair of the attenuated anterior aspect of the capsule as the open approach.

Two types of fixation are commonly used in arthroscopic shoulder repairs: (a) a stapling or tacking device (Fig. 35), and (b) sutures (Fig. 36). The role of tacking devices has evolved from early stapling devices to bioabsorbable tacks.[38,49,81,92] Matthews et al.[49] reported that of 25 shoulders treated with arthroscopic staple capsulorraphy, 67% had good or excellent results at an average follow-up of 36 months. From 1984 to 1989, Lane et al.[38] performed arthroscopic staple capsulorrhaphy on 54 patients, using a ligamentous and capsule repair staple. At an average follow-up of 39 months, 33% of the patients had experienced at least one episode of postoperative instability, and routine radiographs at follow-up demonstrated loose staples in 15% of asymptomatic patients.

TABLE 1. *Summary of recurrence rates cumulated from 50 published series*

Type of procedure	Recurrence rate (%)
Open	
Putti-Platt	3.0
Magnuson-Stack	4.1
Eden-Hybbinette	6.0
Gallie	2.9
DuTolt and Roux	2.0
Bristow-Latarjet	1.7
Bankart	3.3
Anterior capsulolabral reconstruction	3.4
Arthroscopic	4–40[a]

[a] Depending on selection, technique, and follow-up.
From ref. 21, with permission.

The staple repair technique has been associated with an unacceptable incidence of complications related to the use of metal implants adjacent to the joint.[49,92] To overcome this problem, an arthroscopic repair using a bioabsorbable device was developed. This device appeared promising because it seemed technically easier to use than other available methods. Warner et al.,[84] however, noted several technical difficulties in performing the arthroscopic repair using the bioabsorbable tack in a cadaver model. Four technical errors occurred: inadequate abrasion of the scapular neck, inadequate superior and medial shift of the IGHL before placement of the lowest tack, medial placement of the tack relative to the articular margin, and insufficient capture and compression of the capsular tissue by the device. Initial enthusiasm for this technique was dampened by clinical work by Speer et al.[81] They performed arthroscopically assisted repair, using bioabsorbable cannulated tacks, on 52 consecutive patients with recurrent anterior instability of the shoulder. Patients were evaluated at an average follow-up of 42 months. The repair was considered to have failed in 21% of the patients, requiring reoperation.

To avoid the problems posed by staples and tacking devices, suture repair methods have become popular. These methods involve suturing the detached capsulolabral complex to the abraded anterior glenoid rim. There are two basic methods. In the original transglenoid method, sutures are placed through drill holes across the glenoid neck and tied posteriorly. The second method uses implanted suture anchors to fasten the sutures to bone.

Morgan and Bodenstab[53] used two modified Beath pins to spear and gather the detached labrum, then passed a no. 1 PDS suture from anterior to posterior across the glenoid. They tied the sutures together in front, creating a mattress stitch across the anterior aspect of the Bankart lesion, then tied the sutures posteriorly over the thick fascia of the posterior third of the deltoid and infraspinatus. Morgan[52] later reported that, of 175 patients who underwent a transglenoid suture repair with a 1- to 6-year follow-up, 95% had excellent results; there was a 5% failure rate (8 patients). Of the 8 failures, 7 occurred in contact-sport athletes. They concluded that contraindications to arthroscopic repair included patients involved in collision athletics and patients with generalized laxity. Caspari[12] developed a suture punch that allows placement of a no. 1 PDS suture in the anterior capsulolabral complex. Once the damaged tissue has been securely grasped with multiple simple sutures, the sutures are brought out through the anterior opening cannula and threaded through a single pin that is drilled across the anterior superior glenoid to exit posteriorly. The sutures are divided into two groups and tied over the infraspinatus fascia. Caspari[12] noted that 4% of the patients required reoperation and another 4% suffered postoperative subluxation episodes. O'Keefe et al.[58] reinforced the improved results in suture technique over staple and tack techniques. In a dog

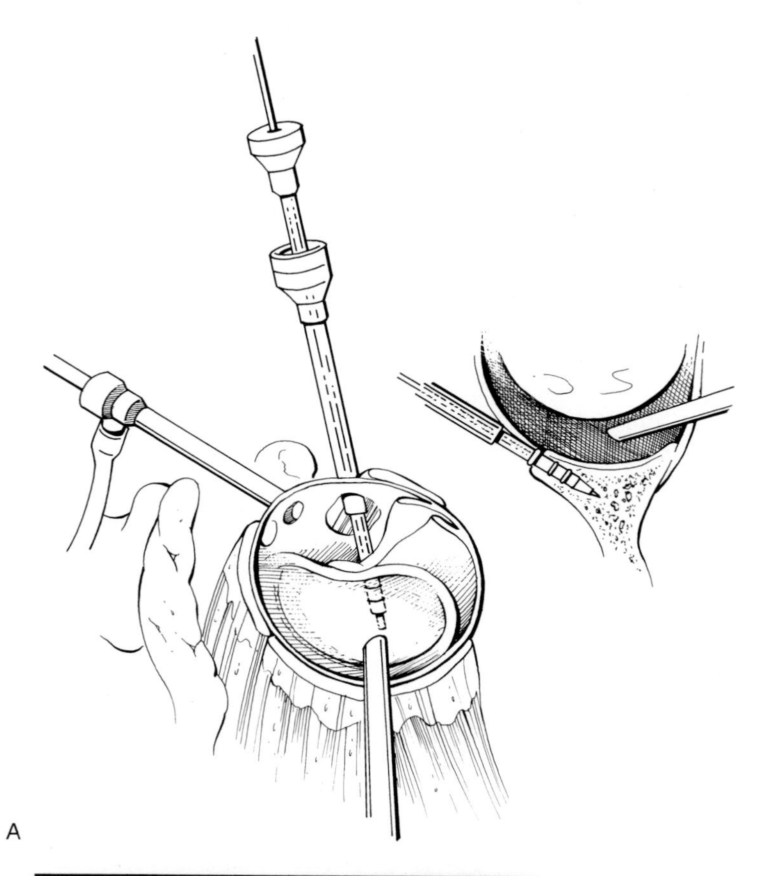

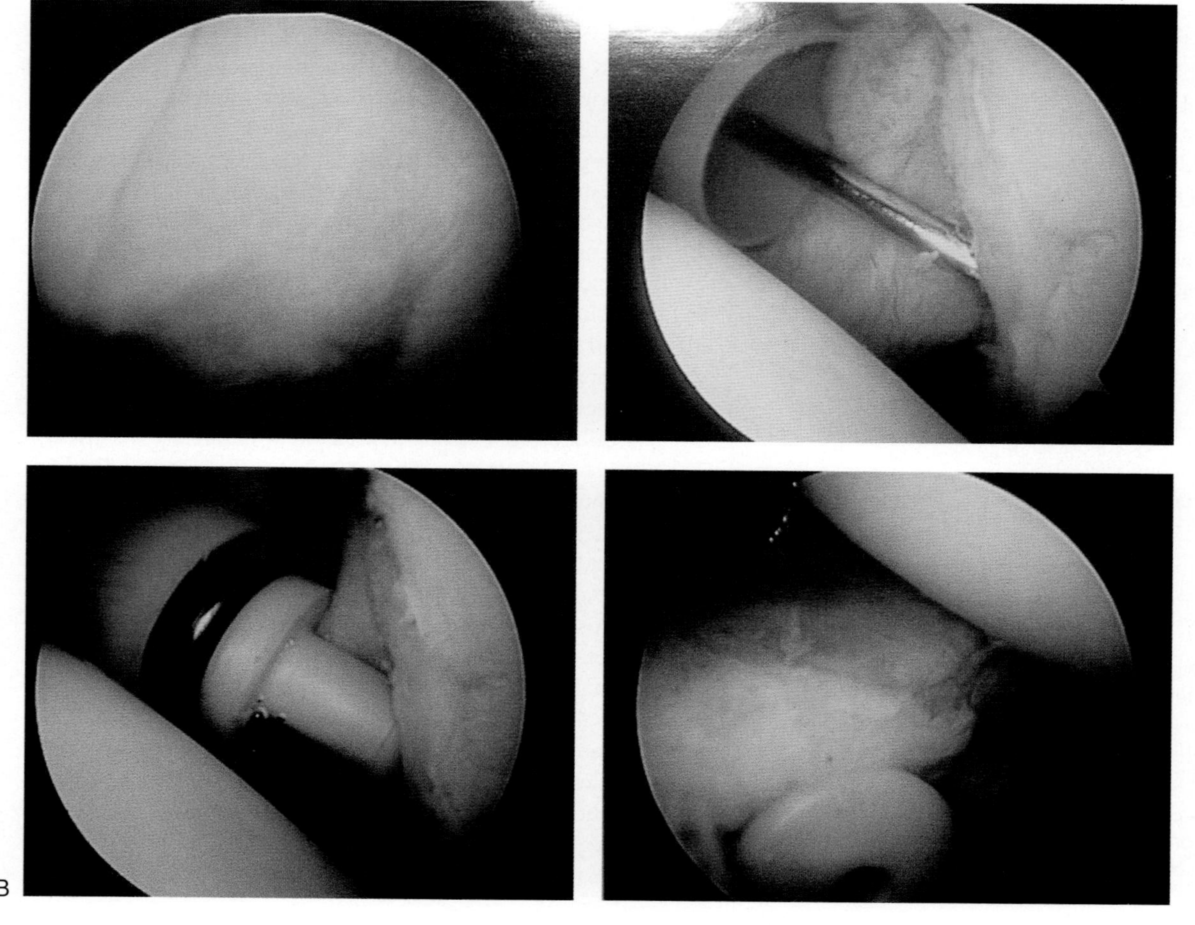

FIG. 35. (A) Arthroscopic procedure for repair of Bankart lesion using bioabsorbable tack. **(B)** Arthroscopic view of an absorbable tack stabilization of an anterior labrum tear (Bankart lesion). (Panel A from ref. 81, with permission.)

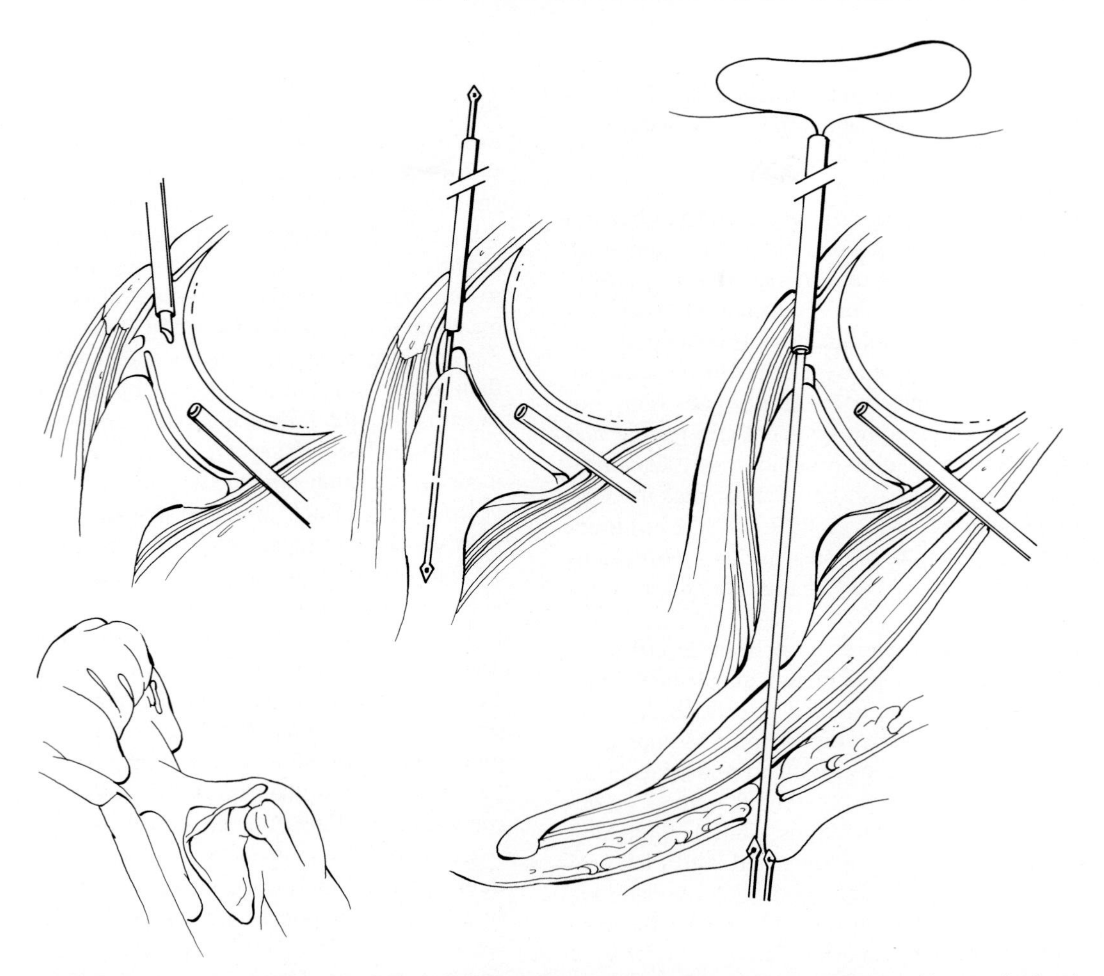

FIG. 36. Transglenoid suture technique of arthroscopic stabilization. (From ref. 60, with permission.)

model, they demonstrated that Bankart lesions repaired by Morgan's suture technique had twice the tensile strength of staple repair. However, the suture repair groups were three times weaker than the undamaged capsulolabral complexes. Recent reports describe less successful results and recommend caution in arthroscopic stabilization. Youssef et al.[91] could not reproduce the results of Caspari[12] in 30 consecutive patients, obtaining a 27% failure rate. Disadvantages of the transglenoid repair include technical difficulty, risk of neurovascular injury, and the potential for loosening of the repair owing to elasticity of the PDS suture.

Snyder and Strafford[79] described using a suture anchor with a no. 2 Ethibond suture and a shuttle system for the repair of Bankart lesions. They also described a method of arthroscopic capsular plication, with a no. 1 Ticron suture, for a patient in whom no Bankart lesion was found. Bacilla et al.[3] performed an arthroscopic repair using nonabsorbable sutures and anchors in 40 consecutive patients. They reported a 93% success rate at 30 months follow-up.

Arthroscopic techniques using staples, tacks, and sutures are not well suited to performing capsular shifts in patients with capsular laxity. The use of nonablative laser treatment to perform capsular shrinkage has recently been studied. In a multiinstitutional trial by Hayashi et al.,[24] a nonablative level of holmium:yttrium-aluminum-garnet (Ho:YAG) laser was applied to the anterior capsule under arthroscopic guidance in patients with glenohumeral instability, but without capsulolabral detachment or full-thickness rotator cuff tears. They reported that the nonablative application of laser shrank the joint capsule, stabilizing the shoulder in most patients. In a rabbit study, Thabit[82] reported laser energy in nonablative levels can significantly alter joint capsule length and its mechanical properties. Although nonablative laser treatment appears to shrink capsular laxity, no long-term clinical study exists to support its use. Heat-controlled devices have been used most recently for thermal capsulorrhaphy. The initial results have been encouraging in patients with microtraumatic subluxation. These techniques should not be used as an isolated procedure if a Bankart lesion is present. They may be considered in conjunction with a repair of the Bankart lesion. Longer term follow-up will be necessary to define the value of these newer techniques.

It has been our experience, as well as that of others, that the stabilization afforded arthroscopically tends to deteriorate over a longer time period, mandating longer-term follow-up of results.

Open Surgical Treatment

The indications for the surgical treatment of recurrent anterior shoulder instability (pain, and limitation of activity after a thorough trial of nonoperative management) are highly subjective.

Although arthroscopic repair of surgical instability has proved to have mixed results, open procedures appear to have a more reliable success rate. A decision to perform surgery and the choice of procedure performed should be individualized based on the pathologic process creating the instability and on the training and experience of the surgeon. Patients with voluntary anterior instability are often poor surgical candidates; they require psychologic testing and may benefit from a rehabilitation program.[70] A trial of prolonged rehabilitation should also be used for patients with generalized ligamentous laxity or those with multidirectional instability. In addition, the presence of a Hill–Sachs lesion or glenoid deficiency may change the surgical approach.

Many open surgical procedures have been described as successful treatments for anterior glenohumeral instability. The major procedures can be divided into three different groups: capsular, subscapularis, and bony. Capsular reattachment procedures, such as the Bankart and Matsen repairs, are based on repairing the "essential lesion," as described by Perthes[64] and Bankart.[6] Subscapularis tightening procedures, such as the Magnuson-Stack and Putti-Platt procedures, are designed to realign and tighten the subscapularis and to limit external rotation. Bony procedures have been developed to augment the bony anterior glenoid. The Bristow procedure provides a bony block and a musculotendinous sling across the anteroinferior glenohumeral joint by transferring the coracoid to the glenoid neck. Other conditions, such as a large Hill–Sachs lesion, may require an osteotomy or an infraspinatus transfer. In Sweden, osteotomies of the proximal humerus have been performed to realign the version of the glenohumeral joint.[85]

Glenoid deficiency may present a unique management problem. An acute glenoid fracture involving greater than one-fourth of the glenoid fossa and associated with shoulder instability is an indication for open reduction of the fragment with screw fixation.[10] A CT scan may be useful in determining fragment size and displacement. Anterior glenoid avulsion fractures are common and require no additional treatment.

Capsular Repairs. Bankart[6] and Perthes[64] described capsular repair by reattaching the detached anterior capsule to the anterior glenoid. Bankart[6] described the repair of the capsule to the bone of the anterior glenoid through the use of drill holes and sutures. The subscapularis muscle, which is carefully divided to expose the capsule, is reapproximated without any overlap or shortening. He reported no evidence of recurrence in 27 consecutive patients.

In describing long-term results with the Bankart procedure, Rowe et al.[69] developed a rating system for repair based on stability, motion, and function (Table 2). Over a 30-year period, they noted a 3.5% recurrence rate in 162 operatively managed shoulders, indicating that the results were excellent in 74% and good in 23%; 69% of the patients had full range of motion. They also noted that a fracture of the rim of the glenoid did not increase the risk of recurrence, but that a moderate to severe Hill–Sachs lesion increased the risk slightly. They performed primary repairs on patients with up to one-fourth of the glenoid fossa avulsed, achieving good to excellent results in all but 1 of 15 patients. They reported that 33% of the patients in throwing sports were able to return to their sports with the same level of proficiency, and that the other 67% could throw a baseball hard, but not with the same velocity as before surgery. There was no evidence of osteoarthritic changes in the 124 patients seen in follow-up.

Rosenberg et al.[68] reported that of 31 patients managed with the Bankart repair, only 13 were normal at follow-up; 14 had minimal degenerative changes, 3 had moderate changes, and 1 had severe degenerative changes (average follow-up, 15 years). Rowe et al.[72] also reported on recurrent anterior dislocation of the shoulder after surgical repair: Of 11 patients with lesions previously repaired by the Bankart procedure, 3 had intact repair at the time of reoperation. The underlying cause of the postoperative instability appeared to be severe laxity of the capsule. The other 8 patients had disruption of the Bankart repair as well as capsular laxity.

Currently, suture anchors (which can simplify the procedure) are commonly used in open Bankart reconstructions. In a follow-up report by Levine et al.,[41] 32 patients underwent this procedure, with no complications from the suture anchor technique. However, there were 2 failures (recurrent anterior dislocations). Hovelius et al.[31] found a 2% redislocation rate after Bankart procedure compared with a 19% redislocation rate with the Putti-Platt procedure. More than one-third of the patients younger than age 25 were dissatisfied with the Putti-Platt procedure. The Bankart repair is frequently modified to adjust for capsular laxity, which makes this the procedure of choice for many orthopedic surgeons.

(1) *Matsen procedure.* In 1989, Thomas and Matsen[83] described a procedure for repairing the anterior glenoid labrum without separating the subscapularis from the capsule (Fig. 37). They recommended detaching the capsule with the subscapularis tendon from the lesser tuberosity and reflecting it medially, exposing the anterior glenoid. A direct repair of the capsule can then be performed by placing suture through the anterior glenoid. The subscapularis can then be reattached without advancement. For patients with capsular laxity, they recommended advancing the subscapularis. At 5.5 years average follow-up, good to excellent results were reported in 97% of patients. Range of motion was maintained with an average of 171 degrees of forward flexion and 84 degrees of external rotation in abduction.

(2) *Rockwood method.* The capsular imbrication procedure (Fig. 38), as described by Wirth et al.[88] and Lusardi et al.,[44] addresses not only the repair of the capsule to the ante-

TABLE 2. *Rating system for Bankart repair*

Scoring system	Units	Excellent (100–90)	Good (89–75)	Fair (74–51)	Poor (50 or less)
Stability					
No recurrence, subluxation, or apprehension	50	No recurrences	No recurrences	No recurrences	Recurrence of dislocation *or*
Apprehension when placing arm in certain positions	30	No apprehension when placing arm in complete elevation and external rotation	Mild apprehension when placing arm in elevation and external rotation	Moderate apprehension during elevation and external rotation	Marked apprehension during elevation or extension
Subluxation (not requiring reduction)	10	No subluxations	No subluxations	No subluxations	
Recurrent dislocation	0				
Motion					
100% of normal external rotation, internal rotation, and elevation	20	100% of normal external rotation; complete elevation and internal rotation	75% of normal external rotation; complete elevation and internal rotation	50% of normal external rotation; 75% of elevation and internal rotation	No external rotation; 50% of elevation (can get hand only to face) and 50% of internal rotation
75% of normal external rotation, and normal elevation and internal rotation	15				
50% of normal external rotation and 75% of normal elevation and internal rotation	5				
50% of normal elevation and internal rotation; no external rotation	0				
Function					
No limitation in work or sports; little or no discomfort	30	Performs all work and sports; no limitation in overhead activities; shoulder strong in lifting, swimming, tennis, throwing; no discomfort	Mild limitation in work and sports; shoulder strong; minimum discomfort	Moderate limitation doing overhead work and heavy lifting; unable to throw, serve hard in tennis, or swim; moderate disabling pain	Marked limitation; unable to perform overhead work and lifting; cannot throw, play tennis, or swim; chronic discomfort
Mild limitation and minimum discomfort	25				
Moderate limitation and discomfort	10				
Marked limitation and pain	0				
Total units possible	100				

From ref. 69, with permission.

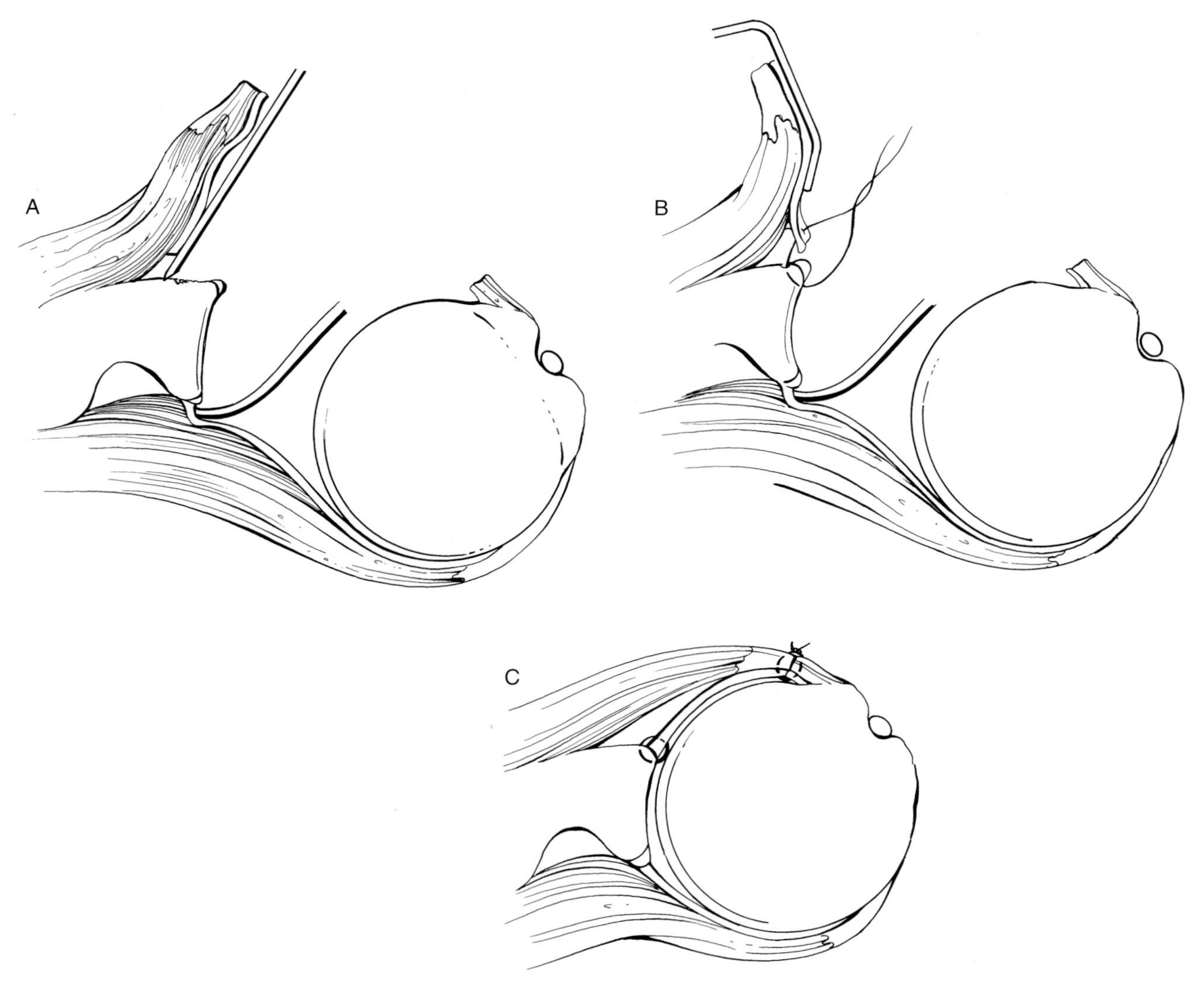

FIG. 37. Matsen procedure: **(A)** The subscapularis is reflected with the capsule, exposing the Bankart lesion. **(B)** After the anterior glenoid neck is roughened with a curette, the Bankart lesion may be repaired. **(C)** The subscapularis is then reattached in its anatomic position to limit loss of external rotation. (From ref. 83, with permission.)

rior labrum, but also the issue of capsular laxity. The subscapularis tendon is divided and reflected off the capsule. The lateral stump of the subscapularis tendon is also reflected from the capsule, exposing the entire capsule. The capsule is then divided vertically midway between its attachment on the glenoid rim and the humeral head. The joint is inspected for labral tear and stripping of the labrum, capsule, and periosteum off their normal attachments on the glenoid rim and the neck of the scapula. If stripping is noted, the capsule is reattached using sutures, followed by imbrication of the anterior capsule. The extent of the anteroinferior capsular laxity determines the degree of imbrication necessary to reduce the glenohumeral joint. In shoulders with a large degree of capsular laxity, the medial aspect of the capsule is often shifted 10 to 15 mm medially and superiorly and is imbricated for 15 to 20 mm by the lateral aspect of the capsule. After this procedure, the lateral aspect of the capsule is "double-breasted" by shifting the lax lateral capsule medially and superiorly and suturing it down to the anterior surface of the medial aspect of the capsule. Lusardi et al.[44] believed that this procedure eliminated laxity and provided added strength to the anterior capsule. Subsequently, the subscapularis tendon is anatomically repaired. In a study of 132 patients,[88] 93% had good or excellent results from this procedure at a minimum follow-up of 2 years. Patients sustained a loss of external rotation of 7 degrees compared with the contralateral side, and there was a 96% success rate on apprehension testing.

(3) *Neer Inferior capsular shift.* Neer and Foster[55] described a capsular shift procedure to address involuntary inferior and multidirectional instability related to capsular laxity (Fig. 39). The goal of this operation is to reduce joint volume. After thorough psychiatric evaluation, followed by initial re-

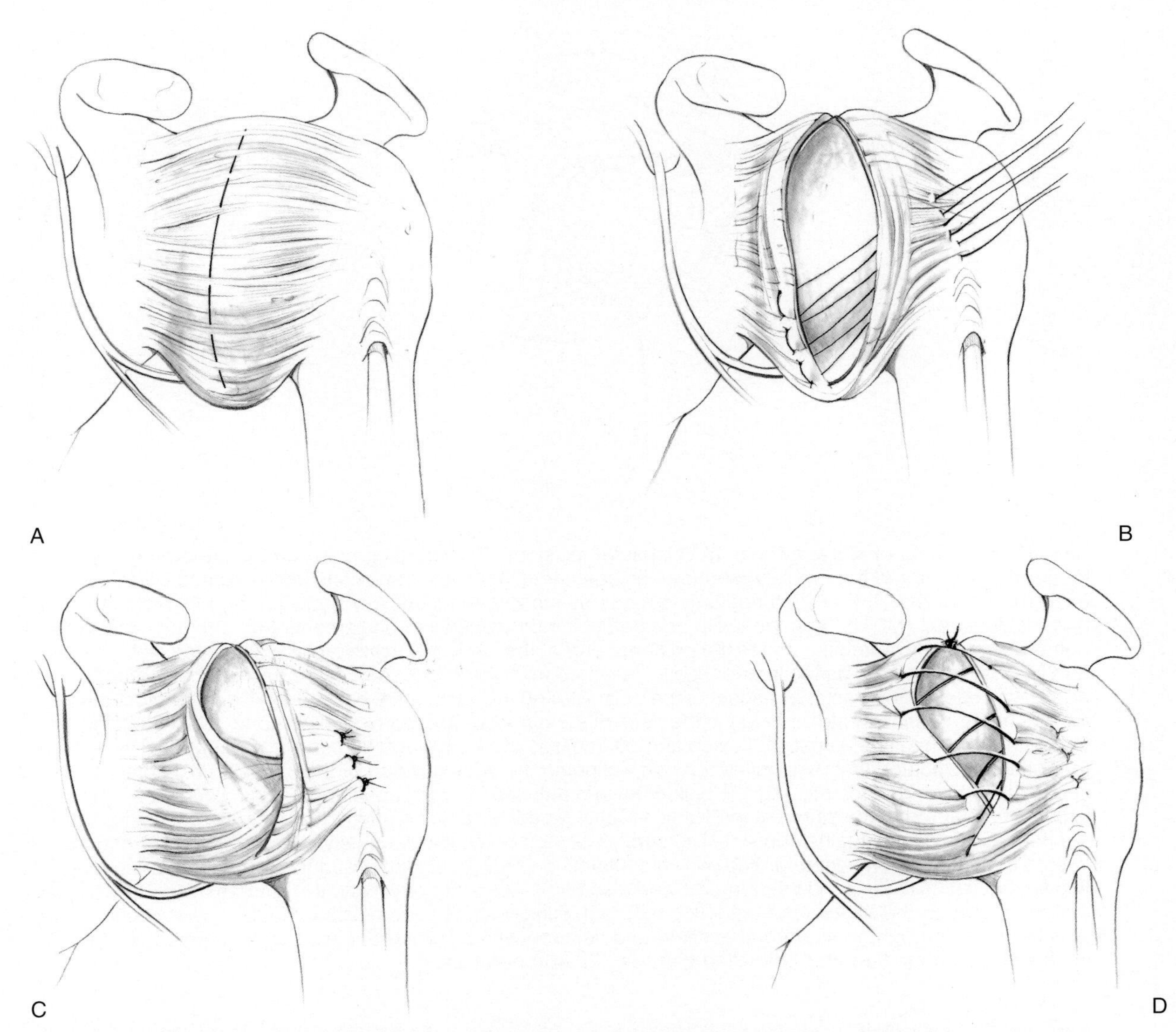

FIG. 38. Rockwood method: **(A)** Division of the capsule vertically midway between the glenoid and humeral attachment. **(B)** The medial aspect of the capsule is overlapped laterally and superiorly under the lateral aspect of the capsule. **(C)** The medial aspect of the capsule is secured under the lateral aspect of the capsule with the arm held in 30 degrees of external rotation, and the lateral aspect of the capsule is advanced superiorly and medially over the medial aspect of the capsule, creating a double thickness of the weakened capsule. **(D)** If a capsular gap occurs, the defect may be repaired by lacing 1-mm–wide Dacron tape across the gap. (From ref. 44, with permission.)

habilitation, a capsular shift is performed, reducing the volume of the inferior portion of the capsule by detaching the capsule from the neck of the humerus and shifting it to the opposite side of the calcar. This maneuver not only obliterates the inferior pouch and capsular laxity on the side of the approach, but also reduces laxity on the opposite side. In a cadaveric study, Lubowitz et al.[43] showed that the inferior capsular shift reduced shoulder volume by 57%. Bigliani et al.[9] performed the Neer capsular shift procedure on 68 shoulders in 63 athletes. There was a 7 degree average loss of external rotation and a 2.9% incidence of recurrent postoperative dislocation. Of the 63 athletes, 92% returned to their sports and 75% of those returned to the same level of competitiveness. All 31 athletes involved in overhead sports returned to their sports (71% at the same level). Of the 10 overhead athletes who were involved primarily in throwing, 5 returned to the same level and 5 returned to throwing, but at a lower effectiveness rate than before surgery. Of the 6 professional or varsity athletes, only 2 returned to the same level of sports. In this series, 31% of the patients had a history of dislocation and had a Bankart lesion. The Bankart lesion is repaired at the time of the capsular shift. The series showed a 96% rate of good or excellent results and a redislocation rate of only 1.5%. No patient had recurrent subluxation.

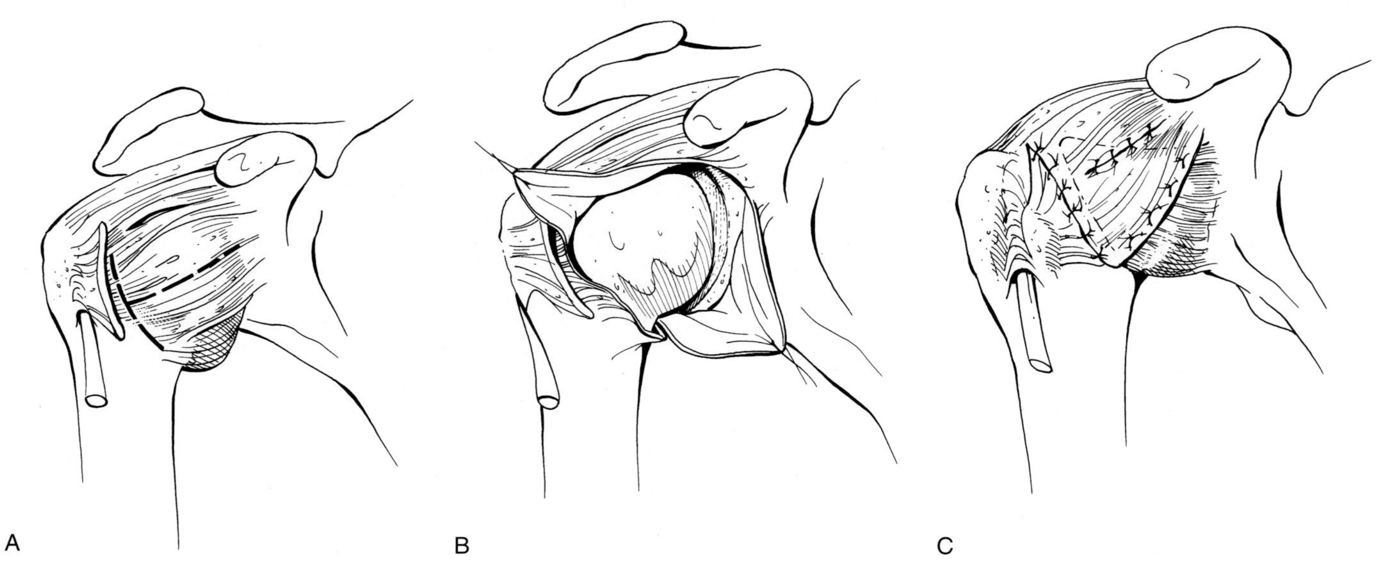

FIG. 39. Neer inferior capsular shift: **(A)** Capsular incisions. The opening between the superior glenohumeral ligament and the medial glenohumeral ligament (which is almost constant) is closed with nonabsorbable sutures. A T-shaped opening is made by incising longitudinally between the middle glenohumeral ligament (MGHL) and the IGHL and detaching the capsule and ligaments from the neck of the humerus anteriorly, inferiorly, and to the posterior part of the neck. **(B)** Preparation of flaps and slot. The arm is externally rotated as the inferior flap is detached from the inferior part of the neck of the humerus, all the way back to the posterior aspect of the neck. During this step, a flat elevator is used to protect the axillary nerve. A shallow slot is made in the neck of the humerus anteriorly and inferiorly. **(C)** Relocating the flaps. The arm is held in slight flexion and 10 degrees of external rotation on the arm board. The inferior flap is relocated first. It is pulled forward to tighten the posterior part of the capsule until posterior subluxation no longer occurs, and it is pulled upward until the inferior capsular pouch is eliminated. The flap is then sutured to the stump of the subscapularis tendon and to the part of the capsule remaining on the humerus to hold it against the slot. The surplus portion of the flap is usually folded over to further reinforce the capsule. The superior flap, which contains the MGHL, is then brought down over the inferior flap so that it acts to suspend the humerus and also reinforces anteriorly. Note the sutures used to close the cleft between the MGHL and the IGHL before making the capsular incision. Finally, the subscapularis tendon is brought to its normal position and secured with nonabsorbable sutures so that it will remain a strong internal rotator. (Modified from ref. 55, with permission.)

When surgical treatment is considered for patients with multidirectional instability, the direction of primary instability and the location of the primary pathology must be determined. In patients with inferior laxity, standard procedures developed for anterior instability may fail. A capsular shift procedure may be required to correct the laxity of the inferior capsule. In patients with anterior and posterior multidirectional instability, overtightening of the capsule can result in subluxation in the direction opposite that of the capsular shift.

(4) *Jobe reconstruction.* The Jobe reconstruction[33,36,37] is a modified anterior capsulolabral shift, in which the subscapularis tendon is split transversely in line with its fibers at the junction of the upper two-thirds with the lower third (Fig. 40). A horizontal anterior capsulotomy is then made in line with the split of the subscapularis tendon. The labrum is left intact if still attached. If it is not, the anterior neck is decorticated and a superior flap is shifted inferiorly, overlapping and reinforcing the inferior flap that was previously shifted superiorly but not medially. Kvitne et al.[37] obtained 97% good or excellent results, with 81% of the patients returning to the same level of competition; 100% of the patients were subjectively satisfied with the operation. At the 2-year follow-up, no complications related to the use of fixation devices had occurred.

Subscapularis Procedures. The current trend in orthopedics is away from subscapularis-based procedures. These procedures have a tendency to decrease external rotation and, although results are excellent in terms of redislocation rates, the patients have higher rates of dissatisfaction and osteoarthritis.

The Putti-Platt operation was described by Osmond-Clark in 1948.[59] This procedure shortens the subscapularis muscle unit by doubling it in a vest-over-pants fashion over the anterior glenohumeral joint. This limits external rotation and causes scarring in the anterior portion of the shoulder. Magnuson and Stack[45] described a procedure that involves transfer of the subscapularis tendon from the lesser to the greater tuberosity across the bicipital groove and 1 cm distally, which is believed to strengthen the anterior

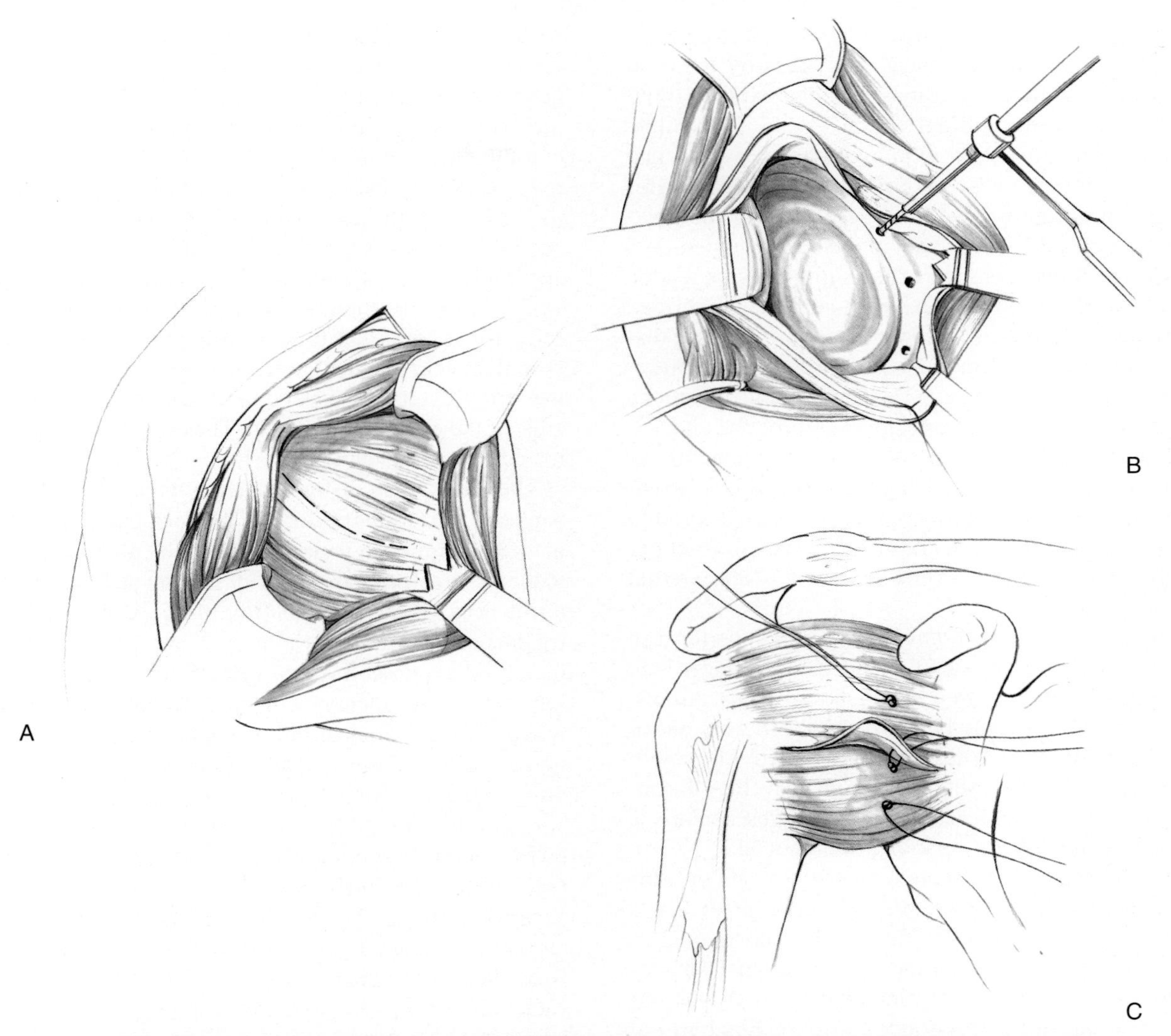

FIG. 40. **(A)** Glenohumeral joint capsule exposure: *Dotted line* indicates site of capsulotomy. **(B)** Suture anchors are placed. **(C)** Superior capsular flap is shifted anteriorly, overlying the inferior flap. (From ref. 36, with permission.)

muscle barrier. As described by Magnuson and Stack, the operation results in 25% to 50% limitation of external rotation. Results of the Putti-Platt procedure show a long-term success rate of approximately 95%,[39,66] but it limits external rotation by 12 to 28.8 degrees. Regan et al.[66] reported that 22% of patients who had a Putti-Platt procedure had to modify throwing (compared with 38% in the Magnuson and Stack study[45]) and that 52% of patients with Magnuson-Stack procedures returned to their preinjury levels of competition.

Bony Procedures. The Bristow procedure, originally described by Helfet[25] and later modified several times,[50] provides a bony block to dislocation by transferring the coracoid with the attached conjoined tendon to the neck of the scapula through an opening in the subscapularis tendon. This also reinforces the capsule with the conjoined tendon. Prevention of dislocation with this procedure has been very good (0% to 4%).[5,42,50,78] Nevertheless, Young and Rockwood[90] reported an overall good to excellent outcome in only 50% of 34 patients treated. A high rate of subluxation and hardware complications have been reported with the modified Bristow procedure; in addition, external rotation is frequently limited and overhead athletes usually cannot return to a highly competitive level.[5,42] Failure of this procedure may be related to its inability to address the detached labrum.

Derotation osteotomies of the humerus for instability have been described by Saha and Das.[75] They noted that the retrotorsion of the upper humerus is converted to relative antetorsion as the arm is raised overhead to 120 degrees. An osteotomy was performed that would align the articular surface of the humerus with the glenoid with the arm in 120 degrees of abduction. Although their early results showed no complications in the initial series, this technique has never become popular in the United States.

The interest in addressing large Hill–Sachs lesions is related to the increased recurrence rate noted by Rowe et al.[69] in patients with these lesions. They noted that 100% of their patients with mild deficits had good to excellent results after Bankart repair, with no recurrences, but that those with moderate and severe defects had 5% poor results. Many procedures have been described for the treatment of a severe Hill–Sachs lesion, including humeral osteotomy[85] and transplantation of the supraspinatus tendon into the head defect.[14] Gerber and Lambert[19] described four patients with locked, chronic posterior shoulder dislocations treated with femoral head allograft reconstruction. In this technique, the humeral head is reduced into the joint with an anterior deltopectoral approach, and the femoral head allograft is fashioned to fit the humeral defect and contoured to restore sphericity as much as possible (Fig 41). With this approach, stability was restored to all patients. The goal of humeral osteotomy is to limit external rotation of the joint while preserving full external rotation of the arm.

The Authors' Preferred Method. We prefer to perform an open modified Bankart repair for all patients younger than 50 years old who are involved in athletic activities. Arthroscopic stabilization is reserved for patients 50 years old or older who are involved in less-demanding activities. With this method, the detached anterior labrum as well as the anterior capsular laxity can be addressed. The subscapularis is not shortened, and external rotation is maintained.

After a diagnostic arthroscopy identifying and confirming the suspected pathology, the patient is placed in a supine position and redraped. The patient is positioned so that the axilla is at the edge of the operating table. The patient's contralateral arm is examined for external rotation; this will be used for comparison with the repaired arm at the conclusion of the repair. A rolled towel is not placed under the shoulder because the presence of the towel places anteriorly directed stress on the humeral head. The surgeon stands facing the patient's axilla, a position that provides control over rotation of the arm.

The coracoid is identified and a 6-cm incision originating on the lateral edge of the coracoid is directed toward the axilla, along the lines of Langer (Fig. 42). Soft-tissue dissection is performed to identify the cephalic vein, which provides the landmark for the deltopectoral interval. The vein should be preserved and may be retracted medially or laterally, depending on the individual anatomy. The conjoined tendon is identified and dissected from the underlying subscapularis muscle (Fig. 43A). It may then be retracted with the pectoralis major muscle, using a Richardson retractor. By externally rotating the arm, improved exposure of the subscapularis muscle is achieved (Fig. 43B). Next, the subscapularis muscle must be separated from the underlying joint capsule. As one moves medially along the subscapularis tendon, it becomes easier to separate from the capsule. We find the best location at which to divide the subscapularis is approximately 2 cm medial to its insertion on the humerus. This provides enough of a cuff stump medially to mark with a suture and later reattach. The tendon is divided in a longitudinal fashion perpendicular to its fibers, being careful not to enter the capsule; the inferior one-fourth should be left intact to protect the axillary nerve. A Cobb elevator may help separate the cuff from the capsule medially. The rotator interval should be inspected and, if an interval exists between the supraspinatus and subscapularis, it should be repaired when reattaching the subscapularis tendon. A blunt-tipped-retractor is then carefully positioned along the anterior scapular neck, just medial to the glenoid rim. At this point, the arm is externally rotated to tighten the capsule, and the edge of the glenoid is palpated. The capsule is incised along the edge of the glenoid (Fig. 44).

The arm is then distracted and a humeral head retractor is placed. The articular surface of the glenoid as well as the glenoid labrum can then be visualized. A Cobb elevator is then used to elevate the anterior labrum and expose the anterior neck of the glenoid (Fig. 45A). This area may be roughened with the elevator. A sharp-tipped retractor is then used to retract the detached labrum medially. We prefer to use suture anchors with no. 2 Ethibond sutures for the repair. Three to four of these anchors are placed at the articular margin of the glenoid. It is important to label the sutures so that they may be placed through the capsule in the correct order (Fig. 45B). One arm of the most inferior suture is placed first in the inferior portion of the lateral capsule, followed by the other sutures, proceeding toward the superior aspect of the glenoid. With the arm in internal rotation, the capsule is tightened by tying the inferior suture first, then proceeding superiorly (Fig. 46). Both arms of each suture are then passed on a free needle through the labrum and the medial capsule, which had previously been reflected (Fig. 47A). They are then tied over the medial capsule to reinforce the repair (Fig. 47B). The arm is then tested for external rotation, and it should equal that of the contralateral side. If acceptable external rotation is not obtained, the repair should be repeated after removal of the fixation devices.

The subscapularis is then repaired anatomically, being careful not to overtighten the tendon. If present, the rotator interval is repaired. The deltopectoral interval is then closed. The skin is closed in a subcuticular fashion. We do not routinely place a drain. The patient is placed in a shoulder immobilizer.

Postoperative Care

The timing of our postoperative rehabilitation protocol is described in Table 3. The patient returns for follow-up at 10 days, at which time the immobilizer is removed and rehabilitation is begun with pendulum exercises, isometric shoulder abduction, and internal rotation exercises. The patient should not proceed to regular activity before 3 months.

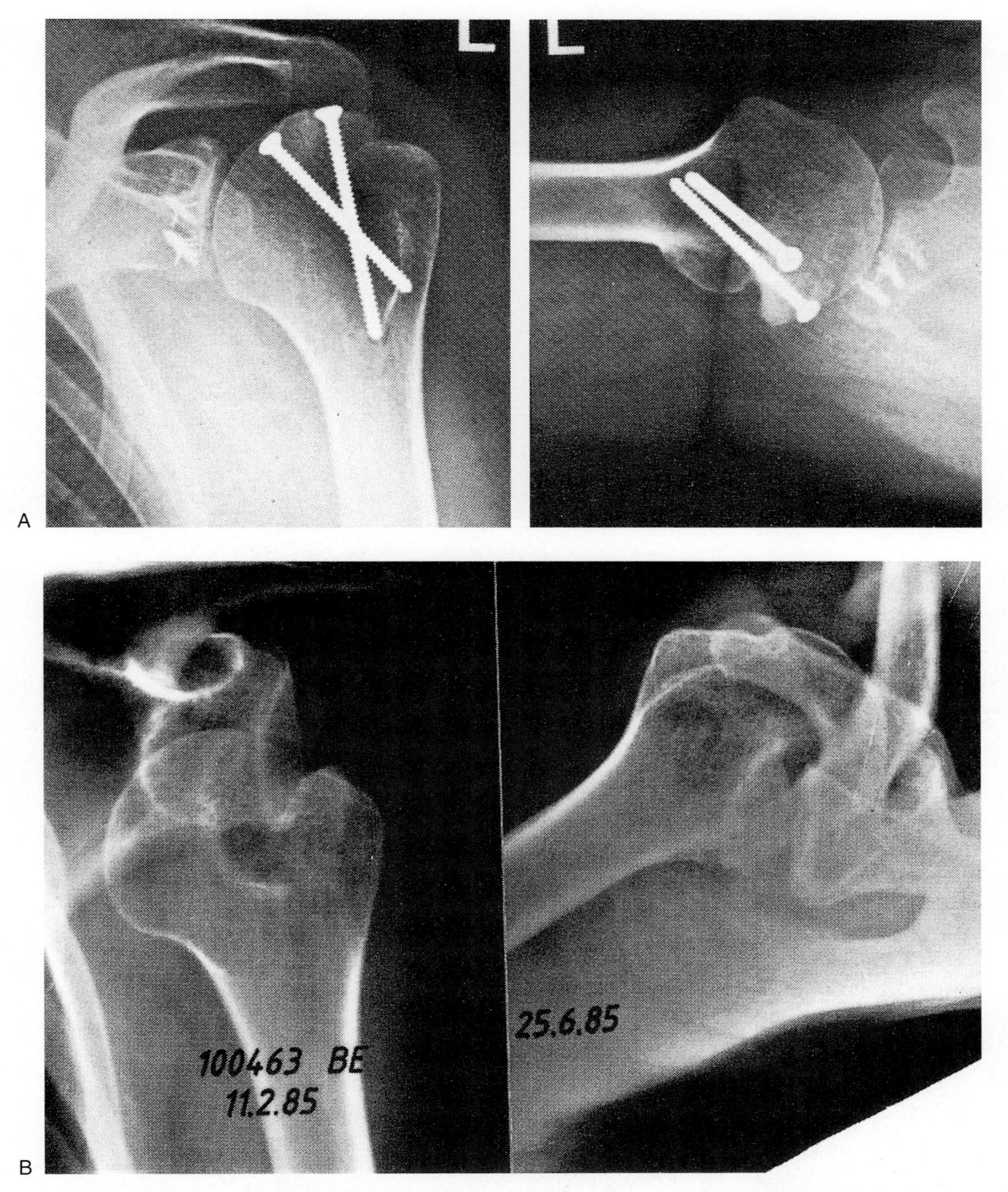

FIG. 41. (A,B) Reconstruction for a chronic anterior dislocation: The allograft is placed into the humeral head defect and the anterior capsular tissues are repaired. (From Gerber C. Chronic locked anterior and posterior dislocations. In: Warner JJ, Iannotti JP, Gerber C, eds. *Complex and revision problems in shoulder surgery*. Philadelphia: Lippincott-Raven, 1997.)

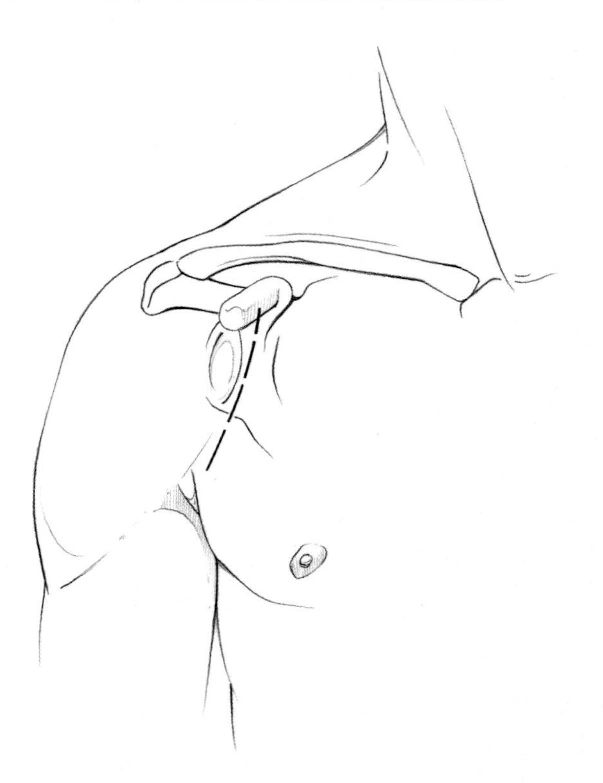

FIG. 42. The incision is based proximally lateral to the coracoid and extends along the lines of Langer.

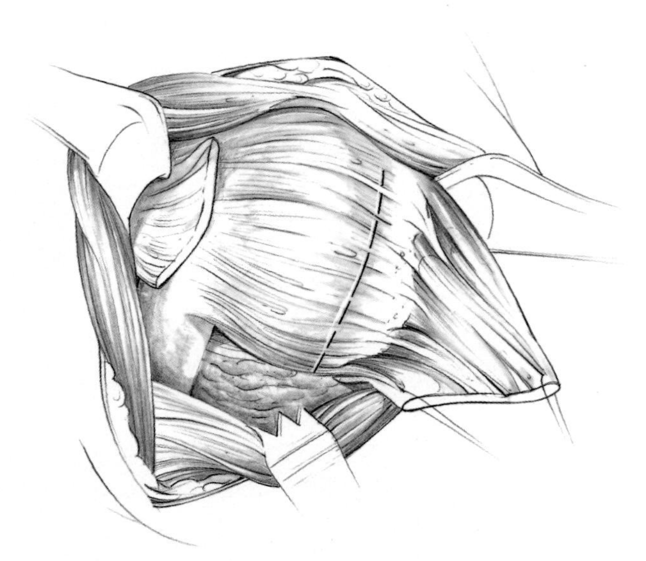

FIG. 44. The capsule is divided along the rim of the glenoid, with the arm in external rotation.

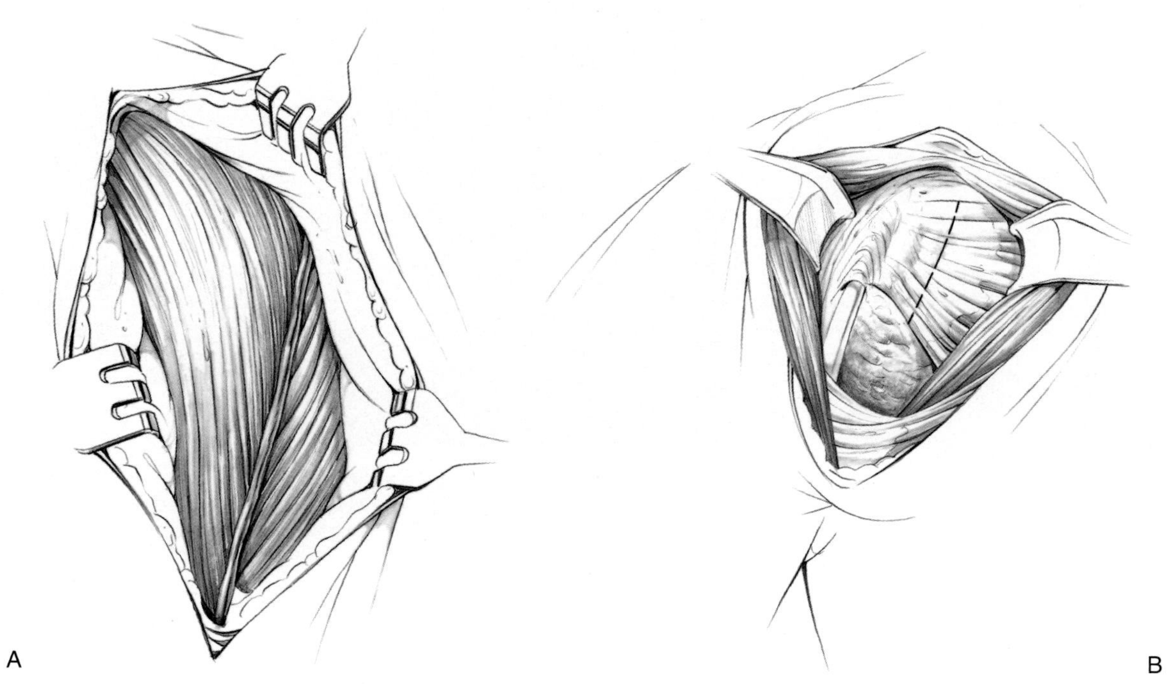

FIG. 43. (A) The conjoined tendon should be retracted medially after a longitudinal incision is made 2 to 3 mm lateral to the tendon. This permits the tendon top to be freely mobile, with minimal trauma to the underlying tissue. **(B)** The subscapularis is divided and reflected from the underlying capsule.

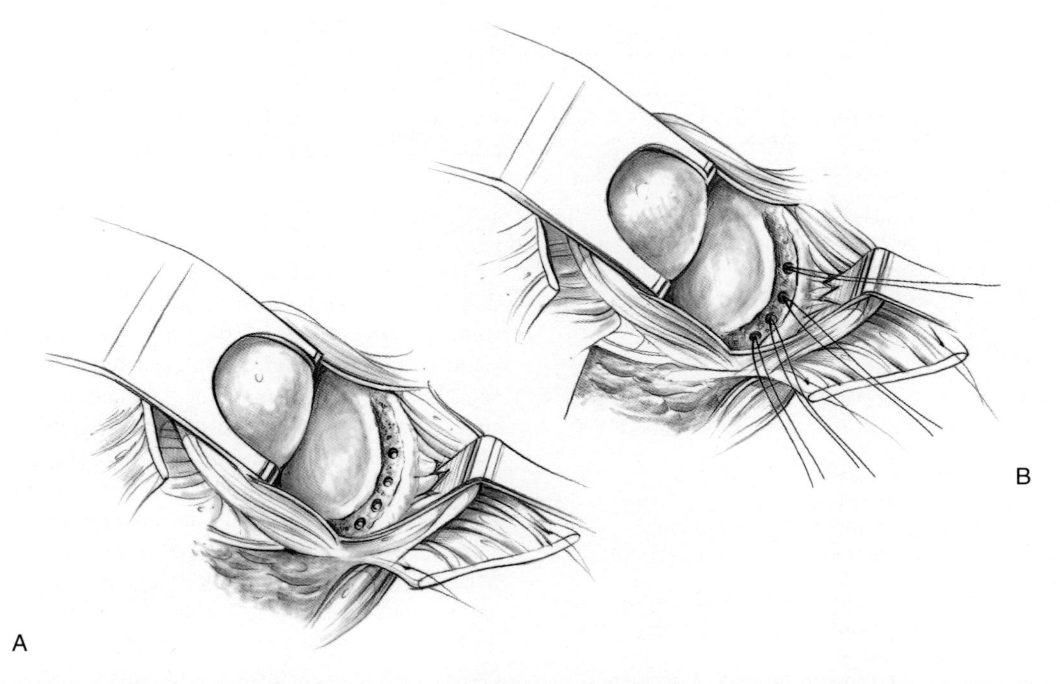

FIG. 45. After a Cobb elevator is used to reflect the soft tissues from the anterior glenoid, **(A)** four holes are drilled, and **(B)** suture anchors are placed.

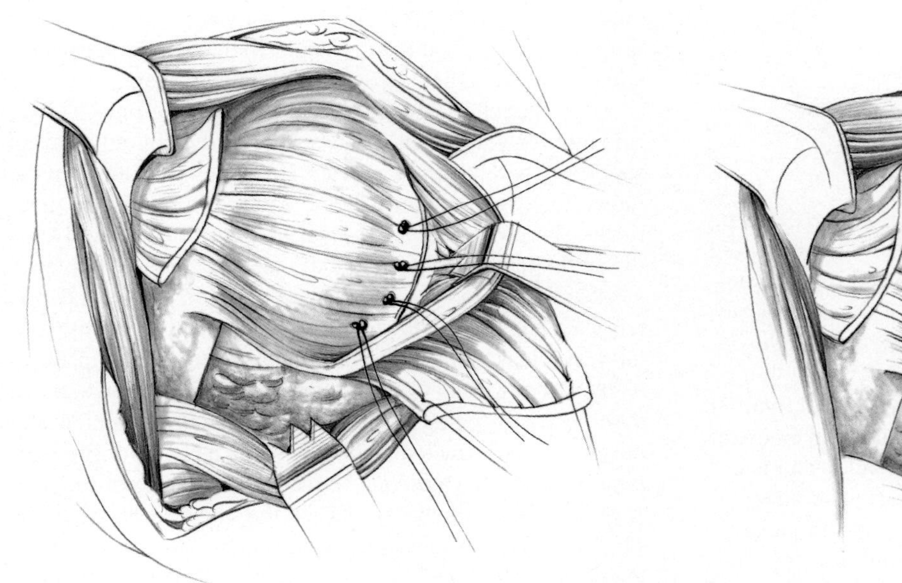

FIG. 46. One strand of the suture is placed through the capsule, and the capsule is shifted superiorly on the neck of the glenoid. The sutures are then tied.

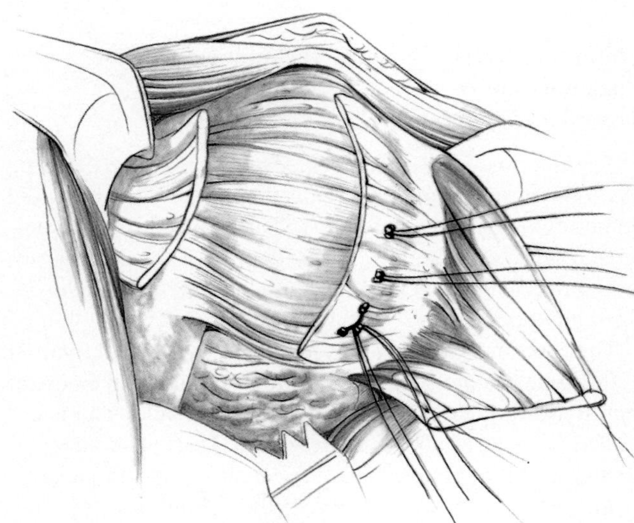

FIG. 47. Both strands of the suture are placed through the medial capsule and tied to reinforce the repair.

TABLE 3. *Postoperative physical therapy protocol*

Time frame	Procedures
0–2 days	Sling can be removed for bathing, dressing, and exercises Active exercises for elbow, wrist, and grip
7–21 days	Wean from sling Pendulum exercises Isometric shoulder abduction and internal rotation exercises
3 weeks	Wall climbing Active assisted ROM, abduction and flexion Continue above
4 weeks	Progressive ROM Active assisted ROM, active ROM, and progressive ROM in flexion, abduction, and internal rotation Progressive resisted exercises Upper body ergometer
6 weeks	Progressive strengthening exercises Isokinetic strengthening when appropriate for patient Isolate external rotation and internal rotation
8–10 weeks	Progressive isokinetic strengthening of internal and external Rotation in increasing ranges of abduction Add isotonic internal and external rotation strengthening
10–12 weeks	Plyoball
3 months	Patient returns to normal activity

ROM, range of motion.

Editors' Preferred Surgical Technique: Anterior Capsulorrhaphy

Superficial Exposure

The anterior approach advocated by the editors is the same for both capsular repair and capsular plication and glenoid bone augmentation procedures. This unified anterior approach allows correction of any degree of anterior capsular–labrum avulsion, capsular laxity, or bone loss that is defined intraoperatively.

The anterior axillary fold is identified by internal rotation of the arm. The incision begins in this anterior skin crease at the inferior border of the pectoralis major tendon and is extended superiorly approximately 6 to 7 cm. The subcutaneous plane is developed along the cephalic vein to the level of the clavicle and within 3 cm of the deltoid insertion site. The investing fascia on the medial side of the cephalic vein is incised over the extent of the subcutaneous dissection, the vein and deltoid muscle are retracted laterally, and the pectoralis major muscle is retraced medially. In heavily muscled patients, incising the upper 1 cm of pectoralis major tendon insertion can facilitate retraction. In many patients, there is a leash of vessels superficial to the clavopectoral fascia that cross over the deltopectoral interval at the level of the tip of the corocoid. These vessels, when necessary, can be ligated to improve exposure. The clavopectoral fascia is incised medial to the corocobrachialis and the short head of the biceps (strap muscles), the musculocutaneous nerve is palpated on the under surface of the muscle to define its location, and these muscle are then retracted medially. In some patients, in whom greater superior exposure is necessary, the corocoacromial ligament can be incised.

Subscapularis Dissection

The structures to be identified are the subscapularis tendon from its bony insertion to its musculotendonous junction, the rotator interval, the long head of the biceps tendon within its groove, and the anterior humeral circumflex vessels. The axillary nerve can be palpated as it courses over the superficial inferior portion of the subscapularis muscle and enters the area under the inferior capsular pouch. The subscapularis tendon is incised with a coagulation Bovie cautery to the level of the capsule. The subscapularis incision begins 1 cm medial to the musculotendinous junction from the upper most portion of the subscapularis, at the rotator interval, and extends inferiorly to the anterior circumflex vessels Fig. 48A. These vessels are not generally ligated, but if more inferior exposure is required, then they can be. At the level of these vessels, the fibers of the subscapularis muscle are bluntly dissected toward the axillary nerve, taking care to protect the nerve from injury. Blunt dissection of the subscapularis at this level will identify the interval between the muscle and capsule. This is more easily accomplished at the inferior portion of the subscapularis than more superiorly where the tendon and capsule are more confluent.

After dissection of the interval between the muscle–capsule inferiorly, the plane of dissection is then bluntly carried superiorly with a narrow elevator. When it is ensured that the interval between the muscle and capsule is developed superiorly, sharp dissection can then be performed laterally between the tendon and capsule to meet the previously placed vertical incision in the tendon (see Fig. 48B). The tendon is retracted medially with traction sutures and the subscapularis muscle is bluntly dissected medially from the capsule to a level 1 cm medial to the glenoid rim. The glenoid rim can then be easily palpated and the subscapularis tendon and muscle can be retracted medial to it with an anterior Bankart-type retractor or Hohmann retractor. Retraction of the subscapularis is facilitated by incising the superior margin of the subscapularis tendon to the glenoid margin, taking care not to cut the underlying capsule or labrum. The entire anterior capsule should now be exposed from the rotator interval to the anterior humeral circumflex vessels. The inferior capsular pouch is then exposed by blunt dissection deep to these vessels and deep to the most inferior portion of the subscapularis tendon. The axillary nerve can now be seen and palpated as it courses over the inferior capsule, and it can be retracted and protected by a blunt retractor. The entire anterior and inferior capsule is now exposed, and the interval between the capsule and lateral stump of the subscapularis tendon is sharply dissected a distance of 5 to 7 mm toward the lesser tuborosity (Fig. 48B).

Lateral Capsulotomy

The arm is placed in the plane of the scapula, 45 degrees abduction, and 45 degrees of external rotation. In this position, the capsule is usually closely applied to the humeral head without any redundancy. If the capsule can be easily pulled away from the humeral head in this arm position, then there is redundancy of the anterior capsular pouch and a capsular shift will likely be necessary. In all anterior procedures, the capsule is incised 5 to 10 mm medial to its insertion on the humeral neck from the rotator interval to the anteroinferior capsular pouch (Fig. 48C). The humeral head is then retracted with a ring retractor and the capsule is retracted medially to inspect the glenoid rim and labrum–capsular attachments. With this exposure, the entire labrum can be examined along with the origin of the biceps tendon, the under surface of the supraspinatus tendon, and the articular surfaces of the glenoid and humeral head. Hill–Sachs lesions can be palpated and, if large, can be seen with extension and internal rotation of the arm.

Repair of the Bankart Lesion

If an avulsion of the capsule and labrum is noted (Bankart lesion), then the lesion is dissected from the glenoid rim medially to the glenoid neck, and the anterior Bankart-type retractor or Hohmann retractor is placed deep to the lesion, thereby exposing the entire anterior glenoid rim. If this exposure is limited by the superior and inferior attachments of the labrum, then additional exposure can be obtained by incision through the rotator interval capsule and labrum at the superior apex of the avulsed labrum. When this is performed, the entire anteroinferior capsule can be retracted medially and inferiorly, because it is hinged on the most inferior extent of the Bankart lesion. The anterior glenoid rim and glenoid are gently decorticated to bleeding bone (Fig. 48D).

Suture anchors are placed at the osteochondral rim of the glenoid. Care is taken not to place these anchors medial to this point (see Fig. 48E). If the glenoid rim has been eroded to a surface that is rounded or flat and even with the glenoid neck, then placement of osseous tunnels is more difficult. When this occurs, but the bone loss is less than 20% of the anterior to posterior glenoid dimension, then bone augmentation is not performed. In this circumstance, the anchors are placed at the margin of the glenoid rim. Two to five suture anchors are placed, with the number of sutures dependent on the size of the lesion. The capsule is then pulled laterally, and the Bankart retractor is placed superficial to the capsule and deep to the subscapularis. The capsule–labrum junction is identified, and both limbs of each suture are passed through this tissue so that when the sutures are tied, the labrum is firmly and anatomically approximated to the glenoid rim (see Fig. 48F). When the labrum and capsule are attenuated, the suture is passed through the labrum and capsule tissue using a "barrel stitch" (see Fig. 48G). With the barrel stitch, the tissue is rolled up, creating a thickened tissue to act as a "new labrum" and as such provide a new "bumper" and restore the concavity of the glenoid fossa.

Lateral Capsular Closure

After completion of the repair of the Bankart lesion, the lateral capsulotomy is closed. The arm is place in the plane of the scapula, 45 to 60 degrees of abduction, and 45 to 60 degrees of external rotation. The arm is held with a sterile intraoperative arm positioner (McConnell arm holder). The capsule is then pulled, with a forceps, laterally and superiorly to simulate closure of the capsule to the capsule on the humeral neck. If there is no capsular redundancy, then the rotator interval and lateral capsule are closed anatomically with nonabsorbable sutures, without any intended shortening of the tissue. The position of the arm is determined by the patient's degree of external rotation in this arm position under anesthesia before making the skin incision, the degree of humeral head anterior translation measured under anesthesia and compared with the normal shoulder, and the degree of generalized ligamentous laxity. In the overhead-throwing athlete, with a Bankart lesion but without generalized ligamentous laxity, the arm is externally rotated to equal the opposite shoulder, and the lateral capsule is closed. When performed in this manner, intraoperative loss of external rotation is approximately 10 to 20 degrees. This intraoperative loss of motion is regained in the postoperative rehabilitation.

If there is mild capsular redundancy noted in the foregoing arm position, then the entire anterior inferior capsule can be shifted superiorly at the rotator interval and sutured. Under the less common circumstance of excessive capsular redundancy and a Bankart lesion, the rotator interval is closed and the capsule is incised between the MGHL and the anterior superior band of the IGHL, taking care not to incise the glenoid labrum. This capsular incision now creates a superior flap (superior glenohumeral ligament and MGHL) and an inferior flap (IGHL and inferior pouch). The arm is positioned in the plane of the scapula at 45 to 60 degrees of abduction and 45 degrees of external rotation. In this arm position, the inferior flap is shifted superiorly, thereby obliterating the inferior capsular pouch. The arm is then placed in 20 degrees of abduction and 35 degrees of external rotation, and the superior flap is shifted inferiorly. The capsular closure is performed with nonabsorbable suture. The extent of the shift and the capsular tightening by this method is determined by the arm position, thereby ensuring that the intraoperative external rotation will be at least 30 degrees measured in neutral abduction and 70 to 90 degrees of external rotation in the abducted position. This technique will avoid overtightening the capsule and ensure reproducible results.

Capsular Shift without a Bankart Repair

The exposure, subscapularis dissection, and lateral capsulotomy for a isolated anterior inferior capsular shift is as de-

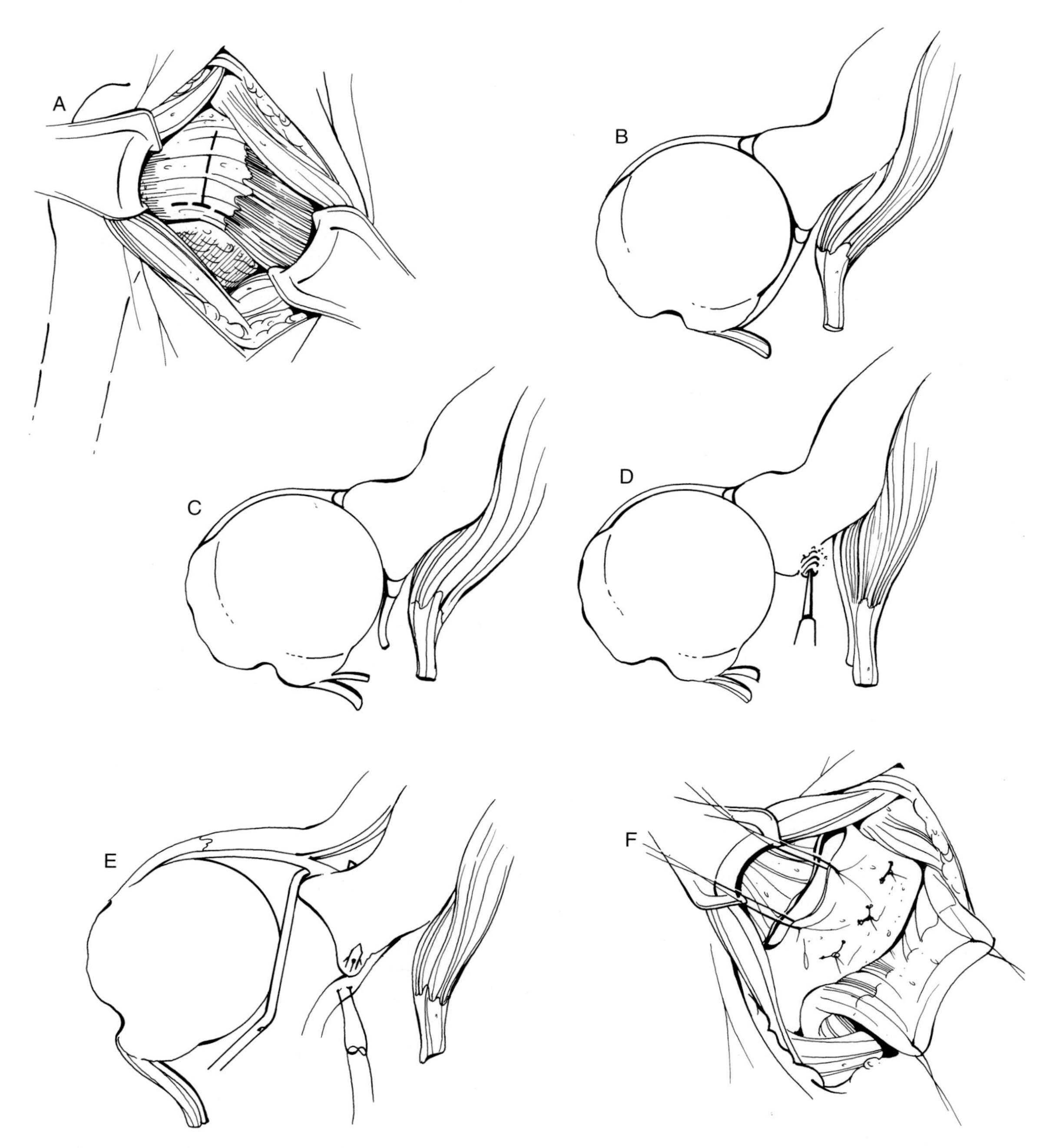

FIG. 48. (A) The subscapularis incision begins 1 cm medial to the musculotendinous junction from the uppermost portion of the subscapularis at the rotator interval, and extends inferiorly to the anterior circumflex vessels. **(B)** The subscapularis is separated from the underlying capsule medially to the glenoid rim and laterally to the lesser tuberosity. The lateral stump of the subscapularis is defined to allow separated closure of the lateral capsule and subscapularis. **(C)** The capsule is then incised 7 to 10 mm from its humeral insertion site from the rotator interval to the inferior capsular pouch. **(D)** The capsule and subscapularis are reflected medially, the glenoid labrum is inspected and, if a Bankart lesion is noted, it is reflected medially and the glenoid rim and neck is decorticated with a burr. **(E)** The suture anchors are placed exactly at the glenoid rim, and both limbs of the sutures are passed through the labrum and capsule. **(F)** The capsule is brought laterally and the limbs of the sutures are tied on the outside of the capsule. *(Continued)*

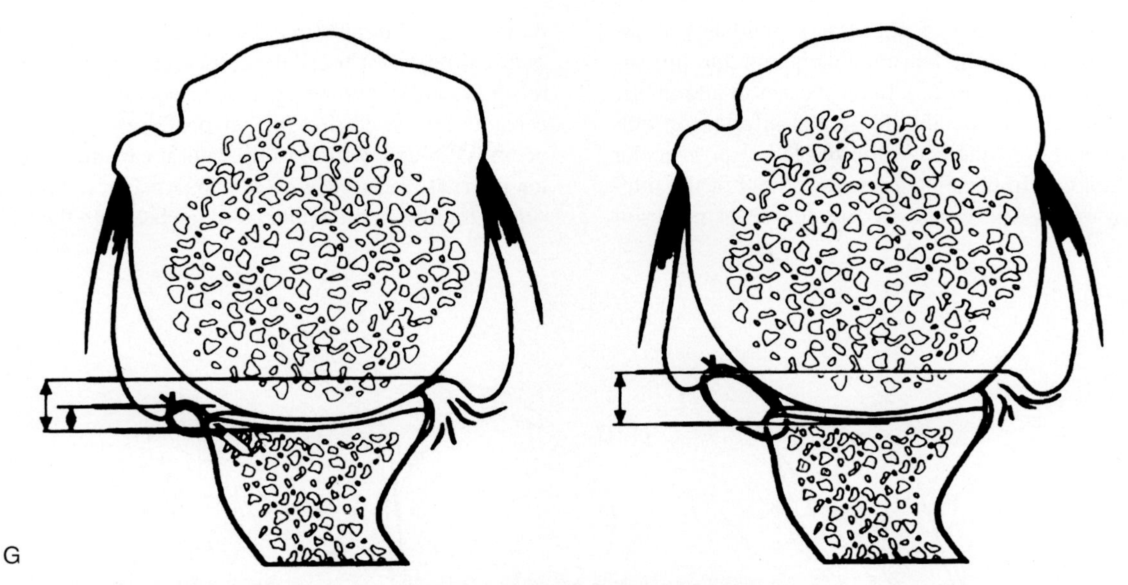

FIG. 48. *(Continued)* **(G)** The goal of the surgery is to repair the capsule and labrum so that a "bumper" effect of the labrum is reconstructed onto the glenoid rim. It, therefore, is necessary to put the anchors at the rim of the glenoid, to pass the suture through the labrum, and if the labrum is attenuated, to use a barrel stitch to gather up the capsule to form a thickened mass of tissue to re-form an anterior bumper.

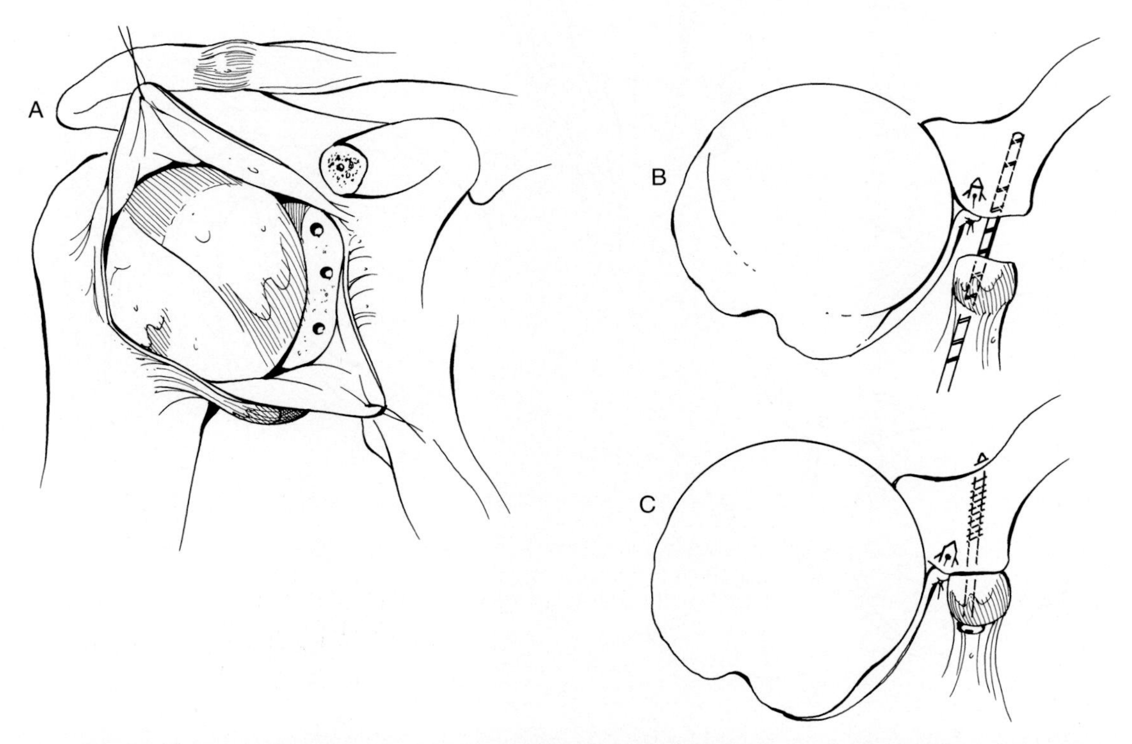

FIG. 49. With moderate glenoid bone loss, an anterior capsulorrhaphy and corocoid transfer are performed. **(A)** The anchors are placed at the glenoid rim and the sutures are passed through the capsule and labrum, but not yet tied. **(B,C)** The glenoid defect is decorticated and the distal 1.5 cm of the corocoid are transferred to the defect and secured with a partially threaded screw.

scribed above. The degree of capsular redundancy is assessed as described, and the labrum attachment and intraarticulator structures are evaluated. In most cases of atraumatic or repetitive microtraumatic anterior, anteroinferior, or multidirectional instability, there is minimal labral or articular cartilage pathology. In these patients, the extent of the inferior capsulotomy is determined by the degree of posterior humeral head translation. The greater the degree of asymmetrical posterior translation, the greater the degree of posterior capsular tightening that is necessary; therefore, the capsulotomy is carried further posterior along the humeral neck. After completion to the lateral capsulotomy, the rotator interval is closed with nonabsorbable sutures. The capsule is incised in the midaxial plane between the MGHL and

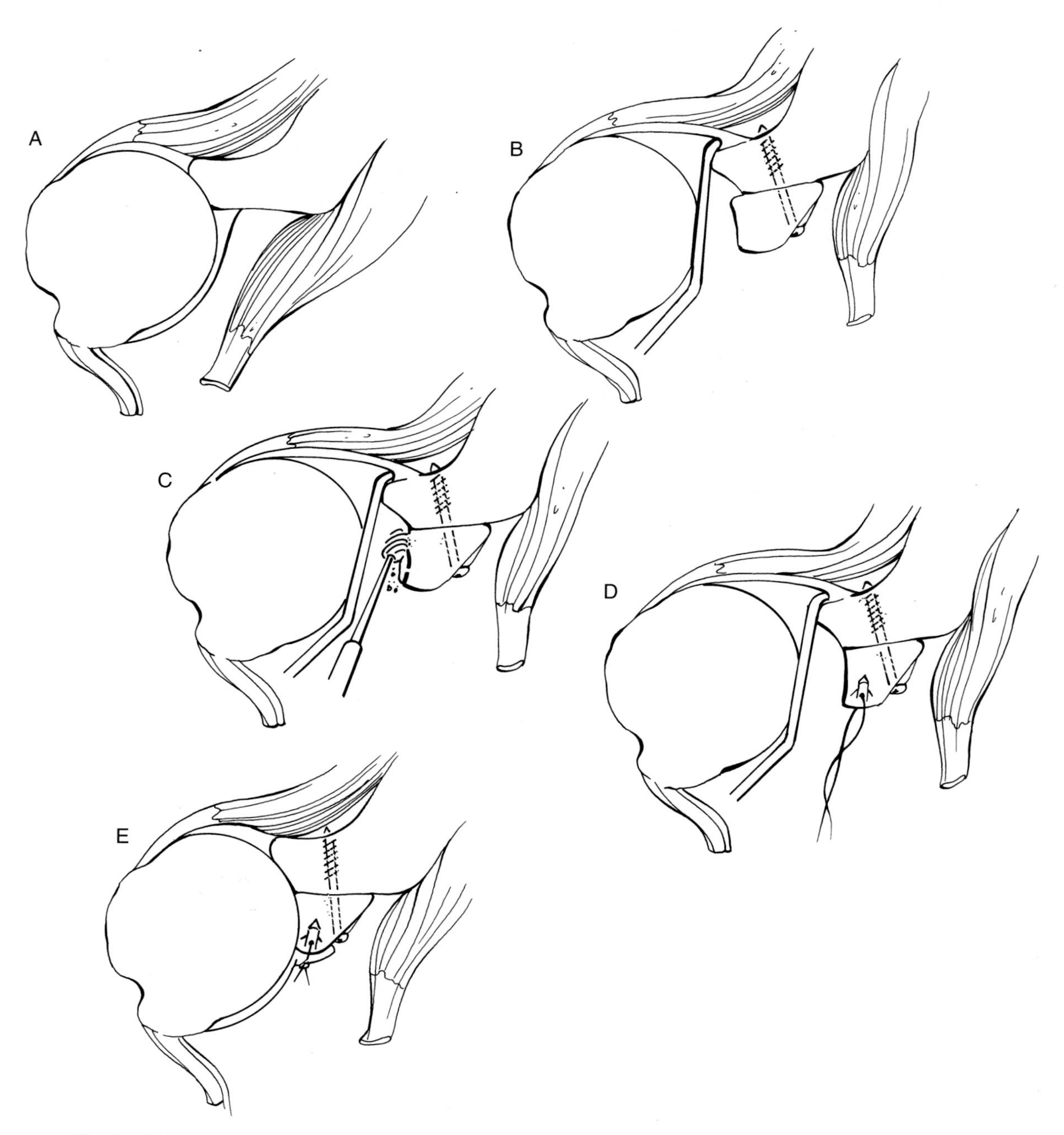

FIG. 50. **(A)** For large anterior glenoid defects an iliac crest graft is used to reconstruct the glenoid defect. **(B)** The defect is decorticated and made flat. A bicortical iliac crest graft is placed with its cancellous surface against the cancellous bone of the defect and secured with two partially threaded screws. **(C)** The position of the graft, which overhangs the face of the glenoid, is burred down to make a smooth contour with the native glenoid. **(D)** Suture anchors are placed into the rim of the graft. **(E)** The limbs of each suture are passed through the capsule and labrum, thereby repairing the ligaments to the new glenoid rim.

the anterior superior band of the IGHL to the labrum, thereby creating superior and inferior capsular flaps. The arm is positioned, and the capsular flaps sutured as described previously.

Subscapularis Closure

Closure of the subscapularis is with nonabsorbable suture without any shortening. In a similar way, the interval between the subscapularis and supraspinatus is closed. A drain is placed in the subdeltoid space. The subcutaneous tissues are closed with absorbable sutures, and the skin is closed with a nonabsorbable monofilament suture using a subcuticular technique. Steri-Strips, a sterile dressing, and a sling are applied, and the patient is reversed from the anesthetic.

Anterior Glenoid Deficiency

There is no consensus about the degree of glenoid bone loss that justifies bone reconstruction of the anterior glenoid. In our practice, we perform a bone reconstruction for cases with approximately 20% loss of the anterior-to-posterior glenoid dimension. In most sized persons, this is approximately 6 mm of bone loss at the anterior inferior aspect of the glenoid margin. Bone loss in the 20% to 30% range can be compensated by using a corocoid transfer; larger defects can be managed using an iliac crest graft.

The exposure, subscapularis dissection, and lateral capsulotomy for the bone augmentation procedures are as described above, with the exception that the skin incision is extended superiorly to the tip of the corocoid. With significant glenoid bone loss, the glenoid defect is burred to a flat surface. Nonabsorbable sutures are placed with suture anchors at the osteochondral junction and passed through the labrum and capsule, but they are not tied (Fig. 49A). The periosteum over the osseous defect is then incised to expose the defect in an extraarticular fashion. The distal 1.5 cm of the corocoid with its attached strap muscles are osteotomized with a right-angle microsaggital saw. The tip of the corocoid is drilled with a 3.2-mm bit in a retrograde fashion and measured with

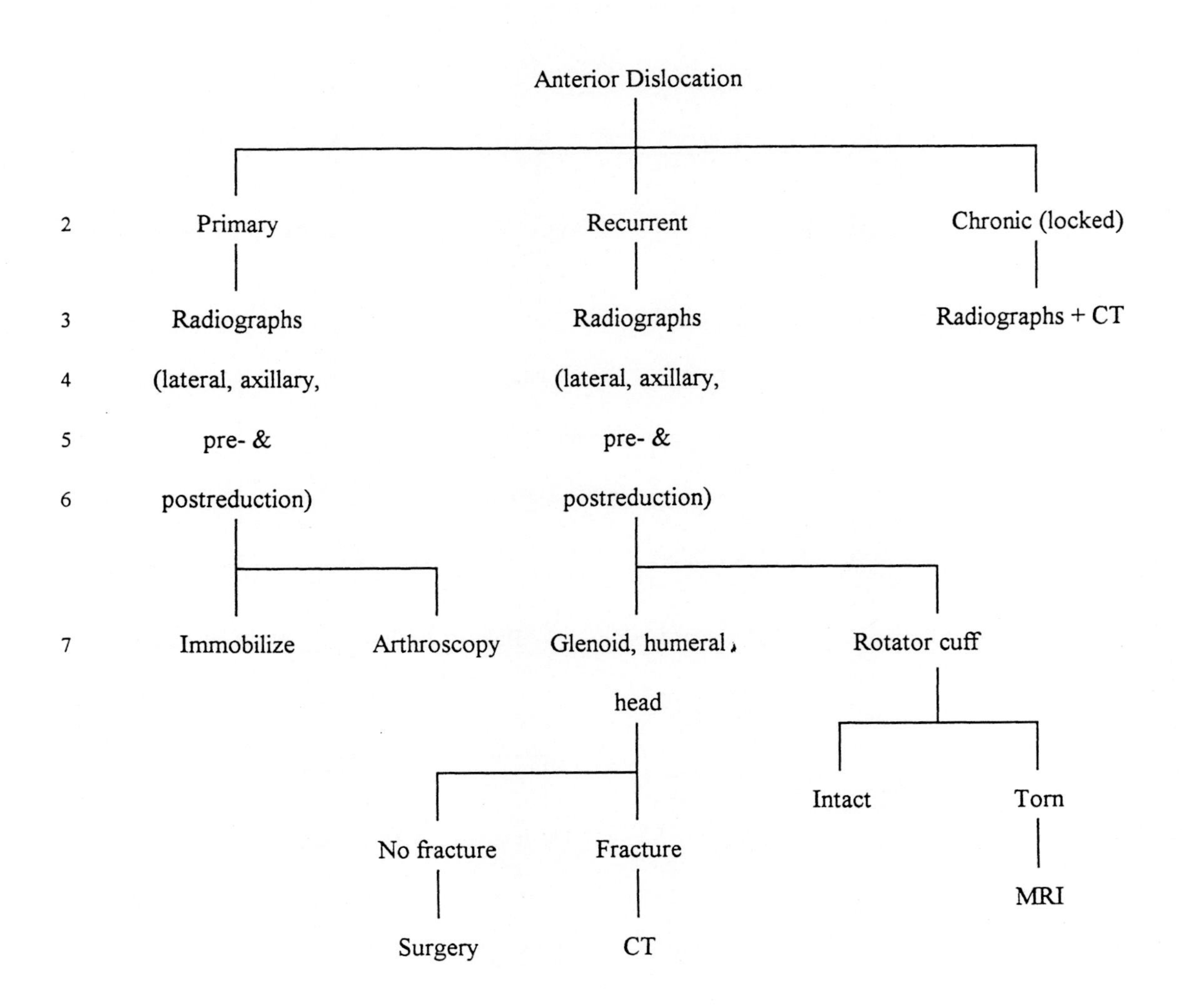

a depth gauge. The drill bit is reversed, the tip of the corocoid is placed into the glenoid defect, the drill is advanced through the posterior glenoid cortex, and the depth of the glenoid hole is measured (see Fig. 49B,C). A partially threaded 4.5-mm cancellous screw is then used to secure the corocoid tip into the glenoid defect. The previously passed capsular sutures are tied, thereby repairing the Bankart lesion to the rim; the corocoid transfer and screw remain extraarticular. The lateral capsular repair can be completed as just described; the technique is based on the degree of capsular redundancy. The subscapularis closure is as described.

For severe bone loss, an iliac crest graft is employed. The exposure, subscapularis dissection, and lateral capsulotomy are as described above. A bicortical iliac crest graft (appropriate size, 1.5 × 2.0 × 1.0 cm) is harvested. The anterior glenoid is decorticated and made flat to receive the flat cancellous surface of the iliac crest graft. The graft is placed so that the cortex of the iliac crest will constitute a new glenoid rim, and so that it slightly overhangs the articular surface of the glenoid. The graft is then secured with two 2.5-mm partially threaded cancellous screws (Fig. 50A,B). With a high-speed burr, the new articulating surface of the graft is contoured to match the level and radius of curvature of the remaining articular cartilage of the glenoid (Fig. 50C). Nonabsorbable sutures are placed at the rim of the iliac crest graft, as described for repair of a Bankart lesion. The lateral capsular and subscapularis closure is as described earlier (Fig. 50D,E).

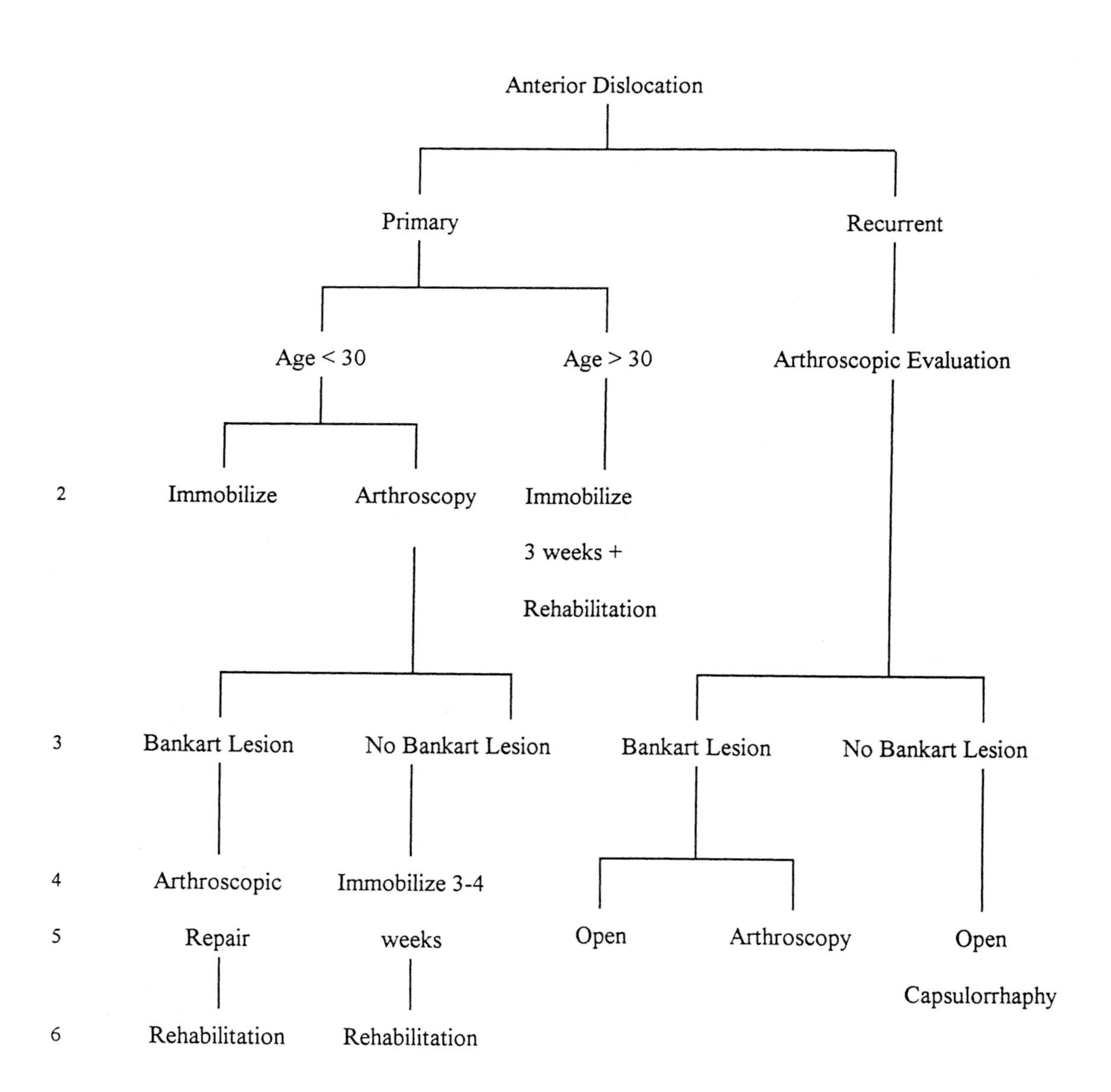

CONCLUSIONS AND SUMMARY

The management of patients with anterior shoulder instability must be based on a thorough knowledge of the etiologic factors associated with the instability and the resulting pathology. The many diagnostic tools available, including history and physical examination, imaging, and arthroscopy, can be invaluable in identifying the location and extent of pathology, and thereby directing treatment.

Stability of the shoulder results from a marvelous harmony of static and dynamic factors. The challenge facing the physician treating anterior shoulder instability is to restore this often delicate balance. The choice of treatment necessary to accomplish this goal will vary according to host factors, specific pathology, and the skill and experience of the surgeon.

REFERENCES

1. Arciero RA, Wheeler JH, Ryan JB, McBride JT. Arthroscopic Bankart repair versus nonoperative treatment for acute, initial anterior shoulder dislocations. *Am J Sports Med* 1994;22:589–594.
2. Aronen JG, Regan K. Decreasing the incidence of recurrence of first time anterior shoulder dislocations with rehabilitation. *Am J Sports Med* 1984;12:283–291.
3. Bacilla P, Field LD, Savoie FH III. Arthroscopic Bankart repair in a high demand patient population. *Arthroscopy* 1997;13:51–60.
4. Baker CL, Uribe JW, Whitman C. Arthroscopic evaluation of acute initial anterior shoulder dislocations. *Am J Sports Med* 1990;18:25–28.
5. Banas MP, Dalldorf PG, Sebastianelli WJ, DeHaven KE. Long-term followup of the modified Bristow procedure [see comments]. *Am J Sports Med* 1993;21:666–671..
6. Bankart ASB. Recurrent or habitual dislocation of the shoulder-joint. *Br Med J* 1923;2:1132–1133.
7. Bankart ASB. The pathology and treatment of recurrent dislocation of the shoulder joint. *Br J Surg* 1938;26:23–29.
8. Bartlett LR, Storey MD, Simons BD. Measurement of upper extremity torque production and its relationship to throwing speed in the competitive athlete. *Am J Sports Med* 1989;17:89–91.
9. Bigliani LU, Kurzweil PR, Schwartzbach CC, Wolfe IN, Flatow EL. Inferior capsular shift procedure for anteriorinferior shoulder instability in athletes. *Am J Sports Med* 1994;22:578–584.
10. Bigliani LU, Pollock RG, Soslowsky LJ, Flatow EL, Pawluk RJ, Mow VC. Tensile properties of the inferior glenohumeral ligament. *J Orthop Res* 1992;10:187–197.
11. Brown LP, Niehues SL, Harrah A, Yavorsky P, Hirshman HP. Upper extremity range of motion and isokinetic strength of the internal and external shoulder rotators in major league baseball players. *Am J Sports Med* 1988;16:577–585.
12. Caspari RB. Arthroscopic reconstruction for anterior shoulder instability. In: Paulos LE, Tibone JD, eds. *Operative techniques in shoulder surgery*. Gaithersburg, MD: Aspen, 1991;57–63.
13. Caspari RB, Geissler WB. Arthroscopic manifestations of shoulder subluxation and dislocation. *Clin Orthop* 1993;291:54—66.
14. Connolly JF. Humeral head defects associated with shoulder dislocations their diagnostic and surgical significance. *Instr Course Lect* 1972; 21:42–54.
15. Di Giovine HM, Jobe FN, Pink M, et al. An electromyographic analysis of the upper extremity in pitching. *J Shoulder Elbow Surg* 1992;1:15–25.
16. Dines DM, Levinson M. The conservative management of the unstable shoulder including rehabilitation. *Clin Sports Med* 1995;14:797–816.
17. Dowdy PA, O'Driscoll SW: Shoulder instability. An analysis of family history. *J Bone Joint Surg [Br]* 1993;75:782–784.
18. Flannigan B, Kursunoglu-Brahme S, Snyder S, Karzel R, Del Pizzo W, Resnick D. MR arthrography of the shoulder: comparison with conventional MR imaging. *AJR Am J Roentgenol* 1990;155:829–832.

18a. Garth WP Jr, Slappey CE, Ochs CW. Roentgenographic dem of instability of the shoulder: apical oblique projection—a te note. *J Bone Joint Surg [Am]* 1984;66:1450–1453.

19. Gerber C, Lambert SM. Allograft reconstruction of segmental def of the humeral head for the treatment of chronic locked posterior dislo cation of the shoulder. *J Bone Joint Surg [Am]* 1996;78:376–382.
20. Grashey R. *Atlas typisher rongenbilder von normalen Menschen*. Munchen: JF Lebmans, 1923.
21. Griffin LY, ed. Chronic shoulder problems in athletes. In: *Orthopaedic knowledge update: sports medicine*. Rosemont, IL: American Academy of Orthopaedic Surgeons, 1994:153–163.
22. Gross ML, Brenner SL, Esformes I, Sonzogni JJ. Anterior shoulder instability in weight lifters. *Am J Sports Med* 1993; 21:599–603.
23. Gusmer PB, Potter HG, Schatz JA, et al. Labral injuries: accuracy of detection with unenhanced MR imaging of the shoulder. *Radiology* 1996; 200:519–524.
24. Hayashi K, Thabit G III, Bogdanske JJ, Mascio LN, Markel MD. The effect of nonablative laser energy on the ultrastructure of joint capsular collagen. *Arthroscopy* 1996;12:474–481.
25. Helfet AJ. Coracoid transplantation for recurring dislocation of the shoulder. *J Bone Joint Surg [Br]* 1958;40:198–202.
26. Hertz H. [Significance of the limbus glenoidalis for the stability of the shoulder joint]. *Wien Klin Wochenschr Suppl* 1984;152:1–23.
27. Hill HA, Sachs MD. The grooved defect of the humeral head. *Radiology* 1940;35:690–700.
28. Hintermann B, Gachter A, Theo van Rens Prize. Arthroscopic assessment of the unstable shoulder. *Knee Surg Sports Traumatol Arthrosc* 1994;2:64–69.
29. Hovelius L. Shoulder dislocation in Swedish ice hockey players. *Am J Sports Med* 1978;6:373–377.
30. Hovelius L, Eriksson K, Fredin H, et al. Recurrences after initial dislocation of the shoulder. Results of a prospective study of treatment. *J Bone Joint Surg [Am]* 1983;65:343–349.
31. Hovelius L, Thorling J, Fredin H. Recurrent anterior dislocation of the shoulder. Results after the Bankart and Putti-Platt operations. *J Bone Joint Surg [Am]* 1979;61:566–569.
32. Jobe FW, Bradley JP. The diagnosis and nonoperative treatment of shoulder injuries in athletes. *Clin Sports Med* 1989;8:419–438.
33. Jobe FW, Giangarra CE, Kvitne RS, Glousman RE. Anterior capsulolabral reconstruction of the shoulder in athletes in overhand sports. *Am J Sports Med* 1991;19:428–434.
34. Jobe FW, Kvitne RS, Giangarra CE. Shoulder pain in the overhand or throwing athlete. The relationship of anterior instability and rotator cuff impingement [published erratum appears in *Orthop Rev* 1989 Dec; 18(12):1268]. *Orthop Rev* 1989;18:963–975.
35. Kiviluoto O, Pasila M, Jaroma H, Sundholm A. Immobilization after primary dislocation of the shoulder. *Acta Orthop Scand* 1980;51: 915–919.
36. Kvitne RS, Jobe FW. The diagnosis and treatment of anterior instability in the throwing athlete. *Clin Orthop* 1993;291:107–123.
37. Kvitne RS, Jobe FW, Jobe CM. Shoulder instability in the overhand or throwing athlete. *Clin Sports Med* 1995;14:917–935.
38. Lane JG, Sachs RA, Riehl B. Arthroscopic staple capsulorrhaphy: a long-term follow-up. *Arthroscopy* 1993;9:190–194.
39. Leach RE, Corbett M, Schepsis A, Stockel J. Results of a modified Putti-Platt operation for recurrent shoulder dislocations and subluxations. *Clin Orthop* 1982;164:20–25.
40. Lephart SM, Pincivero DM, Giraldo JL, Fu FH. The role of proprioception in the management and rehabilitation of athletic injuries. *Am J Sports Med* 1997;25:130–137.
41. Levine WN, Richmond JC, Donaldson WR. Use of the suture anchor in open Bankart reconstruction. A follow-up report. *Am J Sports Med* 1994;22:723–726.
42. Lombardo SJ, Kerlan RK, Jobe FW, Carter VS, Blazina ME, Shields CL Jr. The modified Bristow procedure for recurrent dislocation of the shoulder. *J Bone Joint Surg [Am]* 1976;58:256–261.
43. Lubowitz J, Bartolozzi A, Rubinstein D, et al. How much does inferior capsular shift reduce shoulder volume? *Clin Orthop* 1996;328:86–90.
44. Lusardi DA, Wirth MA, Wurtz D, Rockwood CA Jr. Loss of external rotation following anterior capsulorrhaphy of the shoulder. *J Bone Joint Surg [Am]* 1993;75:1185–1192.
45. Magnuson PB, Stack JK. Recurrent dislocation of the shoulder. *JAMA* 1943;123:889–892.

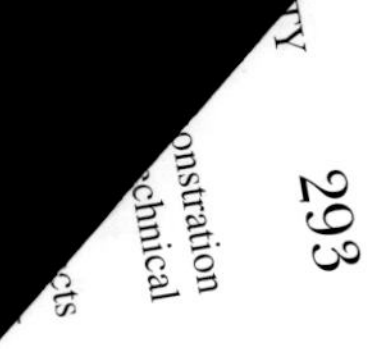

L, Yao L, et al. Labrocapsular ligamentous com- nal anatomy, anatomic variation, and pitfalls of rography. *Radiographics* 1994;14:1211–1223.
C, Rockwood CA Jr. Glenohumeral instabil- Matsen FA III, eds. *The shoulder.* Philadel- 526–622.
Technique and instrumentation for shoulder *ect* 1989;38:169–176.
... Oweida SJ, Spearman J, Helfet DL. Arthro- ... staple capsulorrhaphy for recurrent anterior shoulder instability. *Arthroscopy* 1988;4:106–111.
50. May VR Jr. A modified Bristow operation for anterior recurrent dislocation of the shoulder. *J Bone Joint Surg [Am]* 1970;52:1010–1016.
51. McCauley TR, Pope CF, Jokl P. Normal and abnormal glenoid labrum: assessment with multiplanar gradient-echo MR imaging. *Radiology* 1992;183:35–37.
52. Morgan CD. Arthroscopic transglenoid Bankart suture repair. *Oper Tech Orthop* 1991;1:171–179.
53. Morgan CD, Bodenstab AB. Arthroscopic Bankart suture repair: technique and early results. *Arthroscopy* 1987;3:111–122.
54. Moseley JB Jr, Jobe FW, Pink M, Perry J, Tibone J. EMG analysis of the scapular muscles during a shoulder rehabilitation program. *Am J Sports Med* 1992;20:128–134.
55. Neer CS II, Foster CR. Inferior capsular shift for involuntary inferior and multidirectional instability of the shoulder. A preliminary report. *J Bone Joint Surg [Am]* 1980;62:897–908.
56. Neumann CH, Petersen SA, Jahnke AH. MR imaging of the labral capsular complex: normal variations. *AJR Am J Roentgenol* 1991;157: 1015–1021.
57. Neviaser RJ, Neviaser TJ, Neviaser JS. Anterior dislocation of the shoulder and rotator cuff rupture. *Clin Orthop* 1993;291:103–106.
58. O'Keefe RM Jr, Shea KP, Fulkerson JP. Initial failure strength of arthroscopic Bankart suture and staple repairs [abstr]. *Arthroscopy* 1990;6:158–159.
59. Osmond-Clarke H. Habitual dislocation of the shoulder: the Putti-Platt operation. *J Bone Joint Surg [Br]* 1948;30:19–25.
60. Pagnani MJ, Warren RF. Arthroscopic shoulder stabilization. *Oper Tech Sports Med* 1993;1:276–284.
61. Palmer WE, Caslowitz PL. Anterior shoulder instability: diagnostic criteria determined from prospective analysis of 121 MR arthrograms. *Radiology* 1195;197:819–825.
62. Papilion JA, Shall LM. Fluoroscopic evaluation for subtle shoulder instability [see comments]. *Am J Sports Med* 1992;20:548–552.
63. Pavlov H, Warren RF, Weiss CB Jr, Dines DM. The roentgenographic evaluation of anterior shoulder instability. *Clin Orthop* 1985;194: 153–158.
64. Perthes G. Uber operationen der habituellen schulterluxation. *Dtsche Z Chir* 1906;85:199.
65. Reeves B. Experiments on the tensile strength of the anterior capsular structures of the shoulder in man. *J Bone Joint Surg [Br]* 1968;50: 858–865.
66. Regan WD Jr, Webster-Bogaert S, Hawkins RJ, Fowler PJ. Comparative functional analysis of the Bristow, Magnuson-Stack, and Putti-Platt procedures for recurrent dislocation of the shoulder. *Am J Sports Med* 1989;17:42–48.
67. Rockwood CA Jr. Subluxation of the shoulder the classification, diagnosis, and treatment [abstr]. *Orthop Trans* 1979;4:306.
68. Rosenberg BN, Richmond JC, Levine WN. Long-term followup of Bankart reconstruction. Incidence of late degenerative glenohumeral arthrosis. *Am J Sports Med* 1995;23:538–544.
69. Rowe CR, Patel D, Southmayd WW. The Bankart procedure: a longterm endresult study. *J Bone Joint Surg [Am]* 1978;60:1–16.
70. Rowe CR, Pierce DS, Clark JG. Voluntary dislocation of the shoulder. A preliminary report on a clinical, electromyographic, and psychiatric study of twenty-six patients. *J Bone Joint Surg [Am]* 1973;55:445–460.
71. Rowe CR, Zarins B. Recurrent transient subluxation of the shoulder. *J Bone Joint Surg [Am]* 1981;63:863–872.
72. Rowe CR, Zarins B, Ciullo JV. Recurrent anterior dislocation of the shoulder after surgical repair. Apparent causes of failure and treatment. *J Bone Joint Surg [Am]* 1984;66:159–168.
73. Rozing PM, de Bakker HM, Obermann WR. Radiographic views in recurrent anterior shoulder dislocation. Comparison of six methods for identification of typical lesions. *Acta Orthop Scand* 1986;57: 328–330.
74. Saha AK. The classic. Mechanism of shoulder movements and a plea for the recognition of "zero position" of glenohumeral joint. *Clin Orthop* 1983;173:3–10.
75. Saha AK, Das AK. Anterior recurrent dislocation of the shoulder: treatment by rotation osteotomy of the upper shaft of the humerus. *Indian J Orthop* 1967;1:132–137.
76. Silliman JF, Hawkins RJ. Classification and physical diagnosis of instability of the shoulder. *Clin Orthop* 1993;291:7–19.
77. Simonet WT, Cofield RH. Prognosis in anterior shoulder dislocation. *Am J Sports Med* 1984;12:19—24.
78. Singer GC, Kirkland PM, Emery RJ. Coracoid transposition for recurrent anterior instability of the shoulder. A 20-year follow-up study. *J Bone Joint Surg [Br]* 1995;77:73–76.
79. Snyder SJ, Strafford BB. Arthroscopic management of instability of the shoulder. *Orthopedics* 1993;16:993–1002.
80. Speer KP, Hannafin JA, Altchek DW, Warren RF. An evaluation of the shoulder relocation test. *Am J Sports Med* 1994;22:177–183
81. Speer KP, Warren RF, Pagnani M, Warner JJ. An arthroscopic technique for anterior stabilization of the shoulder with a bioabsorbable tack. *J Bone Joint Surg [Am]* 1996;78:1801–1807.
82. Thabit G. Treatment of unidirectional and multidirectional gelnohumeral instability by an arthroscopic holmium:YAG laser-assisted capsular shift procedure a pilot study. Presented at the Laser Application in Arthroscopy Meeting of the International Musculoskeletal Laser Society, Neuchatel, Switzerland, 1994.
83. Thomas SC, Matsen FA III. An approach to the repair of avulsion of the glenohumeral ligaments in the management of traumatic anterior glenohumeral instability. *J Bone Joint Surg [Am]* 1989;71: 506–513.
84. Warner JJ, Miller MD, Marks P. Arthroscopic Bankart repair with the Suretac device. Part II: experimental observations. *Arthroscopy* 1995; 11:14–20.
85. Weber BG, Simpson LA, Hardegger F, Gallen S. Rotational humeral osteotomy for recurrent anterior dislocation of the shoulder associated with a large Hill–Sachs lesion. *J Bone Joint Surg [Am]* 1984;66: 1443–1450.
86. Wheeler JH, Ryan JB, Arciero RA, Molinari RN. Arthroscopic versus nonoperative treatment of acute shoulder dislocations in young athletes. *Arthroscopy* 1989;5:213–217.
87. Wilk KE, Arrigo C. Current concepts in the rehabilitation of the athletic shoulder. *J Orthop Sports Phys Ther* 1993;18:365–378.
88. Wirth MA, Blatter G, Rockwood CA Jr. The capsular imbrication procedure for recurrent anterior instability of the shoulder. *J Bone Joint Surg [Am]* 1996;78:246–259.
89. Yoneda B, Welsh RP, MacIntosh DL. Conservative treatment of shoulder dislocation in young males [abstr]. *J Bone Joint Surg [Br]* 1982;64: 254—255.
90. Young DC, Rockwood CA Jr. Complications of a failed Bristow procedure and their management. *J Bone Joint Surg [Am]* 1991;73: 969–981.
91. Youssef JA, Carr CF, Walther CE, Murphy JM. Arthroscopic Bankart suture repair for recurrent traumatic unidirectional anterior shoulder dislocations. *Arthroscopy* 1995;11:561–563.
92. Zuckerman JD, Matsen FA III. Complications about the glenohumeral joint related to the use of screws and staples. *J Bone Joint Surg [Am]* 1984;66:175–180.

Disorders of the Shoulder: Diagnosis and Management,
edited by Joseph P. Iannotti and Gerald R. Williams, Jr.
Lippincott Williams & Wilkins, Philadelphia © 1999.

CHAPTER 11

Posterior Instability: Diagnosis and Management

Matthew L. Ramsey and John J. Klimkiewicz

INTRODUCTION

Posterior instability of the shoulder is defined as the symptoms expressed as a result of excessive posterior glenohumeral translation. The symptoms associated with posterior instability may be due to *recurrent subluxation* or acute *dislocation.* Diagnosis depends on the clinical history of instability reported by the patient, reproduction of symptoms during physical examination, as well as the results of diagnostic evaluation.

Acute posterior dislocation is rare in comparison with its anterior counterpart. Recurrent posterior subluxation is the most common form of posterior instability and represents the principal topic of this chapter. Although posterior instability is uncommon in comparison with its anterior counterpart, it is being recognized with increased frequency.[23,29,77] Historically, the literature has been unclear on the distinction between recurrent posterior subluxation and posterior dislocation. This, combined with a limited understanding of the pathophysiology of recurrent posterior subluxation, has resulted in a lack of consensus on its diagnosis and management.

McLaughlin recognized the distinction between (locked) posterior dislocation and recurrent posterior subluxation.[43] Attempts to further classify recurrent posterior subluxation have employed the same terminology as anterior instability. This classification defines instability based on its degree (subluxation, dislocation), origin (traumatic, atraumatic), direction (anterior, posterior, inferior, multidirectional), or patient volition (voluntary, involuntary). In anterior instability, for which the origin and direction of instability often correlate with an underlying pathologic lesion and direct appropriate treatment, these terms are invaluable. The same is not true of posterior instability. Describing posterior instability based on a traumatic or atraumatic basis or as voluntary or involuntary does not necessarily define the underlying pathology or assist in treatment decisions. Regardless of the etiology of posterior instability, the nature of the underlying pathology is not predicted based on current classification schemes. The absence of a classification system that unifies posterior instability has made it difficult to evaluate various treatments and their results.

M. L. Ramsey and J. J. Klimkiewicz: Penn Musculoskeletal Institute, Presbyterian Medical Center, Philadelphia, Pennsylvania 19104.

TABLE 1. *Classification of posterior instability*

Posterior dislocation
Acute posterior dislocation
Chronic (locked) posterior dislocation
Recurrent posterior subluxation
Volitional
Psychogenic
"Learned"
Dysplastic
Glenoid retroversion
Humeral head retrotorsion
Acquired
Soft tissue deficiency
Bony deficiency
Scapulothoracic dysfunction

An anatomically based classification of recurrent posterior subluxation, as opposed to the more traditional etiology-based methods of classification, facilitates treatment by defining the pathologic process that produces the instability. The salient features of this anatomic based classification system are summarized in Table 1.

POSTERIOR DISLOCATION

Acute Posterior Dislocation

Acute posterior dislocations are rare, accounting for approximately 5% of all dislocations. Direct trauma to the front of the shoulder, a posteriorly directed force on an adducted arm (fall on an outstretched hand), and indirect muscle forces (seizure or electrical shock), all can cause posterior dislocation.

Diagnosis

The diagnosis of posterior dislocation should be readily made through a careful history, physical examination, and supporting radiographic studies. Before the advent of radiographs the distinctive presenting features and physical findings of posterior dislocation were described.[13a] The routine use of radiography for injuries of the shoulder should increase the diagnostic accuracy. Unfortunately, nearly half of all posterior dislocations are missed.[29a]

Patients with posterior dislocation typically present with the arm splinted at the side in adduction and internal rotation. The classic physical findings in posterior dislocation include the following (a) limited external rotation of the shoulder with the arm at the side; (b) limited forward elevation of the arm; (c) a void in the anterior aspect of the shoulder; (d) prominence of the coracoid process; and (e) fullness of the posterior aspect of the shoulder. Appreciation of these features is facilitated by examining the shoulder from above. A thorough neurovascular examination before and after shoulder reduction is essential.

Radiographic evaluation for a suspected posterior dislocation includes at least an anteroposterior (AP), scapular lateral, and axillary view of the shoulder. If positioning the patient for a standard axillary radiograph is not possible because of painful abduction, a Velpeau axillary or a trauma axillary radiograph can be obtained. The views are sufficient to diagnose the position of the humeral head and any associated bony lesions (Fig. 1). The classic radiographic features of posterior dislocation include humeral head overlap on the glenoid rim on an AP radiograph, an empty glenoid on axillary or lateral radiograph, fracture of the lesser tuberosity, and a reverse Hill–Sachs lesion.

A computed tomography (CT) scan is recommended when a satisfactory trauma series is difficult to obtain or interpret. If there is any concern about an associated fracture that is not appreciated on the radiographic evaluation, CT scan is helpful in characterizing the fracture pattern.

Treatment

The management of an acute posterior dislocation requires care to avoid further damage to the humeral head. Forceful reduction attempts in the face of a locked dislocation or a nondisplaced fracture risks displacing the humeral head. An

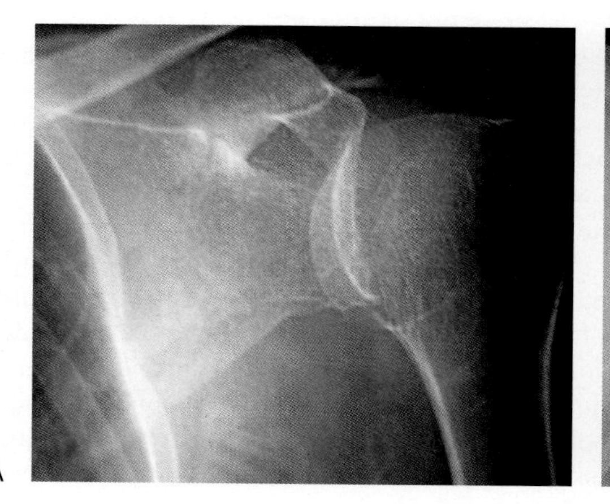
A

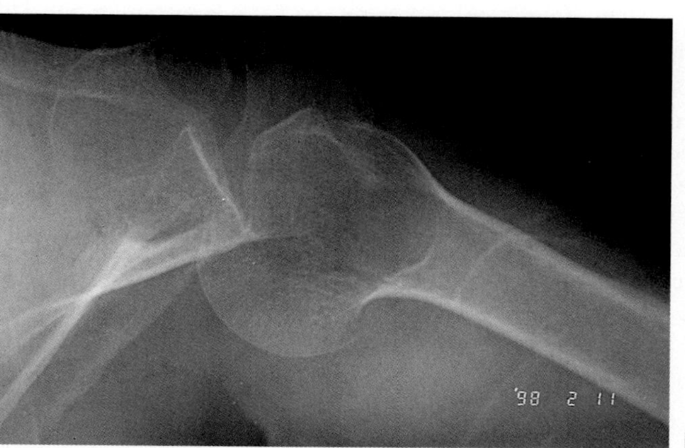

B

FIG. 1. **(A)** Anteroposterior and **(B)** axillary radiograph of a locked posterior dislocation. Note the impression fracture of the humeral head and the nondisplaced anatomic neck fracture (*arrow*).

attempted closed reduction can be attempted if the reverse Hill–Sachs lesion involves 40% or less of the humeral head. The reduction maneuver may require the involvement of an assistant. The arm is flexed to 90 degrees and adducted to disimpact the humeral head from the glenoid rim. The arm should not be externally rotated until the humeral head has cleared the glenoid rim. Lateral traction on the arm assists in disimpacting the humeral head from the glenoid rim. Gentle pressure on the humeral head guides it into the glenoid fossa and provides tactile input on its location relative to the glenoid. Once the humeral head clears the glenoid, the arm is externally rotated and brought down to the side.

The arm is immobilized in a brace, with the arm in slight abduction and neutral to slight external rotation for 4 to 6 weeks. If there is a large (30% to 50%) humeral head defect and the humeral head dislocates with internal rotation when the arm is in neutral (zero degrees of abduction), then consideration should be given to transfer of the subscapularis, bone grafting, or humeral head replacement (see Chap. 13 section on locked posterior dislocation).

RECURRENT POSTERIOR SUBLUXATION

Volitional Recurrent Posterior Subluxation

Voluntary recurrent posterior subluxation describes a group of patients with an underlying conscious or unconscious ability to subluxate their shoulder by using abnormal patterns of muscular activity. In this group of patients there is no initial anatomic pathology in the glenohumeral joint. Over time, stretching of the glenohumeral ligaments can occur such that an involuntary component to the instability develops. Some of these patients have underlying psychiatric disorders as a cause for willful and voluntary posterior subluxation. Rowe labeled these patients habitual dislocators.[62] Habitual dislocators are distinguished from other patients with posterior subluxation, who may have learned how to reproduce their instability, by their willful desire to subluxate their shoulders (Fig. 2). Despite the best intentions of the treating physician, habitual dislocators will frustrate all treatment efforts (operative and nonoperative) because of their abnormal psychologic need to subluxate their shoulder.[62] The overwhelming pathologic process in this group of patients is psychologic and treatment should be directed according to their psychologic needs. Surgical intervention in this group is contraindicated.

A second group of patients can voluntarily reproduce their instability, but they have no underlying psychologic need to do so. This is a learned behavior that over time may develop an involuntary component. It is this involuntary component that is bothersome to the patient and often initiates evaluation by a physician.

Electromyographic evaluation of patients who can voluntarily subluxate their shoulders demonstrate selective inhibition of certain muscle groups that results in an unbalanced force couple, leading to posterior subluxation. Activation of the deltoid and pectoralis major without opposition from the posterior short rotators, resulting in the humeral head being pushed posteriorly, was identified in several patients.[62] Conversely, Pande demonstrated unopposed activation of the posterior short rotators and posterior deltoid that in effect pulls the humeral head posteriorly.[56]

Dysplastic Recurrent Posterior Subluxation

Dysplastic bony architecture of the glenohumeral joint is another uncommon cause of recurrent posterior subluxation.[17] Localized posterior glenoid hypoplasia, increased glenoid retroversion, and increased humeral head retrotorsion are potential causes of recurrent posterior subluxation. Recent investigations have documented a low incidence of abnormal bony architecture in patients with instability and have postulated that developmental bony deformities are rare causes of recurrent posterior subluxation.[24,59,80] Edelson recently reported the incidence of posterior glenoid dysplasia in over 11,000 cadaveric specimens studied. In this group as many as 35% of the specimens had deficiencies in the posteroinferior aspect of the glenoid. Even though this condition may be more prevalent than previously thought, it is impossible to correlate these findings with clinical symptoms of instability.[17]

In the past, the theory that increased glenoid retroversion contributed to recurrent posterior subluxation was supported by radiographic techniques that indirectly measured glenoid retroversion, but are now felt to be inaccurate.[15] The advent of computed tomography (CT) has allowed direct measurement of glenoid geometry and has renewed interest in this area. Recent studies based on CT scan assessment of glenoid version vary widely on the incidence of abnormal glenoid geometry and its contribution to instability. Gerber and Randelli found no correlation between altered glenoid version and instability.[24,59] Conversely, Hurley and Wirth have separately demonstrated increased glenoid retroversion and isolated posterior glenoid hypoplasia, respectively, in all patients with recurrent posterior subluxation reported in their respective series.[33,81] Although the incidence of increased glenoid retroversion or hypoplasia in patients with recurrent posterior subluxation is confused by these conflicting reports, it is clear that increased glenoid retroversion or hypoplasia can contribute in some cases to recurrent posterior instability.[80] The true incidence, however, is unclear.

Although the exact etiology of glenoid hypoplasia is unknown, an abnormality in the formation or development of the proximal (subcoracoid) or inferior centers of ossification may be the cause. As these centers do not appear and ossify until well into the second decade of life, these patients usually do not present with symptoms until their second or third decades.[60] Whereas a CT scan is useful in defining the severity of glenoid hypoplasia, several findings on routine shoulder radiographs have been associated with this condition. Among these include a shallow or irregular glenoid fossa, a prominent coracoid process, an enlarged acromion, hooking of the distal clavicle, an associated hypoplasia of the upper

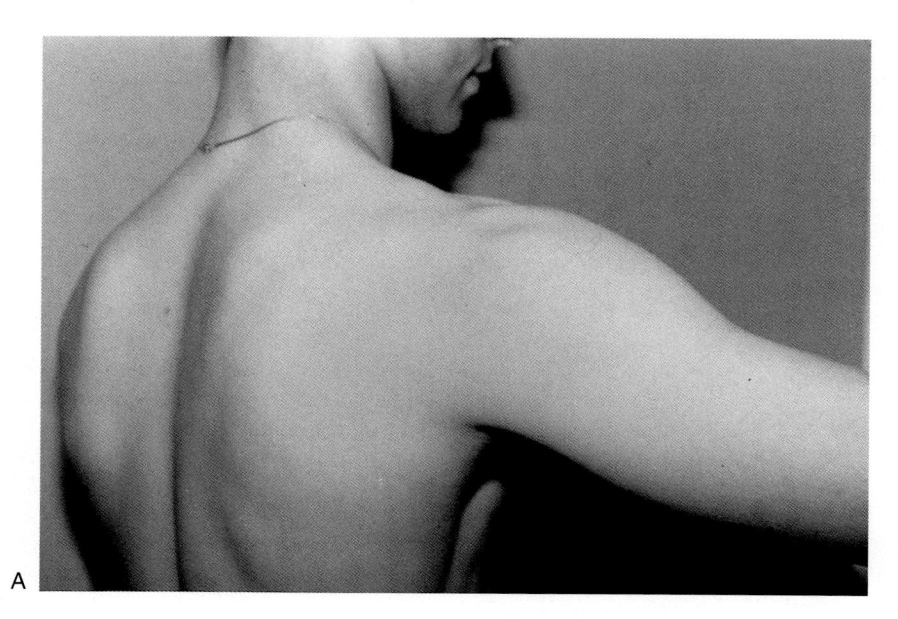

A

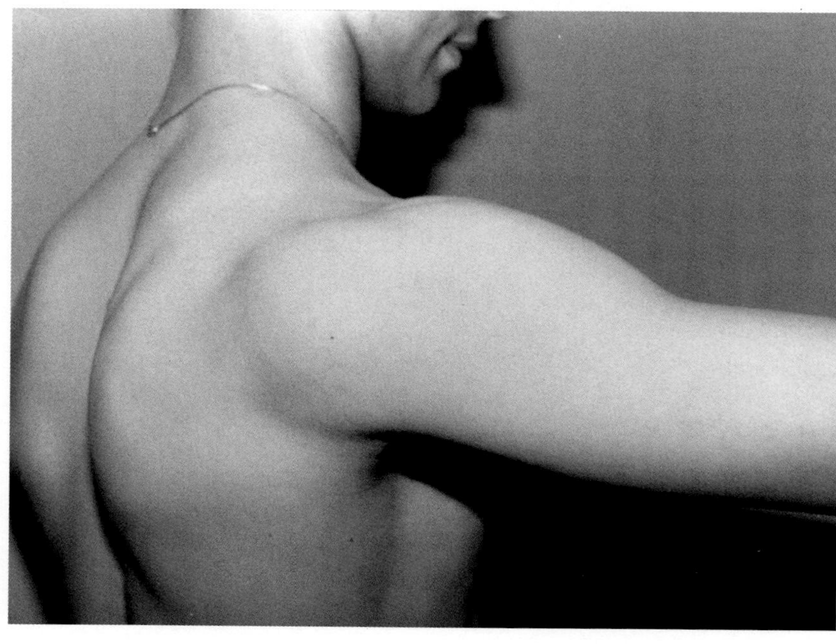

B

FIG. 2. Photograph of a patient **(A)** before and **(B)** after dislocating his shoulder posteriorly with asymmetrical muscular contraction.

ribs, and flattening of the humeral head.[11,15,70] The appearance and the degree of these radiographic findings vary in patients with this condition.

Abnormalities of humeral torsion could lead to glenohumeral instability. Accurate measurement of humeral retrotorsion is difficult. Schutte et al. described a technique for measuring humeral retrotorsion by CT scan.[63] This allows direct measurements of humeral retrotorsion, thereby eliminating the inaccuracy of plain radiographs. Kronberg has documented a correlation between decreased humeral retrotorsion and anterior glenohumeral instability in some patients. However, a relation between increased humeral retrotorsion and recurrent posterior subluxation has not been established.[39]

Reports of proximal humerus rotation osteotomy for the treatment of recurrent posterior subluxation are not supported by radiographic data demonstrating increased humeral retrotorsion.[11,71] The rationale for osteotomy in these series is that patients with recurrent posterior subluxation can provoke symptoms of instability by internal rotation of the arm. Limiting internal rotation through osteotomy was believed to correct the problem by preventing the patient from placing the arm in a position that would incite dislocation.

Acquired Recurrent Posterior Subluxation

The largest group of patients with recurrent posterior subluxation acquires posterior instability as a result of repetitive microtrauma or as a result of a single traumatic event. Traumatic events leading to both osseous and soft-tissue abnormalities can result in subsequent recurrent posterior instability. Because the etiology of this instability is not as crucial to treatment as the underlying pathologic lesion that results in recurrent posterior subluxation, we define acquired recurrent posterior subluxation based upon the anatomic lesion. Lesions of the capsule, labrum, rotator cuff musculature, and glenoid can contribute to recurrent posterior subluxation. The most consistent deficiency relates to redundancy of the posterior capsule. Additionally, dysfunction of normal scapulothoracic mechanics can place the glenohumeral joint at risk for recurrent instability.

Unlike the anterior capsule the posterior capsule is thin. The posterior capsule and the buttress provided by the posterior glenoid labrum are the primary static stabilizers to unidirectional posterior translation. Dynamic posterior stability is conferred by the rotator cuff musculature. The most consistent finding in patients with recurrent posterior subluxation is a patulous posterior capsule.[64] The posterior capsule either stretches over time or tears as a result of single-event trauma and heals in an elongated position, thereby increasing capsular volume. Posterior labral tears have been described with recurrent posterior subluxation; however, they are generally degenerative tears, rather than the rare capsular and labrum avulsion (i.e., reverse Bankart lesion; Fig. 3).[9,21,30,31]

The relation between the anterior soft tissues and posterior stability is referred to as the circle concept of capsuloligamentous stability.[64,65,69,72,78] Several biomechanical studies have investigated the contribution of anterior soft-tissue structures to posterior stability. In a cadaver model, the soft-tissue lesions caused by posterior dislocation have been identified.[46,53] In addition to posterior capsular avulsion and partial or complete tearing of the tendinous portion of the posterior rotator cuff, various lesions of the anterior soft-tissue structures were identified. These included complete anterior capsular avulsion from the humeral neck and tears of the muscular portion of the subscapularis.

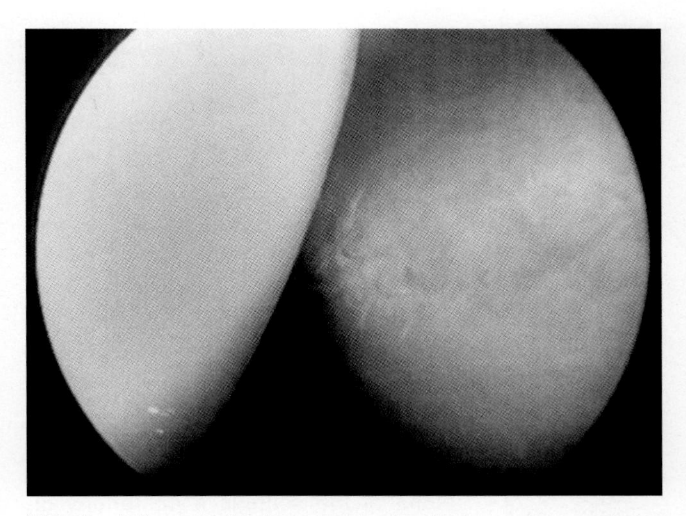

FIG. 3. Arthroscopic photograph of a degenerative posterior labrum in a patient with recurrent posterior instability. Degenerative lesions of the labrum are typical for recurrent posterior instability. True reverse Bankart lesions are rare.

Selective cutting of soft-tissue structures thought to contribute to posterior stability has further defined the role of these anterior and posterior soft tissues to static posterior stability. Increased posterior translation consistently requires a lesion of the posterior capsule, particularly the posterior band of the inferior glenohumeral ligament.[53] Isolated sectioning of the posterior rotator cuff musculature in the absence of a capsular lesion did not increase posterior translation.[54,64] However, when the posterior capsule was sectioned inferiorly, an increase in posterior translation was noted. Subluxation and dislocation occurred only after the anterior capsule and subscapularis tendon were cut.

Several studies have found that the superior capsule (rotator interval capsule) plays an important role in posterior stability.[27,64,66] Sectioning the soft tissues of the rotator interval capsule increased posterior and inferior translation, often to the point of dislocation. Imbrication of the rotator interval increased resistance to posterior and inferior translation.[27]

Acquired posterior subluxation is less commonly caused by posterior glenoid rim deficiency. Although it is uncommon, it does exist and should be investigated with imaging studies if suspected.[21,51,64] The relation between the degree of posterior glenoid erosion and recurrent posterior subluxation has not been established. It seems reasonable to assume that a large posterior glenoid defect will compromise the buttress effect of the glenoid to posterior translation.

In the resting state, the scapula lies on the posterolateral thorax at an angle of 45 degrees.[40] This position on the thorax places the posterior glenoid behind the humeral head, buttressing it against posteriorly directed forces. With shoulder elevation the scapula rotates under the humeral head and provides a platform for glenohumeral motion.[60] A requisite for shoulder stability is that scapulothoracic and glenohumeral rhythm remain synchronous.[12,76]

Dysfunction of scapulothoracic rhythm may compromise the stability of the glenohumeral joint.[76] The serratus anterior muscle plays a key role in scapulothoracic rhythm. Paralysis of this muscle results in scapular winging and loss of power in elevation that potentially may influence glenohumeral stability.[18] Warner et al. used Moire topographic analysis to study patients with glenohumeral instability and demonstrated abnormal scapulothoracic mechanics compared with those of asymptomatic patients.[76] Although no patient demonstrated severe scapular winging, the degree of scapulothoracic dysfunction was variable. In patients with scapular winging from paralysis of the serratus anterior, glenohumeral instability may result from altered scapulothoracic mechanics. In patients with glenohumeral instability and lesser degrees of scapulothoracic dysfunction, it is unclear whether instability is the result of altered scapulothoracic mechanics or the cause of it.

Diagnosis

The most important components in diagnosing recurrent posterior subluxation are a meticulous history and physical examination. Patients typically present with complaints of pain or a sensation of the shoulder dislocating when the arm is placed in a provocative position. The provocative position is variable, but usually includes some degree of flexion, adduction, and internal rotation. An axial load may occasionally be required. In most patients pain is usually limited to episodes of subluxation. Persistent pain is unusual and may be associated with rotator cuff or biceps tendinitis and posterior capsule irritation.[30,73] Pain as a predominant complaint is more common in athletes and may indicate a predisposition to capsular or rotator cuff irritation with overuse during athletic activity.[21,73,74]

A traumatic event initiating recurrent posterior subluxation is not typical. Most often patients cannot recall an initiating event. Over time, with certain activities, they begin to notice shoulder subluxation that readily reduces when the shoulder is taken out of the provocative position. Many of these patients will ultimately learn the position where subluxation occurs and can reproduce the subluxation with specific arm positioning. However, unlike habitual dislocators, patients with nonpsychogenic instability do not voluntarily subluxate their shoulders, unless they are asked to by an examiner, because of the discomfort associated with their instability. In these patients, the most prominent complaint is the involuntary component to the instability that is particularly bothersome and ultimately prompts the patient to seek medical attention.

A

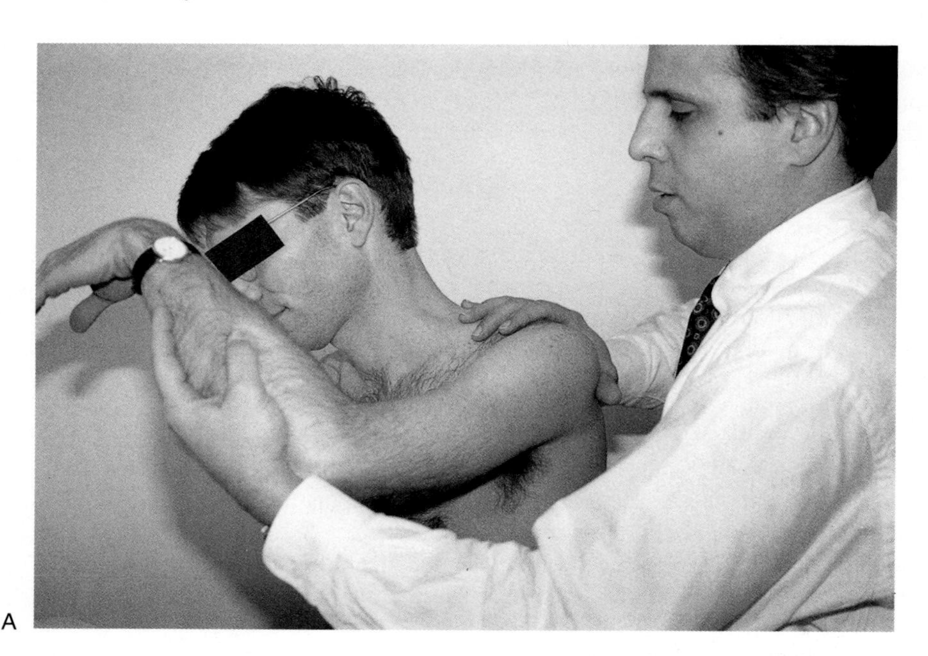

B

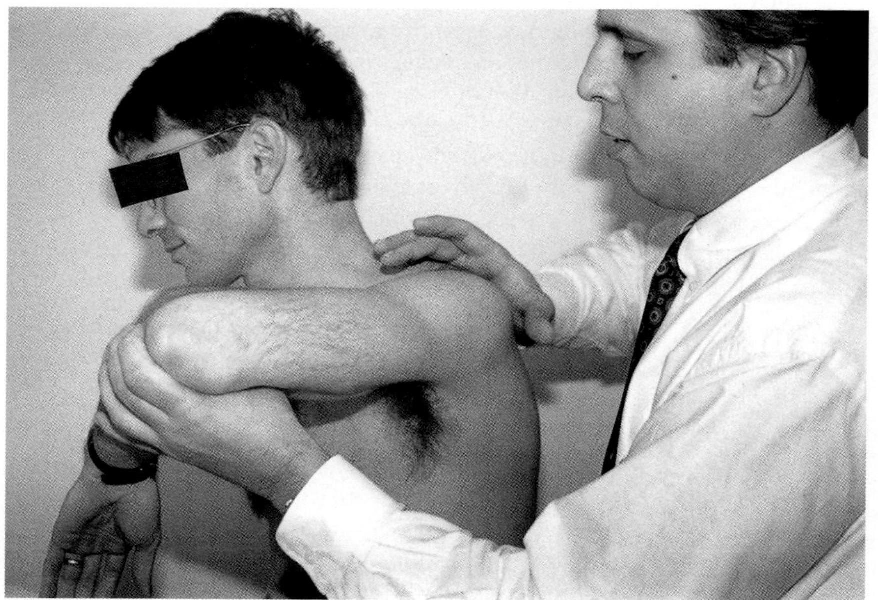

FIG. 4. Seated posterior stress test: The examiner stands to the side of the patient and stabilizes the scapula. With the arm in 90 degrees of forward elevation in the plane of the scapula a posteriorly directed force is applied with the arm in **(A)** external rotation and **(B)** internal rotation. The degree of posterior translation in each position is assessed.

The disability associated with posterior subluxation is variable and is dependent on the severity of the symptoms. As a general rule, activities of daily living and simple work activities are not limited by symptoms of recurrent posterior subluxation.[29–31] Participation in sports, however, is generally more troublesome, and often requires modification or complete elimination of activity. In more severe cases of posterior subluxation (i.e., patients ultimately requiring surgery), activities of daily living and work may be interrupted.[57]

Physical Examination

The physical examination is directed at reproducing the patient's symptoms and defining the character of instability. Range of motion is generally normal in patients who have not had prior surgery. Occasionally, internal and external rotation may be slightly limited. In athletes there is often activity-specific loss of motion. Overhead-throwing athletes often demonstrate increased external rotation, with an associated mild loss of internal rotation.[73,74] It is critical to evaluate scapulothoracic function during the physical examination for scapular winging or disruption of normal scapulothoracic rhythm.

Most patients can demonstrate their subluxation.[29] Once the position of subluxation is demonstrated by the patient, symptoms of instability can usually be recreated by the physician. In patients who cannot demonstrate their instability, the diagnosis of recurrent posterior instability is more difficult.

Testing for posterior subluxation should be performed with the patient in the sitting and supine position. Testing for increased posterior translation must be performed on the opposite side for comparison. It is important to realize that in a normal shoulder, the humeral head can subluxate posteriorly up to 50%.[26,50]

The posterior stress test is performed with the patient seated and the examiner at the affected side (Fig. 4). The scapula is stabilized while the opposite hand positions the arm in flexion, adduction, and internal rotation and applies a posteriorly directed force. If the patient is able to demonstrate subluxation, replacing the arm in this provocative position should recreate the patient's symptoms with posterior stress testing. Otherwise, testing must be performed in varying degrees of flexion (between 90 and 120 degrees), adduction, and internal rotation to determine the arm position where subluxation occurs. With coronal plane extension, the humeral head will relocate into the glenoid fossa. The relocation is sudden and can be felt by the patient and examiner. Most patients with recurrent posterior subluxation have a positive posterior stress test.[21,57] However, apprehension typical of anterior instability is unusual.[29,31] The predominant symptoms are pain or reproduction of instability symptoms.

The load and shift test should be performed with the patient in the sitting and supine positions.[60] In the seated position, with the examiner behind the patient, the scapula is stabilized to minimize scapulothoracic motion (Fig. 5). With the opposite hand, the humeral head is grasped and a centering force is applied. Anterior and posterior translation is assessed and compared with that of the opposite side. We prefer the load and shift test performed in the supine position with the arm in the plane of the scapula, in 45 to 60 degrees of abduction, with varying degrees of rotation from full external to full internal rotation (Fig. 6). Positive testing will result in a reproduction of the patient's symptoms of instability, pain, and crepitation. Side-to-side difference in the amount of internal rotation necessary to obliterate or minimize posterior translation is a clinical measure of residual pathologic capsular laxity.

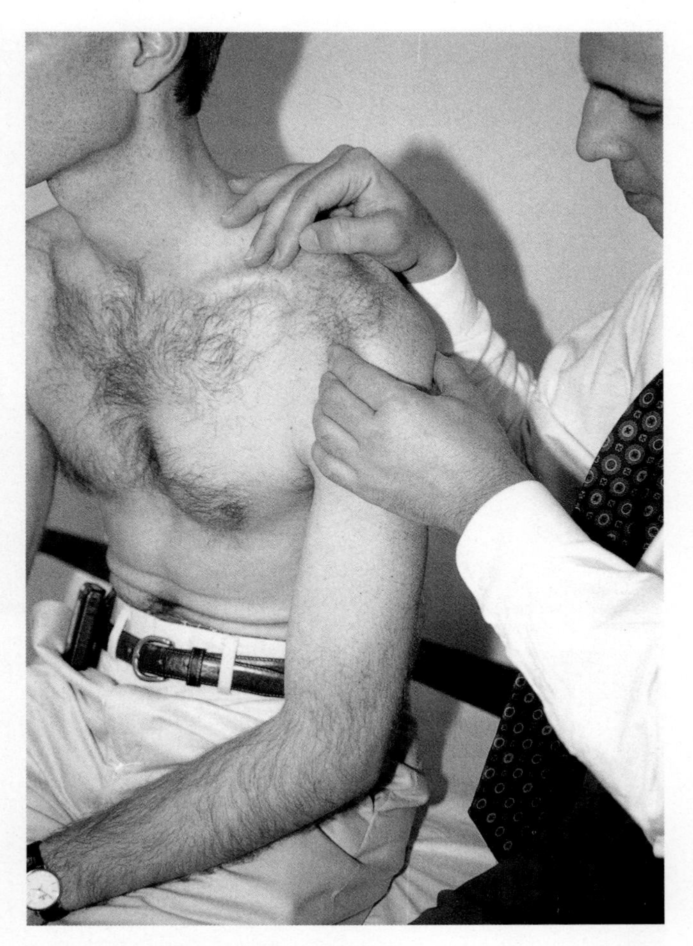

FIG. 5. Seated load and shift test The examiner is seated at the side of the patient. The scapula is stabilized with opposite hand. A centering force is applied to the glenohumeral joint, and the amount of anterior and posterior translation is assessed.

Inferior translation is assessed next by grasping the elbow, with the arm at the side, and applying an inferiorly directed force. Attention to the region below the acromion will show an indentation, indicating a sulcus sign if inferior instability exists, and should be estimated and recorded in centimeter increments (Fig. 7).[60] In most normal patients, passive ex-

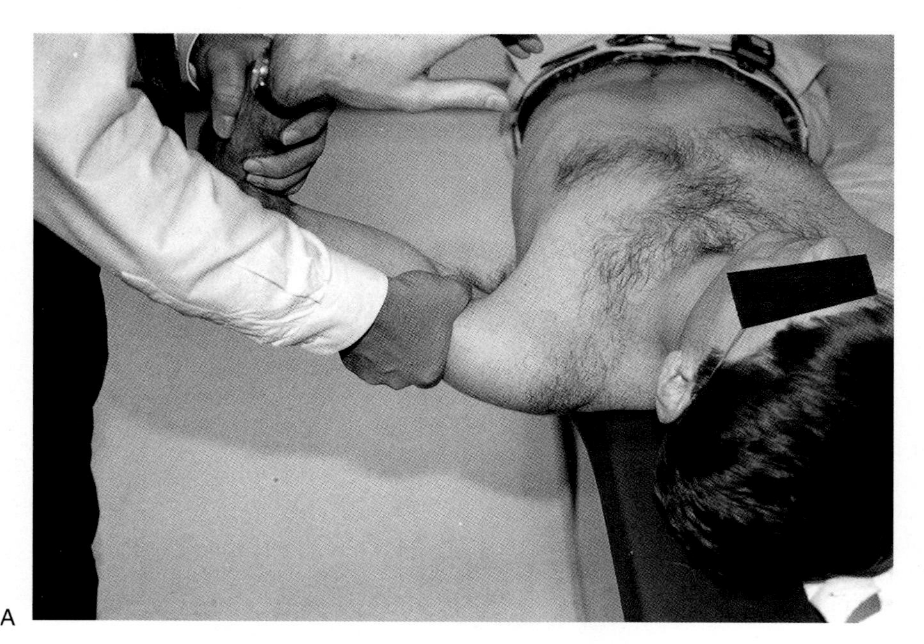

A

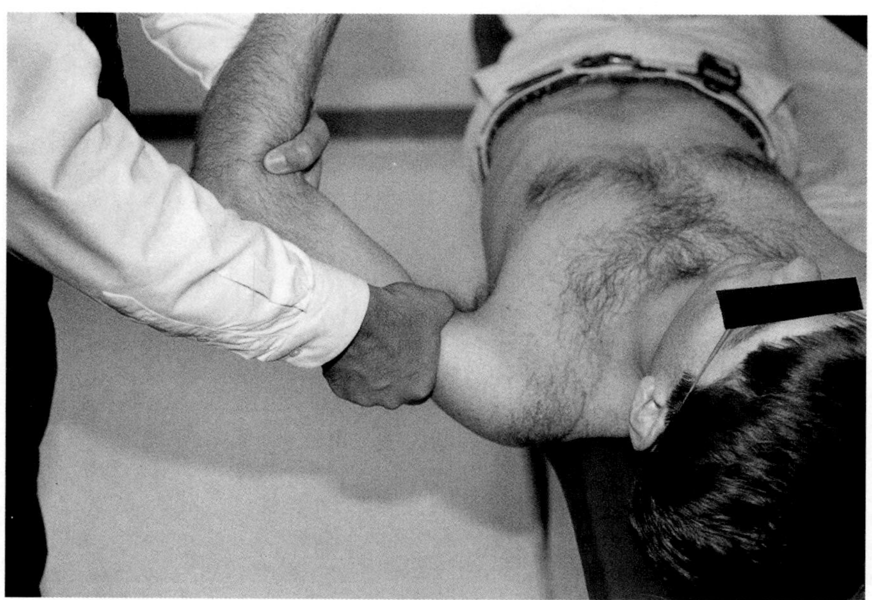

B

FIG. 6. Supine load and shift test: The patient is supine on the examining table. The arm is brought into approximately 90 degrees of forward elevation in the plane of the scapula. A posteriorly directed force is applied to the humerus with the arm in varying degrees of rotation from **(A)** external rotation to **(B)** internal rotation

ternal rotation will cause a decrease in the sulcus sign, which indicates an intact and functioning rotator interval capsule. Asymmetrical loss of this finding supports the diagnosis of a rotator interval lesion and, therefore, would help explain the cause of the instability.

The zone of instability is most often posteroinferior, but can also be straight posterior, or multidirectional. It is important to remember that increased laxity in one direction does not always correlate with, or mean instability. In patients in whom an isolated posterior component of instability exists, the posterior stress test and load and shift tests demonstrate subluxation at approximately 80 to 90 degrees of forward elevation. In the more common instance of a posteroinferior instability, subluxation occurs with more forward elevation (110 to 120 degrees). Additionally, a positive sulcus sign may exist. A sulcus sign that is asymmetrically positive identifies the inferior component of the instability and should raise the suspicion for insufficiency of the rotator interval capsule. In both instances, the degree of subluxation may be exaggerated by simultaneous adduction and external rotation. Rotator interval capsular insufficiency may be an isolated process or, more commonly, a component of multidirectional laxity. In cases of multidirectional laxity with instability primarily manifested in the posteroinferior zone, physical signs of generalized ligamentous laxity (i.e., hyperextension of the elbows, knees, metacarpophalangeal joints, or other) are often present. In addition, there is increased humeral head translation in all directions, but symptoms occur primarily with posterior translation. Distinguishing between these cases of isolated posterior, posteroinferior, and

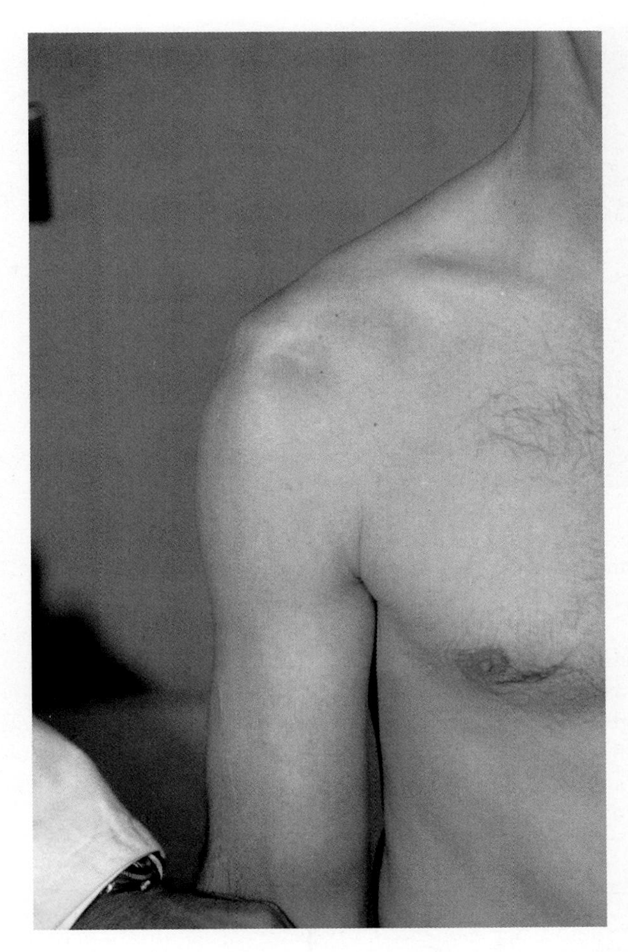

FIG. 7. Sulcus sign: The examiner is seated next to the patient. The forearm is grasped and an inferiorly directed force is applied to the arm in neutral glenohumeral rotation. Attention is directed to the region immediately inferior to the acromion. A positive sulcus sign will reduce with external rotation of the shoulder in a patient with a competent rotator interval capsule.

multidirectional laxity with a primarily posteroinferior component is important in determining treatment options. Depending on the etiology and pattern of instability and the anatomic lesions, the most appropriate treatment may be isolated posterior capsulorrhaphy (reverse Bankart procedure; posteroinferior capsular shift), a bony procedure (bone block or posterior glenoid osteotomy), or an anteroinferior capsular shift combined with rotator interval plication.

Imaging Studies

Routine radiographs of the shoulder should be obtained and include a true anteroposterior (AP) view obtained in the plane of the scapula, a lateral scapular or Y view, and an axillary view. These radiographs may not demonstrate any abnormalities. However, particular attention should be directed toward the axillary radiograph for evidence of calcification of the posterior capsule, fracture or erosion of the posterior glenoid (Fig. 8), or reverse Hill–Sachs defects (Fig. 9).[21,49,51]

Stress axillary radiographs or fluoroscopy are generally not necessary, for the history and physical examination usually clarify the diagnosis. However, in the small group of patients for whom doubt of the diagnosis remains, some authors have found these imaging modalities quite helpful.[15,45,50] Comparison with the unaffected side is recommended, for posterior glenohumeral translation of 50% has been demonstrated in normal shoulders.[26,49]

Advanced-imaging studies are not routinely used, but are considered when the specific pathologic lesion underlying recurrent posterior subluxation is unclear. Computed tomography (CT) excels in its ability to define bony detail. If plain radiographs suggest abnormalities of glenoid version, glenoid hypoplasia, or posterior glenoid erosion, CT or MRI is useful (Fig. 10).[24,59]

Computed arthrotomography was developed to better define intraarticular soft-tissue pathology and to allow assessment of capsular volume. Whereas Bigliani et al. found one-third of CT arthrotomograms to be over- or underread for labral pathology when correlated with findings at surgery, Callaghan found CT arthrotomography to be 100% accurate, sensitive, and specific for posterior labral defects (Fig. 11).[2,8]

Magnetic resonance imaging (MRI) has improved our ability to assess soft-tissue pathology about the shoulder. The advantages of MRI over plain radiographs and CT include no exposure to ionizing radiation, excellent soft-tissue

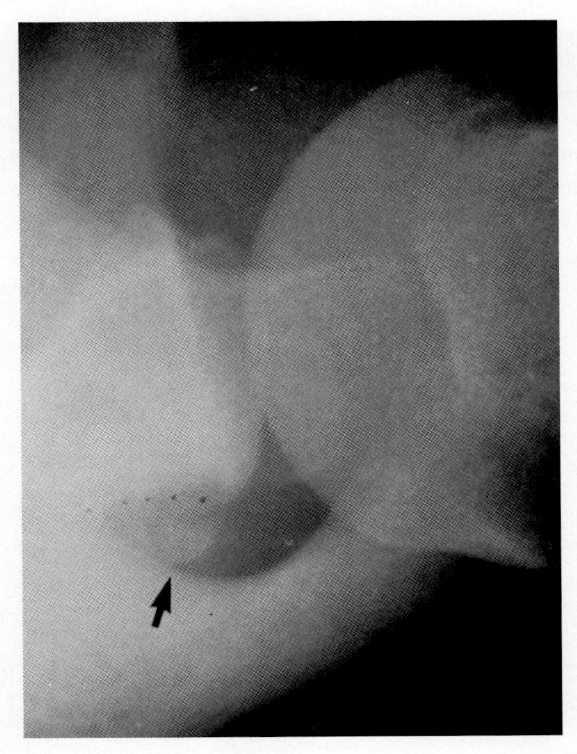

FIG. 8. Axillary radiograph showing fracture of the posterior glenoid rim (*arrow*). The fracture fragment has healed to the posterior glenoid neck.

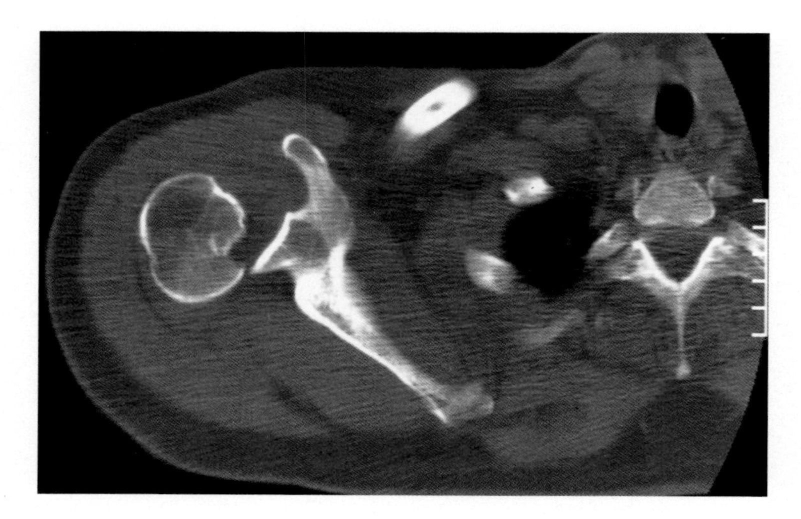

FIG. 9. A CT scan of a large reverse Hill–Sachs lesion.

resolution, noninvasiveness, and ability to image in multiple planes. Numerous studies have shown that MRI is superior to other imaging studies at defining labral and capsuloligamentous pathology.[25,32,34,35,37,67] The posterior capsule inserts directly onto the posterior glenoid labrum not the bony glenoid (Fig. 12). This anatomic relation of the capsulolabral complex often confuses accurate interpretation of MR images. The capsulolabral complex is best demonstrated with the arm in the neutral position. Imaging in external rotation can simulate a labral tear by creating posterior capsular redundancy at the capsulolabral junction.[70] Additionally, in the nondistended joint, the close proximity of the glenohumeral ligaments to the posterior glenoid labrum can be mistaken for a labral tear.[41,47]

Magnetic resonance arthrography (MR arthrography) has been more sensitive at detecting labral pathology than MRI.[10,19] Distention of the joint with contrast affords better visualization of the glenoid labrum and glenohumeral ligaments. Chandnani et al. found that MR arthrography more consistently detects labral tears, detached labral fragments, and labral degeneration than conventional MRI and CT arthrography.[10]

Advanced-imaging techniques have evolved rapidly and afford better definition of intraarticular pathology than do standard radiographic techniques. However, the information obtained can be misleading if not considered in context with the history and physical examination. These studies should be used to confirm the presence of suspected, specific pathologic lesions, rather than as a screening tool.

Examination Under Anesthesia

Before beginning definitive surgical stabilization, examination under anesthesia (EUA) is useful to confirm one's clinical suspicions, even in the most clinically obvious cases of recurrent posterior instability. The sensitivity and specificity of EUA is improved by examining the shoulder in various positions of shoulder elevation and rotation.[13] By placing the arm in 45 to 60 degrees of abduction and varying the degree of humeral rotation, the posterior band of the inferior

A

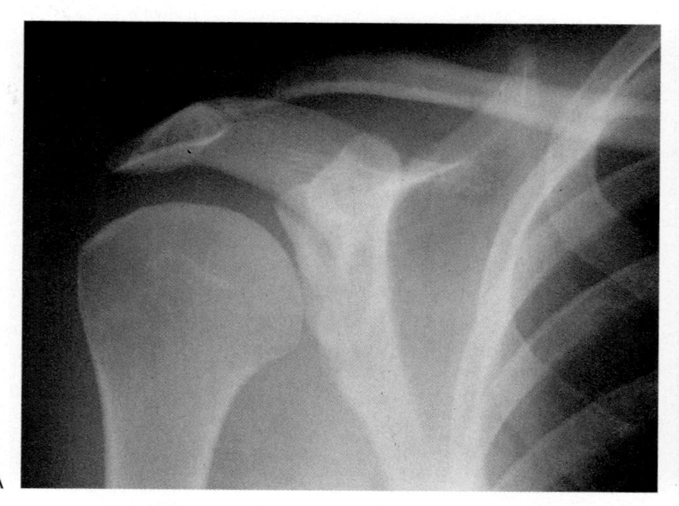

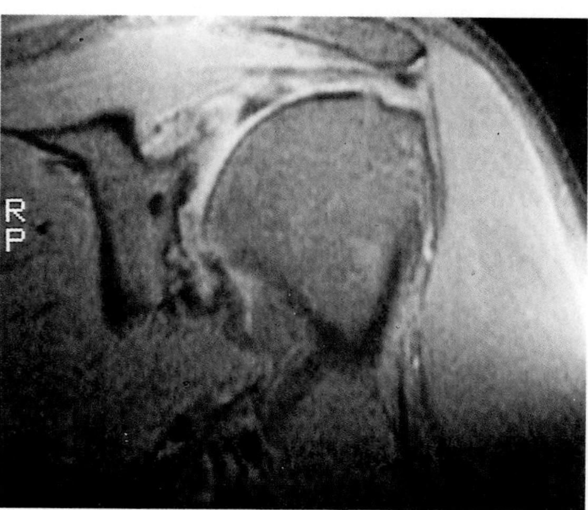

B

FIG. 10. **(A)** Anteroposterior radiograph and **(B)** MRI of a patient with posterior glenoid hypoplasia with increased glenoid retroversion.

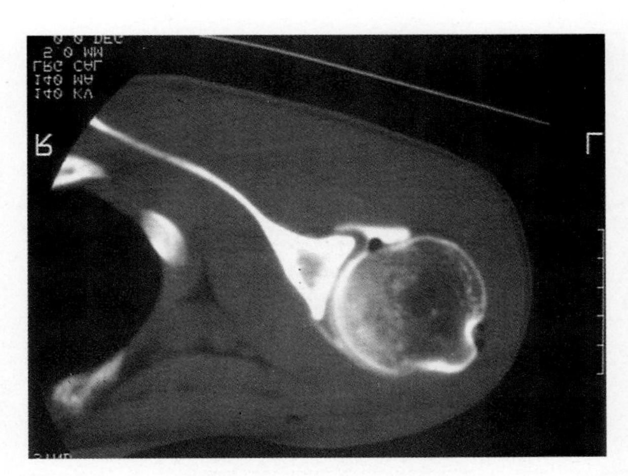

FIG. 11. A CT arthrogram of the shoulder. Intraarticular contrast improves visualization of the glenoid labrum.

glenohumeral ligament and posterior capsule are placed under varying degrees of tension. With the arm in external rotation, the posterior capsular structures are lax allowing posterior translation of the humeral head against a posteriorly directed force. Progressive internal rotation tightens these structures, resulting in capture of the humeral head and elimination of posterior translation against a posteriorly directed force. It is important to note the degree of internal rotation at which posterior translation is minimized. Differences in posterior translation in different arm positions when compared with the opposite shoulder are indicative of posterior capsular insufficiency.

In those circumstances under which a high degree of suspicion exists for posterior subluxation, one may further consider diagnostic arthroscopy after an equivocal examination under anesthesia. Although not as helpful in detecting specific pathologic lesions, such as anterior instability, observation of an incompetent posterior inferior glenohumeral ligament or an excessively redundant posterior capsule may assist one in defining the pathology present before attempting posterior stabilization in special situations.[13]

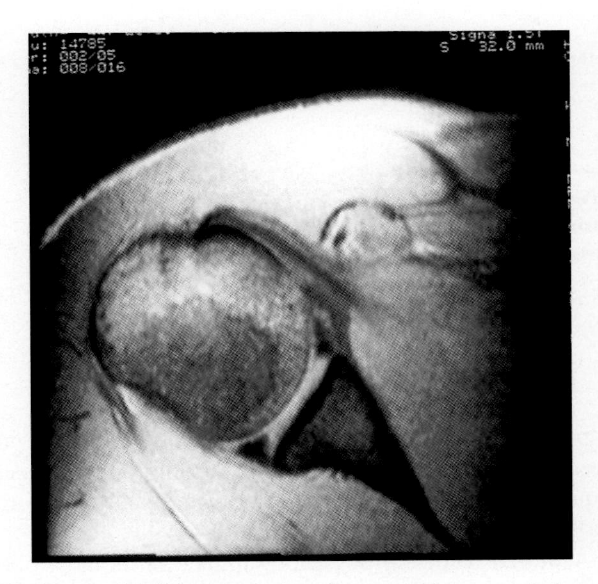

FIG. 12. An MRI demonstrating the posterior capsule inserting on labrum not the glenoid.

TREATMENT

The diagnostic workup along with the treatment algorithm employed by our Shoulder and Elbow Service for recurrent posterior subluxation is summarized in Fig. 13.

Nonoperative

The recommended initial treatment by most authors for symptomatic recurrent posterior subluxation is nonoperative.[7,21,29,42,51,55,57,73] Nonoperative treatment should include activity modification; psychologic counseling for patients with voluntary, psychogenic recurrent posterior subluxation; and a shoulder-strengthening program for the dynamic muscular stabilizers, including the rotator cuff (especially infraspinatus and teres minor), posterior deltoid, and scapular stabilizing muscles. Activity modification is aimed at preventing further injury or stress to the posterior capsule, labrum, or rotator cuff. Activities that place the shoulder in the provocative position of forward elevation, adduction, and internal rotation are best avoided during rehabilitation.

Strengthening is accomplished through resisted external rotation exercises with rubber bands of increasing resistance or free weights, and in time, may progress to isokinetic exercises. It is important to balance the strengthening program with internal rotation exercises. Additionally, periscapular strengthening is vital to reestablish synchronous scapulohumeral rhythm.[44]

Patients who fail a prolonged trial of nonoperative therapy and remain symptomatic should be considered for surgical stabilization. Some authors have found that patients with incapacitating symptoms do poorly with nonoperative management compared with patients with moderate symptoms and suggest early surgical intervention.[4,21] Surgery should be directed at correcting the underlying pathologic lesion causing recurrent subluxation. This underscores the value of an anatomically based classification system, rather than the etiology-based system currently favored.

Surgical Options and Rationale for Surgical Treatment

Numerous posterior procedures have been described for recurrent posterior subluxation. These procedures include posterior capsulorrhaphy, with or without a bone block, posterior bone block alone, glenoid osteotomy, posterior infraspinatus capsular tenodesis, and posteroinferior capsular shift.[1,2,5,6,20,21,36,38,43,45,46,48,51,57,66] Historically, the results of surgery have been poor, with recurrence rates of up to 50% with significant complications.[29,74] The use of proce-

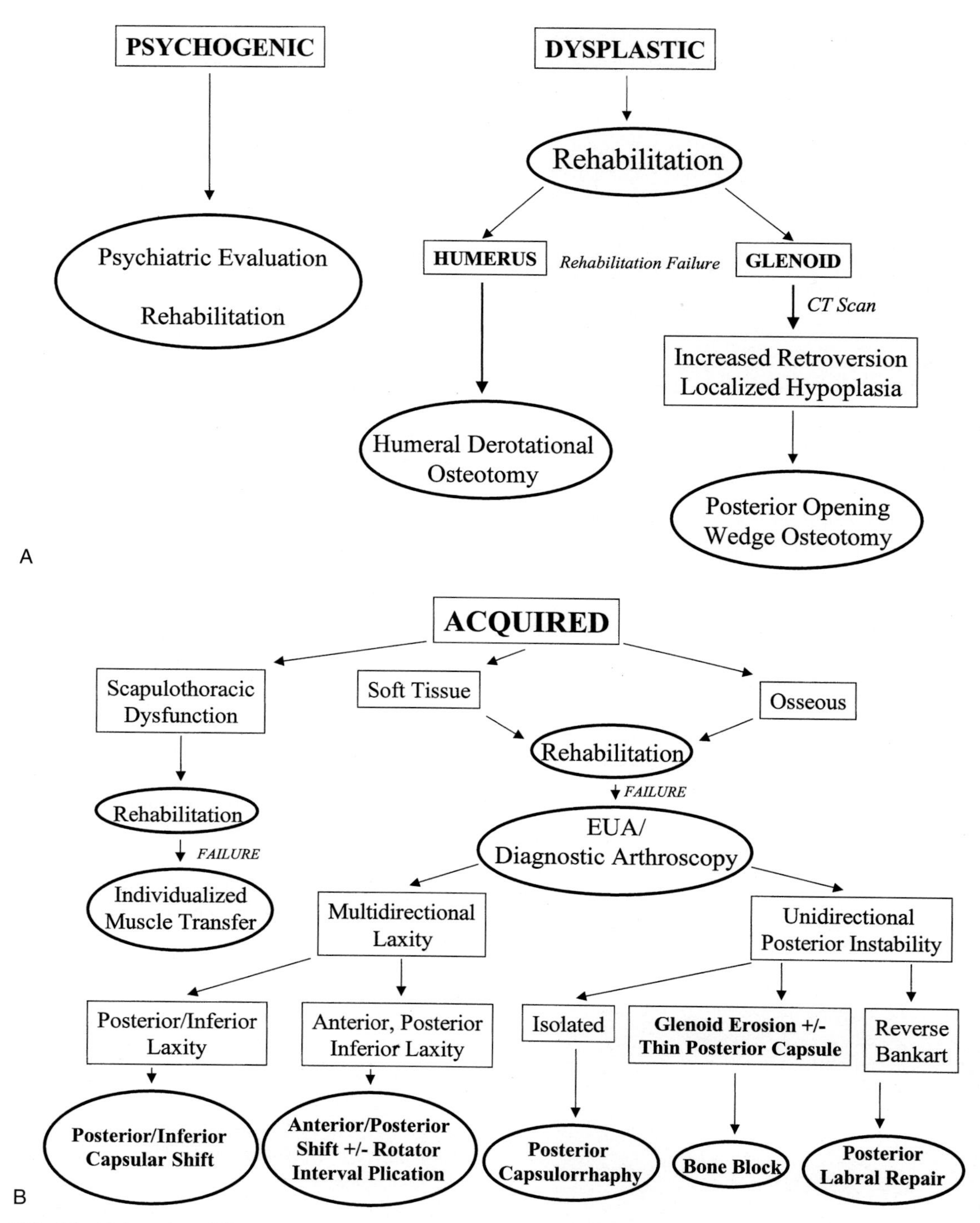

FIG. 13. University of Pennsylvania treatment algorithm for recurrent posterior subluxation. **(A)** Psychogenic and dysplastic recurrent posterior subluxation and **(B)** acquired posterior subluxation.

dures when the pathology of recurrent posterior subluxation was not well understood preoperatively or not completely addressed at surgery no doubt contributed to these poor results. Recently, surgical techniques have been employed that anatomically correct the underlying pathology. This has resulted in more-encouraging results.[3,21] Consequently, the importance of accurately defining the pathologic lesion preoperatively cannot be overstated. The specific surgical techniques are determined by the underlying pathology in each particular case.

Acquired recurrent posterior subluxation is most often caused by soft-tissue deficiency (capsule, labrum, or both), erosion or deficiency of the posterior glenoid, or scapulothoracic dysfunction. A patulous posterior capsule is usually the primary pathologic lesion. If a reverse Bankart lesion coexists with a redundant posterior capsule, a combined repair of the reverse Bankart lesion and posterior capsular plication or shift is necessary. When posterior capsular redundancy or detachment is combined with erosion of the posterior glenoid rim or increased glenoid retroversion (i.e., hypoplasia), the posterior capsular procedure is combined with posterior glenoid bone graft or posterior opening wedge osteotomy, respectively. Posterior bone block may also be indicated for properly performed, but failed capsular procedures, even if the glenoid architecture is normal.

It is critical to determine the direction of instability before surgery. If instability is only posterior, a procedure addressing the redundant posterior capsule is warranted. However, posterior subluxation is often accompanied by varying degrees of inferior and multidirectional laxity. In cases of posteroinferior subluxation when there is no anterior component to the instability pattern and the rotator interval capsule is functionally intact, a posteroinferior capsular shift from a posterior approach should be performed. In patients with multidirectional laxity, the surgical approach depends on the primary location of their symptoms. If their symptoms are directed to the posterior aspect of the shoulder, we prefer to approach these posteriorly and perform a posteroinferior capsular shift. Conversely, anterior symptoms are addressed with an anterorinferior capsular shift. In the rare patient with true multidirectional instability with anterior and posterior symptoms, combined anterior and posterior capsular procedures are performed.

Surgical treatment of scapular winging is beyond the scope of this chapter. However, the importance of restoring scapulothoracic mechanics in controlling posterior instability cannot be overemphasized. Scapular winging can be an important contributor to recurrent posterior subluxation. When caused by long thoracic nerve injury, pectoralis major transfer, alone or in combination with posterior capsulorrhaphy, may be indicated.[58] In these cases, it is often difficult to determine the need for posterior capsulorrhaphy in addition to the pectoralis major transfer. In most instances, pectoralis major muscle transfer alone is sufficient to correct the posterior instability symptoms.

Glenoid or humeral dysplasia is an uncommon cause of posterior subluxation. However, in the presence of glenoid hypoplasia or increased glenoid retroversion, a glenoid osteotomy should be considered.[66] Humeral rotational osteotomy is considered only when there is documented abnormal humeral retrotorsion.[11,71]

Patients with a psychologic cause for recurrent posterior subluxation should be managed with an exercise program combined with psychologic counseling.[62] Surgery is contraindicated as long as the underlying psychologic needs leading the patient to voluntarily subluxate his or her shoulder exist. Surgery should be considered only after their underlying psychologic problems are resolved and the patient still demonstrates symptomatic involuntary recurrent posterior subluxation. Extreme caution is still warranted in performing surgery in this group of patients. If any element of psychogenic posterior subluxation remains, surgery is doomed to failure.

Surgical Technique

Patient Positioning

The patient is positioned in the lateral decubitus position and secured with anterior and posterior posts or a bean bag. The head and neck should be supported in neutral position and the knees and ankles padded. Impervious drapes are placed at the base of the neck and around the axilla, medial to the vertebral border of the scapula, and a minimum of 6 cm medial to the anterior axillary crease (Fig. 14). The arm is prepared and draped free. The arm may be supported anteriorly on a Mayo stand, or an intraoperative sterile shoulder positioner (McConnell Orthopedic Manufacturing Co.; Greenville, TX) may be used.

Surgical Approach

The incision begins at the posterior axillary crease and extends superiorly to the spine of the scapula (Fig. 15). Medial subcutaneous dissection is carried out to the border of the

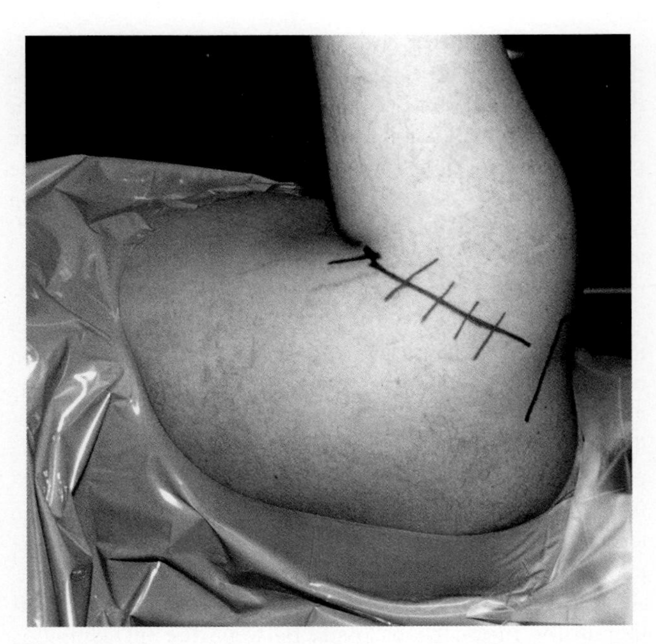

FIG. 14. Intraoperative photograph demonstrating patient positioning and draping in the lateral decubitus position. The shoulder should be draped widely to allow palpation and visualization of topographic structures that will aid in dissection.

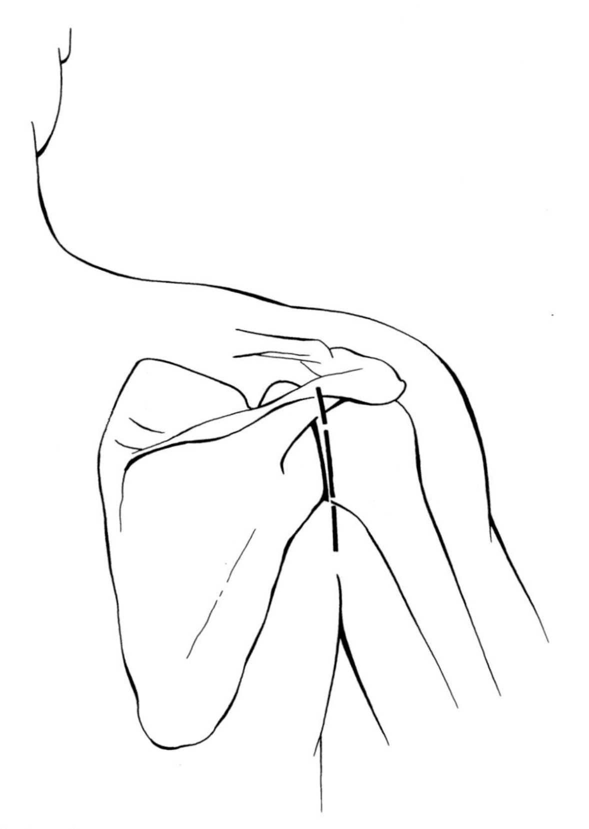

FIG. 15. Drawing of incision for posterior shoulder surgery. A vertical incision is preferred for cosmetic reasons. The incision begins at the spine of the scapula and extends to the posterior axillary crease.

posterior deltoid. The lateral subcutaneous dissection is to the lateral border of the acromion. The fibers of the posterior deltoid are split in that portion of the deltoid that overlies the posterior glenohumeral joint line, from the spine of the scapula distally for a distance of 4 to 5 cm. Blunt dissection of the posterior deltoid fibers is carried deep to the subdeltoid bursa, exposing the underlying infraspinatus and teres minor muscles (Fig. 16). An alternative approach for exposure of the infraspinatus and teres minor muscles is to elevate the posterior deltoid along its inferior margin. Identification of the inferior border of the posterior deltoid allows this margin to be defined. Dissection to the subdeltoid space and abduction of the shoulder facilitate superior retraction of the posterior deltoid. Deep retractors are placed to expose the infraspinatus and teres minor tendons (Fig. 17). Inferior to the teres minor is the quadrangular space that contains the axillary nerve and posterior humeral circumflex vessels.

Exposure of the posterior capsule can be accomplished either in the internervous plane between the infraspinatus (suprascapular nerve) and teres minor (axillary nerve) or within the posterior fat stripe that separates the upper and lower portions of the infraspinatus muscle.[68,79] The fat stripe commonly seen between the upper and lower halves of the infraspinatus muscle is located at the midequator of the glenohumeral joint. Dissection through the infraspinatus fat stripe will place the operative procedure more central within the glenohumeral joint and, thereby, facilitate better exposure of the upper portion of the joint. It is possible to perform posterior capsulorrhaphy through this interval without detaching the infraspinatus insertion, and it is our preferred technique. In this approach, this interval is developed to the posterior capsule (Fig. 18). Dissection superiorly to the supraspinatus tendon and inferiorly to the posteroinferior aspect of the joint is undertaken, and reverse Homan retractors are placed to expose the capsule. Medial dissection along the infraspinatus muscle is limited to 1.5 cm medial to the glenoid margin to avoid injury to the inferior branch of the suprascapular nerve that would denervate the inferior portion of the infraspinatus muscle. Medial exposure is the primary limitation of this approach.

The most extensile exposure of the posterior capsule is obtained by dissecting the interval between the infraspinatus and teres minor. This interval can be extended medially without fear of denervating the infraspinatus (Fig. 19). The infraspinatus muscle and tendon are then bluntly dissected from the underlying capsule. The thickness of the infraspinatus tendon can then be assessed. The midtendinous portion of the infraspinatus tendon is then incised to the level

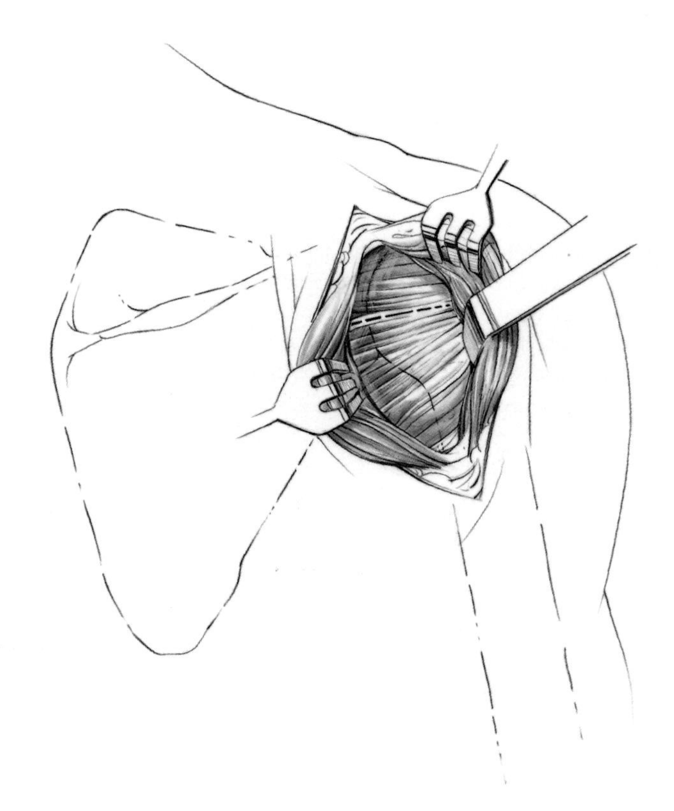

FIG. 16. The longitudinal split in the deltoid should be performed so that the operative field is over the center of the glenohumeral joint, exposing the infraspinatus and teres minor muscles.

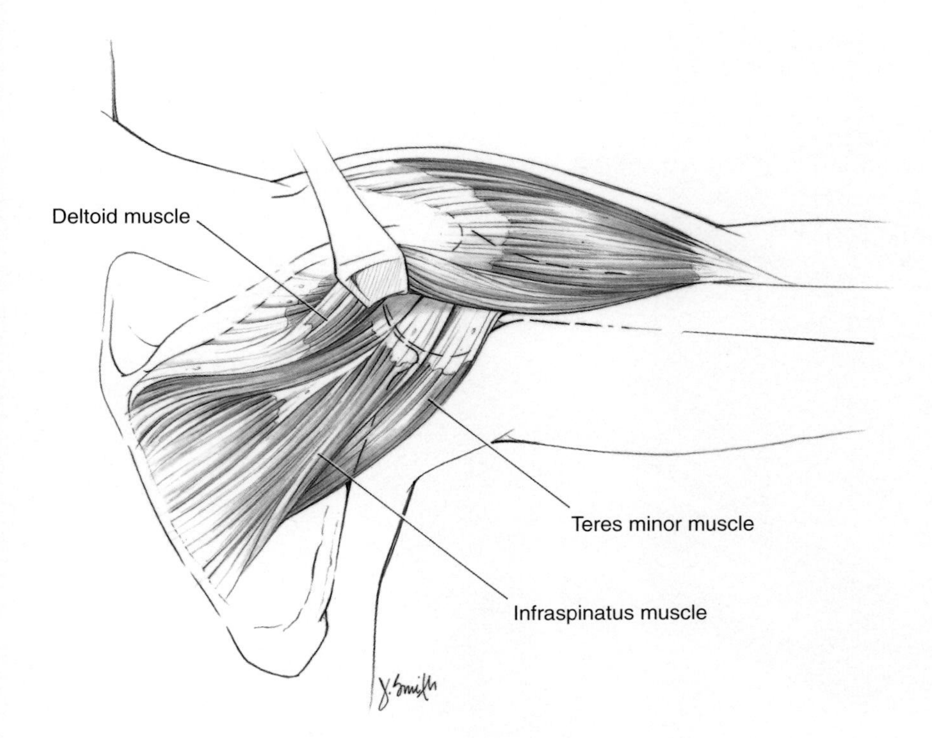

FIG. 17. Superior elevation of the deltoid is an alternative to a deltoid split. The arm must be placed in 90 degrees or more of elevation to allow the deltoid to be retracted cephalad.

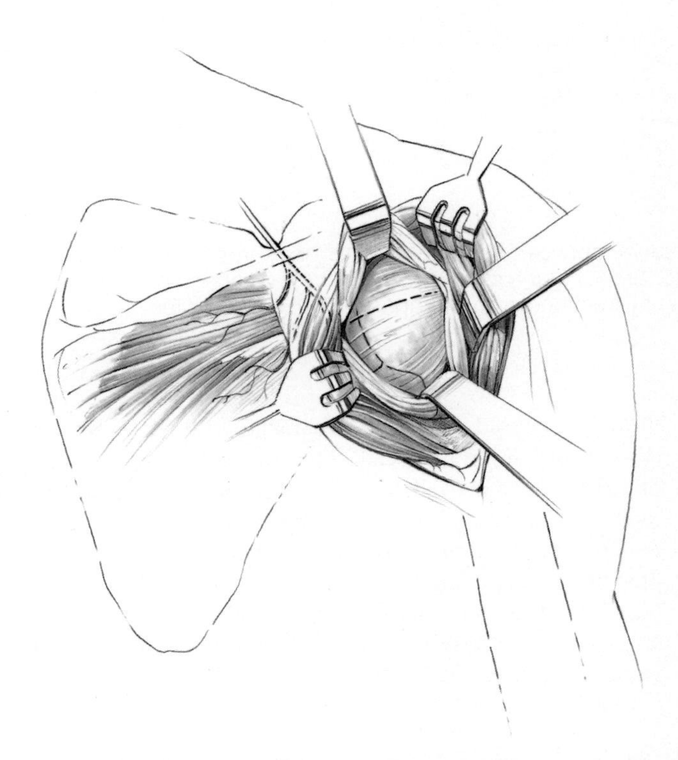

FIG. 18. Posterior capsular exposure through a fat stripe split between the upper and lower portion of the infraspinatus. Medial dissection is limited to 1.5 cm medial to the glenoid so that injury to the inferior branch of the suprascapular nerve is avoided.

of the capsule, approximately 1 cm medial to its humeral attachment. Further blunt dissection is performed to separate the infraspinatus tendon from the capsule superiorly, medial to the glenoid rim and laterally toward the greater tuberosity. The infraspinatus is then reflected medially. Caution should be used in retracting the infraspinatus medial to the glenoid rim to avoid excessive traction on the suprascapular nerve at the spinoglenoid notch. Using a narrow blunt elevator, the posteroinferior capsule is dissected from the underlying teres minor. A narrow, deep blunt retractor is placed deep to the teres minor to expose the posteroinferior capsule.

Posterior Capsulorrhaphy (Author's Preferred Technique)

The capsule is incised in a medial to lateral direction midway between the superior and inferior poles of the glenoid. Traction sutures may be placed in the superoinferior portions of the capsule. A humeral head retractor is inserted, and the glenoid rim is inspected. When a capsular avulsion is not identified then the vertical capsular incision is performed approximately 5 mm medial to the humeral insertion site of the capsule (Fig. 20). The capsulotomy is performed superiorly to the posterior insertion site of the supraspinatus tendon. The inferior extent of the lateral capsulotomy is dependent on the degree of inferior capsular redundancy. In general, the lateral capsulotomy is carried out past the inferior most por-

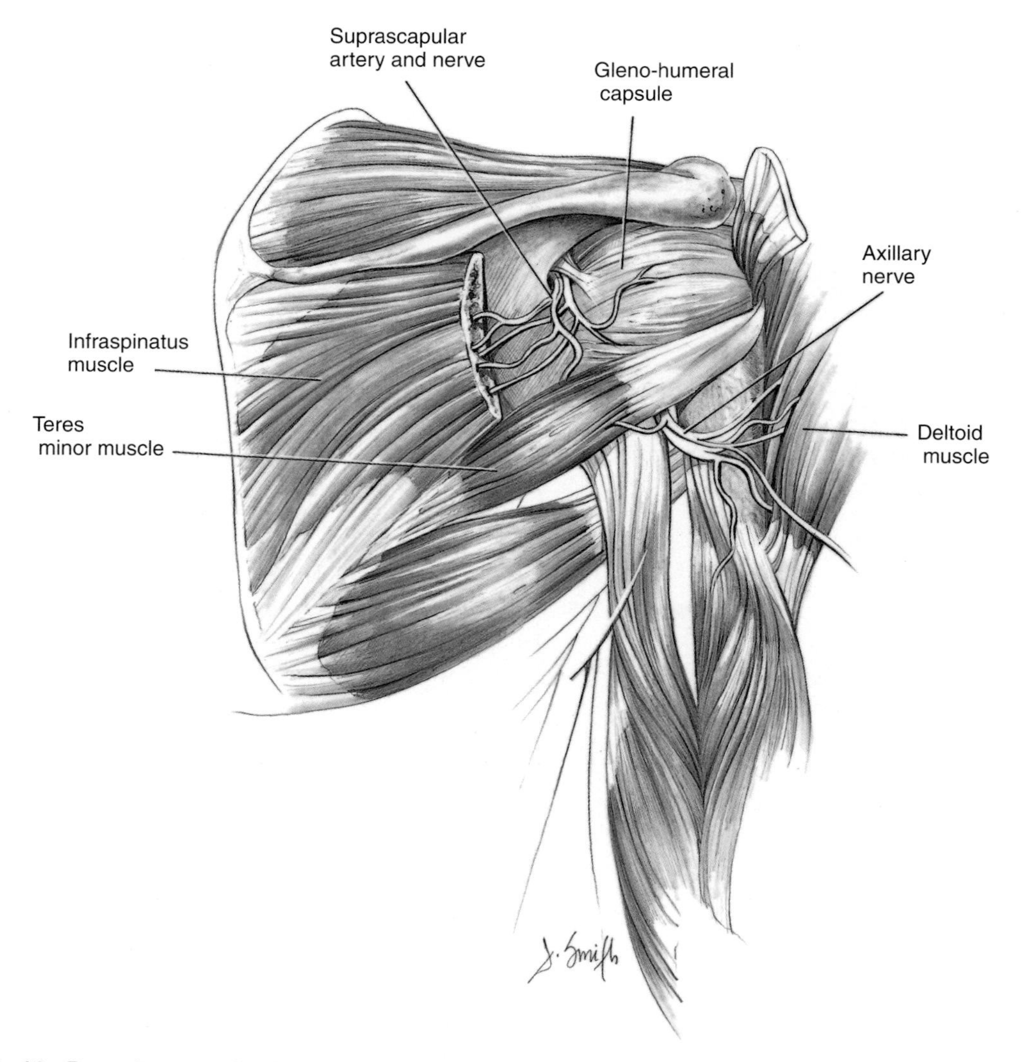

FIG. 19. Posterior capsular exposure through the interval between the infraspinatus and teres minor muscles. This is an extensile exposure to the posterior aspect of the shoulder. Vigorous medial retraction of the infraspinatus should be avoided to prevent traction on the suprascapular nerve at the spinoglenoid notch.

tion of the inferior capsular pouch to the 6:00 o'clock position. The arm is then placed in the plane of the scapula in 45 degrees of abduction and neutral rotation to approximately 15 degrees of external rotation. The inferior leaflet is then shifted superiorly to obliterate the inferior capsular pouch and place the inferior leaflet under slight tension. Lateral capsular closure is accomplished with nonabsorbable sutures. The superior capsular flap is then shifted inferiorly to the point of slight tissue tension.[46] Lateral capsular closure is achieved with nonabsorbable sutures. The interval between the superior and inferior flaps are then closed and reinforced with nonabsorbable sutures (Fig. 21).

If the infraspinatus tendon was cut, it is then closed with slight overlap of the tissue using nonabsorbable sutures. If it was not incised, the infraspinatus is allowed to retract to its normal position and the fascia is closed with absorbable sutures. The deltoid is allowed to retract to its normal position. Absorbable suture is placed in the superficial fascia, and a drain is inserted in the depth of the wound. The subcutaneous tissues are closed with absorbable suture and the skin with nonabsorbable suture using the subcuticular technique. Steri-Strips and a sterile dressing are placed and the arm is positioned in a prefabricated prefitted thoracobrachial orthosis. The arm is positioned slightly posterior to the coronal plane of the thorax in 20 degrees of abduction and 10 degrees of external rotation.

Posterior Labral Repair

The patient positioning and surgical exposure are described on pages 307 and 308. The horizontal capsulotomy is performed, a humeral head retractor is inserted, and the joint is

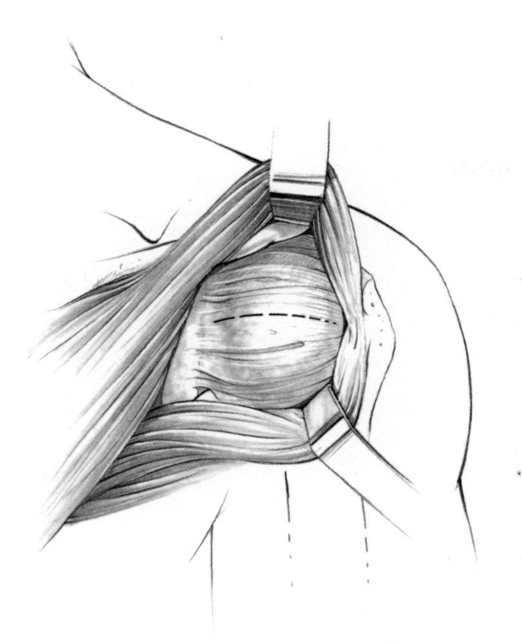

FIG. 20. A horizontal capsulotomy is performed at the midequator of the joint, allowing intraarticular inspection. The lateral vertical limb of the capsulotomy is performed 5 mm medial to the humeral attachment when no posterior labral pathology is noted.

inspected. If a reverse Bankart lesion is identified, the scapular neck must be prepared and the capsule reattached to the glenoid rim. The vertical capsular exposure is made by dissection of the Bankart lesion, thereby reflecting the capsulolabral tissue from the glenoid margin. The posterior glenoid and scapular neck are then decorticated with a curette or power burr. The labrum is reattached to the articular margin of the posterior glenoid using commercially available suture anchors or transosseous tunnels (Fig. 22).

A posteroinferior capsular shift is performed, with repair of the reverse Bankart lesion if excessive posteroinferior capsular redundancy exists. The capsular shift can be performed on the glenoid side when the labrum is repaired or on the humeral side after the labrum is repaired. The humerus is positioned in less external rotation (10 degrees) to avoid overtightening. If the shift is performed on the glenoid side, the capsule and labrum are cut at the midglenoid creating both a superior and inferior flap. The inferior capsular leaflet is then shifted superiorly to obliterate the inferior capsular pouch and place the inferior leaflet under slight tension. The inferior leaflet is repaired to the glenoid margin with suture anchors placed at the glenoid margin. The superior leaflet is subsequently shifted inferiorly to a point of slight tissue tension. The sutures used to secure the inferior leaflet to the glenoid margin are used to secure the superior leaflet (Fig. 23). Infraspinatus closure, skin closure, and bracing are performed as discussed in the foregoing section.

If the capsular shift is performed on the humeral side in the presence of a reverse Bankart lesion, the capsule is incised at the midglenoid level to, but not through, the labrum. The labrum is repaired anatomically (without shift) to the glenoid

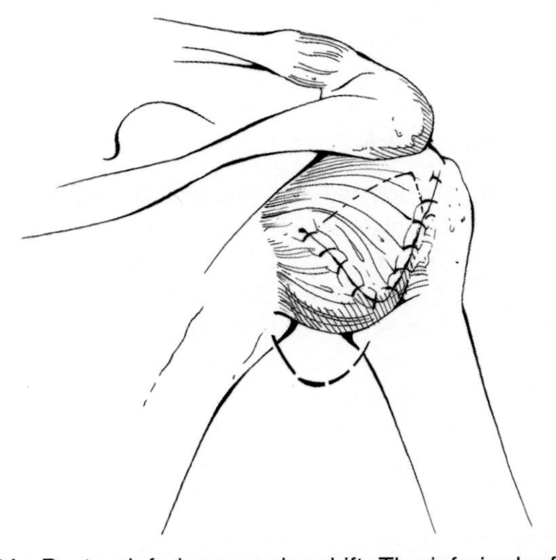

FIG. 21. Posteroinferior capsular shift: The inferior leaflet is shifted superiorly to slight tissue tension with the arm positioned in approximately 45 degrees of abduction and neutral to slight external rotation. The superior leaflet is subsequently shifted inferiorly.

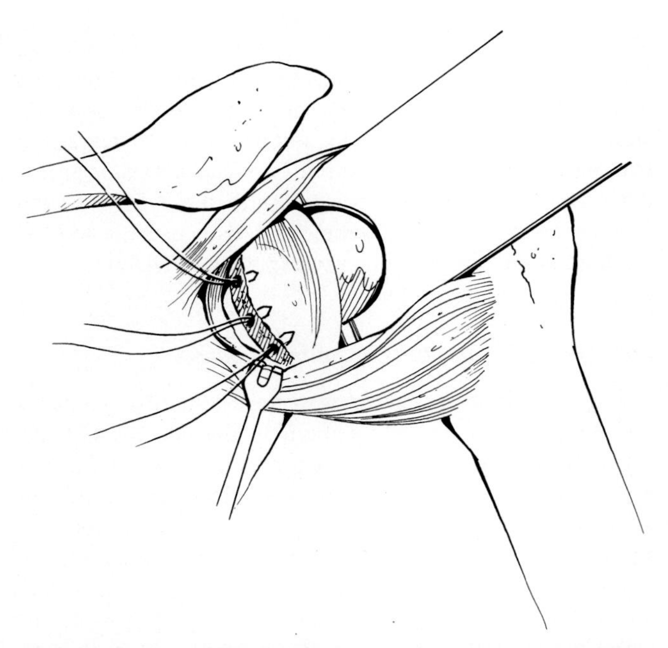

FIG. 22. Posterior labral repair: The horizontal capsulotomy is performed. A humeral head retractor and forked retractor provide exposure to the posterior glenoid neck. The glenoid neck is decorticated and suture anchors or transosseous sutures are placed along the glenoid margin, passed through the detached labral tissue, and tied, thereby reestablishing the normal anatomy of the posterior labrum and glenoid.

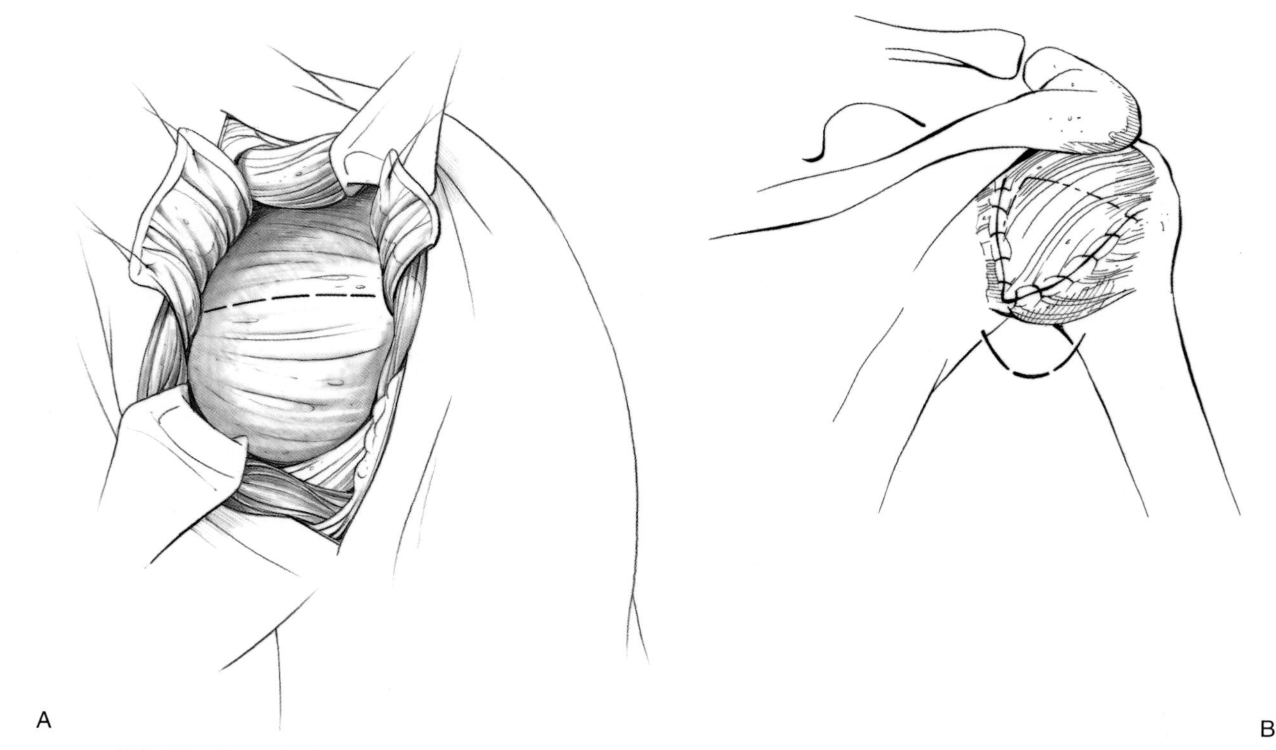

FIG. 23. Posterior labral repair with medial based capsular shift: The horizontal capsulotomy continues through the capsule and labrum. The inferior capsular leaflet and labrum are shifted superiorly to slight tissue tension with the arm in 45 degrees of abduction and neutral to slight external rotation. The superior capsular leaflet and labrum are than shifted inferiorly

margin using suture anchors or transosseous tunnels (see Fig. 22). The capsule is then incised vertically 5 mm medial to its humeral insertion site. The arm is positioned in the position of 45-degrees abduction, and neutral to 10 degrees of external rotation, and a posteroinferior capsular shift procedure is performed, as previously described (see Figs. 20 and 21). This is our preferred technique when a capsular shift is required in the presence of a reverse Bankart lesion.

Posterior Infraspinatus Capsular Tenodesis

Patient positioning and exposure are as described on pages 307 and 308 Once the deltoid is split or elevated, the underlying infraspinatus is exposed. The arm is the placed in neutral position and a 2.5-cm–vertical incision is made through the infraspinatus and underlying capsule, centered on the superior and inferior glenoid margins. This is medial to the insertion of infraspinatus and leaves a lateral cuff of infraspinatus and underlying capsule for tenodesis (Fig. 24). The posterior labral tissue is then identified. If a posterior labral detachment (i.e., reverse Bankart) is found, it is repaired with sutures or a suture-anchoring system, as previously described. The lateral flap of infraspinatus and capsule are then mobilized and secured to the posterior glenoid labrum with nonabsorbable suture, with the arm in slight external rotation (Fig. 25). The remaining portion of infraspinatus and underlying capsule is overlapped over the primary repair with the arm in neutral to slight internal rotation. The deltoid is then allowed to retract back to its normal resting position and the subcutaneous tissue is approximated with absorbable suture. The skin is closed with a nonabsorbable suture in a running subcuticular fashion.[28]

Posterior Bone Block

Patient positioning and exposure is as described on pages 307 and 308. The capsule is incised in the medial lateral direction at the midlevel of the capsule and the joint is inspected. A 2 $\times$ 2-cm, 7- to 10-mm–thick bone graft is obtained from the posterior iliac crest or posterior scapular spine (Fig. 26). The posterior glenoid neck is exposed and the inferior half is decorticated. The capsular–labral attachment to the inferior glenoid is left intact. The cancellous side of the bone graft is placed against the posterior glenoid neck so that it extents to, but not beyond, the posterior glenoid rim (Fig. 27). The bone graft is secured with one or two partially threaded cancellous screws. A burr may be used to contour and trim the bone graft to the level of the posterior glenoid rim after it is secured. The capsule, infraspinatus, and wound are closed as described earlier. If a capsular plication or shift is performed at the time of the bone block procedure and a re-

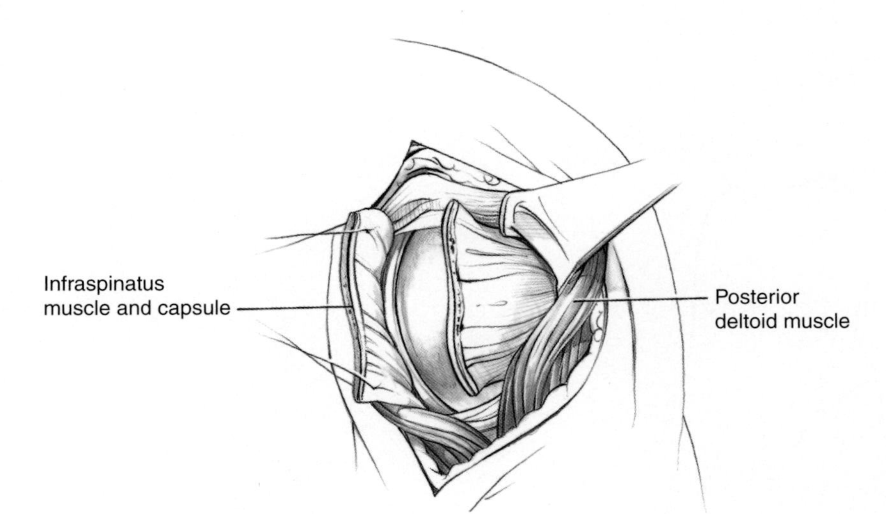

FIG. 24. Posterior infraspinatus capsular tenodesis: The arm is positioned in neutral rotation and the infraspinatus muscle and underlying posterior capsule are incised at, and parallel to, the glenoid rim.

verse Bankart lesion is not present, then a humeral-sided vertical capsulotomy is performed and a capsular shift is carried out as previously described.

Posterior Opening Wedge Glenoid Osteotomy

Patient positioning and exposure is as described on pages 307 and 308. The capsule is incised in a superior-to-inferior direction at the midlevel of the capsule, and the joint is inspected. A straight, flat instrument, such as a osteotome, is placed along the surface of the glenoid fossa. The osteotomy is made parallel to the face of the glenoid surface 10 mm medial to the posterior glenoid rim. The glenoid osteotomy is taken to, but not completely through, the anterior glenoid cortex. Keeping the anterior cortex and periosteum intact is important in keeping the osteotomy stable. The osteotomy is then opened and a cortical bone graft harvested from the spine of the scapula is used to maintain the osteotomy in the open position (Fig. 28). Internal fixation is generally not required, but a small staple may be used if the osteotomy is unstable. If capsular redundancy is present a horizontal capsular incision in the medial-to-lateral direction is performed and a medial based capsular shift is performed. Infraspinatus and wound closure is performed in standard fashion.

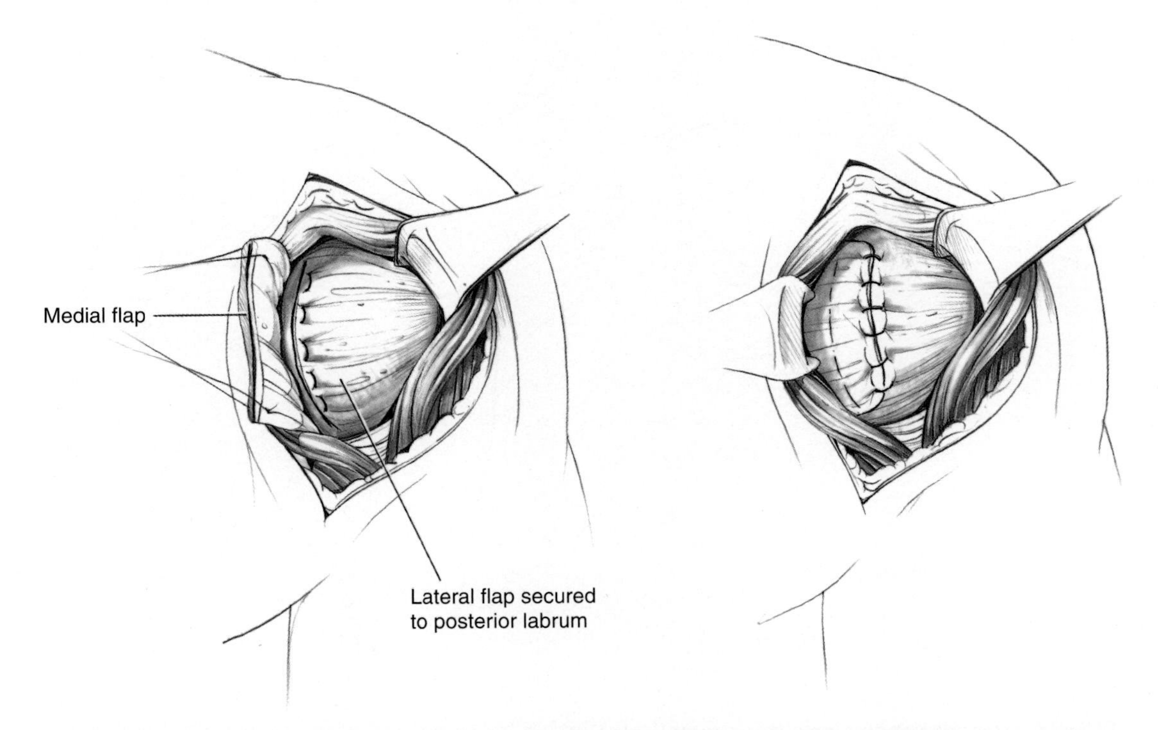

FIG. 25. (A) The arm is placed in slight external rotation and the lateral flap of infraspinatus, and capsule is secured to the posterior labrum. **(B)** The medial flap of infraspinatus and capsule overlaps the lateral flap.

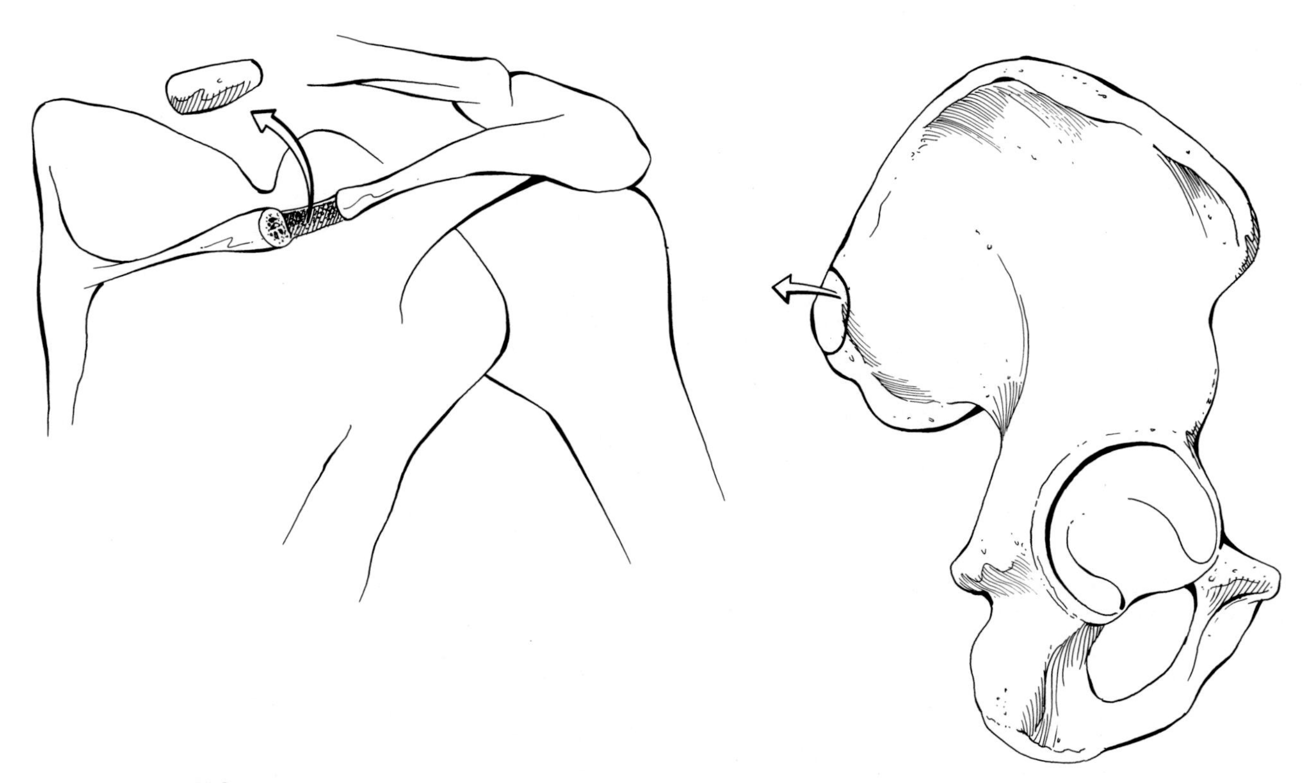

FIG. 26. Bone graft is harvested from **(A)** the scapular spine or **(B)** posterior iliac crest.

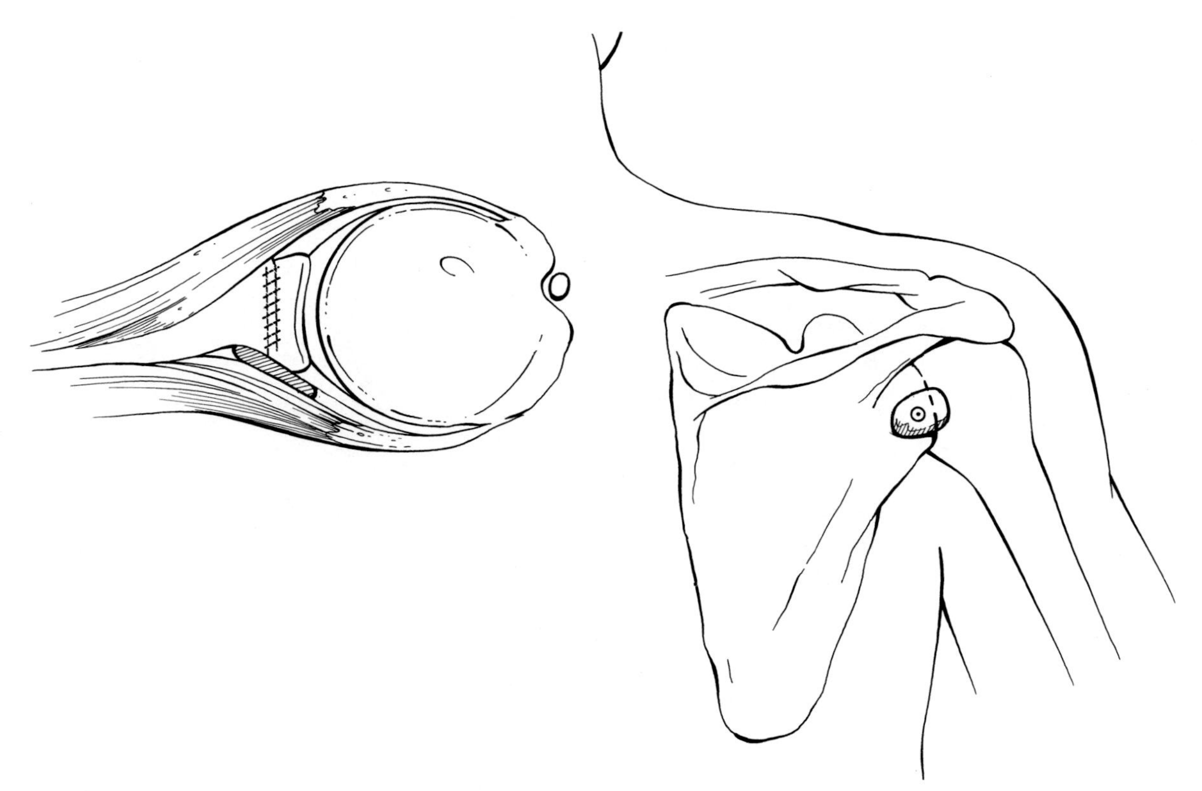

FIG. 27. Posterior bone block: Bone graft is placed just inferior to the equator of the glenoid. Note the graft does not extend posterior to the posterior continuation of the glenoid rim.

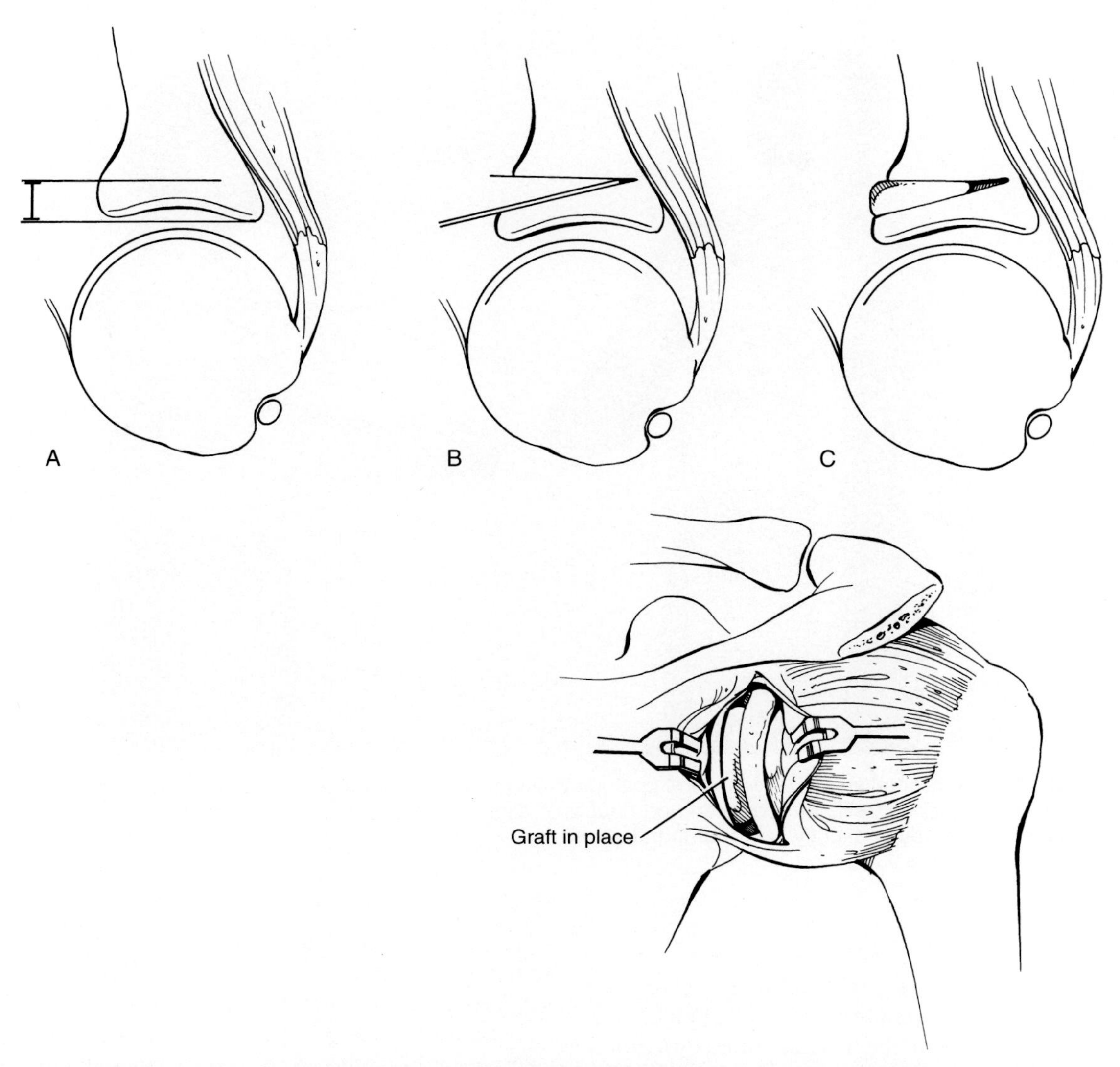

FIG. 28. Posterior opening wedge osteotomy. **(A)** An osteotomy is performed 10 mm medial to the glenoid margin, parallel to the face of the articular surface. **(B)** The osteotomy extends to, but not through, the anterior cortex of the glenoid. **(C)** Bone graft is placed in the opened osteotomy to maintain the relocated position of the articular surface.

POSTOPERATIVE CONSIDERATIONS

Postoperative management after posterior shoulder surgery requires the use of a thoracobrachial orthosis. Prior to surgery patients are fitted for the orthosis with the arm positioned in slight abduction in or slightly posterior to the coronal plane of the body and in neutral to 10 degrees of external rotation (Fig. 29). The prefitted orthosis is applied in the operating room at the conclusion of the surgical procedure.

Immobilization is maintained for a 4- to 6-week period. The time period is determined by the degree of passive motion measured 4 weeks postoperatively. If the shoulder demonstrates inability to internally rotate past the neutral position, the brace is discontinued at 4 weeks. The arm is then kept in a sling for an additional 2 weeks, during which time the patient starts a gentle exercise program. Patients with generalized ligamentous laxity are generally treated with a brace for 6 weeks. During the time that the brace is used the patient is allowed to remove the brace to dress and bathe, as long as the arm is not allowed to internally rotate beyond the neutral position.

After the period of immobilization the patient starts active-assisted supine forward flexion, external rotation, and internal rotation. At 6 to 8 weeks cross-body adduction, active range of motion, and light weight or Theraband progressive resistive exercises are started. Progressive and more aggressive stretches and strengthening are started at 12 weeks after surgery. Total rehabilitation time is generally 16 to 24 weeks for primary capsulorrhaphy surgery. Revision surgery and complex situations, including scapulothoracic reconstruction, may require longer periods for rehabilitation.

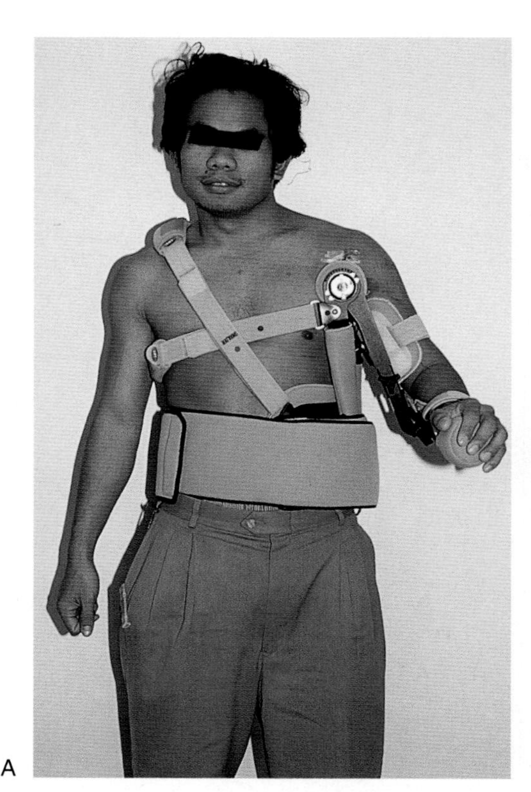

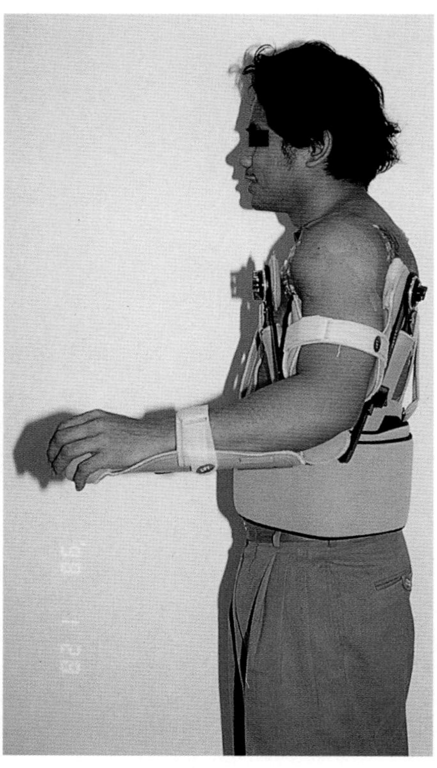

FIG. 29. (A) Frontal and **(B)** side view of postoperative brace positioning after posterior capsulorrhaphy. The arm is placed in slight abduction and neutral to slight external rotation. The arm should be in the plane of the body or slightly posterior to this plane.

RESULTS

The lack of a universally accepted and applied classification system for posterior instability makes interpretation of treatment results presented in the literature more difficult.

Success in treating recurrent posterior subluxation of the shoulder using a nonoperative exercise program is dependent on the amount of disability the patient is experiencing at the time of presentation, as well as on how one judges treatment success or failure. Fronek et al. reports a 63% success rate using nonoperative measures in patients with moderate disability when performing strenuous activities, but who had no interference with activities of daily living on initial presentation.[21] Hurley et al. demonstrated similar improvement in 68% of the patients treated under a similar treatment protocol.[33] Success in both of these clinical investigations was defined as clinical improvement that satisfied the patient to the extent that no further treatment other than maintenance muscular conditioning was required. These patients often demonstrate persistent posterior instability. However, the involuntary subluxations that in many cases prompted them to seek treatment, are significantly improved. These studies combined with the mixed results of surgical intervention warrant the inclusion of nonoperative measures as an initial form of treatment in any algorithm.

At first glance, the results of the surgical treatment of recurrent posterior subluxation are discouraging. This has led some authors to conclude that recurrent posterior subluxation should not be treated surgically.[29] However, a more detailed examination of the literature shows cause for guarded optimism. Historically, confusion over the classification of posterior instability, a poor understanding of the underlying pathophysiology, and the routine use of surgical procedures that failed to address the pathology underlying instability resulted in high surgical failure rates.

The surgical management of recurrent posterior subluxation can be divided into soft-tissue and osseous procedures. Because the cause of posterior instability usually resides in the posterior soft-tissue structures, repairs aimed at reinforcing these deficient structures are more commonly employed. More recently, identification and correction of the specific pathologic lesion has gained favor over so-called nonanatomic repairs.

The most common finding in patients with recurrent posterior subluxation is a patulous posterior capsule. Although treatment of this pathologic lesion depends on the direction of the instability, all anatomic repairs stress a rebalancing of this patulous capsule to restore glenohumeral stability. Fronek and colleagues reported on 24 patients with isolated posterior subluxation treated with posterior capsulorrhaphy with a 91% success rate.[21] The capsular repair is reinforced by the infraspinatus tendon and a posterior bone block if the posterior soft tissues are deficient. Hawkins also favors utilization of the infraspinatus tendon to reinforce the capsular repair posteriorly and reports an 85% success rate.[28,30] In 1980, Neer and Foster introduced the inferior capsular shift in patients for whom there are inferior and posterior components to the instability.[46] Bigliani reported the early results with this procedure in 25 patients with recurrent posterior subluxation, with 88% satisfactory results.[2] Pollock reported longer-term follow-up of this procedure, with an overall satisfactory rate of 80%.[57] Interestingly, several of these failures occurred in patients with revision surgery. Excluding revision cases, the success rate improved to 96%, highlighting the importance of meticulous soft-tissue repair at the first surgery.

Although labral detachment from the posterior glenoid rim is rare in recurrent posterior subluxation, several authors have successfully treated recurrent posterior subluxation with an anatomic labral repair when a reverse Bankart lesion is present. Rowe and Yee performed reverse Bankart repairs on two patients with recurrent posterior subluxation with no recurrence of instability.[61]

Several nonanatomic procedures have been previously described, with mixed results. Among these is the reverse Putti-Platt operation. Dugas et al. treated 18 patients with recurrent posterior subluxation with a reverse Putti-Platt procedure.[14] Satisfactory results were obtained in 16 of 17 patients available for follow-up. Six patients experienced mild loss of motion. Similarly, Hawkins reported good results in his patients undergoing this procedure, but in a separate group of patients, who were originally operated on by other surgeons, he reports a recurrence rate of 83% using this repair. This suggests that success with this procedure may depend on the surgeon's experience.[29] Boyd and Sisk reported nine nonanatomic soft-tissue repairs that were augmented by posterior transfer of the long head of the biceps tendon.[5] All patients reportedly did well without recurrence of instability.The second group of procedures for recurrent posterior subluxation addresses bony pathology by either redirecting abnormal osseous anatomy (glenoid osteotomy or proximal humerus rotational osteotomy) or by augmenting deficient glenoid bone stock or incompetent posterior soft tissues (bone block procedures).

Glenoid osteotomy (glenoplasty), first reported by Scott, is a posterior opening wedge osteotomy of the glenoid neck with interposition of bone graft, thereby redirecting the glenoid more anteriorly.[66] In his original report of three cases, one patient dislocated anteriorly in the early postoperative period and another had recurrent posterior subluxation. Norwood and Terry reported 19 patients with recurrent posterior subluxation, from various causes, treated by glenoid osteotomy.[51] Three patients (16%) continued to experience isolated posterior instability, 4 patients (21%) developed isolated anterior instability, and 2 patients (12%) had multidirectional instability in the postoperative period.

English and McNab advocated an anatomic approach to recurrent posterior subluxation.[16] The surgical results of eight patients were reviewed. All demonstrated increased glenoid retroversion on preoperative radiographs. Four of eight patients were treated with posterior glenoid osteotomy without recurrence. Interestingly, they noted that in patients with ligamentous laxity there was a tendency for the humerus to subluxate anteriorly. More recently, glenoid osteotomy has been successfully employed in patients with localized posterior glenoid hypoplasia and recurrent posterior subluxation.[81]

The role of posterior glenoid opening wedge osteotomy in the treatment of recurrent posterior subluxation is open to many criticisms. Gerber has documented coracoid impingement following posterior glenoid osteotomy.[24] There has been a spectrum of anterior instabilities reported following glenoid osteotomy that range from coracoid impingement to anterior dislocation.[51,66] Posterior glenoid osteotomy is a technically demanding procedure, with the potential for significant complications. Hawkins reported a 41% complication rate with this procedure, including subsequent glenohumeral arthritis in two patients, one caused by intraarticular extension of the osteotomy.[29] Finally, earlier studies that justify glenoid osteotomy based on radiographic evidence of increased glenoid retroversion may have overstated this problem.[15] In the past, the ability to document increased glenoid retroversion by plain radiographs has been questioned. Galinat has recently reported a reproducible means of determining glenoid version from plain radiographs.[22] However, this method was not used in previous studies. Currently, CT scan is the most accurate method of determining glenoid version.

Increased proximal humeral retrotorsion has been implicated as a cause for recurrent posterior subluxation. Rotational osteotomy has been used to treat recurrent posterior subluxation, based on the assumption that increased humeral retrotorsion contributes to posterior instability. However, the relation between humeral retrotorsion and posterior instability has not been established. By limiting internal rotation through proximal humeral rotational osteotomy, it was theorized that posterior instability would subside. Surin reported 12 cases of recurrent posterior instability treated with external rotation osteotomy of the proximal humerus.[71] One patient had pain after osteotomy that was attributed to anterior impingement. A second patient developed recurrent instability. Most patients had significant restriction of external rotation postoperatively. Chaudhuri reported a series of patients who had rotational osteotomy for glenohumeral instability.[11] Only 1 of 16 cases underwent osteotomy for recurrent posterior subluxation. This patient developed postoperative anterior instability requiring muscle transfer.

Another group of bony procedures act to buttress the posterior glenoid with bone graft from the iliac crest or spine of the scapula. Several authors have reported the use of posterior bone block procedures for recurrent posterior instability.[1,36] Ahlgren and colleagues treated five patients with a posterior bone block procedure.[1] Two of five patients had normal shoulders postoperatively, whereas three demonstrated varying degrees of recurrent posterior instability. More commonly, posterior bone block procedures are combined with a posterior capsulorrhaphy or performed for failed posterior soft-tissue procedures.[36,45,75]

CONCLUSIONS

Recurrent posterior subluxation is less common than anterior subluxation, but it is being diagnosed more frequently than in the past. The treatment of recurrent posterior subluxation is dependent on the underlying pathology. An anatomically based classification system facilitates the diagnosis and appropriate treatment plan. The earlier literature on surgical treatment has yielded inconsistent results. More recently, improved recognition of the underlying pathology coupled with more anatomic surgical approaches have resulted in consistently improved results. An algorithm for the evaluation and treatment of posterior instability based upon an anatomic classification is presented.

REFERENCES

1. Ahlgren S, Hedlund T, Nistor L. Idiopathic posterior instability of the shoulder joint: results of operation with posterior bone graft. *Acta Orthop Scand* 1978;49:600–603.
2. Bigliani LU, Endrizzi DP, McIlveen SJ, Flatow EL, Dalsey RM. Operative management of posterior shoulder instability. *Orthop Trans* 1989; 13:232.
3. Bigliani LU, Pollock RG, Endrizzi DP, McIlveen SI, Flatow EL. Surgical repair of posterior instability of the shoulder: long term results. Presented at the 9th combined meeting of the Orthopaedic Associations of the English-Speaking World. Toronto, June, 1992.
4. Bowen MK, Warren RF, Altchek DW, O'Brien SJ. Posterior subluxation of the glenohumeral joint treated by posterior stabilization. *Orthop Trans* 1991;15:764.
5. Boyd HB, Sisk TD. Recurrent posterior dislocation of the shoulder. *J Bone Joint Surg [Am]* 1972;54:779–786.
6. Brewer B, Wubben RC, Carrera GF. Excessive retroversion of the glenoid cavity. A cause of non-traumatic posterior instability of the shoulder. *J Bone Joint Surg [Am]* 1986;68:724–731.
7. Burkhead WZ, Rockwood CA. Treatment of instability of the shoulder with an exercise program. *J Bone Joint Surg [Am]* 19922;74:890–896.
8. Callaghan JJ, McNeisk LM, Dehaven JP, Savory CG. A prospective comparison study of double contrast CT, arthrography, and arthroscopy of the shoulder. *Am J Sports Med* 1988;16:13.
9. Caspari RB, Geissler WD. Arthroscopic manifestations of shoulder subluxation and dislocation. *Clin Orthop* 1993;291:54–66.
10. Chandnani VP, Yeager TD, DeBarardino T, et al. Glenoid labral tears: prospective evaluation with MR imaging, MR arthrography, and CT arthrography. *AJR Am J Roetgenol* 1993;161:1229–1235.
11. Chaudhuri GK, Sengupta A, Saha AK. Rotation osteotomy of the shaft of the humerus for recurrent dislocation of the shoulder: anterior and posterior. *Acta Orthop Scand* 11974;45:193–198.
12. Codman EA. *The shoulder.* Boston: Thomas Todd, 1934.
13. Cofield RH, Nessler JP, Weinstabl R. Diagnosis of shoulder instability by examination under anesthesia. *Clin Orthop* 1993;291:45–53.

13a. Cooper A. On the dislocation of the os humeri upon the dorsum scapula, and upon fractures near the shoulder joint. *Guy's Hosp Rep* 1839;4:265–284.

14. Dugas RW, Scerpella TA, Clancy WG. Surgical treatment of symptomatic posterior shoulder instability. *Orthop Trans* 1990;14:245.
15. Engebretsen L, Craig EV. Radiographic features of shoulder instability. *Clin Orthop* 1993;291:29.
16. English E, Macnab I. Recurrent posterior dislocation of the shoulder. *Can J Surg* 1974;17:147–151.
17. Edelson JG. Localized glenoid hypoplasia. *Clin Orthop* 1995;321: 189–195.
18. Fery A. Results of treatment of anterior serratus paralysis. In: Post M, Morrey BF, Hawkins RJ, eds. *Surgery of the shoulder.* St Louis: Mosby Year-Book, 1990:325–329.
19. Flannigan B, Kursunoglu-Brahme S, Snyder S, Karzel R, DelPizzo W, Resnick D. MR arthrography of the shoulder: comparison with conventional MR imaging. *AJR Am J Roentgenol* 1990;155:829–832.
20. Fried A. Habitual posterior dislocation of the shoulder joint: a case report on 5 operated cases. *Acta Orthop Scand* 1949;18:329.
21. Fronek J, Warren RF, Bowen M. Posterior subluxation of the glenohumeral joint. *J Bone Joint Surg [Am]* 1989;71:205–216.
22. Galinat BJ, Howell SJ, Kraft TA. The glenoid-posterior acromion angle: an accurate method of evaluating glenoid version. *Orthop Trans* 1988;12:727.
23. Gerber C, Ganz R. Clinical assessment of instability of the shoulder. With special reference to anterior and posterior drawer tests. *J Bone Joint Surg [Br]* 1984;66:551–556.
24. Gerber C, Ganz R, Vihn TS. Glenoplasty for recurrent posterior shoulder instability: an anatomic reappraisal. *Clin Orthop* 1987;216:70.
25. Gross ML, Seeger LL, Smith JB, et al. Magnetic resonance imaging of the glenoid labrum. *Am J Sports Med* 1990;18:229–234.
26. Harryman DT, Sildes JA, Clark JM, McQuade KJ, Gibb TD, Matsen FA. Translation of the humeral head on the glenoid with passive glenohumeral motion. *J Bone Joint Surg* 1990;72:1334–1343.
27. Harryman DT, Sidles JA, Harris SL, Matsen FA. The role of the rotator interval capsule in passive motion and stability of the shoulder. *J Bone Joint Surg [Am]* 1992;74:53–66.
28. Hawkins RJ, Bell RH, Lippitt SB. In: Hurley E, ed. *Atlas of shoulder surgery.* St Louis: Mosby, 1996:96–98.
29. Hawkins RJ, Koppert G, Johnston G. Recurrent posterior instability (subluxation) of the shoulder. *J Bone Joint Surg [Am]* 1984;66: 169–174.

29a. Hawkins RJ, Neer CS, Pianta RM, Mendoza FX. Locked posterior dislocation of the shoulder. *J Bone Joint Surg [Am]* 1987;69;9–18.

30. Hawkins RJ, McCormack RG. Posterior shoulder instability. *Orthopedics* 1988;2:101–107.
31. Hawkins RJ, Bell RM. Posterior instability of the shoulder. *AAOS Instr Course Lect* 1989;211–215.
32. Huber DJ, Sauter R, Mueller E, et al. MR imaging of the normal shoulder. *Radiology* 1986;158:405–408.
33. Hurley JA, Anderson TE, Dear W, Andrich JT, Bergfeld JA, Weiker GG. Posterior shoulder instability: surgical versus conservative results with evaluation of glenoid version. *Am J Sports Med* 1992;20:396–400.
34. Iannotti JP, Zlatkin MB, Esterhai JL, Kressel HY, Dalinka MK, Spindler KP. Magnetic resonance imaging of the shoulder. Sensitivity, specificity, and predictive value. *J Bone Joint Surg [Am]* 1991;73: 17–29.
35. Jahnke AH, Petersen SA, Neumann C, Steinbach L, Morgan F. A prospective comparison of computerized arthrotomography and magnetic resonance imaging of the glenohumeral joint. *Am J Sports Med* 1992;20:695–701.
36. Jones V. Recurrent posterior dislocation of the shoulder: report of a case treated by posterior bone block. *J Bone Joint Surg [Br]* 1958;40: 203–207.
37. Kieft GJ, Bloem JL, Rozing PM, et al. MR imaging of recurrent anterior dislocation of the shoulder: comparison with CT arthrography. *AJR Am J Roentgenol* 1988;150:1083–1087.
38. Kretzler HH. Scapular osteotomy for posterior shoulder dislocation. *J Bone Joint Surg [Am]* 1974;56:197.
39. Kronberg M, Brostrom LA. Humeral head retroversion in patients with unstable humeroscapular joints. *Clin Orthop* 1990;260:207–211.
40. Laumann U. Kinesiology of the shoulder joint. In: Kobel R, ed. *Shoulder replacement.* Berlin: Springer-Verlag, 1987.
41. Liou JTS, Wilson AJ, Totty WG, Brown JJ. The normal shoulder: common variations that simulate pathologic conditions at MR imaging. *Radiology* 1993;186:435–441.
42. Matsen FA III. Glenohumeral instability. In: Evarts CM, ed. *Surgery of the musculoskeletal system.* vol 2. New York: Churchill Livingstone, 1983:349–375.
43. McLaughlin HL. Follow-up notes on articles previously published in the journal—posterior dislocation of the shoulder. *J Bone Joint Surg [Am]* 1972;44:1477.
44. Mosley JB, Jobe FW, Pink M, Perry J, Tibone JE. EMG analysis of the scapular muscles during a shoulder rehabilitation program. *Am J Sports Med* 1992;20:128–134.
45. Mowery CA, Garfin SR, Booth R.. Rothman RH. Recurrent posterior dislocation of the shoulder: treatment using a bone block. *J Bone Joint Surg [Am]* 1985;67:777–781.

46. Neer CS, Foster CR. Inferior capsular shift for involuntary inferior and mulitdirectional instability of the shoulder. *J Bone Joint Surg [Am]* 1980;62:897–908.
47. Neumann CH, Petersen SA, Jahnke AH. MR imaging of the labral–capsular complex: normal variations. *AJR Am J Roentgenol* 1991;157: 1015–1021.
48. Nobel W. Posterior traumatic dislocation of the shoulder. *J Bone Joint Surg [Am]* 1962;44:523–538.
49. Norris TR. Diagnostic techniques for shoulder instability. *AAOS Instr Course Lect* 1985;239–257.
50. Norris TR. C-arm fluoroscopic evaluation under anesthesia for glenohumeral subluxation. In: Bateman JE, Welsh RP, eds. *Surgery of the shoulder*. Philadelphia: BC Decker, 1984:22–25.
51. Norwood LA, Terry GC. Shoulder posterior subluxation. *Am J Sports Med* 1984;12:25.
52. Ovesen J, Nielsen S. Posterior instability of the shoulder: a cadavar model. *Acta Orthop Scand* 1986;57:436–439.
53. Ovesen J, Sojbjerg JO. Posterior shoulder dislocation: muscle and capsular lesions in cadavar experiments. *Acta Orthop Scand* 1986;57: 535–536.
54. Ovesen J, Nielsen S. Anterior and posterior shoulder instability: a cadavar study. *Acta Orthop Scand* 1986;57:324–327.
55. Pagnani MJ, Galinat BJ, Warren RF. Glenohumeral instability. In: DeLee J, Drez D, eds. *Orthopaedic sports medicine: principles and practice*.vol 1. Philadelphia: WB Saunders, 1994:580–622.
56. Pande P, Hawkins R, Peat M. Electromyography in voluntary posterior instability of the shoulder. *Am J Sports Med* 1989;17:644–648.
57. Pollock RG, Bigliani LU. Recurrent posterior shoulder instability: diagnosis and treatment. *Clin Orthop* 1993;291:85.
58. Post M. Pectoralis major transfer for winging of the scapula. *J Shoulder Elbow Surg* 1995;4:1–9.
59. Randelli M, Gambrioli PL. Glenohumeral osteometry by computed tomography in normal and unstable shoulders. *Clin Orthop* 1986;208; 151.
60. Rockwood CA, Matsen FA. *The shoulder*. Philadelphia: WB Saunders, 1990.
61. Rowe CR, Yee LBK. A posterior approach to the shoulder joint. *J Bone Joint Surg* 1994;26:580–584.
62. Rowe CR, Pierce DS, Clark JG: Voluntary dislocation of the shoulder: a preliminary report on a clinical, electromyographic, and psychiatric study of 26 patients. *J Bone Joint Surg [Am]* 1973;55:445–460.
63. Schutte JP, Lafayette LA, Hawkins RJ, Chris A. The use of computerized tomography in determining humeral retroversion. *Orthop Trans* 1988;12:727.
64. Schwartz RE, Warren RF, O'Brien SJ, Fronek J. Posterior shoulder instability. *Orthop Clin North Am* 1987;18:409–419.
65. Schwartz RE, O'Brien SJ, Warren RF, Torzilli PA. Capsular restraints to anterior-posterior motion of the shoulder. *Orthop Trans* 1988;12:727.
66. Scott DJ. Treatment of recurrent posterior dislocations of the shoulder by glenoplasty. Report of 3 cases. *J Bone Joint Surg [Am]* 1967;49: 471–476.
67. Seeger LL, Ruszkowski JT, Bassett LW, et al. MR imaging of the normal shoulder. Anatomic correlation. *AJR Am J Roentgenol* 1987;148: 83–91.
68. Shaffer BS, Conway J, Jobe FW, Kvitne RS, Tibone JE. Infraspinatus muscle-splitting incision in posterior shoulder surgery. *Am J Sports Med* 1994;22:113–120.
69. Speer KP, Deng X, Borrero S, Torzilli PA, Altchek DA, Warren RF. Biomechanical evaluation of a simulated Bankart lesion. *J Bone Joint Surg [Am]* 1994;76:1819–1826.
70. Stoller DW. In *Magnetic resonance imaging in orthopaedics and sports medicine*. Philadelphia: JB Lippincott, 1993:511–633.
71. Surin V, Blader S, Markhede G, Sundholm K. Rotational osteotomy of the humerus for posterior instability of the shoulder. *J Bone Joint Surg [Am]* 1990;72:181–186.
72. Terry GC, Hammon D, France P, Norwood LA. The stabilizing function of passive shoulder restraints. *Am J Sports Med* 1991;19:26–34.
73. Tibone JE, Bradley JP. The treatment of posterior subluxation in athletes. *Clin Orthop* 1993;291:124.
74. Tibone J, Ting A. Capsulorrhaphy with a staple for recurrent posterior subluxation of the shoulder. *J Bone Joint Surg.* 1990;72:999–1002.
75. Toumey JW. Posterior recurrent dislocation of the shoulder treated by capsulorrhaphy and iliac bone block. *Lahey Clin Bull* 1948;5:197–201.
76. Warner JJP, Micheli LJ, Arslanian LE, Kennedy J, Kennedy R. Scapulothoracic motion in normal shoulders and shoulders with glenohumeral instability and impingement syndrome. A study using Moire topographic analysis. *Clin Orthop* 1992;285:191.
77. Warren RF. Subluxation of the shoulder in athletes. *Clin Sports Med* 1983;2:339–354.
78. Warren RF, Kornblatt IB, Marchand R. Static factors affecting posterior shoulder stability. *Orthop Trans* 1984;8:89.
79. Wirth MA, Butters KP, Rockwood CA. The posterior deltoid splitting approach to the shoulder. *Clin Orthop* 1993;296:92–96.
80. Wirth MA, Lyons FR, Rockwood CA. Hypoplasia of the glenoid. A review of 16 patients. *J Bone Joint Surg [Am]* 1993;75;1175–1184.
81. Wirth MA, Seltzer DG, Rockwood CA. Recurrent posterior glenohumeral dislocation associated with increased retroversion of the glenoid: a case report. *Clin Orthop* 1994;308:98.

Disorders of the Shoulder: Diagnosis and Management,
edited by Joseph P. Iannotti and Gerald R. Williams, Jr.
Lippincott Williams & Wilkins, Philadelphia © 1999.

CHAPTER 12

Multidirectional Instability: Diagnosis and Management

Frank A. Cordasco and Louis U. Bigliani

INTRODUCTION

In 1980, Neer and Foster introduced the inferior capsular shift for the treatment of involuntary and multidirectional instability of the shoulder. They noted that few papers had been published on the treatment of inferior and multidirectional instability of the glenohumeral joint. Not only was there a relative dearth of information about the management of this problem, but there was little consensus concerning the operative treatment of choice.[57] Before 1980, several authors had recognized the importance of distinguishing this disorder from the more common unidirectional form of instability and recommended a comprehensive trial of strengthening exercises before considering surgical intervention.[3,17,20,70,78] Neer has emphasized the problems encountered when standard procedures used to correct unidirectional anterior or posterior instability are performed in patients with multidirectional instability.[53–55,58] These procedures may fail because they do not reduce the excessive inferior capsular redundancy. Furthermore, excessive tightness created on one side of a hypermobile joint may result in a fixed subluxation or dislocation in the opposite direction, possibly leading to severe glenohumeral arthritis.[2,10,15,23,31,32,34,46–48,58,59,61,64,69,71,72,76,87,88]

F. A. Cordasco: Department of Orthopaedic Surgery, Columbia University, College of Physicians and Surgeons, New York, New York 10033; and St. Lukes–Roosevelt Hospital Center, Columbia–Presbyterian Medical Center, New York, New York 10019.

L. U. Bigliani: Department of Orthopaedic Surgery, Columbia University, College of Physicians and Surgeons, Columbia–Presbyterian Medical Center, New York, New York 10033.

Patients with multidirectional instability have symptomatic glenohumeral subluxation or dislocation in more than one direction: anterior, inferior, and posterior. The primary cause is a loose redundant capsule.[15,53,57,65] This problem is more common than previously recognized.[53,57,85] There is a common misconception that multidirectional instability is limited to young sedentary patients, with generalized ligamentous laxity, bilateral symptoms, and an atraumatic history. Although there is a group of such patients, shoulders with multidirectional instability are often seen in athletic patients, many of whom have had injuries.[53] Repetitive microtrauma, from gymnastics or butterfly swimming, for example, may have selectively stretched out their shoulders so that their other joints may not be lax on examination (Fig. 1). Furthermore, shoulders with multidirectional instability may have Bankart lesions and humeral head impression defects, although less commonly than unidirectional cases resulting from single-event, high-energy trauma.[1,53]

Material property studies of the inferior glenohumeral ligament have disclosed two principal modes of failure: at the glenoid insertion (analogous to a Bankart lesion) and in midsubstance (analogous to capsular stretching or laxity).[9] Significant midsubstance ligament strain before failure was noted even in the specimens that ultimately failed at the glenoid insertion. These findings are consistent with the results of another biomechanical study that demonstrated that a Bankart lesion alone did not increase instability enough to allow anterior dislocation.[74] These studies suggest that reconstructive procedures for shoulder instability must correct capsular laxity as well as the avulsion of the glenohumeral ligaments.

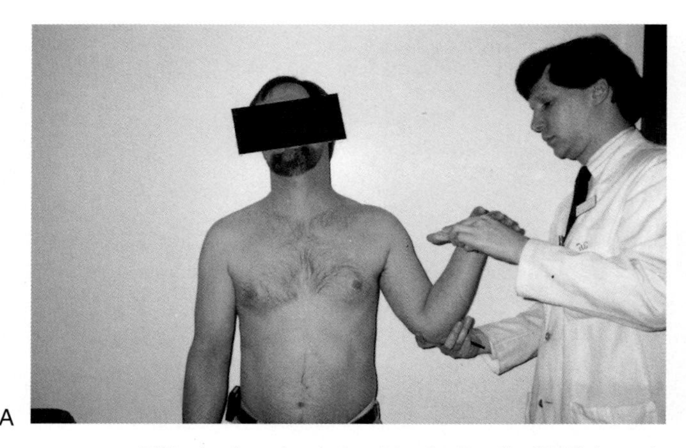
A

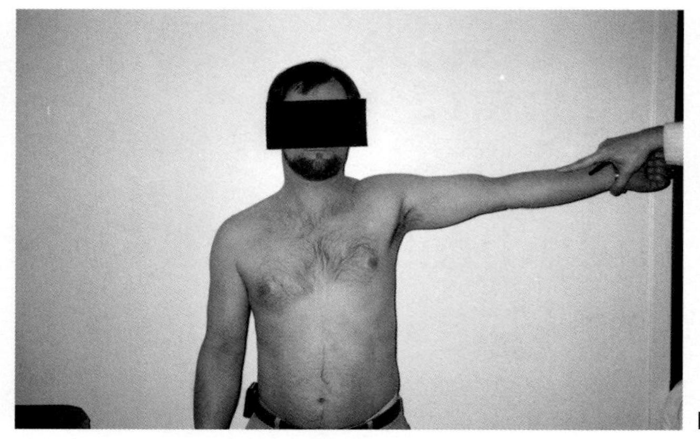
B

FIG. 1. Acquired shoulder laxity. **(Left)** This patient had multidirectional shoulder instability. He has a history of extensive gymnastics during youth, including the rings. Although his shoulders were stretched out over years of repetitive microtrauma, he does not have thumb laxity. **(Right)** He does not have elbow laxity.

Patients with shoulder instability do not always easily separate into clear categories (unidirectional versus multidirectional). This is especially true of athletes, often lax to begin with, who subject their shoulders to repetitive microtrauma on a daily basis, but who also may suffer a superimposed injury. We have found athletes with anterior instability to constitute a spectrum from unidirectional anterior instability to frank multidirectional instability with pronounced inferior capsular laxity, rather than simple discrete groups.[7,15] Accordingly, we have used an inferior capsular shift approach in all cases, modifying the repair so that only as much inferior capsule was shifted as was necessary to reduce the degree of inferior laxity found in each instance.[6,7,15,57]

A methodic approach to the evaluation and treatment of patients with multidirectional instability, addressing the primary pathology within the glenohumeral ligament complex, has led to satisfactory results in a high proportion of cases.[1,8,14,15,23,26,43,48,49,51,53,57,67,68,84,85]

Several investigational techniques are being evaluated.[18,37,59,79] Arthroscopy has been advocated as a diagnostic aid,[52] and a preliminary report of an arthroscopic medial-based capsular shift has demonstrated satisfactory results.[18] The effect of thermal heating on the glenohumeral joint capsule is being investigated and arthroscopic laser contraction of the capsule has been described.[37,79]. The indications for these procedures have yet to be established, and long-term follow-up is unavailable at this time.

CLINICAL PRESENTATION

Patients with multidirectional instability may present in a variety of ways. The patient is often athletic, and swimmers, weight lifters, and gymnasts may be particularly predisposed. The instability episode may have occurred without significant injury and spontaneously reduced or self-reduced. Extremely hypermobile shoulders can become symptomatic without unusual trauma and possibly even from the activities of daily living. A typical presentation is a person with a relatively loose shoulder who stresses it repetitively in athletic activities or work-related events.

There is a subgroup of patients with a family history of hypermobility. Although investigations into the association between connective tissue disorders, such as Ehlers-Danlos syndrome, biochemical abnormalities, and ligamentous laxity syndromes, have been performed, no definitive relationships have been demonstrated.[5,12,19,20,22,40]

The direction of instability may occasionally be determined from the patient's symptom complex. Inferior instability may present with the patient's description of pain associated with carrying heavy suitcases or shopping bags. Occasionally, these symptoms are accompanied by traction paresthesias. Pain associated with pushing open heavy or revolving doors, or use of the arm in a forward flexed and internally rotated position, usually suggests a component of posterior instability, and discomfort in the overhead, abducted, and externally rotated position might generally suggest anterior instability. However, symptoms can be complex, vague, and difficult to sort out.

The physical examination may demonstrate evidence of generalized ligamentous laxity, such as hyperextension at the elbows, the ability to approximate the thumbs to the forearm, hyperextension of the metacarpophalangeal joints, or patellofemoral subluxation. In some of these patients we have noted hypermobile acromioclavicular and sternoclavicular joints, which can be sources of symptoms. Therefore, it is important to examine these joints for tenderness. A significant finding is the sulcus sign (Fig. 2), documenting inferior laxity. Additionally, close inspection of the scapulothoracic articulation should be performed because concomitant scapulothoracic instability may occasionally be present.[33,53] There may be multiple positive findings using the following maneuvers: anterior and posterior load and shift tests, anterior and posterior apprehension tests, fulcrum test, relocation test, Fukuda test, and push–pull or supine stress test.[15,33,53,57,73] The aim is to produce humeral translations anteriorly, posteriorly, or inferiorly (relative to the glenoid) and to document that these translations are reliably accompanied by the patient's report of the usual pain and discomfort.

At times, it can be difficult to determine the primary direction of instability on physical examination. Determining whether the shoulder is moving from a dislocated to a reduced position or from a reduced to a dislocated position can be challenging. Maintaining the fingers of one hand on the coracoid anteriorly and the posterolateral acromion can aid in this determination; consequently, multiple physical examinations are helpful in assessing these patients.

It is important that symptoms be reproduced with such maneuvers, because laxity in and of itself is not an indication for surgical stabilization procedures.[36,53] Biomechanical studies have demonstrated that normal asymptomatic shoulders may show substantial translation on clinical testing.[29] In addition, joint laxity may be remarkable enough to distract the examiner from the primary source of pain, such as a painful acromioclavicular joint or a cervical radiculopathy. Conversely, laxity may be hard to demonstrate, even in a shoulder with multidirectional instability, if pain, muscle spasm, and guarding prevent subluxation. It is helpful to examine the contralateral, asymptomatic shoulder for laxity. If it is extremely loose it may be a clue to the multidirectional nature of the affected side.[53,63]

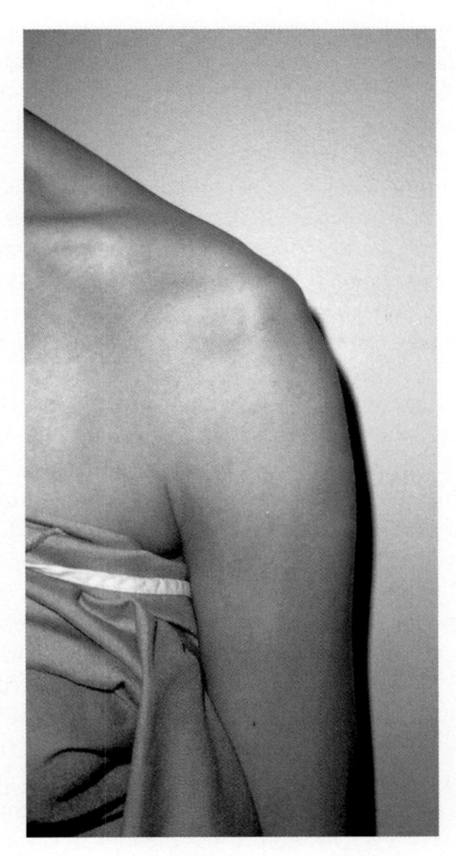

FIG. 2. This 22-year-old female has a 3-plus sulcus sign.

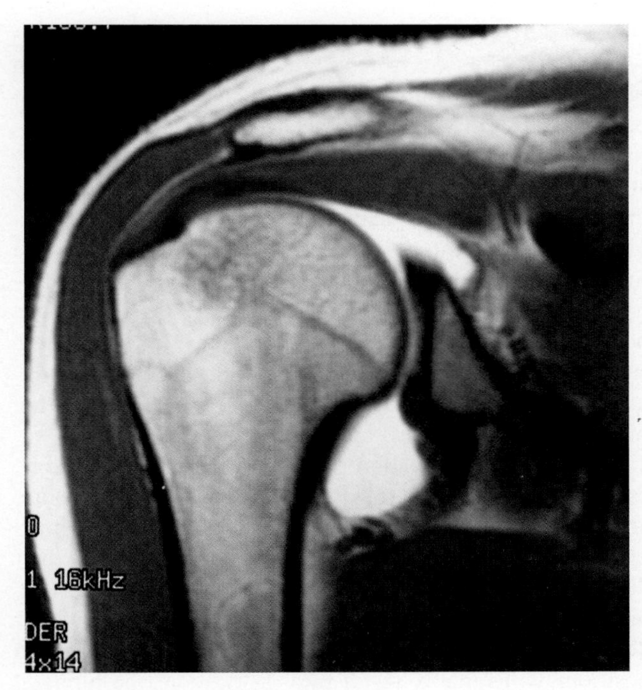

FIG. 3. Saline–gadolinium MRI performed for a 26-year-old woman demonstrating increased capsular volume.

IMAGING STUDIES

Plain radiographs are generally normal, but they should be evaluated for the presence of humeral head defects and glenoid lesions, such as osseous Bankart fragments, reactive bone, or wear. Double-contrast computed tomography (CT) arthrograms may demonstrate an increased capsular volume. Recently, we have been using magnetic resonance imaging (MRI) enhanced with an intraarticular mixture of saline and gadolinium (Fig. 3). This has provided the joint distention necessary to evaluate the capsular volume and the uncommon labral or capsular detachments. Inferior subluxation can be demonstrated by stress radiographs; however, this technique is generally not needed.[39] Cine MRI is currently under investigation, but has the potential to dynamically demonstrate capsular and labral defects in varying positions.[25]

TREATMENT

Once the diagnosis of multidirectional instability has been established, a prolonged course of rehabilitation is instituted with emphasis on strengthening the deltoid and rotator cuff muscles with the arm below the horizontal.[11,41,68] The scapulothoracic stabilizing muscles are strengthened as well. Patients with multidirectional instability may have an associated synovitis and will occasionally develop a secondary impingement syndrome. Nonsteroidal antiinflammatory drugs will be helpful in these instances. At times a subacromial injection of a steroid preparation will provide relief sufficient for the patient to resume his or her exercise regimen.

The role of proprioception in shoulder stability has been

supported by a study demonstrating that athletic individuals with chronic shoulder instability have significant deficits in proprioception and surgical stabilization normalizes proprioceptive sensibility. Because mechanoreceptors must be deformed or loaded to function, they may not be sufficiently stimulated in a lax or injured capsule.[44] Alteration of the normal state of negative intraarticular pressure has also been implicated as potentially affecting the function of the mechanoreceptors and contributing to shoulder instability.[27,28,83] Muscle coordination abnormalities have also been noted in studies of patients with generalized laxity.[42] These studies are supportive of a rehabilitation program that includes neuromuscular adaptation and focuses on improving muscle tone and general coordination.[16,41]

During the rehabilitation program, motivation should be carefully assessed both to be sure that the patient is mature enough to cooperate in the rehabilitative effort required postoperatively as well as to screen out those manipulating their disease for secondary gain.[53,70] Patients with acquired instability may have developed the ability to dislocate the shoulder at will or on command. This is especially true if certain positions will reliably result in a dislocation (the humeral head falls out posteriorly whenever the arm is raised in the forward plane). Such "positional dislocators" may demonstrate this for the examiner, if requested, but otherwise will do their best to avoid such positions. However, these patients must be differentiated from true voluntary dislocators who have underlying psychiatric or behavioral problems and who often use asymmetrical muscle pull to dislocate their shoulder, or even to hold it out, to great dramatic effect.[53,70] To complicate things further, there is a small group of patients who have developed a habitual initiation of improper muscle firing patterns that also produce dislocations by asymmetrical muscle pull. These patients can be unaware of this pattern and may be without psychiatric disturbance. Nevertheless, both groups of "muscular dislocators" are poor candidates for stabilization procedures. Those with psychiatric disturbances need counseling and, for the shoulder, skillful neglect. The group with habitually improper muscle use may be successfully treated with muscle retraining and biofeedback.[4]

If the patient has persistent involuntary instability symptoms that have not responded to conservative treatment, including an exercise regimen as well as the occasional use of antiinflammatory drugs, then surgery is recommended. Surgery may be considered sooner if additional factors, such as a documented glenohumeral ligament avulsion on double contrast CT arthrogram or MRI, are noted.

OPERATIVE TECHNIQUE

The primary pathology in multidirectional instability is the presence of a loose, redundant capsule. This pathologic capsular laxity is directly addressed by the inferior capsular shift procedure, which reduces the volume of the glenohumeral joint anteriorly, inferiorly, and posteriorly. The inferior capsular shift is designed to reduce capsular volume on all sides by thickening and overlapping the capsule on the side of greatest instability and tensioning the capsule on the inferior and opposite sides. For example, in a shoulder that dislocates anteriorly and inferiorly and subluxes posteriorly, an inferior capsular shift would be performed from an anterior approach. The anterior "T" capsulorrhaphy thickens and tightens the anterior capsule. The inferior capsular pouch is obliterated. Finally, shifting the inferior capsule anteriorly, around the humeral neck, tensions the posterior capsule. In addition, the rotator interval is often pathologically widened, and closing this interval (and the associated "cleft" between the superior and middle glenohumeral ligaments, as described by Neer) from an anterior approach, as well as drawing the superior flap of the "T" capsular incision down, tensions the anterosuperior capsule and ligaments.

Neer believed that the rotator interval between the supraspinatus and subscapularis and the deeper cleft between the superior and middle glenohumeral ligaments was widened in patients with multidirectional instability. He described closing it before shifting the superior flap inferiorly "to act as a sling against inferior subluxation."[57] Recent studies of the rotator interval confirm its important role in instability, and substantiate the importance of addressing this area at the time of reconstructive surgery, as described by Neer.[21,30,60,84] The inferior capsular shift corrects the redundant inferior pouch associated with inferior instability in the abducted arm, and the widened rotator interval responsible for inferior instability in the adducted arm. This concept has been supported by subsequent biomechanical and clinical studies.[7–9,21,27–30,60,62,66,67,74,75,80–84] Thus, the soft tissues are balanced in a systematic way to meet the pathology actually present.

The capsular attenuation or redundancy may be addressed in three ways. The capsular approach to the joint may be lateral (humeral), as described by Neer,[57] intermediate (middle), as advocated by Wirth and colleagues,[86] or medial (glenoid), as described by Altchek and associates.[1] We prefer the lateral capsular incision because it offers several advantages. The capsule is shaped similar to a cone or funnel, with a broader insertion and surface area on the humeral side. Therefore, more capsule can be shifted because the tissue can be shifted a greater distance and reattached to a broader insertion. This is particularly consequential in patients whose shoulders have significant inferior redundancy or a patulous capsule. The lateral capsular incision also affords relative protection to the axillary nerve if the shoulder is maintained in a position of external rotation and adduction during the dissection, for the nerve is more medial in this situation.[6,15,53] Additionally, in the unusual instance of capsular tears at the humeral insertion, a lateral approach facilitates diagnosis and repair. The intermediate (middle) incision in the capsule has been recommended because it is thought to be technically easier than a medial approach, improves medial visualization of the glenoid rim, and allows "double-breasting" of the glenohumeral ligaments.[86] A pri-

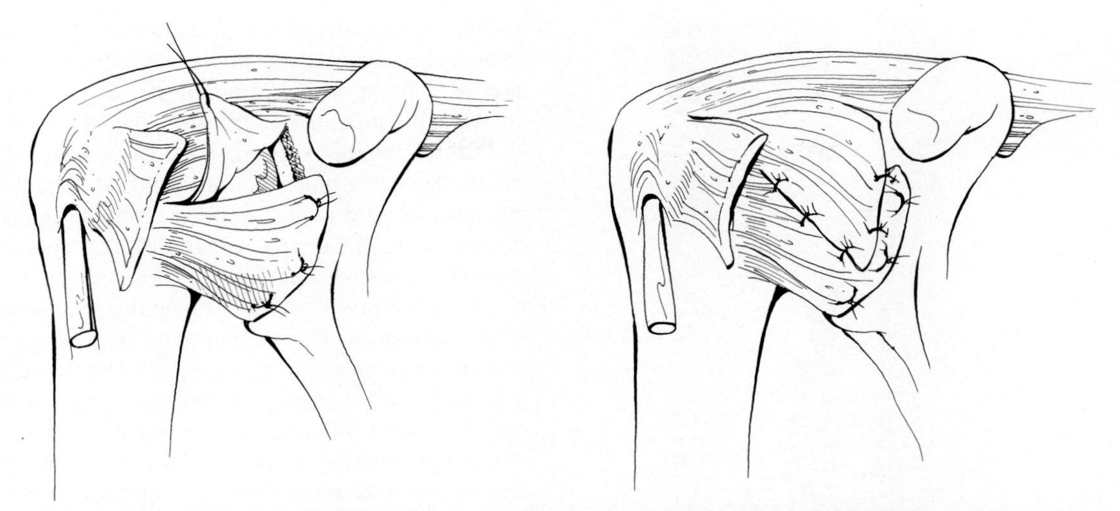

FIG. 4. T-plasty modification of the Bankart procedure. **(Left)** A superior shift of the inferior flap and suture to the glenoid margin. **(Right)** The superior flap is to be advanced anteriorly to make a better layered closure. (From ref.1, with permission.)

mary disadvantage is that inferior dissection must be done with great care as injury to the axillary nerve is quite possible. The medial (glenoid) approach to the capsule (Fig. 4) has the advantage of facilitating repair of the capsule and labrum to bone when a concomitant Bankart lesion is present.[1] It may be more difficult to shift as much capsule from a medial (glenoid) approach, and the rare humeral avulsion of the glenohumeral ligaments would be less accessible than with a lateral (humeral) approach.

AUTHORS' PREFERRED METHOD

An interscalene regional block is the anesthesia of choice when possible. Some infiltration of the skin and subcutaneous tissues of the axilla aid in comfort because of overlap with thoracic segmental nerves. The patient is placed in the beach chair position, and all bony prominences are carefully padded to avoid skin and neurovascular compromise. Head and neck positioning is greatly simplified in an awake patient under regional anesthetic. However, if the patient is asleep, hyperextension or hyperflexion of the cervical spine is avoided by securing the head and neck in a stable position. The upper extremity is prepared and draped from the sternum, base of neck, and medial border of the scapula, with the upper extremity free. Prophylactic antibiotics are administered intravenously.

The examination under anesthesia is then performed. One disadvantage of the interscalene regional anesthetic is the inability to examine the contralateral shoulder under anesthesia. Biomechanical studies have contributed to the fund of knowledge on the static stabilizers of the glenohumeral joint, and this has aided in the performance of the examination under anesthesia.[9,13,27–30,36,62,66,74,75,80–83] Because different portions of the capsule and ligament system are brought into play in different arm positions, the glenohumeral joint is stressed anteriorly, posteriorly, and inferiorly in adduction, 45 degrees of abduction, 90 degrees of abduction, and internal and external rotation. Usually, the direction of greatest instability has been determined preoperatively after the assessment of the history, multiple repeat examinations of both shoulders, plain radiographs, and any additional imaging studies such as a double-contrast CT arthrogram or MRI. It is rare to change the approach intraoperatively on the basis of the examination under anesthesia.

This technique is usually performed from one surgical approach, anterior or posterior. Over the years we have found that most of our inferior capsular shifts have been approached from the anterior side. The capsulorrhaphy is reinforced on the side of the direction of greatest instability, which is also the side chosen for the approach.[6,8,15,53] Sometimes it is difficult to decide on the best side for the approach; our method for this determination is outlined in the algorithm in Table 1. Essentially, the side that dislocates takes precedence over lesser degrees of instability. Shoulders that dislocate both an-

TABLE 1. *Treatment algorithm*

Indications for approach (anterior vs. posterior)	
Anterior approach:	Anterior: subluxation + posterior: stable or subluxation
	Anterior: dislocation + posterior: stable or subluxation or dislocation
Posterior approach:	Anterior: stable + posterior: subluxation or dislocation
	Anterior: subluxation + posterior: dislocation

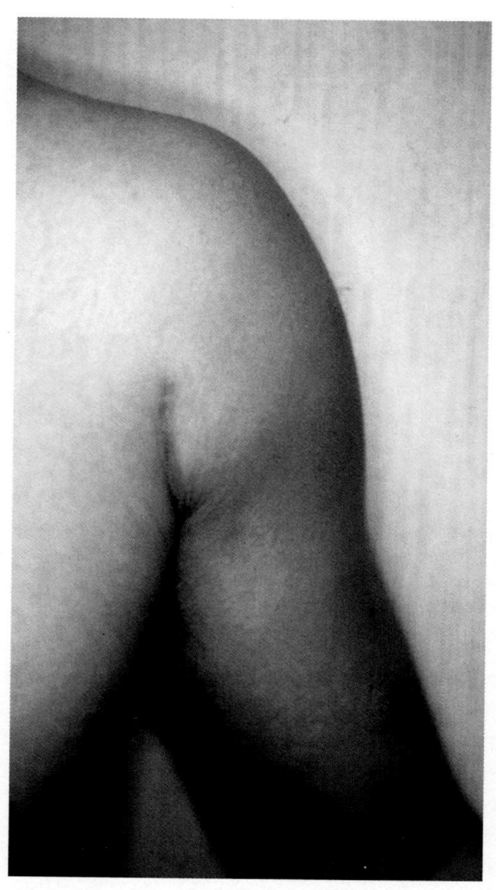

FIG. 5. The skin incision begins at a point midway between the tip of the coracoid and the inferior border of the pectoralis major and extends to the inferior border of the pectoralis major, concealed within the anterior axillary skin crease.

teriorly and posteriorly should be approached from the anterior side. Cooper and Brems have preferred to approach all cases from the anterior aspect of the shoulder.[14]

An extended axillary skin incision is made, as described by Leslie and Ryan.[45] This is a concealed incision within the axillary crease skin folds and begins at a point midway between the tip of the coracoid and the inferior border of the pectoralis major and extends to the inferior border of the pectoralis major (Fig. 5). The incision is taken through the subcutaneous tissues to the level of the deltopectoral interval. Careful hemostasis is obtained with the use of the needle tip electrocautery. The subcutaneous tissues are mobilized superiorly to the inferior aspect of the clavicle and anteroinferior acromion. The cephalic vein is mobilized with the deltoid laterally, and retractors are placed beneath both the pectoralis major for medial retraction and the deltoid for lateral retraction. The superior third of the pectoralis major insertion may be taken down if needed and tagged for later repair. The long head of the biceps tendon is carefully protected during this maneuver.

Next, the clavipectoral fascia is incised lateral to the strap muscles, which are gently retracted. Osteotomizing the coracoid or incising the strap muscles may place the musculocutaneous nerve at risk and is not necessary for exposure. The arm is then placed in a slight degree of external rotation to facilitate identification of the superior and inferior borders of the subscapularis. After excising any overlying subdeltoid bursa, the lesser tuberosity is identified. A small wedge of the anterior portion of the coracoacromial ligament may be excised to facilitate visualization of the superior border of the subscapularis tendon.

The importance of the subscapularis muscle cannot be overemphasized, and meticulous care throughout the approach and repair is imperative.[38,50] The subscapularis tendon is generally incised approximately 1 cm medial to its insertion on the lesser tuberosity. The incision is oriented from superior to inferior, perpendicular to the tendon fibers, and extends from the rotator interval superiorly to the lower border of the subscapularis inferiorly (Fig. 6). The anterior humeral circumflex vessels are cauterized to prevent bleeding. The subscapularis tendon is elevated from the underlying capsule. Stay sutures are placed in the subscapularis tendon, which is retracted medially. A stay suture is placed in the rotator interval for later repair. The remaining lateral insertion of the subscapularis is elevated (undercut) from the underlying capsule. This facilitates differentiating the capsular and subscapularis flaps so that they may be later individually repaired. The surgeon must be cognizant of the position of the axillary nerve, because it courses quite close to the inferior portion of the capsule and is at less risk with the humerus in adduction and external rotation (Fig. 7). We have found the "tug test" (Fig. 8) to be quite helpful in locating the anterior aspect of the axillary nerve.[24] If the vertical incision is too far medial, muscle fibers may be damaged thereby compromising the subscapularis repair. Wirth and Rockwood have recommended preservation of the inferior portion of the subscapularis in an effort to protect the axillary nerve and anterior humeral circumflex vessels.[86] An anatomic study has demonstrated that 40% of the subscapularis tendon insertion into the proximal humerus is inferior to the anterior humeral circumflex vessels.[38] Neglecting to release the inferior subscapularis will severely compromise the inferior capsular dissection and may limit the ability to shift the inferior capsule superiorly. Although the possibility of compromise to humeral head vascularity has been suggested, Steinmann and associates found no significant reduction following ligation of the anterior humeral circumflex artery.[77] There is collateral circulation from the posterior humeral circumflex vessels to the ascending branch of the anterior humeral circumflex vessels.

The lateral (humeral) approach to the capsule begins 5 mm medial to its humeral insertion. The incision starts at the level of the rotator interval. As the inferior aspect is approached, the arm is maintained in external rotation to avoid injury to the axillary nerve. Stay sutures are placed in the capsule as it is mobilized (Fig. 9). As the humerus is externally rotated and flexed, the capsule is incised around the neck of the humerus, extending as far posteriorly as neces-

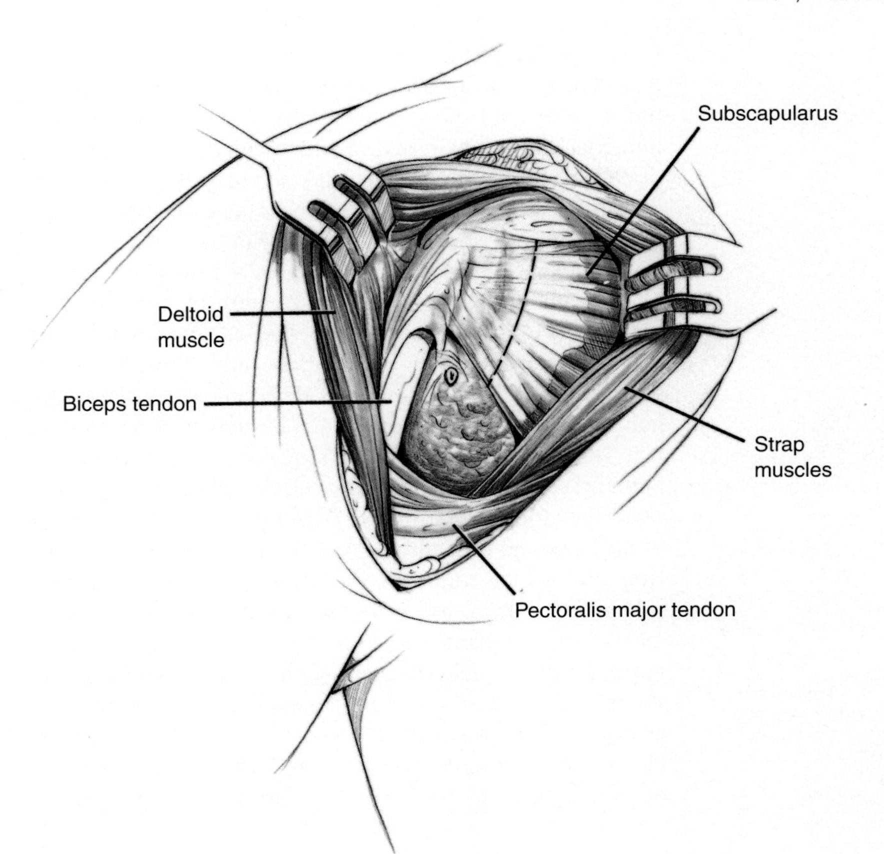

FIG. 6. Subscapularis tendon identification begins superiorly at the level of the rotator interval and inferiorly in the region of the anterior humeral circumflex vessels. The incision begins 1 cm medial to the lesser tuberosity.

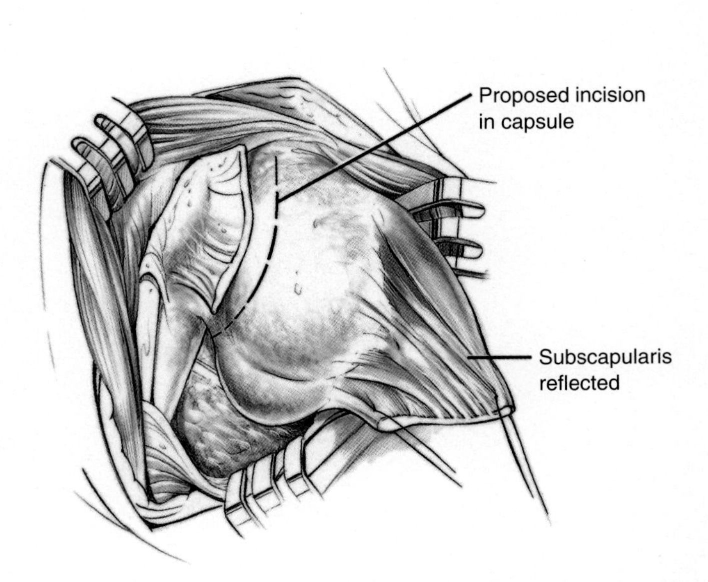

FIG. 7. The capsular incision is performed 5 mm medial to the lateral cuff of subscapularis tendon as the arm is maintained in external rotation and adduction to avoid injury to the axillary nerve.

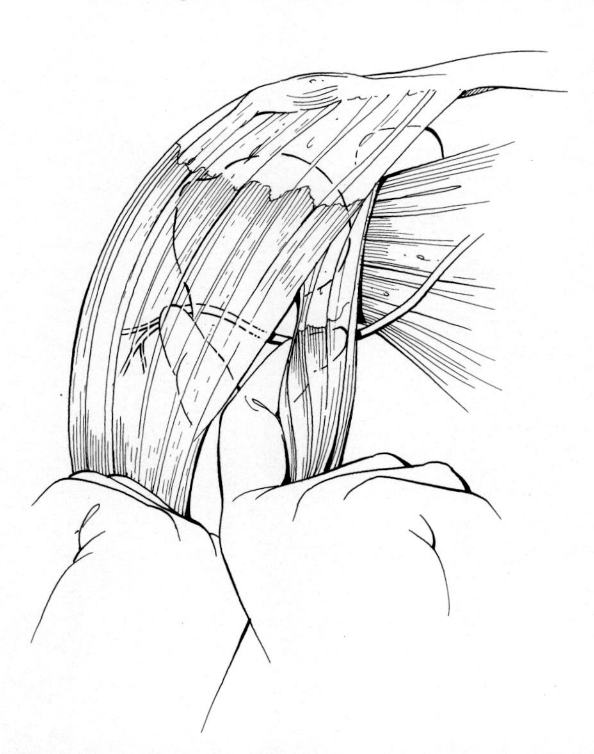

FIG. 8. The "tug test": One finger is placed on the axillary nerve at the front of the subscapularis, and the other finger under the deltoid on the anterior branch. A gentle tug applied by either finger will be transmitted to the other finger and is usually easily palpable.

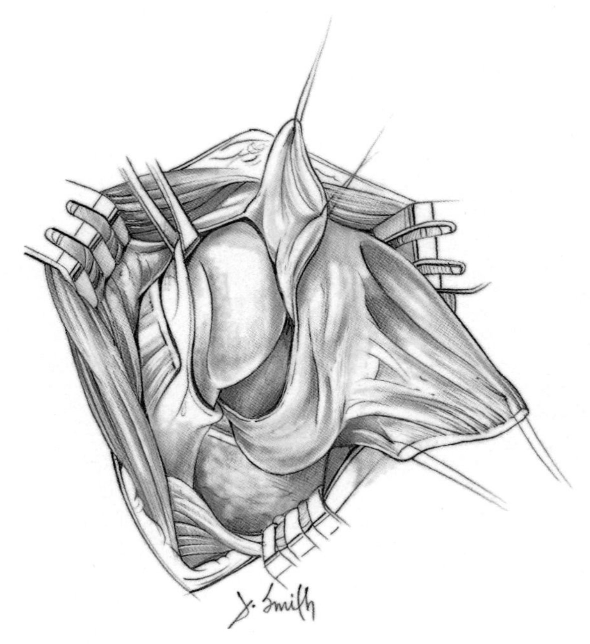

FIG. 9. Stay sutures are placed In the capsule as it is incised, and progressive external rotation facilitates inferior dissection.

sary, depending on the degree of instability. A finger may be placed in the inferior pouch to assess how large it is and how much redundant capsule needs to be released from the humerus before repair. In a shoulder with classic multidirectional instability, the capsule is taken down all the way to the posterior capsule, which can then be tensioned as the detached inferior capsule is shifted anteriorly.

A Fukuda ring retractor (Tiemann Co, Hauppage, NY) is placed, and the joint is inspected carefully. Intraarticular pathology, loose bodies, and articular cartilage defects are noted. It is at this stage that special steps are added as the pathology indicates. If there is detachment of the glenohumeral ligament complex (Broca-Perthes-Bankart lesion), it is repaired. Although less frequently observed, glenohumeral ligament detachments do occur in patients with multidirectional instability.[1,15,53] Sutures through drill holes in the bone and or suture anchors may be used for fixation. Both ends of the suture are passed through the medial capsule and tied down to secure the capsule, labrum, and ligaments to the roughened anterior glenoid neck (Fig. 10). Bone grafting is rarely required for patients with multidirectional shoulder instability.[53] If there is anterior glenoid bone deficiency involving more than 25% of the glenoid articular surface (secondary to erosion from multiple previous dislocations or from prior fracture), a bone graft may be performed.

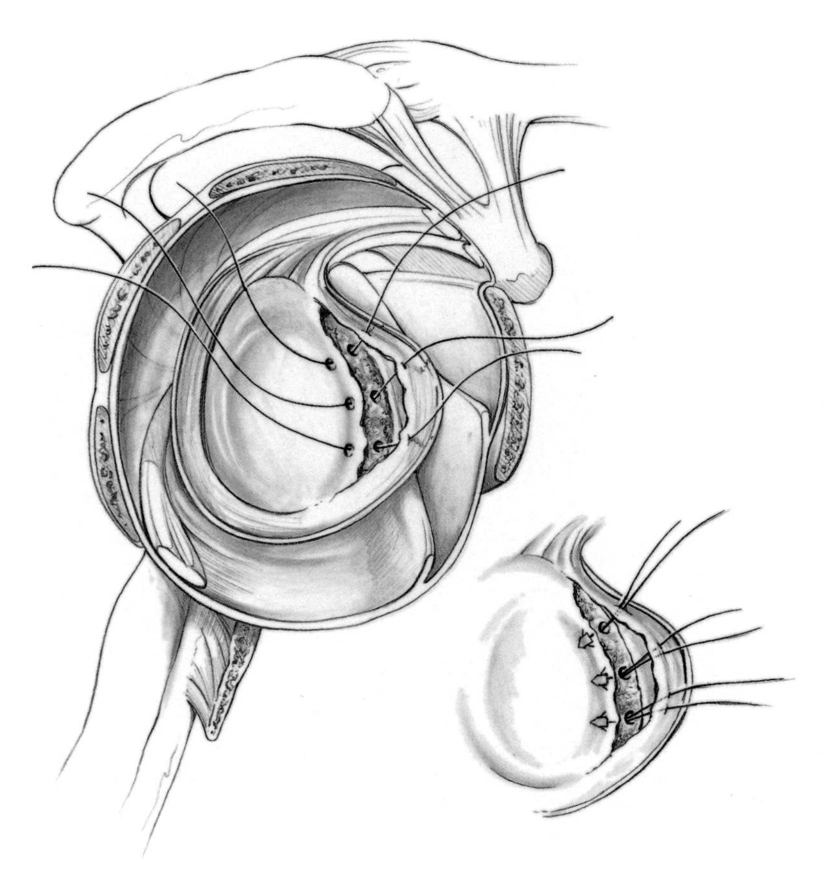

FIG. 10. A capsulolabral avulsion from the bony neck of the glenoid should be repaired before any attempt at capsulorrhaphy or shifting of the anterior capsule. Bone sutures or suture anchors can be used.

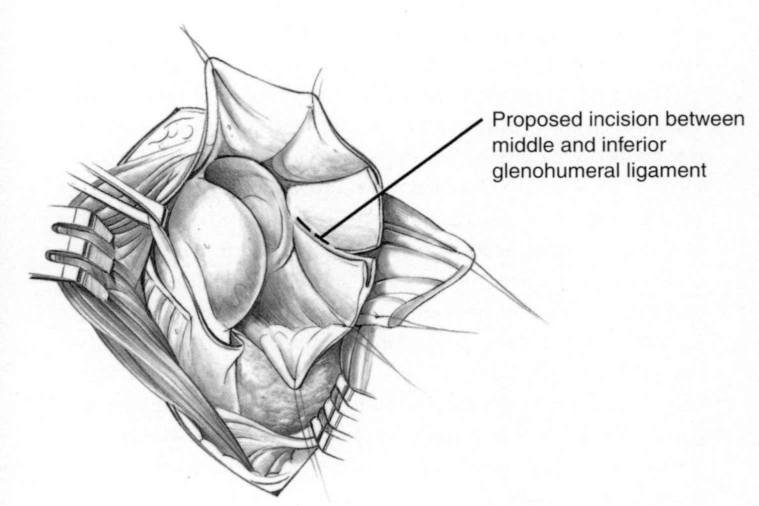

FIG. 11. The capsule is incised horizontally in a "T" fashion between the middle and inferior glenohumeral ligaments.

After carefully evaluating the joint, the capsule is incised horizontally in a "T" fashion. This is generally performed between the middle and inferior glenohumeral ligaments (Fig. 11). The superior flap thus has the superior and middle glenohumeral ligaments, whereas the inferior flap consists of the three portions of the inferior glenohumeral ligament. At this time the inferior capsular flap should be mobilized superiorly. The pouch should be obliterated, and this can be evaluated by placing a finger inferiorly and placing traction on the sutures in a superior direction. If there is any remaining subscapularis muscle on the inferior part of the capsule, there may be difficulty mobilizing this flap superiorly. Shifting the inferior capsular flap should effectively eliminate the redundant inferior pouch and tension the posterior capsule. The bone of the humerus just lateral to the articular margin is freshened to facilitate healing. The "T" incision allows adjustment of mediolateral and superoinferior tension independently, which can be especially helpful in athletes in whom restriction of motion needs to be avoided.

The capsule is repaired in general with the arm in approximately 25 to 45 degrees of external rotation and 20 to 45 degrees of abduction. This is modified based on the requirements of the individual patient, examination of the contralateral shoulder, and hand dominance. We repair the dominant shoulders of throwers in relatively more external rotation (45 to 60 degrees) and abduction (45 to 70 degrees). The repair is performed beginning with the inferior flap, which is shifted superiorly (Fig. 12). The sutures are placed in a simple interrupted manner progressing superiorly, repairing the inferior flap to the lateral stump of capsular insertion. Occasionally, when the quality of the capsular tissue remaining on the humerus is poor, sutures through humeral bone or suture anchors are used. Next, the superior cleft is repaired in a simple interrupted manner, closing the enlarged rotator interval when present. The arm is then placed in 20 to 45 degrees of external rotation and 20 degrees of abduction, and the superior capsular flap is shifted inferiorly and repaired (see Fig. 12).

The subscapularis muscle is reattached to its insertion in an anatomic manner. It is not transferred laterally. If release of the pectoralis major insertion was necessary, it is repaired using nonabsorbable sutures. The deltopectoral interval is closed with absorbable sutures in an interrupted simple manner, and the skin is closed in a running subcuticular fashion.

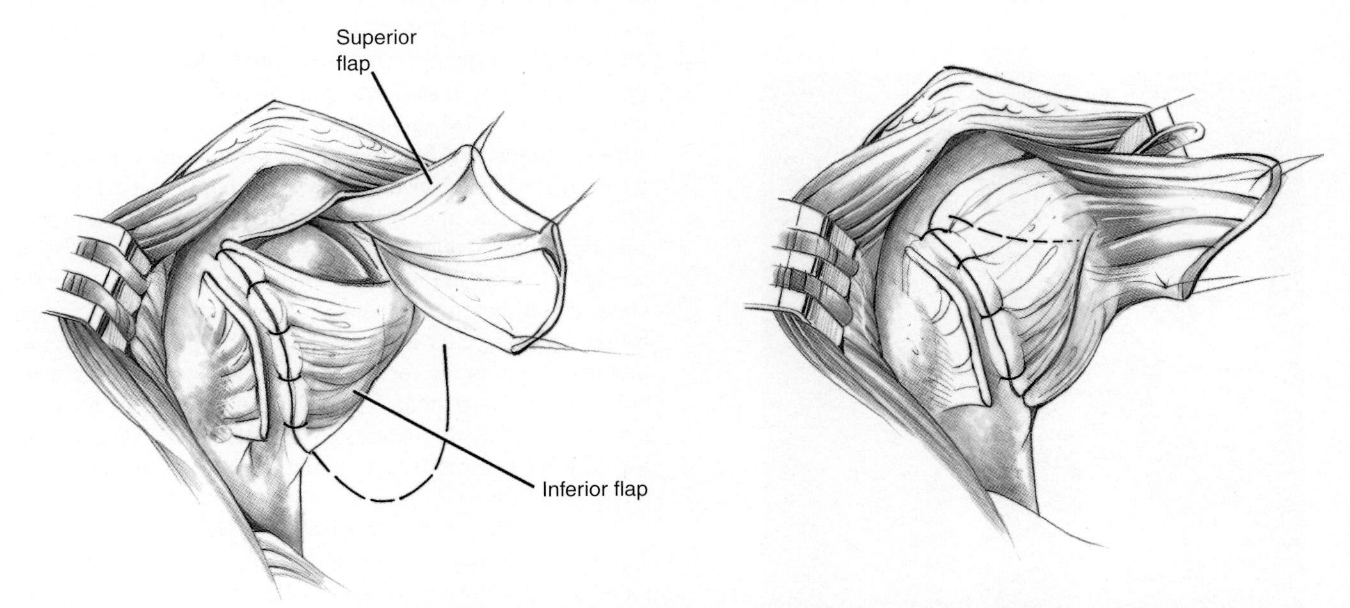

FIG. 12. The capsular shift begins as the inferior flap of the capsule is shifted superiorly and repaired to the lateral cuff of capsule. After repair of the superior cleft, the superior capsular flap is then shifted inferiorly and repaired.

In recent years we have found that most of our inferior capsular shifts for the treatment of multidirectional instability have been performed from an anterior approach. Because there is another chapter on posterior instability in this text, we refer the interested reader to previously published work for details about the posterior approach.[6,53,57]

REHABILITATION

Patients who have multidirectional instability, without associated posterior dislocations, are protected in a sling for 6 weeks, but after 10 days the arm is removed from the sling for exercises, including isometrics and external rotation to 10 degrees and forward elevation to 90 degrees. From 2 to 4 weeks external rotation is increased to 30 degrees and forward elevation to 120 degrees, and isometric strengthening is added. From 4 to 6 weeks external rotation is increased to 40 degrees and forward elevation to approximately 140 degrees, and resistive exercises are begun. After 6 weeks, external rotation is increased to 60 degrees and forward elevation to 160 degrees. After 3 months, external rotation may be progressed. Strengthening begins with the arm in neutral below 90 degrees. As the rehabilitation progresses, more dynamic strengthening exercises are introduced. These exercises include the use of medicine balls in various sizes and weights, as well as plyometric exercises.[16,41]

For those patients with multidirectional instability and associated posterior dislocations, a special brace that holds the arm in a slightly abducted position with neutral rotation is used (Fig. 13). The arm is immobilized in this brace for 6 weeks; only gentle isometric exercises and supervised elbow range of motion are allowed during that time. At 6 weeks the brace is discontinued, and range of motion exercises are gradually introduced. At 12 weeks, postoperatively progressive strengthening is instituted on an individualized basis.

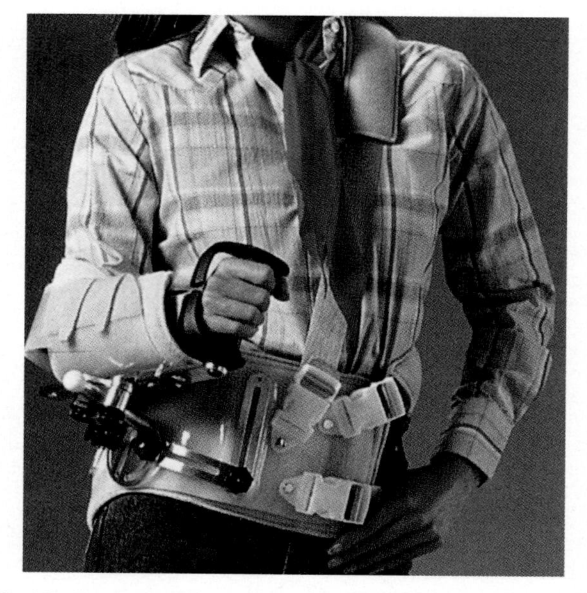

FIG. 13. Brace utilized during the early postoperative period in patients with multidirectional instability and associated posterior dislocations.

These are general protocols and are modified on an individual basis as indicated. For example, the dominant shoulder of throwers would be progressed more quickly, particularly with reference to external rotation. The objective is to regain motion over several months, because progression that is too quick may lead to recurrent instability. This is especially true in patients with some degree of generalized ligamentous laxity and in younger patients in late adolescence. Careful and frequent postoperative follow-up is necessary, because patients who are not progressing quickly enough may need an accelerated program, whereas those who are regaining motion too quickly may need to be slowed down. Return to contact sports is generally restricted until 9 to 12 months have elapsed.

RESULTS

Since 1980 several investigators have reported on the treatment of patients with multidirectional instability.[8,14,31,43,51,53,85] Operative management using the inferior capsular shift has been quite successful. Neer's initial report in a series of 32 patients noted only 1 unsatisfactory result.[57] One decade later he reported "more than one hundred additional inferior capsular shifts have been done with similar satisfactory results."[53] Cooper and Brems reviewed their series of 43 shoulders in 38 patients with a minimum 2-year follow-up after inferior capsular shift. Thirty-nine of 43 shoulders (91%) were rated by the patients as satisfactory, with no recurrent instability. Postoperatively, recurrent symptomatic instability developed in 4 patients (11%). Two of these patients required subsequent revision inferior capsular shifts, and 1 of those later required a humeral head replacement for arthritis. The latter patient had a prior Bristow procedure. They concluded that the inferior capsular shift procedure provided satisfactory objective and subjective results. Failures and recurrences of symptomatic instability generally occurred in the early postoperative period, less than 2 years after surgery. Their findings did not demonstrate a deterioration of the results with follow-up to 6 years.[14] Our service reported the results after inferior capsular shift for classic multidirectional instability in 52 shoulders. Average follow-up of 5 years was present, and all patients were immobilized in a brace for 6 weeks. Satisfactory results were noted in 94% of patients.[8] Hawkins and associates have reported less favorable results in a series of 31 patients followed for 2 to 5 years. Just under 40% of the patients (12) went on to failure.[35]

Altchek and Warren reported their results following a T-plasty modification of the Bankart procedure for multidirectional instability in 42 shoulders. The patient population differed somewhat in that 38 of the 42 cases had a Bankart lesion or detachment of the labrum and glenohumeral ligament complex. Patient satisfaction was rated excellent for 40 (95%) of the shoulders. The average loss of external rotation was 5 degrees. They noted that throwing athletes found they were unable to throw a ball with as much speed as before the operation. Additionally, 7 of 42 shoulders (16%) demonstrated 2 plus or greater posterior instability postoperatively. There were 4 cases of symptomatic recurrent instability, 1 anterior and 3 posterior, and 1 patient required a posterior stabilization 2 years postoperatively.[1]

The results following capsular shift procedures for patients with anteroinferior instability were satisfactory.[7,67] Our service has published preliminary results after 75 inferior capsular shifts performed in young athletes. Eighty-nine percent were able to return to their major sport, whereas 73% maintained the same level of competitiveness. Seven patients (9.3%) reported a single episode of probable subluxation that was not followed by recurrent instability and did not affect the final result, whereas two patients (2.7%) had dislocation postoperatively, and both cases were associated with a traumatic episode. The average loss of external rotation was 7 degrees.[7] Our experience using the inferior capsular shift in 171 anterior repairs has been reported.[67] The cause was primarily traumatic in 122 shoulders (71%), repetitive microtrauma in 22 (13%), and atraumatic in 27 (16%). The direction of instability was unidirectional (anterior) in 50 (29%), bidirectional (anterior and inferior) in 87 (51%), and multidirectional (anterior, inferior, and posterior) in 34 (20%). At follow-up averaging 5 years (range, 2 to 13 years), 97 (57%) were rated excellent, 61 (36%) good, 4 (2%) fair, and 8 (5%) poor. Seven shoulders (4%) had recurrent instability. The cause (traumatic, atraumatic, or acquired) and direction (anterior versus anteroinferior versus multidirectional) of the instability were not found to influence the rate of success.[67]

CONCLUSIONS

The operative treatment of choice for patients with multidirectional instability has become the inferior capsular shift since the landmark article by Neer and Foster in 1980.[57] Anatomy deforming procedures, bony procedures, muscle transfers, and procedures designed for unidirectional instability have fallen into disfavor.[8,14,15,23,32,34,43,48,53,61,64,67,69,72,76,84,87,88]

Turkel et al. demonstrated that anterior glenohumeral stability is provided by varying regions of the capsule, depending on arm position.[80] Similarly, Warner et al. demonstrated that inferior humeral translation is restrained by the anterosuperior capsule and ligaments with the arm at the side, and by the inferior capsule and ligaments with the arm in abduction.[82,84] This is consistent with the clinical findings of Neer and Foster,[57] who described inferior humeral translation with the arm at the side and with the arm in abduction in patients with multidirectional instability and emphasized reducing redundant capsular volume on all sides at the time of surgical reconstruction. Isolated tensioning of the anterosuperior capsular structures and rotator interval has been proposed to treat the inferior component of instability.[21,60] Although preliminary results are favorable, the role for these variations in technique has not yet been established.

The capsular shift procedure eliminates laxity in the rotator interval, anterosuperior capsule, and anteroinferior capsule, and can be continued around the humeral neck to reduce as much laxity in the posteroinferior and posterior capsule as is actually found. Thus, it is a highly versatile procedure allowing precise soft-tissue balancing on several sides of the joint. Because of the shifting of load between different capsular regions, as shown by Turkel et al.,[80] the capsular shift affords stability in varying functional positions while preserving motion and is especially useful in the reconstruction of the unstable athletic shoulder.

The advantage of a versatile surgical approach to shoulder instability is that the surgeon is not committed to any one technique at the start. Varying degrees of instability can be dealt with precisely using a utility approach. We have found that overlap syndromes are especially common in overhead athletes given their associated repetitive stress and injury. Thus, rather than there being two discrete groups, unidirectional and multidirectional, there is a spectrum of varying amounts of inferior and posterior laxity on which, for example, a traumatic anterior stress may be superimposed. We have found the inferior capsular shift approach very valuable, allowing precise takedown of as much inferior capsule as is actually needed on an individual basis to eliminate a redundant pouch. Thus, one can perform only a modified shift, essentially an anterior capsulorrhaphy, if anterior instability is found,[6,7,56,67] or a full inferior capsular shift for classic multidirectional instability.[8,57] Additionally, when a labral or ligamentous detachment is encountered, it can be repaired to the medial glenoid rim to anchor the capsule before shifting the capsular flaps. In this way, both elements of capsular damage may be addressed. The inferior capsular shift procedure is a versatile and reliable treatment for patients with multidirectional shoulder instability.

REFERENCES

1. Altchek DW, Warren RF, Skyhar MJ, Ortiz G. T-plasty modification of the Bankart procedure for multidirectional instability of the anterior and inferior types. *J Bone Joint Surg [Am]* 1991;73:105–112.
2. Arendt EA. Multidirectional shoulder instability. *Orthopedics* 1988;11: 113–120.
3. Bateman JE, ed. *The shoulder and neck*, ed 2. Philadelphia: JB Lippincott, 1978:475–564.
4. Beall MS Jr, Diefenbach G, Allen A. Electromyographic biofeedback in the treatment of voluntary posterior instability of the shoulder. *Am J Sports Med* 1987;15:175–178.
5. Belle RM. Collagen typing in multidirectional instability of the shoulder. *Orthop Trans* 1989;13:680–681.
6. Bigliani LU. Anterior and posterior capsular shift for multidirectional instability. *Tech Orthop* 1989;3:36–45.
7. Bigliani LU, Kurzweil PR, Schwartzbach CC, et al. Inferior capsular shift procedure for anterior inferior shoulder instability in athletes. *Am J Sports Med* 1994;22:578–584.
8. Bigliani LU, Pollock RG, Owens JM, et al. The inferior capsular shift procedure for multidirectional instability of the shoulder. *Orthop Trans* 1994;17:576.
9. Bigliani LU, Pollock RG, Soslowsky LJ, Flatow EL. The tensile properties of the inferior glenohumeral ligament. *J Orthop Res* 1992;10: 187–197.

10. Bigliani LU, Weinstein DM, Glasgow MT, Pollock RG, Flatow EL. Glenohumeral arthroplasty for arthritis after instability surgery. *J Shoulder Elbow Surg* 1995;4:87–94.
11. Burkhead WZ, Rockwood CA. Treatment of instability of the shoulder with an exercise program. *J Bone Joint Surg [Am]* 1992:74:890–896.
12. Carter C, Sweetnam R. Recurrent dislocations of the patella and of the shoulder. Their association with familial joint laxity. *J Bone Joint Surg [Br]* 1960;42:721–727.
13. Cofield RH, Nessler JP, Weinstabl R. Diagnosis of shoulder instability by examination under anesthesia. *Clin Orthop* 1993;291:45–53.
14. Cooper RA, Brems JJ. The inferior capsular shift procedure for multidirectional instability of the shoulder. *J Bone Joint Surg* 1992;74: 1516–1521.
15. Cordasco FA, Pollock RG, Flatow EL, Bigliani LU. Management of multidirectional instability. *Oper Tech Sports Med* 1993;1:293–300.
16. Cordasco FA, Wolfe IN, Wootten ME, Bigliani LU. An electromyographic analysis of the shoulder during a medicine ball rehabilitation program. *Am J Sports Med* 1996;24:386–392.
17. Depalma AF, ed. *Surgery of the shoulder*, 2nd ed. Philadelphia: JB Lippincott, 1973:403–432.
18. Duncan R, Savoie FH III. Arthroscopic inferior capsular shift for multidirectional instability of the shoulder: a preliminary report. *Arthroscopy* 1993;9:24–27.
19. Emery RJ, Mullaji AB. Glenohumeral joint instability in normal adolescents: incidence and significance. *J Bone Joint Surg [Br]* 1991;73: 406–408.
20. Endo H, Takigawa T, Takata K, et al. A method of diagnosis and treatment for loose shoulder. *Cent Jpn J Orthop Surg Trauma* 1971;14: 630–632.
21. Field LD, Warren RF, O'Brien SJ, Altchek DW, Wickiewicz TL. Isolated closure of rotator interval defects for shoulder instability. *Am J Sports Med* 1995;23:557–563.
22. Finsterbush A, Pogrund H. The hypermobility syndrome: musculoskeletal complaints in 100 consecutive cases of joint hypermobility. *Clin Orthop* 1982;168:124–127.
23. Flatow EL. Multidirectional instability. In: Bigliani LU, ed. *The unstable shoulder*. Park Ridge, IL: American Academy of Orthopaedic Surgeons, 1996:79–90.
24. Flatow EL, Bigliani LU. Locating and protecting the axillary nerve in shoulder surgery: the tug test. *Orthop Rev* 1992;21:503–505.
25. Friedman RJ, Bonutti PM, Genez B, Norfray JF. Cine magnetic resonance imaging of the glenohumeral joint. *Orthop Trans* 1993–1994;17: 1018–1019.
26. Foster CR. Multidirectional instability of the shoulder in the athlete. *Clin Sports Med* 1983;2:355–368.
27. Gibb TD, Sidles JA, Harryman DT II, McQuade KJ, Matsen FA III. The effect of capsular venting on glenohumeral laxity. *Clin Orthop* 1991;268:120-127.
28. Habermeyer P, Schuller U, Wiedemann E. The intra-articular pressure of the shoulder: an experimental study on the role of the glenoid labrum in stabilizing the joint. *Arthroscopy* 1992;8:166–172.
29. Harryman DT, Sidles JA, Harris SL, Matsen FA. Laxity of the normal glenohumeral joint: a quantitative in vivo assessment. *J Shoulder Elbow Surg* 1992;1:66–76.
30. Harryman DT, Sidles JA, Harris SL, Matsen FA. The role of the rotator interval capsule in passive motion and stability of the shoulder. *J Bone Joint Surg [Am]* 1992:74:53–66.
31. Hawkins RJ, Abrams JS, Schutte J. Multidirectional instability of the shoulder: an approach to diagnosis. *Orthop Trans* 1987;11:246.
32. Hawkins RJ, Angelo RL. Glenohumeral osteoarthrosis. *J Bone Joint Surg [Am]* 1990;72:1193–1197.
33. Hawkins RJ, Bokor DJ. Clinical evaluation of shoulder problems. In: Rockwood CA, Matsen FA, eds. *The shoulder*. Philadelphia: WB Saunders, 1990:167–171.
34. Hawkins RH, Hawkins RJ. Failed anterior reconstruction for shoulder instability. *J Bone Joint Surg [Br]* 1985;67:709–714.
35. Hawkins RJ, Kunkel SS, Nayak NK. Inferior capsular shift for multidirectional instability of the shoulder: 2–5 year follow-up. *Orthop Trans* 1991;15:765.
36. Hawkins RJ, Schutte JP, Janda DH, Huckell GH. Translation of the glenohumeral joint with the patient under anesthesia. *J Shoulder Elbow Surg* 1996;5:286–292.
37. Hayashi K, Thabit G III, Massa KL, et al. The effect of thermal heating on the length and histologic properties of the glenohumeral joint capsule. *Am J Sports Med* 1997;25:107–112.
38. Hinton MA, Parker AW, Drez D, Altchek D. An anatomic study of the subscapularis tendon and myotendinous junction. *J Shoulder Elbow Surg* 1994;3:224–229.
39. Jalovaara P, Myllyla V, Paivansalo M. Autotraction stress roentgenography for demonstration anterior and inferior instability of the shoulder joint. *Clin Orthop* 1992;284:136–143.
40. Jerosch J, Castro WH. Shoulder instability in Ehlers-Danlos syndrome: an indication for surgical treatment? *Acta Orthop Belg* 1990;56: 451–453.
41. Kennedy K. Rehabilitation of the unstable shoulder. *Oper Tech Sports Med* 1993;1:311–324.
42. Kronberg M, Brostrom L-A, Nemeth G. Differences in shoulder muscle activity between patients with generalized joint laxity and normal controls. *Clin Orthop* 1991;269:181–192.
43. Lebar RD, Alexander AH. Multidirectional shoulder instability: clinical results of inferior capsular shift in an active-duty population. *Am J Sports Med* 1992;20:193–198.
44. Lephart SM, Warner JJP, Borsa PA, Fu FH. Proprioception of the shoulder joint in healthy, unstable, and surgically repaired shoulders. *J Shoulder Elbow Surg* 1994;3:371–380.
45. Leslie JT Jr, Ryan TJ. The anterior axillary incision to approach the shoulder joint. *J Bone Joint Surg [Am]* 1962;44:1193–1196.
46. Lusardi DA, Wirth MA, Wurtz D, Rockwood CA. Loss of external rotation following anterior capsulorrhaphy of the shoulder. *J Bone Joint Surg [Am]* 1993;75:1185–1192.
47. MacDonald PB, Hawkins RJ, Fowler PJ, Miniaci A. Release of the subscapularis for internal rotation contracture and pain after anterior repair for recurrent anterior dislocation of the shoulder. *J Bone Joint Surg [Am]* 1992;74:734–737.
48. Mallon WJ, Speer KP. Multidirectional instability: current concepts. *J Shoulder Elbow Surg* 1995;4:54–64.
49. Marberry TA. Experience with the Neer inferior capsular shift for multidirectional shoulder instability. *Orthop Trans* 1988;12:747.
50. McCann PD, Cordasco FA, Ticker JB, et al. An anatomic study of the subscapular nerves: a guide for the electromyographic analysis of the subscapularis muscle. *J Shoulder Elbow Surg* 1994;3:94–99.
51. Mizuno K, Itakura Y, Muratsu H. Inferior capsular shift for inferior and multidirectional instability of the shoulder in young children: report of two cases. *J Shoulder Elbow Surg* 1992;1:200–206.
52. Mok DW, Fogg AJ, Hokan R, et al. The diagnostic value of arthroscopy in glenohumeral instability. *J Bone Joint Surg [Am]* 1990;72:698–700.
53. Neer CS II. *Shoulder reconstruction*, Philadelphia: WB Saunders, 1990:273–341.
54. Neer CS II. Involuntary inferior and multidirectional instability of the shoulder. Etiology, recognition, and treatment. In: Stauffer ES, ed. American Academy of Orthopaedic Surgeons *Instructional Course Lectures XXXIV*. St Louis, MO: CV Mosby, 1985:232–238.
55. Neer CS II. Recent concepts in dislocation and subluxation. In: Takagishi N, ed. *The shoulder: proceedings of the 3rd international conference on surgery of the shoulder*. Tokyo, Japan: Professional Postgraduate Services, 1987:7–12.
56. Neer CS II, Fithian TF, Hansen PE, et al. Reinforced cruciate repair for anterior dislocations of the shoulder. *Orthop Trans* 1985;9:44.
57. Neer CS II, Foster CR. Inferior capsular shift for inferior and multidirectional instability of the shoulder: a preliminary report. *J Bone Joint Surg [Am]* 1980;62:897–908.
58. Neer CS II, Perez-Sanz JR, Ogawa K. Causes of failure in repairs for recurrent anterior dislocations. Presented at New York Orthopaedic Hospital Alumni Annual Meeting. In: Neer CS II, ed. *Shoulder reconstruction*. Philadelphia: WB Saunders, 1990:279.
59. Nobuhara K, Ikeda H. Glenoid osteotomy for loose shoulder. In: Bateman JE, Welsh RP, eds. *Surgery of the shoulder*. Philadelphia: BC Decker, 1984:100–103.
60. Nobuhara K, Ikeda H. Rotator interval lesion. *Clin Orthop* 1987;223: 44–50.
61. Norris TR, Bigliani LU. Analysis of failed repair for shoulder instability–A preliminary report. In: Bateman JE, Welsh RP, eds. *Surgery of the shoulder*. Philadelphia: BC Decker, 1984:111–116.
62. O'Brien SJ, Neves MC, Arnockzky SP, Warren RF. The anatomy and histology of the inferior glenohumeral ligament complex of the shoulder. *Am J Sports Med* 1990; 18:449–456.
63. O'Driscoll SW, Evans DC. The incidence of contralateral shoulder in-

stability in patients treated for recurrent anterior instability: an epidemiological investigation. *Orthop Trans* 1991;15:762.
64. O'Driscoll SW, Evans DC. Long term results of staple capsulorrhaphy for anterior instability of the shoulder. *J Bone Joint Surg [Am]* 1993;75: 249–258.
65. Ozaki J. Glenohumeral movements of the involuntary inferior and multidirectional instability. *Clin Orthop* 1989;238:107–111.
66. Pagnani MJ, Warren RF. Stabilizers of the glenohumeral joint. *J Shoulder Elbow Surg* 1994:3:173–190.
67. Pollock RG, Owens JM, Nicholson GP, et al. The anterior inferior capsular shift procedure for anterior glenohumeral instability: technique and long-term results. *Orthop Trans* 1993–1994;17:1109.
68. Rockwood CA. Management of patients with multidirectional instability of the shoulder. *Orthop Trans* 1994;18:328.
69. Rockwood CA, Gerber C. Analysis of failed surgical procedures for anterior shoulder instability. *Orthop Trans* 1985;9:48.
70. Rowe CR, Pierce DS, Clark JG. Voluntary dislocation of the shoulder: a preliminary report on a clinical electromyographic and psychiatric study of twenty-six patients. *J Bone Joint Surg [Am]* 1973;55:445–460.
71. Rowe CR, Zarins B, Ciullo JV. Recurrent anterior dislocation of the shoulder after surgical repair: apparent causes of failure and treatment. *J Bone Joint Surg [Am]* 1984;66:159–168.
72. Samilson RL, Prieto V. Dislocation arthropathy of the shoulder. *J Bone Joint Surg [Am]* 1983;65:456–460.
73. Silliman JF, Hawkins RJ. Classification and physical diagnosis of instability of the shoulder. *Clin Orthop* 1993;291:7–19.
74. Speer KP, Deng X, Borrero S, et al. Biomechanical evaluation of a simulated Bankart lesion. *J Bone Joint Surg [Am]* 1994;76:1819–1826.
75. Speer KP, Deng X, Torzilli PA, Altchek DA, Warren RF. Strategies for an anterior capsular shift of the shoulder: a biomechanical comparison. *Am J Sports Med* 1995;23:264–269.
76. Steinmann SR, Flatow EL, Pollock RG, et al. Evaluation and surgical treatment of failed shoulder instability repairs. *Orthop Trans* 1992;16: 727.
77. Steinmann SR, Gaccione DR, McGee TH, Higgins D, Cammarata A, Hughes S. The effect of anterior shoulder reconstruction on humeral head vascularity. *Orthop Trans* 1994–1995;18:1066.
78. Thompson FR, Moga JJ, Fielding JW. Unusual habitual shoulder dislocations: combined operative repair. Audiovisual presentation at the Annual Meeting of the American Academy of Orthopaedic Surgeons, New York, 1965.
79. Thabit G III. Laser-assisted capsular shift for the treatment of glenohumeral instability. *Orthopaedics* 1994;3:10–12.
80. Turkel SJ, Panio MW, Marshall JL, et al. Stabilizing mechanisms preventing anterior dislocation of the glenohumeral joint. *J Bone Joint Surg [Am]* 1981;63:1208–1217.
81. Warner JJP, Caborn DNM, Berger R, Fu FH, See M. Dynamic capsuloligamentous anatomy of the glenohumeral joint. *J Shoulder Elbow Surg* 1993;2:115–133.
82. Warner JJP, Deng X, Warren RF, Torzilli PA. Static capsuloligamentous restraints to superior–inferior translation of the glenohumeral joint. *Am J Sports Med* 1992;20:675–685.
83. Warner JJP, Deng X, Warren RF, Torzilli PA, Obrien SJ. Superior-inferior translation in the intact and vented glenohumeral joint. *J Shoulder Elbow Surg* 1993;2:99–125.
84. Warner JJP, Johnson D, Miller M, Caborn DNM. Technique for selecting capsular tightness in repair of anterior–inferior shoulder instability. *J Shoulder Elbow Surg* 1995;4:352–364.
85. Welsh RP, Trimmings N. Multidirectional instability of the shoulder. *Orthop Trans* 1987;11:231.
86. Wirth MA, Blatter G, Rockwood CA. The capsular imbrication procedure for recurrent anterior instability of the shoulder. *J Bone Joint Surg [Am]* 1996;78:246–259.
87. Young DC, Rockwood CA. Complications of a failed Bristow procedure and their management. *J Bone Joint Surg [Am]* 1991;73:969–981.
88. Zuckerman JD, Matsen FA III. Complications about the glenohumeral joint related to the use of screws and staples. *J Bone Joint Surg [Am]* 1984;66:175–180.

Disorders of the Shoulder: Diagnosis and Management,
edited by Joseph P. Iannotti and Gerald R. Williams, Jr.
Lippincott Williams & Wilkins, Philadelphia © 1999.

CHAPTER 13

Treatment of Locked Anterior and Posterior Dislocations of the Shoulder

Sean M. Griggs, G. Brian Holloway, Gerald R. Williams Jr., and Joseph P. Iannotti

INTRODUCTION

Dislocations of the shoulder account for approximately 45% of the dislocations seen in the major joints.[16] In 1974, Cave et al.[5] presented the demographics of a large series of shoulder dislocations. In their series, anterior dislocations accounted for 84% of glenohumeral dislocations, acromioclavicular dislocations for 12%, sternoclavicular dislocations for 2.5%, and posterior dislocations for 1.5%. Although these injuries are common and are readily diagnosed by careful physical examination and by obtaining the appropriate radiographic examination, the evaluating physician can sometimes miss them.

The true incidence of chronic dislocations of the shoulder is unknown. This is partially due to the lack of consistent criteria for defining what time frame should be used to declare a dislocation to be chronic. In the literature, the definition for chronic has ranged from as early as 24 hours to as late as 6 months.[12,29,30] In 1968, Schulz wrote, "unrecognized dislocations need not be old to be troublesome."[30] In Schulz and colleagues report on 61 shoulder dislocations they used the time frame of 24 hours to define a chronic dislocation. Although their data are biased toward an early definition of chronic, this study did provide useful epidemiological data. In their review of both anterior and posterior dislocations, they found the following: (a) 50% had associated fractures about the joint, (b) 33% had neurologic injury (5 of the 17 posterior dislocations and 18 of the 44 anterior dislocations), and (c) 28% of the dislocations were posterior. They also re-

S. M. Griggs: Park Plaza Hand and Upper Extremity Center, Houston, Texas 77004.
G. B. Holloway: Knoxville Orthopaedic Clinic, Knoxville, Tennessee 37909.
G. R. Williams, Jr. and Joseph P. Iannotti: Department of Orthopaedic Surgery, Hospital of the University of Pennsylvania, Philadelphia, Pennsylvania 19104.

ported that seizures were the cause of 29% of the dislocations. Eleven of the 18 dislocations caused by seizures had associated fractures. Fifty percent of seizure-caused injuries were posterior dislocations.

In 1982, Rowe and Zarins[29] proposed that the injury be at least 3 weeks old to define it as chronic. They presented 23 patients with 24 dislocations: 14 were posterior, 8 were anterior, 1 was inferior, and 1 was superior. Remarkably, 79% of the posterior dislocations that they evaluated were missed by the original treating physician. To determine how often chronic dislocations were seen by the average orthopedist, Rowe and Zarins surveyed 208 New England orthopedic surgeons.[29] Their survey found that 50% of orthopedic surgeons in practice for 5–10 years had seen a chronic dislocation, that 70% of those in practice for 10–20 years had seen this injury, and that 90% of orthopedic surgeons in practice for over 20 years had seen at least one chronic dislocation. Based on their survey, 65% of chronic dislocations were anterior and 35% were posterior. This survey, as well as the relatively few clinical series reporting these injuries, attests to the rarity of chronic shoulder dislocations.

The purpose of this chapter is to help the reader develop an algorithm to approach the treatment of locked dislocations of the shoulder. We use the term *locked dislocation*, instead of chronic dislocation, because we feel the treatment algorithm should include the treatment of acute injuries as well as chronic injuries. The time from injury is an important factor in determining which treatment is likely to be effective. In this chapter, we define *chronic* as any dislocation that has been present for at least 3 weeks. Injuries that are more than 3 weeks old are unlikely to be reduced with a closed manipulation and will require operative intervention. Injuries that are more than 6 months old are apt to have significant loss of articular cartilage viability and will likely require joint replacement.

In this chapter, we will also review the literature pertaining to the outcomes obtained from the suggested treatments given for locked dislocations of the shoulder. The number of series reported in the literature is small and the number of patients in each report ranges from a single case report to 61 patients.[10–12,15,22,26,29–33] Therefore, there are only a few patients whose outcomes can be evaluated for each suggested treatment. Also, the outcome data from earlier series are marred by a lack of a consistent method for reporting functional results. More recent authors have tried to correct this problem by using both subjective and objective grading methods. It is difficult to compare the results among these studies. The results reported in the early literature will be discussed in terms of satisfactory versus unsatisfactory, and when available, more objective outcome measurements will be reported.

POSTERIOR LOCKED DISLOCATION

Although posterior dislocations account for approximately 1.5% of shoulder dislocations, they account for most chronic locked dislocations of the glenohumeral joint. In 1982, Rowe and Zarins[29] reported that 11 of the 14 locked posterior dislocations that they evaluated, in a referral practice, were unrecognized by the initial treating physician. It is estimated that more than 60% of posterior dislocations of the glenohumeral humeral joint are missed at the time of initial evaluation.[12,29]

There are many reasons that these injuries may be missed on initial evaluation. Posterior dislocations of the shoulder usually occur from either seizures or violent trauma. These patients may present to the emergency department with more urgent medical problems, and the normal-appearing posture of the posteriorly dislocated shoulder leads to the injury being overlooked. Patients with these injuries may present with a near–normal-appearing shoulder contour, holding the injured arm in the common guarding position of internal rotation with the elbow at the side. Another reason the injury may be overlooked is due to inadequate radiographic evaluation at the time of the presentation. In posterior dislocations of the glenohumeral joint, the humeral head can dislocate directly posterior to the glenoid. This can result in a near normal appearing anteroposterior radiograph of the shoulder (Fig. 1).

History

Patients presenting with chronic posterior dislocations of the shoulder usually have a history of major trauma, such as a motor vehicle accident or fall from a height, or they have a history of a convulsive episode from either an intrinsic seizure disorder or an electrical shock. They initially have substantial pain in the shoulder, with a loss of use of the arm. The initial severe discomfort often resolves to a tolerable level within a few weeks of the injury, and the patient will begin to use the shoulder for waist level activities of daily living. Many times, this slow resolution of pain and the return of limited function are mistaken for the process of recovery by the patient or the treating physician. There are multiple reports of patients with locked posterior dislocations being sent to therapy with the diagnosis of a frozen

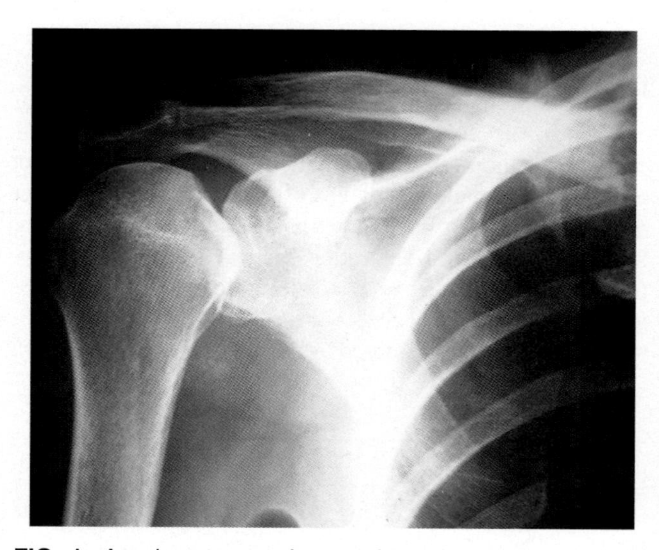

FIG. 1. An almost normal-appearing anteroposterior radiograph of the shoulder in a patient with a chronic posterior dislocation.

shoulder, only to later be given the correct diagnosis once treatment fails.[12,29,30]

Once the diagnosis of a locked posterior dislocation is made, it is important for the physician to evaluate these patients' functional status. Surprisingly these patients may adapt sufficiently enough to the limitations of motion and discomfort produced by the injury to have few perceived functional limitations. The patient may have been referred to the office because of concerns of the previous treating physician or by a well-meaning family member and not because they were concerned about their disability. It is also important to obtain a past medical history to determine if there are any important medical problems that would influence the choice of treatment.

Physical Examination

Unlike patients with an anterior dislocation of the shoulder, the patient with a posterior dislocation can appear, at first glance, to have a normal shoulder. These injuries, when chronic, may cause minimal discomfort to the patient, and many patients with long-standing dislocations learn to adapt their activities to minimize the effect of the lost motion in the involved shoulder. It is also important to examine both shoulders, for these injuries can be bilateral.

The patient should be examined with the entire shoulder exposed to allow adequate visual inspection. The contour of the shoulders is best visualized by standing behind and slightly superior to the patient. The dislocated shoulder will appear to have less fullness anteriorly. While standing behind the patient, the examiner should palpate both shoulders, noting any asymmetry between the anterior deltoid and the coracoid processes. If the shoulder is dislocated posteriorly, the coracoid of the involved shoulder may be more prominent, and there will be a loss of the normal anterior contour of the shoulder.

Loss of external rotation beyond neutral is almost pathognomonic of a locked posterior dislocation of the shoulder. Limitation of glenohumeral abduction to less than 60 degrees is also usually present (Fig. 2). With long-standing dislocations in which the humeral head is locked onto the glenoid, the windshield wiper effect of the glenoid against the humeral head during motion can create a large enough defect to permit surprisingly functional motion. It is important to evaluate active range of motion in these patients. The physician should make note of the discomfort experienced by the patient while moving the extremity in their adapted functional range of motion. This will be important when determining the treatment path for the older, debilitated patient.

In cadaver studies, posterior dislocations of the shoulder have been associated with disruptions of the rotator cuff.[25] The true incidence of cuff lesions is unknown. Gerber states that he has seen three such lesions in the patients on whom he has operated.[10] The muscles of the rotator cuff, therefore, should be examined for any evidence of atrophy or disruption. A thorough examination of the remainder of the extremity must also be done to rule out any associated neurovascular injuries.[8] Schulz reported that 5 of the 17 posterior dislocations that he evaluated had an associated nerve injury.[30]

Radiographic Evaluation

Plain radiographs will confirm the clinical diagnosis of a posterior dislocation of the shoulder only if the appropriate views are obtained. Hawkins and colleagues showed that in 50% of the cases that they evaluated, the diagnosis could not be made with certainty based solely on an anteroposterior radiograph taken with the beam directed at 90 degrees to the plane of the scapula.[12] The diagnoses could be made in all patients when an axillary lateral radiograph was obtained. It is therefore imperative that any injury of the shoulder have,

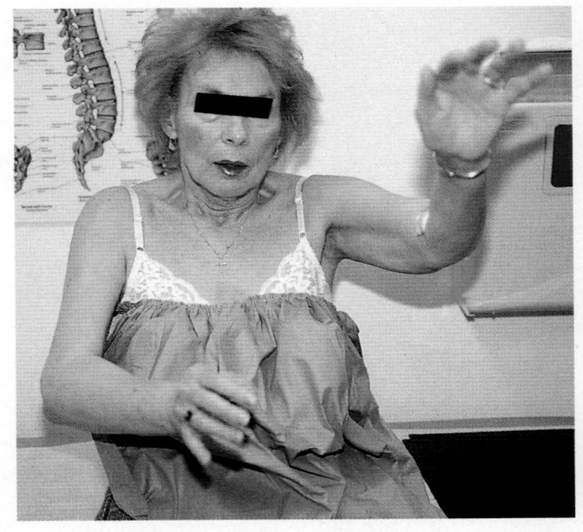

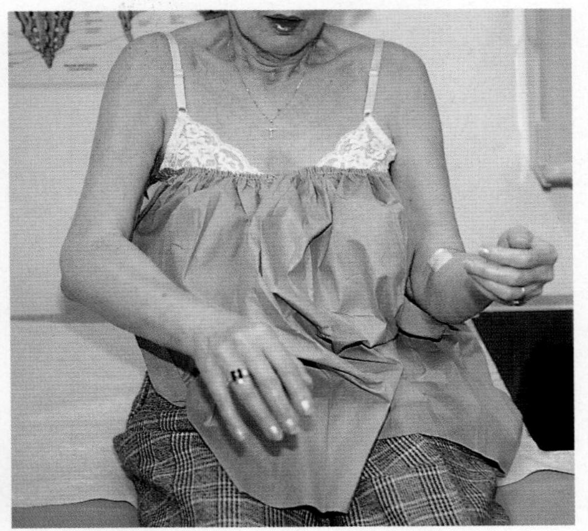

FIG. 2. Clinical photographs of a patient with a locked posterior dislocation of the shoulder: **(A)** loss of forward elevation; **(B)** loss of external rotation.

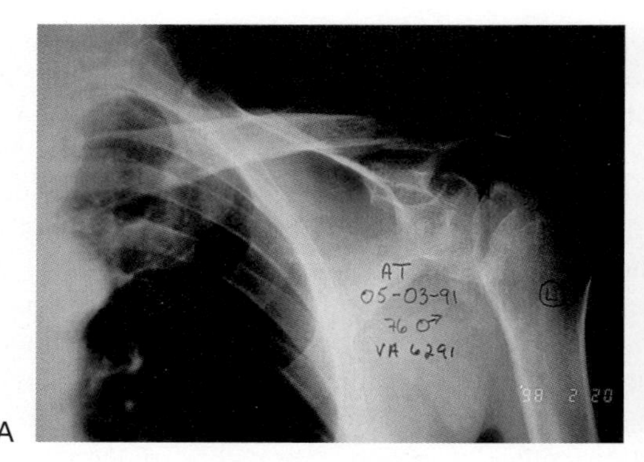

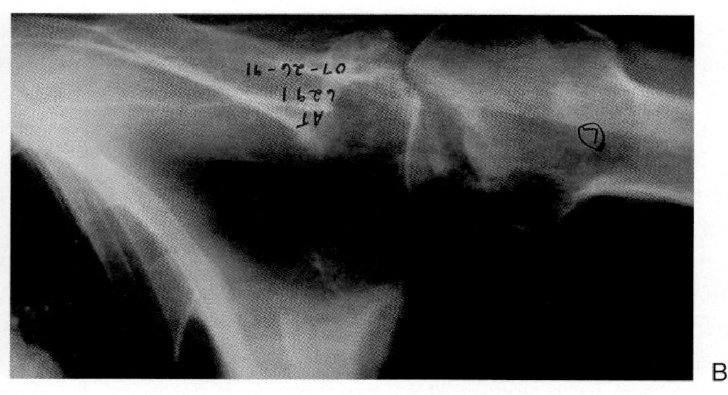

A B

FIG. 3. (A) An anteroposterior radiograph showing a posterior dislocation of the humeral head; **(B)** the axillary lateral radiograph of the same patient confirming the direction of the dislocation.

at a minimum, an anteroposterior and axillary lateral radiograph taken of the shoulder (Fig. 3A and 3B).

In the setting of a locked posterior dislocation, a true anteroposterior radiograph in the plane of the scapula and an axillary lateral radiograph should be obtained. These views will permit evaluation of the glenohumeral joint and are essential for preoperative planning. The axillary view will show the extent of glenoid wear and the amount of humeral head impaction that invariably is present with the locked posterior dislocation (see Fig. 3B).

These radiographs should also be evaluated for any evidence of associated fractures of the humerus and glenoid. In the series reported by Schulz,[30] Hawkins,[12] and Wilson,[33] 50% of posterior dislocations had an associated fracture of the humeral neck or tuberosities. The presence of these injuries will influence the surgeon's choice of treatment, especially if an attempt at closed reduction is contemplated in a dislocation less than 6 weeks from the time of injury. In the patient with a more chronic dislocation, these fractures may have developed into a malunion or a nonunion, and this will add further challenges to successful treatment (Fig. 4).

The axillary lateral radiograph is important for preoperative evaluation of the impaction fracture of the humeral head. This fracture is invariably found to be present. By dividing the arc of the impacted surface of the humeral head and comparing it with the length of the arc created by the articular surface of the humeral head in its preinjury state, the surgeon can estimate the percentage of the humeral head involved in the impaction (Fig. 5). This information is essential for preoperative planning and helps the surgeon determine if there is the need to obtain a computed tomography (CT) scan.

If the area of impaction is measured to be greater than 20% of the humeral head surface, or if there is any question of a fracture involving the glenoid, then a CT scan should be obtained. This scan should be used to evaluate the amount of humeral head and glenoid erosion[18,23] (Fig. 6). The CT scan, if obtained, should also be used to evaluate the remaining bone quality of the humeral head.[10] Changes in the appearance of

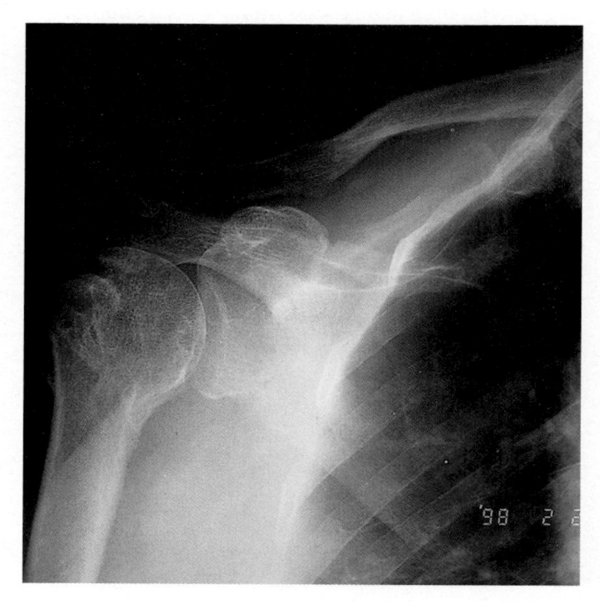

FIG. 4. An AP radiograph of a shoulder that is posteriorly dislocated. A malunion of the tuberosity can be seen.

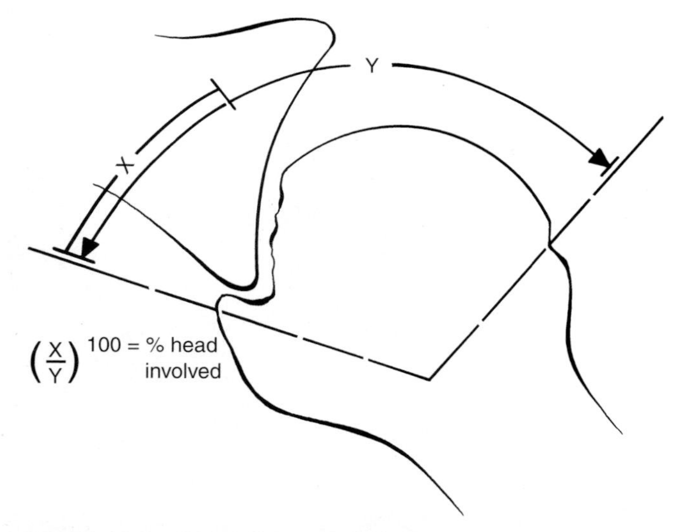

FIG. 5. The percentage of the head involved can be determined by measuring the arc of the area of impaction and dividing by the arc of the intact humeral head. This number is then multiplied by 100 to give the percentage of the head involved.

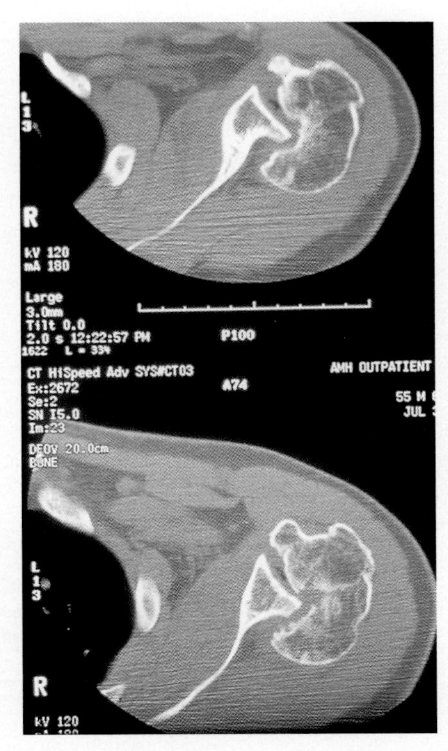

FIG. 6. Computed tomograghy can provide valuable information. Here, it shows a posterior fracture–dislocation, with evidence of glenoid wear and osteopenia.

the remaining head, such as thinning of the subchondral bone and loss of the normal trabecular architecture, indicate the presence of osteopenia. This information will prepare the surgeon for the possibility of the shoulder requiring replacement, and the patient's consent can be obtained for this procedure.

Many patients are referred to our office after having undergone a magnetic resonance imaging (MRI) study. If this is so, we use the axial cuts of the MRI to determine the size of the humeral tear defect (Fig. 7). In this scenario, we do not obtain a CT scan because it would not be cost-effective. There are really no added benefits from MRI studies, and a CT scan is preferred.

An electromyogram (EMG) should be obtained if there is any evidence of nerve injury. An arteriogram is needed if there is any evidence of vascular compromise.

Treatment Choice and Preoperative Planning

The first step to choosing the proper treatment of these patients is to have an understanding of the patients' perceived disability and their general health and ability to undergo a surgical procedure. These patients must also be able to understand and comply with the postoperative rehabilitation of the shoulder. In general, if the patient has low demands on the shoulder, has adapted his or her activities to cope with the limitations of the shoulder, or has pain that is easily controlled, then he or she should be considered for conservative treatment. Inability to follow the directions of rehabilitation will also affect the choice of treatment. Patients who are considered a high risk for surgery, owing to medical problems, should also be treated conservatively.

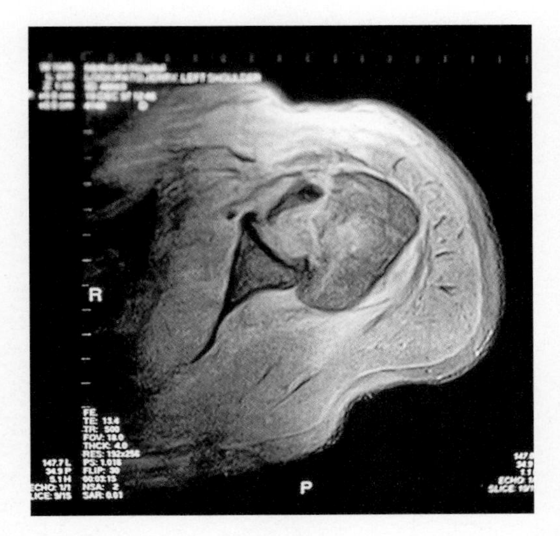

FIG. 7. An MRI scan obtained before referral can also be used to evaluate the humeral head defect and glenoid. An axial cut is shown. We prefer CT scan, owing to the better visualization of the bony architecture.

Once the patient is deemed a surgical candidate, the surgeon will need to decide on the most appropriate procedure for the patient. This is determined by the patient's age, the time from the initial injury, the demands on the shoulder, and the available bone stock present in the shoulder. Here, bone stock refers not only to the amount of bone loss because of the injury, but also to the intrinsic quality of the bone. If a patient is felt to have significant osteopenia, the surgeon must be prepared to perform an arthroplasty. The duration of the dislocation also influences the choice of treatment. Generally, the more chronic the injury the more likely that there will be disuse osteopenia, loss of the articular surface's structural integrity, or both. Reduction of an osteopenic head with poor articular cartilage viability will inevitable lead to an early failure requiring a second procedure. Hawkins[12] and Rowe[29] suggest that any injury of longer than 6 months duration may have irreversible damage to the articular surfaces. Patients with long-standing dislocations are also more likely to have erosion of the glenoid rim, requiring reconstruction and prosthetic arthroplasty. A preoperative CT scan will help determine whether this will be needed.[23]

If the injury is relatively fresh (defined as less than 3 weeks), there is a possibility that the defect in the humeral head can be disimpacted and bone grafted. In this circumstance, the patient must give consent for the possibility of a bone graft and should be positioned and draped appropriately at the time of the procedure.

With the foregoing preoperative evaluation, the patient can be placed into a "likely" treatment group. The surgeon, however, must be prepared to move along the treatment algorithm (Fig. 8). The goals are to have a general treatment

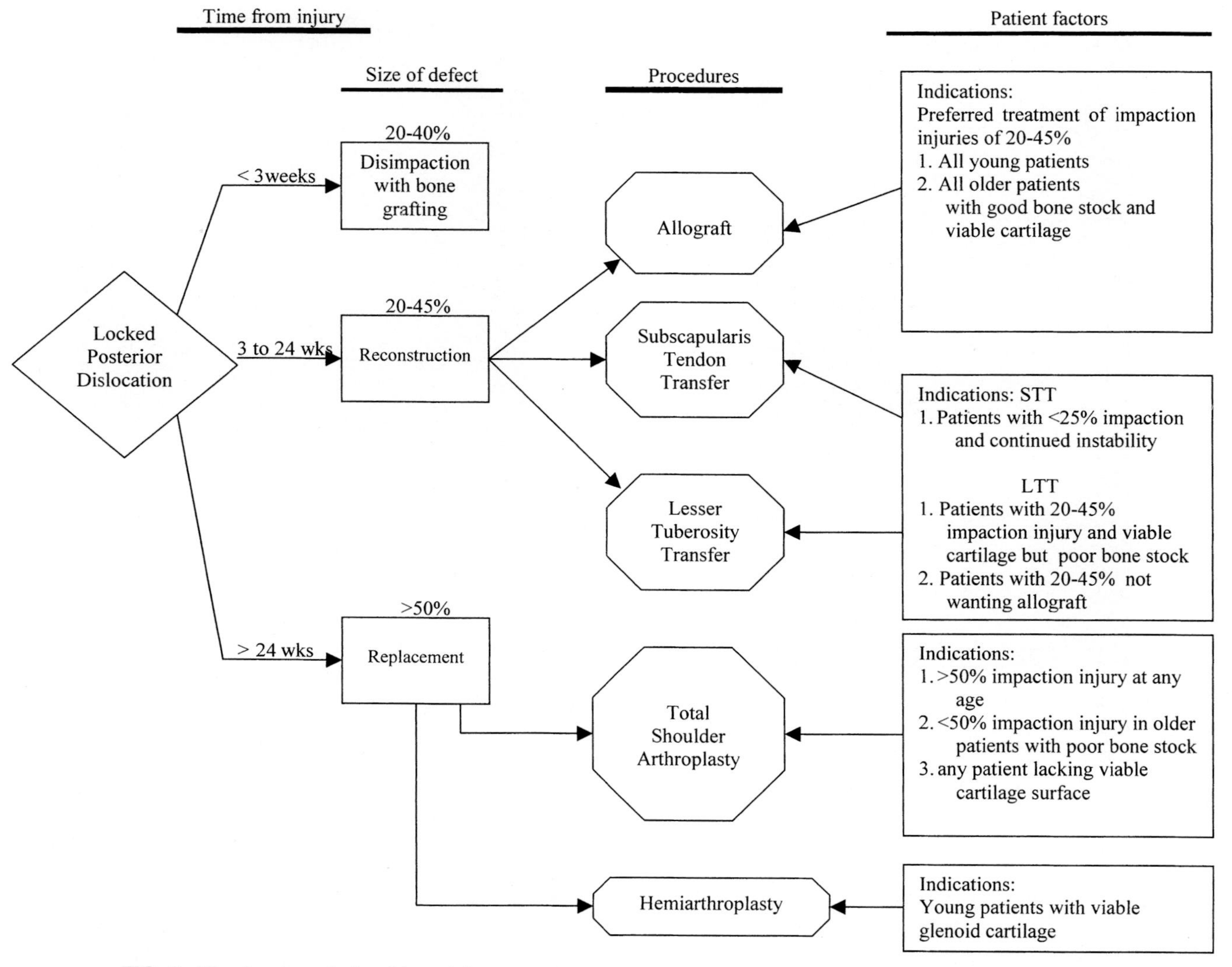

FIG. 8. The treatment algorithm giving our approach to the surgical treatment of locked posterior dislocations.

plan before surgery, an understanding of which choices are available, and the knowledge required to make the correct intraoperative surgical decision.

Treatment Options

For the purposes of preoperative evaluation, we will use 3 weeks to define a chronic injury.[12,29] Three weeks is chosen because after this time it becomes difficult to perform a successful closed reduction. The time from injury also influences the quality of the bone and cartilage present at the time of surgery. Each of these factors affects the choice of treatment and outcome.

Nonoperative Treatment

Nonoperative treatment includes the skillful neglect of chronic injuries of longer than 3 weeks duration. For patients who have minimal pain and do not perceive their limited motion as disabling, or for patients who are at high risk for surgery owing to medical or mental illnesses, skillful neglect can be an acceptable treatment option. Some patient profiles for this method of treatment are the following: an elderly patient with low demands on the extremity, with relatively mild pain, and an adapted lifestyle; a patient medically at risk for surgical treatment; or a patient mentally unable to comply with postoperative rehabilitation. These patients are best treated with supportive measures to control pain and with future evaluation if they develop worsening of their symptoms or deterioration in the function of the extremity.

Closed Reduction

The criteria for choosing a patient who will be suitable for an attempt at closed reduction are the following: the patient can be of any age, the injury should be less than 3 weeks old, the impaction injury to the humeral head must be less than 25%, and the humerus must have no other fractures present.

If these criteria are met, the patient may undergo an attempt at closed reduction.

The closed reduction is best performed under scalene block or general anesthesia.[6] The patient is placed supine and gentle traction is applied to the humerus in line with the long axis of the body. Gentle adduction and flexion is then applied. The humerus is gently externally rotated, and pressure is applied to the humeral head in a posterior to anterior direction. With this technique, the shoulder should reduce.

Once the joint is reduced, the humerus should be internally rotated to evaluate the shoulder for stability. The humerus is internally rotated and the point of instability noted. This position is the "danger zone" for dislocation. Patients who have no instability with the humerus internally rotated enough to place the hand on the abdomen are considered to have a stable injury. This is unlikely to occur with a chronic posterior dislocation, but may occur for acute injuries. If the shoulder is stable with the arm in internal rotation, the patient is immobilized in an orthosis. The humerus is held at the side in neutral rotation with the shoulder extended a few degrees.

Rehabilitation of the shoulder is begun day 2 after injury. The patient is allowed unlimited external rotation and is allowed to perform isometric strengthening of the shoulder girdle. The brace is removed after 4 weeks, and the patient is encouraged to use the shoulder as tolerated. The patient is not allowed to bring the arm behind the trunk (maximum internal rotation) for 6 weeks. Lifting more than 5 lb above the plane of the chest is discouraged for 6 weeks. Heavy labor is discouraged for 3 months.

If closed reduction is successful, a good outcome is to be expected. Hawkins et al.[12] reported excellent results in the three patients whose shoulders could be reduced and were stable after reduction. Schulz et al.[30] reported satisfactory results in the three posterior dislocations that they were able to reduce. All six of these shoulders were reduced within 4 weeks of injury.

If after closed reduction the shoulder remains unstable and dislocates with internal rotation at a point before the hand reaches the abdomen, the patient should be placed in a prefabricated splint. The shoulder should be slightly extended and the humerus should be externally rotated 20 degrees from neutral. The patient is then further evaluated to determine why the shoulder continues to be unstable. A CT scan should be obtained to evaluate the glenoid for fracture and to reassess the size of the humeral head defect.[19] If a CT scan was obtained before closed reduction and the cause for instability after reduction can be determined, open surgical intervention is performed at that time.

If a fracture of the glenoid is present, but well reduced with the arm in the splint, the patient continues to be treated conservatively. Weekly follow-up radiographic evaluation is required until early fracture union occurs. This usually takes 6 weeks. During this period of immobilization, the patient is allowed to externally rotate the humerus passively, and after 3 weeks is allowed to internally rotate to within 20 degrees of the danger zone, as determined at the time of reduction. At 6 weeks, the patient is allowed full passive range of motion and is allowed to progress with active motion as pain permits. Strengthening is not started until 10 to 12 weeks.

If the glenoid fracture is displaced or unstable, the patient will require an open reduction with internal fixation of the glenoid as described in Chapter 23. If the humeral head impaction fracture is the cause of continued instability and involves less than 45% of the articular surface, then the patient will need to undergo open repair of the humeral head defect. If there are fractures present of the tuberosities or humeral neck, the reduction should be performed under general anesthesia. Because there is a risk of displacing these fractures during closed reduction, the humeral neck or tuberosity fractures should undergo percutaneous pin fixation before any attempt at reduction (see Chapter 24).[13] If the fractures are displaced, then the fractures should be treated as outlined in Chapter 24.

Open Reduction

Open reduction of locked posterior dislocations will be required if the injury is more than 3 weeks old, if the shoulder is unstable after closed reduction, or if the impacted area of the humeral head involves greater than 25% of the articular surface. The best treatment of these injuries will be determined by the following factors: (a) the size of the humeral head defect, (b) the amount of time from injury, (c) the patient's age, (d) the amount of post traumatic arthritis present, and (e) the quality of the humeral head bone stock. Most articles addressing the treatment of locked posterior dislocations has used the size of the humeral head impaction injury to determine the approach to treatment.[10–12,22,24,29,30] The other factors listed are also important in determining the final choice of treatment.

Note that these injuries are rare, and the number of reported patients treated with each method is small; therefore, it is impossible to draw any statistical conclusions from the data presented in the literature regarding the treatment of these injuries. The surgeon should choose the method with which he or she is most comfortable.

Impaction of 20–45% of the Humeral Head: Disimpaction and Bone Grafting

This method of treatment is best reserved for an acute injury (less than 3 weeks old) with a humeral head defect that involves less than 45% of the articular surface. The patient must have adequate bone stock to provide for secure fixation and must have structurally intact articular cartilage to be considered for this procedure. It is ideal for use in the younger patient, but may also be effectively used in older patients with good bone stock. The patient is positioned and the ipsilateral iliac crest is prepared and draped, so that bone graft can be obtained if needed.

The standard deltopectoral approach is used. The axillary nerve is always identified and protected. The ascending branch of the anterior humeral circumflex artery is identified and protected in procedures where the humeral head will be preserved. The subscapularis tendon is incised 1 cm from its insertion and dissected from the underlying capsule. This may be difficult, owing to the scarring caused by the injury. It is important to maintain or repair the coracohumeral and superior glenohumeral ligament at their attachment sites, because they provide posterior stability. A vertical capsulotomy is then performed, and the joint is debrided of any scar tissue. Once the articular surfaces are identified, an evaluation of the injury is performed. The glenoid is inspected for fracture or articular injury. The humeral head is reduced by placing a Cobb elevator into the site of impaction and using it to lever the head over the glenoid rim. The posterior labrum and capsule are inspected. In the majority of shoulders with posterior dislocations, there is an avulsion of the capsule as a sleeve of tissue. Unlike the Bankart lesion seen with anterior dislocations, the injury to the posterior labrum and capsule does not always need to be reattached to the glenoid.[10,12]. Usually, it is only necessary to roughen up the posterior aspect of the glenoid with a curved curette, with the expectation that the capsule will heal to its origin. The impacted region of the humeral head and the remaining intact humeral head are inspected. A determination is made as to whether the cartilage surface at the site of impaction can be salvaged. If the articular surface can be salvaged, then disimpaction with bone grafting is performed as follows (Fig. 9).

Disimpaction of the articular cartilage with its underlying subchondral bone is performed by creating a bone window in the greater tuberosity directly opposite the impacted area (Fig. 9A). This will require internal rotation of the humerus to create the window and to disimpact the fracture through it. The surgeon will have to externally rotate the humerus to visualize the progression of the disimpaction of the articular defect. Once the window is created, a bone tamp or the blunt end of a 10-mm drill is placed into the window and impacted toward the defect opposite it (Fig. 9B). This will disimpact

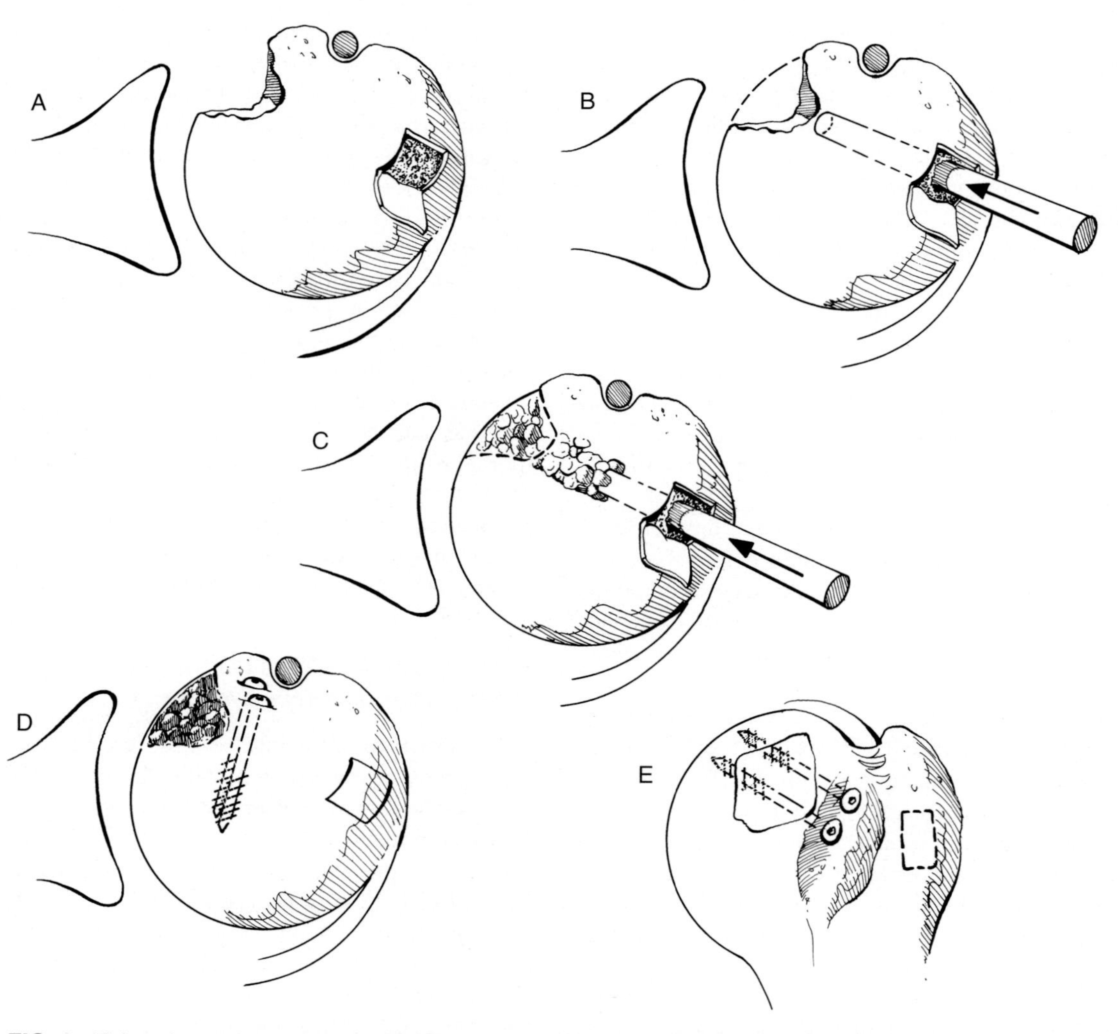

FIG. 9. This schematic represents the technique of disimpaction and bone grafting of injuries less than 3 weeks old: **(A)** A bone window is made in the greater tuberosity opposite the fracture; **(B)** a bone tamp is used to disimpact the area; **(C)** cancellous autograft is packed into the defect to support the area; and **(D,E)** fixation is provided to shore up the area of grafting.

the humeral head defect in its central portion. Once the articular surface's contour is properly restored centrally, a small curved osteotome placed into the bone tunnel can be used to lever the edges of the defect, if needed. After the area is disimpacted, a void will have been created below the area of the fracture. This void is filled by packing the area with cancellous bone. The bone tamp is used to pack the defect (Fig. 9C). Once the void is filled, the cortical window is closed. Attention is then turned to fixation of the fragments. Any loose areas of articular surface are fixed with bioabsorbable k wires placed through the articular surface. Collapse of the disimpacted area is prevented by placing parallel screws along the articular margin and aiming them just inferior to and across the area of disimpaction (Fig. 9D and E). Placed in this fashion, these screws act as a lattice to support the area of the grafting. This will help to prevent collapse. The bone graft must be of good quality and adequate quantity. Cancellous bone should therefore be obtained from the iliac crest. Allograft bone is less desirable, but it can be used if indicated.

After the fragments are secured, the shoulder is taken through a range of motion in internal rotation. The position in which the grafted area comes into contact with the glenoid is noted. This position should be avoided postoperatively until the graft has consolidated, which usually requires at least 6 weeks. The anterior capsule is closed side-to-side and overtightening of the capsule is avoided. The subscapularis is reattached anatomically, and the wound is closed. Humeral internal rotation is avoided during closure. The patient is placed into a postoperative brace in neutral to 20 degrees of external rotation. If the defect is not repairable by this method, the patient is treated by either transfer of the subscapularis tendon into the defect, by allograft reconstruction or hemiarthroplasty.

Rehabilitation is the same as that for closed reduction, with a few exceptions. The patient is not allowed internal rotation into the danger zone as determined intraoperatively for 6 weeks and, therefore, must wear the brace for 6 weeks. Gentle passive external rotation, as well as isometric exercises, is started on postoperative day 2.

Gerber has reported success with this technique.[10] No clinical series has been reported in the English literature.

Open Reduction with Transfer of the Subscapularis Tendon or Transfer of the Lesser Tuberosity

To successfully perform either subscapularis transfer or transfer of the lesser tuberosity, the patient must have adequate bone stock to securely hold either sutures or screws. The articular surface of the remaining intact humeral head must be structurally viable. Any patient with a dislocation of the shoulder present for over 3 weeks is at risk of having irreversible cartilage damage at the site of impaction. This would make disimpaction and grafting less effective and transfer of the subscapularis or lesser tuberosity a better consideration.

In patients without radiographic evidence of osteoarthritis, the determination of the structural integrity of the articular surface is made at the time of arthrotomy. If the shoulder has been dislocated for more than 6 months, the possibility of the shoulder requiring a shoulder arthroplasty must be discussed with the patient, and the prosthesis must be available at the time of surgery. Older patients with significant loss of cartilage or bone stock should be placed in the arthroplasty group. In younger patients, an attempt to preserve the joint should be made.

Transfer of the Subscapularis

This procedure should be considered for small humeral head defects (<25%). The approach used to perform the subscapularis transfer is the same as that used for performing an arthroplasty, with the exception that the tendon of the subscapularis is released from its insertion. The joint is exposed and debrided of scar tissue. The humeral head is reduced, as described earlier. The articular cartilage is evaluated and the size of the defect is confirmed visually. If the articular cartilage of the intact humeral head is intact and the defect is small (<25%), then transfer of the subscapularis is undertaken. If the remaining articular cartilage is not significantly damaged and the defect size is between 25% and 45%, a transfer of the lesser tuberosity or osteochondral allograft is considered. If the articular surface of the remaining humeral head is not intact or the defect is larger than the anticipated 45%, the patient is moved into the arthroplasty group. Arthroplasty is also performed if the bone in the intact portion of the humeral head is markedly osteoporotic.

For transfer of the subscapularis, the same approach as that described for disimpaction with grafting is used. Any adhesions to the subscapularis are released from its anterior and posterior surfaces. The posterior rim of the glenoid is inspected for the presence of any significant erosion that would preclude stability without reconstruction. The humeral head is reduced and the posterior glenoid is abraded to prepare a healing bed for the posterior capsule. The defect in the humeral head is then cleared of all scar tissue until a bed of cancellous bone is prepared. With use of transosseous drill holes that are placed into the base of the defect, the subscapularis is secured into the defect. After the transosseous stitch is placed and the subscapularis is pulled into position, the shoulder is taken through a full range of motion. If the shoulder dislocates despite the repair, then the defect should be considered too large for this technique, and either an allograft or arthroplasty should be performed. If the shoulder is stable, then the sutures are tied and the wound is closed. The patient is then placed in a prefabricated splint, with the arm held at the side in 20 degrees of external rotation.

Transfer of the Lesser Tuberosity

The standard deltopectoral approach is used, and the biceps tendon is identified. The rotator cuff interval is identified and released sharply. This allows access to the superior aspect of the lesser tuberosity, which will help visualize the articular side of the osteotomy. Once the lesser tuberosity is identified, it is osteotomized. Care must be taken to not include the medial wall of the bicepital grove in the osteotomy, because this will result in subluxation of the biceps tendon and thereby require tenodesis. The amount of lesser tuberosity to be taken is determined by the size of the defect to be filled with the bone fragment. Once the lesser tuberosity osteotomy is complete, the freed tuberosity is secured with a traction stitch. With traction applied, the subscapularis and the underlying capsule are dissected as one layer away from the anterior surface of the glenoid. The subscapularis must be freed of any adhesions, if return of its function is to be expected. The joint is debrided of any scar tissue. The articular surfaces are then evaluated for viability. The posterior rim of the glenoid is inspected for the presence of any significant erosion that would preclude stability without reconstruction. The posterior glenoid is roughened with a curved curette to produce a cancellous bed. The area of the impaction is debrided of fibrous tissue and any articular cartilage. A fresh bed of cancellous bone must be present before fixation of the lesser tuberosity. The lesser tuberosity is then secured into the defect with two cancellous lag screws at 90 degrees to the plane of the osteotomy. The humerus is internally rotated to assess the stability of the shoulder. If the shoulder is stable, the wound is closed and the patient is placed in a prefabricated splint with the arm externally rotated to 20 degrees. The shoulder should be stable after this procedure. If dislocation continues, then the defect should be considered too large for this procedure, and the patient should be considered for prosthetic arthroplasty.

Rehabilitation

Patients with subscapularis or lesser tuberosity transfer are immobilized in the brace for 4 weeks. The patient is allowed to begin passive external rotation and abduction of the shoulder on postoperative day 2. At this time, the patient also begins isometric strengthening of the external rotators of the shoulder.

At 4 weeks, the brace is removed and the patient is allowed full motion of the shoulder. Active internal rotation is discouraged until week 6. At this point, gentle active internal rotation and light strengthening of the shoulder girdle muscles are commenced. More strenuous activity is not allowed for an additional 6 weeks.

McLaughlin[22] was the first to report the use of the subscapularis tendon transfer technique in the treatment of locked posterior dislocations of the humeral head. He reported using this technique in four patients and found the results to be satisfactory in the two patients with sufficient follow-up. Rowe and Zarins[29] reported satisfactory results in their two patients treated by subscapularis transfer.

In 1982, Hawkins et al.[12] reported on 9 patients who had been treated with subscapularis transfer and reported excellent results in 4 of the patients they had treated with this procedure. The average range of motion obtained in these patients was 165 degrees of active forward elevation, 40 degrees of external rotation, and internal rotation to the level of the 12th thoracic vertebra. The remaining 5 patients were referred to them after already having undergone subscapularis transfer by the referring physician. These patients were therefore considered failures and were treated with a different procedure.

Hawkins et al.[12] and Neer[24] advocated transfer of the lesser tuberosity for patients with humeral head defects involving 20% to 45% of the articular surface. Neer developed the lesser tuberosity transfer procedure and had treated 4 patients using this technique.[12] All 4 patients were reported to have excellent results. The average range of motion in these 4 patients was 160 degrees of active forward elevation, 45 degrees of external rotation, and internal rotation to the 12th thoracic vertebra.

Gerber[10,11] has argued against this method because he feels that it distorts the anatomy of the proximal humerus. He argues that this would cause revision to an arthroplasty to be difficult if the tuberosity transfer were to fail. Therefore, he advocates the use of an allograft to reconstruct defects of this size. Of note, no patient treated by Neer required a revision operation after transfer of the lesser tuberosity. However, his follow-up of these patients was limited at a range of 2 to 9 years.[12]

Allograft Reconstruction

In 1996, Gerber[11] reported on the use of allografts to treat the humeral head defects associated with chronic locked posterior dislocations of the shoulder. He recommended using this technique in patients whose shoulder had been dislocated at least 4 weeks and had defects involving up to 50% of the humeral head.[10,11] He advised against the use of this technique if there was significant osteoporosis present in the remaining portion of the humeral head. A suitable fresh frozen allograft must be available for this type of reconstruction. A size-matched fresh-frozen humeral head allograft is best suited for obtaining the graft. If this is not available, a fresh-frozen femoral head will suffice. This procedure should be reserved for the younger patient and for the older patient with good bone stock whose dislocation has been present for less than 6 weeks. A CT scan is invaluable in helping to determine if significant osteopenia is present.

The exposure is the same as previously described for transfer of the subscapularis tendon. Again, a vertical capsulotomy should be used, so that the insertion of the coracohumeral ligament and the superior glenohumeral ligament are preserved or repaired. After the capsulotomy is completed, the joint is inspected and debrided of scar tissue. If the cartilage and bone quality are sufficient, then the reconstruction is performed. If the quality of either tissue is poor, then an arthroplasty is performed. The posterior aspect of the glenoid neck should be roughened before placement of the graft.

Instead of curretting the base of the humeral head defect, an osteotome or oscillating saw is used to cut a wedge out of

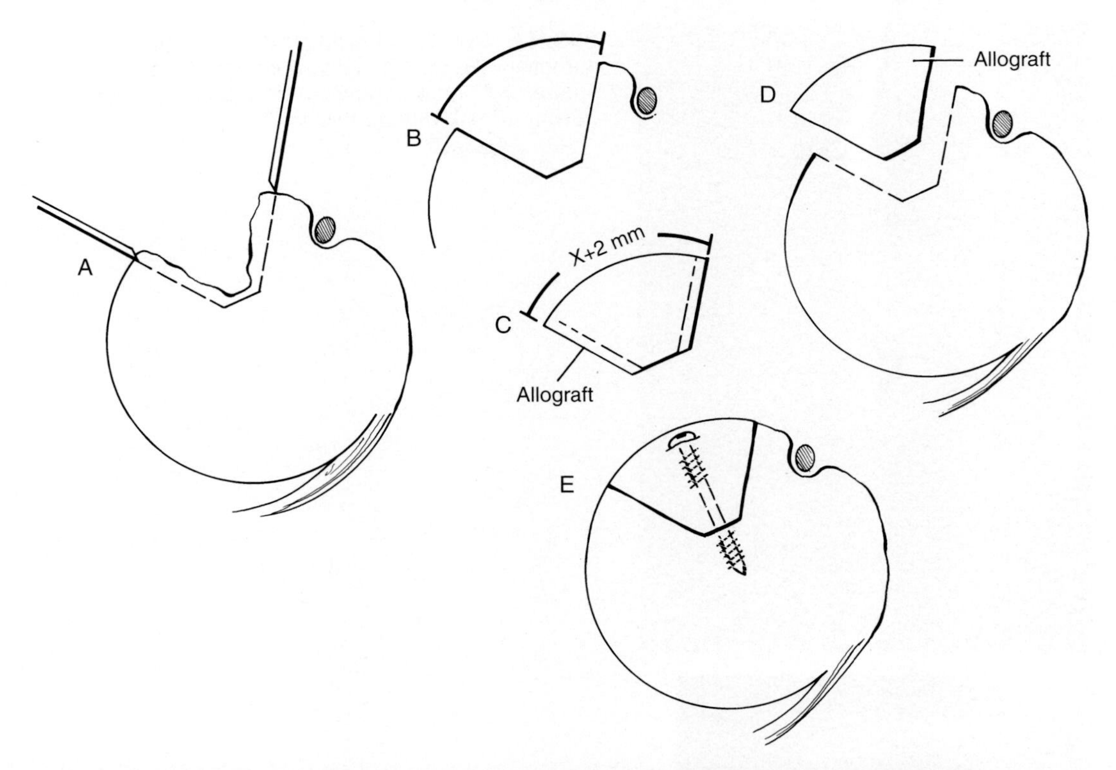

FIG. 10. This schematic represents the technique of allograft reconstruction: **(A)** The edges of the defect are prepared sharply; **(B)** the defect is measured; **(C)** a suitable surface of the allograft is used to cut a wedge 2 mm larger than the defect; **(D)** the allograft is impacted into place; **(E)** the allograft is fixed into position with a cancellous screw.

the humeral head, which includes the edges of the defect (Fig. 10A). Once this is done, the breadth of the excised wedge, as well as its depth, should be ascertained (Fig. 10B). The allograft head should then be inspected for a surface that will match the contour of the humeral head at its defect. An oscillating saw is then used to cut a wedge from the allograft that is approximately 2 mm wider than the width of the true defect (Fig. 10C). This will permit impaction of the allograft into the defect, creating a press fit (Fig. 10D). If the press fit is secure, no further fixation is required. If there is concern about the security of the graft, then the graft should be fixed with one or two countersunk cancellous lag screws or Herbert screws (Fig. 10E; Fig. 11). With the graft in place, the shoulder is then taken through a full range of motion. The shoulder should be stable, with no further tendency for dislocation. If the shoulder is unstable, this can be remedied by either imbrication of the posterior capsule or by postoperative immobilization of the shoulder in a stable position. It is Gerber's belief that the posterior capsule avulsion or redundancy need not be addressed by formal posterior capsulorrhaphy, because his experience has shown that the muscular and capsular tension about the shoulder will return with proper rehabilitation.[10] The subscapularis is repaired anatomically and the wound is closed. The patient is immobilized in a prefabricated brace in neutral rotation for 6 weeks.

Rehabilitation is similar to that following subscapularis tendon transfer, with the exception of the additional 2 weeks of immobilization.

Allograft reconstruction of articular surface defects has been an efficacious and safe treatment for articular surface defects in weight-bearing joints.[20,21] Gerber has used these data to support the use of allografts in the reconstruction of defects in the humeral head. He also supports this opinion with the argument that the shoulder is typically a non–weight-bearing joint; therefore, it should put fewer demands on the allograft. In 1996, Gerber[11] presented the preliminary results in 4 patients treated for locked posterior dislocations of the humeral head using allograft reconstruction. Three of the patients had satisfactory results, with an average score of 95% of that of an age- and sex-matched normal population. This scoring was based on the system of Constant and Murley.[7] The follow-up period for these 3 patients was more than 5 years from the time of the procedure. The one poor result was in a patient who developed avascular necrosis and collapse of the head after 6 years from the time of surgery. It was felt that this development was related to the patient's history of alcohol abuse and not to the reconstruction. Gerber later stated that he has had similar results in an additional 6 patients.[10] He did, however, stress that this procedure should not be used if the patient's bone was osteoportic by CT scan or by examination at the time of surgery.

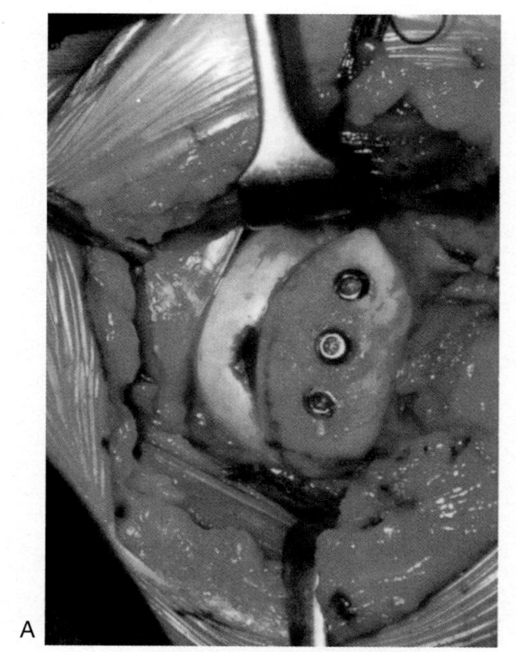

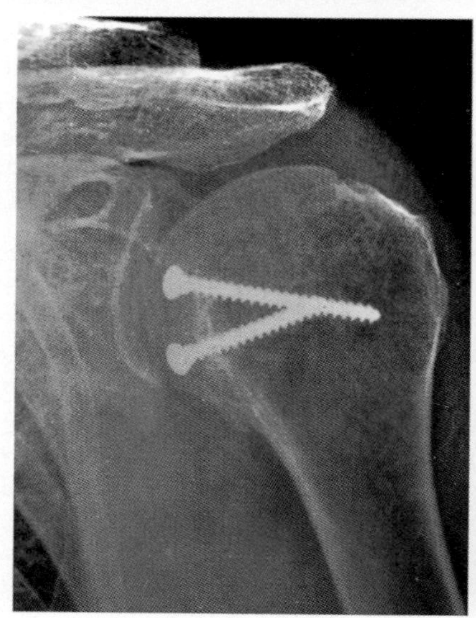

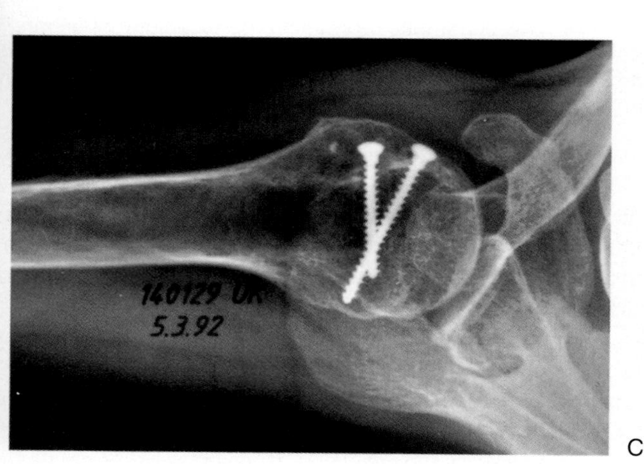

FIG. 11. **(A)** Clinical example of an allograft reconstruction; **(B)** an AP radiograph; and **(C)** an axillary lateral radiograph showing the results at 5 years. (From ref. 10, with permission.)

The results of allograft reconstruction given by Gerber's small series are similar to those shown with the other humeral head-preserving techniques. This technique allows preservation of near-normal kinematics in the shoulder joint and preserves the normal anatomy of the proximal humerus. We agree with Gerber and believe that, if at all possible, allograft reconstruction should be performed as the treatment of choice in young patients and in older patients with adequate bone stock and intact articular cartilage on the remaining portion of the humeral head.

Hemiarthroplasty and Total Shoulder Arthroplasty

Indications for either a hemiarthroplasty or a total shoulder arthroplasty are a defect measuring more than 50% of the articular surface of the humeral head, severe articular cartilage damage, marked osteopenia, or erosion of the glenoid rim, leading to instability (see Figs. 3 and 6).

The choice of whether to use a hemiarthroplasty versus a total shoulder arthroplasty depends on the condition of the glenoid surface. Relative to the condition of the articular cartilage, it stands to reason that if the humeral head has been dislocated for a long enough time to have irreversible changes to the humeral head articular cartilage, then the glenoid cartilage is likely to require resurfacing. If the glenoid has significant wear, then bone grafting of the glenoid defect may be required. On the other hand, if the dislocation has not been present long enough to irreversibly damage the cartilage of the glenoid, then a hemiarthroplasty is preferred (Fig. 12). The standard deltopectoral approach is used. The tuberosities should not be osteotomized if at all possible. If a malunion of the neck is present, an osteotomy of the neck may be required.

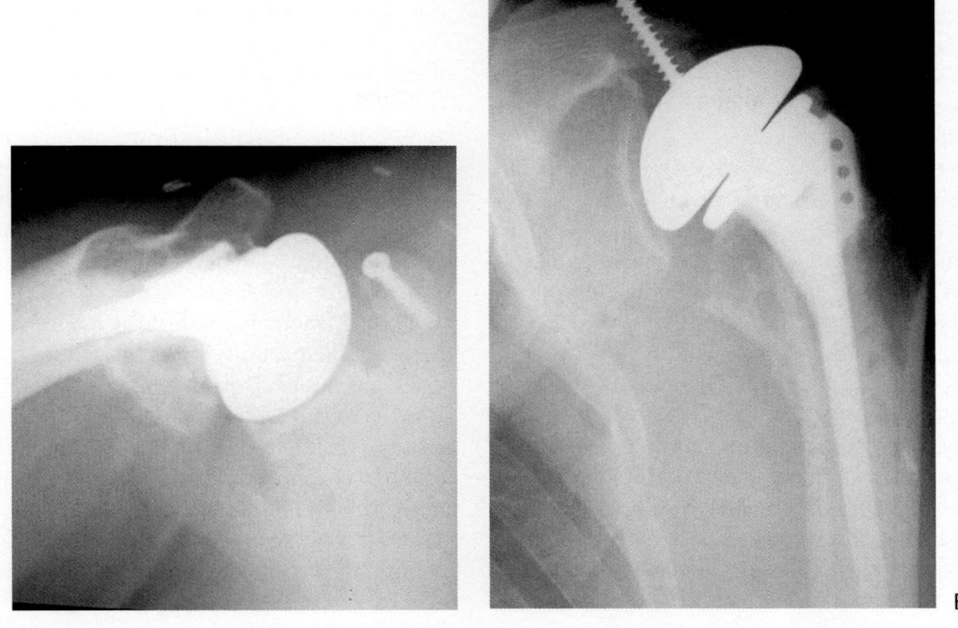

FIG. 12. Radiographs taken 2 years after a hemiarthroplasty was performed on the patient whose CT scan is shown in Fig. 6.

An osteotomy of the neck is preferred because it allows placement of the humeral component into correct rotational alignment, which restores more normal anatomy. In some cases, the humeral prosthetic should be placed in significantly less retroversion (zero degrees) to compensate for the change in the soft-tissue balance caused by the dislocation. In general, the more chronic the injury is, the less retroversion is used. Hawkins and Neer[12] reported that, with experience, they felt that they could dial-in the precise amount of version required to restore immediate joint stability. The humeral head is sized to be equal to the patient's normal head size. Oversizing of the humeral head must be avoided, to compensate for the patulous posterior capsule. This will overstuff the joint and make subscapularis closure difficult. Once the trials are in place, the shoulder is taken through a full range of motion to determine joint stability. Because the posterior capsule may be patulous as a result of the injury, posterior capsular plication may be necessary. Stability of the joint must be evaluated intraoperatively, as well as in the early postoperative period. Active contraction of the rotator cuff in the awake patient will improve shoulder stability. This may correct subtle intraoperative instability, but will not correct for gross instability. If the joint is unstable and posterior capsularrhaphy was already performed, we recommend the use of a brace to hold the arm in neutral to 20 degrees of external rotation during the postoperative period.

Rehabilitation

If the shoulder is stable after total shoulder arthroplasty, the patient does not require bracing. The patient is allowed to perform range of motion exercises by postoperative day 3, and by 2 weeks active and light resistive exercises are added. No heavy use of the extremity is allowed for 3 months. If at the time of surgery the shoulder was found to be unstable despite plication of the posterior capsule, then the arm is immobilized in neutral rotation for 6 weeks. On postoperative day 1, the patient is allowed gentle active external rotation and is allowed isometric strengthening of the external rotators and deltoid. These exercises are performed in the brace. The brace is removed at 6 weeks, and the patient is allowed full motion of the joint. He or she is also started on muscle conditioning exercises at that time.

Hawkins and colleagues[12] remedied the tendency for posterior dislocation in patients undergoing prosthetic arthroplasty by changing the rotation of the humeral component. During the early period of their study, they suggested that the humeral component be placed in neutral rotation if the dislocation had been present for longer than 6 months, and in 20 degrees of retroversion if the dislocation had been present for less than 6 months. With more experience, the authors stated they felt that they could adjust the precise degree of version to restore immediate stability. By using this technique, they were able to obtain satisfactory results in 11 of 16 patients. Their best results were seen in patients who had been treated with primary total shoulder arthroplasty (TSA), which was available only during the later part of their patient series. Of the 6 patients who underwent primary TSA, 5 showed excellent results and had an average active forward elevation of 152 degrees, external rotation of 40 degrees, and internal rotation to the level of the 12th thoracic vertebra. The 1 failure had a postoperative dislocation and refused further treatment. These results led them to recommend TSA as the procedure of choice in the treatment of chronic locked posterior dislocations in patients not felt to be candidates for humeral head preservation. Others have also advocated changing the version of the humeral component to control the tendency towards redislocation.[24,26] It is Gerber's recommendation that the normal axis of rotation be re-created whenever treating a chronic posterior dislocation with an arthroplasty.[10] He felt that this would lead to more normal joint kinematics than would be seen if the humeral component was placed in excessive anteversion. To prevent postoperative instability, he recommended soft-tissue releases of the posterior capsule, the subscapularis, and the anteroinferior capsule. It was his belief that with postoperative immobilization and properly modified rehabilitation, the soft tissues would rebalance toward their normal tensions. He states that the release of these tissues may require the use of a brace for 6 weeks after the surgery. No clinical outcome data are available for the patients that he has treated with this technique. Gerber does concur with Hawkins and Neer that TSA is the treatment of choice in patients with long-standing dislocations.

CHRONIC LOCKED ANTERIOR DISLOCATION

Although many of the same principles used in the diagnosis and treatment of posterior dislocations are employed in the diagnosis and treatment of anterior dislocations, anterior dislocations have unique characteristics that require a distinct approach to diagnosis, treatment, and rehabilitation. For instance, an anterior dislocation leaves the arm in relative abduction and external rotation. If the arm remains locked in this position, the patient will be unable to reach the mouth and will be unable to perform daily care activities. In contrast, posterior dislocations leave the arm in the more functional position of adduction and internal rotation. The position of the arm is the most likely reason that the functional outcome in patients with neglected anterior dislocations yields a poorer result than the results seen in chronic posterior dislocations. This difference in function was in fact shown to be present in Rowe and Zarins' 1982 series of seven patients with chronic, untreated shoulder dislocations.[29] In this study, they found that the 3 patients with untreated posterior dislocations scored better in objective and subjective testing of shoulder function than the 4 untreated anterior dislocations.

Classic teaching would lead one to believe that chronic posterior dislocations are more common than chronic anterior dislocations. However, in 1982, Rowe and Zarins polled 208 orthopedic surgeons and asked if they had treated a chronic dislocation of the shoulder.[29] Interestingly, they found that 65% of the missed shoulder dislocations treated in this series were anterior, compared with 35% for posterior. The larger number of missed anterior dislocations likely occurs as a result of the proportionally larger rate of occurrence of acute anterior dislocations, compared with posterior dislocations. As a percentage of the type of injury, posterior dislocations are more frequently missed, but the number of acute posterior dislocations is relatively small.

History

As with posterior dislocations of the shoulder, anterior dislocations of the shoulder may result from trauma or a convulsive episode. Classically, seizures have been related to the occurrence of posterior dislocations of the shoulder; however, anterior dislocations have been reported to occur in one-half of all dislocations caused by a seizure.[3,30] Clinical suspicion should, therefore, be raised in any seizure disorder patient who has shoulder pain or a diagnosis of a frozen

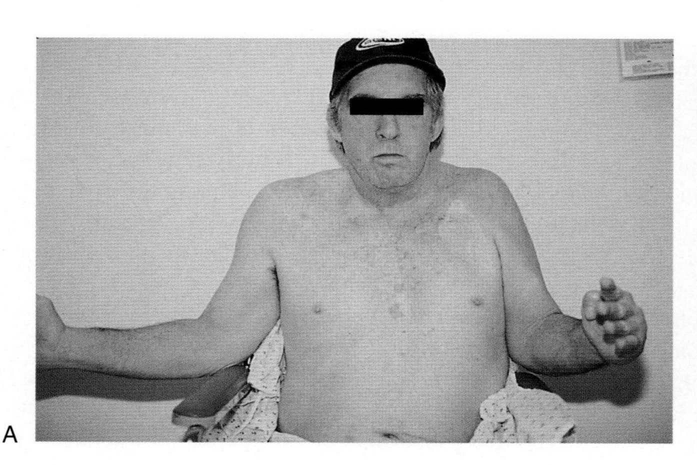

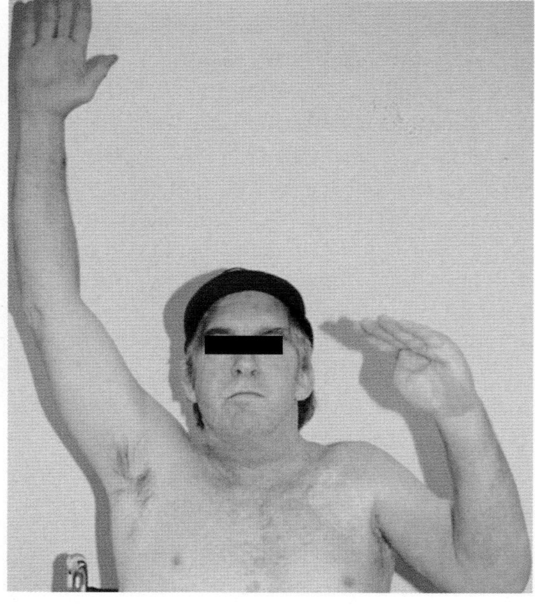

FIG. 13. Clinical photographs of a multiply injured trauma patient who presented with a chronic locked anterior dislocation: **(A)** He has severe limitation of rotation, with a marked amount of pain. **(B)** The severe loss of forward elevation made reaching his face very difficult.

shoulder that is not responding to therapy. Patients suffering from a multiple trauma can often have a shoulder injury that is overlooked because of the severity of other injuries (Fig. 13). Thorough repeat examinations of the trauma patient on a daily basis are necessary to avoid unrecognized injuries.

Physical Examination

The physical examination of a patient with a chronic locked anterior dislocation of the shoulder will reveal severe limitation of rotation. The patient will be seen to hold the arm away from the body in external rotation, which frequently causes the arm to be dysfunctional. Pain with chronic dislocations is variable and may be relatively mild after a long-standing dislocation. Figure 14 shows the clinical photographs of a patient who was misdiagnosed as having a shoulder contusion that was later felt to have developed into a frozen shoulder. After 3 months of failed treatment, the diagnosis of an anterior shoulder dislocation was confirmed after obtaining the appropriate radiographs (Fig. 15).

A thorough neurovascular examination should be performed on any shoulder dislocation. Schulz et al. showed in their series that 40% of anterior dislocations had an associated neurologic injury.[30] In a prospective evaluation using EMG, de Laat and colleagues found evidence of a nerve injury in 45% of patients after an acute dislocation of the shoulder or fracture of the humeral neck. Electromyography should be performed to document any suspected brachial plexus or axillary nerve injury before surgical correction of the deformity. There have also been reports of damage or rupture of the axillary artery with anterior dislocations of the shoulder.[1,17]

Radiographic Evaluation

Radiographic evaluation of the locked anterior dislocation should include an AP and lateral view of the shoulder in the plane of the scapula, as well as an axillary lateral view (see Fig. 15). As with locked posterior dislocations, the axillary lateral view will help determine the extent of humeral head impaction, as well as the integrity of the glenoid. Advanced radiographic techniques, such as CT, add valuable information relative to bone loss in the humeral head and glenoid (Fig. 16). Preoperative determination of bone quality is important for surgical planning where an allograft may be needed for reconstruction of a large Hill–Sachs lesion. Associated fractures of the proximal humerus have been seen in up to 50% of these injuries and should be carefully ruled out.[30]

Intraoperative Findings

Chronic anterior dislocations of the shoulder are characterized by intraoperative findings different from those seen in posterior dislocations. In anterior locked dislocations, the humeral head compression fracture is found in the posterolateral aspect of the head (the classic Hill–Sachs lesion[14]). In contrast to posterior dislocations, anterior dislocations commonly have glenoid loss as well as humeral head deficiency. The anteroinferior aspect of the glenoid cavity may become deficient from chronic wear against the posterolateral aspect of the humeral head (Fig. 17). In locked posterior dislocations, the posterior capsule and labrum are usually avulsed from the glenoid as a contiguous sleeve and are not felt to require reattachment to the glenoid during repair. In contrast, reattachment of the anteroinferior capsular structures and glenoid labrum to the glenoid is very important in the recreation of a stable shoulder after reduction of a locked anterior dislocation.

The neurovascular structures are also at a much greater risk during surgical reconstruction of chronic anterior dislocations than with posterior dislocations. With a chronic anterior dislocation, the brachial plexus and axillary vessels may become scarred to the anterior aspect of the subscapularis muscle, making soft-tissue dissection difficult. The axillary nerve is frequently stretched and scarred to the inferior

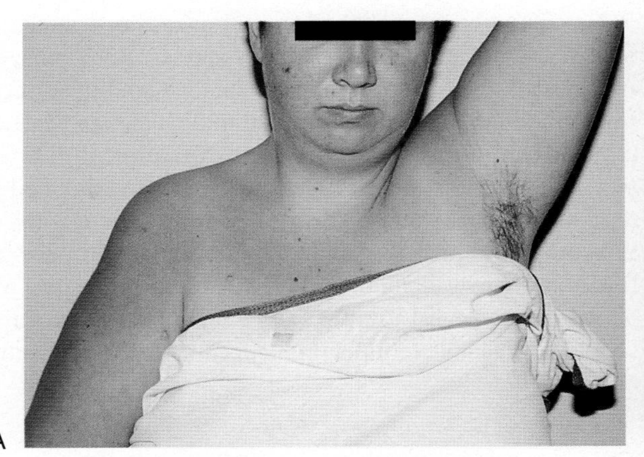
A

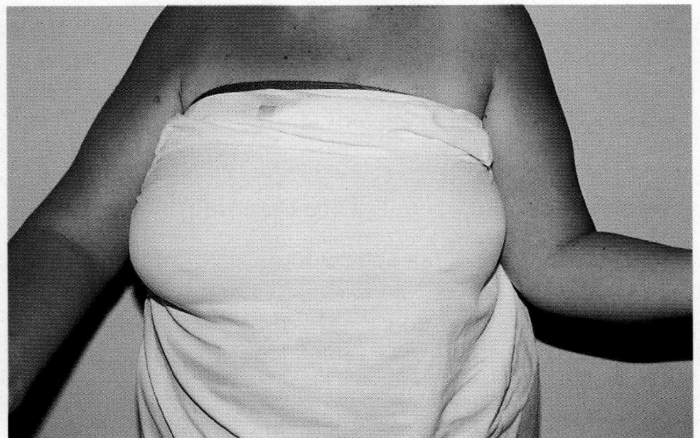
B

FIG. 14. Clinical photographs of a patient misdiagnosed with a shoulder contusion after a fall: **(A)** Marked limitation of forward elevation of the right arm was both active and passive, secondary to a locked anterior dislocation with an associated axillary nerve palsy. **(B)** The loss of rotation of the right arm is depicted in this photograph. (Courtesy of Jeffrey S. Noble, M.D., Akron, Ohio.)

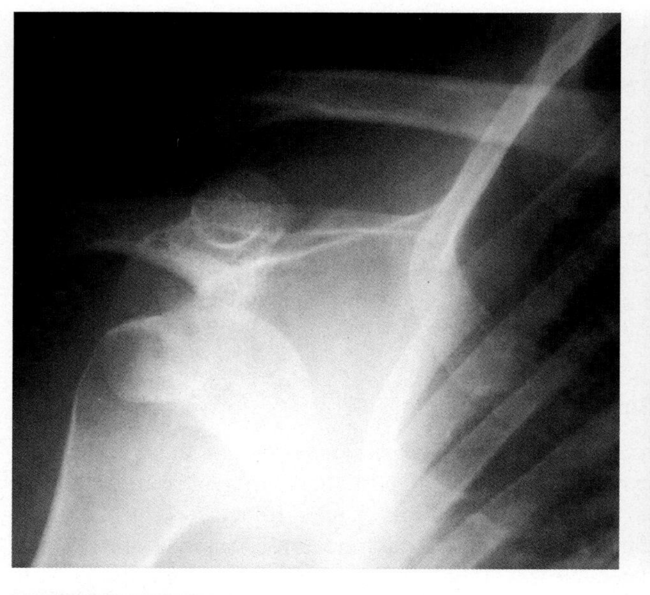

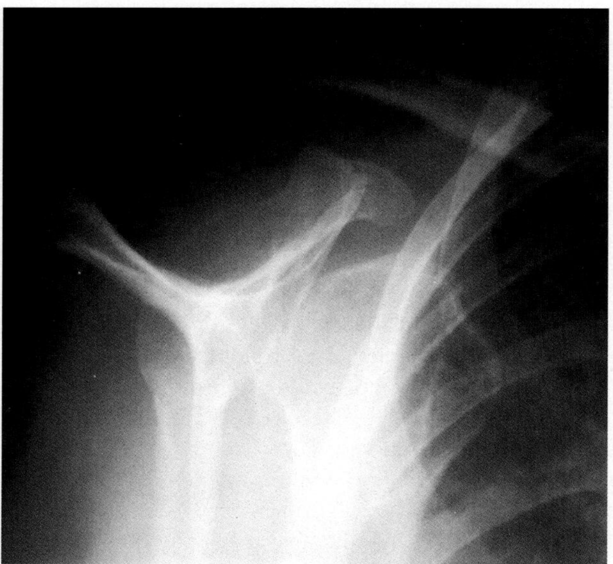

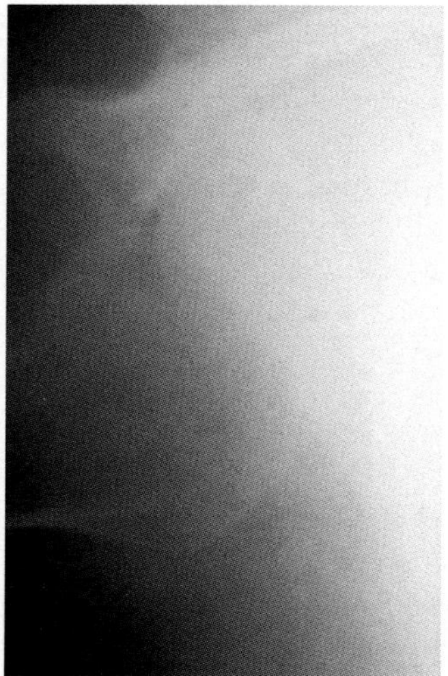

FIG. 15. Clinical radiographs of the patient in Fig. 14 with a locked anterior dislocation: **(A)** scapular AP; **(B)** scapular lateral; and **(C)** axillary views confirmed the diagnosis. (Courtesy of Jeffrey S. Noble, M.D.)

aspect of the subscapularis muscle, placing the nerve at risk during open reduction. As always, the axillary nerve must be identified and protected throughout the procedure. Neuropraxias are not uncommon after open reduction of a chronic anterior dislocation. Recovery is to be expected, as long as the nerve is gently protected and not transected.[30]

Treatment Choice and Preoperative Planning

As with the treatment of locked posterior dislocations, the treatment options for locked anterior dislocations range from benign neglect to total shoulder arthroplasty. The treatment of choice will depend on the size of the defect, the time from injury, the condition of the humeral head and glenoid, and the patient's medical status. The surgeon must develop an algorithmic approach to the treatment of these injuries, so that the proper preoperative plan can be made and the surgeon can move along the algorithm if intraoperative findings require a change of treatment (Fig. 18).

Nonoperative

Nonoperative treatment is an option in the treatment of locked anterior dislocations of the shoulder. Benign neglect may be the treatment of choice in patients with little discomfort and minimal functional limitation. It is also indicated in patients not felt to be medically fit for surgical intervention.[9,10,29,30] Although the functional results of untreated anterior shoulder dislocations are inferior to the results obtained after reduction, some patients have a surprisingly functional range of motion (Fig. 19). Patients treated with benign neglect must usually have a functional contralateral shoulder to be able to function independently in their activities of daily living.

Closed Reduction

The success of closed reduction is very unlikely in a locked anterior dislocation more than 3 weeks old.[10,30] Be-

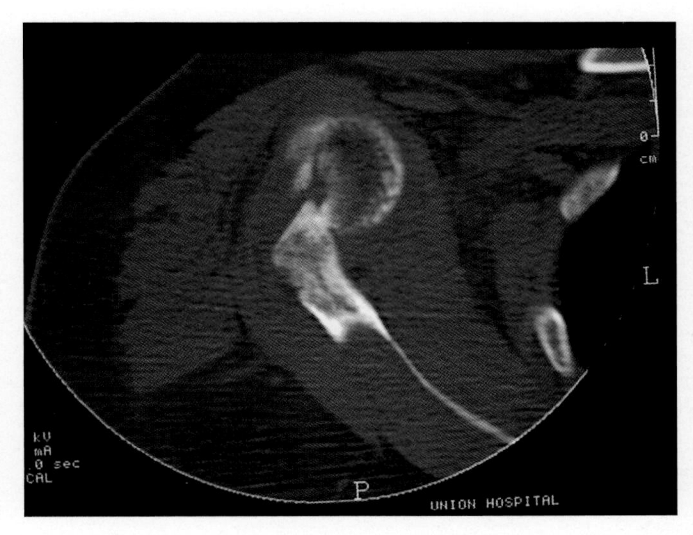

FIG. 16. CT scan of the patient in Figs. 14 and 15 with a locked anterior dislocation. The glenoid was relatively preserved, with a Hill–Sachs lesion of approximately 25%. (Courtesy of Jeffrey S. Noble, M.D.)

cause the incidence of vascular injuries reported with closed reductions performed in the setting of a chronic injury is high, we do not recommend an attempt at closed reduction if the injury is older than 3 weeks.[4] This holds especially true for older patients. If a closed reduction is to be attempted, careful evaluation of preoperative radiographs must be done to ensure that there is not an associated fracture of the tuberosities, humeral neck, or glenoid. If an associated fracture is present, it should be addressed, as described in the treatment of locked posterior dislocations. To perform a closed reduction, slow gentle traction under general anesthesia or scalene block is required. Torque on the arm must be kept to a minimum to prevent humeral fracture.

Open Reduction

If the impaction fracture of the humeral head involves more than 25% of the articular surface or the dislocation is more than three weeks old, the patient will require an open reduction to treat the dislocated shoulder. As previously stated, surgical exposure in chronic anterior dislocations requires careful handling of soft tissues to prevent damage to the neurovascular structures. The anterior labrum and glenoid will also require special attention to regain stability after reduction.

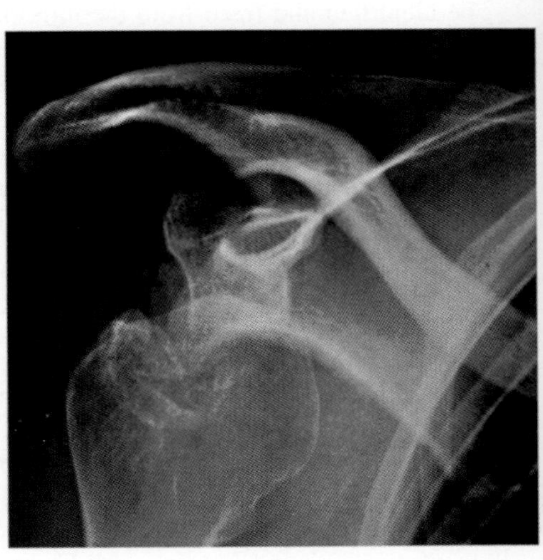

A

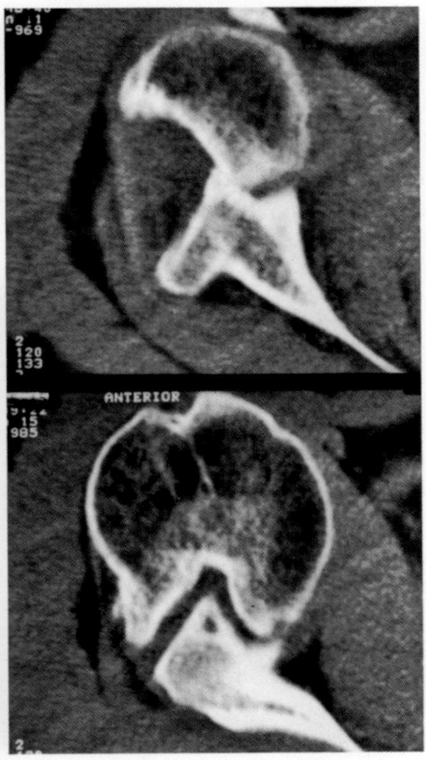

B

FIG. 17. Right shoulder of a bilateral, locked anterior dislocation: There are severe changes seen on the humerus and the glenoid by **(A)** conventional radiographs and **(B)** CT scan. (From ref. 10, with permission.)

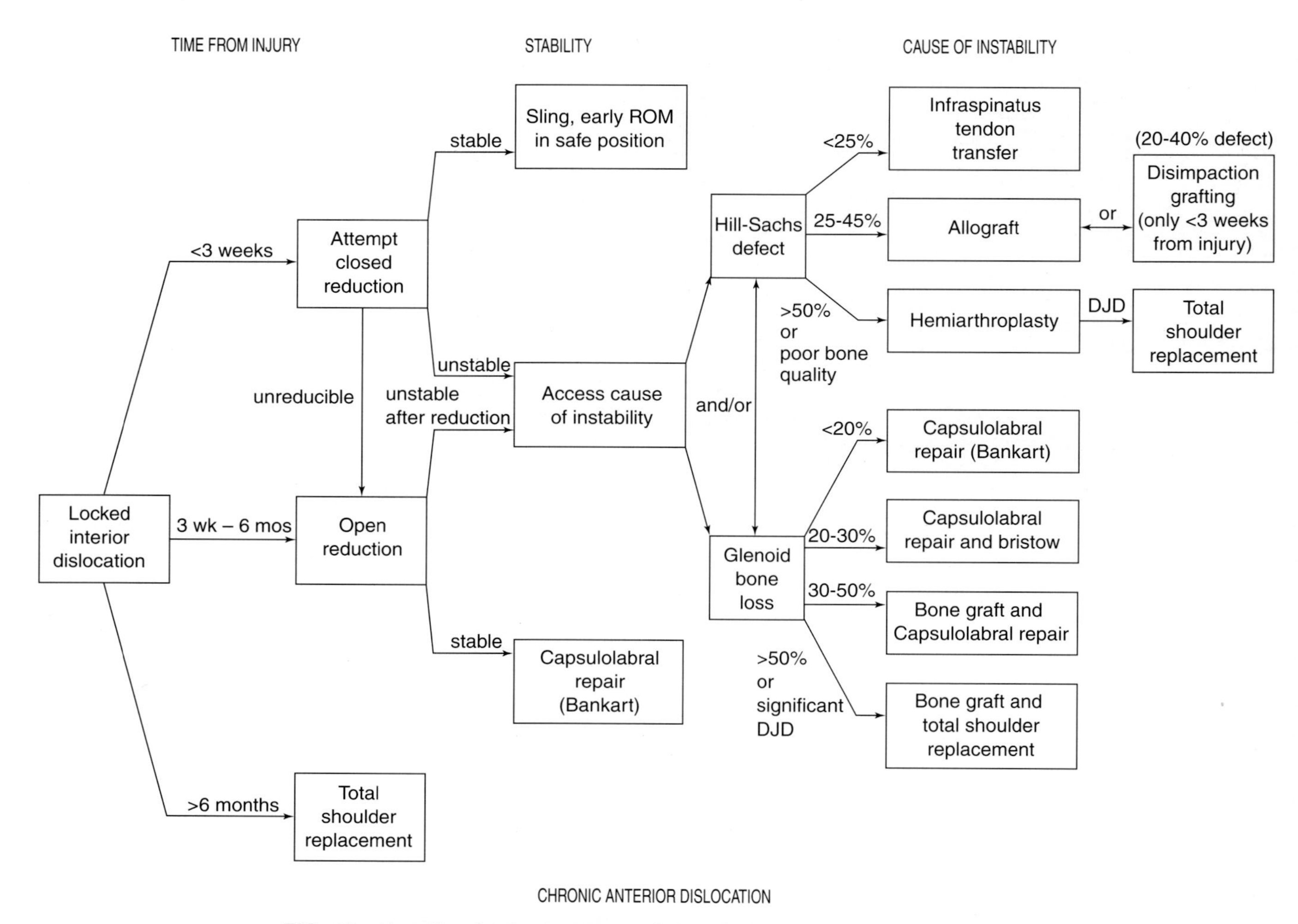

FIG. 18. Algorithm for the treatment of chronic, locked anterior dislocations.

We will first describe the surgical approach to the shoulder, and then we will discuss the surgical management of the capsulolabral complex and the deficient glenoid. This will then be followed by a discussion of the surgical options for treatment of the humeral head defect.

Surgical Approach

A long deltopectoral approach is employed for anterior dislocations. The incision extends from just proximal to the coracoid to just medial to the deltoid insertion. An osteotomy of the coracoid process with its attached conjoined tendon is often necessary to aid in exposure of the medially displaced humeral head. If an osteotomy is necessary, the coracoid should be predrilled and the hole tapped before the osteotomy. This will ensure anatomic alignment of the coracoid at the time of reduction. At the time of closure, the coracoid is fixed with a partially threaded cancellous screw. After the osteotomy is complete, the conjoined tendon is reflected medially to allow identification of the neurovascular structures. These structures must be gently retracted to avoid injury. Release of the superior portion of the pectoralis major tendon is helpful to gain access to the inferior portion of the subscapularis tendon and axillary nerve.

The subscapularis is then carefully dissected. Its anterior surface must be freed of any adhesions to ensure that the brachial plexus is not adherent to it. The axillary nerve must be identified and freed from the inferior border of the subscapularis. For chronic dislocations requiring extensive dissection in this area, the axillary artery is at high risk of injury and may require repair. A vascular surgeon on stand-by is suggested in case severe bleeding occurs. This added precaution is particularly important in older persons, in whom the vascular tissue tends to be more friable and at greater risk for tearing during dissection. Once free of adhesions, the entire subscapularis tendon is released laterally at its insertion into the lesser tuberosity.

The next step in the approach is the capsulotomy. The capsulotomy is performed by releasing the capsule from its humeral insertion. This is in contrast to the vertical capsulotomy performed during the approach to the posteriorly dislocated shoulder. The anterior capsule is attenuated by the dislocated humeral head. The inferior capsule, on the other hand, is contracted and tethers the humeral neck to the an-

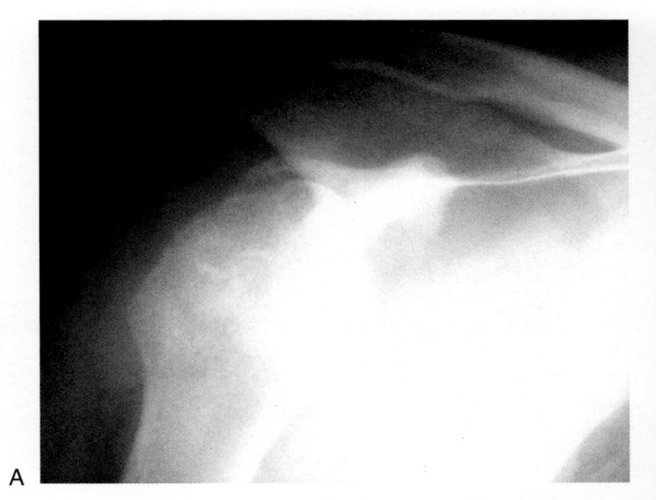

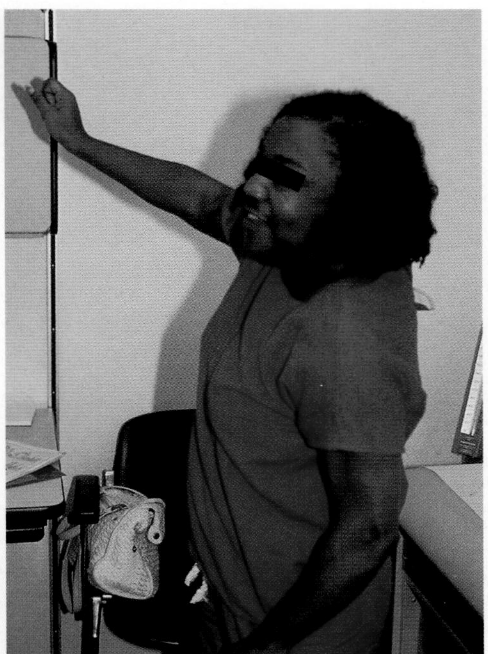

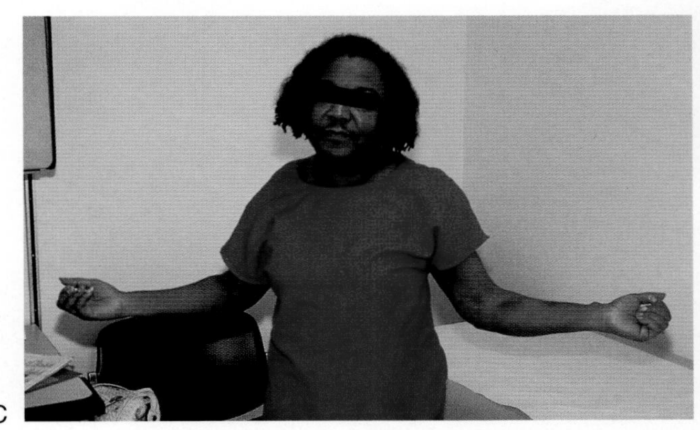

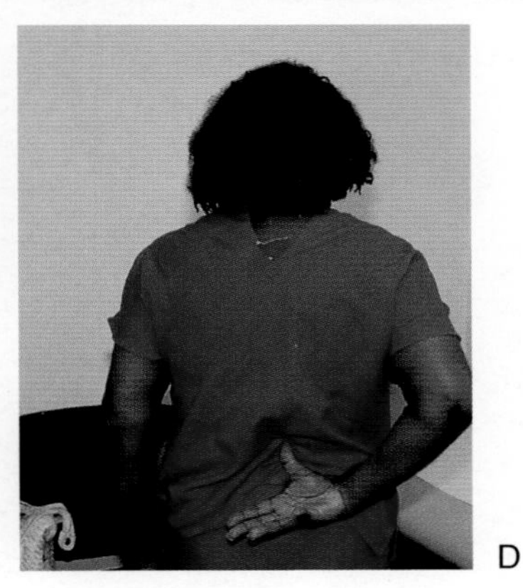

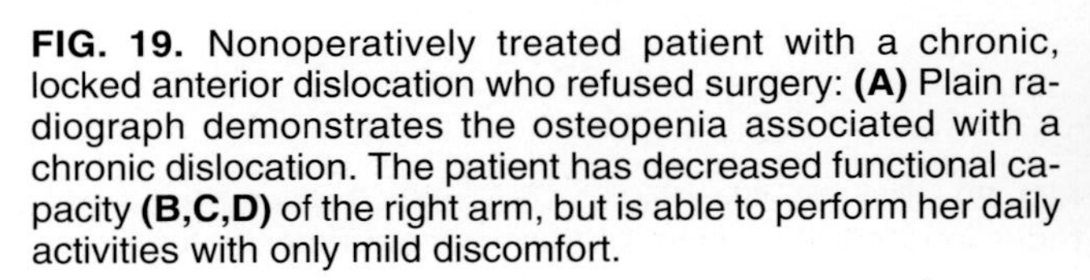

FIG. 19. Nonoperatively treated patient with a chronic, locked anterior dislocation who refused surgery: **(A)** Plain radiograph demonstrates the osteopenia associated with a chronic dislocation. The patient has decreased functional capacity **(B,C,D)** of the right arm, but is able to perform her daily activities with only mild discomfort.

teroinferior glenoid.[9] Before releasing the inferior capsule, the axillary nerve must be clearly identified and retracted to prevent injury. Once take-down of the capsule is performed, a Cobb elevator can be used to reduce the humeral head. Scar and granulation tissue must be debrided from the glenoid to allow reduction.

Once reduction is obtained, a posterior capsulotomy is performed along the glenoid margin. This maneuver allows internal rotation of the arm and helps prevent the tendency toward redislocation caused by the tight posterior capsule. A humeral head retractor is often required to allow access to the posterior capsule. After the capsulotomy is completed, a Cobb elevator is used to ensure that the capsule is free from the posterior aspect of its glenoid insertion.

Locked anterior dislocations of the shoulder require reconstruction of the anteroinferior capsulolabral complex (the Bankart lesion[2]), as described by Rowe in 1981.[28] A soft-tissue Bankart lesion can be repaired with suture anchors placed onto the glenoid margin (Fig. 20). A bony Bankart lesion requires fixation of the bony fragment and its attached labrum back onto the glenoid. If there is marked loss of the glenoid surface by erosion, then a reconstruction of the glenoid may be required.

Glenoid Reconstuction

In cases of glenoid bone loss, a bone graft may be required to reconstruct the anterior glenoid rim. Smaller defects involving less than 20% of the glenoid surface may be reconstructed with a capsulolabral repair, reinforced with a Bristow procedure. If the lesion involves greater than 30% of the glenoid, then reconstruction with a tricortical iliac crest bone graft is required.

Smaller defects of less than 20% of the glenoid surface can be reconstructed with a Bankart repair to the remaining glenoid rim, followed by reinforcement with an anterior bone block procedure, such as a Bristow procedure. A standard Bankart repair is performed, using suture anchors to

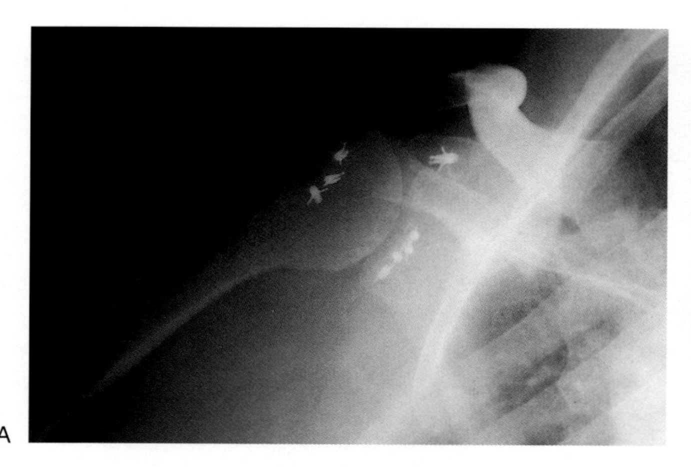
A

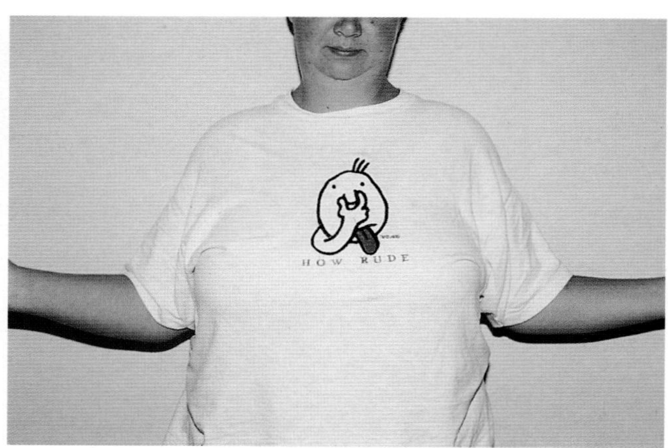

C

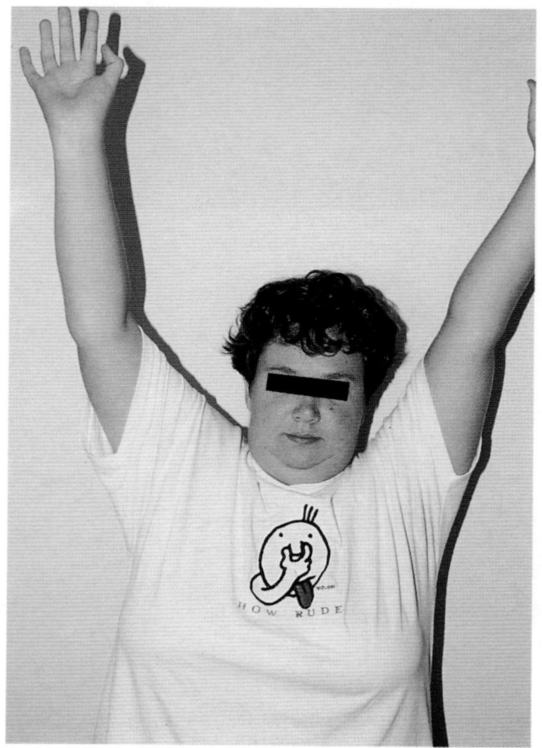

B

FIG. 20. The patient in Figs. 14, 15, and 16 was reduced with an open reduction and take-down of the coracoid process for exposure: **(A)** Postreduction radiograph reveals a concentric reduction of the glenohumeral joint with repair of the capsulolabral complex. Follow-up clinical radiographs show excellent return of **(B)** forward elevation and **(C)** rotation after return of the axillary nerve. (Courtesy of Jeffrey S. Noble, M.D.)

reattach the capsulolabral complex to the margin of the remaining glenoid. The tip of the coracoid with its attached conjoined tendon is then fixed in an extraarticular fashion to the anteroinferior portion of the glenoid with a bicortical screw (Fig. 21). This bone block acts as a secondary restraint to anterior translation. The capsule and subscapularis tendon are then repaired in typical fashion.

A tricortical iliac crest bone graft is often required for reconstruction of the glenoid surface, if there is bone loss involving 30% to 50% of the glenoid surface. The reconstruction must create a stable surface for the humeral head to articulate.

Reconstruction is performed by first exposing the anterior glenoid by subperiosteal dissection. A burr is used to roughen the anterior glenoid to create an adequately flat surface for grafting. The size of the defect is then estimated, and a size-matched corticocancellous piece of iliac crest is harvested. The cortical surface of the graft is placed flush with the articular surface of the glenoid. The graft is then fixed to the anterior glenoid by partially threaded cancellous screws. The screws are placed parallel to the joint surface in a lagged fashion and in an anteroposterior direction. The donor graft is fashioned with a burr to allow a smooth transition from the glenoid cartilage to the graft reconstruction. The anteroinferior capsulolabral complex is then attached to the graft, using suture anchors (Fig. 22).

In the presence of degenerative arthritis or defects involving more than 50% of the glenoid surface, a total shoulder replacement is the treatment of choice. In this instance, the resected humeral head is used to reconstruct the glenoid, as

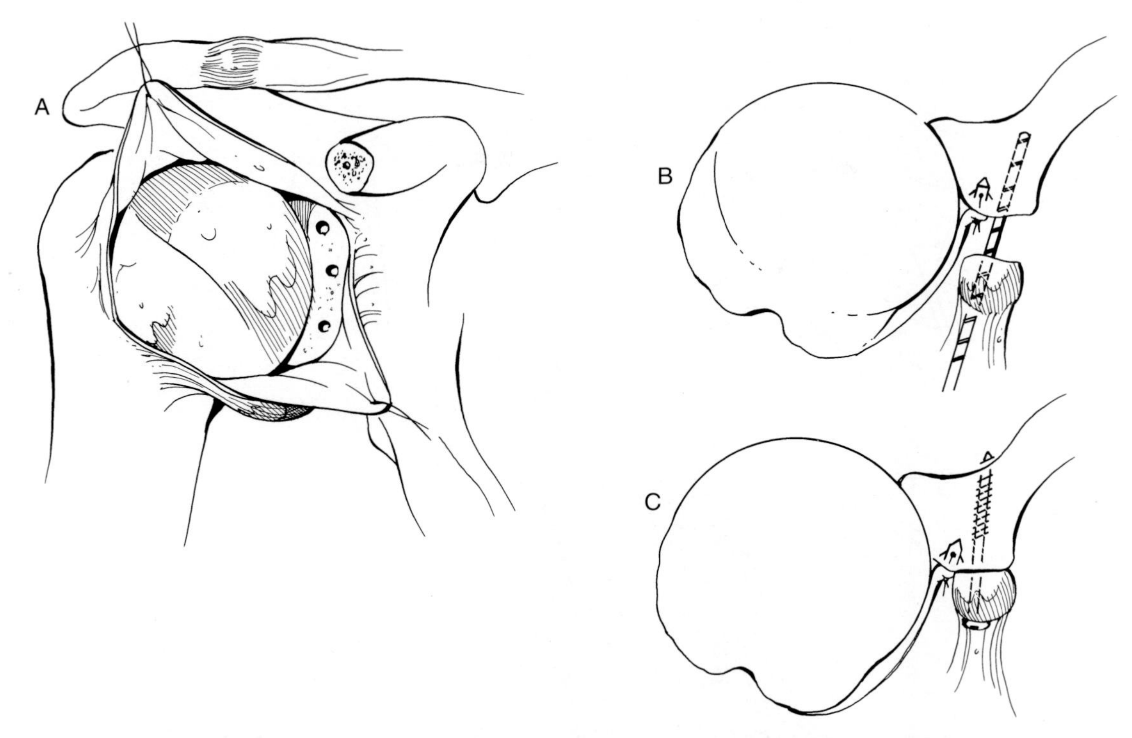

FIG. 21. With moderate glenoid bone loss, an anterior capsulorrhaphy and corocoid transfer are performed. **(A)** The anchors are placed at the glenoid rim and the sutures are passed through the capsule and labrum, but not yet tied. **(B,C)** The glenoid defect is decorticated and the distal 1.5 cm of the corocoid are transferred to the defect and secured with a partially threaded screw.

described for the iliac crest reconstruction. This reconstructed surface is used to support the glenoid component in a total shoulder replacement.

Postoperative rehabilitation for glenoid reconstruction is centered around protecting the anterior glenoid. A sling is worn for approximately 6 weeks and external rotation and motions posterior to the plane of the scapula are avoided.

Reconstruction of the Humeral Head Defect

As seen in the treatment of locked posterior dislocations of the shoulder, the choice of treatment will greatly depend on the size of the humeral head impaction fracture and the time from injury. Small Hill–Sachs lesions involving less than 25% of the humeral head often do not require attention. However, if the shoulder remains unstable after reduction, then transfer of the infraspinatus tendon may be required to obtain stability.

Defects larger than 25% of the humeral head need to be addressed, if the reduction of the humeral head is to be maintained. If the defect involves between 25% and 45% of the articular surface, the choices for treatment are the following: disimpaction with bone grafting, if the injury is less than 3 weeks old and there is adequate bone stock; allograft reconstruction, if the injury is more than 3 weeks old and the bone stock is adequate; or shoulder arthroplasty, if there is marked osteopenia or articular cartilage wear. Any defect involving more than 50% of the humeral head should be treated with an arthroplasty.

Transfer of the Infraspinatus Tendon (Defects Less Than 25%)

The glenohumeral joint is exposed, as described previously. The shoulder is reduced and the size of the defect confirmed. The shoulder is then taken through a range of motion, and the position of instability is noted. If the shoulder is unstable at less than 90 degrees of abduction and 90 degrees of external rotation, an infraspinatus transfer is performed through a posterior approach. The Hill–Sachs defect is debrided and the infraspinatus is released from its insertion and reattached into the base of the defect by transosseous sutures.

Postoperative rehabilitation is centered around early passive motion that avoids the position of recurrent dislocation. In anterior dislocations, the position to avoid is motion posterior to the plane of the scapula, such as abduction and external rotation. On postoperative day 1, pendulums and supine forward elevation with the arm in internal rotation are begun. After 6 weeks, the patient is allowed to begin stretching in external rotation and abduction. Strengthening is reserved for approximately 10 to 12 weeks after surgery, and after a full stable range of motion is obtained.

Disimpaction and Bone Grafting

If the humeral head defect involves between 20% and 40% of the humeral head and the injury is less than 3 weeks old, then disimpaction and bone grafting can be attempted. The indications and intraoperative evaluation of the humeral

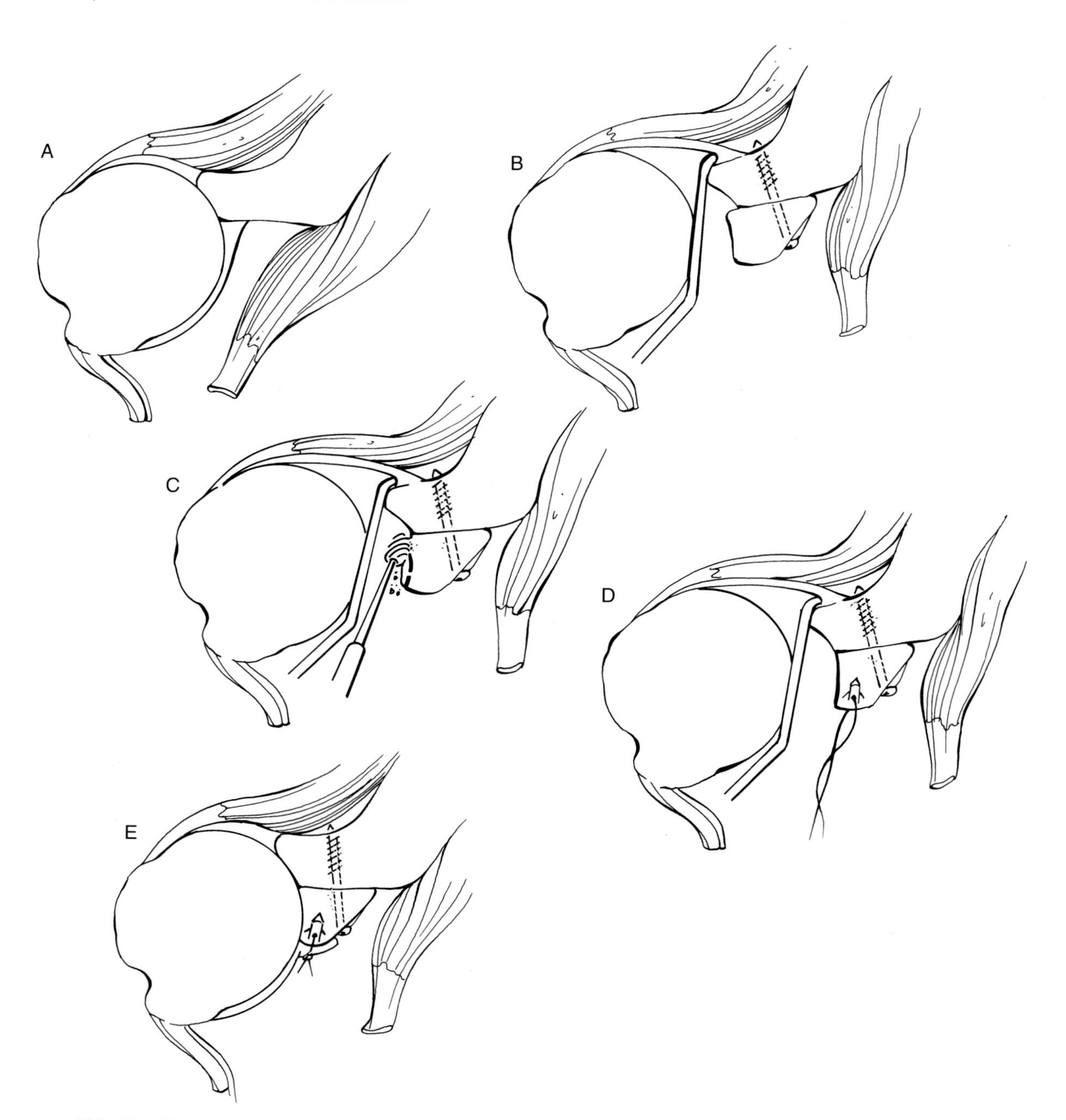

FIG. 22. (A) For large anterior glenoid defects an iliac crest graft is used to reconstruct the glenoid defect. **(B)** The defect is decorticated and made flat. A bicortical iliac crest graft is placed with its cancellous surface against the cancellous bone of the defect and secured with two partially threaded screws. **(C)** The position of the graft, which overhangs the face of the glenoid, is burred down to make a smooth contour with the native glenoid. **(D)** Suture anchors are placed into the rim of the graft. **(E)** The limbs of each suture are passed through the capsule and labrum, thereby repairing the ligaments to the new glenoid rim.

head are similar to those described for the posterior locked dislocation. In treating the Hill–Sachs lesion, the cortical window is created in the lesser tuberosity. Disimpaction and bone grafting are then carried out as described in Fig. 9.

The patient is placed in a sling for 3 weeks. Rehabilitation is begun on postoperative day 1. Gentle range of motion is begun, with care taken to avoid placing the arm in a position that would place stress on the disimpacted area. The positions to avoid should be determined at the time of surgery. In general, these will be abduction and external rotation. These motions should be avoided for approximately 6 weeks, until the graft has had time to consolidate.

Allograft Reconstruction

If the Hill–Sachs lesion involves between 25% and 45% of the humeral head, then allograft reconstruction can be performed. For this technique to be successful, the patient must have good bone stock and a suitable articular cartilage. Historically, defects of this size have been addressed with infraspinatus transfer into the defect, cancellous bone grafting of the defect, or humeral head replacement. More recently, however, Gerber has reported success treating this type of defect with allograft reconstruction[10] (Fig. 23). He stresses that allograft reconstruction requires good bone stock in the remaining humeral head to prevent collapse. Dislocations of more than 6 months often have poor bone stock, and collapse of the humeral head following reduction is common.[9,27] If osteopenia is present, then humeral head replacement would be the better option in these patients.

Allograft reconstruction of a posterolateral Hill–Sachs lesion from an anterior approach requires extensive exposure. To allow access to the posterior aspect of the humeral head, the entire subscapularis insertion needs to be detached. The ascending branch of the anterior circumflex humeral artery must be protected to prevent vascular compromise to the humeral head. The capsule must then be released around its circumference, and the coracoacromial ligament must be released. The arm can then be brought into adduction and extension to gain access to the posterior head.[10] The allograft is fashioned to fit the defect and is fixed into place with 3.5-mm cortical screws.

Postoperatively, the patient is placed in a sling. Rehabilitation consists of gentle pendulums and passive supine elevation, with avoidance of external rotation beyond zero degrees for 6 weeks. At 6 weeks, the patient is allowed full motion of the shoulder and light strengthening is begun. No heavy lifting is allowed for 3 months.

Gerber has reported good results in a small series of pa-

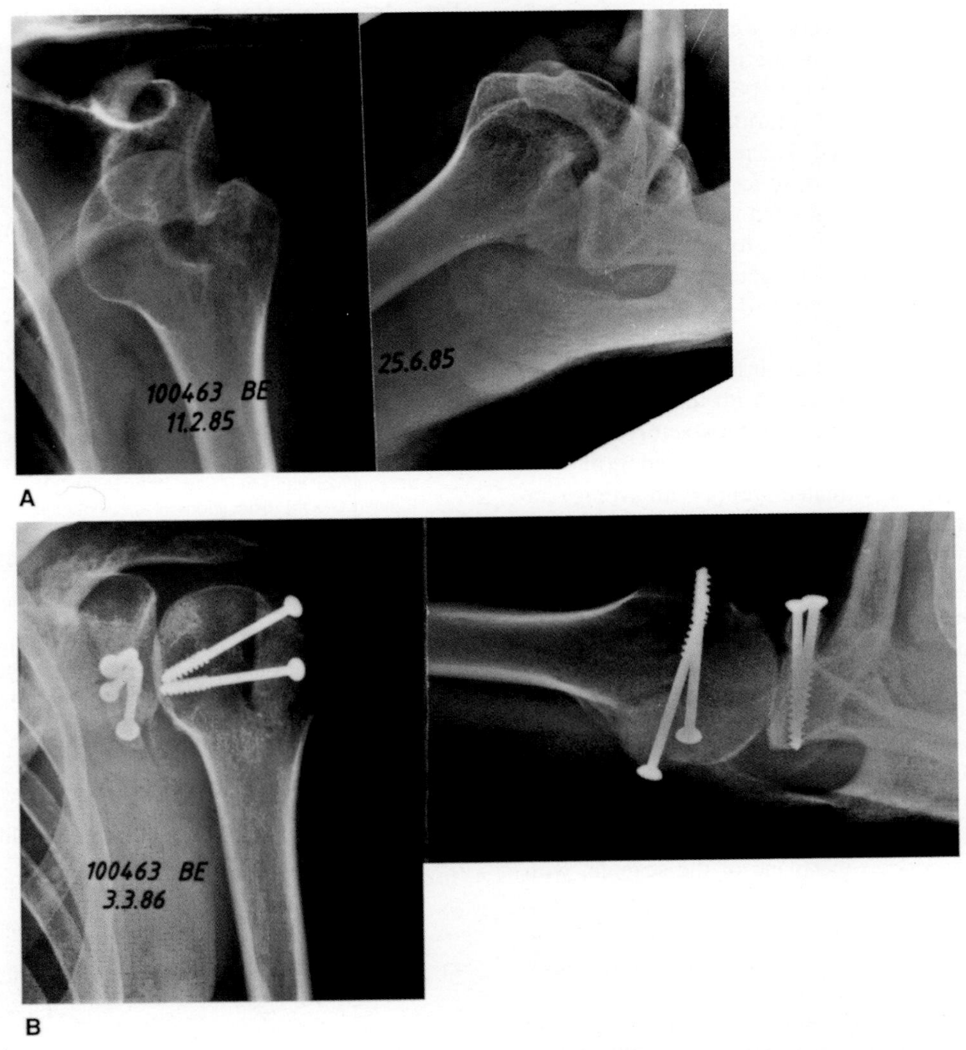

FIG. 23. Radiographs of a patient with **(A)** a severe humeral head defect that was reconstructed with **(B)** an allograft and the glenoid augmented with a modified Bristow bone block. (From ref.10, with permission.)

tients treated with this procedure. Postoperative elevation averaged 145 degrees with a Constant score averaging 70%.[10]

Prosthetic Reconstruction

In patients with greater than 50% involvement of the articular surface of the humeral head, shoulder arthroplasty is the treatment of choice. Arthroplasty is also the treatment of choice in patients with marked osteopenia or loss of articular surface integrity, owing to the chronic nature of their injury. Some authors have actually reported collapse of the articular surface of the humeral head after reduction of a long-standing dislocation.[9,27] Therefore, a humeral head replacement will often be needed for dislocations that are older than six months.

When performing a humeral head replacement to treat a locked anterior dislocation, the surgeon should attempt to place the prosthesis in approximately 30 degrees of retroversion. Therefore, if the glenoid is deficient, it must be reconstructed, as described in the section on glenoid reconstruction, using autograft bone from the resected head. If the defect in the glenoid is larger than 50% of the glenoid surface or the remaining glenoid is arthritic, then placement of a glenoid component is required. The resected humeral head can be used as bone graft to reconstruct the glenoid.

Any rotator cuff tears encountered during prosthetic replacement should be repaired.[9,27] The rotator cuff aids in stability of the shoulder and prevents superior migration of the humeral head. The repair is performed after the head is excised and before prosthetic fixation.

Flatow and colleagues reported on nine chronic anterior dislocations of the shoulder treated with total shoulder replacement with four excellent, four satisfactory, and one unsatisfactory result.[9] The surgically treated group far outscored the nonsurgically treated group, with average active forward elevation to 147 degrees and average active external rotation to 69 degrees. All were able to function well with activities of daily living.

Some authors suggest that the version of the prosthesis can be adjusted to compensate for the chronic dislocation and aid in preventing a recurrent dislocation.[9,26] Pritchett and Clarke reported a series of 7 patients for whom the retroversion was increased 30 to 50 degrees, with no episodes of recurrent dislocation. All patients improved with five good and two poor results.[26]

Postoperative rehabilitation is instituted on day 1. Gentle range of motion anterior to the plane of the scapula, with avoidance of provocative positions, is performed for 4 to 6 weeks.[29] If the shoulder remains unstable at the end of the procedure, then the shoulder can be immobilized in a sling for 3 weeks to allow the soft tissues to scar.[9] After 3 weeks, the sling is removed and gentle range of motion is begun. In this scenario, the position of instability is avoided for 6 weeks. No heavy activity is allowed for 3 months.

Resection of the Humeral Head

Resection is undertaken only for intractable pain in a shoulder that can not be reconstructed. In Rowe and Zarins's series, three out of four resections resulted in only fair results.[29] Although reported series are small, resection is inferior to nonoperative treatment, as far as functional outcome is concerned.

SUMMARY

Locked dislocations of the shoulder are rare injuries. Because of this, there are only a small number of series addressing the management of these difficult injuries. In this chapter, we have attempted to summarize the treatment recommendations given in the literature and the results obtained using each method. We have added to this information our own approach to the treatment of locked dislocations of the shoulder. For injuries involving less than 20% or more than 50% of the humeral head, the choice of treatment is rather straightforward. However, injuries involving 20% to 50% of the humeral head require that the surgeon understand the benefits and limitations of each of the treatments discussed. The percentages given for determining which treatment to use, as well as the time from injury listed, are only meant to serve as a guide during decision making. The surgeon must make his or her surgical choice based on the individual patient factors discussed and on the findings at the time of surgery.

REFERENCES

1. Antal C, Conforty B, Engelberg M. Injuries to the axillary artery due to anterior dislocation of the shoulder. *J Trauma* 1973;13:564–566.
2. Bankart ASB. The pathology and treatment of recurrent dislocation of the shoulder joint. *Br J Surg* 1939;26:23–29.
3. Bennett G. Old dislocations of the shoulder. *J Bone Joint Surg [Am]* 1936;18:594–606.
4. Calvert J, Leroy M, Lacroix L. Luxations de l'epaule et lesions vasculaires. *J Chir* 1942;58:337–346.
5. Cave E, Burke JF, Boyd RJ. *Trauma management*. Chicago: Year Book Medical Publishers, 1974.
6. Conn R, Cofield RH, Byer DE, Linstromberg JW. Interscalene block anaesthesia for shoulder surgery. *Clin Orthop* 1987;216:94–98.
7. Constant CR, Murley AHG. A clinical method of functional assessment of the shoulder. *Clin Orthop* 1987;214:160–164.
8. de Laat EA, Visser CP, Coene LN, Pahlplatz PV, Tavy DL. Nerve lesions in primary shoulder dislocations and humeral neck fractures. A prospective clinical and EMG study. *J Bone Joint Surg [Br]* 1994;76:381–383.
9. Flatow E, Miller SR, Neer CS. Chronic Anterior dislocation of the shoulder. *J Shoulder Elbow Surg* 1993;2:2–10.
10. Gerber C. Chronic, locked anterior and posterior dislocations. In: Warner JJ, Iannotti JP, Gerber C, eds. *Complex and revision problems in shoulder surgery*. Philadelphia: Lippincott–Raven, 1997:99–113.
11. Gerber C, Lambert SM. Allograft reconstruction of segmental defects of the humeral head for the treatment of chronic locked posterior dislocation of the shoulder. *J Bone Joint Surg [Am]* 1996;78:376–382.
12. Hawkins RJ, Neer CS II, Pianta RM, Mendoza FX. Locked posterior dislocation of the shoulder. *J Bone Joint Surg [Am]* 1987;69:9–18.

13. Hersche O, Gerber C. Iatrogenic displacement of fracture–dislocations of the shoulder. A report of seven cases. *J Bone Joint Surg [Br]* 1994; 76:30–33.
14. Hill H, Sachs MD. The grooved defect of the humeral head. A frequently unrecognized complication of dislocations of the shoulder joint. *Radiology* 1940;35:690–700.
15. Kavanaugh J. Posterior shoulder dislocation with ipsilateral humeral shaft fracture. *Clin Orthop* 1978;131:168–172.
16. Kazar B, Relovszky E. Prognosis of primary dislocation of the shoulder. *Acta Orthop Scand* 1969;40:216–224.
17. Kirker J. Dislocation of the shoulder complicated by rupture of the axillary vessels. *J Bone Joint Surg [Br]* 1952;34B:72–73.
18. Kirtland S, Resnick D, Sartoris DJ, Pate D, Greenway G. Chronic unreduced dislocations of the glenohumeral joint: imaging strategy and pathologic correlation. *J Trauma* 1988;28:1622–1631.
19. Kummel B. Fractures of the glenoid causing chronic dislocation of the shoulder. *Clin Orthop* 1970;69:189–191.
20. Mankin H, Doppelt S, Tomford W. Clinical experience with allograft implantation: the first ten years. *Clin Orthop* 1983;174:69–86.
21. McDermott A, Langer F, Pritzker KPH, Gross AE. Fresh small-fragment osteochondral allografts: long term follow-up study on first 100 cases. *Clin Orthop* 1985;197:96–102.
22. McLaughlin HL. Posterior dislocation of the shoulder. *J Bone Joint Surg [Am]* 1952;34A:584–590.
23. Mullaji A, Beddow FH, Lamb GHR. CT measurement of glenoid erosion in arthritis. *J Bone Joint Surg [Br]* 1994;76B:384–388.
24. Neer CS II. *Shoulder reconstruction*. Philadelphia: WB Saunders, 1990.
25. Ovesen J, Söjbjerg JO. Posterior shoulder dislocation: muscle and capsular lesions in cadaver experiments. *Acta Orthop Scand* 1986;57: 535–536.
26. Pritchett JW, Clark JM. Prosthetic replacement for chronic unreduced dislocations of the shoulder. *Clin Orthop* 1987;216:89–93.
27. Rowe C. *Dislocations of the shoulder*. New York: Churchill Livingston, 1988.
28. Rowe CR, Zarins B. Recurrent transient subluxation of the shoulder. *J Bone Joint Surg [Am]* 1981;63:863–872.
29. Rowe CR, Zarins B. Chronic unreduced dislocations of the shoulder. *J Bone Joint Surg [Am]* 1982;64:494–505.
30. Schulz TJ, Jacobs B, Patterson RL Jr. Unrecognized dislocations of the shoulder. *J Trauma* 1969;9:1009–1023.
31. Scougall S. Posterior dislocation of the shoulder. *J Bone Joint Surg [Br]* 1957;39:726–732.
32. Tanner MW, Cofield RH. Prosthetic arthroplasty for fractures and fracture–dislocations of the proximal humerus. *Clin Orthop* 1983;179: 116–128.
33. Wilson J, McKeever FM. Traumatic posterior (retroglenoid dislocation of the humerus. *J Bone Joint Surg [Am]* 1949;31:160–172.

Disorders of the Shoulder: Diagnosis and Management,
edited by Joseph P. Iannotti and Gerald R. Williams, Jr.
Lippincott Williams & Wilkins, Philadelphia © 1999.

CHAPTER 14

Complications of Instability Surgery

Mark D. Lazarus and Dan Guttmann

The only way to prevent complications, is to not perform surgery.[133]

INTRODUCTION

Rarely do we as surgeons proceed as confidently as when we operate for recurrent instability. For traumatic instability, a surgeon can confidently inform his patient that his or her chances of returning to near normal function are greater than 90%. When instability surgery fails, however, that surgical confidence can deflate as fast as a punctured balloon. Faced with the patient who has suffered multiple failures of instability surgery, we as surgeons can become thoroughly humbled. This chapter will explore the common causes of failure after instability surgery, how to avoid these failures, and techniques for recovery.

M.D. Lazarus: Department of Shoulder and Elbow Surgery, Albert Einstein Medical Center, and Department Orthopaedic Surgery, Temple University Medical School, Philadelphia, Pennsylvania 19141.

D. Guttmann: Department of Orthopaedic Surgery, Albert Einstein Medical Center, Philadelphia, Pennsylvania 19141.

OPEN REPAIRS FOR ANTERIOR INSTABILITY

Recurrent anterior glenohumeral instability occurs most often following a significant traumatic incident and is often referred to as recurrent traumatic instability. This traumatic event usually takes place with the arm in an abducted, extended, and externally rotated position. Glenohumeral dislocation reproduced in the laboratory demonstrates a severe and explosive event, supporting the destructive pathology noted in the shoulders of these patients. As many as 84% to 97% of these patients will have avulsions of the anteroinferior capsulolabral complex from the glenoid rim (the so-called Bankart or Perthes lesion).[9,90,92,125,144] The surgical correction, therefore, usually involves an attempt to repair this defect (the Bankart repair). A wide array of factors can be responsible for failure of this repair (Table 1).

Recurrence of Instability

Incidence

The most common complication reported after repair for anterior instability is recurrence of instability.[21,58,

TABLE 1. *Causes of failure of open anterior instability repairs*

Recurrence of instability	Subscapularis failure
Loss of motion	Hardware complications
Capsulorrhaphy arthropathy	Neurovascular injury

[106,121,128,168] The exact rate of instability recurrence depends on the specific surgical correction employed at the time of the index procedure, but ranges from 3% to almost 50%.[11,91,92]

Etiology

Numerous causes may be responsible for recurrence of instability after previous surgical repair (Table 2). Although discussed individually, several of these situations may coexist in the same patient. In the patient with instability recurrence, the revision surgeon must consciously rule out each of these causes before choosing a course of action.

Incorrect Diagnosis

In an ideal world, every patient with recurrent traumatic anterior instability would present to the surgeon with a radiograph demonstrating the dislocation. In the absence of a radiograph, the patient would give a clear history of instability events directly related to positioning the arm in abduction, extension, and external rotation. Unfortunately, as is usually true in medicine, patients rarely read the textbook before giving their history. Deciding on the direction of instability, or differentiating unidirectional traumatic from multidirectional instability, can sometimes be a confusing task, and the diagnosis should be made by thorough history, examination, and radiographic analysis.

Accurate determination of the direction of instability is crucial for obtaining satisfactory results after instability surgery. Even Hippocrates recognized the importance of performing the corrective procedure at the precise location of instability and the worsening that might result from misdiagnosis:[1]

> For many physicians have burned the shoulders subject to dislocation, at the top of the shoulder, at the anterior part where the head of the humerus protrudes, and a little behind the top of the shoulder; these burnings, if the dislocation of the arm were upward, or forward, or backward, would have been properly performed; but now, when the dislocation is downward, they rather promote then prevent dislocations.

TABLE 2. *Etiology of recurrent instability after anterior repair*

Decision-making errors	Anatomic factors
Incorrect diagnosis	Glenoid concavity defect
Incorrect surgical procedure	Residual capsular laxity
Voluntary instability	Anterior capsular deficiency
Surgical errors	Hill–Sachs lesion
Technical error	
Other	
Severe recurrent trauma	

If a patient with recurrent anterior instability is incorrectly diagnosed as having posterior instability, a posterior repair would result in continued or worsened anterior instability.[11,21,06,78,92,168] Subsequent appropriate anterior repair would result in an excessively tight shoulder. Similarly, if an anterior repair is performed, but the true diagnosis is multidirectional or posterior instability, posterior displacement may be worsened (Fig. 1).

Hawkins and Hawkins reviewed cases of recurrent instability after surgical repair and attempted to retrospectively assign a cause to the repair failure.[58] In 12 of 31 patients, the authors believed that the primary cause of surgical failure was in the diagnosis, usually a confusion of direction of instability or type of instability. McAuliffe et al., in an analysis of 36 patients with failed instability repairs, found that 15 of those patients had recurrence secondary to misdiagnosis.[95] Norris and Bigliani determined that 9 of 42 patients with recurrent instability were incorrectly diagnosed, including 4 who underwent surgery on the incorrect side of the shoulder.[107] Rockwood and Gerber thought that the cause of recurrent, postoperative instability in 68% of 57 reported patients was failure to recognize multidirectional instability.[121]

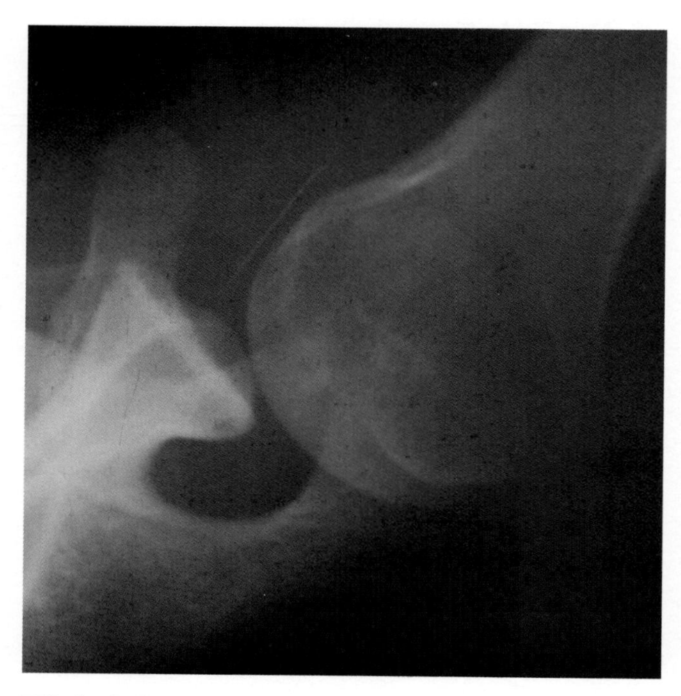

FIG. 1. Axillary radiograph of a 24-year-old man who underwent a Putti-Platt procedure for presumed recurrent anterior instability when the true diagnosis was recurrent posterior instability. Symptomatic posterior instability was worsened by the anterior repair. (Courtesy Douglas T. Harryman II, University of Washington Medical Center, Seattle, WA.)

Finally, Burkhead and Richie analyzed 23 patients with postoperative instability and determined that, for 5 of 23, the diagnosis of multidirectional instability had been missed.[21]

Surgery for glenohumeral instability will also result in failure if the underlying diagnosis is not instability.[107] Through recent teachings, we have correctly become more alert to the potential of instability as a cause of shoulder pain in the young population. However, not all shoulder pain in the young patient indicates occult instability. Unless the diagnosis of glenohumeral instability is truly indicated by history and physical examination and is demonstrated by an examination under anesthesia, instability surgery should not be performed.

Incorrect Surgical Procedure

In most patients with recurrent anterior instability, the pathologic defect is a tear of the anteroinferior glenoid labrum and origin of the inferior glenohumeral ligament, necessitating a repair of this defect to provide stability.[9,90,92,125,144] In the literature, however, more than 150 different operative procedures have been described in the treatment of recurrent traumatic anterior instability. As a general rule, these alternative procedures do not address the inherent pathology and are associated with a greater likelihood of instability recurrence.[67,91,92] Although surgeries that involve bone blocks, subscapularis reefing, and musculotendinous slings may be technically easier than a Bankart repair, these procedures do not address the pathologic anatomy; therefore, they have higher rates of postoperative instability.

Rowe et al. reviewed the results of surgical correction after a prior failure of instability surgery.[128] In 84% of their patients, they found residual, unrepaired Bankart lesions at the time of revision surgery. With revision surgery, usually a Bankart repair, they were able to restore stability in 92% of patients. Hawkins and Hawkins found residual anteroinferior labral detachments in most of their patients who underwent surgery for recurrence of instability.[58].

Revising non-Bankart instability operations can often be a formidable challenge. These procedures are all usually accomplished through an anterior deltopectoral approach. If a surgeon is contemplating revision surgery when he did not perform the index procedure, review of the operative note from that index procedure is crucial to determine the nature of the index operation and possible difficulties revision might entail. Radiographs should also be evaluated for hardware and other hints as to the index operation.

Particular note is made of revision of procedures that involve transfer of the coracoid process (Bristow and Laterjet operations). Young and Rockwood described in detail the surgical difficulties encountered in revising a failed Bristow procedure.[166] Specifically, loss of normal anatomic landmarks, extensive scar formation, and subscapularis deficiency all made surgery difficult. Matsen has coined the phrase "lighthouse of the shoulder" to describe the coracoid process, meaning that the coracoid can guide a surgeon between the "safe" lateral side of the conjoined tendon and the "suicide" medial side.[90] Revision surgery without this lighthouse, as in after coracoid transfer procedures, is technically demanding and dangerous.

Surgical results after a previous Bristow operation may also be less gratifying than after other surgical procedures. For those patients with recurrent instability, Young and Rockwood obtained good or excellent results in 8 of 13.[166] Because of the associated problems of scar formation, hardware problems, and articular degeneration, the overall success rate at revision surgery was only 50%.

Technical Error

As much as we all wish to perform the perfect surgery in each and every case, there are times when the procedure does not proceed exactly as anticipated. The goal of the Bankart procedure is repair of the anterior glenoid labrum and inferior glenohumeral ligament (IGHL) to the glenoid rim. Although the surgeon may set out to perform a Bankart repair, difficulty with the exposure or unfamiliarity with the anatomy may result in the surgical goals being left unaccomplished.

It may be difficult to initially determine the cause of recurrence of instability in these cases. The index operative note may describe a Bankart-type repair as intended. With the increased use of suture anchors during Bankart-type repairs, the location of the anchors on a radiograph can be of assistance (Fig. 2). If the integrity of the anteroinferior glenoid labrum and IGHL are not restored, a Bankart repair was not accomplished and instability recurrence is predictable.

Technical errors leading to instability recurrence also plague non-Bankart repairs. For the Bristow procedure, correct placement of the transferred coracoid tip is essential to success.[66] If the coracoid tip is secured too medial or superior on the glenoid neck, recurrent instability would be expected. If the procedure is to be successful, the transferred coracoid process must be placed at the anteroinferior quadrant to act as a bone block against anteroinferior humeral translation. A surgeon cannot rely on the "sling" of conjoined tendon to prevent humeral subluxation.[129]

Failure to Restore Glenoid Concavity

The shoulder is often described as inherently unstable owing to the shallow glenoid fossa. Relative to the acetabulum, the glenoid fossa is shallow. However, just as a golf ball on a tee, the humeral head gains a great degree of stability from its position within a concave glenoid fossa, and should actually be considered inherently stable. Howell and Galinat determined the depth of the glenoid fossa to be 9 mm in the superior to inferior direction and 5 mm in the anteroposterior direction.[68] Half of the depth was attributed to the effect of the glenoid labrum, with the other half coming from the

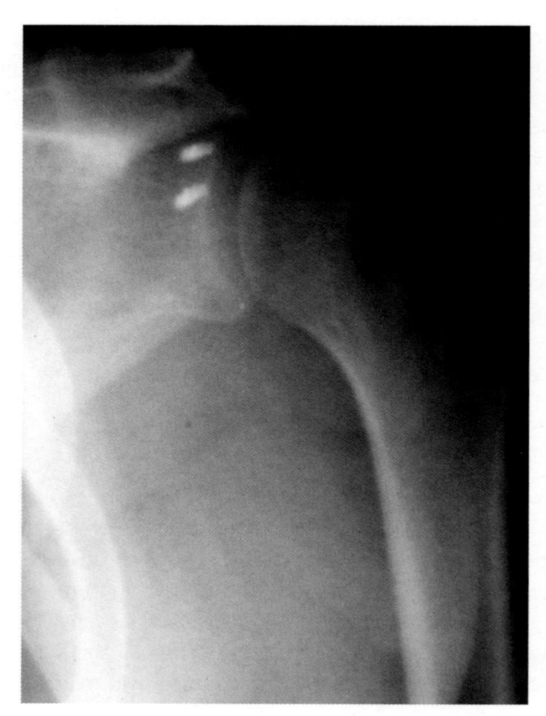

FIG. 2. Radiograph of a 19-year-old man who had two previous "Bankart" repairs for recurrent, traumatic anterior instability. Placement of suture anchors in this superior position is unlikely to result in repair of the inferior glenohumeral ligament origin.

combined effect of the bony glenoid structure and the peripherally thickened chondral surface. This depth confers a great deal of stability to the glenohumeral articulation.

Even without ligamentous support, glenoid concavity plays a surprisingly effective role in providing glenohumeral stability. Lippitt et al. defined the *concavity–compression* mechanism of glenohumeral stability as the combined stabilizing effect of a spherical humeral head contained in a deep glenoid fossa, held there by muscular compressive action.[84] These investigators used a graphic representation, referred to as the glenoidogram, to define glenoid depth. The glenoidogram demonstrates that lateral displacement of the humeral head is first necessary before anterior translation can occur (Fig. 3). They also used the *stability ratio*, a factor defined by Fukuda et al. as the humeral translating force required to cause a glenohumeral dislocation divided by the humeral compressive load maintaining stability, multiplied by 100, to analyze the effectiveness of glenoid concavity in promoting stability.[35] Normal glenoids were noted to have significant concavity, equating with an ability to provide a tremendous stabilizing effect (stability ratios as high as 63%). Excising the glenoid labrum caused a reduction in the stability ratio of approximately 20%.

To relate the concept of concavity–compression more directly to the diagnosis of recurrent traumatic anterior instability, Lazarus et al. measured glenoid concavity and stability ratios before and after creation of an anteroinferior glenoid chondral–labral defect.[79] This defect was designed to be similar to that which might be found after numerous anterior glenohumeral dislocations (Fig. 4). This investigation demonstrated significant reduction in the effectiveness of concavity–compression after creation of the instability defect. Glenoid concavity and stability ratios could be normalized with a simulated surgical reconstruction of the glenoid concavity (Fig. 5).

Failure to reconstruct normal glenoid concavity during an instability repair is a cause of instability recurrence. The normal glenoid labral attachment is directly to the glenoid rim. Instability repairs that result in a capsulolabral repair to the glenoid neck and not to the glenoid rim fail to restore the normal glenoid architecture and can result in surgical failure. This type of repair is more commonly seen with the use of auxiliary fixation devices, particularly tacks, staples, and suture anchors (Fig. 6). Either because of their size or because of the surgeon's reluctance to place these devices near the articular surface, use of these tools can result in medial placement and subsequent inadequate repair. Although the in-

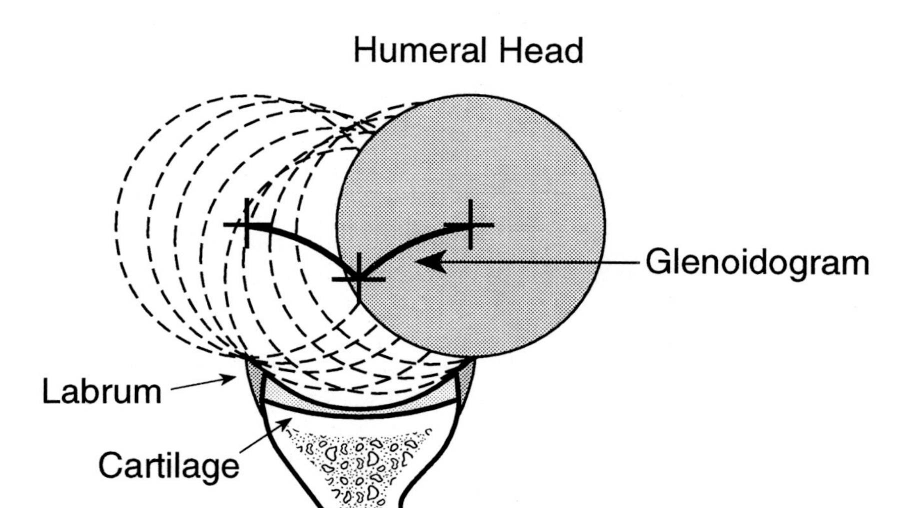

FIG. 3. The "glenoidogram" defines the glenohumeral stabilizing effect of glenoid concavity. For the humeral head to translate anteriorly, posteriorly, or inferiorly out of the glenoid, it must initially move laterally, against the stabilizing force of the rotator cuff.

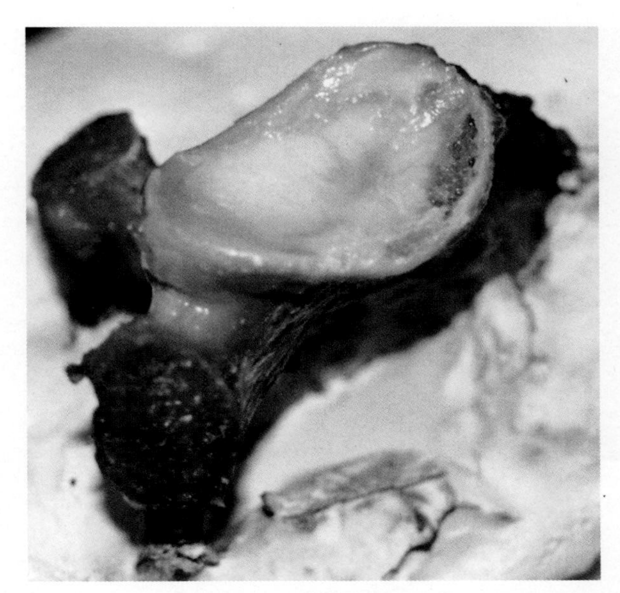

FIG. 4. Surgically created anteroinferior glenoid labral and chondral defect to simulate the findings of glenoid concavity loss in recurrent, traumatic anterior instability.

tegrity of the IGHL may be restored with this type of repair, normal glenoid concavity is diminished and the concavity–compression mechanism of stability is impaired (Fig. 7).

Revision surgery in cases of medial capsulolabral repair requires an attempt to restore normal glenoid anatomy and depth. Usually, the anterior capsular complex is found healed to the neck of the glenoid and requires mobilization. Care is taken to preserve the thickness of the glenoid labrum and capsular tissue. Once this tissue is freed from the glenoid neck, traditional repair to the rim of the glenoid is accomplished. We recommend the technique of Thomas and Matsen.[144] A standard deltopectoral approach is used with a low axillary incision. Scar and adhesions between the overlying deltoid, acromion, and conjoined tendon and the underlying rotator cuff and humeral head are mobilized. Often these adhesions are extremely thick and require sharp incision. Care should be taken not to be too superficial and risk injury to the axillary nerve as it travels on the deep surface of the deltoid. Scar on the superficial surface of the subscapularis should be excised only up to the lateral border of the conjoined tendon. Subscapularis mobilization is completed after complete incision of the tendon.

The subscapularis and capsule are sharply incised as a single unit, approximately 1 cm medial to the lesser tuberosity. A small elevator can be passed through the rotator interval and deep to the subscapularis and capsule before incision, to gauge the combined thickness, protect the long head of the biceps, and protect the underlying humeral articular surface. After capsulotomy, the subscapularis can be completely mobilized by using traction sutures to pull the tendon laterally and cause adhesions on the undersufface of the conjoined tendon to present themselves lateral to the tendon.

Upon capsulotomy, capsulolabral repair to the glenoid neck is found. This repair is mobilized by either a small periosteal elevator or sharp dissection. The anterior, nonarticular glenoid surface is burred, using the burr to contour a new glenoid rim (Fig. 8A). Three to four bone tunnels are created using a 1.5-mm wire-passer burr and a 3-0 angled curette. Each of these holes is filled with a no. 2 Polydek suture, passed with a no. 5 curved Mayo needle (see Fig. 8B). Finally, the trailing medial edge of capsule is repaired with simple suture passes, taking care to mobilize the capsule superiorly with repair (see Fig. 8C). The subscapularis and capsulotomy are closed end-to-end. We prefer an "all inside" repair performed through transosseous bone tunnels in the anterior glenoid rim because we believe this type of repair has a bunching effect on the labrum, further enhancing anterior glenoid concavity.[90,92,144] Capsulolabral repair with suture anchors can also be successful, as long as the anchors are placed directly on the glenoid rim. Typically in these situations, repair of the capsule and labrum to its true anatomic position is successful in achieving glenohumeral stability.

Postoperatively, these patients are managed as a primary instability repair. A sling is worn for 3 weeks, the patient removing the sling five times each day to perform supine active-assisted forward elevation to 90 degrees and external rotation to neutral. At 3 weeks postoperative, the sling is discontinued, and full motion is permitted. At 6 weeks postoperative, resistance exercises are begun, including rotator cuff strengthening and scapular stabilization. Noncontact athletics are permitted at 3 months postoperative, with full contact at 6 months.

Larger concavity defects occur with fracture of the glenoid rim. It has been well reported that glenoid rim fractures are associated with recurrent anterior instability.[11,63,75,92] Treatment options in the face of a glenoid rim fracture include excision of the fragment and capsulolabral

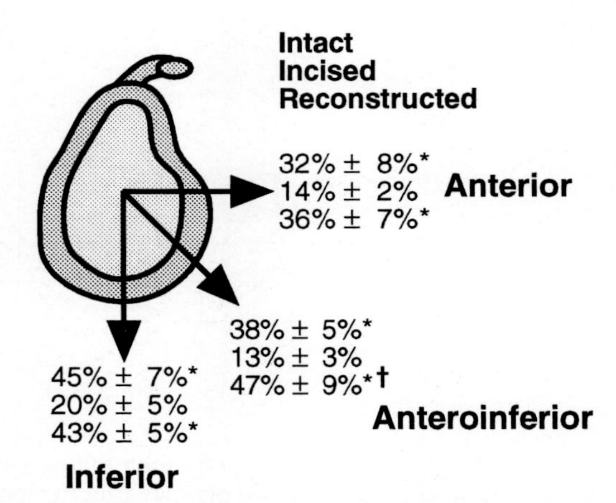

FIG. 5. Stability ratios (humeral translating force/compressive load × 100) for intact specimens, those with surgically created anteroinferior chondral–labral defects, and those surgically reconstructed. Notice that, by restoring and even enhancing glenoid concavity, stability ratios can be corrected (*$P < 0.0001$ vs. incised, $P < 0.0001$ vs. intact).

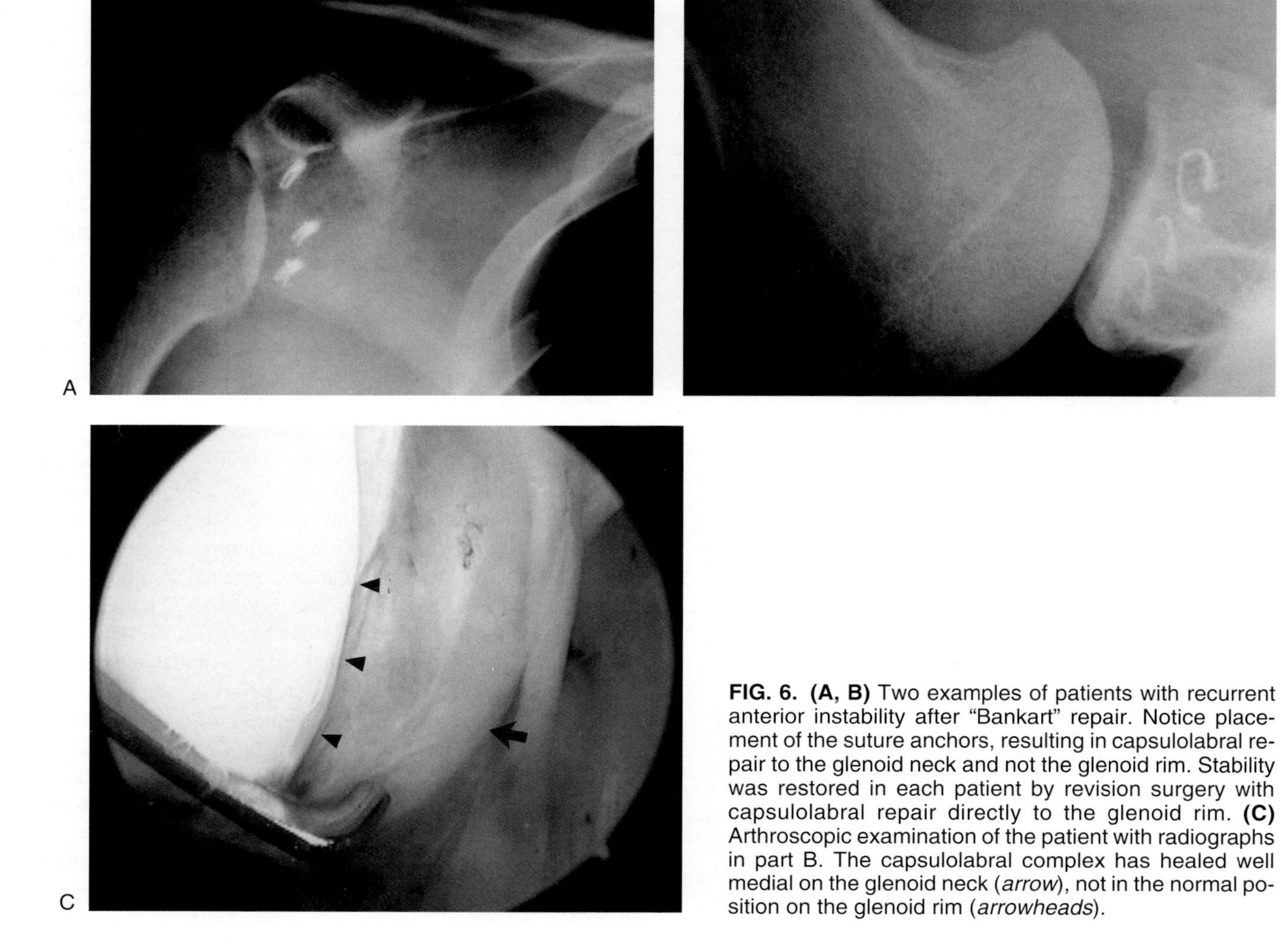

FIG. 6. (A, B) Two examples of patients with recurrent anterior instability after "Bankart" repair. Notice placement of the suture anchors, resulting in capsulolabral repair to the glenoid neck and not the glenoid rim. Stability was restored in each patient by revision surgery with capsulolabral repair directly to the glenoid rim. **(C)** Arthroscopic examination of the patient with radiographs in part B. The capsulolabral complex has healed well medial on the glenoid neck (*arrow*), not in the normal position on the glenoid rim (*arrowheads*).

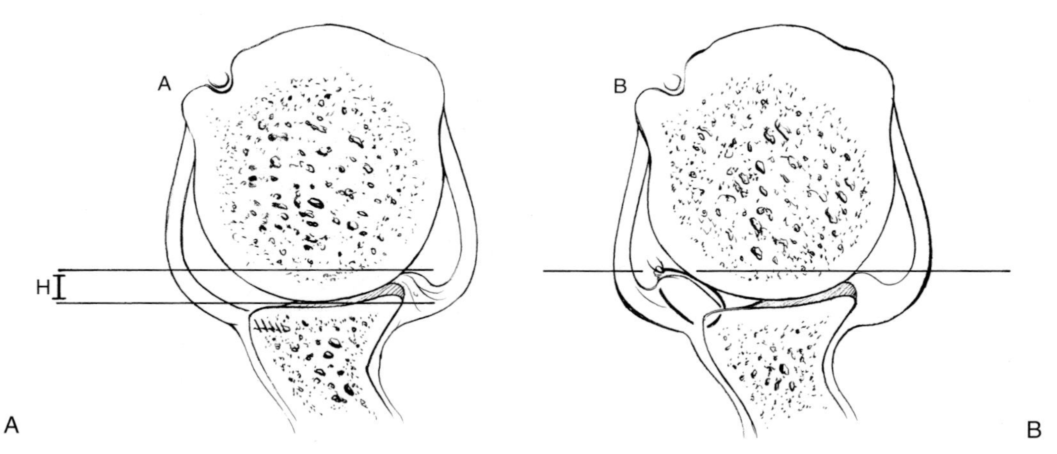

FIG. 7. (A) Capsulolabral repair to the glenoid neck fails to restore normal glenoid concavity. **(B)** Capsulolabral repair to the glenoid articular margin restores normal glenoid concavity.

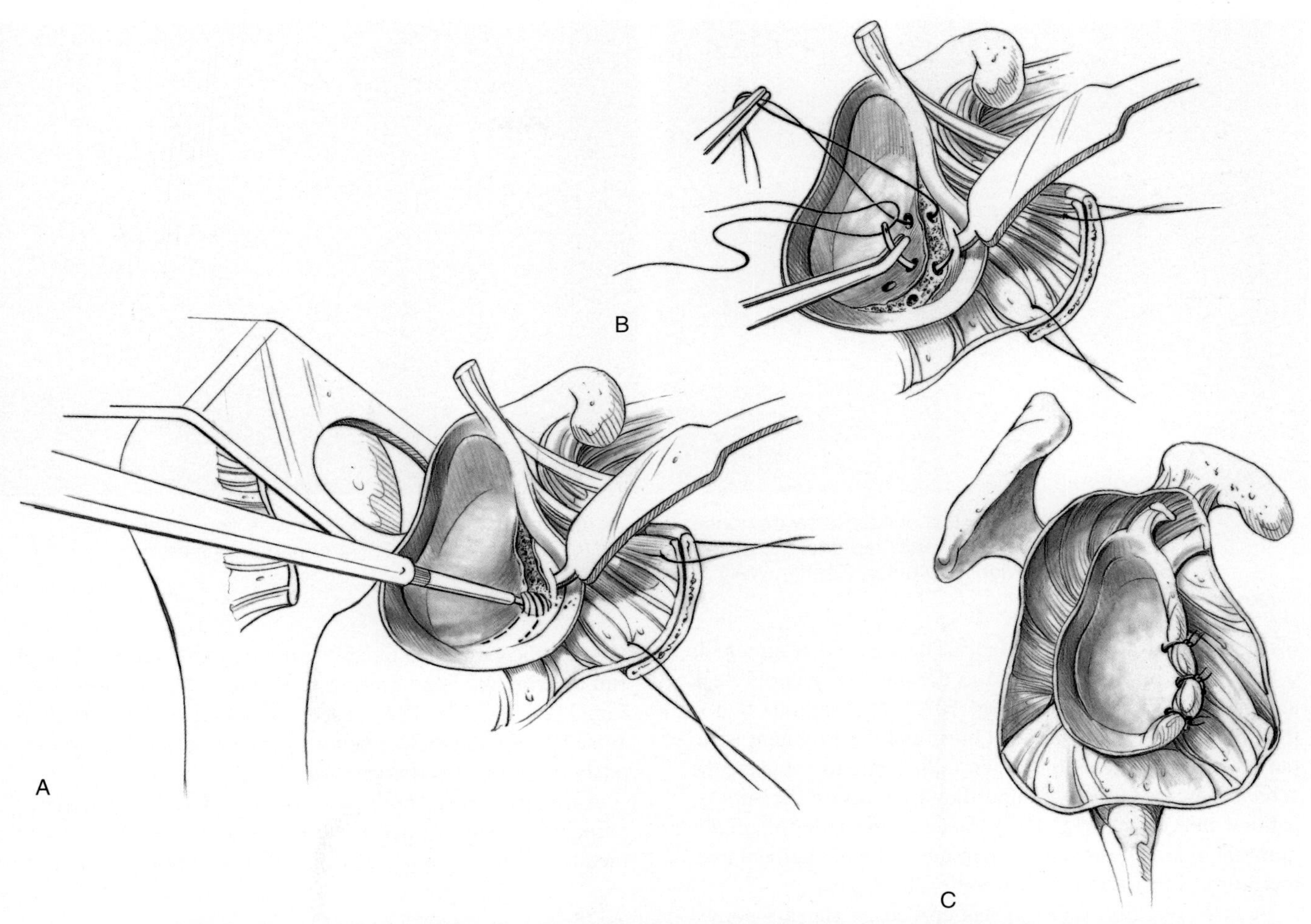

FIG. 8. **(A)** The previous medial capsulolabral repair is elevated from the glenoid neck. A high-speed burr is then used to create a lip to the typically rounded anterior glenoid rim. **(B)** Bone tunnels are made in the glenoid rim and each receives a no. 2 braided, nonabsorbable suture. **(C)** By passing the sutures in simple fashion (all-inside technique), the labrum is bunched on the glenoid rim, restoring glenoid concavity.

repair to the remaining glenoid rim versus direct internal fixation of the anterior glenoid fragment. Most authors recommend repair of the fragment if it constitutes more than 25% of the glenoid width.[11,168]

Failure to account for and reconstruct an anterior glenoid rim fracture can be a cause of instability recurrence after surgery[11] (Fig. 9A). Gerber has reported work on the effect of loss of the anteroinferior glenoid rim on stability.[38] Instead of measuring the percent loss of the glenoid rim, he recommends measuring the shortest distance from the glenoid rim just superior to the defect to the intact rim at the inferior aspect of the defect. In his study, if this distance was greater that 15 mm, the stability to translational force was decreased by over 60%. More importantly, the stability could not be corrected by ignoring the osseous lesion and repairing the capsule and labrum into the defect.

The accurate preoperative evaluation of a potential clinically significant osseous glenoid lesion is critical. Special radiographic studies, including a Garth view and West Point axillary view should be obtained. A computed tomography (CT) scan may be needed to adequately visualize and size a glenoid rim defect. Glenoid rim fractures of less than 25% of the articular width can be effectively treated by simple repair of the capsulolabral complex into the defect. If the defect involves more than 25% to 30% of the glenoid articular width, however, it must be repaired or reconstructed for successful revision surgery.

If, during revision surgery, the residual bone fragment appears viable, direct internal fixation of the fragment should be performed (see Fig. 9B). In these situations, we alter the standard Bankart approach by dividing the subscapularis and capsule as two distinct layers. The subscapularis is divided approximately 1 cm medial to the lesser tuberosity. Then, using sharp dissection or an electrocautery, the subscapularis tendon is elevated, in a medial direction, from the underlying capsule. The tendon must be freed in a medial direction past the glenoid rim fragment. The anterior capsule is then incised, allowing visualization

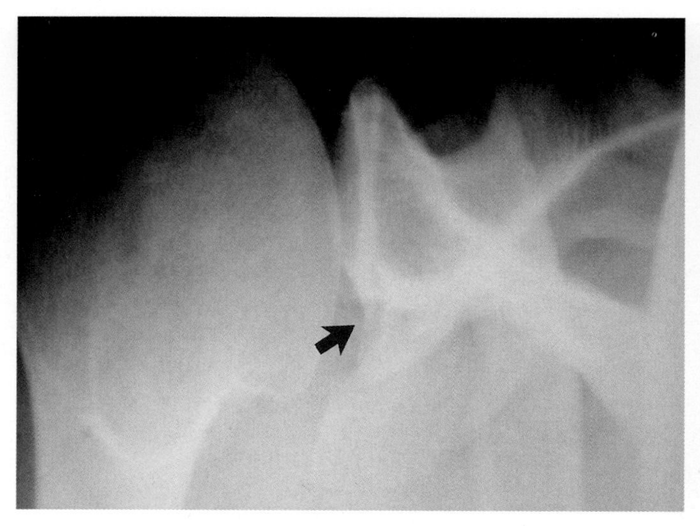

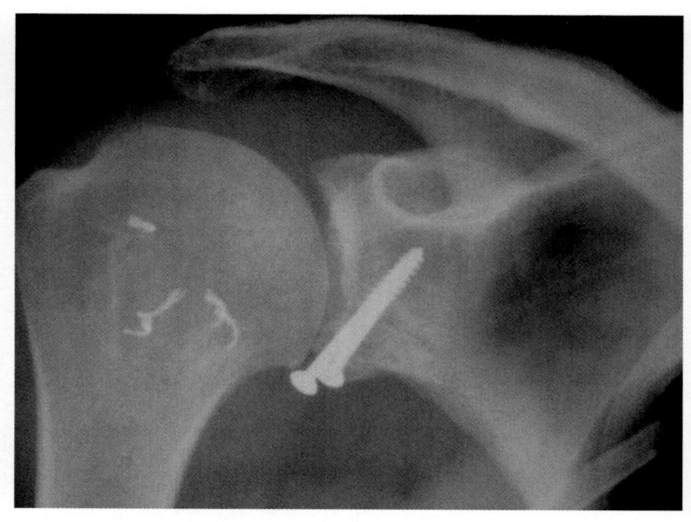

FIG. 9. **(A)** Garth apical oblique view demonstrating a large anteroinferior glenoid osseous defect (*arrow*). **(B)** Same patient after repair of the osseous lesion. (Courtesy Douglas T. Harryman II, University of Washington Medical Center, Seattle, WA.)

of the glenoid articular surface. The glenoid fragment is usually found partially healed to the anterior glenoid neck and requires mobilization (Fig. 10A). The osseous bed is then prepared by a high-speed burr, and the fragment is repaired with bicortical lag screws, taking care to not leave the screws long posteriorly where they may injure the suprascapular nerve (see Fig. 10B). Usually the anterior glenohumeral ligaments are attached to the osseous fragment and, therefore, are restored with union of the repair.

If, however, the fragment has eroded or appears nonviable, the glenoid rim must be reconstructed. Gerber has discussed reconstruction of the glenoid rim by placement of autogenous iliac crest graft, secured with bicortical screws, and fashioned to match the curvature of the native glenoid.[38] In a preliminary report, he found the technique restored stability in 12 of 13 patients, with the final patient having questionable recurrence of subluxation only. The only patients who developed progressive degenerative change were those who had some degree of degeneration preoperatively.

Our preference in these difficult situations is to use autogenous bone to fashion a graft for the rim, similar to Gerber. The surgical approach is as described earlier. The remaining atrophic glenoid fragment is excised, taking care to preserve the full length of the anterior capsuloligamentous structures. A pine cone burr is used to freshen and prepare the bed. A tricortical graft is harvested from the iliac crest. With a pine cone burr, the graft is fashioned to approximately conform to the curvature of the glenoid. Sutures of no. 2 Polydek are placed under the graft for later capsulolabral repair (Fig. 11A). The graft is then secured with bicortical lag screws, taking care to closely observe the articular surface for screw penetration and to not leave the screws long posteriorly where they may irritate the suprascapular nerve. Finally, the pine cone burr is again used to complete fashioning of the graft in situ (see Fig. 11B). With use of the previously placed sutures, the capsule is repaired directly to the native glenoid rim, leaving the bone graft in an extracapsular position (see Fig. 11C; Fig. 12). The subscapularis and capsule are then closed side-to-side. The postoperative regimen is as previously described for Bankart repair.

An alternative to bone grafting is a Bristow or Laterjet coracoid transfer. Either of these procedures would be technically easier than bone grafting of the anterior glenoid rim.

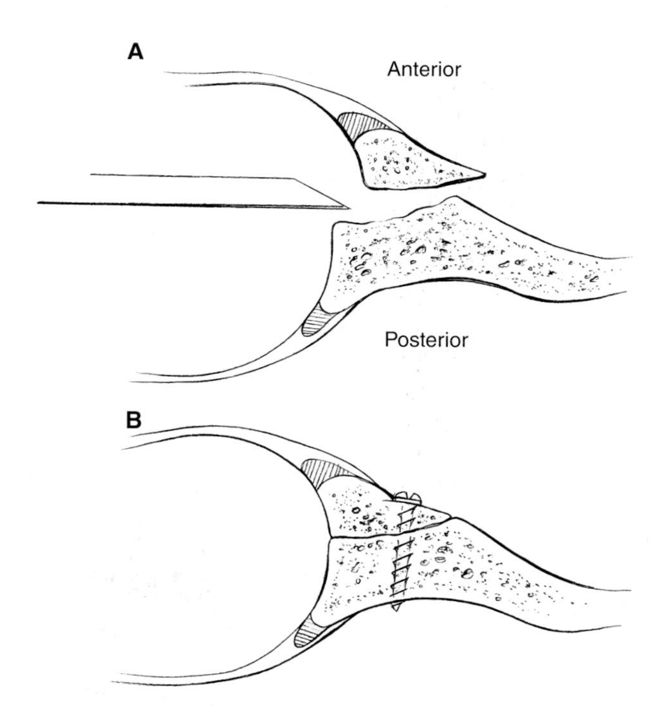

FIG. 10. **(A)** For repair of a large osseous Bankart lesion, the bone fragment is mobilized from its partially healed position on the anterior glenoid neck. **(B)** Fixation is by two 3.5-mm bicortical lag screws or 4.0-mm cannulated screws.

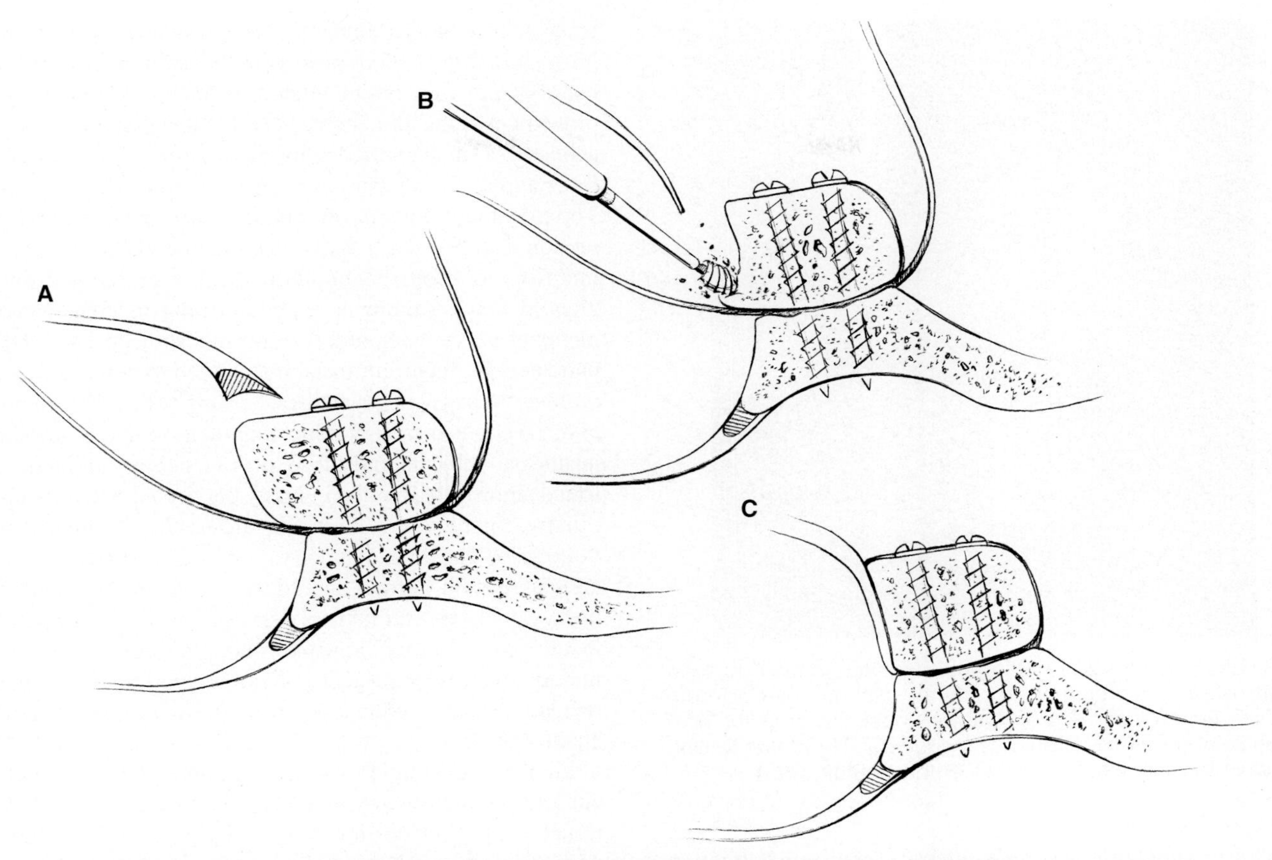

FIG. 11. **(A)** For a large osseous Bankart lesion that requires grafting, a tricortical graft is taken from the iliac crest and applied to a prepared bed on the anterior glenoid neck. Sutures are placed under the graft for later capsular repair. **(B)** The graft is burred to conform to the curvature of the normal glenoid. **(C)** When burring is completed, the anterior capsule is repaired over the graft using the previously placed sutures. This repair leaves the graft in an extracapsular, supportive position.

Coracoid transfer procedures, however, provide only a block to dislocation and do not reestablish the glenoid curvature, thereby leaving the patient susceptible to continued anterior subluxation.

Residual, Abnormal Anteroinferior Capsular Laxity

In the science of shoulder instability, there is currently ongoing debate over the presence or absence of plastic deformation of the IGHL in patients with recurrent traumatic anterior instability and, if present, its clinical significance. Bigliani et al. recently demonstrated plastic deformation of the IGHL before the ultimate failure by avulsion from the glenoid rim during stress to failure of the IGHL complex.[17] Reeves had previously confirmed these findings in older cadaveric shoulders, but found isolated capsular avulsion without plastic deformation in shoulders of younger cadavers, within the age group most likely to suffer recurrent traumatic anterior instability.[117] Recently, McMahon et al. presented work that demonstrated capsulolabral avulsion in 8 of 12 cadaveric shoulders when the application of stress was performed with the arm positioned in the critical abducted and externally rotated position.[97] More importantly, even in these older, cadaveric shoulders that are clinically and biomechanically notorious for capsular injury, the amount of plastic deformation of the anterior capsule was only 2.3 mm, a finding of questionable clinical significance.

These studies leave in question the occurrence of stretch of the IGHL as a component of recurrent traumatic anterior instability. In addition, if such plastic deformation was confirmed in the laboratory, the clinical significance is still unclear. For instance, a period of immobilization after initial dislocation might be expected to lead to scar and contracture of interstitial IGHL injury, not lengthening. Also, if a concomitant Bankart lesion was present, repeated dislocations would be expected to occur with less stress applied to the interstitial fibers of the IGHL.

Several authors have blamed residual capsular laxity as the cause of recurrent anterior instability after Bankart repair.[21,58,95,121,128,160,166,168] At the time of revision surgery, the presence of a redundant or patulous anteroinferior capsule was noted by these investigators. This finding was purely observational and no specific measurements were recorded. Rowe et al. describe a method whereby the arm is

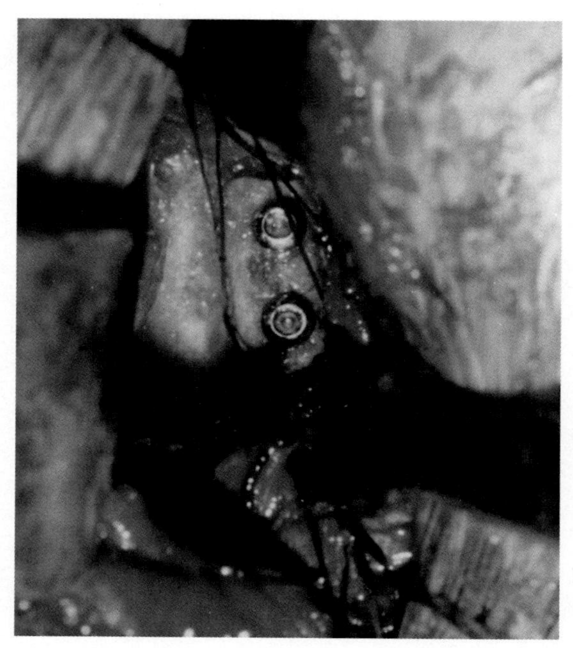

FIG. 12. Intraoperative photograph of autogenous iliac crest graft used to reconstruct an anterior osseous glenoid deficiency. Note placement of sutures under the graft for later capsulolabral repair. (Courtesy Douglas T. Harryman II, University of Washington Medical Center, Seattle, WA.)

placed in adduction and in 90 degrees of external rotation and the anteroinferior capsule is grabbed with a clamp and pulled upward.[128,168] If the capsule can be mobilized greater than 1 cm, this indicates residual capsular laxity. All of these authors described some type of capsular shifting or imbricating procedure as an integral component of the revision repair.

The difficulty in judging residual capsular redundancy, however, is differentiating capsular stretch from normal capsular laxity. Speer et al., in a recent study on the biomechanical effects of a Bankart tear, found only minor increases in anterior humeral translation after creation of a Bankart lesion.[138] This result seems to indicate that plastic deformation of the IGHL is a necessary component of recurrent traumatic anterior instability. Humeral translation and humeral instability, however, are two properties that are not only different, but also they may not be related. Humeral *translation* is the movement of the humeral head across the glenoid fossa in response to a small applied translational force (for instance, the force applied by an examiner during a drawer or sulcus test). The maximum amount of humeral translation in a given direction is a shoulder's *laxity*. Glenohumeral *instability* is the inability to keep the humeral head centered within the glenoid fossa. Lippitt et al., performing in vivo measurements of laxity in shoulders of normal subjects and those of patients with recurrent instability, failed to demonstrate differences in laxity between these groups[82] (Fig. 13). Hawkins et al., who used radiographic examination under anesthesia in normal subjects and those with unstable shoulders, also found significant overlap in laxity between the two groups.[60] Finally, Sperber et al. found no differences in intracapsular volume or capsular elasticity in unstable shoulders when compared with normal shoulders.[142] Therefore, whether or not residual capsular laxity exists as a cause of postoperative instability remains controversial. Moreover, the exact method by which a surgeon can intraoperatively differentiate residual capsular redundancy from normal capsular laxity is equally unclear.

Finally, glenohumeral dislocation under load does not occur as a gradual event, as replicated by measuring translational laxity, but occurs as a sudden and explosive event, with minimal translation before the moment of sudden dislocation (Fig. 14). The absence of significant translation before the moment of dislocation implies that glenohumeral articular congruity and glenoid concavity are the major determinants of glenohumeral stability, with ligamentous integrity serving as the final checkrein against dislocation.[32,79,84,90,137] The clinical significance of relating laxity measurements to glenohumeral instability, therefore, is unknown.

Most cases of recurrent traumatic anterior instability are attributable to the presence of an anteroinferior capsulolabral avulsion from the glenoid rim and are successfully managed by repair of this defect without any further capsular tensioning.[9,90–92,144] There are situations, however, for which true

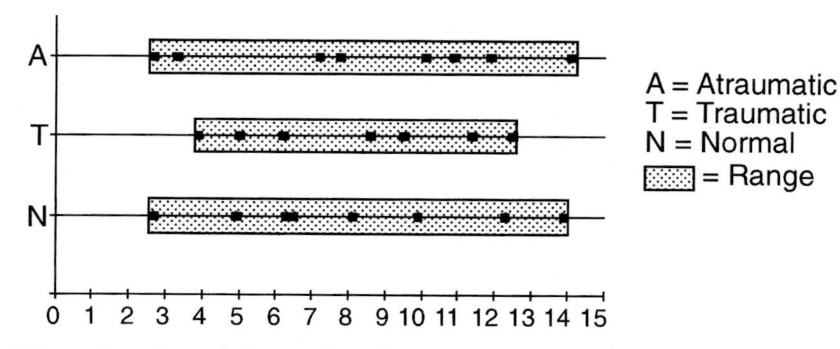

FIG. 13. In vivo laxity to anterior drawer test in normal subjects and patients with either traumatic or atraumatic instability. Notice the significant overlap in laxity between these groups. (Permission from Lippincott Publishers, ref. 82.)

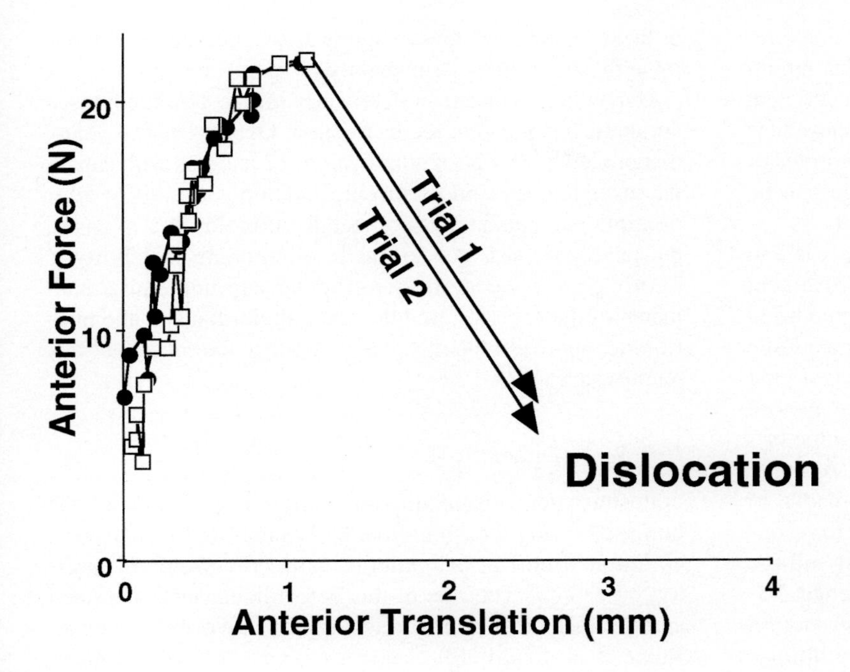

FIG. 14. Translation before dislocation in a loaded, cadaveric shoulder. Even in an older, cadaveric shoulder, there is minimal humeral translation before the explosive moment of dislocation. (Permission from JBJS, ref. 90.)

and demonstrable clinical instability exists, yet either a Bankart tear is not present or the tear appears too small to account for the patient's degree of instability. In these cases, some plication or shifting of the anteroinferior capsule may be necessary to restore stability. However, considering the unavoidable capsular tightening that occurs simply by repairing a Bankart lesion and side-to-side closure of a capsulotomy, combined with the typical postoperative scarring and contracture of the anterior soft tissues, residual or unrepaired anterior capsular laxity as a cause of postoperative instability should be considered a diagnosis of exclusion.

Residual capsular laxity as a cause of recurrence of instability after surgical repair should be considered in the following situations:

1. When true and clinically demonstrable glenohumeral instability was present at the time of the index operation and either no or a small Bankart tear was noted at entrance into the glenohumeral joint
2. When an appropriate and technically correct Bankart repair was performed at the time of the index operation and, at revision surgery, that repair is still intact despite true and clinically demonstrable instability
3. When obvious and large differences in translation on anterior drawer testing compared with the patient's contralateral shoulder are present in the absence of a large Bankart tear
4. When either no or a small Bankart tear is present in the patient with a history of repetitive microtrauma, such as throwing, swimming, or gymnastics

When other causes of instability recurrence are ruled out and one or more of the above conditions exist, stability can be restored by an anteroinferior capsular shift.[3,92,160] There are several descriptions in the literature on the technique of capsular shift, and the exact procedure is not critical (see Chapter 12). What is important is to contract the excessively lax anterior and inferior capsule without overtightening the shoulder.

Anterior Capsular Deficiency

One reason for the wonderful results after primary instability surgery is tissue quality. Typically, patients requiring surgery for recurrent traumatic anterior instability have thick, healthy anterior capsular tissue, that permits a robust repair. After repeated attempts at anterior repair, however, the anterior glenohumeral capsule may become a thin, attenuated remnant, incapable of being repaired. Preoperative workup may reveal subscapularis deficiency in these individuals (discussed later). In these difficult cases, the surgeon needs both a specific plan of attack as well as availability of alternatives to the usual capsuloligamentous repair.

Revision surgery begins by defining the humeroscapular motion interface, that plane between the underlying rotator cuff and the overlying deltoid, acromion, and conjoined tendon.[90] Initially, the surgeon may be fooled by the intact and often thickened clavipectoral fascia. However, this fascia will not move as one with the humerus during humeral rotation, being clearly differentiated from the subscapularis. All scar and adhesions within this interface are excised and the axillary and musculocutaneous nerves are located. At this juncture, the amount and quality of the subscapularis and anterior capsule can be assessed. A Joker or Freer elevator can be passed through the rotator interval and deep to the combined anterior capsule and subscapularis to gauge the combined thickness of these structures.

Occasionally, when incising the clavipectoral fascia, it instantly becomes clear that the anterior capsule and subscapularis are completely deficient. In these situations, reconstruction of the capsule is necessary. Capsular reconstruction begins by identifying the interval between deficient and normal capsule. Typically, the posteroinferior capsule is normally present. By performing a limited posteroinferior capsular shift, this normal posteroinferior capsule can be mobilized to reconstruct the anteroinferior quadrant.

Gallie and LeMesurier recommended use of fascia lata to reconstruct the anterior glenohumeral capsule as a treatment for recurrent instability.[36] This technique has been modified by Harryman to reconstruct the superior (SGHL) and middle (MGHL) glenohumeral ligaments[78] (Fig. 15). Using a pine cone burr (4 mm diameter), holes are created in the glenoid and the humeral head, these holes corresponding to the origin and insertion sites of the SGHL and MGHL. A single strip of autograft tendon is passed from lateral to medial to recreate the SGHL and then from medial to lateral to reconstruct the MGHL. With the humeral head reduced and the arm in neutral rotation, the reconstruction is tightened. Patients must be aware that they will have permanent motion restrictions, sacrificing normal motion range for stability. Postoperatively, a sling is placed for 3 weeks, with abduction and external rotation isometrics being the only exercise program. After 3 weeks, the sling is removed three to five times each day for gentle supine active-assisted forward elevation and external rotation exercises. Particularly with external rotation, patients are shown the neutral rotation point and are cautioned against attempting to stretch beyond this range. At 6 weeks postoperative, the sling is discontinued, and a gentle rotator cuff and scapular strengthening program is begun. No lifting of greater than 10 lb (4.5 kg) is permitted for 6 months. In addition, patients with heavy-labor occupations or those involved in contact sports are encouraged to discontinue these activities permanently.

Harryman's current preference is to use semitendinosus autograft for ligament reconstruction. Over the past 4 years, this procedure has been employed in 17 patients with capsular insufficiency and recurrent, disabling instability after multiple attempts at anterior stabilization. In 70% of cases, the procedure was successful in eliminating instability.[78] Thorough knowledge of the scapular and humeral attachments of the superior, middle, and anterior band of the inferior glenohumeral ligaments is essential to the success of this reconstruction.[147]

Hill–Sachs Deformity

Posterolateral osteochondral impression fracture of the humeral head, the so-called Hill–Sachs deformity, is a common finding in patients with recurrent instability.[64,65,91,92,156] The role of this defect in causing continued anterior instability after surgical repair, however, is unclear. Rowe et al. found Hill–Sachs lesions in 76% of shoulders that had recurrence of instability after surgical repair.[128] Previously, Rowe and colleagues had noted a slightly higher incidence of redislocation in those patients who had moderate or severe Hill–Sachs deformities[125].

It is rare for a humeral head defect to play an isolated role in recurrent anterior instability. The combination of a large humeral head defect and a glenoid rim defect, however, dramatically decreases the amount of humeral rotation necessary to engage the osteochondral lesion onto the anterior glenoid rim, potentially leading to glenohumeral dislocation (Fig. 16). A surgeon who is considering the effect of a

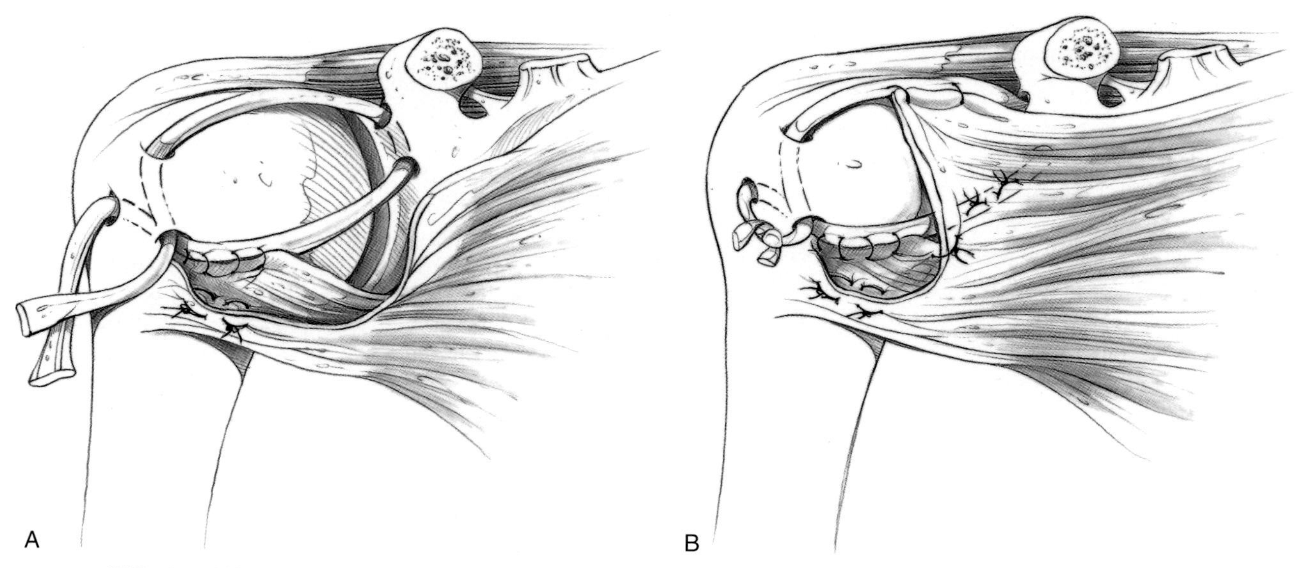

FIG. 15. (A) Technique to reconstruct severe loss of anterior subscapularis and capsular tissue. The posteroinferior capsule is shifted to reconstruct the anteroinferior quadrant. Autogenous tendon graft is then woven through drill holes in the glenoid and humerus. This graft recreates the superior and middle glenohumeral ligaments. **(B)** The graft is secured with the glenohumeral joint located and the arm in neutral rotation. Remnant subscapularis tendon can be secured to the shifted capsule and the tendinous autograft.

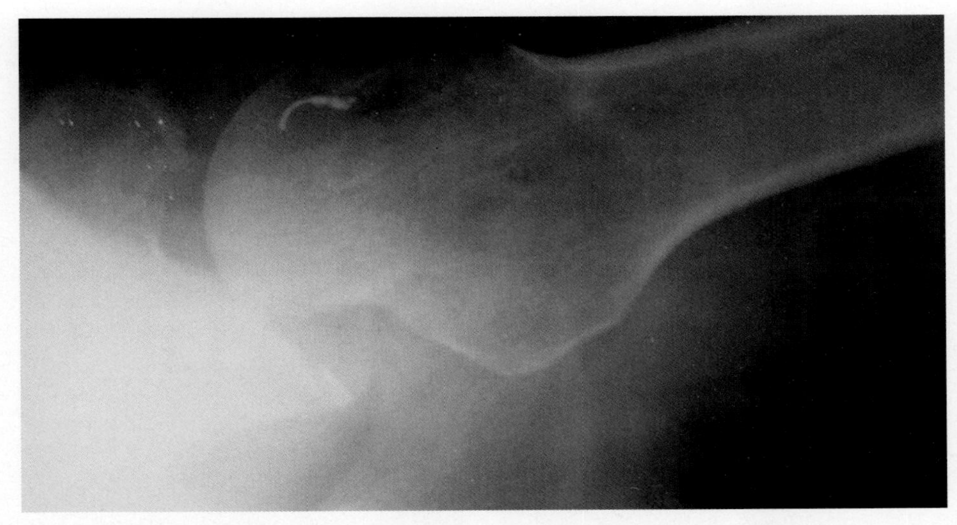

FIG. 16. Axillary radiograph of a 26-year-old man with continued anterior instability after a Bankart repair and capsular shift procedure. The combination of a large Hill–Sachs deformity and osseous Bankart lesion results in contact of the Hill–Sachs lesion with the glenoid rim with minimal glenohumeral rotation.

Hill–Sachs lesion should obtain a CT scan preoperatively to measure the dimensions of the defect to help select the most appropriate surgical option.

At surgery, when a posterior Hill–Sachs lesion comes in contact with the anterior glenoid rim before terminal external rotation, several solutions exist. The simplest and often the most effective answer is to limit the patient's external rotation by a slight imbrication of the capsule or subscapularis. Surprisingly little decrease in external rotation is required to exclude the Hill–Sachs lesion from contact. Each centimeter of capsular or tendinous shortening diminishes humeral rotation by approximately 20 degrees.[52]

Another method to account for a large Hill–Sachs lesion is to render the defect extraarticular. Connolly has reported transfer of the infraspinatous with a portion of the greater tuberosity into the defect, thereby leaving the lesion extraarticular.[24] Subsequently, with humeral external rotation, the lesion can no longer contact the anterior glenoid rim.

Humeral osteotomy has also been described as a method of treating a large Hill–Sachs defect. Weber et al. have reported humeral rotational osteotomy as a treatment for severe posterolateral humeral head defects, the goal being to rotate the Hill–Sachs lesion away from potential glenoid contact.[156] They reported a redislocation rate of 5.7% after this procedure, but it is important to recognize that they include subscapularis shortening as part of their technique.

On rare occasions, the posterolateral humeral defect will be so severe that it involves more than 40% of the articular surface of the head. In this situation, the lesion will contact the anterior glenoid with minimal external rotation. To preserve any glenohumeral external rotation while providing stability, some extension of the humeral articular surface is required. Gerber et al. have reported on the successful treatment of a reverse Hill–Sachs deformity with placement of an osteochondral allograft into the defect.[41] We have had some success in the treatment of large Hill–Sachs deformities by reconstruction of the defect using an osteochondral femoral head allograft (Fig. 17). In rare cases, a humeral hemiarthroplasty may be indicated.

Voluntary Instability

In 1973, Rowe et al. published their comprehensive and classic description of voluntary glenohumeral instability.[126] In that study, patients with underlying psychiatric dysfunction did poorly with all types of treatment. For most patients, a rehabilitation program for muscle strength and coordination was recommended.

In any patient for whom multiple surgical reconstructions have failed to provide stability, voluntary instability should be considered. It is important to recognize, however, that having the ability to volitionally subluxate or dislocate the shoulder does not necessarily place a patient in this category.[34,59,150] Warren separates volitional instability into positional and muscular types.[150] The positional group can cause an instability event by arm movement. The muscular group can cause instability by simple muscle contraction. Surgery in this second group is unlikely to be successful. Neer has long discussed the difference between the patient who can cause an instability event and the one who either has great secondary gain in the event or who has a desire to cause instability.[102,150] It is in this second group that surgery should be avoided.

Severe Traumatic Event

The literature is somewhat unclear about the role of trauma in causing failure of an instability repair. Some investigators have found recurrent trauma in the face of an ad-

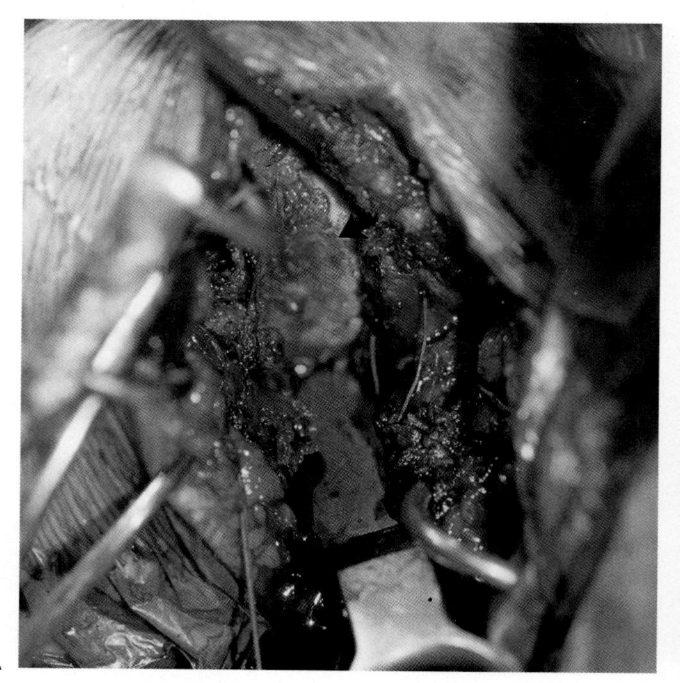
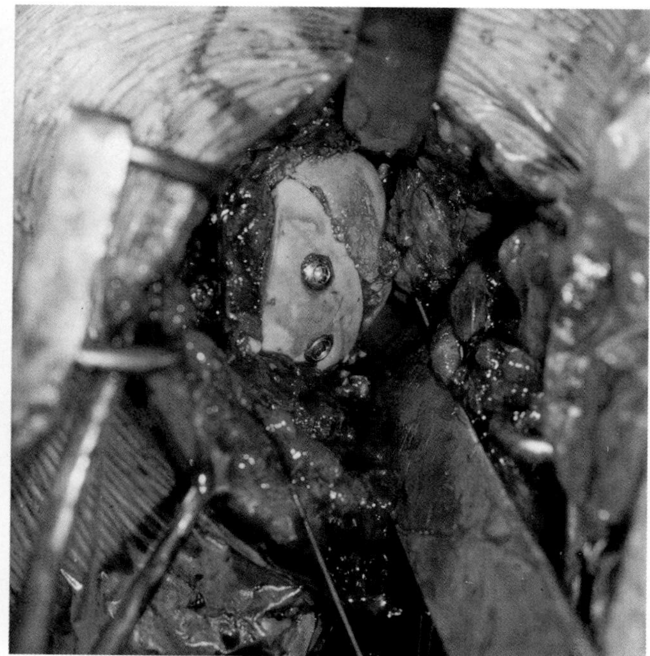
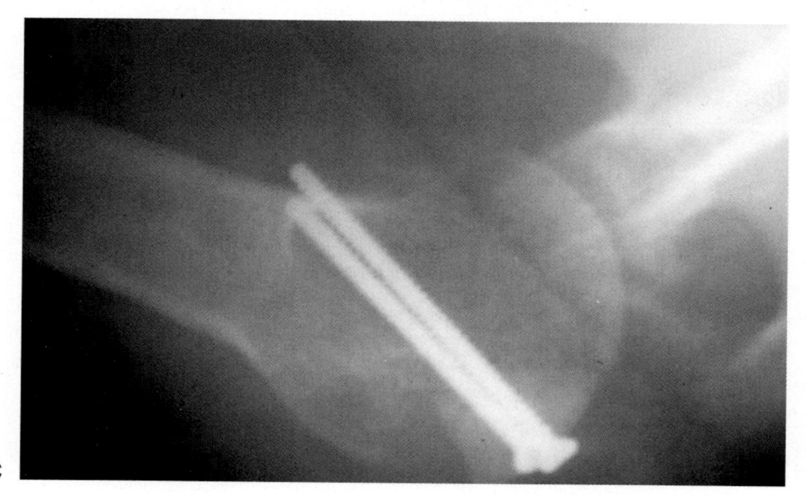

FIG. 17. (A) Intraoperative photograph of a large Hill–Sachs lesion (*arrow*) seen through a posterior approach. The normal humeral articular surface (*medial*) is to the right. **(B)** Reconstruction of the Hill–Sachs lesion with placement of an osteochondral allograft. **(C)** Postoperative radiograph demonstrating extension of the humeral articular surface by the allograft.

equate index repair to be a significant cause of instability after repair.[21,58] Others have determined that failure of instability repair typically occurs secondary to a failure of diagnosis or technique, not secondary to trauma.[95,128]

Clearly, if significant force is applied to the hand or arm while in a vulnerable abducted, extended, and externally rotated position, failure of even the strongest of repairs can occur. Trauma as the sole cause of failure, however, should be a diagnosis of exclusion. Only when misdiagnosis and persistent structural pathology are ruled out can significant trauma be blamed for instability recurrence.

Loss of Motion

Possibly the most common nonphysiologic outcome after surgery for recurrent traumatic instability, but infrequently reported as an actual complication, is loss of motion. In fact, limiting external rotation to a certain value is often stated as a desired surgical goal.[92] Often, some imbrication or "shifting" of the anterior capsule is recommended to correct presumed plastic deformation. If, however, a normal length or fibrotic, shortened capsule is imbricated at the time of Bankart repair, motion restriction will occur.

Limitation of a patient's normal, physiologic glenohumeral external rotation may have serious consequences. Minor deficits in external rotation can lead to a decrease in a patient's ability to assume the late-cocking position and, therefore, can decrease the velocity of a throw or serve.[61,85,146] Major reductions in external rotation can have disastrous consequences. Harryman et al. described obligate humeral translation, whereby the tightened anterior capsule at terminal external rotation forces the humeral head to translate posteriorly.[54] Hawkins and Angelo reported on seven patients in whom previous Putti-Platt procedures with overtightening of the anterior structures resulted in glenohumeral arthritis.[55] When the anterior structures are too tight, obligate humeral translation occurs with minimal external rotation, forcing the humeral head in a posterior direction and creating a shear force on the posterior glenoid, resulting in articular degeneration. This degenerative process, which Matsen has referred to as capsulorrhaphy arthropathy, is not only related to the Putti-Platt procedure, but can also be seen in any patient who has nonphysiologic, asymmetrical tightening of the capsule or rotator cuff tendon unit.[90]

The treatment for an excessively tight anterior capsulorrhaphy is to reverse the altered biomechanics. Specifically, abnormally shortened anterior soft tissues must be lengthened. If the original surgical procedure involved an imbrication or transfer of the subscapularis, a subscapularis release can be performed as described by MacDonald, et al.[88] The technique begins with release of the subscapularis from its insertion (original or transferred). The humerus is then externally rotated to the desired position. With external rotation, the subscapularis tendon is drawn medially. At the point of desired external rotation, the subscapularis tendon is repaired to the underlying glenohumeral capsule.

If capsular contracture is also anticipated or if greater than 20 degrees of rotational correction is necessary, a coronal Z-plasty of the combined subscapularis and anterior capsule is required.[90,102] The technique is begun by passing a small elevator through the rotator interval and posterior to the anterior glenohumeral capsule to gauge the combined thickness of the subscapularis and capsule. Using sharp dissection and beginning approximately 1 cm medial to the lesser tuberosity, the superficial subscapularis tendon is cut in a longitudinal fashion until 50% of the combined subscapularis–capsular thickness is divided. Then, in the coronal plane, the superficial subscapularis is elevated off the underlying deep capsule. This coronal division is taken medially to a point just lateral to the palpable glenoid rim. The deep layer is then longitudinally incised, making sure to remain lateral to the glenoid labrum. The medial capsulolabral glenoid attachment should not be disturbed during this technique. At arthrotomy, debridement of osteophytes, loose bodies, and hypertrophic synovium can be accomplished. By repairing the lateral edge of the superficial flap to the medial edge of the deep, as much as 2 cm of length (40 degrees of rotation) can be gained. To date, we know of no patient who has redeveloped anterior instability regardless of the amount of external rotation gained by this method.

Capsulorraphy Arthropathy

Repeated attempts at external rotation against anterior capsular restriction may lead to capsulorraphy arthropathy.[55,90] Typical findings are severe glenohumeral destruction, eccentric posterior glenoid wear, and posterior subluxation. For established capsulorraphy arthropathy with subluxation, subscapularis lengthening and joint debridement is unlikely to provide any longstanding benefit. If symptoms warrant, the most successful treatment is shoulder arthroplasty. Because of the tendency towards posterior glenoid deficiency and subluxation, humeral hemiarthroplasty alone may lead to continued posterior subluxation. Therefore, despite the often young age of these unfortunate patients, total shoulder replacement is usually indicated.

Bigliani et al. reported on 17 patients who underwent shoulder arthroplasty for end-stage capsulorraphy arthropathy.[18] The average time between instability repair and arthroplasty was 16 years. At a mean follow-up of 3 years, 77% of patients obtained a satisfactory result. Although these results are good, they are less than what would be expected after arthroplasty for osteoarthritis. Specific surgical problems were distorted anatomy, anterior soft-tissue contracture, and posterior glenoid deficiency.

Subscapularis Failure

Rupture of the subscapularis after an anterior instability repair is increasingly recognized as a cause of surgical failure and postoperative disability.[47,169] Patients usually present with pain that fails to subside postoperatively, weakness, tenderness over the lesser tuberosity, apprehension, and possibly recurrent instability. Physical examination reveals an increase in passive external rotation relative to the normal side, weakness or pain on active internal rotation, and inability to perform a lumbar lift-off test as described by Gerber.[39] The diagnosis can be made on physical examination alone but, if uncertainty remains, magnetic resonance imaging (MRI) may be helpful. Usually the patient will give a history of persistent postoperative pain that fails to abate during the normal rehabilitation period or a traumatic event in the early postoperative period that initiates symptoms.

The initial step in the management of subscapularis repair failure is prophylaxis. Greis et al. have questioned whether early, aggressive mobilization after instability surgery may lead to an increase in subscapularis failure.[47] Motion exercises within the first 3 to 6 weeks after instability repair should not be performed to the point of tension on the subscapularis repair.

Mobilization and repair of the ruptured subscapularis tendon can be a challenging undertaking, especially if the patient presents late after subscapularis failure.[169] The subscapularis tendon will often retract under the conjoined tendon where it adheres to the surrounding tissues. Subsequent attempts at mobilization can be extremely hazardous to important neurovascular structures. Also, the upper, middle, and lower subscapular nerves usually insert more lateral than would be expected.[23,167] Dissection medially on the superficial surface of the subscapularis may result in denervation.

Repair of the ruptured subscapularis, once it is adequately mobilized, can also be formidable. If sufficient quality tendon tissue remains on the muscle and bone insertion, direct tendinous repair is performed. If the lower half of the subscapularis tendon remains intact, it is separated from any re-

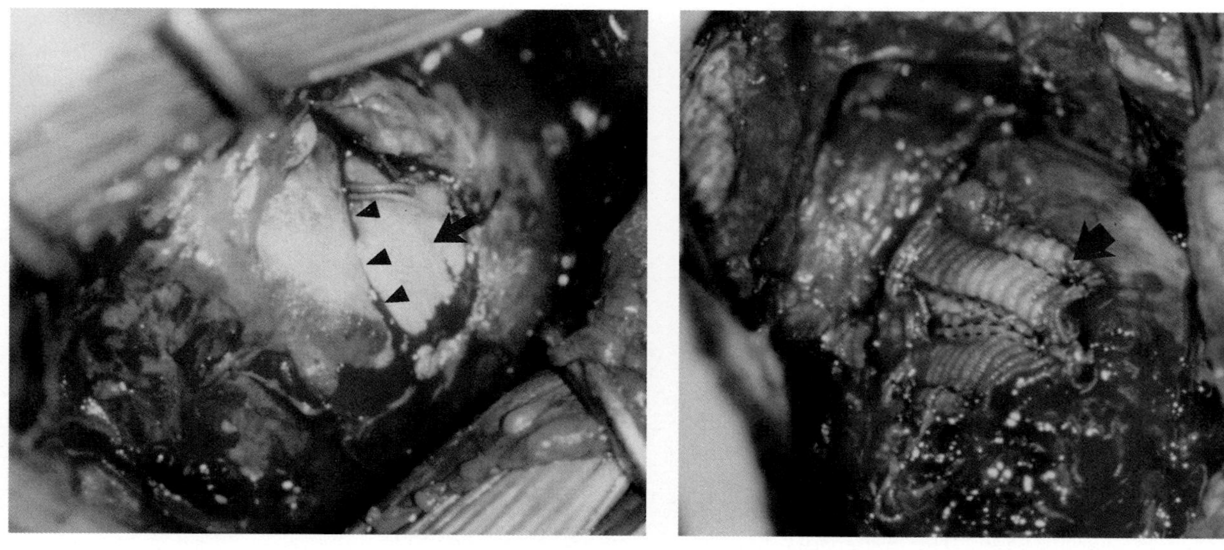

FIG. 18. (A) Intraoperative photograph of the left shoulder of a patient who had failure of the subscapularis repair after a previous Bankart repair. The *arrowheads* demonstrate the retracted subscapularis edge with the arrow showing the underlying exposed humeral head. **(B)** Repair of the subscapularis and reinforcement of thin tissue with a Dacron graft (*arrow*).

maining capsule and transferred superiorly. Usually, the humeral side has only a remnant of tissue and repair of the tendon through bone tunnels at the articular margin adjacent to the lesser tuberosity is required. On occasion, we have found patients who have extremely poor subscapularis tissue. In these circumstances, we have reinforced the subscapularis repair with a Dacron graft (Fig. 18). The Dacron is used primarily to protect and augment the tendon repair or reinforce large defects. We do not use the graft to span a full-thickness defect, but only to reinforce thin tissue.

The optimal treatment of an irreparable, full-thickness subscapularis defect is controversial. Wirth et al. have recommended superior transfer of the clavicular head of the pectoralis major to restore stability, with excellent results.[161] Because the pectoralis major and subscapularis share many actions, we have not chosen to use this transfer, for fear of further weakening these functions. In addition, the pectoralis major has an anterior force vector on the humeral head, as opposed to the posteriorly directed vector of the subscapularis. The pectoralis, therefore, while providing anterior soft tissue, does not provide a stabilizing vector. If the patient's problem is anterior tissue loss, an irreparable subscapularis, and recurrent instability, we resort to an anterior autograft tendinous weave, as discussed previously.

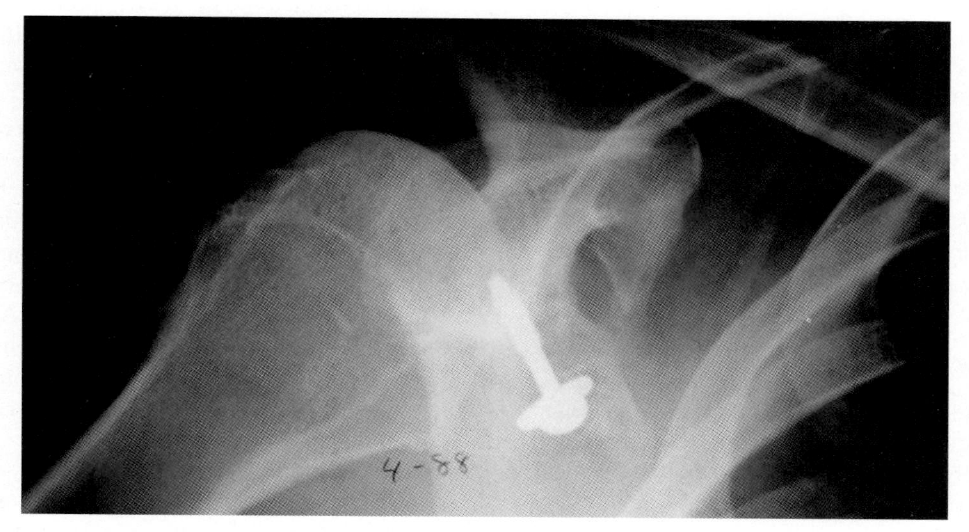

FIG. 19. A 26-year-old man, 3 years after a Bristow reconstruction. He developed recurrent dislocations and was noted to have a loose screw and coracoid nonunion. (Courtesy Frederick A. Matsen III, University of Washington Medical Center, Seattle, WA.)

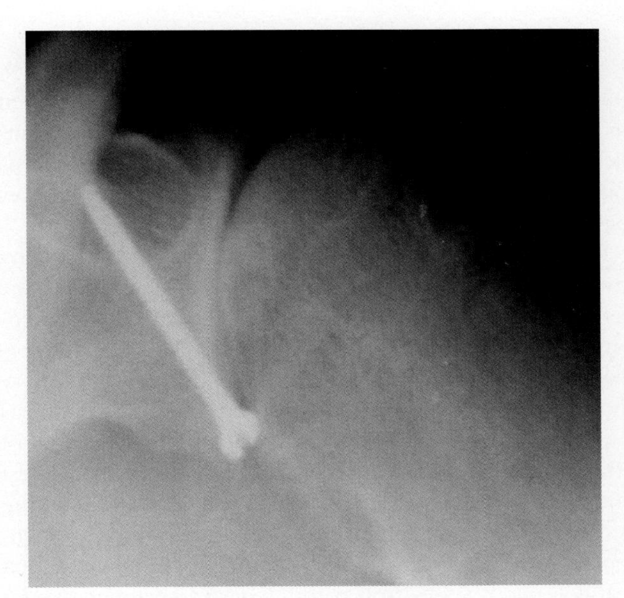

FIG. 20. A 36-year-old man, 12 years after a Bristow reconstruction, presented with increased pain and decreased range of motion. The screw head has begun to erode the humeral articular surface.

Hardware Complications

Any foreign object placed within the vicinity of the glenohumeral joint has the potential to loosen and migrate. The great range of the glenohumeral joint and significant soft-tissue tensile loads put enormous demands on any fixation device. Hardware failure or loosening can be seen at any point in the postoperative period, from within weeks to years after surgery. Metal that was safely away from the articular surfaces at placement can later become a constant articular gouge during glenohumeral motion. More seriously, loose hardware in the shoulder can migrate significant distances to threaten vital structures.

The largest series in the literature of problems in the shoulder after placement of hardware was reported by Zuckerman and Matsen.[170] Screws and staples placed to secure a transferred coracoid or plicate an anterior capsule were usually at fault. Most of the patients required reoperation and 41% percent had significant chondral injury noted at reoperation. Norris and Bigliani noted "avoidable" hardware complications in 40% of the patients in their series of failed instability repairs.[107] In particular, coracoid screws placed during the Bristow operation have caused problems.[8,30,70,108,170] (Figs. 19 and 20).

The simplest method of preventing complications of hardware is to not use it at all. All anatomic repairs for anterior instability can be performed without implanted devices. Although metal suture anchors may shorten operative time and are safe in virtually all cases, they are not without risk; anchors can loosen or become prominent, hastening chondral degeneration.

If the patient requires revision surgery, creating strong bone tunnels in an anterior glenoid that has been filled with suture anchors can be a formidable challenge. Often, suture anchors are placed medial to the anatomic glenoid rim. During revision, we have had success using the residual bone defect after removal of the suture anchor as the nonarticular side of the bone tunnel for suture placement. We will often place a small amount of cancellous autograft into the remaining defects (Fig. 21). Fracture of the glenoid rim, however, is a greater risk during revision surgery requiring anchor removal.

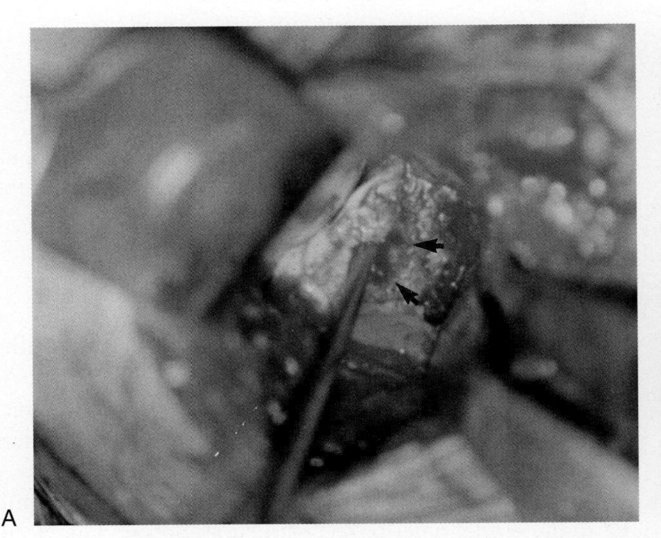

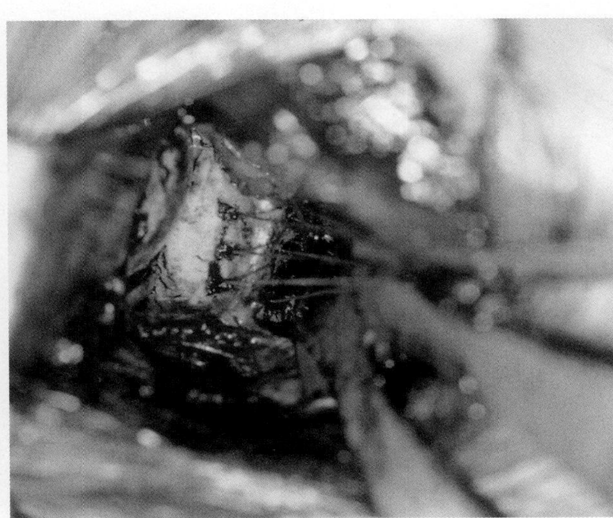

FIG. 21. (A) Intraoperative photograph of a right shoulder during revision Bankart surgery after previous suture anchor repair. Because of their location and size, the suture anchors required removal, leaving large osseous defects in the anterior glenoid neck (*arrows*). **(B)** The osseous defects were used as the nonarticular side of the bone tunnels and a nonabsorbable, braided suture has been passed for capsulolabral repair. The defects are then packed with cancellous graft.

Neurovascular Injury

Anterior instability surgery may jeopardize the anterior neurovascular structures. Richards et al. have reported on neurologic injury after anterior instability surgery, specifically Putt-Platt and Bristow operations.[120] The most common nerve involved was the musculocutaneous nerve, with the axillary second (Fig. 22). Flatow has performed anatomic dissections of the musculocutaneous nerve and found the nerve to enter the conjoined tendon as near as 2 cm to the coracoid process.[31] The nerve, therefore, is particularly at risk during procedures that involve coracoid osteotomy or transfer.

Because of its direct relation to the inferior glenohumeral capsule, the axillary nerve is at particular risk during instability surgery.[86] Richards reported two axillary nerve injuries in his series, one of these caused by a suture around the nerve.[120] The single best way to avoid injuring the axillary nerve is to constantly be sure of its location. We always directly localize the nerve after incision of the clavipectoral fascia, as recommended by Rockwood.[92] Throughout the procedure the nerve is palpated and localized. Finally, before closure, the nerve is once again palpated or visualized. This final step is critical in postoperative decision making should the patient awake with an axillary nerve palsy. If the nerve was palpably or visually intact at the end of the procedure, the surgeon can be much more comfortable with a provisional diagnosis of neuropraxic injury and may wait for recovery.

Ho and Cofield recently reported an incidence of neurologic injury in patients undergoing instability surgery of 8.2%.[62] These were predominantly neuropraxic injuries of the brachial plexus. All patients showed signs of neurologic recovery by 3 months after surgery and, at a mean of 8.4 years follow-up, 19 of 24 patients had complete recovery. We advocate an open-blade retractor with a spring lock mechanism that will release before undue tension is placed on the brachial plexus, although this method will not completely prevent neuropraxic injury.[52] If the procedure lasts longer than expected, the retractor should be occasionally released to restore blood flow to the brachial plexus.

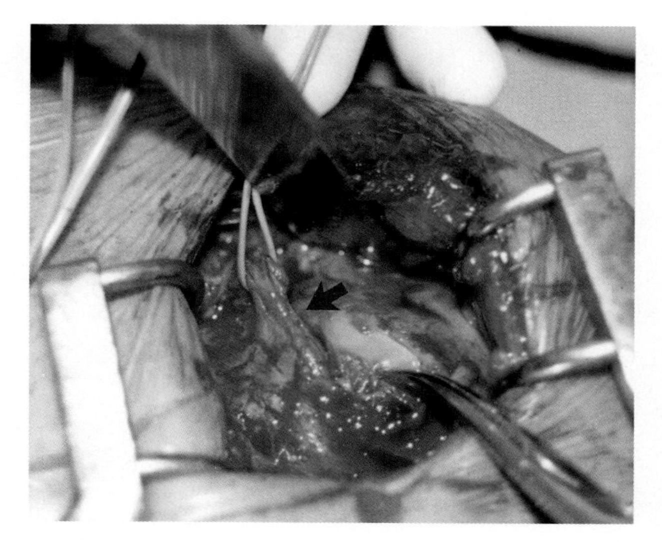

FIG. 22. A 28-year-old man with complete absence of musculocutaneous nerve function after a reported revision Bankart repair with capsular shift. On exploration, a subscapularis repair suture (hemostat) was found around the musculocutaneous nerve (*arrow*).

If postoperative examination reveals a mononeuropathy involving the axillary or musculocutaneous nerve, and the nerves were not palpated and known to be intact before closure, an electromyography study (EMG) should be performed immediately. EMG within the first 24 hours of injury should be able to demonstrate axonotmesis. If axonotmesis is confirmed, immediate nerve exploration with removal of offending suture or nerve repair is indicated. Because most injuries are neuropraxic, any mononeuropathy involving nerves that were palpably intact at closure or any polyneuropathy can be treated with observation. Neurologic deficit that does not reverse itself within 6 weeks postoperative requires an EMG. If the EMG is consistent with neuropraxic injury, further observation is appropriate and, as demonstrated by Ho and Coefield, clinical signs of neurologic recovery should become obvious by 3 months.[62] Should the findings be consistent with axonal interruption, however, immediate exploration with possible repair or cable graft is necessary.

Vascular injuries secondary to instability surgery are exceedingly rare. Most of the reports in the literature concern late axillary artery problems secondary to loose Bristow screws.[8,30,70] Both Artz et al. and Iftikhar et al. described axillary artery pseudoanuerysms caused by loose Bristow screws. The diagnosis was initially made clinically by neurologic loss associated with the compressive effects of the pseudoanuerysm, with the diagnosis confirmed by arteriography. In both of their reports, despite prompt diagnosis and exploration, permanent neurologic loss ensued.

OPEN REPAIRS FOR POSTERIOR INSTABILITY

The causes of failure after posterior instability repair mimic those of anterior repairs. There are, however, several failure mechanisms unique to posterior repairs (Table 3).

Recurrence of Instability

The causes of recurrent posterior glenohumeral instability as well as the best surgical correction remain uncertain. As would then be expected, the results of surgery for unidirectional posterior instability are variable and often much less gratifying than those for anterior instability.

Many of the causes for postoperative instability are similar to those after anterior reconstruction. Specifically, accurate diagnosis is critical. Because recurrent anterior instability is much more common in frequency than recurrent posterior, it is easy to misdiagnose a posterior dislocator simply on a statistical basis (see Fig. 1). On the other hand, if the

TABLE 3. *Causes of failure of open posterior repair*

Recurrence of instability
Degenerative arthritis
Coracoid impingement syndrome

true diagnosis is multidirectional or even anterior instability, posterior repair may accentuate the underlying problem.

The actual incidence of recurrent instability after open posterior repair has been reported as extremely variable and dependent on the index procedure. Surgical procedures for posterior instability can be divided into osseous, soft-tissue, or combination. The most common osseous procedure performed is posterior glenoid osteotomy. Scott reported the use of posterior glenoid osteotomy to treat recurrent posterior instability.[130] In his initial report of three patients, one of the three suffered from anterior instability postoperatively. When using a similar technique, Kretzler reported a recurrence rate of posterior instability of 14%.[74] In 1984, Hawkins et al. reported a recurrence of instability rate of 41% after posterior glenoid osteotomy, posterior capsular plication, and infraspinatous imbrication.[59]

Soft-tissue reconstructions have an even more widely reported recurrence rate. Boyd and Sisk reported their results of posterior capsular imbrication, with and without posterior transfer of the long head of the biceps tendon, and found no recurrences at longer than 2 years postoperative.[19] Hurley and colleagues, on the other hand, reported a recurrence of instability rate of 72% after soft-tissue reconstruction for posterior instability.[69] When Hawkins et al. reviewed their cases of posterior capsular and infraspinatous imbrication, they found a recurrence rate of 83%.[59] Regardless of the technique used, the overall recurrence rate in that study was 50%. Tibone and Ting reported recurrence of instability in 6 of 20 patients who underwent staple posterior capsulorrhaphy.[145]

Some investigators, however, have reported better results and lower recurrence rates with posterior instability repairs. Fronek et al. reported 11 patients who underwent posterior capsulorraphy with or without posterior bone block and found recurrence of instability in only 1 of those patients.[34] Bigliani and colleagues reported the results of posteroinferior capsular shift in 35 patients with posterior instability.[16] At a mean follow-up of 5 years, only 4 patients suffered from recurrence.

Hawkins used CT scan to analyze shoulders after posterior glenoid osteotomy.[57] He noted several potential complications, including under correction of version, intraarticular fracture, graft extrusion, and osteoarthritis. The rate of instability recurrence was 17%.

The exact rate of recurrence of posterior instability after surgical repair remains unknown. Much of the difficulty lies in differences in diagnosis and the wide variety of available surgical techniques. What is clear, however, is that recurrence of instability is more common after posterior repair than after anterior.

Given the wide variety of surgical procedures used to treat posterior instability, an exact cause of recurrence is likely to be elusive. As with anterior instability, assuring an accurate diagnosis is critical, including unidirectional versus multidirectional as well as anterior versus posterior. Most importantly, voluntary instability must be excluded. In cases of recurrence, a CT scan is indicated to accurately evaluate glenoid version. If greater than 20 degrees of retroversion is found, a posterior glenoplasty is indicated as part of the revision procedure. In addition, given the high rate of recurrence of posterior instability, glenoplasty should be combined with a posterior capsulorraphy. Postoperatively, these patients should be maintained in a spica cast for 6 weeks, with a cuff strengthening program to follow. Although gently forward elevation and external rotation stretching is permitted, patients are counseled not to stretch to obtain internal rotation range.

Degenerative Joint Disease

The technique of posterior glenoid osteotomy is fraught with difficulty. Of particular note is the possibility of extension of the osteotomy into the articular surface. The classic technique is described as ending at the anterior glenoid neck such that the glenoid can be "cracked" open and hinged on the anterior cortex. Unfortunately, it is dangerously easy to enter the joint with the osteotomy cut or for the crack to propagate into the joint (Fig. 23). Entrance into the glenoid articular surface will predispose the shoulder to arthritic degeneration.

Johnston et al. described a case of glenohumeral arthritis requiring total shoulder arthroplasty in a patient 5 months after posterior glenoid osteotomy.[72] The authors blamed possible intraarticular extension of the osteotomy as the cause of the rapidly progressive chondral degeneration. Hawkins et al. reported avascular necrosis of an isolated posterior glenoid rim fragment after extension of the osteotomy into the joint.[59] Hawkins noted osteoarthritis in 1 of 12 patients after posterior glenoid osteotomy.[57]

The treatment of glenohumeral degeneration after posterior glenoid osteotomy is difficult. Ultimately, most of these patients will require total shoulder arthroplasty, regardless of their young age. Technically, restoring normal glenoid component version may require posterior support, including bone grafting.

Coracoid Impingement Syndrome

Posterior glenoid osteotomy is a recommended surgical option in the treatment of recurrent posterior instability. Theoretically, if the glenoid version is overcorrected, the humeral head will have a tendency toward anteromedial orientation. This nonphysiologic alignment can result in contact between the anterior humeral head and the coracoid process, the so-called coracoid impingement syndrome.

Gerber et al. reported a combined clinical and anatomic

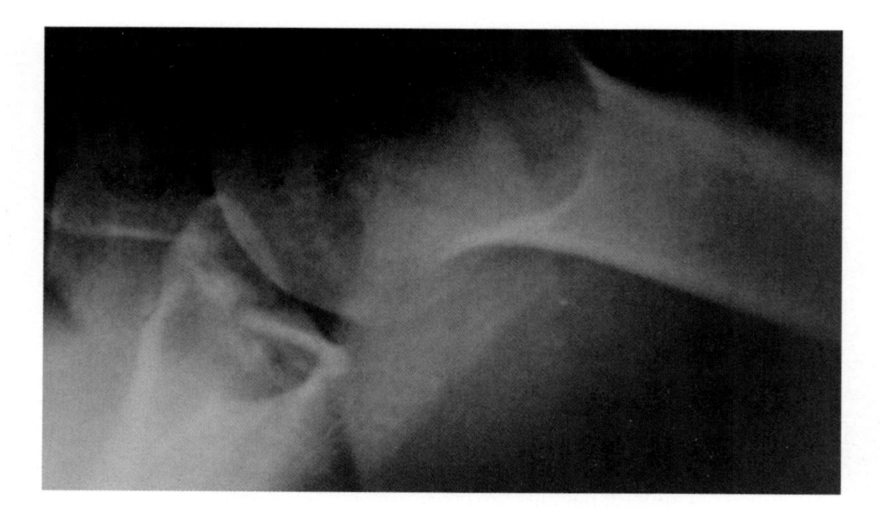

FIG. 23. Intraarticular extension of a posterior glenoid osteotomy. This patient is at increased risk for necrosis of the isolated posterior glenoid fragment or for glenohumeral degeneration.

study on the consequences of posterior glenoid osteotomy.[40] They presented a case report of significant, symptomatic coracoid impingement after glenoid osteotomy treated with resection of the inferolateral aspect of the coracoid process. In a corresponding anatomic study, 13 cadaveric shoulders displayed evidence of coracoid impingement after posterior glenoid osteotomy. Humeral contact against the coracoid and coracoacromial ligament was effectively relieved in the cadaveric shoulders by resection of the coracoacromial ligament and inferolateral coracoid process.

OPEN REPAIRS FOR MULTIDIRECTIONAL INSTABILITY

The literature on the surgical treatment of multidirectional instability is not as vast as that for traumatic instability. Yet, many of the complications that plague surgery for traumatic instability are analogous to those for multidirectional.

Recurrence of Instability

Overall, the rate of instability recurrence after capsular shift for an appropriate diagnosis of multidirectional instability is low. In 1980, Neer and Foster reported 40 patients who had undergone capsular shift for multidirectional instability, with only 1 patient suffering a recurrence.[103] Altchek et al. described recurrent instability (posterior) in 1 patient of 40 who underwent a T-plasty Bankart repair for multidirectional instability (anterior and inferior).[3] Cooper and Brems reported recurrence in 4 of 39 patients after capsular shift.[25]

The causes of instability recurrence after capsular shift can be divided into mechanical and biologic. The capsular shift procedure is predicated on decreasing capsular volume in the appropriate regions, as defined by the patient's instability pattern. Preferential imbrication of one side of the capsule may result in instability in the opposite direction in patients with circumferential multidirectional instability.[3] To correctly perform a capsular shift for patients unstable anteriorly, inferiorly, and posteriorly, the inferior humeral capsule must be released well past the inferior humeral margin, back to the posteroinferior quadrant. With subsequent superior capsular shift, anterior, inferior, and posterior capsules will all be equally tightened.

Although past investigators have concentrated on reducing the inferior capsular pouch, more recent attention has been directed toward the superior capsule, particularly in the treatment of inferior instability. Basmajian and Bazant hypothesized the primary importance of the superior capsule in preventing inferior instability.[12] Rowe and colleagues reported the presence of a defect in the rotator interval in patients with recurrent subluxations.[127] Recent basic science has further defined the rotator interval capsule (coracohumeral ligament and superior glenohumeral ligament) as the primary inferior stabilizer of the adducted shoulder,[53,154] and other investigators have noted the clinical importance of rotator interval repair.[105] Considering these data, imbrication of the rotator interval should be considered an integral aspect of the capsular shift procedure.

Of all the patients referred to our clinic with a diagnosis of recurrent instability after capsular shift procedure for multidirectional instability, the most common direction of persistent instability is inferior. This pattern of instability is also extremely disabling because carrying is a significant aspect of activities of daily living. Often, these patients can have dramatic sulcus signs even with stress by gravity alone (Fig. 24). Sometimes, because of repeated attempts at capsular shift, the patients are overtightened in the anterior and posterior directions, yet continue to display instability in the inferior direction, caused by uncorrected incompetence of the rotator interval (Fig. 25). Revision surgery, therefore, needs to primarily address this defect. We will usually imbricate the rotator interval capsule with the glenohumeral joint held located and the arm in approximately 20 degrees external rotation. If the degree of inferior instability is severe, less external rotation is applied, sacrificing external rotation at the side for stability.

Recurrence of instability after capsular shift can also occur in the anterior or posterior directions. If the patient in-

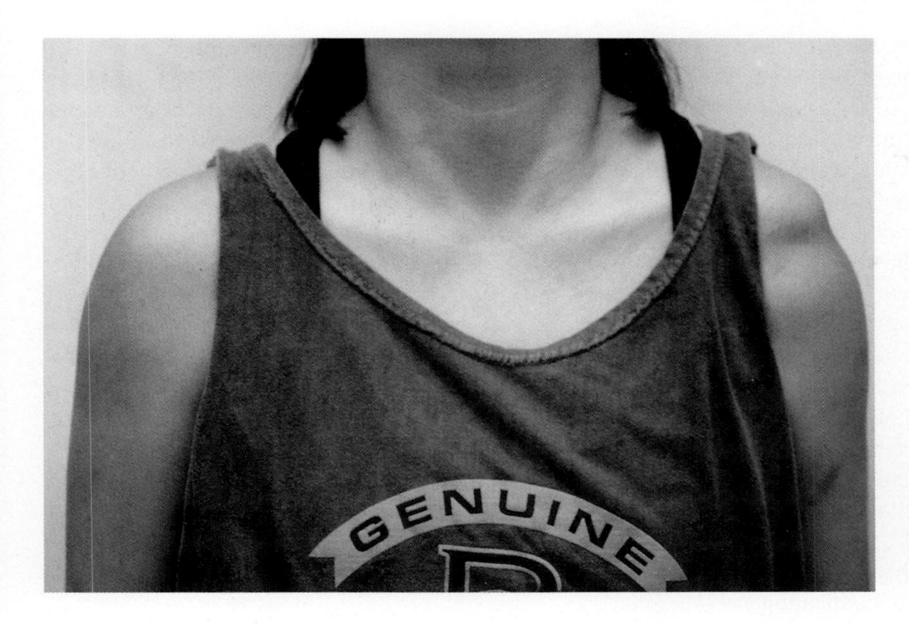

FIG. 24. A 24-year-old woman after six previous surgical stabilization attempts. She has continued inferior instability, even to gravity stress. (Courtesy Frederick A. Matsen III, University of Washington Medical Center, Seattle, WA.)

deed has recurrent multidirectional instability, consideration should be given to combined anterior and posterior approaches at the time of revision. Neer and Foster suggested this strategy in their initial description of the inferior capsular shift procedure for multidirectional instability.[103] Specifically, they recommended Bankart repair, if necessary, through an anterior approach, with a concomitant posterior approach for capsular shift. The technique is also useful, however, in the absence of a Bankart lesion. Through the posterior approach, complete access is gained to the posterior and posteroinferior capsule. From anteriorly, the anteroinferior, anterior, and rotator interval capsular regions can be addressed.

Postoperatively, these patients are placed in a shoulder spica cast, with the arm positioned in the neutral "gunslinger position," but with the entire humerus and shoulder girdle superiorly displaced. This cast is maintained for 6 weeks, with the patient performing abduction and external rotation isometrics in the cast. At 6 weeks postoperative, the cast is removed and a sling is placed. The patient is permitted to re-

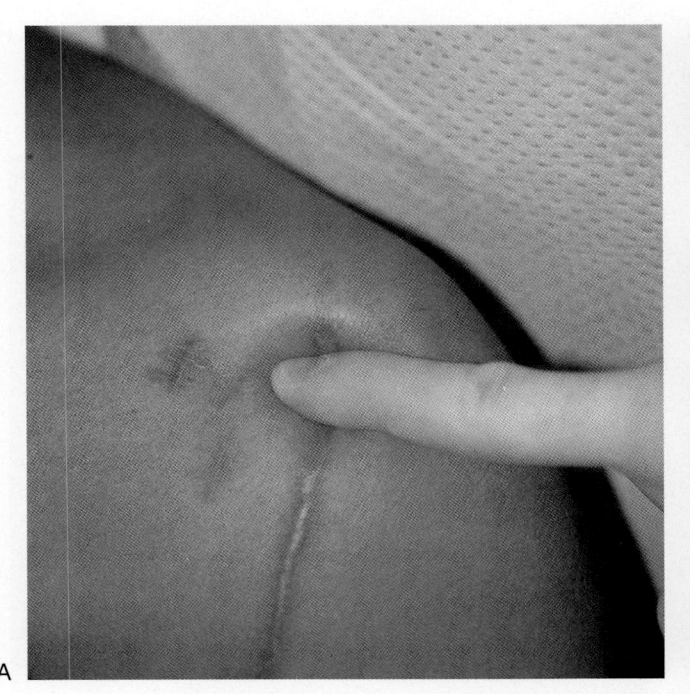
A

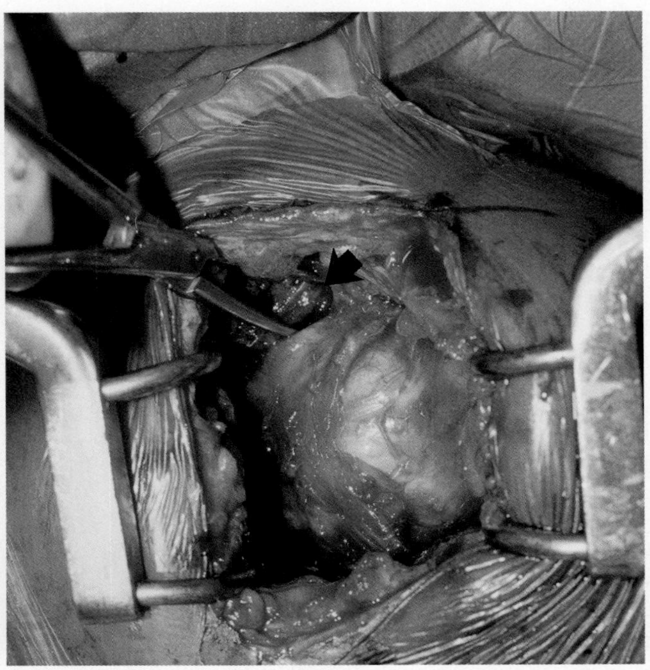
B

FIG. 25. (A) Persistent inferior instability in a patient who had undergone four previous capsular shift procedures. The rotator interval was not addressed in any of the previous surgeries. **(B)** Intraoperative photograph of the same patient. The rotator interval capsule was noted to be completely deficient and the interval was widened (*arrow*).

move the sling for activities of daily living, but they are encouraged to wear the sling for activities during which the arm may be expected to hang to gravity. At 10 weeks postoperative, the patient is begun on a gentle, supine, active-assisted motion program, rotator cuff strengthening against resistance, and a scapular stabilization and balancing program. Contact athletics and heavy lifting are restricted for 1 year.

Despite our mechanical knowledge of the ligamentous support of the glenohumeral joint, multidirectional instability is not a pure mechanical problem. It has long been recognized that patients with multidirectional instability are often systemically ligamentously lax. Neer and Foster discussed not only an increase in capsular volume, but abnormal capsular compliance in these individuals.[103] McNab and McNab reported on the poor-healing potential in patients with multidirectional instability, implying an overall collagen defect in this disorder. In a recent report, Rodeo et al. found that, in patients with multidirectional instability, there was a decreased cysteine content of the capsule, possibly indicating a higher prevalence of less stiff collagen type III. In addition, the skin of these patients had smaller collagen fibril diameters, again suggesting an underlying defect of collagen.[123]

Patients with recurrence of instability after capsular shift often appear to have abnormal healing. Skin incisions seem to be wider than usual. The patient may say that they had "opening" of the incision in the initial postoperative period, indicating wound dehiscence. On revision surgery, the amount of deltopectoral and humeroscapular interface scarring appears minimal, and can often be divided by finger dissection. Most importantly, the capsuloligamentous structures are almost always attenuated and deficient. Occasionally, this deficiency may also include the subscapularis tendon and may extend to the point of tissue absence.

We as surgeons do not yet have a good method of overcoming the biologic deficiency in these patients. We tend to treat these patients in a manner similar to that discussed earlier for traumatic instability with anterior capsular deficiency. The surgical approach begins by defining the humeroscapular interface and judging the presence and amount of anterior subscapularis and capsular tissue. In cases of anterior deficiency, we resort to an autologous tendon graft to reconstruct anterior capsuloligamentous defects. (see Fig. 15).

End-Stage Instability

Rarely, a patient will continue to suffer from disabling glenohumeral instability despite numerous attempts at surgical reconstruction. Although this condition can occur after any type or direction of instability, it is most common with multidirectional instability. These persons usually have impairment of most if not all of their stabilizing mechanisms, including loss of glenoid concavity, absence of capsuloligamentous restraint, severe Hill–Sachs lesions, and severe scapulohumeral dysfunction.

Richards et al. have reported the results of glenohumeral arthrodesis for patients with terminal instability.[119] After fusion, four of six patients with atraumatic instability had not only poor results, but also continued to have the sensation of episodic instability, despite clinical and radiographic evidence of solid fusion. In patients with end-stage instability, we have also resorted to arthrodesis when all other reconstructive methods have failed (Fig. 26). Many patients with atraumatic instability are prone to also have problems of the scapulothoracic joint, particularly ptotic posturing, pseudowinging, and snapping scapulae. In this population, glenohumeral arthrodesis initiates or worsens scapulothoracic symptoms. Regretfully, despite the high incidence of continued symptoms, glenohumeral arthrodesis remains the only surgical option for the treatment of end-stage instability.

ARTHROSCOPIC REPAIRS

Over the past two decades shoulder arthroscopy has developed from a diagnostic tool into a valid treatment option for the management of shoulder instability. Arthroscopic repair offers the potential advantages of quicker surgery, with less surgical morbidity; decreased postoperative pain; more selective anatomic repair, without violating the normal adjacent soft tissues; and recovery of more normal range of motion.[7,45,155] The shoulder, however, has been identified as the joint with the highest rate of arthroscopic complications.[27,134,135] Some of the previously mentioned complications of open instability repair apply equally, if not more so, to arthroscopic surgery. Arthroscopic repairs are also subject to unique complications specific to the repair method (Table 4).

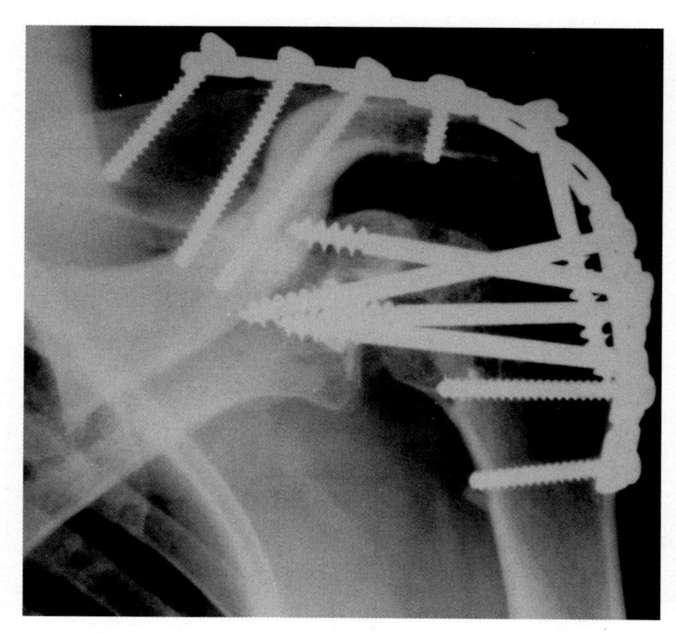

FIG. 26. Glenohumeral arthrodesis for end-stage instability.

TABLE 4. *Causes of failure after arthroscopic repair*

Recurrence of instability
Loss of motion
Neurovascular injury
Hardware complications

Recurrence of Instability

Incidence

The literature is extremely varied on the recurrence rate of glenohumeral instability after arthroscopic repair. Much of the variability probably relates to the wide array of different arthroscopic repair techniques, differences in surgeons' experience, and short follow-up. When viewed as a whole, the reported recurrence rate of instability after arthroscopic repair ranges from zero to 69%. Overall, the rate of recurrence of instability is higher after arthroscopic repair when compared with open.[7,13,43–45,56,76,81,100]

Arthroscopic techniques for shoulder instability can be divided into several main categories: metal fixation such as screws or staples, absorbable devices, suture-based repairs, and laser treatment. Each technique offers unique advantages. However, each can also result in unique complications and causes for instability recurrence.

Initial arthroscopic Bankart repairs were performed by staple capsulorraphy. Johnson's staple repair technique, which formed the basis for many other subsequent approaches, had an initial failure rate of 21%.[71] This high recurrence rate was somewhat related to allowing patients early range of motion postoperatively. The failure rate was cut by a third with immobilization for 4 weeks postoperatively. Other authors, however, continued to report high recurrence rates after arthroscopic staple capsulorraphy.[20,26,48,56,71,77,93,116,134,158,159]

As a response to the problems of staple capsulorraphy, other investigators developed arthroscopic suture techniques,[7,13,22,28,33,37,43,44,76,99,100,104,113,124,149,157,165] based on the transglenoid open Bankart repair procedures of Reider and Inglis.[118] Some initial reports listed failure rates using this suture technique at less than 8%, but these rates have ranged from zero to as high as 69% in both short and long-term follow-up.[7,13,22,33,37,43–45,81,99,100,118,132,155,164] Many studies have shown excellent short-term results (no recurrence of dislocation or subluxation) using the transglenoid technique in acute dislocators.[13,100] Recurrence rates, however, can be fairly significant after this technique. Landsiedle, using the same technique, showed 14% postoperative dislocation over 24 to 60 months (no mention of subluxation).[76] Manta's recent review of 38 shoulders, stabilized with the arthroscopic transglenoid suture technique, demonstrated a 10% failure rate at 2 years and a 40% failure rate at a minimum 5 years of follow-up.[89] As reported by others, however, the rate of recurrent instability may be as high as 69%.[81]

The other common method of arthroscopic instability repair involves use of suture anchors, either absorbable or permanent.[112,139,140,151,152,155] The most common absorbable fixation device is the Suretac (Acufex Microsurgical, Mansfield, MA), composed of polyglyconate polymer. Although the device loses its strength as it resorbs, it acts as a temporary compressive fixation for what is thought to be a sufficient time to allow healing of the capsulolabral separation.[112,139] Use of this device has resulted in exceptionally low rates of recurrence if surgery is performed after initial dislocation.[7] However, even in experienced hands, the overall rate of instability recurrence is approximately 21%.[141] Speer and colleagues have recently published results of arthroscopically assisted repair of the anterior aspect of the labrum with the use of a bioabsorbable tack. Their reported failure rate of 21% (11 patients) included 4 secondary to traumatic and 7 resulting from atraumatic reinjury.[141]

Causes of Recurrent Instability after Arthroscopic Repair

The higher rate of recurrence of instability after arthroscopic procedures when compared with open ones may simply reflect our comparing apples and oranges. Specifically, most currently performed arthroscopic techniques do not recreate the classic Bankart repair and, therefore, direct comparison may not be accurate. As such, the causes of instability recurrence after arthroscopic repair are not necessarily the same as those after open repair (Table 5).

Incorrect Diagnosis

Some of the reasons for instability recurrence after arthroscopic repair are similar to those after open repair. For instance, accurate diagnosis is essential to obtain a good outcome. For all techniques of arthroscopic repair, a high recurrence rate has been reported in patients with multidirectional instability. Manta et al. found a high failure rate of transglenoid repair in females (70%), particularly those with multidirectional instability.[89] Landsiedle attributed failures

TABLE 5. *Factors affecting recurrence of instability after arthroscopic repair*

Incorrect diagnosis	Recurrence of Bankart tear
	Early mobilization
Anatomic factors	Strength of repair
Defects of glenoid concavity	
Residual capsular laxity	
Rotator interval defect	
Unrecognized humeral avulsion of glenohumeral ligament (HAGL)	

to poor suture technique and poor patient selection, including those patients with nontraumatic dislocation and the absence of a Bankart or Hill–Sachs lesion.[76] Warner et al. suggested that success of the procedure may improve by selecting only patients with unidirectional, traumatic, anterior instability who have a discrete Bankart lesion and well-developed ligamentous tissue.[152] Speer and colleagues have commented that their high rate of recurrence (21%), when compared with open procedures for instability, was related to an underestimation of the degree of overall capsular laxity at the time of initial arthroscopic treatment in those patients with atraumatic instability.[141]

Recurrence of Bankart Tear

Either failure of healing of the Bankart lesion or recurrence may lead to postoperative instability. Warner and colleagues recently sought to clarify the issue of Bankart repair healing by analyzing a group of patients who underwent a "second-look" arthroscopy to evaluate and treat pain or recurrent instability following arthroscopic Bankart repair with the Suretac device. Second-look arthroscopy was performed at an average of 9 months, for recurrent instability in seven patients, pain in six, and pain and stiffness in two. In the seven patients with recurrent instability, the Bankart repair was completely healed in three (43%), partially healed in one (14%), and had recurred in three (43%). In the remaining eight cases with stable shoulders, the Bankart repair had completely healed in five cases (62.5%) and partially healed in three patients (37.5%).[152]

Defects of Glenoid Concavity

As with open repair, failure to correct defects of glenoid concavity will result in higher rates of surgical failure. Multiple authors have noted worse results after arthroscopic repair in the presence of either an osseous lesion of the anterior glenoid rim or severe labral deficiency.[46,89,113,149] Transglenoid suturing may be unable to account for these defects. In addition, if suture anchors are not placed directly on the rim of the glenoid, this technique also will not restore deficiencies of concavity (see Fig. 7). Although not documented, enhanced ability to restore concavity through an open technique may be partly responsible for the better results of open surgery.

Warner and colleagues analyzed eight cadaver shoulders that underwent arthroscopic repair of an experimental Bankart lesion using the Suretac device.[151] These shoulders were then dissected to reveal the placement of the Suretac and the adequacy of the Bankart lesion repair. There were several technical errors that occurred, including medial placement of the Suretac relative to the articular margin. As noted earlier, medial anchor placement fails to adequately restore glenoid contour and concavity and may lead to instability recurrence.

Residual Capsular Laxity

Failure to address residual capsular laxity has been thought to be an important cause of recurrent instability after arthroscopic repair. Guanche and colleagues have reported a 27% revision rate in arthroscopic cases that did not address capsular laxity as compared with 8% in open cases.[49] Both Manta et al. and Landsiedle et al. reported worse results in those patients with hyperlaxity.[76,89] Manta, Pagnani and Walch all documented failure to definitively address inferior laxity as a contributing factor to failure.[89,113,149] Speer and colleagues have recently reported on arthroscopic reoperations for recurrent anterior instability, in which seven of eight patients had completely healed Bankart lesions. In these patients, the anteroinferior aspect of the capsule was felt to be patulous in each patient.[141]

To correct presumed residual capsular laxity, Hardy et al. used laser-assisted capsular shrinkage (LACS) together with labral repair by either anterior reattachment (REVO screws, Linvatec, USA) or transglenoid suture.[50] None of the patients were reported to have had a recurrence of instability at an average follow-up of 1 year. Although this study would suggest a role for residual capsular laxity as a cause of postoperative instability, both comparison studies and longer follow-up are necessary.

As discussed in the section on failures of open instability repairs, normal shoulders can have a great degree of capsular laxity, and the significance of residual and unrepaired capsular laxity remains unclear (see Fig. 13). Moreover, the exact techniques used to differentiate excessive capsular laxity from normal laxity are unknown and are difficult to perform even in the open setting. Because we do not arthroscope normally lax shoulders, we do not know how many normals would have arthroscopic signs of persistent laxity. Although it is easy to blame persistent laxity as a cause for failure after arthroscopic repair, it remains to be proved that residual laxity after arthroscopic repair is abnormal. Laxity does not necessarily equal instability; therefore, persistent laxity as a cause for instability is a diagnosis of exclusion.

Rotator Interval Defect

During open repair, the rotator interval is usually sutured during closure. For patients with inferior instability, imbrication of the interval is recommended. Failure to address a rotator interval defect in the patient with inferior instability can lead to recurrence (see Fig. 25). Assessing and addressing the rotator interval arthroscopically, however, is difficult. It may be that failure to address the rotator interval is a cause for postoperative instability.

Speer et al. performed arthroscopic evaluation of eight patients with recurrence of instability after previous arthroscopic Bankart repair. In seven of the eight patients, the Bankart repair had healed. An open lesion of the rotator interval was seen in five of these seven patients.[141]

The Humeral Avulsion of Glenohumeral Ligaments Lesion

Avulsion of the capsulolabral complex at the glenoid (Bankart lesion), is a well-known cause of anterior shoulder instability. Wolf and colleagues have reported on the importance of recognizing a lesser known entity, the humeral avulsion of glenohumeral ligaments (HAGL). They arthroscopically evaluated 64 shoulders with the diagnosis of anterior instability. Six shoulders had HAGL lesions (9.3%), 11 shoulders had generalized capsular laxity (17.2%), and 47 shoulders had Bankart lesions (73.5%). In patients with documented anterior instability without a demonstrable Bankart lesion, a HAGL lesion should be ruled out. This lesion is readily recognized arthroscopically, and its appropriate repair can restore anterior stability.[63] Failure to address a HAGL lesion may result in persistence of instability.

Strength of Repair

Because recurrence of the Bankart lesion has been demonstrated as a cause of failure after arthroscopic repair, fixation strength of the repair technique probably plays some role in lesion healing. Arthroscopic repair techniques have varied in their ability to accomplish a robust fixation.

McEleny and others looked at the initial failure strength of eight repair techniques using a previously described canine model of Bankart repair. Intact capsule-to-bone complexes failed at the bony interface at 236 N. Traditional Bankart repair failed at 122.1 N (two sutures) and 74.7 N (one suture), Acufex TAG rod (Acufex Microsurgical, Mansfield, MA) at 143.5 N (two sutures) and 79.8 N (one suture), transglenoid suture technique (two sutures) at 166.6 N, Mitek GII (Mitek, Norwood, MA) (one suture) at 96.4 N, Zimmer Statak (Zimmer Inc, Warsaw, IN) (one suture) at 95.2 N, and Acufex bioabsorbable Suretac at 82.2 N. The two-suture repairs were statistically equivalent in strength to each other, as were the one-suture repairs and the Suretac device. Two-suture repairs were significantly stronger than one-suture repairs ($P < 0.01$). In the single-suture specimens, failure occurred by suture breakage in 46% (18 of 39) of specimens and soft-tissue failure around the suture in 54% (21 of 39). Failure in the two-suture techniques occurred primarily by soft-tissue failure (23 of 25). No device broke or pulled out of bone.[96]

Shall evaluated three mechanical soft tissue fixation devices (SuperAnchor, Suretac, and the Instrument Makar [IM] Bioabsorbable Staple) in a cadaveric model by examining ultimate tensile failure and modes of failure in simulated Bankart repairs. He attempted to realistically evaluate the strengths of soft-tissue reattachment procedures at the anterior glenoid under worst-case conditions—load to failure. The mean load at failure for the SuperAnchor was 217.32 N; for the IM Staple, 132.32 N; and for the Suretac, 122.37 N. The load at failure for the SuperAnchor was statistically greater ($P < 0.001$) than the IM Staple and Suretac. There was no statistical difference between load at failure for the Suretac and the IM Staple. The most common failure mode for the Mitek was suture breakage (71%). Anchor pullout from bone was the most common failure mode for the IM Staple (75%) and Suretac (94%).[131]

In a labral repair model, Gohkle and colleagues compared the strength of suture-anchor repair to the standard Bankart procedure and the intact anterior capsule.[42] The mean load at failure for the suture anchor repairs varied from 90 to 115 N and was lower than in the standard Bankart procedure (127 N). All suture anchors demonstrated similar holding strength with the exception of an absorbable wedge ($P < 0.05$).[42]

Loutzenheiser and Harryman have recently demonstrated that some failures may relate to the challenge of tying secure knots arthroscopically. Many knots tied arthroscopically commonly consist of an initial slip knot to remove slack, and a series of half-hitches. Half-hitches, instead of square throws, are difficult to avoid and result when asymmetrical tension is applied to the suture strands. For this reason, the security of knots tied arthroscopically may not be equivalent to square knots and a greater rate of failure may occur. The most secure knot configurations were achieved by reversing the half-hitch throws and alternating the posts. These knots performed significantly better than all other knots tested ($P < 0.002$). Thus the surgeon can control the holding capacity and minimize suture loop displacement by properly alternating the tying strands and reversing the loop when placing the hitches.[87]

The importance of strength of fixation of suture anchor repair in the Bankart reconstruction is unknown because we do not stress these patients early on in the healing process. Because failure of Bankart repair is a complication of arthroscopic repair, however, strength of fixation may play a role in this repair failure.

Early Mobilization

Because the fixation strength is probably less after arthroscopic than after open repair, the period of postoperative immobilization likely plays an important role in preventing recurrence of instability. Johnson determined that he could cut his recurrence rate (of about 20%) after arthroscopic staple capsulorraphy by one-half if he increased the period of postoperative immobilization from less than 3 weeks to 4 weeks.[71] Three to 4 weeks of strict immobilization has also been recommended by other investigators.[2,22,100] Limiting early trauma is also thought to be extremely important. If the patient desires to return to contact sports, a 6-month delay has been reported to lower the rate of instability recurrence.[136]

Loss of Motion

It has become increasingly evident that shoulder motion, especially external rotation, need not be sacrificed for stability. In theory, by not incising the subscapularis or violating the humeroscapular motion interface, arthroscopic repair offers the potential for better preservation of glenohumeral motion than does open repair.

After arthroscopic Bankart repair, most patients can anticipate a reliable return of motion that is nearly symmetrical with that of the contralateral shoulder.[143] Arciero treated 25 patients by arthroscopic Bankart repair using a cannulated bioabsorbable fixation device. Nineteen patients with an average follow-up of 19 months had an average loss of external rotation of 3 degrees.[6] Warner and Warren reported on 26 patients with a minimum of 24-month follow-up, treated with the Suretac device, who had an overall recurrence rate of 8%. They noted an average loss of external rotation of 7 degrees, with 5 of 8 throwing athletes and 4 of 4 swimming athletes being able to return to their premorbid level of athletic participation.[155] Finally, Uribe and Hechtman reported on 11 young athletes with acute anterior Bankart lesions treated with the transglenoid suture repair. When using the Rowe scale there were 9 excellent and 2 good results. All eventually achieved full external rotation in adduction and 90 degrees of abduction compared with the opposite side.[148]

Wall and colleagues reported their postoperative protocols commonly expect normal motion by 10 to 12 weeks in nonthrowing athletes and 6 to 8 weeks in throwing athletes. If after these time periods, there is restricted motion, especially external rotation less than 10 degrees or abduction below 90 degrees, there is cause for concern. If aggressive physical therapy fails to regain motion, manipulation under anesthesia or arthroscopic release may be employed. The authors describe using an anterior release for limitations of external rotation and axillary pouch release for abduction contractures, sometimes using electrocautery or lasers as an adjunct. For lesser degrees of motion restriction, they will wait 6 months to treat arthroscopically.[150]

Neurovascular Injury

Neurovascular injury has been an infrequent, but potentially devastating complication of arthroscopic instability repair. These complications can be separated into those resulting from positioning and setup, portal placement, or suturing techniques.

Positioning

Shoulder arthroscopy has classically been performed in either the lateral decubitus or beach chair position. The lateral decubitus position has a potential disadvantage in that the necessary use of a traction device may endanger the brachial plexus.[153] Andrews and others have recommended that longitudinal traction of 15 lb (6.8 kg) be applied with the patient in the lateral decubitus position and with the arm in 15 degrees of forward flexion and 70 degrees of abduction.[5] Traction setup used for shoulder arthroscopy in the lateral position should not exceed 15 lb, with 10 lb usually being sufficient. Careful attention to excessive shoulder abduction and extension should be paid to prevent potential neuropraxia.[15,150] It is recommended that traction be maintained at less than 20 lb (9.1 kg) to minimize the risk of neuropraxias.[122] The beach chair position has been used by many surgeons, and no episodes of brachial plexus nerve palsy have been reported. There is one case report of a hypoglossal nerve palsy, thought to result from change in position of the head and subsequent compression beneath the angle of the mandible.[101]

The reported rate of neuropraxia after shoulder arthroscopy has ranged from zero to 30%.[5,73,111,115,122,134,135] Small reported on a prevalence of less than 0.1% neurologic complications. These included three brachial plexus traction injuries (two subsequent to arthroscopic anterior staple capsulorraphy) and one axillary nerve injury (during an arthroscopic anterior acromioplasty).[134] Ogilvie-Harris and Wiley reported 1 transient musculocutaneous nerve palsy after a total of 439 shoulder arthroscopies, a prevalence of 0.2%.[111] Andrews and Carson reported on 3 neurologic injuries, 1 musculocutaneous neuropraxia and 2 involving the ulnar nerve, after 120 arthroscopies, a prevalence of 3%.[4] Klein cited a prevalence of transient paresthesias of about 10%; however, no specific numbers were given.[73] Pitman reported on 2 transient neuropraxias in 20 patients, 1 involving the lateral antebrachial cutaneous nerve and the other with diffuse hypoesthesia of the lateral aspect of the arm and forearm with paresis of the wrist extensors.[115]

Klein and colleagues studied the strain on the brachial plexus that results from traction loads applied at various arm positions and correlated this with visibility through the arthroscope. They mounted strain gauges to the upper trunk, lateral cord, median nerve, and radial nerve of five fresh human cadavers. Each cadaver was placed in a lateral decubitus position, with the head fixed in a neutral position, as for shoulder arthroscopy, and the strain on the plexus was measured as a function of arm position and traction load. A final cadaver was used to determine the accessibility and visibility in the arthroscope at each of the arm positions. At a given flexion angle, increasing abduction was associated with decreasing strain. At a given abduction angle, increasing flexion resulted in decreased strain. The minimum overall strain was noted at 90 degrees of flexion and 0 degree of abduction. Visibility at this position was limited. Klein concluded that the ideal arthroscopic position is a combination of two positions that would maximize visibility while minimizing strain to the nerves. These two positions are 45 degrees of forward flexion and 90 degrees of abduction in combination with 45 degrees of forward flexion and 0 degree of abduction.[73]

Somatosensory evoked potentials (SEPs) were recorded by Pitman during shoulder arthroscopy in 20 patients to monitor the musculocutaneous nerve, ulnar nerve, and either the median or radial nerve. In all 20 cases, abnormal SEPs of the musculocutaneous nerve were demonstrated. In 16 patients, this was produced on initial joint distention, and in 15 patients, by traction; in 11, by longitudinal traction of greater than or equal to 12 lb; and in 6 by perpendicular traction of greater than or equal to 7 lb. In 10 patients, there were varying combinations of median, ulnar, and radial nerve involvement. There were 2 cases of clinical neuropraxia in this series. One resolved in 24 hours and 1 in 48 hours. Pitman concludes that there is a real potential for neurologic damage during shoulder arthroscopy and that the musculocutaneous nerve is the most vulnerable. Factors responsible include joint distention, excessive traction, extravasation of fluid, and tension on the musculocutaneous nerve as it was stretched over the humeral head with the shoulder in extension, abduction, and external rotation.[115]

Because most neurologic insults are neuropraxic-type injuries, the initial approach should be observation. If no nerve recovery is seen by 3 weeks, one should consider an EMG, and then serial EMGs based on the clinical examination. In neuropraxic injury, the surgeon should expect neurologic function to be fully recovered by approximately 3 months.

Portal Placement

Knowledge of the local anatomy is essential in portal placement. Matthews and others reported on 1 proximal median nerve palsy in 47 shoulder arthroscopies, a prevalence of 2%. The presumed etiology was injury during anterior portal placement.[94] For anterior portals staying superior and lateral to the coracoid within the "safe triangle" avoids injury to the musculocutaneous nerve.[94,110] Wolf has done cadaveric studies describing an anteroinferior portal that lies 1.5 to 4 cm from the musculocutaneous nerve, and provides a more useful working angle for stabilizing the anteroinferior labral ligamentous complex. This distance increases with adduction, thus he recommends placing this portal with the arm in less than 30 degrees of abduction.[93,162]

Laceration of the cephalic vein may also occur during anterior portal placement. Ligation is indicated, and meticulous hemostasis intraarticularly is essential to prevent hemarthrosis. The use of epinephrine in the irrigating fluid, proper joint distention, and hypotensive anesthesia may also aid in controlling bleeding.[15]

Suturing Techniques

Arthroscopic stabilization procedures can be complicated by neurovascular injury. The most notorious of these complications is injury to the suprascapular nerve during transglenoid suturing. Mologne reported the clinical outcome of arthroscopic labral reconstruction using a transglenoid suture technique in 49 shoulders.[98] Suprascapular nerve palsy occurred in three cases (6%).

Bigliani and colleagues studied the course of the suprascapular nerve and its distance from fixed scapular landmarks in 90 cadaveric shoulders. In an additional 15 cadavers, three pins were passed at various angles in an anterior to posterior direction through the middle of the glenoid neck just inferior and lateral to the base of the coracoid process. The distance between the exit site on the posterior glenoid neck and the suprascapular nerve at the base of the scapular spine was recorded for each pin. Inferiorly directed pins were the furthest from the suprascapular nerve and averaged 16 mm. On the basis of these data, a relative safe zone was described in the posterior glenoid neck.[14] Morgan recommends the anterior starting point for transglenoid drilling should be at the two o'clock position (right shoulder) and directed 30 degrees inferior to the transverse plane and 15 degrees medial to the plane of the glenoid to minimize injury to the suprascapular nerve.[100]

In patients undergoing transglenoid drilling, the presence of suprascapular nerve injury postoperatively should signal a prompt workup. An EMG may be indicated in the first 24 hours to rule out axonotmesis. If no recovery is seen in 24 to 48 hours, early exploration should be considered.

Hardware Complications

Complications of Staples

Numerous hardware problems have been seen after arthroscopic staple capsulorraphy. The earliest staples were made malleable so that they would not break. This proved to be a problem in that they were easily bent by forceful direction change during insertion. Subsequent generations were less malleable and thus the complication of staple loosening (usually as a result of reinjury or dislocation), impingement, breakage, and eventual migration was seen.[71]

Another staple complication involved placement of the staple in an incorrect perpendicular orientation to the anterior glenoid. Even if oriented correctly, the staple may be placed only partly (one tine only) in bone or be placed too deep into the bone, thus amputating the glenohumeral ligaments or cutting into the labrum. If placed too superior, the staple may end up in the coracoid process. The staple head may also cause irritation to the subscapularis tendon. Placement of the metallic staple at the anterior glenoid margin may cause erosion of the humeral head cartilage.[71]

Biologic Response to Absorbable Implants

Abnormal biologic response to absorbable suture anchors has been infrequently reported, but can be of great clinical significance. Warner et al. reported two cases of biopsy of the repair site on "second-look" arthroscopy 6 to 8 months after labral repair using the Suretac device, a polyglyconate absorbable suture anchor. The authors found residual polyglyconate polymer debris surrounded by a histiocytic infiltrate.[152]

Edwards and colleagues have reported on adverse reactions to the Suretac absorbable anchor in five of their patients. All patients complained of increasing pain and loss of shoulder motion. They all required arthroscopic lavage and debridement of the intracapsular synovitis. Nonspecific granulomatous reactions were identified histologically in all cases and no organisms were grown from the operative specimens. One specimen had a dense inflammatory response surrounding refractile material (presumably particles of the Suretac).[29]

By definition, absorbable devices erode from a biologic response. If this response becomes exaggerated, clinical implications may result. Although clinically significant reaction to polyglyconate anchors has been infrequent, it clearly can occur. As seen with other biomaterials, the extent of the biologic reaction is usually material-specific. Whether or not clinically significant reactions will occur with the next generation of absorbable suture anchors remains to be seen. Poly-L-lactic acid has recently been studied and demonstrated no significant abnormal reaction in an animal.[10]

Any patient who develops symptoms of worsening pain, decreasing motion, increasing warmth, or erythema within 4 to 6 weeks of surgery, should have an infection workup. In addition, one should consider an early arthroscopic exploration with removal of residual anchor debris and synovectomy.

Miscellaneous Complications

Fluid extravasation into the adjacent tissues is a very common complication of shoulder arthroscopy. This fluid may increase compartment pressures in the arm, potentially leading to compartment syndrome. Lee and colleagues measured the intramuscular deltoid pressure using a slit catheter. Although they found that the intramuscular pressure became transiently elevated during the arthroscopic procedures, in every case the pressures promptly returned to normal levels within 30 minutes postoperatively. The clinical swelling and tenseness remained for a longer period. Despite a sometimes alarming amount of swelling during shoulder arthroscopy, intramuscular pressure elevations were only sustained for a short time and returned to normal levels very quickly after the cessation of fluid infusion.[80] There are several ways to

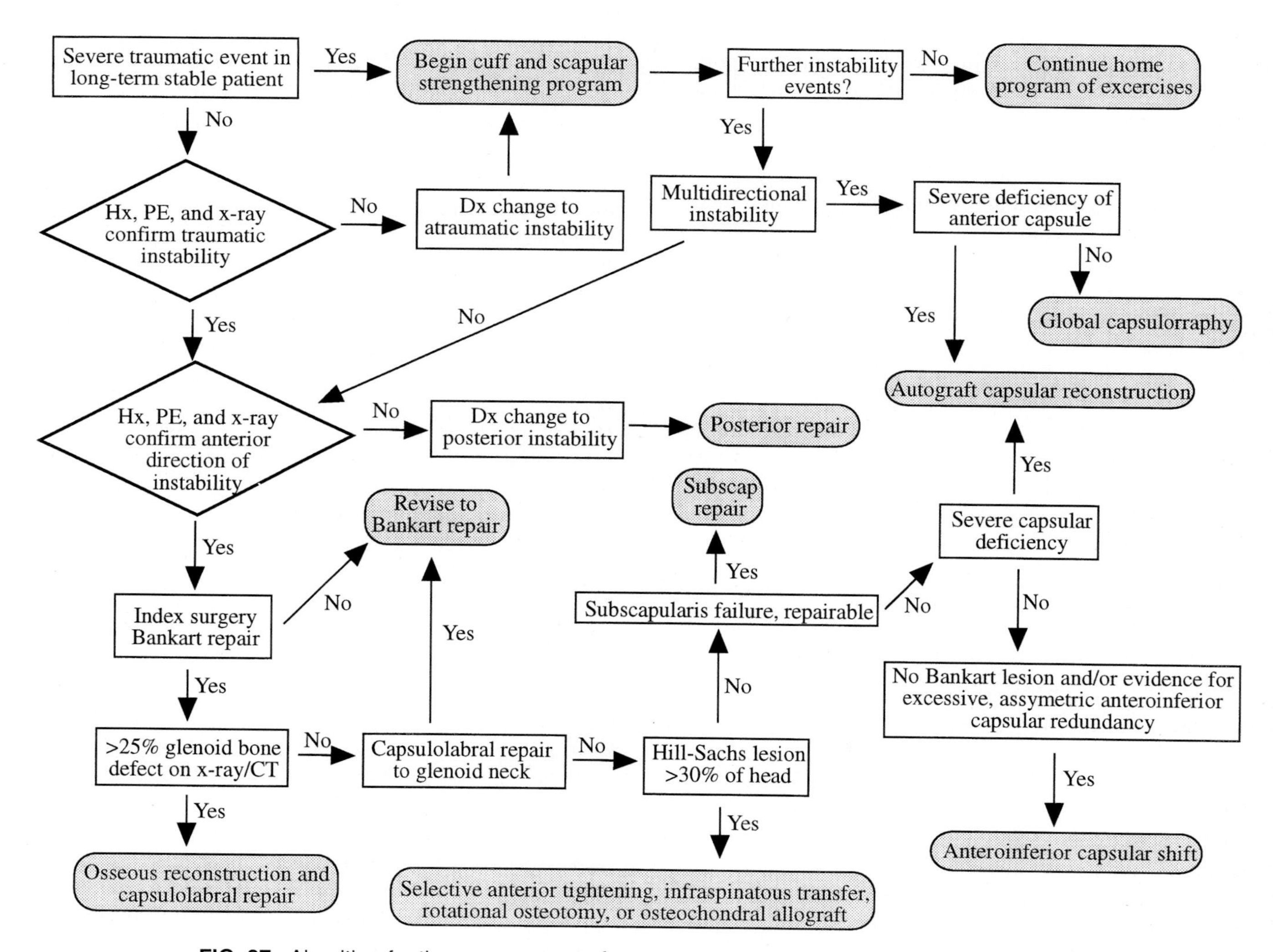

FIG. 27. Algorithm for the management of recurrent instability after previous surgical repair.

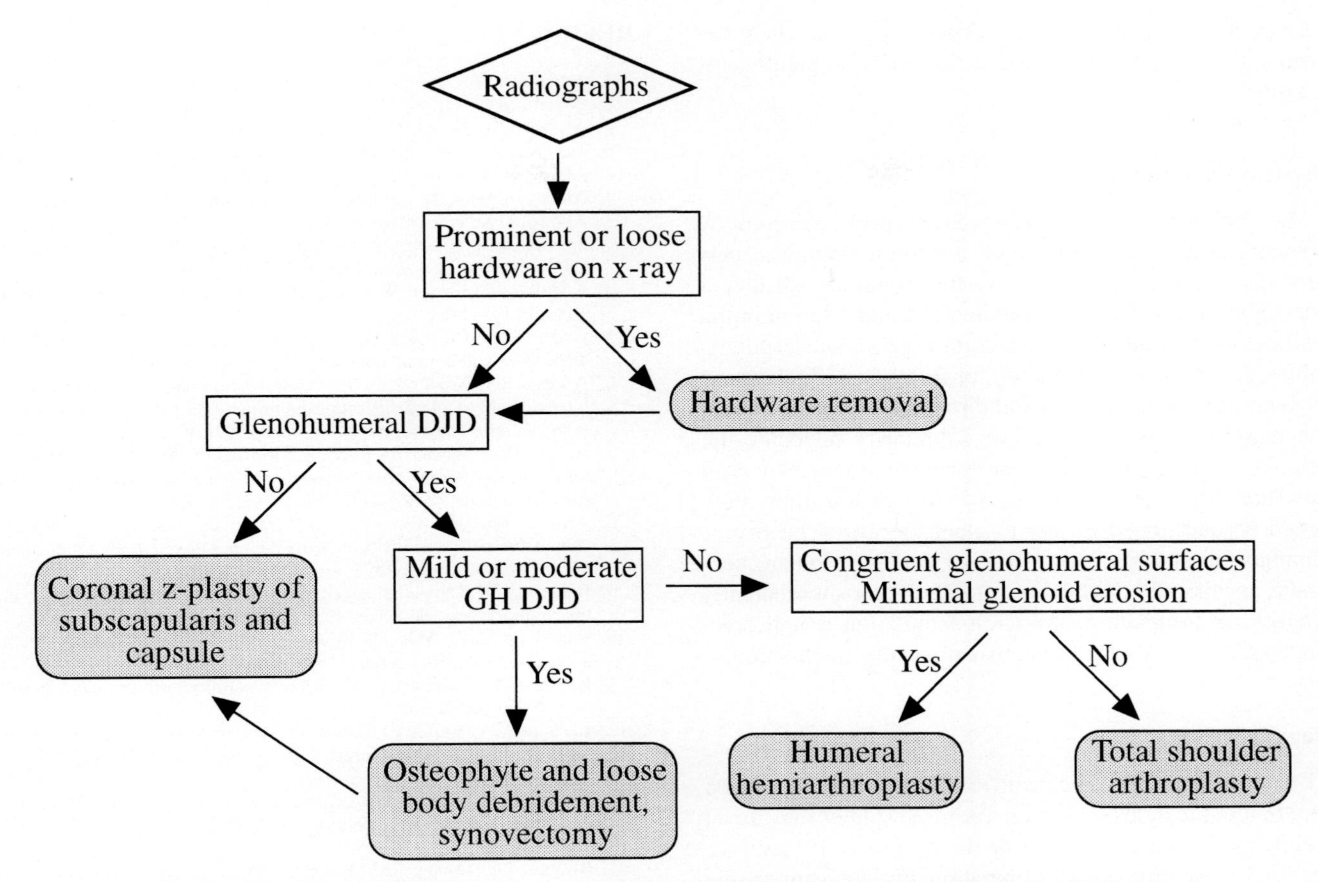

FIG. 28. Algorithm for the management of motion loss (external rotation less than neutral) after previous instability repair.

control this extravasation, including making small, tight portals around cannulas, decreasing operative time, and careful monitoring of fluid inflow pressures.[71] Case reports of compartment syndrome have been presented.[114]

Injury to the rotator cuff is also a possible consequence of incorrect portal placement. These punctures may produce permanent rotator cuff defects. Creating a cuff defect is best avoided by making the superior portal with the arm adducted and the posterior portal with the arm adducted and internally rotated.[109]

PATIENT EVALUATION AFTER FAILED INSTABILITY REPAIR

It is clear that "failure of instability surgery" encompasses multiple diagnoses. A careful and thorough approach is necessary to elucidate the problem and arrive at the appropriate treatment plan, particularly if the problem is recurrent instability or motion loss (Figs. 27 and 28).

History

The most important aspect of the patient history is questioning about the initial instability event. It is clear from the literature that failure of diagnosis is the most common cause of error. The patient, therefore, should be questioned about the activity that caused initial dislocation, the position of the arm at the time of dislocation, and the severity of the initial trauma. The physician should question about subsequent instability events, again determining arm position during these incidents. A history of contralateral shoulder instability may indicate multidirectional instability.

The patient should be questioned in detail about current symptoms. Once the unique feeling of instability is defined for the patient as such, it is a feeling that is never forgotten, that sensation forming the basis for the apprehension test. The patient should be questioned as to whether they still feel unstable. Did they have a period after the operation when they were improved? Was there a significant postoperative traumatic event? Which humerothoracic positions are associated with instability events?

In cases of stiffness, the degree of functional impairment should be assessed. The patient should be questioned on the difficulty with activities of daily living, sporting activities, and hobbies. Attempt to ascertain the degree of patient compliance with their index postoperative rehabilitation.

Operative notes from prior procedures should be obtained. Those notes should be reviewed to determine the exact approach used and intervals incised as, in cases of postsurgical contracture, these locations are likely to contain the most adhesions. Knowing the technique of prior repair can help determine the cause of failure in situations of postoperative instability.

Physical Examination

The shoulder should be observed for prior incisions. A thorough examination for range of motion should be performed. Severe limitation of external rotation indicates a "too-tight" repair. Increased passive external rotation in the position of humerothoracic adduction suggests subscapularis failure. A complete examination for instability is necessary, concentrating on laxity tests and directions of apprehension. The patient should be asked to voluntarily dislocate the shoulder. If they are able to perform this maneuver with muscular contraction and not by arm positioning, they should be questioned further to elucidate a true history of voluntary instability. Tests of rotator cuff function are necessary, specifically the lumbar lift-off test for subscapularis integrity. A complete neurologic examination is indicated, concentrating on axillary and musculocutaneous function.

Diagnostic Tests

Every attempt should be made to obtain radiographs taken from before the index operation, for these studies may assist in either confirming or correcting the diagnosis. If hardware was used at the time of index operation, initial postoperative radiographs should be reviewed and compared with recent studies. In our practice, new radiographs including a true scapular anteroposterior view in both internal and external humeral rotation, an axillary lateral, a West Point lateral, and a Garth apical oblique view are obtained. If the plain radiographic studies indicate an osseous glenoid deformity or a Hill–Sachs lesion, a CT scan is used to further define these abnormalities. An MRI scan is usually not needed in cases of failed instability, although it may be helpful in defining subscapularis failure in the face of an equivocal examination. If there is any examination evidence for neurologic dysfunction, EMG studies should be performed.

SUMMARY

Evaluating and treating the patient who has had a failed instability repair can be a daunting task. A complete evaluation is needed to define the problem and determine appropriate solutions. The most important technique that will result in an excellent result from revision surgery is assuring the exact diagnosis. Once that diagnosis is confirmed, the appropriate surgical intervention can be applied. At revision, the surgeon should be prepared for a complete range of pathology, from soft-tissue contractures and adhesions to osseous and soft-tissue deficiencies. The goal in treatment is to restore stability and motion with minimal alteration to normal anatomy.

REFERENCES

1. Adams F. *The genuine works of hippocrates.* New York: William Wood and Co., 1886.
2. Altchek DW, Skyhar MJ, Warren RF. Shoulder arthroscopy for shoulder instability. In: Barr JS, Jr, eds. *Instructional course lectures*, The American Academy of Orthopaedic Surgeons. Park Ridge, IL: The American Academy of Orthopaedic Surgeons, 1989;38:187–198.
3. Altchek DW, Warren RF, Skyhar MJ, et al. T-Plasty modification of the Bankart procedure for multidirectional instability of the anterior and inferior types. *J Bone Joint Surg [Am]* 1991;73:105–112.
4. Andrews JR, Carson WG. Shoulder joint arthroscopy. *Orthopedics* 1983;6:1157–1162.
5. Andrews JR, Carson WGJ, Ortega K. Arthroscopy of the shoulder: techniques and normal anatomy. *Am J Sports Med* 1984;12:1–7.
6. Arciero RA, Taylor DC, Snyder RJ, Uhorchak JM. Arthroscopic bioabsorbable tack stabilization of initial anterior shoulder dislocations: a preliminary report. *Arthroscopy* 1995;11:410–417.
7. Arciero RA, Wheeler JH, Ryan JB, McBride JT. Arthroscopic Bankart repair versus nonoperative treatment for acute, initial anterior shoulder dislocations. *Am J Sports Med* 1994;22:589–594.
8. Artz T, Huffer JM. A major complication of the modified Bristow procedure for recurrent dislocation of the shoulder. *J Bone Joint Surg [Am]* 1972;54:1293–1296.
9. Bankart ASB. The pathology and treatment of recurrent dislocation of the shoulder joint. *Br J Surg* 1939;26B:23.
10. Barber FA, Deck MA. The in vivo histology of an absorbable suture anchor: a preliminary report. *Arthroscopy* 1995;11:77–81.
11. Barron OA, Bigliani LU. Revision instability surgery. *Clin Sports Med* 1995;14:955–972.
12. Basmajian JV, Bazant FJ. Factors preventing downward dislocation of the adducted shoulder joint. *J Bone Joint Surg [Am]* 1959;41:1182–1186.
13. Benedetto KP, Glotzer W. Arthroscopic Bankart procedure by suture technique: indications, technique, and results. *Arthroscopy* 1992;8:111–115.
14. Bigliani LU, Dalsey RM, McCann PD, April EW. An anatomical study of the suprascapular nerve. *Arthroscopy* 1990;6:301–305.
15. Bigliani LU, Flatow EL, Deliz ED. Complications of shoulder arthroscopy. *Orthop Rev* 1991;20:743–751.
16. Bigliani LU, Pollock RG, McIlveen SJ, Endrizzi DP, Flatow EL. Shift of the posteroinferior aspect of the capsule for recurrent posterior glenohumeral instability. *J Bone Joint Surg [Am]* 1995;77:1011–1020.
17. Bigliani LU, Pollock RG, Soslaws LJ. Tensile properties of the glenohumeral ligament. *J Orthop Res* 1992;10:187–197.
18. Bigliani LU, Weinstein DM, Glasgow MT, Pollock RG, Flatow EL. Glenohumeral arthroplasty for arthritis after instability surgery. *J Shoulder Elbow Surg* 1995;4:87–94.
19. Boyd HB, Sisk TD. Recurrent posterior dislocation of the shoulder. *J Bone Joint Surg [Am]* 1972;54:779–786.
20. Burger RS, Shengel D, Bonatus T, et al. Arthroscopic staple capsulorraphy for recurrent shoulder instability. *Orthop Trans* 1990;14:596–597.
21. Burkhead WZ Jr, Richie MF. Revision of failed shoulder reconstruction. *Contemp Ortho* 1992;24:126–133.
22. Caspari R, Savoie FH. Arthroscopic reconstruction of the unstable shoulder: the Bankart repair. In: McGinty J, ed. *Operative arthroscopy*. New York: Raven Press, 1991:507–516.
23. Checchia SL, Doneux SP, Martins MG, Meireles FS. Subscapularis muscle enervation: the effect of arm position. *J Shoulder Elbow Surg* 1996;5:214–218.
24. Connolly JF. Humeral head defects associated with shoulder dislocations—their diagnostic and surgical significance. In: MacAusland, Jr, eds. *Instructional course lectures*. The American Academy of Orthopaedic Surgeons. St Louis: Mosby, 1972;21:42–54.
25. Cooper RA, Brems JJ. The inferior capsular-shift procedure for multidirectional instability of the shoulder. *J Bone Joint Surg [Am]* 1992;74:1516–1521.
26. Coughlin L, Rubinovich M, Johansson J, et al. Arthroscopic staple capsulorraphy for anterior shoulder instability. *Am J Sports Med* 1992;20:253–256.
27. DeLee JC. Complications of arthroscopy and arthroscopic surgery: results of a national survey. *Arthroscopy* 1985;1:214.

28. Duncan R, Savoie FH. Arthroscopic inferior capsular shift for multidirectional instability of the shoulder: a preliminary report. *Arthroscopy* 1993;9:24–27.
29. Edwards DJ, Hoy G, Saies AD, Hayes MG. Adverse reactions to an absorbable shoulder fixation device. *J Shoulder Elbow Surg* 1994;3: 230–233.
30. Fee HJ, McAvoy JM, Dainko EA. Pseudoaneurysm of the axillary artery following a modified Bristow operation. *J Cardiovasc Surg* 1978;19:65–68.
31. Flatow EL, Bigliani LU, April EW. An anatomic study of the musculocutaneous nerve and its relationship to the coracoid process. *Clin Orthop* 1989;244:166–171.
32. Flatow EL, Soslowsky LJ, Ateshian GA, et al. Shoulder joint anatomy and the effect of subluxations and size mismatch on patterns of glenohumeral contact. *Orthop Trans* 1991;15:803–804.
33. Foster CR. Arthroscopic shoulder reconstruction for instability. *Orthop Trans* 1994;18:192.
34. Fronek J, Warren RF, Bowen M. Posterior subluxation of the glenohumeral joint. *J Bone Joint Surg [Am]* 1989;71:205–216.
35. Fukuda K, Chen C, Cofield RH, Chao EYS. Biomechanical analysis of stability and fixation strength of total shoulder prostheses. *Orthopedics* 1988;11:141–149.
36. Gallie WE, LeMesurier AB. Recurring dislocation of the shoulder. *J Bone Joint Surg [Am]* 1948;30B:9–18.
37. Geiger DF, Hurley JA, Tovey JA, et al. Results of the arthroscopic versus open Bankart suture repair. *Orthop Trans* 1993;17:973.
38. Gerber C. Symposium on shoulder instability. American Academy of Orthopaedic Surgeons Annual Meeting. San Francisco, CA, 1997.
39. Gerber C, Farron A. Isolated tears of the subscapularis tendon. American Shoulder and Elbow Surgeons Annual Open Meeting. Orlando, FL, 1995.
40. Gerber C, Ganz R, Vinh TS. Glenoplasty for recurrent posterior shoulder instability. *Clin Orthop* 1987;216:70–79.
41. Gerber C, Lambert SM. Allograft reconstruction of segmental defects of the humeral head for the treatment of chronic locked posterior dislocation of the shoulder. *J Bone Joint Surg [Am]* 1996;78:376–382.
42. Gohlke F, Schneider P, Siegel K, Balzer C. Tensile strength of various anchor systems in surgical correction of instability of the shoulder joint. *Unfallchirurg* 1993;96:546–50.
43. Goldberg BJ, Nirschl RP, McConnell JP, Pettrone FA. Arthroscopic transglenoid suture capsulolabral repairs: preliminary results. *Am J Sports Med* 1993;21:656–665.
44. Grana W, Buckeley P, Yates C. Arthroscopic Bankart suture repair. *Am J Sports Med* 1993;21:348–353.
45. Green MR, Christensen KP. Arthroscopic versus open Bankart procedures: a comparison of early morbidity and complications. *Arthroscopy* 1993;9:371–374.
46. Green MR, Christensen KP. Arthroscopic Bankart procedure: two- to five-year followup with clinical correlation to severity of glenoid labral lesion. *Am J Sports Med* 1995;23:276–281.
47. Greis PE, Dean M, Hawkins RJ. Subscapularis tendon disruption after Bankart reconstruction for anterior instability. *J Shoulder Elbow Surg* 1996;5:219–222.
48. Gross RM. Arthroscopic shoulder capsulorraphy: does it work? *Am J Sports Med* 1989;17:495–500.
49. Guanche C, Quick D, Sodergren K, et al. Arthroscopic versus open reconstruction of the shoulder in patients with isolated Bankart lesions. *Am J Sports Med* 1996;24:144–148.
50. Hardy P, Thabit GR, Fanton GS, Blin JL, Lortat-Jacob A, Benoit J. Arthroscopic management of recurrent anterior shoulder dislocation by combining a labrum suture with antero-inferior holmium:YAG laser capsular shrinkage. *Orthopade* 1996;25:91–93.
51. Harryman DTD, Ballmer FP, Harris SL, Sidles JA. Arthroscopic labral repair to the glenoid rim. *Arthroscopy* 1994;10:20–30.
52. Harryman DT II. Common surgical approaches to the shoulder. In: Eilert RE, ed. *Instructional course lectures*. Park Ridge, IL: American Academy of Orthopaedic Surgeons, 1992:3–11.
53. Harryman DT II, Sidles JA, Harris SL, Matsen FA III. The role of the rotator interval capsule in passive motion and stability of the shoulder. *J Bone Joint Surg [Am]* 1992;74:53—66.
54. Harryman DT II, Sidles JA, Matsen FA III. The role of the coracohumeral ligament in range of motion and obligate translation in the shoulder. *Orthop Trans* 1990;14:727.
55. Hawkins R, Angelo R. Glenohumeral osteoarthrosis: a late complication of the Putti-Platt Repair. *J Bone Joint Surg [Am]* 1990;72: 1193–1197.
56. Hawkins RB. Arthroscopic stapling repair for shoulder instability: a retrospective study of 50 cases. *Arthroscopy* 1989;5:122–128.
57. Hawkins RH. Glenoid osteotomy for recurrent posterior subluxation of the shoulder: assessment by computed axial tomography. *J Shoulder Elbow Surg* 1996;5:393–400.
58. Hawkins RH, Hawkins RJ. Failed anterior reconstruction for shoulder instability. *J Bone Joint Surg [Br]* 1985;67:709–714.
59. Hawkins RJ, Koppert G, Johnston G. Recurrent posterior instability (subluxation) of the shoulder. *J Bone Joint Surg [Am]* 1984;66: 169–174.
60. Hawkins RJ, Schutte JP, Janda DH, Huckell GH. Translation of the glenohumeral joint with the patient under anesthesia. *J Shoulder Elbow Surg* 1996;5:286–292.
61. Hill JA, Lombards SJ, Kerlan RK, et al. The modified Bristow-Helfet procedure for recurrent anterior subluxations and dislocations. *Am J Sports Med* 1981;9:283–287.
62. Ho E, Cofield RH. Neurologic complications after shoulder stabilization procedures. American Academy of Orthopaedic Surgeons 64th Annual Meeting. San Francisco, CA, 1997.
63. Hopkinson WJ, Ryan JB, Wheeler JH. Glenoid rim fracture and recurrent shoulder instability. *Comp Orthop* (March/April) 1989;36–45.
64. Hovelius L. Anterior dislocation of the shoulder in teenagers and young adults. Five-year prognosis. *J Bone Joint Surg [Am]* 1987;69: 393.
65. Hovelius L, Eriksson K, Fredin H, et al. Recurrences after initial dislocation of the shoulder: results of a prospective study of treatment. *J Bone Joint Surg* 1983;65:343–349.
66. Hovelius L, Korner G, Lundberg B, et al. The coracoid transfer for recurrent dislocation of the shoulder. Technical aspects of the Bristow-Laterjet procedure. *J Bone Joint Surg [Am]* 1983;65:924–936.
67. Hovelius L, Thorling GJ, Fredin H. Recurrent anterior dislocation of the shoulder. Results after the Bankart and Putti-Platt operations. *J Bone Joint Surg [Am]* 1979;61:566–569.
68. Howell SM, Galinat BJ. The glenoid–labral socket. A constrained articular surface. *Clin Orthop* 1989;243:122–125.
69. Hurley JA, Anderson TE, Dear W, Andvish JT, Bergfeld JA, Weiker GG. Posterior shoulder instability: surgical vs. non-surgical results. *Orthop Trans* 1987;11:458.
70. Iftikhar TB, Kaminski RS, Silva I Jr. Neurovascular complications of the modified Bristow procedure. *J Bone Joint Surg [Am]* 1984;66: 951–952.
71. Johnson LI, ed. *Diagnostic and surgical arthroscopy of the shoulder*. St Louis: Mosby-Year Book, 1993.
72. Johnston GH, Hawkins RJ, Haddad R, Fowler PJ. A complication of posterior glenoid osteotomy for recurrent posterior shoulder instability. *Clin Orthop* 1984;187:147–149.
73. Klein AH, et al. Measurement of brachial plexus strain in arthroscopy of the shoulder. *Arthroscopy* 1987;3:45–52.
74. Kretzler HH. Scapular osteotomy for posterior shoulder dislocation. *J Bone Joint Surg [Am]* 1974;56:197–200.
75. Kummel BM. Fractures of the glenoid causing chronic dislocation of the shoulder. *Clin Orthop* 1970;69:189–191.
76. Landsiedle F. Arthroscopic therapy of recurrent anterior luxation of the shoulder by capsular repair. *Arthroscopy* 1992;8:296–304.
77. Lane JG, Sachs RA, Riehl B. Arthroscopic staple capsulorrhaphy: a long-term follow-up. *Arthroscopy* 1993;9:190–194.
78. Lazarus MD, Harryman DT II. Failed anterior instability repairs. In: Warner JP, Iannotti JP, Gerber C, eds. *Complex and revision problems in the shoulder*. New York: Raven Press, 1996.
79. Lazarus MD, Sidles JA, Harryman DT II, Matsen FA III. The effect of a chondral–labral defect on glenoid concavity and glenohumeral instability: a cadaver model. *J Bone Joint Surg [Am]* 1996;78:94–102.
80. Lee YF, Cohn L, Tooke SM. Intramuscular deltoid pressure during shoulder arthroscopy. *Arthroscopy* 1989;5:209–212.
81. Leutzow WF, Atkin DM, Sachs RA. Arthroscopic versus open Bankart repair of the shoulder for recurrent anterior dislocations. American Academy of Orthopaedic Surgeons Annual Meeting, Orlando, FL, 1995.
82. Lippitt SB, Harris SL, Harryman DT II, Sidles JA, Matsen FA III. In vivo quantification of the laxity of normal and unstable glenohumeral joints. *J Shoulder Elbow Surg* 1994;3:215–223.

83. Lippitt SB, Harryman DT II, Sidles JA, Matsen FA III. Diagnosis and management of AMBRI syndrome. *Tech Orthop* 1991;6:61–73.
84. Lippitt SB, Vanderhooft E, Harris SL, Sidles JA, Harryman DT II, Matsen FA III. Glenohumeral stability from concavity-compression: a quantitative analysis. *J Shoulder Elbow Surg* 1993;2:27–35.
85. Lombardo SJ, Kerlan RK, Jobe FW, Carter VS, Blazina ME, Shields CL Jr. The modified Bristow procedure for recurrent dislocation of the shoulder. *J Bone Joint Surg [Am]* 1976;58:256–261.
86. Loomer R, Graham B. Anatomy of the axillary nerve and its relation to inferior capsular shift. *Clin Orthop* 1989;243:100–105.
87. Loutzenheiser TD, Harryman DTN, Yung SW, France MP, Sidles JA. Optimizing arthroscopic knots. *Arthroscopy* 1995;11:199–206.
88. MacDonald PB, Hawkins RJ, Fowler PJ, Miniaci A. Release of the subscapularis for internal rotation contracture and pain after anterior repair for recurrent anterior dislocation of the shoulder. *J Bone Joint Surg [Am]* 1992;74:734–737.
89. Manta JP, Pettrone FA. Increased failure rate with long-term arthroscopic shoulder stabilization. *Complications Orthop* 1996;19–27
90. Matsen FA III, Harryman DT II, Sidles JA, Lippitt SL. *Practical evaluation and managment of the shoulder*. Philadelphia: WB Saunders, 1994.
91. Matsen FA III, Thomas SC. Glenohumeral instability. In: Evarts CM, ed. *Surgery of the musculoskeletal system*. New York: Churchill Livingstone, 1990:1439–1469.
92. Matsen FA III, Thomas SC, Rockwood CA. Anterior glenohumeral stability. In: Rockwood CA, Matsen FA III, eds. *The shoulder*. Philadelphia: WB Saunders, 1990:547–551.
93. Matthews LS, Vetter WL, Oweida SJ, Spearman J, Helfet DL. Arthroscopic staple capsulorrhaphy for recurrent anterior shoulder instability. *Arthroscopy* 1988;4:106–111.
94. Matthews LS, Zarins B, Michael RH, et al. Anterior portal selection for shoulder arthroscopy. *Arthroscopy* 1985;1:33–39.
95. McAuliffe TB, Pangayatselvan T, Bayley I. Failed surgery for recurrent anterior dislocation of the shoulder. *J Bone Joint Surg [Br]* 1988; 70:798–801.
96. McEleney ET, Donovan MJ, Shea KP, Nowak MD. Initial failure strength of open and arthroscopic Bankart repairs. *Arthroscopy* 1995; 11:426–431.
97. McMahon PJ, Dettiing J, Sandusky MD, Peatman TW, Tibone JE, Lee TQ. Shoulder instability: a multidisciplinary study of the glenoid origin of the anterior band of the inferior glenohumeral ligament. American Shoulder and Elbow Surgeons 13th Annual Meeting. San Francisco, CA, 1997.
98. Mologne TS, Lapoint JM, Morin WD, Zilberfarb J, O'Brien TJ. Arthroscopic anterior labral reconstruction using a transglenoid suture technique. Results in active-duty military patients. *Am J Sports Med* 1996;24:268–274.
99. Morgan CD. Arthroscopic transglenoid Bankart suture repair. *Oper Tech Orthop* 1991;1:171–179.
100. Morgan CD, Bodenstab AB. Arthroscopic Bankart suture repair: technique and early results. *Arthroscopy* 1987;3:111–122.
101. Mullins RC, Drez DJ, Cooper J. Hypoglossal nerve palsy after arthroscopy of the shoulder and open operation with the patient in the beach-chair position. A case report. *J Bone Joint Surg [Am]* 1992;74: 137–139.
102. Neer CS II. *Shoulder reconstruction*. Philadelphia: WB Saunders, 1990.
103. Neer CS II, Foster CR. Inferior capsular shift for involuntary inferior and multidirectional instabliity of the shoulder. *J Bone Joint Surg* 1980;62:897–907.
104. Neviaser TJ. The anterior labroligamentous periosteal sleeve avulsion lesion: a cause of anterior instability of the shoulder. *Arthroscopy* 1993;9:17–21.
105. Nobuhara K, Ikeda H. Rotator interval lesion. *Clin Orthop* 1987;223: 44–50.
106. Norris TR. Complications following anterior instability repairs. In: Bigliani LU, ed. *Complications of shoulder surgery*. Baltimore: Williams & Wilkins, 1993:98–116.
107. Norris TR, Bigliani LU. Analysis of failed repair for shoulder instability—a preliminary report. In: Bateman JE, Welsh RP, eds. *Surgery of the shoulder*. Philadelphia: BC Decker, 1984:111–116.
108. Norris TR, Bigliani LU. Complications following the modified Bristow procedure for shoulder instability. *Orthop Trans* 1987;11: 232–233.
109. Norwood LA, Fowler HL. Rotator cuff tears: a shoulder arthroscopy complication. *Am J Sports Med* 1989;17:837–841.
110. Nottage WM. Arthroscopic portals: anatomy at risk. *Orthop Clin North Am* 1993;24:19–26.
111. Ogilvie-Harris DJ, Wiley AM. Arthroscopic surgery of the shoulder. A general appraisal. *J Bone Joint Surg [Br]* 1986;68:201–207.
112. Pagnani MJ, Warren RF. Arthroscopic shoulder stabilization. *Oper Tech Sports Med* 1993;1:276–284.
113. Pagnani MJ, Warren RF, Altchek DW. Arthroscopic shoulder stabilization using transglenoid sutures: four year minimum follow-up. American Academy of Orthopaedic Surgeons Annual Meeting, Orlando, FL, 1995.
114. Peek R, Haynes DW. Compartment syndrome as a complication of arthroscopy: a case report and a study of interstitial pressures. *Am J Sports Med* 1984;12:464–468.
115. Pitman MI. The use of somatosensory evoked potentials for the detection of neuropraxia during shoulder arthroscopy. *Arthroscopy* 1988;4: 250–255.
116. Rao JP, Tovey JE, Zoppi A, et al. Comparison of arthroscopic capsulorraphy for anterior shoulder instability. *Orthop Trans* 1993;17: 972–973.
117. Reeves B. Experiments on the tensile strength of the anterior capsular structures of the shoulder in man. *J Bone Joint Surg [Br]* 1968;50: 858–865.
118. Reider B, Inglis AE. The Bankart procedure modified by the use of Prolene pull-out sutures. *J Bone Joint Surg [Am]* 1982;64:628–629.
119. Richards RR, Beaton D, Hudson AR. Shoulder arthrodesis with plate fixation: functional outcome analysis. *J Shoulder Elbow Surg* 1993;2: 225–239.
120. Richards RR, Hudson AR, Bertoia, JT, et al. Injury to the brachial plexus during Putti-Platt and Bristow procedures: a report of eight cases. *Am J Sports Med* 1987;15:374–380.
121. Rockwood Jr CA, Gerber C. Analysis of failed surgical procedures for anterior shoulder instability. *Orthop Trans* 1985;9:48.
122. Rodeo SA, Forster RA, Weiland AJ. Neurologic complications due to arthroscopy. *J Bone Joint Surg [Am]* 1993;75:917–926.
123. Rodeo SA, Hannafin SK, Bhargava MM, Warren RF. Analysis of collagen and elastic fibers in shoulder capsule in shoulder instability. The American Orthopaedic Society for Sports Medicine. San Francisco, CA, 1997.
124. Rose DJ. Arthroscopic suture capsulorraphy for anterior shoulder insatbility. *Orthop Trans* 1990;14:597.
125. Rowe C, Patel D, Southmayd W. The Bankart procedure: a long term, end results study. *J Bone Joint Surg [Am]* 1978;60:6–11.
126. Rowe CR, Pierce DS, Clark JG. Voluntary dislocation of the shoulder. A preliminary report on a clinical, electromyographic, and psychiatric study of twenty-six patients. *J Bone Joint Surg [Am]* 1973;55: 445–460.
127. Rowe CR, Zarins B. Recurrent transient subluxation of the shoulder. *J Bone Joint Surg [Am]* 1981;63:863–872.
128. Rowe CR, Zarins B, Ciullo JV. Recurrent anterior dislocation of the shoulder after surgical repair. *J Bone Joint Surg [Am]* 1984;66: 159–168.
129. Schauder KS, Tullos HS. Role of the coracoid bone block in the modified Bristow procedure. *Am J Sports Med* 1992;20:31–34.
130. Scott DJ. Treatment of recurrent posterior dislocations of the shoulder by glenoplasty. *J Bone Joint Surg [Am]* 1967;49:471–476.
131. Shall LM, Cawley PW. Soft tissue reconstruction in the shoulder. Comparison of suture anchors, absorbable staples, and absorbable tacks. *Am J Sports Med* 1994;22:715–718.
132. Shea KP, Lovallo JL. Scapulothoracic penetration of a Beath pin: an unusual complication of arthroscopic Bankart suture repair. *Arthroscopy* 1991;7:115–117.
133. Sherman OH. Arthroscopy-no problem surgery. *J Bone Joint Surg [Am]* 1986;68:256–265.
134. Small NC. Complications in arthroscopy: the knee and other joints. Committee on complications of the Arthroscopy Association of North America. *Arthroscopy* 1986;2:253–258.
135. Small NC. Complications in arthroscopy performed by experienced arthroscopists. *Arthroscopy* 1988;4:215–221.
136. Snyder SJ, Strafford BB. Arthroscopic management of instability of the shoulder. *Orthopedics* 1993;16:993–1002.
137. Soslowsky LJ, Bigliani LU, Flatow EL. Articular geometry of the glenohumeral joint. *Clin Orthop* 1992;285:181–190.

138. Speer KP, Deng X, Borrero S, Torzilli PA, Altchek DA, Warren RF. Biomechanical evaluation of a simulated Bankart lesion. *J Bone Joint Surg [Am]* 1994;76:1819–1826.
139. Speer KP, Pagnani M, Warren RF. Arthroscopic anterior shoulder stabilization: 2–5 year follow-up using a bioabsorbable tac. *J Shoulder Elbow Surg* 1995;4(suppl):54.
140. Speer KP, Warren RF. Arthroscopic shoulder stabilization. A role for biodegradable materials. *Clin Orthop* 1993;67–74.
141. Speer KP, Warren RF, Pagnani M, Warner JP. An arthroscopic technique for anterior stabilization of the shoulder with a bioabsorbable tack. *J Bone Joint Surg [Am]* 1996;78:1801–1806.
142. Sperber A, Wredmark T. Capsular elasticity and joint volume in recurrent anterior shoulder instability. *Arthroscopy* 1994;10:598–601.
143. Swenson TM, Warner JJ. Arthroscopic shoulder stabilization. Overview of indications, technique, and efficacy. *Clin Sports Med* 1995;14:841–862.
144. Thomas SC, Matsen FA III. An approach to the repair of glenohumeral ligament avulsion in the management of traumatic anterior glenohumeral instability. *J Bone Joint Surg [Am]* 1989;71:506–513.
145. Tibone J, Ting A. Capsulorraphy with a staple for recurrent posterior subluxation of the shoulder. *J Bone Joint Surg [Am]* 1990;72: 999–1002.
146. Torg, Balduini, Bonci C, et al. A modified Bristow Helfet May procedure for recurrent dislocation and subluxation of the shoulder. *J Bone Joint Surg [Am]* 1987;69:904–913.
147. Turkel S, Panio M, Marshall J, et al. Stabilizing mechanisms preventing anterior dislocation of the glenohumeral joint. *J Bone Joint Surg [Am]* 1981;63:1208–1217.
148. Uribe JW, Hechtman KS. Arthroscopically assisted repair of acute Bankart lesion. *Orthopedics* 1993;16:1019–1023.
149. Walch G, Boileau P, Levigne C, Mandrino A, Neyret P, Donell S. Arthroscopic stabilization for recurrent anterior shoulder dislocation: results of 59 cases. *Arthroscopy* 1995;11:173–179.
150. Wall MS, Warren, RF. Complications of shoulder instability surgery. *Clin Sports Med* 1995;14:973–1000.
151. Warner JJ, Miller MD, Marks P. Arthroscopic Bankart repair with the Suretac device. Part II: Experimental observations. *Arthroscopy* 1995; 11:14–20.
152. Warner JJ, Miller MD, Marks P, Fu FH. Arthroscopic Bankart repair with the Suretac device. Part I: Clinical observations. *Arthroscopy* 1995;11:2–13.
153. Warner JJP. Recurrent anterior instability: arthroscopic repair. In: Bigliani, LU, ed. *The unstable shoulder: monograph series.* Rosemont, IL: American Academy of Orthopaedic Surgeons, 1996.
154. Warner JJP, Deng X-H, Warren RF, Torzilli PA. Static capsuloligamentous restraints to superior–inferior translation of the glenohumeral joint. *Am J Sports Med* 1992;20:675–685.
155. Warner JJP, Warren RF. Arthroscopic Bankart repair utlizing a cannulated absorbable fixation device. *Oper Tech Orthop* 1991;1: 192–198.
156. Weber BG, Simpson A, Hardegger F. Rotational humeral osteotomy for recurrent anterior dislocation of the shoulder associated with a large Hill–Sachs lesion. *J Bone Joint Surg [Am]* 1984;66:1443.
157. Weber SC. A prospective evaluation comparing arthroscopic and open treatment in the management of recurrent anterior glenohumeral dislocation. *Orthop Trans* 1991;15:763.
158. Wiley AM. Arthroscopy for shoulder instability and a technique for arthroscopic repair. *Arthroscopy* 1988;4:25–30.
159. Wilson, FD, Adams G, Hile LE, et al. Arthroscopic treatment of the recurrent dislocating shoulder. *Orthop Trans* 1993;17:973.
160. Wirth M, Blatter G, Rockwood C. The capsular imbrication procedure for recurrent anterior instability of the shoulder. *J Bone Joint Surg [Am]* 1996;78:246–258.
161. Wirth MA, Seltzer DG, Rockwood CA. Jr. Replacement of the subscapularis with the pectoralis muscles in anterior shoulder instability. American Shoulder and Elbow Surgeons Annual Open Meeting. Orlando, FL, 1995.
162. Wolf EM. Anterior portals in shoulder arthroscopy. *Arthroscopy* 1989;5:20—1–208.
163. Wolf EM, Cheng JC, Dickson K. Humeral avulsion of glenohumeral ligaments as a cause of anterior shoulder instability. *Arthroscopy* 1995;11:600–607.
164. Wolf EM, Wilk RM, Richmond JC. Arthroscopic Bankart repair using suture anchors. *Oper Tech Orthop* 1991;1:184–191.
165. Wolin PM. Arthroscopic glenoid labrum suture repair. *Orthop Trans* 1990;14:597.
166. Young DC, Rockwood CA Jr. Complications of a failed Bristow procedure and their management. *J Bone Joint Surg [Am]* 1991;73: 969–981.
167. Yung SW, Lazarus MD, Harryman DT II. Practical guidelines to safe surgery about the subscapularis. *J Shoulder Elbow Surg* 1996;5: 467–470.
168. Zarins B, Rowe CR, Stone, JW. Shoulder instability: management of failed reconstructions. In: Barr JS, Jr, eds. *Instructional Course Lectures.* Rosemont, IL: American Academy of Orthopaedic Surgeons, 1989;38:217–230.
169. Ziegler DW, Harryman DT II, Matsen FA III. Subscapularis insufficiency in the previously operated shoulder. American Shoulder and Elbow Surgeons 12th Open Meeting. Atlanta, GA, 1996.
170. Zuckerman JD, Matsen FA II. Complications about the glenohumeral joint related to the use of screw and staples. *J Bone Joint Surg [Am]* 1984;66:175–180.

PART III

Frozen Shoulder

Disorders of the Shoulder: Diagnosis and Management, edited by Joseph P. Iannotti and Gerald R. Williams, Jr. Lippincott Williams & Wilkins, Philadelphia © 1999.

CHAPTER 15

Diagnosis, Classification, and Management of the Stiff Shoulder

Frances Cuomo

INTRODUCTION

Frozen shoulder is one of the most common, yet one of the most poorly understood disorders of the glenohumeral joint. This is primarily due to confusing terminology, difficulty defining and differentiating it clearly from other conditions with similar symptoms and findings but with distinctly different etiologies, and the inability of physicians to agree on the exact definition of frozen shoulder syndrome. Frozen shoulder syndrome comprises a group of conditions with different underlying etiologies. Initially, periarthritis of the shoulder was used as an all encompassing term to describe painful shoulders for which the symptoms could not be explained on the basis of arthritis of the glenohumeral joint.[34] Codman described the disorder known as frozen shoulder as a "condition difficult to define, difficult to treat, and difficult to explain from the point of view of pathology."[26] The terms adhesive capsulitis and periarthritis of the shoulder are used at times with a meaning synonymous with frozen shoulder. In this chapter, a working definition of *frozen shoulder* is suggested: frozen shoulder is a condition of uncertain etiology characterized by significant restriction of both active and passive shoulder motion that occurs in the absence of a known intrinsic shoulder disorder.[141] Previous authors have defined primary frozen shoulder as an idiopathic condition and secondary frozen shoulder as one associated with a known intrinsic, extrinsic, or systemic pathology.[72] Although this is most likely a worthwhile distinction, it is probably inappropriate to include all intrinsic, extrinsic, and systemic etiologies as secondary frozen shoulder. Intrinsic disorders such as rotator cuff pathology should be considered separately, for they represent a known underlying disorder or condition that results in the clinical picture of frozen shoulder. Extrinsic disorders, such as cervical radiculopathy or intrathoracic conditions, and systemic disorders, such as diabetes mellitus or hypothyroidism, should be considered together yet separate from the intrinsic disorders, for they more closely resemble the primary or idiopathic condition. This schema is shown in Fig. 1.

In this chapter only primary frozen shoulder will be discussed, reviewing pathophysiology, evaluation, operative and nonoperative management, as well as complications. Secondary frozen shoulder associated with intrinsic conditions will not be discussed because, in these situations, treatment approaches are directed primarily at correction of the underlying disorder, which is critical to the alleviation of the symptoms of frozen shoulder. Exclusion criteria for primary frozen shoulder, therefore, include patients with glenohumeral arthritis, fractures, dislocations, cervical spondylosis, neuromuscular disease, and referred pain from an intrathoracic source. Intrinsic shoulder pathology, such as subacromial impingement, calcific tendinitis, and postsurgical stiffness, therefore, is also excluded from this review and will be discussed elsewhere in the text.

F. Cuomo: Shoulder Service, New York University Hospital for Joint Diseases, New York, New York 10003.

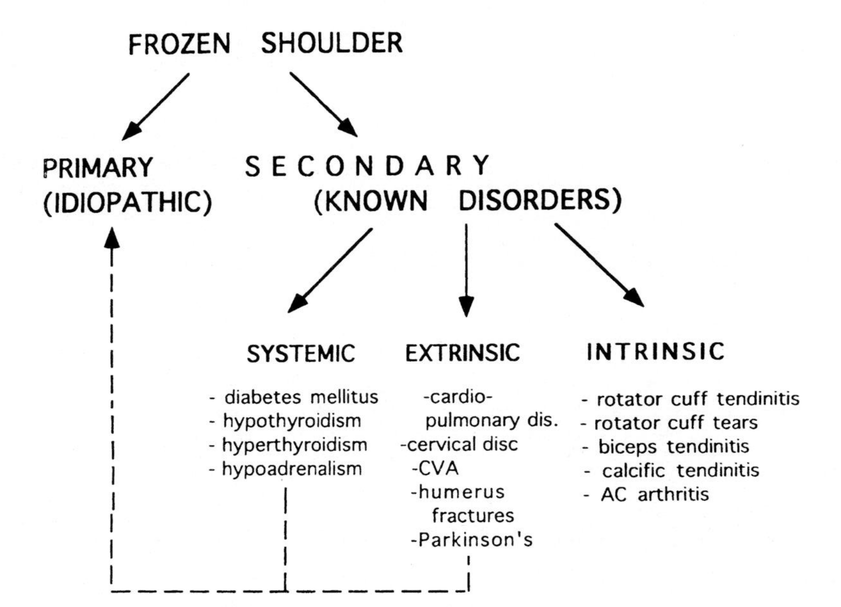

FIG. 1. Proposed pathways for the development of frozen shoulder syndrome.

SURGICAL ANATOMY AND BIOMECHANICS

When considering frozen shoulder syndrome, it is important to include the overall shoulder girdle complex, consisting of the glenohumeral joint, acromioclavicular and sternoclavicular joints, as well as the scapulothoracic articulation. Scapulothoracic and glenohumeral movements occur simultaneously as the arm is used away from the side.[53] The normal glenohumeral to scapulothoracic ratio is 2:1, with the most elevation attributed to the glenohumeral joint.

The inherently loose articulation of the normal shoulder is a necessary anatomic feature that permits the large range of motion required for normal shoulder function. The glenohumeral joint is enclosed entirely by the joint capsule. The capsule of the shoulder is normally a loose structure of which the surface area is almost twice that of the humeral head.[57] The stability of this joint is maintained further by osseous, static, and dynamic stabilizers. It is a nonconstrained articulation, with the larger humeral head having nearly perfect congruity with the smaller osseous glenoid. To enhance the surface area of this loose articulation, the fibrous glenoid labrum is attached around the periphery of the glenoid. The dynamic stabilizers of the joint consist of the rotator cuff musculature. The primary function of the rotator cuff muscles is to create compression of the convex humeral head into the matched concavity of the glenoid fossa. The capsuloligamentous structures are the primary static stabilizers and are responsible for the stability of the joint, mainly at the extreme positions of rotation and translation, as they are normally lax during most shoulder rotations. The capsule attaches around the perimeter of the glenoid and extends across to attach to the anatomic neck of the humerus, except inferiorly where the attachment is about 1 cm distal to the articular margin. There are numerous areas within the capsule that are thickened secondary to attachment or confluence with local structures. The tendons of the rotator cuff adjacent to the joint capsule thicken the capsule anteriorly, superiorly, and posteriorly. In addition, the superior, middle, and inferior glenoid humeral ligaments will present further areas of thickening of the joint capsule.[9,10,12,32,38] The inferior capsule, however, is not supported by adjacent muscles and tendons, thereby leaving a lax double fold of capsule that forms the inferior or axillary recess. This potential space of the axillary pouch formed by the redundant fold of capsule is normally present while the arm is at the side, but the pouch disappears and the capsule becomes taut as the arm is brought up into forward elevation or abduction allowed by the stretch of the inferior capsule. Superiorly, there is a triangular-shaped region between the anterior border of the supraspinatus tendon and the superior border of the subscapularis tendon known as the rotator interval. The ligamentous components of this region are the superior glenohumeral ligament and the coracohumeral ligament. Review of classic descriptions of the coracohumeral ligament describe it as a dense, fibrous structure originating on the lateral surface of the coracoid process at its base and inserting into the greater and lesser tuberosities adjacent to the bicipital groove.[32]

At arthroscopy or arthrography, several recesses may be identified in the normal shoulder. Anteriorly, a synovial recess is often present between the superior and middle glenohumeral ligaments, known as the rotator cleft, also known as the subscapular bursa. There is a posterior outpouching of the capsule also, just deep to the infraspinatus muscle, known as the infraspinatus bursa. There is an inferior recess of redundant capsule forming a pouchlike fold when the arm is at the side. The synovial membrane is also a structure that has been implicated in the frozen shoulder process. This structure lines the capsule and is in continuity with the surrounding bursae and recesses. The synovium invests the long head of the biceps and passes deep to the transverse humeral ligament in the bicipital groove. The biceps tendon sheath may extend for a distance of 5 cm beyond the transverse ligament, distal into the bicipital groove, especially when the arm is in abduction, the arm position where the least amount of biceps tendon is intraarticular.[80,81]

During normal motion of the shoulder, the tightening and loosening of the glenohumeral ligaments and capsule encircling the humeral head is accompanied by lengthening and shortening of the rotator cuff and deltoid muscle.[131] These structures, working in concert, allow the normal 2:1 glenohumeral to scapulothoracic ratio necessary for elevation of the arm. In the pathologic state of frozen shoulder syndrome, Nicholson noted the scapula usually moved excessively in upward rotation to compensate for the loss of glenohumeral motion. On clinical examination, he consistently found the inferior glide of the humerus to be the most restricted of the accessory movements of the shoulder.[94] Numerous investigators have described the pathologic findings associated with frozen shoulder in an attempt to offer explanation for the observed microscopic capsular changes.[26,72,74,75,82,86,87,101,108,121] Much of our current understanding of the pathology of frozen shoulder is due to the work of J. S. Neviaser, who coined the term "adhesive capsulitis" to describe an avascular, tense capsule that was markedly adherent to the humeral head and associated with decreased joint volume and synovial fluid. The histologic changes were consistent with chronic inflammation, fibrosis, and perivascular infiltration in the subsynovial layer, with the synovial layer remaining uninvolved.[87]

Simmonds theorized that a chronic inflammatory reaction caused by a degeneration of the supraspinatus tendon resulted in the capsular changes seen in frozen shoulder. He described a local hyperemia within the joint capsule, as observed earlier by Neviaser.[121] He thought that the tight, fibrotic characteristics of the capsular tissue extended out into the soft tissues around the shoulder.

From intraoperative findings of gross contracture of the rotator cuff, McNab postulated that the primary lesion was in the cuff itself, with subsequent contracture of the capsule and coracohumeral ligament. He confirmed a region of constant hypovascularity in the supraspinatus tendon, called the critical zone by Codman,[26] and theorized that this was responsible for the initial cuff degeneration.[108] The localized degeneration of the collagen was then theorized to induce an autoimmune response. McNab felt that the round cell infiltrate found in the capsule at open surgical release of the shoulder could be interpreted as an autoimmune response. Further reports have failed to identify any statistically significant clinical or laboratory evidence for an immunologic basis for this condition.[72,80] Lundberg confirmed the absence of intraarticular adhesions in his operative observations at cinearthrography.[71,72,102] Although on histologic examination the synovial cells were largely unchanged, Lundberg did report finding a more compact, dense collagen layer within the shoulder capsule. The glycosaminoglycans' distribution in the shoulder capsule had the characteristics of a repair action.[73]

Ozaki and associates[101] described the role of contracture of coracohumeral ligament and the rotator interval in the pathogenesis of frozen shoulder. These investigators found fibrotic hyalinization and fibrinoid degeneration in these structures. Neer[84–86] also reported the importance of coracohumeral ligament contracture, but he stressed that it was unlikely that any one anatomic structure or pathologic process was responsible for causing the entire symptom complex associated with frozen shoulder. The normal rotator interval contains elastic membranous tissue and, as a result, enhances the range of motion of the glenohumeral joint. The coracohumeral ligament helps strengthen this region and acts as a suspensory ligament of the humeral head. The long head of the biceps is located beneath the rotator interval. In patients with chronic severe adhesive capsulitis, the pathologic findings in the coracohumeral ligament and in the rotator interval are extremely important. These structures are contracted and can be converted into a thick fibrous cord that holds the humeral head tightly against the glenoid fossa and restricts glenohumeral movement in all directions.

Much of the information on the gross and microscopic pathologic findings has been derived from operative observation and autopsy studies. DePalma described the fibrous capsule, synovial tissue, and rotator cuff as thickened fibrotic and contracted around the humeral head. The folds in the capsule and the synovial membrane along the inferior aspect of the humeral head were obliterated.[31]

Recent arthroscopic evaluation of patients with arthrographically documented adhesive capsulitis is believed by some authors to involve four stages of the disease. Stage I, the preadhesive stage, is seen in patients with minimal or no limitation of motion. There is a fibrinous synovial inflammatory reaction that is detectable only by arthroscopy. This reinforces the need to obtain arthroscopic evaluation of any patient who is treated by decompression for an impingement syndrome. In stage II, acute adhesive synovitis, there is proliferative synovitis and early adhesion formation. The adhesions are seen well in the dependent folds extending to the humeral head. Stage III, the stage of maturation, has less synovitis with loss of the axillary fold. In stage IV, the chronic stage, adhesions are fully mature and markedly restrictive.[93]

PATHOPHYSIOLOGY

Numerous pathologic mechanisms have been proposed to explain the cause of frozen shoulder, but all remain largely theoretic. The syndrome of frozen shoulder was first described by Duplay in 1896. He introduced the term "scapulohumeral periarthritis," and felt that the initiating lesion was an obliteration of the subdeltoid bursa.[34]

Myer,[83] from a study of postmortem specimens, suggested that the initiating lesion was a breakdown on the intraarticular portion of the biceps tendon. His observations were supported subsequently by Pasteur[104] and Lippman[65] and more recently by DePalma.[30] Codman, however, believed that the changes in the biceps tendon were of little etiologic significance.[26]

McLauglin, one of the earliest investigators to describe the changes in the rotator cuff, stressed the importance of contracture of the subscapularis in the development of the syndrome.[77,78] Bateman reported his observations on the development of a hypertrophic inflammatory synovitis associated with intraarticular adhesions.[4] Several investigators have proposed an autoimmune basis for frozen shoulder.[5,19,20,21,46] Although some clinicians have reported a high incidence of human leukocyte antigen B27 in patients with frozen shoulder,[20] others have not confirmed this association.[58,95,115,126] In later studies, serum immunoglobulin A (IgA) levels were significantly lower in patients with frozen shoulder, and the immune complex and C-reactive protein levels were increased.[5,19,21] In general, however, sufficient evidence to support immunologic therapy has been lacking.

A relation to myofascial pain syndrome has been proposed. A syndrome of active trigger points about the shoulder, specifically within the subscapularis muscle, has been suggested as a possible cause of frozen shoulder syndrome.[127] *Trigger points* are defined as locally tender, self-sustaining, hyperirritable foci located in the skeletal muscle or its associated fascia. The trigger points are also characteristically related to a zone of referred pain when the trigger is stimulated. Once activated, perpetuating factors may be responsible for the chronicity of pain. Another characteristic of the myofascial pain syndrome is palpable bands of muscle fibers that undergo a local twitch response when the trigger point is stimulated with a snapping palpation.[12,122,137]

Travell and others theorized that the subscapularis trigger points exert an influence on the sympathetic vasomotor activity, leading to hypoxia of the periarticular tissues. It is further theorized that the hypoxia leads to a local proliferation of fibrous tissue about the shoulder capsule, resulting in the clinical picture of frozen shoulder syndrome.[83,127] A biochemical basis for frozen shoulder has been proposed. Lundberg, in his analysis of the capsules from patients with frozen shoulder, found an increase in glycosaminoglycans and a decrease in glycoprotein content. These biochemical changes in the capsule, however, are consistent with the process of fibrosis, and they may represent the effect of frozen shoulder, rather than its cause.[70,72]

Neurologic dysfunction has been postulated to be a cause of frozen shoulder syndrome. In 1959, Kopell[60] proposed suprascapular compression neuropathy as a possible cause of frozen shoulder, but electromyography (EMG) and nerve conduction studies have not supported this theory. Others have suggested that frozen shoulder is a result of autonomic dysfunction and represents a form a reflex sympathetic dystrophy.[114] Sufficient evidence to support these hypotheses has not been provided.

Bunker et al. prospectively studied 50 patients with the diagnosis of primary frozen shoulder. These authors were able to identify increased serum lipid levels in these patients compared with those of age- and sex-matched control subjects. The fasting serum triglyceride and cholesterol levels were significantly elevated in the frozen shoulder group. Increased serum triglyceride levels have also been found in patients with diabetes as well as Dupuytren's disease, suggesting that hyperlipidemia may be the common thread that links these three disorders.[22,23]

Various endocrine disorders are associated with frozen shoulder. In particular, patients with diabetes mellitus manifest a much greater incidence of frozen shoulder than their nondiabetic counterparts. Bridgman found that the incidence of frozen shoulder in 800 diabetic patients was 10.8%, compared with 2.3% in 600 nondiabetic controls.[15] A second study identified abnormal glucose tolerance test results for 28% of patients with frozen shoulder, compared with 12% in age- and sex-matched controls with other rheumatologic conditions.[64] Frozen shoulder has also been reported to occur with increased incidence among patients with thyroid disorders,[11,37] as well as those with hypoadrenalism,[136] or corticotropin deficiency.[24]

Trivial trauma has been postulated to be an important factor, particularly when it is followed by a prolonged period of immobilization.[30,106] This does seem to be the sequence of events in some patients who develop frozen shoulder. The association of frozen shoulder with major trauma to the shoulder or other parts of the upper extremity is recognized. The association with minor trauma that may be forgotten is difficult to document and may be overlooked.[26,78] Most patients who sustain minimal trauma, even when combined with a period of immobilization, do not develop frozen shoulder. This has led some investigators to conclude that there are some patients who possess a "constitutional" predisposition to develop a frozen shoulder. Support for this theory is provided by the significant incidence of bilateral frozen shoulders.[20,72,96,110,139]

The role of psychologic factors has been considered in the development of frozen shoulder. Some investigators have suggested that a certain personality structure, coupled with untoward life events and inappropriate responses to stress, may serve as a predisposing or precipitating factor for its development.[27,37,68,114] Coventry chose the term periarthritic personality to describe one component of a three-part theory on the pathogenesis of frozen shoulder in a group of patients with painful stiff shoulders. He observed that most patients had "a peculiar emotional constitution in which they were unable to tolerate pain, expected others to get them well, and refused to take any personal initiative in their recovery."[27] Other studies, however, have found no evidence for a characteristic personality disorder.[96,139] It would appear, therefore, that a specific periarthritic personality type is difficult to identify. The role of psychologic factors should be considered, at best, a secondary factor in the management of these patients.

Fibromatosis has also been implicated in the causation of frozen shoulder syndrome. The pathomechanics are believed to be found in fibrous tissue contracture formed in response to cytokines, lymphocyte, or monocyte products. Platelet-derived growth factor is a potent mytogenic polypeptide for mesenchymal cells. Immunocytochemistry was performed with monoclonal antibodies on the rotator ligaments excised from 12 patients with resistant frozen shoulder. Bunker and Anthony report that the pathologic process is active fibroblastic proliferation accompanied by some transformation to a smooth-muscle phenotype (myofibroblasts). The fibroblasts lay down collagen that appears as a thick nodular band or fleshy mass. These appearances are reportedly very similar to those seen in Dupuytren's disease of the hand, with no inflammation and no synovial involvement. The contracture acts as a checkrein against external rotation, causing a loss of both active and passive movement.[22]

Frozen shoulder associated with a known underlying disorder is considered to be secondary, and this group includes intrinsic, extrinsic, or systemic disorders. Intrinsic shoulder abnormalities include rotator cuff tendinitis, rotator cuff tears, tendinitis of the long head of the biceps tendon, calcific tendinitis, and acromioclavicular arthritis. Extrinsic disorders, which represent pathologic conditions remote from the shoulder region, include ischemic heart disease and myocardial infarction,[79,139] pulmonary disorders including tuberculosis,[55] chronic bronchitis, emphysema,[119] and tumor,[29] cervical disc disease and radiculopathy,[3,56,139] cerebral vascular hemorrhage,[14,17] previous coronary artery bypass graft surgery,[122] previous breast surgery, lesions of the middle humerus,[123] and central nervous system disorders, such as Parkinson's disease.[113] Systemic disorders represent generalized medical conditions that are known to occur in association with frozen shoulder. Such conditions and poor prognostic indicators include diabetes mellitus, hypothyroidism, hyperthyroidism, and hypoadrenalism.

Epidemiologically, the exact prevalence and incidence of frozen shoulder are not known, but the cumulative risk of at least one episode of frozen shoulder has been estimated to be a minimum of 2%.[72] It is most frequently found in patients between the fourth and sixth decades of life, and it is more common in women than men.[3] The nondominant extremity appears to be more commonly involved, with most reported cases being described as affecting the left side.[30,65,72] Bilateral involvement occurs in 6% to 50% of cases, although only 14% of these bilateral cases manifest simultaneously.[3,5,21,72,114] When a history of bilateral involvement is identified, the possibility of a constitutional predisposition should be explored.[4,72,114] The same shoulder is rarely involved again with adhesive capsulitis.[5,6]

There is significant controversy over the natural history of frozen shoulder relative to both objective and subjective outcomes. Historically, frozen shoulder has been touted as a condition for which "recovery is always sure and may be confidently expected."[26] Several investigators using a variety of treatment methods have reported that a high percentage of affected patients achieve full range of motion.[26,40,65] In addition, they have found complete or near complete symptomatic relief.[40,46] More recent investigations have questioned the early optimistic reports, finding measurable restriction at follow-up in 39% to 76% of patients[18,25,79,82,110] and persistent symptoms in up to 45%.[5,106]

The time course of adhesive capsulitis has been described as classically lasting 18 to 24 months.[5] Recent studies have challenged this commonly held belief. Reeves noted that the mean duration of symptoms was 30 months.[110] Patients describing themselves as functionally recovered tend to underestimate their loss of motion.[20] Reeves described some restriction in shoulder motion in more than 50% of patients in a 5- to 10-year follow-up, but functional impairment was identified in only 7%.[110] Clark found 42% of patients had persisting limitations of motion after 6 years of follow-up.[25] Binder, in a prospective study, noted that 90% of patients did not regain the minimum range of motion when matched for age and sex with a controlled group 6 months after diagnosis.[5] He also reported that 40% of patients failed to regain a minimum range of motion when matched for age and sex with a controlled group when followed for a minimum of 3 years. In a retrospective study, performed by Schaffer et al., of a carefully selected group of frozen shoulder patients, almost half remained symptomatic many years after the onset of symptoms, and up to 56% had residual restriction in one or more planes.[119]

Despite the subjective and objective outcome of this disorder, there seems to be widespread agreement on the seeming lack of significant or frequent functional disability documented at cessation of treatment. Regardless of objective restriction or the presence of symptoms, few patients are reportedly functionally restricted to any significant degree.[5,25,66,110] The lack of correlation between subjective and objective findings has been noted consistently.[5,7,18,25,46,82] Symptomatic patients frequently have no measurable restricted range of motion in any plane. Conversely, those patients with the most significant motion restriction were often pain-free. Whether this is due to adaptation to such restriction, or restriction in motion is unimportant for daily living activities is an unresolved issue. According to Neer, however, the presence of such restriction depends on the functional demands of the patient. Even in the active patient, the presence of 150 degrees of active elevation, 50 degrees of external rotation, and internal rotation to the eighth thoracic vertebra is probably sufficient for normal function.[86] In Schaffer's report of an older population whose functional demands were surely less than the aforestated, the degree of restriction tolerated in any plane was certainly even greater. The author states that the preeminent importance of forward flexion and elevation in daily activities superseded the findings of restriction predominantly in the abducted and externally rotated positions, which resulted in little functional impairment.[119]

In general, the natural history of frozen shoulder is uncertain, and additional randomized, prospective studies are needed. Difficulty exists in performing these studies owing to the ethical dilemma of assigning patients to an untreated group.

EVALUATION

Because frozen shoulder represents a symptom complex, rather than a specific diagnostic entity, a careful clinical history is crucial for making the diagnosis. Patients with this condition will often report a gradual loss of function, associated with vague discomfort of varying levels of intensity about the shoulder, after minimal or no trauma at all. The symptoms usually begin insidiously and are often worse at night. One should inquire about whether or not the pain is exacerbated with use, if the pain is present at rest, and if there is pain that interrupts sleep. Overhead and internal rotation or behind the back activities become especially difficult to perform as motion is diminished. These symptoms closely resemble those found in rotator cuff pathology, thereby mandating a careful physical examination to consider frozen shoulder as the primary condition, or one that is secondary to a specific shoulder problem. The patient should be asked to describe how the shoulder condition limits his or her function as well as its duration. The physician needs to inquire about risk factors, especially diabetes and thyroid disorders, for these may adversely affect the outcome. Among diabetic patients the rate of frozen shoulder is much higher than in the normal population, with bilateral presentation in as many as 77% of those cases; therefore, a careful history of the opposite upper extremity is required.[117] Patients who have taken insulin for more than 10 years have a significantly higher incidence of ongoing disability than other patients, despite treatment. An inquiry relative to specific occupational duties is made because frozen shoulder is more common in patients with sedentary occupations than in manual laborers.

As the shoulder stiffens, there is a progressive loss of glenohumeral motion. The most significant loss usually is in external rotation, with a smaller loss of abduction and internal rotation.[17] The patient may report the functional restrictions as difficulty using the arm above chest level, reaching to the side, or in the movement of putting on a coat. Loss of internal rotation is exhibited by functional restrictions in dressing or performing personal hygiene activities. There may be discomfort over the acromioclavicular joint, which can be secondary to increased scapulothoracic motion. Pain at the endpoint of restricted shoulder motion is characteristic.

Physical Examination

Physical examination of the cervical spine, opposite shoulder, and trunk should always be performed to exclude any associated abnormality or pathology. The clinical hallmark is the limitation of active and passive range of motion of the glenohumeral joint (Fig. 2). When the scapula is stabilized by the examining physician's hand, it becomes apparent that the primary limitation is in the shoulder joint. Determine the limits of motion caused by firm endpoints, not just muscular guarding, which often occurs secondary to pain. Pain may be absent when the shoulder is moved within its free range, depending on the stage of presentation. Both active and passive motion losses must be recorded and compared because concomitant conditions, such as a rotator cuff tear, can result in loss of active motion in a shoulder that is also stiff owing to adhesions. The examiner must be careful to identify and control compensatory motions to measure only pure glenohumeral motion. Patients with glenohumeral stiffness often exhibit relatively good motion owing to increased scapulothoracic motion or trunk lean. Active shoulder elevation is measured in the plane of the scapula, with the patient seated, and is referenced to the patient's thorax not to a line vertical to the floor. This eliminates compensatory movement, such as associated trunk tilt or increased scapulothoracic contribution to overall motion. External rotation as well as internal rotation along the thoracic and lumbar vertebrae are measured with the arm at the side. A firm endpoint is often appreciated, with pain at the extremes of motion. There has been little consensus about the degree of restriction of shoulder motion needed to make the diagnosis of frozen shoulder.[5,6] In general, external rotation, abduction, and internal rotation are the most affected.

Passive motion should then be evaluated with the patient in the supine position, restricting excessive scapulothoracic movement and eliminating lumbar or trunk tilt, thereby providing a more accurate assessment of pure glenohumeral motion. Passive forward elevation, external rotation at the side, and internal and external rotation at 90 degrees of abduction, as well as a cross-chest adduction are measured.

Localized areas of tenderness especially about the rotator cuff, biceps tendon, and acromioclavicular (AC) joint should be assessed in addition to a complete neurologic examimation. Specific patterns of motion loss are also noted relative to the etiology of the stiffness. For example, primary adhesive capsulitis is usually associated with global motion loss, whereas postsurgical or posttraumatic stiffness may present with loss of motion in all planes, or it may be a more discrete limitation of motion affecting some planes while relatively sparing others. Recognition of these different patterns of motion loss is important in determining the etiology as well as planning the nonoperative and possibly operative treatment program. Motion loss often correlates with the location of a capsular contracture. Isolated areas of pathology within the capsule will have varying clinical presentations. For example, limitation of external rotation with the arm in the abducted position is usually associated with scarring in the anteroinferior region of the capsule, as opposed to limitation of external rotation in the adducted shoulder, which is associated with contracture in the anterosuperior capsular region in the rotator interval.[85,87,101] Limitation of internal rotation in adduction and abduction is associated with scarring in the posterior capsule, which is also reflected in loss of horizontal cross-chest adduction.[45] Extraarticular contractures, such as those ensuing from subdeltoid or subacromial bursitis and the impingement process, as well as subscapularis entrapment, can also cause scarring between tissue planes and contribute to global motion loss.

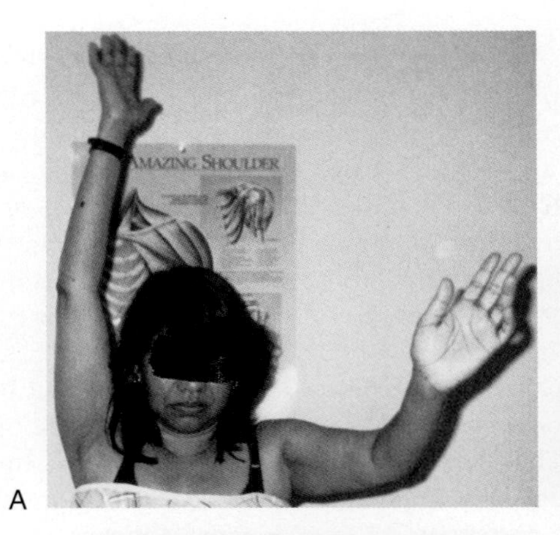

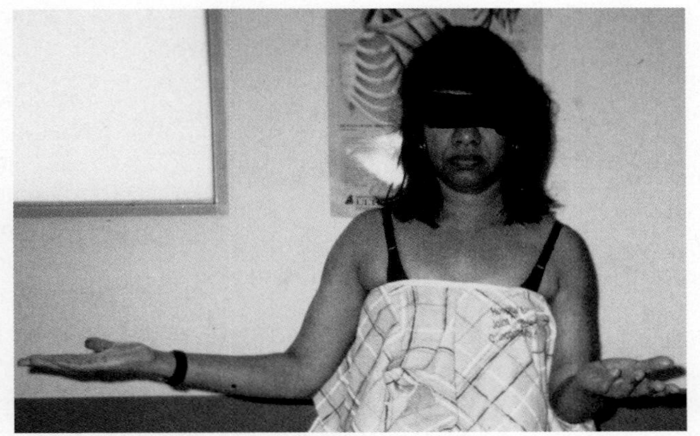

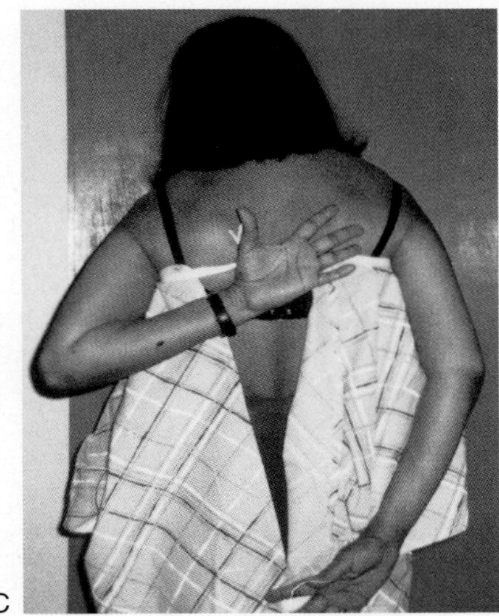

FIG. 2. (A–C) Globally restricted active and passive range of motion demonstrated by loss of forward elevation, external and internal rotation, respectively.

On completion of the physical examination the most helpful additional test that can be performed within the office setting is that of the lidocaine injection test. This is not limited only to the subacromial space, but also can be applied to the AC joint, depending on the presence or absence of the impingement signs as well as AC joint tenderness and pain on cross chest-adduction. In a subacromial disorder, an injection of 10 mL of 1% lidocaine into this region will reveal true active motion as opposed to pain-inhibited motion. When the pain is eliminated, one must record the postinjection increase in motion that helps differentiate loss caused by impingement versus true motion loss from soft-tissue contracture. In an individual with limited motion secondary to pain from rotator cuff pathology, an increase in forward elevation will be noted as well as relief of pain. This is in contrast to the patient with a true soft-tissue contracture in which limited passive and active motion will persist despite anesthetic in the subacromial space.

Laboratory and Imaging Studies

Routine hematologic testing, although the results are usually normal, should include a complete blood cell count, chemistry profile, rheumatoid factor test, and serology. The erythrocyte sedimentation rate is elevated in as many as 20% of patients.[5,6] No specific tests are diagnostic. There remains ongoing controversy about the significance of the reported increased levels of immune complexes in patients with adhesive capsulitis.[20,21,57] Fasting serum triglyceride and cholesterol levels have also been significantly elevated in those patients with frozen shoulder syndrome, compared with age- and sex-matched controlled subjects.[23]

Bulgen and associates reported on 40 patients with clinical signs of frozen shoulder who had shown an increase in immune complex levels, including C-reactive protein and impaired cell-mediated immunity. Tests to measure these values 8 months following the onset of the shoulder disorder revealed a tendency for the values to return to normal levels.[21] With the exception of disuse osteopenia, radiographic findings are usually negative. Significant findings, however, may aid in the identification of an underlying intrinsic disorder, and a complete set of radiographs consisting of scapular anteroposterior films in neutral, external, and internal rotation, as well as supraspinatus outlet and axillary views should be obtained. These views give excellent visualization of the proximal humerus and surrounding soft tissues. The axillary view will help exclude dislocation, fracture, and locking osteophytes. Confirmation of a normal glenohumeral joint is often obtained by plain radiography in patients with primary frozen shoulder. Disuse osteoporosis is often evident, especially in patients who present with the clinical features of reflex sympathetic dystrophy. Minor degenerative changes of the humeral head in the area of the greater tuberosity or a narrowing of the subacromial space have also been reported with incidences of 19% and 12%, respectively.[18]

Technetium scanning has been used in the evaluation of frozen shoulder. Findings of increase uptake, although nonspecific, are probably secondary to hypervascularity. Wright and colleagues noted a favorable association between an increased pertechnetate uptake about the shoulder and rapid response to corticosteroid injections.[139] Bender and associates observed that over 90% of their patients had an increased uptake on the diphosphonate scans, with 29% having more than a 50% increase in uptake compared with the opposite shoulder. These authors, however, could not find any association between the bone scan findings and the duration of symptoms, the initial severity of the disease, the arthrographic findings, or the eventual recovery.[7]

The early descriptions of the characteristic shoulder arthrography findings in frozen shoulder by Neviaser have allowed a better understanding of the underlying shoulder joint pathology, without having to resort to surgical exposure. He described as typical the combination of a decreased joint volume, an irregular joint outline, and variable filling in the bicipital tendon sheath at arthrography.[91] The reduction in the shoulder joint capsule capacity to less than 10 to 12 mL and the variable lack of filling of the axillary fold and subscapular bursa are the currently accepted characteristic findings.[1,47,69,90,91] Since the time of this classic description, arthrography has been used as a standard diagnostic technique to confirm frozen shoulder. This technique reveals at least a 50% reduction of shoulder joint volume and a boxlike appearance of the joint cavity.[7,114] The shoulder joint volume capacity of patients with frozen shoulder is noted to be only 5 to 10 mL, as compared with that of normal shoulders of 20 to 30 mL.[39,40,57,69,114] The findings during arthrography include a tight, thickened capsule,[40,57,90] and loss of the axillary recess, the subcoracoid folds, and the subscapular bursa.[47,69,89,106] Binder and coworkers noted that, although arthrography is useful in the diagnosis of frozen shoulder, arthrographic findings do not indicate the type of onset (i.e., primary or secondary), or the rate or extent of recovery.[7] Other authors confirm that such findings also have not had any predicted value in terms of disease severity or prognosis.[54,69]

Lundberg, as well as other authors, has used arthrography to document tearing of the joint capsule during manipulation under anesthesia.[1,72] Tears of the capsule allow dye to escape into the extracapsular space, but no tears of the rotator cuff tendons themselves following manipulation under anesthesia were noted in an extensive study by Lundberg.[72]

TREATMENT

The overall goal in the treatment of patients with frozen shoulder is to relieve pain and restore motion and function. Before formulating a treatment plan, the clinician should have an appreciation for the usual disease course of a frozen shoulder. Reeves described this condition as consisting of three phases. The painful phase is characterized by diffuse shoulder pain and progressive stiffness. This phase lasts 3 to 9 months and is reportedly followed by the stiffening or frozen phase. During this phase the pain is diminished and a more comfortable, but severely restricted, range of motion exists. This interval usually lasts 4 to 12 months. In the final phase, the thawing phase, motion and function gradually improve over the next 12 to 42 months, although to a variable degree.[110] Ideally, efforts should be directed toward prevention of this syndrome by identifying the patients at risk and initiating early intervention. This is best accomplished by emphasizing early motion in potential secondary cases (after trauma and surgery) whenever possible. Unfortunately, most patients present with an already painful stiff shoulder. The clinician must design a treatment plan that is individualized and based on the severity and chronicity of the patients symptoms, as well as previous therapeutic efforts. As in other medical conditions for which the pathophysiology is poorly understood, many different forms of treatment are used empirically in the management of frozen shoulder syndrome. Treatment is continuously modified, depending on the individual's response to a particular treatment modality.

The first objective in the treatment of patients with frozen shoulder syndrome is pain relief. This is essential, for it permits patients to more readily participate in an exercise program aimed at restoring motion and recovering function. Efforts to obtain pain relief by rest, analgesia, or transcutaneous electrical nerve stimulation (TENS), are useful in the early stages of this syndrome.[6,114] The routine use of narcotics should be avoided because they carry a risk of dependency and nonsteroidal antiinflammatory medications can be equally effective, although there have been no controlled studies to document their efficacy compared with placebo.[33,52,111] Nonsteroidal antiinflammatory medications are often used empirically, but when questioned, patients found the nonsteroidal agents less helpful than nonsalicylate anagelsics[6]. Oral corticosteroids have also been recommended for the treatment of frozen shoulder, but there exists little evidence to support their routine use.[6,9,10,35,88]

Many medical practitioners prefer the intraarticular injection of steroids, accompanied by local analgesics and gentle active motion, especially in the freezing stage of frozen shoulder[18,47,69] Local intraarticular and subacromial corticosteroid injections have been used to relieve pain, but less frequently to improve motion in patients with frozen shoulder.[2,18,28,62,88,107,112,116] They may be particularly helpful in the early phase of the condition, when pain prevents the patient from actively participating in rehabilitation. Hollingworth reported that injection of corticosteroid directly into the anatomic site of the lesion produced pain relief and at least 50% improvement in range of motion in 26% of cases studied.[50] Adversely, Quigley[106] and Neviaser[89] report the belief that steroids cannot affect established scars, contractures, or adhesions, but Quigley felt that they may reduce pain if administered in conjunction with manipulation.

Paired injections have also been used in a study by Richardson, who reported the results of a blind, controlled multicenter study of 37 patients afflicted with frozen shoulder syndrome who received two injections of 25 mg of prednisolone acetate, one into the bursa and one into the glenohumeral joint, on the initial visit and again at 2 weeks. These patients were compared with controls receiving injections of normal saline. Richardson also noted the inability of most physicians to successfully inject into the markedly retracted shoulder joint.[112] It is thought by several authors that an arthrogram is better used to determine the anatomic landmarks for subsequent intraarticular injections. A technically satisfactory arthrogram could not be achieved in 12% of their patients.[134]

Murnaghan and colleagues also compared regional infiltration of the shoulder joint capsule with 25 mL of hydrocortisone acetate with injections of 2% lidocaine in the absence of a control group. The authors found both treatments to be beneficial, but the hydrocortisone failed to offer any significant advantage.[81]

The use of intraarticular injections, in summary, has theoretical merits and is reported with various results, but in general, the evidence is equivocal. In patients with moderately stiff shoulders for whom pain is a major impediment to exercise, an intraarticular injection repeated on one or two occasions, if necessary, seems to be justified.[82] Steroid injections have not been shown to improve the rate of return of shoulder motion.[72,107] Although steroid injections have been reported to be beneficial in some respects, their use should be limited owing to the potentially deleterious side effects on the connective tissue.

Nonoperative Treatment

Patients with frozen shoulder should be placed on an exercise program with the aim of maintaining and regaining range of motion (Fig. 3). Indications for treatment of the frozen shoulder in general are based on the chronicity and etiology of the stiffness. Nonoperative treatment is indicated for those primary or secondary frozen shoulders with stiffness of less than 6 months and or no previous treatment. Each patient should begin an active-assisted range of motion exercise program complying with gentle, passive, stretching exercises. These exercises should be performed four to five times daily, including forward elevation, internal and external rotation, and cross-body adduction. They can be performed standing or sitting, but are most readily performed in the supine position. It is most important to perform four or five short sessions per day, lasting for 5 to 10 minutes, rather than one long session because the shoulder will become stiff again in between each session. It is important to perform these exercises gently, but it needs to be stressed that at each session the arm should be pushed slightly past the point of pain, otherwise no progress in the range of motion would be expected. Forward elevation may be assisted by using the opposite arm or a pulley to pull the arm up over head, external rotation is aided with a cane while the patient is lying supine and holding the arm at the side, and external rotation is performed by pulling the arm up behind the back with the assistance of the opposite arm or a towel. Using the opposite extremity, the affected limb is stretched to its limit and slightly past it, held in place for a count of 5 to 10 seconds and then brought to a resting position. Periods of rest in between each session are necessary to relieve muscle tension and pain.

To encourage continued exercises, daily bar charts are helpful to document progress because small improvements in range of motion might otherwise be unnoticed by the patient, especially those who are easily discouraged. Local modalities consisting of heat at the initiation of the exercise session and ice at its conclusion may be helpful to increase flexibility and reduce inflammation, respectively. These modalities are certainly not curative, but can aid in decreasing discomfort, which will allow greater ease in performing the exercises.

Forward elevation of the shoulder is performed with the extremity in the plane of the scapula as it is grasped either at the wrist or behind the elbow and pushed upward gradually. This is best performed supine to keep compensatory factors, such as trunk tilt, to a minimum. A pulley can also be used to accomplish this motion, which is best performed seated with the back of the patient to the pulley. Similarly, cross-body adduction is performed as the affected extremity is pulled across the chest toward the contralateral shoulder. This maneuver assists in stretching the posterior portion of the capsule, which is of utmost importance in obtaining internal rotation. External rotation is performed supine with the elbow close to the body. A stick is held in the hand with the elbow flexed to 90 degrees and is used to rotate the affected extremity away from the body. Internal rotation is performed by pulling the wrist of the affected extremity into extension first behind the back then bringing the hands up between the shoulder blades. It may also be assisted with a towel or by grasping a door handle behind the back and performing a deep knee bend. In the early stages of the exercise program one should start with simple stretching, such as Codman's pendulum exercise to gently loosen and relax the shoulder. The patient bends at the waist, balances with the good arm and allows the stiff side to swing with gravity in a circular motion with the hand turned inward and then outward. Overly forceful stretching exercises are contraindicated in the early phases of the frozen shoulder syndrome and may exacerbate symptoms. Constant reassurance from the physician is necessary to promote continued compliance.

The physical therapist plays a major role as a teacher, explaining to the patient that it will take time to resolve symptoms and that pain will decrease as motion improves. When-

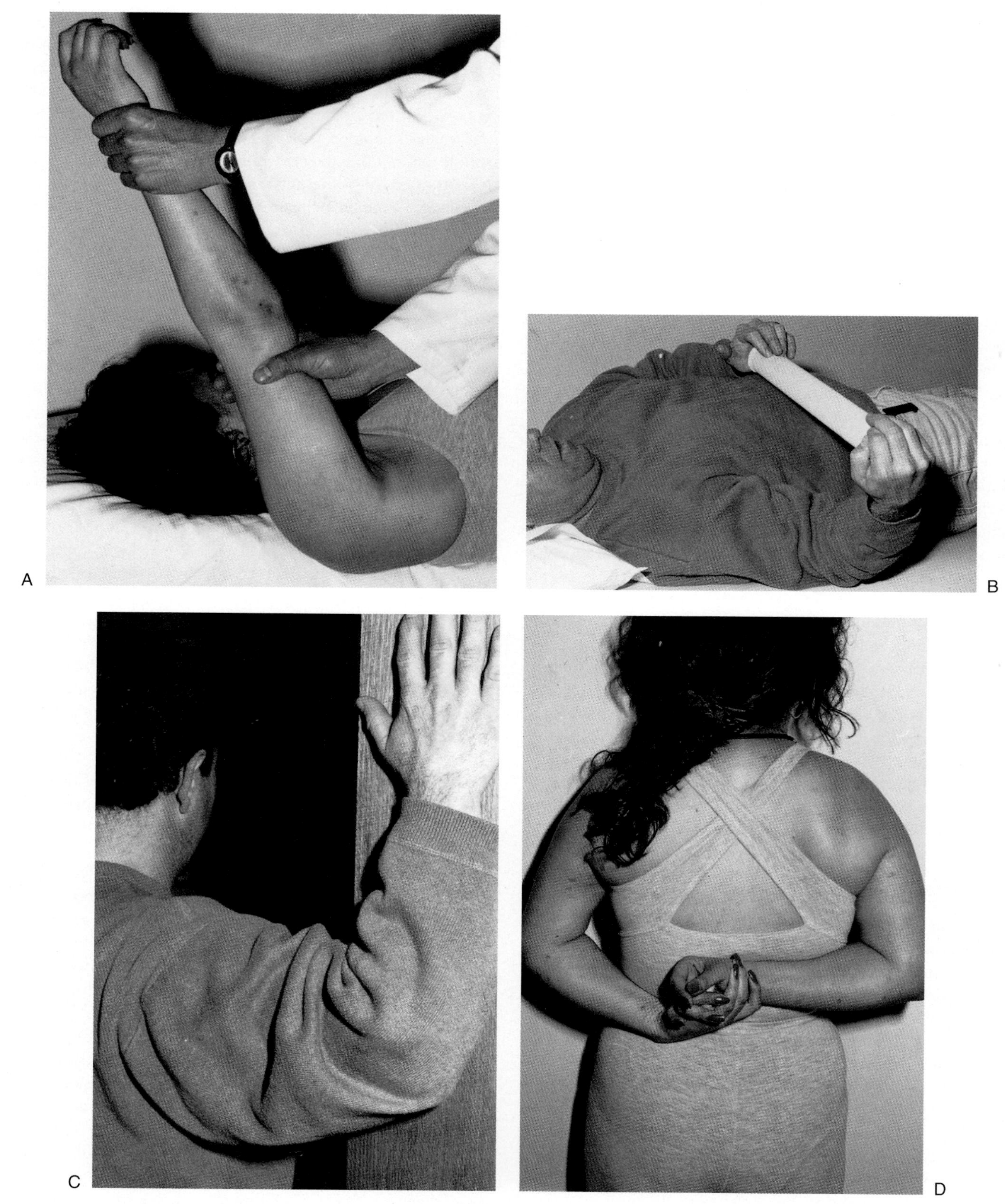

FIG. 3. (A–D) Passive stretching exercises performed for overhead elevation, external rotation at side, 90 degrees of abduction, and internal rotation behind back.

ever possible, the therapy program should be performed under the supervision or in addition to a physical therapist on a weekly basis. The patient should be instructed that the success or failure of the therapy largely depends on their compliance in performing the exercises as directed, not only with the therapist but four or five times daily on their own. In a closely supervised physical therapy program, most patients will improve with time, although it may take months. Thus, in most cases, more invasive treatment is generally not required.

Capsular Distention or Brisment

The method of capsular distention, referred to as distention arthrography or brisment, has been advocated as a means of expanding the contracted capsule.[1,36,39,51,69,100] This procedure involves injecting fluid into the glenohumeral joint in sufficient enough volume to generate pressures high enough to cause capsular disruption that is evidenced by significant decrease in the pressure necessary to continue injection. This procedure has been performed in a variety of ways; with injection of contrast as part of an arthrogram;[39,69,100,110] with injection of saline and local anesthetic, such as hydraulic distention;[36] and arthroscopically.[51] As with all other methods of treatment for frozen shoulder syndrome the reported results have been variable and difficult to interpret because the procedure often is combined with other procedures such as manipulation or corticosteroid injections, and the experience has been limited. The addition of these other variables makes it difficult, if not impossible, to compare reports. A recent article by Rizk examined 16 patients with adhesive capsulitis of the shoulder treated in an open trial of capsular distention with intraarticular injection of 30 mL of fluid containing 8 mL of 1% lidocaine, 2 mL of corticosteroid, and 20 mL of radiocontrast material. A capsular tear during arthrography occurred in all cases, usually at the subscapular bursa or subacromial bursa, as documented by extravasations in either of these areas. Rupture at the distal bicipital sheath occurred in two patients and was not associated with pain relief. Thirteen of 16 patients experienced immediate pain relief and increased shoulder mobility. This improvement was maintained over a follow-up interval of 6 months. Given these results the authors felt that disruption of the contracted capsule by hydraulic distention seemed to be the mechanism for achieving symptomatic relief in adhesive capsulitis.[115]

Manipulation under Anesthesia

No aspect of adhesive capsulitis of the shoulder is more varied or controversial than treatment. Manipulation under general anesthesia results in rapid return to normal range of motion in some cases, but several authors have found that, although manipulation shortens the time during which the shoulder range of motion is extremely restricted, the overall course of the disease remains unchanged.[72,82] Timing of manipulation is also controversial, but advocates suggest manipulation for patients who do not obtain 90 degrees of passive forward elevation and show little or no progress after 3 to 6 months of supervised physical therapy. This procedure has been a successful method of improving the range of motion of frozen shoulders that have not responded to a rehabilitation program or that exhibit progression of stiffness while undergoing conservative treatment.[46–48,66,92,102,103,126] Manipulation should be performed in a gentle, controlled manner to avoid complications. Complications that have been reported include humeral fracture, glenohumeral dislocation, rotator cuff tears, and radial nerve injuries. Manipulation is contraindicated in those patients with severe osteopenia in which fracture is a high risk, those with reflex sympathetic dystrophy, and in patients when stiffness is secondary to a previous surgery or fracture. Manipulation is ill-advised in these situations owing to increased risk of fracture, disruption of the soft-tissue repair, nerve injuries such as brachial plexus traction, palsies, and postmanipulation instability. Patients who will be unable or unwilling to cooperate with the required postmanipulation exercise program are also contraindicated for this procedure. It is important to emphasize that treatment of primary adhesive capsulitis should not be considered while the patient is experiencing severe pain in addition to motion loss, for this may represent the inflammatory phase of the disease. Neviaser and Neviaser have pointed out that any surgical treatment in this stage will likely exacerbate the patient's motion loss by increasing capsular injury. It is important to wait until pain is present only at the end range of motion, indicating that the active inflammatory process has resolved. Any type of operative or manipulative intervention during this inflammatory phase has the potential to worsen symptoms.[92]

Manipulation can be performed either under general or regional anesthesia. The anesthetic technique is an extremely important aspect of the overall treatment. There must be complete muscle paralysis during the procedure. The advantage of regional anesthesia (i.e., interscalene block) is that it allows direct observation of the recovered motion by the patient and the more effective, immediate use of continuous passive motion and physical therapy. It also has the benefit of eliminating the subsequent pain after manipulation that interferes with therapy in the immediate postoperative period. Therefore, it is recommended that an interscalene block with a long-acting agent such as bupivacaine be used. The block may be administered either as a single percutaneous injection or by the placement of indwelling interscalene catheter.[16,105] If a single block is performed it may be repeated in the morning on the first and second post-operative days for continued pain relief and ease of therapy. This will greatly decrease the patients' requirement for narcotics while increasing their tolerance to physical therapy and continuous motion. Use of 0.5% bupivacaine as a single block will provide anesthesia for approximately 12 hours. If an interscalene catheter is used, a continuous slow drip of bupivacaine is administered.

The patient is placed supine along the edge of the operating table with the scapula stabilized along its axillary border, allowing more isolated and controlled glenohumeral movement of the involved extremity. Manipulation into forward elevation is carried out first. The humerus is grasped close to the axilla to diminish the lever effect. With gradual traction and flexion, there is usually a palpable and audible release of adhesions. This maneuver usually results in rupture of the inferior portion of the capsule.[60,91] The arm is then stretched across the patient's chest into adduction to stretch the posterior capsule and aid in returning internal rotation. The arm is then brought down to the side of the body while holding it in the supracondylar area of the distal humerus to avoid spiral fracture of the humerus, two-finger pressure only is placed on the forearm rotating the humerus externally, taking care to avoid injury to the elbow ligaments. This maneuver releases anterior capsular adhesions. The arm is then manipulated at 90 degrees of scapular plane abduction, with further external rotation performed in this plane to stretch the anteroinferior capsule (Fig. 4). Continuing with the arm in scapular plane abduction, internal rotation is performed holding the arm at the proximal humeral level to release the posterior capsule. The arm is then stretched across the patient's chest into adduction to further release the posterior capsule. Further stretch of the inferior capsule is obtained with increased abduction in the scapular plane. While maintaining internal rotation, the arm is lowered to the patient's side with the elbow extended and the forearm pronated to complete the posterior capsule release. All rotational maneuvers must be performed carefully holding the arm in the supracondylar or proximal humeral areas to decrease the risk of fracture. The object of a manipulation under anesthesia is for the recovered motion to be symmetrical with the uninvolved side.

Postmanipulation rehabilitation is of paramount importance in maintaining the motion gained. Immediately following manipulation, the patient is met in the recovery room by the therapist to initiate the therapeutic exercise program. It is particularly helpful if regional anesthesia has been used because a long-acting block permits exercise without discomfort. Continuous passive motion machines have also been used after manipulation, but there have been no long-term, controlled studies to verify their efficacy. In my own experience these machines help continue motion within a somewhat functional range, but fail to stress the shoulder to the extreme limits of overhead elevation as well as external rotation. They are also cumbersome and difficult to set up for external rotation and in changing positions from the bedside to a seated position.

After discharge from the hospital, the premanipulation exercise program is continued, but on a more frequent basis. If a good range of motion was obtained initially, but is then lost, Harryman has suggested repeating the procedure, especially within the first 3 to 4 weeks after the initial manipulation.[43] However, this has not been necessary in my experience.

A prospective clinical study was performed by Bulgen and coworkers examining the evaluation of three treatment regimens for frozen shoulder, including intraarticular steroids, mobilization, and ice therapy as compared with no treatment at all. In this prospective study of 42 patients followed for 8 months, the authors stated that there was little long-term advantage in any of the treatment regimens, but that the steroid injections may have been of benefit for pain and range of movement in the early stages of the condition.[18]

Manipulation of the shoulder has been advocated as a safe and effective means of enabling these patients to return to functional motion about the shoulder area. Haggart and coworkers looked at 97 patients treated with manipulation of the shoulder.[41] They found that 95% had excellent or good

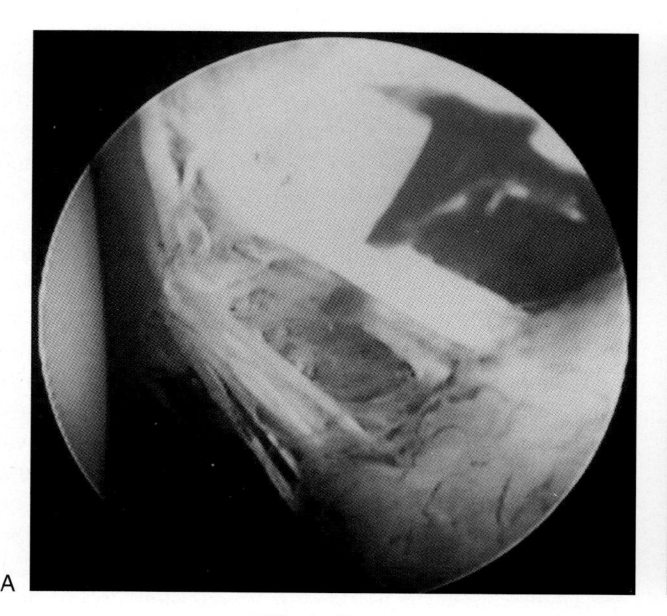
A

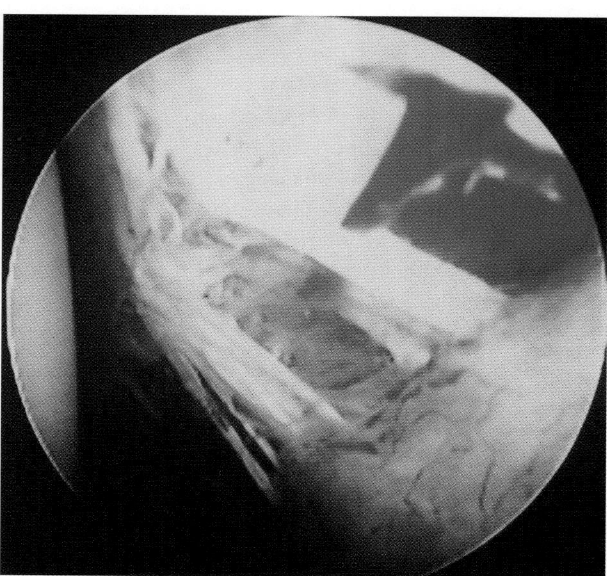
B

FIG. 4. Torn labrum and capsule in inferior axillary pouch postmanipulation.

results with 4 to 9 years of follow-up. Harmon reported 400 manipulated shoulders.[42] On three separate follow-up studies 2 to 3 years postmanipulation, he found that there was full painless motion in 64% to 94% of the patients. In a study by Hill and Bogumill, 9 of 12 (75%) of the patients with frozen shoulder syndrome had painless full range of motion of the shoulder at the time of follow-up postmanipulation, whereas 3 of 12 (25%) continued to complain of minimal aching about the shoulder joint after vigorous activity, but did not feel that this was impairing their ability to function. All of the patients felt they were able to perform satisfactorily at their job, during activities of daily living, and during recreational activities. Five out of 6 of the patients (83%) were not working prior to their shoulder problems, but returned to work within an average of 3 months after the manipulation. Those patients who were working before their shoulder problems were back to work within 1 month of manipulation. These authors state that manipulation was found to be a safe means of treating adhesive capsulitis and significantly shortened the course of the disease. Manipulation in these patients allowed them to return to a normal life style and to work much sooner than the reported natural history of this condition would indicate.[48]

Arthroscopic Release

Although conservative management, with or without, manipulation performed with the patient under anesthesia is the generally effective treatment strategy for frozen shoulder syndrome, considerable interest has been shown in arthroscopic surgical procedures for this disorder. Arthroscopy has been used in the evaluation and treatment of frozen shoulder. Arthroscopy may provide some diagnostic information (e.g., labral tears, and partial- or full-thickness rotator cuff tears), that is not identified during the clinical evaluation.[51,76] Arthroscopy has been used as a means of capsular distention.[11,51,135] However, the potential benefit of this procedure is difficult to evaluate, because it is usually combined with manipulation or other forms of treatment.[76,135] Arthroscopy not only allows identification of associated pathology, but also permits its treatment, including debridement of intraarticular adhesions, subacromial decompression, removal of calcific deposits, and treatment of acromioclavicular arthritis.

Although most patients with primary frozen shoulder syndrome respond to physical therapy in nonoperative measures, some will require closed manipulation to achieve and maintain sufficient improvement in motion. A small percentage of those patients will continue to have motion loss that is refractory even to manipulation of the shoulder under anesthesia. Perhaps the most significant potential benefit of arthroscopy in the treatment of frozen shoulder is the possibility of releasing contracted structures in those patients with resistant cases. It is usually performed in association with some type of manipulation. This procedure allows precise, selective capsular release, thereby avoiding the potential morbidity associated with an open procedure. It has the advantage of allowing more immediate, aggressive active and passive range of motion than after open release.

The role of arthroscopy in the treatment of frozen shoulder, with few large studies in the literature, has fewer experts in decided disagreement over its usefulness.[13,51,92,99,109] In clinical trials arthroscopy has proved important in delineating the pathology present in frozen shoulder, as well as documenting the results of closed manipulation,[13,94,109] but recommendations for its widespread use are conflicting. Some believe strongly that it has no use in the treatment of adhesive capsulitis,[28] whereas others use this technique to assist with distention of joint,[51] or to visualize and treat associated lesions in the shoulder joint after manipulation.[13]

The primary indication for arthroscopic capsular release is a failed attempt at closed manipulation. It has also been used in the postoperative shoulder, such as after rotator cuff repair. In these patients, subacromial decompression and a selective capsular release can be performed, lessening the chance of fracture or retearing of the rotator cuff. Patients with full-thickness rotator cuff tears may also be candidates for arthroscopic capsular release, for it may decrease the chance for tear that can occur with closed manipulation, provided the source of the stiffness is felt to be intracapsular. This procedure should be avoided in patients who are sensitive to significant fluid shifts, and in those in whom extensive extraarticular adhesions are suspected such as posttraumatic or selected surgical procedures.[43,130] The latter patients are often better treated with an open release. Arthroscopic release is also abandoned if the surgeon cannot identify a discreet subscapularis tendon superiorly. If this structure cannot be identified, the procedure must be converted to an open release because failure to curtail the arthroscopic release in this situation can result in the division of the subscapularis tendon as well as the anterior capsule. Arthroscopy, whether as an adjunct to manipulation or in the form of arthroscopic release, is reserved for patients with frozen shoulder whose symptoms do not improve with an adequate course of physical therapy and home exercise program. In general, I do not suggest this treatment before pursuing a minimum course of 6 months of stretching exercises with the patient plateauing relative to motion over a 2-month period.

The operative technique involves three basic components: anesthesia, preferably by interscalene brachioplexus block regional anesthesia; manipulation of the shoulder, performed either before, during, or after the third portion of component of this triad, which is arthroscopic release. The interscalene block has been safe and well tolerated in my experience as well as in the experience of others.[16]

The procedure is performed with the patient in the beach chair position for both an anterior and posterior capsule release. A lateral decubitus position is also used by some surgeons who prefer the added joint distraction produced when traction is applied to the arm in this position. The arthroscope is inserted through a standard posterior viewing portal and carefully slid intraarticularly over the humeral head because a more inferior passage is difficult owing to inadequate joint distention. It is always difficult to insert the arthroscope into a stiff shoulder, for capsular contracture and decreased joint volume are problematic. Articular injury from forceful insertion of the arthroscope is certainly a concern. Chondral damage can be avoided by gently inserting the arthroscope over the humeral head, rather than taking a more inferior approach. Some surgeons have recommended the use of a 3.9-mm–diameter arthroscope such as that used for small joint arthroscopy in the wrist, although I have used the standard 30-degree 5.5-mm arthroscope without difficulty. The problem of entering a stiff joint with the arthroscope can be completely avoided by manipulation before arthroscopic insertion, thereby increasing the available space.[92,99,109] If the joint has been previously manipulated it is lavaged of blood. A systematic inspection is then undertaken to determine the site and severity of inflammation as well as to visualize the location of the ruptured structures after manipulation. The biceps tendon is the first anatomic landmark that should be identified. It marks the upper edge of the rotator interval which is formed by the anterior edge of the supraspinatus and the superior border of the subscapularis tendon.[45] This region is usually composed of a thick band of scar tissue that may obscure the normally visible upper edge of the subscapularis tendon.

A second anterior working portal is established through which a variety of instruments can be passed to begin the release, which is generally performed in the midcapsule. This portal is placed just beneath the biceps tendon and the capsular scar tissue is divided with the use of an electrocautery device and a motorized shaver (Fig. 5). The capsular division begins superiorly just inferior to the biceps tendon and continues inferiorly until the discrete upper edge of the subscapularis is encountered. This is the area of the rotator interval including the coracohumeral ligament and anterosuperior capsule which is aggressively divided and debrided with a shaver. The electrocautery may be used through the anterior portal to detach the coracohumeral ligament from its coracoid attachment. This is especially important if resistance to external rotation with the arm at the side persists after closed manipulation. Both Neer[85] and Ozaki[101] have shown that such a release performed through an open approach is successful in restoring external rotation in shoulders with refractory frozen shoulder syndrome.

With partial release having been performed, the humeral head more easily moves inferiorly and laterally allowing more space in the joint for the arthroscope to be moved about. At this point one has the option to perform a manipulation to restore motion in all planes if this has not been obtained before manipulation and in conjunction with the release of the rotator interval region. The electrocautery can be used to incise the anterior glenohumeral ligaments. This maneuver allows the motorized shaving instrument to perform more efficiently in excising the tissue. The release proceeds from superior to inferior, including the inferior axillary portion of the capsule. The arm is frequently manipulated during the procedure using the same maneuver as described previously to assess the adequacy of release. External rotation in adduction is usually restored with almost no manipulation force. If there continues to be minimal or no improvement of motion in the remaining planes, the remainder of the anteroinferior capsule is released. Capsular release is performed from the midcapsular region and extended inferiorly to obtain external rotation in abduction. Some surgeons have expressed concern about the risk to the axillary nerve with capsular release, and this certainly warrants caution.[105] The subscapularis can act as a buffer in the adducted position as it is interposed between the anteroinferior capsule in the axillary nerve when the arm is in the adducted position. Care is taken to avoid releasing in the axillary pouch region with this technique. A restriction in cross-body adduction and internal rotation generally indicates further constriction in the posterior capsule warranting posterior capsular release. In these cases the viewing and working portals are switched and a posterior capsular release is performed in a similar fashion.

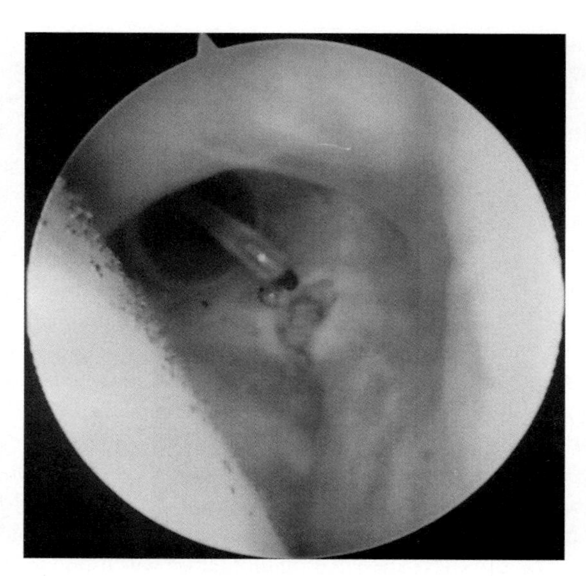

FIG. 5. Arthroscopic view during release of contracted capsule and glenohumeral ligaments with eletrocautery in anterior portal.

A small subset of patients may have an isolated posterior capsular contracture characterized by motion loss primarily limited to internal rotation, cross-chest, or horizontal adduction and flexion, with relative preservation of external rotation. This type of posterior capsular contracture has been implicated in impingement-type pain and may result in nonoutlet-type impingement caused by increased anterosuperior translation during shoulder elevation and internal rotation. This condition is treated with posterior capsular release to restore lost motion and normal kinematics.[132]

The posterior capsular release is also performed in a beach chair position with the arthroscope placed through a cannula in the anterosuperior portal, and the posterior portal is used as the operative portal. Again, either with electrocautery or a motorized shaver, posterior capsular release is performed from just posterior to the biceps tendon down to the posterior inferior rim of the glenoid. The arthroscopic release of the posterior capsule must be performed just at the glenoid rim; the infraspinatus is quite superficial and there is risk of dividing the infraspinatus tendon if the capsular division is performed more laterally. Division of the infraspinatus as a strong, external rotator, would potentially weaken external rotation by creating a tear within this tendon.

Inspection of the subacromial space is then performed, with release of bursal adhesions also undertaken at this time as needed. If impingement secondary to the coracoacromial ligament is noted, incision or excision of the hypertrophy ligament may be performed. Associated lesions, such as calcific deposits and acromioclavicular arthritis, that may have been the underlying cause of the development of stiffness should be simultaneously addressed arthroscopically. Acromioplasty may also be performed if this is deemed to be the cause of the stiffness, with the caution that excessive surgical debridement can possibly produce more adhesions. The goal is to obtain motion that is symmetrical with the contralateral or unaffected side. One must understand that the arthroscopic technique performed is tailored to fit the precise pathology encountered in each patient.

The technique of arthroscopic release in conjunction with manipulation is not indicated in the treatment of every stiff shoulder. For example, shoulders with stiffness on the basis of scarring between the subscapularis, strap muscles, and deltoid (such as those who have undergone previous surgery) cannot be adequately addressed with this form of treatment and are candidates for open release when they remain sufficiently symptomatic. Moreover, patients with severe osteoporosis are not suitable candidates either, based on the risk of fracturing the humerus during manipulation.

Segmuller et al.[118] reviewed the results of patients who underwent an arthroscopic release of the inferior capsule, reproducing in a controlled fashion a traumatic disruption of the inferior capsule commonly caused by manipulation with the patient under anesthesia. The authors reviewed a purely arthroscopic treatment of what they termed adhesive capsulitis. The outcome of 26 shoulders was assessed with an average follow-up of 13.5 months. The release was performed in a lateral decubitus position with the arthroscope in the posterior portal. In all cases the arthroscope was unable to pass into the anterior portion of the joint, and the posterior inferior portal was established under direct vision with the needle used as a guide. This portal was placed into the inferior recess approximately 5 cm inferior to the posterior corner of the acromion. A cutting diathermy knife was used to divide the inferior capsule from the 3:00 o'clock position anteriorly to the 9:00 o'clock position posteriorly. Capsular biopsies were also performed. Traction was then released and the arm brought into full abduction, with an occasional minor breakdown of adhesions reported. After traction was reestablished, the arthroscope was used to obtain hemostasis and explore the anterior aspect of the joint. In patients with limited internal rotation, the middle glenohumeral ligament was divided. Invariably a proliferative synovitis was found just in the area beneath the biceps tendon insertion, and a limited synovectomy was performed. Subsequently, the subacromial space was inspected and, at the end of the procedure, 1 mL of betamethasone and 10 mL of 0.5% bupivacaine with epinephrine was instilled into both the glenohumeral and subacromial spaces. In the recovery room the patients received intensive physiotherapy and further daily physiotherapy was continued after discharge from ambulatory surgery. According to the constant scoring system, 87% of patients had achieved a good or excellent result when compared with the contralateral normal shoulder score. A total of 88% of patients were very satisfied with the procedure, and no operative complications had occurred.[118]

Pollock et al.[105] reported on the use of arthroscopy in treatment of resistant frozen shoulder, combining the technique of manipulation under interscalene brachioplexus block anesthesia followed by arthroscopic examination and debridement of the glenohumeral joint in the subacromial space. The authors state the addition of the athroscope allowed identification and treatment of the associated pathology, such as impingement lesions and secondary subacromial space inflammation, calcific deposits, and acromioclavicular arthritis. Range of motion was also increased by arthroscopically guided sectioning of the coracohumeral ligament. This treatment regimen yielded overall satisfactory results in 25 of 30 shoulders (83%). The authors note that a subgroup of diabetic patients fared less well than other groups, with only 64% satisfactory results.[105]

Treatment of the resistant frozen shoulder was reviewed relative to manipulation versus arthroscopic release by Ogilvie-Harris. Arthroscopy was performed in 40 patients who had persistent pain, stiffness, and functional loss for at least 1 year without improvement despite conventional nonoperative treatment for frozen shoulder syndrome. In the first 20 patients, manipulation was performed in conjunction with an arthroscopy either before or afterward. In the second 20 patients, the contracted structures were divided through arthroscopic release. The arthroscopic division portion of the procedure was performed in four sequential steps: (a) resection of the inflammatory synovium in the interval between the subscapularis and supraspinatus (i.e., the rotator interval); (b) progressive division of the anterior superior glenohumeral ligament and anterior capsule; (c) division of the subscapularis tendon but not muscle; (d) division of the inferior capsule. The results were assessed independently on the basis of pain, stiffness, and function. With a follow-up varying from 2 to 5 years it was noted that patients treated with arthroscopy and manipulation did as well as the patients treated with arthroscopic division alone for restoration of range of motion. However, the patients in the arthroscopic division group had significantly better pain relief and restoration of function. Fifteen of 20 patients treated with arthroscopic division had an excellent result, compared with 7 of 18 patients treated with arthroscopy and manipulation.

Initially, diabetic patients did not perform as well, but the outcome was similar to patients without diabetes in the long-term. The authors state that if, after a suitable waiting time (at least 1 year) and adequate nonsurgical treatment, the patient continues to report significant pain, loss of motion, and functional impairment, arthroscopic division of the rotator interval and anterior structures offered the patient a better chance of a long-term excellent result. The authors stressed that patients with diabetes, in particular, should be considered for this form of management in preference to treatment by manipulation.[98] Warner et al. reported the results of arthroscopic release in 23 patients with idiopathic adhesive capsulitis with the use of interscalene regional anesthesia followed by repeated nerve blocks or continuous infusion through an interscalene catheter. The authors reported significant improvements in range of motion, including a mean improvement to flexion of 49 degrees, external rotation at the side improved 42 degrees, and internal rotation improved a mean of eight spinous process levels. The authors did combine the release with varying amounts of closed manipulation throughout the procedure, which was felt to require much less force than when performed alone. Complications were not discussed.[130]

Open Release

Open surgical release is reserved for patients who fulfill one or more of the following criteria: (a) significant osteopenia, previous fracture with posttraumatic stiffness, such that closed manipulation might carry an increased risk of fracture either through the osteoporotic bone or through the previous fracture site; (b) failed closed manipulation or failed arthroscopic release, despite compliance with the post-operative rehabilitation program; (c) failure of a prolonged nonoperative trial for greater than or equal to 6 months; (d) attempted manipulation or arthroscopic release that was unsuccessful in regaining range of motion; (e) previous surgical repairs that prohibit manipulation or are at risk for disruption (i.e., previous rotator cuff repair); (f) cases in whom the adhesions are felt to be primarily extraarticular. In general, the goal of this procedure is to release contracted structures so that the range of motion can be increased while maintaining glenohumeral stability. The objective is to release both intra- and extraarticular contracted structures. The advantage of an open surgical release is that it can free up both sides of the joint without risk of soft-tissue or bony injury.

Open releases generally have been successful, but experience and reports of large series have been limited.[59,67,73,85,86] Although the major advantage of this procedure is that it affords the surgeon the opportunity to accurately locate and release contracted structures under direct vision, the major disadvantage of an open release includes postoperative pain, which can interfere with initiating motion. When performing an open release it is critical to identifying the tissues that are contracted and to determining how the release should increase range of motion. The structures usually released include subacromial and subdeltoid bursal adhesions,[59,101] the coracohumeral ligament and rotator interval,[59,63,84,86,101] a complete perilabral capsular release performed circumferentially or selectively around the glenoid, and the subscapularis,[6,98] which is often lengthened and then released 360 degrees and securely repaired to maintain anterior stability. After these structures are released, the surgeon should address the degree of motion regained and the necessity for further dissection.

After either general or interscalene block anesthesia, a deltopectoral incision is used, and the open procedure is begun with the release of adhesions between the deltoid, acromion, coracoacromial ligament, coracoid, and strap muscles from the underlying rotator cuff. Extensive scarring through all layers of the dissection is identified. Adhesions between the deltoid and the humerus are sharply released. This must be done with care because the axillary nerve travels approximately 3 cm distal to the lateral board of the acromion on the under surface of the deltoid. This dissection is made easier with the shoulder in the abducted position, which allows the deltoid to become lax and more easily retracted. Dissection in this area may be done sharply or bluntly, taking care to stay lateral to the coracoid in an attempt to avoid injury to the musculocutaneous nerve. One continues to gently dissect under the deltoid and avoid entering the muscle laterally to prevent injury to the axillary nerve. Internal rotation of the arm while gently retracting the deltoid muscle will allow release of the subdeltoid adhesions in an anterior to posterior manner until the deltoid can move freely over the proximal humerus when the arm is rotated. Within the subacromial space the coracoacromial ligament is either incised or excised, the subacromial space may be filled with dense scar adhesions between the rotator cuff and the acromion, which will most likely require sharp release.

The conjoined tendon is then separated from the scarred area joining it to the underlying subscapularis and retracted medially. This can usually be accomplished with the combination of blunt and sharp dissection. It is essential to keep the dissection lateral to the base of the coracoid process to prevent injury to the neurovascular structures, especially the musculocutaneous nerve.

The coracohumeral ligament and rotator interval are then released by identifying the superior border of the subscapularis and dissecting the supraspinatus and subscapularis from the coracoid bluntly or sharply as needed. The rotator interval is released extending from the humerus to the coracoid.[85,86,101] As the dissection proceeds from superficial to deep within these tissue layers, the shoulder may be gently manipulated at this point to regain further motion. If there is still marked limitation of external rotation owing to scarring in the interval between the subscapularis and the capsule, the options of splitting the subscapularis between its fibers and elevating it off the capsule, versus a coronal plane lengthening of the subscapularis tendon, are available. The coronal Z-plasty of the subscapularis tendon is begun with a vertical incision in the superficial fibers of the tendon at its lesser tuberosity insertion. The subscapularis is then separated from the underlying remaining tendon and capsule and reflected medially. The superficial half of the tendon remains attached to the muscle, with the remaining deep half divided at the glenoid and remaining attached to the lesser tuberosity. The deepened or remaining tendon and capsule are then incised from the labrum medially. The orientation of the coronal dissection can be guided by determining the thickness of the scarred tendon and capsular tissue once the rotator interval region has been opened. The subscapularis is usually entrapped in scar tissue. To achieve full mobility, it may be necessary to visualize and dissect the axillary nerve. With the nerve adequately visualized and protected, the subscapularis can be released circumferentially on its superior, inferior, deep, and superficial surfaces.

At this point, if abduction and internal rotation are still limited, the inferior and posterior capsules can be released. This can be done selectively or circumferentially, depending on the degree and pattern of stiffness. The release is performed just lateral to the labrum and proceeds from anterosuperior to anteroinferior and then from posteroinferior to posterosuperior, as needed. If the posterior capsule needs to be released it is most easily visualized by placing a humeral head retractor to displace the humeral head posteriorly within the joint in addition to a blunt retractor beneath the inferior capsule to protect the axillary nerve. After the release of all contracted structures, the lateral end of the superficial subscapularis is sutured to the deep end of the tendon and capsule, with the arm in maximum external rotation that would allow secure closure of the Z-plasty with nonabsorbable suture. Each centimeter of length gained from the lengthening increases external rotation by approximately 20 degrees (Fig. 6). Range of motion is assessed again to determine where there is tension on the soft-tissue repair and thus define a "safe zone" for early pass of range of motion and rehabilitation.

The results of open release of recalcitrant chronic adhesive capsulitis of the shoulder and the role of contracture of the coracohumeral ligament and rotator interval were evaluated in a study by Ozaki et al. Seventeen patients who failed to improve with standard nonoperative measures underwent open release through an anterolateral incision. Release concentrated on the hypertrophied coracohumeral ligament and contracted tissues within the rotator interval at operation. The major cause of restricted glenohumeral movement was contracture of these structures. Histological study revealed fibrosis, hyalinization, and fibrinoid degeneration in the contracted connective tissues, as well as fibrosis of the subsynovial tissue and absence of the synovial cell layer on the joint side of the rotator interval. Once release had been performed within the rotator interval, the glenohumeral joint was then gently manipulated through a full range of motion, also mobilizing the biceps tendon within its groove.

Immediately postoperatively active mobilization of the shoulder was begun. At an average follow-up of 6.8 years,

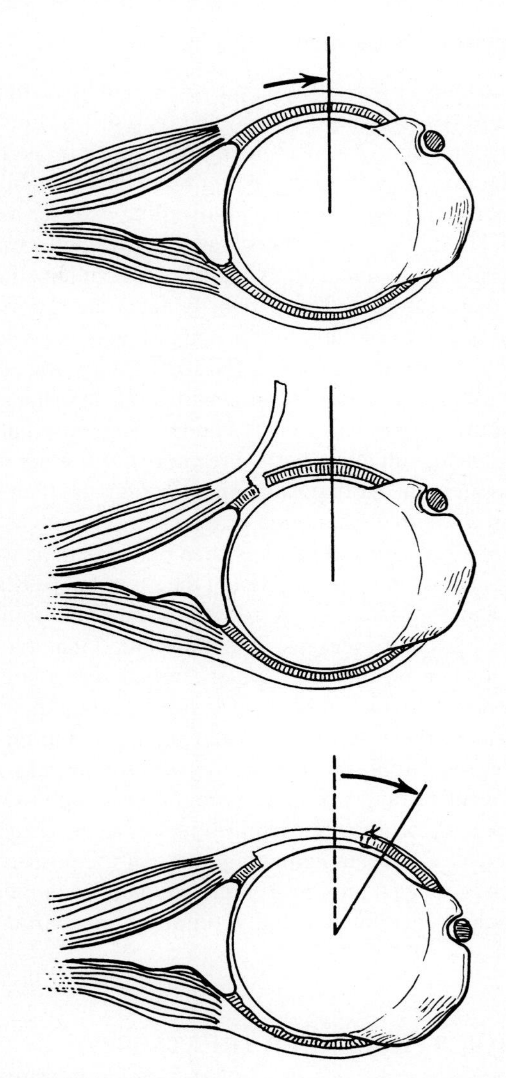

FIG. 6. Contracted subscapularis and anterior capsule **(top)** limit external rotation. This condition is treated by incising the subscapularis from the lesser tuberosity laterally **(middle)** and suturing it to the medial end of the capsule which is transected close to the glenoid **(bottom)**. This release results in substantial lengthening of these structures. Each centimeter of length gained increases external rotation by approximately 20 degrees.

16 patients were reported to have full range of motion, with 1 presenting with a slight limitation of motion. The authors state that they felt the essential changes in the tissue at the time of surgery that are productive of chronic adhesive capsulitis, such as fibrosis, hyalinization, and fibrinoid degeneration of the contracted connective tissues, a decrease in the number of synovial cells in addition to the absence of the synovial cell layer on the joint side of the rotator interval, may be related to an intrinsic disorder of collagen. They report that this procedure is logical and simple, and they recommend an open operative release of the contracted structures, especially the hypertrophied coracohumeral ligament and rotator interval, in patients in whom the shoulder does not respond to nonoperative therapy.[101]

Postoperative Treatment

Immediately after arthroscopic release, the patient should be met in the recovery room by the therapist to initiate the exercise program. A repeat manipulation can be performed later the same day if a long-acting block has been administered or the following day if an indwelling catheter has been placed, but this has been unnecessary in my hands. Continuous passive motion machines can be used, but have failed to prove there efficacy. The patient is encouraged to use the arm for activities of daily living, and a sling is not worn. Exercises are performed four to five times daily for approximately 10 to 15 minutes at a time with a self-assisted stretching exercise program as well as a pulley. Supervised physical therapy on an outpatient basis three to five times per week is also begun in the early postoperative period and then slowly decreased as time and motion progresses.

When a soft-tissue repair has been performed, as with the Z-plasty lengthening in the front of the shoulder, passive motion is again initiated, but restricted for internal rotation behind the back and excessive external rotation that may place undue tension on the subscapularis repair. Intraoperatively the position at which resistance is felt and the repair is observed to be under tension is noted and is used to guide the postoperative limits of motion. After 4 to 6 weeks an aggressive active range of motion program is begun as well as continued stretching, following both the arthroscopic and open releases. The strengthening phase of the postoperative regimen is delayed until nearly full and pain-free motion has been achieved, which usually requires approximately 3 months.

AUTHOR'S PREFERRED TREATMENT

My approach has always been to make a thorough initial assessment, obtaining a complete history of shoulder symptomatology as well as other associated medical conditions that may contribute to the cause of the frozen shoulder. After a careful preliminary diagnostic workup, as previously discussed, I insist on accurate scapular anteroposterior, lateral, as well as axillary radiographs of the shoulder. If any symptom seems to be related to the cervical spine, then radiographs of this area are also reviewed. An underlying cause is always sought and an attempt is made to determine whether the presentation is that of a primary or secondary frozen shoulder. If a secondary frozen shoulder is diagnosed, concurrent treatment of the precipitating factor is also started when possible.

After range of motion is recorded, an assessment is made of whether pain is restricted to just the extreme of motion or throughout the entire range. If pain is persistent throughout, analgesics such as antiinflammatory medications are added to the treatment regimen. I have not found the use of intraarticular steroid injections beneficial in my patient population. A careful explanation is given to the patient on the effect of immobilization of the arm against the side and the importance of light use and passive exercises. The aim of reestablishing external rotation and elevation to eliminate the pain caused by stiffness is explained.

At the time of the initial visit I begin gentle pendulum exercises as well as a stretching program. The patient is advised to perform these exercises three to five times daily preceeded by low heat and to advance them according to the amount of stiffness and pain. Passive forward elevation is performed by assisting the arm with the unaffected side up overhead in a supine or seated position. This may also be done with a pulley as well as reaching the arm up to a solid object that is just beyond reach and then having the patient lower themselves and sustain a moderate stretch adjusted to tolerance for 5 to 10 seconds. External rotation stretch is performed in the supine position with the elbow flexed to 90 degrees rotating the arm out to the side with a stick or cane. Internal rotation is performed with either the assistance of a cane or the opposite arm behind the back, at which time the affected side is pushed into hyperextension and then pulled up behind the back flexing the elbows. Adduction is performed also by pulling the involved extremity across the chest with the assistance of the uninvolved side. Short exercise sessions of 5 to 10 minutes are repeated throughout the day. I feel these have been most effective. In the early time frame, little attempt is made to progress strengthening exercises because I think the main focus should be on stretching, until an acceptable range of motion has been achieved. A supervised physical therapy program can also be instituted in conjunction with the home exercise program. This is best instituted in those patients with severe stiffness and a long history of shoulder pain, often after failed treatment. This nonoperative stretching approach can be continued as long as any improvement continues to occur. It is important for the physician to supervise the program, checking the range of motion at intervals and discussing goals of therapy with the therapist and patient until recovery of range of motion is complete and the patient is comfortable.

At the next visit, usually 6 to 8 weeks later, the patient is again examined and progress recorded. The exercises are reviewed and refined as needed. As pain subsides, more aggressive stretching can be instituted. If other etiologies of the frozen shoulder syndrome become apparent as treatment progresses, then confirmation and treatment of this source is begun. For example, if impingement-type pain seems to be present in the overhead position, a subacromial lidocaine and possibly steroid injection for diagnosis and treatment, respectively, can be given. Unless a rotator cuff tear is suspected or other concern over diagnosis and pathology is present, an MRI is rarely used in a diagnostic workup of frozen shoulder syndrome.

If the patient with a significant deficiency in motion reaches a plateau, at which time no further improvement in range of motion occurs within 4 to 6 months, closed manipulation or arthroscopic versus open release are discussed, with the previously noted indications and contraindications. Regardless of the method of treatment chosen, frozen shoulder patients usually require 1 full year of either nonoperative treatment or postoperative follow-up to maximize their recovery.

COMPLICATIONS

In most patients frozen shoulder runs a self-limited course with most of the complications encountered with this disorder being iatrogenic. Potential complications of manipulation include fractures of the proximal humerus and shaft, dislocation of the glenohumeral joint and recurrent instability, rotator cuff tears or tear extension, and injuries to the brachial plexus. Additional complications after arthroscopic or open release include axillary nerve injury, as well as recurrent stiffness secondary to extensive surgical dissection.

The primary objective in the treatment of frozen shoulder is to increase the range of motion. This should be taken into account when deciding on a rational approach for the treatment of the complications incurred while managing this problem. Iatrogenic fractures of the proximal humerus and shaft present an exceptionally difficult problem. These necessitate stabilization with internal fixation in such a way as to permit early shoulder range of motion and prevent the ensuing stiffness that is so likely to occur after fracture and immobilization.

Rotator cuff tears or tear extension that occur after manipulation are also a possible cause of failure. Although this may rarely occur, these tears usually heal spontaneously, provided that it is not superimposed on an impingement tear.[87] Extension of previously existing impingement tears would necessitate open repair that may either be performed at the time of manipulation, with special attention to postoperative range of motion to prevent recurrent stiffness, or after successful maintenance of motion the patient could be reevaluated and a treatment program established directed at repair of the rotator cuff.

The long overhead suspension of the arm after manipulation, which has been advocated by some surgeons, can be a source of neurologic injury.[90] Traction injuries of the brachioplexus and peripheral nerves have been reported after closed manipulation of the shoulder.[8] These injuries usually are neuropraxias that can recover spontaneously over time. It is critical to maintain passive motion while the nerves are recovering to avoid recurrent stiffness. Although a sling should be used to prevent excessive traction on the plexus while it is recovering, it should be removed for physical therapy and home exercise sessions. The patient and the physical therapist need to be made aware of the problem so that extremes of range of motion, particularly forward elevation and abduction, are avoided to prevent further nerve injury. The diagnosis of middle and lower plexus injuries can be made almost immediately with somatosensory-evoked potentials. Diminished sensory nerve action potentials at 5 days after the injury may also be helpful in diagnosing an early plexopathy. Definitive electrodiagnostic studies can be performed 3 weeks after the injury to evaluate the extent of nerve damage and the potential of recovery.

REFERENCES

1. Andren L, Lundberg BJ. Treatment of rigid shoulders by joint distension during arthrography. *Acta Orthop Scand* 1965;36:45.
2. Barry H, Fernandes I, Bloom B, et al. Clinical study comparing acupuncture, physiotherapy, injection, oral anti-inflammatory therapy in shoulder cuff lesions. *Curr Med Res Opin* 1980;7:121.
3. Baslund B, Thomsen BS, Jensen EM. Frozen shoulder: current concepts. *Scand J Rheum* 1990;19:321.
4. Bateman JE. *The shoulder and neck*, 2nd ed. Philadelphia: WB Saunders, 1978.
5. Binder A, Bulgen DY, Hazleman BL. Frozen shoulder: a long-term prospective study. *Ann Rheum Dis* 1984;43:361.
6. Binder A, Hazleman BL, Parr G, et al. A controlled study of oral prednisolone in frozen shoulder. *Br J Rheumatol* 1986;25:228.
7. Binder AI, Bulgen DY, Hazleman BL, et al. Frozen shoulder: an arthrographic and radionuclear scan assessment. *Ann Rheum Dis* 43: 365, 1984.
8. Birch R, Jessop J, Scott G. Brachial plexus palsy after manipulation of the shoulder. *J Bone Joint Surg [Br]* 1991;73:172.
9. Bland JH, Merrit JA, Boushey DR. The painful shoulder. *Semin Arthritis Rheum* 1977;7:21.
10. Blockey NJ, Wright JK, Kellgren JH. Oral cortisone therapy in periarthritis of the shoulder: a controlled trial. *Br Med J* 1954;1:1455.
11. Bowman CA, Jeffcoate WJ, Pattrick M, et al. Bilateral adhesive capsulitis, oligoarthritis and proximal myopathy as presentation of hypothyroidism. *Br J Rheum* 1988;27:62.
12. Bowen MK, Deng XH, Warner JP, et al. The effect of joint compression on stability of the glenohumeral joint. *Trans Orthop Res Soc* 1992;17:289.
13. Bradley JP. Arthroscopic treatment for frozen capsulitis. *Oper Tech Orthop* 1991;1:248–252.
14. Braun RM, West F, Mooney V, et al. Surgical treatment of the painful shoulder contracture in the stroke patient. *J Bone Joint Surg [Am]* 1971:53:1307.
15. Bridgman JF. Periarthritis of the shoulder and diabetes mellitus. *Ann Rheum Dis* 1972;31:69.
16. Brown AR, Weiss R, Greenberg C, et al. Interscalene block for shoulder arthroscopy: comparison with general anesthesia. *Arthroscopy* 1993;9:295–300.
17. Bruckner FE, Nye CJ. A prospective study of adhesive capsulitis of the shoulder (frozen shoulder) in a high risk population. *Q J Med* 1981;50:191.
18. Bulgen DY, Binder A, Hazleman BL, et al. Frozen shoulder: prospective clinical study with an evaluation of three treatment regimens. *Ann Rheum Dis* 1983;43:353.
19. Bulgen DY, Binder AI, Hazleman BL, et al. Immunological studies in frozen shoulder. *J Rheumatol* 1982;9:893.
20. Bulgen DY, Hazleman BL, Voak DL. HLA-B27 and frozen shoulder. *Lancet* 1976;1:1042.
21. Bulgen DY, Hazleman BL, Ward M, et al. Immunological studies in frozen shoulder. *Ann Rheum Dis* 1978;37:135.
22. Bunker TD, Anthony PP. The pathology of frozen shoulder. A Dupuytren-like disease. *J Bone Joint Surg [Br]* 1995;77:677–683.
23. Bunker TD, Esler CNA. Frozen shoulder and lipids. *J Bone Joint Surg [Br]* 1995;77:864–866.
24. Choy EH, Corhill M, Gibson T, et al. Isolated ACTH deficiency presenting with bilateral frozen shoulder. *Br J Rheum* 1991;30:226.
25. Clarke GR, Willis LA, Fish WW, et al. Preliminary studies in measuring range of motion in normal and painful stiff shoulders. *Rheum Rehabil* 1975;14:39.
26. Codman EA. Rupture of the supraspinatus tendon and other lesions in or about the subacromial bursa. In: *The shoulder*. Boston: Thomas Todd, 1934.
27. Coventry MB. Problem of painful shoulder. *JAMA* 1953;151:177.
28. Dacre JE, Beeney N, Scott DL. Injections and physiotherapy for the painful stiff shoulder. *Ann Rheum Dis* 1989;48:322.
29. Demaziere A, Wiley AM. Primary chest wall tumor appearing as frozen shoulder: review and case presentations. *J Rheumatol* 1991;18: 911.

30. DePalma AF. Loss of scapulohumeral motion (frozen shoulder). *Ann Surg* 1952;135:193.
31. DePalma AF. *Surgery of the shoulder*, 2nd ed. Philadelphia: JB Lippincott, 1973:455–468.
32. DePalma AF, Gallery G, Bennett GA. Variational anatomy and degenerative lesions of the shoulder joint. In: Blount WP, ed. *Instructional Course Lectures*. Ann Arbor, MI: American Academy of Orthopaedic Surgeons, 1949:255–281.
33. Duke O, Zeclear E, Grahame R. Anti-inflammatory drugs in periarthritis of the shoulder: a double blind, between-patient study of naproxen versus indomethacin. *Rheumatol Rehabil* 1981;20:54.
34. Duplay ES. De la periarthrite scapulohumerale et des raideurs de l'epaule qui en son la Consequence. *Arch Gen Med* 1872;20:513–542.
35. Ehrlich M, Carp SP, Berkowitz SS, et al. ACTH and cortisone in periarthritis of the shoulder ("frozen shoulder"). *Ann Rheum Dis* 1951; 10:485.
36. Fareed DO, Gallivan WRJ. Office management of frozen shoulder syndrome: treatment with hydraulic distension under local anesthesia. *Clin Orthop* 1989;242:177.
37. Fleming A, Dodman S, Beer TC, et al. Personal in frozen shoulder. *Ann Rheum Dis* 1975;35:456.
38. Flood V. Discovery of a new ligament. *Lancet* 1829;671–672.
39. Gilula L, Schoenecker PL, Murphy WAW. Shoulder arthrography as a treatment modality. *AJR Am J Roentgenol* 1978;131:1047.
40. Grey RG. The natural history of "idiopathic" frozen shoulder. *J Bone Surg* 1978;60:564.
41. Haggart GE, Dignam RJ, Sullivan T. Management of the "frozen" shoulder. *JAMA* 1956;161:1219–1222.
42. Harmon PH. Methods and results in the treatment of 2,580 painful shoulder. *Am J Surg* 1958;95:527–544.
43. Harryman DT II. Shoulders: frozen and stiff. *Instr Course Lect* 1993; 42:247.
44. Harryman DT, Sidles JA, Clark JM, et al. Translation of the humeral head on the glenoid with passive glenohumeral motion. *J Bone Joint Surg* 1990;72:1334–1343.
45. Harryman DT, Sidles JA, Harris SL, et al. The role of the rotator interval capsule in passive motion and stability of the shoulder. *J Bone Joint Surg* 1992;74:53–66.
46. Hazleman BL. The painful stiff shoulder. *Rheumatol Phys Med* 1972; 11:413.
47. Helbig B, Wagner P, Dohler R. Mobilization of frozen shoulder under general anesthesia. *Acta Orthop Belg* 1983;49:267.
48. Hill JJ, Bogumill HL. Manipulation in the treatment of frozen shoulder. *Orthopedics* 1988;9:1255–1260.
49. Hill JJ Jr, Bogumill H. Manipulation in the treatment of frozen shoulder. *Orthopedics* 1988;11:1255.
50. Hollingworth GR, Ellis R, Hattersley TS. Comparison of injection techniques for frozen shoulder pain: results of a double-blind, randomized study. *Br J Med* 1983;287:1339–1341.
51. Hsu SY, Can KM. Arthrographic distension in the management of frozen shoulder. *Int Orthop* 1991;15:79.
52. Huskisson EC, Bryans R. Diclofenac sodium in treatment of the painful stiff shoulder. *Curr Med Res Opin* 1983;8:350.
53. Inmann VT, Saunders JB, Abbott LC. Observations on the shoulder. *J Bone Joint Surg* 1944;26:1–30.
54. Itoi E, Tabata S. Range of motion and arthrography in the frozen shoulder. *J Shoulder Elbow Surg* 1992;1:106.
55. Johnson JT. Frozen shoulder syndrome in patients with pulmonary tuberculosis. *J Bone Joint Surg [Am]* 1959;41:877.
56. Kamieth H. Rontgenkefunde der Halswerbesaule und der Schulter bie der Periarthritis Humerscapularis undihre einordnung in die pathogenese diser Erkrankung. [Radiography of the cervical spine in shoulder periarthritis]. *Z Orthop* 1965;100:162.
57. Kessel L, Bayley I, Young A. The frozen shoulder. *Br J Hosp Med* 1981;25:334–339.
58. Kessel L, Bayley I, Young A. The upper limb: the frozen shoulder. *Br J Hosp Med* 1981;25:334.
59. Kieras DM, Matsen FA III. Open release in the management of refractory frozen shoulder. *Orthop Trans* 1991;15:801.
60. Kopell AP, Thompson WAL. Pain and the frozen shoulder. *Surg Gynecol Obstet* 1959;109:279.
61. Kraft GH, Johnson EW, Laban MM. The fibrositis syndrome. *Arch Phys Med Rehabil* 1968;49:155–162.
62. Lee M, Haq AM, Wright V, et al. Periarthritis of the shoulder; a controlled trial of physiotherapy. *Physiotherapy* 1973;59:312.
63. Leffert RD. The frozen shoulder. *Instr Course Lect* 1985;34:199.
64. Lequesene M, Dang N, Bensasson M, et al. Increased association of diabetes mellitus and capsulitis of the shoulder and shoulder–hand syndrome. *Scand J Rheumatol* 1977;6:53.
65. Lippman RK. Frozen shoulder: periarthritis: bicipital tenosynovitis. *Arch Surg* 1943;47:283.
66. Lloyd-Roberts GG, French PR. Periarthritis of the shoulder: a study of the disease and its treatment. *Br Med J* 1959;1:1996.
67. Lusardi DA, Wirth MA, Wurtz D, et al. Loss of external rotation following anterior capsulorrhaphy of the shoulder. *J Bone Joint Surg* 1993;75:1185–1192.
68. Lorenz TH, Musser MJ. Life, stress, emotions, and the painful stiff shoulder. *Ann Arthritis Med* 1952;37:1232.
69. Loyd JA, Loyd HM. Adhesive capsulitis of the shoulder: arthrographic diagnosis and treatment. *South Med J* 1983;76:879.
70. Lundberg BJ. Glycosaminoglycans of the normal and frozen shoulder joint capsule. *Clin Orthop* 1970;69:279.
71. Lundberg BJ. Pathomechanics of the frozen shoulder and the effect of brisement force. In: Bayley J, Kessel L, eds. *Shoulder surgery* Berlin-Heidelberg: Springer-Verlag, 1982:109–110.
72. Lundberg BJ. The frozen shoulder: clinical and radiographical observations. The effect of manipulation under general anesthesia: structure and glycosaminoglycan content of the joint capsule. *Acta Orthop Scand [Suppl]* 1969;119:1–59.
73. MacDonald PB, Hawkins RJ, Fowler PJ, et al. Release of the subscapularis for internal rotation contracture and pain after anterior repair for recurrent anterior dislocaiton of the shoulder. *J Bone Joint Surg* 1992;74:734–737.
74. Macnab I. Rotator cuff tendinitis. *Ann Coll Surg Engl* 1973;53:271.
75. Macnab I. Rotator cuff tendonitis. In: McKibbon GT, ed. *Recent advances in orthopaedics*. Edinburgh: Churchill Livingstone, 1975.
76. McGraw JW, Turba JE. Frozen shoulder. Treatment by arthroscopy and manipulation. *Orthop Trans* 1989;13:661.
77. McLaughlin HL. Lesions of the musculotendinous cuff of the shoulder. *J Bone Joint Surg* 1944;26:31.
78. McLauglin HL. On the "frozen shoulder." *Bull Hosp Joint Dis Orthop Inst* 1951;12:383.
79. Mintner WT. The shoulder–hand syndrome in coronary disease. *J Med Assoc Ga* 1967;56:45.
80. Mosley HF. *Shoulder lesions*. Springfield, IL: Charles C Thomas, 1945:66.
81. Murnaghan GF, McIntosh D. Hydrocortisone in painful shoulder: a controlled trial. *Lancet* 1955;269:798–800.
82. Murnaghan JP. Frozen shoulder. In: Rockwood CAJ, Matsen FA, eds. *The shoulder*. Philadelphia: WB Saunders, 1990:837.
83. Myer AW. Chronic functional lesions of the shoudler. *Arch Surg* 1937;35:646.
84. Neer CS, Satterlee CC, Dalsy R, et al. On the value of the coracohumeral ligament release. *Orthop Trans* 1985;34:199.
85. Neer CS, Satterlee CC, Dalsy R, et al. The anatomy and potential effects of contracture of the corachohumeral ligament. *Clin Orthop* 1992;280:182–185.
86. Neer CS II. Frozen shoulder. In: Neer CS, ed. *Shoulder reconstruction*. Philadelphia: WB Saunders, 1990:422.
87. Neviaser JS. Adhesive capsulitis of the shoulder: study of pathological findings in periarthritis of the shoulder. *J Bone Joint Surg* 1945;27: 211.
88. Neviaser JS. Adhesive capsulitis of the shoulder (the frozen shoulder). *Med Times* 1962;90:783.
89. Neviaser JS. Adhesive capsulitis and the stiff and painful shoulder. *Orthop Clin North Am* 1980;11:327.
90. Neviaser JS. Arthrography of the shoulder joint. *J Bone Joint Surg* 1962;44:1321–1330.
91. Neviaser RJ. Painful conditions affecting the shoulder. *Clin Orthop* 1983;173:63.
92. Neviaser RJ, Neviaser TJ. The frozen shoulder: diagnosis and management. *Clin Orthop* 1987;223:59.
93. Neviaser RJ, Neviaser TJ. The frozen shoulder diagnosis and management. *Clin Orthop* 1987;223:59–64.
94. Nicholson GG. The effects of passive joint mobilization on pain and hypomobility associated with adhesive capsulitis of the shoulder. *Orthop Sports Phy Ther* 1985;6:238–246.
95. Noy S, Dekel S, Orgad S, et al. HLA-B27 and frozen shoulder. *Tissue Antigens* 1981;17:251.

96. Oesterreicher W, Van Dam G. Social and psychological researches into brachialgia and periarthritis. *Arthritis Rheum* 1964;7:670.
97. Ogilvie-Harris DJ, Biggs DJ, Fitsialos DP, et al. The resistant frozen shoulder. Manipulation versus arthroscopic release. *Clin Orthop* 1995;319:238–248.
98. Ogilvie-Harrris DJ, Wiley AM. Arthroscopic surgery of the shoulder. *J Bone Joint Surg* 1986;68:201–207.
99. Ogilvie-Harris DJ, Wiley AM. Arthroscopic surgery of the shoulder: a general appraisal. *J Bone Joint Surg [Br]* 1986;68:201.
100. Older MW, McIntyre JL, Lloyd GJ. Distention arthrography of the shoulder joint. *Can J Surg* 1976;19:203.
101. Ozaki J, Nakagawa Y, Sakurai G. Recalcitrant chronic adhesive capsulitis of the shoulder: role of contracture of the coracohumeral ligament and rotator interval in pathogenesis and treatment. *J Bone Surg [Am]* 1989;71:1511.
102. Parker RD, Froimson AL, Winsburg DD, et al. Frozen shoulder. Part I. Chronology, pathogenesis, clinical picture and treatment. *Orthopedics* 1989;12:869.
103. Parker RD, Froimson AI, Winsburg DD, et al. Frozen shoulder. Part II. Treatment by manipulation under anesthesia. *Orthopedics* 1989; 12:989.
104. Pasteur F. Sur une forrme nouvelle de periarthralgia et d'ankylose de l'epaule. *J Radiol Electrol Med Nucl* 1934;18:327.
105. Pollock RG, Duralde YA, Flatow EL, et al. The use of arthroscopy in the treatment of frozen shoulder. *Clin Orthop* 1994;304:30–36.
106. Quigley TB. Checkrein shoulder, a type of "frozen" shoulder: diagnosis and treatment by manipulation under and ACTH or cortisone. *Clin Orthop* 1982;164;4.
107. Quin CE. "Frozen shoulder": evaluation of treatment with hydrocortisone injections and exercises. *Ann Phys Med* 1965;8:22.
108. Rathbun JB, Macnab. the microvascular pattern of the rotator cuff. *J Bone Joint Surg [Br]* 1970;52:540.
109. Reeves B. Arthroscopic changes in frozen and post-traumatic stiff shoulder. *Proc R Soc Med* 1966;59:827–830.
110. Reeves B. The natural history of the frozen shoulder syndrome. *J Rheumatol* 1975;4:193.
111. Rhind V, Downie WW, Bird HA, et al. Naproxen and indomethacin in periarthritis of the shoulder. *Rheumatol Rehabil* 1982;21:51.
112. Richardson AT. Enest Fletcher lecture: the painful shoulder. *Proc R Soc Med* 1975;68:731.
113. Riley D, Lang AE, Blair RD, et al. Frozen shoulder and other shoulder disturbances in Parkinson's disease. *J Neurol Psychiatry* 1989;52: 63.
114. Rizk TE, Pinals RD. Frozen shoulder. *Semin Arthritis Rheum* 1982; 11:440.
115. Rizk TE, Pinals RS. Histocompatibility type and racial incidence in frozen shoulder. *Arch Phys Med Rehabil* 1984;65:33.
116. Roy S, Oldham R. Management of painful shoulder. *Lancet* 1976;1: 1322.
117. Sattar MA, Lugman WA. Periarthritis: another duration-related compication of diabetes mellitus. *Diabetes Care* 1985;8:507–510.
118. Segmuller HE, Taylor DE, Hagan CS, et al. Arthroscopic treatment of adhesive capsulitis. *J Shoulder Elbow Surg* 1995;4:403–408.
119. Shaffer B, Tibone JE, Kerlan RK. Frozen shoulder: a long-term follow-up. *J Bone Joint Surg [Am]* 1993;74:738.
120. Shaw DK, Deutsch DT, Bowling RJ. Efficacy of shoulder range of motion exercise in hospitalized patients after coronary artery bypass graft surgery. *Heart Lung* 1989;18:364.
121. Simmonds FA. Shoulder pain, with particular reference to the "frozen shoulder." *J Bone Joint Surg [Br]* 1949;31B:426.
122. Simmons DB. Myofascial pain syndromes: where are we? where are we going? *Arch Phys Med Rehabil* 1988;69:209–212.
123. Smith CR, Binder AI, Paice EW. Lesions of the midshaft of the humerus presenting as shoulder capsulitis. *Br J Rheumatol* 1990;29: 386.
124. Steinbrocker I, Argyros TG. Frozen shoulder: treatment by local injection of depot corticosteroids. *Arch Phys Med Rehabil* 1974;55:209.
125. Stodell MA, Sturrock RD. Frozen shoulder. *Lancet* 1981;2:527.
126. Thomas D, Williams RA, Smith DS. The frozen shoulder: a review of manipulative treatment. *Rheumatol Rehabil* 1980;19:173.
127. Travell JG, Simmons DG. *Myofascial pain and dysfunction: trigger point manual*. Baltimore: Williams & Wilkins, 1983:410–424.
128. Warner JP. Frozen shoulder: diagnosis and management. *Am Acad Orthop Surg* 1997;5:130–140.
129. Warner JP, Allen A, Marks PH, et al. Arthroscopic release for chronic refractory adhesive capsulitis of the shoulder. *J Bone Joint Surg* 1996; 78:1808–1816.
130. Warner JP, Allen AA, Marks P, et al. Arthroscopic release of refractory capsular contracture of the shoulder. Video presentation, American Academy of Orthopaedic Surgeons, 62nd Annual Meeting, Orlando, FL, 1995.
131. Warner JP, Coborn DNM, Berger R, et al. Dynamic capsuloligamentous anatomy of the glenohumeral joint. *J Shoulder Elbow Surg* 1933; 2:115–133.
132. Warner JP, Ianotti JP. Treatment of a stiff shoulder after posterior capsulorrhapy. *J Bone Joint Surg* 1996;78:1419–1421.
133. Watson JR. Simple treatment of the stiff shoulder. *J Bone Joint Surg [Br]* 1963;45:207.
134. Weiss JJ, Ting YM. Arthrography assisted intra-articular injection of steroids in the treatment of adhesive capsulitis. *Arch Phys Med Rehabil* 1979;59:285–287.
135. Wiley AM. Arthroscopic appearance of frozen shoulder. *J Arthrosc Rel Surg* 1991;7:138.
136. Wohlgethan JR. Frozen shoulder in hyperthyroidism. *Arthritis Rheum* 1987;30:936.
137. Wolfe F. Fibrositis, fibromyalgia and musculoskeletal disease: the current status of fibrositis syndrome. *Arch Phys Med Rehabil* 1988;69: 527–531.
138. Wright MG, Richards AJ, Clark MB. 99-M pertechnetate scanning in capsulitis. *Lancet* 1975;2:1265.
139. Wright V, Haq AM. Periarthritis of the shoulder: I. Aetiological considerations with particular reference to personality factors. *Ann Rheum Dis* 1976;35:213.
140. Young A. Immunological studies in the frozen shoulder. In: Bayley J, Kessel L, eds. *Shoulder surgery*. Berlin-Heidelberg: Springer-Verlag, 1982:110–113.
141. Zuckerman JD, Cuomo F. Frozen shoulder. In: Matsen FA, Fu F, Hawkins RJ, eds. *The shoulder: a balance of mobility and stability*. Rosemont, IL: American Academy of Orthopaedic Surgeons, 1993: 253.

PART IV

Glenohumeral Joint: Arthritis and Related Disorders

Disorders of the Shoulder: Diagnosis and Management,
edited by Joseph P. Iannotti and Gerald R. Williams, Jr.
Lippincott Williams & Wilkins, Philadelphia © 1999.

CHAPTER 16

Pathophysiology, Classification, and Pathoanatomy of Glenohumeral Arthritis and Related Disorders

David N. Collins

D. N. Collins: Department of Orthopaedic Surgery, University of Arkansas for Medical Sciences, Little Rock, Arkansas 72205.

INTRODUCTION

Regardless of the cause or the location of the joint, the pathologic changes of arthritis have the greatest effect on the articular cartilage and underlying bone. Initially, the soft-tissue involvement includes only the synovium, but later it may involve, both directly and indirectly, the joint capsule, ligaments, and adjacent tendons. The progression of arthritis is not only influenced by the existing disease processes, but also by the extent and rate of joint loading by mechanical forces.

The predominant clinical feature of arthritis is pain. For most major joints, this is on the basis of the intraarticular changes of arthritis. Unlike other joints, however, the shoulder is more often affected by periarticular soft-tissue disorders, which may coexist with glenohumeral arthritis and influence its clinical course. The functionally important musculotendinous cuff, along with the capsule and supporting ligaments, may undergo secondary changes as a result of glenohumeral joint arthritis. These include muscular weakness, pathologic musculotendinous shortening, and attenuation of ligamentous tissue. With articular disease progression and the associated direct or indirect involvement of the unique soft-tissue envelope of the glenohumeral joint, the clinical effect will be profound.

The glenohumeral arthritides and associated disorders can be among the most challenging diagnoses. The clinician is required to use the acquired skills of careful history-taking, thorough physical examination, and prudent use of cost-effective testing. Glenohumeral arthritis and allied conditions include osteoarthritis, posttraumatic arthritis, arthritis of dislocation, osteonecrosis, rheumatoid arthritis, crystalline arthritis, noninfectious inflammatory arthritis, and rotator cuff tear arthropathy.

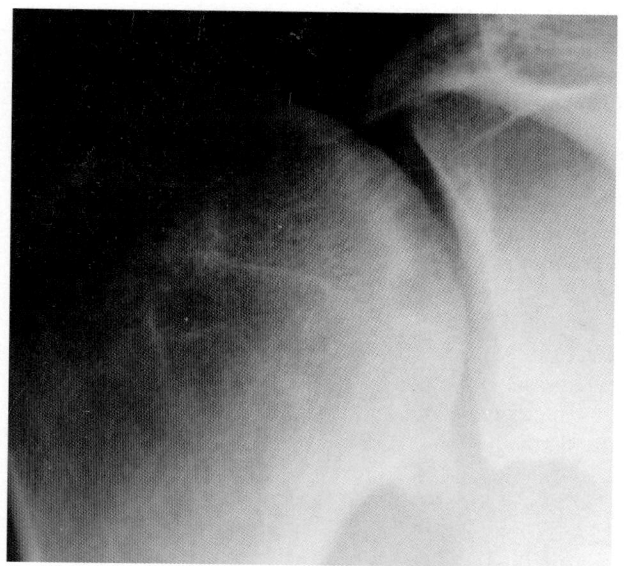

A

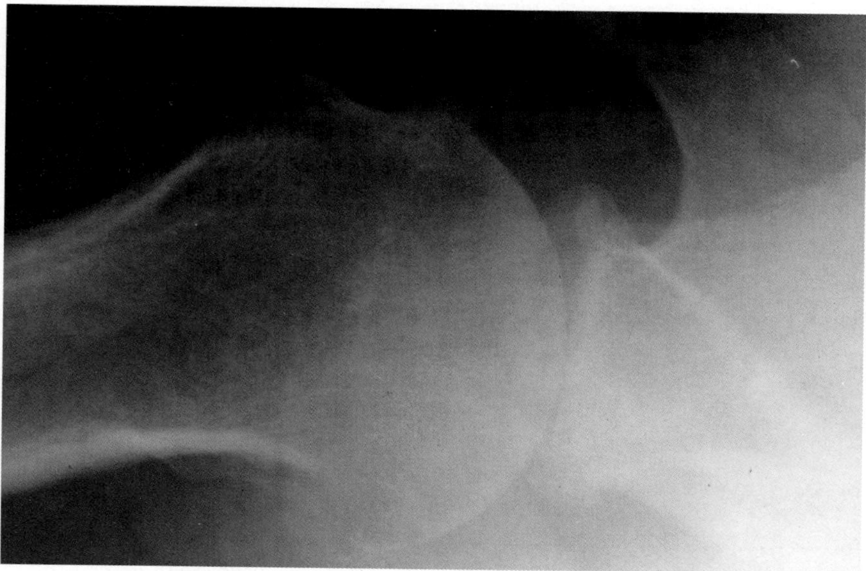

B

FIG. 1. (A) True anteroposterior view of the glenohumeral joint and **(B)** transaxillary lateral view, adequately demonstrating moderately severe osteoarthritis.

Shoulder pain is not only a very common symptom that clinicians are asked to evaluate, but also the chief complaint of patients with glenohumeral arthritis. Acute traumatic shoulder pain is reviewed elsewhere in this textbook. This chapter will highlight the major causes of glenohumeral arthritis and profile the characteristics of each disorder.

Clinical Presentation

Although the shoulder is no less susceptible than other diarthrodial joints to arthritic conditions, arthritis is not a typical cause of shoulder pain. Probably as few as 5% to 10% of patients with shoulder pain have arthritis as a part of a polyarticular systemic disease, or a monarticular disease process. Painful dysfunction is more often a disorder of one or more of the soft-tissue elements of the shoulder.

There exist more than 100 different types of arthritis. They may be defined as inflammatory or degenerative, polyarticular or monarticular, and acute or chronic. Distinction is made from historical factors, physical findings, radiographic analysis, and tissue sampling, including synovial fluid analysis and serum studies.

The predominant symptom of patients with arthritis is pain, usually intensifying with use and interfering with sleep. Shoulder motion is restricted by synovial membrane inflammation and increased fluid production. The synovium and capsule are richly innervated structures easily irritated by distention from the accumulation of synovial fluid. Exacerbation of discomfort with rotary movement with the elbow at the side is a characteristic physical finding of an inflammatory condition of the glenohumeral joint. Degenerative conditions are more tolerant of passive range of motion. Tenderness over the posterior joint line, as noted by Neer,[212] is notable in glenohumeral osteoarthritis. Tenderness lateral and inferior to the coracoid process is very suggestive of an inflammatory disease. It is commonly not elicited in rotator cuff disease or noninflammatory conditions.

Imaging

Green and Norris have provided an excellent review of imaging strategies to be employed for patients with glenohumeral arthritis.[91] Initial evaluation of the painful shoulder will almost always include plain radiographs.[145] The most commonly employed views for the orthopaedic surgeon are the true anteroposterior (AP) of the glenohumeral joint orthogonal to the plane of the scapula and the transaxillary lateral. Glenohumeral arthritis is easily distinguished from other soft-tissue conditions and is classified based on features identified on plain films (Fig. 1).[266] These include alignment and relation of the humerus to the glenoid and acromion process, the width of the articular cartilage, osseous erosions, productive changes including osteophytes, and the presence of soft-tissue swelling and calcification.

Distinction of the articular cartilage space is best made when the x-ray beam is directed tangent to the joint surface. For the shoulder, this requires accurate patient, shoulder, and extremity positioning. Once the plane has been determined, the humerus can be externally rotated to approximately 35 degrees (Fig. 2). This will profile the load-bearing portion of the articular surface so that the earliest narrowing does not escape detection, and it is also the position favoring visualization of marginal humeral head osteophytes.[146] Apple et al. have suggested a weighted abduction Grashey shoulder method as a more sensitive means of detection of loss of articular cartilage.[6a] When the disease is more advanced, positioning the humerus in external rotation is difficult and cannot be done exclusive of the position of the scapula (Fig. 3). For Nelson and colleagues, plain radiography, as opposed to magnetic resonance imaging (MRI), computed tomography (CT) arthrogram, and ultrasonography, was most useful for the diagnosis of osteoarthritis.[222]

Although shoulder arthrography is most useful for detection of rotator cuff tears, the articular surfaces and contours of the synovial lining of the joint can be easily visualized.[311] The arthrographic features may be enhanced by the use of poly- or computed tomography.[285] Filling defects may be observed in the cartilaginous surfaces and the thickness of the residual cartilage estimated. Magnetic resonance arthrography using gadopentetate dimeglumine may offer a more sensitive method for detection of intraarticular abnormalities.[156,233] These techniques, for practical purposes, are rarely employed by us for the routine assessment of glenohumeral arthritis.

Ultrasound study of the glenohumeral articulation has a very limited, yet undefined, role in the evaluation of the articular surfaces.

Although generally not required for the diagnosis of articular disorders, a CT scan can be quite helpful to delineate the

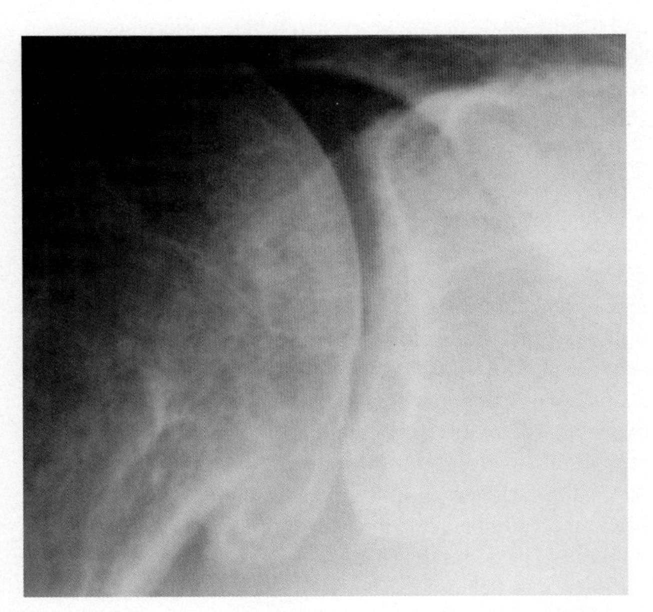

FIG. 2. Humerus in 35 degrees of external rotation, profiling the articular surface in the true anteroposterior plane of the scapula.

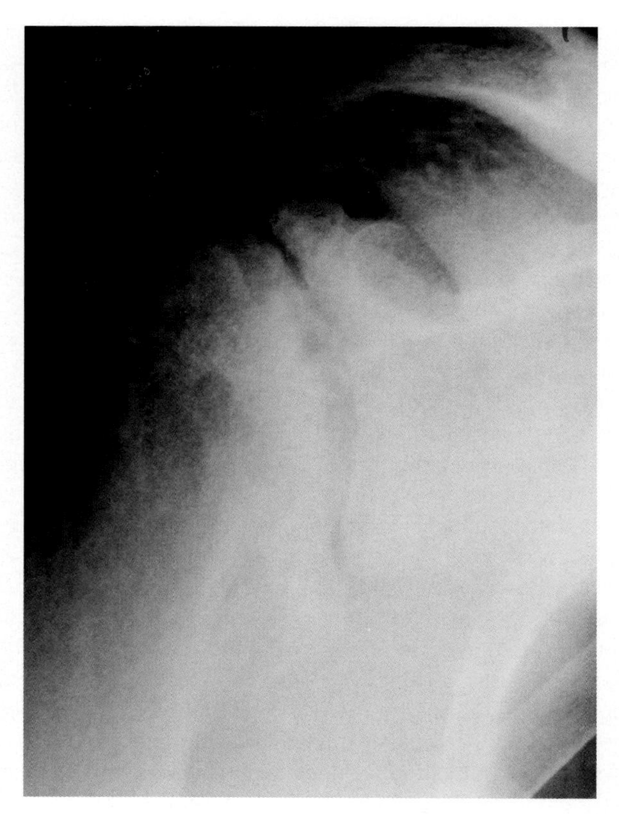

FIG. 3. More advanced osteoarthritis, requiring total rotation of the humerus with the torso, a result of fixed internal rotation contracture of the glenohumeral joint.

extent of bone involvement and assess glenoid orientation (Fig. 4).[79,207] Glenohumeral morphology can be detailed, as can the quality and quantity of the glenoid. CT scanning will also help detect subtle cortical erosions, deposits of calcium, and the presence of newly formed bone. A more accurate assessment of glenohumeral relations may be realized by CT when extreme stiffness or deformity does not allow the shoulder to be positioned for optimal plain film study.

Perhaps the best-imaging study for detecting early chondral injury or damage is MRI, even though assessment of the articular cartilage can be technically challenging. Hayes stated that an accurate MRI scan of articular cartilage requires good spatial resolution for the detection of small defects, good subject contrast and image contrast for the detection of signal intensity changes in articular cartilage, and reliable distinctions for the detection of signal intensity changes in articular cartilage, and reliable distinction between articular cartilage and adjacent subchondral bone and joint fluid.[113] Broderick's study drew attention to the tendency for cartilage abnormalities to be underestimated with MRI when compared with arthroscopic observations.[19]

There is now, however, a consensus that normal articular cartilage can be imaged by MRI, perhaps to the extent of "zonal" analysis.[37,198,234,272] Three-dimensional imaging data can provide information about joint surface topography utilizing refined techniques.[8,25,235,236,258,309] Quantitative MRI is under investigation as a means of earlier detection and as a tool for monitoring the response of the articular cartilage to treatment.[100]

With few exceptions, scientific studies of MRI of articular cartilage involve the knee.[14,37,95,99,119,191,235,258] Huber, in one of the earliest published reports on MRI of the normal shoulder, cited the failure of MRI to effectively define articular cartilage.[123] The literature was replete with studies of MRI of the shoulder that had assessed features of the rotator cuff and capsulolabral morphology in impingement and instability disorders, respectively, and rarely mentioned the findings of the glenohumeral articular cartilage. Recent monographs and textbooks concerned with MRI of the shoulder and shoulder imaging inadequately address arthritis imaging by MRI, particularly the articular cartilage changes.[292,316,338] The preferred timing, sequences, and technical parameters have not been determined with uniform success, and are evolving.[118] Therefore, MRI applications for glenohumeral articular disorders are not yet as extensive as for the knee. Zlatkin has stated that MRI is rarely required to assess patients for glenohumeral osteoarthritis alone.[337] MRI arthrography utilizing gadolinium may prove to be an effective technique to enhance the articular surfaces.[156]

A shortcoming of conventional radiographs is failure to detect soft-tissue details, although in some cases swelling can be identified. Joint effusions may be suspected on plain films, but are best evaluated by ultrasound, CT, or MRI. The MRI is probably the most useful, accurate, reliable and expensive.[316,327]

In normal shoulders, the MRI findings show only a thin rim of joint fluid around the biceps tendon sheath and narrow bands in the axillary recess and subscapularis bursa.[286] The volume has been observed to be increased with age.[286] Accumulation of glenohumeral joint fluid is abnormal; usually, it is related to rotator cuff tears or osteoarthritis (Fig. 4).[286] The intravenous administration of gadopentetate dimeglumine will enhance the MR image of joint fluid, although the response is slower and less vigorous than synovium.[326]

Use of MRI allows direct visualization of inflammatory synovitis and synovial proliferation within the joint, as well as its penetration into the adjacent bone and periarticular soft tissues (Fig 4).[261,328] Contrast enhancement with the use of gadolinium provides a more specific assessment of synovitis or pannus.[154,261] The rate and intensity of synovial enhancement may vary, depending on the activity of the synovium as a reflection of the activity of the disease process, as well as the image timing.[326]

Radionuclide isotope uptake in tissue reflects the rate and extent of blood flow through the tissue and, in bone, is a measure of bone metabolism, especially osteoblastic activity. Scintigraphy, in particular triple-phase bone scan, may prove useful in distinguishing soft-tissue inflammation from osteoarticular changes.[87,179,315] It is very sensitive, but it does not distinguish acute inflammatory disease from bone and joint sepsis.[314] Technectium scans have been used to confirm the presence of rheumatoid arthritis before the appearance of

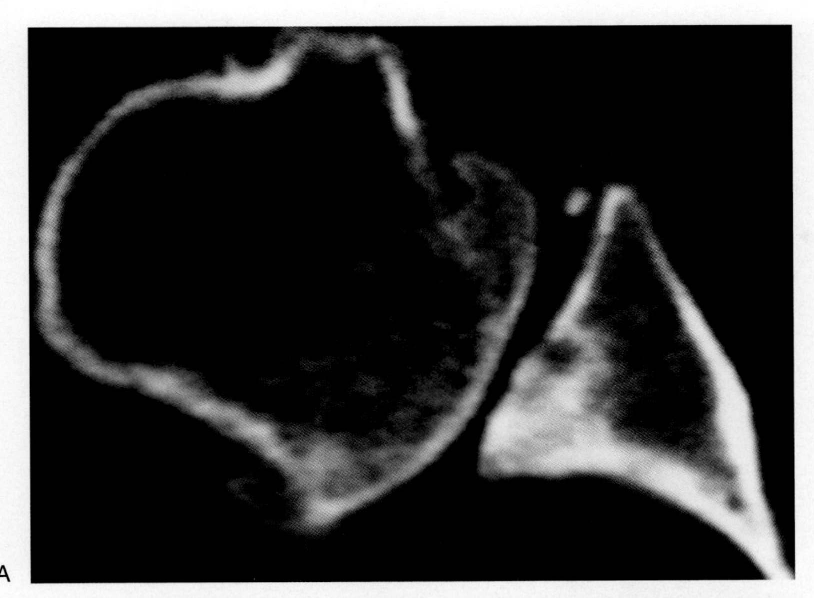

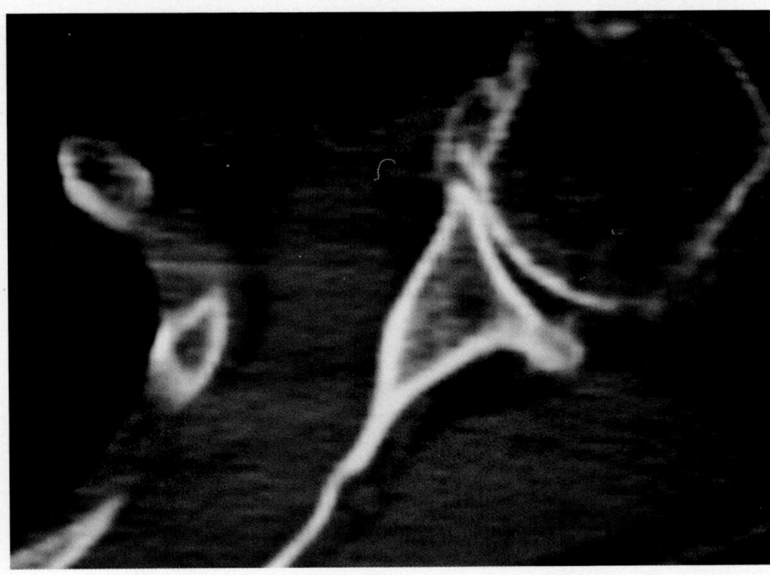

FIG. 4. **(A)** CT scan of osteoarthritis showing posterior glenoid erosion and articular cartilage narrowing, preservation of the anterior cartilage, peripheral osteophyte formation, and an anterior loose body. **(B)** A more unusual pattern with preservation of posterior cartilage, wear of the anterior cartilage, and peripheral osteophytes. This could only be appreciated by CT scan. *(continued)*

radiographic abnormalities.[61] Indium-111 chloride has been used for detection of rheumatoid arthritis as well as following the course of disease activity.[276,291] Immune complex scintigraphy holds promise for monitoring disease activity and response to treatment.[50,148] MRI may have clinical application in the early detection of rheumatoid arthritis, its staging, and the assessment of treatment outcomes.[11,20,335] Uptake defects can exist in osteonecrosis, and can be enhanced with single-photon emission computed tomography (SPECT) images.[313,322] White cell-labeled scans are useful when an infectious disease process is being considered.[315,319]

Laboratory

Serum studies may be helpful, but only rarely can a diagnosis be obtained from this information alone. Complete blood count, autoantibodies (rheumatoid factor [RF] and antinuclear antibody [ANA]), uric acid and acute-phase reactant measurements, erythrocyte sedimentation rates (ESR), and C-reactive protein (CRP) are most often performed as an initial-screening battery and most helpful when the diagnosis is in question.[280] Acute-phase reactants are serum proteins formed in the liver and include coagulation, transport, complement, and miscellaneous reactive proteins. Their production is accelerated in the presence of inflammatory states and tissue necrosis.[161] The ESR is a rough, indirect quantification of their serum levels. The CRP level has been used more recently. Both are serum markers that reflect the extent or degree of inflammation and can be used for assessment of disease activity or response to treatment over time.[36] CRP levels (normally less than 1 mg/dl) may exhibit moderate elevation (1–10 mg/dl) in most connective tissue diseases; marked elevation (more than 10 mg/dl) may signify an acute bacterial infection such as septic arthritis.[201]

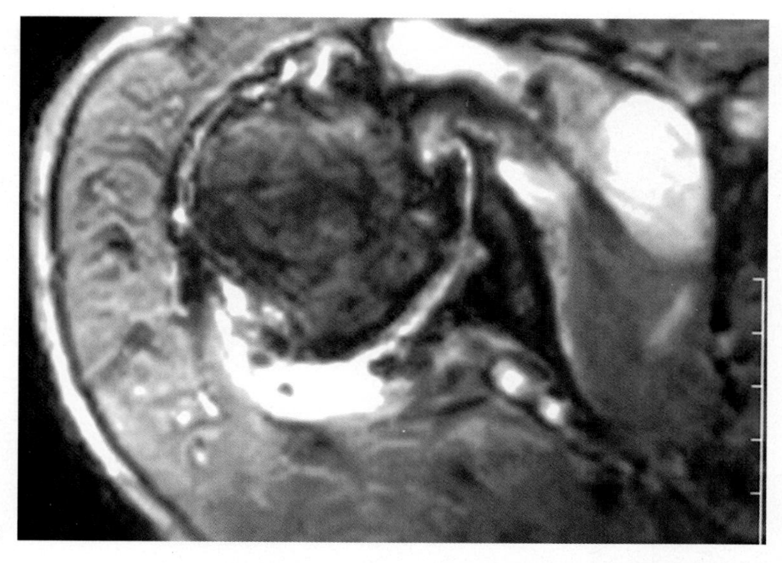

C

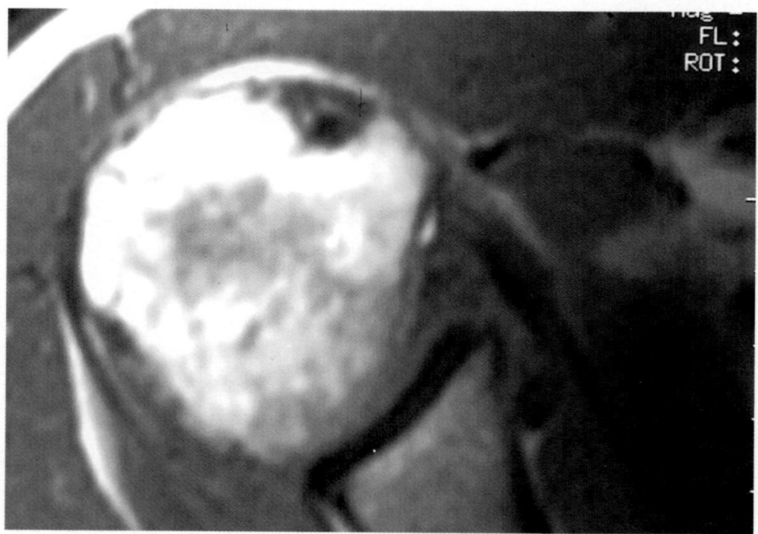

D

FIG. 4. *Continued.* **(C)** MRI demonstrating abnormal accumulation of joint fluid in advanced glenohumeral osteoarthritis. **(D)** MRI of glenohumeral, pigmented villonodular synovitis, seen here obliterating the joint space.

Clinically detectable effusions are uncommon in most arthritides. When present or suspected, however, a fluid sample should be obtained. It should also be obtained at any time the patient's history, physical examination, and radiographs support the diagnosis of arthritis, but a diagnosis has yet to be determined.[83] The findings of joint fluid analysis have been shown to change a clinically suspected diagnosis, and often treatment, in 20% of samplings.[65]

Arthrocentesis of the shoulder can be performed from the anterior or posterior approach. Anteriorly, the tip of the coracoid process is palpated. After locally instilled anesthesia, an 18- or 21-gauge spinal needle is passed through the deltoid muscle at a point approximately 1.5 cm inferior and 1.5 cm lateral to the tip of the coracoid process. The cephalic vein is nearby and may be inadvertently punctured. Entry into the joint is gained with passage through the subscapularis muscle and the joint capsule. Posteriorly, the point of entry is two- to three-finger breadths inferior and one- to two-finger breadths medial to the posterolateral corner of the acromion process. Directed toward the coracoid process, the needle will penetrate the deltoid and infraspinatus muscles to enter through the capsule into the joint.

As much fluid as possible is withdrawn and its volume is determined. It is characterized as shown in Table 1.[38] The gross characteristics are noted. These include viscosity and color, which is normally clear and yellowish tinged. The fluid is typically not bloody, although blood tinging may suggest a traumatic tap or the existence of a pathologic lesion.

Fluid in normal joints is present in quantities that may preclude sampling by arthrocentesis. Recht detected fluid in 14 of 20 shoulders by MRI in 12 asymptomatic young volunteers; in none was more than 2 ml evident.[259] If the joint fluid is obtained, the white count is less than 200, predominantly monocytic as opposed to polymorphonuclear, and there are no red cells.[83]

TABLE 1. *Synovial fluid analysis*

	Normal	Noninflammatory	Inflammatory	Pyogenic	Nonpyogenic
Gross analysis					
Volume	1–4 mL	Increased	Increased	Increased	Increased
Color	Clear, pale yellow	Yellow (xanthochromic)	Yellow-green, white	Yellow, white, gray	Variable
Clarity/turbidity	Transparent	Transparent	Transparent to opaque	Opaque, purulent	Variable
Viscosity	Very high	High	Low	Very low/variable	Decreased/variable
Mucin clot	Good (tight)	Good/fair	Fair/poor (friable)	Poor (friable)	Fair/poor
Spontaneous clot	None	Often	Often	Often	Variable
Microscopic analysis					
Leukocytes	<200	200–2,000	2,000–50,000	15,000–200,000	10,000–20,000
Neutrophils	<25%	<25%	25%–75%	>75%	50%–75%
Organism stains	Negative	Negative	Negative	Positive	Variable
Predominant cell types	Mononuclear	Mononuclear	Polymorphonuclear	Polymorphonuclear	Polymorphonuclear
Chemical analysis					
Fluid/serum glucose	1:1	0.8–1.0	0.5–0.8	<0.5	<0.5
Protein (g/dL)	<2.5	<2.5	2.5–8.0	2.5–8.0	2.5–8.0
Lactic acid	Plasma	Plasma	>Plasma	>Plasma	>Plasma
Culture	Negative	Negative	Negative	Positive	Positive

From ref. 38, with permission.

Additional joint fluid types have been noted.[83] Noninflammatory fluid has a white cell count usually less than 2000.[38] The fluid is transparent or nearly so. This type of fluid can be seen in trauma, osteoarthritis, systemic lupus erythematosus (SLE), sarcoid, and hypothyroidism.

Inflammatory fluid may show varying degrees of clarity and color. The white cell count is more than 2,000, but usually not more than 50,000.[38] This is commonly seen in rheumatoid arthritis, gout, and possibly some infectious disorders. It is also associated with Reiter's syndrome, ankylosing spondylitis, psoriatic arthritis, and juvenile rheumatoid arthritis.

Pyogenic fluid is opaque or grossly purulent. The white cell count exceeds 50,000, often higher, and is predominantly polymorphonuclear cells.[38] This is typical of infectious arthritis and, in some cases, gout or other very inflammatory arthritides.

Nonpyogenic fluid has variable characteristics. The white blood cell count is usually fewer than 20,000.[38] Additionally, joint fluid can be characterized as hemorrhagic. This will occur in cases of trauma, hemophilia, and other bleeding disorders.

The fluid should routinely be examined for calcium pyrophosphate and uric acid crystals that are further characterized by polarized light microscopy. Gout crystals are pointed and negatively birefringent.[82,241] Calcium pyrophosphate crystals are rhomboid, and positively birefringent.[82,241]

Synovial fluid glucose levels are normally approximately 20 mg/dL less than the serum. Lower concentrations may be observed in joint sepsis. Synovial fluid protein is often increased in inflammatory disease. Appropriate organism stains and cultures should be obtained.

OSTEOARTHRITIS

Definition

Recognized as the most common of all arthritis, osteoarthritis is an irreversible, slowly progressive arthropathy characterized by the focal loss of articular cartilage, with hypertrophic reaction in the subchondral bone. Its cause is unknown. Although it does not seem to be a single disease, common features are found during the evolution of the disorder as it arises in a number of different conditions.

Incidence

The occurrence of osteoarthritis at the glenohumeral joint is much less common than at the hip or knee. Its incidence increases with age, and it is the site with the oldest average age of onset.[48,136] Difficulty in determining the early diagnosis, the timing of its onset, and the absence of longitudinal data make estimates of the prevalence of osteoarthritis and its incidence imprecise.

DePalma had an early interest in the aging shoulder and carefully studied its morphologic aspects.[53,55] On the glenoid side, from his study of cadavers, ranging in age from 14 to 87, he determined that the degenerative process reached its maximum by the sixth decade. The most significant changes seemed to be located at the superior aspect of the glenoid. At the glenoid site of labral attachment, particularly in the anterior and anteroinferior regions, there was a marginal proliferation of bone and cartilage. This was believed to be secondary to traction forces applied to the soft tissues in these areas, with a resultant functional response to stress loading. Over time, a generalized thickening of the synovial membrane was observed. This occurred secondary to proliferation of the fibrous stromal elements in the synovial areas, resulting in an increased number of villous projections. On the humeral side, articular surface changes were never profound. The changes were certainly never equal to those seen on the glenoid side and were felt to be attributable to the mismatch of the humeral to glenoid surface area (4:1).

Cadaver studies by others have confirmed the relative absence of humeral cartilage thinning with increasing age.[192,237] Petersson radiographically reviewed the glenohumeral joint spaces in normal persons and concluded that, with age alone, the joint space does not decrease.[239]

Pathogenesis

Age is the greatest factor for the development of primary (idiopathic) arthritis in all joints.[17,240] Ethnicity and race have bearing on the incidence, and a genetic predisposition is possible.[143,240] Bone density may play a role, as noted by the apparent inverse relation between osteoarthritis and osteoporosis.[152] There are no special associations in glenohumeral arthritis, except a coexistence of degenerative changes of the rotator cuff.[26,146]

Pathophysiology

For details on the pathophysiology of osteoarthritis in general, the reader is referred to major textbooks of rheumatology and recent monographs discussing osteoarthritis.[142,150,189] Most epidemiologic, clinical, and in vivo data come from studies of osteoarthritis of the large weight-bearing joints, the hip and the knee, as opposed to the glenohumeral joint.

Osteoarthritis may not be so much a disorder of the articular cartilage, but a response within the joint as an organ that ultimately fails.[254] Stresses applied to the joint exceed its capacity to repair what initially may be reversible changes.

Normal cartilage is maintained in homeostasis by the repair capacity of chondrocytes within the cartilaginous matrix. One hypothesis for the initiation of osteoarthritis is that altered mechanical forces initiate metabolic activity change within the chondrocytes.[90,98,132,277] Presuming that, normally, a feedback mechanism exists between the regulation of activity and mechanical stimulation, an imbalance of cartilage activity may result when the mechanical signal, or its transduction mechanism, is changed. The precise mechanism is unknown, but Mow and and others suggest that the process is mediated by altered chondrocyte activity. A cascade of events leads to the formation of a structurally impaired and weakened matrix that has irreversibly changed load–response characteristics.[206] As a result, the capacity for cartilage to repair appears to fail, a dysfunction that ultimately leads to its loss.

The major forces on articular cartilage result from contractions of the muscles that impart stability and motion to the joint.[260] Although the glenohumeral joint in normal persons is not truly weight bearing, the forces across the joint are not insignificant: 0.9 × body weight when the arm is held between 60- and 90-degrees abduction.[245,246] Factors of load magnitude, its direction and duration, as well as the distance between the point of application and the joint, may influence the force applied to the articular cartilage.

In addition to normal load, a depletion of articular cartilage may occur from joint trauma. Whereas chronic overloading of normal joints or subtle changes in joint mechanics may evolve slowly into osteoarthritis, significant joint injuries may precipitate significant osteoarthritis within a short time. An analogy for the shoulder would be the fate of the glenohumeral joint with glenoid hypoplasia, compared with one sustaining a comminuted displaced intraarticular glenoid fracture that resulted in an unfavorable malunion.[329]

Repetitive stresses may play a role, depending on the type of force transmitted to the joint. Articular cartilage can withstand significant shear forces without incurring irreversible damage.[172] Harryman showed a wide variety of measurable translation in normal shoulders, implying an internal shear component during physiologic glenohumeral motion.[106]

The thickness of articular cartilage is unfavorable for effective shock absorbancy.[253] Impact loading forces are thereby delivered to the subchondral bone and the surrounding joint soft tissues.[115,253] The major bone load is transmitted to and attenuated by the cancellous subchondral trabeculae and the interposed fluid marrow elements.[225,252] This concept may help explain the observation concerning the inception of osteoarthritis predominantly on the glenoid side: less surface area, less cancellous bone volume.[52,256]

Acute ligamentous injuries alter the mechanics and biologic properties of the joint, especially its articular cartilage. The most extensively studied animal model for this condition has been the canine anterior cruciate ligament transection.[5,93,290] The mechanical and biomechanical components combine to progressively change the articular cartilage, not unlike that known to occur in osteoarthritis in the humans.[16]

Impact loading by mechanisms of trauma results in a more rapid or sudden increase in the force acting upon the articular cartilage. Experimental studies have demonstrated cellular changes with increased hydration and increased cellular activity, suggesting a repair or a remodeling capacity.[62,310] The overall affect is a weakening of the cartilage.

Just as there are conditions that alter joint load applied to normal cartilage, there are those that alter cartilage metabolism, rendering it vulnerable to physiologic loading alone. Primary disturbances in cartilage metabolism may occur in disorders such as hemochromatosis (iron), ochronosis (homogentistic acid), Wilson's disease (copper), gout (urate crystals), and calcium pyrophosphate dihydrate deposition disease, that result in the deposition of metabolic by-products into the articular cartilage matrix.[193,204,278,283] Degeneration of the cartilage as a result of loss of its compliance, or chondrocyte injury, leads to osteoarthritis. Endocrine disorders, such as acromegaly, may also influence the quality of the cartilage.[13] Skeletal dysplasias may predispose the joint to increased susceptibility to mechanical forces.[334]

At the same time certain catabolic activities within the joint are taking place in the cartilage, anabolic activities are under way, especially remodeling and hypertrophy of bone. Increased subchondral bony plate density or sclerosis is observed radiographically.[27] The tidemark advances with new bone formation in the basal layers of the calcified zone. Cartilage which is supported by this abnormally dense bone is exposed to more intense stresses, in itself, contributing to the cartilage degradation. Degeneration of the cartilage decreases its capacity to distribute stress, and causes higher peak stresses in the subchondral bone. Focal pressure necrosis of bone may occur.[195] In response to these changes in stress, additional bone is laid down.

Defects sometimes develop within the exposed subchondral bone plate. If there is excessive intraarticular pressure, fluid may be forced through these defects and into the subchondral marrow spaces.[164,263] Increasing accumulations of pressurized fluid, coupled with the secondary resorption of surrounding trabeculae, may result in the formation of cysts contiguous with the joint surface.[228] New bone formation may occur in areas that are loaded. The osteophytes enlarge the joint surface and may be covered by newly formed hyaline and fibrocartilaginous cartilage.[17,21] Intraarticular bodies, formed from fragmentation of surface cartilage or bone, may float in the joint or become sessile, maintaining potential for enlargement.[196]

Pathoanatomy

Damage to the joint and reaction to it may result in an early, subclinical stage of arthritis that may exist for years or decades. The degeneration takes the form of thinning and softening of the articular cartilage. Surface fibrillation and, in the deeper layers, fissures and vertical clefts develop as the cartilage succumbs, exposing subchondral bone. Fibrocartilaginous repair may take place.

The synovium thickens in response to the joint debris produced by the reactive changes in the articular cartilage and bone. Villous hypertrophy with random synovial cell hyperplasia may characterize the membrane. It may be filled with cartilage fragments and foreign body giant cells.[21] Loose or sequestered osteocartilaginous bodies may be seen.[21] The subsynovial region stroma may be filled with a mild chronic inflammatory reaction.[88]

The gross pathologic findings of glenohumeral osteoarthritis are fairly consistent and have been characterized by Neer.[208,212,221] Thinning or absence of the cartilage of the humeral head is most pronounced in a position corresponding to 60 to 90 degrees of abduction, the area of maximum joint reaction force.[128] The normally convex humeral head flattens. The exposed bone becomes eburneous and sclerotic, acquiring a marblelike appearance, often stippled with small reddish-brown vascular proliferations and fibrocartilaginous plugs (Fig. 5). Osteophytes appear circumferentially at the margin of the articular surface of the humeral head, resulting in its apparent enlargement (Fig. 6). The large inferomedial osteophytes, which have been termed "the goat's beard" by

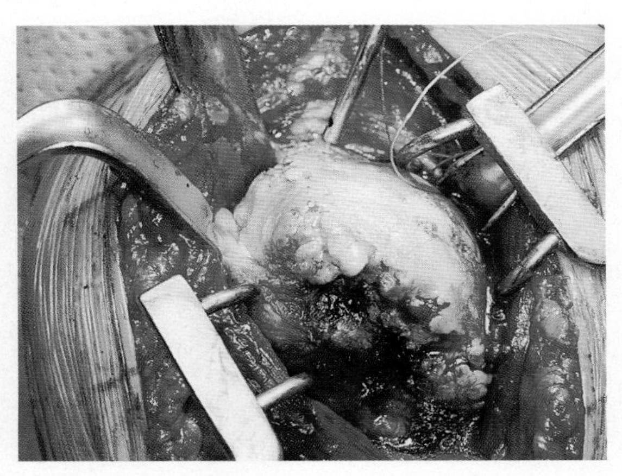

FIG. 5. Osteoarthritis: Humeral head at the time of total shoulder arthroplasty. Flattening and enlargement of the humeral head is seen. Large proliferative osteophytes are noted circumferentially with predominance inferomedially, the "goat's beard." Punctate cystic lesions dot the eburneous bone. The biceps tendon and rotator cuff are intact.

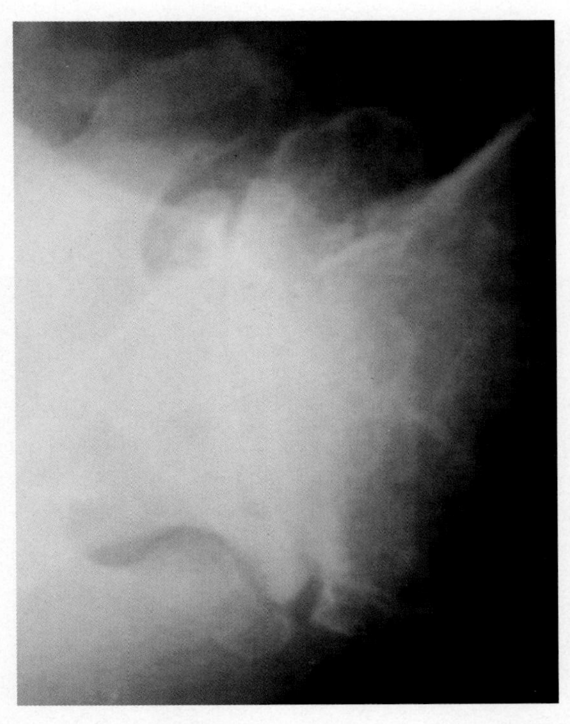

FIG. 6. Osteoarthritis: Axillary lateral view with enlargement and flattening of the humeral head. There is concentric erosion of the glenoid.

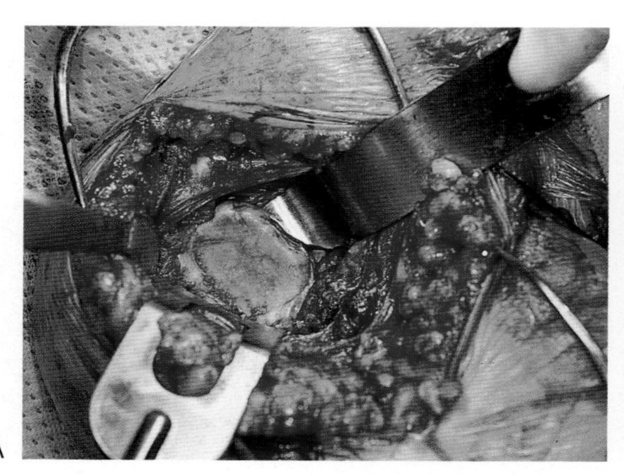

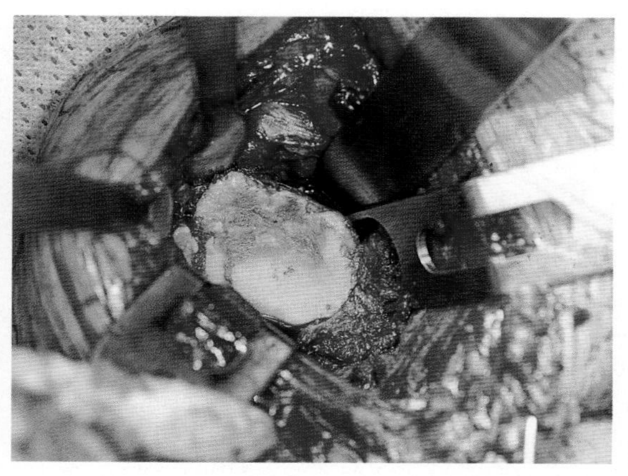

FIG. 7. Osteoarthritis: Glenoids at the time of total shoulder arthroplasty demonstrating **(A)** demarcation between intact anterior cartilage and posterior eburneous subchondral bone. Peripheral osteophytes are seen. **(B)** Significant circumferential osteophyte formation.

Matsen, may envelope and tension the adjacent capsule, contributing to limitations of external rotation (see Fig. 5).[181] Subchondral cysts are often present on the glenoid as well as the humeral head.

The rotator cuff and the biceps tendon long head are intact in 89% to 95% of cases.[32,33,214,221] Neer believed their integrity and capability to generate essential glenohumeral compressive forces are a prerequisite for the development of osteoarthritis.[214] He further believed that an enlarged osteoarthritic head helps prevent upward migration, resulting in fewer impingement-type rotator cuff tears.[214] Rupture of the biceps tendon long head can rarely occur, but the mechanism is in response to the presence of spurs in the intertubercular groove and not by the process of impingement against the coracoacromial arch.[214]

Although primary glenohumeral osteoarthritis usually begins on the glenoid, the glenoid cartilage is typically spared anteriorly (Fig. 7).[256] The wear is more pronounced posteriorly, and a true crista (Fig. 8) may be formed as a demarcation between intact articular cartilage and exposed subchondral bone. Disease progression favors excessive glenoid bone erosion posteriorly with resultant posterior humeral head subluxation. This stretches and attenuates the posterior capsule while the anterior capsule significantly thickens and contracts. Peripheral osteophytes may "enlarge" the glenoid (see Figs. 7B and 9). Osteocartilaginous bodies, either loose or attached, seek the recesses of the synovial cavity, especially the subscapularis bursa (Fig. 10). They may enlarge and become intimately attached to the adjacent bony structures, significantly distorting the normal anatomy. The soft-tissue envelope tightens further as it drapes over the osteocartilaginous bodies and osteophytes.

The same findings are observed in secondary osteoarthritis. In addition, in cases of ochronosis, the characteristic blackening of the articular cartilage caused by homogentistic acid deposition is noted.

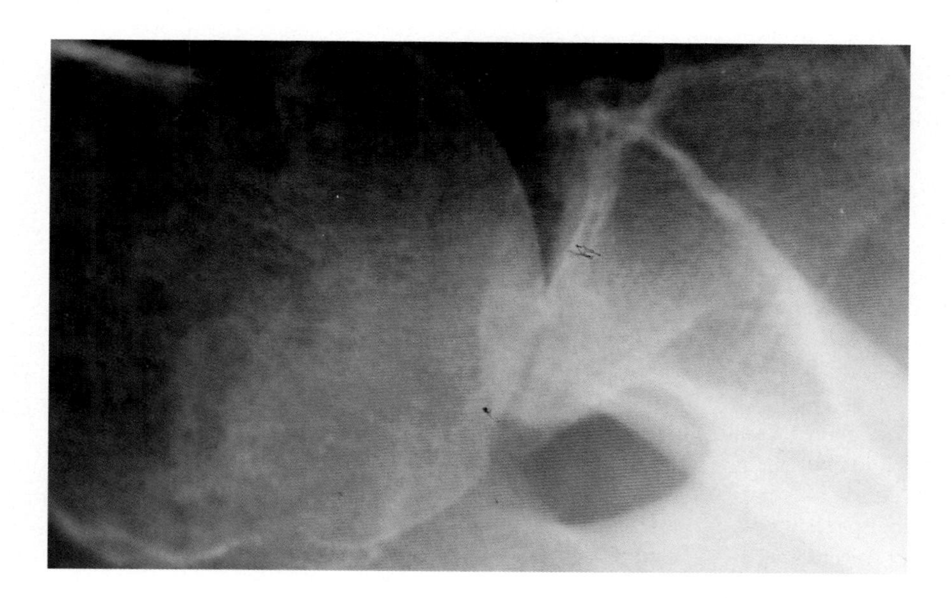

FIG. 8. Osteoarthritis: Axillary lateral view demonstrating preservation of the anterior cartilage, posterior subluxation of the humeral head, and preferential wear of the posterior aspect of the glenoid.

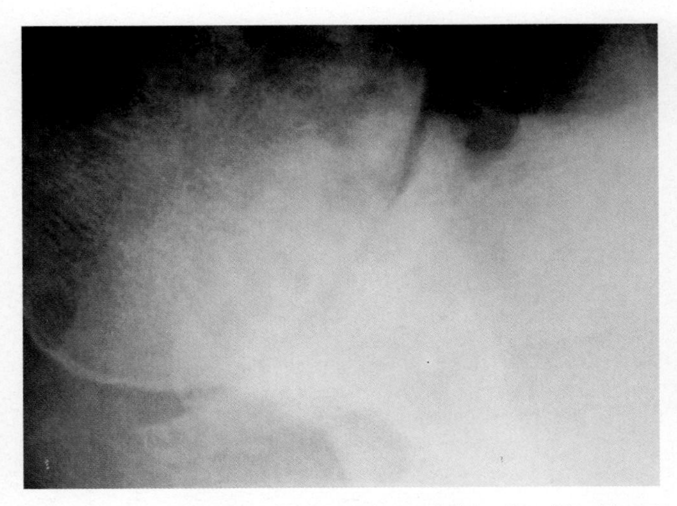

FIG. 9. Osteoarthritis: Enlargement of the glenoid without evidence of significant preferential posterior wear.

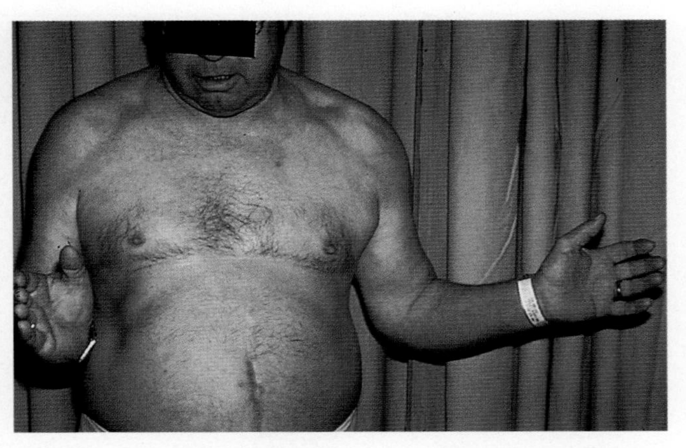

FIG. 11. Osteoarthritis: Significant loss of external rotation is seen before total shoulder arthroplasty.

Clinical Evaluation

Patients may present for evaluation and treatment by age 40 to 50.[6] Their primary complaints are shoulder pain and loss of range of motion. More than 50% of patients are unable to sleep on the affected side and cannot perform common functional tasks.[184] Unremitting progression of the disease process will lead to more intense symptoms, failure of conservative management measures, and consideration for surgical treatment. The gender distribution is equal for this active and generally healthy subset of patients.[214] The dominant arm is involved to a greater extent than the nondominant arm.

Generalized atrophy of the shoulder is often notable, especially when the disorder is unilateral. Early in the disease, motion changes are minimal and difficult to detect, unless the most sensitive testing position—supine—is used. As the glenohumeral changes become more advanced, motion of the soft tissues is restricted, with a significant diminution of external rotation (Fig. 11). This is a more sensitive test of intraarticular activity than is the loss of elevation. A specific point of localized tenderness is over the posterior joint line, more easily elicited as the humeral head becomes subluxed with advancing disease. Attempts at active and passive motion are painful and may produce catching and squeaking sounds from the rough glenohumeral articulation. Synovial thickening and a large joint effusion may be palpable in thin individuals.

Imaging

Plain films are most helpful for making the diagnosis of osteoarthritis, but probably underestimate the extent of pathologic osteoarticular changes.[256] The AP view of the humeral articulation to the scapular plane and a high quality axillary lateral view are all that is needed. They enable one to ascertain joint orientation, the amount of erosion of the glenoid, humeral head position, and the extent of disease activity. Because of soft-tissue contractures or pain, optimum films are sometimes not possible to obtain. In those instances, a CT scan will prove extremely useful in assessing glenoid morphology, glenohumeral relations, the presence of osteocartilaginous bodies, and the determination of the volume of the glenoid vault (Fig. 12). Other findings of os-

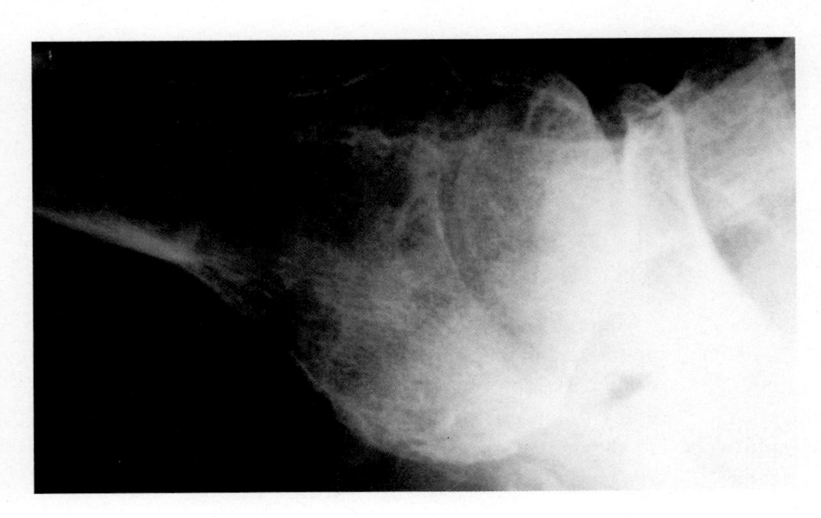

FIG. 10. Osteoarthritis: Multiple osteocartilaginous bodies are seen in the posterior aspect of the glenohumeral joint.

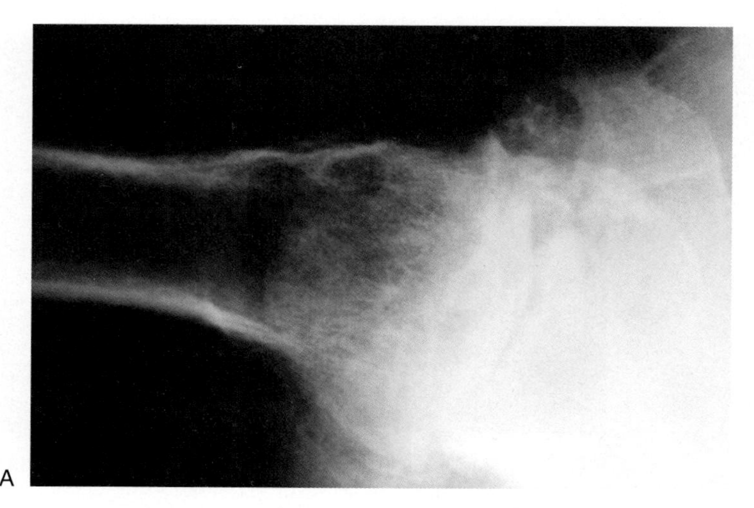

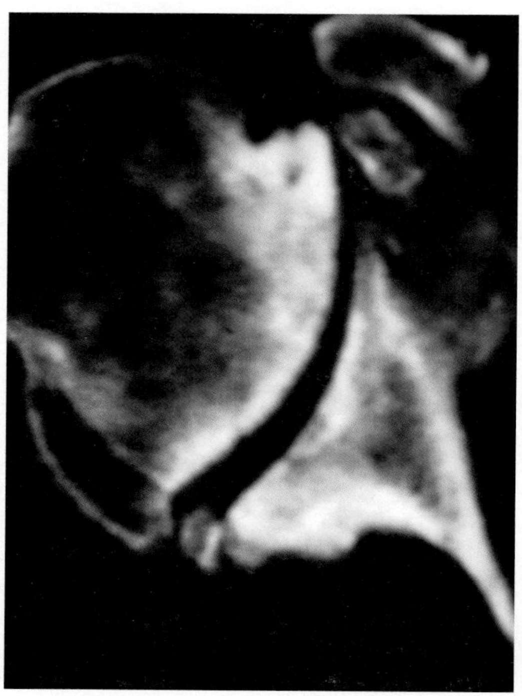

FIG. 12. **(A)** Osteoarthritis: Findings on axillary lateral view may fail to define the pathoanatomy with accuracy. **(B)** Significant deformity noted on CT scan. Loose bodies have attached to the anterior glenoid. External rotation limitation can be appreciated, due to contact of the posterior humeral head and osteophyte against the glenoid.

teoarthritis are densification of subchondral bone, subchondral cysts, and peripheral osteophytes along the glenoid margins and adjacent to the articular surface of the humeral head, especially inferiorly. The humeral head may be flattened and enlarged.

Laboratory

Laboratory studies are rarely helpful in the evaluation of primary osteoarthritis. Blood studies and synovial fluid analysis may help identify an underlying cause of secondary osteoarthritis. Synovial fluid levels of biochemical markers (aggrecan-aggregates) of catabolic activity within the articular cartilage enable the detection of all stages of glenohumeral osteoarthritis, with a high degree of accuracy.[256] The identification of the disorder before radiographic changes are present may prove extremely useful to expand treatment options and to monitor disease progression and response to treatment.[256]

Adjunctive Diagnostic Tests

Arthroscopy of the glenohumeral joint can improve the diagnostic accuracy when the clinical diagnosis is suspected and the radiographs do not show advanced stages.[66,256]

POSTTRAUMATIC ARTHRITIS

Major articular surface incongruities that exist at the completion of intraarticular fracture healing will inevitably lead to the deterioration of the joint quality (Fig. 13). Tolerance of any joint to withstand minor variations in surface contact are dependent on many factors: surface geometry, surface area, specific load-bearing characteristics, and the integrity

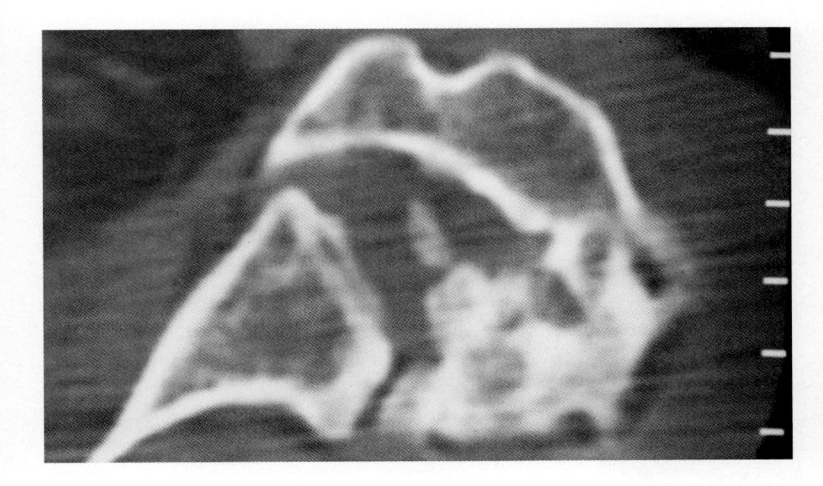

FIG. 13. Posttraumatic osteoarthritis: Changes resulting from proximal humerus fracture, demonstrating joint incongruity and loss of humeral articular surface.

of associated joint-supporting soft tissues. The discrepancy in the surface area of the humeral head and the glenoid is assurance that a small portion of the humeral head is in contact with the glenoid at any moment. It would appear, therefore, that a significant glenoid articular surface step-off or gap would have far greater influence on the development of posttraumatic arthritis than a corresponding one on the humeral side. Extraarticular fractures of the proximal humerus (surgical neck) may result in reorientation of the articular segment relative to the shaft or relative to the glenoid (Fig. 14). Up to 45 degrees of angulation are seemingly well tolerated without significant posttraumatic arthrosis or functional impairment.[209]

In many instances, the precise cause of posttraumatic osteoarthritis cannot be determined. Varying combinations of joint incongruity from malunion, joint instability from adjacent soft-tissue injuries, circulatory disturbance, and intraarticular fibrosis will have a bearing on the fate of the joint (Fig. 15). Zyto reported a 64% incidence of osteoarthritis in patients sustaining displaced four-part proximal humerus fractures and 25% for three-part fractures.[340] One of the more common forms of posttraumatic arthritis is that seen following glenohumeral instability.[121] This is further discussed in the next section.

Chronic dislocations will result in disturbances of circulation and malnourishment of the articular cartilage surfaces (Fig. 16). The absence of stress to the underlying bone results in softening. Rapid deterioration of the joint is seen following closed and open reduction of these chronic dislocations, unless the surface abnormalities have been addressed.[112,251,271]

Proximal humerus fractures and their sequelae are given

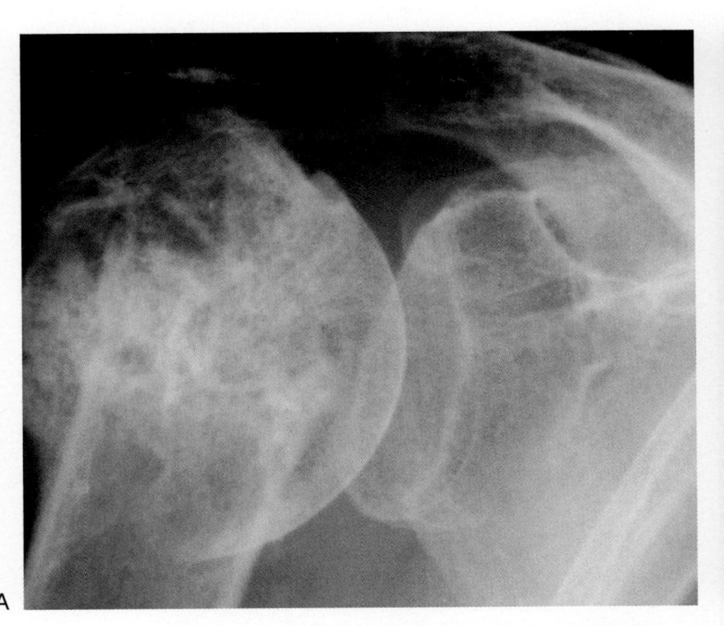

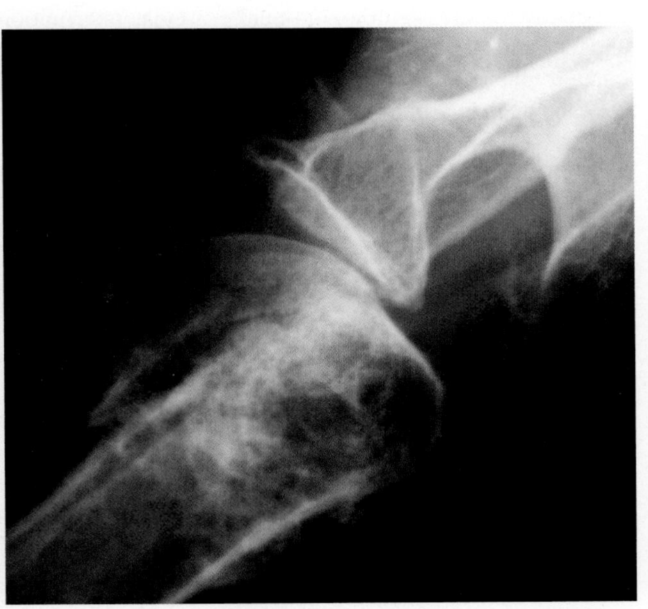

A B

FIG. 14. (A,B) Posttraumatic arthritis. Proximal humeral malunion with distortion of proximal humeral anatomy. Early arthritic changes are observed. Dysvascular changes are not present in the articular segment.

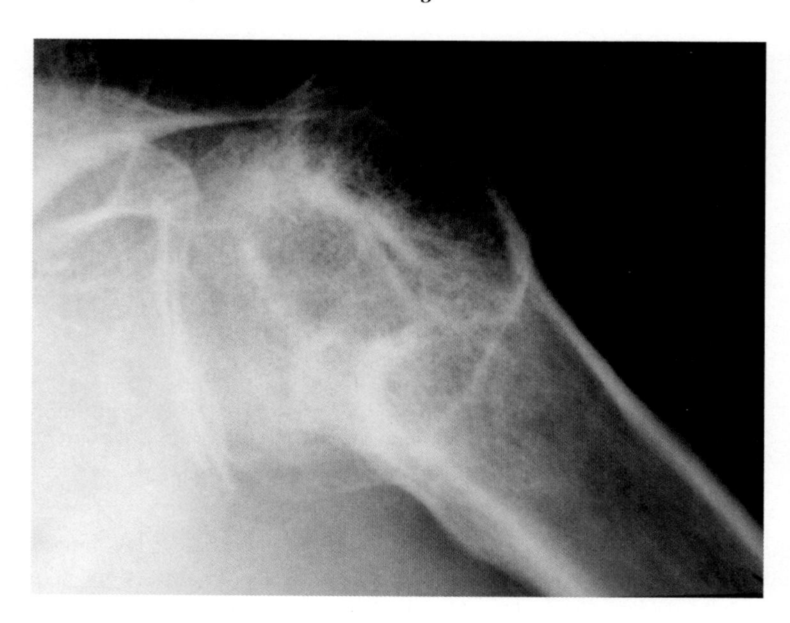

FIG. 15. Posttraumatic arthritis: Malunited proximal humerus fracture leading to advanced disease.

consideration in the section "Osteonecrosis." This may be the most common complication of proximal humerus fracture that will lead to posttraumatic arthritis. Proximal humerus nonunions may result in the formation of fibrous ankylosis of the glenohumeral joint, predisposing to posttraumatic arthritis.

ARTHRITIS OF DISLOCATION

Definition

Glenohumeral joint dislocations occur more frequently than any other major joint dislocation. Acute complications related to the initial dislocation include fracture, musculotendinous rupture, neurologic injury, vascular interruption, and recurrent glenohumeral instability. A late debilitating sequela to glenohumeral instability and its surgical treatment was, in one form, first appreciated by Hindmarsh and, in another, initially observed by Neer.[116,220] The term "dislocation arthropathy" was coined and included those occurrences of glenohumeral arthritis with a well-documented history of glenohumeral dislocation, often in patients having undergone surgical treatment (Fig. 17).[221,274]

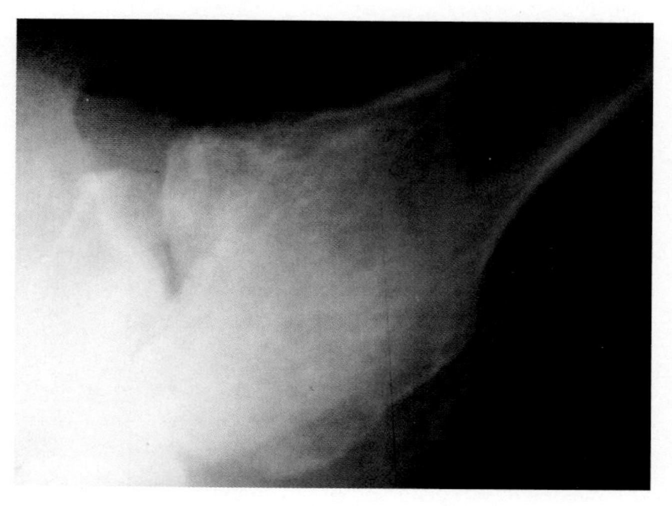

FIG. 16. Posttraumatic arthritis: Chronic locked posterior dislocation with gross incongruity of the glenohumeral joint.

Incidence

The incidence of this disorder has not been accurately established. Hovelius et al. performed a 10-year prospective study of patients younger than the age of 40 to assess the outcome of a primary anterior dislocation of the shoulder treated with closed reduction, both with and without immobilization.[121] The incidence of dislocation arthropathy was 20%. The degree of involvement was mild in 11% and severe in 9%.

By far the most common cause of arthritis of dislocation is iatrogenic. Termed capsulorrhaphy arthropathy, its incidence cannot be accurately determined.

Pathogenesis

Hovelius's data suggested no relation between dislocation arthropathy and the number of recurrent dislocations or the treatment rendered, either operative or nonoperative.[121] This study pointed out further that advanced glenohumeral arthritis may occur even after a single anterior glenohumeral dislocation treated without surgery.

Morrey prudently observed that looseness of the joint played a role in the development of surgical failures after the performance of a unidirectional repair.[202] Factors shared by these patients included a positive family history, occurrence of bilateral glenohumeral instability, and the coexistence of posterior instability in the shoulder that was operated on. Neer introduced the term "multidirectional instability," perhaps for the same subset of patients.[220] He was also the first

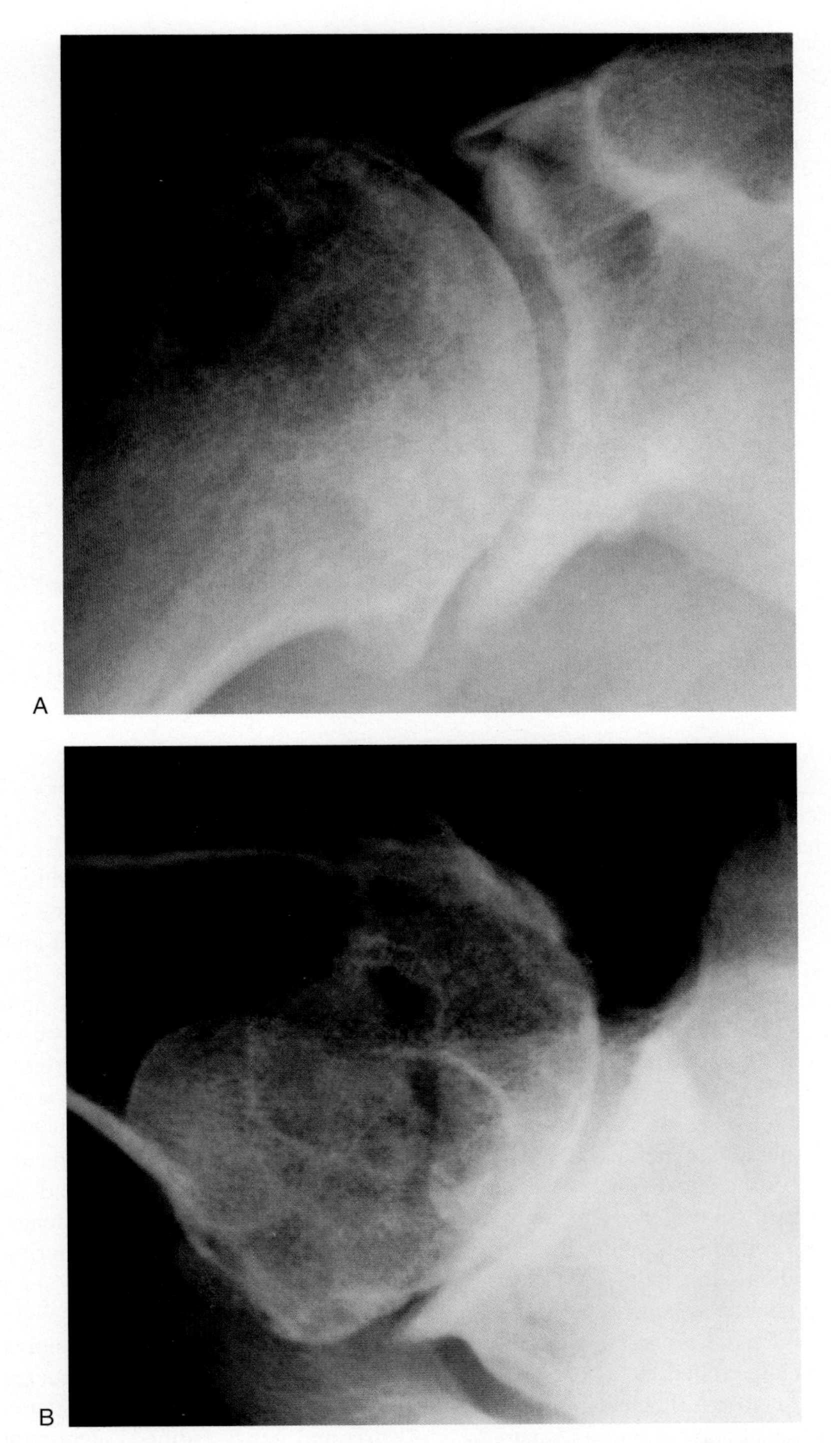

FIG. 17. (A,B) Arthritis of dislocation: The sequelae to two previous surgeries including anterior stabilization and subsequent staple removal.

to draw the association between the disorder and arthritis of dislocation.[221] It was his belief that multidirectional instability existed on the basis of lax ligaments, repeated minor injuries, or a combination of both. The most frequent cause of multidirectional instability was felt to be an acquired laxity, explained on a heritable basis. The initial instability episode in this group of patients most often occurred without high forces, major injury, or significant associated injuries. Typically, if a dislocation was present, it reduced spontaneously or required minimal, usually self-manipulative effort. Generalized ligamentous laxity was often recognized. Examination of the contralateral shoulder revealed excessive anterior and posterior translations, as well as inferior translation, as evidenced by the "sulcus sign." The presence of this so-called sulcus sign was pathognomonic for multidirectional laxity. Neer concluded that "by far the most frequent etiologic mechanism for the development of arthritis of recurrent dislocation is a 'standard' operative procedure intended to remedy recurrent unidirectional dislocations that is unsuspectingly performed on a loose, multidirectional shoulder."[215] He observed that the "procedures displace(d) the humeral head in a loose shoulder away from the side of the repair, creating a fixed subluxation. The subluxed head wears unevenly on the glenoid, and arthritic changes can develop surprisingly fast."[215]

It was actually Hindmarsh, however, who first implicated the role of stabilization surgery in the production of moderate to severe glenohumeral arthritis.[116] A variety of surgical procedures performed in an attempt to stabilize the glenohumeral joint and prevent recurrences led to glenohumeral arthritis.[109,110,124,175,177,221,223,226,302,324] When a unidirectional repair, such as the Putti-Platt,[122] Eden-Hybinette-Lange,[324] Magnuson-Stack,[274] Bristow,[120,174,295,333] Du-Toit,[226,274,296,339] or Bankart,[122,223,274] was performed to eliminate instability recurrences, the stage was set for further glenohumeral joint deterioration.

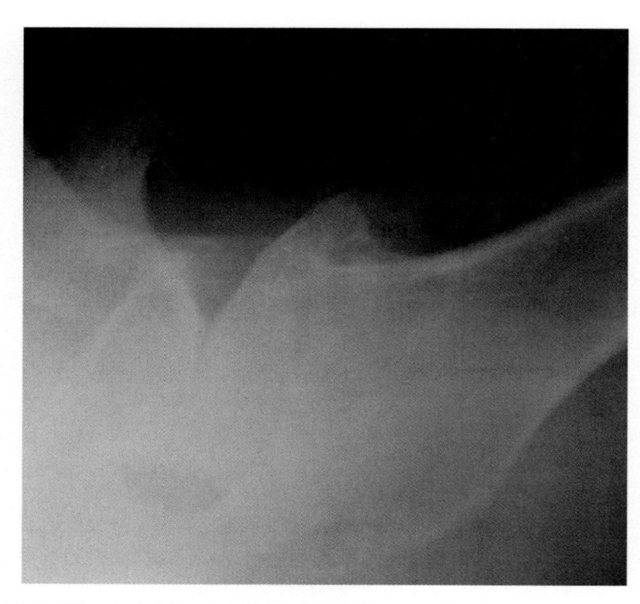

FIG. 18. Arthritis of dislocation: The result of recurrent posterior glenohumeral instability. Note significant posterior humeral subluxation and eccentric wear of the posterior two-thirds of the glenoid.

Pathophysiology

The more widespread recognition of this late sequela to instability reconstruction has led to hypotheses about its mechanism. When unidirectional surgery is imposed on a multidirectional lax glenohumeral joint, glenohumeral biomechanics are altered.[220] This occurrence has been assigned predominant responsibility for the development of the arthritis of dislocation. Even in the presence of normal laxity, a unidirectional repair, resulting in excessive tightening of the soft tissues, forces the humeral head in the direction opposite that of the repair.[106,110] When this is performed for anterior instability, there is a significant limitation of external rotation. As external rotation is performed, contact compression and shear forces at the glenohumeral articulation increase. This results in translation of the humeral head posteriorly, with a shift in the center of rotation. Eccentric loading forces are concentrated on a smaller glenoid surface area with deterioration in the quality and quantity of articular cartilage.[76,299] Over time, there is a progressive development of glenohumeral degenerative changes. Those procedures that transpose bone to create a blockade carry the additional risk of humeral articular surface scraping against the bone or metal hardware fixation devices.[9,120,174,324,336]

Samilson noted that the occurrence of arthritis was much more common after posterior glenohumeral dislocation (Fig. 18).[274] This was thought to be because of the delay in diagnosis and treatment of posterior glenohumeral dislocation, especially chronic occurrences. In Samilson's series, the number of dislocations was not determinant of the severity of glenohumeral joint arthrosis. Of the group of patients with moderate to severe arthrosis, 71% had experienced only one glenohumeral instability event. In this same group of patients, 26% had recurrent instability. No correlation was recognized in the presence of a Hill–Sachs or bony Bankart lesion. Those patients who were slightly older at the time of their index glenohumeral instability event had more severe arthrosis. In Bigliani's study, 7 of 17 patients continued to have instability in the presence of arthropathy.[12]

The pathophysiologic process that leads to dislocation arthropathy after one or more glenohumeral dislocations is less clear. A more severe arthritis existing in patients with a single dislocation suggests a direct relation between the forces dissipated to the articular cartilage and the restraining soft tissues. In so-called "tight" shoulders, higher forces may be necessary for traumatic dislocation, whereas more lax shoulders require less force. The development of postdislocation arthrosis may result from recurrent episodes of instability because eccentric loading during pathologic translocation transmits greater shear and compression forces at the articular interface. It is possible that surface imperfections and impression fractures of the humeral head could further damage the articular cartilage with each successive dislocation event. The resultant accumulations of particulate joint debris and newly formed osteocartilaginous loose bodies could theoretically contribute a third body wear mechanism. These detrimental effects could coexist and become additive in their potential for joint destruction.

Pathoanatomy

The pathology encountered is often dependent on the index stabilization operation. In general, excessive scarring and adhesions are the predominant finding.[12] Operations involving greater manipulation of the soft tissues, such as the

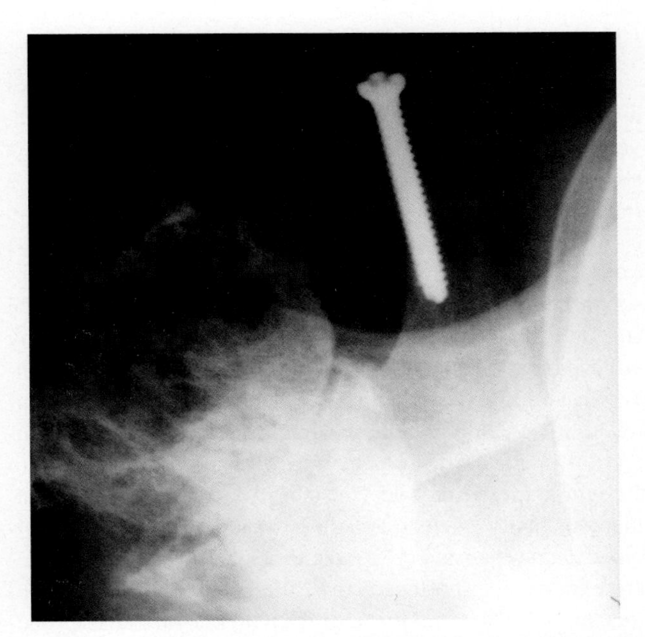

FIG. 19. Arthritis of dislocation: Capsulorrhaphy arthropathy with significant deterioration of the glenohumeral articulation, total loss of joint space, and secondary changes within the humeral head.

Bristow procedure, often result in encasement of all anterior soft-tissue structures, sometimes including the axillary nerve.[12] The subcoracoid, subacromial, and subdeltoid planes of motion are usually scarred. The subscapularis musculotendinous unit will be contracted, as is the anterior joint capsule. Occasionally, the subscapularis integrity will be preserved, such as in a Magnuson-Stack procedure.[178]

The articular surface contours may appear normal with simply posterior subluxation and instability of the humeral head. More often, the glenoid articular surface involvement is quite significant (Fig. 19). The anterior glenoid cartilage may be reasonably preserved, whereas the more posterior cartilage demonstrates thinning and erosion to subchondral bone. In advanced cases, posterior glenoid bone erosion and loss is observed. The humeral head shows concomitant wear changes. The penetration of metallic fixation devices into the intraarticular space may be observed, with associated articular surface changes (Fig. 20).[9,226,336,339]

When operative care has not been rendered, the findings are essentially those of glenohumeral osteoarthritis. Preferential glenoid wear or humeral head subluxation may be observed in the direction of the instability. Variable soft-tissue changes may exist.

Clinical Evaluation

The patient, often younger than 40 years of age, usually presents to the surgeon for evaluation many years (average 16) after the glenohumeral stabilization operation or the index dislocation occurrence.[12,18,110,221] Most these patients have not had interval recurrences or symptoms. Within 2 to 3 years of presentation, shoulder symptoms have begun to evolve. At the time of the evaluation, the chief complaints are related to intense, often disabling pain. Almost all patients have had long-standing limitation of range of motion, many with the development of an internal rotation contracture. Moderate to severe functional disability is present secondary to pain and altered range of motion. Some have had multiple surgical procedures.

The physical examination of these patients is consistent. They are usually younger, healthy-appearing men, often muscular with the exception of the affected shoulder. One or more scars may be present, frequently hypertrophic. For those who have undergone anterior reconstructions, the coracoid is often prominent. When viewed from overhead, the prominence of the posteriorly subluxated humeral head may produce posterior fullness. Examination from the side may demonstrate a posterior attitude to the arm as it hangs at the side. Focal tenderness is often present at the posterior joint line. Active and passive glenohumeral joint motions produce crepitation. Examination of the contralateral shoul-

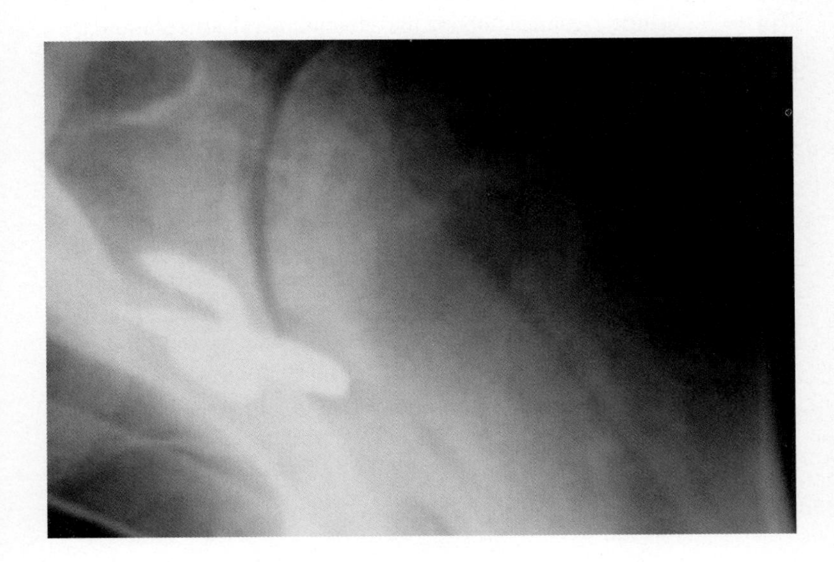

FIG. 20. Arthritis of dislocation: Degenerative changes of the glenohumeral joint following prior anterior stabilization. Metallic staples are noted to be intraarticular with secondary effect upon the humeral head.

der will often demonstrate signs of multidirectional laxity including a positive jerk test, positive drawer testing, and a positive sulcus sign. Limitation of external rotation of the symptomatic shoulder is often pronounced; the more advanced the arthrosis, the more significant the loss of external rotation. Samilson noted 62 degrees of external rotation with mild involvement, 23 degrees of external rotation with moderate involvement, and 14 degrees of external rotation with severe involvement.[274] This compared with 72 degrees on the contralateral side. Hawkins observed an average of −5 degrees of external rotation,[110] and Bigliani identified 17 patients with an average external rotation of −2 degrees.[12]

Imaging

Conventional imaging studies that include a true AP view of the glenohumeral joint and an axillary lateral view are often all that are needed. The CT scan is helpful when a high quality axillary lateral cannot be obtained; MRI examination is unnecessary.

The humeral head is usually posteriorly subluxed, with eccentric wear of the glenohumeral joint cartilage. Posterior glenoid erosion may be extreme. The additional findings of glenohumeral osteoarthritis are often severe. Signs of previous surgery also include the presence of periarticular and, sometimes, intraarticular metal fixation devices (Fig. 21). Osteopenia from disuse may be present.

Laboratory

Specific laboratory investigation is not necessary.

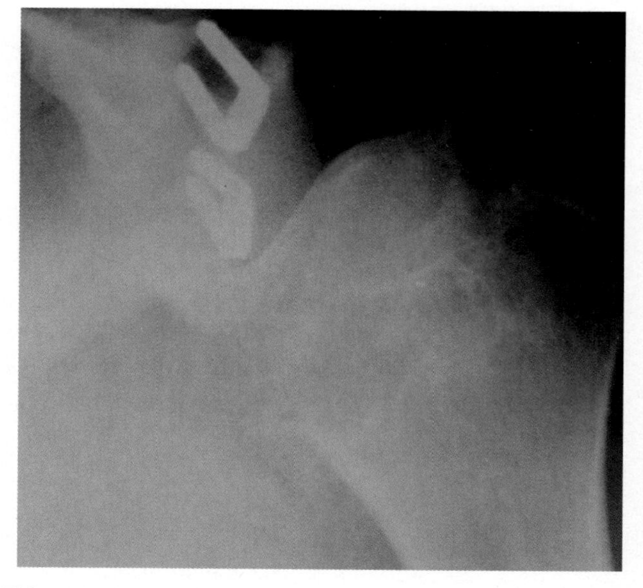

FIG. 21. Arthritis of dislocation: Grossly altered glenohumeral articulation with large osteophyte formation, anteroinferior subluxation of the humeral head, and intraarticular placement of metallic fixation devices.

Clinical Significance

A single common cause does not exist for the arthritis of dislocation. Nonoperative treatment was successful in preventing recurrences in 52% of patients in Hovelius's study.[121] Nearly one-fourth of the patients with more than 2 recurrences "spontaneously" stabilized. His study also showed that glenohumeral arthropathy can result from the trauma of a single dislocation without recurrences. The subset of patients treated nonoperatively was not exposed to the surgical risk factors predisposing to capsulorrhaphy arthropathy. When operative treatment for instability is rendered, additional risks of some degree are inevitably entailed. It is incumbent that the diagnosis of the extent and direction of instability be accurately established. Failure to recognize multidirectional instability and generalized ligamentous laxity can lead to a disastrous outcome when a unidirectional repair is performed, especially if the soft tissues are excessively shortened. It is, therefore, important not to treat all glenohumeral instabilities with one operative procedure. The direction of instability must be determined and the appropriate side stabilized appropriately. The surgeon should be familiar with the complications related to the use of metal and avoid the circumstances that place the glenohumeral joint at high risk for penetration.[176,339] Arthroscopic evaluation and treatment of glenohumeral instability may traumatize the joint from direct damage to the articular surfaces with the scope, instrumentation, and fixation devices.

Natural History

With few exceptions, available data have not permitted prospective evaluation of consistently homogeneous groups of patients with glenohumeral instability.[121] It appears that an increased risk of arthritis is not seen in voluntary subluxation of the glenohumeral joint in children.[125]

The work of Edelson identified skeletal specimens with findings of instability.[64] Coexistent findings of diffuse arthritic changes about the glenohumeral articulation were not observed. The data did not support the concept of prophylactic stabilization to prevent arthritic changes from developing. Hovelius's study would lend support to this concept, for a number of shoulders, even after one or more recurrences, stabilized over time without surgery.[121] Inappropriate stabilization in these cases may have led to the unnecessary development of dislocation arthropathy.

The natural history of established arthritis of dislocation is the progressive development of severe wear and, ultimately, glenoid deficiency (Fig. 22). Prevention would have the greatest influence on this destructive entity of the glenohumeral joint. Accurate diagnosis of the unstable shoulder and, when necessary, appropriate surgical treatment are mandatory. Early recognition of the condition plays a role if the joint is to be surgically salvaged without implant arthroplasty.[175,177]

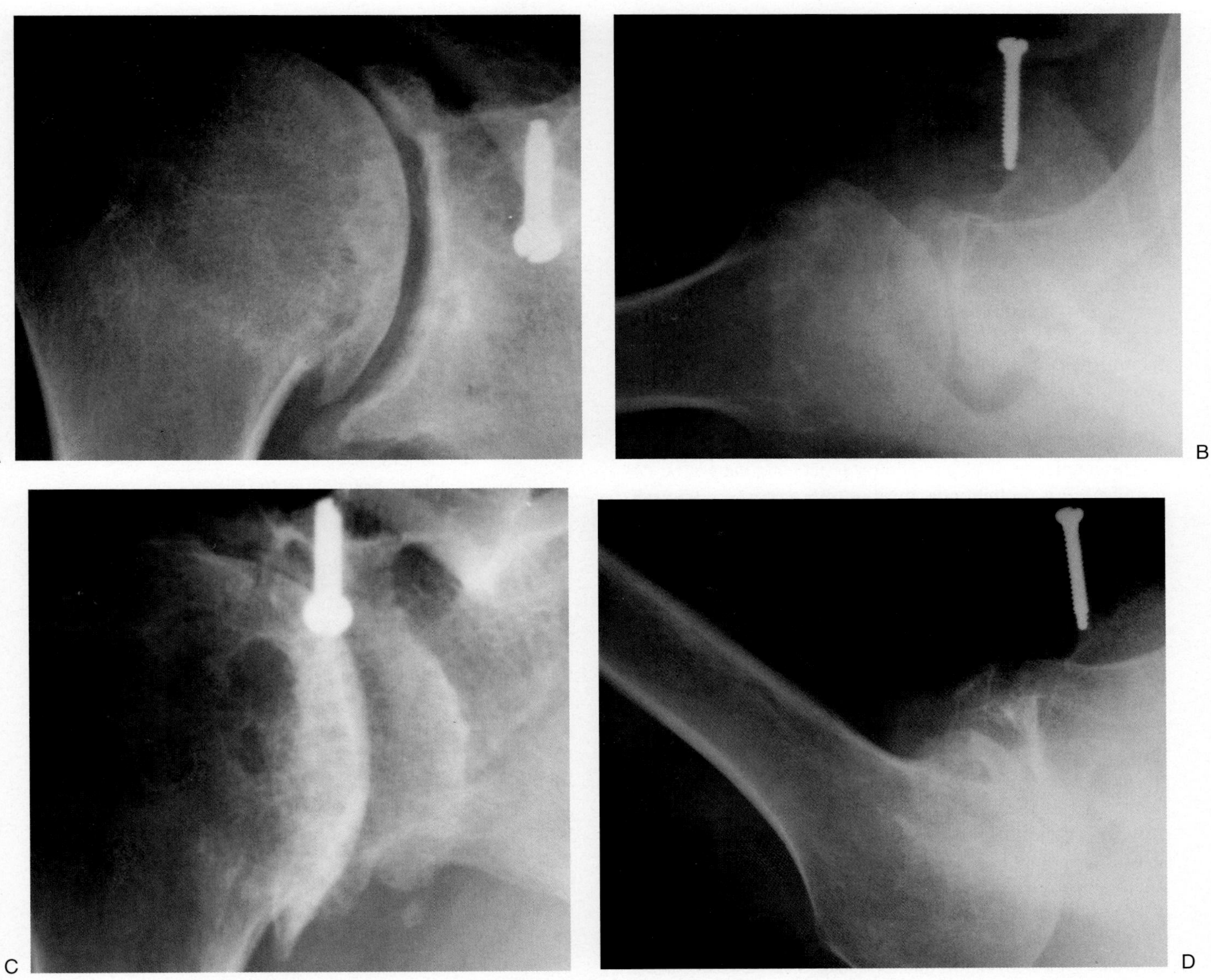

FIG. 22. **(A,B)** Arthritis of dislocation: Ten-year interval following anterior stabilization procedure with moderate glenohumeral arthritis. **(C,D)** Now 18-year interval depicting further progression, with the formation of increased subchondral density, subchondral cysts, osteophytes, and loose bodies. Significant posterior wear and subluxation are seen.

OSTEONECROSIS

Definition

Osteonecrosis, sometimes termed avascular necrosis or aseptic necrosis, is simply bone death, both the osteocytes and the marrow contents. However, it is the bone's failure of repair that leads to destructive changes within the joint. The earliest reports of implant arthroplasty for the shoulder includes patients with osteonecrosis after proximal humerus fracture or dislocations.[159,218]

Osteonecrosis of the humeral head is best classified as traumatic or atraumatic. Fractures of the proximal humerus or fracture dislocations involving the glenohumeral joint place the articular segment of the proximal humerus at risk for osteonecrosis. The atraumatic category includes those occurrences of osteonecrosis that result from disease processes.

Incidence

The incidence of posttraumatic osteonecrosis has been difficult to determine. Factors including the severity of the fracture, the amount of displacement and, to some extent, the type of treatment rendered will have influence on the occurrence of posttraumatic osteonecrosis. The incidence of osteonecrosis is highest after three- and four-part fractures, but can also occur after certain two-part fractures.[78,84,97,152,158,170,230,304] Closed treatment of displaced three-part fractures has resulted in a 3% to 14% avascular necrosis rate.[97] In four-part fractures treated closed, the incidence has ranged from 13% to 34%.[84,97,151,210,242,288,301,305,340] For any method of treatment, anatomic neck fracture occurrences approach 100%.[54,129,209,210]

It has been suggested that operative treatment carries a higher risk of osteonecrosis because of the wide surgical exposure necessary to provide for adequate internal fixation.[304] The incidence of avascular necrosis in three-part fractures that have been treated operatively ranges from 12% to 34%.[97,111,157,205,304] Four-part fractures treated with open reduction and internal fixation have a much higher rate of avascular necrosis and malunion.[97,130,157,158,210,230,275,301,304,305,307] Neer believes the incidence to be as high as 90%.[210]

The incidence of atraumatic osteonecrosis cannot be determined. It is probably the third or fourth most common indication for glenohumeral implant arthroplasty.

TABLE 2. *Etiology of osteonecrosis*

Relationship clearly established
Traumatic
Proximal humerus fractures
Chronic glenohumeral dislocations
Nontraumatic
Dysbaric disorders
Gaucher's disease
Sickle cell
Radiation
Relation probable
Traumatic
Repetitive injury
Nontraumatic
Steroids
Alcohol ingestion
Cushing's disease
Lipid metabolism disorders
Fatty liver
Pancreatitis
Organ transplants (renal)
Systematic lupus erythematosus
Osteomalacia
Lymphoma
Cytotoxic drugs

Pathogenesis

Some common causes of osteonecrosis and their relation to the disorder are summarized in Table 2. Proximal humerus fractures and dislocations have most clearly been established to jeopardize the circulatory integrity of the humeral head.

Neer's classification of proximal humerus fractures and glenohumeral fracture dislocations gave better understanding of the pathomechanics and the prognosis following treatment of these injuries.[209] He cited the importance of the vascularity of the articular segment and the relation of the articular segment to other parts of the proximal humerus and to the glenoid.

When the proximal humerus fractures, the wider the displacement of the articular segment from the shaft or from the tuberosities, the higher the incidence of osteonecrosis. More than 80% of the proximal humerus fractures are minimally displaced, according to Neer's criteria, keeping them at low risk for osteonecrosis (Fig. 23).[211]

Disturbance of microcirculation can be the result of elevated intraosseous and interstitial pressures, such as with marrow hypertrophy, infiltration, or replacement.[126] Venous congestion as a mechanism has been popularized.[127] Although most of this information has come from studies of the femoral head, there is less knowledge of the specific occurrences within the humeral head.[200] Occlusion of the microcirculation may take place also by infiltration of hematopoietic marrow spaces with metabolic by-products.

Thrombosis of vessels may occur in vascular disorders or coagulopathies. Embolization phenomena with vasoocclusion occur in sickle cell disorders (sickled cells),[29,30,49,134,289] caisson disease (nitrogen bubbles),[28,133,140] and possibly microscopic lipid droplets.[75,135,320] Repetitive trauma may play a role.[144]

Steroid ingestion is the predominant identifiable risk factor.[42] The precise mechanism of occurrence is unknown.[44,45,321] There is alteration in serum lipid content and concentration with associated fatty change within the liver. Systemic fat emboli may occur.[74,135] Osteonecrosis may follow short-term use as well as intraarticular injections.[6,43,70,165,308]

L'Bisolata reviewed a series of patients who had symptoms for 9 years.[169] The shortest interval from the completion of steroids to the onset of symptoms was 1 year. The shortest course of steroids was 1 week. In Cruess's study, the interval to the development of symptoms was not less than 6 months from the onset of steroid ingestion, the longest interval being 18 months.[43] L'Bisolata observed that 76% of patients using steroids developed osteonecrosis at sites other than the shoulder: the hip and knee, most commonly.[169]

Other causes of osteonecrosis include sickle cell disease and other hemoglobinopathies, Gaucher's disease, excessive alcohol ingestion, decompression sickness, pancreatitis, familial hyperlipidemia, renal or other organ transplants, lymphoma, gout, Cushing's disease, radiation, chemotherapy, myxedema, peripheral vascular disease, pregnancy, systemic lupus erythematosus, and idiopathic.

Pathophysiology

The blood supply of the proximal humerus plays a critical role in the development of posttraumatic avascular necrosis; the incidence is not uncommon after displaced fractures of this region (Fig. 24). Most of the blood supply to the humeral head derives from the anterior humeral circumflex artery through its ascending branch.[163,203,257,268] Entry into the humeral head is in the region of the biceps groove. The ar-

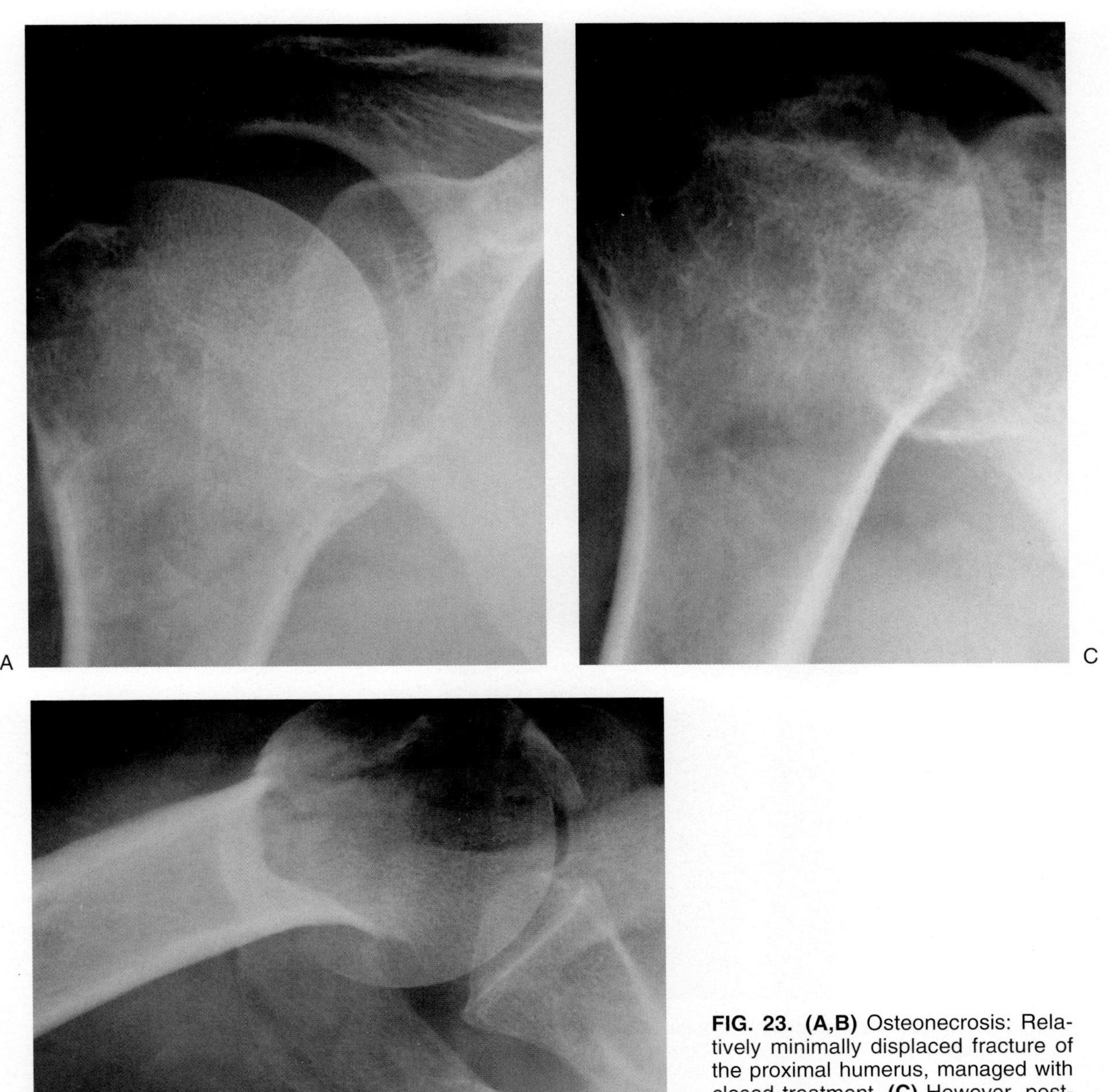

FIG. 23. (A,B) Osteonecrosis: Relatively minimally displaced fracture of the proximal humerus, managed with closed treatment. **(C)** However, posttraumatic segmental osteonecrosis developed, requiring hemiarthroplasty reconstruction.

cuate artery is the intraosseous communication that arborizes and becomes the major blood supply to the head (Fig. 25).[85] Collateral circulation, normally not present to a great extent in the shoulder, will become insufficient if the fragments are widely displaced. The posterior humeral circumflex artery through rotator cuff attachments will provide a small amount of collateral flow. In addition, the more anterior portion of the cuff will receive other branches of the anterior humeral circumflex, which provides collateral circulation for the articular segment.[203,257,268]

It is likely that the event of circulatory arrest leading to humeral head osteonecrosis occurs at the moment of injury. Forceful manipulative attempts at reduction or surgical intervention may further disturb precarious circulation to the articular segment. Although commonly felt to favor prevention of osteonecrosis in the hip, the effect of prompt reduction and stabilization on the incidence of osteonecrosis is unknown. Because the vascular supply plays such a critical role in proximal humerus fractures, classifications based on this fact alone have evolved, allowing prognosis after injury and treatment.[129]

Whereas the underlying diagnosis in femoral head osteonecrosis is often elusive and determined to be idiopathic, the cause of nontraumatic osteonecrosis of the humeral head is often identifiable. Despite the etiologic factors involved in the development of osteonecrosis, a common pathway is fol-

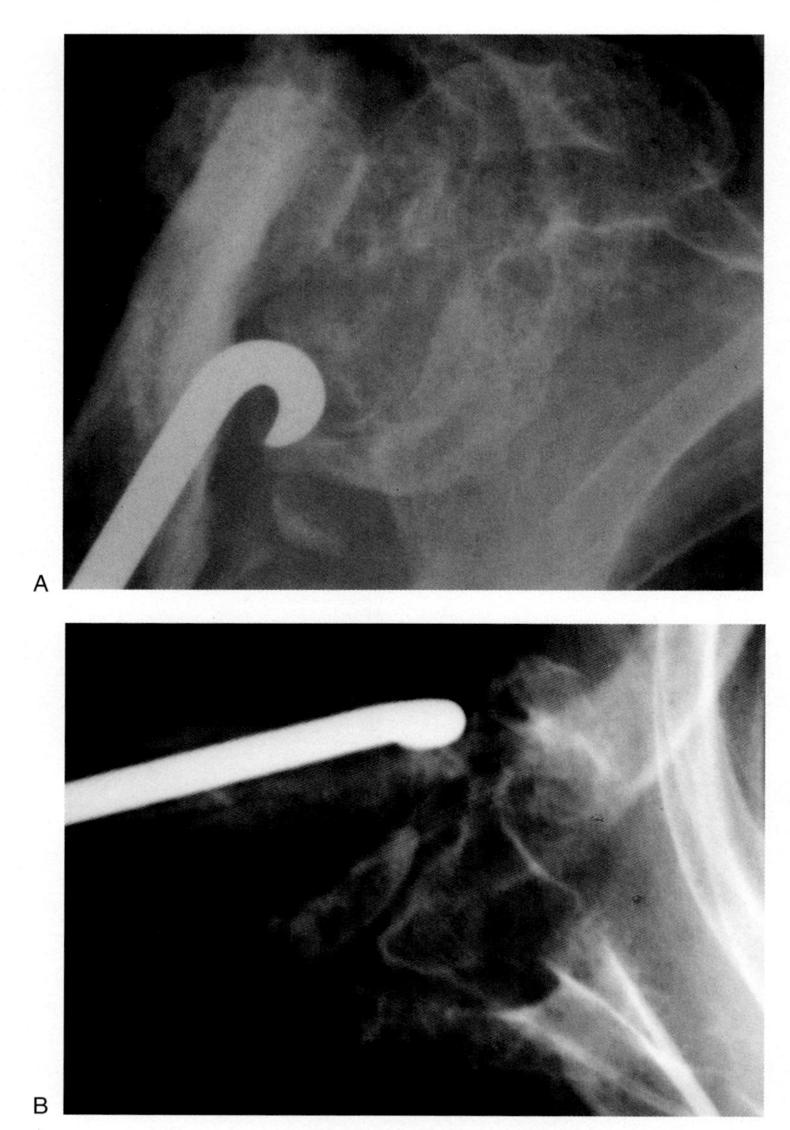

FIG. 24. (A,B) Osteonecrosis: Displaced comminuted fracture of the proximal humerus, treated by ORIF, resulting in total resorption of the avascular articular segment.

lowed as the disease process evolves. Unlike the usual arthritides that begin with the involvement of the articular cartilage, osteonecrosis initially involves the subchondral cancellous bone in the portion of the humeral head under the greatest load. Later, the articular surface may be altered and, eventually, more extensive damage extends to the glenoid.

Osteonecrosis from disease processes probably results from repetitive insults leading up to a threshold of vascular embarrassment. The resultant ischemia of the marrow elements and osteocytes eventually leads to infarction. Pain may or may not be present at this stage. Discomfort may be related to increased intra-osseous pressure in the absence of collapse of the articular surface. What role increased intraosseous pressure plays at this point is uncertain, although its presence has been clearly documented.[73,155]

Pathoanatomy

The repair process is initiated soon after the initial vascular insult. The response is vascular ingrowth in attempt to remove necrotic marrow and to rebuild necrotic bone. The repair process is on-going even continuing in the presence of vascular insults. Continued stress on viable bone resulting in microfractures, trabecular collapse, and compression may establish a front impenetrable by the repair granulation tissue. At the time of collapse, the overlying subchondral bone and cartilage remain intact. Initially, this occurs in the area of maximum joint reaction force and creates a gap which, radiographically, is known as the "crescent sign." With further loading, there is complete segmental failure with incongruity of the subchondral bone.

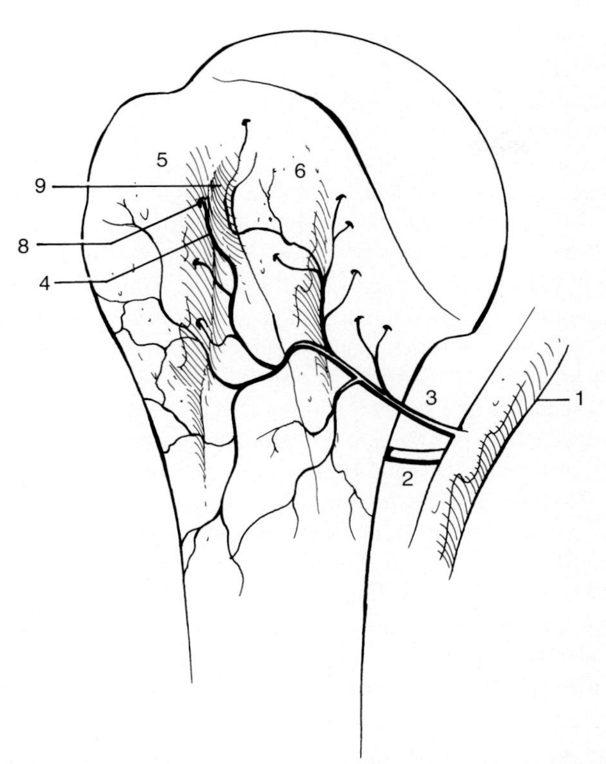

FIG. 25. Graphic representation of the anterior aspect of the humeral head depicting the arterial vascularization: 1) Axillary artery, 2) Posterior circumflex artery, 3) Anterior circumflex artery, 4) Anterolateral branch of the anterior circumflex artery, 5) Greater tuberosity, 6) Lesser tuberosity, 7) Constant site of entry of the anterolateral branch into bone, 8) Intertubercular groove. (From Gerber C, Schneeberger A, Vinh TS. The arterial vascularization of the humeral head. J Bone Joint Surg [Am] 1990;72:1489, with permission)

Articular surface damage may take place even though the cartilage remains viable (Fig. 26). Depending on the extent of involvement, the humeral head undergoes progressive secondary degeneration. As a result of bearing against the morphologically altered humeral head, the glenoid eventually develops osteoarthritic changes.

Clinical Evaluation

The chief complaint of patients with osteonecrosis is pain. The onset is usually insidious and discomfort is not initially severe. In sickle cell disorders, the clinical distinction between a crisis, bone or synovial infarction, and incipient osteonecrosis may be extremely difficult.[282]

Shoulder pain may later intensify with progressive involvement of the head or owing to alterations of the articular surface. Not only will there be an intense synovial response, but mechanical symptoms of locking or catching ensue. Early in the disease, the shoulder range of motion is maintained with guarding at the extremes. Gradually, the range diminishes to that required for essential functional tasks, later accompanied by atrophy and weakness. Crepitation of articular origin can be elicited as the shoulder actively or passively rotates.

Imaging

Imaging studies include tomography, MRI, and CT to assess the amount of humeral head involvement, bone loss, and the distortion of underlying anatomy. McCallum offered a classification scheme that separated humeral head, neck, and shaft involvement from juxtaarticular lesions.[185] In the latter, the earliest findings were dense areas with an intact cortex. Spherical segmental opacities and linear opacities were noted. When structural failure occurred, a translucent subcortical band could be seen. Later, the articular cartilage would collapse and the cortex would be separated. The final stage was osteochondrosis.

The radiographic progression of the disease has been more recently staged according to the system of Ficat and Arlet, as modified by Cruess (Fig. 27).[43,44,72] Stage I includes subtle changes within the humeral head. Pain may or may not be present. The plain films show that the humeral head is round, with some mottling present: MRI examination will pick up this early finding. Stage II is the development of focal sclerosis without collapse. The anteroposterior view of the

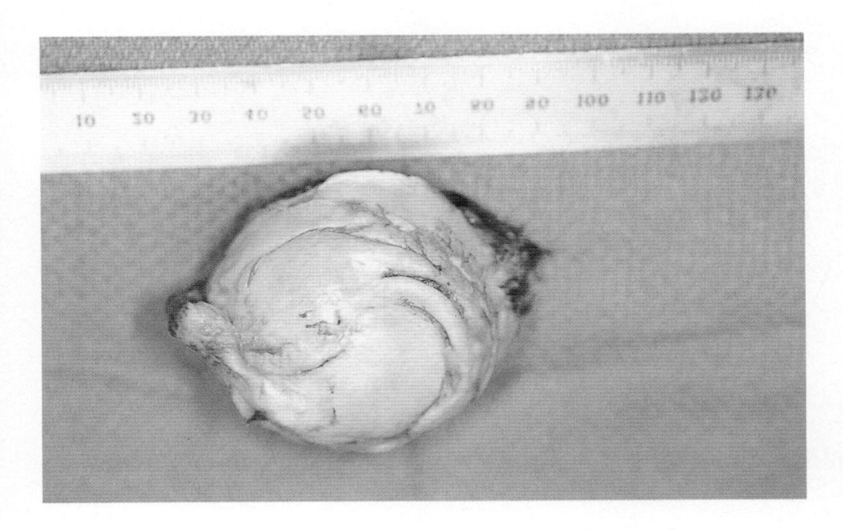

FIG. 26. Osteonecrosis: Humeral head osteonecrosis at the time of hemiarthroplasty reconstruction. The viable cartilaginous surface is irregular and collapsed.

humerus in external rotation is often diagnostic at this stage, as is the MRI. The cartilage surface can be round, but there is some ballotability of the affected segment. Stage III is the development of collapse or a crescent sign (Fig. 28). There is no displacement of the articular surface more than 1 or 2 mm. The cartilage may loosen as a flap, creating symptoms of internal derangement. At this point, the glenoid is normal. Stage IV results in a displaced cartilaginous flap, accompanied by humeral head softening and collapse (Fig. 29). Stage V is wear of the cartilage and the bone of both the glenoid and humerus. The joint becomes incongruent with secondary degenerative changes (Fig. 30).

Laboratory

Laboratory studies may be important for the detection of underlying diseases.

Natural History

The necrotic segment size may vary in traumatic occurrences of osteonecrosis. Smaller areas of involvement may be sufficiently revascularized and stabilized before the stage of collapse. Larger necrotic segments remain isolated from incoming circulation, inevitably progressing to collapse and eventual head destruction. Sometimes, however, the glenohumeral joint congruity will be preserved, allowing maintenance of adequate function.[170,205]

Almost three-fourths of patients with atraumatic osteonecrosis will have progression of their disease to the extent that will require surgery, or will result in significant pain or disability.[43,45,264] At the time of presentation, 20% of patients in L'Bisolata's series required surgery on the basis of pain alone.[169] Thirty-four percent responded initially to conservative care for an average period of 2 years, and then required surgery. Forty-six percent responded to conservative care for an average of 10 years. Half of these patients were satisfied and half were unsatisfied with their outcome. At 4.5 years after presentation, 80% of Rutherford's patients with stage II and III disease had no clinical progression.[273] In a follow-up study at the same institution, Hattrup and Cofield remarked that the need for shoulder arthroplasty was dependent on the underlying diagnosis and the extent and Cruess stage of humeral head involvement.[108] At a 3-year interval, traumatic

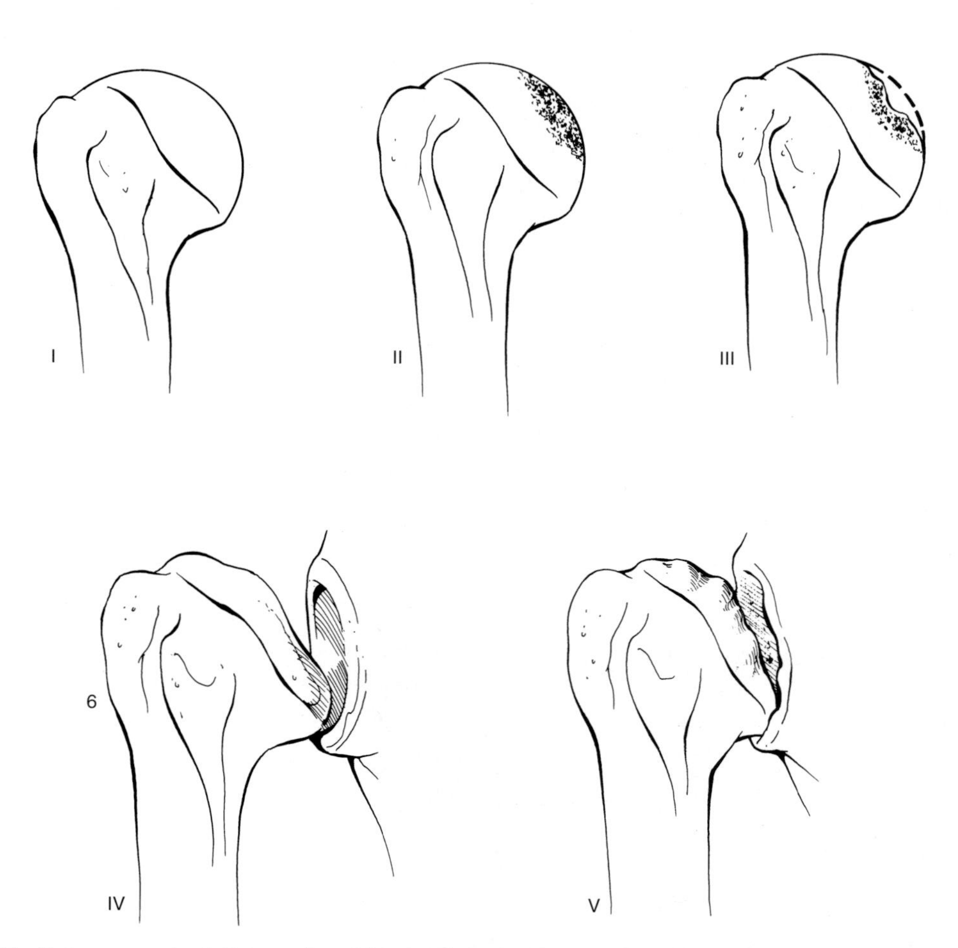

FIG. 27. Osteonecrosis: Artist-rendered figure of staging system for humeral head osteonecrosis. (Modified from Cofield RH. Osteonecrosis. In: Friedman RJ, ed. *Arthroplasty of the shoulder*. New York: Thieme, 1994:174).

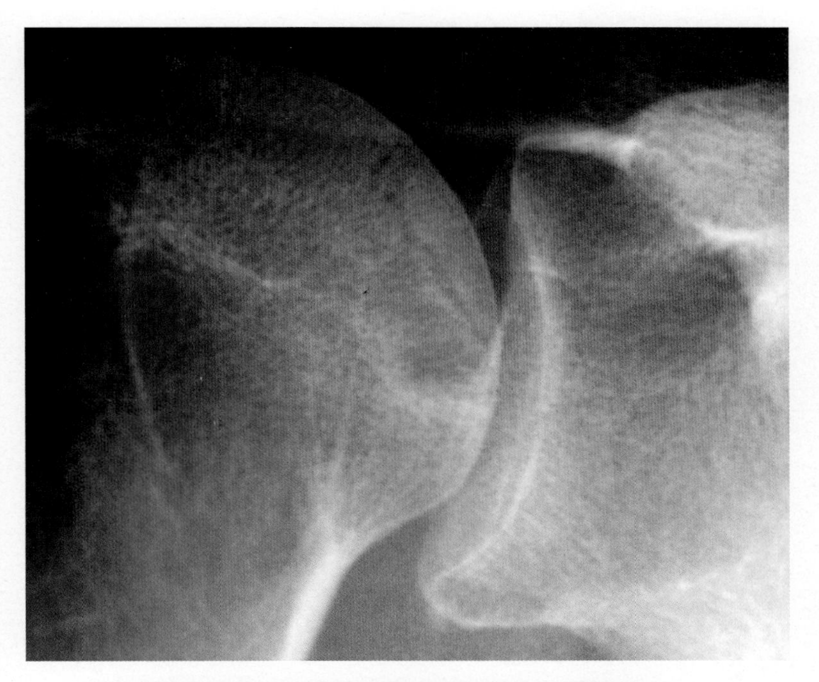

FIG. 28. Osteonecrosis: Stage III. A "crescent sign" is seen. There is preservation of the subchondral articular margin.

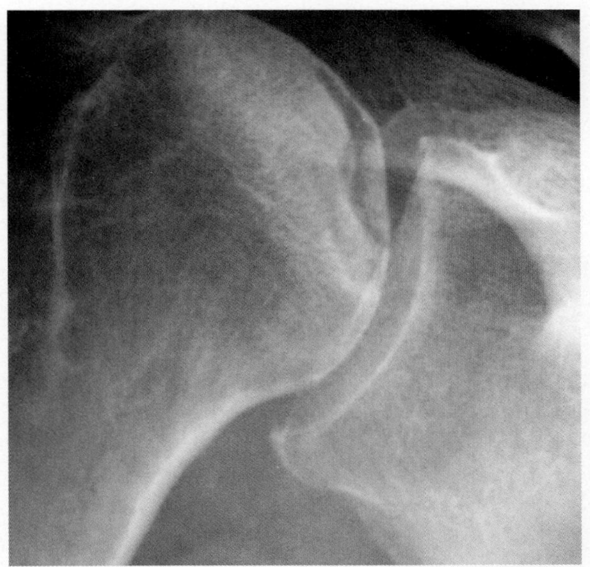

A

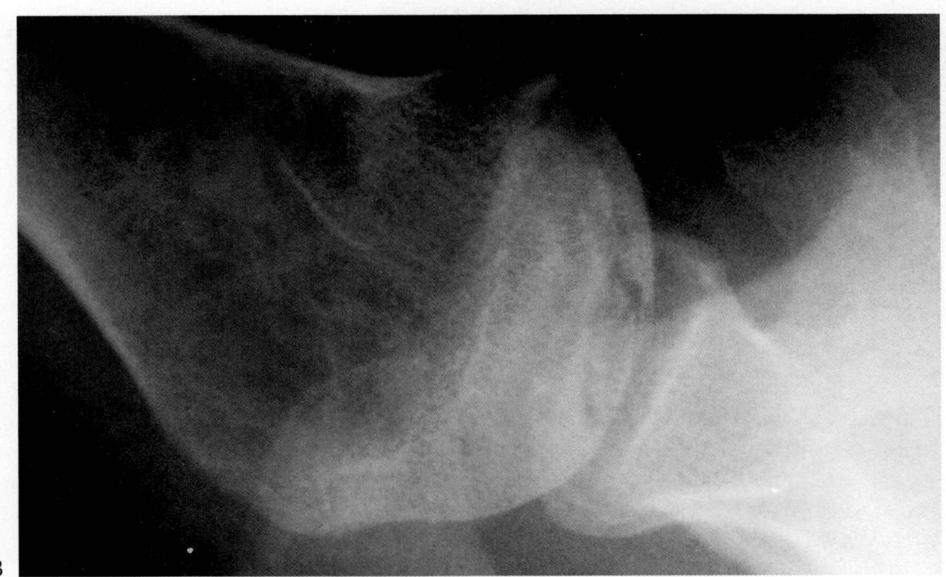

B

FIG. 29. (A,B) Osteonecrosis: Stage IV osteonecrosis of the humeral head with localized collapse and irregularity of the articular surface.

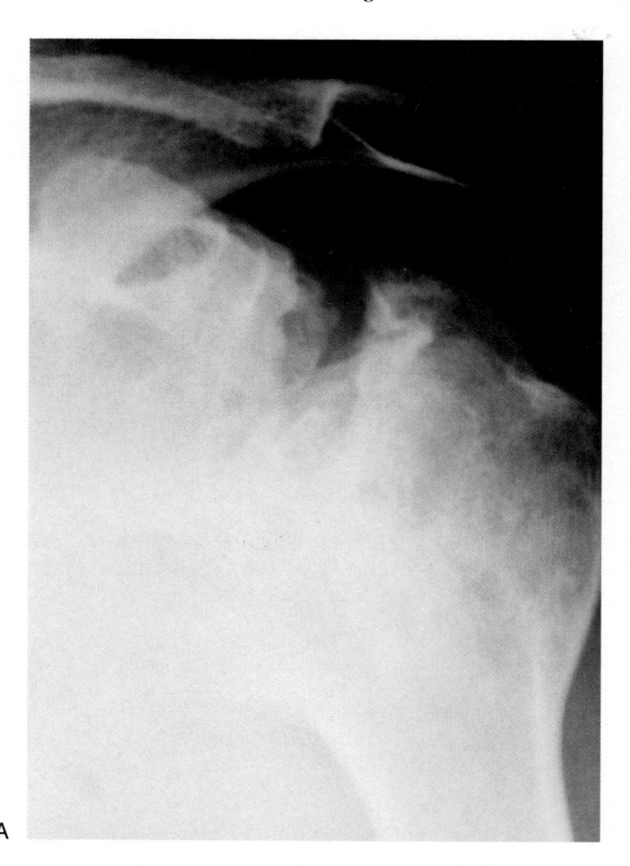

A

FIG. 30. (A,B) Osteonecrosis: Stage V. Secondary changes following proximal humerus osteonecrosis.

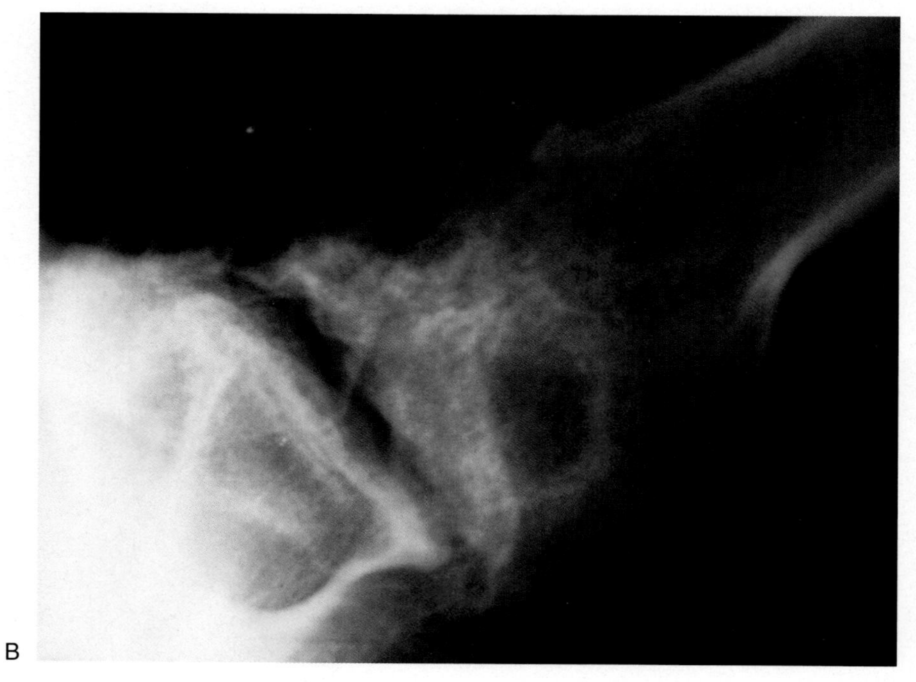

B

etiology versus steroid intake was more likely to result in surgical treatment, 80% versus 43%. Three-fourths of patients initially treated nonoperatively continued to be pain-free, or have only moderate discomfort, almost 9 years after diagnosis.

Clearly, radiographic progression is commensurate with a poor outcome. This is particularly true with radiographic stage III, or greater, and evidence of disease progression. L'Bisolata et al. observed that poor outcomes were more common in women than in men and patients with steroid-induced disease had a better prognosis.[169]

RHEUMATOID ARTHRITIS

Definition

Rheumatoid arthritis is a systemic autoimmune disorder of unknown etiology. It is believed to occur in individuals who are genetically predisposed in response to an arthritogenic agent or antigen. Although its effects may be systemic, its major distinctive feature is chronic, often symmetrical erosive synovitis of the peripheral joints.

Incidence

The incidence of rheumatoid arthritis is approximately 20:100,000 to 40:100,000 adults. Women have a two- to threefold greater risk, and the disease is more prevalent with advancing age.[117]

The shoulder is invariably involved, usually as a clinical feature of progressive disease.[92] It is not commonly one of the first manifestations of the disease; never is it the only one. Its presence is usually bilateral.

The actual incidence of glenohumeral involvement, depending on which patient group is selected or studied, ranges from 20% to 90%.[41,238] The incidence is 50% to 60% when polyarticular rheumatoid disease exists.[265,300] The incidence is highest in patients undergoing surgical intervention, whereas shoulder occurrences are much less frequent with those patients who manifest minor symptoms of the disease.

It may be the first joint to be involved in approximately 4% of the cases with rheumatoid arthritis.[107] When it is the presenting joint, the illness soon becomes systemic and polyarticular. Therefore, only rarely can rheumatoid arthritis account for a chronic monarthritis of the shoulder.

Pathogenesis

Although connective tissue, wherever it is present, is susceptible to the effects of rheumatoid disease, its greatest effect is on the internal aspects of the joint, especially the synovial membrane. A single primary cause has not been determined.[109,197] Infectious agents, autoimmunity, and heritable factors, their activities perhaps interrelated, are being investigated.[109,197] Rheumatoid factor (IgM) may be found in 3% of healthy people. Its role in rheumatoid arthritis may be to amplify rheumatoid inflammation, but it does not appear to serve as a primary etiologic agent or as a trigger.[280]

Pathophysiology

The exact sequence or cause of events leading to symptomatic rheumatoid arthritis has not been determined. The initial pathologic event appears to be activation and injury of subsynovial microvascular endothelial cells.[159,281] In the subsynovial areas around small capillaries, tissue macrophages process and present antigen to T lymphocytes.[131,249] These cells, as well as B-cell lymphocytes and their products—cytokines and immunoglobulins—proliferate in a poorly restrained manner. The normally flimsy, one- to two-cell–thick lining layer and sublining synovial membrane may thicken by as much as 100 times through the process of hypertrophy and activation of the connective tissue stroma.[232] Joint fluid volume increases with activation and proliferation of the synovial cells. Inflammatory cells and chemical mediators of inflammation accumulate and weaken the supporting soft-tissue structures of the synovium.

The synovitis resembles both tumor growth and wound healing, relying on new blood vessel proliferation—angiogenesis—to sustain its expansion.[160,303] These abnormal cells develop abrasive qualities that take on the behavior of malignancy and advance onto the adjacent cartilage and bone.[69] This tissue, which continues to proliferate, develops invasive properties, and bears resemblance to granulation tissue, is known as pannus.[105] Whether its initiation is pathologic or reparative has not been clarified.[105] It can invade adjacent tendons, tendon sheaths, ligaments, bone, and articular cartilage. As the cartilage is eroded, breaks in the underlying bone may develop. Cysts may form and subsequently coalesce into large subchondral defects with potential for collapse in areas of greatest load.

Pathoanatomy

Crossan identified three pathologic phases of synovial inflammation. Exudative, infiltrative, and degradative.[40] The exudative phase begins at the articular cartilage margin. There is increase in capillary permeability, initially with the efflux of fluid into the interstitial space. The infiltrative phase is marked by the escape and movement of cells into the subsynovial and periarticular tissues. Monocytes and lymphocytes invade the inflamed synovium when earliest biopsies are obtained. The development of lymphoid follicles may occur, but they rarely have germinal centers. When this takes place, an increased number of plasma cells follow. Multinucleated giant cells may exist in the subsynovial layers. The activated synovial surface appears villous and papillary as different portions exist in different stages of development. The degradation phase begins with peripheral marginal injury to the avascular hyaline cartilage. The result is disorganization and loss of the intercellular matrix, yielding to limited repair attempts by fibrosis. Chondrocyte and matrix loss results in cartilage thinning. Pannus may undermine the subchondral and marginal bone and result in osteoclastic bone destruction, observed as the periarticular erosion seen on radiographs.

The entire shoulder structure may become involved in the rheumatoid process. Earliest changes are in the adjacent soft tissue, including the subacromial bursa, rotator cuff tendons, and the long head of the biceps. In the early stages, the rotator cuff is vulnerable to infiltration by rheumatoid synovium. This may result in attenuation or rupture of the cuff and the formation of subacromial bursal effusions. From 20% to 50% of patients acquire full-thickness tears,[67] and a smaller number, partial-thickness tears.[80,213,221] In patients undergoing total shoulder arthroplasty for rheumatoid arthritis, approximately one-third will have a full-thickness rotator cuff tear.[80,221,250] Arthrography fails to demonstrate up to one-third of intertubercular grooves, implying biceps tendon stenosis within the canal.[56] In later stages, when destruction of the humeral articular cartilage is prominent, up to two-thirds of the biceps tendons rupture.[231] Poor bone quality, subchondral cysts, and soft-tissue contractures are often recognized.

The characteristic erosions of glenohumeral rheumatoid arthritis occur in the superior aspect, medial to the greater tuberosity at the synovial reflection, and correspond to the most common site of rotator cuff tearing. The humeral head may ascend with secondary erosive changes owing to glenohumeral incongruity. A classification of shoulder disease in 100 patients with rheumatoid arthritis undergoing lower extremity surgery described these changes.[40] Forty percent of shoulders initially manifested only erosive changes, often involving the acromioclavicular joint. The humeral head remained spherical, and the glenohumeral articulation remained normal. In 40%, proximal subluxation of the humeral head occurred. In half of these, the acromiohumeral interval was less than 6 mm as a result of significant soft-tissue damage. The humeral head remained spherical and the glenoid preserved in approximately one-half of the cases. End-stage disease occurred in the remaining 20%. The humeral head was destroyed with associated destructive changes of the glenoid. Resorption was a common feature. The acromiohumeral interval was significantly diminished, and there were gross distortions in glenohumeral relations.

Clinical Evaluation

The symptoms and manifestations of glenohumeral rheumatoid arthritis usually have an insidious onset and slow progression. Adaptive and compensatory mechanisms by the elbow and wrist enable most patients to maintain their functional status while the disease progressively takes its toll on the glenohumeral joint and soft tissues. As a result, advanced changes are often manifest at initial presentation. The shoulder symptoms typically do not correlate with the general severity or activity of the disease.

Pain is the most common symptom reported by patients with glenohumeral rheumatoid arthritis. The pain may be intense, even before radiographically advanced changes of severe bone loss, osteopenia, erosions, and humeral head translocations are observed. Unlike other involved joints, night pain is more typical when the shoulder is involved. Patients sense an awareness of stiffness. Functional loss may occur early in the disease.

The physical findings include those related to inflammation: tenderness, often diffuse, but sometimes more localized to the joint line posteriorly, as well as the infracoracoid region corresponding to the anterior joint line. There may be increased overlying cutaneous warmth when compared with the adjacent areas. Erythema is not common. Swelling from a glenohumeral joint effusion may be present, although not always prominent. More often, the swelling is observed superiorly in the subacromial bursa from an extension of articular fluid through a defect in the rotator cuff. Atrophy of the shoulder girdle may be present, although the presence of swelling and effusions may make recognition more difficult. Motion restriction may be attributable to several causes. Reflex activity limitations because of discomfort will accompany most conditions that cause pain. Active range of motion losses and weakness may occur because of rotator cuff tears. Some motion loss may be noted from weakness because of muscle atrophy. Joint capsule contractures may inhibit both active and passive range of motion. Large effusions and articular surface changes may contribute to diminished range of motion.

Imaging

Larsen presented the first radiographically refined and standardized grading system for the radiographic severity of rheumatoid arthritis.[166] This method was applied to multiple small and large joints, including the shoulder (Table 3).

Radiographically, Neer has identified three clinical types of rheumatoid glenohumeral arthritis.[216] The dry type is characterized by loss of the joint space, formation of subchondral cysts, sclerosis, and marginal osteophytes, not unlike osteoarthritis (Fig. 31). Marginal erosions are infrequent. Patients have more difficulty mobilizing the shoulder involved with this type of rheumatoid arthritis. A wet type results from the proliferation of exuberant granulation tissue at the articular margins (Fig. 32). Marginal erosions, sometimes quite large, are characteristic of this pattern. The proximal humeral architecture, altered by a gradual loss of humeral head and tuberosity contours, acquires a "pointed appearance." The wet and resorptive phase is the most destructive, characterized by "centralization" (Fig. 33). This

TABLE 3. *Larsen radiographic staging for rheumatoid arthritis*

Grade	Description	Anatomical findings
0	Normal	
I	Slight abnormality	One or more: periarticular soft-tissue swelling, periarticular osteoporosis, slight joint space narrowing
II	Definite early abnormality	Erosion and joint space narrowing
III	Medium destructive abnormality	Erosion and joint space narrowing
IV	Severe destructive	Erosion and joint space narrowing; bone deformity
V	Mutilating	Disappearance of original articular surfaces; gross deformity

From ref. 166, with permission.

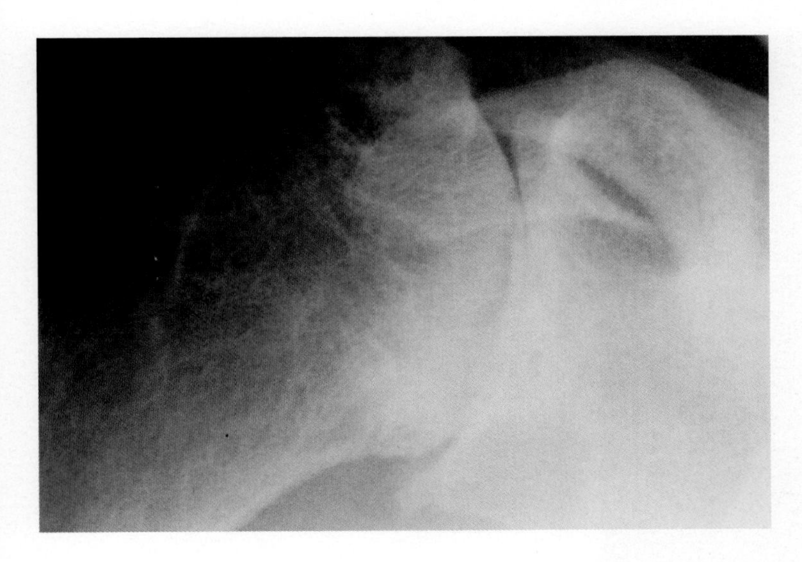

FIG. 31. Rheumatoid arthritis: Dry type, characterized by loss of joint space, sclerosis, and marginal osteophytes.

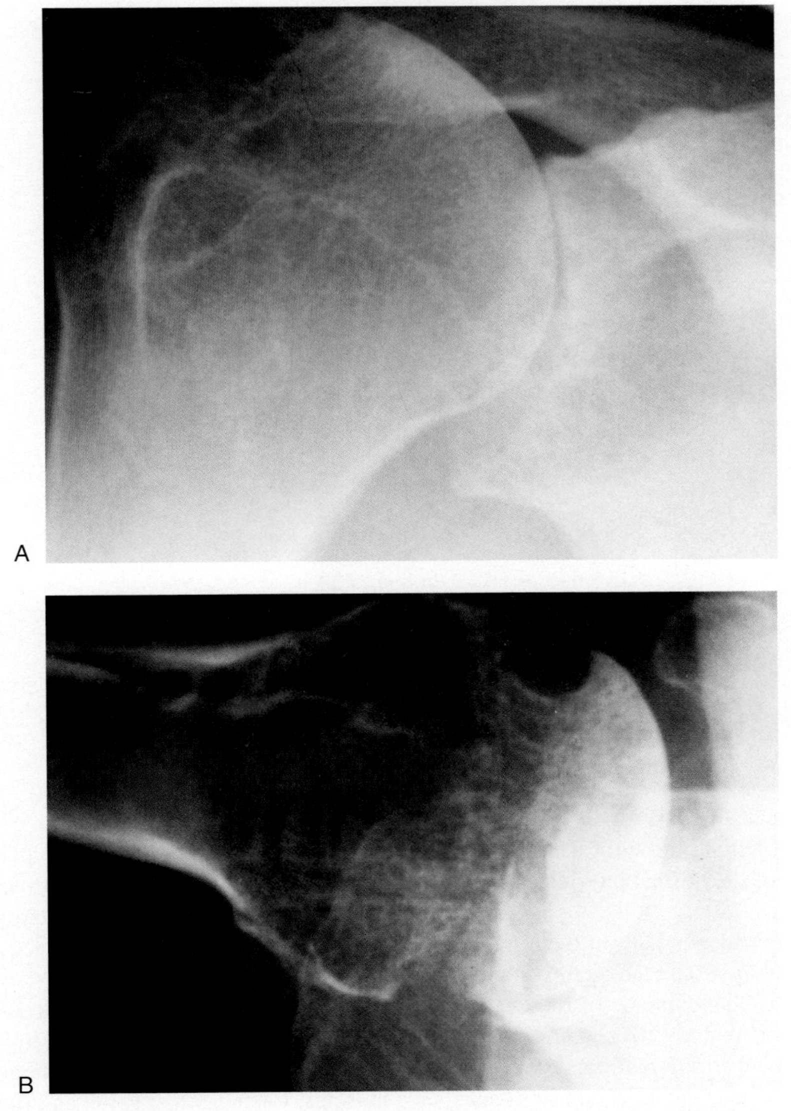

FIG. 32. (A,B) Rheumatoid arthritis: Wet type, with large erosions characteristically found at synovial attachment sites.

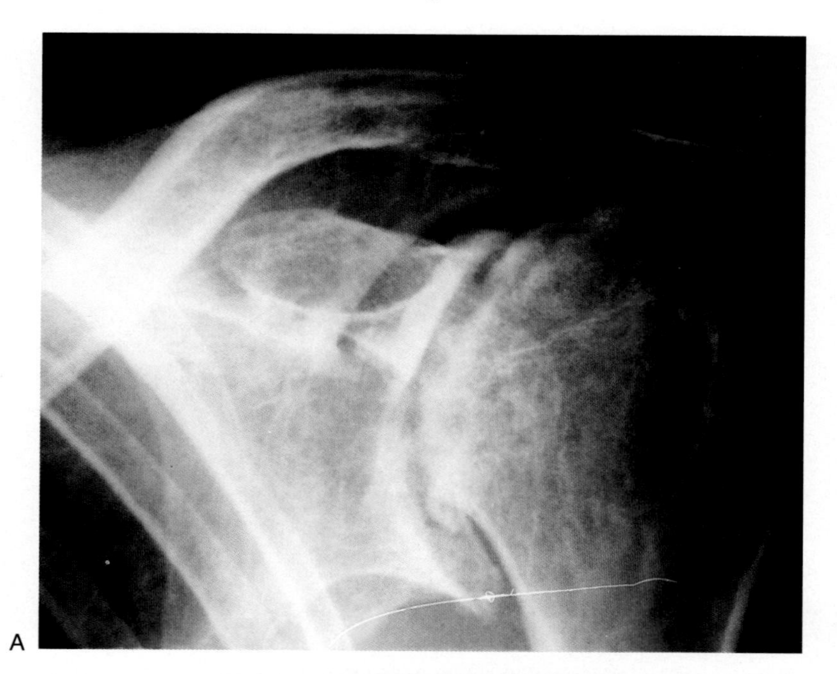

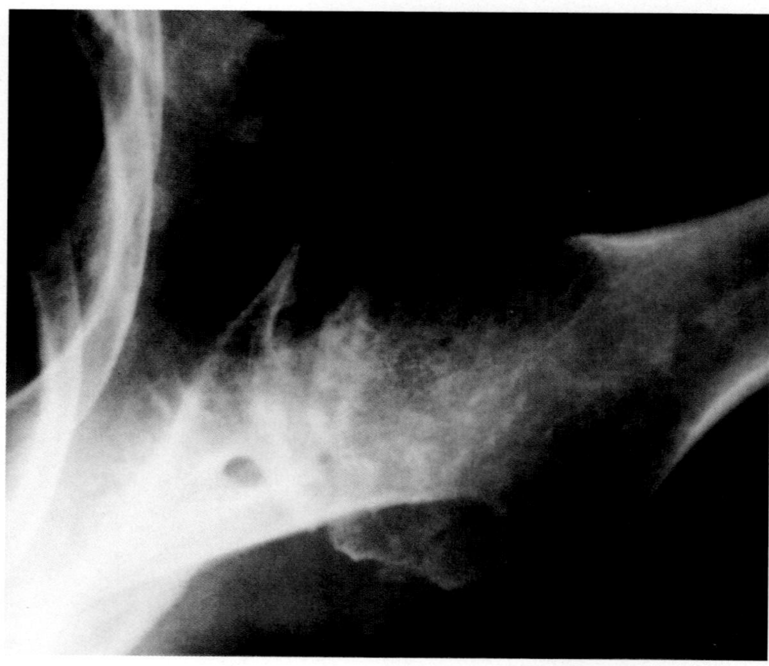

FIG. 33. Rheumatoid arthritis: **(A,B)** Wet and resorptive type. Subchondral cyst formation and erosion of the glenoid and humeral head. (*continued*)

phenomenon evolves in response to a rapid and severe articular cartilage and bone loss. Medial migration with the loss of bone mass results in a loss of the normal physical contour of the shoulder (Fig. 34).

The radiographic findings are dependent on the duration and extent of the disease, and may reflect the quality of medical management. Symmetry is characteristic of rheumatoid arthritis. The initial radiographic features may be normal, but later, because of disuse or local inflammation, osteopenia may be observed (Fig. 35). Osseous erosions appear at sites of synovial tissue concentrations, most commonly the anatomic neck, superior and medial to the greater tuberosity. With the gradual concentric loss of articular cartilage, and erosion of the subchondral bony plates, the glenoid and the humeral head move closer together (Fig. 36). In rare instances, osteophytes may secondarily occur. Invasive biceps tenosynovitis may produce surface erosions of the intertubercular groove.

The position of the humeral head relative to the glenoid and to the acromion is controlled by several factors. Initially, there may be ascent of the humeral head because of weak muscles. Later, with attrition and rupture of the rotator cuff, the acromiohumeral interval narrows further. During the end-stages of disease, the acromiohumeral interval may be-

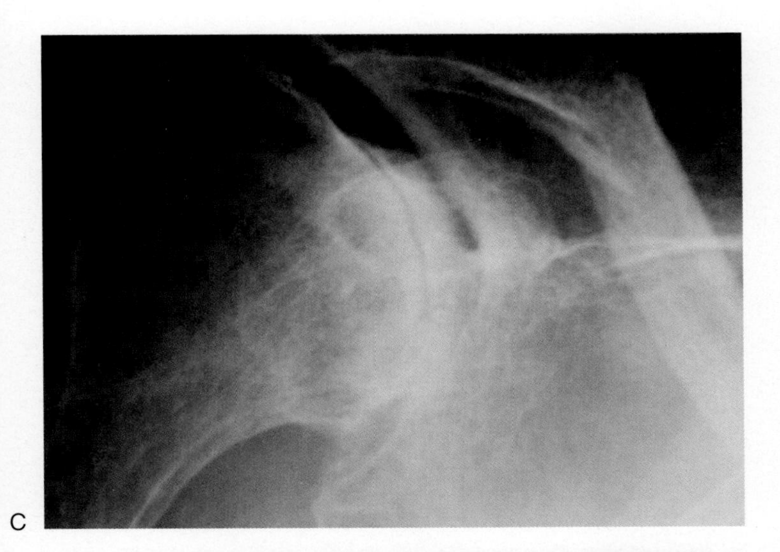
C

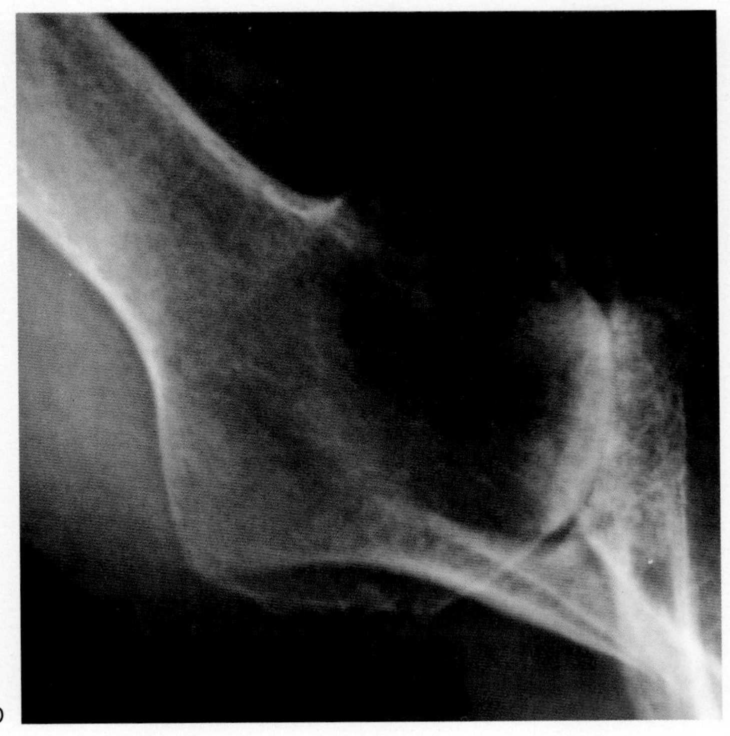
D

FIG. 33. (*continued*) **(C,D)** More severe involvement with advanced centralization of the joint is noted with generalized loss of the glenoid.

come obliterated with the formation of a new acromiohumeral articulation. At this point, gross destruction of the glenohumeral articulation may be observed. Large cysts, subchondral sclerosis, and secondary osteoarthritis may develop (Fig. 37). There may be overall centralization of the joint due to extreme glenoid erosion (Fig. 38). The humeral head may resorb and collapse onto the glenoid (Fig. 39).

Computed tomography scanning will help to better define the extent of the erosions and cyst formation within the humeral head and glenoid.[4] A determination of the volume and orientation of the glenoid vault can be made in preparation for arthroplastic reconstruction.[79] Significant centralization may result in a wafer-thin glenoid, which would yield to the preparation and placement of a prosthetic glenoid component. Mullaji noted that only one-half of the surface area of the rheumatoid glenoid was supported by sufficient bone.[207] Humeral bone quality in rheumatoid arthritis may be underestimated by CT.[4]

Arthrography can be used to discriminate an acute rheumatoid flare from a full-thickness rotator cuff tear. When there is significant stiffness, adhesive capsulitis can be assessed. Chronic synovitis is often diagnosed on the basis of filling defects within the joint. Distension of the biceps tendon sheath may be observed.[56]

An MRI scan can accurately determine the presence of synovial fluid, estimate its volume, and trace the extent of its dissection through the periarticular tissues. The rotator cuff integrity and quality can be assessed. In the rheumatoid

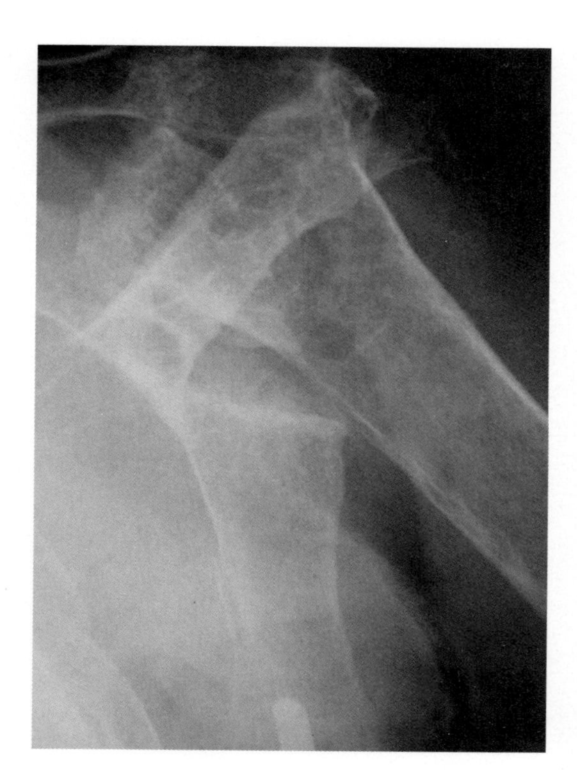

FIG. 34. Rheumatoid arthritis, end-stage, with total distortion of glenohumeral anatomy.

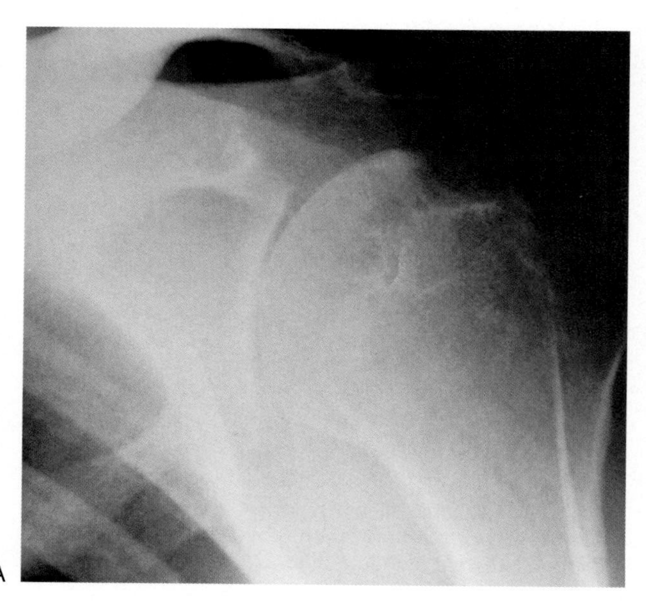

A

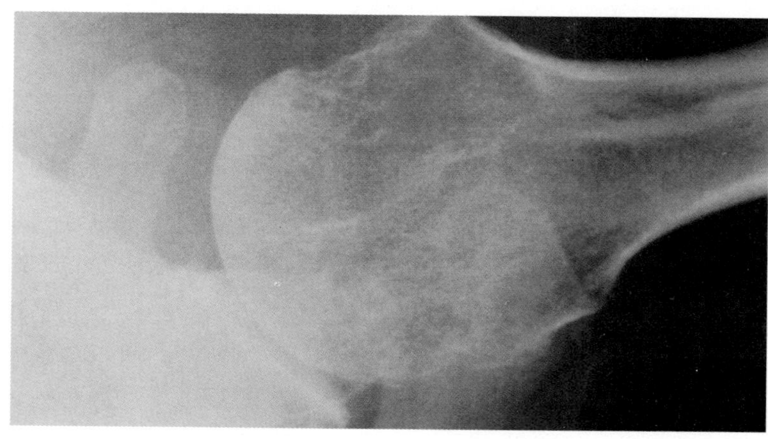

B

FIG. 35. (A,B) Rheumatoid arthritis: Early disease with preservation of the glenohumeral articular surface; periarticular osteoporosis, particularly in the humeral head.

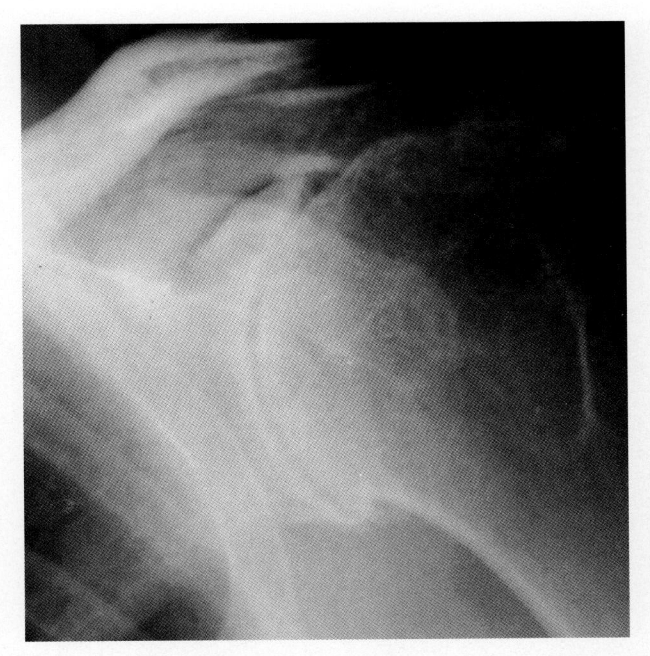

FIG. 36. Rheumatoid arthritis: Concentric loss of the articular space and osteopenia. Erosions are not prominent.

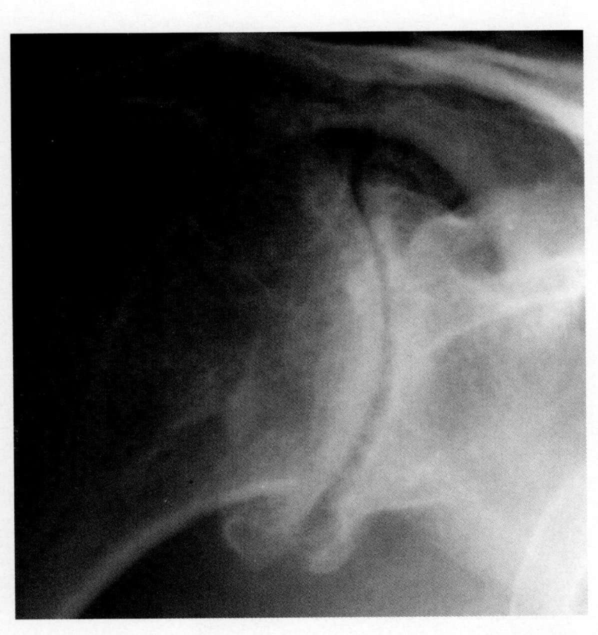

FIG. 37. Rheumatoid arthritis: Secondary osteoarthritic changes are present.

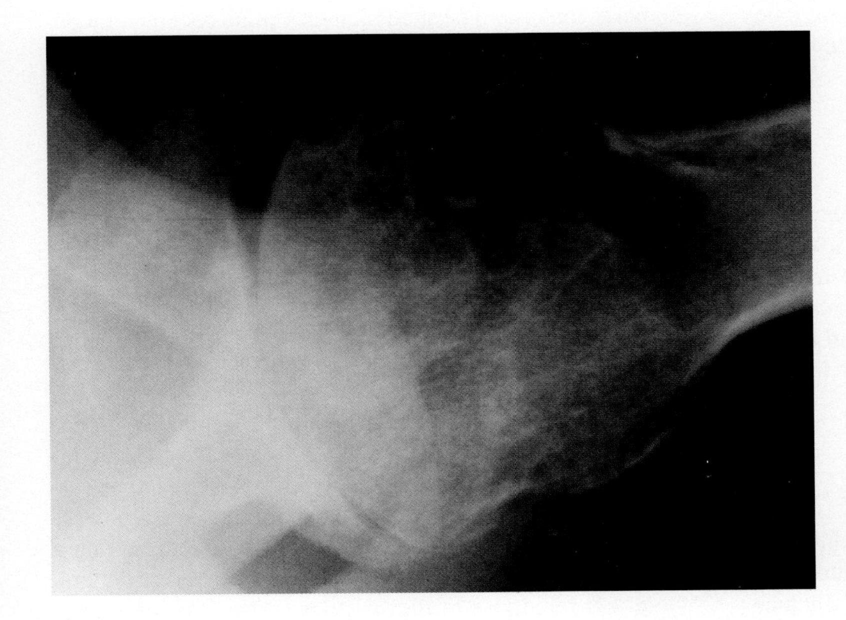

FIG. 38. Rheumatoid arthritis: The morphology of the humeral head is satisfactorily preserved. There is significant "centralization."

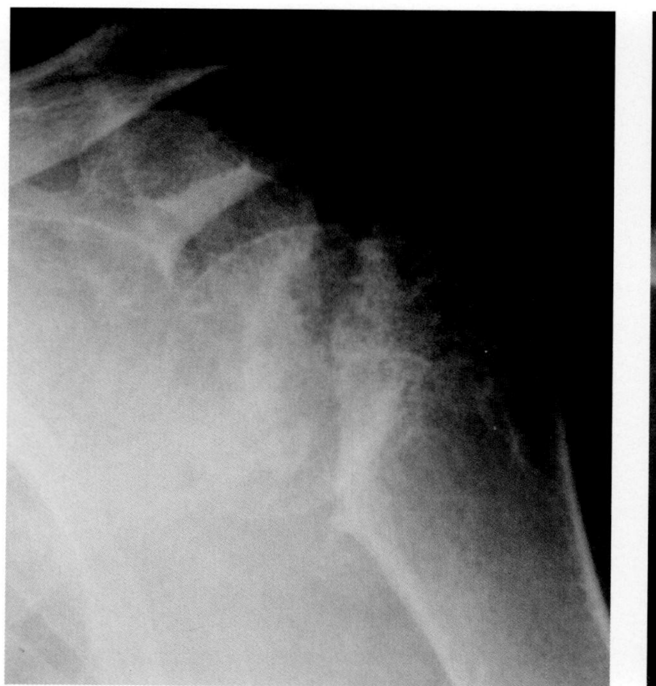

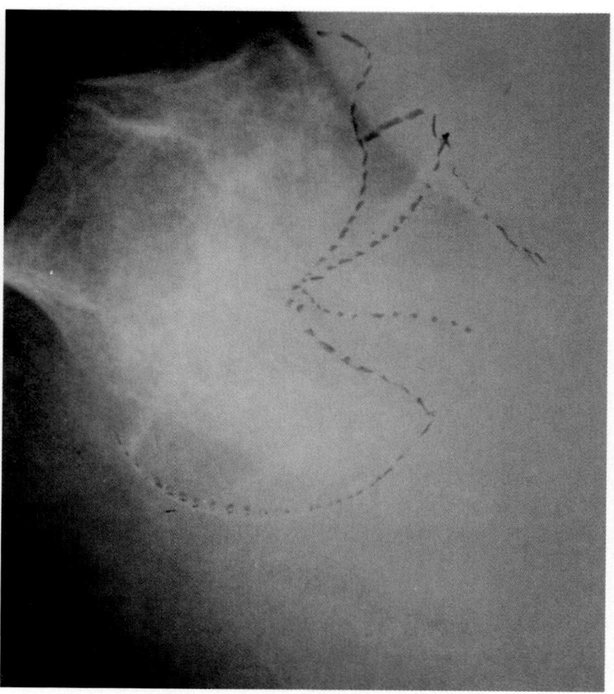

A B

FIG. 39. (A,B) Rheumatoid arthritis: Significant osteopenia is observed. There has been collapse of the humeral head in the absence of significant trauma, in essence, a pathologic fracture dislocation.

knee, subchondral cyst contents and dimensions may become more apparent with MRI, their detection dependent on size, location, and perhaps biologic activity.[244]

Laboratory

Blood work may detect anemia, but generally there is a normal WBC. Rheumatoid factor is positive in 75% to 90% of cases.[7,330] Acute-phase reactants (ESR, CRP) may be present and elevated.[10] Their usefulness may be more appropriate for monitoring the activity of rheumatoid arthritis.[229] Synovial fluid analysis is confirmatory for inflammation.

Natural History

The rate of progression of rheumatoid disease involvement of the shoulder is unknown. Three main patterns of shoulder involvement have been suggested.[40] These include acute rotator cuff tear, progressive cuff attrition, and medial head displacement. In a few patients, acute rotator cuff tear occurs. This is usually the result of acute synovitis that has involved the synovium adjacent to the insertion of the supraspinatus tendon. The synovium will infiltrate the adjacent tendon, with resultant spontaneous rupture. Progressive cuff attrition is the result of end-stage disease. With progressive muscular and tendinous weakening, there is ascent of the humeral head and diminution in the available acromiohumeral interval. The glenohumeral joint becomes incongruous and develops progressive erosion. Glenohumeral deformity soon follows. Medial head displacement is rarely an early event. Only when there has been significant cuff attrition and proximal migration does medial head displacement occur. A significant toll is taken on the articular and subchondral osseous tissues. Pannus formation within the glenoid fossa results in a significant loss of supporting bone stock. As the shoulder comes under load, the forces progressively collapse the weakened glenoid. Repair cannot keep pace with the mechanical overload of the weakened glenoid. The humeral head assumes a more medial position as the glenoid gradually disappears.

Neer pointed out the pathologic variations in glenohumeral rheumatoid arthritis.[216] A low-grade type of involvement showed the slow development of articular surface changes and bone loss. An intermediate type was associated with the formation of osteophytes, indicating a response to the on-going process. In the most severe pattern, there was rapid loss of the articular space, and collapse of the underlying bone, with narrowing of the acromiohumeral interval.

CRYSTALLINE ARTHRITIS

Calcium Pyrophosphate Dihydrate Deposition Disease

Calcium pyrophosphate dihydrate (CPPD) deposition disease is a disorder of the articular tissues resulting from the liberation and deposition of calcium pyrophosphate dihydrate crystals. A prerequisite for diagnosis of the disorder is identification of the deposition of CPPD crystals into fibrocartilage and hyaline cartilage. The relation between CPPD and osteoarthritis is unclear, but notably strong.[71] Unlike gout, there is not a metabolic disturbance. The incidence of clinically symptomatic disease is at least half that of classic gout, with the knee most commonly involved, followed by the wrist, then the shoulder.[58] Okazaki reported an incidence of up to 50%[227]

Incidence

CPPD deposition disease does not favor one gender. Clinically, 2 stages of the disorder have been recognized.[60] First is the occurrence of acute attacks of synovitis precipitated by the liberation, accumulation, and reactivity from calcium pyrophosphate crystals within the intraarticular space. Termed "pseudogout," these attacks clinically resemble gout.[154] Often the acute events are imposed on a joint with chronic arthropathy. Patients present with an acute severely painful shoulder with motion limitation. Tenderness, swelling, and increased warmth overlying the joint may be appreciated. Fever is not uncommon. If left untreated, symptoms may persist for weeks. A familial form is common in the shoulder.[103]

CPPD arthropathy will evolve from repeated attacks and the accumulation of deposition pyrophosphate crystals within the articular cartilage. Secondary degenerative arthritis will develop, accompanied by chronic pain. A propensity for elderly women is recognized with this form.[194]

Pathogenesis

The mechanism of crystal shedding into the joint is unclear. The association of trauma, infection, or illness has not been established, but there may be a predisposition for joints with degenerative changes. McCarty proposed six types including sporadic, pseudorheumatoid arthritis (multiple joints), pseudoosteoarthritis, asymptomatic, chondrocalcinosis, and neuropathic-like.[186] Occurrences at the time of surgery are not uncommon. An increasing incidence with age suggests that the disorder may be a part of the aging process.

Chondrocytes within the articular cartilage possess enzyme systems capable of regulating pyrophosphate and CPPD concentrations within the cartilage.[332] If chondrocyte damage occurs, normal pyrophosphate homeostasis is disturbed. The crystal form accumulates and is liberated into the joint when concentrations exceed a critical threshold. A synovial inflammatory response ensues: chemotactic factors are released and propagated by polymorphonuclear phagocytosis. Further articular cartilage damage leads to the additional release of calcium pyrophosphate crystals.

Imaging

The disorder may present incidentally on plain radiographs (Fig. 40A). Known as chondrocalcinosis, these opacities in articular and fibrocartilage are observed in CPPD as well as diabetes, hyperparathyroidism, hemochromatosis, ochronosis, gout, and hypophosphatation syndromes.[103] Radiographs of CPPD arthropathy are essentially comparable with osteoarthritis (see Fig. 40B).

Laboratory Findings

Although laboratory workup might include screening serum studies for the foregoing disorders, the diagnosis is made on the basis of synovial fluid analysis. The fluid is often thicker than normal and, at times, turbid; especially in elderly women. At other times, recurrent hemarthroses may exist.[194] It may be indistinguishable from purulent joint fluid. The cell count is representative of inflammatory fluid. Characteristic rhomboid-shaped positively birefringent crystals are identified (Fig. 41). Some are intracellular, following engulfment by polymorphonuclear cells.

Gout

Gout is a disease characterized by hyperuricemia and resultant accumulation of sodium urate crystals within tissues and joints. The clinical manifestations of gout caused by urate crystal accumulations include acute and chronic arthritis, tophi—tissue deposits of crystals—and nephropathy.

Incidence

The incidence is difficult to determine because of the relapsing–recurring nature of the disorder. Males significantly outnumber females. It is the most common inflammatory arthropathy in men older than 40 years of age and peaks in the fifth decade.[270] Ninety percent of initial acute attacks of gout are monarticular and rarely involve the glenohumeral joint, unless widespread disease is present.[96,141] In some reports, glenohumeral involvement is not even mentioned. When it is affected, it is rarely early in the disease. It may be the presenting joint in a postoperative flare and in postmenopausal women. Glenohumeral occurrences are much more common in elderly patients, particularly those taking diuretics.[15]

Pathogenesis

Uric acid is the end product of purine catabolism. Humans, as a species, lack the enzyme uricase that governs the degradation of uric acid to allantoin.[35] This conversion is necessary to eliminate the highly insoluble uric acid in the form of the highly soluble compound allantoin. In human tissues, therefore, urate metabolism does not exist, necessitat-

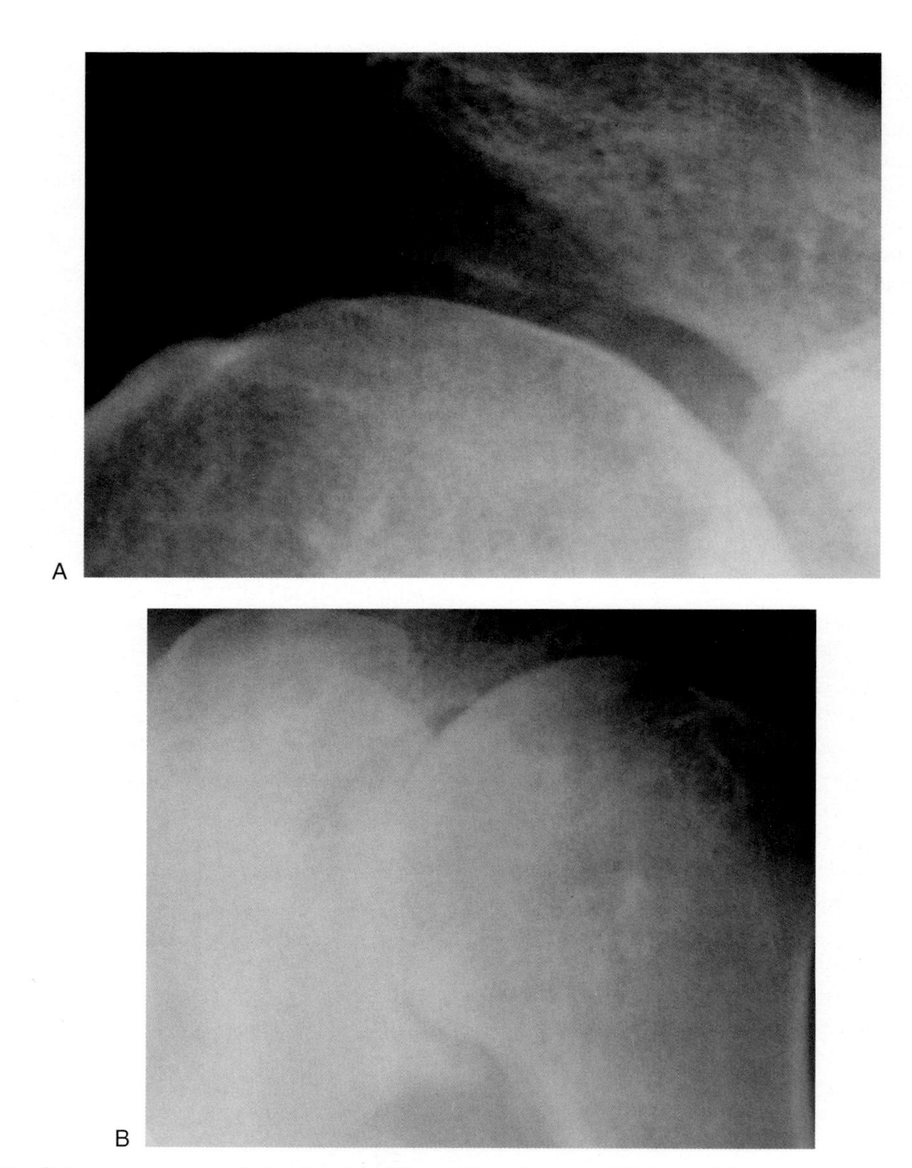

FIG. 40. Calcium pyrophosphate dihydrate deposition disease: **(A)** Crystal deposition is observed in the articular cartilage of the humeral head. **(B)** Progressive deterioration of the glenohumeral articulation is seen.

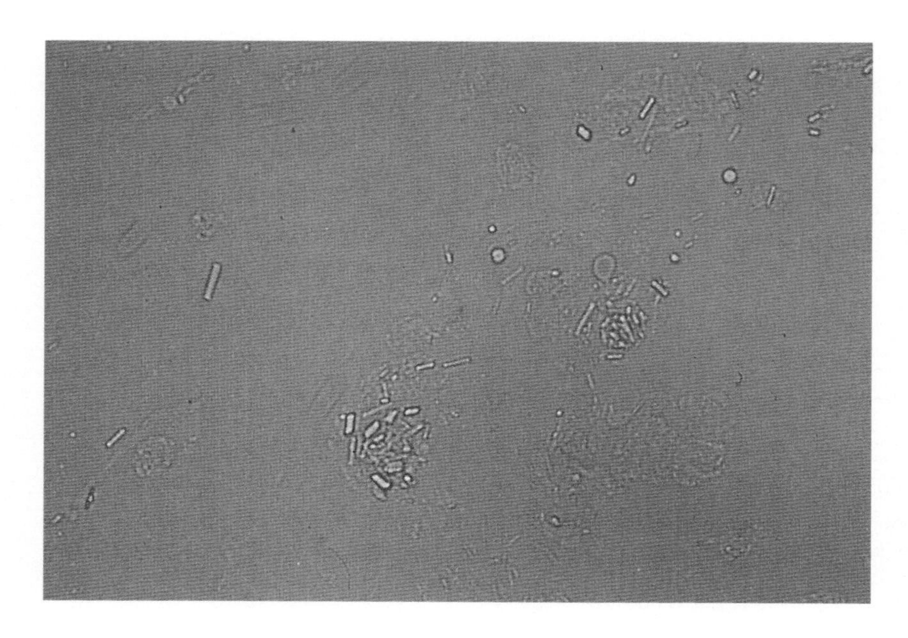

FIG. 41. Calcium pyrophosphate dihydrate deposition disease: Rhomboid-shaped, positively birefringent crystals.

ing elimination. Two-thirds of uric acid disposition is by the kidney and approximately one-third is by the gut by bacterial oxidation.[35] Hyperuricemia may be the result of overproduction or undersecretion. Overproduction results from increased synthesis or, much less commonly, alterations in the purine metabolic pathway. The elimination capacity of the kidney is exceeded with supersaturation of serum with uric acid. Up to 90% of cases are the result of deficits of renal excretion.[171]

Most evidence supports the concept of crystal formation in acute attacks of gouty arthritis.[188,287] The mechanisms leading to precipitation of urate crystals are still not well understood. Serum and synovial fluid urate concentrations typically, but not always, are at supersaturated levels.[187] Underlying joint disorders may favor urate crystallization.[306] Proteoglycan concentration, cation (Na^+, Ca^+) concentration, synovial fluid dynamics and pH, intraarticular temperature, as well as other local factors, may play a role.[139,173,293,294,323] Liberation of monosodium urate crystals may also be explained on the basis of tophi present in the synovium.[149] These result from uric acid precipitation caused by increasing circulatory levels. Polymorphonuclear cells invade the synovium, target and then phagocytose the crystals.

Whether the crystal–white blood cell interreaction takes place within the joint or within the synovium, a common pathway ensues. Mediators of inflammatory response, including chemotactic factors, lysozymes, collagenase, oxygen radicals, and prostaglandins, all are released. The synovium is stimulated and proliferates; an acute inflammatory cellular infiltrate rapidly develops. When the joint has been subject to repeated attacks, a local foreign body reaction ensues with the synovium and results in the local resorption of the adjacent cartilage and bone. Radiographically, this is what is seen as the "punched-out" lesions without an associated bony response.

The pathology of the tophi is a chronic foreign body granuloma around a urate crystal. The tophi are often encapsulated. There is an associated inflammatory reaction that involves monarticular cells and giant cells.

Clinical Presentation

With glenohumeral joint involvement, patients will present with an acute onset of shoulder pain. They may previously have had symptoms attributable to gout in another joint. These patients are often obese, most are men and, sometimes, have excessively ingested alcohol. A previous history of renal dysfunction may be obtained, and diuretics may be in use. Occasionally, there is an abrupt reduction in serum uric acid, as might occur with hyperuricemic treatment or the cessation of alcohol ingestion. These factors will result in the dissolution of uric acid from disrupted tophi.[149]

Physical findings of acute gouty arthritis include decreased range of motion of the shoulder, overlying warmth, tenderness, and perhaps, swelling. Occasionally, these patients will have fever. Chronic gout often exists in the presence of secondary arthritis, the symptoms of which have been discussed earlier.

Imaging

Plain radiographs are usually unremarkable, unless there have been repeated attacks. In such cases, radiographs will show juxtaarticular osteopenia and perhaps juxtaarticular tophi. Sharply outlined erosions, punched-out with sclerotic margins and overhanging edges, will be present. Chronic arthropathy from gout results in secondary osteoarthritis and is indistinguishable radiographically (Fig. 42).

Laboratory

Only a minor fraction of individuals with elevated serum uric acid levels will develop symptomatic gout. Therefore, the diagnosis cannot be made on the basis of uric acid alone. Sometimes, leukocytosis is present. Synovial fluid analysis is diagnostic, with the presence of monosodium urate crystals, often intracellular, visualized with a polarizing microscope. The needle-like crystals are negatively birefringent (Fig. 43).

Apatite Deposition Disease

This disorder, sometimes known as apatite gout, has been described by many authors.[57,81,137,190,284] It is associated with the presence of intraarticular hydroxyapatite crystals. The link between the crystals, arthropathy, and osteoarthritis is unclear. There is a predisposition for large joints. McCarty popularized the condition as "Milwaukee shoulder."[190]

It typically involves the shoulder and occurs in older women.[24] Hydroxyapatite crystals do not excite the same degree of synovial response as do sodium urate crystals.[24] As a result, over a period of weeks or months, chronic mild discomfort typically evolves. Physical examination is characterized by a boggy effusion and limitation of motion. This is associated with radiologic soft-tissue calcification, ascent of the humeral head, and destruction of the glenohumeral relations. Joint fluid often contains debris as well as calcium crystals, but relatively few inflammatory cells, predominantly monocytes.[59] Blood-stained fluid is common.[190] The effusion may rupture into the adjacent soft-tissue planes, creating additional symptoms and signs, sometimes interpreted as venous occlusive disease.[331] A rotator cuff tear is common. The calcium hydroxyapatite crystals are not seen by light microscopy because of their size. They require alizarin red S staining of the synovial fluid preparation.[114] Electron microscopy may be more reliable, but is generally less available. Synovial collagenases and neutral proteases are present in high concentrations, indicative of underlying enzymatic

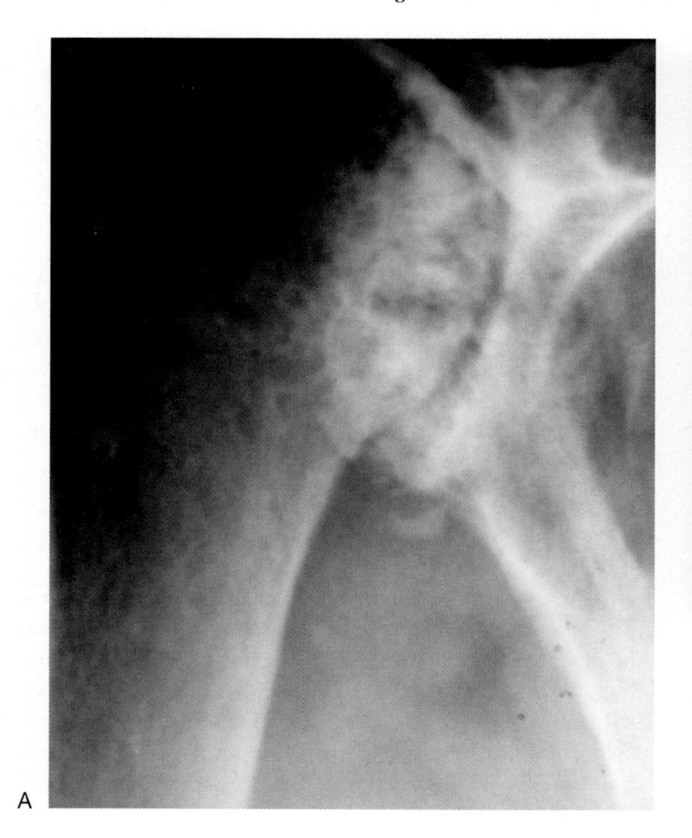

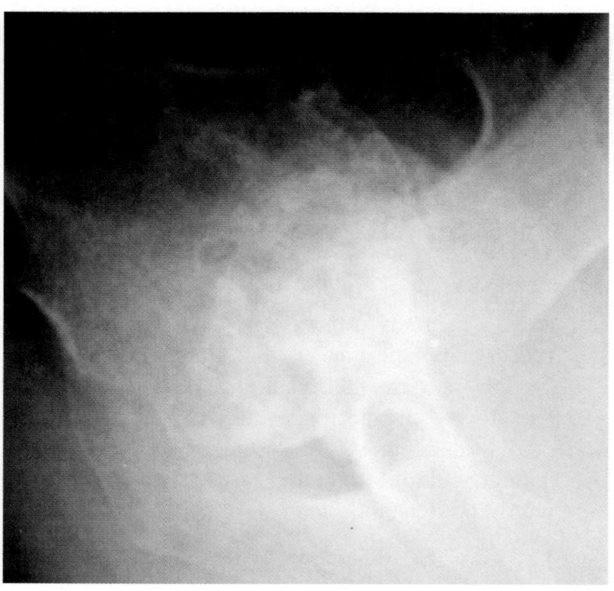

FIG. 42. (A,B) Gout: Arthropathy with loss of glenohumeral joint cartilage and subchondral cyst formation.

action.[101] Further discussion will be given to this entity in the next section.

ROTATOR CUFF TEAR ARTHROPATHY

A special condition originating in the tendinous socket of the shoulder, which leads to arthritic changes in the glenohumeral joint, has been recognized clinically for over a century.[2,3,297,298] It is characterized by recurrent, often hemorrhagic, effusions, containing biochemically active enzymes; the complete absence of the rotator cuff; advanced degenerative glenohumeral joint changes with humeral head collapse; and erosion of the acromion process, the acromioclavicular joint, and the distal clavicle. McCarty and associates in 1981 recognized this clinical entity and it became popularized as the Milwaukee shoulder.[81,102,190] Neer and others in 1982 recognized a subset of patients with similar clinical and radiographic findings, and coined the term "cuff arthropathy."[219]

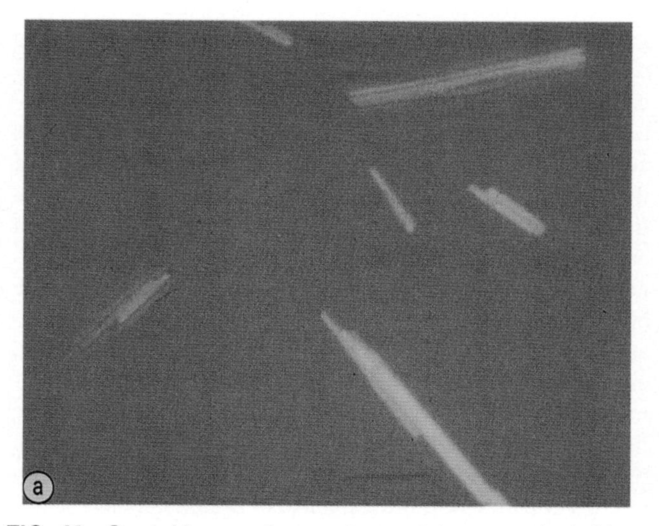

FIG. 43. Gout: Monosodium urate crystals—negatively birefringent.

The pathogenic role of calcium phosphate crystals (hydroxyapatite) in the deterioration process was touted by McCarty.[190] Neer, on the other hand, believed that glenohumeral instability resulted from the massive rotator cuff tearing, with resultant impaired cartilage nutrition, bone softening, collapse, and bone destruction.[214,219] Its genesis continues to be a source of debate and speculation.

Milwaukee shoulder is also known as apatite gout. It is characteristically found in older female patients. Often, their symptoms are bilateral and have been chronic for many years, with periodic exacerbations of more intense discomfort. Physical examination is remarkable for atrophy, weakness, and a shoulder effusion. Synovial fluid analysis by electron microscopy or alizarin red is diagnostic but difficult, and usually not necessary. Imaging studies will demonstrate full-thickness rotator cuff tears.

The destruction of the osteoarticular elements of the shoulder appears to result from the progressive formation of a massive, irreparable, rotator cuff tear and its mechanical sequelae.[181,219] Joint debris and biomechanical products of an active synovial lining also play a role in disease progression. Their presence is the likely result of glenohumeral instability, a consequence of losing rotator cuff integrity.

Progressive narrowing of the acromiohumeral interval by ascent of the humeral head is a prominent feature of rotator cuff arthropathy. With the loss of the stabilizing effect of the rotator cuff, the humeral head displaces upward.

On the basis of their anatomic positioning, the musculotendinous units of the rotator cuff serve as glenohumeral joint compressors; as opposed to acting as humeral head depressors. The force generated by the muscles pulls the humeral head into the concavity of the glenoid and serves as its primary stabilizer. The creation of this efficient fulcrum enables the humeral head to resist the upward force vector of the contracting deltoid muscle. By this mechanism, the hand can be placed overhead or away from the body. An entirely intact rotator cuff is not necessarily required, many patients are capable of overhead mobility with full-thickness defects. The arm can be elevated, as long as there is sufficient muscle activity for compressive stabilization of the humeral head.

A secondary humeral head-stabilizing system includes the acromion, coracoid process, coracoacromial ligament, and the distal clavicle. This coracoacromial archway is the final functional restraint to superior humeral head migration, when the primary stabilizing system has failed.[168]

Pathophysiology and Pathoanatomy

Muscular weakness and degenerative tendon fiber failure are age-related changes that inevitably occur within the rotator cuff.[31,183] Initially, only the supraspinatus tendon is involved. Eventually, further interstitial tendon fiber failure, often clinically interpreted as tendonitis, may lead to partial- and, later, full-thickness tears of the supraspinatus. With continuing activity, the tear may enlarge as adjacent fibers are loaded beyond their elastic limit, and it predictably extends to involve the infraspinatus and, later, the subscapularis. Subtle superior humeral head migration occurs as the concavity compression forces diminish. Initially, this phenomenon is satisfactorily tolerated in terms of comfort and presents little or no functional deficit.

Once the superior forces have exceeded the medially directed forces, abrasive contact occurs against each side. Impingement of the rotator cuff tissue against the acromion accelerates the loss of tendinous tissue. When the cuff tendon tissue superior to the humeral head axis of rotation has vanished, contracture of the lower half of the cuff and the deltoid will create a fixed "boutonniere" deformity of the humeral head against the coracoacromial arch.[138] As a result of the increased friction against the nonarticular and nonconforming undersurface of acromion, the articular surface of the humerus begins to wear.

In response to increased pressure, tensioning of the coracoacromial ligament may result in the formation of an anterior or inferior acromial traction spur. This bony projection may potentially gouge the underlying tendinous tissue and articular cartilage, inducing further damage. In response to load, the acromion process develops the characteristic changes of eburnation and erosion, whereas the coracoacromial ligament may hypertrophy. When the primary stabilizers have failed, limited although purposeful function may be maintained, in spite of the unopposed action of the deltoid, by the secondary stabilization within the coracoacromial arch.[168] Although initially adequate, further articular cartilage degradation and further rotator cuff tendon damage are incurred.

This disorder does not spare the glenohumeral articulation. As a failure of containment, the humeral head subluxes superiorly with force concentration on the narrower superior glenoid. An even greater demand is placed on the primary and secondary stabilizers. Articular surface wear is accelerated and is soon followed by a collapse and degradation of the underlying subchondral bone of the humeral head.

When articular cartilage fragments and underlying areas of softened, and often nonviable, bone are exposed, particulate debris is shed into the joint.[101,190] In response, the synovium proliferates with the development of large effusions, often contained only by a weakened, and sometimes surgically altered, deltoid muscle. "Subcutaneous effusions" may evolve as the fluid herniates through the soft-tissue pathways of least resistance. Sometimes, the fluid accumulates superior to the acromioclavicular joint; recognized as the "geyser sign" on shoulder arthrogram.[39]

Rotator cuff arthropathy is not likely an obligate end-stage of the so-called impingement syndrome and rotator cuff tendon failure. As long as the humeral head can be maintained concentrically opposed to the glenoid by the balanced action of residual intact columns of anterior and posterior cuff, the shoulder is protected from the requisite instability that may lead to rotator cuff arthropathy.[22] A limited degree of superior subluxation of the humeral head can apparently be tolerated without progressively erosive changes of the bony surfaces.

Clinical Evaluation

When presenting for evaluation, patients with rotator cuff arthropathy complain bitterly of unrelenting pain. For years before the acute and intolerable exacerbation, the disorder has been in slow evolution with periodic exacerbations. Not only is the pain felt in the depth of the shoulder, it is often referred to the deltoid insertion. Weakness, crepitation, and sudden sharp pain often limits the attempted use of the extremity for lifting or overhead activities. Significant night pain exists. Minor traumatic experiences are common, and patients will often deny a history of major shoulder injury. Although symptoms may exist bilaterally, one shoulder is often more significantly affected. One or more arthrocenteses accompanied by corticosteroid instillation may have been performed. The typical patient is a woman and is older than 70 years of age.

The disorder is characterized by physical findings indicative of the chronic nature of the disorder. Atrophy of the spinati and, sometimes the deltoid musculature, is prominent. Sometimes, a large effusion will obscure the presence of atrophy. A superiorly subluxed humeral head may rest directly beneath the deltoid muscle anterior to the acromion process. Profound weakness results in a significant restriction in active range of motion. Restraints to passive movement include pain, contracture, and glenohumeral incongruity. Invariably, crepitation, arising from many different sources, often indistinguishable, will be present. The physical findings may exist bilaterally.

Imaging

Sophisticated imaging studies are unnecessary to diagnose rotator cuff tear arthropathy or to adequately identify the pathology (Fig. 44). Plain films represent the most cost-effective means of evaluation, as well as the most accurate. Osteopenia, superior migration of the humeral head, narrowing or obliteration of the acromiohumeral interval, and severe erosions of the glenohumeral joint are the characteristic findings. Osteophytes, irregular cystic formation, subchondral sclerosis, and loss of tuberosity prominence may also be seen. The glenohumeral joint takes on the appearance of the hip.[182] "Acetabularization" results from sculptured erosion of the acromion, superior glenoid, and coracoid bone, and contact of the humeral head against the coracoacromial arch.[182] Likewise, reciprocal "femoralization" of the proximal humerus includes tuberosity round-off and loss of the bicipital groove, resulting in a large spherical head.[182]

Laboratory

Synovial fluid analysis is usually not necessary. Routine demonstration of calcium phosphate crystals is extremely difficult, requiring special-staining techniques, or electron microscopy.

OTHER ARTHROPATHIES

Rheumatoid Arthritis of the Elderly

This condition presents typically in older persons (Fig. 45). Involvement is most often confined to the shoulders and wrists. Over a 4- to 6-month course, it can become very disabling. The rheumatoid factor is negative and ESR is elevated.

Juvenile Rheumatoid Arthritis

The shoulder is not typically involved early in the various forms of juvenile rheumatoid arthritis (JRA). When juvenile spondylitis or the polyarticular form exits, shoulder involvement is more likely, up to 25%. It is less common in the pauciarticular form. Typically, when the patients are seropositive, a rapidly destructive and severe glenohumeral involvement can be observed.[269]

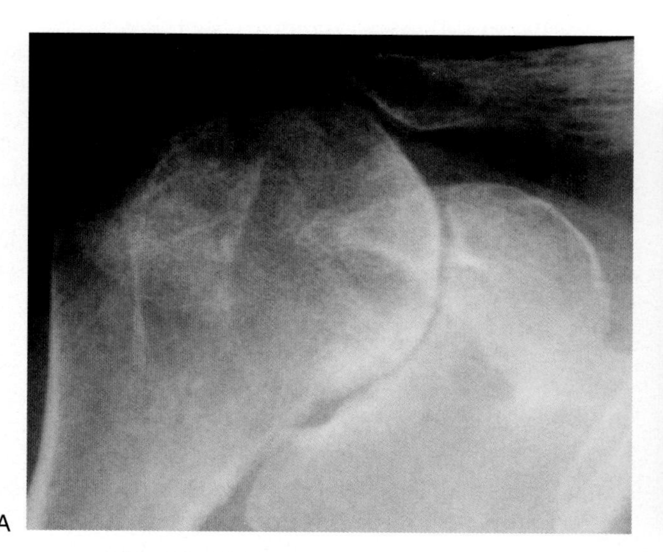
A

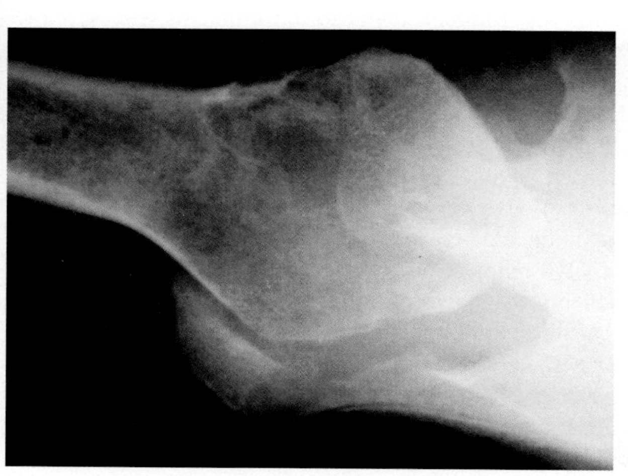
B

FIG. 44. (A,B) End-stage rotator cuff arthropathy with significant superior glenoid erosion into the acromioclavicular joint and insufficiency fracture of the acromion process.

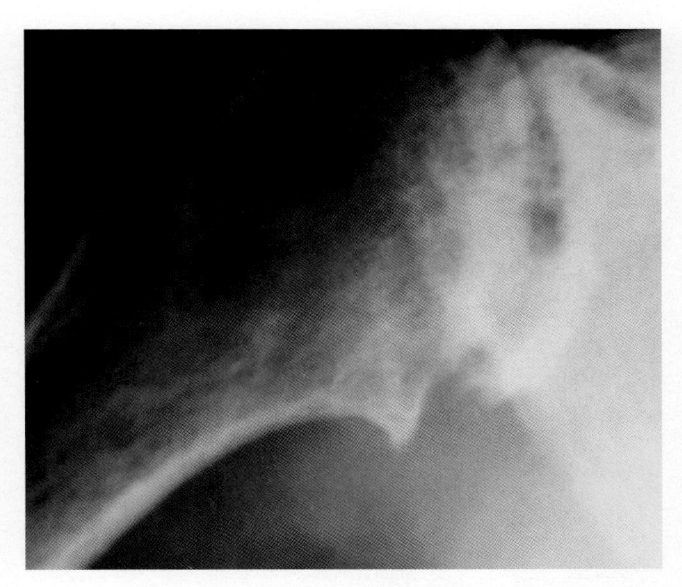

FIG. 45. Rheumatoid arthritis of the elderly.

Adult Still's disease, a rare inflammatory disease accompanied by polyarthritis with features similar to the systemic form of JRA, may affect the shoulder in up to 43% of cases at the time of presentation (Fig. 46).[47,51,248] Thirty percent to 50% of patients with more chronic arthropathy will have glenohumeral involvement.[166,248]

Rheumatoid Syndrome

Neer identified a select group of patients who manifested symptoms, signs, and radiologic changes consistent with rheumatoid arthritis.[217] Members of this group were almost exclusively women between the ages of 35 and 55. The involvement spared other joints and was almost always confined to the shoulder. Bilaterality was common; involvement was of the dry low-grade type. The rheumatoid factor was positive. Radiographic changes include glenohumeral joint space loss, cysts, and sclerotic changes (Fig. 47). Progressive disease over a short time was observed.

Spondyloarthropathies

The axial joints are typically involved, including the shoulder. Involvement of the shoulder typically occurs somewhat early in the disease process. Entities such as psoriatic arthritis, enteropathic arthritis, and ankylosing spondylitis are known to involve the shoulder.[77,180] Psoriatic arthritis involves the shoulder in 30% to 50%. A rapidly destructive form of glenohumeral change can occur, particularly in psoriasis.

In ankylosing spondylitis, the frequent involvement of the hip and shoulder (50%), although clinically mild, follows the presence of spinal disease.[147] Sometimes, the first symptoms are in the shoulder. Bilateral involvement is common. The radiographic changes include osteoporosis, joint space narrowing, and bone exostosis (Fig. 48).[262] The "hatchet sign", a characteristic destructive abnormality, involves the superior lateral aspect of the humeral head.[267] Rotator cuff tear often accompanies this lesion.

Reiter's disease may present as an acute arthritic attack, often following an enteric or urogenital infection. There may be an associated fever. There appears to be some genetic susceptibility. Acute shoulder pain will occur in 8%.[318] Seventy percent of patients are HLA-B27 positive. The shoulder is not involved to the extent of the subtalar, ankle, and hip joints. If the attack of Reiter's disease is protracted, patients are more likely to have shoulder involvement.[318] Clinically,

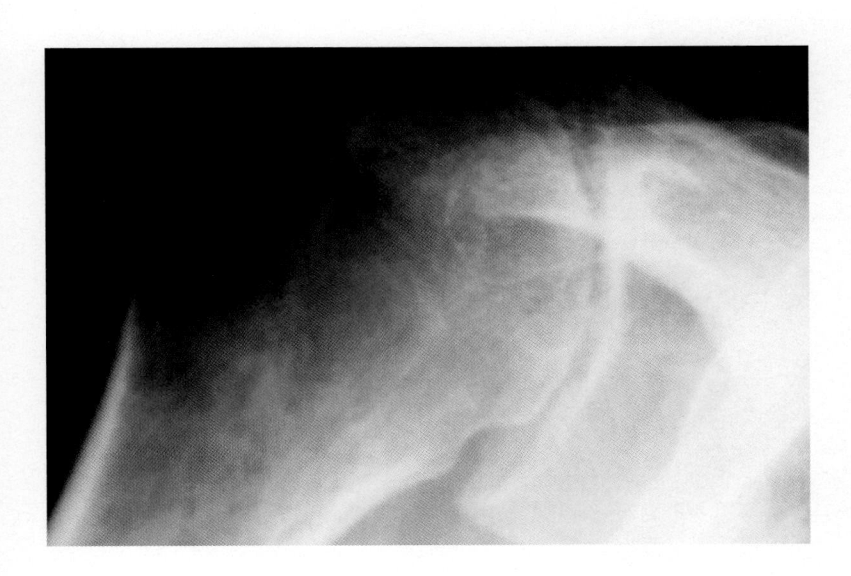

FIG. 46. Adult-onset Still's disease with distortion of the glenohumeral articulation and moderately severe glenohumeral arthritis.

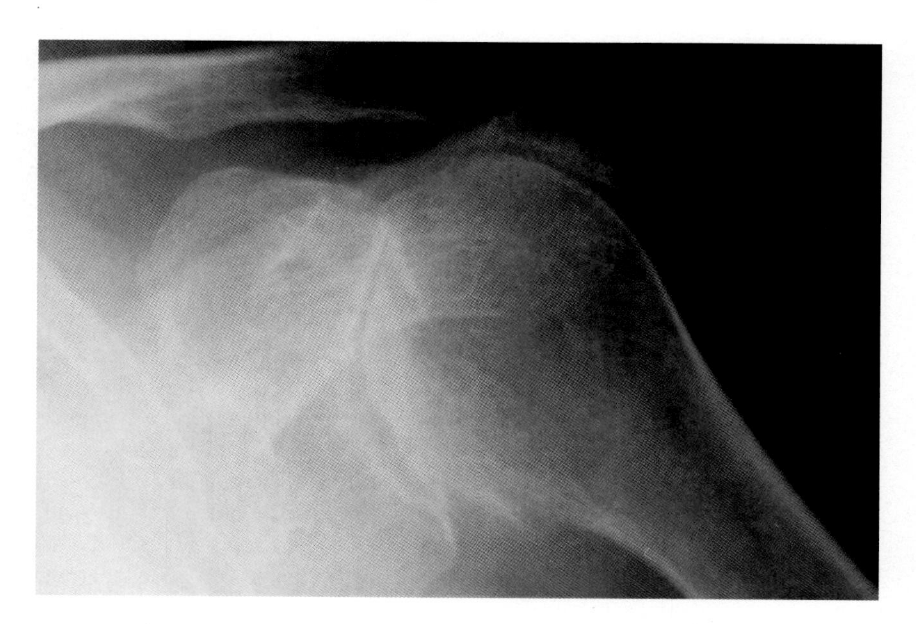

FIG. 47. Rheumatoid syndrome with a "dry type" appearance to the glenohumeral articulation.

this cannot be distinguished from other seronegative arthropathies.

Enteric arthritis parallels the activity of the inflammatory bowel disease.[199] Shoulder involvement occurs in 5% to 10% and is usually associated with sacroiliitis and spondylitis.

Erythema nodosum may result from sarcoid, tuberculosis, drug ingestion, inflammatory bowel disease, Behcet's disease, and beta-hemolytic streptococcal infections. Acute shoulder involvement can be as high as 36%.[312]

Patients with sarcoid disease will develop arthritis in 16% to 25% of cases. One-fourth of these patients will have shoulder involvement.[94,325]

Systemic lupus erythematosus (SLE) and other connective tissue diseases may have significant shoulder involvement, but these occurrences are uncommon. Sixty percent to 90% of SLE patients will develop arthritis, the most common manifestation of the disease.[162] Osteonecrosis occurs in 10% to 52%, not always associated with steroid ingestion.[1] Amyloid deposition disease will involve the shoulder in 68% of cases.[46] Usually, this is not related to glenohumeral destruction; but a problem in the soft tissues.[138] Osteopenia with associated joint destruction is a very late phenomenon.[34]

Arthropathy associated with hemochromatosis can affect the shoulder.[63,104,255] Ochronosis arthropathy affecting the

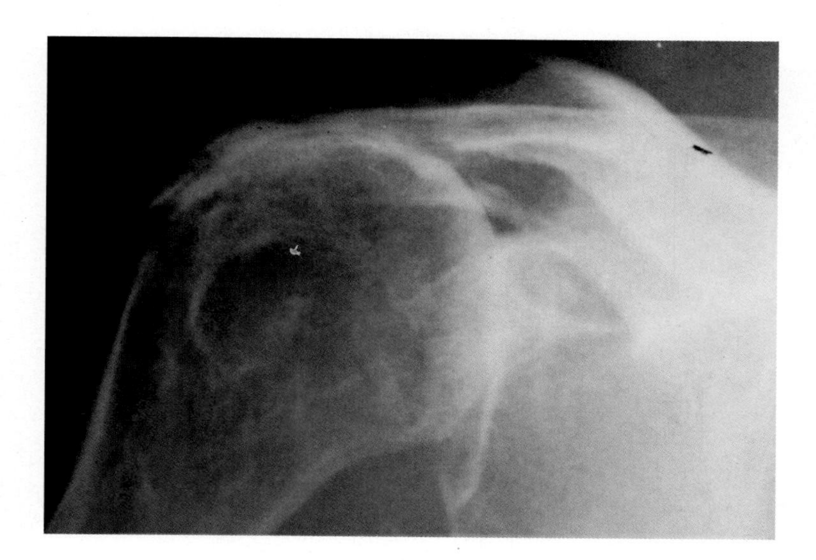

FIG. 48. Ankylosing spondylitis with accompanying loss of the rotator cuff.

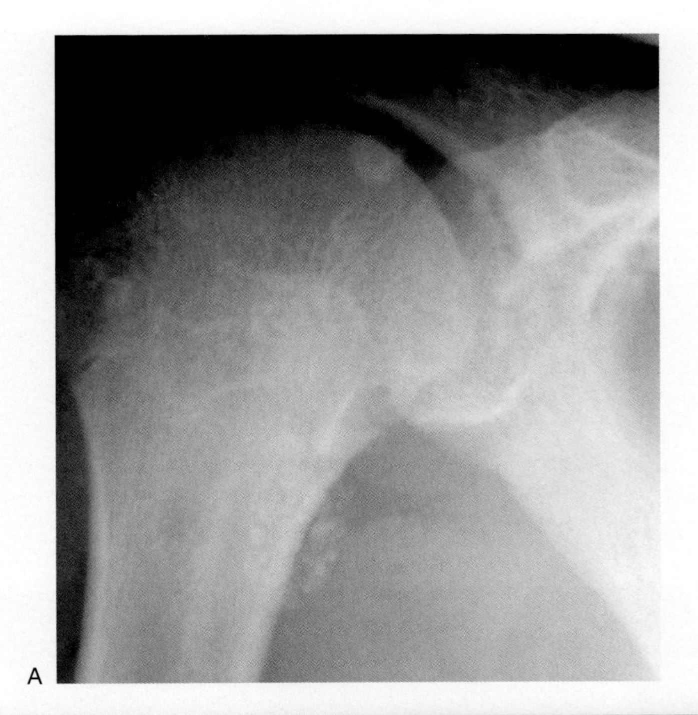

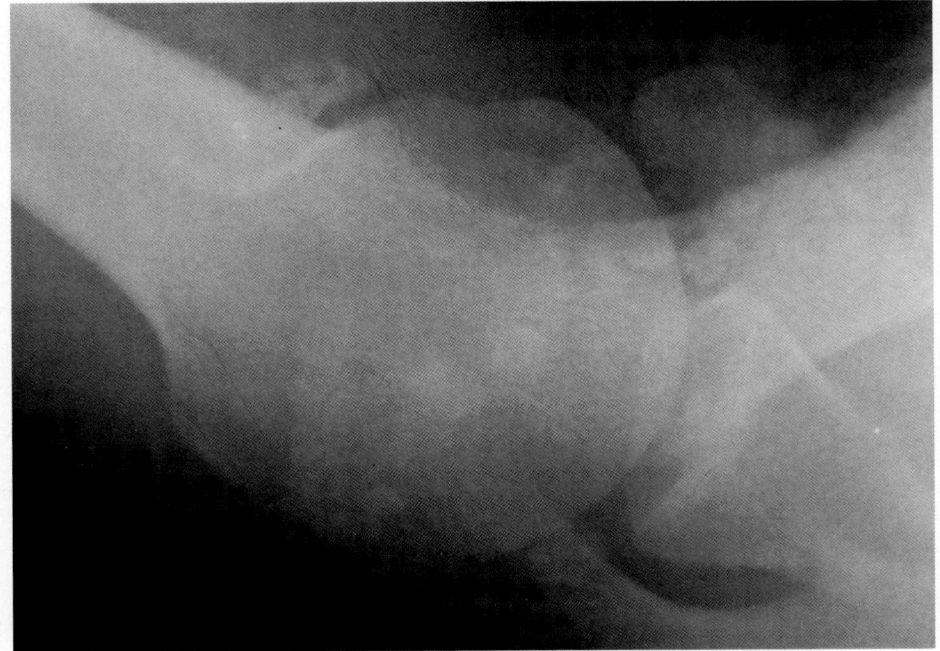

FIG. 49. (A,B) Synovial osteochondromatosis.

spine and hips precedes shoulder involvement by many years.[89] Acromegaly can result in peripheral joint arthropathy, most commonly occurring in large joints, including the shoulder.[13,243] Articular cartilage hypertrophy, a condition unique to this disorder and prone to degeneration, leads to eventual osseous disruption. Glenohumeral arthropathy has also been observed as a sequela to hyperparathyroidism and hemophilia.[68,244]

Polymyalgia rheumatica is a pain and stiffness syndrome that commonly affects the elderly. It may be difficult to distinguish from late-onset rheumatoid arthritis.[86] Constitutional symptoms include fever, malaise, and weight loss. Symmetrical shoulder involvement is common, sometimes expressed as synovitis, although large effusions are uncommon.

Synovial chondromatosis, a cartilaginous metaplasia of synovium, rarely affects the glenohumeral joint (Fig. 49)

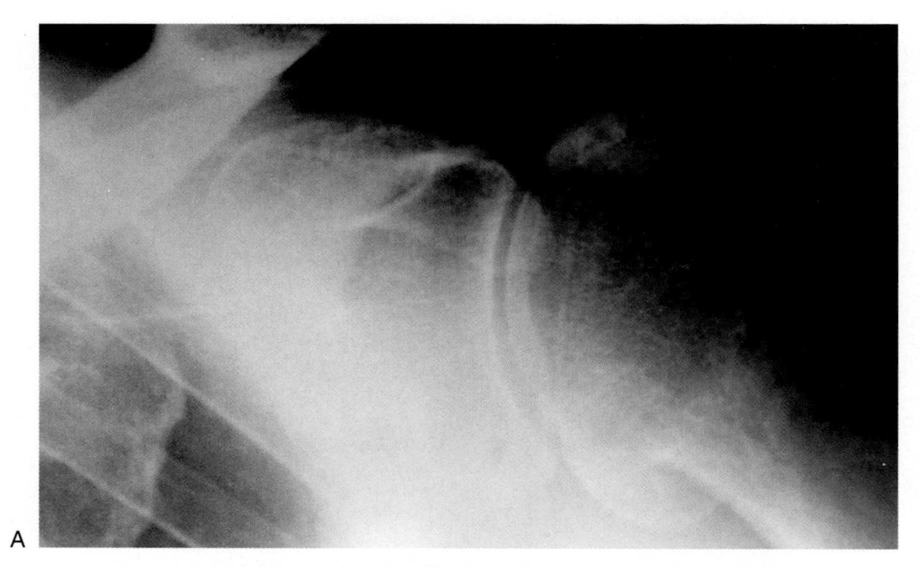

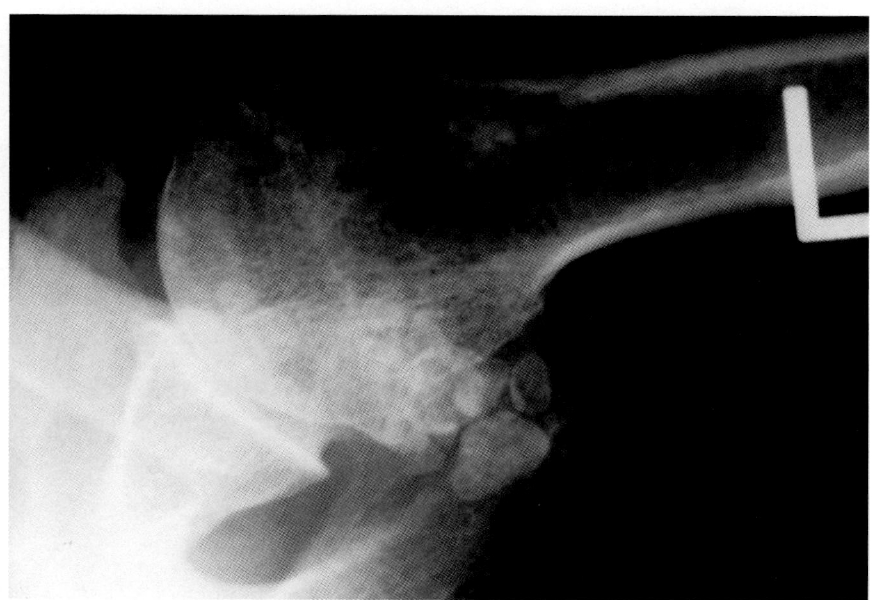

FIG. 50. (A,B) Synovial osteochondromatosis with early degenerative changes of the glenohumeral articulation.

Secondary arthropathy associated with coarse intraarticular crepitation can follow years of intermittent or continuous pain (Fig. 50).[247,317]

REFERENCES

1. Abeles M, Urman JD, Rothfield NF. Aseptic necrosis of the bone in SLE. *Arch Intern Med* 1978;138:750–754.
2. Adams R. *Illustrations of the effects of rheumatic gout or chronic rheumatic arthritis on all of the articulations: with descriptive and explanatory statements.* London: John Churchill and Sons, 1857;1–31.
3. Adams R. *A treatise of rheumatic arthritis of all the joints*, 2nd ed. London: John Churchill and Sons, 1983;1–568.
4. Albertsen M, Egund N, Jonsson E, Lidgren L. Assessment of CT of the rheumatoid shoulder with surgical correlation. *Acta Rheumatol* 1994;35:164–168.
5. Altman RD, Tenenbaum J, Latta L, et al. Biomechanical and biochemical properties of dog cartilage in experimentally induced osteoarthritis. *Ann Rheum Dis* 1984;43:83–90.
6. Anderton JM, Heim R. Multiple joint osteonecrosis following short-term steroid therapy. *J Bone Joint Surg [Am]* 1982;64:139–141.

6a. Apple AS, Pedowitz RA, Speer KP. The weighted abduction Grashey shoulder method. *Radiol Technol* 69(2): 151–156.

7. Arnett FC, Edworthy SM, Block DH, et al. The American Rheumatoid Association 1987 revised criteria for the classification of rheumatoid arthritis. *Arthritis Rheum* 1988;31: 315–324.
8. Ateshian GA, Soslowsky JL, Mow VC. Quantification of articular surface topography and cartilage thickness in knee joints using stereophotogrammetry. *J Biomech* 1991;24:761–776.
9. Bach BF. Arthroscopic removal of painful Bristow hardware. *Arthroscopy* 1990;6:324–326.
10. Ballou SP, Kushner I. In: Kelley WN, Harris ED Jr, Ruddy S, Sledge CB, eds. *Textbook of rheumatology*, 5th ed. Philadelphia: WB Saunders, 1997:699–705.
11. Beltran J, Caudill JL, Herman LLA, et al. Rheumatoid arthritis: MR imaging manifestations. *Radiology* 1987;165:153–157.

12. Bigliani LU, Weinstein DM, Glasgow MT, Pollock RG, Flatow EL. Glenohumeral arthroplasty for arthritis after instability surgery. *J Shoulder Elbow Surg* 1995;4:87–94.
13. Bluestone R, Bywaters E, Hartog M, Holt P, Hyde S. Acromegalic arthropathy. *Ann Rheum Dis* 1971;30:243–258.
14. Bongartz G, Bock E, Horbach T, Requardt H. Degenerative cartilage lesions of the hip—magnetic resonance evaluation. *Magn Reson Imaging* 1989;7:179–186.
15. Borg E, Rasker J. Gout in the elderly, a separate entity? *Ann Rheum Dis* 1987;46:72–76.
16. Brandt KD, Braunstein EM, Visco DM, et al. Anterior (cranial) cruciate ligament transection in the dog: a bona fide model of osteoarthritis, not merely of cartilage injury and repair. *J Rheumatol* 1991;18: 436–446.
17. Brandt K, Fife RS. Ageing in relation to the pathogenesis of osteoarthritis. *Clin Rheum Dis* 1986;12:117–130.
18. Brems JJ. Shoulder replacement in arthritis of dislocation. *Orthop Trans* 1989;13:235.
19. Broderick LS, Turner PA, Renfrew DL, Snitzen TJ, Huff JP, Harris C. Severity of articular cartilage abnormality in patients with osteoarthritis: evolution with fast spin-echo MR versus arthroscopy. *Am J Roentgenol* 1994;162:99–103.
20. Brown DG, Edwards NL, Greer JM, et al. Magnetic resonance imaging in patients with inflammatory arthritis of the knee. *Clin Rheumatol* 1990;9:73–83.
21. Bullough PG. The pathology of osteoarthritis. In: Moskowitz RW, Howell DS, Goldberg VM, et al., eds. *Osteoarthritis diagnosis and medical/surgical management*, 2nd ed. Philadelphia: WB Saunders, 1992:39–69.
22. Burkart SS. Flouroscopic comparison of kinematic patterns in massive rotator cuff tears. A suspension bridge model. *Clin Orthop* 1992;284: 144–152.
23. Campion GV, McCrae F, Alwan W, et al. Idiopathic destructive arthritis of the shoulder. *Semin Arthritis Rheum* 1988;17:232–245.
24. Cawston T, Dieppe P, Mercer E, et al. Milwaukee shoulder—synovial fluid contains no active collagenase. *Br J Rheumatol* 1987;26: 311–312.
25. Chan WP, Lang P, Chieng PU, et al. Three-dimensional imaging of the musculoskeletal system: an overview. *J Formosan Med Assoc* 1991;90:713–722.
26. Chard M, Hazleman B. Shoulder disorders in the elderly. *Ann Rheum Dis* 1987;46:684–689.
27. Christensen SB. Osteoarthritis changes in bone, cartilage and synovial membrane in relation to bone scintigraphy. *Acta Orthop Scand Suppl* 1985;214:1–43.
28. Chryssanthou CP. Dysbaric osteonecrosis: etiological and pathogenic concepts. *Clin Orthop* 1978;130:94–106.
29. Chung SMK, Alavi A, Russell MO. Management of osteonecrosis in sickle-cell anemia and its genetic variants. *Clin Orthop* 1978;130: 158–174.
30. Chung SMK, Ralston EL. Necrosis of the humeral head associated with sickle cell anemia and its genetic variants. *Clin Orthop* 1971;80: 105–107.
31. Codman ET. *The shoulder. Rupture of the supraspinatus tendon and other lesions in or about the subacromial bursa*. Boston: Thomas Todd, 1934.
32. Cofield RH. Total shoulder arthroplasty: associated disease of the rotator cuff, results, complications. In: Bateman JE, Welsh RP, eds. *Surgery of the shoulder*. Philadelphia: BC Decker, 1984:229–233.
33. Cofield RH. Unconstrained total shoulder prosthesis. *Clin Orthop* 1983;173:97–108.
34. Cohen AS, Canoso JJ. Rheumatological aspects of amyloid disease. *Clin Rheum Dis* 1975;1:149–161.
35. Cohen MG, Emerson BT. Gout. In: Klippel JH, Dieppe PA, eds. *Rheumatology*. St Louis: Mosby, 1994:7.12.1–12.16.
36. Cohick CB, Furst DE, Quagliata S, et al. Analysis of elevated serum interleukin-6 levels in rheumatoid arthritis: correlation with erythrocyte sedimentation rate or C-reactive protein. *J Lab Clin Med* 1994; 123:721–727.
37. Cole PR, Jasani MK, Wood B, et al. High resolution, high field magnetic resonance imaging of joints: unexpected features in proton images of cartilage. *Br J Radiol* 1990;63:907–909.
38. Collins DN, Nelson CL. Infections of the hip. Table 31-2. In: Steinberg MD, ed. *The hip and its disorders*. Philadelphia: WB Saunders, 1991:657.
39. Craig EV. The geyser sign and torn rotator cuff: clinical significance and pathomechanics. *Clin Orthop* 1984;191: 213–215.
40. Crossan JF. Pathology of the rheumatoid shoulder. In: Watson MS, ed. *Surgical disorders of the shoulder*. Edinburgh: Churchill Livingston, 1991:195–202.
41. Crossan JF, Vallance R. The shoulder joint in rheumatoid arthritis. In: Bayley I, Kessel L, eds. *Shoulder surgery*. New York: Springer-Verlag, 1982:131–143.
42. Cruess RL. Corticosteroid-induced osteonecrosis of the humeral head. *Orthop Clin North Am* 1985;16:789–796.
43. Cruess RL. Experience with steroid-induced avascular necrosis of the shoulder and etiologic considerations regarding osteonecrosis of the hip. *Clin Orthop* 1978;130:86–93.
44. Cruess RL. Osteonecrosis of bone: current concepts as to etiology and pathogenesis. *Clin Orthop* 1986;208:30–39.
45. Cruess RL. Steroid-induced avascular necrosis of the head of the humerus. Natural history and management. *J Bone Joint Surg [Br]* 1976;58:313–317.
46. Curran JF, Ellman MH, Brown NL. Rheumatologic aspects of painful conditions affecting the shoulder. *Clin Orthop* 1983;173:27–37.
47. Cush JJ, Medsger TA Jr, Christy WC, Herbert DC, Cooperstein LA. Adult-onset Still's disease: clinical course and outcome. *Arthritis Rheum* 1987;30:186–194.
48. Cushnaghan J, Dieppe PA. Study of 500 patients with limb joint osteoarthritis. I. Analysis by age, sex and distribution of symptomatic joint sites. *Ann Rheum Dis* 1991;50:8–13.
49. David HG, Bridgman SA, Davies SC, Hine AL, Emery RJH. The shoulder in sickle-cell disease. *J Bone Joint Surg [Br]* 1993;75B: 538–545.
50. de Bois HMW, Arndt JW, Tak PP, et al. ^{99m}Tc labeled polyclonal human immunoglobulin G scintigraphy before and after intra-articular knee injection of triamcinolone hexacetonide in patients with rheumatoid arthritis. *Nucl Med Commun* 1993;14:883–887.
51. Del Paine DW, Leek JC. Still's arthritis in adults: disease or syndrome? *J Rheumatol* 1983;10:758–762.
52. DePalma AF. Arthritides of the synovial joints of the shoulder. In: Depalma AF, ed. *Surgery of the shoulder*, 3rd ed. Philadelphia: JB Lippincott, 1983:305.
53. DePalma AF. Biologic aging of the shoulder. In: DePalma AF, ed. *Surgery of the shoulder*, 3rd ed. Philadelphia: JB Lippincott, 1983: 211–241.
54. DePalma AF, Cautilli RA. Fractures of the upper end of the humerus. *Clin Orthop* 1961;20:73–93.
55. DePalma AF, Gallery G, Bennett GA. Variational anatomy and degenerative lesions of the shoulder joint. *Instr Course Lect* 1949;6: 255–281.
56. DeSmet AA, Ting YM, Weiss JJ. Shoulder arthrography in rheumatoid arthritis. *Diagn Radiol* 1975;116:601–605.
57. Dieppe PA, Huskisson EC, Crocker P, Willoughby DA. Apatite deposition disease: a new arthropathy. *Lancet* 1976;1: 266–269.
58. Dieppe PA, Alexander GM, Jones H, Doherty M, Scott DG. Pyrophosphate arthropathy: a clinical and radiological study of 105 cases. *Ann Rheum Dis* 1982;41:371–376.
59. Dieppe PA, Doherty M, Macfarlane D, Hutton C, Bradfield J, Watt I. Apatite associated destructive arthritis. *Br J Rheumatol* 1984;23: 84–91.
60. Doherty M, Dieppe PA. Clinical aspects of calcium pyrophosphate dihydrate crystal deposition. *Rheum Dis Clin North Am* 1988;14: 395–414.
61. Domljan C, Dodig D. The value of early and late ^{99m}Tc methylene diphosphonate scintigrams of hands in patients with rheumatoid arthritis and other inflammatory rheumatic diseases. *Z Rheumatol* 1984;45:444–447.
62. Donohue JM, Buss D, Oegema TR Jr, et al. The effects of indirect blunt trauma on adult canine articular cartilage. *J Bone Joint Surg [Am]* 1983:65:948–957.
63. Dymock IW, Hamilton EBD, Laws JW, Williams R. Arthropathy of hemochromatosis. *Ann Rheum Dis* 1970;29:469–476.
64. Edelson JG. Bony changes of the glenoid as a consequence of shoulder instability. *J Shoulder Elbow Surg* 1996;4:293–298.
65. Eisenberg JM, Schumacher RH, Davidson PK, Kaufmann L. Usefulness of synovial fluid analysis in the evaluation of joint effusions. *Arch Intern Med* 1984:144;715–719.
66. Ellman H, Harris E, Kay SP. Early degenerative joint disease simulat-

ing impingement syndrome: arthroscopic findings. *Arthroscopy* 1992; 8:482–487.
67. Ennevaara K. Painful shoulder joint in rheumatoid arthritis: a clinical and radiological study of 200 cases with special reference to arthrography of the glenohumeral joint. *Acta Rheumatol Scand* 1967;(11): 1–116.
68. Epps CH Jr. Painful hematologic conditions affecting the shoulder. *Clin Orthop* 1983;173:38–43.
69. Fassbender HG, Simmling-Annefield M. The potential aggressiveness of synovial tissue in rheumatoid arthritis. *J Pathol* 1983;139:399–406.
70. Fast A, Alon M, Weiss S, Ser-Aviv FR. Avascular necrosis of bone following short-term dexamethasone therapy for brain edema. *J Neurosurg* 1984;61:983–985.
71. Felson DT, Anderson JJ, Naimark A, et al. The presence of chondrocalcinosis in the elderly and its association with knee osteoarthritis: the Framingham study. *J Rheumatol* 1989;16:1241–1245.
72. Ficat RP, Arlet J. Necrosis of the femoral head. In: Hungerford DS, ed. *Ischemia and necrosis of bone*. Baltimore: Williams & Wilkins, 1980: 53–75.
73. Ficat RP, Arlet J. Necrosis of the femoral head. In: Hungerford DS, ed. *Ischemia and necrosis of bone*. Baltimore: Williams & Wilkins, 1980: 29–52.
74. Fisher DE. The role of fat embolism in the etiology of corticosteroid-induced avascular necrosis: clinical and experimental results. *Clin Orthop* 1978;130:68–80.
75. Fisher DE, Bickel W II. Corticosteroid-induced avascular necrosis: Clinical study of 77 patients. *J Bone Joint Surg [Am]* 1971;53: 859–873.
76. Flatow EL, Soslowsky LJ, Ateshian GA, et al. Shoulder joint anatomy and the effect of subluxations and size mismatch on patterns of glenohumeral contact. *Orthop Trans* 1991;15:803–804.
77. Fournie B, Railhac J-J, Monod P, et al. The enthesopathic shoulder. *Rev Rheum Mal Osteoartic* 1987;54:447–451.
78. Fourrier P, Martini M. Post-traumatic avascular necrosis of the humeral head. *Int Orthop* 1977;1:187–190.
79. Friedman RJ, Hawthorne KB, Genez BM. The use of computerized axial tomography in the measurement of glenoid version. *J Bone Joint Surg [Am]* 1992;74:1032–1037.
80. Friedman RJ, Thornhill TS, Thomas WH, Sledge CB. Nonconstrained total shoulder replacement in patients who have rheumatoid arthritis and class-IV function. *J Bone Joint Surg [Am]* 1989;71:494–498.
81. Garancis J, Cheung H, Halverson P, McCarty D. Milwaukee shoulder—association of microspheroids containing hydroxyapatite crystals, active collagenase and neutral protease with rotator cuff defects III. Morphologic and biochemical studies of an excised synovium showing chondromatosis. *Arthritis Rheum* 1981;24:484–491.
82. Gatter RA. Use of the compensated polarized microscope. *Clin Rheum Dis* 1977;3:91–103.
83. Gatter RA, Schumacher HR. *A practical handbook of joint fluid analysis*. 2nd ed. Philadelphia: Lea & Febiger, 1991.
84. Geneste R, et al. Closed treatment of fracture–dislocations of the shoulder joint. *Rev Chir Orthop* 1980;66:383–386.
85. Gerber C, Schneeberger AG, Vinh TS. The arterial vascularization of the humeral head. *J Bone Joint Surg [Am]* 1990;72:1486–1494.
86. Gibson T, Grahame R. Acute arthritis in the elderly. *Age Ageing* 1973; 2:3–13.
87. Gilday DL, Paul DJ, Paterson J. Diagnosis of osteomyelitis in children by combined blood pool and bone imaging. *Radiology* 1975;117: 331–335.
88. Goldenberg DL, Egan MS, Cohen AS. Inflammatory synovitis in degenerative joint disease. *J Rheumatol* 1982;9:204–209.
89. Grantham A, Neer CS II. Alkaptonuric ochronosis. *NY Orthop Hosp Bull* 1960;4:11.
90. Gray ML, Pizzanelli AM, Grodzinsky AJ, et al. Mechanical and physiochemical determinants of the chondrocyte biosynthetic response. *J Orthop Res* 1988;6:777–792.
91. Green A, Norris TR. Imaging techniques for glenohumeral arthritis and glenohumeral arthroplasty. *Clin Orthop* 1994;307:7–17.
92. Gschwend N, Kentsch A. Arthritic disorders. Surgery of the rheumatoid shoulder. In: Bateman JE, Welsh PR, eds. *Surgery of the shoulder*. Philadelphia: BC Decker, 1984:269–280.
93. Guilak F, Ratcliffe A, Lane N, et al. Mechanical and biochemical changes in the superficial zone of articular cartilage in a canine model of osteoarthritis. *J Orthop Res* 1994;12:474–484.
94. Gumpel JM, Johns CJ, Shulman LE. The joint disease of sarcoidosis. *Ann Rheum Dis* 1967;26:194–205.
95. Gylys-Morin V, Hajek PC, Sartons W, Resnick D. Articular cartilage defects: detectability in cadaver knees with MR. *Am J Roentgenol* 1987;148:1153–1157.
96. Hadler NM, Franck NA, Bress NM, Robinson DR. Acute polyarticular gout. *Am J Med* 1974;56:714–719.
97. Hagg O, Lundberg B. Aspects of prognostic factors in comminuted and displaced proximal humerus fractures. In: Bateman JE, Welsh RP, eds. *Surgery of the shoulder*. Philadelphia: BC Decker, 1984:51–59.
98. Hall AC, Urban JP, Gehl KA. The effects of hydrostatic pressure on matrix synthesis in articular cartilage. *J Orthop Res* 1991;9:1–10.
99. Hall F, Wyshak G. Thickness of articular cartilage in the normal knee. *J Bone Joint Surg [Am]* 1980;62:408–413.
100. Hall LD, Tyler JA. Can quantitative magnetic resonance imaging detect and monitor the progression of early arthritis? In: Kuettner KE, Goldberg VM, eds. *Osteoarthritic disorders*. American Academy of Orthopaedic Surgery, 1995:67–84.
101. Halverson PB, Cheung HS, McCarty DJ, Garancis J, Mandel N. Milwaukee shoulder—association of microspheroids containing hydroxyapatite crystals, active collagenase and neutral protease with rotator cuff defects II. Synovial fluid studies. *Arthritis Rheum* 1981;24: 474–483.
102. Halverson PB, McCarty DJ, Cheung AS, Ryan LM. Milwaukee shoulder syndrome: 11 additional cases with involvement of the knee in 7 (basic calcium phosphate crystal deposition disease). *Semin Arthritis Rheum* 1984;14:36–44.
103. Hamilton EBD. Diseases associated with calcium pyrophosphate deposition disease. *Arthritis Rheum* 1976;19:353–357.
104. Hamilton EBD, Bomford AB, Laws JW, Williams R. The natural history of arthritis in idiopathic haemochromatosis. Progression of the clinical and radiological features over ten years. *Q J Med* 1981;50: 321–329.
105. Harris ED Jr. Mechanisms of disease: rheumatoid arthritis—pathology and implications for treatment. *N Engl J Med* 1990;322: 1277–1289.
106. Harryman DT Jr, Sidles JA, Clark JM, McQuade KJ, Gibb TD, Matsen FA III. Translation of the humeral head on the glenoid with passive glenohumeral motion. *J Bone Joint Surg [Am]* 1990;72: 1334–1343.
107. Haskard DO, Grahame R. Management of chronic inflammatory arthropathy. In: Watson MS, ed. *Surgical disorders of the shoulder*. New York: Churchill-Livingston, 1991:203–215.
108. Hattrup SJ, Cofield RH. Osteonecrosis of the humeral head. Natural history. Presented at American Shoulder and Elbow Surgeons 13th Open Meeting. San Francisco, California. February 16, 1997.
109. Hawkins RH, Hawkins RJ. Failed anterior reconstruction for shoulder instabilty. *J Bone Joint Surg [Br]* 1985;67:709–714.
110. Hawkins RJ, Angelo RL. Glenohumeral osteoarthritis: a late complication of Putt-Platt repair. *J Bone Joint Surg [Am]* 1990;72: 1193–1197.
111. Hawkins RJ, Bell RH, Gurr K. The three-part fracture of the proximal part of the humerus. *J Bone Joint Surg [Am]* 1986;68:1410–1414.
112. Hawkins RJ, Neer CS II, Pianta RM, Mendoza FX. Locked posterior dislocation of the shoulder. *J Bone Joint Surg [Am]* 1987;69:9–18.
113. Hayes CW, Conway WF. Evaluation of articular cartilage: radiographic and cross sectional imaging techniques. *Radiographics* 1992; 12:409–428.
114. Hernando, P, Reginato A, Schumacher H. Alizarin red S staining as a screening test to detect compounds in synovial fluid. *Arthritis Rheum* 1983;26:191–200.
115. Hill AV. Production and absorption of work by muscle. *Science* 1960; 131:897.
116. Hindmarsh J, Lindberg A. Eden-Hybinett's operation for recurrent dislocation of the humeroscapular joint. *Acta Orthop Scand* 1967;38: 459–478.
117. Hochberg MC. Adult and juvenile rheumatoid arthritis: current epidemiologic concepts. *Epidemiol Rev* 1981;3:27–44.
118. Holder J, Loredo RA, Longo C, Truddell D, Yu JS, Resnick D. Assessment of articular cartilage thickness of the humeral head: MR—anatomic correlation in cadavers. *Am J Roentgenol* 1995;165: 615–620.
119. Holder J, Trudell D, Pathria MN, Resnick D. Width of the articular cartilage of the hip: quantification by using fat-suppression spin-echo MR imaging in cadavers. *Am J Roentgenol* 1992;159:351–355.

120. Hovelius L, Akemark-nark C, Allorektsson B, et al. Bristow-Laterjet procedure for recurrent anterior dislocation of the shoulder: a 2–5 year follow-up on the results of 112 cases. *Acta Orthop Scand* 1983;54: 284–290.
121. Hovelius L, Augustine B, Fredin H, Johansson O, Norlin R, Thorling J. Primary anterior dislocation of the shoulder in young patients. *J Bone Joint Surg [Am]* 1996;78:1677–1684.
122. Hovelius L, Thorling J, Fredin H. Recurrent anterior dislocation of the shoulder: results after the Bankart and Putti-Platt operations. *J Bone Joint Surg [Am]* 1979;61:566–569.
123. Huber DJ, Sauter R, Mueller E, Requardt H, Webe H. MR imaging of the normal shoulder. *Radiology* 1986:158;405–408.
124. Huber HM. Incidence of recurrence and osteoarthritis after rotational humeral osteotomy according to Weber. *J Bone Joint Surg [Br]* 1992; 74(supp):7.
125. Huber H, Gerber C. Voluntary subluxation of the shoulder in children. *J Bone Joint Surg [Br]* 1994;76:118–122.
126. Hungerford DS, Lennox DW. The importance of increased intraosseous pressure in the development of osteonecrosis of the femoral head: implications for treatment. *Orthop Clin North Am* 1985;16: 635–654.
127. Hungerford DS, Zizic TM. Alcoholism associated ischemic necrosis of the femoral head. *Clin Orthop* 1978;130:144–153.
128. Inman VT, Saunders JB, Abbott LC. Observations on the functions of the shoulder joint. *J Bone Joint Surg* 1944;26:1–30.
129. Jakob RP, Kristiansen T, Mayo K, et al. Classification and aspects of treatment of fractures of the proximal humerus. In: Bateman JE, Welsh RP, eds. *Surgery of the shoulder*. Philadelphia: BC Decker, 1984:330–343.
130. Jakob RP, Miniaci A, Anson PS, Jaberg H, Osterwalder A, Ganz R. Four-part valgus impacted fractures of the proximal humerus. *J Bone Joint Surg [Br]* 1991;73:295–298.
131. Janossy G, Panayi GS, Duke O, Bofill M, Poulter LW, Goldstein G. Rheumatoid arthritis: a disease of T-lymphocyte/macrophage immunoregulation. *Lancet* 1981;2:839–842.
132. Jones IL, Klamfeldt A, Sandstrom T. The effect of continuous mechanical pressure upon the turnover of articular cartilage PGs in vitro. *Clin Orthop* 1982;165:283–289.
133. Jones JP Jr, Behnke AR Jr. Prevention of dysbaric osteonecrosis in compressed-air workers. *Clin Orthop* 1978;130:118–128.
134. Jones JP Jr, Engleman EP. Osseous avascular necrosis associated with systemic abnormalities. *Arthritis Rheum* 1966;9:728–736.
135. Jones JP Jr, Sakovich L. Fat embolism of bone. *J Bone Joint Surg [Am]* 1966;48:149–164.
136. Jurmain RD. The pattern of involvement of appendicular degenerative joint disease. *Am J Phys Anthropol* 1980;53:143–150.
137. Kahan A, Amor B, Benhamou C. Rapidly progressive idiopathic chondrolysis simulating tuberculosis of the shoulder. *J Rheumatol* 1983;10:291–293.
138. Katz GA, Peter JB, Pearson CM, Adams WJ. The shoulder pad sign: a diagnostic feature of amyloid arthropathy. *N Engl J Med* 1973;288: 354–355.
139. Katz WA. Role of proteoglycans in the development of gouty arthritis. In: Kelly WN, Weiner IM, eds. *Uric acid*. (*Handbook experimental pharmaceutics*). Berlin:Springer-Verlag, 1978;51: 347–377.
140. Kawashima M, Torisu T, Hayashi K, Kitano M. Pathological review of osteonecrosis in divers. *Clin Orthop* 1978;130:107–117.
141. Kelley WN, Fox IH. Gout and related disorders of purine metabolisn. In: Kelley WN, Harris ED, Ruddy S, Sledge CB, eds. *Textbook of rheumatology*. Philadelphia:WB Saunders, 1985:1359–1398.
142. Kelley WN, Harris ED Jr, Ruddy S, Sledge CB, eds. *Textbook of rheumatology*, 5th ed. Philadelphia: WB Saunders, 1997.
143. Kellgren JH, Lawrence JS, Bier F. Genetic factors in generalized osteoarthrosis. *Ann Rheum Dis* 1963;22:237–255.
144. Kenzora JE, Glimcher MJ. Accumulative cell stress: the multifactorial etiology of idiopathic osteonecrosis. *Orthop Clin North Am* 1985;16: 669–679.
145. Kernwein GA. Roentgenographic diagnosis of shoulder dysfunction. *JAMA* 1965;194:179–183.
146. Kerr R, Resnick D, Pineda C, Haghighi P. Osteoarthritis of the glenohumeral joint: a radiologic–pathologic study. *Am J Roentgenol* 1985; 144:967–972.
147. Khan MA, Kushner I. Diagnosis of ankylosing spondylitis. In: Cohen AS, ed. *Progress in clinical rheumatology*, Vol 1. Orlando: Grune & Stratton, 1984:145–178.
148. Kinne RW, Becker W, Schwab J, et al. Comparison of ^{99}MTc labeled specific murine CD-4 monoclonal antibodies and nonspecific human immunoglobulin for aging inflamed joints in rheumatoid arthritis. *Nucl Med Commun* 1993;14:667–675.
149. Kirk JA. The painful shoulder. *NZ Med J* 1977;151–153.
150. Klippel JH, Dieppe PA, eds. *Rheumatology*. St Louis: Mosby, 1994.
151. Knight, RA, Mayne JA. Comminuted fractures and fracture–dislocations involving the articular surface of the humeral head. *J Bone Joint Surg [Am]* 1957;39:1343–1355.
152. Knight SM, Ring EFJ, Bhalla AK. Bone mineral density and osteoarthritis. *Ann Rheum Dis* 1992;51:1025–1026.
153. Kohn NN, Hughes RE, McCarty DJ, Faires JS. The significance of calcium pyrophosphate crystals in the synovial fluid of arthritic patients: the "pseudogout syndrome." II. Identification of crystals. *Ann Intern Med* 1962;56:738–745.
154. Konig H, Sieper J, Wolf KJ. Rheumatoid arthritis: evaluation of hypervascular and fibrous pannus with dynamic MR imaging enhanced with Gd-DTPA. *Radiology* 1990;176:473–477.
155. Koo HH, Kim R, Cho SH, Song HR, Lee G, Ko GH. Angiography, scintigraphy, intraosseous pressure, and histologic findings in high-risk osteonecrotic femoral heads with negative magnetic resonance images. *Clin Orthop* 1994;308:127–138.
156. Kramer J, Recht MP, Imhof H, et al. Postcontrast MR arthrography in assessment of cartilage lesions. *J Comput Assist Tomogr* 1994;18: 218–224.
157. Kristiansen B, Christensen SW. Plate fixation of proximal humerus fractures. *Acta Orthop Scand* 1986;57:320–323.
158. Kristiansen B, Christensen SW. Proximal humeral fractures. Late results in relation to classification and treatment. *Acta Orthop Scand* 1987;58:124–127.
159. Krueger FJ. A vitallium replica arthroplasty on the shoulder. A case report of aseptic necrosis of the proximal end of the humerus. *Surgery* 1951;30:1005–1011.
160. Kulka JP, Bocking D, Ropes MW, et al. Early joint lesions of rheumatoid arthritis. *Arch Pathol* 1955;59:129–150.
161. Kushner I. Regulation of the acute phase response by cytokines. *Prospect Biol Med* 1993;36:611–622.
162. Lahita RG. Clinical presentation of systemic lupus erythematosus. In: Kelley WN, Harris ED Jr, Ruddy S, Sledge CB, eds. *Textbook of rheumatology*, 5th ed. Philadelphia: WB Saunders, 1997:1028–1039.
163. Laing PG. The arterial supply of the adult humerus. *J Bone Joint Surg [Am]* 1956;38:1105–1116.
164. Landells JW. The bone cysts of osteoarthritis. *J Bone Joint Surg [Br]* 1953;35:643–649.
165. Laroche M, Arlet J, Mazieres B. Osteonecrosis of the femoral and humeral heads after intraarticular corticosteroid injections. *J Rheumatol* 1990;17:549–551.
166. Larsen A, Dale K, Eek M. Radiographic evaluation of rheumatoid arthritis and related conditions by standard reference film. *Acta Radiol Diagn* 1977;18:481–491.
167. Larson EB. Adult Still's disease. Evolution of a clinical syndrome and diagnosis, treatment, and follow-up of 17 patients. *Medicine* 1984;63: 82–91.
168. Lazarus MD, Harryman DT II, Yung SW, Sidles JA. Anterosuperior humeral displacement: limitation by the coracromial arch. *J Shoulder Elbow Surg* 1996;5(2 of part 2 supp):57.
169. L'Bisolata JL, Pagorani MJ, Warren RF, Dines, DM. Humeral head osteonecrosis: clinical course and radiographic predictors of outcomes. *J Shoulder Elbow Surg* 1996;5:355–361.
170. Lee CK, Hansen HR. Post-traumatic avascular necrosis of the humeral head in displaced proximal humeral fractures. *J Trauma* 1981;21: 788–791.
171. Levinson D, Becker MA. Clinical gout and pathogenesis of hyperuricemia. In: McCarty DJ, Koopman WJ, eds. *Arthritis and allied conditions*. Philadephia: Lea & Febiger, 1993:1773–1806.
172. Linn FC, Radin EL. Lubication of animal joints. III. The effect of certain chemical alterations of the cartilage and lubricant. *Arthritis Rheum* 1968;11:674–682.
173. Loeb JN. The influence of temperature on the solubility of monosodium urate. *Arthritis Rheum* 1972;15:189–192.
174. Lombardo SJ, Kerlan RK, Jobe FW, Cartar VS, Blazina ME, Shields CL. The modified Bristow procedure for recurrent dislocation of the shoulder. *J Bone Joint Surg [Am]* 1976;58:256–261.
175. Lusard DA, Wirth MA, Wurtz D, Rockwood CA Jr. Loss of external

rotation following anterior capsulorrhaphy of the shoulder. *J Bone Joint Surg [Am]* 1993;75:1185–1192.
176. Lyons FR, Rockwood CA. Migration of the pins used in operations on the shoulder. *J Bone Joint Surg [Am]* 1990;72:1262–1267.
177. MacDonald PB, Hawkins RJ, Fowler PJ, Miniaci A. Release of the subscapularis for internal rotation contracture and pain after anterior repair for recurrent anterior dislocation of the shoulder. *J Bone Joint Surg [Am]* 1992;74:734–737.
178. Magnuson PB, Stack JK. Recurrent dislocation of the shoulder. *JAMA* 1943:123;889–892.
179. Majd M, Frankel RS. Radionuclide imaging in skeletal inflammatory and ischemic disease in children. *Am J Roentgenol* 1976;126: 832–841.
180. Marks SH, Barnett M, Calin A. Ankylosing spondylitis in women and men: a case control study. *J Rheumatol* 1983;10:624–628.
181. Matsen FA III, Lippit SB, Sidles JB, Harryman DT II. *Practical evaluation and management of the shoulder*. Philadelphia: WB Saunders, 1994:198.
182. Matsen FA III, Lippit SB, Sidles JB, Harryman DT II. *Practical evaluation and management of the shoulder*. Philadelphia: WB Saunders, 1994:219.
183. Matsen FA III, Lippit SB, Sidles JB, Harryman DT II. *Practical evaluation and management of the shoulder*. Philadelphia: WB Saunders, 1994:118–120.
184. Matsen FA III, Ziegler DW, DeBartolo SE. Patient self-assessment of health status and function in glenohumeral degenerative joint disease. *J Shoulder Elbow Surg* 1995;4:345–351.
185. McCallum RI, Walder DN. Bone lesions in compressed air workers with special reference to men who worked in the Clyde Tunnel. *J Bone Joint Surg [Br]* 1966;48:207–235.
186. McCarty DJ Jr. Calcium pyrophosphate dihydrate deposition disease. *Arthritis Rheum* 1975;19:275–285.
187. McCarty DJ Jr. Gout without hyperuricemia. *JAMA* 1994;271: 302–303.
188. McCarty DJ Jr. Phagocytosis of urate crystals in gouty spinal fluid. *Am J Med Sci* 1962;243:288–295.
189. McCarty DJ Jr, Koopman WJ, eds. *Arthritis and allied conditions*, 12th ed. Philadelphia: Lea & Febiger, 1993.
190. McCarty DJ Jr, Halverson P, Carrera G, Brewer B, Kozin F. Milwaukee shoulder: association of microspheroids containing hydroxyapatite crystals, active collagenase and neutral protease with rotator cuff deficits. 1. Clinical aspects. *Arthritis Rheum* 1981;24:464–491.
191. McCauley TR, Kier R, Lynch KJ, Joki P. Chondromalacia patellae: diagnosis with MR imaging. *Am J Roentgenol* 1992;158: 101–105.
192. Meachim G. Effect of age on the thickness of adult articular cartilage at the shoulder joint. *Ann Rheum Dis* 1971;30: 43–47.
193. Menerey KA, Eider W, Brewer GJ, et al. The arthropathy of Wilson's disease: clinical and pathologic patterns. *J Rheumatol* 1988;15: 331–337.
194. Menkes C, Simon F, Delrieu F, Forest M, Delbarre F. Destructive arthropathy in chondrocalcinosis articularis. *Arthritis Rheum* 1976;19: 329–348.
195. Milgram JW. Morphologic alterations in the subchondral bone in advanced degenerative arthritis. *Clin Orthop* 1983;173: 293–312.
196. Milgram JW. The classification of loose bodies in human joints. *Clin Orthop* 1977;124:282–291.
197. Mitchell OM. Epidemology. In: Utsinger PD, Zvaifler NJ, Ehrlich EG, eds. *Rheumatoid arthritis*: etiology, diagnosis and treatment. Philadelphia: JB Lippincott, 1985:133–150.
198. Modl JM, Sether LA, Haughton VM, et al. Articular cartilage: correlation of histologic zones with signal intensity at MR imaging. *Radiology* 1991;181:853–855.
199. Moll JM. Inflammatory bowel disease. *Clin Rheum Dis* 1985;11: 87–111.
200. Mont MA, Maar DC, Urquhart MW, Lennox D, Hungerford DS. Avascular necrosis of the humeral head treated by core decompression. *J Bone Joint Surg [Br]* 1993;75:785–788.
201. Morley JJ, Kushner I. Serum C-reactive protein levels in disease. *Ann NY Acad Sci* 1982;389:406–418.
202. Morrey BF, Janes JM. Recurrent anterior dislocation of the shoulder: long term follow-up of the Putti-Platt and Bankart procedures. *J Bone Joint Surg [Am]* 1976;58:252–256.
203. Moseley HF. The arterial pattern of the rotator cuff of the shoulder. *J Bone Joint Surg [Br]* 1963;45:780–789.
204. Moskowitz RW. Introduction. In: Moskowitz RW, Howell DS, Goldenberg VM, et al., eds. *Osteoarthritis, diagnosis and medical/surgical management*, 2nd ed. Philadelphia: WB Sanders, 1992:1–7.
205. Mouradian WH. Displaced proximal humeral fractures. Seven years' experience with a modified Zickel supracondylar device. *Clin Orthop* 1986;212:209–218.
206. Mow VC, Setton, LA, Guilak F, Ratcliffe A. Mechanical factors in articular cartilage and their role in osteoarthritis. In: Kuettner KE, Goldberg V, eds. *Osteoarthritic disorders*. Monterey, CA: American Academy of Orthopaedic Surgery Symposium, 1994:147–173.
207. Mullaji AB, Beddow FH, Comb GHR. CT measurement of glenoid erosion in arthritis. *J Bone Joint Surg [Br]* 1994;76: 384–388.
208. Neer CS II. Degenerative lesions of the proximal humeral articular surface. *Clin Orthop* 1961;20:116–125.
209. Neer CS II. Displaced proximal humeral fractures. Part I. Classification and evaluation. *J Bone Joint Surg [Am]* 1970;52:1077–1089.
210. Neer CS II. Displaced proximal humeral fractures. Part II, Treatment of three-part and four-part displacement. *J Bone Joint Surg [Am]* 1970;52:1090–1103.
211. Neer CS II. Fractures and dislocations of the shoulder. Part I: Fractures about the shoulder. In: Rockwood CA Jr, Green DP, eds. *Fractures*, 2nd ed. Philadelphia: JB Lippincott, 1984:675–721.
212. Neer CS II. Replacement arthroplasty for glenohumeral osteoarthritis. *J Bone Joint Surg [Am]* 1974;56:1–13.
213. Neer CS II. The shoulder. In: Kelley WN, Harris ED Jr, Ruddy S, Sledge CB, eds. *Textbook of rheumatology*, 4th ed. Philadelphia: WB Saunders, 1993:1808–1822.
214. Neer CS II. *Shoulder reconstruction*. Philadelphia: WB Saunders, 1990:143–271.
215. Neer CS II. *Shoulder reconstruction*. Philadelphia: WB Saunders, 1990:202–208.
216. Neer CS II. *Shoulder reconstruction*. Philadelphia: WB Saunders, 1990:273–362.
217. Neer, CS II. The rheumatoid shoulder. In: Cruess RL, Mitchell NS, eds. *Surgery of rheumatoid arthritis*. Philadelphia: JB Lippincott Company, 1971:117–125.
218. Neer CS II, Brown TH Jr, McLaughlin HL. Fracture of the neck of the humerus with dislocation of the head fragment. *Am J Surg* 1953;85: 252–258.
219. Neer CS II, Craig EV, Fukuda H. Cuff tear arthropathy. *J Bone Joint Surg [Am]* 1983;65:1232–1244.
220. Neer CS II, Foster CR. Inferior capsular shift for involuntary inferior and multidirectional instability of the shoulder. A preliminary report. *J Bone Joint Surg [Am]* 1980;62:897–908.
221. Neer CS II, Watson KC, Stanton FJ. Recent experience in total shoulder replacement. *J Bone Joint Surg [Am]* 1982;64:319–337.
222. Nelson MC, Leather GP, Nirschl RP, Pettrone FA, Freedman MT. Evaluation of the painful shoulder: a prospective comparison of magnetic resonance imaging, computerized tomographic arthrography, ultrasonography and operative findings. *J Bone Joint Surg [Am]* 1991; 73:707–716.
223. Norris TR, Bigliani LU. Analysis of failed repair for shoulder instability: a preliminary report. In: Bateman JE, Welsh RP, eds. *Surgery of the shoulder*. Philadelphia: BC Decker, 1984:111–116.
224. Nussbaum AJ, Doppman JL. Shoulder arthropathy in primary hyperparathyroidism. *Skeletal Radiol* 1982;9:98–102.
225. Ochoa JA, Heck DA, Brandt KD, Hillberry BM. The effect of intertrabecular fluid on femoral head mechanics. *J Rheumatol* 1991;18: 580–584.
226. O'Driscoll SW, Evans DC. Longterm results of staple capsulorrhaphy for anterior instability of the shoulder. *J Bone Joint Surg [Am]* 1993; 75:249–258.
227. Okazaki T, Saito T, Mitomo T, Siota Y. Pseudogout: clinical observations and chemical analyses of deposits. *Arthritis Rheum* 1976;19: 293–305.
228. Ondrouch AS. Cysts formation in osteoarthritis. *J Bone Joint Surg [Br]* 1963;45:755–761.
229. Otterness IG. The value of C-reactive protein measurement in rheumatoid arthritis. *Semin Arthritis Rheum* 1994;24:91–104.
230. Paavolainen P, Bjorkenheim J-M, Slatis P, Paukku P. Operative treatment of severe proximal humerus fractures. *Acta Orthop Scand* 1983; 54:374–379.
231. Pahle JA. Experiences with synovectomy of the shoulder. In: Lettin AWF, Peterson C, eds. *Rheumatoid arthritis surgery of the shoulder*. Basel: Karger, 1989:12:31–39.

232. Pahle JA, Kvarnes L. Synovectomy of the shoulder. In: Friedman RL, ed. *Arthroplasty of the shoulder*. New York: Thieme, 1994:113–125.
233. Palmer WE, Caslowitz PL, Chew FS. MR arthrography of the shoulder: normal intra-articular structures and common abnormalities. *AM J Roentgenol* 1995;164:141–146.
234. Paul PK, Jasani MK, Sebok D, et al. Variation in MR signal intensity across normal human knee cartilage. *JMRI* 1993;3:569–574.
235. Peterfy CG, Majumdar S, Lang P, et al. MR imaging of the arthritic knee: improved discrimination of cartilage, synovium and effusion with pulsed saturation transfer and fat-suppressed T1-weighted sequences. *Radiology* 1994;191:413–419.
236. Peterfy CG, van Dijke CF, Janzen DL, et al. Quantification of articular cartilage in the knee by pulsed saturation transfer and fat-suppressed MRI: Optimization and validation. *Radiology* 1994;192: 485–491.
237. Petersson CJ. Degeneration of the glenohumeral joint. *Acta Orthop Scand* 1983;54:277–283.
238. Petersson CJ. Painful shoulders in patients with rheumatoid arthritis. *Scand J Rheumatol* 1986;15:275–279.
239. Petersson CJ, Raedlulnd-Johnell J. Joint space in normal glenohumeral radiographs. *Acta Orthop Scand* 1983;54:274–276.
240. Peyron JG. The epidemiology of osteoarthritis. In: Moskowitz RW, Howell DS, Goldberg VM, Makhin HJ, eds. *Osteoarthritis*: diagnosis and management. Philadelphia: WB Saunders, 1984:9–27.
241. Phelps P, Steele AD, McCarty DJ. Compensated polarized light microscopy. *JAMA* 1968;203:508–512.
242. Pilgaard S, Och Ostger A. Four-segment fractures of the humeral neck. *Acta Orthop Scand* 1973;44:124.
243. Podgorski M, Robinson B, Weissberger A, et al. Articular manifestations of acromegaly. *Aust NZ J Med* 1988;18:28–35.
244. Poleksic L, Zdravkovic D, Jablankov D, Watt I, Bacic G. Magnetic resonance imaging of bone destruction in rheumatoid arthritis: comparison with radiography. *Skeletal Radiol* 1993;22: 577–580.
245. Poppen NK, Walker PS. Forces at the glenohumeral joint in abduction. *Clin Orthop* 1978;135:165–170.
246. Poppen NK, Walker PS. Normal and abnormal motion of the shoulder. *J Bone Joint Surg [Am]* 1976;58:195–201.
247. Porcellini G, Campi F, Burnetti E. Osteoarthritis caused by synovial chondromatosis of the shoulder. *J Shoulder Elbow Surg* 1994;3: 404–406.
248. Pouchot J, Sampalis JS, Beaudet F, et al. Adult Still's disease: manifestations, disease course and outcome in 62 patients. *Medicine* 1991; 70:118–136.
249. Poulter LW, Janossy G. The involvement of dendritic cells in chronic inflammatory disease. *Scand J Immununol* 1985;21:401–407.
250. Preston L. *The surgical management of rheumatoid arthritis*. Philadelphia: WB Saunders, 1968.
251. Pritchett JW, Clark JM. Prosthetic replacement for chronic unreduced dislocations of the shoulder. *Clin Orthop* 1987;216:89–93.
252. Radin EL. Mechanical factors in the etiology of osteoarthritis. In: Peyron JG, ed. *Epidemiology of osteoarthritis*. Paris: Ciba-Geigy, 1981: 136–139.
253. Radin EL, Paul IL. Does cartilage compliance reduce skeletal impact loads? The relative force attenuating properties of articular carilage, synovial fluid, peri-articular soft-tissues and bone. *Arthritis Rheum* 1970;13:139–144.
254. Radin EL, Schaffler M, Gibson G, Tashman S. Osteoarthritis as a result of repetitive trauma in osteoarthritic disorders. In: Kuettner KE, Goldberg VM, eds. *Osteoarthritis*. Rosemont, IL: American Academy of Orthopaedic Surgery, 1995: 197–204.
255. Rand JA, Sim FH. Total shoulder arthroplasty for the arthropathy of hemochromatosis: a case report. *Orthopedics* 1981;4:658–660.
256. Ratcliffe A, Flatow EL, Roth N, Saed-Nejad F, Bigliani LU. Biomechanical markers in synovial fluid identify early osteoarthritis of the glenohumeral joint. *Clin Orthop* 1996;330:45–53.
257. Rathbun JB, Macnab I. The microvascular pattern of the rotator cuff. *J Bone Joint Surg [Br]* 1970;52:540–553.
258. Recht MP, Krammer J, Marcelis S, et al. Abnormalities of articular cartilage in the knee: analysis of available MR techniques. *Radiology* 1993;187:473–478.
259. Recht MP, Krammer J, Petersilge CA, et al. Distribution of normal and abnormal fluid collections in the glenohumeral joint: implications for MR arthrography. *JMRI* 1994;4:173–177.
260. Reilly DT, Mertnes M. Experimental analysis of the quadriceps muscle force and patellofemoral joint reactive forces for various activities. *Acta Orthop Scand* 1972;43:126–137.
261. Reiser MF, Naegele M. Inflammatory joint disease: static and dynamic gadolinium-enhanced MR imaging. *JMRI* 1993;3:307–310.
262. Resnick D. Patterns of peripheral joint disease in ankylosing spondylitis. *Radiology* 1974;110:523–532.
263. Rhaney K, Lamb DW. The cysts of osteoarthritis of the hip. A radiologic and pathologic study. *J Bone Joint Surg [Br]* 1955;37:663–675.
264. Rindell K. Muscle-pedicle bone graft in revascularization of aseptic necrosis of the humeral head. *Ann Chir Gynecol* 1987;76:283–285.
265. Riordan J, Dieppe P. Arthritis of the glenohumeral joint. *Baillieres Clin Rheumatol* 1989;3:607–625.
266. Rogers LF, Hendrix RW. The painful shoulder. *Radiol Clin North Am* 1988;26:1359–1371.
267. Rosen PS. A unique shoulder lesion in ankylosing spondylitis: clinical comment. *J Rheumatol* 1980;7:109–110.
268. Rothman RH, Parke WW. The vascular anatomy of the rotator cuff. *Clin Orthop* 1965;41:176–186.
269. Rothschild BM. Severe generalized (Charcot-like) joint destruction in juvenile rheumatoid arthritis. *Clin Orthop* 1981;155:75–80.
270. Roubenoff R. Gout and hyperuricemia. *Rheum Dis Clin North Am* 1990;16:539–50.
271. Rowe CR, Zavins B. Chronic unreduced dislocations of the shoulder. *J Bone Joint Surg [Am]* 1982;64:494–505.
272. Rubenstein JD, Kim JK, Morava-Protzner I, et al. Effects of collagen orientation on MR imaging characteristics of bovine cartilage. *Radiology* 1993;188:219–226.
273. Rutherford CS, Cofield RH. Osteonecrosis of the shoulder. *Orthop Trans* 1987;11:239.
274. Samilson RL, Preito V. Dislocation arthropathy of the shoulder. *J Bone Joint Surg [Am]* 1983;65:456–460.
275. Schai P, Inhoff A, Preiss S. Comminuted humeral head fractures: a multicenter analysis. *J Shoulder Elbow Surg* 1995;4:319–330.
276. Schmerling RS, Parker JA, Johns WD, et al. Measurement of joint inflammation and rheumatoid arthritis with ^{111}In chloride. *Ann Rheum Dis* 1990;49:88–92.
277. Schneiderman R, Keret D, Maroudas A. Effects of mechanical and osmotic pressure on the rate of glycosaminoglycan synthesis in the human adult femoral head cartilage: an in vitro study. *J Orthop Res* 1986;4:393–408.
278. Schumacher HR. Hemochromatosis and arthritis. *Arthritis Rheum* 1964;7:41–50.
279. Schumacher HR, ed. *Primer on rheumatic disease*, 10th ed. Atlanta: Arthritis Foundation, 1993:64.
280. Schumacher HR, ed. *Primer on rheumatic disease*, 10th ed. Atlanta: Arthritis Foundation, 1993:87.
281. Schumacher HR. Synovial membrane and fluid morphologic alterations in early rheumatoid arthritis: microvascular injury and virus-like particles. *Ann NY Acad Sci* 1975:256:39–64.
282. Schumacher HR, Andrews R, McLaughlin G. Arthropathy in sickle cell disease. *Ann Intern Med* 1973;78:203–211.
283. Schumacher HR, Holdsmith OE. Ochronotic arthropathy. I: clinopathologic studies. *Semin Arthritis Rheum* 1977;6:207–246.
284. Schumacher HR, Tse R, Reginato A, Miller J, Maurer K. Hydroxyapatite-like crystals in synovial fluid cell vacuoles: a suspected new cause for crystal induced arthritis. *Arthritis Rheum* 1976;19:821.
285. Schuman WP, Kilcoyne RF, Matsen FA, Rogers JV, Mack LA. Double contrast computed tomography of the glenoid labrum. *Am J Roentgenol* 1983;141:581–584.
286. Schweitzer MD, Magbalon MJ, Fenlin JM, Frieman BG, Ehrlich S, Epstein RE. Effusion criteria and clinical importance of glenohumeral joint fluid: MR imaging evaluation. *Radiology* 1995;194:821–824.
287. Seegmiller JE, Howell RR, Malawista SE. Inflammatory reaction to sodium urate: its possible relationships to the genesis of acute gouty arthritis. *JAMA* 1962;180:469–475.
288. Seeman WR, Siebler G, Rupp HG. A new classification of proximal humerus fractures. *Eur J Radiol* 1986;6:163–167.
289. Sennara H, Gorry F. Orthopedic aspects of sickle cell anemia and allied hemoglobinopathies. *Clin Orthop* 1978;130:154–157.
290. Setton LA, Mow VC, Muller FJ, et al. Mechanical properties of canine articular cartilage are significantly altered following transection of the anterior cruciate ligament. *J Orthop Res* 1994;12:451–463.
291. Sewell KL, Ruthazer R, Parker JA. The correlation of ^{111}In joint scans with clinical synovitis and rheumatoid arthritis. *J Rheumatol* 1993;20: 2015–2019.

292. Shankman S, Beltran J. MRI of the shoulder. *Curr Prob Diagn Radiol* 1995;24(6):201–228.
293. Simkin PA. Role of local factors in the precipitation of urate crystals. In: Kelley WN, Weiner M, eds. *Uric Acid.* (*Handbook Experimental Pharmaceutics*, vol 51). Berlin: Springer-Verlag, 1978:379–395.
294. Simkin PA, Pizzorno JE. Transynovial exchange of small molecules in normal human subjects. *J Appl Physiol* 1974;36:581–587.
295. Singer GC, Kirkland PM, Emery RJ. Coracoid transpositions for recurrent anterior instability of the shoulder. A 20-year follow-up study. *J Bone Joint Surg [Br]* 1995;77:73–76.
296. Sisk TD, Boyd HB. Management of recurrent anterior dislocation of the shoulder: DuToit-type or staple capsulorrhaphy. *Clin Orthop* 1974;103:150–156.
297. Smith RW. Observations upon chronic rheumatoid arthritis of the shoulder—I. *Dublin Q J Med Sci* 1983;15:1–16.
298. Smith RW. Observations upon chronic rheumatoid arthritis of the shoulder—II. *Dublin Q J Med Sci* 1983;15:343–358.
299. Soslowsky KJ, Flatow EL, Bigliani LU, Pawluk RJ, Ateshian GA, Mow VC. Quantitation of in situ contact areas at the glenohumeral joint: a biomechanical study. *J Orthop Res* 1992;10:524–534.
300. Souter WA. The surgical treatment of the rheumatoid shoulder. *Ann Acad Med Singapore* 1983;12:243–255.
301. Stableforth PG. Four-part fractures of the neck of the humerus. *J Bone Joint Surg [Br]* 1984;66:104–108.
302. Steinmann SR, Flatow EL, Pollock RG, Glasgow MD, Gigliani LR. Evaluation and surgical treatment of failed shoulder instability repairs. *Orthop Trans* 192;16:727.
303. Stevens CR, Blake DR, Merry P, et al. A comparative study by morphometry of the microvasculature in normal and rheumatoid synovium. *Arthritis Rheum* 1991;34:1508–1513.
304. Sturzenegger M, Fornaro E, Jakob RP. Results of surgical treatment of multifragmented fractures of the humeral head. *Arch Orthop Trauma Surg* 1982;100:249–259.
305. Sven-Hansen H. Displaced humeral fractures. A review of 49 patients. *Acta Orthop Scand* 1974;45:359–364.
306. Tak HK, Cooper SM, Wilcox WR. Studies on the nucleation of monosodium urate at 37 degrees centigrade. *Arthritis Rheum* 1980;23: 574–580.
307. Tanner MW, Cofield RF. Prosthetic arthroplasty for fractures and fracture dislocations of the proximal humerus. *Clin Orthop* 1983;179: 116–128.
308. Taylor LJ. Multifocal avascular necrosis after short-term high-dose steroid therapy. A report of three cases. *J Bone Joint Surg [Br]* 1984; 66:431–433.
309. Tervonen O, Dietz MJ, Carmichael SW, Ehman RL. MR imaging of knee hyaline cartilage: evaluation of two- and three-dimensional sequences. *JMRI* 1993;3:663–668.
310. Thompson RC Jr, Oegema TR Jr, Lewis LJ, et al. Osteoarthritic changes after acute transarticular load: an animal model. *J Bone Joint Surg [Am]* 1991;73:990–1001.
311. Tirman RM, Nelson CL, Tirman WS. Arthrography of the shoulder joint: state of the art. *Diagn Imaging* 1981;17:19–76.
312. Truelove LH. Articular manifestations of erythema nodosum. *Ann Rheum Dis* 1960;19:174–180.
313. Tumeh SS. Scintigraphy in the evaluation of arthropathy. *Radiol Clin North Am* 1996;34(2):215–231.
314. Tumeh SS, Tohmeh AG. Nuclear medicine techniques in septic arthritis and osteomyelitis. *Rheum Dis Clin North Am* 1991;17:559–583.
315. Tumeh SS, Tohmeh AG. Nuclear medicine technology. *Radiol Clin North Am* 1991;17:559–583.
316. Tyson LL. Imaging of the painful shoulder. *Curr Prob Diagn Radiol* 1995;24(3):109–140.
317. Varma BP, Ramakrishna YJ. Synovial chondromatosis of the shoulder. *Aust NZ J Surg* 1976;19:151–158.
318. Vartiainen J, Hurri L. Arthritis due to *Salmonella typhimurium. Acta Med Scand* 1964;175:771–776.
319. Verlooy H, Mortelmans L, Verbruggen A, et al. Tc-99m HM-PAO labelled leukocyte scanning for detection of infection in orthopedic surgery. *Prog Clin Biol Res* 1990;355:181–187.
320. Volpin G. Synovial chondromatosis of the shoulder. *Am Surg* 1986; 46:422–424.
321. Wang G, Moga DB, Richemer WG, et al. Cortisone-induced bone changes and its response to liquid clearing agents. *Clin Orthop* 1978; 130:81–85.
322. Weber DA. Options in camera technology for the bone scan: role of SPECT. *Semin Nucl Med* 1988;18:78–89.
323. Wilcox WR, Khalef A. Nucleation of monosodiuim urate crystals. *Ann Rheum Dis* 1975;34:332–339.
324. Wildner M, Wimmer B, Reichelt A. Osteoarthritis after the Eden-Hybbinette-Lange procedure for anterior dislocation of the shoulder: a 15-year follow up. *Int Orthop* 1994:18;280–283.
325. Williams MJ. Sarcoidosis presenting with polyarthritis. *Ann Rheum Dis* 1961;20:138–143.
326. Winalski CS, Aliabadi P, Wright JR, et al. Enhancement of joint fluid with intravenously administered gadopentate dimeglumine: technique, rationale, and implications. *Radiology* 1993;187:179–185.
327. Winalski CS, Mulkern RV, Utz PJ, et al. In vivo T2 relaxation times of synovium and joint fluid in rheumatoid arthritis: optimization of nonenhanced MR imaging. *Radiology* 1994;193(P):206.
328. Winalski CS, Palmer WE, Rosenthal DI, Weissman BN. Magnetic resonance imaging of rheumatoid arthritis. *Radiol Clin North Am* 1996;34(2):243–258.
329. Wirth MA, Lyons FR, Rockwood CA Jr. Hypoplasia of the glenoid. *J Bone Joint Surg [Am]* 1993;75:1175–1183.
330. Wolfe F, Cathey MA, Roberts FK. The latex test revisited: rheumatoid factor testing in 8,287 rheumatic disease patients. *Arthritis Rheum* 1991;34:951–960.
331. Woolf AD, Cawston T, Dieppe P. Idiopathic haemorrhagic rupture of the shoulder in destructive disease of the elderly. *Ann Rheum Dis* 1986;45:498–501.
332. Wortman RI, Karas B, McCarty DJ. Cartilage nucleoside triphosphate pyrophosphohydrolase. II. Role in extracellular pyrophosphate generation and nucleoside metabolism. *Arthritis Rheum* 1985;28:413–418.
333. Wouters JMGW, van de Putte LBA. Adult-onset Still's disease; clinical and laboratory features, treatment and progress of 45 cases. *Q J Med* 1986;61:1055–1065.
334. Wynne-Davies R, Gormley J. The prevalence of skeletal dysplasias: an estimate of their minimum frequency and the number of patients requiring orthopaedic care. *J Bone Joint Surg [Br]* 1985;67:133–137.
335. Yanagawa A, Takano K, Nishioka K, et al. Clinical staging and gadolinium-DTPA enhanced images of the wrist in rheumatoid arthritis. *J Rheumatol* 1993;20:781–784.
336. Young DC, Rockwood CA. Complications of failed Bristow procedure and their management. *J Bone Joint Surg [Am]* 1991;73: 969–981.
337. Zlatkin MB. Other glenohumeral joint disorders. In: Zlatkin MB, ed. *M.R.I. of the shoulder*. New York: Raven Press, 1991:131–165.
338. Zlatkin MB, ed. *M.R.I. of the shoulder*. New York: Raven Press, 1991.
339. Zuckerman JD, Matsen FA. Complications about the glenohumeral joint related to the use of screws and staples. *J Bone Joint Surg [Am]* 1984;66:175–180.
340. Zyto K, Kronberg M, Brostrom L-A. Shoulder function after displaced fractures of the proximal humerus. *J Shoulder Elbow Surg* 1995;4:331–336.

Disorders of the Shoulder: Diagnosis and Management,
edited by Joseph P. Iannotti and Gerald R. Williams, Jr.
Lippincott Williams & Wilkins, Philadelphia © 1999.

CHAPTER 17

Biomechanics of the Glenohumeral Joint: Influence on Shoulder Arthroplasty

Gerald R. Williams, Jr. and Joseph P. Iannotti

INTRODUCTION

The goals of prosthetic reconstruction of the glenohumeral joint are to relieve pain and to improve shoulder function. Assuming that the rotator cuff is intact or can be repaired and that soft-tissue contractures can be corrected, these goals are most likely to be realized if the implant chosen results in anatomic reconstruction of the articular surfaces which restores normal glenohumeral rotational and translational motion. The surgical goals of anatomic articular reconstruction and normal postoperative glenohumeral kinematics may not be attainable. However, as our knowledge of normal articular anatomy, normal articular kinematics, and prosthetic articular kinematics continues to grow, implant design is evolving toward increasingly anatomic joint replacements with potentially improved biomechanical performance.

Several anatomic and biomechanical factors have been identified that may have an effect on prosthetic design. Important anatomic factors include humeral head size, humeral head shape, humeral head offset, humeral neck-shaft angle, glenoid size and shape, glenoid offset, and lateral glenohumeral offset. Biomechanical factors that may influence prosthetic design and performance include glenohumeral articular conformity, glenohumeral articular constraint, periarticular muscular forces, ligamentous restraints, normal glenohumeral kinematics, and prosthetic kinematics. The purposes of this chapter are to review the current knowledge of the relevant anatomic and biomechanical factors that potentially influence glenohumeral prosthetic design and to discuss the possible effects that variations in these design parameters may have on prosthetic performance.

G. R. Williams, Jr., and J.P. Iannotti: Department of Orthopaedic Surgery, Hospital of the University of Pennsylvania, Philadelphia, Pennsylvania 19104.

ANATOMIC FACTORS

Humeral Head Size

Given the assumption that the humeral head is a sphere, the volume (i.e., size) of the articular segment is determined by the humeral head radius of curvature and humeral head thickness or neck length (Fig. 1). Humeral head radius, humeral head thickness, and humeral head size are all variable. Mean humeral head radius is approximately 24 mm, with a range of 19 to 28 mm (Fig. 2).[16,31] Mean humeral head thickness is approximately 19 mm, with a range of 15 to 24 mm (Fig. 3).[16,31] Both humeral head radius and thickness correlate strongly with humeral shaft length and patient

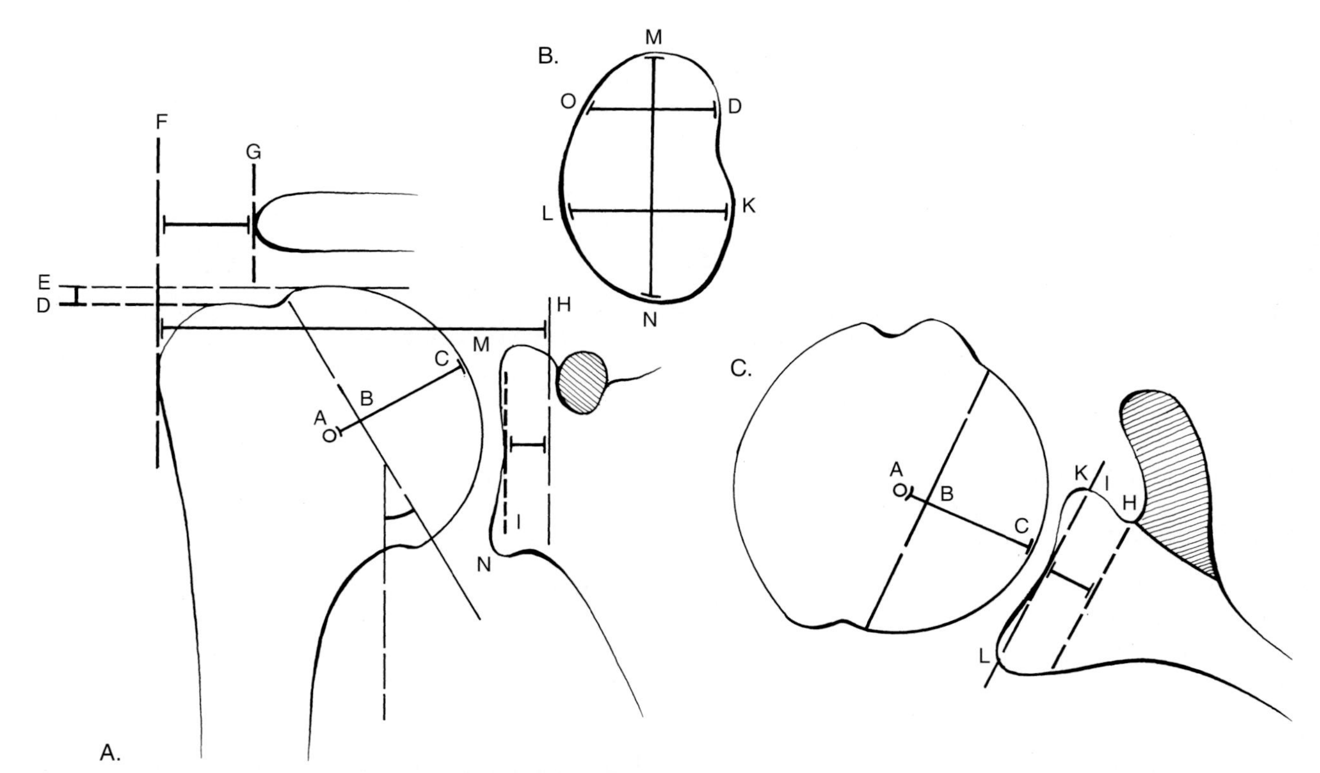

FIG. 1. Normal glenohumeral relations depicted in **(A)** the coronal plane include *(A)* humeral head center, *(AC)* humeral head radius of curvature, *(BC)* humeral head thickness or neck length, α humeral neck-shaft angle, *(HF)* lateral glenohumeral offset, *(FG)* greater tuberosity to acromion distance, *(DE)* greater tuberosity to humeral head distance, *(MN)* superoinferior glenoid dimension, and *(HI)* glenoid offset. **(B)** The glenoid dimensions measured in the sagittal plane include *(MN)* the superoinferior dimension, *(OP)* the anteroposterior dimension of the upper half, *(KL)* and the anteroposterior dimension of the lower half. **(C)**The glenohumeral relations in the axial plane include *(A)* the humeral head center, *(AC)* the humeral head radius of curvature, *(BC)* the humeral head thickness or neck length, *(KL)* the anteroposterior dimension of the glenoid, and *(HI)* the glenoid offset. (From ref. 17, with permission.)

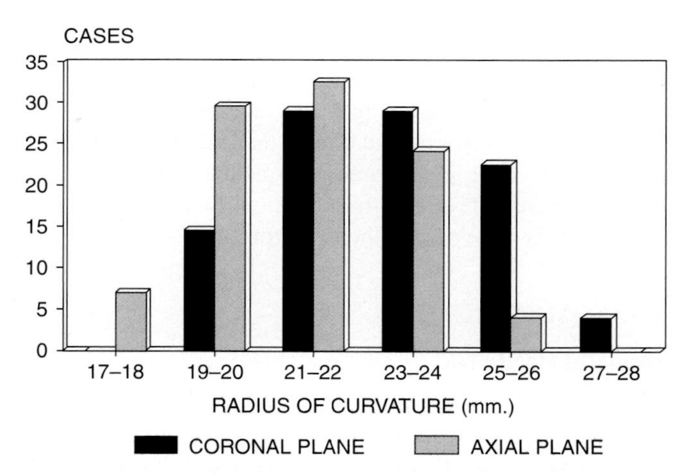

FIG. 2. Humeral head radius of curvature fits a gaussian distribution with a mean of 23 to 24 mm and a range of approximately 19 to 28 mm. Note that the axial plane radius is slightly smaller than the coronal plane radius. (From ref. 17, with permission.)

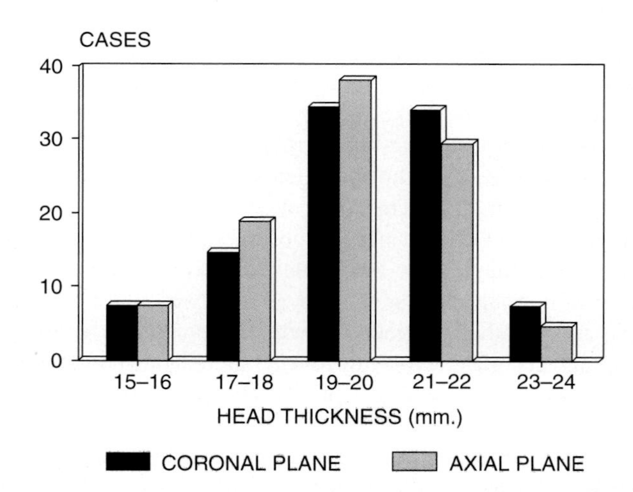

FIG. 3. Humeral head thickness also demonstrates a bell-shaped distribution with a mean of 19 mm and a range of 15 to 24 mm. (From ref. 17, with permission.)

height.[16,31] However, the ratio of humeral head thickness to humeral head radius of curvature is remarkably constant at approximately 0.7 to 0.9, regardless of patient height or humeral shaft size.[16,31] The surface arc of the humerus available for contact with the glenoid is directly proportional to the ratio of humeral head thickness to humeral head radius and is, therefore, also relatively constant, irrespective of humeral shaft length or patient height.[31]

Humeral Head Shape

The assumption that the humeral head is spherical is only partially accurate. The central 80% of the articular surface is spherical, with the coronal plane and axial plane radii of curvature being equal.[1,7,16,27] However, in the peripheral 20% of the articular surface, the radius of curvature in the axial plane is, on average, 2 mm less than in the coronal plane (see Fig. 2). Therefore, the peripheral 20% of the humeral articular surface is elliptical, with the ratio of the axial plane radius to the coronal plane radius being 0.92.[16]

Humeral Head Offset

The center of the humeral head does not coincide with the projected center of the humeral shaft. Alternatively, the point in the proximal humeral metaphysis that corresponds to the center of the humeral head (assuming that the humeral head is a sphere) does not lie on a line projected proximally into the humeral metaphysis from the central axis of the intramedullary canal of the humeral diaphysis.[3,5,28,31,35] The distance between the center of the humeral head and the central axis of the intramedullary canal is defined as the *humeral head offset*.[3,5,31,35] Although humeral head offset is undoubtedly three-dimensional, it is commonly described in two planes, coronal and axial. Similar to most other proximal humeral anatomic parameters, reported humeral head offsets are variable.[3,5,28,31,35] In the coronal plane, the humeral head offset is approximately 7 to 9 mm medial to the central axis of the intramedullary canal; in the axial plane, the humeral head offset is 2 to 4 mm posterior to the central axis of the intramedullay canal (Fig. 4).[3,5,31,35]

Humeral head offset is correlated with humeral head radius and humeral head thickness. However, for a given humeral head radius, humeral head thickness, and humeral head offset in the coronal and axial planes, the location of the humeral articular surface may vary relative to angle of rotation about the central intramedullary axis (i.e., humeral retroversion) and superoinferior translation along the central intramedullary axis (i.e., head to greater tuberosity height). Humeral retroversion averages 20 to 30 degrees, with a wide range of approximately 20 to 55 degrees.[5,25,31,35] The vertical distance between the highest point of the humeral articular surface and the highest point of the greater tuberosity (i.e., head to greater tuberosity height) is approximately 8 mm and shows a relatively small range of interspecimen variability.[16,31]

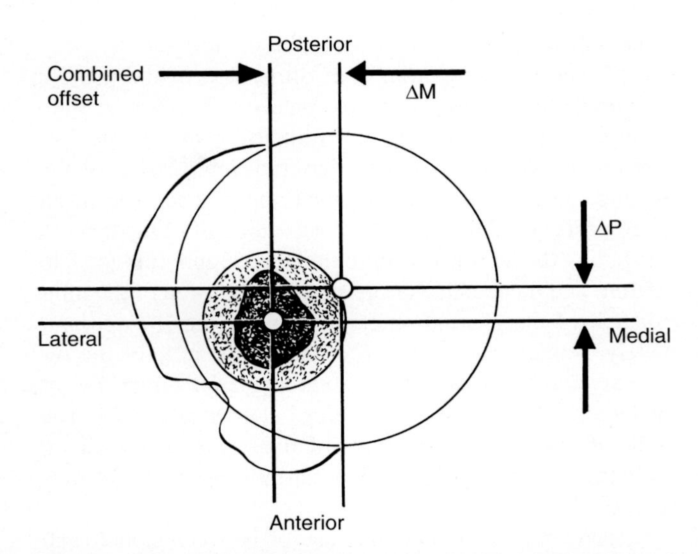

FIG. 4. This axial plane radiograph reveals the combined posterior and medial humeral head offset relative to the central axis of the intramedullary canal. (From ref. 5, with permission.)

Humeral Neck-Shaft Angle

The *neck-shaft angle* is defined as the angle subtended by the central intramedullary axis of the humeral shaft and the base of the articular segment (see Fig. 1). The average neck-shaft angle is 40 to 45 degrees.[5,16,28,31] However, more importantly, humeral neck-shaft angle demonstrates significant individual variation with a range of 30 to 55 degrees.[5,16,28,31] One study has shown a correlation between humeral head radius and neck-shaft angle, with larger humeral heads demonstrating larger neck-shaft angles (Fig. 5).[16]

Glenoid Size and Shape

The size and shape of the articular surface of the glenoid can be defined by its linear superoinferior and anteroposte-

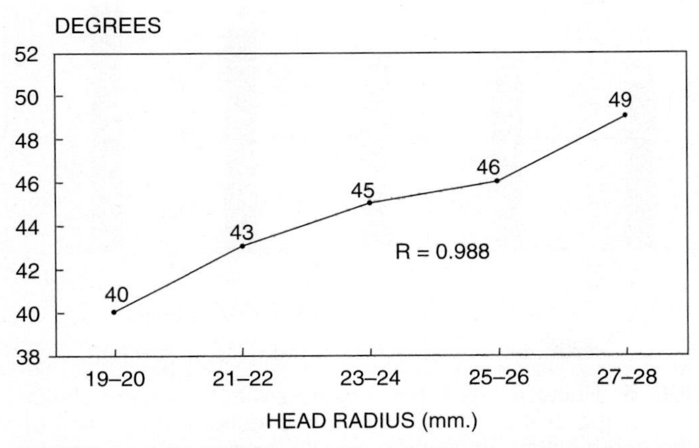

FIG. 5. Humeral neck-shaft angle correlates with humeral head size. (From ref. 17, with permission.)

rior dimensions, as well as by its radius of curvature (see Fig. 1).[16,28] The mean superoinferior dimension of the glenoid (excluding the labrum) is approximately 39 mm (range 30 to 48 mm).[16] The anteroposterior dimension of the superior half of the glenoid is shorter than the inferior half of the glenoid, resulting in a pear-shaped appearance. The mean anteroposterior dimension of the superior half of the glenoid (excluding the labrum) is approximately 23 mm (range 18 to 30 mm) and the mean anteroposterior dimension of the inferior half of the glenoid (excluding the labrum) is approximately 29 mm (range 21 to 35 mm).[16] The ratio of the superoinferior dimension to the anteroposterior dimension of the larger, inferior half of an average glenoid is 1 : 0.7.[16] The humeral head radius correlates with the size of the glenoid in both the superoinferior and anteroposterior dimensions (Fig. 6).[16]

Controversy exists about the relation between glenoid and humeral articular radius of curvature.[16,24,28,38] This controversy exists because of differences in measuring techniques, differences in sample sizes, and large individual variations in anatomy. The thickness of the articular cartilage of the glenoid increases toward the periphery of the articular surface and must be included when measuring the glenoid radius of curvature.[38] However, even when the articular cartilage is included in the measurement, the radius of curvature of the glenoid articular surface does not equal the radius of the humeral articular surface in all specimens.[16,24,28,38] Iannotti and colleagues[16] observed that, on average, the glenoid radius of curvature in the coronal plane was 2.3-mm larger than the coronal plane humeral radius of curvature in the same specimen. Soslowsky and coworkers[38] reported a difference between humerus and glenoid radii of curvature of less than 2 mm in 88% of specimens and less than 3mm in all specimens. Kelkar and associates[24] reported a mean humeral radius of curvature that was 2 mm less than the mean glenoid radius of curvature.

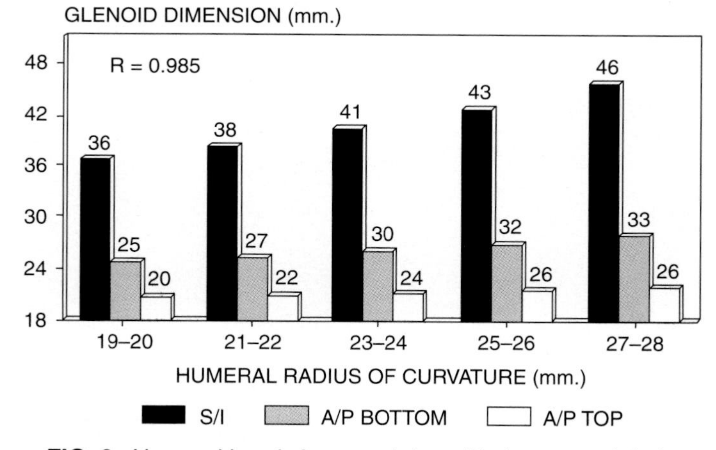

FIG. 6. Humeral head size correlates with the superoinferior dimension of the glenoid, the anteroposterior dimension of the upper half of the glenoid, and the anteroposterior dimension of the inferior half of the glenoid. (From ref. 17, with permission.)

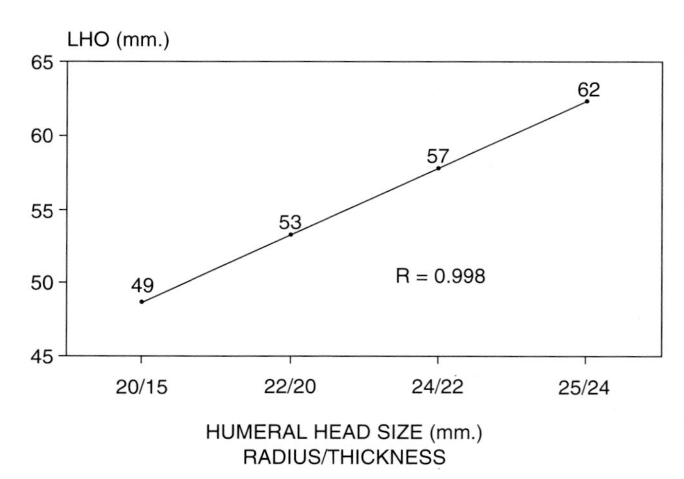

FIG. 7. Lateral glenohumeral offset is defined as the distance from the base of the coracoid process to the lateral aspect of the greater tuberosity and is correlated with humeral head size. (From ref. 17, with permission.)

Glenoid Offset

The *glenoid offset* is defined as the perpendicular distance between the base of the coracoid process and the deepest portion of the glenoid articular surface (see Fig. 1). This distance determines the location of the glenohumeral joint line and is not correlated with humeral or patient size. The average glenoid offset is approximately 2 mm (range −5.0 to +5.0 mm).[16]

Lateral Glenohumeral Offset

The *lateral glenohumeral offset* can be defined as the perpendicular distance from the base of the coracoid process to the most lateral extent of the greater tuberosity (see Fig. 1).[16] The distance from the most lateral extent of the greater tuberosity to the lateral edge of the acromion process correlates with the lateral glenohumeral offset and is easily measured intraoperatively (see Fig. 1). Lateral glenohumeral offset is important in shoulder function because it determines capsular tension, resting length of the rotator cuff muscles, and the moment arm for the deltoid muscle. Lateral glenohumeral offset averages approximately 54 to 57 mm (range 43 to 68 mm) and the distance from the greater tuberosity to the lateral margin of the acromion process averages 17 mm (range 15 to 21 mm).[16] Because the glenoid offset is less than 5 mm in all normal shoulders, it has little effect on lateral glenohumeral offset.[16] However, both lateral glenohumeral offset and greater tuberosity to acromion distance correlate with humeral head size and patient height (Fig. 7).[16]

BIOMECHANICAL FACTORS

Glenohumeral Articular Conformity

Conformity of the articular surfaces refers to the difference between the radii of curvature of the humerus and glenoid. Congruent or conforming articulations are characterized by glenoid and humeral surfaces with equal radii of curvature. Incongruent or nonconforming articulations exist when the humerus and glenoid radii of curvature are not equal. In the normal shoulder, the components of the articulating surfaces include the humeral articular cartilage, glenoid articular cartilage, and the glenoid labrum. The humeral articular cartilage is uniform in thickness throughout the entire articulating surface. The glenoid articular cartilage is thicker at the periphery than in the center.[15] The glenoid labrum extends the arc of the articular cartilage and deepens the glenoid socket, but does not change the radius of curvature of the glenoid surface. The articular cartilage and glenoid labrum are deformable without permanent loss of shape. Therefore, for practical purposes, normal glenohumeral joints can be considered to be conforming if the humeral head radius of curvature is equal to or larger than the glenoid radius of curvature.[19] Normal glenohumeral joints are considered to be nonconforming when the humeral head radius is less than the glenoid radius.[19]

Conformity or congruence of the normal glenohumeral articulation is variable, as mentioned earlier in the section on glenoid size and shape.[16,19,24,28] In most specimens reported, the humeral head radius is within 2 to 3 mm of the glenoid radius.[16,19,24,28] However, even small amounts of articular incongruence or nonconformity have important implications for glenohumeral kinematics during active motion.[19]

Glenohumeral Articular Constraint

Constraint is defined as the ability of the articular surfaces to resist translational motion of the humerus on the glenoid. The most extreme example of a constrained articulation is one in which the glenoid and humeral components are mechanically coupled to one another. In normal shoulders, where the glenoid and humerus are obviously not mechanically coupled, articular constraint is a function of the percentage of the humeral head covered by the glenoid. Articular constraint is correlated with glenoid wall height or, alternatively, socket depth, and is independent of articular conformity. In other words, different articulations may have equal conformities but different constraints, and vice versa (Fig. 8).

The normal glenoid is more constrained (i.e., has greater depth) in the superoinferior direction than in the anteroposterior direction.[15,28] Additionally, the depth of the normal glenoid is contributed to equally by the articular cartilage and the glenoid labrum.[15] In the superoinferior and anteroposterior dimensions, the glenoid articular cartilage and labrum combine to yield a socket that is 9 mm and 5 mm deep, respectively.[15] Glenoid depth can also be thought of in terms of coverage of the humeral head.[28] In the superoinferior direction, the glenoid covers approximately a 65-degree arc of the humeral surface, compared with a 50-degree arc of coverage in the anteroposterior direction.[28]

Periarticular Muscular Forces

The interactions between the many muscles that control motion of the shoulder girdle are extremely complex and beyond the scope of this chapter. However, in a simplified sense, the deltoid muscle provides power movement to the glenohumeral joint, while the rotator cuff muscles compress the humeral head into the glenoid socket to provide a steering and stabilizing function.[4,11,32–34,37,40] In a normal shoulder, the sheer force imparted by the deltoid and other large muscles is counterbalanced by the axial or compressive force imparted by the rotator cuff. This results in decreased humeral translation and increased joint stability.[26] Pathologic conditions that result in altered rotator cuff function, such as certain forms of glenohumeral arthritis, may exhibit altered glenohumeral kinematics because of muscular imbalance between the rotator cuff and deltoid.

Ligamentous Restraints

The glenohumeral ligaments are thickenings of the joint capsule that are somewhat variable in their appear-

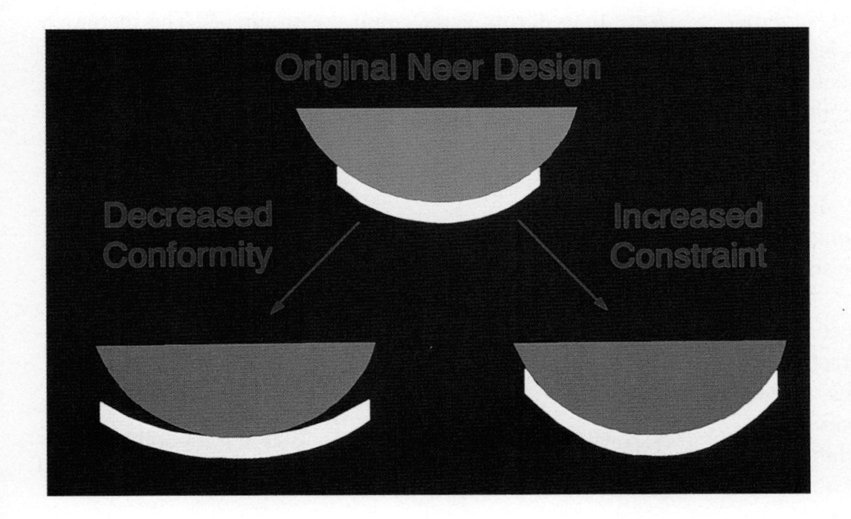

FIG. 8. Conformity refers to the difference between the humeral head radius and the glenoid radius. Constraint is determined by glenoid wall height and is independent of conformity. Two articulations may have identical conformity and different constraints and vice versa.

ance.[6,10,30,39,41] They act as checkreins to excessive rotation or translation of the humeral head at the extremes of glenohumeral motion.[6,30,41] The ability of various ligaments to control glenohumeral motion depends on their location within the capsule as well as the arm position. The rotator interval capsule occupies the gap between the upper portion of the subscapularis and the anterior border of the supraspinatus. It consists of the superior glenohumeral ligament and coracohumeral ligament.[8,14,42,43] The rotator interval capsule is primarily responsible for limiting external rotation and inferior subluxation of the humerus with the arm at the side.[8,14,42,43] The middle glenohumeral ligament limits external rotation and anterior subluxation of the humerus with the arm in midabduction.

The inferior glenohumeral ligament consists of an anterior band, axillary pouch, and posterior band.[29,39] It is taut in abduction and thereby limits the degree of abduction as well as inferior translation of the humeral head in full abduction. The anterior band tightens in combined abduction and external rotation, thereby limiting the amount of abduction and external rotation possible as well as anterior translation with the arm in this position.[29,39,41] The posterior band is taut in abduction and internal rotation; it limits the amount of simultaneous abduction and internal rotation possible and also limits posterior humeral translation with the arm in this position.[29,39,41] The anterior and posterior bands can be made even more taut by passively positioning the abducted humerus posterior and anterior to the scapular plane, respectively.

Tension in any of the glenohumeral ligaments will cause obligate translation in the opposite direction. For example, tension in the anterior band of the inferior glenohumeral ligament will result in posterior translation of the humeral head.[12,14] Pathologic conditions that result in capsular contracture, such as glenohumeral arthritis, may lead to altered humeral rotation and translation because of premature capsular tightening.

Normal Kinematics

Glenohumeral motion comprises translation and rotation of the humerus on the glenoid. When the humerus is moved from one point in space to another, the motion occurs as a combination of rotation and translation. The percentage of that motion that occurs as rotation is variable and depends on the rotator cuff forces, capsular tension, and joint conformity.[19] If the motion were purely rotation, the shoulder would be considered strictly a "ball-in-socket" joint. Conversely, if the motion were entirely translation, the shoulder would be considered a planar joint.

Humeral head translation during active joint positioning, with a normal rotator cuff and no capsular contracture, is variable but small.[19,22–24] Under these conditions, glenohumeral motion approaches ball-in-socket kinematics. Anteroposterior translation and superoinferior translation are approximately 2 mm (Fig. 9).[19] Rotation occurs about a relatively fixed point that is located within 1 to 3 mm of the geometric center of the humeral head.[22–24] Although the translations are small, they are correlated with conformity of the articular surfaces. Nonconforming joints exhibit more translation during active motion than conforming joints (Fig. 10).[19]

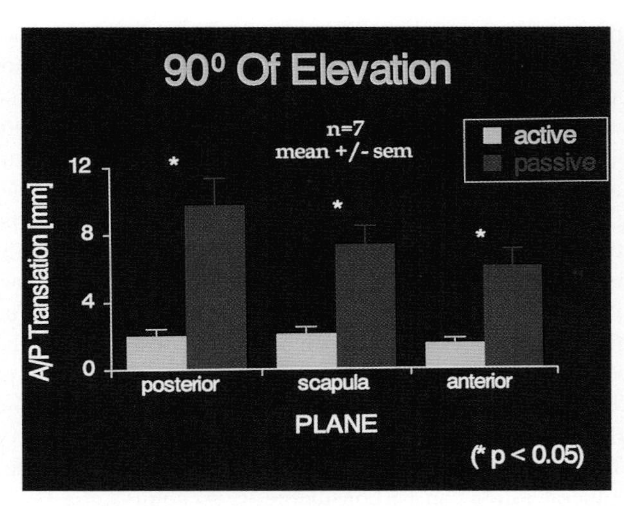

FIG. 9. This figure depicts anteroposterior humeral translation during both active and passive positioning from maximum internal to maximum external rotation at 90 degrees of total elevation (i.e., 60 degees glenohumeral and 30 degrees scapular) in, 30 degrees anterior to, and 30 degrees posterior to the scapular plane. Note that anteroposterior humeral translation is small (2 mm) during active joint positioning and large (8 mm) during passive joint positioning.

Humeral head translation during passive joint positioning with a nominal centering force is much larger than during active joint positioning with normal rotator cuff forces and is independent of joint conformity (see Figs. 9 and 10).[12,14,19] Anteroposterior passive translation is approximately 8 mm, fourfold greater than active translations.[19] Passive superoinferior translation is approximately 4 mm, twofold greater than active translation (see Fig. 9).[19]

The range of motion achievable during passive joint positioning, with only a nominal centering force applied, is much larger than during active joint positioning.[19] The increased humeral translation observed during passive joint position-

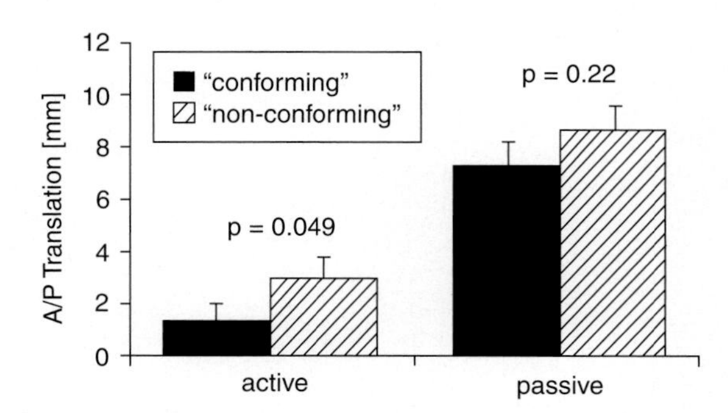

FIG. 10. Nonconforming joints have significantly greater translation during active joint positioning than conforming joints. (From ref. 20, with permission.)

ing occurs at the extremes of rotational motion not achievable during active joint positioning. In fact, if passive and active humeral translations are compared over the same range of motion (i.e., midrange), the difference is insignificant (Fig. 11).[19] Moreover, the increased passive translations that occur at the extremes of motion correlate with increased ligament length (i.e., tension) on the side of the joint opposite the translation.[19] For example, anterior translation with the humerus in 90 degrees of elevation in the scapular plane occurs with increasing internal rotation and is associated with increasing length of the posterior band of the inferior glenohumeral ligament.[19]

Prosthetic Kinematics

In general, the relations between active translations, passive translations, joint conformity, and ligament length observed in the normal shoulder are also present in the prosthetically reconstructed shoulder.[20] Humeral head translations observed during active joint positioning are small (0.3 to 1.7 mm) and are strongly correlated with component conformity (Fig 12).[20] Humeral head translations during passive joint positioning are large (5 to 9 mm) and independent of joint conformity.[20] The increased passive translations that occur at the extremes of motion are correlated with increasing length of the capsule (i.e., ligament) on the opposite side of the joint to the translation.[20] The degree of radial mismatch that produces a kinematic pattern of active motion that most closely resembles the natural joint is unknown and likely to vary from individual to individual. However, in one study of seven cadaver shoulders, radial mismatch of approximately 4 mm produced active translations that most closely resembled the specimen mean before prosthetic arthroplasty (see Fig. 12).[20]

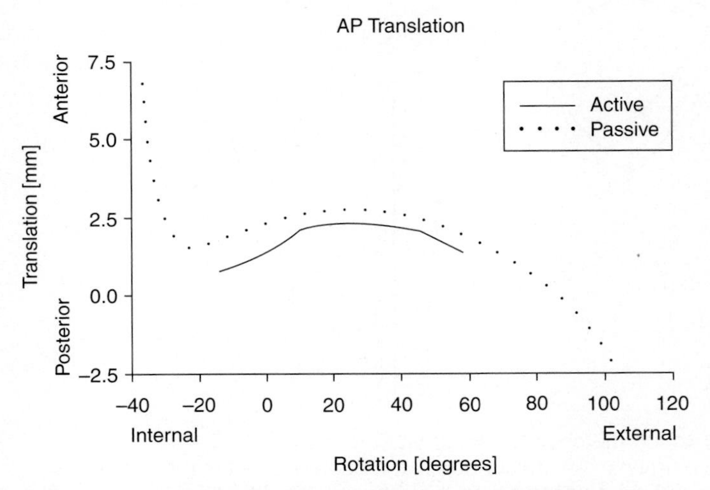

FIG. 11. This representative plot of translation versus range of motion demonstrates that the increased translations seen during passive joint positioning occur at the extremes of rotation not achievable during active joint positioning. Humeral head translations during active and passive joint positioning over the same range of rotation are not significantly different. (From ref. 20, with permission.)

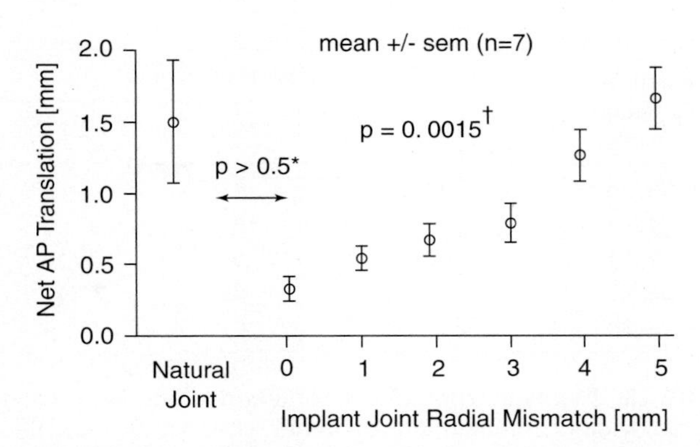

FIG. 12. Humeral head translation during active joint positioning following prosthetic arthroplasty is correlated strongly with component conformity. (From ref. 21, with permission.)

IMPLICATIONS FOR PROSTHETIC DESIGN

The ability of a particular prosthetic design to achieve anatomic reconstruction of the glenoid and humeral articular surfaces and to restore normal glenohumeral kinematics is obviously limited by the ability of the surgeon to restore soft-tissue balance and correct any bony deficiencies. Certainly, prosthetic design alone cannot overcome pathology that is too severe to be corrected. Moreover, the choice of implant cannot substitute for skillful surgical technique. However, assuming that all other variables are equal, the implant that is able to place a humeral head of the same size as the normal head, in exactly the same position on the humeral metaphysis as the normal head, in articulation with a glenoid component that anatomically restores both the location and inclination of the joint line has the best opportunity for restoring normal glenohumeral kinematics.

Anatomic Factors

Eighty-five percent of all humeral heads can be reconstructed to within 2 mm of their natural dimensions with eight head sizes (Fig. 13).[16] Maintaining the ratio of humeral head radius to humeral head thickness to a narrow range will allow maximization of humeral surface area available for contact.[16] Except in unusual situations with extraordinary bone loss or soft-tissue deficiency, humeral heads with small radii of curvature and large thicknesses (or vice versa) are undesirable. Heads with inappropriately large neck lengths for their radius of curvature have a larger volume than the natural head that was removed and will result in overstuffing of the joint, increased soft-tissue tension, and decreased range of motion or subscapularis rupture.[13]

Modular humeral systems offer some advantages over one-piece designs. The ability to place any humeral head on any humeral body results in less inventory. In addition, if revision is required, the head can be removed without removing the body.[36] However, modularity is also accompanied by some potential disadvantages. First, the head and body can become disassembled.[9] Second, in some designs, there is a

Radius of Curvature *(mm)*	Thickness *(mm)*		
	15–17	18–20	21–24
19–20	10	3	2
21–22	7	18	3
23–24	0	9	18
25–26	0	8	14
27–28	0	0	4

FIG. 13. Eighty-five percent of all humeral head sizes are defined by eight combinations of humeral head radius and thickness. Note that humeral head sizes with large radii but small thicknesses, and vice versa, are not frequently encountered in normal shoulders. (From ref. 17, with permission.)

large gap between the body of the implant and the head. This results in loss of available articular surface and potential contact between nonarticular portions of the proximal humerus and the glenoid component (Fig. 14).[17,31] If this gap is combined with beveling of the edge of the humeral head, thus creating a nonspherical implant, loss of available articular surface can be substantial.[2]

The normal variability of the humeral neck-shaft angle creates some difficult choices for prosthetic design. Implants with fixed neck-shaft angles can result in an anatomic reconstruction of the articular surface only if its neck-shaft angle matches the neck-shaft angle of the natural humerus in which it is being implanted. Differences in neck-shaft angle between the implant and the natural humerus cannot be corrected by changing humeral head thickness, radius, or offset without placing the articular surface of the head in a nonanatomic location or changing head volume.[31] If the neck-shaft angle of the implant is less than that of the natural humerus (i.e., varus cut), the position of the prosthetic humeral head will be too low on the humeral metaphysis and the greater tuberosity will be too high (Fig. 15). If the prosthetic neck-shaft angle is more than that of the natural humerus (i.e., valgus cut), the articular surface will be located superior and lateral to the anatomic location. Furthermore, the joint will contain the volume of the remaining natural head as well as the added volume of the prosthetic head. This overstuffing cannot be avoided by decreasing the humeral head size without also decreasing the surface area available for contact.[31]

Ideally, the prosthetic humeral head should be placed in the center of the cut surface of the humeral metaphysis. Because the center of the humeral head often does not coincide with the central axis of the intramedullary canal of the humeral diaphysis, the prosthetic humeral head must also be offset relative to the intramedullary canal. This requires that the prosthetic humeral head be offset relative to the prosthetic humeral body, or that the prosthetic head and body together be offset relative to the intramedullary canal. The latter scenario can be accomplished by undersizing the prosthetic humeral body and cementing it in the intramedullary canal so that the head and body are centered on the cut surface of the metaphysis, rather than within the intramedullary canal. The former situation can be accomplished through prosthetic design by providing a coupling mechanism, such as an offset taper, between the humeral head and body that allows the surgeon multiple placement options of the head on the body.

The consequences of nonanatomic placement of the humeral head relative to the humeral diaphysis are unknown. However, several potential problems can be identified. First,

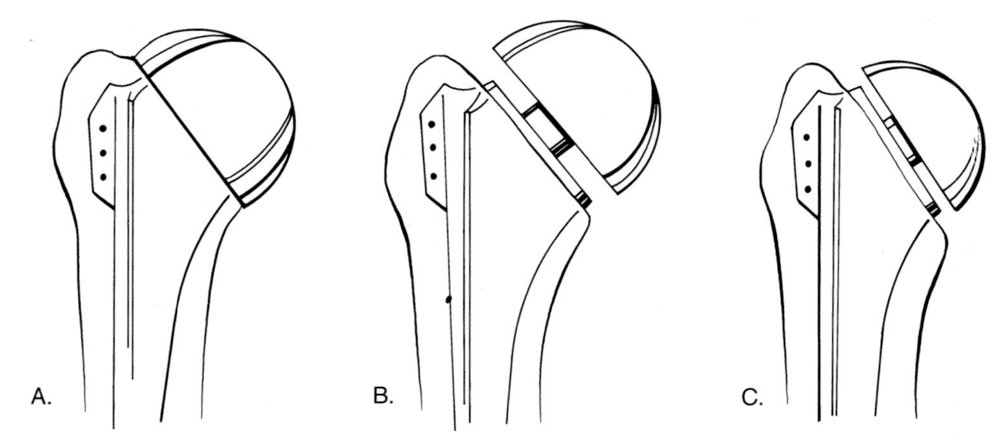

FIG. 14. (A) A prosthesis, the neck-shaft angle of which matches the neck-shaft angle of the native humerus and the articular surface of which rests flush against the cut surface of the humerus, offers the most anatomic reconstruction with maximal surface area for contact with the glenoid. **(B)** A modular prosthesis that has a large gap between the head and the collar can overstuff the joint and also lead to internal component impingement because of diminished surface area for contact, even if the neck-shaft angle and head size are anatomic. **(C)** If the prosthesis is undersized to account for the gap between the head and the body, the tuberosity to head distance is altered (i.e., the greater tuberosity is prominent), and the surface area available for glenoid contact is diminished.

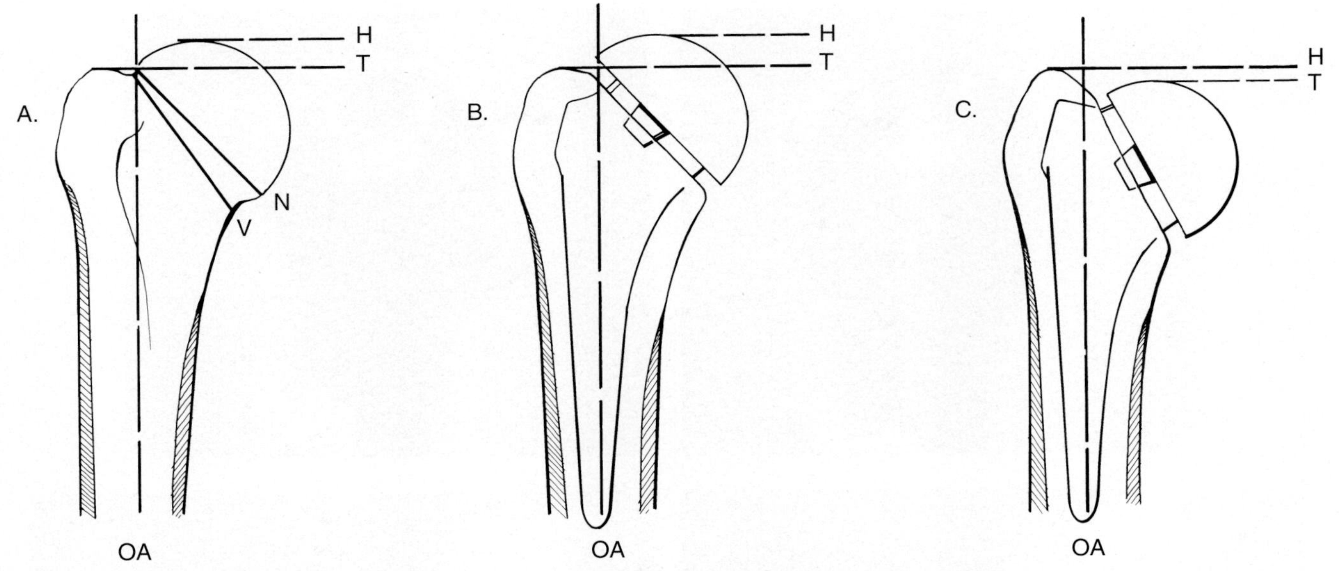

FIG. 15. (A) The greater tuberosity to head distance *(HT)* can be altered by the type of humeral osteotomy performed—normal *(N)* or varus *(V)*. **(B)** If the neck-shaft angle of the prosthesis matches the neck-shaft angle of the native humerus, the humerus undergoes a normal cut *(N)*, and the prosthetic humeral head is the appropriate size, the greater tuberosity to head distance will be anatomically reconstructed. However, **(C)** if the prosthesis has a neck-shaft angle that is less than the neck-shaft angle of the native humerus and calls for a varus cut *(V)*, the greater tuberosity to head distance will be less and may even become negative, even if the head is anatomically sized.

if the prosthetic humeral head is malpositioned anteriorly on the humeral metaphysis, the edge of the implant could overhang the anterior cortex of the humeral metaphysis and produce excessive tension on the subscapularis repair (Fig. 16).[17] In addition, the anteriorly displaced humeral head will leave the posterior portion of the metaphysis uncovered. When the humerus is placed in abduction and external rotation, this uncovered humeral metaphysis may impinge against the posterosuperior glenoid and interfere with further motion or cause damage to the glenoid component (see Fig. 16). Inferior malposition of the humeral head results in a decreased or reversed greater tuberosity to humeral head distance. When the humeral head is then centered within the glenoid, the greater tuberosity may impinge against the acromion or coracoacromial ligament (Fig. 17). As mentioned, these are potential complications of humeral malposition that require verification with further study.

The number of glenoid sizes required to fit all glenoids is probably fewer than the number of humeral head sizes required to fit all humeri. However, if articular mismatch is considered to be important and is to remain constant, a matching glenoid must be available for every humerus. If articular mismatch were to remain within a narrow range, rather than constant, fewer glenoids would be necessary.

The shape of the glenoid component should be based on the shape of the natural glenoid. The bone of the natural glenoid should support the prosthetic glenoid component in its entirety. A pear-shaped component would seem to offer the best opportunity to provide the largest amount of glenoid articular surface without overhanging the anterior or posterior margins of the superior portion of the natural glenoid. If the anteroposterior dimensions of the superior and inferior portions of the glenoid component are equal (i.e., the component is oval), the humeral head may articulate against the unsupported anterosuperior and posterosuperior portions of the component. This may result in bending moments at the component rim, which could stress the component anchoring point or deform the rim. In addition, the increased anteroposterior dimension of the superior portion of an oval glenoid component may facilitate contact between the edges of the component and nonarticular portions of the proximal humerus.

The concept of nonarticular portions of the prosthetic humerus contacting the glenoid component has been mentioned as a potential consequence of nonanatomic reconstruction. In the nonprosthetic shoulder, this phenomenon has been termed internal glenoid impingement.[17] Nonanatomic prosthetic designs may result in component impingement.[17] Nonanatomic features that may predispose to the development of internal component impingement include decreased humeral surface area, increased glenoid anteroposterior size, nonanatomic humeral head placement, and an oval-shaped glenoid. These potentially predisposing factors are especially relevant when glenohumeral motion following prosthetic replacement is normal or near normal. In the presence of diminished glenohumeral motion, internal

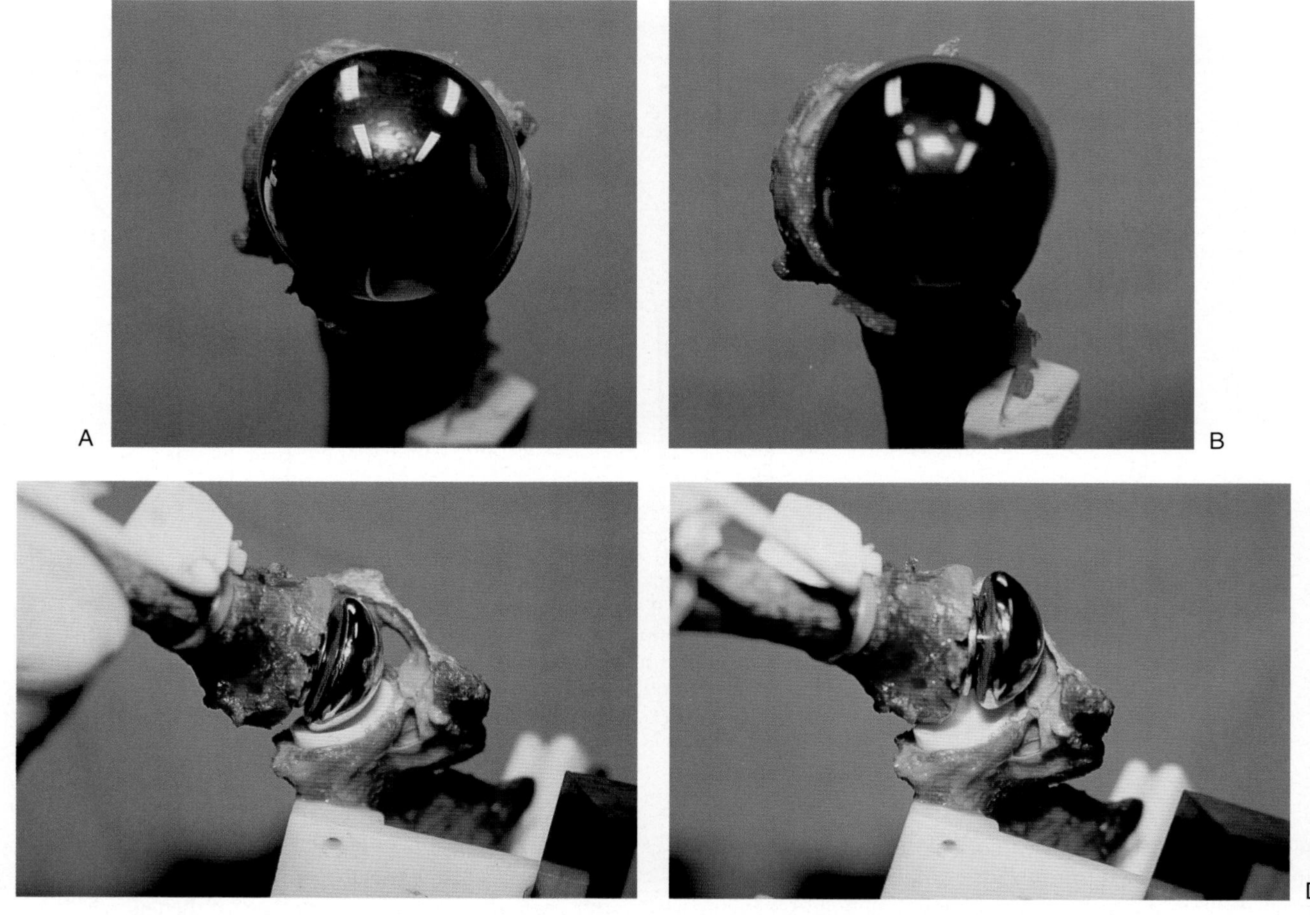

FIG. 16. (A) Ideally, the prosthetic humeral head should be positioned in the center of the cut surface of the humeral metaphysis. **(B)** If the humeral head is offset anteriorly relative to the metaphyseal center, it may overhang the anterior cortex of the humeral metaphysis and place tension on the subscapularis repair. **(C)** A head that is centered on the metaphysis allows full abduction and external rotation without impingement of the nonarticular portion of the humerus against the glenoid component. **(D)** An anteriorly offset humeral head leaves the posterior portion of the metaphysis uncovered, which can impinge against the glenoid component when the arm is positioned in abduction and external rotation.

component impingement may occur only with large deviations in prosthetic sizing or placement.

Biomechanical Factors

Elastic deformation of the glenoid articular cartilage and labrum in the normal shoulder can accommodate the small humeral head translations observed during active motion with a normal rotator cuff and no capsular contracture. Polyethylene does not have the same loading characteristics as articular cartilage and labrum. In a completely conforming articulation, humeral translation can occur only with subluxation of the humeral component and subsequent rim loading. This rim loading may result in permanent deformation of the glenoid component, unusual wear of the glenoid component, or rocking of the glenoid anchoring points.

Strain patterns on the surface of the keel of a cemented glenoid component are dependent on articular conformity.[18] As a simulated humeral head is translated across the glenoid surface, from the anterior rim to the posterior rim, strain along the anterior surface of the keel starts out as mildly compressive and reaches a maximum compressive strain when the humeral head reaches the midpoint of the glenoid. As the humeral head continues to translate posteriorly, the strain becomes increasingly tensile until it reaches a maximum at the posterior glenoid rim (Fig. 18). The maximum tensile strain increases with increasing conformity, indicating the presence of an increasing bending moment. However, the maximum compressive strain observed when the humeral head is at the midpoint of the glenoid increases with decreasing conformity.[18] The clinical significance of these alterations in component strain is not currently known.

The force required for dislocation of a prosthetic glenohumeral joint with a constant joint reaction force is a function of component constraint (i.e., wall height), not component conformity.[21] If wall height and joint reaction force

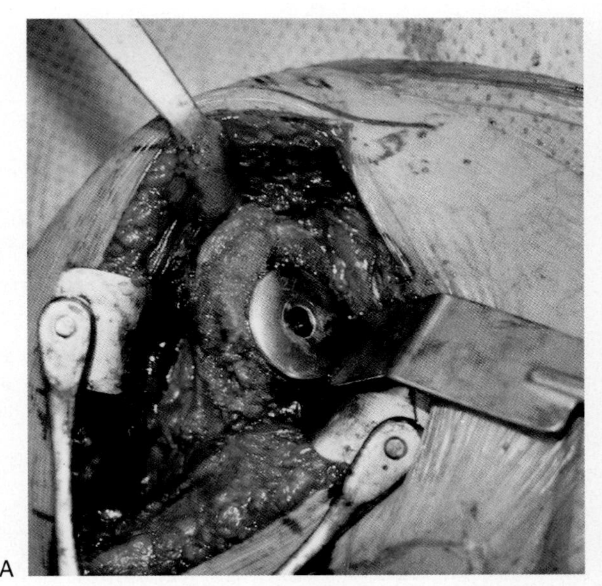

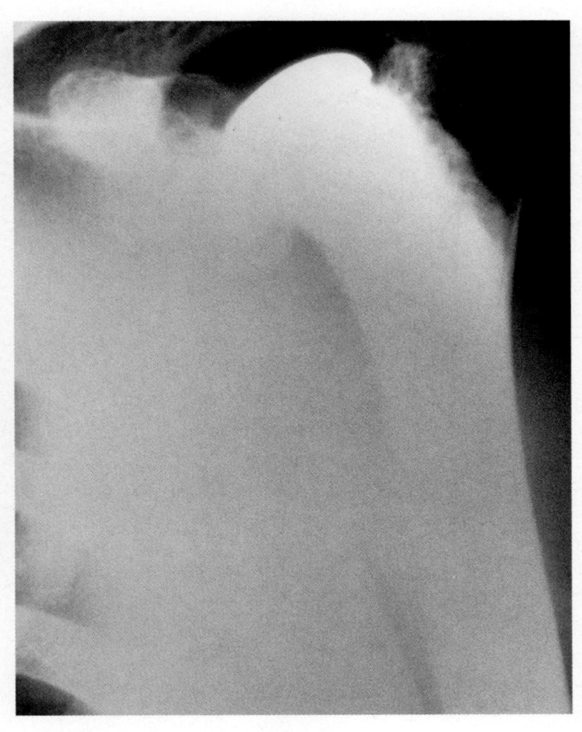

FIG. 17. **(A)** Inferior placement of the humeral stem intraoperatively may occur from a number of causes, most commonly a varus cut. **(B)** This will lead to a reversed greater tuberosity to head distances and potential subacromial impingement.

remain constant, the force required for dislocation of the prosthetic components remains the same, regardless of conformity. As articular conformity decreases, the amount of humeral translation permitted before the glenoid wall is encountered increases. However, continued translation to the top of the glenoid rim requires the same force, irrespective of decreasing component conformity (Fig. 19).[21]

Articular nonconformity of prosthetic components seems desirable if reproduction of normal glenohumeral kinematics is a goal of prosthetic reconstruction. However, the ideal amount of articular mismatch is unknown. There is probably an acceptable range of articular nonconformity. Too much nonconformity may decrease contact area and increase contact stresses to a level that could threaten the integrity of polyethylene. In addition, given the small dimensions of the natural glenoid, a glenoid component that is both excessively flat and small enough to fit on the surface of the natural glenoid will have a diminutive wall height and may be prone to instability. Conversely, too little nonconformity limits humeral translation and encourages glenoid component rim loading. This results in increased tensile strain at the anchoring point of the glenoid component and may lead to increased component wear, peripheral component deformation, or early loosening.

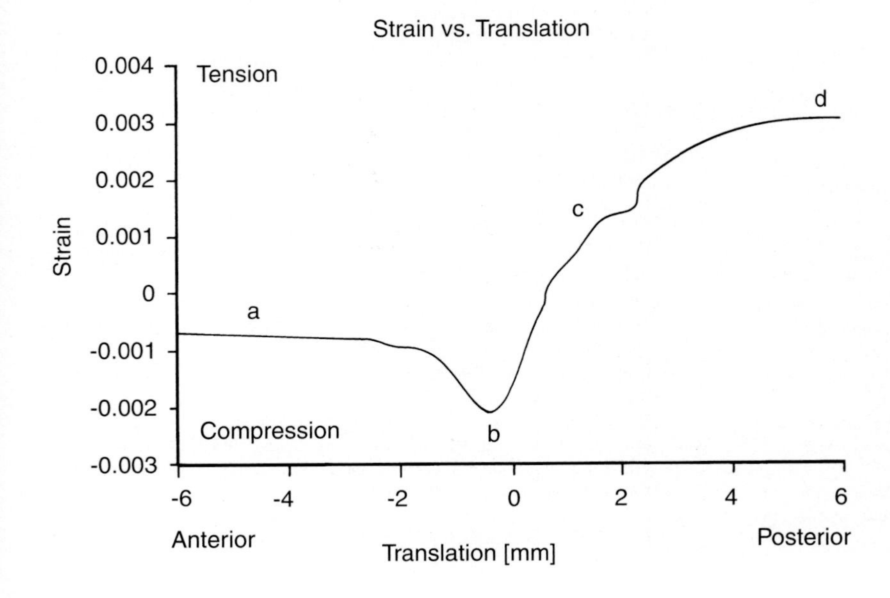

FIG. 18. As the humeral head is translated from the anterior glenoid rim to the posterior glenoid rim, strain on the anterior surface of the keel changes. The strain begins as a compressive strain that increases to a maximum when the humeral head is positioned over the deepest portion of the glenoid component. The strain reverses and becomes tensile and reaches a maximum tensile strain when the humeral head reaches the posterior glenoid rim. Increasing component conformity is associated with an increase in maximum tensile strain. Decreasing component conformity is associated with increasing maximum compressive strain.

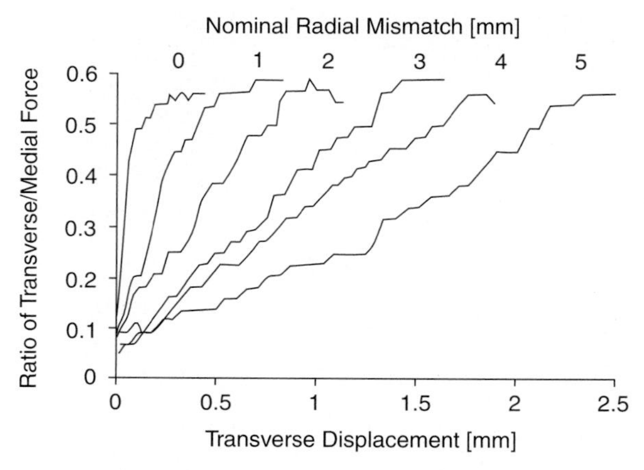

FIG. 19. This graph plots force versus transverse displacement as a function of conformity. As component conformity decreases, there is more humeral head translation permitted for the same normalized displacement force ratio. However, the force required for maximum displacement (i.e., dislocation force) does not change appreciably. (From ref. 22, with permission.)

SUMMARY

Glenohumeral component design should be based on known anatomic and biomechanical relations of the normal shoulder. The goals of prosthetic reconstruction of the glenohumeral joint should continue to be anatomic reconstruction of the articular surfaces with restoration of normal glenohumeral kinematics. Given the severe soft-tissue and occasional osseous abnormalities that are encountered in patients with glenohumeral arthritis, this goal may not be attainable. Prosthetic designs that most closely mimic normal anatomy and allow the most intraoperative flexibility in prosthetic sizing and placement are likely to improve our chances of attaining these goals. However, shoulder replacement is and always will be a technique-dependent process. No prosthetic implant can substitute for good surgical technique.

REFERENCES

1. Amstutz HC, Hoy ALS, Clarke IC. UCLA anatomic total shoulder arthroplasty. *Clin Orthop* 1981;155:7–20.
2. Ballmer FT, Lippitt SB, Romeo AA, Matsen FA III. Total shoulder arthroplasty: some considerations related to glenoid surface contact. *J Shoulder Elbow Surg* 1994;3:299–306.
3. Ballmer FT, Sidles JA, Romeo AA, Matsen FA III. Humeral head prosthetic arthroplasty: surgically relevant geometric considerations. *J Shoulder Elbow Surg* 1993;2:296–304.
4. Bassett RW, Browne AO, Morrey BF, An KN. Glenohumeral muscle force and moment mechanics in a position of shoulder instability. *J Biomech* 1990;23:405–415.
5. Boileau P, Walch G. The three-dimensional geometry of the proximal humerus. Implications for surgical technique and prosthetic design. *J Bone Joint Surg [Br]* 1997;79:857–865.
6. Clark JM, Harryman DT II. Tendons, ligaments, and capsule of the rotator cuff. *J Bone Joint Surg [Am]* 1992;74:713–725.
7. Clarke IC, Gruen TAW, Hoy AS, Hirschowitz D, Maki S, Amstutz HC. Problems in gleno-humeral surface replacements—real or imagined? *Eng Med* 1979;8:161–175.
8. Cooper DE, O'Brien SJ, Arnoczky SP, Warren RF. The structure and function of the coracohumeral ligament: an anatomic and microscopic study. *J Shoulder Elbow Surg* 1993;2:70–77.
9. Cooper RA, Brems JJ. Recurrent disassembly of a modular humeral prosthesis. *J Arthroplasty* 1991;6:375–377.
10. DePalma AF, Gallery G, Bennett CA. Variational anatomy and degenerative lesions of the shoulder joint. In: W. Blount, ed. *American Academy of Orthopaedic Surgeons Instructional Course Lectures*. Ann Arbor: JW Edwards, 1949:255–281.
11. Flatow EL. Prosthetic design considerations in total shoulder arthroplasty. *Semin Arthroplasty* 1995;6:233–244.
12. Freedman L, Munro RR. Abduction of the arm in the scapular plane: scapular and glenohumeral movements. *J Bone Joint Surg [Am]* 1966; 48:1503–1510.
13. Harryman DT II, Sidles JA, Clark JM, McQuade KJ, Gibb TD, Matsen FA III. Translation of the humeral head on the glenoid with passive glenohumeral motion. *J Bone Joint Surg [Am]* 1990;72:1334–1343.
14. Harryman DT II, Sidles JA, Harris SL, Lippitt SB, Matsen FA III. The effect of articular conformity and the size of the humeral head component on laxity and motion after glenohumeral arthroplasty. *J Bone Joint Surg [Am]* 1995;77:555–563.
15. Harryman DTI, Sidles JA, Harris SL, Matsen FAI. The role of the rotator interval capsule in passive motion and stability of the shoulder. *J Bone Joint Surg [Am]* 1992;74:53–66.
16. Howell SM, Galinat BJ. The glenoid–labral socket: a constrained articular surface. *Clin Orthop* 1989;243:122–125.
17. Iannotti JP, Gabriel JP, Schneck SL, Evans BG, Misra S. The normal glenohumeral relationships. *J Bone Joint Surg [Am]* 1992;74:491–500.
18. Jobe CM, Iannotti JP. Limits imposed on glenohumeral motion by joint geometry. *J Shoulder Elbow Surg* 1995;4:281–285.
19. Karduna AR, Williams GR, Iannotti JP, Williams JL. Total shoulder arthroplasty biomechanics: a study of the forces and strains at the glenoid component. *J Biomech Eng* 1998;120:92–99.
20. Karduna AR, Williams GR, Williams JL, Iannotti JP. Kinematics of the glenohumeral joint: influences of muscle forces, ligamentous constraints, and articular geometry. *J Orthop Res* 1996;14:986–993.
21. Karduna AR, Williams GR, Williams JL, Iannotti JP. Glenohumeral joint translations before and after total shoulder arthroplasty. A study in cadavera. *J Bone Joint Surg [Am]* 1997;79:1166–1174.
22. Karduna AR, Williams GR, Williams JL, Iannotti JP. Joint stability after total shoulder arthroplasty in a cadaver model. *J Shoulder Elbow Surg* 1997;6:506–511.
23. Kelkar R, Flatow EL, Bigliani LU, Mow VC. The effects of articular congruence and humeral head rotation on glenohumeral kinematics. *Adv Bioeng* 1994;28:19–20.
24. Kelkar R, Newton PM, Armengol J, et al. Glenohumeral kinematics. *J Shoulder Elbow Surg* 1993;2:S28.
25. Kelkar R, Newton PM, Armengol J, et al. Three-dimensional kinematics of the glenohumeral joint during abduction in the scapular plane. *Trans Orthop Res Soc* 1993;18:136.
26. Kronberg M, Brostrom LA, Soderlund V. Retroversion of the humeral head in the normal shoulder and its relationship to the normal range of motion. *Clin Orthop* 1990:113–117.
27. Lippitt SB, Vanderhooft JE, Harris SL, Sidles JA, Harryman DT, Matsen FA. Glenohumeral stability from concavity-compression: a quantitative analysis. *J Shoulder Elbow Surg* 1993;2:27–35.
28. Maki S, Gruen T. Anthropometric study of the gleno humeral joint. *Trans Orthop Res Soc* 1976;1:173.
29. McPherson EJ, Friedman RJ, An YH, Chokesi R, Dooley RL. Anthropometric study of normal glenohumeral relationships. *J Shoulder Elbow Surg* 1997;6:105–112.
30. O'Brien SJ, Neves MC, Arnoczky SP, et al. The anatomy and histology of the inferior glenohumeral ligament complex of the shoulder. *Am J Sports Med* 1990;18:449–456.
31. O'Connell PW, Nuber GW, Mileski RA, Lautenschlager E. The contribution of the glenohumeral ligaments to anterior stability of the shoulder joint. *Am J Sports Med* 1990;18:579–584.
32. Pearl ML, Volk AG. Coronal plane geometry of the proximal humerus relevant to prosthetic arthroplasty. *J Shoulder Elbow Surg* 1996;5:320–326.
33. Perry J. Anatomy and biomechanics of the shoulder in throwing, swimming, gymnastics and tennis. *Clin Sports Med* 1983;2:247–270.
34. Poppen NK, Walker PS. Normal and abnormal motion of the shoulder. *J Bone Joint Surg [Am]* 1976;58:195–201.
35. Poppen NK, Walker PS. Forces at the glenohumeral joint in abduction. *Clin Orthop* 1978;135:165–170.

36. Roberts SN, Foley AP, Swallow HM, Wallace WA, Coughlan DP. The geometry of the humeral head and the design of prostheses. *J Bone Joint Surg [Br]* 1991;73:647–650.
37. Shaffer BS, Giordano CP, Zuckerman JD. Revision of a loose glenoid component facilitated by a modular humeral component. *J Arthroplasty* 1990;5:S79–S81.
38. Soslowsky LJ, Carpenter JE, Bucchieri JS, Flatow EL. Biomechanics of the rotator cuff. *Orthop Clin North Am* 1997;28:17–30.
39. Soslowsky LJ, Flatow EL, Bigliani LU, Mow VC. Articular geometry of the glenohumeral joint. *Clin Orthop* 92;285:181–190.
40. Turkel SJ, Panio MW, Marshall JL, Girgis FG. Stabilizing mechanisms preventing anterior dislocation of the glenohumerl joint. *J Bone Joint Surg [Am]* 1981;63:1208–1217.
41. Walker PS, Poppen NK. Biomechanics of the shoulder joint during abduction in the plane of the scapula. *Bull Hosp Joint Dis* 1977;38: 107–111.
42. Warner JJP, Caborn DNM, Berger R, Fu F, Steel M. Dynamic capsuloligamentous anatomy of the glenohumeral joint. *J Shoulder Elbow Surg* 1993;2:115–133.
43. Warner JJP, Deng X, Warren RF, Torzilli PA, O'Brien SJ. Superoinferior translation in the intact and vented glenohumeral joint. *J Shoulder Elbow Surg* 1993;2:99–105.
44. Warner JJP, Deng X-H, Warren RF, Torzilli PA. Static capsuloligamentous restraints to superior-inferior translation of the glenohumeral joint. *Am J Sports Med* 1992;20:675–685.

Disorders of the Shoulder: Diagnosis and Management,
edited by Joseph P. Iannotti and Gerald R. Williams, Jr.
Lippincott Williams & Wilkins, Philadelphia © 1999.

CHAPTER 18

Alternatives to Replacement Arthroplasty for Glenohumeral Arthritis

John G. Skedros, Peter J. O'Rourke, Joshua M. Zimmerman, and Wayne Z. Burkhead, Jr.

INTRODUCTION

Although a century has passed since the French surgeon Pean performed the first prosthetic shoulder arthroplasty,[54] shoulder implants with predictable results have become available only in the past 20 years. Consequently, many other surgical procedures and nonsurgical interventions have been developed—and many still have a role today—for the treatment of patients with symptomatic glenohumeral arthritis. In most cases prosthetic arthroplasty is the optimal surgical option for patients with moderate to severe disease; however, in a small percentage of these cases, glenohumeral arthrodesis or resection arthroplasty are appropriate surgical alternatives. Arthroscopic debridement and capsular release are viable options in some patients with pain or stiffness associated with mild arthritis. On the horizon are techniques for transplanting autologous osteochondral tissue or genetically engineered cartilage. However, it is only after the failure of nonsurgical treatment that surgical interventions should be considered. Furthermore, there may be patients for whom surgery is contraindicated, even though they may have substantial shoulder pain (e.g., patients who have excessive risk of perioperative mortality or who are too young or active to consider replacement). For these patients, it is imperative that the practitioner fully explore alternatives to arthroplastic interventions. Specific alternatives to replacement arthroplasty discussed include physical therapy and other nonoperative interventions, arthroscopic debridement, capsule release, synovectomy, periarticular osteotomy, corrective osteotomy, resection arthroplasty, interpositional arthroplasty, and shoulder arthrodesis (see Treatment Algorithms I and II).

J. G. Skedros: Department of Orthopaedic Surgery, Ogden Clinic, Ogden, Utah 84403.
P. J. O'Rourke, J. M. Zimmerman and W. Z. Burkhead Jr.: Department of Orthopaedic Surgery, W. B. Carrell Memorial Clinic, Dallas, Texas 75204.

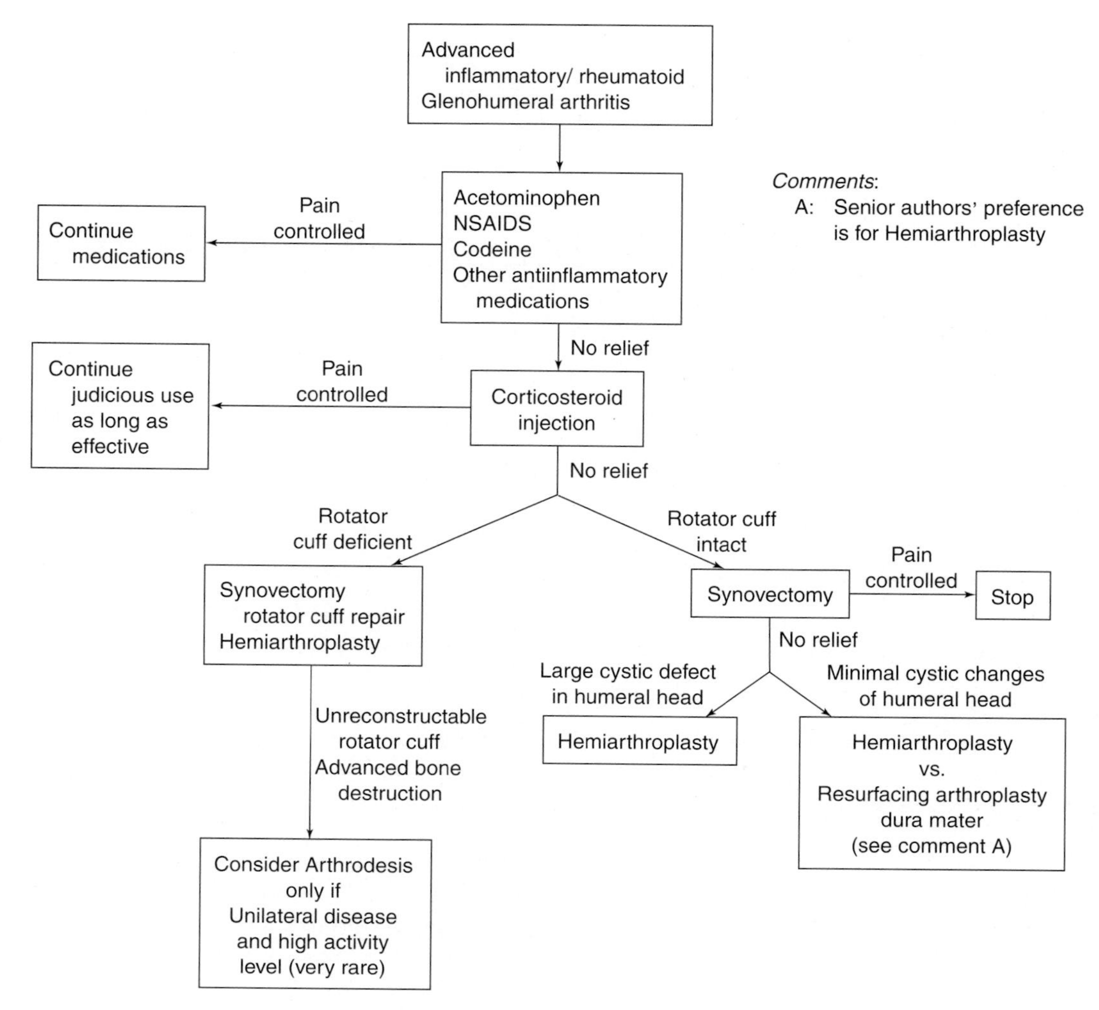

I. Algorithm for treatment of inflammatory arthritides.

Noninflammatory and Inflammatory Arthritides of the Shoulder

Distinguishing osteoarthritis from rheumatoid arthritis and other inflammatory arthritides is important because the following interventions that are discussed may not be similarly effective in treating shoulders with these disorders.

Osteoarthritis

The relative importance of factors that control the development of symptoms in osteoarthritis (OA) is still disputed.[24,25] Although roentgenographic features seen in this disease primarily result from the loss of articular cartilage and changes in the adjacent bone,[96] this disease process affects all periarticular tissues.[12,53,86] To some extent this may explain the poor correlation between clinical symptoms and roentgenographic changes in various arthritic joints in some patients.[14,53] Many patients with this disease have mechanical, inflammatory, and psychologic components to their pain.[22] The shoulder joint is an uncommon site of primary OA, except in elderly women.[20] However, in relatively young individuals, OA of the shoulder may be seen as a consequence of trauma.[84] Specifics of the pathoanatomy of this diagnosis have been detailed by Neer.[64]

Rheumatoid Arthritis and Other Inflammatory Arthritides

Glenohumeral joint involvement is common in patients with rheumatoid arthritis (RA), and is usually part of a polyarthropathy. Laine and associates of Finland defined the spectrum of shoulder disease in 277 hospitalized patients with RA.[47] Glenohumeral arthritis was detected in 47% of patients and many of these also had symptoms arising from the coracoacromial arch. Of note, 16 (6%) patients, with a mean age of 31 years, had shoulder arthralgia without demonstrable roentgenographic changes. Petersson reported on a series of 105 patients with RA, 91% of whom reported shoulder problems.[73] Thirty-one percent of these patients had such severe shoulder disability that they considered it to be their main problem.

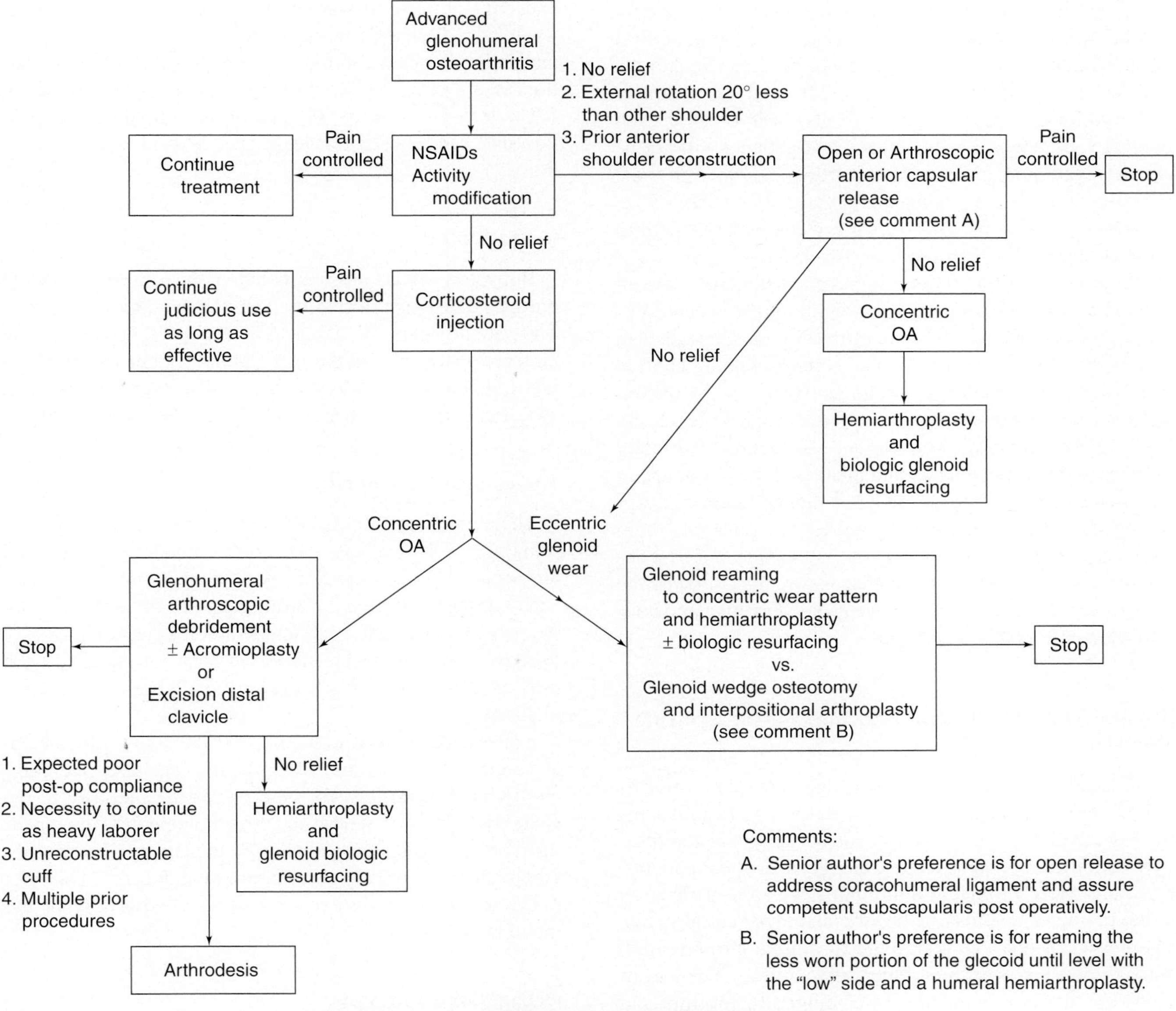

II. Algorithm for treatment of glenohumeral osteoarthritis.

Patients with symptomatic RA of the shoulder are typically women who are between 35 to 55 years of age and are rheumatoid factor positive. The destructive process may be quite advanced before significant symptoms are noted.[18] In addition to loss of motion, two common complaints in patients with RA are fatigue and muscle weakness. Rotator cuff defects occur in approximately 25% of these patients.[30,88] According to Pollock and associates[76] the treatment of choice in rotator cuff deficiency in moderately to severely painful rheumatoid shoulders is humeral hemiarthroplasty with cuff repair. We also recommend repair of symptomatic cuff defects when glenohumeral arthritis is minor; this facilitates future reconstructive procedures. In many respects, surgical management of rotator cuff tear arthropathy is similar to that of cuff-deficient rheumatoid shoulders.[76] Synovectomy of the rheumatoid shoulder joint, which can be effective in treating some patients with effusive disease, will be discussed later in this chapter.

Many symptomatic patients with early stages of arthritis, regardless of etiology, will benefit from noninvasive forms of therapy.

NONOPERATIVE TREATMENT

Education

An explanation of the arthritic process and its probable future implications is an important first step in treating all patients. This helps ensure that patients' expectations are consistent with their prognosis. Education and encouragement also promote compliance with appropriate exercise and the avoidance of detrimental activities. The goals of treatment and anticipated improvements are also discussed at each clinical visit. Typically this means that patients will not be able to regain previous levels of sporting and other physical activities. If a patient is a manual laborer, then the early realization that she or he will be unable to continue in their previous occupation will facilitate early retraining.

Patients with arthritis are taught how to interpret symptoms so they can provide information important in determining appropriate therapy. They contribute to the exercise plan and assume responsibility for its implementation. The patient's active contribution to treatment fosters a sense of control over the effects of the disease. An insightful essay by R. E. Jones[43] discusses how patient satisfaction is strongly influenced by the personality and manner of the physician, as well as the quality of the physician–patient relationship. Applying the basic principles discussed by Jones will help physicians teach these patients how to manage and best enjoy the highest quality of life that is possible through the technologic achievements of present-day operative and nonoperative orthopedic interventions.

Physical Therapy: General Principles for the Arthritic Shoulder

Although nearly all patients with glenohumeral arthritis will benefit from physical therapy, those who benefit most have decreased range of motion and weakness in the presence of minor roentgenographic findings. In some patients, especially those with painful inflammatory arthropathies, an initial period of rest may be beneficial. However, an excessive period of rest can contribute to muscle atrophy, joint contractures, and worsened functional abilities. The aim of physical therapy is to increase range of motion and strength.[55] But, therapy should not be considered a failure if the result is only the maintenance of the existing range of motion. Exercises are designed specifically for the needs of each patient—this includes gentle passive motion and isometric strengthening.[55] Preferential strengthening of specific muscle groups is especially beneficial for patients with mild OA whose symptoms are exacerbated by instability.[23,36]

Although acting in nearly diametric ways, heat and cold are therapeutically useful when employed at appropriate times in chronic and acute phases of inflammatory pain. Cold treatment is useful in treatment of acute inflammatory flare-ups; the analgesic effects have been attributed to the ability of cold to depress the excitability of nerve fibers and muscle spindles, thereby increasing the pain threshold.[51,98] Cutaneous vasoconstriction and resulting reduction in blood flow reduce edema even in deeper tissues.

When inflammatory pain is chronic, then the application of heat, usually in the dry form, is useful in temporizing pain and enhancing joint motion by increasing tissue elasticity.[3,50,52,98] Increased tissue metabolic activity also accompanies the increased blood flow resulting from vasodilatation. Heat can be delivered superficially by using hot packs, hot water, or convective fluid therapy, while therapeutic ultrasound can be used for deeper penetration (see later section).

Hydrotherapy

Buoyancy effects of water help to reduce stress exerted on muscles and joints during therapeutic shoulder exercises.[87] The patient's exertion can also be regulated because of the direct relation between the speed of movement and the resistance encountered. Adjustments in water temperature and agitation enhance the beneficial effects of hydrotherapy.

Therapeutic Ultrasound

The clinical usefulness of therapeutic ultrasound is based primarily on its capacity to increase blood circulation and temperature in deep tissues. Tissue temperature can be elevated at depths up to 5 cm from the point of application on the patient's skin, and peak temperatures occur in bone.[48,49] When the treatment objective is to heat muscle tissue, the most effective modality currently available is shortwave diathermy.[98]

Application of heat and cold, hydrotherapy, ultrasound, and range of motion and strengthening exercises are commonly used modalities for helping restore mobility to the stiff shoulder.[45,55,87] These and other nonoperative therapeutic interventions are contraindicated in patients who have severe pain and a rapidly deteriorating condition.[98] This scenario could imply concomitant sepsis, especially in the rheumatoid patient.

Occupational Therapy

Functional limitations are second only to pain in frequency of complaints of patients with glenohumeral arthritis. Impaired ability to dress and effect personal hygiene are particular problems. Occupational therapists can assist these patients by providing assistive devices and by teaching alternative ways to accomplish these tasks. For patients who desire to continue their gainful employment, analysis of job requirements is helpful in identifying problematic work practices.

Medications and Local Injections

Local anesthetic injections are of great value in diagnosing shoulder conditions by localizing the anatomic site of the pain generators. Appropriate steroid injections can also have tremendous therapeutic value.[8,35] Although the use of intraarticular steroids can be effective in abating symptoms in joints afflicted with RA, they are generally of comparatively limited value in OA, typically providing relatively short-term relief of symptoms.

Dacre et al.[21] studied the results of local steroid injections or physiotherapy in treating patients with painful or stiff rheumatoid shoulders. The study design was prospective, randomized, and observer-blinded. Sixty consecutive patients of similar age, sex, diagnosis, and disease severity were allocated into three groups to receive either local steroids, 6 weeks of physiotherapy, or both. Assessments of pain and shoulder movement were made initially, at 6 weeks and at 6 months. Results showed that physiotherapy alone was just as effective as local steroid injections or a combination of these 2 methods. In the uncomplicated case, a local steroid injection was the most cost-effective treatment.

Oral analgesics, such as salicylates, acetaminophen, and codeine, can be very effective in treating arthritic pain. The role of nonsteroidal antiinflammatory drugs (NSAIDs) in treating patients with symptomatic inflammatory arthropathies is well established.[44] However, for use in OA it is controversial whether NSAIDs are any better than simple analgesia.[24] NSAIDs may have deleterious effects on articular cartilage in addition to the risk of untoward effects on gastric, renal, and liver function, which are particular problems in elderly patients.[24,44] Nevertheless, in a randomized trial examining pain relief in patients with OA of the knee treated with NSAIDs versus simple analgesics, NSAIDs were clearly superior in providing better quality of life and pain relief at the time of true inflammation.[71]

Chronic Pain Management

Management of patients with intractable shoulder pain, without mechanical cause, can be difficult. They may be best treated initially with a trial of interventions managed by a team of specialists trained in treating chronic pain. These specialists can manage depression, manipulate medication intake, inject trigger points, perform nerve blocks, and administer other modalities. A neurologic workup is also often necessary to rule out cervical radiculopathy, brachial plexopathy, reflex sympathetic dystrophy, or other disorders.

OPERATIVE TREATMENT

Arthroscopic Debridement

Arthroscopic debridement or lavage for arthritis has been successfully used in the weight-bearing joints of the lower limb, particularly the knee.[38,70] In many cases, this may be the result of a strong placebo effect.[63] In contrast to the knee, the benefits of, and indications for, arthroscopic debridement in the shoulder are not as clear, although most orthopedic surgeons know of anecdotal evidence suggesting that this can benefit some patients. In some cases, arthroscopy will reveal previously unrecognized grade 2 to 4 osteochondral lesions.[37] Cofield reported[16] that in 8 patients with glenohumeral arthritis the use of arthroscopy confirmed or modified the diagnosis, or altered the course of treatment, in all cases. Ellman et al. reported[28] on 18 patients who underwent shoulder arthroscopy for impingement syndrome and, at surgery, were found to have coexisting glenohumeral degenerative joint disease, which was not apparent during preoperative, clinical, and roentgenographic evaluation.

Generally, results of arthroscopic debridement for OA of the shoulder depend on the extent of degenerative changes.[40,66–68] Ogilvie-Harris and Wiley[66] reviewed 54 patients with OA of the shoulder who were followed for 3 years. When degenerative changes were mild, successful outcome occurred in two-thirds of cases; and when changes were severe, successful outcome occurred in only one-third of cases. An additional group of patients who did well were those who had debridements of degenerative labral tears. There are also several reported cases in whom synovial chondromatosis of the shoulder, associated with arthritic changes, has been adequately treated by arthroscopic debridement.[19,81,103]

Anecdotal experience suggests that if exposed bone is present, then abrasion arthroplasty may be of value.[40] However, this is unproved. It is unlikely that debridement without capsule release or manipulation will result in a significant increase in motion.[99] Debridement can also be used to treat some cases of aseptic necrosis of the humeral head, for which small early lesions can be debrided with removal of any coexisting loose bodies.[33,40,41]

In another study, a group of 27 patients, with a primary diagnosis of degenerative joint disease of the glenohumeral joint, underwent arthroscopic debridement.[98] Average follow-up was 30 months (range 9 to 63), and their average age was 42 years (range 27 to 72). These patients presented with moderate to severe pain and had failed conservative treatment. The average time from onset of symptoms to surgical treatment was 24 months (range 3 to 60). Arthroscopic treatment included simple joint lavage, loose body removal, debridement of degenerative cartilage, debridement of labral or soft tissue, and subacromial space bursectomy. Although there were no significant changes in range of motion, a significant improvement in pain relief and function was obtained. Overall, there were 78% satisfactory results (excellent and good) and 22% unsatisfactory (fair and poor). There were no surgical complications. Sixty-seven percent of the patients involved in recreational sports (unspecified) were able to return to their previous activities. Of the unsatisfactory results, some pain relief was obtained in all patients for a minimum of 8 months before deterioration. Additional surgical treatment had been recommended for 11% of the patients. These authors concluded that in patients with mild glenohumeral osteoarthritis, with concentricity maintained, arthroscopic debridement is a useful procedure.

In contrast, Norris and Green[65] were less enthusiastic about the usefulness of arthroscopic debridement in the glenohumeral joint. In their series of patients only a small percentage obtained any long-lasting pain relief. They concluded that arthroscopic debridement did not alter the natural history of glenohumeral arthritis. It is possible that the addition of a subacromial bursectomy in the patients of Weinstein et al.[99] may have been responsible for some of the difference in these 2 studies.

The efficacy of subacromial decompression in providing pain relief in the face of established glenohumeral arthritis has been demonstrated in two recent studies. Simpson and Kelley[85] performed an acromioplasty and bursectomy in 24 patients with rheumatoid arthritis with radiographic evidence of advanced glenohumeral disease. They were able to achieve good pain relief and improved range of motion in 19 of these patients. Ellowitz et al.[29] also evaluated the results of subacromial decompression in a group of 21 patients who were noted to have Outerbride grade IV osteoarthritic changes in the glenohumeral joint on preliminary arthroscopic evaluation. They reported uniformly good results and concluded that subacromial decompression provided adequate pain relief in this group of patients. Given the foregoing information, the value of isolated glenohumeral arthroscopic debridement for the treatment of degenerative arthritis remains to be proved, but it may be an effective temporizing procedure in a select group of patients. In our current practice, we seldom recommend arthroscopic glenohumeral debridement as an isolated procedure.

Capsule Release

In 1990, Hawkins and Angelo[32] recognized OA in ten patients (11 shoulders) who had had Putti-Platt capsulorrhaphies for anterior shoulder instability. They hypothesized that this resulted from excessive stress imparted to the cartilage during the abnormal glenohumeral motion caused by the excessively tight anterior capsule imbrication. In seven shoulders the complication was treated successfully with periodic administration of NSAIDs, supplemented by gentle range of motion exercises and occasional mild analgesic medications. The remaining four shoulders were treated operatively; two of these received nonconstrained total shoulder replacements. All four of these shoulders received anterior capsule releases for improving motion and decreasing abnormal forces on the glenohumeral joint. Hawkins and Angelo expected that this procedure would improve pain and retard the degenerative process in the two cases where it was done without resurfacing arthroplasty. With this rationale, we suggest that in similar cases in whom mild to moderate OA is associated with limited motion, especially external rotation, capsular release should be considered.

Ogilvie-Harris and Wiley[66] reported that in 54 patients with OA of the shoulder who were treated with arthroscopic debridement, 14 had an associated frozen shoulder. In these cases severely restricted motion was restored either by cutting or removing adhesions, or by manipulation. In general, if there was more than 20 degrees loss of passive motion, compared with the opposite shoulder, then an arthroscopic capsular release was performed.

Surgical and Medical Synovectomy

Beneficial effects of synovectomy in the treatment of inflammatory arthropathies of some joints are well established.[18,46,100,101] The knee has historically been considered one of the most appropriate joints for this procedure, and open synovectomy was the means by which this was accomplished.[46,70,90] An early reported case of synovectomy in the shoulder was in 1965 when Wilkinson and Lowry reported on a series of 69 synovectomies, 1 of which was in a shoulder, and was done without the arthroscope.[100]

In proliferative synovitis of the shoulder, surgical synovectomy gives good pain relief and increased mobility and function.[69] Open synovectomy of the shoulder is no longer considered absolutely necessary unless carried out in conjunction with debridement of cystic bone lesions,[91] extensive disease,[73] rotator cuff repair,[66] or osteotomy (see later discussion); otherwise arthroscopic synovectomy is adequate.[13]

Synovectomy done early in the inflammatory disease process will slow its progression; however, the procedure may need to be repeated several times, but it is associated with low morbidity. Although abnormal synovium may regrow after synovectomy for rheumatoid arthritis,[72] patients typically enjoy a relatively pain-free period with improved function.

In an attempt to better evaluate the results of open surgical synovectomy in late stages of rheumatoid disease, Tressel et al.[95] reviewed 75 cases in 53 patients with average follow-up of 6 years. Only 4% of shoulders had early-stage disease. Swelling and motion improved in approximately 70% and pain was diminished in approximately 50%, irrespective of the site and degree of joint destruction (Fig. 1; Table 1). Overall, 75% of patients were satisfied with their results. The best outcomes were obtained when the shoulder joint alone was involved and the poorest outcome occurred with more extensive soft tissue involvement (e.g., adjacent bursa and rotator cuff).

TABLE 1. *Results of open synovectomy in late-stage rheumatoid disease*

Direction of motion	Stages I and II ($n=20$)	Stage III ($n=44$)	Stage IV ($n=11$)
Flexion beyond 90°	85%	66%	45%
Abduction beyond 90°	70%	52%	66%
Internal rotation beyond 20°	75%	66%	80%

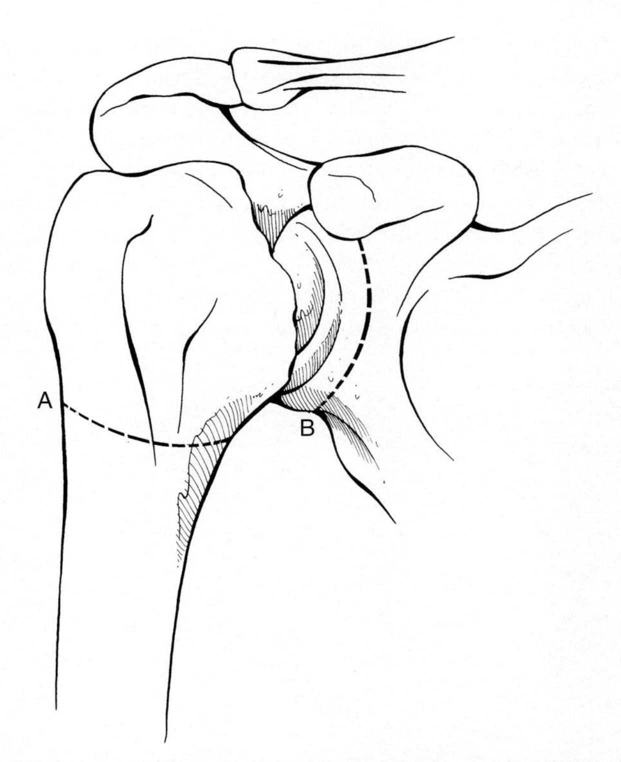

FIG. 1. Schematic representation of the Benjamin double osteotomy. **(A)** Humeral osteotomy. **(B)** Glenoid osteotomy. (Reproduced with permission from: Jaffe R, Learmonth ID. Benjamin double osteotomy for arthritis of the gleno-humeral joint. In: Lettin AFW, Petersson C, eds. *Rheumatoid Arthritis Surgery of the Shoulder*. Rheumatology. Basel: Karger. 1989;12:52–59.)

In the early effusive stages of inflammatory shoulder disease or in OA with synovitis, synovectomy can also be accomplished medically by the use of sclerosing agents or radiocolloids such as yttrium 90.[59,89] Yet these methods have an overall success rate of only about 50% and, similar to surgical synovectomy, often require multiple treatments. Radiocolloid synovectomy should be considered in patients who are not medically stable for arthroscopic shoulder synovectomy. In a study using yttrium 90 on various joints, Stucki et al.[89] reported poor results in the shoulder and suggested that this may be due to established pathologic involvement of the all-important rotator cuff, which would not be influenced by synovectomy.

Periarticular Osteotomy

Although uncommonly performed in the United States, periarticular osteotomy is a well-established treatment for symptomatic degenerative joint disease associated with biomechanically abnormal articulations. In addition to abnormal transarticular force transmission, subchondral venous hypertension may be one of the causal factors in the symptoms associated with OA in these patients.[10] This hypothesis resulted in the development of osteotomies for decreasing venous pressure in joints afflicted with OA. Other suggested benefits of such osteotomies may be the enhancement of local perfusion that, presumably, accompanies healing of the osteotomy.

On the basis of these principles and noted benefit in arthritic knees, Benjamin described a double osteotomy for the arthritic shoulder.[6] An anterior approach is used, and the subscapularis is incised medial to its insertion, exposing the neck of the glenoid. The glenoid is osteotomized 5 to 10 mm medial to the articular surface. The posterior cortex is not cut, but it is manually cracked so that the posterior periosteum maintains position and stability. Transverse osteotomy of the humeral neck is then performed just distal to the capsule, again the posterior cortex is cracked to preserve the posterior periosteal hinge (Fig. 1). The osteotomies are not fixed. Passive shoulder movements are started within a week. Although the suggested benefit of reducing venous pressure is supported by data showing venous hypertension near osteoarthritic joints, the double osteotomy is more commonly used in the treatment of RA, despite the lack of similar data.

In Benjamin's series of 16 patients, the procedure was performed for OA in 4 cases, adult RA in 10 cases, and adult or juvenile RA in 2 cases.[7] Average patient age was 51 years; average time to evaluation was 2 years and 11 months. All of these patients reported substantial pain relief and had an average of 50 degrees increase (range 10 to 150 degrees) in active abduction. The increased motion was from both scapulothoracic and glenohumeral joints. When using this double osteotomy for arthritic shoulders, Jaffe and Learmonth[39] reported similar improvement in pain and active motion in 32 shoulders of 28 patients followed up for 8 to 72 months (mean 35 months). Twenty-seven patients had rheumatoid arthritis, 4 had degenerative arthritis, and 1 had avascular necrosis. Tillmann and Braatz, however, achieved less improvement in their series of 24 surgeries carried out entirely for RA.[92,94] This discrepancy may be the consequence of the mixed diagnoses or the lower mean age (about 9 years) of patients in the study of Jaffe and Learmonth.[39] With this procedure, long-term maintenance of pain relief and motion has been less than ideal.[61,94] Most authors suggest that this procedure should be reserved for relatively young patients with severe RA, and for patients with limited functional goals, poor rehabilitative capacity, or poor compliance. In contrast, interpositional arthroplasty (see later discussion) is recommended for patients with good bone stock, an intact rotator cuff, and an ability to comply with the postoperative regimen.[94]

In general, periarticular osteotomy is not commonly performed and has not been reported by other surgeons in peer-reviewed publications. This is probably because endoprosthetic replacement provides more consistent pain relief and improvement in motion, and has a low reoperation rate.[18]

Corrective Osteotomies for Dysplasia and Acquired Deformities

Humeral osteotomy has been described for correcting rotational deficits and abnormal shoulder biomechanics associated with malunited fractures and glenohumeral instability. In theory, this procedure abates the early development of degenerative joint disease in the these conditions. External derotation osteotomy of the humerus is also effective in relieving pain in selective cases of shoulder rheumatoid arthritis associated with internal rotation contractures.[1]

It has been suggested that posterior glenohumeral instability may, occasionally, result from increased retroversion of the glenoid.[9,26,36] However, there is no documented evidence clearly showing that this leads to the development of degenerative disease of the glenohumeral joint. Radiographic projection-effect error may also errantly demonstrate significant (more than −7 degrees) glenoid retroversion. In some symptomatic individuals with significant retroversion or fixed subluxation, and early eccentric glenohumeral arthritis, osteotomy of the scapular neck may be an

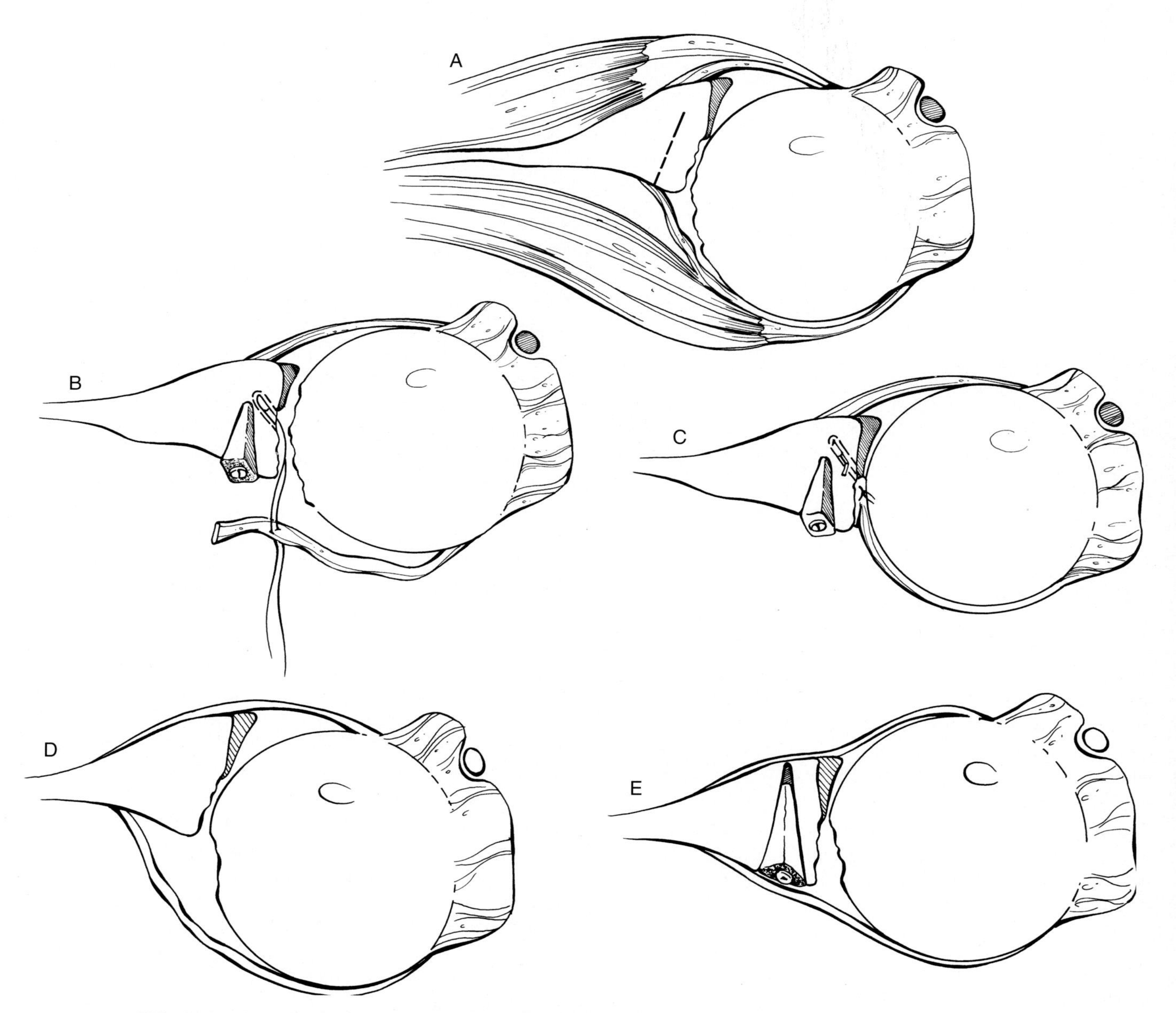

FIG. 2. Interposition arthroplasty with wedge osteotomy for eccentric glenohumeral wear. **(A)** Posterior subluxation: The *dotted line* demonstrates depth and direction of osteotomy; **(B)** proper position of iliac crest wedge graft and placement of suture anchor in glenoid; **(C)** final construct with interposed posterior capsule in area of eccentric wear; **(D)** symmetrical posterior eccentric wear with posterior subluxation of the humeral head and "relative" redundancy of the posterior capsule. **(E)** The osteotomy is carried out to the anterior cortex, and the anterior periostomy capsule sleeve is kept intact to improve stability of the glenoid fossa. The wedge is opened and bone is grafted with an opening posterior wedge. The capsule is tightened and the head is recentered. (From ref. 37, with permission.)

effective treatment by correcting the abnormal biomechanics of the joint (Fig. 2).[37] Complications of these osteotomies include infection, nonunion, and arthritis secondary to glenoid penetration by metal hardware.

Destructive osteoarthritic changes in the glenohumeral joint have rarely been described in patients who have glenoid hypoplasia.[75,77] Although glenoid hypoplasia is very uncommon, progressive degenerative joint disease, which can be quite symptomatic, develops in a small percentage of patients.[102] Nearly all patients can be managed with a specific rehabilitation program for the shoulder.[102]

Resection Arthroplasty

The reluctance of most surgeons to undertake shoulder arthroplasty for glenohumeral arthritis in younger high-demand patients resulted in the development of techniques for resecting, debriding, or reshaping the articular surfaces of the glenohumeral joint. Resection of the humeral head has been advocated in the past as a treatment for severe fracture or sepsis; but only occasionally for degenerative or inflammatory arthropathies.[18] After humeral head resection, chondroid tissue forms between the remaining humeral head and the glenoid. The pseudarthrosis formed is important in achieving a good functional result.

Rather than resecting the humeral head, some authors have reduced its diameter.[92] If stability is a concern, then adjustments in the version of the newly fashioned head can also be made. For example, in situations of rotator cuff deficiency, increasing retroversion by some 10 degrees can reduce the chance of dislocation. However, the results of this procedure have not been reported in peer-reviewed publications by these or other surgeons.

Glenoidectomy has also been advocated for treatment of the painful arthritic shoulder.[31,97] Gariepy described resecting 7 to 8 mm of the glenoid surface, leaving a new flat surface. More recently, this has been carried out, albeit with more limited bone resection, in conjunction with a humeral hemiarthroplasty and biologic interpositional arthroplasty over the glenoid fossa (Fig. 3).[11] Glenoidectomy is probably performed relatively infrequently because of both the limited indications for its use and the greater predictability of prosthetic replacement.

Interpositional Arthroplasty

The use of biologic tissue to form an interpositional arthroplasty has been successful in treating some patients with arthritic joints. In the shoulder this technique was first

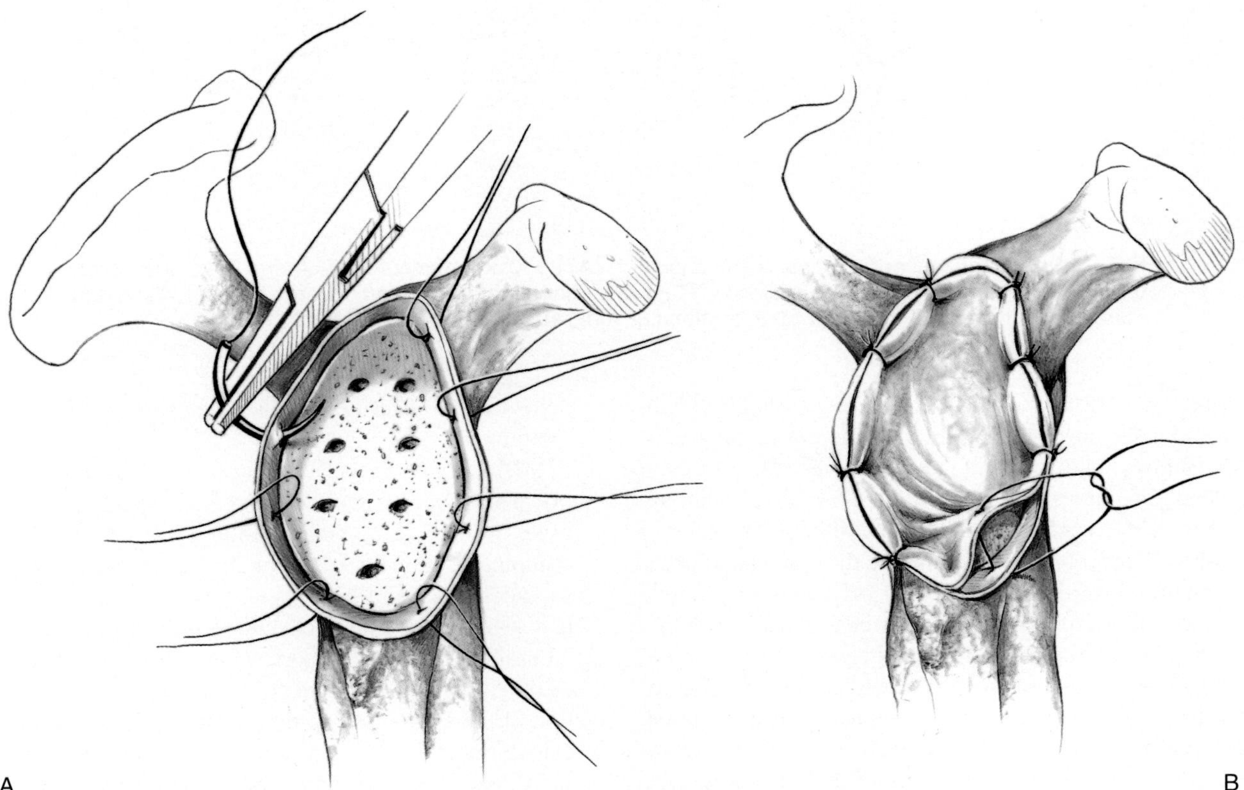

FIG. 3. (A) Preparation of the glenoid, showing marginal suture placement and central drill holes to enhance incorporation of the graft. **(B)** Final glenoid construct demonstrating graft material sutured to the glenoid surface. A suture anchor placed in the central glenoid helps to firmly appose the graft. (From ref. 11, with permission.)

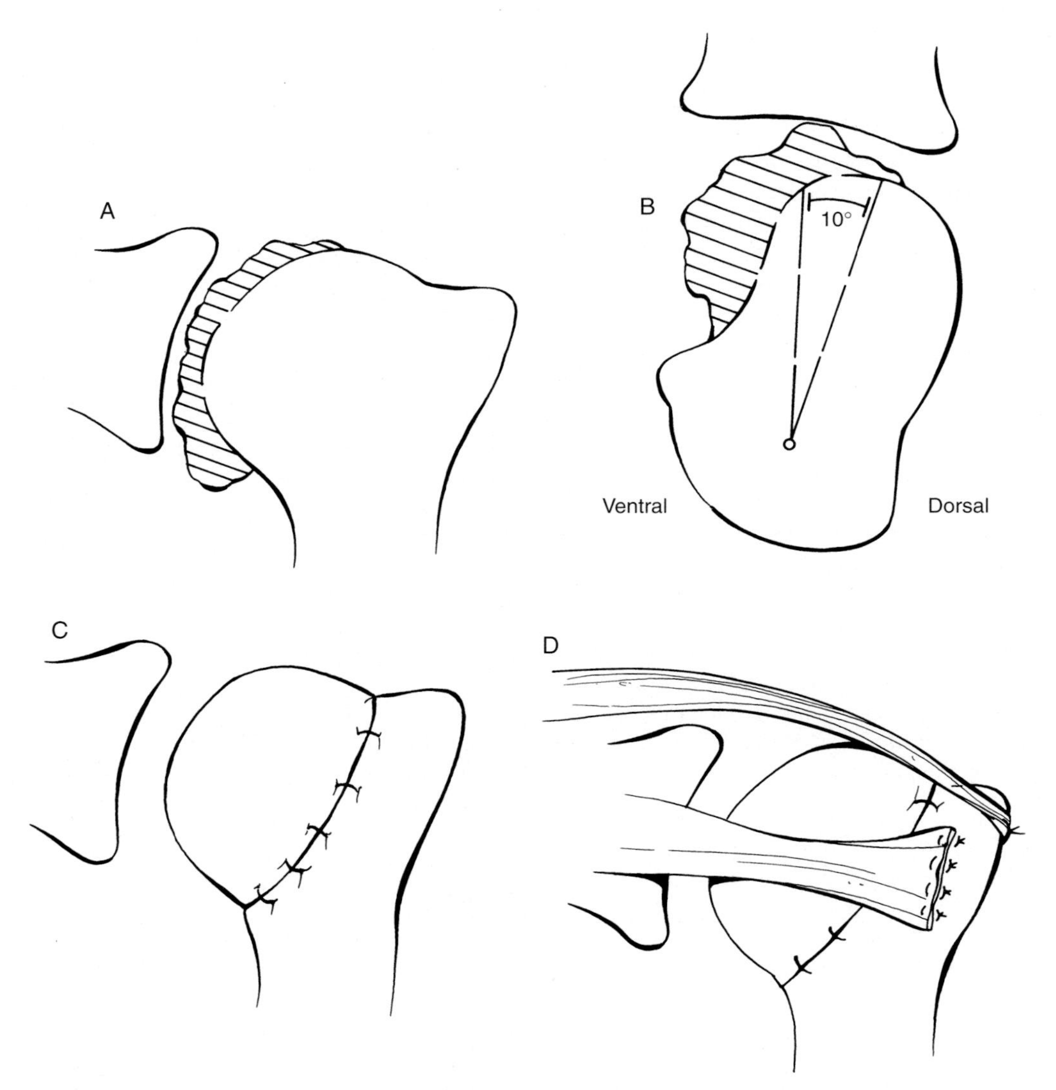

FIG. 4. Interpositional arthroplasty of the shoulder: **(A)** bony deformity of the humeral head seen in anteroposterior view; **(B)** axillary lateral view; **(C)** newly shaped humeral head covered by lyophylized dura mater; **(D)** refixation of the rotator cuff tendons. (From ref. 93, with permission.)

described in 1918 by Baer who used a pig's bladder.[4] Tillmann and associates[93,94] described an interpositional arthroplasty using lyophilized dura mater to cover the surfaces of the glenohumeral articulation (Fig. 4). A transacromial approach is used to expose the glenohumeral joint. The anterior two-thirds of the rotator cuff, including the cranial half of the infraspinatus insertion, is dissected off the bone. After a complete synovectomy, the humeral head is reshaped to a smaller radius of curvature that facilitates reconstruction of the usually deficient rotator cuff; retroversion is also increased by 10 degrees to reduce the chance of dislocation. Lyophylized dura mater is then sutured around the circumference of the reshaped head. The rotator cuff is then reattached under appropriate tension. A 4- to 10-year follow-up in 29 patients showed good pain relief and approximately an average of 80-degree–increased range of movement in combined flexion and abduction. During the course of follow-up there was no deterioration in either pain relief or range of motion.

Miehlke and Thabe[60] evaluated the results of interpositional arthroplasty performed on 32 shoulders and evaluated at an average of 20-months follow-up. The diagnosis was rheumatoid arthritis in 29 of the 32 cases. Twenty-seven shoulders had mild or no pain, 3 had moderate pain, and 2 had severe pain. Range of motion improved in all cases. In 23 of the 32 cases, a rotator cuff tear was present and subsequently repaired. Complications included 3 cases of dislocation of the lateral part of the acromion. (The acromion was osteotomized in the surgical approach.) One case was revised, and the other remained asymptomatic and was not treated. The third case had an associated rotator cuff tear in addition to acromial dislocation; ultimately arthrodesis was performed for biomechanical instability resulting from severe muscular deficit.

Milbrink and Wigren[61] have described a modification of the procedure of Tillman and Braatz[92] in which the glenoid and humeral head of rheumatoid shoulders are covered with a biologic membrane. If necessary, the surface of the glenoid may be smoothed. A sheet of lyophylized dura mater is folded and sutured at the fold to the posterior wall of the glenohumeral joint capsule. The remaining portions of the graft are then sutured, one to the rim of the glenoid and the other over the humeral head. Results reported in ten patients with late-stage shoulder RA at 6 months to 1 year follow-up showed very good pain relief and improvement in range of motion. There was also significant improvement in strength by the end of the first postoperative year. But it is important to emphasize that the follow-up in this study averaged only approximately 6 months.

The main indication for modern techniques of shoulder interpositional arthroplasty is in the rheumatoid patient who has late-stage disease and a well-preserved rotator cuff, and who is capable of complying with postoperative rehabilitation. Contraindications include the presence of large cysts in the humeral head or major defects in the rotator cuff.

Shoulder Arthrodesis

Although advances in the development of shoulder prosthetic arthroplasty have greatly reduced the indications and frequency of shoulder arthrodesis as a primary procedure, arthrodesis remains an excellent salvage procedure in a small percentage of patients with glenohumeral arthritis.[5,78,80,82] Indications for glenohumeral arthrodesis include recurrent or indolent infection, severe soft-tissue deficiency including massive rotator cuff tear and coracoacromial deficiencies, poor function of the deltoid, brachial plexus palsy, or persistent symptomatic instability. It is also a viable option in multiply operated on patients. Patients with both neurogenic pain (e.g., owing to brachial plexus injury) and glenohumeral pain (caused by arthritis) will not have relief of neurogenic pain with a shoulder arthrodesis. However, if function is improved, then the neurogenic pain is generally better tolerated by the patient.[79,80]

In times past, shoulder arthrodesis, coupled with spica immobilization, did not predictably produce solid fusion and was not tolerated well by individuals at risk for surgical complications.[2,15,17,18] However, with the use of internal fixation, autogenic and allogenic bone graft material, and aggressive medical management, glenohumeral fusion is more predictable in these patients.[2] The procedure is contraindicated for a patient who cannot cooperate with the program of rehabilitation.[80] Sufficient motion of the scapulothoracic muscles and strength of the trapezius and serratus anterior muscles are important for good function of the arthrodesed shoulder.[58,79]

In a review of a series of 71 shoulder arthrodeses performed for a variety of conditions, Cofield and Briggs[15] reported a pseudarthrosis rate of 4%. Other potential complications include reflex sympathetic dystrophy, acromioclavicular joint arthritis, infection, and failure of the internal fixation. In a review of a series of 41 arthrodeses carried out solely for rheumatoid arthritis, Rybka et al.[82] reported that 90% of shoulders had solid bony fusion at 6-years–average follow-up (range 6 months to 20 years). The remaining shoulders had not yet achieved fusion or had fibrous ankylosis. The range of scapulothoracic movement improved by an average of 60% (includes active abduction plus sagittal flexion). Results were rated as excellent or good in 68%, and fair in the remaining 32%.

Current techniques for shoulder arthrodesis are described by Richards in Chapter 19. We also use these techniques.

AUTHORS' PREFERENCE

Illustrative Cases

For the younger patient who is significantly debilitated as a result of glenohumeral arthritis, we prefer to avoid prosthetic arthroplasty whenever possible. This is not always possible, as will be illustrated by one of the cases described in the following.

Case 1

A 43-year-old male prison officer presented with pain in his dominant right shoulder. Although he had played college football as a linebacker, he denied any history of shoulder trauma. He had progressive right shoulder pain for several years. His past medical history was not significant.

On examination he had a slightly reduced range of motion in his symptomatic right shoulder: 170-degrees flexion, 40-degrees external rotation, and internal rotation to the T-12 vertebra; as compared with the left shoulder showing 180-degrees flexion, 60-degrees external rotation, and internal rotation to T-8. There was significant crepitation with glenohumeral motion. Manual muscle testing showed good strength of the rotator cuff muscles. Roentgenograms demonstrated severe glenohumeral osteoarthritis, with multiple loose bodies (Fig. 5A).

The patient was very active and desired to continue working in his occupation, maintaining his current level of duties. Initial treatment included intraarticular steroid injections and a gentle exercise program. Symptomatic relief was temporary. Therefore, surgical treatment options were discussed and included arthroscopic lavage–debridement with removal of loose bodies, versus open debridement and cheilectomy with coronal Z-lengthening of the subscapularis, versus biologic resurfacing procedure. He opted for the biologic resurfacing, for it was felt that this would offer the best possibility of continuing his current occupation.

Surgery

A long deltopectoral incision was used. The subscapularis was incised in a single layer from its humeral attachment to expose the joint. Multiple loose bodies were removed and

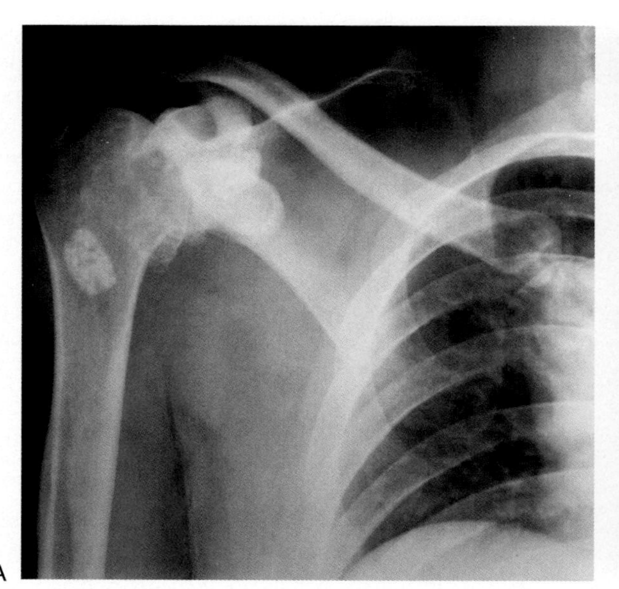

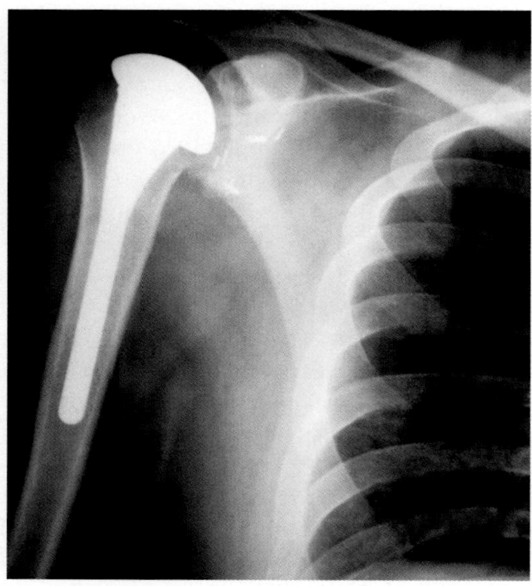

FIG. 5. (A) Preoperative anteroposterior roentgenogram showing complete loss of joint space and osteophyte formation. **(B)** One-year postoperative roentgenogram showing hemiarthroplasty and reconstitution of apparent joint space, demonstrating maintenance of interpositional graft.

osteophytes were debrided. With the use of reamers, the diameter of the humeral head was then reduced to 48 mm. This exposed a 2 × 3-cm cyst in the head. An attempt was made to fill the cyst with morcellized bone graft, but the resulting surface was not deemed strong enough to support forces that would be applied to this region. Therefore, the humerus was prepared for a standard hemiarthroplasty.

Using a burr, the glenoid was reamed to bleeding subchondral bone and multiple drill holes were made on the reamed surface. A 5 × 15-cm fascia lata autograft was harvested from the thigh. The graft was folded and the edges sutured together. The two-layer graft was then secured to the margins of the glenoid using simple transosseus sutures. A suture anchor was used to appose the center of the graft to the central glenoid.

An uncemented humeral hemiarthroplasty (Select Shoulder; Sulzer Orthopedics, Austin, TX) was then performed. The subscapularis was repaired using a combination of suture anchors and transosseus sutures (see Fig. 5A,B). Postoperative recovery was uneventful. The limb was placed in an upper limb immobilizer for approximately 1 week. The patient was then started on pendulum, pulley, and stick exercises. At 6 weeks, external rotation and range of motion exercises were started. At 8 weeks a gentle strengthening program was commenced with the addition of internal rotation exercises at 10 weeks.

Postoperative Results

By 4½ months after surgery, the patient had resumed work, during the course of which he was required to subdue a prisoner. This was achieved by rendering the prisoner unconscious with a punch, using his arm that had been operated on. Radiographs of the shoulder 1 year postoperatively demonstrated a preserved joint space and satisfactory component position (see Fig. 6B).

It is now more than 2 years after his surgery, and he has range of motion of 160-degrees flexion, 45-degrees external rotation, and internal rotation to T-12. Currently, he is pain-free and reports minimal functional limitations because of his shoulder.

Case 2

A 24-year-old right-hand dominant male office worker presented with pain in his right shoulder. Four years previously he had shoulder surgery for recurrent, symptomatic posterior subluxation. Surgery consisted of a glenoid osteotomy for glenoid hypoplasia and a posterior capsular reconstruction. A severe postoperative infection developed and proved difficult to eradicate, persisting for 9 months. Pain and limitations in activities of daily living progressively worsened. Even light office work was painful. He was regularly taking NSAIDS and simple analgesics with intermittent courses of narcotics, but pain relief was always incomplete and of short duration.

On examination there was atrophy of the supraspinatus, infraspinatus, trapezius, and deltoid muscles. A bony fullness was noted at the posterior aspect of the shoulder and the coracoid was prominent anteriorly. Range of motion was painful and restricted to 80-degrees flexion, 60-degrees abduction, 20-degrees external rotation, and internal rotation to the sacroiliac joint. Muscle weakness (3/5 to 3+/5) was noted in abduction, external rotation, and elevation in the plane of the scapula. Tinel's sign was mildly positive at both the thoracic outlet and inlet.

Electromyography demonstrated a suprascapular nerve palsy and brachial plexus traction neuritis. Roentgenograms revealed marked destruction of the humeral head and glenoid (Fig. 6A,B). An MRI scan showed no obvious foci of residual infection. Selective injections into the glenohumeral and acromioclavicular joints and subacromial space showed that most of the pain was relieved with the glenohumeral injection.

In view of the patient's age and shoulder muscle atrophy, a glenohumeral arthrodesis was recommended as the best surgical option for abating symptoms and improving function.

Surgery

The incision used extended from the spine of the scapula, across the anterior aspect of the acromion, and down to the anterior aspect of the humerus. The deltoid was detached from the scapular spine and acromion. The axillary nerve was preserved. The rotator cuff tendons were excised. A burr was used to expose bleeding subchondral bone of the humeral head, glenoid, and the undersurface of the acromion.

With interfragmentary screws, the humeral head was fixed to the glenoid in a position of 30-degrees flexion, 30-degrees abduction, and 30-degrees internal rotation. A 4.5-mm dynamic compression plate (Synthes; Wayne, PA) was then applied, spanning across the spine of the scapula to the anterior aspect of the humeral head (see Fig. 6C). The acromioclavicular joint was excised and the deltoid was reattached with suture through drill holes.

Postoperative Results

Postoperative recovery was uneventful, and intraoperative fluid and tissue cultures showed no evidence of infection. At 3-weeks postoperation, gradual passive mobilization was commenced. By 7 weeks the range of scapulothoracic movement was 75-degrees of flexion, 65-degrees of abduction, 30-degrees of external rotation, and internal rotation to the hip pocket. Unfortunately, during the rehabilitation phase, reflex sympathetic dystrophy developed. This has since resolved. At 1-year postoperation, the fusion is solid and the metal hardware has been removed. The patient reports good use of his arm.

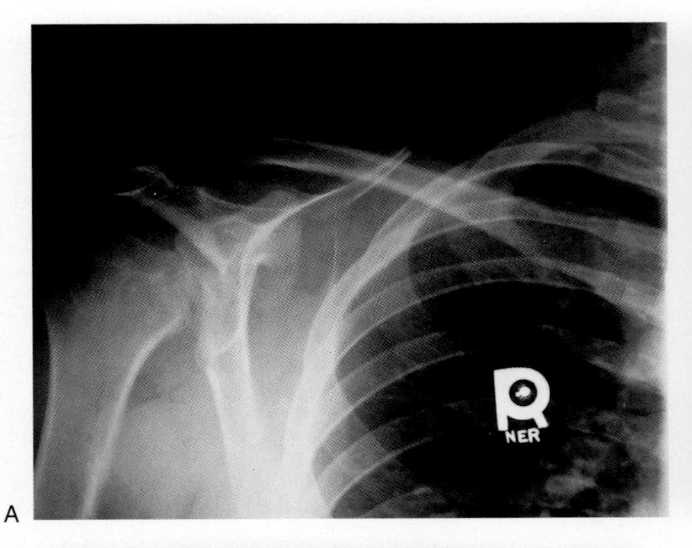

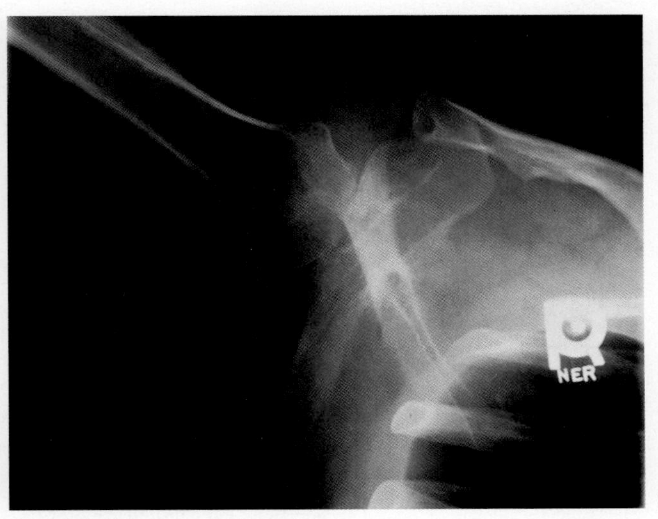

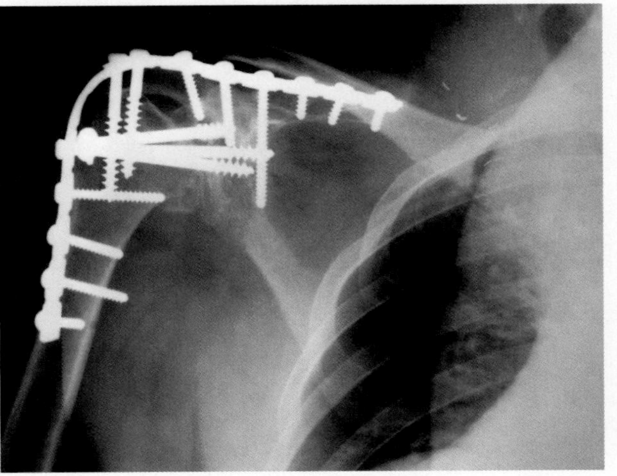

FIG. 6. (A) Preoperative anteroposterior roentgenogram showing collapse of humeral head and poor articular congruity. **(B)** Preoperative axillary lateral view demonstrates posteriorly subluxed humeral head. **(C)** Postoperative anteroposterior view showing shoulder arthrodesed with reconstruction plate and transarticular screws.

REFERENCES

1. Allieu Y, Lussiez P, Desbonnet P, Benichou M. External derotation osteotomy of the humerus in rheumatoid arthritis. In: Lettin AFW, Petersson C, eds. *Rheumatoid arthritis surgery of the shoulder. Rheumatology*. Basel: Karger, 1989;12:60–67.
2. Arntz CT, Matsen FA, Jackins S. Surgical management of complex irreparable rotator cuff deficiency. *J Arthroplasty* 1991;6:363–367.
3. Backlund L, Tiselius P. Objective measurement of joint stiffness in rheumatoid arthritis. *Acta Rheum Scand* 1967;13:275–288.
4. Baer WS. Arthroplasty with the aid of animal membrane. *Am J Orthop Surg* 1918;16.
5. Barton NJ. Arthrodesis of the shoulder for degenerative conditions. *J Bone Joint Surg [Am]* 1972;54:1759–1764.
6. Benjamin A. Double osteotomy of the glenoid. *Scand J Rheumatol* 1974;3:65.
7. Benjamin A, Hirschowitz D, Arden GP. The treatment of arthritis of the shoulder joint by double osteotomy. *Int Orthop* 1979;3:211–216.
8. Blair B, Rokito AS, Cuomo F, Jarolem K, Zuckerman JD. Efficacy of injections of corticosteroids for subacromial impingement syndrome. *J Bone Joint Surg [Am]* 1996;78:1685–1689.
9. Brewer BJ, Wubben RC, Carrera GF. Excessive retroversion of the glenoid cavity. *J Bone Joint Surg [Am]* 1986;68:724–731.
10. Brookes M, Helal B. Primary osteoarthritis, venous engorgement and osteogenesis. *J Bone Joint Surg [Br]* 1968;l50:493–504.
11. Burkhead WZ Jr, Hutton KS. Biologic resurfacing of the glenoid with hemiarthroplasty of the shoulder. *J Shoulder Elbow Surg* 1995;4: 263–270.
12. Byers PD, Contepomi CA, Farkas TA. A postmortem study of the hip joint including the prevalence of the features of the right side. *Ann Rheum Dis* 1970;29:15–31.
13. Caspari RB. Shoulder arthroscopy: a review of the present state of the art. *Contemp Orthop* 1982;4:523–530.
14. Cobb S, Merchange WR, Rubin T. The relation of symptoms to osteoarthritis. *J Chronic Dis* 1957;5:197–204.
15. Cofield RH, Briggs BT. Glenohumeral arthrodesis. Operative and long term functional results. *J Bone Joint Surg [Am]* 1979;61: 668–677.
16. Cofield RH. Arthroscopy of the shoulder. *Mayo Clin Proc* 1983;58: 501–508.
17. Cofield RH. Degenerative and arthritic problems of the glenohumeral joint. In: Rockwood CA, Matsen FA, eds. *The shoulder*, vol 1. Philadelphia: WB Saunders, 1990:678–749.
18. Cohen S, Jones R. An evaluation of the efficacy of arthroscopic synovectomy of the knee in rheumatoid arthritis. *J Rheumatol* 1987;14: 452–455.
19. Covall D, Fowble C. Arthroscopic treatment of synovial chondromatosis of the shoulder and biceps tendon sheath. *Arthroscopy* 1993; 9:602.
20. Cushnaghan J, Dieppe PA. Study of 500 patients with limb osteoarthritis. 1. Analysis by age, sex and distribution of symptomatic joint sites. *Ann Rheum Dis* 1991;50:8–13.
21. Dacre JE, Beeney N, Scott DL. Injections and physiotherapy for the painful stiff shoulder. *Ann Rheum Dis* 1989;48:322–325.
22. Davis MA, Ettinger WH, Neuhaus JM, Barclay JD, Segal MR. Correlates of knee pain among US adults with and without radiographic knee osteoarthritis. *J Rheumatol* 1992;19:1943–1949.
23. Dean MT, Burkhead WZ Jr. Nonoperative treatment of anterior shoulder instability. *Sport Med Arthrosc Rev* 1993;1:202–209.
24. Dieppe P. Drug treatment of osteoarthritis. *J Bone Joint Surg [Br]* 1993;75:673–674.
25. Dieppe P. Therapeutic targets in osteoarthritis. *J Rheumatol Suppl* 1995;22:136–139.
26. Edelson JG. Localized glenoid hypoplasia. An anatomic variation of possible clinical significance. *Clin Orthop* 1995;321:189–195.
27. Ellman H. Shoulder arthroscopy: current indications and techniques. *Arthrosc Indications Tech* 1988;11:45–51.
28. Ellman H, Harris E, Kay SP. Early degenerative joint disease simulating impingement syndrome: arthroscopic findings. *J Arthrosc Rel Surg* 1992;8:482–487.
29. Ellowitz AS, Rosas R, Rodosky MW, Buss DD. The benefit of arthroscopic decompression for impingement in patients found to have unsuspected glenohumeral osteoarthritis. Presented at American Academy of Orthopaedic Surgeons Annual Meeting, February 1997.
30. Ennevaara K. Painful shoulder joint in rheumatoid arthritis: a clinical and radiological study of 200 cases with special reference to arthrography of the glenohumeral joint. *Acta Rheumatol Scand Suppl* 1967;2: 1–108.
31. Gariepy R. Glenoidectomy in the repair of the rheumatoid shoulder. *J Bone Joint Surg Proc [Br]* 1977;59:122.
32. Hawkins R, Angelo R. Glenohumeral osteoarthrosis: a late complication of Putti-Platt repair. *J Bone Joint Surg [Am]* 1990;72:1193–1197.
33. Hayes JM. Arthroscopic treatment of steroid-induced osteonecrosis of the humeral head. *J Arthrosc Rel Surg* 1993;5:218–221.
34. Hertling D. Autobilization techniques of the extremity. In: Kessler RM, Hertling D, eds. *Management of common musculoskeletal disorders*. Philadelphia: Harper & Row, 1983:178–191.
35. Hollingworth GR, Ellis RM, Hattersley TS. Comparison of injection techniques for shoulder pain: results of a double blind, randomized study. *Br Med J* 1983;287:1339–1341.
36. Hurley JA, Anderson TE, Dear W, Andrish JT, Bergfeld JA, Weiker GG. Posterior shoulder instability. Surgical versus conservative results with evaluation of glenoid version. *Am J Sports Med* 1992;20: 396–400.
37. Iannotti JP, Naranja RJ Jr, Warner JJP. Surgical management of shoulder arthritis in the young and active patient. In: Warner JJP, Iannotti JP, Gerber C, eds. *Complex and revision problems in shoulder surgery*. Philadelphia: Lippincott–Raven, 1997:289–302.
38. Jackson RW. Current concepts review arthroscopic surgery. *J Bone Joint Surg [Am]* 1983;65:416–420.
39. Jaffe R, Learmonth ID. Benjamin double osteotomy for arthritis of the gleno-humeral joint. In: Lettin AFW, Petersson C, eds. *Rheumatoid arthritis surgery of the shoulder. Rheumatology*. Basel: Karger. 1989; 12:52–59.
40. Johnson LL. Arthroscopic abrasion arthroplasty historical and pathologic perspective: present status. *J Arthrosc Rel Surg* 1986;2:54–69.
41. Johnson LL. Synovial conditions. In: *Arthroscopic surgery: principles and practice*, 3rd ed. St Louis: Mosby, 1986:1239–1296.
42. Johnson LL. *Diagnostic and surgical arthroscopy of the shoulder*. St Louis: Mosby, 1993:239–248.
43. Jones RE. Taking care of the patient with total hip replacement. *Tech Orthop* 1990;4:1–4.
44. Kaplan SR, Lally EV. Part 1: steroids, NSAIDs, gold and D-penicillamine, and antimalarials. Decision points in the management of rheumatoid arthritis. *J Musculoskeletal Med* 1986;46–50.
45. Kessler RM, Hertling D. Joint mobilization techniques. In: Kessler RM, Hertling D, eds. *Management of common musculoskeletal disorders*. Philadelphia: Harper & Row, 1983:128–177.
46. Laine VA. Early synovectomy in rheumatoid arthritis. *Annu Rev Med* 1967;18:173–184.
47. Laine VAI, Vainio KJ, Pekanmaki K. Shoulder affections in rheumatoid arthritis. *Ann Rheum Dis* 1954;13:157–160.
48. Lehmann JF, DeLateur BJ, Warren CG, Stonebridge JS. Heating produced by ultrasound in bone and soft tissue. *Arch Phys Med Rehabil* 1967;48:397–401.
49. Lehmann JF, DeLateur BJ, Warren CG, Stonebridge JB. Heating of joint structures by ultrasound. *Arch Phys Med Rehabil* 1968;49: 28–30.
50. Lehmann JF, DeLateur BJ. Therapeutic heat. In: Lehmann JF, ed. *Therapeutic heat and cold*. Baltimore: Williams & Wilkins, 1990: 417–589.
51. Lehmann JF, DeLateur BJ. Cryotherapy. In: Lehmann JF, ed. *Therapeutic heat and cold*. Baltimore: Williams & Wilkins, 1990:590–632.
52. Lehmann JF, DeLateur BJ. Application of heat and cold in the clinical setting. In: Lehmann JF, ed. *Therapeutic heat and cold*. Baltimore: Williams & Wilkins, 1990:633–644.
53. Lloyd-Roberts GC. The role of capsular changes in osteoarthritis of the hip. *J Bone Joint Surg [Br]* 1953;35:627–642.
54. Lugli T. Artificial shoulder joint by Pean (1893). The facts of an exceptional intervention and prosthetic method. *Clin Orthop* 1978;133: 215–218.
55. Mahowald ML, Krug H, Steveken MNE, Ytterberg SR. Exercise and other physical therapies of rheumatoid arthritis. *J Musculoskeletal Med* 1990;7(6):52–68
56. Matsen FA, Thomas SC, Rockwood CA. Glenohumeral instability. In: Rockwood CA, Matsen FA, eds. *The shoulder*, vol 1. Philadelphia: WB Saunders, 1990:526–622.
57. Matthews LS, LaBudde JK. Arthroscopic treatment of synovial diseases of the shoulder. *Shoulder Arthrosc Rel Surg* 1993:24:101–109.

58. May VR Jr. Shoulder fusion. *J Bone Joint Surg [Am]* 1962;44:65–76.
59. Menkes CJ, Millet B. Synoviorthesis of the shoulder joint in rheumatoid arthritis. In: Lettin AFW, Petersson C, eds. *Rheumatoid arthritis surgery of the shoulder. Rheumatology*. Basel: Karger, 1989;12: 46–51.
60. Miehlke RK, Thabe H. Resection interposition arthroplasty of the rheumatoid shoulder. In: Lettin AFW, Petersson C, eds. *Rheumatoid arthritis surgery of the shoulder. Rheumatology*. Basel: Karger, 1989; 12:73–76.
61. Milbrink J, Wigren A. Resection arthroplasty of the shoulder. *Scand J Rheumatol* 1990;19:432–436.
62. Mitchell N, Shepard N. The effect of synovectomy on synovium and cartilage in early rheumatoid arthritis. *Clin Orthop* 1972;89:178.
63. Moseley JB Jr, Wray NP, Kuykendall D, Willis K, Landon G. Arthroscopic treatment of osteoarthritis of the knee: a prospective, randomized, placebo-controlled trial. Results of a pilot study. *Am J Sports Med* 1996;24:28—34.
64. Neer CS II. Replacement arthroplasty for glenohumeral osteoarthritis. *J Bone Joint Surg [Am]* 1974;56:1–13.
65. Norris T, Green A. Arthroscopic treatment of glenohumeral osteoarthritis. Presented at Annual Meeting of American Shoulder and Elbow Surgeons, 1997.
66. Ogilvie-Harris DJ, Wiley AM. Arthroscopic surgery of the shoulder. A general appraisal. *J Bone Joint Surg [Br]* 1986;68:201–207.
67. Ogilvie-Harris DJ. Arthroscopy and arthroscopic surgery of the shoulder. *Semin Orthop* 1987;2:246–258.
68. Ogilvie-Harris DJ, D'Angelo G. Arthroscopic surgery of the shoulder. *Sports Med* 1990;9:120–128.
69. Pahle JA. Experiences with synovectomy of the shoulder. In: Lettin AFW, Petersson C, eds. *Rheumatoid arthritis surgery of the shoulder. Rheumatology*. Basel: Karger, 1989;12:31–39.
70. Paradies LH. Synovectomy for rheumatoid arthritis of the knee. *J Bone Joint Surg [Am]* 1975;57:95–100.
71. Parr G, Darekar B, Fletcher A, Bulpitt CJ. Joint pain and quality of life: results of a randomized trial. *Br J Clin Pharmacol* 1989;27: 235–242.
72. Patzakis MJ, Mills DM, Bartholomew BA, Clayton ML, Smyth CJ. A visual, histological, and enzymatic study of regenerating rheumatoid synovium in the synovectomized knee. *J Bone Joint Surg [Am]* 1973; 55:287–300.
73. Petersson CJ. The shoulder joint in chronic polyarthritis. [German] *Orthopade* 1986;15:297–303.
74. Petersson CJ. Shoulder surgery in rheumatoid arthritis. *Acta Orthop Scand* 1986;57:222–226.
75. Pettersson H. Bilateral dysplasia of the neck of scapula and associated anomalies. *Acta Radiol Diagn* 1981;22:81–84.
76. Pollock RG, Reliz ED, McIlveen SJ, Flatow EL, Bigliani LU. Prosthetic replacement in rotator cuff-deficient shoulders. *J Shoulder Elbow Surg* 1992;1:173–186.
77. Resnick D, Walter RD, Crudale AS. Bilateral dysplasia of the scapular neck. *AJR Am J Roentgenol* 1982;139:387–389.
78. Richards RR, Waddell JP, Hudson AR. Shoulder arthrodesis for the treatment of brachial plexus palsy. *Clin Orthop* 1985;198:250–258.
79. Richards RR, Sherman RMP, Hudson AR, Waddell JP. Shoulder arthrodesis using a pelvic-reconstruction plate. *J Bone Joint Surg [Am]* 1988;70:416–421.
80. Richards RR. Redefining indications and problems of shoulder arthrodesis. In: Warner JJP, Iannotti JP, Gerber C, eds. *Complex and revision problems in shoulder surgery*. Philadelphia: Lippincott–Raven, 1997:319–338.
81. Richman JD, Rose DJ. The role of arthroscopy in the management of synovial chondromatosis of the shoulder. A case report. *Clin Orthop* 1990;257:91–93.
82. Rouholamin E, Wootton JR, Jamieson AM. Arthrodesis of the shoulder following brachial plexus injury. *Injury* 1991;22:271–274.
83. Rybka V, Raunio P, Vainio K. Arthrodesis of the shoulder in rheumatoid arthritis. A review of forty-one cases. *J Bone Joint Surg [Br]* 1979;61:155–158.
84. Samilson RL, Prieto V. Dislocation arthropathy of the shoulder. *J Bone Joint Surg [Am]* 1983;65:456–460.
85. Simpson NS, Kelley IG. Extra-glenohumeral joint shoulder surgery in rheumatoid arthritis: the role of bursectomy, acromioplasty, and distal clavicle excision. *J Shoulder Elbow Surg* 1994;3:66–69.
86. Sokoloff L. *The biology of degenerative joint disease*. Chicago: Chicago University Press, 1969.
87. Speer KP, Cavanaugh JT, Warren RF, Day L, Wickiewicz TL. A role for hydrotherapy in shoulder rehabilitation. *Am J Sports Med* 1993;21: 850–853.
88. Stegers M, Tahira S, Miehlke RK. Involvement of the shoulder in rheumatoid arthritis. In: Lettin AFW, Petersson C, eds. *Rheumatoid arthritis surgery of the shoulder. Rheumatology*. Basel: Karger, 1989; 12:24–30.
89. Stucki G, Bozzone P, Treuer E, Wassmer P, Felder M. Efficiency and safety of radiation synovectomy with yttriun-90: a retrospective long term analysis of 164 applications in 82 patients. *Br J of Rheumatol* 1993;32:383–386.
90. Swett PP. Synovectomy in chronic infectious arthritis. *J Bone Joint Surg* 1923;5:110–121.
91. Takenaka R, Fukatsu A, Matsuo S, Ishikawa K, Toriyama T, Kawahara H. Surgical treatment of hemodialysis-related shoulder arthropathy. *Clin Nephrol.* 1992;38:224–230.
92. Tillmann K, Braatz D. Results of resection arthroplasty and the Benjamin Double Osteotomy. In: Kolbel R, Helbig B, Blauth W, eds. *Shoulder replacement*. Berlin: Springer-Verlag, 1987:47–50.
93. Tillmann K, Braatz D. Resection interposition arthroplasty of the shoulder in rheumatoid arthritis. In: Lettin AFW, Petersson C, eds. *Rheumatoid arthritis surgery of the shoulder. Rheumatology*. Basel: Karger, 1989;12:68–72.
94. Tillmann K, Braatz D, Ruther W, Backer J. Osteotomy and resection arthroplasty of the shoulder. In: Friedman RJ, ed. *Arthroplasty of the shoulder*. New York: Thieme Medical, 1994:126–133.
95. Tressel W, Kohler G, Mohing W. Synovectomy of the shoulder joint in rheumatoid arthritis. In: Lettin AFW, Petersson C, eds. *Rheumatoid arthritis surgery of the shoulder. Rheumatology*. Basel: Karger, 1989; 12:40–45.
96. Trueta J. Degenerative arthritis. In: Trueta J, ed. *Studies of the development and decay of the human frame*. Philadelphia: WB Saunders, 1968:335–361.
97. Wainwright D. Glenoidectomy in the treatment of the painful arthritic shoulder. *J Bone Joint Surg [Br]* 1996;57:377.
98. Warren CG. The use of heat and cold in the treatment of common musculoskeletal disorders. In: Kessler RM, Hertling D, eds. *Management of common musculoskeletal disorders*. Philadelphia: Harper & Row, 1983:115–127.
99. Weinstein D, Bucchieri J, Pollock R, et al. Arthroscopic debridement of the shoulder for osteoarthritis. *Arthroscopy*. 1993;9:366.
100. Wilkinson MC, Lowry JH. Synovectomy for rheumatoid arthritis. *J Bone Joint Surg [Br]* 1965;47:482–488.
101. Wilkinson MC. Synovectomy for rheumatoid arthritis. *Clin Orthop* 1974;100:125–142.
102. Wirth MA, Lyons FR, Rockwood CA Jr. Hypoplasia of the glenoid. A review of 16 patients. *J Bone Joint Surg [Am]* 1993;75:1175–1184.
103. Witwity T, Uhlmann R, Nagy MH, Bhasin VB, Bahgat MM, Singh AK. Case report. Shoulder rheumatoid arthritis associated with chondromatosis, treated by arthroscopy. *J Arthrosc Rel Surg* 1991;7: 233–236.

Disorders of the Shoulder: Diagnosis and Management,
edited by Joseph P. Iannotti and Gerald R. Williams, Jr.
Lippincott Williams & Wilkins, Philadelphia © 1999.

CHAPTER 19

Glenohumeral Arthrodesis

Robin R. Richards

OPTIONS

The advent of total shoulder arthroplasty and the refinement of other reconstructive procedures have narrowed the indications for glenohumeral arthrodesis.[33] Nevertheless, arthrodesis of the glenohumeral joint continues to provide a valuable method of shoulder reconstruction for specific indications.[13,17,53] Although the procedure is infrequently performed, it reliably provides patients with a stable, strong shoulder. Albert first attempted glenohumeral arthrodesis in 1881. Since then a voluminous literature has evolved outlining different indications for the procedure and a variety of surgical techniques for performing glenohumeral arthrodesis. Controversies have developed in the literature about the indications for the procedure and the optimum position for glenohumeral arthrodesis.[2,46] More recently, discussion has arisen of the functional results that can be achieved with the procedure.[10] In this chapter I will address the complex and revision problems and then discuss the complications and the results of glenohumeral arthrodesis.

Arthrodesis is an important method of shoulder reconstruction. The procedure has stood the test of time and continues to deserve a place in the shoulder surgeon's armamentarium. For certain specific indications it provides the best method of restoring function to the shoulder.

INDICATIONS

Glenohumeral arthrodesis can effectively restore shoulder function to highly selected patients. Successful glenohumeral arthrodesis reliably results in a strong and stable

R. R. Richards: Division of Orthopaedic Surgery, Department of Surgery, University of Toronto and Division of Orthopaedic Surgery, Department of Surgery, St. Michael's Hospital, Toronto, Ontario, Canada M5C 1R6.

shoulder. However, the procedure sacrifices all rotation through the glenohumeral joint. Wherever possible shoulder arthroplasty is preferable to glenohumeral arthrodesis, if for the particular patient there is a choice between the two procedures (Fig. 1). Shoulders can be fused if an arthroplasty fails, although fusion in this situation is a technical challenge. The indications for surgery in the author's personal series are illustrated in Fig. 2.

Paralysis

All authors agree that the presence of a flail shoulder is an indication for glenohumeral arthrodesis. Patients with anterior poliomyelitis, severe proximal root and irreparable upper trunk brachial plexus lesions, and some patients with isolated axillary nerve paralysis are candidates for glenohumeral arthrodesis.[43] These patients have good function in their elbows and hands, but are unable to optimize their upper extremity function because of their inability to place their hand in space. If such a patient has good function in the periscapular musculature, particularly the trapezius, levator scapula, and serratus anterior, glenohumeral arthrodesis stabilizes the extremity and allows effective hand function.[40] Such patients can then fully utilize their upper extremity potential and can work effectively at bench level. In addition, many patients with flail shoulders develop inferior subluxation of the glenohumeral joint owing to periarticular paralysis (Fig. 3). This condition is uncomfortable and, in some patients, frankly painful. Such patients often find that they must keep their arm in a sling to avoid injuring it. Painful inferior subluxation of the shoulder provides another indication for stabilization of the glenohumeral joint.

Patients who have the combination of a flail shoulder and flail elbow need both shoulder and elbow reconstruction. In this situation, glenohumeral arthrodesis combined with elbow flexorplasty improves the result of the elbow flexorplasty. Without shoulder stabilization elbow flexion tends to drive the humerus posteriorly, resulting in shoulder extension, rather than elbow flexion. Arthrodesis of the shoulder in some flexion and abduction helps eliminate the effect of gravity and optimizes the result that can be achieved with the elbow flexorplasty. Patients with flail shoulders often have a tendency to internally rotate their upper extremity to their chest when some function remains in the powerful internal rotators of the shoulder (pectoralis major, latissimus dorsi) and no function remains in the external rotators. Shoulder stabilization either in the form of arthrodesis or a L'Episcopo tendon transfer reduces this undesirable tendency.[40]

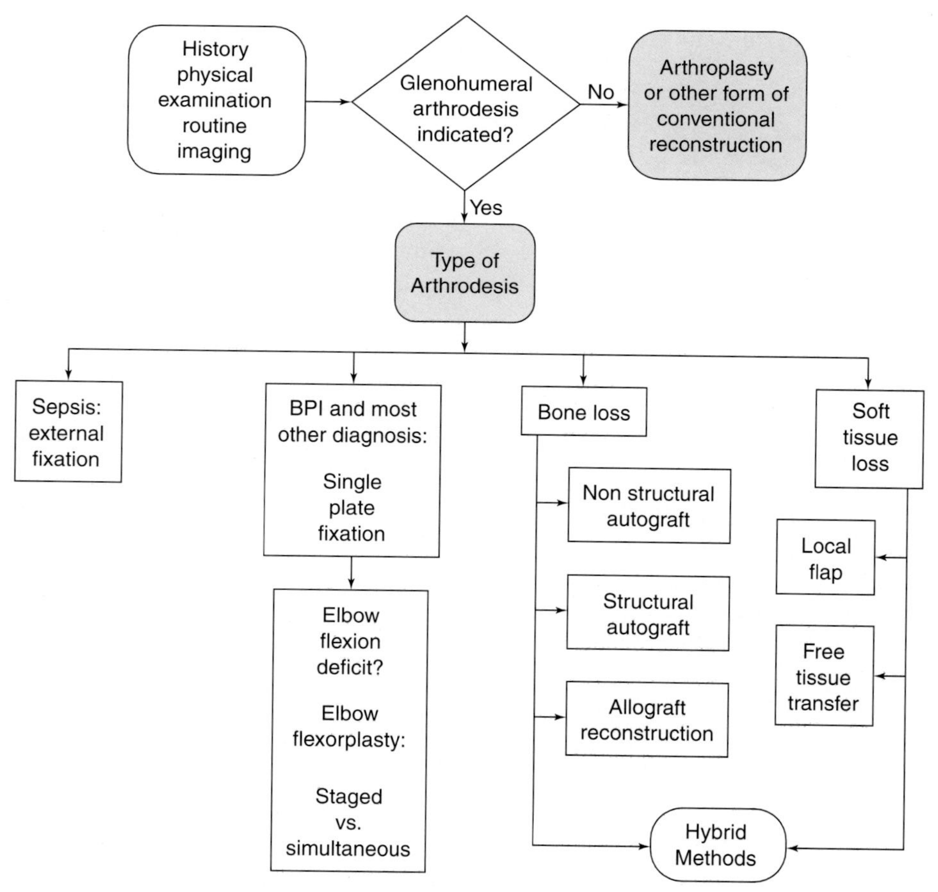

FIG. 1. Algorithm for evaluation and management of patients presenting to be considered for glenohumeral arthrodesis.

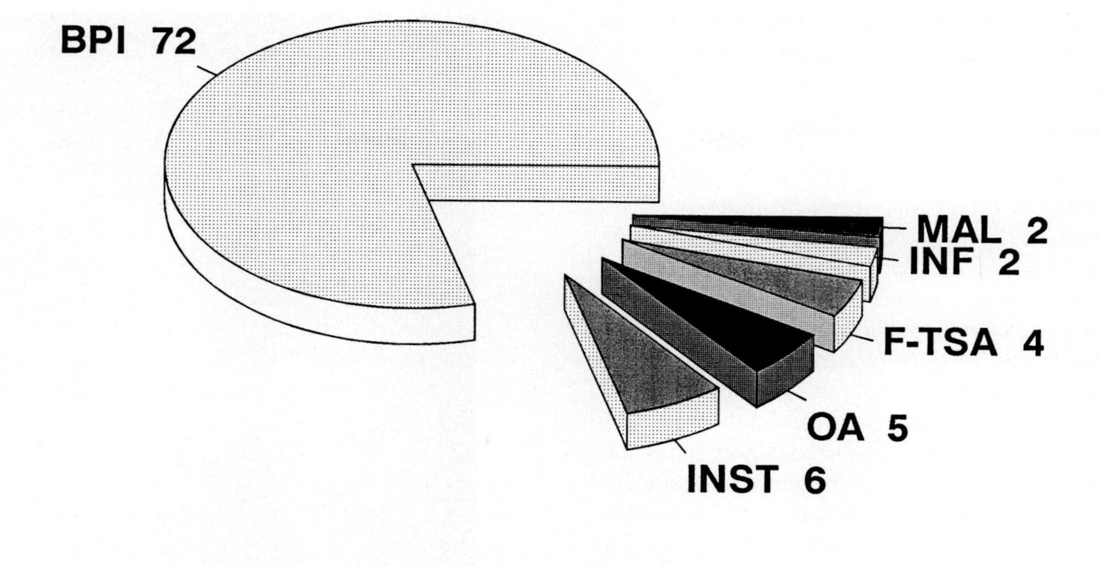

FIG. 2. Indications for glenohumeral arthrodesis in the author's personal series.

There is a wide degree of variability in the disability caused by axillary nerve paralysis, and I have seen many patients who have virtually full motion following paralysis of the axillary nerve, providing the rotator cuff musculature is undisturbed (endurance is never normal). Patients with isolated paralysis of the axillary nerve can be treated by either muscle or tendon transfer or glenohumeral arthrodesis. Numerous reports exist in the literature on the value of muscle and muscle tendon transfer to restore shoulder function following paralysis of the axillary nerve.[16] It is generally agreed that multiple transfers are necessary to restore deltoid function and that significant problems can occur with gliding of transfers over the acromion. It is often necessary to harvest autogenous tissue, such as fascia lata, to prolong the transfers, and the process of rehabilitation is challenging following such procedures. In my experience such transfers are indicated primarily for pediatric patients and adult patients who have only partial paralysis of the axillary nerve.[16] However, pediatric patients do well with glenohumeral arthrodesis, and some authors feel they are better able to adapt to the procedure.[26] If total paralysis of the axillary nerve is present and significant limitation of shoulder function ensues, I would recommend glenohumeral arthrodesis, recognizing that the alternative of muscle transfers may be available in carefully selected patients. Glenohumeral arthrodesis is useful in such patients, provided their symptoms justify the procedure.

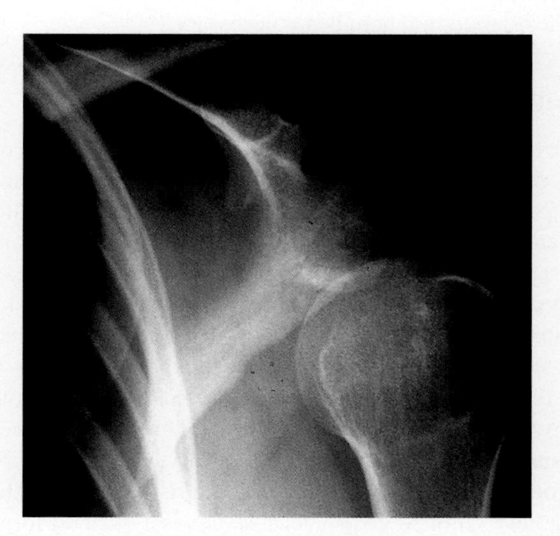

FIG. 3. Severe inferior subluxation of the glenohumeral joint in a patient with brachial plexus palsy. The patient is severely disabled, in spite of good hand and wrist function, because he is unable to position the hand in space.

Reconstruction Following Tumor Resection

En bloc resection of periarticular malignant tumors often requires sacrifice of the rotator cuff or the deltoid, or both. If the resection requires sacrifice of these tissues, reconstruction of the shoulder with an arthroplasty is inadvisable owing to the high risk of instability if an unconstrained prosthesis is used and the certainty of loosening if a constrained prosthesis is used. Glenohumeral arthrodesis is the procedure of choice to reconstruct the shoulder following wide resection of periarticular malignancies. Specific techniques have been recommended for glenohumeral arthrodesis following tumor resection.[25] These include the use of specialized fixation devices and bone-grafting techniques. Vascularized bone grafts and massive allografts are sometimes necessary because of the large defects created by tumor resection.[23] These techniques will be discussed later.

Shoulder Joint Destruction by Infection

Destruction of the shoulder joint by septic arthritis remains an indication for glenohumeral arthrodesis. In the past, tuberculous arthritis was a common indication for glenohumeral arthrodesis. Worldwide, this condition remains prevalent, although in the Western world it has become extremely uncommon. Septic arthritis continues to occur, and when it does, the shoulder joint can be destroyed with resultant pain and limitation of function. Most surgeons would agree that in a young patient with shoulder dysfunction for this reason arthrodesis of the shoulder, as opposed to total shoulder arthroplasty, would be indicated. Although total shoulder arthroplasty can be performed in patients with a remote history of sepsis, if there is a recent history of sepsis or if the patient is young, arthrodesis provides a more satisfactory alternative.

Failed Total Shoulder Arthroplasty

The author has seen several patients who have had multiple unsuccessful shoulder arthroplasties. Although the results of shoulder arthroplasty are generally good, there are some patients in whom loosening, sepsis, and implant breakage occur. These patients often have severe loss of humeral and glenoid bone stock (Fig. 4). In this situation the surgeon must choose between attempting a repeat revision of the shoulder arthroplasty and obliteration of the shoulder joint by arthrodesis. The results of revision total shoulder arthroplasty are suboptimal when compared with the results of primary arthroplasty for other reasons. The decision between these two alternatives must be made on the basis of the patient's age, the presence or absence of sepsis, the bone stock that remains in the proximal humerus and glenoid, the symptoms the patient is experiencing, the quality and function of the rotator cuff and the deltoid, and the technical experience and expertise of the surgeon. In several patients who were significantly disabled I have carried out glenohumeral arthrodesis following failed total shoulder arthroplasty and found it to be a gratifying procedure. It is my belief that glenohumeral arthrodesis must be considered when the reconstructive surgeon is confronted with a patient with a history of multiple failed total shoulder arthroplasties.

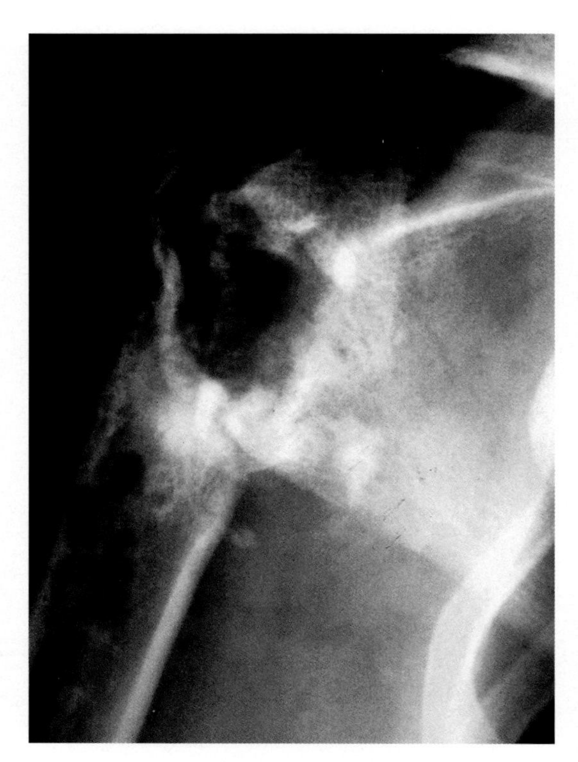

FIG. 4. Excision arthroplasty of the glenohumeral joint after several failed total shoulder arthroplasties. The patient is disabled by severe unremitting pain with any activity. Glenohumeral arthrodesis is indicated to provide the patient with a stable, relatively painless shoulder.

Shoulder Instability

Virtually all patients with shoulder instability can be treated by soft-tissue or bony reconstructive procedures to stabilize the glenohumeral joint. Rarely, a patient will present with chronic shoulder instability after multiple attempts at surgical stabilization. If every surgical therapeutic alternative has been exhausted, the patient's shoulder remains symptomatically unstable, and the patient does not wish to wear a thoracobrachial support, arthrodesis can be indicated to restore shoulder stability. In this situation careful assessment of the patient's psychologic makeup must be carried out and one must be certain the patient has a full understanding of the implications of the procedure. Much has been written about the difficulties in managing such patients and further elaboration here is not necessary.[41,47]

Rotator Cuff Tear

Severe shoulder dysfunction can result from massive rotator cuff tears.[1] Most rotator cuff tears can be managed by coracoacromial decompression and repair of the cuff. In patients who have massive rotator cuff tears that cannot be repaired, some authors have reported good results with debridement of the cuff tear and coracoacromial decompression.[44] Long-standing rotator cuff tears can lead to cuff tear arthropathy as reported by Neer.[34] Neer reports that this difficult pathologic entity can be treated by prosthetic arthroplasty with cuff reconstruction. This is predicated on the surgeon's ability to repair the cuff by cuff transfer or the use of exogenous materials. Neer reports that such patients must have "limited goals" because this is a difficult form of reconstruction. Glenohumeral arthrodesis should be kept in mind as a possible alternative form of reconstruction in such patients when the technical skill of the surgeon or the available tissues do not permit cuff reconstruction and the patient is sufficiently symptomatic to exchange the loss of glenohumeral motion for the relief of pain. In my experience, this situation rarely, if ever, develops.

Malunion

Glenohumeral arthrodesis is rarely indicated for posttraumatic deformity. Most patients with posttraumatic deformities, such as osteonecrosis of the humeral head, chronic fracture dislocations, tuberosity impingement, or a malunion of the proximal humerus, are best treated by shoulder reconstruction using either osteotomy, arthroplasty, or a combination of both. If these procedures are not possible, then glenohumeral arthrodesis can be considered.

Osteoarthritis

The presence of glenohumeral osteoarthritis in an otherwise normal shoulder is an indication for total shoulder arthroplasty. However, almost all patients with glenohumeral osteoarthritis are of sufficient age that they are excellent candidates for total shoulder arthroplasty. If the patient were to develop osteoarthritis at a relatively young age, then glenohumeral arthrodesis might be considered,[3] particularly if the patient was a laborer and modified work was not available to him or her. The results of total shoulder arthroplasty are so much superior, that in our experience the operation is rarely indicated for patients with this diagnosis.

Rheumatoid Arthritis

Patients with rheumatoid arthritis affecting the glenohumeral joint commonly have multiple problems in their upper extremity. Glenohumeral arthrodesis is recognized as a procedure that can decrease pain arising in the glenohumeral joint.[19,37,48] Obliteration of glenohumeral motion has a negative influence on the upper extremity function. Frequently both upper extremities are involved. It is our belief that patients with rheumatoid arthritis are much more effectively treated by total shoulder arthroplasty.[14] Favorable reports of the combination of shoulder and elbow arthroplasty have appeared in the literature, and I would advocate this method of reconstruction for such patients.

CONTRAINDICATIONS TO GLENOHUMERAL ARTHRODESIS

Glenohumeral arthrodesis should not be performed if an alternative method of shoulder reconstruction is available. Many patients are amenable to arthroplastic reconstruction that preserves glenohumeral motion and has greater potential to restore function. Glenohumeral arthrodesis places a significant functional demand on the patient, requires a major effort on the part of the patient to rehabilitate the shoulder following surgery and to strengthen the thoracoscapular musculature. The procedure is contraindicated in a patient who cannot cooperate with such a program of rehabilitation; consequently, I have not performed glenohumeral arthrodesis on elderly patients. Similarly, the procedure is contraindicated in any patient with a progressive neurologic disorder who may experience paralysis or weakness of the trapezius, levator scapula, or serratus anterior. Glenohumeral arthrodesis relies on these muscles to motor the extremity, and significant weakness will grossly impair shoulder function following the procedure.

RESULTS

Review of Literature

Many techniques for glenohumeral arthrodesis have been reported. Some authors have used extraarticular arthrodesis, others have reported on methods of intraarticular arthrodesis, and still others have combined the two methods. In reviewing the literature it is apparent that internal fixation has been employed more and more frequently in recent years. Historically most authors have recommended external immobilization, although recently reports of glenohumeral arthrodesis without external immobilization have appeared.[22,43] I will now discuss extraarticular arthrodesis, intraarticular arthrodesis, the use of internal fixation, and the use of external fixators.

Extraarticular Arthrodesis

Extraarticular arthrodesis is primarily a historical procedure used before the antibiotic era to treat tuberculous arthritis. This treatment method was used to avoid entering the tuberculous joint and to obliterate motion at the joint without activating and spreading the infection. Watson-Jones[52] described a technique utilizing a Cubbin's approach[10a] to the shoulder, decorticating the superior and inferior surfaces of the acromion. A bone flap was then cut into the greater tuberosity and both the clavicle and the acromion were osteotomized. The arm was abducted and the acromion positioned to lie between the two edges of the bone flap in the proximal humerus. A spica cast was applied for 4 months.

Putti[36] described a technique whereby the spine of the scapula and the acromion were exposed subperiosteally. The spine of the scapula was detached, the acromion split, and the medial and lateral portions and the upper end of the humerus exposed. The lateral surface of the humerus was split similar to the method described by Watson-Jones and the spine of the scapula driven down into the humerus with the arm abducted. Spica cast immobilization was necessary following this procedure. Neither Watson-Jones' nor Putti's technique were truly extraarticular because the shoulder joint was usually entered when creating the split in the proximal humerus.

Brittain[6] described a true extraarticular arthrodesis. This arthrodesis used a large tibial graft that was placed between the medial humerus and the axillary border of the scapula. The graft was maintained in position by its "arrow" shape (the pointed end was inserted into the humerus and the opposite, notched, end into the axillary border of the scapula). The graft was stabilized by its shape and adduction of the arm, which produced a compressive force along the long axis of the graft. DePalma[12] reports that the failure rate of the arthrodesis was high owing to fracture of the long tibial graft.

Intraarticular Arthrodesis

Gill[15] combined intraarticular and extraarticular arthrodesis. Gill used a U-shaped incision centered 2 cm below the acromion combined with a downward limb to the incision. Gill denuded the superior and inferior surface of the acromion and excised the rotator cuff. The glenoid fossa was decorticated as was the cartilaginous surface of the humeral head. An osseous flap was elevated from the anterolateral surface of the humerus, and a wedge-shaped slice of bone, with its base superiorly, was removed from the humerus. The arm was then abducted and impacted onto the acromion. The position was maintained by suture of the capsule and rotator cuff to the periosteum on the superior surface of the acromion. This technique is predicated on the assumption that it is desirable to fuse the glenohumeral joint in a large amount of abduction. This can be desirable in children when internal fixation is not used because, with time, the amount of abduction decreases. The technique is undesirable in adults owing to the likelihood of excessive abduction being retained following arthrodesis.

Makin[27] has reported on a method of glenohumeral arthrodesis in children that preserves the growth potential of the proximal humeral epiphysis. Makin fused the shoulder in 80 to 90 degrees of abduction, fixing the humerus to the glenoid with Steinman pins inserted first into the humerus in a proximal-distal direction and then driven in the reverse direction into the glenoid. Makin followed his children to adult life and noted that there was only a small loss in humeral length and no change in position of the fused shoulder. He recommended this technique, stating that this amount of abduction was necessary to maintain the growth potential of the proximal humeral epiphysis. I have had no experience with this technique. If this amount of abduction was maintained, the shoulder would be dysfunctional in adulthood.

Moseley[30] reported division of the rotator cuff insertion and excision of the intraarticular portion of the biceps tendon. Moseley advocated suture of the biceps tendon into the bicipital groove after division of its origin. This is an important step to remember in those patients who have functioning biceps, to avoid the unsightly cosmetic deformity identical with that seen in rupture of the long head of the biceps tendon and to avoid the small loss of elbow flexor power and greater loss of supinator strength that is associated with this pathologic condition. The author performs a biceps tenodesis during glenohumeral arthrodesis in all patients who have a functional biceps. Moseley denuded the inferior surface of the acromion as well as the articular cartilage of the humeral head and glenoid fossa. This is an important step in performing glenohumeral arthrodesis because the humeral head presents such a small area to the glenoid across which fusion can occur.

Beltran et al.[5] performed glenohumeral arthrodesis through an anterior approach. They osteotomized the coracoid and created a tunnel that crossed the humerus and entered the glenoid cavity. They utilized a screw for internal fixation and in addition used a Cloward reamer to position a fibular graft from the proximal humerus into the infraglenoid area. Other techniques for glenohumeral arthrodesis have been described by May[28] and Davis and Cottre.[11]

Internal Fixation

A variety of methods of internal fixation have been advocated for glenohumeral arthrodesis. It is generally agreed that internal fixation is desirable because it maintains the position of the arthrodesis and can decrease the length of time that plaster immobilization is necessary to obtain an arthrodesis. Makin advocates the use of Steinman pins in children who are undergoing glenohumeral arthrodesis at an early age. Carroll[7] reported on the use of a wire loop to maintain the position of glenohumeral arthrodesis. Carroll advocated the use of 22-gauge wire passed through the head of the humerus and the anterosuperior lip of the glenoid. He employed this method of arthrodesis in 15 patients, and all patients achieved solid bony union between the third and fourth month following surgery. Carroll notes that it was possible to manipulate the shoulder following surgery and change the position of the arthrodesis. As time has gone by most authors have advocated more rigid forms of internal fixation. At present, few surgeons would use a wire loop as a method of internal fixation when performing glenohumeral arthrodesis.

Other authors have reported the use of screws to obtain fixation during glenohumeral arthrodesis. May[28] use a single stabilizing wood screw crossing the humerus and entering the glenoid fossa. Davis[11] used a similar technique and added a muscle pedicle bone graft that was fixed in place with wood screws. Cofield[10] and Leffert[24] also report on the use of compression screw fixation without the use of a plate. Beltran[5] developed a special fixation device using a screw bolt and washer to obtain glenohumeral arthrodesis. In addition, Beltran used an acromiohumeral screw and a fibular graft as methods of internal fixation.

The ASIF group first advocated the use of plate fixation in 1970. They described this method of arthrodesis as not requiring supplementary plaster immobilization. The AO/ASIF group advocated the use of two plates for internal fixation.[31] The first plate was applied along the spine of the scapula and then bent down over the humerus, maintaining a position of 70 degrees of abduction between the vertebral border of the scapula and the humerus. The object of this position was to obtain a clinical position of 50 degrees of abduction, 40 degrees of internal rotation, and 25 degrees of flexion. They anchored this plate to the scapula with a long screw placed down through the plate, the acromion, and into the neck of the glenoid (Fig. 5). They also noted that fixation could be improved by the insertion of two long screws inserted through the plate, the humeral head, and into the glenoid. "If necessary," a second plate applied posteriorly was advocated to improve the internal fixation. I have rarely found it necessary to use two plates when performing glenohumeral arthrodesis.

Kostuik and Schatzker[22] have reported on the use of the ASIF technique. They did not use external immobilization postoperatively and reported good results in their patients. Riggins[43] reported on shoulder fusion without external immobilization in 1976. Both the AO group and Riggins supplemented their arthrodeses with bone grafts. Riggins treated four patients with the use of a plate for internal fixation. Two of the patients had above-elbow amputations. The arthrodesis was successful in each case.

My colleagues and I have reported on the results of a modified method of glenohumeral arthrodesis using internal fixation in 14 adult patients with brachial plexus palsy.[38] We first used a single 4.5 AO/ASIF dynamic compression (DC) plate applied over the spine of the scapula onto the shaft of the humerus. We advocate placement of two cancellous compression screws passing through the plate and the proximal humerus into the glenoid first to achieve compression at the glenohumeral arthrodesis site. The plate is anchored to the scapula with a long screw passing through the spine of the scapula into the area of the coracoid base. Anchorage of the plate by this method, as opposed to the AO method which inserts the screw into the glenoid neck, provides good fixation, yet leaves room for the large compression screws in the glenoid, which are felt to be more important in obtaining arthrodesis. Initially, we advocated the use of a postoperative spica cast because adult patients with brachial plexus injuries generally have significant osteoporosis, poor muscular control, and decreased proprioception, resulting from their neurologic injury. Bone grafts were not used in this series, and no nonunions occurred. More recently, we have begun to use thermoplastic thoracobrachial orthoses when performing glenohumeral arthrodesis and no longer use a spica cast (see following discussion).

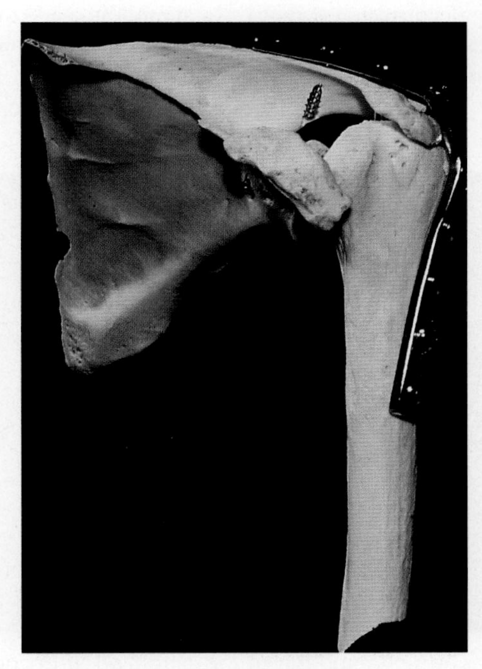

FIG. 5. Appearance of the humerus and scapula after glenohumeral arthrodesis with a single plate. Screws have been passed from the spine of the scapula, through the plate into the area of the coracoid base. Excellent fixation in the scapula can be obtained with this technique.

Recently, we have reported a modification of the technique described in 1985.[39] The current technique uses a malleable plate for internal fixation. In the modified procedure a single ten-hole 4.5 AO pelvic reconstruction plate is used for internal fixation. This plate, although weaker than the 4.5 DC plate, is much easier to contour in the operating room and is much less prominent as it passes over the acromion onto the shaft of the humerus. None of the 11 patients whose shoulders were fused by this method complained of plate prominence. Fusion was obtained in each instance without failure of the internal fixation device. External cast immobilization was used for 6 weeks postoperatively. Plate prominence can also be decreased postoperatively by notching the acromion laterally where the plate crosses this structure.

External Fixation

Charnley[8] reported a method of compression arthrodesis of the shoulder utilizing two Steinman pins. The first Steinman pin was inserted posterosuperiorly into the base of the acromion and then into the main mass of the scapula just proximal to the glenoid. The second pin was inserted posterolaterally in relation to the shaft of the humerus and perpendicular in relation to the axis of the humerus to transfix the region of the surgical neck. A compression apparatus was then applied to the two pins. After application of the compression apparatus a plaster spica cast was applied and worn for an average of 4.8 weeks. After removal of the pins and compression clamps a second plaster cast was applied for an average of 5.3 weeks. Other methods of external fixation have been reported.[18,21,32,49]

Currently, the indications for glenohumeral arthrodesis using external fixation are limited. I have used this method occasionally in patients with active septic arthritis of the shoulder and in patients with massive trauma resulting in bone and soft-tissue loss. I have utilized pins placed through the clavicle and acromion and a second set of pins inserted in a separate plane into the spine of the scapula and neck of the glenoid. Two half-frames are then constructed to stabilize the shoulder. The two half frames can be cross-connected for increased stability. This technique is desirable if there is an open, infected wound draining from the shoulder joint. This method allows dressing changes and care of the soft tissues without the increased dissection and soft-tissue disruption necessary to place an internal fixation device. If the soft-tissue envelope improves, internal fixation can be performed later.

AUTHOR'S PREFERRED TREATMENT

Position of Arthrodesis

A wide variety of different positions for glenohumeral arthrodesis have been advocated in the literature. Perusal of the literature reveals that no two authors agree on exactly the same optimum position for glenohumeral arthrodesis. There was sufficient controversy in the literature that the American Orthopaedic Association established a committee to determine, among other things, the optimum position for glenohumeral arthrodesis. This committee reported in 1942[2] and concluded that the optimum position for glenohumeral arthrodesis was 45 to 50 degrees abduction (measured from the vertebral border of the scapula), forward flexion from the plane of the scapula 15 to 25 degrees, and 25 to 30 degrees of internal rotation. This report caused a great deal of controversy in the literature following its publication. Part of the controversy revolved around the method of measurement of abduction. Some authors recommended using the angle formed by the vertebral border of the scapula and the axis of the humerus to determine abduction, whereas others argued that the angle between the arm and the side of the body was more appropriately measured (clinical abduction).

Rowe noted in 1974 that the amount of abduction that had been recommended was excessive for adults.[46] This position had been recommended primarily for patients who were having their shoulders fused as children in whom internal fixation was not used. In this situation, the amount of abduction present at the time of surgery was commonly lost during the period required for arthrodesis to become secure, as well as during continued growth. If the same position were used in adults, excessive scapular winging would occur and the scapula would not comfortably rest at the side. Furthermore, Rowe noted that the measurement of clinical abduction was more practical and recommended this method, rather than measuring abduction from the vertebral border of the scapula. Rowe recommended that the arm be placed nearer the center of gravity of the body, with enough abduction to clear the axilla and sufficient flexion and internal rotation to bring the hand to the midline of the body.

Other authors have recommended a variety of positions for glenohumeral arthrodesis. All authors agree that abduction and forward flexion are desirable. Most have recommended internal rotation. In my opinion, the optimum position for glenohumeral arthrodesis is one that brings the hand to the midline anteriorly so that with elbow flexion the mouth can be reached. The amount of abduction should not be excessive so that the arm can rest comfortably at the side. I recommend a position of 30-degrees abduction (measured clinically), 30-degrees forward flexion, and 30-degrees internal rotation. The so-called 30-30-30 position is easily obtained in the operating room and usually provides patients with the ability to reach their mouth, their front pocket, and their back pocket. It must be recognized that the position cannot be measured exactly at the time of surgery. I have found in my series of shoulder arthrodeses that it is usually possible to arthrodese the shoulder within 10 degrees of the foregoing position.

Technique

The patient is placed in the semisitting position.[4] The arm is free draped. An incision extends from the spine of the scapula to the anterior acromion and down the anterior aspect of the shaft of the humerus. Uematsu has recommended a posterior approach when performing glenohumeral arthrodesis.[51] Other authors have described arthroscopically assisted glenohumeral arthrodesis.[29] The deltoid muscle is detached from the anterior acromion and its fibers are split distally. Because deltoid function is not present in patients with brachial plexus palsy undergoing glenohumeral arthrodesis, denervation of the muscle is not usually a concern. If deltoid function is present, the incision should be curved over to the deltopectoral interval and the shoulder approached in this fashion. By using this approach, deltoid bulk will be maintained and the patient will experience a more satisfactory cosmetic result. Sparing the deltoid may prevent the development of pain from neuromata arising from the axillary nerve postoperatively. The rotator cuff is resected. The undersurface of the acromion and the humeral head are decorticated (Fig. 6). An attempt is made to obtain arthrodesis of both the glenohumeral and acromiohumeral articulations because the glenoid fossa offers such a small area for fusion with the humeral head. Decortication of the

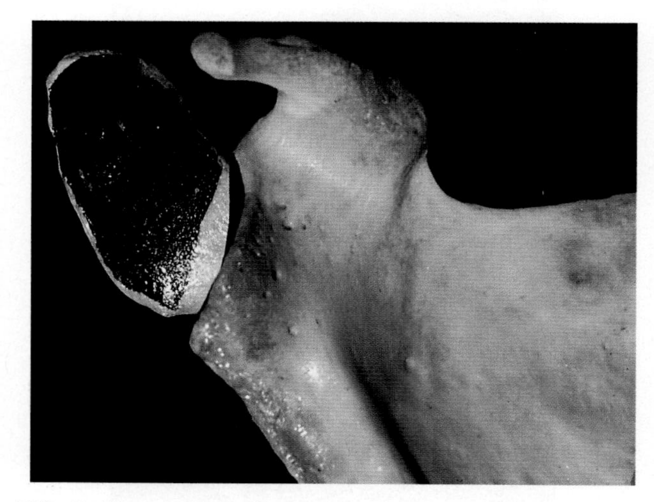

FIG. 6. The undersurface of the acromion is decorticated (*shaded area*). Decortication of the acromion provides a much larger area across which fusion can occur. When the arm is placed in the "30-30-30" position the superior aspect of the humerus, when it is brought proximally, abuts against the undersurface of the acromion.

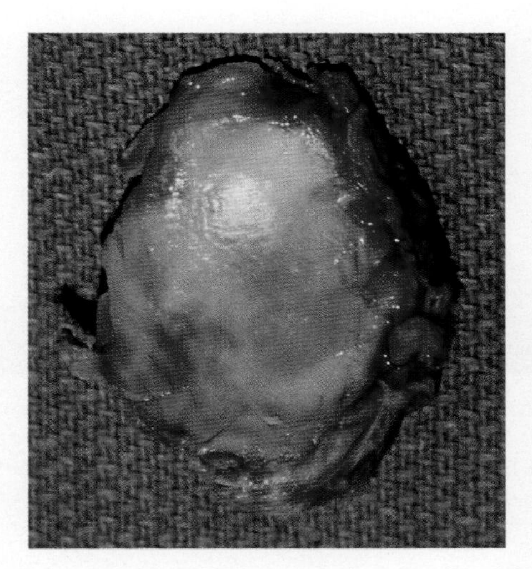

FIG. 7. The glenoid articular surface, the glenoid labrum, and the underlying subchondral bone are resected. This is most easily accomplished with a curved osteotome.

undersurface of the acromion increases the potential fusion area. The articular surface of the glenoid, the glenoid labrum, and the subchondral bone are resected with a curved osteotome (Fig. 7). A ten-hole 4.5-mm pelvic reconstruction plate is used for internal fixation during the procedure (Fig. 8).

After resection of the rotator cuff and decortication of the joint surfaces, the shoulder is supported in 30-degrees flexion, 30-degrees abduction, and 30-degrees internal rotation. Abduction is measured from the side of the body. This method of measurement does not accommodate for individual variations in muscle mass or body fat. However, clinical experience has shown it to be accurate within 10 degrees in any plane. The humeral head is brought proximally to appose the decorticated undersurface of the acromion. When the humerus is abducted and flexed 30 degrees, the humeral head apposes both the undersurface of the acromion and the glenoid fossa (Fig. 9). The position is maintained by supporting the arm with sterile folded sheets. An assistant is assigned to maintain the position while the plate is contoured. Thirty degrees of internal rotation brings the hand to the midline. I have not found it necessary to measure abduction radiographically.

Handheld bending irons are used to contour the plate along the spine of the scapula, over the acromion, and down onto the shaft of the humerus (Figs. 10 and 11). The malleable nature of the plate allows precise intraoperative contouring of the implant to the specific local anatomy in any given patient. The plate must be gently bent 60 degrees over the acromion and twisted 20 to 25 degrees just distal to the bend to appose the shaft of the humerus. The reconstruction plate has holes that allow angulation of the screws as they are passed through the plate.

The screws passing through the plate and the humeral head into the glenoid fossa are inserted first (Fig. 12). Two (usually) or three (sometimes) screws can be inserted in this fashion. If the glenoid is dysplastic only one screw can be used. These screws compress the arthrodesis site. A screw should be directed next from the spine of the scapula into the base of the coracoid process. Because of the cortical bone in

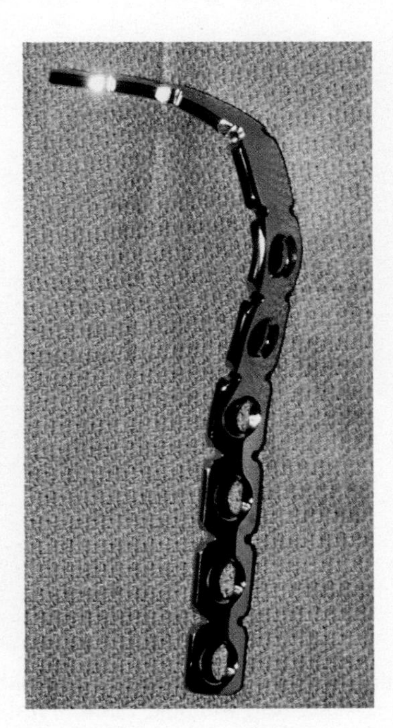

FIG. 8. Specially modified 4.5 pelvic reconstruction plate used for shoulder arthrodesis. The plate is bent as it crosses the acromion and twisted just past the bend. The plate can be easily bent in all planes with the handheld bending irons.

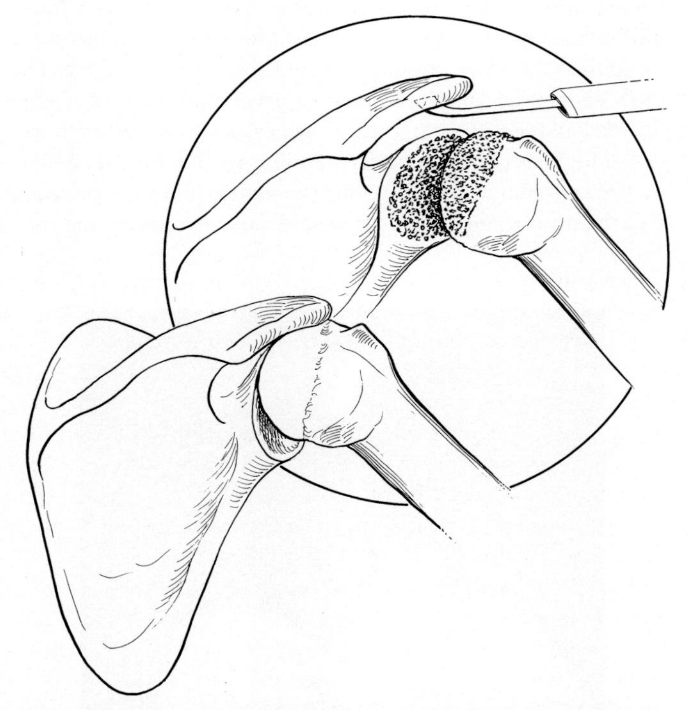

FIG. 9. The glenoid, humeral head, and undersurface of the acromion are decorticated and shaped so that the humeral head has the greatest surface area contact. This technique increases the likelihood of a solid fusion.

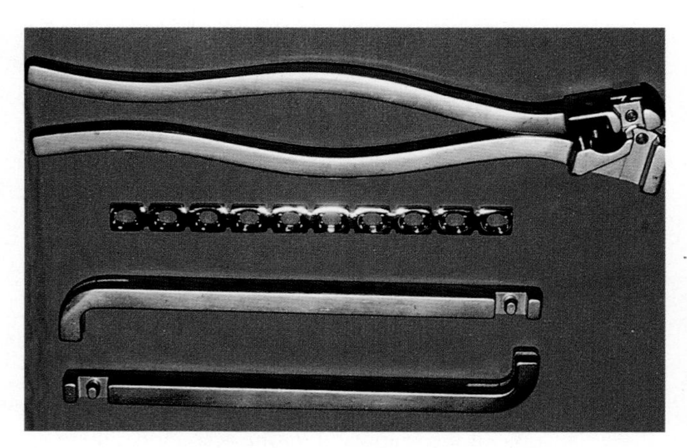

FIG. 10. Handheld plate press and bending irons used to contour the pelvic reconstruction plate intraoperatively.

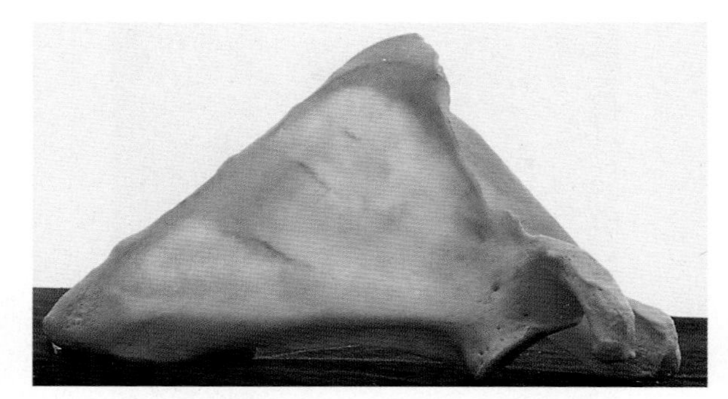

FIG. 12. Transluminated scapula: There is little bone available for fixation in the scapula except in the area of the glenoid and coracoid base. Apart form the borders of the scapula, these are the only areas that do not transluminate.

this region, care must be taken not to break the drill bit when drilling into the scapula. Another cancellous screw is placed across the acromiohumeral fusion site, and the remaining holes of the plate are secured with cortical screws (Figs. 13 and 14). The acromion is not osteotomized, for it is used to augment fixation of the scapula to the humerus. Creating a notch in the lateral acromion may reduce plate prominence in this area (Fig. 15). Autogenous bone graft is not used routinely. If there is deficiency of the glenoid or humerus, a bone graft should be used. This is often the situation when the procedure is performed for failed total shoulder arthroplasty (see later discussion).

The arm of the patient is supported postoperatively with a pillow and swathe. A thermoplastic thoracobrachial orthosis is applied 24 hours postoperatively (Fig. 16). If possible the orthosis can be fabricated preoperatively and then adjusted in the postoperative period as necessary. The orthosis is worn for 6 weeks postoperatively. During this time it can be removed for short periods while the patient showers, providing the arm is supported. Six weeks postoperatively the patient is examined radiographically, and the stability of the fusion is tested manually in a gentle fashion.

If there is no radiographic sign of loosening of the internal fixation after 6 weeks, the patient's arm is placed in a sling (Fig. 17). Gentle range of motion exercises are allowed until radiographic union is achieved. It is difficult to be certain when fusion occurs radiographically because the fixation is sufficiently rigid that very little callus forms around the arthrodesis site. Muscle strengthening is encour-

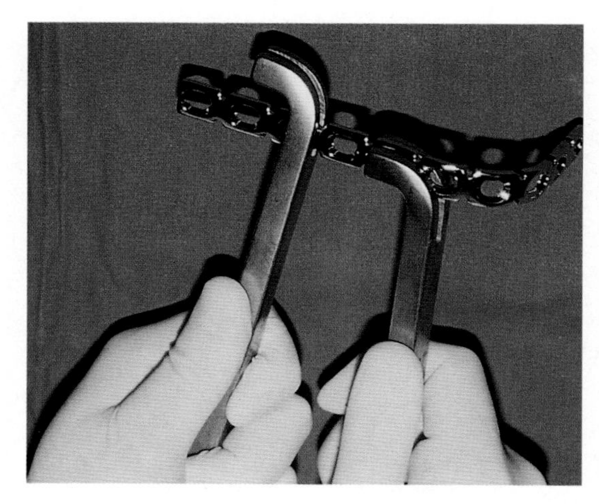

FIG. 11. Plate must usually be contoured in the sagittal plane to appose the surface of the underlying humerus.

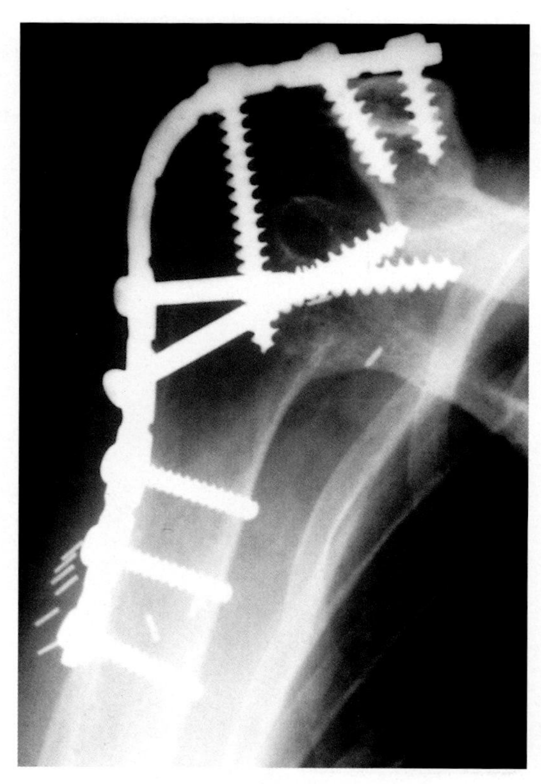

FIG. 13. Anteroposterior (AP) radiograph following glenohumeral arthrodesis with a single plate. Two screws have been inserted into the glenoid to provide fixation. These screws are inserted first to compress the arthrodesis site and augment the fixation by interdigitation of the cancellous bone surfaces.

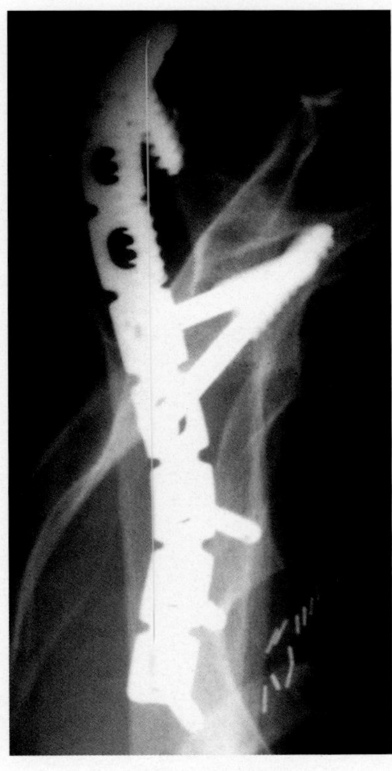

FIG. 14. Lateral radiograph following glenohumeral arthrodesis with a single plate. The plate has been contoured in the sagittal plane to appose the surface of the humeral shaft.

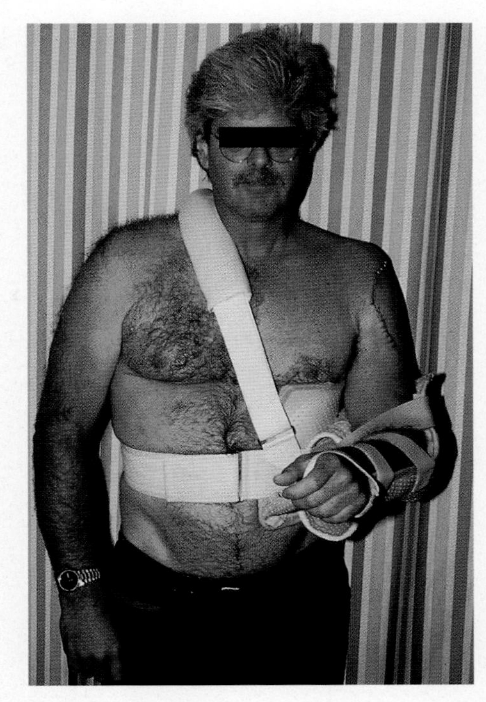

FIG. 16. Patient wearing a thermoplastic thoracobrachial orthosis a few days following glenohumeral arthrodesis. The orthosis can be constructed preoperatively and adjusted in the immediate postoperative period. The orthosis is worn full-time for 6 weeks and part-time (when out of the house) for another 6 weeks postoperatively.

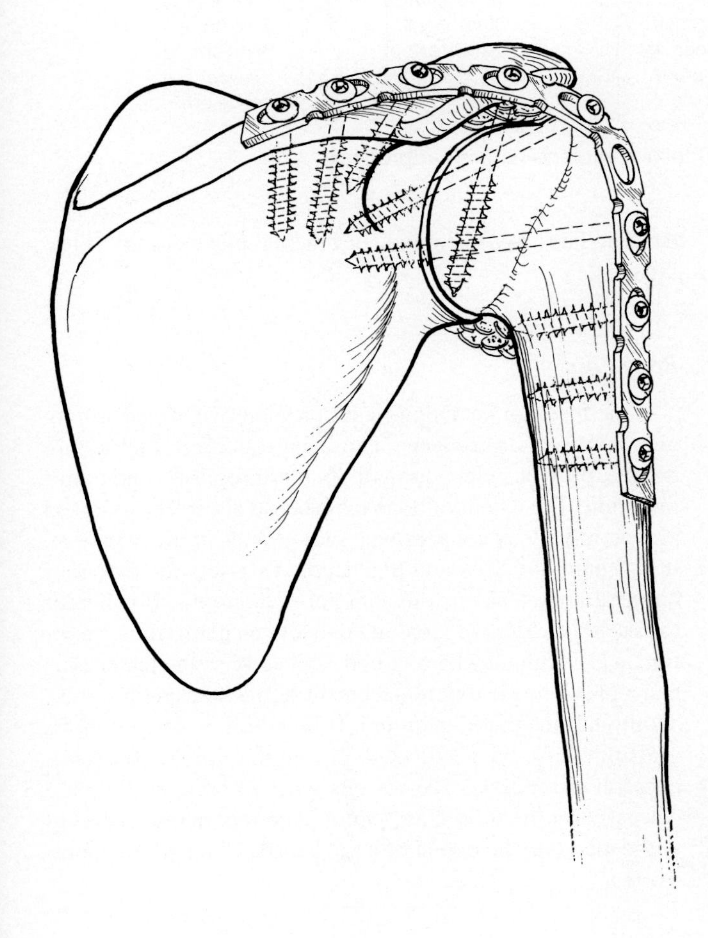

FIG. 15. Drawing of a ten-hole AO/ASIF reconstruction plate applied to stabilize the arthrodesis. The humeral head contacts the acromion and the glenoid, and there is cancellous bone graft packed into the interval between the inferior humeral neck and the glenoid.

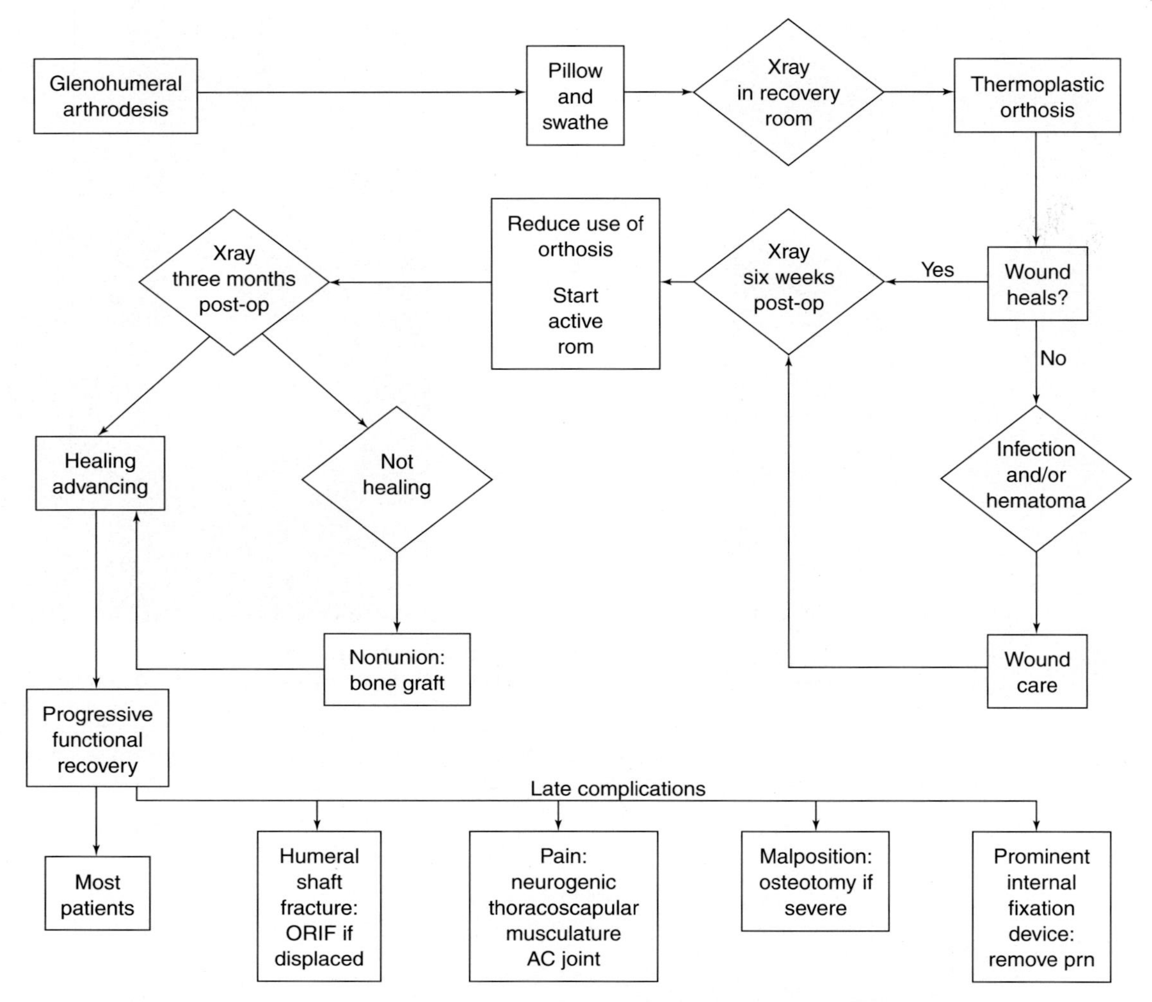

FIG. 17. Algorithm for management following glenohumeral arthrodesis.

aged after removal of the thermoplastic thoracobrachial orthosis, but return to strenuous activity is delayed for at least 16 weeks postoperatively. Thoracoscapular strengthening and mobilization exercises can usually be started 3 months following surgery.

Special Problems

Elbow Flexorplasty

Some forms of elbow arthroplasty can be performed at the time of glenohumeral arthrodesis. If arthrodesis of the shoulder and elbow flexorplasty can be accomplished under one anesthetic, morbidity and the time required for rehabilitation can be decreased. Pectoralis major tendon transfer is an example of a form of elbow flexorplasty that can be performed at the time of glenohumeral arthrodesis (Figs. 18 and 19). When performing this type of flexorplasty at the same time as glenohumeral arthrodesis, it is important to not set the tension on the transfer until the position of the shoulder has been secured with a plate. This type of reconstruction can accomplish a great deal for the patient with a flail elbow and shoulder who has a favorable type of brachial plexus injury (Figs. 20 and 21).

Bone Loss

Bone loss can be a significant problem when performing glenohumeral arthrodesis. The usual etiologic factors are trauma, previous glenohumeral joint arthroplasty, and tumor resection. The extent of bone loss should always be assessed preoperatively by conventional radiographs in every patient. It is usually possible and practicable to assess the extent of humeral bone loss on conventional radiographs. It is harder to assess the extent of glenoid bone loss on plain films; therefore, a CT scan may be required. Certainly, if the patient has had a previous glenoid replacement or has a scapular tumor, additional imaging is required. If bone loss is present, bone grafting must be performed in conjunction with glenohumeral arthrodesis. The various types of bone grafting are discussed in the following section, and the method selected will depend on the extent of bone loss determined preoperatively.

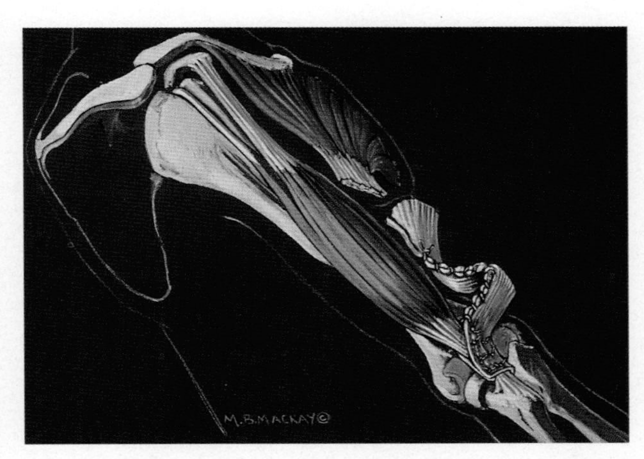

FIG. 18. Simultaneous glenohumeral arthrodesis and elbow flexorplasty. A tube of fascia lata harvested from the opposite thigh is sewn to the biceps tendon distally. The fascia lata is passed subcutaneously proximally to the area of the pectoralis major insertion.

Bone Grafting

Routine bone grafting is advocated by some authors during glenohumeral arthrodesis. The AO/ASIF group recommend prophylactic bone grafting at the termination of a plate if a plate is used for internal fixation. Of Cofield's 71 patients 11 had autogenous bone grafts at the time of their initial procedure.[10] Richards et al. obtained successful arthrodesis without primary bone grafts in patients with significant osteoporosis.[24] I do not routinely use bone grafts in adults when performing glenohumeral arthrodesis. Bone grafting is indicated to fill large defects in patients who are undergoing glenohumeral arthrodesis for complex and revision problems. Bone grafting is also indicated following tumor resection. If large defects have been created following such resection, free vascularized bone grafts may be indicated. Nonunion of shoulder arthrodeses should be treated by revision of the arthrodesis combined with bone grafting.

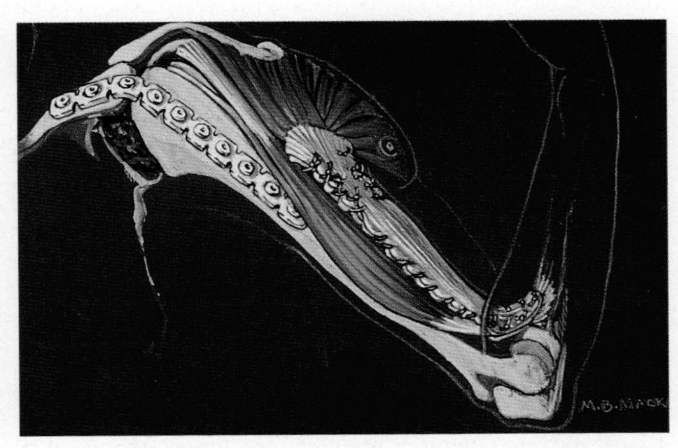

FIG. 19. After stabilization of the glenohumeral arthrodesis with a plate, the fascia lata is sewn at the appropriate tension to the pectoralis major tendon. Patients are treated in a thermoplastic orthosis as described in the foregoing.

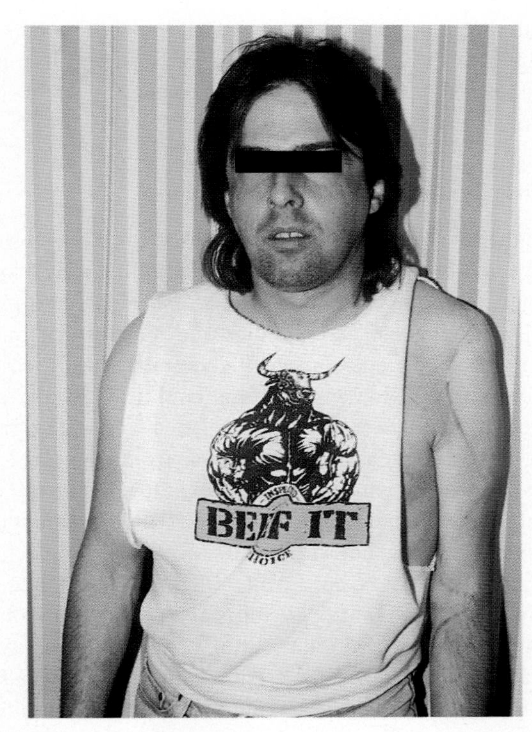

FIG. 20. Male patient with an irreparable lesion of the brachial plexus a few months following simultaneous glenohumeral arthrodesis and elbow flexorplasty using fascia lata to the pectoralis major tendon.

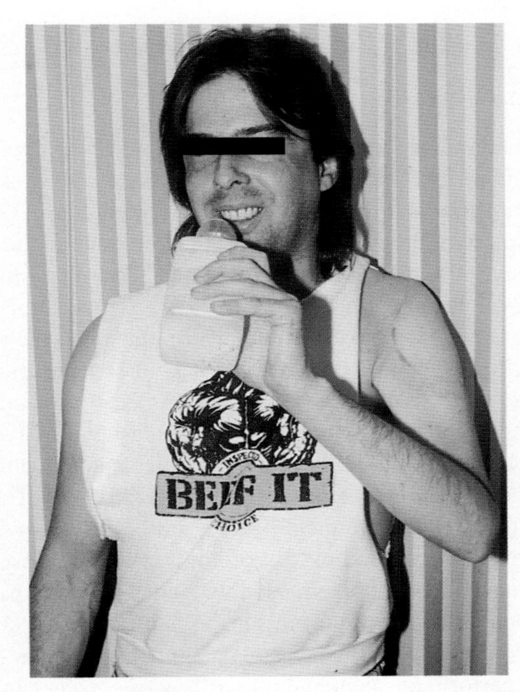

FIG. 21. The patient can actively flex his elbow through a functional range. The pectoralis major tendon transfer is seen as a web in the anterior axillary fold.

An attempt must be made to obtain rigid internal fixation during the arthrodesis. This method of treatment has, in my own experience, been successful when used.

Nonstructural Autogenous Bone Grafting

Autogenous bone grafting can be used to provide osteoinductive and osteoconductive material at or in the arthrodesis site to increase the likelihood of successful fusion. Some authors routinely use cancellous bone harvested from the humeral head when performing glenohumeral arthrodesis. In complex and revision cases the humeral head usually is not present, and it is necessary to look elsewhere for autogenous bone. My preference is to harvest bone from the inner aspect of the iliac crest when a nonstructural autogenous graft is required. This is conveniently performed with the patient in the semisitting position unless the patient is obese, in which case the bone graft must be harvested with the table extended and the position changed after closure of the iliac crest wound. I resect the superior and inner cortex of the iliac crest with a sagittal saw. A Capener gauge is then used to excavate strips of cancellous bone. If large amounts of bone are required, it may be necessary to use both iliac crests. If the patient has had previous surgery in these areas, a bone graft can be harvested from the posterior aspect of the iliac crest, although the position of the patient must be changed intraoperatively. Alternatively, nonstructural autogenous bone can be obtained from the greater trochanter or provided by morselized rib grafts.

Structural Autogenous Bone Grafting

Structural autogenous bone grafting uses an anatomically intact bone graft, such as a full-thickness iliac crest or fibular strut graft. Following unsuccessful glenohumeral joint arthroplasty there is a significant defect relating to the often extensive resection of the humeral head and excavation of the proximal humerus. A full-thickness (tricortical) iliac crest graft can be harvested and incorporated into the fusion mass (Fig. 22). I have placed such grafts underneath the plate with screws passing through the plate, the tricortical iliac crest bone graft, and into the glenoid. Such a graft will maintain the contour of the shoulder and provide autogenous osteoconductive tissue across which fusion can occur. The disadvantage of an anatomically intact graft is prolonged time required for incorporation. Accordingly, when such a graft is used, it should be supplemented with small chips of cancellous bone. It is usually necessary to harvest the cancellous bone from the other iliac crest. I have not used fibular grafts when performing glenohumeral arthrodesis except in conjunction with a vascularized fibular graft. Nonvascularized fibular grafts consist of dense cortical bone, have a limited biologic (but initially a good structural) potential, and probably should not be used in isolation.

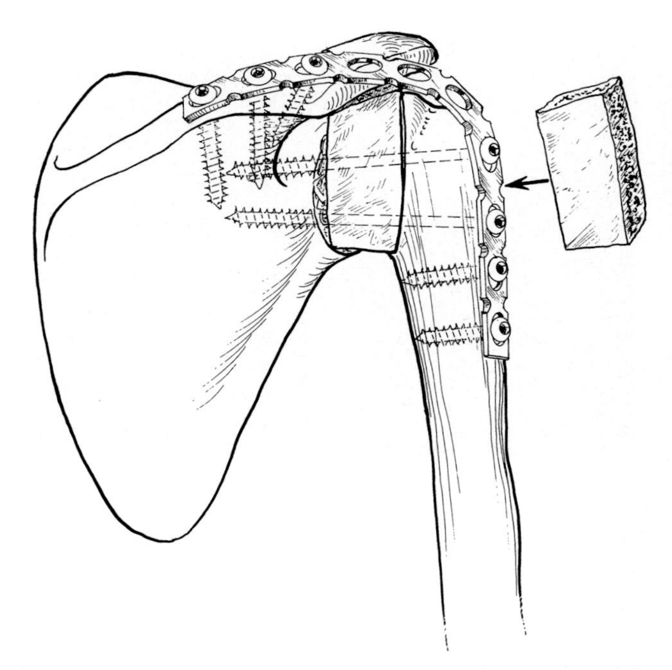

FIG. 22. A corticocancellous block of autogenous iliac crest graft can be used to promote a fusion in the setting of proximal humeral deficiency, as may occur after a failed arthroplasty procedure.

Vascularized Autogenous Bone Grafting

Vascularized autogenous bone grafting has the advantage of providing tissue with great biologic potential. The conventional wisdom is that when the surgeon is faced with an intercalary defect that is larger than 6 cm, a vascularized bone graft should be considered. Following tumor resection, intercalary defects of this magnitude are common, and I have used vascularized fibular bone grafts in this situation. The bone grafting is performed in conjunction with plate fixation. My preference is to use a very long heavy plate spanning the entire intercalary defect (Fig. 23). The vascularized fibular bone graft should be fixed in position with a minimum amount of internal fixation at each bony juncture. Vascularized fibular bone grafts of up to 25 cm can be used to span very large defects. The vascular anastomosis is performed between the peroneal and its vena comitantes and a branch of either the axillary or the brachial artery. Vascularized fibular bone grafts should be supplemented with chips of autogenous bone at each juncture to maximize the likelihood of fusion occurring.

Vascularized full-thickness iliac crest bone grafts can be used to provide both bone and soft tissue. The use of such a bone graft creates a significant donor deficit, but can be considered if a bone and soft-tissue defect coexist. The shape of the iliac crest limits its usefulness somewhat for long intercalary defects, although the graft can be osteotomized to straighten it. Alternatively, vascularized iliac crest bone grafts can be used in conjunction with a nonvascularized fibular graft or an allograft.

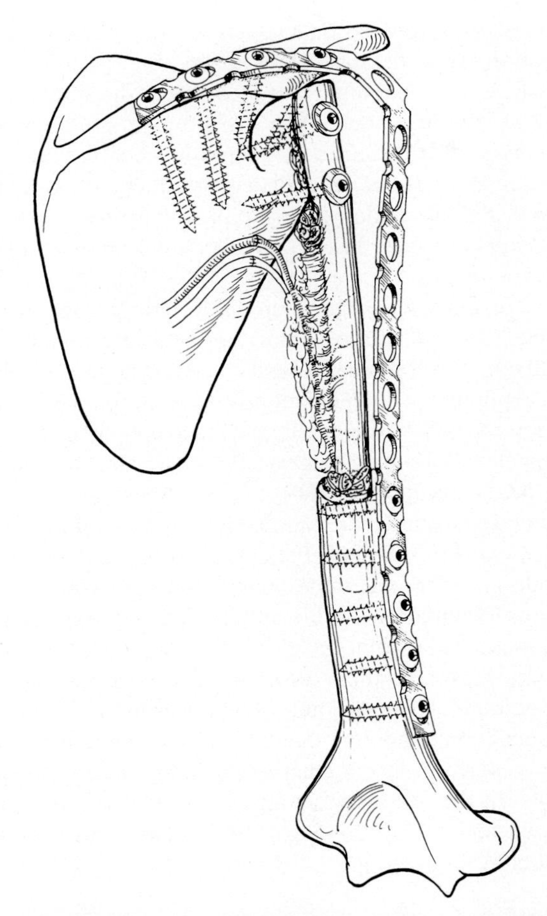

FIG. 23. Drawing of the technique of vascularized fibular graft used to span a deficiency of the proximal humerus. Cancellous bone graft has been placed at both ends of the fibular graft.

Allograft Reconstruction

Allograft reconstruction can be considered in conjunction with bone grafting when performing glenohumeral arthrodesis for complex and revision cases.[9] It is my preference, wherever possible, not to use allograft bone if autogenous bone is available. For instance, if bone grafting is required to supplement a vascularized fibular graft, I would consider using the contralateral fibula or iliac crest graft to supplement the vascularized fibular graft in preference to an allograft. At times, allograft must be used owing to the nonavailability of autogenous bone. Both structural and nonstructural allograft bone can be used. More commonly, allograft is used in conjunction with a large implant to perform an arthroplastic reconstruction following tumor resection. This is discussed elsewhere in Chapter 33.

Soft-Tissue Loss

Soft-tissue loss can be caused by trauma or the necessity to resect soft tissue to obtain clear margins following tumor resection. The most common soft-tissue deficiency about the shoulder relates, the rotator cuff. Isolated rotator cuff deficiency does not require special consideration and, in fact, our conventional method of glenohumeral arthrodesis involves resection of the rotator cuff in its entirety.

Local Flap Techniques

If deltoid resection is required for tumor ablation or if the deltoid has been lost as a result of trauma, consideration should be given to augmentation of the soft-tissue envelope. In particular, it is important to have well-vascularized muscle surrounding the arthrodesis site. The presence of good muscle coverage is associated with enhanced bone formation and enhanced revascularization of autogenous dysvascular or avascular bone as seen following bone grafting,[42] Fortunately, both local and free flap techniques are available to provide a stable soft-tissue envelope about the shoulder. The latissimus muscle provides a local source of autogenous tissue that can be rotated to cover the shoulder. The entire latissimus muscle can be elevated on its vascular pedicle and rotated easily to cover the shoulder. The latissimus has an excellent blood supply, and most surgeons are familiar with its dissection. The flap can be rotated as either a pure muscle flap or as a myocutaneous flap, depending on the patient's requirements. If the nerve supply to the latissimus is kept intact it can also be used as a flexorplasty, as described by Zancolli.[54] The requirement to use a latissimus flap in this manner might be seen following trauma to the shoulder and proximal humerus resulting in the loss of biceps function. Other local flaps about the shoulder are less reliable. The latissimus flap should be considered to be the mainstay of treatment when soft tissue is required locally.

Free Tissue Transfer

If a latissimus flap cannot be used, consideration can be given to a free tissue transfer. Such a transfer is required relatively infrequently about the shoulder. The trapezius should not be used to cover a soft-tissue defect following glenohumeral arthrodesis. Good function of the trapezius is required to motor the shoulder girdle following arthrodesis, and its anatomy should not be disturbed.

"Hybrid" Methods of Reconstruction

Complex and revision problems about the shoulder require special techniques when performing glenohumeral arthrodesis. In some cases a combination of techniques is required and such hybrid methods of treatment are in the patient's best interest when faced with complex bone and soft-tissue deficits. For instance, following tumor resection, it may be necessary to perform a vascularized fibular bone graft, a pedicled latissimus muscle flap, autogenous iliac crest bone grafting, and a pectoralis major to scapular transfer (owing to long thoracic nerve palsy) to stabilize the shoulder girdle and provide enough tissue that arthrodesis can occur. The timing and staging of such complex procedures must be assessed on an individual basis.

PERSONAL SERIES

The author has performed 91 glenohumeral arthrodeses. The ages have ranged from 19 to 64. Seventy-two patients were operated on for irreparable lesions of the brachial plexus, 6 patients for recalcitrant shoulder instability, 5 patients for osteoarthritis, 4 patients for failed total shoulder arthroplasties, and 2 patients for sepsis. The technique used was that of combined glenohumeral and acromiohumeral arthrodesis, as described earlier. In the author's home community tumor surgery is almost exclusively performed by colleagues at the Mount Sinai Hospital. Accordingly, I have had less experience with glenohumeral arthrodesis for this indication.

Results

Solid arthrodesis has usually been obtained with the primary procedure. Two patients developed only an acromiohumeral fusion and one of these patients developed a broken screw. This patient had a secondary bone-grafting procedure. Infection occurred in only one case. Clinical examination showed all shoulders to be fused within 10 degrees of the desired position. We have not used special techniques to assess the position of the arthrodesis.[20] Eighteen patients have required surgery for plate removal, and two patients sustained fractures of the humerus distal to the plate.

Activities of Daily Living

In a review of 33 patients we assessed functional outcome in detail.[41] The patients ability to perform specific activities of daily living (ADLs) following their glenohumeral arthrodesis were ranked ordered as follows:

Working at waist level 29
Getting dressed 29
Sleeping 27
Lifting bags 25
Using knife 25
Washing face 25
Reaching front pocket 23
Working at shoulder level 21
Doing up buttons 21
Reaching opposite axilla 20
Eating 17
Managing toileting 13
Reaching back pocket 11
Bathing 7
Washing back 6
Doing hair 5

The ability to perform ADLs was heavily dependant on the adequacy of hand function in patients with brachial plexus injuries. Regression analysis revealed the underlying indication (preoperative diagnosis) for glenohumeral arthrodesis to be the single best predictor of the ability of patients to perform their ADLs following glenohumeral arthrodesis. The patient's compensation board status was also a predictor of outcome. Patient satisfaction was highest in those patients undergoing the procedure for a brachial plexus injury, osteoarthritis, and failed total shoulder arthroplasty.

Five patients who had neurogenic pain preoperatively continued to complain of significant neurogenic pain postoperatively. Several other patients who had compensable injuries continued to complain of postoperative pain in spite of solid arthrodesis. Most patients can reach both their front and back pockets following surgery, and many have returned to fairly heavy occupations. These occupations have included tool and dye manufacture, gardening, heavy equipment operation, and brick laying. Patients who had glenohumeral arthrodesis for compensable injuries did not return to their previous occupations. The author has not experienced acromioclavicular joint problems following glenohumeral arthrodesis. Some authors recommend excision arthroplasty of the acromioclavicular joint following arthrodesis in an effort to maximize shoulder motion[35]. I have not found it necessary to perform this adjunctive procedure in my series of patients. In the following paragraphs I will discuss fusion, function, and pain following glenohumeral arthrodesis in more detail.

Fusion

Fusion rates following glenohumeral arthrodesis are high. Most older series do not report any nonunions. Recent series that have used internal fixation devices report high union rates. It is often difficult to judge radiographic union in patients who have had internal fixation. The internal fixation device commonly obscures the arthrodesis site, and rigid internal fixation prevents the formation of periarticular new bone. Because I routinely use rigid internal rotation I tend to arbitrarily discontinue or decrease external immobilization by 6 or 8 weeks. The shoulder is examined clinically and, assuming that the patient is comfortable, the patient is placed in a sling at this time. Any attempt to actively mobilize the thoracoscapular musculature is avoided until at least 3 months after arthrodesis. By using this method of postoperative rehabilitation I have found delayed union or nonunion to be distinctly uncommon.

Function

The amount of improvement in shoulder function following arthrodesis is dependent on the function that was present preoperatively. Patients who have flail shoulders experience a significant improvement in glenohumeral function following arthrodesis because they can actively position their extremities in space (Fig. 24). Shoulder subluxation is relieved,

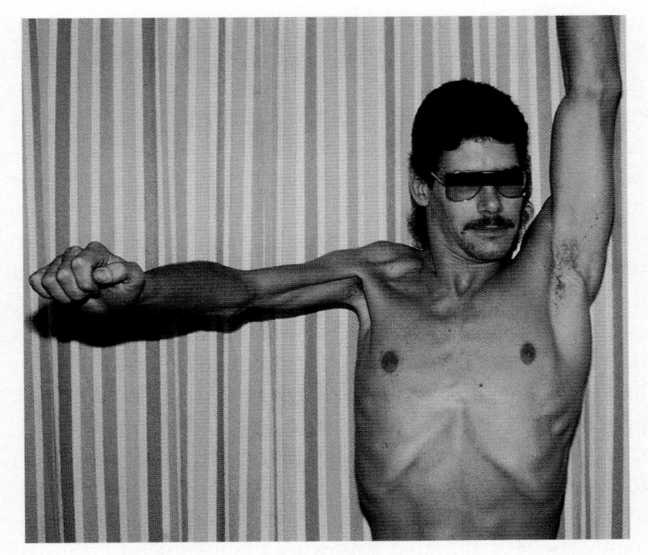

FIG. 24. Range of shoulder elevation following glenohumeral arthrodesis. Most patients recover approximately two-thirds the normal range of motion following glenohumeral arthrodesis. The procedure effectively prevents glenohumeral rotation.

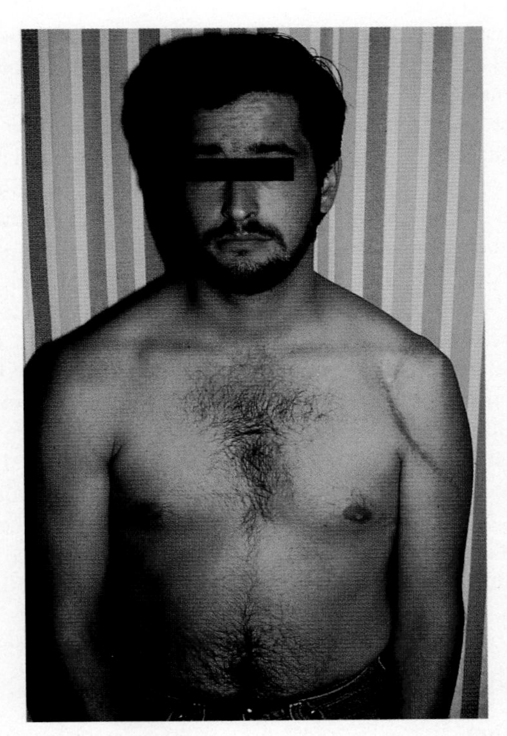

FIG. 25. An AP clinical photograph of patient following successful glenohumeral arthrodesis in the functional position. The arm can drop comfortably to the side even through thoracoscapular movement even though the glenohumeral joint has been arthrodesed in the 30-30-30 position.

and function is significantly improved. Most, but not all, patients can use their extremity to lift, dress, tend to personal hygiene, eat, and comb their hair (Figs. 25 and 26). In Cofield's series, hair combing was the most difficult task to perform following arthrodesis of the glenohumeral joint.[10]

Pain

Pain relief is not universal following glenohumeral arthrodesis. In fact, some pain is commonly present in patients whose shoulders have been successfully arthrodesed. The presence of moderate to severe pain following successful glenohumeral arthrodesis is difficult to explain, but occurs not infrequently. It is thought that such pain is related to the contiguous soft tissues. Glenohumeral arthrodesis places a substantial amount of strain on the periscapular musculature and requires the patient to make a profound functional adjustment. Pain surrounding successful fusions has also been reported following hip and knee arthrodesis. Most patients experience less pain with longer follow-up periods, and this suggests that with time the periscapular musculature adjusts to the changes imposed on it by glenohumeral arthrodesis.

Patients with neurogenic pain caused by brachial plexus injury will not experience pain relief following glenohumeral arthrodesis. Shoulder function is improved in these patients, but they should understand fully that the procedure is being performed to improve function and not to relieve pain. It has been our impression that if function is improved, such neurogenic pain is generally better tolerated by the patient. Therefore, we concentrate on the restoration of limb function, rather than on relief of pain by neurosurgical means.

Acromioclavicular Joint Pain

Acromioclavicular joint pain has been reported following glenohumeral arthrodesis.[35] Some methods of glenohumeral arthrodesis require osteotomy of the acromion. Such os-

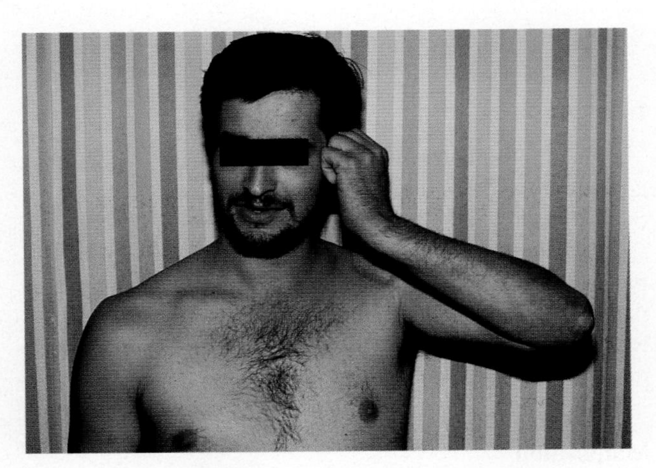

FIG. 26. Most patients can reach their mouth, their ear, their front pocket, and the side of their hip following glenohumeral arthrodesis.

teotomies disturb the normal acromioclavicular relation. If pain arises from the acromioclavicular joint postoperatively, excision arthroplasty is indicated if local injections confirm that the pain is arising from the acromioclavicular joint. Some authors have reported anecdotally that excision arthroplasty of the acromioclavicular joint improves motion following glenohumeral arthrodesis.[35] In our experience, acromioclavicular joint pain is rare following glenohumeral arthrodesis when the acromion is left in the anatomic position. Therefore, I do not recommend acromial osteotomy to approximate the acromion to the superior surface of the humeral head. I do advocate moving the humerus proximally to appose both the acromiohumeral and glenohumeral arthrodesis sites. The glenoid presents a small surface to the humeral head across which arthrodesis can occur. This is why decortication of the undersurface of the acromion as well as the glenoid and humeral head is advocated. The presence of a broader surface across which arthrodesis can occur is desirable, and it is believed that this increases the arthrodesis rate.

COMPLICATIONS

Nonunion

Nonunion following glenohumeral arthrodesis is surprisingly infrequent in view of the magnitude of the procedure, the high stresses across the arthrodesis site and the difficulty of postoperative immobilization. In spite of these difficulties nonunion is reported surprisingly infrequently in the literature. In Cofield's series of 71 shoulder arthrodeses only 3 patients went on to nonunion.[10] All 3 patients' shoulders were successfully fused following a second operative procedure. If nonunion occurs following glenohumeral arthrodesis, a repeat operation with revision of the internal fixation device is indicated. Bone grafting should be used to augment the arthrodesis site if a nonunion has occurred. I have seen a few patients who have obtained an acromiohumeral fusion, but have not fused solidly at the glenohumeral joint. In 1 such patient the internal fixation device failed and bone grafting was necessary.

Infection

Infection is relatively uncommon following glenohumeral arthrodesis owing to the excellent vascularity of the periarticular tissues. Infection following glenohumeral arthrodesis should be treated with surgical drainage and the appropriate parenteral antibiotics. The internal fixation should not be removed if it is providing stability at the arthrodesis site. An attempt should be made to obtain solid arthrodesis before removal of any fixation device.

Malposition

Excessive abduction of the extremity during glenohumeral arthrodesis can place a substantial strain on the thoracoscapular musculature. Adult patients have great difficulty adapting to positions of greater than 45 degrees of abduction. Hyperabduction at the arthrodesis site causes significant winging of the scapula for the arm to drop to the patient's side. Indeed, in some patients the arm will not approximate the trunk if the shoulder has been arthrodesed in too much abduction. Women in particular are unhappy with the cosmetic appearance of a shoulder that has been fused in too much abduction owing to the significant prominence of the scapula that is created when the arm is adducted.

Fusion of the shoulder in too much internal rotation can occur. If this occurs the patient cannot easily bring his or her hand to the mouth and cannot reach either their front or back pocket. Rotational osteotomy of the humerus may be necessary for patients whose extremities have been positioned in too much internal rotation. I have performed three such osteotomies for this indication. Suprascapular nerve entrapment has been reported following glenohumeral arthrodesis.[50]

Prominence of the Internal Fixation Device

Many patients who have had internal fixation devices applied over the spine of the scapula have significant skin tenderness in the area of the appliance. This can be particularly troublesome when the patient must wear a prosthetic harness, and skin irritation and ulceration has been reported.[38] Cofield[10] reports a significant incidence of tenderness over the internal fixation device, which required its removal in 17 of his patients. My experience has been similar, although use of a malleable reconstruction plate has decreased skin tenderness and made the need for removal of internal fixation less frequent.[39] The development of appliances specifically designed for glenohumeral arthrodesis is likely to decrease the incidence of tenderness of the skin overlying internal fixation devices even further.

Fracture of the Humerus

Fracture of the humerus at the distal end of the internal fixation device is sufficiently common that the AO group have recommended prophylactic bone grafting of this area.[31] Cofield[10] reports a fracture in the fused extremity occurring in 10 of his 71 patients. This complication has occurred in our series as well in association with significant trauma to the arthrodesed shoulder. If an unstable fracture does occur at the end of the internal fixation device, I advocate removal of the device together with internal fixation of the fracture if the arthrodesis has solidly healed. If the fracture is relatively undisplaced, it can be treated by closed means, but in our experience this is uncommon (Fig. 27).

SUMMARY

Glenohumeral arthrodesis remains an important procedure that should be part of every shoulder surgeon's arma-

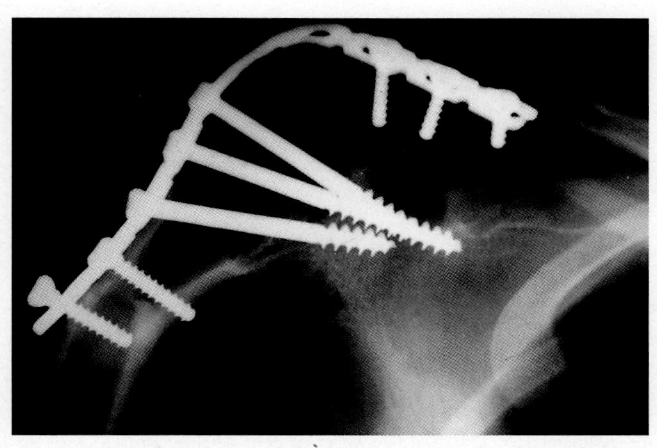

FIG. 27. Fracture of the humerus at the end of the plate. This particular patient had a solid glenohumeral arthrodesis when he fell onto his arthrodesed arm. The fracture is minimally displaced in this case and can be treated nonoperatively, unless further displacement were to occur.

mentarium. The procedure is indicated for patients with paralytic disorders, those who require en bloc resection of their glenohumeral joint together with the rotator cuff or deltoid for tumor, and those whose shoulder joints have been destroyed by septic arthritis. The procedure has been useful in a few patients with failed total shoulder arthroplasties and shoulder instability. It is rarely indicated for patients with rotator cuff tears, periarticular malunions, osteoarthritis, or rheumatoid arthritis.

Although a variety of different positions for glenohumeral arthrodesis has been advocated in the literature, my recommendation is a position of 30-degrees abduction (measured clinically), 30-degrees flexion, and 30-degrees internal rotation. This position brings the hand to the midline anteriorly so that, with elbow flexion, the patient can reach his or her mouth. With the shoulder fused in this position the arm drops comfortably to the side. I recommend fusion of both the acromiohumeral and glenohumeral articulations and the use of internal fixation when performing glenohumeral arthrodesis. Complications following glenohumeral arthrodesis are relatively infrequent and most can be dealt with successfully if they do occur.

The improvement in shoulder function following glenohumeral arthrodesis is dependant on the patient's preoperative shoulder function. Patients with flail shoulders experience a significant improvement in function. Patients with significant mechanical pain in the glenohumeral joint experience relief following the procedure. Glenohumeral arthrodesis does not relieve neurogenic pain and requires a significant functional adjustment on the part of patients who have had the procedure. Glenohumeral arthrodesis is primarily indicated to restore function. Bone grafting is routinely used for complex and revision procedures. The procedure is contraindicated in any patient with a progressive neurologic disorder affecting the periscapular musculature.

ACKNOWLEDGMENTS

The author acknowledges the assistance of Mrs. Kim Mason in preparing the references.

REFERENCES

1. Earns CT, Matsen F, Jacking S. Surgical management of complex irreparable rotator cuff deficiency. *J Arthroplasty* 1991;6:363–370.
2. Barr J, Freiberg JA, Colonna PC, Pemberton PA. A survey of end results on stabilization of the paralysed shoulder. Report of the Research Committee of the American Orthopaedic Association. *J Bone Joint Surg* 1942;24:699–707.
3. Barton NJ. Arthrodesis of the shoulder for degenerative conditions. *J Bone Joint Surg [Am]* 1972;54:1759–1764.
4. Bateman JE. *The shoulder and neck*, 2nd ed. Philadelphia: WB Saunders, 1978:273–274.
5. Beltran JE, Trilla JC, Barjan R. A simplified compression arthrodesis of the shoulder. *J Bone Joint Surg [Am]* 1975;57:538–541.
6. Brittain HA. *Architectural principles in arthrodesis*, 3rd ed. Edinburgh: E & L Livingstone, 1952.
7. Carroll RE. Wire loop in arthrodesis of the shoulder. *Clin Orthop* 1957; 9:185–189.
8. Charnley J, Houston JK. Compression arthrodesis of the shoulder. *J Bone Joint Surg [Br]* 1964;46:614–620.
9. Cheng EY, Gebhardt MC. Allograft reconstructions of the shoulder after bone tumor resections. *Orthop Clin* 1991;22:37–48.
10. Cofield RH, Briggs BT. Glenohumeral arthrodesis. *J Bone Joint Surg [Am]* 1979;61:668–677.

10a. Cubbins WR, Callahan JJ, Scuderi CS. The reduction of old or irreducible dislocations of the shoulder joint. *Surg Gynecol Obstet* 58: 129, 1934.

11. Davis JB, Cottrell GW. A technique for shoulder arthrodesis. *J Bone Joint Surg [Am]* 1962;44:657–661.
12. DePalma AF. *Surgery of the shoulder*, 3rd ed. Philadelphia: JB Lippincott, 1983:132–143.
13. De Velasco PG, Cardoso MA. Arthrodesis of the shoulder. *Clin Orthop* 1973;90:178–182.
14. Freidman RJ, Ewald FC. Arthroplasty of the ipsilateral shoulder and elbow in patients who have rheumatoid arthritis. *J Bone Joint Surg [Am]* 1987;69:661–666.
15. Gill AB. A new operation for arthrodesis of the shoulder. *J Bone Joint Surg* 1931;13:287.
16. Goldner JL. Muscle–tendon transfers for partial paralysis of the shoulder girdle. In: Evarts CMC, ed. *Surgery of the musculoskeletal system*. New York: Churchill Livingstone, 1983:167–184.
17. Hawkins RJ, Neer CS. A functional analysis of shoulder fusions. *Clin Orthop* 1987;223:65–76.
18. Johnson CA, Healy WL, Brooker AF Jr, Krackow KA. External fixation shoulder arthrodesis. *Clin Orthop* 1986;211:219–223.
19. Jonsson E, Brattstrom M, Lidgren L. Evaluation of the rheumatoid shoulder function after hemiarthroplasty and arthrodesis. *Scand J Rheum* 1988;17:17–26.
20. Jonsson E, Lidgren L, Rydholm U. Position of shoulder arthrodesis measured with Moire photography. *Clin Orthop* 1989;238:117–121.
21. Kocialkowski A, Wallace WA. Shoulder arthrodesis using an external fixation. *J Bone Joint Surg [Br]* 1991;73:180–181.
22. Kostiuk JP, Schatzker J. Shoulder arthrodesis—AO technique. In: Bateman JE, Welsh RP, eds. *Surgery of the shoulder*. Philadelphia: CV Mosby, 1984:207–210.
23. Kumar VP, Satku SK, Mitra AK, Pho RW. Function following limb salvage for primary tumors of the shoulder girdle. Ten patients followed 4 (1–11) years. *Acta Orthop Scand* 1994;65:55–61.
24. Leffert RD. *Brachial plexus injuries*. New York: Churchill Livingstone, 1985:193–210.
25. Macdonald W, Thrum CB, Hamilton SGL. Designing an implant by CT scanning and solid modelling: arthrodesis of the shoulder after excision of the upper humerus. *J Bone Joint Surg [Br]* 1986;68:208–212.
26. Mah JY, Hall JE. Arthrodesis of the shoulder in children. *J Bone Joint Surg* 1990;72:582–586.
27. Makin M. Early arthrodesis for a flail shoulder in young children. *J Bone Joint Surg [Am]* 1977;59:317–321.

28. May VR. Shoulder fusion: a review of fourteen cases. *J Bone Joint Surg [Am]* 1962;44:65–76.
29. Morgan CD, Casscells CD. Arthroscopic-assisted glenohumeral arthrodesis. *Arthroscopy* 1992;8:262–266.
30. Mosely HF. Arthrodesis of the shoulder in the adult. *Clin Orthop* 1961; 20:156–162.
31. Muller ME, Allgower AM, Willenegger H. *Manual of internal fixation*, 2nd ed. Berlin: Springer-Verlag, 1979.
32. Nagano A, Okinaga S, Ochiai N, Kurokawa T. Shoulder arthrodesis by external fixation. *Clin Orthop* 1989;247:97–100.
33. Neer CS II, Watson KC, Stanton FJ. Recent experience in total shoulder replacement. *J Bone Joint Surg [Am]* 1982;64:319–337.
34. Neer CS II, Craig EV, Fukada H. Cuff tear arthropathy. *J Bone Joint Surg [Am]* 1983;65:416–419.
35. Pipkin G. Claviculectomy as an adjunct to shoulder arthrodesis. *Clin Orthop* 1967;54:145–160.
36. Putti V. Arthrodesis for tuberculosis of the knee and shoulder. *Chir Organi Mov* 1933;13:217.
37. Raunio P. Arthrodesis of the shoulder joint in rheumatoid arthritis. *Reconst Surg Traumatol* 1981;18:48–54.
38. Richards RR, Waddell JP, Hudson AR. Shoulder arthrodesis for the treatment of brachial plexus palsy. *Clin Orthop* 1985;198:250–258.
39. Richards RR, Sherman RMP, Hudson AR, Waddell JP. Shoulder arthrodesis using a modified pelvic reconstruction plate: a review of eleven cases. *J Bone Joint Surg [Am]* 1988;70:416–421.
40. Richards RR. Operative treatment for irreparable lesions of the brachial plexus. In: Gelberman RH. *Operative nerve repair and reconstruction*. Philadelphia: JB Lippincott, 1991:1303–1328.
41. Richards RR, Beaton DE, Hudson AR. Shoulder arthrodesis with plate fixation: a functional outcome analysis. *J Shoulder Elbow Surg* 1993:2: 225–239.
42. Richards RR, Schemitsch EH. The effect of muscle flap coverage on bone blood flow following devascularization of segment of tibia: an experimental investigation in the dog. *J Orthop Res* 1989:32:366–369.
43. Riggins RS. Shoulder fusion without external fixation. *J Bone Joint Surg [Am]* 1976;58:1007–1008.
44. Rockwood CA, Burkhead WZ. The management of patients with massive rotator cuff defects by acromioplasty and radical cuff debridement. Presentation to the Orthopaedic Associations of the English Speaking World. Washington, DC, May 1987.
45. Rouholamin E, Wootton JR, Jamieson AM. Arthrodesis of the shoulder following brachial plexus injury. *Injury* 1991;22:271–274.
46. Rowe CR. Re-evaluation of the position of the arm in arthrodesis of the shoulder in the adult. *J Bone Joint Surg [Am]* 1974;56:913–922.
47. Rowe CR, Pierce DS, Clark JG. Voluntary dislocation of the shoulder. A preliminary report on a clinical, electromyographic and psychiatric study of twenty-six patients. *J Bone Joint Surg [Am]* 1973;55:445–460.
48. Rybka V, Raunio P, Vainio K. Arthrodesis of the shoulder in rheumatoid arthritis: a review of forty-one cases. *J Bone Joint Surg [Br]* 1979; 61:155–158.
49. Schrader HA, Frandsen PA. External compression arthrodesis of the shoulder joint. *Acta Orthop Scand* 1983;54:592–595.
50. Sjostrom L, Mjoberg B. Suprascapular nerve entrapment in an arthrodesed shoulder. *J Bone Joint Surg [Br]* 1992;74:470–471.
51. Uematsu A. Arthrodesis of the shoulder: posterior approach. *Clin Orthop* 1979;139:169–173.
52. Watson-Jones R. Extra-articular arthrodesis of the shoulder. *J Bone Joint Surg* 1933;15:862–871.
53. Wilde AH, Brems JJ, Boumphrey FR. Arthrodesis of the shoulder: current indications and operative technique. *Orthop Clin North Am* 1987; 18:463–472.
54. Zancolli E, Mitre H. Latissimus dorsi transfer to restore elbow flexion. An appraisal of eight cases. *J Bone Joint Surg [Am]* 1973;55: 1265–1275.

Disorders of the Shoulder: Diagnosis and Management, edited by Joseph P. Iannotti and Gerald R. Williams, Jr. Lippincott Williams & Wilkins, Philadelphia © 1999.

CHAPTER 20

Prosthetic Arthroplasty for Glenohumeral Arthritis with an Intact or Repairable Rotator Cuff: Indications, Techniques, and Results

Thomas Schenk and Joseph P. Iannotti

INTRODUCTION

History

The first replacement arthroplasty of the glenohumeral joint dates to 1893 when a French Surgeon, Pean, used a platinum and rubber implant to replace the proximal one-half of the humerus in a patient suffering from tuberculous arthritis of the shoulder.[57] The implant required removal approximately 2 years later for persistent, uncontrollable infection. Additional materials used in replacement of the proximal humerus predating the modern era of shoulder arthroplasty included fibular autografts, resurfacing grafts of fascia lata, and ivory and acrylic prostheses.[1,50,53,77]

The modern era of shoulder arthroplasty was founded in the early 1950s, when prosthesis design sought to replicate the anatomic shape of the humeral head. The specific geometries of the earliest nonconstrained components were derived from measurements taken from cadaveric humeri.[54,61] In 1951 Krueger reported the implantation of the first anatomically designed humeral head prosthesis for a patient with aseptic

T. Schenk and J. P. Iannotti: Department of Orthopaedic Surgery, Hospital of the University of Pennsylvania, Philadelphia, Pennsylvania 19104.

necrosis.[54] The short-term results of this single surgery demonstrated promise, with relief of pain and favorable function being achieved. At the same time, Neer, being prompted by his observation of the unsatisfactory results of conventional surgical treatments for proximal humeral fracture–dislocations, was designing his first anatomic prosthesis, which was introduced in a report in 1953.[61] In 1955 Neer described the use of his second prosthesis, a redesigned vitallium humeral head replacement (Neer I prosthesis) in 12 cases, including patients with acute four-part proximal humeral fractures or proximal humeral fracture–dislocations and patients with avascular necrosis from prior fractures.[62] The short-term results in which 11 of 12 patients were free from pain provided momentum furthering the application of humeral head replacement surgery. In 1964 Neer published a follow-up report in which the indications for the procedure expanded to include patients with degenerative arthritis of the glenohumeral joint.[63] With a follow-up ranging from 2 to 11 years, results remained favorable and supported the use of a humeral head replacement for acute trauma, posttraumatic arthritis, and both inflammatory and noninflammatory degenerative arthritis.

In the early 1970s, several authors reported on the implantation of a polyethylene glenoid component for the humeral head prosthesis to articulate with and, as such, the age of total shoulder arthroplasty arrived.[33,52,65,95] Neer designed a new humeral head prosthesis (Neer II prosthesis) for implantation with any of his glenoid component designs or as a humeral head replacement independent of a glenoid (Fig. 1). The Neer II system has been the most widely used and reported shoulder resurfacing implant to date.

Since the time of these original works, many component designs have come and gone. In broad terms, three basic designs of total shoulder arthroplasty have been used: constrained, semiconstrained, and nonconstrained prostheses.

Constrained total shoulder arthroplasty conceptionally seemed desirable because of the inherent stability achieved at the articulating surfaces and the belief that with the maintenance of a stable fulcrum of rotation the deltoid would be able to assume the role of the rotator cuff in a cuff-deficient shoulder. A variety of designs was introduced, most of which used a fixed fulcrum ball-and-socket type construction (Fig. 2). Neer and Averill designed three constrained prosthetic systems, each with a modification to improve on the previous design.[71] In 1974 Neer abandoned the use of any constrained prosthesis because of dissatisfaction with mechanical failure and his realization that these designs would not solve the problem of an inadequate rotator cuff.[69] Although pain relief was satisfactory in many cases of constrained total shoulder arthroplasty, these designs lost popularity owing to relatively high rates of component mechanical failure, disassembly, and loosening at the bone–implant fixation sites.[27,55,75,76]

Semiconstrained glenoid components or hooded glenoid components were designed to articulate with anatomic humeral head components for patients with rotator cuff-deficient shoulders. These glenoid components were modified with a rooflike extension or hood at the superior rim[67] (Fig. 3). The purpose of the hooded modification was to block superior translation of the humeral head from superiorly directed displacement forces inherent to rotator cuff defi-

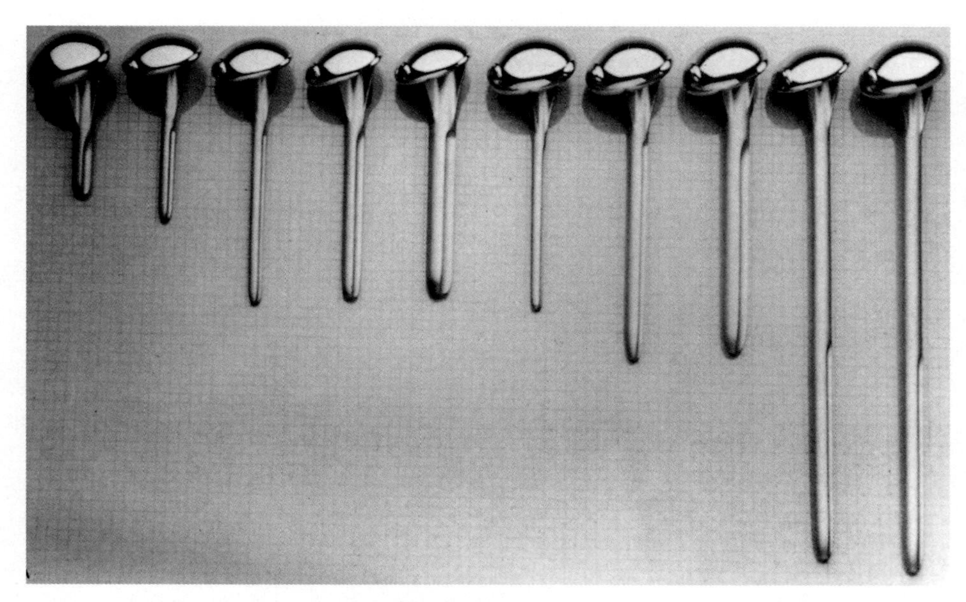

FIG. 1. The Neer II system nonconstrained prosthetic arthroplasty system. Humeral components with two diameters of stem, two lengths of head, and three lengths of stems; standard polyethylene component; standard metal-backed component; revision 300% glenoid component. (From ref. 71, with permission.)

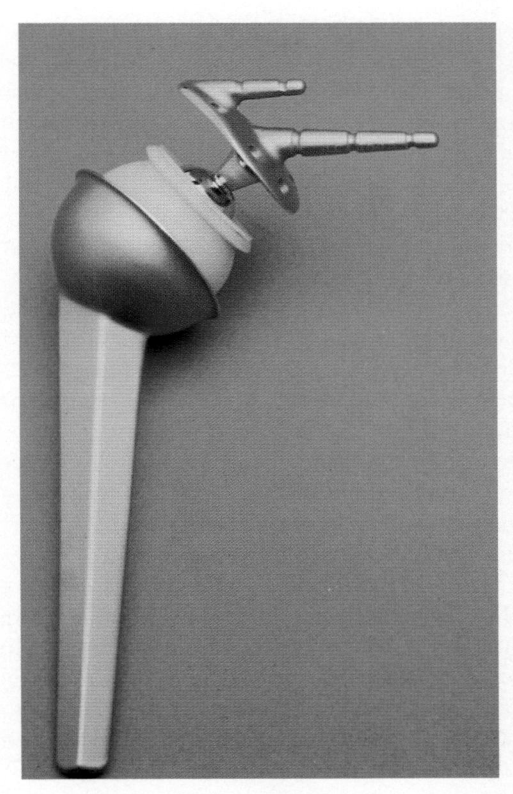

FIG. 2. A constrained total shoulder design with a reversed ball-in-socket articulation

ciency. In theory the semiconstrained design should allow the deltoid to independently achieve greater degrees of arm elevation. In the few articles that report on the use of semiconstrained prostheses, improvements in active arm elevation, if they occurred at all, were not dramatic, although pain relief was satisfactory.[17,32] The need of revision surgery and number of complications were higher than in nonconstrained designs.[17,32,34]

Nonconstrained prostheses have been designed to closely replicate normal bony anatomy to allow the surgeon to restore a close approximation of normal anatomic relations. The percentage of good and excellent results and number of complications of nonconstrained shoulder arthroplasty now appear to have had little change since the earliest reports, despite an evolution of component design features and component options. If we assume that the surgeon's decision making, the surgeon's technical skill, and postoperative rehabilitation are adequate, the results of shoulder arthroplasty are most dependent on the status of the soft-tissue structures (rotator cuff tendon integrity, capsular elasticity and competency, rotator cuff and deltoid strength.) surrounding the bony glenohumeral joint and that varies depending on the underlying diagnosis. As constrained and semiconstrained prostheses have rare, if any, indications for use currently, the subject of this chapter will concentrate solely on nonconstrained total shoulder and humeral head replacement surgery.

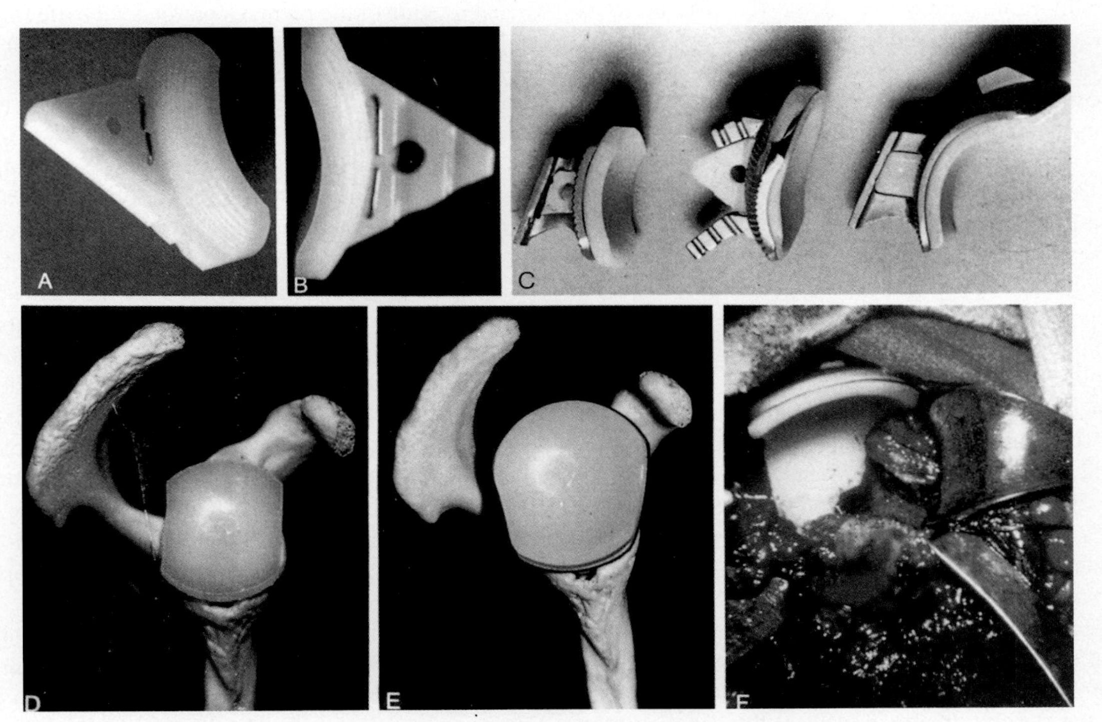

FIG. 3. **(A)** The initial Neer glenoid component; **(B)** the modified all-polyethylene component; **(C)** the Neer initial design of the metal-backed glenoid components showing **(D)** the standard surface area glenoid; **(E)** the 200% surface area glenoid; and **(F)** the 600% surface area glenoid. (From ref. 71, with permission.)

Indications

The indications for joint resurfacing arthroplasty of the shoulder are similar to other joint arthroplasties. Total shoulder replacement or humeral head replacement surgery is indicated when pain and shoulder dysfunction are the result of structural damage to the glenohumeral articular surfaces and when nonoperative management fails to sufficiently relieve patient symptoms. The primary expected gain from shoulder arthroplasty is pain relief. Secondary goals are improvements in motion and shoulder function, although these are more dependent on additional factors that vary from case to case. The ability of a well-performed shoulder arthroplasty to restore premorbid function is variable and depends on the achievement of pain relief, the condition and reconstructability of the rotator cuff, and the adequacy of postoperative rehabilitation. Replacement shoulder arthroplasty for stiffness alone without pain is rarely indicated (but can be performed), for the goals of such surgery cannot be met as predictably. Contraindications to shoulder arthroplasty include active infection, neuropathic arthropathy, and neurologic deficit involving both the rotator cuff and deltoid musculature. Isolated rotator cuff tears are not a contraindication to joint arthroplasty as long as deltoid function is preserved.

Results

It is difficult to compare the results of shoulder arthroplasty from multiple publications and often difficult to assess the results within individual publications for several reasons. Data for pain, motion, function, patient satisfaction, and overall results have not been reported between publications with uniform methods. Factors such as method of component fixation and the status of the rotator cuff vary from report to report as well. Patients within a publication often represent a mixed group from whom the results of several diagnostic categories are tallied together and reported as a single data point. At times, results of patients receiving a humeral head replacement are not separated from patients receiving a nonconstrained total shoulder arthroplasty.

Neer noted that the main factors that influenced the overall results—the condition of the rotator cuff and deltoid musculature and the required details of surgery—varied depending on the diagnostic category being addressed.[67] As such, Neer emphasized the importance of grouping patients to diagnostic categories when assessing the results of total shoulder arthroplasty.

Neer reported his results using an overall results-grading system that subdivided patients into two categories.[67] Depending on the status of the rotator cuff and deltoid musculature and the stability of the implant at the completion of surgery, patients were assigned to either a full-rehabilitation category or a limited-goals rehabilitation category. A patient was assigned to a full-rehabilitation category if the muscles were intact and functioning, or were detached but capable of recovering function after repair, and component stability was verified intraoperatively.[67] Clinical results for full-rehabilitation patients were graded as either excellent, satisfactory, or unsatisfactory, depending on the degree of patient satisfaction, pain relief, strength, and motion. An excellent result required that the patient had no pain or slight pain, had active abduction within 35 degrees of normal and 90% of normal external rotation, and was satisfied with the result. A satisfactory result was achieved if the patient had no pain, slight pain, or moderate pain only with vigorous activities; active abduction of more than 90 degrees and 50% of normal external rotation; and was satisfied with the procedure. An unsatisfactory rating required failure to achieve any of these criteria.

A limited-goals rehabilitation category was assigned if the muscles were detached and not capable of recovering function after repair because of fixed contracture or denervation, or if the stability of the implant was judged to be problematic.[67] Clinical results for the limited-goals category were graded as either satisfactory or unsatisfactory, depending on patient satisfaction, pain relief, and restoration of limited, but useful, shoulder function. A satisfactory result required no pain, slight pain, or moderate pain only with vigorous activity and active abduction of more than 70 degrees and external rotation of more than 20 degrees.

The grading system of Neer is perhaps the most rigorous of all such systems. As an example, if a patient is completely satisfied with their result yet only achieves 80% of the external rotation of the normal, contralateral extremity, only a satisfactory result can be granted, despite that external rotation is, say, 35 degrees, compared with 45 degrees in the contralateral extremity, and allows the patient to engage in all activities performed premorbidly. Thus, aside from an overall results perspective, it is valuable to understand the results of shoulder arthroplasty for the various categories (pain, motion, function, and patient satisfaction) separately.

Pain relief is the most predictable benefit of total shoulder arthroplasty and appears to vary little between diagnostic categories. Approximately 90% of patients can be expected to attain good or excellent pain relief. When inadequate pain relief occurs, the source is often explained by an identified intraoperative or postoperative complication. More common reasons for inadequate pain relief include glenoid component loosening, malpositioning of the components, improper soft-tissue balancing, rotator cuff tears, and inadequate postoperative rehabilitation. In our experience it is uncommon for inadequate postoperative pain relief to lack explanation.

Range of motion has been a difficult area of assessment because only recently has a standardized system for measuring motion been recognized.[78] Assuming the arthroplasty was technically well performed, postoperative rehabilitation has been adequate, and the patient is well motivated, active range of motion most directly correlates with the status of the rotator cuff and deltoid musculature. Osteoarthritis and osteonecrosis rarely have rotator cuff tears and most consistently obtain the greatest motion for which full or close to full active range of motion is not unusual postoperatively.[4,20,45,67] Gains in motion in rheumatoid arthritis patients are more variable, and several factors are likely responsible. The severity of disease varies and often affects other joints that interfere with the ability to rehabilitate the shoulder. The quality of the rotator cuff tissue is often compromised, being either atrophic or possessing tears of variable size and thickness.[20,51,58] In general, the longer the disease process persists, the more atrophic the deltoid musculature becomes and the greater the rotator cuff involvement. Therefore, it should be anticipated that rehabilitation in rheumatoid patients will require more time.[67,69] The functional results of nonconstrained total shoulder arthroplasty have been obtained by measuring the patient's ability to perform specific tasks of daily living. Most functional grading systems include activities that require varying degrees of forward elevation of the arm, with many being performed at waist level and fewer being performed at shoulder level or higher. Functional evaluation systems vary from report to report, making comparison between studies difficult. In the publications in which patients are separated into groups, based on diagnosis, functional scores are consistently higher in osteoarthritis than in rheumatoid arthritis. Functional scores tend to be lower for arthroplasty performed for old trauma.[3,4,67] The functional results of shoulder arthroplasty are dependent on both pain relief and gains in active range of motion. A patient who does not obtain gains in motion, but has less pain, is more inclined to use the extremity in functional activities within the range of motion available to him or her. This is especially so in patients who require only low-demand use of the extremity within limited arcs of motion. However, if significant gains in active range of motion are also achieved, the patient can participate in a broader spectrum of functional activities.

Our review of the literature yielded over 40 publications reporting the results of nonconstrained shoulder arthroplasty. These reports consistently demonstrate favorable overall results with approximately 90% of procedures being rated as good or excellent at short- and midterm follow-up periods. The results of all comparable reports for nonconstrained total shoulder arthroplasty (various nonconstrained component designs) have been placed in table format for the purpose of comparison and tabulating averages (Table 1). With the exception of one report, the long-term results of total shoulder arthroplasty have not been documented.[94]

To date only one long-term follow-up report of total shoulder arthroplasty has been performed. Torchia and Cofield followed 89 Neer total shoulder arthroplasties clinically and radiographically for a mean of 12.2 years (range 5 to 17 years).[94] Patients represented three diagnostic categories: osteoarthritis, rheumatoid arthritis, or traumatic arthritis. Twelve shoulders were allocated to a limited-goals rehabilitation category because of major tears of the rotator cuff. When comparing Cofield's previous report, which included patients in the most recent study, pain relief appears to decline with longer follow-up: 72 shoulders (81%) were without moderate or severe pain as compared with the previous report in 1984 (mean follow-up of 3.8 years) for which 92% of shoulders were free of moderate or severe pain.[20,94] Gains in active forward elevation and external rotation do not appear to deteriorate over time, for these were similar in both reports. Radiographic evidence of definite glenoid loosening increased from 11% in Cofield's previous report to 44% in the recent long-term follow-up study. Loss of pain relief and glenoid component loosening appear to be closely associated because 13 of 17 (76%) shoulders with moderate or severe pain had radiographic evidence of definite glenoid loosening, whereas only 7 of 41 (17%) shoulders without pain had radiographic evidence of such loosening. Twenty-three shoulders (30%) achieved unsatisfactory overall results according to Neer's criteria. Included in the unsatisfactory results category were 8 complications necessitating component removal including: loosening, fracture, instability, or infection. Only 7 of the 12 shoulders (58%) assigned to the limited-goals category achieved satisfactory results with long-term follow-up. Additional reports are required to establish firmly the long-term results of total shoulder arthroplasty.

Plain film evaluation has shown the prevalence of glenoid radiolucent lines to range between 30% and 80% at various periods of follow-up.[4,11,20,67] However, the high prevalence of radiolucent lines has not correlated strongly with the presence of symptoms. As such, the significance of these lines remains a controversial subject. Of 46 reoperations performed at the Mayo Clinic between 1976 and 1988 addressing complications of nonconstrained total shoulder arthroplasty, 13 (28%) were for glenoid loosening.[22] As in the Mayo Clinic article most articles report that the most common complication of total shoulder arthroplasty is glenoid component loosening. The need for reoperation for this problem was summarized from 19 reports (1,413 procedures) by Brems.[14] At an average of 5-years follow-up, radiolucent lines were present in 546 (38.6%) procedures, and in 42 (2.9%) reoperation was required for glenoid component loosening. The rate of radiolucent lines requiring revision glenoid surgery was 7.7% (42 of 546). Therefore, relatively few of these radiolucencies became symptomatic at midterm follow-up. The incidence of radiographic evidence of glenoid component loosening appears to increase with longer periods of follow-up.[16,94]

OSTEOARTHRITIS

Preoperative Evaluation

A correct diagnosis of osteoarthritis of the shoulder is usually arrived at with little difficulty if a thorough history and physical examination have been performed and a set of appropriate, high-quality plain radiographs have been obtained. The details of the information obtained during preoperative

TABLE 20-1. *Clinical results of total shoulder arthroplasty for comparable publications*

Author	No. in series	Age (mean)	Follow-up; yr (mean and range)	Osteoarthritis	Rheumatoid arthritis	Old trauma	AVN	No or slight pain	Moderate or severe pain	Patient satisfaction	Gains in forward elevation (degrees)	Gains in external rotation (degrees)
Averill[2] (1980)	57	—	2.7 (1–5.5)	10	40	1	3	55 (96%)	2 (4%)	96%	30	—
Clayton[18] (1982)	8	—	2	2	6	—	—	7 (88%)	1 (12%)	—	22	16
Thornhill[99] (1983)	150	60 (18–86)	3.6 (1–8.3)	25	106	2	2	136 (91%)	14 (9%)	—	—	—
Bade[3] (1984)	27	50	4.5 (2–7.3)	3	13	3	5	25 (93%)	2 (7%)	—	—	—
Cofield[20] (1984)	73	56 (22–75)	3.8 (2–6.5)	31	29	13	—	67 (92%)	6 (8%)	92%	44	26
Barret[24] (1987)	50	59 (24–81)	3.5 (2–7.5)	33	11	6	—	44 (88%)	6 (12%)	94%	29	33
Settergen[87] (1987)	71	55	7.5 (5–11)	30	30	11	—	64 (90%)	7 (10%)	93%	44	—
Frich[40] (1988)	50	59 (31–78)	2.25 (1–3.5)	8	35	7	—	46 (92%)	4 (8%)	—	—	—
Brenner[15] (1989)	51	59 (88–88)	5.6 (2–10.8)	25	25	1	—	46 (90%)	4 (10%)	90%	36	23
Hawkins[45] (1989)	70	69	3.3 (2–8.6)	29	34	—	—	64 (91%)	6 (6%)	—	60	18
Roper–Day[81] (1990)	25	60	5	5	18	2	—	25 (100%)	—	—	30	21
Fenlin[35a] (1994)	47	62	4.5	22	17	5	2	41 (87%)	6 (13%)	—	35	18
	Total = 679	Total mean = 59.3	Total mean = 4.1	Percent of total 34.1%	Percent of total 55.4%	Percent of total 8.4%	Percent of total 2.1%	Group average = 91.3%	Group average = 8.7%	—	Average gain = 40.3°	Average gain = 23°

[a] One patient had a humeral head replacement for rotator cuff tear arthropathy and was included in the authors results
AVN, avascular necrosis.

evaluation, especially for the physical examination and radiographic evaluation, often influence surgical technique. One should keep in mind the need to exclude other anatomic sources that can be variably responsible for the patient's experience of shoulder pain and that may persist postoperatively, despite a well-performed shoulder arthroplasty. For example, the provocation of symptoms distal to the neck during cervical spine evaluation (cervical ranges of motion, Spurling's test, or others) requires careful interpretation and possibly further diagnostic testing.[90] A glenohumeral intraarticular injection of 10 mL of 1% lidocaine can be diagnostically useful to help sort out the relative contribution of cervical pathology versus glenohumeral arthritis to shoulder pain.

Acromioclavicular (AC) arthritis can coexist with osteoarthritis of the shoulder, although, more often than not it is a radiographic finding that is asymptomatic. If tenderness is elicted at the AC joint, pain localizes to the AC joint during forced crossed-body adduction of the arm, and radiographs confirm AC degenerative arthritis, a distal clavicle excision at the time of shoulder arthroplasty should be considered. These findings on physical examination should be at least partially eliminated with an AC intraarticular injection of 2 to 3 mL of 1% lidocaine to indicate the need to add a distal clavicle excision to the procedure.

The coexistence of impingement and osteoarthritis is controversial and difficult to document confidently. Impingement signs can be invalidated because limited motion related to osteoarthritis may block the ability to place the arm within impingement arcs of glenohumeral motion. Furthermore, pain related to osteoarthritis within impingement arcs of motion often occurs simultaneously. Information that influences the decision to perform an acromioplasty includes radiographic evidence or intraoperative palpation of a significant acromial spur or the presence of a full-thickness reparable rotator cuff tear. The need to perform an acromioplasty in an osteoarthritic shoulder is infrequent.

Evaluation of the rotator cuff status on physical examination in osteoarthritis rarely raises suspicion for the presence of a rotator cuff tear. Neer's belief that the rotator cuff must be intact to develop the compressive forces required to produce primary osteoarthritis in shoulders subjected to ordinary activities[71] is at least supported by the reported low prevalence of rotator cuff tears in osteoarthritic shoulders. It is often difficult to determine whether weakness on strength testing is related to the status of the rotator cuff, pain inhibition, or chronic disuse. Significant atrophy within the supraspinatus or infraspinatus fossa should be investigated, especially if plain film evaluation does not suggest rotator cuff tear arthropathy. Such atrophy may be related to chronic rotator cuff tears, dysfunction of the suprascapular nerve, or possibly chronic disuse. Depending on one's clinical suspicion, significant atrophy may require a magnetic resonance imaging (MRI) scan of the shoulder or an electromyogram (EMG) to differentiate causation.

Preoperative assessment of limited external rotation often dicatates the use of specific subscapularis-lengthening techniques to ensure improved external rotation postoperatively. In our practice, if external rotation is at least 20 degrees, the subscapularis tendon is released in a standard fashion 1 cm medial to its insertion, and is repaired at the end of the procedure at its physiologic length, tendon end-to-tendon end. When external rotation is between −20 to 20 degrees of external rotation, the entire length of the tendon is released subperiosteally, starting at the lateral aspect of the lesser tuberosity, and is repaired to the humeral osteotomy site, a more medial location. When external rotation is less than −20 degrees, a Z-plasty coronal release of the tendon can be performed, with subsequent end-to-end tendon repair increasing the tendon length. A Z-plasty lengthening has been deemed appropriate in less than 2% of our cases involving primary osteoarthritis.

Axillary lateral radiographs should be carefully interpreted to detect the presence and extent of asymmetric posterior glenoid bone loss and an estimate of glenoid version. If a significant amount of retroversion or glenoid bone loss is determined on plain radiographs, a preoperative computed tomography (CT) scan can be obtained to further define bony anatomy. This information may dictate the use of special techniques for restoring normal glenoid version or for addressing glenoid bone deficiency. An axillary radiograph will show whether the humeral head is subluxated posteriorly. If significant posterior subluxation is identified, one should anticipate the possible need to surgically shorten the posterior capsule for achieving soft-tissue balancing.

Preoperative assessment for the presence of dental disease is important to minimize the risk of infective seeding before attempting any joint arthroplasty. Patients who have poor dentition or a history of dental infection should undergo preoperative dental evaluation and possible tooth extraction(s).

Surgical Approach

Surgery can be performed under general anesthesia or an interscalene (regional) block.[13] Ranges of glenohumeral motion are evaluated in the anesthetized extremity to confirm the preoperative assessment and the extent to which capsular release will be needed to restore motion. The surgical table is converted to a modified beach chair position. The surgical shoulder must be positioned off the edge of the table to afford unobstructed arm extension. Placement of a small folded towel under the patient's scapula will deliver the glenoid more anteriorly, allowing better glenoid exposure and providing stabilization of the scapula. The patient's head must be supported and stabilized in neutral position. Special headrests (e.g., Mayfield neurosurgical or McConnell) have been designed to simplify this task. The operative shoulder is then sterilely prepared and draped free. Before making the incision prophylactic intravenous antibiotic(s) are administered.

An anterior deltopectoral surgical approach is used.[47] The incision follows a straight line which begins superiorly at the clavicle, extends inferiorly over the tip of the coracoid process, and continues across the anterior arm toward the insertion of the deltoid (Fig. 4). The cephalic vein is dissected and the deltopectoral interval is developed, retracting the deltoid and the cephalic vein laterally and the pectoralis major medially. The cephalic vein may undergo less stretch or injury if it is dissected laterally and retracted medially with the pectoralis major. The superior 1 to 2 cm of the pectoralis major tendon is released near its insertion site with electrocautery to improve exposure of the inferior glenohumeral joint (Fig. 5). Care must be taken with this release to avoid injuring the biceps tendon, which lies immediately deep and medial to the pectoralis insertion site. It is generally not necessary to repair the pectoralis tendon.

The clavipectoral fascia is incised along the lateral edge of the conjoined tendon up to the coracoacromial ligament. In osteoarthritis with an intact rotator cuff a full or partial release of the coracoacromial ligament can be performed to improve exposure. The coracoacromial ligament should be preserved or repaired when large rotator cuff tears are encountered to preserve a restraint against superior translation of the humeral head. In these cases the CA ligament is released at the base of the coracoid process and repaired to it at the time of wound closure. With the clavipectoral fascia incised, a modified Taylor retractor or reverse Howman retractor can be easily placed over the superolateral aspect of the humeral head in the lateral aspect of the subacromial space to retract the deltoid. One must be careful to not lever on the acromion for fear of fracture, especially in the presence of osteopenic bone.

The conjoined tendon is retracted medially with a broad medium-sized blunt retractor. The musculocutaneous nerve penetrates the lateral coracobrachialis muscle between 3.1 and 8.2 cm distal to the tip of the coracoid process.[36] The position of the axillary nerve should be identified along the anterior surface of the subscapularis muscle, deep to the conjoined tendon.[79] This is especially important in cases with complex deformities or scar tissue formation (e.g., old trauma or revision surgery). The axillary nerve crosses the inferolateral border of the subscapularis 3 to 5 mm medial to its musculotendinous junction and has an intimate anatomic relation with the inferior capsule.[56]

The anterior humeral circumflex artery and veins are visualized at the inferior one-third of the subscapularis tendon and are isolated, ligated, and divided. The medial division will be retracted with the released subscapularis tendon.

The subscapularis tendon is released with electrocautery at one of two standard locations. If the patient has approximately 20 degrees or more of external rotation, the tendon can be divided 1 cm medial to its attachment site on the lesser tuberosity and subsequently reattached, tendon-to-tendon, at its physiologic length (Fig. 6A). If external rotation is less than 20 degrees, we prefer dissection of the tendon directly off the lesser tuberosity, beginning at its most lateral site of insertion (see Fig. 6B).[79] With this technique the tendon will achieve a relative lengthening when it is reattached to a more medial location at the anterior humeral osteotomy site. A coronal Z-plasty lengthening can be used for severely limited external rotation (−20 to −30 degrees; see Fig. 6C,D). Because this technique halves the thickness of the subscapularis tendon, the tendon is weakened. As a general rule, 1 cm of tendon lengthening achieves 20 degrees of additional external rotation regardless of the technique.[71]

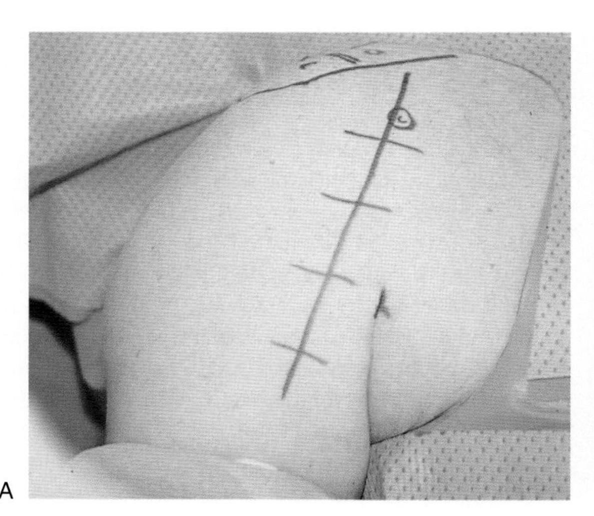
A

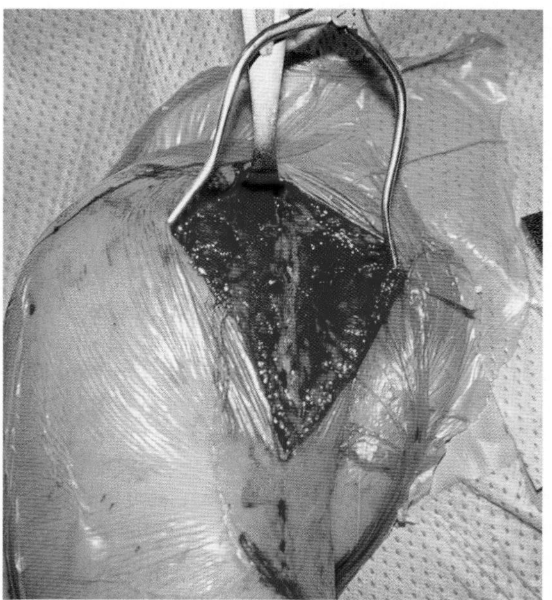
B

FIG. 4. (A) The skin incision for a routine total shoulder arthroplasty is centered over the deltopectoral interval and the tip of the corocoid. The incision begins near the lateral third of the clavicle and extends near the deltoid tuberosity. **(B)** The cephalic vein is exposed and may be dissected medially with the pectoralis major or laterally with the deltoid. The latter technique is generally preferred.

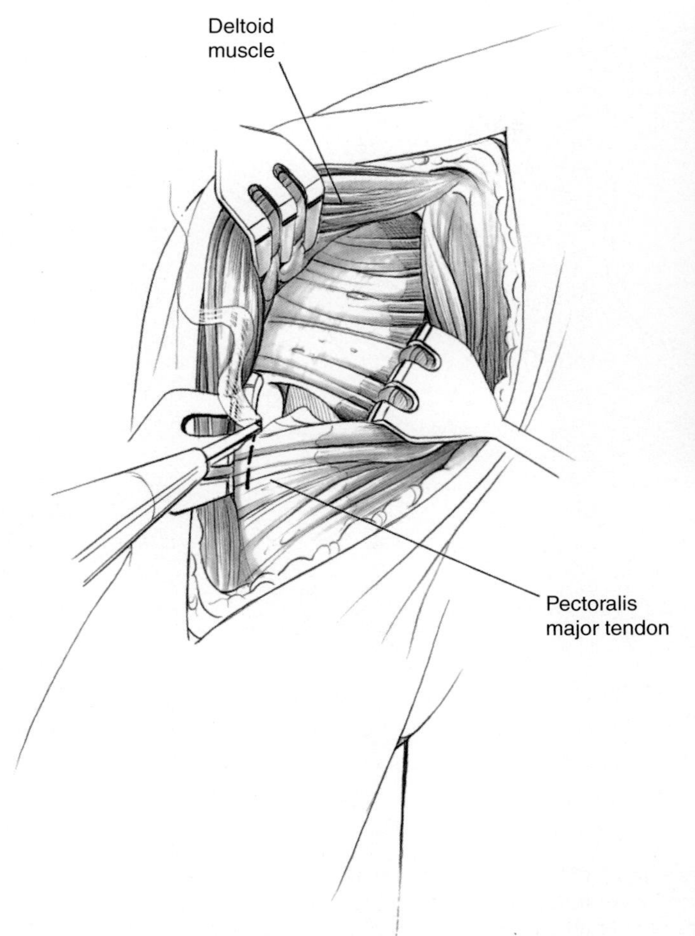

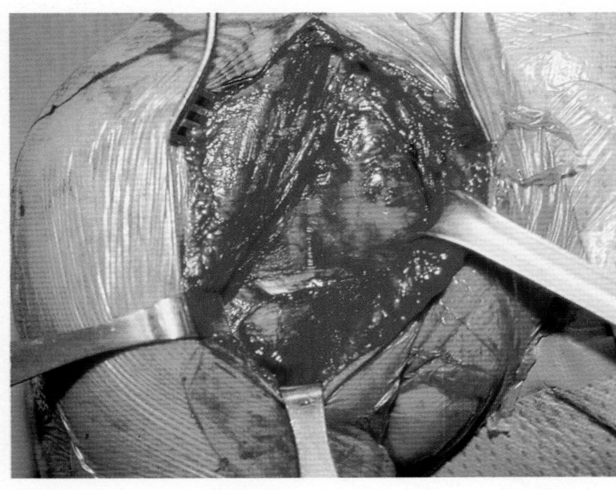

FIG. 5. (A & B) The deltopectoral interval is dissected and the upper 1 to 2 cm of the pectoralis major insertion site is incised.

It may be difficult to maintain the subscapularis tendon and glenohumeral capsule as separate layers during the subscapularis release. Usually, the subscapularis can be dissected from the capsule, but if there is capsular contracture it is necessary to separate the 2 layers to mobilize the subscapularis and achieve maximum external rotation. Regardless, the subscapularis must be freed of adhesions circumferentially for optimum lengthening and unrestricted gliding.[24] Release of the subscapularis tendon should include the capsule on the deep surface, the base of the coracoid process, and the rotator interval capsule superiorly, and the conjoined tendon superficially (Fig. 7). Care must be taken when releasing the capsule inferiorly because of the proximity of the axillary nerve. The axillary nerve, which is relatively protected by externally rotating and slightly flexing the adducted arm, should be definitively protected by the placement of a small blunt retractor between it and the humeral neck. The anterior capsular release must reach at least the 6:00 o'clock position in all cases for the humeral head to be dislocated, and in most cases a more extensive release inferiorly and posteriorly is required to regain passive motion.

Humeral Preparation

Patients with osteoarthritis possess a ring of osteophytes of variable size following the articular margin of the humeral head. This osteophyte ring must be removed carefully, leaving the native humeral neck undisturbed. Osteophytes should be removed with a rongeur and a small curved osteotome before performing the humeral osteotomy (Fig. 8). The location of the axillary nerve must be realized and protected. Greater ease of dislocating the proximal humerus and more accurate soft-tissue balancing are achieved once the osteophytes are removed.

In some arthroplasty systems the neck shaft angle is prescribed by the prosthetic design. In these systems an extramedullary or intramedullary cutting guide is used. The height of the cut is determined by the insertion site of the supraspinatus tendon. The amount of retroversion is determined by the degree of rotation of the arm. To achieve a correct humeral osteotomy the saw blade (or osteotome) must be oriented with reference to three alignments: medullary canal axis, height, and version. For an extramedullary system the stem of the humeral osteotomy guide should align with the medullary canal axis to prevent varus or valgus po-

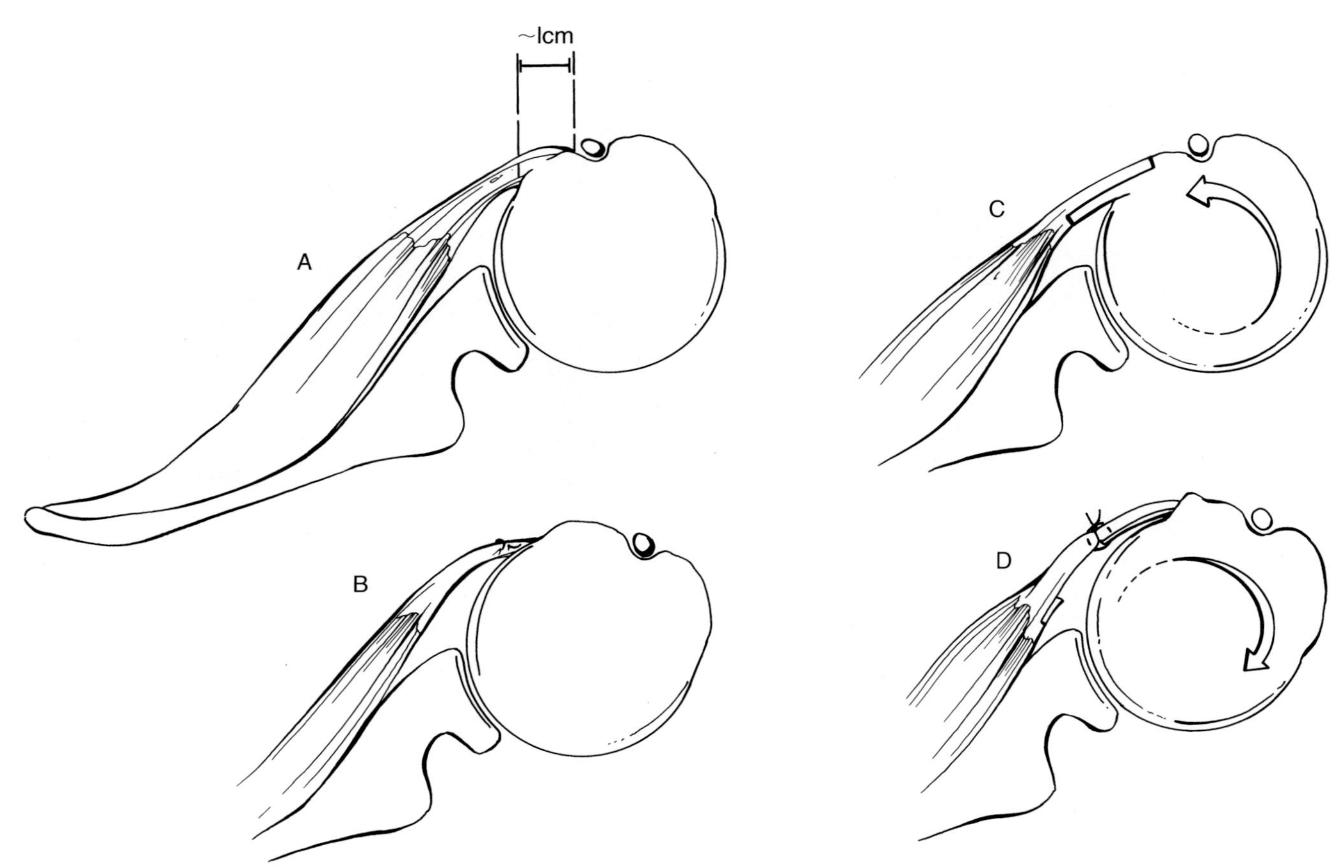

FIG. 6. **(A)** Subscapularis tenotomy for shoulders with 20 degrees or more of external rotation. **(B)** Subperiosteal dissection of the subscapularis from the lesser tuberosity. Later closure of the subscapularis to the osteotomy surface of the humerus will medialize (lengthen) the insertion site and, thereby, improve passive external rotation. **(C,D)** Coronal Z-plasty of the subscapularis for lengthening it is performed when there is severe loss of external rotation.

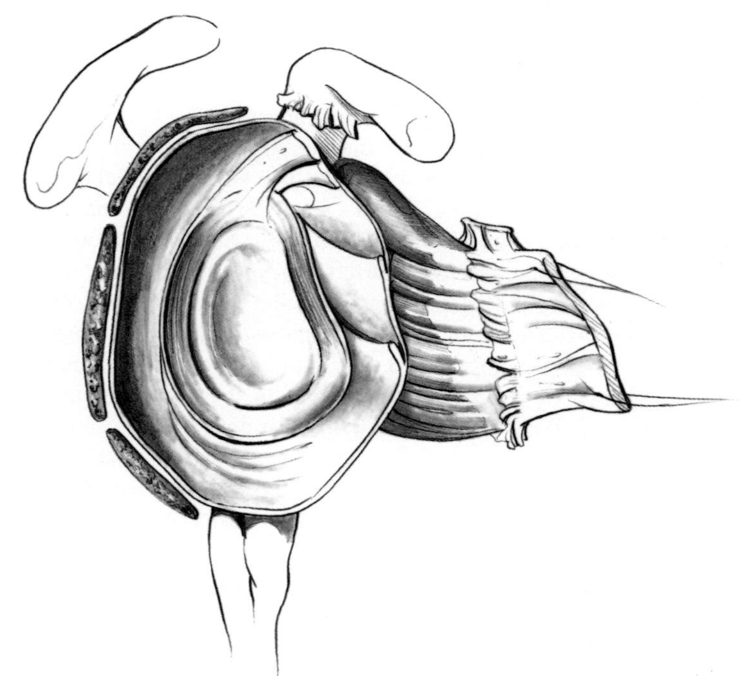

FIG. 7. Circumferential release of the subscapularis is necessary in all cases where there is restriction of external rotation. Circumferential release requires that the capsule be separated from the subscapularis, the rotator interval is released to the glenoid, the coracohumeral ligament is released from the base of the corocoid, and any scar tissue superficial to the subscapularis tendon and muscle is removed.

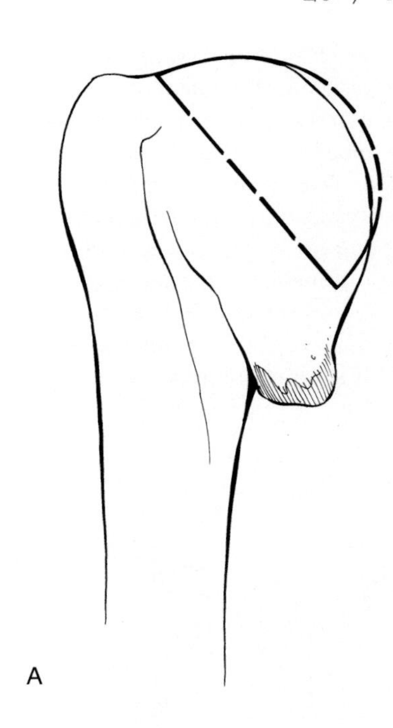

FIG. 8. (A-C) In osteoarthritis a large osteophyte is often present and will obscure the normal location of the anatomic neck. This osteophyte should be removed circumferentially before making the humeral osteotomy. Removal of the humeral osteophyte and capsular release to the posteroinferior portion of the humeral neck is always necessary. This will allow complete dislocation of the humeral head when the arm is maximally externally rotated and extended. Also, this will permit the humeral osteotomy to be made at the anatomic neck and in anatomic version.

A

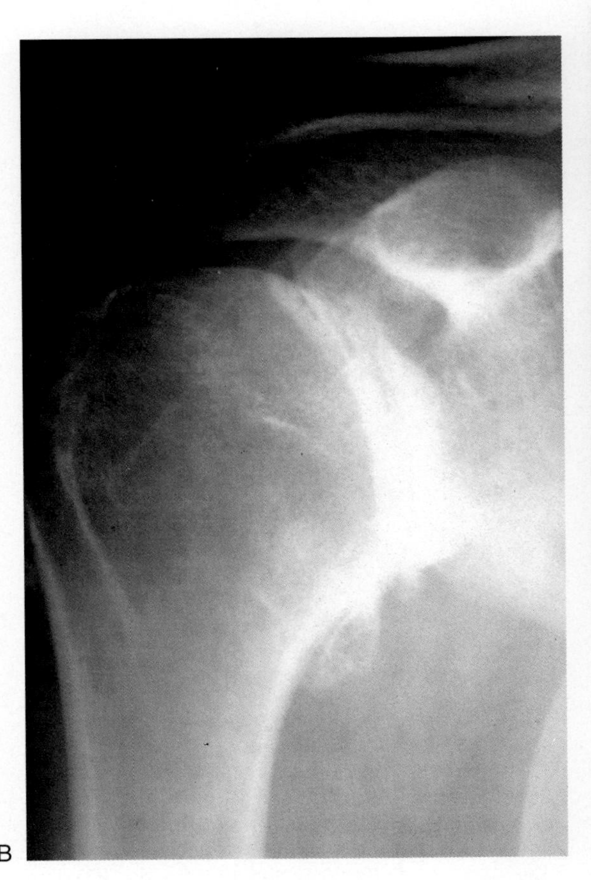

B

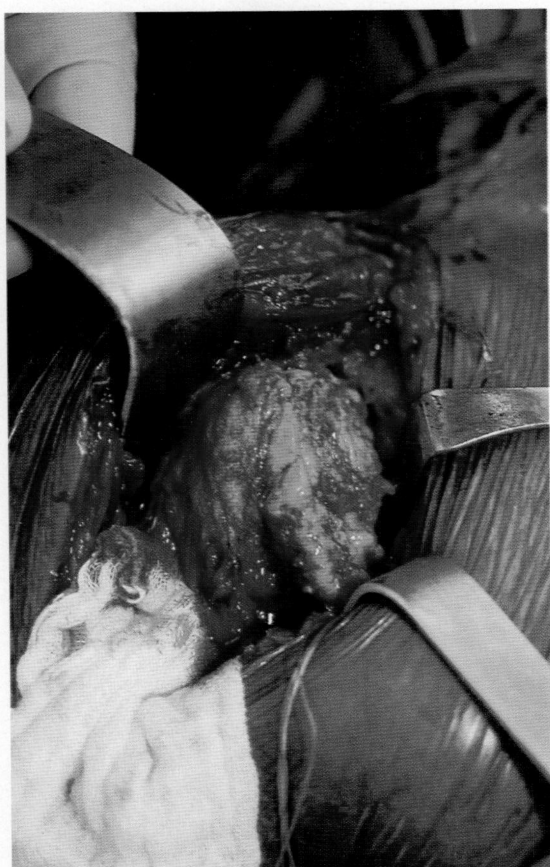

C

sitioning. Correct alignment is achieved by laying the stem of the humeral osteotomy guide parallel to the axis of the shaft of the humerus (Fig. 9A,B). The osteotomy guide should aim distally between the midpoint of the palpated medial and lateral epicondyles of the distal humerus[71] (see Fig. 9B). Some shoulder systems have the option of first placing a guide down the intramedullary canal to which an osteotomy guide is assembled and a humeral osteotomy is performed. In other systems the humeral head is cut along the anatomic neck without a guide and the prosthetic system allows for variation in the neck shaft angle (see Fig. 9C).

The height, that is, the proximal to distal relation of the guide, is adjusted to resect the thickness of the humeral head articular surface. A narrow retractor is placed under the biceps tendon just medial to the insertion site of the supraspinatus tendon. With gentle retraction the space between the supraspinatus tendon and lateral edge of the articular cartilage can be defined. The lateral extent of the osteotomy should exit just medial to the supraspinatus tendon. The superior-most point of the humeral articular surface averages a distance of 8 $\pm$ 3.2 mm cephalad to the top of the greater tuberosity.[49] It is critically important to reestablish a

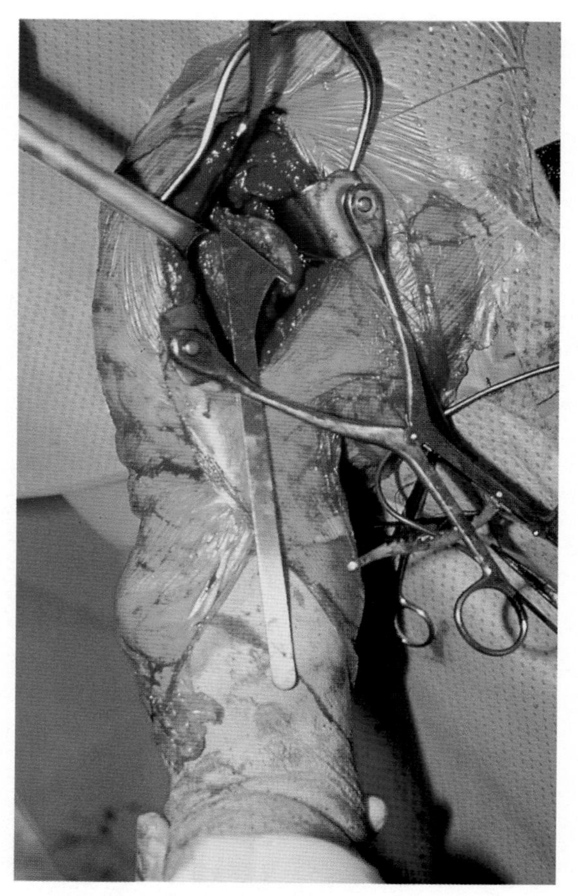
A

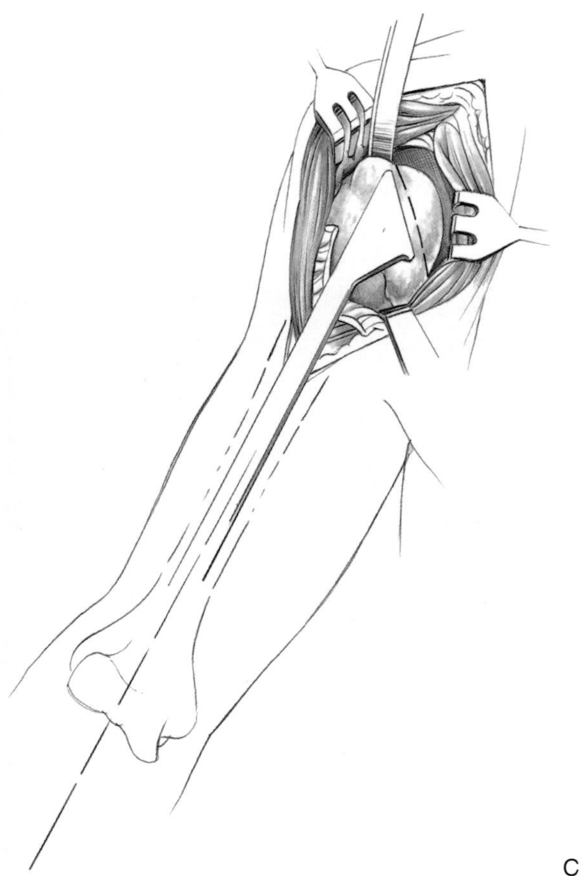
C

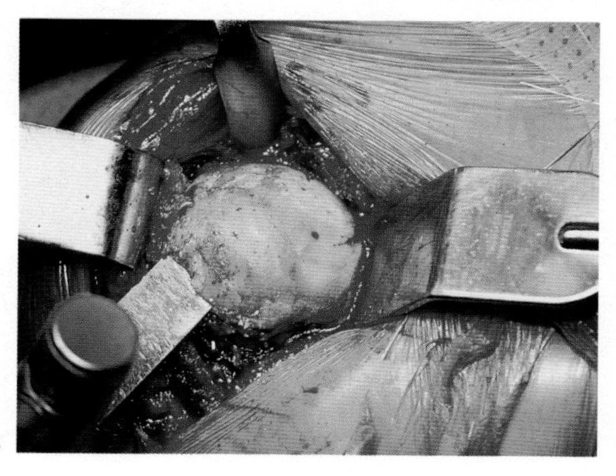
B

FIG. 9. (A,B) An extramedullary-cutting guide is placed at the top of the supraspinatus insertion site to determine the height of the osteotomy, and the long axis of the guide is aligned along the lateral shaft of the humerus. The osteotomy is made along the flat surface of the guide thereby defining the neck shaft angle of the prosthesis. **(B)** The version is determined by the rotation of the arm. The angle of the epicondylar axis and the osteotomy surface will determine prosthetic version. **(C)** The humeral osteotomy may be made along the anatomic neck without a cutting guide. The prosthetic system must then allow for variation in neck shaft angle between individuals.

close approximation of this relation. When too much bone is resected by placing the osteotomy guide too distally, the greater tuberosity will be too superior relative to the superior-most point of the replaced humeral head, and the cuff attachment site may be compromised. Inferior humeral head placement will also occur with an abnormal (varus) decrease in the neck shaft angle. As a result, the greater tuberosity may impinge against the acromion when the patient actively elevates the arm. If too little bone is resected by placing the guide too proximally, excessive height of the implanted humeral component can lead to excessive soft-tissue tension (an overstuffed joint). Overstuffing results in increased loads being borne by the glenoid component, decreased ranges of motion, and pain. Overstuffing of the joint can occur if component sizing is not accurate (Fig. 10). A second surgical procedure to revise these errors will likely be needed should they go unrecognized at the index procedure.

The humeral head is rotated so that the articular margin is perpendicular to the floor and the head is osteotomized in anatomic retroversion, which is usually between 30 and 35 degrees. The version of the humeral osteotomy is on occasion changed to compensate for altered glenoid version or situations of soft-tissue imbalance. For example, in shoulder arthroplasty for chronic locked posterior dislocation, the osteotomy is performed in smaller degrees of retroversion to compensate for the imbalance created in the stretched-out posterior soft tissues to minimize the tendency for postoperative posterior instability.[67] One must realize that the attachment of the posterior rotator cuff limits the extent that one can compensate in the direction of increasing degrees of retroversion. If this is not realized the posterior cuff could be detached. In general, to achieve a stable arthroplasty the combined version of the humeral osteotomy and the resurfaced glenoid should be a sum of 40 degrees of retroversion. For example, if the glenoid is in 20 degrees of retroversion, the humeral osteotomy should be performed in 20 degrees of retroversion, giving a combined retroversion of 40 degrees.[71]

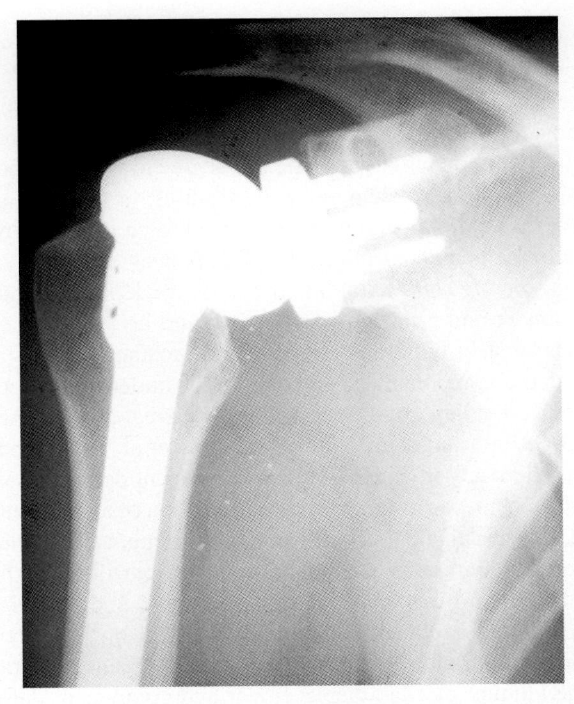

FIG. 10. An example of an overstuffed, total shoulder arthroplasty. The distance between the greater tuberosity and acromion is excessive. Overstuffing in this case is due to a high humeral osteotomy, too large of a humeral head, and a lateralized glenoid joint line (thick glenoid component).

The proximal humerus is delivered into the anterior wound with external rotation and extension. Posterior osteophytes on the humeral neck that have not yet been removed may become locked on the posterior rim of the glenoid, preventing this maneuver. Usually this can be resolved by placing a straight, flat retractor (Darrach retractor, shoe-horn retractor, or the like) inside the glenohumeral joint beyond the posterior glenoid rim. The smooth metallic surface can then be used as a skid for rotating and gliding on the posterior humeral neck. The remaining osteophytes should be removed with a rongeur or osteotome.

A 6- to 8-mm medullary rasp is started 5 to 7 mm posterior to the biceps groove at the upper-most portion of the humeral osteotomy surface.[7] A rasp or currete is passed vertically through the cancellous bone of the osteotomy site in line with the axis of the humeral shaft to identify the medullary canal (Fig. 11). Sequential reaming is done with progressively larger reamers until mild resistance is felt. The endosteal cortex should not be thinned or notched. While reaming, a slight lateral force is maintained to avoid an inherent tendency toward varus reaming.[24] The cancellous bone of the metaphysis can then be prepared according to the specifications of the particular shoulder arthroplasty system being used. A series of rasps are generally provided for this procedure. A trial component is implanted and tested for axial and rotational stability. At times, the lateral fin of the prosthesis will impinge against lateral cortical bone during the final 3 cm of prosthesis seating. Should this occur, it is necessary to create a notch in the lateral cortex at the biceps groove for the fin to fit in. If this notch is not created in such cases the component could potentially angulate into varus.

Glenoid Preparation

The trial articular head component is removed and the glenoid is exposed. The trial humeral stem component is left in place to protect the prepared proximal humerus from injury from retractors. A humeral head retractor is positioned behind the posterior rim of the glenoid and the proximal humerus is retracted posteriorly. Narrow, pointed retractors are carefully placed just outside the superior, anterior, and inferior margins of the glenoid. The glenoid labrum is excised sharply at its peripheral edge anteriorly, inferiorly, and posteriorly. The superior labrum is excised carefully to preserve the insertion site of the long head of the biceps tendon,

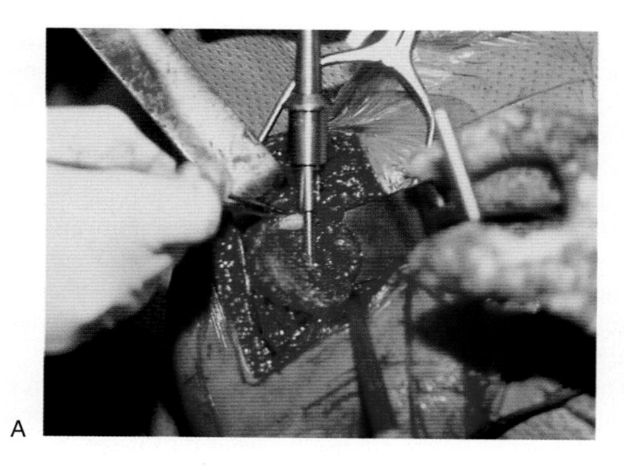
A

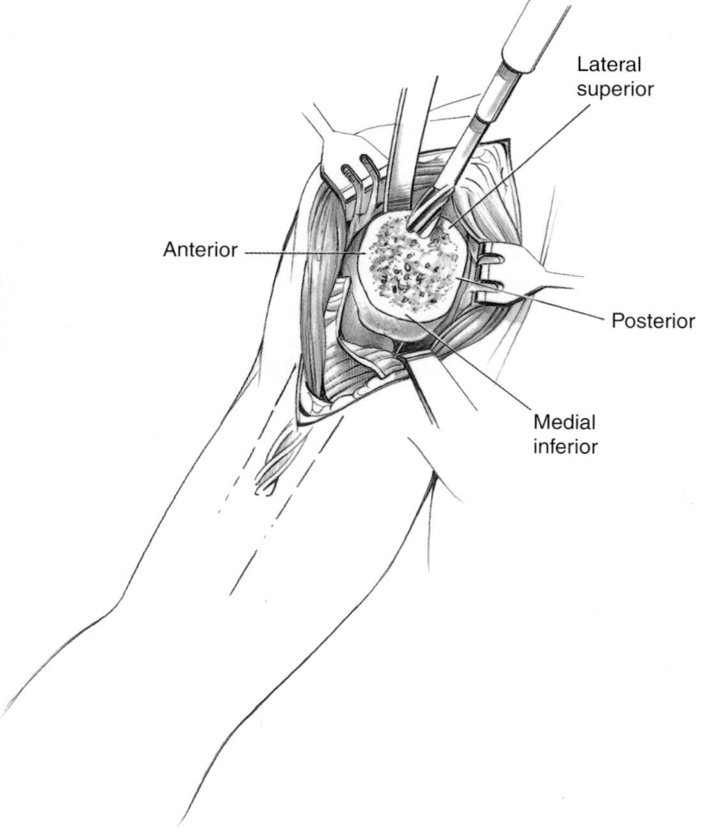

FIG. 11. (A,B) The humeral shaft is prepared for the humeral stem. A narrow canal reamer is placed in the center of the anterior posterior dimension of the osteotomy surface. In most cases the site of entry is 5 to 7 mm posterior to the biceps groove.

unless the tendon is to be tenodesed because of advanced degeneration.

It is important to understand the particular bony geometry of the glenoid in each case. A normal glenoid offers minimal bone for prosthesis support and fixation and even less in most disease states. In many cases of osteoarthritis the humeral head will be posteriorly subluxated and the posterior rim of the glenoid will be worn, both to a variable degree.[67]

The principles of glenoid resurfacing are consistent from case to case despite variation in glenoid component designs and fixation techniques. The back of the glenoid component should *precisely match the surface area of the bony glenoid.* Too large a component leaves its periphery unsupported and increases the risk of component loosening. Additionally, an oversized glenoid component can be impinged on by the proximal humerus at the extremes of motion. It is important to recognize that glenoid osteophytes can add area to the glenoid articular surface eccentrically. Osteophytes may mislead the surgeon into creating drill holes for pegged components or the slot for keeled components in an eccentric position relative to the entrance of the glenoid neck. This error can result in perforating the cortex of the glenoid neck, resultant bone cement extravasation with possible thermal nerve injury, and suboptimal glenoid component fixation. Preoperatively the degree of osteophyte formation can be estimated from radiographs, and excessive nonstructural osteophytes should be excised. The anterior rim and neck of the glenoid should be palpated and visualized to determine glenoid version and locate the position of the glenoid neck. Such evaluation will help guide the degree to which glenoid version should be changed with reaming or burring and where the central position of the glenoid fossa is located relative to the bony confines of the glenoid neck.

An exacting congruent fit between the back of the glenoid component and prepared bone bed should be achieved. An incongruent fit between host bone and prosthesis leaves areas of the component unsupported and, under physiologic eccentric-loading conditions, allows for greater component deformations and displacements. Collins et al. performed a cadaveric study in which glenoid component deformity and displacement was tested with the application of an off-center load, comparing glenoid surfaces that were prepared by three different techniques: simple removal of cartilage with a curette, hand-burring the osseous surface, and spherical reaming with a reamer that matched the back of the glenoid component's radius of curvature.[25] A significant reduction in the amount of edge displacement and component deformity was observed in glenoids that had been prepared with spherical reaming.

Ideally, the prepared *glenoid surface will have approximately neutral version.* It is not always possible nor wise to restore glenoid version to neutral. With mild changes in glenoid version (less than 1 cm of eccentric bone loss), it is easiest to lower the high side with eccentric glenoid reaming or power burring. When addressing greater degrees of altered version with this technique, one must be wary of the untoward effects of resecting too much bone. One must bear in mind that the paucity of glenoid bone affords only a little opportunity for modification. The glenoid pedicle can be narrowed to such an extent that enough bone stock is not available for implanting a glenoid component. The subchondral bone plate, which stabilizes the back of the glenoid prosthesis, can be compromised with excessive efforts to level the glenoid face. Bone removal in excess of 1 cm to correct glenoid version is discouraged. Additionally, the surgeon must bear in mind that the glenoid surface faces 5 to 10 degrees superiorly,[84,86] and excessive bone removal either superiorly, especially in the presence of superior erosion, or inferiorly must be avoided.

Fixation of the glenoid component must achieve *immediate stability*. Although a variety of components (cemented, noncemented, all polyethelene, and metal backed) is available, the most commonly used is an all polyethelene design with multiple pegs or a keel for implantation with polymethylmethacrylate cement. This design and method of fixation has demonstrated a low rate of failure at 5- to 10-year follow-up.[20,28,67]

When the glenoid surface is prepared with reaming, a hole must be created in the articular surface that centers over the entrance to the glenoid neck (Fig. 12). The hub of the reamer is inserted into the prepared hole and reaming is performed to create a surface that congruently matches the back of the glenoid prosthesis. If a pegged component is chosen, then several drill holes will be created according to the manufacturer's drill guide system (Fig. 13). The drill holes are inspected with a small curved hemostat to detect whether the cortex of the glenoid neck has been perforated. If a perforation is found it is plugged with bone taken from the osteotomized humeral head and a smaller amount of bone cement will be used. When a perforation occurs at a superficial depth it may not be possible to obtain cement fixation for that particular peg.

If a keeled component is chosen, a rectangular slot will need to be made in the glenoid surface that centers over the entrance of the glenoid neck. We use a power burr to create the rectangular perforation and to excavate the least amount of cancellous bone in the glenoid neck to fully accept the keel. Neer has remarked that inferior osteophytes must be accounted for when determining the superoinferior relation for positioning the glenoid component.[71] The base of the coracoid process superiorly serves as a landmark with which the superior level of the slot should align. A small amount of cancellous bone can be removed from the base of the coracoid process with a small curved curette for bone cement to lock into.[71]

A trial glenoid component is inserted and checked for coverage and congruency of fit. The trial glenoid should be tested digitally for unwanted rocking motion. Imperfections in the reamed surface, if found, are addressed to ensure congruency. Pegged component techniques require unobstructed glenoid exposure. If the glenoid exposure is suboptimal, it may not be possible to complete the steps necessary for placing a pegged component. Therefore, it is wise to be versed in the techniques for implanting keeled component designs.

The glenoid bone is debrided of blood clot and loose bone fragments with pulsatile lavage. A dry bone bed will optimize cement penetration into the cancellous interstices. A variety of hemostatic agents can be used to dry the cancellous bone bed. Sponges soaked with either epinephrine, thrombin, or hydrogen peroxide are commonly used. The bone cement is mixed and is ready for injection through a cardiac syringe when it has reached the late liquid phase. The sponge is removed from the glenoid just before the cement is injected. The cement is pressurized digitally, and excess cement is removed (Fig. 14). The component is seated firmly in place and constant pressure is maintained until the cement has hardened. Excess cement is removed once the component is seated. It is most undesirable to have cement resting between the prepared glenoid face and the back of the component. Such cement is likely to fragment and displace, which leaves areas of the back of the glenoid component unsupported and prone to loosening.

Although the presence of radiolucent lines at the glenoid component fixation interface has not directly correlated with symptoms or the need for revision surgery, good surgical technique should theoretically minimize their early appearance. Brems et al. noted that radiolucent lines were present on postoperative recovery room radiographs in 69% of patients.[11] As well, the presence or absence of lucent lines was statistically correlated with specific surgeons who had different habits of bone preparation. Thus, meticulous bone drying and cementing technique is essential.

Component Sizing and Trial Reduction

The humeral head retractor is removed and the proximal humerus is delivered into the anterior wound with extension, adduction, and external rotation. When using modular humeral head components, a wide range of neck lengths are available for a given head size allowing control over myofascial tension. If inadequate myofascial tension is restored the shoulder is prone to instability, especially inferiorly. On the other hand, excessive myofascial tension creates an overstuffed joint, with loss of passive motion. It is best to perform the needed elements of a circumferential soft-tissue release and then achieve correct soft-tissue balance by trying various prosthetic head sizes. After a correct soft-tissue release, the head size chosen should closely approximate the size of the normal premorbid humeral head in both radius of curvature and neck length.

Ranges of motion and glenohumeral translations are tested to determine if soft-tissue balance and myofascial ten-

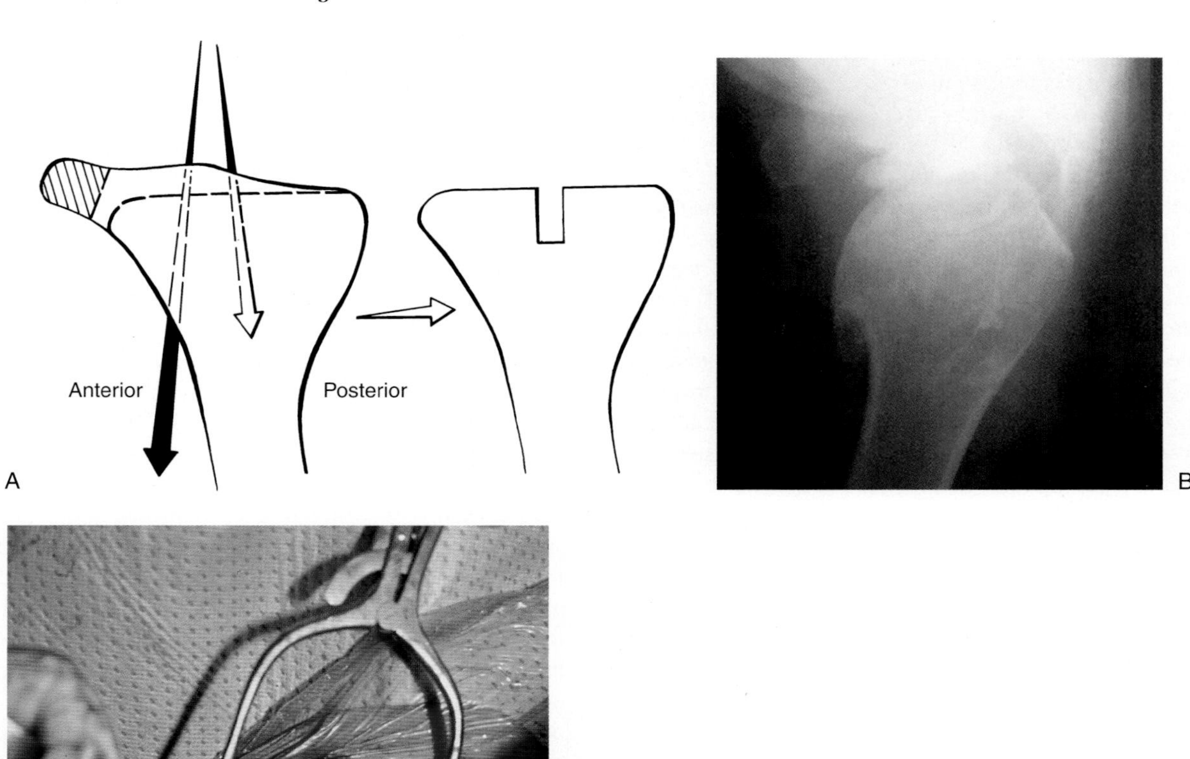

C

FIG. 12. (A,B) With 1 cm of posterior glenoid erosion, or less, the anterior half of the glenoid can be reamed to change version to a more neutral position. **(C)** A central hole is made in the glenoid, and a power reamer can be used to achieve intimate contact between the back of the prosthesis and the glenoid component. It is important that the central hole be placed centrally within the glenoid vault.

sion are appropriate. Anterior stability should be observed during external rotation to 40 degrees with the arm at the side. Next, with the subscapularis tendon approximated to the anterior osteotomy site using a small tenaculum, the arm should achieve approximately 35 to 40 degrees of external rotation without undue subscapularis tension. The arm should achieve approximately 140 degrees of elevation and greater than 20 degrees of internal rotation in the 90-degree abducted position. If internal rotation in the 90-degree abducted position is less than 20 degrees, a posterior capsular release is indicated. Posterior capsular release is performed by removing the trial humeral component, placing the arm in neutral rotation, and using a bone hook to laterally distract the proximal humerus from the glenoid. In this way the posterior capsule is placed under tension and is exposed at the glenoid margin for capsular release. If the posterior capsule is released, care is taken to avoid penetrating the posterior rotator cuff tendons that lie immediately behind the capsule. Posterior laxity should allow the humeral head to be posteriorly translated approximately 50% of the anteroposterior diameter of the glenoid face with digital pressure. On release of the posterior translating force, the humeral head should spontaneously reduce, otherwise excessive posterior laxity exists. Excessive posterior translation is addressed by performing a vertical posterior capsular incision and a pants-over-vest imbrication with no. 2 nonabsorbable sutures.

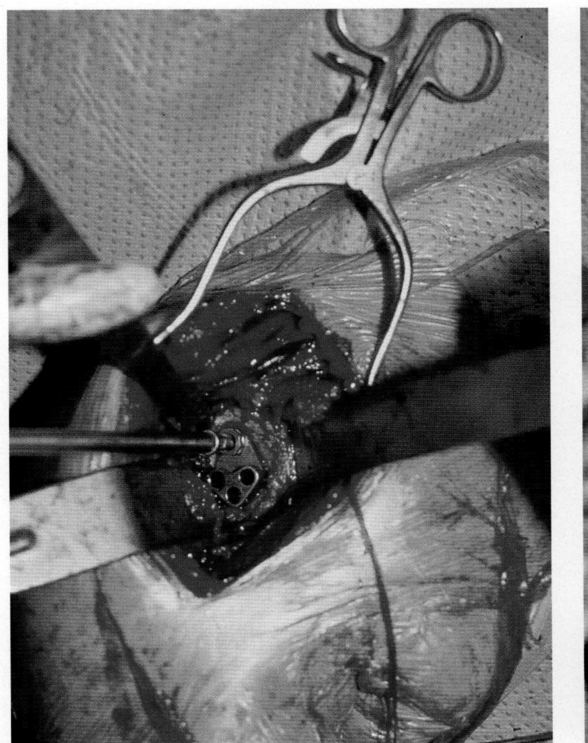

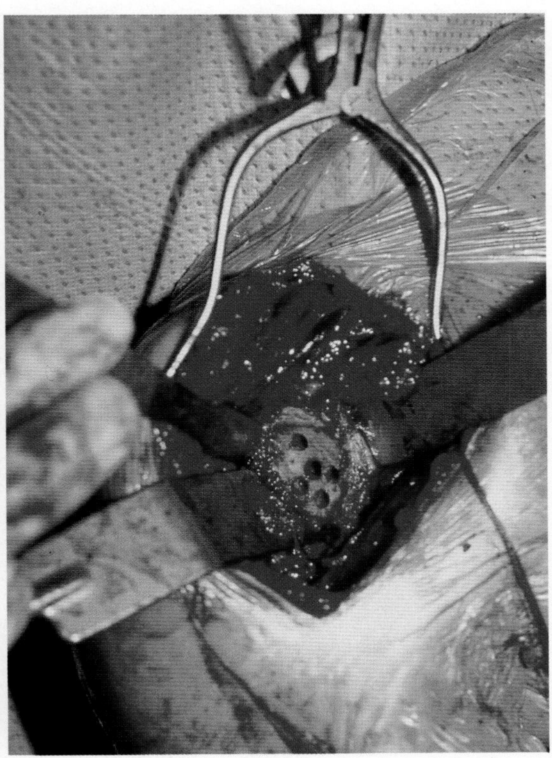

A B

FIG. 13. (A,B) The guide system for fixation of the glenoid system is then used. In this system multiple pegs are used for glenoid fixation. In other systems a keel or screws are used for fixation.

Closure

Before implanting the final humeral component, rotator cuff tears, when found, are repaired (see Special Techniques section). If the subscapularis tendon is to be reattached to the anterior humeral osteotomy site, three or four drill holes must be made adjacent to the osteotomy site and loops of suture material passed through them. These loops of free suture will be used to pull the subscapularis tendon sutures through the drill holes, allowing a reattachment of tendon to bone (Fig. 15). Depending on the prosthetic design, the final humeral prosthesis can be stably implanted with press fitting in most patients with osteoarthritis. In certain situations, such as large degenerative proximal humeral cysts, cement fixation is used because a stable press-fit cannot be achieved. In some prosthetic designs, cemented fixation is recommended and necessary to avoid late loosening. The final humeral component is now seated in correct position. If a modular system is used, the Morse taper articulating surfaces must be thoroughly cleaned and dried. The components are assembled and tamped using a mallet and impactor to secure the head in place. Depending on how the subscapularis tendon was initially detached, it is either repaired tendon-to-tendon with either nonabsorbable 1-mm–Dacron-tape suture or no. 2 braided nonabsorbable sutures to the osteotomy site. Several configurations for passing the suture material through the subscapularis tendon can be selected. We prefer a modified Mason–Allen or Kessler suture configuration. The axillary nerve can be palpated to ensure its intactness. The wound is thoroughly irrigated, suctioned, and final hemostasis is obtained. Wound closure over suction drainage is performed according to the surgeon's preference. Skin closure is with a subcuticular technique.

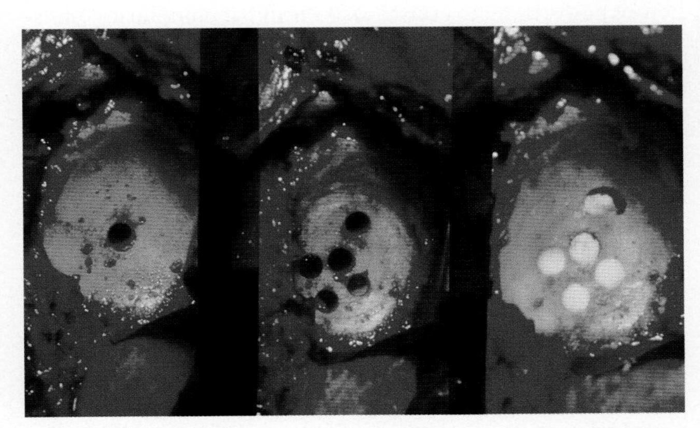

FIG. 14. The fixation holes are irrigated with pulsatile lavage and homeostasis achieved. Each fixation hole is pressurized with cement, and the component is inserted.

Postoperative Rehabilitation

The outcome following shoulder arthroplasty is as much dependent on the ability of the surgeon to perform a techni-

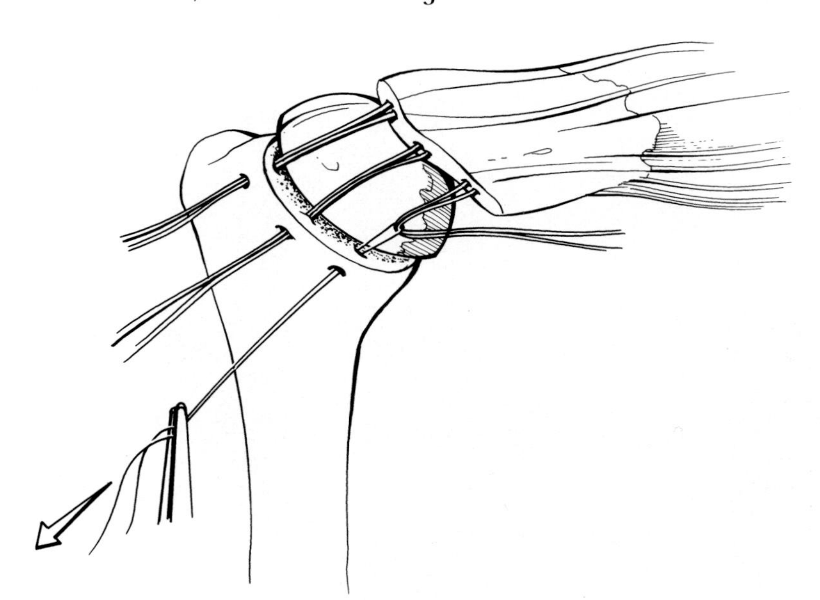

FIG. 15. The technique for repair of the subscapularis will be dependent on the technique by which the tendon was incised. For tendon removed by subperiosteal dissection from the lesser tuberosity, the tendon is repaired to the osteotomy surface by transosseous sutures using 1-mm–Dacron sutures. The sutures are passed through the tendon using a modified Mason–Allen or Kessler technique.

cally excellent procedure as it is the adequacy of postoperative rehabilitation. It should be understood that no one single postoperative rehabilitation program is appropriate for all patients. The specific exercises chosen, the way in which exercises are modified, and the rate of progression during rehabilitation must be dictated by the surgeon to address the specific needs of each patient. In particular, the rehabilitation program should be modified depending on the surgeon's intraoperative assessment of the stability of the components and the quality of soft-tissue and bone repairs. For example, if a rotator cuff repair is performed, the exercises must allow for healing of the repair before initiating active range of motion and strengthening exercises. If a tendency toward posterior instability is identified the surgeon should delay or even eliminate internal rotation stretching exercises to minimize the chances of postoperative instability. Maximum benefit following shoulder arthroplasty may take up to 6 months to 1 year.

The initial goal of rehabilitation is to obtain passive motion to prevent early intra- and extraarticular adhesion formation while protecting the subscapularis tendon repair from detachment. Rehabilitation is begun the first or second postoperative day in the hospital's physical therapy department. Range of motion exercises for the hand, wrist, and elbow joints are performed to prevent stiffness and minimize swelling. Shoulder mobility is addressed with pendulum exercises, supine passive forward elevation, and, using a stick (or dowel), supine passive external rotation exercises with the arm at the side. In our practice, we like the patient to achieve at least 120 degrees of supine passive forward elevation before hospital discharge. The amount of external rotation allowed for the first 6 postoperative weeks is determined intraoperatively on completion of the subscapularis repair. The surgeon determines a safe range of external rotation intraoperatively by noting the maximal degree of external rotation possible before causing undue tension at the subscapularis reattachment site. In a typical case of osteoarthritis with an adequate, circumferential subscapularis release, the safe zone of external rotation is usually between 30 and 45 degrees.

The arm is initially taken through the supine passive exercises by the physical therapist, but ultimately, the patient learns to use the hand of the nonoperative upper extremity to move the surgical arm passively for forward elevation and to control the stick used for external rotation. The patient can more accurately perform true passive exercises independently of another person's assistance in the supine position because the effect of gravity is lessened. If the patient cannot perform the exercises independently, a family member or friend can assist the patient after hospital discharge. At times, however, the patient may need the assistance of a physical therapist in an outpatient setting or of an in-home visiting physical therapist. Administration of analgesics and application of moist heat (e.g., a hot water bottle) 30 minutes before performing exercises will diminish pain during physical therapy.

A sling is provided postoperatively to be used during sleep and when the patient is away from home in the community. The patient is encouraged to progressively use the arm in the plane in front of the body for simple tasks (e.g., eating, putting on makeup, buttoning a shirt, and other such activities). To protect the subscapularis repair the patient must obey the limit on external rotation and not perform activities that require lifting of more than 1 to 2 lb. The patient continues performing the exercises learned during hospitalization at home.

At 10 to 14 days postoperatively the skin closure suture is removed and the patient is encouraged to use the arm in light activities within arcs of motion that are limited by pain. Active arm extension exercise using a stick or dowel and passive internal rotation exercise with the arm at the side are added to the exercise program. During this first postoperative visit the patient is given a pulley device to be used in a seated position for increasing passive arcs of forward elevation. Driving a motor vehicle with an automatic transmission is generally allowed at 4 weeks postoperatively, as long as narcotic analgesics are not required for pain other than sleep.

The patient returns to the office 6 weeks postoperatively and strengthening exercises are initiated and stretching exercises are modified. Exercises for strengthening internal and external rotation with the arm at the side are performed against the resistance of Therabands. Therabands come in six levels of increasing resistance. The patient should progress every 2 to 3 weeks in sequence to the next Theraband of higher resistance. However, not all patients should be expected to progress through all six levels of increasing resistance. Strengthening for the anterior, middle, and posterior thirds of the deltoid are similarly performed with Therabands as separate exercises. The strengthening program is continued for a minimum of 6 to 10 weeks. Additional exercises using light free weights for both concentric and eccentric contractions can be added as needed to optimize strengthening at 3 to 4 months postoperatively. Also at the 6-week follow-up, passive crossed body adduction stretching is initiated to stretch the posterior capsule. Depending on the patient's progress, stretching exercises may need to be modified at this point to help achieve the final degrees of end ranges of motion. The concept of moving the arm passively in the supine position is changed to placing the arm against an immovable object (e.g., door frame, wall, table, or other) in the standing position and moving or rotating the body to cause passive glenohumeral stretching.

The indications for antibiotic prophylaxis to prevent bacterial seeding of the replaced glenohumeral joint are controversial. It is our practice to use prophylactic antibiotic coverage for all subsequent surgeries, oscopy procedures, and dental extractions or root canals. Any identified infection (e.g., urinary tract infection; UTI) must be treated promptly.

Results

The main difference between osteoarthritis and other diagnoses following total shoulder arthroplasty is that, in osteoarthritis, good to excellent functional recovery and improved motion are more predictable. The main reason for this difference is the presence of good rotator cuff tendon tissue and the infrequency of rotator cuff tears in osteoarthritis. In Neer's series, 36 patients achieved excellent results, 3 satisfactory results, and no unsatisfactory overall results.[67] The average gains in active elevation and external rotation were 77 and 51 degrees, respectively. Cofield reported mean active abduction following total shoulder arthroplasty of 141 degrees in osteoarthritis, 109 degrees in posttraumatic arthritis, and 104 degrees in rheumatoid arthritis.[20]

SPECIAL TECHNIQUES

Rotator Cuff Repair

Preoperative Evaluation

During arthroplasty for osteoarthritis full-thickness rotator cuff tears are encountered in approximately 5% to 10% of cases.[20,67] When discovered in osteoarthritis, in our experience, tear size is usually small (less than 1 cm) or occasionally medium (less than 3 cm).[21] Large tears should alert the surgeon to consider a missed diagnosis of rotator cuff tear arthropathy. In rheumatoid arthritis the percentage of cases with full-thickness cuff tears ranges between 20% and 42%, but rotator cuff disease is seen in a significantly higher percentage of patients.[4,20,42,45,51,67]

Detecting the presence of rotator cuff tears on physical examination is difficult because weakness is often related to either pain inhibition, stiffness, or chronic disuse, and subacromial crepitation is difficult to differentiate from glenohumeral crepitation. Plain radiographs can show indirect evidence of large rotator cuff tears. Loss of rotator cuff tendon integrity and its role as a humeral head depressor can be inferred from narrowing of the acromial–humeral distance (less than 5 mm) on AP radiographs. MRI can accurately depict the presence and size of rotator cuff tears and also show the degree of tendon retraction and the extent of associated muscle atrophy. However, the additional expense of an MRI scan is not easily justified for all routine cases. A shoulder MRI can be helpful in preoperative planning in selected patients in whom a large cuff defect is suspected based on the clinical examination, radiographs, or type of arthritis. Use of MRI or arthrography is helpful in patients who require additional preoperative counseling for the likely expectations of functional recovery after shoulder arthroplasty.

Indications and Techniques

Because the rotator cuff performs multiple important tasks (dynamic glenohumeral stability, humeral head depression, secondary power for moving the arm), all reparable full-thickness rotator cuff tears encountered at the time of shoulder arthroplasty should be repaired. Visualization of the rotator cuff tissues and biceps tendon is improved once the humeral head is osteotomized. The rotator cuff should be inspected before preparation of the glenoid fossa, because if a massive, irreparable tear is identified, it is generally agreed that a glenoid component should not be implanted.

Standard techniques of rotator cuff repair are used. The torn rotator cuff tendon must be mobilized with dissection on its superficial (bursal) surface and deep (capsular) surface. Placement of several nonabsorbable sutures in the rotator cuff tissue is used to pull traction on to facilitate mobilization. Care must be taken when using dissection to mobilize the supraspinatus tendon medial to the glenoid rim for fear of injuring the suprascapular nerve. Also, dissection inferior to the teres minor tendon places the axillary nerve at risk. If the retracted rotator cuff tendons are tethered by a contracted glenohumeral capsule, the capsule should be divided sharply just outside the glenoid rim from inside the joint. Additional releases often required to fully mobilize the supraspinatus tendon include the rotator interval capsule, the coracohumeral ligament, and around the superior, lateral, and inferior aspects of the base of the coracoid process. A small rim (1 to 3 mm) of the torn edge of the rotator cuff tendon is sharply excised to expose healthy tendon tissue for repair. The rotator cuff tendons are repaired to the osteotomy surface on the greater tuberosity.

Nonabsorbable heavy sutures are passed into the rotator cuff tendon for repair. The rotator cuff is approximated to the greater tuberosity at the time of trying the humeral heads. When the correct component size is determined, bone tunnels are made through the osteotomy surface and out the lateral cortex of the greater tuberosity at least 2 cm distal to the superior edge of the tuberosity. The repair sutures are passed through the bone tunnels, the final prosthetic component is inserted, and the repair sutures are pulled, delivering the torn rotator cuff edge to the osteotomy surface, and are tied. If the rotator cuff tear has a longitudinal component, it is repaired side-to-side with inverted nonabsorbable sutures. Postoperative rehabilitation is modified to allow for healing of rotator cuff tissue. During the first 6 weeks, range of motion exercises are only performed passively. Also, the patient is instructed not to move the arm actively away from the side. During this time, frequent evaluation of the patient's passive range of motion is necessary to prevent postoperative stiffness. For large rotator cuff tears we use postoperative abduction bracing.

The biceps tendon is also inspected at the time of arthroplasty and is tenodesed if degeneration has resulted in loss of approximately 50% of its cross-sectional diameter or rupture is imminent because of poor tissue quality. The technique of biceps tenodesis requires excision of the tendon from its insertion at the superior glenoid tubercle and shortening it to the level at which it will be tenodesed. The residual humeral stump of the released superior pectoralis tendon is a convenient soft-tissue anchor for tenodesing the biceps tendon with several heavy nonabsorbable sutures.

Glenoid Deficiency

Preoperative Evaluation

Glenoid bone stock deficiency accompanies many of the diagnoses for which total shoulder arthroplasty is indicated. Frequently, glenoid bone loss occurs *asymmetrically*, with either the anterior, posterior, or inferior halves of the glenoid remaining relatively preserved. Asymmetrical bone loss alters glenoid version and is associated with radiographic evidence of subluxation or dislocation of the humeral head. Posterior glenoid erosion is typical of osteoarthritis and arthritis after anterior instability repairs. Anterior erosion, which is less common, is seen in arthritis after posterior instability repairs and in chronic, unreduced anterior dislocations. Superior glenoid bone loss is associated with superior subluxation of the humeral head and occurs in rotator cuff deficiency. Symmetrical bone loss medializes the glenoid fossa with little or no effect on glenoid version. It is seen almost exclusively in patients with inflammatory arthritis. Complex glenoid deficiency is seen in patients who have had prior tumor resection, fractures, or bony dysplasia involving the glenoid fossa. Additionally, glenoid bone volume can be replaced by large, cavitating subchondral cysts in a variety of diagnoses.

In any candidate for shoulder arthroplasty glenoid version and the degree of glenoid bone loss must be critically evaluated on plain radiographs. An accurate axillary lateral radiograph is the most useful view for making this assessment (Fig. 16); CT scans with 2-mm cuts most accurately depict bony architecture and are indicated when plain films are inadequate or demonstrate significant bone loss that would result in a greater surgical challenge. Such radiographic information will help guide the surgeon's decision making as to whether the amount of bone available is sufficient to implant a glenoid component and, if sufficient, how much eccentric glenoid reaming can be safely performed. Radiographic information is also used to determine whether bone grafting is required to recreate a glenoid fossa to support a glenoid component and whether this challenge is even feasible.

For practical purposes of glenoid preparation it is reasonable to conclude that normal glenoid version lies close to zero degrees (neutral). A recent well-controlled study assessed glenoid version using CT in 63 normal subjects who had normal plain radiographs.[43] These subjects had a mean and standard deviation of 2 ± 5 degrees of anteversion (range: 14 degrees of anteversion to 12 degrees of retroversion). Only 3 patients had greater than 6 degrees of retroversion. Twenty shoulders with severe arthritic changes (10 osteoarthritis, 8 rheumatoid arthritis, and 2 gouty arthritis) had a mean of 11 degrees of retroversion, with a range of 2 degrees of anteversion to 32 degrees of retroversion.

Obligatory contracture or elongation of the glenohumeral capsule and rotator cuff tendons accompany the bony changes of glenoid deficiency. Rotator cuff deficiency and occasionally corcoacromial arch (anterior acromion, coracoacromial ligament, and coracoid process) deficiency are associated with superior glenoid erosion. During the physical examination the competency of the rotator cuff tendons, the capsule, and the coracoacromial arch must be evaluated. Limited passive motion occurs secondary to soft-tissue contracture or articular incongruity–osteophytosis. Limited active motion can relate to muscle weakness, rotator cuff deficiency, soft-tissue contracture, articular incongruity–osteophytosis, or pain inhibition. Superior translation of the humeral head during initial degrees of active forward elevation often indicates incompetency of the coracoacromial arch; namely, the coracoacromial ligament. Such examination can help the surgeon anticipate the particular elements of soft-tissue reconstruction. For example, in osteoarthritis

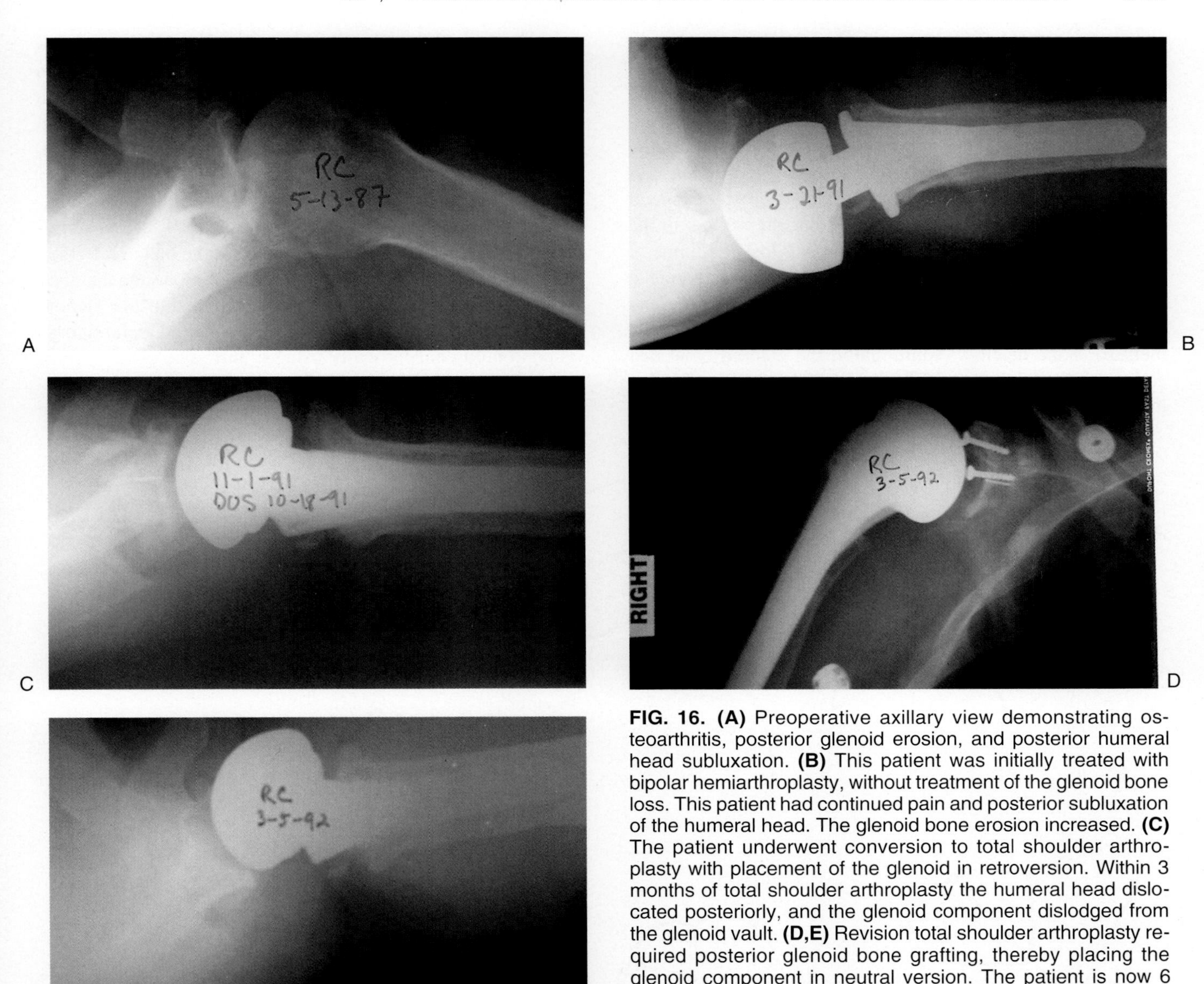

FIG. 16. (A) Preoperative axillary view demonstrating osteoarthritis, posterior glenoid erosion, and posterior humeral head subluxation. **(B)** This patient was initially treated with bipolar hemiarthroplasty, without treatment of the glenoid bone loss. This patient had continued pain and posterior subluxation of the humeral head. The glenoid bone erosion increased. **(C)** The patient underwent conversion to total shoulder arthroplasty with placement of the glenoid in retroversion. Within 3 months of total shoulder arthroplasty the humeral head dislocated posteriorly, and the glenoid component dislodged from the glenoid vault. **(D,E)** Revision total shoulder arthroplasty required posterior glenoid bone grafting, thereby placing the glenoid component in neutral version. The patient is now 6 years after this revision total shoulder arthroplasty, with excellent prosthetic stability and painless shoulder function.

with significant posterior glenoid erosion, the contracture of the anterior capsule and subscapularis muscle–tendon unit will pose a significant restriction to external rotation. The posterior capsule may be found intraoperatively to have undergone significant lenthening as a consequence of posterior subluxation. The surgeon must be familiar with techniques of releasing, lengthening, and shortening (imbricating) soft-tissue components to achieve soft-tissue balance in cases of glenoid deficiency.

Bone Grafts: Indications and Techniques

Fortunately, most candidates for total shoulder arthroplasty have only a mild degree of glenoid bone loss. In these patients a well-balanced, stable component can be achieved by lowering the high side with eccentric glenoid reaming and hand burring, placing the humeral component in somewhat greater or lesser degrees of retroversion to compensate for residual degrees of altered glenoid version, and performing correct soft-tissue releases or, rarely, soft-tissue tightening techniques (see Standard Case: Osteoarthritis).

Glenoid bone grafting is indicated for significant (generally more than 1-cm) asymmetrical or focal glenoid bone deficiency that cannot be managed with asymmetrical glenoid reaming or burring and altering the version of the humeral component in patients who have good quality rotator cuff tendon tissue (whether intact or reparable). Contraindications to glenoid bone grafting are insufficient glenoid bone stock from severe erosion, rotator cuff tear arthropathy, or rotator cuff tissue that is likely incapable of functioning as a humeral head depressor because of poor quality. Glenoid bone grafting is a most technically demanding procedure and is rarely indicated during shoulder arthroplasty.

Glenoid exposure must allow the native bone to be contoured precisely, the graft fit to be well visualized, and the accurate placement of screws for fixation. A corticocancellous bone graft can be obtained from the osteotomized humeral head, the scapular spine, the coracoid process, or the iliac crest. For most cases of glenoid bone loss the humeral head or iliac crest is preferred so an adequately sized piece of bone can be obtained. The glenoid is contoured with a burr to bleeding bone to provide a favorable biologic environment for bone healing. Additionally, the glenoid bone bed and corticocancellous graft should be shaped to optimize mechanical stability. This can be achieved by burring the bone bed to create a stepwedge with two healing surfaces oriented perpendicularly (Fig. 17). The bone graft is then shaped precisely to both maximize the area of contact with host bone and to restore the dimensions of the glenoid such that the glenoid component will lie flush against a congruent, reconstructed glenoid fossa (see Fig. 17).

Small fragment screws are used to fix the graft under compression, preferably, with cortical purchase. If screws are inserted through the articulating surface of the bone graft, they must be countersunk. Screws must be oriented such that they will not block the insertion of the keel within the glenoid neck. The slot is created after the reconstructed glenoid fossa is contoured concentrically using a burr. The glenoid component is cemented in place. Soft-tissue releases of the capsule and rotator cuff tendons are especially needed in these

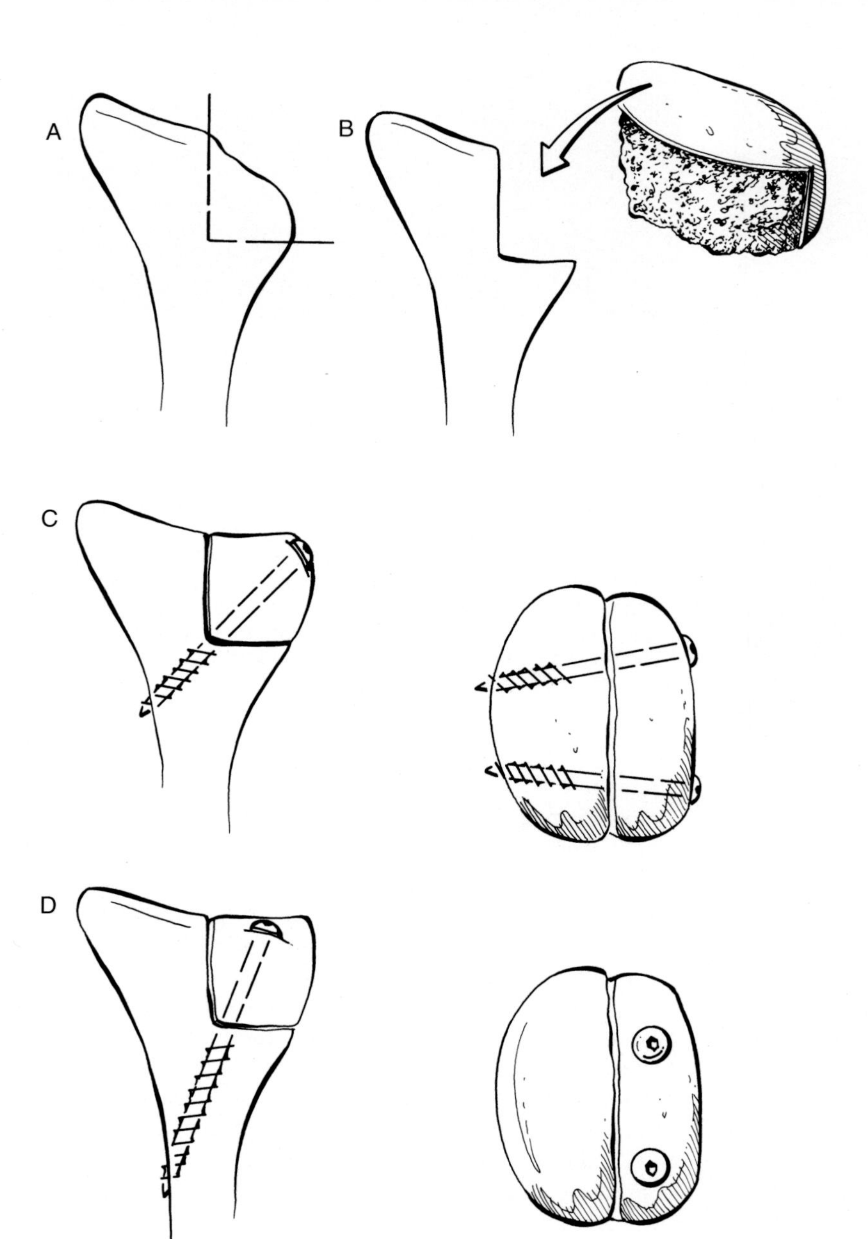

FIG. 17. (A-D) Technique for glenoid bone grafting: The deepest portion of the defect is defined. The glenoid defect is then cut to be symmetrical with a step configuration. The bone graft may be obtained from the humeral head, iliac crest, or bone bank. The graft is fashioned to fit into the defect, secured with two small fragment, partially threaded cancellous screws. The graft may be trimmed in situ if necessary with a burr or reamer. It may be necessary to insert the screws though a separate posterior stab wound or formal deltoid-splitting approach.

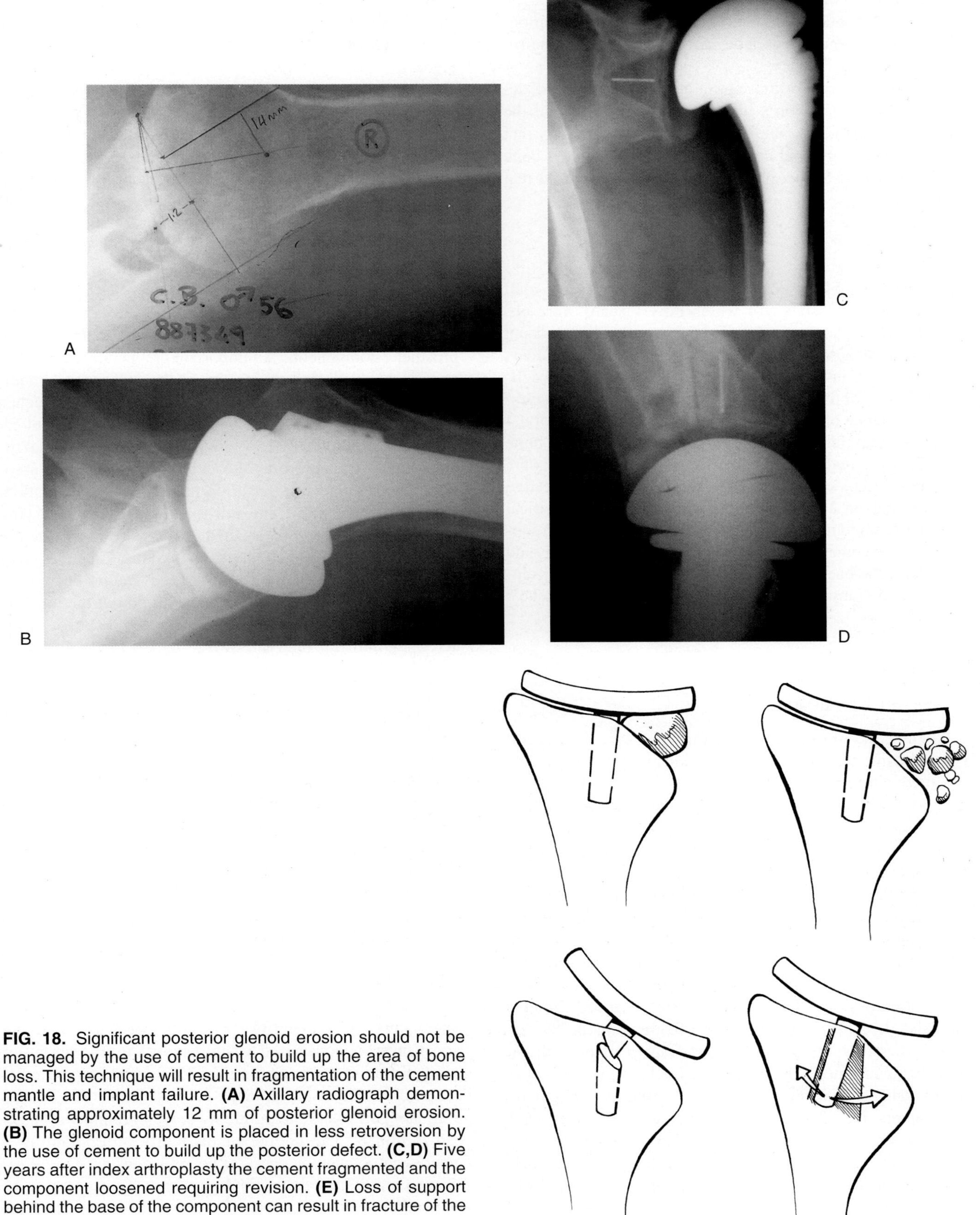

FIG. 18. Significant posterior glenoid erosion should not be managed by the use of cement to build up the area of bone loss. This technique will result in fragmentation of the cement mantle and implant failure. **(A)** Axillary radiograph demonstrating approximately 12 mm of posterior glenoid erosion. **(B)** The glenoid component is placed in less retroversion by the use of cement to build up the posterior defect. **(C,D)** Five years after index arthroplasty the cement fragmented and the component loosened requiring revision. **(E)** Loss of support behind the base of the component can result in fracture of the implant.

cases because additional soft-tissue tension is created as the insertion of a bone graft lateralizes the joint line. Additionally, lateralization increases the difficulty of performing rotator cuff repairs.

The postoperative exercise program will be modified, depending on the surgeon's judgment of the stability of the glenoid reconstruction. In instances of revision surgery that address a loose glenoid component with a nonunited bone graft, extraction of the glenoid component is often all that can be done.

Results

In Neer and Morrison's series of 463 consecutive total shoulder arthroplasties (for which no CT scans were obtained) only 2 patients could not have a glenoid component implanted because of deficient bone.[70] Nineteen shoulders required large, internally fixed bone grafts for glenoid deficiency. None of the glenoid components had clinical loosening or evidence of migration at an average follow-up of 4.4 years. Postoperative radiographs demonstrated the bone grafts to be united to the glenoid fossa. Clinical results were excellent in 16, satisfactory in 1, and achieved the desired limited goals in 2. These authors warned that asymmetrical bone loss should never be compensated by building up a support of bone cement. Such a construct of cement loosens and dislodges, the back of the glenoid component is left unsupported, and component loosening or keel fractures ensue[80] (Fig. 18).

RHEUMATOID ARTHRITIS

Preoperative Evaluation

Rheumatoid arthritis is a systemic, polyarticular disease often causing pain and dysfunction at multiple joints. The destructive inflammatory process affects not only the articular surfaces, but also, to varying degrees, the periarticular soft tissues. The timing and technique of glenohumeral arthroplasty must consider specific characteristics of rheumatoid pathology.

The indications for shoulder arthroplasty for rheumatoid arthritis are the same as those for osteoarthritis, with pain relief and improved function being the primary and secondary goals, respectively. However, the timing of shoulder arthroplasty in the rheumatoid patient is a more critical issue because oftentimes there are multiple joints involved simultaneously. If additional joints are being considered for reconstructive surgery, appropriate staging of procedures must be determined. The timing of shoulder arthroplasty is individualized, depending on a careful consideration of multiple factors, including patient age, ambulatory status, level of dependence on others, and extent of involvement and disease progression at each articulation. As a general guideline the joint causing the greatest amount of pain and disability is operated on first.

Before administering a general anesthetic, the cervical spine must be evaluated for instability and treated appropriately. The use of ambulatory aids must be prohibited for at least 3 months following shoulder arthroplasty to allow healing of the subscapularis reattachment and rotator cuff tears, if repaired. Thus, indicated lower extremity surgery should be performed before shoulder arthroplasty if it can potentially eliminate the use of ambulatory aids. When the ipsilateral elbow is involved, the most symptomatic joint should be operated on first. If the elbow and shoulder are equally involved, the order of procedures is controversial. One report showed greater functional improvement of the upper extremity when symptoms at the shoulder and elbow were equivalent and elbow arthroplasty was performed first.[41] Humeral stem length of both the shoulder and elbow prostheses should be considered relative to the length of the humeral medullary canal to ensure adequate room for both prosthetic components. An important preoperative consideration is the condition and function of the rotator cuff. Shoulders affected by rheumatoid arthritis have a high incidence of rotator cuff disease. In Cofield's series only 5 of 29 rheumatoid shoulders were classified as having a normal rotator cuff.[20] The spectrum of rotator cuff involvement associated with rheumatoid arthritis includes cuff attenuation, friability, and partial- and full-thickness tears of varying size. Full-thickness rotator cuff tears have been reported in 20% to 42% of patients with rheumatoid disease undergoing shoulder arthroplasty.[20,42,67,92] With advancing degrees of rotator cuff involvement, superior migration of the humeral head is observed on plain radiographs as a decrease in the acromial–humeral interval. Severe narrowing of the acromial–humeral interval is a clue that the rotator cuff may be irreparably torn.

Rheumatoid patients often have poor bone quality. This is partly related to osteopenia of disuse and the use of corticosteroids. As a result, the risk of iatrogenic humeral shaft fractures during arthroplasty is increased. As the disease progresses extensive erosion of both the glenoid and humerus often occurs. Glenoid erosion is more dramatic in rheumatoid arthritis than in osteoarthritis and tends to occur centrally or centrally and superiorly.[20] The glenoid fossa may erode medially to the base of the coracoid process. This finding has been termed a *protrusio glenoidale*[89] (Fig. 19). In such situations the implantation of a glenoid component is often precluded.

Once the disease process destroys the articular surfaces, further loss of glenoid bone stock and further deterioration of rotator cuff tendon integrity can be anticipated. This ongoing threat must be considered when deciding on the timing of surgical intervention. Continuing to defer surgery can increase the difficulty of shoulder reconstruction. The quality of rotator cuff tissue and the ability to repair rotator cuff tears can diminish. The degree of difficulty of implanting a glenoid component increases as bone loss ensues. Disuse results in significant deltoid atrophy, slowing progress with postoperative rehabilitation. The overall functional result can be compromised.

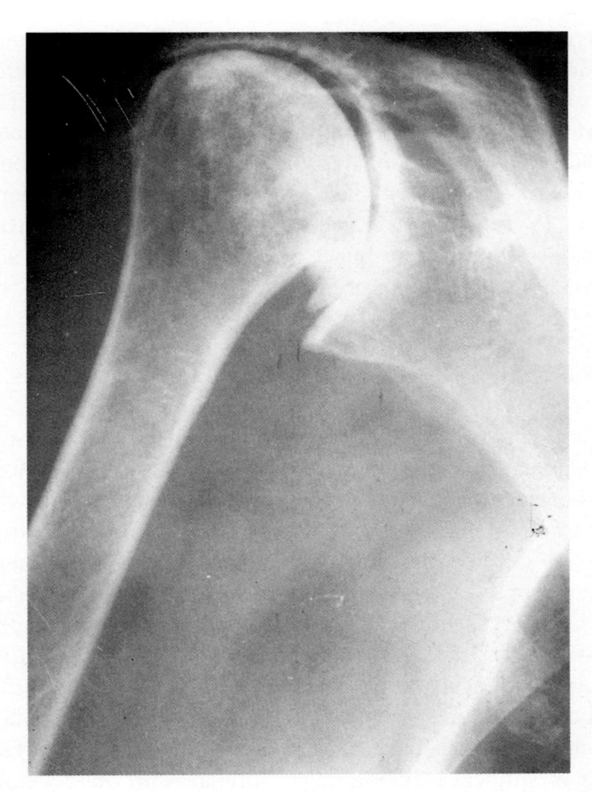

FIG. 19. Central glenoid erosion can be severe with superior migration of the humeral head. Glenoid component placement in this case is not recommended. The humeral head migrates centrally and there is a significant decease in the lateral glenohumeral offset.

Some patients with rheumatoid arthritis meet indications for total shoulder arthroplasty at a young age. Such patients have long-term needs for their prostheses. With longer periods of use the risk of component loosening and the need of revision surgery increases. The survivorship of total shoulder arthroplasty in this select group of patients has not yet been clarified. It may be that because these patients generally place less demand on their shoulders prosthesis longevity will be excellent. Nevertheless, this issue should be discussed with any young candidate for total shoulder arthroplasty.

Technical Considerations

Although the technique of nonconstrained shoulder arthroplasty in treating rheumatoid arthritis is similar to that of osteoarthritis, aspects of rheumatoid pathology influence the procedure. The skin is often very thin and fragile, especially in patients taking corticosteroids. The surgeon must handle the skin delicately to avoid wound-healing problems. The subscapularis tendon is often too thin to allow Z-plasty lengthening when correcting for limited external rotation. Our preference is to achieve lengthening of the subscapularis tendon by reattaching it through drill holes to the humeral osteotomy site. It is advisable to release the subscapularis tendon and anterior capsule as a single layer to preserve more tissue substance for holding suture material during reattachment of the subscapularis tendon. The anterior capsule can be released near the glenoid margin from inside the joint to achieve a release of the subscapularis tendon on its deep surface. When rotator cuff tears are identified, every effort should be made to preserve the coracoacromial ligament. The CA arch may serve an increasingly important role as a superior restraint, years from the time of the index procedure, should rotator cuff function worsen secondary to deteriorating tissue quality, new rotator cuff tears, or failure of rotator cuff repairs.

Because of the increased risk of fracture, the humeral shaft must be maneuvered with care, especially when dislocating the proximal humerus for humeral preparation. Excessive arm manipulation (rotational forces), humeral reaming, or humeral impaction should be avoided.[8] When the cortex of the humeral shaft is particularly thin it is wise to ream the canal more gently. Thin humeral cortices dictate the use of cemented stems. Bone quality and quantity are often insufficient to safely use press-fit fixation.

The amount of glenoid destruction is highly variable. Reaming or hand burring the glenoid fossa easily becomes too aggressive because of poorer bone quality. Subchondral cysts must be curetted and either filled with bone graft or cement so that structural support for the component is not compromised by areas of void.

If reparable rotator cuff tears are encountered, standard techniques of rotator cuff repair are employed (see Special Techniques: Rotator Cuff Repair). The postoperative exercise program is modified to allow for rotator cuff healing. When the humeral head is superiorly subluxated in the presence of irreparable rotator cuff tears, a humeral head replacement is implanted without a glenoid component, as in rotator cuff tear arthropathy.

Results

There are relatively few articles reporting the results of shoulder arthroplasty exclusively for rheumatoid arthritis. Many of the articles that evaluate several diagnostic categories do not separate the results of rheumatoid patients. It should be remembered that the extent of involvement of rheumatoid arthritis is highly variable. In terms of the musculoskeletal system, the spectrum ranges from patients with essentially isolated shoulder arthritis who function independently, to patients with severe, crippling, multiple joint involvement of both the upper and lower extremities, who are completely dependent on others for basic living needs. Also, a broad spectrum of inflammatory destruction is evident that affects the soft-tissues and the osseous elements of the shoulder. Thus, in any reporting for rheumatoid arthritis, a degree of patient heterogeneity is implicit. The strength of conclusions drawn must be understood in light of the variable degree of rheumatoid involvement within individuals of a study population.

Despite known differences in the severity of involvement, satisfactory pain relief is consistently achieved. Nearly all published series report greater than 90% of patients obtaining good or excellent pain relief at short- and midterm follow-up. [20,40,42,45,51,58,67] The presence of rotator cuff tears has not been shown to adversely affect attainment of pain relief.[45,58] Additionally, patients with severe rheumatoid involvement (class IV function) achieve pain relief comparable with that of patients with less severe involvement.[42] The most frequent findings associated with less than satisfactory pain relief include glenoid component loosening, failure of rotator cuff repairs, or the occurrence of postoperative rotator cuff tearing.[3,15,20,40] Rarely has inadequate pain relief been unexplainable.[20,40]

Significant improvement in active range of motion is not as consistent as is the achievement of pain relief. Postoperative active forward elevation or abduction averages 90 degree and strongly correlates with the condition of the rotator cuff.[3,4,20,42,45,51,58] In Cofield's report, when the rotator cuff was normal or minimally affected (5 patients) average postoperative active abduction was 143 degrees, when the cuff was thin and scarred (17 patients) average active abduction was 102 degrees, and when a rotator cuff repair was performed for major tears (full-thickness tear running at least the width of the supraspinatus tendon) active abduction averaged 66 degrees (6 patients). [20] The average gain in active abduction for the entire rheumatoid group was 46 degrees. McCoy et al. reported 82 degrees of postoperative elevation in 18 patients with intact cuffs and 67 degrees in 11 patients with cuff disease of which several had rotator cuff repairs.[58] The extent to which accomplishing a rotator cuff repair affects motion postoperatively is unknown, but generally, the greater the extent of rotator cuff disease, the less are the expectations with postoperative active forward elevation.

As opposed to forward elevation, postoperative external rotation improves consistently. Postoperative external rotation averages approximately 35 degrees.[4,20,42,45,51,58] External rotation is influenced to great extent by the adequacy of the anterior capsule and subscapularis tendon releases and by the presence of a functional posterior rotator cuff. Additionally, postoperative immobilization to protect rotator cuff repairs and poor cooperation with postoperative rehabilitation negatively influence gains in range of motion.

Functional gains for performing activities of daily living occur in essentially all patients who obtain satisfactory pain relief.[4,20,42,45,51,58,67] The surgeon must appreciate that rheumatoid patients often are limited to a sedentary lifestyle because of polyarticular or systemic involvement and the ability to perform high-demand activities with the shoulder in the premorbid rheumatoid patient is unusual. Thus, premorbid function is often restored in patients who obtain significant pain relief and improved arcs of rotational motion. The ability to perform activities at or above shoulder level postoperatively is variable, as opposed to osteoarthritis patients, and correlates to the status of the rotator cuff. Patients with poor or absent function of the rotator cuff whether occurring because of large cuff tears, irreparable cuff tears, poor cuff tendon quality, or a combination of these are often incapable of placing the hand higher than the mouth.[42,71] The severity of disease also appears to be an independent factor influencing the functional results of arthroplasty. Functional scores for patients with the severest degree of involvement, class IV function, were not significantly different from shoulders that had an intact or attenuated rotator cuff and those in which a minor or major tear had been repaired.[42]

ARTHRITIS OF INSTABILITY

Preoperative Evaluation

The diagnostic category referred to as arthritis of instability became established in the early 1980s.[66] Of patients who have at least one episode of shoulder dislocation and subsequently develop glenohumeral arthritis, two categories have been recognized: one, patients who have undergone instability surgery (often referred to as postcapsulorrhaphy arthropathy), and two, patients who have not. The first group, with a history of instability surgery, comprises the majority of patients represented in the published literature. Such publications have focused on the identification of factors of surgical technique that correlate with the development of glenohumeral arthritis. Identified surgical factors include overtightening during soft-tissue instability repairs on the side of the glenohumeral joint being addressed (anterior or posterior); use of unidirectional instability repairs in the face of multidirectional instability, resulting in fixed subluxation of the humeral head toward the lax unaddressed side of the glenohumeral joint; the use of metallic fixation devices (e.g., screws or staples) that impinge on the glenohumeral articular interface because of inaccurate placement or subsequent hardware migration (Fig. 20); and the use of bone grafts that constrain the articulation (Fig. 21). [6,12,46,66,96]

The second group, without instability surgery, has been described in three publications to date.[48,71,85] In Neer's series 8 of 61 patients (14%) and in Samilson's review 16 of 74 patients (22%) with a history of a single or recurrent shoulder dislocations and subsequent osteoarthritis had no surgical intervention.[71,85] Recently, Hovelius et al. reported prospectively on 247 primary shoulder dislocations followed for 10 years.[48] Arthropathy was defined according to the system described by Samilson and Prieto: mild (osteophytes smaller than 3 mm on the humeral head), moderate (osteophytes between 3 and 7 mm on the humeral head or the glenoid rim), or severe (osteophytes of larger than 7 mm, with or without articular incongruity).[85] Of 106 shoulders that had had only one shoulder dislocation and no surgery performed, 11 (10%) had mild and 6 (6%) had moderate or severe radiographic evidence of arthropathy. Thus, the occurrence of a single episode of shoulder dislocation is not an innocuous event. Of the 39 shoulders that had had two or more dislocations and no surgery, 5 (13%) had mild and 5 (13%) had moderate or severe radiographic evidence of arthropathy. Of

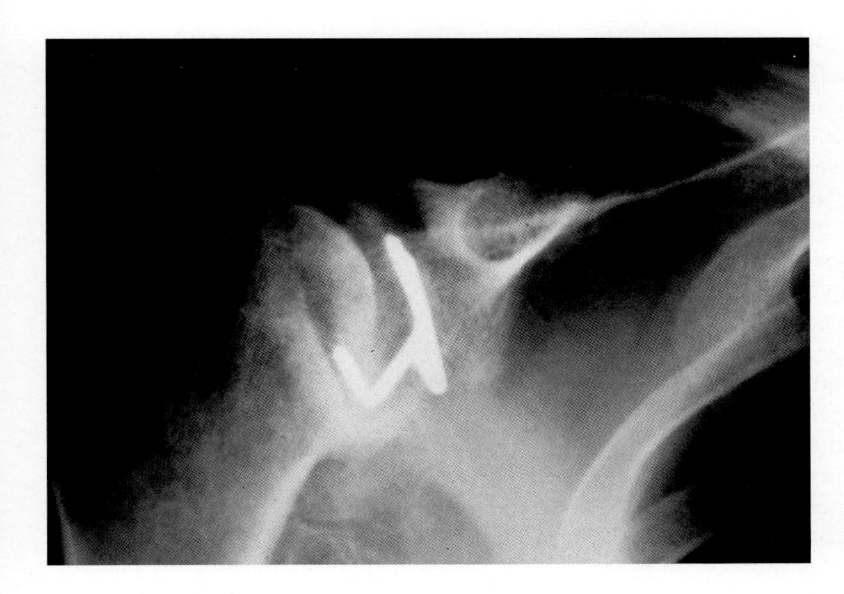

FIG. 20. Postcapsulorrhaphy arthropathy caused by implant abrasion.

the 53 shoulders that had had two or more dislocations and surgical stabilization, 6 (11%) had mild and 6 (11%) had moderate or severe radiographic evidence of arthropathy. Of the 10 shoulders that had had only one recurrent dislocation, 1 (10%) had mild and 1 (10%) had moderate or severe arthropathy. The occurrence of one recurrent shoulder dislocation had essentially an equal incidence of mild and moderate or severe arthropathy as those of patients who had surgical stabilization or had not had surgical stabilization and had two or more recurrent dislocations.

Unfortunately, arthritis of instability tends to develop at a young age. When arthritis is sufficiently symptomatic at

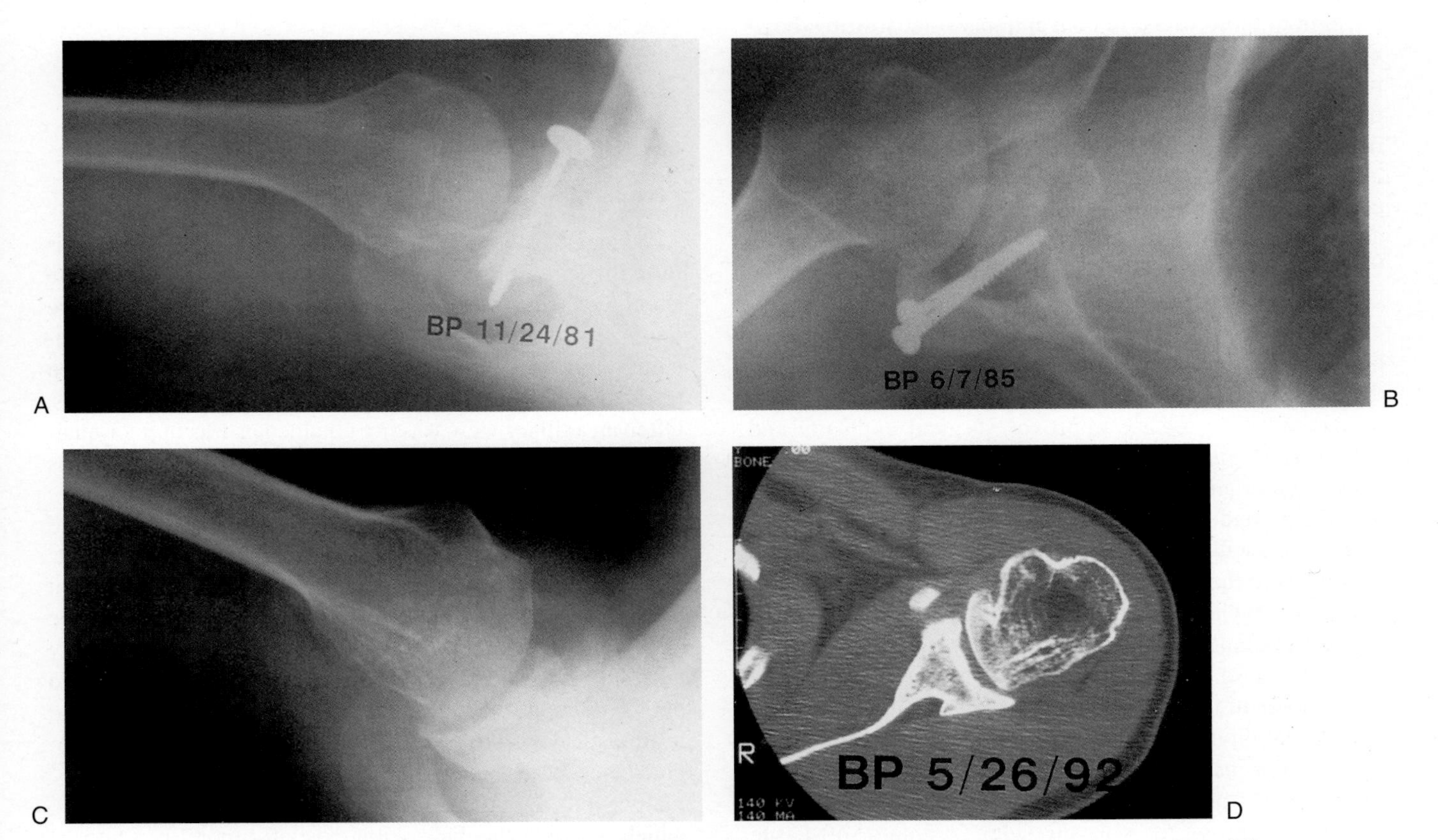

FIG. 21. **(A)** Patient with multidirectional instability initially treated with a Bristow procedure in 1981, **(B)** continued with instability, having a posterior bone block procedure in 1985. The patient continued to have pain, and **(C)** in 1992 demonstrated degenerative arthritis. **(D)** The CT scan demonstrated degenerative arthritis and a constrained articulation owing to a laterally placed bone graft.

early radiographic stages (minimal evidence of joint space narrowing or osteophytosis) patients may be benefited by open capsular release, with subscapularis lengthening if there is significant loss of external rotation. Indications for shoulder arthroplasty are the same as those for conventional osteoarthritis despite younger patient age. Delaying shoulder arthroplasty for as long as possible, as is often the thinking in young patients who are candidates for total knee or total hip replacement arthroplasty, increases the difficulty of surgery and could negatively influence the ultimate result. The surgeon must bear in mind that the longer surgery is delayed the farther the disease process progresses. Soft-tissue contractures and muscle atrophy worsen. As eccentric glenoid wear continues, glenoid bone stock loss and glenoid version changes progress; the difficulty of implanting a stable, well-positioned glenoid component only increases. Moreover, a delay in surgical treatment deprives a patient of the benefits during more productive and active years of life.

Patients with significant atrophy of deltoid or spinati fossa musculature may have nerve dysfunction from previous injury or surgery. In questionable cases an EMG can be obtained preoperatively.

Technical Considerations

Many of the anatomic alterations of arthritis of instability are akin to those found in conventional osteoarthritis; however, several specific technical challenges can be anticipated, oftentimes related to previous surgery. Metallic fixation devices from prior surgery that are prominent, unstable in bone, involve articular surfaces, are free in soft tissues, or interfere with placement of either the humeral or glenoid components should be removed. Stable hardware that is well anchored in bone and does not involve articular surfaces can be left in place, especially if its removal is deemed to require significant bone or soft-tissue destruction.

Because of prior surgery it is not infrequent for adhesions between the deep deltoid fascia and the superficial surface of the rotator cuff tendons to require extensive release by sharp dissection. This release improves surgical exposure and helps restore glide between these tissue interfaces. Patients with previous anterior instability repairs invariably have significant limited external rotation.[46] Usually, the subscapularis tendon will require lengthening by repairing it through drill holes to the humeral osteotomy site or, in more severe cases, by a Z-plasty lengthening. Dense adhesions should be released circumferentially around the subscapularis tendon.

The humeral head is almost invariably in a position of fixed subluxation (subluxated posteriorly from previous anterior instability repairs or subluxated anteriorly from previous posterior instability repairs). As a result, the capsular tissue can have considerable volume on the side of subluxation and contraction on the opposite side. To obtain soft-tissue balance and component stability it is usually necessary to perform a capsular release to correct for excessive tightness and occasionally necessary to perform a capsular imbrication to reduce excessive capsular volume. A complete circumferential capsular release (capsulotomy) is often required when the head is centrally located. Eccentric glenoid bone loss is a consistent feature of arthritis of instability and special techniques for correction of glenoid bone loss may be required.

Results

Bigliani et al. performed 12 total shoulder arthroplasties and 5 humeral head replacements in 17 patients with postcapsulorrhaphy arthropathy.[6] With the outcome criteria of Neer, ten excellent, three satisfactory, and five unsatisfactory results were reported. Patient age averaged 43 years and follow-up 2.9 years. Only one patient had moderate to severe pain. Forward elevation improved an average of 37 degrees and external rotation 53 degrees. Because of posterior glenoid wear the humeral component was usually placed in 5 to 10 degrees less retroversion. Brems reported pain relief in all of his 18 patients who underwent total shoulder arthroplasty for postcapsulorrhaphy arthropathy.[12] Patient age averaged 44 years and follow-up averaged 29 months. Forward elevation increased an average of 40 degrees and external rotation 50 degrees. Motion and function were less reliably improved compared with patients with conventional osteoarthritis. Glenoid bone grafting was not performed in any patient in the foregoing two series.

CHRONIC DISLOCATION

Preoperative Evaluation

When an accurate axillary radiograph is obtained there is little difficulty in diagnosing a shoulder dislocation. Acute shoulder dislocations are occasionally missed in multiple trauma patients for whom attention is diverted to life threatening-injuries. Otherwise, long-standing dislocations often result because of failure to obtain the necessary radiographs. Often an axillary view was not obtained or was of poor quality at the initial evaluation. Occasionally, a dislocation is chronic because the patient neglects to seek timely care.

Arthroplasty for long-standing dislocations is indicated over other surgical procedures when there is sufficient alteration of the humeral head shape, or when there is sufficient damage to the articular cartilage. Neer observed that chronic anterior dislocations of 6 weeks to 9 months duration usually have a preserved humeral head and, thus, are amenable to open reduction.[71] If the dislocation exceeds 1 year, the head is almost always too soft and the articular cartilage too atrophied; hence, replacement of the head is usually preferable.[71] Flatow et al. commented that softening of the humeral head, which occurs if the dislocation exists for more than 6 to 12 months, causes the head to flatten on reduction into the glenoid fossa.[37]

Neer stated that posterior dislocations are invariably associated with humeral articular surface impression fractures that vary in size.[71] When the impression fracture involves 50% or more of the articular surface, his preference was to replace the humeral head. In addition, Hawkins et al. favored arthroplasty for posterior dislocations of 6 months or longer duration because of loss of humeral head cartilage viability.[44] Long-standing dislocations can be associated with glenoid cartilage atrophy, which may require the implantation of a glenoid component. Technical difficulties of glenoid replacement should be anticipated because of associated eccentric glenoid bone loss. Preoperative CT scans are of great value in defining the details of the bony anatomy; plain films are of value, but are often inadequate on their own (Fig. 22). Additional information is obtained at the time of surgery when the condition of the cartilage is directly visualized.

Technical Considerations

A generous, if not complete, release of the pectoralis major tendon is required for adequate exposure and to achieve a reduction. Because of relative immobility the tissue planes between the deep surface of the deltoid and underlying rotator cuff become adhesed with scar tissue. Restoration of glide between these two interfaces is essential in restoring functional range of motion. The capsule and overlying rotator cuff can become so fibrosed together that differentiation of the two layers is impossible.[82] Many times the humeral head will not reduce until the subscapularis tendon is detached. The subscapularis should be released either directly off the lesser tuberosity to retain as much length as possible or with a Z-plasty lengthening. If the proximal humerus cannot be relocated, the humeral articular surface may need to be osteotomized or removed in pieces to bring the humeral shaft in line with the glenoid. Soft-tissue contracture and scar formation make identification of the axillary nerve difficult and pose increased risk of iatrogenic nerve injury.[82]

The glenoid fossa will often need debridement of fibrous granulation tissue.[82] This tissue can be so abundant that the humeral head or shaft resists relocation until it is removed. The decision to implant a glenoid component depends on the condition of the glenoid cartilage and must take into account the degree of bone loss.

Altering the version of the humeral component will offset the tendency for postoperative instability.[37,44,67,74] The humeral component is placed in greater degrees of retroversion for anterior dislocations. Increased degrees of anteversion are used for posterior dislocations. Hawkins et al. used 20 degrees of retroversion for posterior dislocations of less than 6 months duration and neutral version for posterior dislocations of longer durations.[44] Soft-tissue balancing for stability and mobility often requires a capsular release on the opposite side of the dislocation. This may require both anterior and posterior approaches. Stretched-out capsular tissue on the side of the dislocation may need to be plicated if a tendency for dislocation or excessive translations are identified with the trial components in place. Before wound closure, ranges of motion and translations should be tested again to

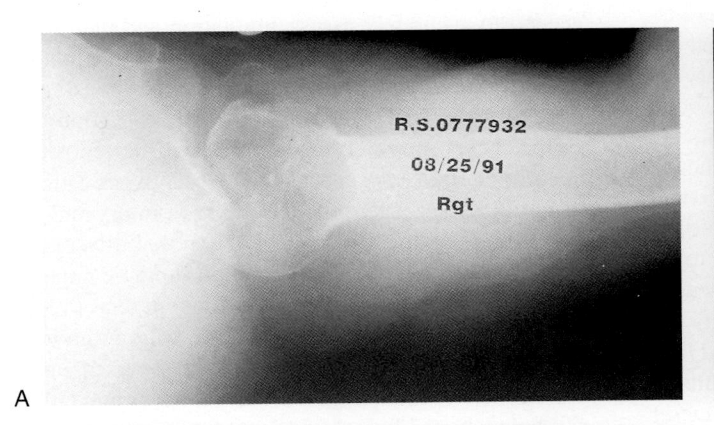

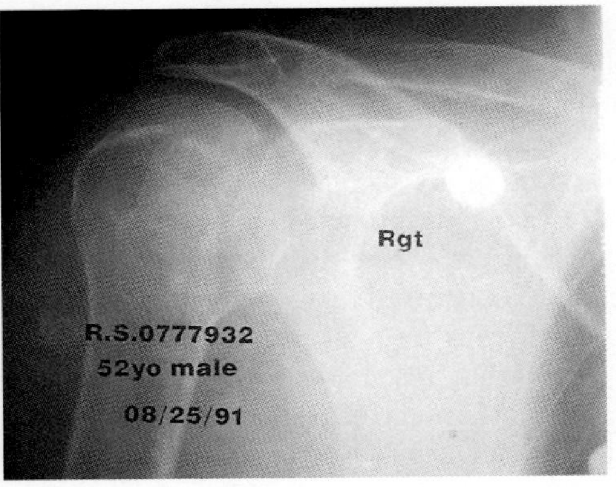

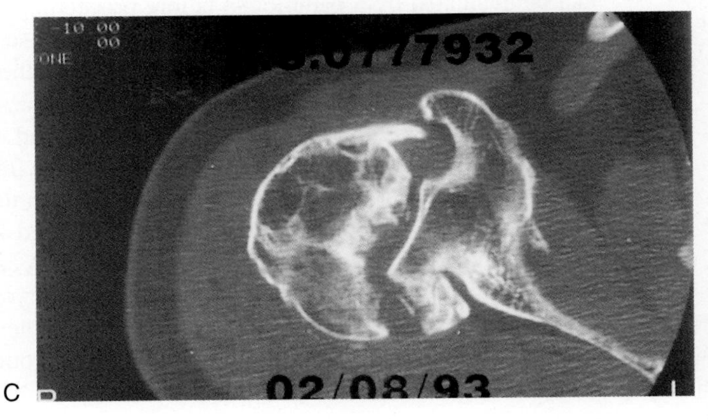

FIG. 22. (A-C) The AP and axillary views of a chronic posterior dislocation. Two years later the CT scan of the same patient demonstrated further degenerative changes and fragmentation of the humeral head, with chronic posterior dislocation.

ensure that all tendencies toward redislocation have been addressed.

Results

To date, the results of shoulder arthroplasty for longstanding dislocations have been reported for only a few patients.[37,44,74,82] In all reports arthroplasty was indicated because of the severity of damage to the articular surfaces. Rowe et al. reported one fair, one good, and one excellent result in three patients treated with shoulder arthroplasty for chronic dislocations.[82] Their system of rating results allocates a possible 30 points for pain relief, 40 points for motion, and 30 points for function. Prichett and Clark treated four anterior and three posterior chronic dislocations with humeral head replacement surgery.[74] Five good and two fair results were reported according to the rating system of Rowe et al.[82] These authors stressed that the expectations following surgery for motion and function should not be as high as for shoulder arthroplasty for more common diagnoses, but that pain relief was predictably good.

Hawkins et al. reported on nine patients with chronically locked posterior dislocations treated with humeral head replacement surgery.[44] Three patients were considered failures because they ultimately required the implantation of a glenoid component for persistent pain. All three obtained pain relief after glenoid component implantation. The remaining six patients, who were followed from 2 to 14 years, had mild or no pain, no limitations with activities of daily living, and on average could elevate and externally rotate the arm 140 and 30 degrees, respectively. An overall results-grading system was not used in the study. Six additional patients followed for 1 to 8 years were treated with primary total shoulder replacement of which two had glenoid bone grafting performed. The results for pain relief, function, and motion for five of six patients were similar to the hemiarthroplasty group. The one exception was a patient who had an immediate postoperative dislocation and refused further treatment. Additionally, six patients were considered to be inappropriate for any form of surgical management because of either poor health, inactivity, or insufficient disability.

When using the criteria of Neer, Flatow et al. reported four excellent, four satisfactory, and one unsatisfactory results in nine patients treated with shoulder arthroplasty (one humeral head replacement and eight total shoulder replacements) for chronic anterior dislocations.[37] Follow-up averaged 3.9 years. Four patients required glenoid bone grafting and two patients had simultaneous rotator cuff repairs.

NONUNIONS AND MALUNIONS

Preoperative Considerations

Shoulder arthroplasty for malunions or nonunions of the proximal humerus are usually very challenging reconstructive procedures. The preoperative evaluation is more extensive because there are more elements of associated pathology that require identification and definition. Associated pathology can be categorized as being related to the bony or the soft-tissue structures. The effects of prior surgical intervention, if undertaken, may influence both categories.

Bony pathology can be either isolated or combinations of malunions or nonunions of the tuberosities, the surgical neck, the anatomic neck, or articular surface. Posttraumatic articular surface incongruity may be related to head collapse secondary to avascular necrosis, head-splitting fractures, attritional changes of articular cartilage from chronic unreduced dislocations, Hill–Sachs or reverse Hill–Sachs lesions from an initial event or recurring events of dislocation, or hardware from prior surgery that impinges on the articular interface. The soft-tissue pathologies most commonly encountered include dense adhesion formation between the deep surface of the deltoid and superficial surface of the rotator cuff tendons, rotator cuff tears, either because of preexisting cuff disease or cuff tearing at the time of injury, significant rotator cuff and capsular contractures, and neurologic injury with associated muscular atrophy related to either the initial event of trauma or prior surgery. Anterior deltoid denervation, failure of subscapularis tendon reattachments, and failure of anterior deltoid origin reattachments should be specifically sought in patients having undergone prior surgery.

Additional preoperative testing may be indicated. In some cases standard plain film evaluation including an AP view in the plane of the scapula and an axillary lateral view is sufficient for preoperative planning. In proximal humeral malunions additional views in various degrees of rotation may be needed to accurately assess angulation and plan for corrective osteotomies. Preoperative CT scanning is often obtained in cases of nonunited or malunited tuberosities to assess the need of tuberosity osteotomies and the condition of the recipient bone on which tuberosities will be repositioned. If neurologic injury is suspected an EMG examination should be performed to determine the extent of injury and the prognosis for neurologic recovery. The possibility of infection complicating malunion or nonunion must be considered in patients who have undergone previous surgery. Preoperative hematologic studies and an aspiration arthrogram for culture and cell count can help verify the presence of infection.[30] Additionally, intraoperative frozen sections and Gram stains can be evaluated by a pathologist before proceeding with a definitive reconstructive procedure. If the results of such examinations document or are strongly suggestive of the presence of infection, a debridement of soft tissue, bone, and a resection of the articular portion of the humeral head is performed and long-term antibiotics are initiated. If the implantation of a prosthesis is planned for a later date, an antibiotic-impregnated bone cement spacer that is fashioned in the shape of a humeral endoprosthesis can be inserted. A cement spacer can help prevent further contracture of the myofacial sleeve, potentially maintain better function during the interval between staged procedures, and deliver antibiotics directly to the debrided, infected tissue bed[19].

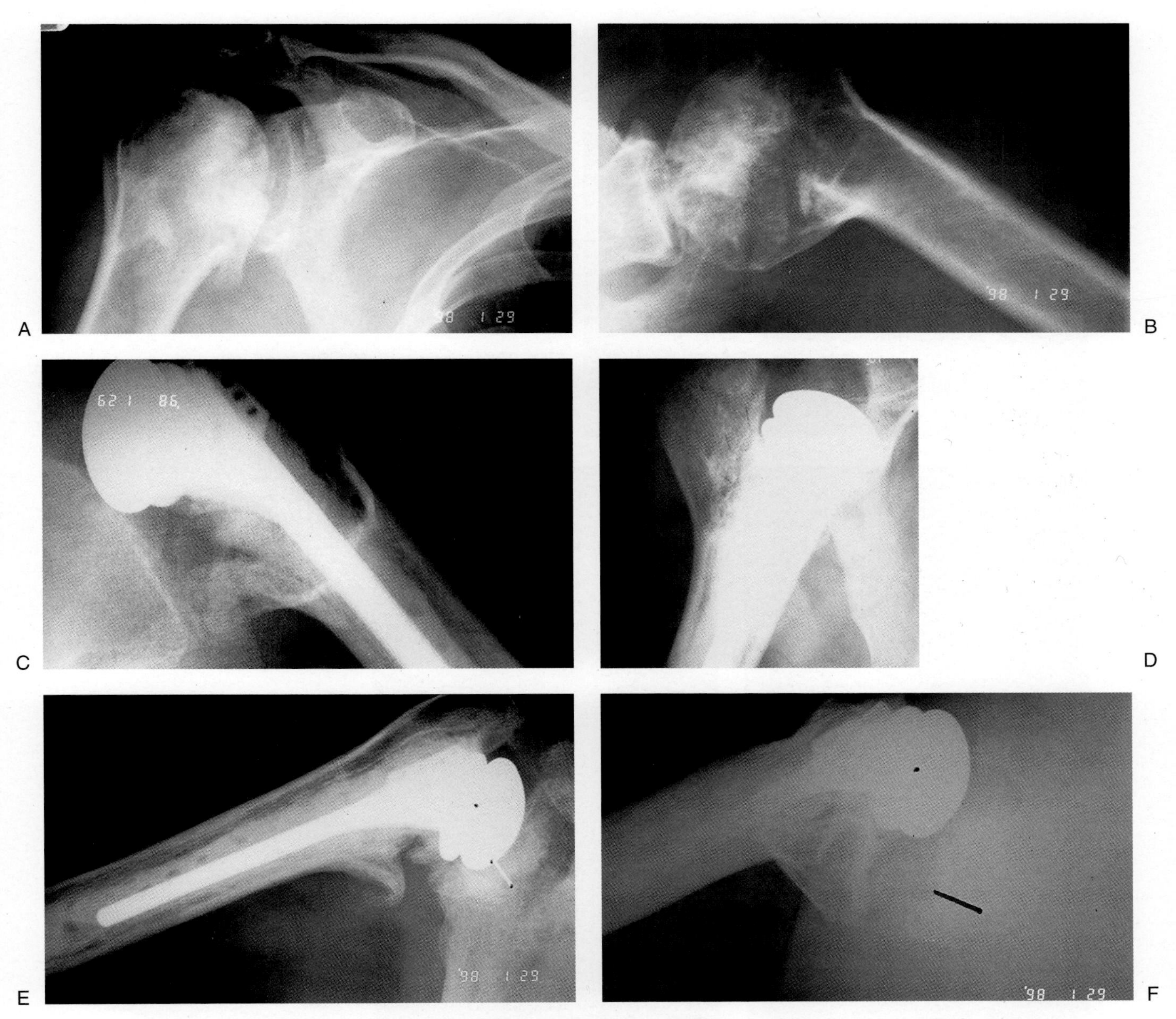

FIG. 23. (A,B) Patient with a four-part malunion, who was **(C,D)** treated initially with hemiarthroplasty without tuberosity osteotomy. The head is undersized and the tuberosity is prominent both superiorly and posteriorly. The shoulder is painful and is dislocated anteriorly. The greater tuberosity impinges on the CA arch and the posterior glenoid is levering the humeral head anteriorly out of the glenoid. **(E,F)** Because of persistent pain, a glenoid component is placed and the humeral component and malunited greater tuberosity are left in place. The humeral component is chronically dislocated for 2 years. (*continued*)

The main indication for humeral head replacement surgery for malunions or nonunions is pain that is caused by humeral articular incongruity. Total shoulder arthroplasty is performed when concomitant glenoid articular defects are present. Other factors may also indicate shoulder arthroplasty as the best surgical option. For example, for surgical neck nonunions, a humeral head replacement is sometimes chosen, despite the presence of intact articular surfaces, because either a small humeral head fragment size or poor bone quality precludes the use of internal fixation.

The expected results in terms of pain relief are generally good; however, gains in motion and function are often less than those achieved for more common diagnostic categories.[30,31,68,72] Because of associated pathology and degree of technical challenge, shoulder arthroplasty for malunions and nonunions is frequently undertaken with the expectations of achieving limited goals. The patient must be apprised of such expectations to make an informed decision. Despite striking radiographic findings, some patients with malunions or nonunions have relatively little pain and disability, especially in low-demand or elderly patients.[71] Surgical intervention is not justified in such patients.

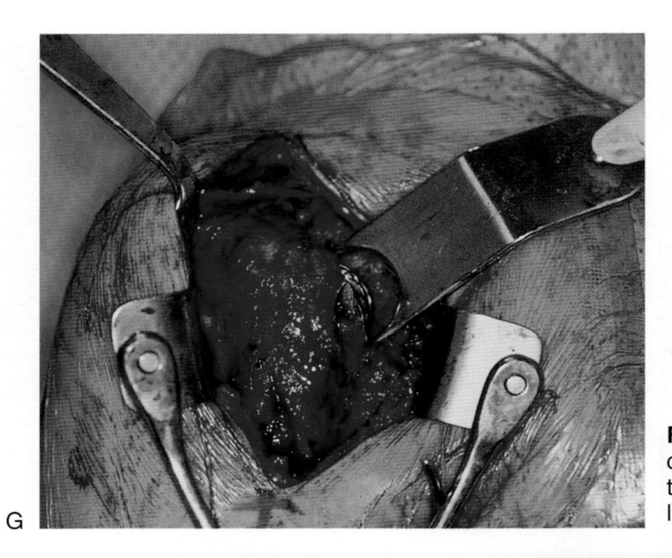

G

FIG. 23. (*continued*) **(G)** Revision arthroplasty required a complete circumferential capsulectomy, tuberosity osteotomy, removal of all components, **(H,I)** placement of a larger-sized head and glenoid component and ORIF of the

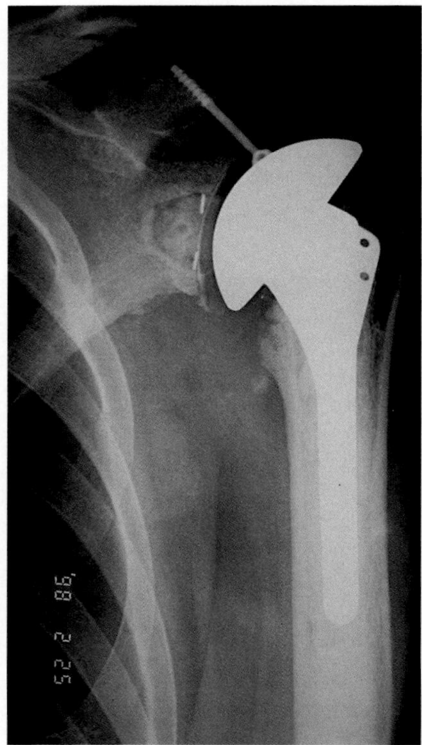

H

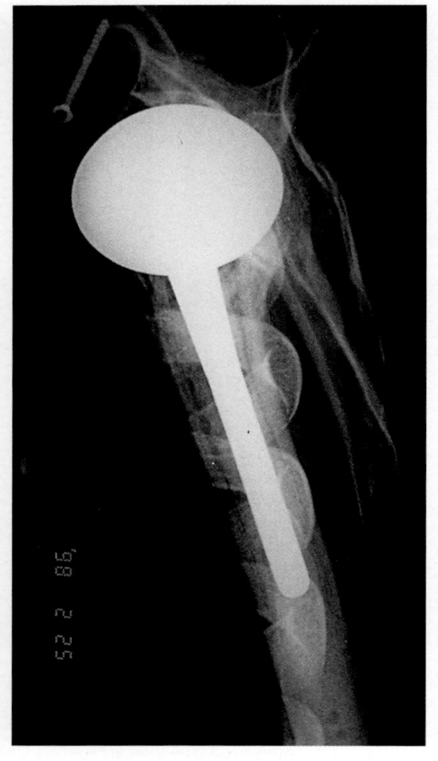

I

Technical Considerations

An extended deltopectoral approach from the lateral third of the clavicle to the deltoid insertion is often needed. Further exposure can be obtained by performing a coracoid osteotomy or detaching a portion of the anterior deltoid origin. One should anticipate additional effort to sufficiently release adhesions and contracted tissue for adequate exposure. The entire subdeltoid space and the superficial and deep surfaces of the rotator cuff tendons must be released. Usually, the capsule is so contracted that its release is performed with no intention of its repair. Sometimes a posterior deltoid-splitting approach is needed to address specific pathology that cannot be accessed through the deltopectoral approach. Thus, draping should be wide enough to allow for a posterior approach. For example, a posterior approach may be needed to osteotomize a malunited greater tuberosity or to mobilize a nonunited, significantly displaced greater tuberosity; to facilitate the osteotomy of a malunitied humeral head; or less commonly, to repair the posterior capsule for persistent posterior instability.

The technical principles of tuberosity malunions and nonunions during shoulder arthroplasty are similar. There must be sufficient quantity and quality of tuberosity and recipient proximal humeral bone, as well as sufficient mobility of the attached components of the rotator cuff, for accurate repositioning to obtain stable tuberosity fixation and anticipate bony union. Malunited tuberosities can mechanically block arcs of glenohumeral motion. Malunions of the greater tuberosity may block external rotation if healed in a prominent position posteriorly, or they can impinge against the anterior acromion during elevation of the arm if healed superiorly (Fig. 23). Lesser tuberosity malunions tend to block internal rotation at the anterior glenoid rim or coracoid process. In general, when a tuberosity is malunited a centimeter from its usual position, a block to rotation occurs.[30] When indicated, malunited tuberosities are osteotomized for repositioning. Care must be taken to retain an appropriate amount of tuberosity bone for fixation and to avoid iatrogenic detachment of the rotator cuff tendons. An osteotomized malunited tuberosity must be of sufficient length to ensure contact with the humeral shaft when repositioning. Once the tuberosity is freed, the attached rotator cuff is mobilized using the needed complement of rotator cuff release techniques. The main difference between malunions and nonunions of the tuberosities is that in nonunions there is generally more rotator cuff retraction and, thus, more difficulty in achieving needed rotator cuff mobilization.

If both tuberosities are being reattached three to four heavy nonabsorbable sutures are used to link the tuberosities to one another through the holes in the fin of the humeral component. Additional sutures are passed through the tuberosities and through drill holes in the proximal humeral shaft. These sutures assist in delivering the tuberosities inferiorly to assure contact with the humeral shaft. Impingement of the tuberosities against the acromion during arm elevation will be avoided by ensuring that the tuberosities are fixed below or within the confines of the prosthetic humeral head. Cancellous bone graft is used judiciously to fill in areas of void at the bony healing surfaces.

Postoperative physical therapy is individualized depending on the stability of tuberosity fixation. A maximal range of motion that does not cause undue tension to the reconstructed tuberosities or rotator cuff repairs (safe range of motion) is determined before wound closure. Passive range of motion exercises are initiated the day after surgery and are maintained until tuberosity union is achieved (usually, 6 to 8 weeks). Tanner and Cofield found that functional results of shoulder arthroplasty were negatively influenced by the need for tuberosity reconstruction.[91] Dines et al. reported better results in patients who did not require tuberosity osteotomy as compared with those who did.[30]

In chronic injuries that involve a *nonunion* of the *surgical neck*, arthroplasty is indicated for humeral articular incongruity or because poor bone quality or small humeral head fragment size precludes the use of internal fixation (Fig. 24). In cases deemed appropriate for arthroplasty, one typically finds a significant degree of resorption of the proximal fragment and proximal migration of the shaft segment.[71] Accurate reconstruction of humeral length will restore appropriate deltoid myofascial tension and lessen the risk of postoperative shoulder instability. The residual humeral articular surface is osteotomized or, if very soft, is removed with a rongeur. If the tuberosities are intact or healed the greater and lesser tuberosities will require osteotomies at the bicipital groove to create in essence a four-part fracture to allow more accurate repositioning. Fibrous granulation tissue is debrided at the surgical neck nonunion site and the medullary canal of the humeral shaft is prepared as in acute fractures for a cemented prosthesis. Excess bone cement above the level of the shaft fragment is removed before hardening. Cancellous bone graft is packed around the proximal prosthesis to create a bed for the tuberosities. The tuberosities are fixed as previously mentioned with heavy nonabsorbable suture material. Cancellous bone graft is impacted at any additional gaps existing between bone surfaces that must unite. The use of a modular component that provides several humeral neck lengths is beneficial when the myofascial envelope requires tension adjustment.

Malunions involving the *surgical neck* usually occur in varus and apex anterior angulation. Decreased abduction and forward elevation occurs progressively with increasing angulation at the malunion site. Varus angulation can position the greater tuberosity cephalad to the articular surface of the humeral head resulting in painful impingement. When the articular surfaces are intact an osteotomy with internal fixation can be performed if clinically indicated. Osteotomy of surgical neck malunions followed by internal fixation is most appropriate for young patients with two- or three-part injuries, provided there is no avascular necrosis, joint incongruity, or poor bone quality. Arthroplasty for surgical neck malunions is indicated when the articular surface is incongruous or poor bone quality precludes adequate internal fixation (Fig. 25).

If tuberosity position blocks glenohumeral motion, as determined by intraoperative range of motion testing, tuberosity osteotomy and repositioning should be performed. If a surgical neck malunion has mild to moderate angulation, it sometimes is possible to implant the humeral component without an osteotomy. In such situations a modified short-stemmed humeral component sometimes can be cemented in situ, being centered within the tuberosities. However, as angulation of the malunion increases so does the need to both reestablish the alignment of the medullary canal axes proximally and distally to accept a standard humeral component stem length and reposition the tuberosities through osteotomies. It may be difficult to mobilize the rotator cuff tendons sufficiently to reattach the tuberosities. Thus, it is critical for the surgeon to simultaneously judge the affect of repositioning the articular surface with a prosthesis and the ability of osteotomized tuberosities to reach their reattachment sites.

Results

Norris and Turner reported a series of four elderly patients with surgical neck nonunions who achieved satisfactory pain relief and function with cemented hemiarthroplasty using local bone graft from the discarded humeral head fragment.[72]

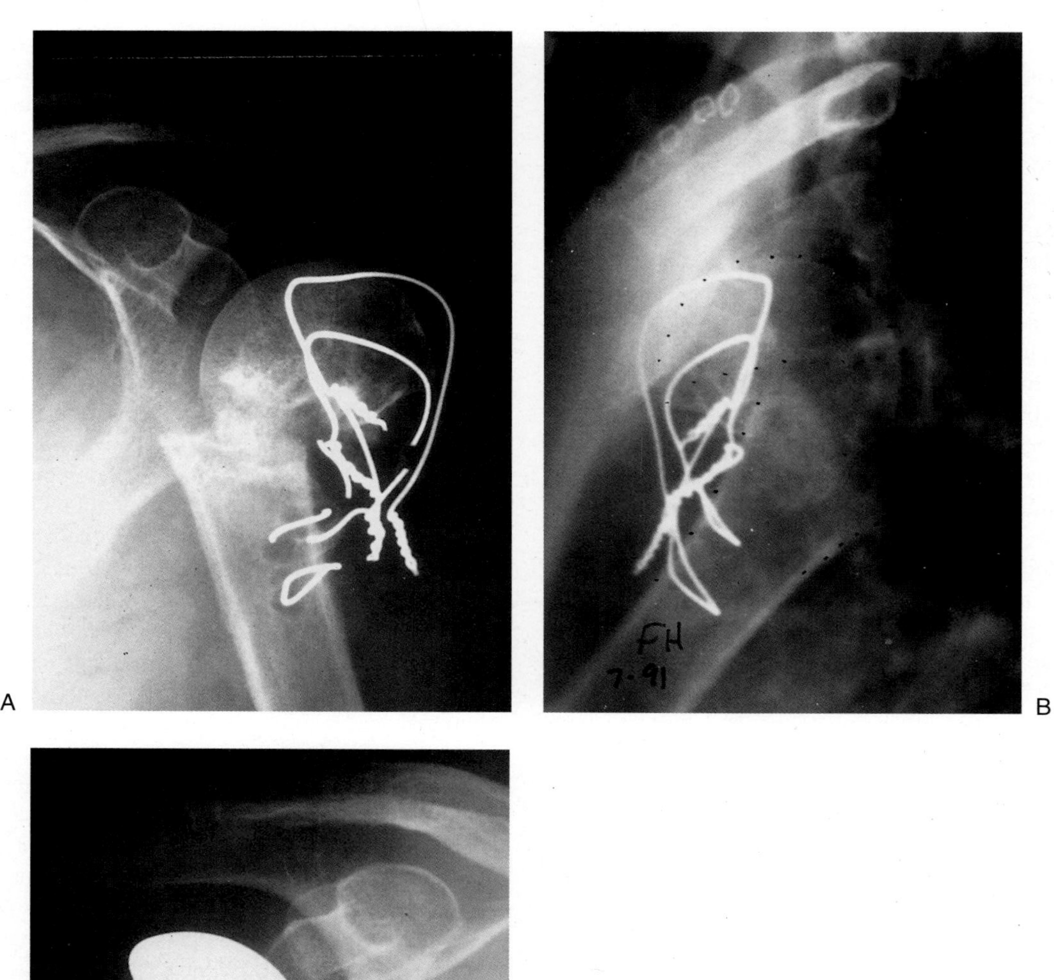

C

FIG. 24. **(A,B)** A long-standing surgical neck nonunion with bone resorption at the nonunion site, fractures hardware, and osteoporosis in a 75-year-old woman. **(C)** Therefore, this nonunion was treated with hemiarthroplasty, rather than revision ORIF.

No complications were reported. Frich et al. found increased pain scores and less forward elevation in patients treated with arthroplasty for surgical neck nonunions as compared with a group treated with arthroplasty for acute surgical neck fractures.[39] Neer noted patients treated with arthroplasty for nonunions who had good deltoid and rotator cuff muscles achieved the best results, and patients with impaired rotator cuff or deltoid muscles generally achieved satisfactory pain relief and function only with the arm at the side.[71]

The results of prosthetic replacement of three- and four-part malunions or nonunions do not approach those of prosthetic treatment for similar acute fractures.[5,39,59] Pain relief is usually achieved, but range of motion and strength are often limited. Frich et al. found better pain relief in four-part fractures treated early with arthroplasty than in those treated after a surgical delay, which in their series was of at least 4 months duration.[39] Of 11 patients with chronic four-part fractures treated with prosthetic replacement, only 1 had a

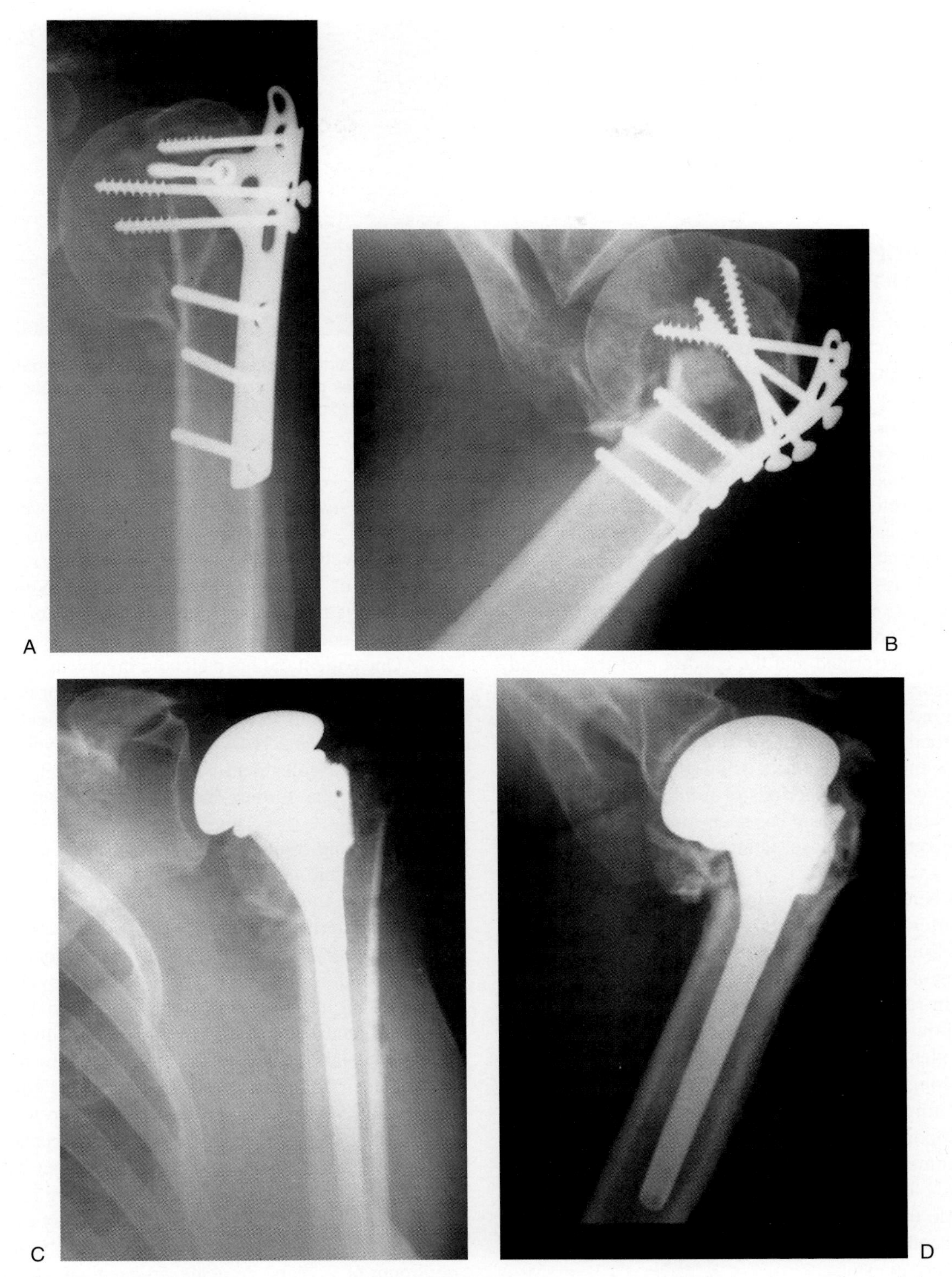

FIG. 25. (A,B) Surgical neck varus malunion and degenerative arthritis of the glenohumeral articulation treated with **(C,D)** total shoulder arthroplasty.

good result, compared with 3 excellent results and 6 good results in the 15 patients treated early with replacement. In nine cases of chronic three-part fractures no excellent or good results were achieved. A high incidence of instability was identified in the delayed surgery group, which was attributed to the increased difficulty in obtaining soft-tissue tensioning, including rotator cuff reconstruction. Norris et al. also reported problems with instability with delayed prosthetic replacement.[73] Frich and coworkers found that infection related to a primary attempt at internal fixation compromised results when surgical revision was required to implant a prosthesis and demonstrated that, overall, a failed primary nonarthroplasty surgical procedure reduced the likelihood of a good result with subsequent arthroplasty.

Thus, one should give serious consideration toward prosthetic replacement for acute, displaced fractures involving the surgical neck and tuberosities of the proximal humerus.

HEMIARTHROPLASTY VERSUS TOTAL SHOULDER ARTHROPLASTY

The results of humeral head replacement surgery at midterm follow-up have been favorable.[63,65] However, more recently, the results for specific diagnostic categories have been improved on with glenoid resurfacing.[9,23,67,97] Common diagnoses for which glenoid resurfacing is indicated, assuming bone stock is sufficient and large irreparable rotator cuff tears are not encountered, include osteoarthritis, inflammatory arthritis, and arthritis of instability. In cases of shoulder arthroplasty for old trauma there usually is evidence of more than minimal glenoid surface involvement to indicate glenoid resurfacing.

The decision to implant a glenoid component should be based on the diagnosis for which the joint resurfacing arthroplasty is being performed and the condition of the glenoid surface as depicted on preoperative radiographs and inspection at the time of surgery. In our experience, pain relief is better with total shoulder arthroplasty when there is glenoid cartilage loss and glenoid bone erosion (Fig. 26). This is particularly true with longer periods of follow-up. Conversion to total shoulder arthroplasty has been successful, in our experience, in returning these patients to painless shoulder function.

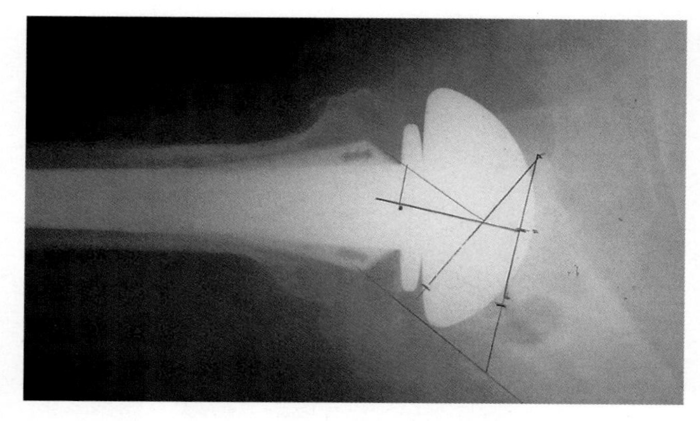

FIG. 26. Painful hemiarthroplasty with asymmetrical glenoid erosion. This patient was converted to total shoulder arthroplasty with excellent pain relief.

Potential benefits of preserving the glenoid surface include a shorter and technically less-demanding operative procedure, eliminating the possible need of revision surgery for loosening of the glenoid component, and reasonably predictable pain relief and improved function (at short- and midterm follow-up).[10,63,65] The potential detriments of preserving the glenoid include incomplete pain relief or failure to achieve long-lasting pain relief, necessitating revision surgery to implant a glenoid component.[9,23] Modular humeral components are distinctly advantageous when converting a humeral head replacement to a total shoulder arthroplasty.[88] The modular head is easily disassembled allowing ample exposure to the glenoid fossa. Without this feature an adequate exposure will require removal of the entire humeral component.

The results of hemiarthroplasty for avascular necrosis or acute fractures are generally good or excellent.[3,9,26,29,60,64,83] There appears to be no current rationale for resurfacing the glenoid when it is found to be in good condition in a disease process, such as avascular necrosis or acute fractures of the proximal humerus, that have no or only a minimal affect on the glenoid fossa if caught early. Five shoulders that underwent humeral head replacement for steroid-induced osteonecrosis involving only the humeral head were evaluated by Cruess.[29] At follow-up, which ranged from 1 to 6 years postoperatively, all patients had satisfactory relief of pain, and range of motion approached normal. Similar results were reported by Rutherford and Cofield for 11 humeral head replacements in similar patients with avascular necrosis.[83] One patient did have glenoid involvement, but to such an extent that a glenoid component could not be implanted. No or slight pain was experienced by 10 patients and active abduction averaged 161 degrees postoperatively. Advanced stages of avascular necrosis that secondarily involve the glenoid articular surface should undergo total shoulder replacement.

Encouraging results of humeral head replacement for osteoarthritis were reported by Neer in 1974.[65] Forty-six procedures were followed for an average of 6 years. According to Neer's criteria 20 achieved excellent, 20 satisfactory, and 6 unsatisfactory results. Of the 6 unsatisfactory ratings, overlapping conditions that influenced the final overall outcome were present in 4 patients, including a massive rotator cuff tear, an infection, a case of poliomyelitis with preoperative shoulder instability, and a case complicated by a psychiatric disturbance. Patient satisfaction included 27 who were enthusiastic, 15 who were satisfied, and 4 who were dissatisfied with the results of the surgery. Of the 28 patients treated for primary osteoarthritis none had significant pain postoperatively. In 1982 Neer reported encouraging results for total shoulder replacement surgery for a variety of diagnostic categories.[67] Of 40 osteoarthritic shoulders, followed for a minimum of 2 years, 36 achieved excellent, 3 satisfactory, and 1 unsatisfactory overall results. Since then, Neer's general recommendations have been that humeral head replacement without a glenoid component should be considered when the glenoid fossa is in good condition or when glenoid bone stock is so deficient that a glenoid component cannot predictably achieve stable fixation.[71]

Cofield et al. reported on 35 humeral head replacements for osteoarthritis with an average follow-up of 9.3 years.[23]

Nine shoulders (26%) required conversion to total shoulder arthroplasty for pain at an average of 6 years postoperatively. Two patients had revision within 2 years of the index procedure, 2 patients between 2 and 4 years, and 5 after 4 years. All 9 patients achieved pain relief following glenoid component implantation. These authors concluded that humeral head replacement should be used sparingly in patients with osteoarthritis, because pain relief tends to deteriorate with longer periods of follow-up. Zuckerman et al. followed 39 osteoarthritic shoulders treated with humeral head replacement surgery for an average of 39 months.[97] Moderate to severe pain was present in 7 shoulders (18%) postoperatively. These authors concluded that humeral head replacement should be considered in young patients, but total shoulder arthroplasty will usually be the procedure of choice for glenohumeral arthritis.

Rheumatoid arthritis is a unique diagnostic category because when large irreparable rotator cuff tears or insufficient glenoid bone stock is encountered the implantation of a glenoid component is generally not recommended because of the relatively high risk of glenoid component loosening.[38] Boyd et al. compared results of rheumatoid patients treated with humeral head replacement and total shoulder arthroplasty with an average follow-up of 44 months.[9] Forty-six of 95 patients (48%) treated with total shoulder arthroplasty, as compared with 8 of 27 patients (29%) treated with humeral head replacement, achieved complete pain relief. Additionally, gains for active range of motion were higher, as was patient satisfaction, in patients receiving total shoulder arthroplasty. Total shoulder arthroplasty was recommended as the procedure of choice for rheumatoid arthritis.

Neer's series of total shoulder arthroplasties in 43 rheumatoid patients, followed for an average of 37 months without massive rotator cuff deficiency, yielded 28 excellent, 12 satisfactory, and 3 unsatisfactory results.[67] According to Neer's criteria the unsatisfactory results occurred solely because of poor active forward elevation (being less than 90 degrees) as opposed to pain or component failure.[67] In the absence of irreparable rotator cuff tears or severe glenoid erosion precluding the use of a glenoid component, most authors concur that total shoulder arthroplasty is the procedure of choice in rheumatoid patients.[9,28,94,97]

REFERENCES

1. Albee FH. Restoration of shoulder functioning in cases of loss of head and upper portion of humerus. *Surg Gynecol Obstet* 1921;32:1–19.
2. Averill RM, Sledge CB, Thomas WH. Neer total shoulder arthroplasty. *Orthop Trans* 1980;4:287.
3. Bade HA III, Ranawat CS, Warren RF, et al. Long term results of Neer total shoulder replacement. In: Bateman JE, Welsh RP, eds. *Surgery of the shoulder*. St Louis: CV Mosby, 1984:294–302.
4. Barrett WP, Franklin JL, Jackins SE, et al. Total shoulder arthroplasty. *J Bone Joint Surg [Am]* 1987;69:865–872.
5. Bigliani LU. Fractures of the shoulder. Part I: fractures of the proximal humerus. In: Rockwood CA, Green DP, Bucholz RW, eds. *Fractures in adults*. Philadelphia: JB Lippincott, 1991:884–886.
6. Bigliani LU, Weinstein DM, Glasgow MT, et al. Glenohumeral arthroplasty for arthritis after instability of the shoulder. *J Shoulder Elbow Surg* 1995;4:87–94.
7. Boileau P, Walch G. The combined offset (medial and posterior) of the humeral sphere. *J Shoulder Elbow Surg* 1994;3:S65.
8. Bonutti PM, Hawkins RJ. Fracture of the humeral shaft associated with total replacement arthroplasty of the shoulder. *J Bone Joint Surg [Am]* 1992;74:617–618.
9. Boyd AD, Thomas WH, Scott RD, Sledge CB, Thornhill TS. Total shoulder arthroplasty versus hemi-arthroplasty. *J Arthroplasty* 1990;5: 329–336.
10. Boyd AD, Thornhill TS. Glenoid resurfacing in shoulder arthroplasty. In: Friedman RJ, ed. *Arthroplasty of the shoulder*. New York: Thieme, 1994:306–316.
11. Brems JJ, Wilde AH, Borden LS, Boumphrey FRS. Glenoid lucent lines. *Orthop Trans* 1986;10:231.
12. Brems JJ. Shoulder replacement in arthritis of dislocation. *Orthop Trans* 1989;13:235.
13. Brems JJ, Yoon HJ, Tetzlaff J. Interscalene block anesthesia and shoulder surgery. *Orthop Trans* 1990;14:250.
14. Brems J. The glenoid component in total shoulder arthroplasty. *J Shoulder Elbow Surg* 1993;2:47–54.
15. Brenner BC, Ferlic DC, Clayton ML, et al. Survivorship of unconstrained total shoulder arthroplasty. *J Bone Joint Surg [Am]* 1989;71: 1289–1296.
16. Brostrum L, Kronberg M, Wallensten R. Should the glenoid be replaced in shoulder arthroplasty with an unconstrained Dana or St. George prosthesis? *Ann Chir Gynaecol* 1992;81:54–57.
17. Brownlee RC, Cofield RH. Shoulder replacement for rotator cuff arthropathy. *Orthop Trans* 1986;10:230.
18. Clayton ML, Ferlic DC, Jeffers PD. Prosthetic arthroplasties of the shoulder. *Clin Orthop* 1982;164:184–191.
19. Codd TP, Yamaguchi K, Pollock RG, Flatow EF, Bigliani LU. Infected shoulder arthroplasties: treatment with staged reimplantation vs. resection arthroplasty. *J Shoulder Elbow Surg* 1996;5:S5.
20. Cofield RH. Total shoulder arthroplasty with the Neer prosthesis. *J Bone Joint Surg [Am]* 1984;66:899–906.
21. Cofield RH, Lanzer WL. Pathology of rotator cuff tearing and methods of tendon repair. *Orthop Trans* 1985;9:42.
22. Cofield RH, Edgerton BC. Total shoulder arthroplasty: complications and revision surgery. *Instr Course Lect* 1990;39:449–462.
23. Cofield RH, Frankle MA, Zuckerman JD. Humeral head replacement for glenohumeral arthritis. *Semin Arthroplasty* 1995;6:214–221.
24. Collins DN, Harryman DT, Lippitt SN, Jackins SE, Matsen FA III. The technique of glenohumeral arthroplasty. *Tech Orthop* 1991;6:43–59.
25. Collins D, Tencer A, Sidles J, Matsen F. Edge displacement and deformation of glenoid components in response to eccentric loading. The effect of preparation of the glenoid bone. *J Bone Joint Surg [Am]* 1992; 74:501–507.
26. Compito CA, Self EB, Bigliani LU. Arthroplasty and acute shoulder trauma: reasons for success and failure. *Clin Orthop* 1994;307:27–36.
27. Couglin MJ, Morris JM, West WF. The semiconstrained total shoulder arthroplasty. *J Bone Joint Surg [Am]* 1979;61:574–581.
28. Craig EV. Total shoulder replacement. *Orthopedics* 1988;11:125–136.
29. Cruess RL. Steroid-induced avascular necrosis of the head of the humerus. *J Bone Joint Surg [Br]* 1976;58:313–317.
30. Dines DM, Klarren RF, Altchek DW, Moeckel B. Posttraumatic changes of the proximal humerus: malunion, nonunion, and osteonecrosis. Treatment with modular hemiarthroplasty or total shoulder arthroplasty. *J Shoulder Elbow Surg* 1993;2:11–21.
31. Duralde XA, Flatow EL, Pollock RG, Nicholson GP, Self EB, Bigliani LU. Operative treatment of nonunions of the surgical neck of the humerus. *J Shoulder Elbow Surg* 1996;5:169–180.
32. Ellman H, Jinnah R, Amstutz HC. Experience with the DANA hooded component for cuff deficient shoulder arthroplasty. *Orthop Trans* 1986; 10:217.
33. Engelbrecht E, Stellbrink G. Totale Schulterendoprosthese Modell St. George. *Chirurgie* 1976;47:525–530.
34. Faludi DD, Weiland AJ. Cementless total shoulder arthroplasty: preliminary experience with thirteen cases. *Orthopedics* 1983;6:431–437.
35. Fenlin JM, Ramsey ML, Allardyce TJ, Frieman BG. Modular total shoulder replacement: design rationale, indications, and results. *Clin Orthop* 1994;307:37–46.
36. Flatow EL, Bigliani LU, April EX. An anatomical study of the musculocutaneous nerve and its relationship to the coracoid process. *Clin Orthop* 1989;244:166–171.

37. Flatow EL, Miller SR, Neer CS II. Chronic anterior dislocations of the shoulder. *J Shoulder Elbow Surg* 1993;2:2–10.
38. Franklin JL, Barrett WP, Jackins SE, Matsen FA III. Glenoid loosening in total shoulder arthroplasty. Association with rotator cuff deficiency. *J. Arthroplasty* 1988;3:39–46.
39. Frich LH, Sojbjerg JO, Sneppen O. Shoulder arthroplasty in complex acute and chronic proximal humeral fractures. *Orthopedics* 1991;14: 949–954.
40. Frich LH, Moller BN, Sneppen O. Shoulder arthroplasty with the Neer Mark-II prosthesis. *Arch Orthop Trauma Surg* 1988;107:110–113.
41. Friedman RJ, Ewald FC. Arthroplasty of the ipsilateral shoulder and elbow in patients who have rheumatoid arthritis. *J Bone Joint Surg [Am]* 1987;69:661–666.
42. Friedman FJ, Thornhill TS, Thomas WH, Sledge CB. Nonconstrained total shoulder replacement in patients who have rheumatoid arthritis and class-IV function. *J Bone Joint Surg [Am]* 1989;71:494–498.
43. Friedman RJ, Hawthorne KB, Genez BM. Evaluation of glenoid bone loss with computerized tomography. *J Bone Joint Surg [Am]* 1992;74: 1032–1037.
44. Hawkins RJ, Neer CS II, Pianta RM, Mendoza FX. Locked posterior dislocation of the shoulder. *J Bone Joint Surg [Am]* 1987;69:9–18.
45. Hawkins RJ, Bell RH, Jallay B. Total shoulder arthroplasty. *Clin Orthop* 1989;242:188–194.
46. Hawkins RJ, Angelo RL. Glenohumeral osteoarthrosis: a late complication of the Putti-Platt repair. *J Bone Joint Surg [Am]* 1990;72: 1193–1197.
47. Hoppenfeld S, De Boer P. *Surgical exposures in orthopaedics.* Philadelphia: WB Saunders, 1990:1–23.
48. Hovelius L, Augustini GBG, Fredin OH, et al. Primary anterior dislocation of the shoulder in young patients: a ten-year prospective study. *J Bone Joint Surg [Am]* 1996;78:1677–1684.
49. Iannotti JP, Gabriel JP, Schneck SL, Evans BG, Misra S. The normal glenohumeral relationships. An anatomical study of one hundred and forty shoulders. *J Bone Joint Surg [Am]* 1992;74:491–500.
50. Jones L. Reconstructive operation for nonreducible fractures of the head of the humerus. *Ann Surg* 1933;97:217–225.
51. Kelly IG, Goster RS, Fisher WD. Neer total shoulder replacement in rheumatoid arthritis. *J Bone Joint Surg [Br]* 1987:69;723–726.
52. Kenmore PI, MacCartee C, Vitek B. A simple shoulder replacement. *J Biomed Mater Res* 1974;8:329–330.
53. Konig F. Uber die Immplantation von Elfen Hein Zum Eustatz von Knochen und Gelenkenden Brums Beitr. *Klin Chir* 1914;85:613.
54. Krueger FJ. A vitallium replica arthroplasty on the shoulder: a case report of aseptic necrosis of the proximal end of the humerus. *Surgery* 1951;30:1005–1011.
55. Lettin AWF, Copeland SA Scales JF. The Stanmore total shoulder replacement. *J Bone Joint Surg [Br]* 1982;64:47–51.
56. Loomer R, Graham B. Anatomy of the axillary nerve and its relation to the inferior capsular shift. *Clin Orthop* 198;243:100–105.
57. Lugli T. Artificial shoulder joint by Pean (1893). The facts of an exceptional intervention and the prosthetic method. *Clin Orthop* 1978; 133:215–218.
58. McCoy SR, Warren RF, Bade HA, Ranawat CS, Inglis AE. Total shoulder arthroplasty in rheumatoid arthritis. *J Arthroplasty* 1989;4: 105–113.
59. McGuigan FX, Norris TR, Sharkey PF. Delayed shoulder arthroplasty for cases of failed outcome in complex fractures of the proximal humerus. *Orthop Trans* 1992–1993;16:823.
60. Moeckel BH, Dines DM, Warren RF, Altchek DW. Modular hemiarthroplasty for fractures of the proximal humerus. *J Bone Joint Surg [Am]* 1992;74:884–889.
61. Neer CS II, Brown TH Jr, McLaughlin HL. Fracture of the neck of the humerus with dislocation of the head fragment. *Am J Surg* 1953;85: 252–285.
62. Neer CS II. Articular replacement for the humeral head. *J Bone Joint Surg [Am]* 1955;37:215–228.
63. Neer CS II. Followup notes on articles previously published in the journal. Articular replacement for the humeral head. *J Bone Joint Surg [Am]* 1964;46:1607–1610.
64. Neer CS II. Displaced proximal humerus fractures. Part II. Treatment of 3-part and 4-part fracture displacement. *J Bone Joint Surg [Am]* 1970;52:1090–1103.
65. Neer CS II. Replacement arthroplasty for glenohumeral osteoarthritis. *J Bone Joint Surg [Am]* 1974;56:1–13.
66. Neer CS II, Foster CR. Inferior capsular shift for involuntary inferior and multidirectional instability of the shoulder. *J Bone Joint Surg [Am]* 1980;62:897—908.
67. Neer CS II, Watson KC, Stanton JF. Recent experience in total shoulder replacement. *J Bone Joint Surg [Am]* 1982;64:319–336.
68. Neer CS. Nonunion of the surgical neck of the humerus. *Orthop Trans* 1983;7:389.
69. Neer CS II. Unconstrained shoulder arthroplasty. In: Bateman JE, Welsh RP, eds. *Surgery of the shoulder.* St Louis: CV Mosby, 1984: 240–245.
70. Neer CS II, Morrison DM. Glenoid bone-grafting in total shoulder arthroplasty. *J Bone Joint Surg [Am]* 1988;70:1154–1162.
71. Neer CS II. *Shoulder reconstruction.* Philadelphia: WB Saunders, 1990:143–247.
72. Norris TR, Turner JA. Surgical treatment of nonunion of the upper humerus shaft fracture in the elderly. *Orthop Trans* 1985;9:1985.
73. Norris TR, Turner JA, Bovil D. Nonunion of the upper humerus: an analysis of the etiology and treatment in 28 cases. In: Post M, Morrey BF, Hawkins RJ, eds. *Surgery of the shoulder.* St. Louis: Mosby Year-Book, 1990:63–70.
74. Pritchett JW, Clark JM. Prosthetic replacement for chronic unreduced dislocations of the shoulder. *Clin Orthop* 1987;217:89–93.
75. Post M. Haskell SS, Jablon M. Total shoulder replacement with a constrained prosthesis. *J Bone Joint Surg [Am]* 1980;62:327–335.
76. Post M. Constrained arthroplasty of the shoulder. *Orthop Clin North Am* 1987;18:455–462.
77. Richard A, Judet R, Rene L. Acrylic prosthetic reconstruction of the upper end of the humerus for fracture-luxations. *J Chir* 1952;68:537–547.
78. Richards RR, An K-N, Bigliani LU, et al. A standardized method for the assessment of shoulder function. *J Shoulder Elbow Surg* 1994;3: 347–352.
79. Rockwood CA II. The technique of total shoulder arthroplasty. *Instr Course Lect* 1990;39:437–447.
80. Rodowsky MW, Weinstein DM, Pollock RG, Flatow EL, Bigliani LU, Neer CS II. On the rarity of glenoid component failure. *J Shoulder Elbow Surg* 1995;4:S13–14.
81. Roper BA, Paterson JM, Day WH. The Roper-Day total shoulder replacement. *J Bone Joint Surg [Br]* 1990;72:694–697.
82. Rowe CR, Zarins B. Chronic unreduced dislocations of the shoulder. *J Bone Joint Surg [Am]* 1982;64:494–505.
83. Rutherford CS, Cofield RH. Osteonecrosis of the shoulder. *Orthop Trans* 1987;11:239.
84. Saha AK. Dynamic stability of the glenohumeral joint. *Acta Orthop Scand* 1971;42:491–505.
85. Samilson RL, Prieto V. Dislocation arthropathy of the shoulder. *J Bone Joint Surg [Am]* 1983;65:456–460.
86. Sarrifian SK. Gross and functional anatomy of the shoulder. *Clin Orthop* 1983;213:11–19.
87. Settergren CR, Cofield RH. Total shoulder arthroplasty: five to ten year assessment. *Orthop Trans* 1987;11:238.
88. Shaffer BS, Giordano CP, Zuckerman JD. Revision of a loose glenoid component facilitated by a modular humeral component: a technical note. *J Arthroplasty* 1990;5S:79–81.
89. Souter WA. The surgical treatment of the rheumatoid shoulder. *Ann Acad Med Singapore* 1983;12:243–255.
90. Spurling RG, Scoville WB. Lateral rupture of the cervical intervertebral discs. A common cause of shoulder and arm pain. *Surg Gynecol Obstet* 1944;78:350–358.
91. Tanner MW, Cofield RH. Prosthetic arthroplasty for fractures and fracture-dislocations of the proximal humerus. *Clin Orthop* 1983;179: 116–128.
92. Thomas BJ, Amstutz HC, Cracchiolo A. Shoulder arthroplasty for rheumatoid arthritis. *Clin Orthop* 1991;265:125–128.
93. Thornhill TS, Karr MJ, Averill RM, et al. Total shoulder arthroplasty: the Brigham experience. *Orthop Trans* 1983;7:497.
94. Torchia ME, Cofield RH. Long-term results of Neer total shoulder arthroplasty. *Orthop Trans* 1994–1995;18:977.
95. Zippel J. Vollstandiger schultergelenkersatz aus kunstoff und metall. *Biomed Tech* 1972;17:87–91.
96. Zuckerman JD, Matsen FA III. Complications about the glenohumeral joint related to the use of screws and staples. *J Bone Joint Surg [Am]* 1984;66:175–180.
97. Zuckerman JD, Cofield RH. Proximal humeral prosthetic replacement in glenohumeral arthritis. *Orthop Trans* 1986;10:231–232.

Disorders of the Shoulder: Diagnosis and Management,
edited by Joseph P. Iannotti and Gerald R. Williams, Jr.
Lippincott Williams & Wilkins, Philadelphia © 1999.

CHAPTER 21

Shoulder Arthroplasty: Massive Cuff Deficiency

John M. Fenlin, Jr. and Barbara Frieman

INTRODUCTION

Any discussion of the unique and variable problems associated with treatment of glenohumeral arthritis and massive rotator cuff deficiency must be based on an awareness of the continuing evolution of the understanding of the underlying pathology. The history of shoulder arthroplasty, although relatively short, continues to evolve. Understanding the impact of massive cuff deficiency on the outcome of shoulder arthroplasty is still an area of some debate. In this chapter the evolution of our understanding of the pathology, and the treatment of glenohumeral arthritis with massive cuff deficiency, and current recommendations will be outlined.

HISTORY

In 1934 Codman[1] detailed his experience with rotator cuff disease. He theorized that full-thickness supraspinatus tears can gradually extend with time and multiple minor traumas. Codman was the first to postulate that the ultimate result of massive cuff deficiency is a host of pathologic changes in the glenohumeral joint. In addition to describing rupture of multiple rotator cuff tendons and the long head of the biceps tendon, Codman also described glenohumeral articular damage, erosion of the tuberosities, thinning and sclerosis of the acromion, accumulation of intraarticular fluid, and superior migration of the humerus.

Adams[2] in 1873 described a form of "chronic rheumatic arthritis," both localized and generalized, with examples of gross pathology of the shoulder. The generalized form was later defined as "rheumatoid arthritis." The localized form of chronic rheumatoid arthritis of the shoulder is similar to the "Milwaukee shoulder" described by McCarty in 1981.[3] Neer[4] in 1983 described "cuff tear arthropathy" as an entity unique to the shoulder joint with pathology similar to that of Milwaukee shoulder syndrome.

Milwaukee shoulder syndrome was described as a disease localized to the shoulder joint found in elderly women.[3,5,6] Full-thickness rotator cuff tendon defects were always present in association with a large noninflammatory joint effusion. Hydroxyapatite crystals within microspheroids, activated collagenase, and neutral proteases were present in the joint fluid. Shoulder instability, with severe glenohumeral joint destruction, synovial hypertrophy, and the presence of other basic calcium phosphate crystals, characterized this distinctive arthropathy of the shoulder in later reports.[7,8] The etiology of this disease is unknown, but the rheumatologic literature stresses the role of the basic calcium phosphate crystals in the pathology of the disease. The soft-tissue and bony destruction is thought to be a result of the crystalline arthropathy.[9] Cuff tear arthropathy, although similar in pathology and presentation to crystalline arthropathy, was felt to result from nutritional and mechanical factors related to the instability of the glenohumeral joint caused by massive rotator cuff tendon tearing. Neer thought that the resultant constellation of physical and chemical joint pathology was a direct result of wear debris caused by joint instability.[4,11] It is still debatable whether crystalline arthropathy and cuff tear arthropathy are the same disease or different entities.

Rheumatoid arthritis of the glenohumeral joint when associated with massive cuff deficiency can present in a fashion similar to cuff tear arthropathy. Although there is the added pathology of a destructive pannus, poor quality soft

J. M. Fenlin, Jr. and B. Frieman: Department of Orthopaedic Surgery, Jefferson Medical College, Walnut Street, Philadelphia, PA 19107.

tissues, and bone destruction caused by the rheumatoid pathology, there is the overlap of instability and wear debris from cuff deficiency, much like cuff tear arthropathy. An understanding of the mechanical problems associated with massive cuff deficiency in all these entities is critical to their surgical treatment, regardless of their pathologies.

Throughout the evolution of prosthetic design, it was recognized early that massive cuff deficiency from any cause created unique problems. In patients with massive cuff deficiency, postoperative, clinical function was significantly lower, and complications of loosening and component failure were higher than in normal patients.[12–14,17,18,21,29] Semiconstrained and constrained designs attempted to compensate for cuff deficiency with superior constraints.[13–16] These prostheses had a high rate of loosening and failure.[17–24] Although unconstrained designs had the best results[25,26] in these cases, eccentric glenoid loading caused by continued superior migration of the humeral head resulted in glenoid loosening and asymmetrical wear.[27,28] Superior spacer blocks or various types of resurfacing of the acromion to prevent humeral migration met with little success.[19]

Leaving the glenoid component out and using hemiarthroplasty have been reported to give results that are superior to those from any type of total shoulder arthroplasty in patients with massive cuff deficiency.[30–32] Normal-sized hemiarthroplasty does not restore the normal humeral length, lateral offset, or center of rotation of the premorbid anatomy. However, many authors report good results using it. The use of an oversized humeral head for hemiarthroplasty does accomplish the restoration of normal joint alignment, and better functional results have been reported using a modular prosthesis.[33,34]

Another treatment option used before the development of more adequate prostheses was glenohumeral arthrodesis. Unfortunately, although arthrodesis is a reliable procedure, elderly patients with osteopenic bone are not ideal candidates for this procedure. Because of patient satisfaction with hemiarthroplasty, arthrodesis is less frequently used now than it had been in the past.[35–37]

CLINICAL PRESENTATION AND EVALUATION OF PATIENTS

Patients with massive cuff deficiency and glenohumeral arthritis tend to be elderly, with female preponderance and dominant arm involvement. Pain in the affected shoulder is intensified by use, but also is present at rest, and is the primary complaint. Weakness and inability to use the arm are always present, but are usually less bothersome than the pain. Patients with massive rotator cuff tears without arthritis have similar complaints. Differentiating between the impingement pain of rotator cuff deficiency and the glenohumeral pain of arthritis can be difficult clinically. Patients with rotator cuff deficiency alone should be treated with a different treatment protocol. Thus, differentiating the two sources of pain is clinically important in determining the appropriate treatment for any particular patient.

Patients with massive cuff tears without arthritis are frequently middle-aged, and preponderantly male. Impingement pain occurs with active elevation of the arm into the impingement zone. Abduction to 90 degrees will aggravate impingement pain. Full external or internal rotation while abducted will usually aggravate this pain. These painful impingement maneuvers are usually accompanied by some acromial crepitus. The pain is localized under and around the acromion in the area of the subdeltoid and subacromial bursa.

Radiographs of shoulders with massive rotator cuff tears without arthritis show sclerosis and possibly thinning of the acromion (Fig. 1). There can be anterior and lateral acromial spur formation. The humeral tuberosities can be sclerotic and have exostoses. The joint space should not be narrowed and the articular surfaces of both the humeral head and glenoid should be relatively normally shaped. There is usually some superior translation of the humeral head.

Patients with both massive cuff deficiency and glenohumeral arthropathy have a slightly different presentation. They are more likely older, more likely female, and usually have more pain at rest. The pain is aggravated immediately upon initiation of motion in any direction. The contraction of

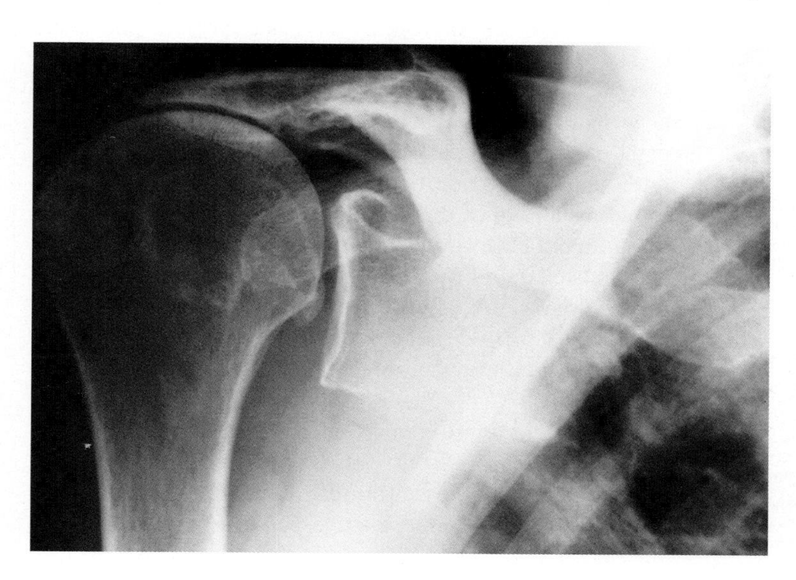

FIG. 1. Radiograph of a patient with massive cuff tear, superior migration of the humeral head, and sclerois of the acromion.

the deltoid causes an increase in joint contact forces and thus initiates pain immediately. The pain can increase further in the impingement zone, and crepitus can be present with any motion. One test that is helpful in differentiating glenohumeral arthritis pain is active eccentric lowering of the arm from 60 degrees of abduction to 0 degrees of abduction. During this maneuver pain and crepitus signal glenohumeral arthritis. Compression of the humeral head against the glenoid by the examiner can also cause pain and crepitus. The pain in these patients may be in the same distribution as in patients with massive cuff tears, but they also complain of pain in the glenohumeral articulation medially over both the anterior and posterior aspects of the joint. Instability testing with anterior and posterior translation of the humeral head can also produce this more medial type pain. In many patients, a large effusion may be obvious to the examiner.

Radiographs in cuff tear arthropathy show advanced glenohumeral arthropathy. There can be superior (Fig. 2) erosion of the glenoid called "acetabularization." The humeral head is more eroded with the appearance of "femoralization" from erosion and flattening of the tuberosities. There is a false facet on the superior glenoid (acromion). The acromion may be extremely thin with stress fractures present. The joint space is frequently totally obliterated with subchondral sclerosis on both the glenoid and humeral surfaces. Superior migration and medialization are marked. However, if the arm is relaxed and dependent during the radiographic examination, the subacromial narrowing may not be appreciated on radiographs (Fig. 3).

Magnetic resonance imaging is not necessary to confirm the diagnosis of cuff tear arthropathy. However, it can be helpful in excluding other diagnoses such as osteomyelitis

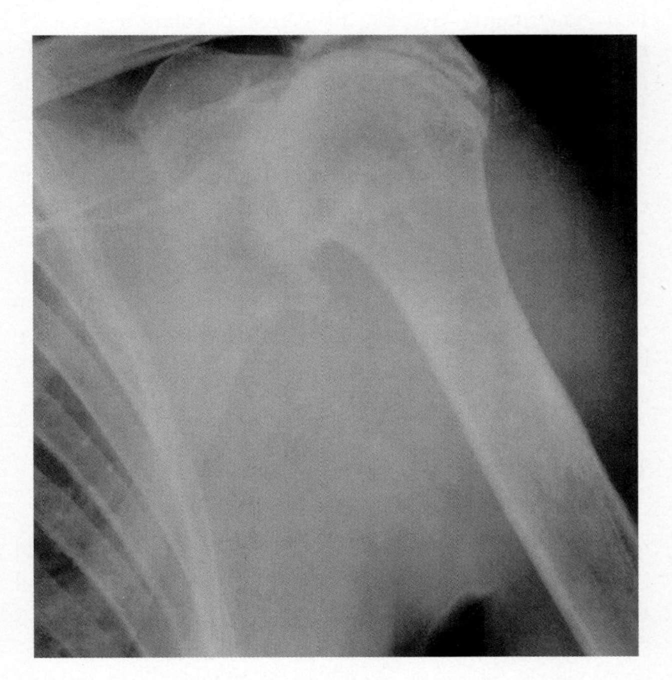

FIG. 2. Anteroposterior radiograph of a patient with rotator cuff arthropathy demonstrating the typical acetabularization of the glenoid and corocoacromial arch. The humerus is articulating with the false glenoid facet and the acromion.

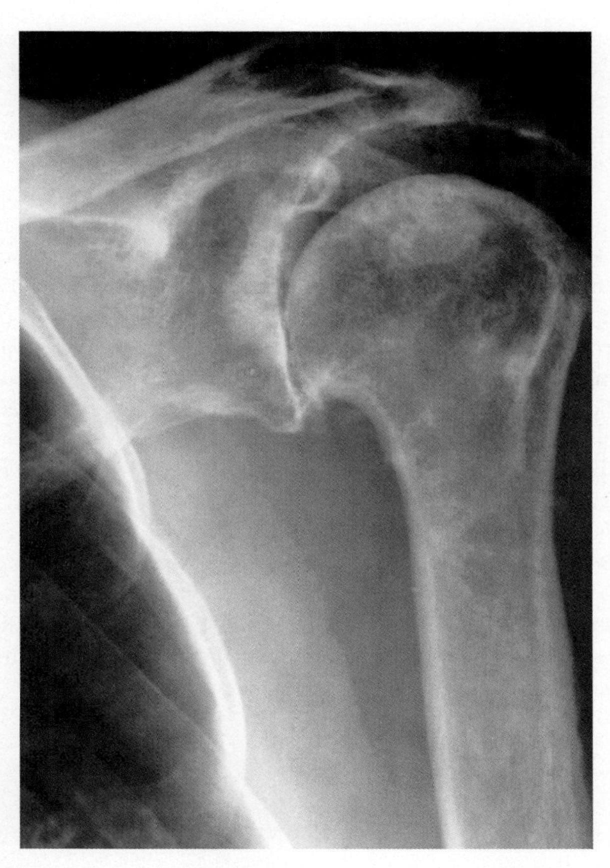

FIG. 3. The same patient, and same radiographic view as Fig. 2 with deltoid relaxed.

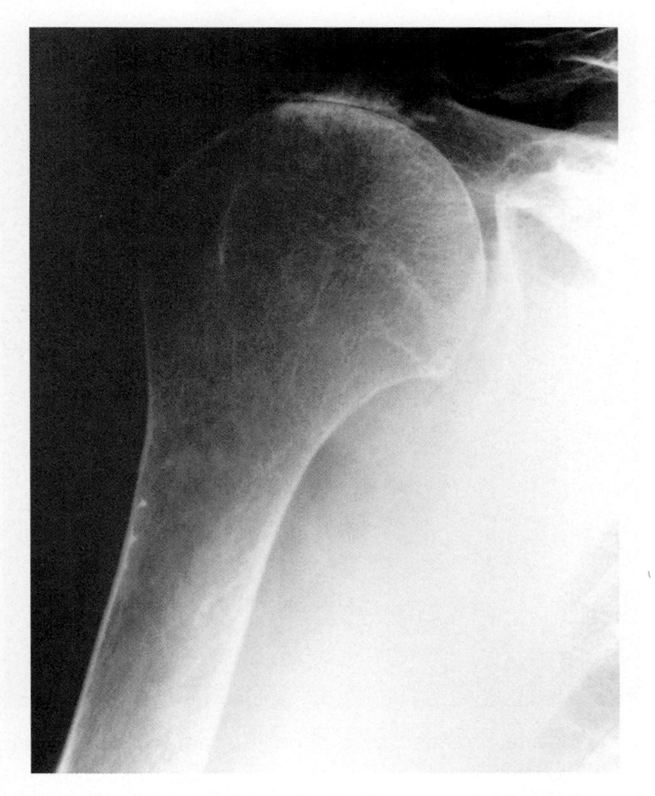

FIG. 4. Radiograph of a patient with rheumatoid arthritis and rotator cuff imcompetence.

and sepsis. Rheumatoid arthritis with massive cuff deficiency can have a similar radiographic appearance to that of cuff tear arthropathy (Fig. 4). Magnetic resonance imaging can indicate pannus and bony scalloping that are not always easily visualized on plain radiographs (Figs. 5 and 6).

In patients with suspected massive cuff tears, with only mild evidence of glenohumeral arthritis, magnetic resonance imaging can size the cuff tear and show retraction. Muscle atrophy of the rotator cuff muscles is frequently present in massive chronic tears and may predict a poor result for the primary repair. The articular cartilage is usually not well delineated on magnetic resonance imaging; however, occasionally, articular defects are seen. When defects are present, the patient should be examined carefully for symptoms and signs of glenohumeral pain before any attempt is made to repair the rotator cuff tendons.

Arthrograms can show large vacuous intraarticular spaces in advanced cuff tear arthropathy. The so-called geyser sign is present when the acromioclavicular joint communicates with the glenohumeral articular space. In such advanced disease states, an arthrogram should not be necessary to confirm the diagnosis.

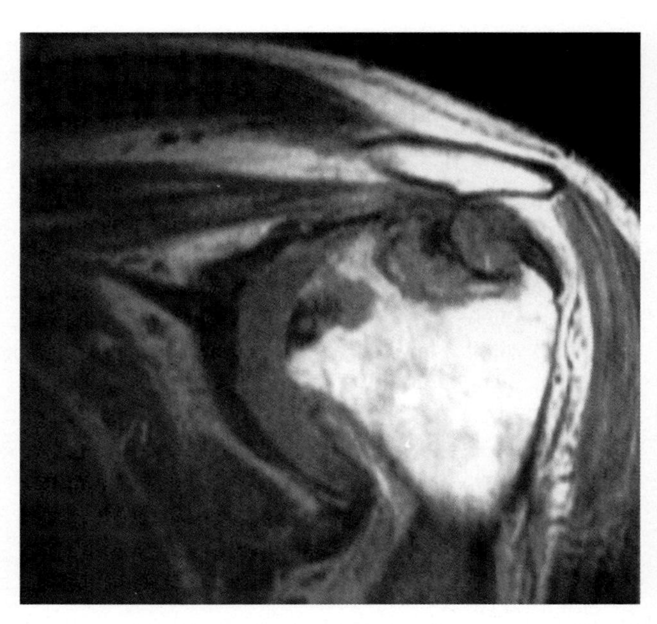

FIG. 6. An MRI of rheumatoid arthritis demonstrates pannus invading the humeral head and thinning of the incompetent rotator cuff.

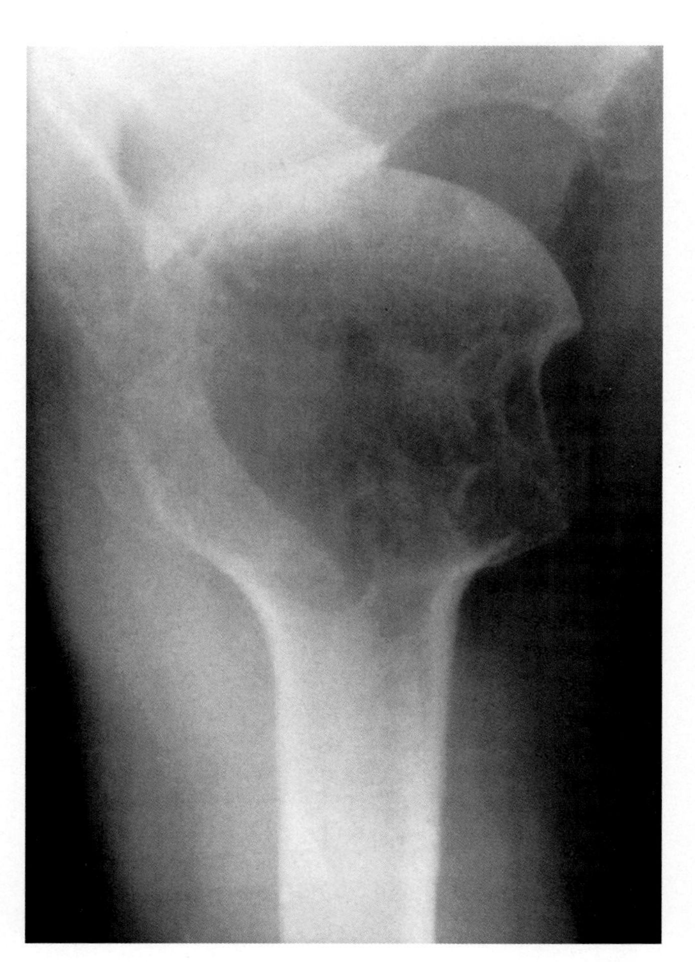

FIG. 5. The pannus has eroded the metaphysics of the humeral head.

Before determining treatment, care must be taken to exclude other diagnoses. A neuropathic or Charcot joint can cause rapid severe arthropathy of the glenohumral joint similar to cuff tear arthropathy. Therefore, all patients must have a careful neurologic examination. Blood testing for diabetes is usually routinely done in these patients. Electromyographic testing should be done in patients with any neurologic abnormality. Because this patient population is elderly, coexistent degenerative disease of the cervical spine is common. Magnetic resonance imaging can diagnose a spinal cord syrinx or myelomalacia, which can cause neuropathic arthropathy.

Low-grade chronic infections in the glenohumeral joint can also cause a rapid severe arthropathy with all the hallmarks of cuff tear arthropathy. When infection is suspected aspiration and culture should delineate the diagnosis. Magnetic resonance imaging and open biopsy can be used when aspiration alone is not diagnostic. Technetium and indium bone scans may not always differentiate inflammatory arthritides from infectious arthritides.

TREATMENT OPTIONS

Unlike other arthritic disorders of the shoulder, glenohumeral arthritis with massive cuff deficiency does not tend to lead to stiffness. In fact, instability of the glenohumeral joint is a prominent part of the pathology. Passive range of motion tends to be maintained even when patients do not actively elevate their shoulder above the waist level, or actively externally rotate their shoulder.

As with other arthritides, pain is the most prominent complaint in these patients. Pain control consists of rest, antiinflammatory agents, and exercises to maintain the strength of any remaining intact cuff muscles and to maintain as much active motion as possible. Weakness, loss of active range of motion, and pain usually worsen with time. Therefore, long-term nonoperative treatment should be reserved for patients who are poor surgical risks, or those who refuse surgery. The elderly population now has maintained an active lifestyle into their aged years. Loss of a dominant arm can severely handicap patients' abilities to care for themselves. Surgery to maintain function and control pain can be a key for elderly patients to function independently. Aggressive surgical approach for even aged patients may be the best treatment to allow continued independence.

As has been mentioned, a glenohumeral arthrodesis has been used successfully to treat the pain and regain stability in patients with massive cuff deficiency and glenohumeral arthritis. Currently, arthrodesis is used as the first choice of treatment only in patients who have some contraindication for arthroplasty. Deltoid detachment, weakness or paralysis, glenohumeral infection, neuropathic arthropathy, and brachial plexus damage with paralysis, all are contraindications to shoulder arthroplasty. Patients with these problems should be considered candidates for shoulder fusion. The status and possible reconstruction of the opposite shoulder need to be considered before determining final treatment. Patients with bilateral disease and massive cuff deficiency bilaterally may benefit from arthrodesis on one shoulder for strength, and arthroplasty on the other shoulder for mobility. In patients with rheumatoid arthritis or other generalized arthritis, all joints must be considered. The need for a cane or other assistive device, for instance, may make arthrodesis of the shoulder a more reasonable treatment than arthroplasty.

The coracoacromial arch is made up of the acromion, the coracoid, and the coracoacromial ligament. These structures can be deficient as a result of a disease process, or a previous surgery. The most common disease that affects these structures is rheumatoid arthritis. The acromion can become deficient after surgery owing to overzealous acromioplasty or acromionectomy. In patients with massive cuff tear arthropathy the coracoacromial arch is the passive restraint to anterosuperior dislocation of the humeral head; therefore, loss of continuity of the corocoacromial arch is a relative contraindication to shoulder arthrosplasty in patients with massive cuff tear deficiency. Attempts to reconstruct the coracoacromial arch have been only marginally successful. Humeral head replacement in the face of a deficient coracoacromial arch and massive cuff deficiency can result in an anterosuperior dislocation of the humeral prosthesis, with a loss of function. Arthrodeisis of the shoulder joint in this instance can create a more stable, and a more functional shoulder. Shoulder arthrodesis is a difficult procedure to perform when bone stock is of poor quality, or when bone is absent (see Chapter 19). Elderly patients do not tolerate the long periods of immobilization necessary to assure fusion. Furthermore, arthrodesis is associated with a significant failure rate, which may necessitate reoperation and continued immobilization. Whenever possible, glenohumeral arthrodesis should be considered a reconstructive procedure for patients with unique circumstances, or for patients who have failed arthroplasty.[38]

Unconstrained total shoulder arthroplasty has a high failure rate in patients with massive cuff deficiency because of continued instability. Transferring tissue, grafting, or repairing massive cuff defects over a humeral prosthesis does not replace an intact, functioning rotator cuff, and usually leads to failure. Positioning both components so that the loading of the glenoid is symmetrical can be very difficult (Fig. 7). Constrained and semiconstrained shoulder prostheses fail rapidly in these patients. Most authors no longer recommend glenoid resurfacing in patients with massive cuff deficiency.[27] With time, the humerus will continue to migrate superiorly with associated wear of the acromion, leading to eccentric glenoid loading and loosening. Hemiarthroplasty has been the most successful arthroplasty performed in patients with massive cuff deficiency. The pain relief, although not as complete as in total shoulder arthroplasty, has been adequate. Continued instability and weakness can be present after hemiarthroplasty, especially if the humeral head is small. The coracoacromial arch must be intact to prevent superior dislocation. The hemiarthroplasty articulates with the coracoacromial arch and the superior glenoid. The deltoid muscle is the soft-tissue envelope that contains the hemiarthroplasty and must be intact and functional for the hemiarthroplasty to function.

Oversizing the humeral head to fill the soft-tissue envelope can improve the function and stability of the hemiarthroplasty. An oversized humeral head effectively lengthens and lateralizes the humerus (Fig. 8). This approach regains some of the normal tension and length of the deltoid muscle envelope. The center of rotation of the glenohumeral joint is normalized by increasing the length and lateral offset. The prosthesis replaces the space vacated by the missing cuff tissue and this reestablishes the normal tension on the deltoid muscle (Fig. 9). The mechanical advantage of the deltoid is restored, which increases the potential function of the muscle. The oversized humeral head fits over the tuberosities much like an umbrella overhanging the bone. This allows articulation between the humeral head with the acromion and the superior glenoid in full abduction. The tuberosities themselves never articulate with the coracoacromial arch because of the prominence of the prosthesis. The increase in prosthetic surface area available for articulation increases the stability of the joint. In rotator cuff tear arthropathy the soft-tissue envelope is the deltoid muscle and some remnants of subdeltoid bursa. With most of the rotator cuff tissue absent, and erosion of the coracoacromial arch and centralization of the glenoid, there is a large cavity to fill.

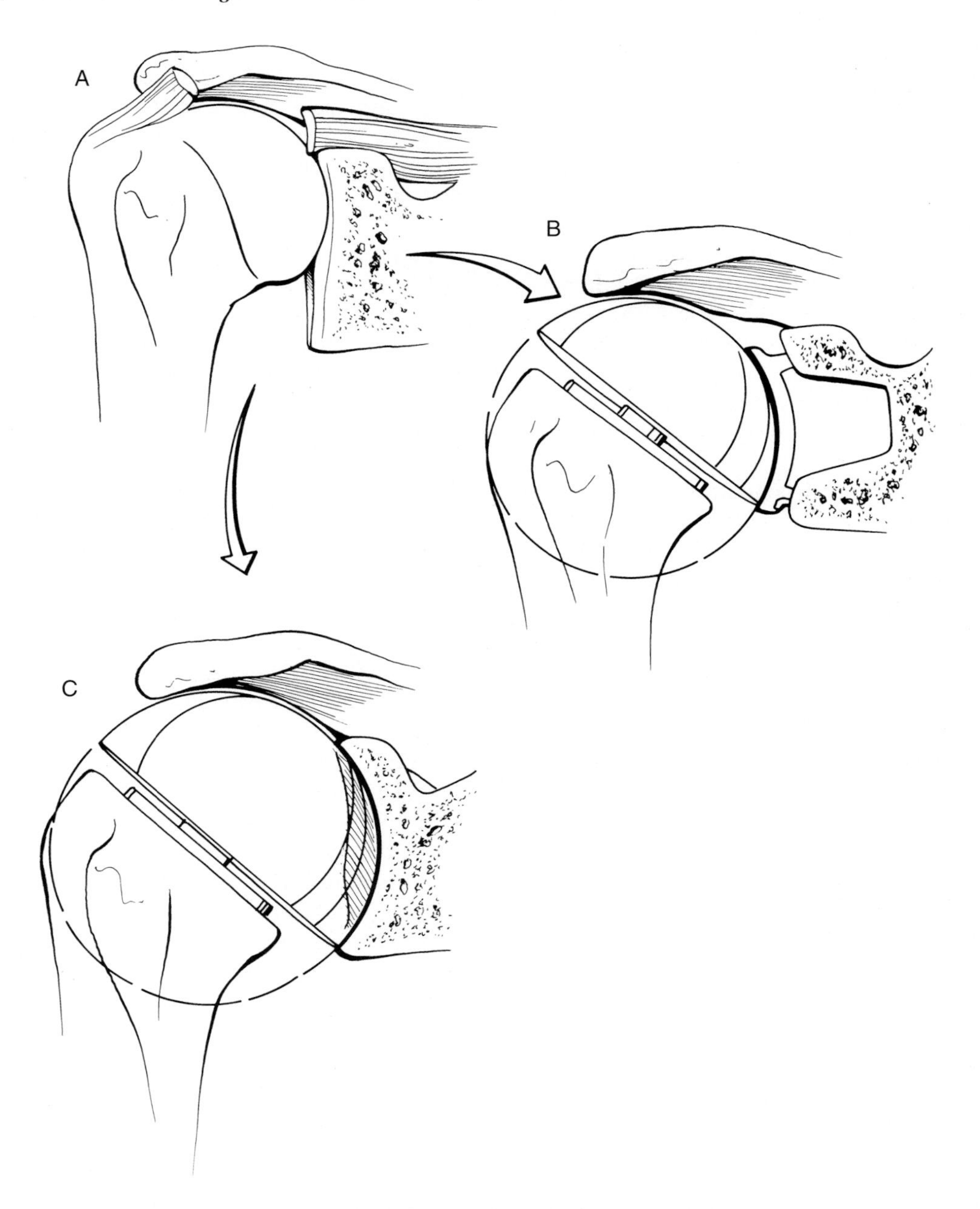

FIG. 7. (A) Superior subluxation with pseudofacet on superior glenoid. **(B)** Simultaneous congruous articulation with acromion on glenoid component is almost impossible to achieve. **(C)** Simultaneous congruous articulation with acromion and glenoid with slight reshaping is easier and avoids potential for glenoid loosening.

Sizing, therefore, is critical to the success of hemiarthroplasty when an oversized humeral head prosthesis is used. In our experience overstuffing the joint causing potential stiffness and loss of function has not been a problem.[33] The prosthesis should articulate with the coracoacromial arch and the superiorly eroded glenoid and should place the deltoid soft-tissue envelope under some tension. A prosthesis that is larger than the anatomic humeral head should still allow posterior subluxation of about 50% of the diameter of the prosthesis posteriorly as Arntz et al.[30] advise. Some authors prefer an anatomically sized hemiarthroplasty, rather than an oversized hemiarthroplasty, to avoid overstuffing the joint. Good to excellent results have been reported using humeral hemiarthroplasties of more anatomic size.

Loss of deltoid function, loss of continuity of the coracoacromial arch, paralysis of the shoulder girdle, infection, and neuropathic arthropathy are all contraindications to hemiarthroplasty. The absence of glenoid bone stock is not a

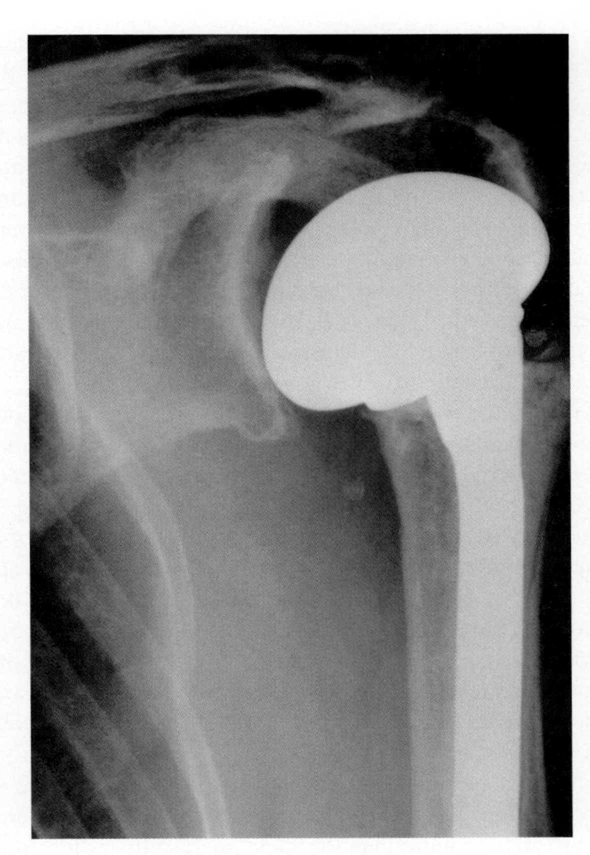

FIG. 8. After hemiarthroplasty the prosthesis replaces the humeral head and articulates with the acromion and the eroded superior glenoid.

contraindication. The humeral prosthesis can articulate with the acromion and function comfortably, even in the face of stress fractures of the acromion.[10,30,33,34]

PREFERRED TREATMENT METHOD

Large-head hemiarthroplasty is our preferred treatment in patients with glenohumeral arthritis and massive cuff deficiency. Patients must have an intact functional deltoid and intact coracoacromial arch, including an intact coracoacromial ligament, to be considered for hemiarthroplasty. Patients unable to perform rehabilitation or those who have uncontrolled seizures or spasticity are poor candidates.

We previously reported upon a series of 13 patients treated with a large-head hemiarthroplasty who were followed up for more than 1 year. Successful relief of pain was achieved in 12 of 13 cases. Active range of motion was maintained or improved in all but 1 patient. Only 1 patient was disappointed in the results of his surgery, and all patients would elect to have the surgery again. Instability did not occur in any of these patients. The functional results of large-head or any type of hemiarthroplasty are unpredictable in rotator cuff tear arthropathy. However, pain relief, the primary goal of surgery, is a predictable result.[33]

SURGICAL TECHNIQUE

Most patients are operated upon with interscalene block anesthesia. The patient is placed on the operating table in the beach chair position with the arm draped free and rested upon an independent mobile arm board. A standard deltopectoral incision is used. A thin pseudocapsule distended with fluid is often encountered anteriorly in the region of the

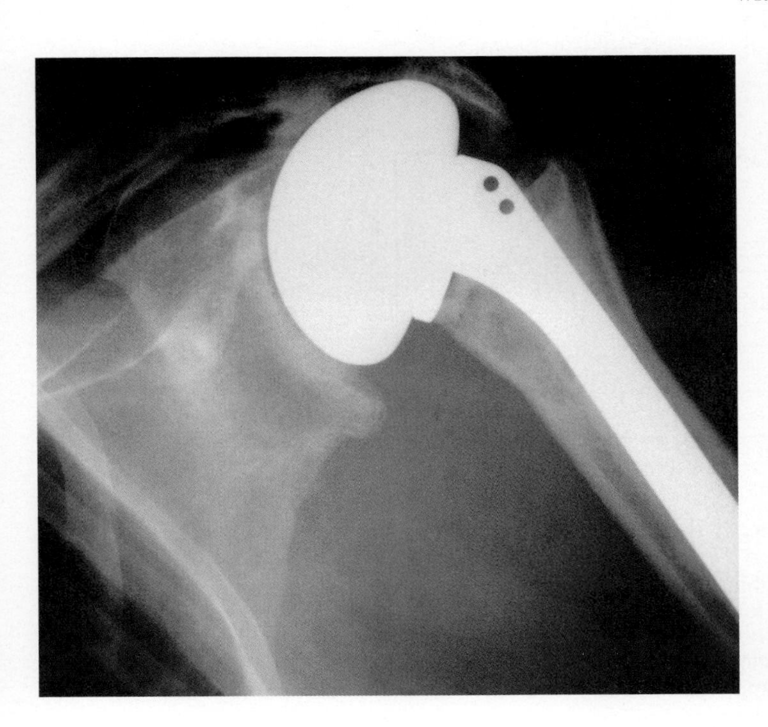

FIG. 9. The deltoid contraction demonstrates the active articulation of the prosthesis.

subscapularis. An incision is made in the pseudocapsule to drain the fluid from the joint, and to allow digital inspection of the joint through the opening. Any residual functional rotator cuff tendon insertions are identified at this time so that they will be preserved in the further dissection. Usually, the lower one-third or one-half, of the subscapularis is intact, and the teres minor is intact. If more than one-half of the subscapularis remained intact, and its insertion interfered with resection of the head and neck and installation of the prosthesis, then as much of the subscapularis as required would be released from its bony insertion (never divide the tendon in its substance). This subscapularis tendon would be reattached to its bony insertion with a dacron tape after installation of the prosthesis.

The resection of the head and neck is as generous as possible, preserving the residual rotator cuff and capsular insertions. The neck shaft angle is dictated by the neck shaft angle of the chosen prosthesis. The version angle is determined by the capsular insertions anteriorly and posteriorly.

The tendon of the long head of the biceps is often ruptured or medially displaced. If present, tendonesis is performed to the anterior lateral humeral shaft. The humeral shaft is then carefully sized with hand reamers to avoid fracture. The bone most often is osteopenic with a wide-open medullary canal, and does not lend itself to a press fit. To date, cement has been used in every case in our series. A cement restrictor plug is placed 1 cm distal to the tip of the prosthetic stem. The cement is injected into the humerus in the liquid state and the humeral prosthesis inserted by hand, not impacted with mallet to avoid potential splitting of the humeral shaft.

The coracoacromial arch is not disturbed. The coracoacromial ligament is always left intact and is the only remaining restraint to anterosuperior dislocation in the severely cuff-deficient patients. The acromion is usually thinned 50% or more. In three cases in our series multiple stress fractures were encountered in the acromion. These fractures were left undisturbed and seemed to tolerate the larger smooth surface of the prosthesis well. Two of these patients did not have significant residual pain. One patient, however, was considered a failure, and was the only failure in the series. The failure, however, was as a result of having fallen and sustaining a glenoid fracture with a posterior subluxation several months postoperatively. In all other cases the under surface of the acromion was a very smooth polished surface that could not be improved. Every effort should be made not to weaken the corcoacromial arch, or to destabilize any pseudarthroses that are encountered.

The glenoid is often eroded centrally, forming a pseudofacet on the superior one half of the glenoid. (The pseudofacet is usually sclerotic, and quite dense.) Marginal osteophytes often widen the articular surface, creating a pseudosocket. This pseudosocket is not disturbed in that it is a major stabilizer of the glenohumeral articulation in the absence of a functional capsule and rotator cuff. On a few occasions we have done minor reshaping of the glenoid by contouring the ridge between the original glenoid and the pseudofacet with a pineapple burr. Very minimal bone was removed so as not to destabilize the socket, nor to expose cancellous bone.

There has been considerable misunderstanding relative to the concept of "large-head hemiarthroplasty." The humeral head is nothing more than the standard 26-mm–radius prosthesis that has an extended neck length (Fig. 10). As the neck length (head height) is increased with a constant radius, the area of coverage of the prosthesis on the humerus increases very rapidly. As the size of the coverage area increases, the prosthesis becomes too bulky; therefore, the margins of the prosthesis need to be pared down to more functional limits. Simply put, these are 26-mm–radius humeral heads with extended neck lengths.

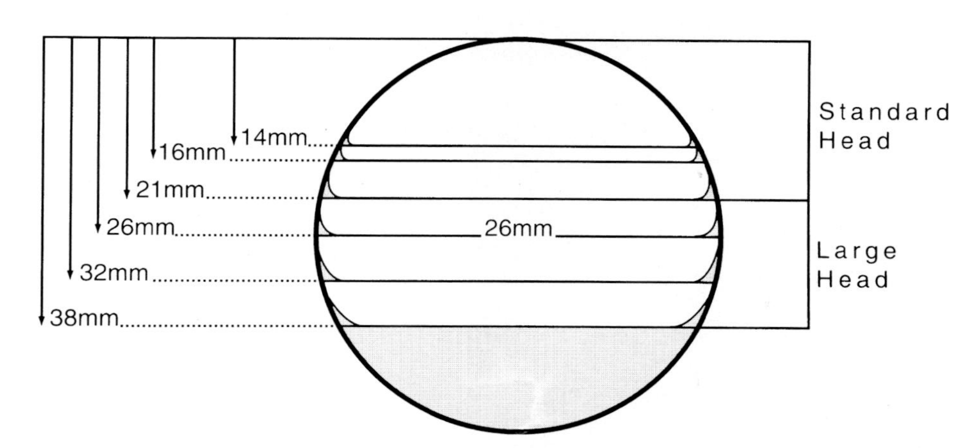

FIG. 10. "Large-head hemiarthroplasty" is nothing more than the standard 26-mm–radius prosthesis that has an extended neck length. As the neck length (head height) is increased with a constant radius, the area of coverage of the prosthesis on the humerus increases very rapidly. As the size of the coverage area increases, the prosthesis becomes too bulky; therefore, the margins of the prosthesis need to be pared down to more functional limits. Simply put, this is a 26-mm–radius humeral head with an extended neck length.

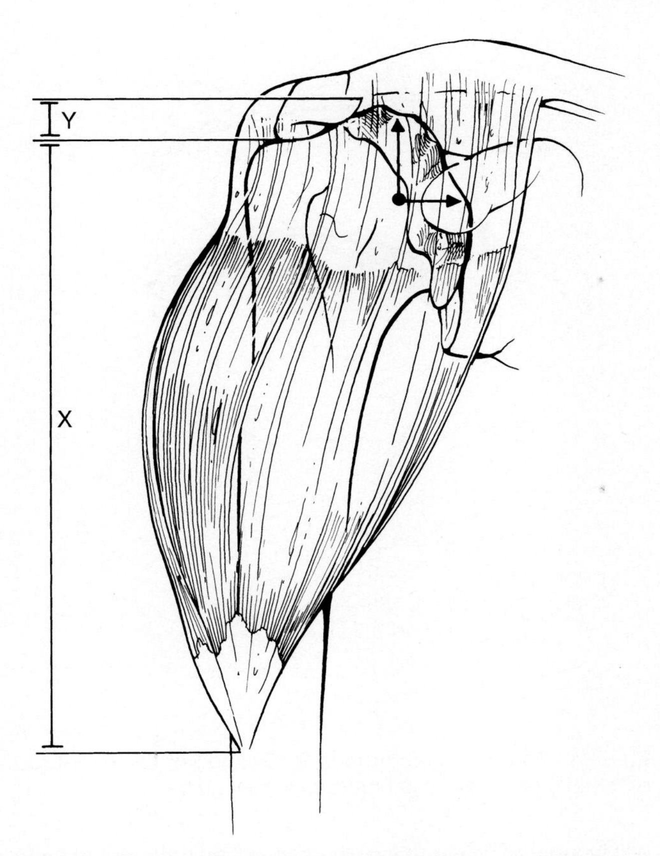

FIG. 11. In rotator cuff tear arthropathy, there is medial and superior displacement of the center of rotation of the glenohumeral joint. The deltoid muscle loses its normal convex contour resulting in "dimpling" from humeral shortening and centralization.

In rotator cuff tear arthropathy, there is medial and superior displacement of the center of rotation of the glenohumeral joint (Fig. 11). The deltoid muscle loses its normal convex contour, resulting in dimpling from the humeral shortening and centralization. When viewed from the lateral side (Fig.12) the diseased glenohumeral joint shows the superior subluxed humeral head articulating with the coracoacromial arch. Again, the deltoid muscle loses its normal convex contour and is dimpled anterolaterally, and posteriorly because of the loss of bone and centralization of the joint. The large head of the prosthesis reapproximates the volume of the joint, which has been lost by erosion of the cartilage and bone, and retraction of the soft tissues (Fig.13). Lateralization of the center of rotation of the joint is also accomplished by the increased humeral head size. The deltoid envelope is tightened by lengthening the humerus. The distance between the acromion and the greater tuberosity is improved, and the space previously occupied by the rotator cuff tendons is filled with the large head hemiarthroplasty. (see Fig. 6). The anteroposterior contour, and the width of the deltoid, are also restored. There is a congruous articulation of the oversized prosthetic head with the coracoacromial arch and restoration of humeral length (Fig.14). Therefore, the large-head hemiarthroplasty improves the mechanical advantage of the deltoid envelope by increasing its functional length in all planes and reestablishing the center of rotation near its normal position. The enlarged size of the hemiarthroplasty also contributes to stability by applying tension to the soft-tissue envelope.

The tension should be no greater, and is usually less than that of a normal joint. Overstuffing of the joint is almost impossible in advanced rotator cuff tear arthropathy. If the prosthesis can not be subluxed by 50% posteriorly in neutral rotation, it may be too tight.

Clinically, the surgeon should attempt to choose the size of prosthesis that fills the void created by abnormal erosion of the glenoid and coracoacromial arch (see Fig. 11). A nearly congruous fit of the large-head hemiarthroplasty with the coracoacromial arch will result in an improved center of rotation of the joint (Fig. 13).

Once the proper size is chosen, the final prosthesis is reduced. The deltoid falls in place and the incision is closed cosmetically. There is no attempt to repair the rotator cuff tendons unless part of the subscapularis had to be removed to gain access to the proximal humerus. If the subscapularis does need to be repaired, it should be repaired to bone. The deltopectoral interval does not require closure. A soft drain is used for 24 hours.

In the recovery room, the patient is started on passive range of motion exercises. Passive supine elevation with a pulley, and passive external rotation within the limits of the subscapularis repair are started immediatly. After 2 weeks

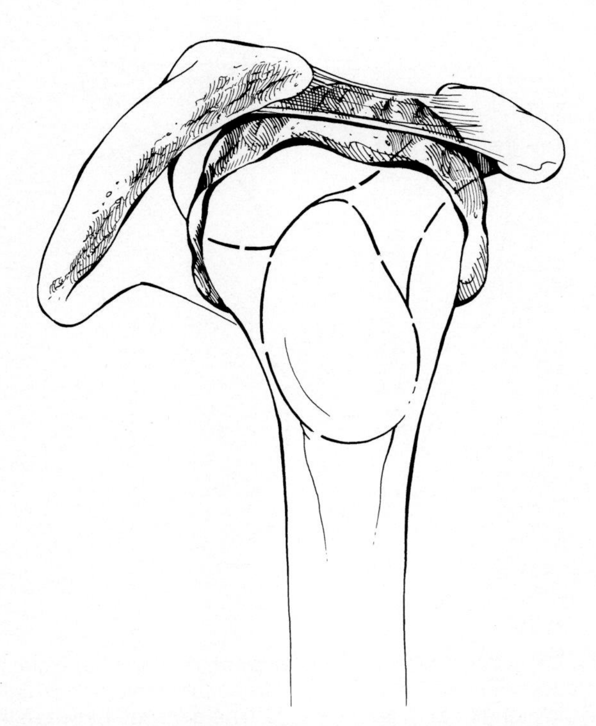

FIG. 12. The diseased glenohemeral joint slows the superior subluxed humeral head articulating with the coracoacromial arch.

the pulley is used to regain full forward elevation against gravity. At 4 weeks, passive internal and external rotation is started. Active elevation in the supine position is started at 4 to 6 weeks and continued for the next several months. Active internal and external rotation in the supine position is also started at 4 to 6 weeks, and continued for the next several months. The prosthesis should articulate with the acromion and the eroded glenoid in a nearly concentric arch (see Fig. 13). Usually, at 4 tó 5 months postoperatively, patients are able to actively flex to approximately 50 to 70 degrees against gravity. At this point further progress and strengthening may be difficult. However, strength will increase up to a year or more after surgery if the patients are aggressive with an exercise program. Eccentric lowering from full forward flexion to 90 degrees, and active elevation from 90 degrees back to full elevation can be extremely helpful in regaining deltoid strength and improving active range of motion. If there is any feeling of instability in the early postoperative period, exercising in the plane of the scapula rather than in neutral rotation can help maintain stability while continuing to improve deltoid strength. It is very important to continue exercises for at least 1 year postoperatively to maximize the final functional result.

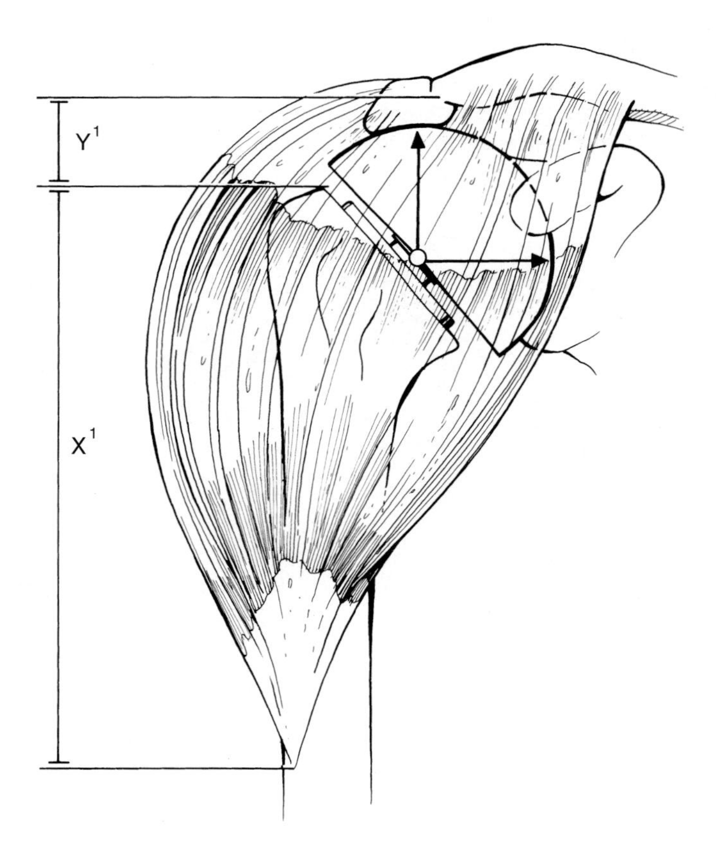

FIG. 13. Lateralization of the center of rotation of the joint by increased humeral head size. The deltoid envelope is tightened by lengthening the humerus. The distance between the acromion and the greater tuberosity is improved, and the space previously occupied by the rotator cuff tendons is filled with the large-head hemiarthroplasty.

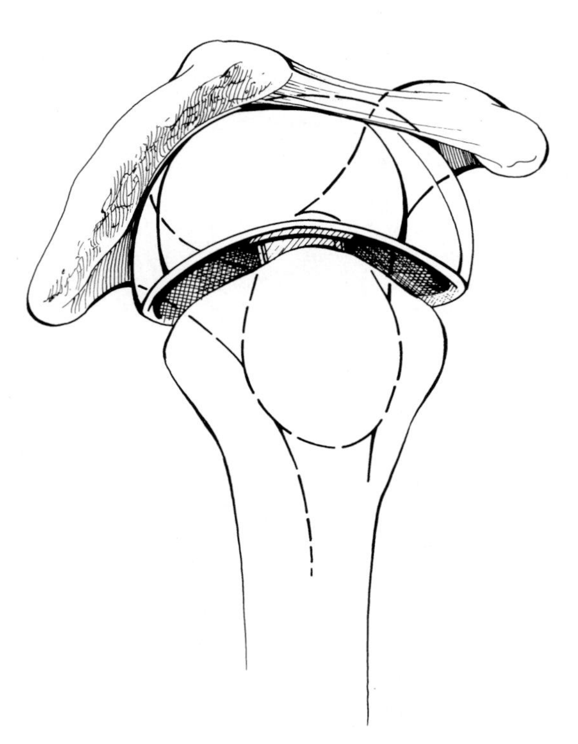

FIG. 14. There is a congruous articulation of the oversized prosthetic head with the coracoacromial arch.

The goal of rehabilitation is to strengthen the deltoid and remaining shoulder girdle muscles to maximize function. Pain relief with hemiarthroplasty is usually quite good. The active function of the shoulder correlates significantly with patient compliance with the exercise program. Weakness in external rotation is always persistent, but forward flexion and abduction can be surprisingly strong.

In summary, superior mechanical instability and the loss of the normal center of rotation of the glenohumeral joint found in rotator cuff tear arthropathy create stresses across the joint that preclude total shoulder arthroplasty. In this unique set of circumstances, hemiarthroplasty with a longer neck length (head height) can restore some of the soft-tissue tension that has been lost and result in a more stable functional construct. Both anatomically sized and enlarged sized hemiarthroplasty will relieve pain without high risk of loosening. Because pain relief is the goal of surgical treatment, satisfactory results can be achieved with either procedure. Large-head hemiarthroplasty theoretically should improve function as well as relieve pain, but adequate studies are still pending.

REFERENCES

1. Codman EA. *The shoulder: rupture of the supraspinatus tendon and other lesions in or about the subacromial bursa.* Boston: T. Todd, 1934.
2. Adams R. *A treatise of rheumatic gout or chronic rheumatic arthritis of all the joints*, 2nd ed. London: John Churchill and Sons, 1873:1–568.
3. McCarty DJ, Halverson PB, Carrera GF, Brewer BJ, Kogin F. "Milwaukee shoulder": association of microspheroids containing hydroxyapatite crystals, active collagenase and neutral protease with rotator cuff defects. I. Clinical aspects. *Arthritis Rheum* 1981;24:464–473.

4. Neer CS II, Craig EV, Fukuda H. Cuff tear arthropathy. *J Bone Joint Surg [Am]* 1983;65:1232–1244.
5. Halverson PB, Cheung HS, McCarty DJ, Garancis J, Mandel N. "Milwaukee shoulder": association of microsperoids containing hydroxyapatite crystals, active collagenese and neutral protease with rotator cuff defects. II Synovial fluid studies. *Arthritis Rheum* 1981:24:474–483.
6. Garancis JC, Cheung HS, Halverson PB, McCarty DJ. "Milwaukee shoulder": association of microspheroids containing hydroxyapatite crystals, active collagenase, and neutral protease with rotator cuff defects. III Morphological and biochemical studies of the excised synovium showing chondromatosis. *Arthritis Rheum* 1981;24: 484–491.
7. Halverson PB, McCarty DJ, Cheung HS, et al. Milwaukee shoulder syndrome: eleven additional cases with involvement of the knee in seven (basic calcium phosphate crystals deposition disease). *Semin Arthritis Rheum* 1984;14:36–44.
8. Dieppe PA, Docherty M, Macfarlane DG, et al. Apatite associated destructive arthritis. *Br J Rhematol* 1984;23:84–91.
9. Altman R, Asch E, Bloch D, et al. Development of critieria for the classification and reporting of osteoarthritis. *Arthritis Rheum* 1986;29: 1029–1049.
10. Neer CS, Bigliani LU, Hawkins RJ. Rupture of the long head of the biceps related to subacromial impingement. *Orthop Trans* 1977;1:111.
11. Neer CS II. Replacement arthroplasty for glenohumeral osteoarthritis. *J Bone Joint Surg [Am]* 1974;56:1–13.
12. Neer CS II, Watson KC, Stanton FJ. Recent experience in total shoulder replacement. *J Bone Joint Surg [Am]* 1982;64:319–337.
13. Amstutz HC, Sewhoy AL, Clarke IC. UCLA anatomic total shoulder. *Clin Orthop* 1981;155:7–20.
14. Amstutz HC, Thomas BJ, Kalso JM, et al. The Dana total shoulder arthropathy. *J Bone Joint Surg [Am]* 1988;74:1174–1182.
15. Faludi DD, Weiland AJ. Cementless total shoulder arthroplasty: preliminary experience with thirteen cases. *Orthopeadics* 1982;6: 431–437.
16. McElwain JP, English F. The early results of porous coated total shoulder arthroplasty. *Clin Orthop* 1987;218:217–224.
17. Ellman H, Jinnah R. Experience with the Dana hooded component for cuff deficient shoulder arthroplasty. *Orthop Trans* 1986;10:217.
18. Figgie HC III, Inglis AC, Goldberg VM, et al. An analysis of factors affecting the long term results of total shoulder arthroplasty in inflammatory arthritis. *J Arthroplasty* 1988;3:39–46.
19. Clayton ML, Ferlic DC, Jeffers PD. Prosthetic arthroplasty of the shoulder. *Clin Orthop* 1982;164:184–191.
20. Lettin AWF, Copeland SA, Scales JT. The Stanmore total shoulder replacement. *J Bone Joint Surg [Br]* 1982;64:47–51; int replacement. *Orthop Clin North Am* 1975;6:565–583.
21. Thomas BJ, Amstutz HC, Cracchiolo A. Shoulder arthroplasty for rheumatoid arthritis. *Clin Orthop* 1991;265:125–128.
22. Post M, Haskell SS, Jablon M. Total shoulder replacement with a constrained Richards, R. shoulder arthrodesis. Presented at ninth combined meeting of orthopaedic prosthesis. *J Bone Joint Surg [Am]* 1980;62: 327–335.
23. Post M, Jablon M. Constrained total shoulder arthroplasty. Long term follow-up observations. *Clin Orthop* 1983;173:109–116.
24. Fenlin JM. Total glenohumeral joint replacement. *Orthop Clin North Am* 1975;6:565–583.
25. Post M. Constrained arthroplasty: its uses and misuse: *Semin Arthroplasty* 1990;2:151–159.
26. Loughlin MJ, Morris JM, West WF. The semiconstrained total shoulder arthroplasty, *J Bone Joint Surg [Am]* 1979;61:574–581.
27. Franklin JL, Barrett WP, Jackins SF, Matsen FA. Glenoid loosening in total shoulder arthroplasty: association with rotator cuff deficiency. *J Arthroplasty* 1988;3:39–46.
28. Bonutti PM, Hawkins RJ. Component loosening in unconstrained shoulder arthroplasty. *Semin Arthroplasty* 1990;2:124–128.
29. Hawkins RJ, Bell RH, Jallay B. Total shoulder arthroplasty. *Clin Orthop* 1989;242:188–194.
30. Arntz CT, Jenkins S, Matsen FA. Prosthetic replacement of the shoulder for the treatment of defects in the rotator cuff and the surface of the glenohumeral joint. *J Bone Joint Surg [Am]* 1993;75:485–491.
31. Pollack RG, Delig ED, McIlveen SJ, Flatow EL, Bigliani LN. Prosthetic replacement in rotator cuff deficient shoulder. *J Shoulder Elbow Surg* 1992;1:4:173–186.
32. Boyd AD, Thomas WH, Scott RD, Sledge CB, Thornhill TS. Total shoulder arthrophasty versus hemiarthroplasty. *J Arthroplasty* 1990;5: 329–336.
33. Frieman BG, Allardyce TJ. Hemiarthroplasty in rotator cuff tear arthropathy. *Oper Tech Orthop* 1994;4:253–257.
34. Field LD, Zubinski SJ, Dines DM, Warren RF, Altchek DW. Hemiarthroplasty of the shoulder for rotator cuff arthropathy. *J Shoulder Elbow Surg* 1997;6:118–23.
35. Rowe CR. Arthrodesis of the shoulder used in treating painful conditions. *Clin Orthop* 1983;173:92–96.
36. Wilde AH, Brems JJ, Boumphrey FR. Arthrodesis of the shoulder. *Orthop Clin North Am* 1987;18:463–472.
37. Hawkins RJ, Neer CS II. A functional analysis of shoulder fusions. *Clin Orthop* 1987;223:65–76.
38. Flatow EL, Connor PM, Levine WN, Arroyo JS, Pollock RG, Bigliani LU. Coracoacromial arch reconstruction for anterosuperior instability. ASES, 13th open meeting, San Francisco, CA. Feb. 2–16, 1997.
39. Richards R. Shoulder arthrodesis. Presented at ninth combined meeting of orthopaedic associations of the English speaking world. Toronto, Canada, 1992.
40. Burkhead WZ, Hutton KS. Biologic Resurfacing of the glenoid with hemiarthroplasty of the shoulder. *J Shoulder Elbow Surg* 1995;4: 4263–4270.

Disorders of the Shoulder: Diagnosis and Management,
edited by Joseph P. Iannotti and Gerald R. Williams, Jr.
Lippincott Williams & Wilkins, Philadelphia © 1999.

CHAPTER 22

Complications of Shoulder Arthroplasty

Robert H. Cofield, Win Chang, and John W. Sperling

INTRODUCTION

Outcomes of shoulder arthroplasty can be adversely affected by several situations. It is useful to separate the less than optimal result from a complication. Following surgery, without developing a complication, patients can have more than expected residual pain, a smaller arc of movement, or a decrease in strength.

There are a number of categories of complications. One useful way is to consider them in four categories. First, a condition can exist along with glenohumeral arthritis such as a chronic dislocation or a rotator cuff tear, and this can either persist or recur in the postoperative period. Second, the healing process may be altered; for example, lack of subscapularis tendon healing leading to weakness of internal rotation or anterior shoulder instability, or too intense a healing process such as a periarthritic inflammatory response leading to joint stiffness. Third, there are rather general complications for most musculoskeletal surgery such as the medical complications that occur in an older-aged group, wound problems, infections, nerve injuries, and intraoperative fractures. Finally, in a fourth category are complications that are rather specific to arthroplasty, including periprosthetic fracture in the postoperative period or loosening of a component from its attachment to bone.

It is probably better to consider the complications of total shoulder arthroplasty and humeral head replacement (hemiarthroplasty) separately, for the frequency of complications is different and the nature of the complications varies. However, it will be useful to compare and contrast one against the other.

There is extensive literature on this subject; however, complications are often addressed obliquely in the materials presented, with only a few articles concentrating on a specific complication or complications per se. By collating this literature one can glean quite nicely the types and frequency of complications, but there is less information about the nuances of each type of complication and treatment recommendations. Thus, we have chosen not only to detail the information in various patient series and to outline the fewer articles addressing a specific complication but also to present the materials developed over time at our institution that can be analyzed in some depth.

TYPES AND FREQUENCIES OF COMPLICATIONS

Literature

We identified 22 patient series published since 1980 on unconstrained total shoulder arthroplasty.[1,2,4–6,10,13,14,18,19,23–25,28,34,40,45,52,53,57,58,65] Combined, these series have reported on 1,183 total shoulder arthroplasties. The authors identified 23 different complications. The total number of

R. H. Cofield: Department of Orthopedics, Mayo Medical School, Mayo Clinic and Mayo Foundation, Rochester, Minnesota 55905.
W. Chang: Somers Orthopaedic Surgery and Sports Medicine Group, Somers, New York 10589.
J. W. Sperling: Department of Orthopedic Surgery, Mayo Clinic and Mayo Foundation, Rochester, Minnesota 55905.

complications was 123 for a relative percentage of 10.4%—assuming one complication occurred in each of the shoulders having a complication. Certainly some shoulders had two or more complications, so the number of shoulders having a complication would be somewhat less than 10%. Only rotator cuff tearing, instability, and glenoid loosening occurred in more than 1% of shoulders reported (Table 1).

We identified 20 patient series reporting on hemiarthroplasty of the shoulder that have been published since 1980.[3,6,8,10,16,21,26,29,30,33,36–38,48,53,54,56,58,63,69] These included reports on 498 shoulders. Nineteen different complications were identified and 78 total complications were reported, for relative frequency of complications of 15.7%—assuming only one complication occurred in each shoulder (Table 2). Six complications occurred at a frequency of 1% or more. These included glenohumeral instability, painful glenoid arthritis, humeral tuberosity nonunion, rotator cuff tearing, nerve injury, and infection.

TABLE 2. *Complications of H.H.R.*[a]

Complication	No.	(%)[b]
Instability	14	(2.8)
Glenoid arthritis	12	(2.4)
Tuberosity nonunion	9	(1.8)
Rotator cuff tear	9	(1.8)
Nerve injury	8	(1.6)
Infection	5	(1.0)
Intraoperative fracture	3	(0.6)
Humeral loosening	3	(0.6)
Wound problems	2	(0.4)
Tuberosity malposition	2	(0.4)
Hematoma	2	(0.4)
Perioperative death	2	(0.4)
Postoperative fracture	1	(0.2)
Heterotopic ossification	1	(0.2)
Impingement	1	(0.2)
Reflex dystrophy	1	(0.2)
Acromioclavicular pain	1	(0.2)
Pain, unexplained	1	(0.2)
Stiffness	1	(0.2)
Totals = 19	78	(15.7)

[a] 20 series since 1980/498 shoulders studied.
[b] Relative percentages of each complication, assuming one complication occurred in each of the shoulders having a complication.

The Mayo Clinic Experience

Total Shoulder Arthroplasty

Four hundred nineteen Neer total shoulder arthroplasties were performed in 369 patients by the senior author (RHC) between December 1975 and December 1989. To examine the type and frequency of complications encountered, all medical records were reviewed irrespective of the length of follow-up. The mean length of follow-up was 4.9 years and ranged from 21 days to 14.3 years. Eighty-seven shoulders were followed less than 2 years, 138 from 2 to 5 years, 126 from more than 5 years to 10 years, and 68 from more than 10 years to 15 years. Average patient age was 62.4 years (range 17 to 87 years). There were 213 women and 156 men. Diagnosis included osteoarthritis in 161, rheumatoid arthritis in 128, posttraumatic arthritis in 47, rotator cuff arthropathy in 37, humeral head osteonecrosis in 17, failed humeral head prosthesis in 15, failed total shoulder arthroplasty in 7, shoulder fusion in 4, and excision arthroplasty in 3. In addition to the shoulders with the previous reconstructive procedures mentioned, there were 47 other previous surgical procedures. These included rotator cuff surgery in 24, internal fixation for fractures in 18, and a shoulder stabilization procedure in 5. Twelve shoulders had more than one of these procedures.

TABLE 1. *Complications of TSA*[a]

Complication	No.	(%)[b]
Rotator cuff tear	23	(1.9)
Instability	18	(1.5)
Glenoid loosening	15	(1.3)
Intraoperative fracture	15	(0.9)
Malposition	7	(0.6)
Nerve injury	7	(0.6)
Infection	5	(0.4)
Humeral loosening	4	(0.3)
Postoperative fracture	4	(0.3)
Wound problem	4	(0.3)
Wire breakage	3	(0.3)
Impingement	3	(0.3)
Tuberosity non-union	3	(0.3)
Pain, unexplained	3	(0.3)
Reflex dystrophy	2	(0.2)
Hematoma	2	(0.2)
Component dissociation	2	(0.2)
Extruded cement	2	(0.2)
Heterotopic ossification	1	(0.1)
Stiffness	1	(0.1)
Spacer dislocation	1	(0.1)
Intraoperative death	1	(0.1)
Pulmonary embolism	1	(0.1)
Totals = 23	123	(10.4)

[a] 22 series since 1980/1183 shoulders studied.
[b] Relative percentages of each complication, assuming one complication occurred in each of the shoulders having a complication.

Preoperative shoulder subluxation was present in 63 shoulders. Subluxation was both anterior and superior in 31, superior in 15, posterior in 14, and both anterior and inferior in 3. Intraoperatively 216 shoulders had rotator cuff disease. Ninety-eight had noticeably thin rotator cuff tissue (72 in rheumatoid arthritis), 58 had a rotator cuff tear less than 3 cm in the longest diameter, and 60 had rotator cuff tearing greater or equal to 3 cm in the longest diameter. Forty-one had a variable degree of glenoid bone deficiency and 16 had some deficiency of the bone of the proximal humerus. Two hundred fifty-eight of the glenoid components were all high-density polyethylene and 161 had metal backing. Two hundred and eleven humeral head components were of the larger size and 208 of the smaller size. Three hundred sixty-two humeral stems were press-fitted and 57 were cemented in place.

The complications were defined according to time of occurrence, with early complications occurring within 90 days of surgery and late complications occurring after this period of time. The complications were also divided into medical and surgical groups. Each medical complication was identified as minor, requiring little or no treatment, or major, requiring significant medical intervention or being life-threatening. Surgical complications were classified as minor when there was no compromise of outcome and little or no treatment was needed, or as major when the final result was compromised or reoperation was required.

The Kaplan-Meier method was used to estimate the survivorship data. Log rank tests were used to compare individual survivorships. The Cox proportional hazard model was used to test the association of continuous variables with survivorship and to perform multivariate analysis of survival of the prosthetic surgery. The chi-square test was used to test differences between discreet variables. A P value of less than 0.05 was considered significant.

There were 15 medical complications in 10 patients (2.7%). All medical complications occurred early: 5 were cardiac, 4 were a deep venous thrombosis, 3 were pulmonary embolism, and 1 each was a hypertensive crisis, a cerebral ischemic event, and acute pancreatitis. Eight complications, occurring in 5 patients, were considered to be major complications.

Surgical complications occurred in 90 shoulders of 90 patients. There were 5 intraoperative complications including proximal humeral fracture in 3, glenoid fracture in 1, and axillary nerve laceration in 1. A total of 152 postoperative complications occurred in the remaining 85 shoulders (Table 3). Fifty-two occurred early and 100 occurred late (Table 4). Twenty-seven of the complications were considered to be minor, 35 were considered to be major, and an additional 95 were considered to be major and required reoperation (Table 5).

Of the 90 shoulders in 90 patients (21%) having one or more surgical complications, in 16 (4%) the complication was minor, in 29 (7%) the complication was major, and in 45 (11%) the complication was major and required reoperation. The time from surgery to the development of a complication was affected by diagnosis, with patients in the cuff tear arthritis, revision procedure, and osteonecrosis groups faring worse. In general, complications increased in frequency over time (Fig. 1). Reoperations were also affected by diagnosis and related to time (Fig. 2). Again those in the cuff tear arthritis, revision procedure, and osteonecrosis groups had more frequent reoperations.

Risk factors for any complication and for specific compli-

TABLE 3. *Postoperative Surgical Complications*

Complication	No.	(%)
Subluxation	44	(11)
Rotator cuff tear	33	(8)
Glenoid loosening	19	(5)
Brachial plexopathy	11	(3)
Dislocation	10	(2)
Humeral loosening	9	(2)
Infection (deep)	6	(1)
Impingement	5	(1)
Dysesthesias	5	(1)
Infection (superficial)	4	(1)
Hematoma	2	(0.5)
Reflex dystrophy	2	(0.5)
Tuberosity non-union	1	(0.2)
Long head of biceps rupture	1	(0.2)
Total	152	

TABLE 4. *Timing of Postoperative Surgical Complications*

Complication	Early[a]	Late
Subluxation	16	28
Rotator cuff tear	11	22
Glenoid loosening		19
Brachial plexopathy	11	
Dislocation		10
Humeral loosening		9
Infection (deep)		6
Impingement		5
Dysesthesias	5	
Infection (superficial)	4	
Hematoma	2	
Reflex dystrophy	2	
Tuberosity non-union	1	
Long head of biceps rupture		1
Totals	52	100

[a] Early ≤90 days, late >90 days postoperative.

TABLE 5. *Severity of Surgical Complications*

Complication	Minor[a]	Major	Reoperation
Subluxation	1	11	32
Rotator cuff tear	5	11	17
Glenoid loosening		2	17
Brachial plexopathy	3	8	
Dislocation			10
Humeral loosening			9
Infection (deep)			6
Impingement	5		
Dysesthesias	5		
Infection (superficial)	2		2
Fracture	3	1	
Hematoma	1		1
Reflex dystrophy		2	
Nerve laceration			1
Tuberosity non-union	1		
Long head of biceps rupture	1		
Totals	27	35	95

[a] See text for definitions.

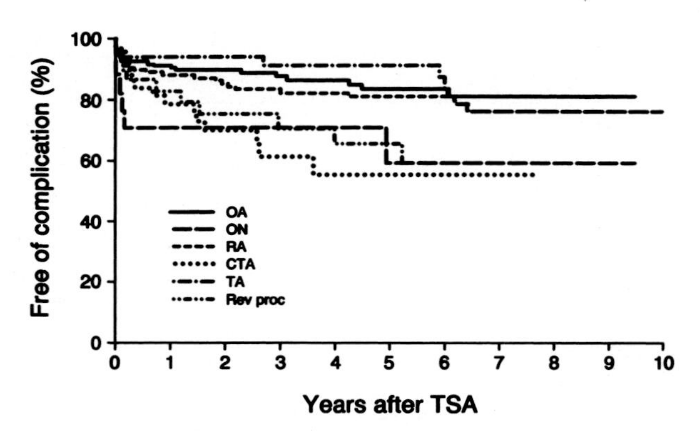

FIG. 1. Time to first complication by diagnosis.

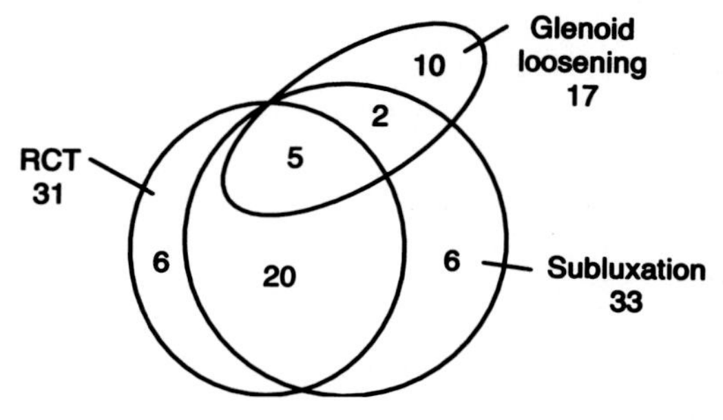

FIG. 3. Relation of rotator cuff tear, shoulder instability, and symptomatic glenoid loosening in primary TSA.

cations were carefully studied. Statistically significant risk factors ($P<0.05$) for developing a complication after total shoulder arthroplasty included the diagnosis of cuff tear arthropathy, preexisting rotator cuff disease, and previous shoulder surgery. Risk factors for postoperative shoulder instability, subluxation, or dislocation, included older age, increased preoperative range of external rotation, preexistent rotator cuff disease, and small prosthetic humeral head size. Significant risk factors for postoperative rotator cuff tearing including the diagnosis of cuff tear arthropathy, preexisting rotator cuff disease, and a history of previous major shoulder reconstruction. Only the diagnosis of cuff tear arthropathy was a significant risk factor for glenoid loosening. Glenoid loosening otherwise was spread evenly among the other diagnostic groups. Seemingly there was a relation between rotator cuff tearing, shoulder instability, and symptomatic glenoid loosening in those shoulders undergoing a primary total shoulder arthroplasty as illustrated in the Venn diagram (Fig. 3).

It seems clear relative to total shoulder arthroplasty that if one focuses on identifying complications and includes all patients in the follow-up period, the frequency of complications is somewhat greater than the 10% recorded in the literature and may well approach 20% as indicated in our series. It is also clear that there are many different complications, many of lower frequency, contributing to the overall complication rate. The three major complications are without question postoperative instability, rotator cuff tearing, and glenoid loosening.

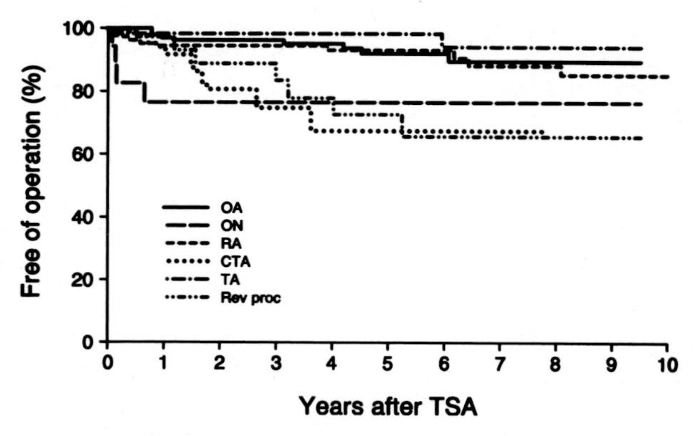

FIG. 2. Reoperation by diagnosis.

Hemiarthroplasty

We have analyzed our hemiarthroplasties in two groups. The first group includes those with glenohumeral arthritis—either osteoarthritis or rheumatoid arthritis. Between July 1977 and March 1983, 77 shoulders were so treated in 74 patients.[20] Six patients with six surgically treated shoulders were lost to follow-up and four others died before evaluations were complete. This resulted in 67 shoulders in 64 patients forming the basis of the review. There were 35 shoulders in 35 patients with osteoarthritis and 32 shoulders in 29 patients with rheumatoid arthritis. Follow-up evaluation averaged 9.3 years and ranged from 2 to 14.1 years. There were only three complications: 1 patient developed a hematoma requiring surgical evacuation; the second had a humeral shaft fracture at the time of surgery, which was treated with internal fixation using a long-stemmed component and cerclage, and the fracture healed. The third complication was a brachial plexus traction injury that recovered without residual symptomatology. In evaluating these complications we considered the brachial plexopathy a minor complication, the humeral fracture a major complication, and the hematoma a major complication requiring reoperation.

The outcomes of humeral head replacements performed for acute proximal humeral head fractures and chronic proximal humeral head fractures between 1979 and 1995 were also reviewed, focusing on complications.[50] Twenty-eight replacements were performed in 26 patients with acute fractures and 55 hemiarthroplasties were performed in 55 patients for problems that arose following initial treatment for a proximal humeral fracture or fracture–dislocation. Again, all patients were included to be sure that every complication was recognized during the follow-up period. In the acute group follow-up averaged 56 months, ranging from 2 to 184 months, whereas in the chronic group follow-up averaged 57 months ranging from 5 to 156 months. The complications identified for these acute and chronic fracture groups are displayed in Table 6. One is immediately impressed that these are much greater in number and many more types of compli-

TABLE 6. *Complications of Herniarthroplasty for Fractures*[a]

Complication	Acute (No. = 28)	Chronic (No. = 55)	Totals (No. = 83)
Instability	2	10	12
Glenoid arthritis	2	7	9
Rotator cuff tear	2	4	6
Infection	3	3	6
Tuberosity non-union	2	2	4
Fracture		3	3
Implant malposition		3	3
Implant loosening	1	2	3
Tuberosity malunion		2	2
Reflex dystrophy	1		1
Totals	13	36	49

[a] Adapted from Muldoon MP, Cofield RH. Complications of Humeral Head Replacements for Proximal Humeral Fractures. Amer. Acad. Orthop. Surg. *Instructional Course Lectures.* 1997;46:15–24.

cations arose when compared with hemiarthroplasty done for the elective treatment for shoulder arthritis.

SPECIFIC TYPES OF COMPLICATIONS

The six significant and most common complications will be individually presented. Material will generally be arranged in the following sequence: the recognition and evaluation of the complication with a classification system if one is applicable; reference to the frequency of the complication as presented in the literature; identification of specific literature for the complication; notation of materials included in pertinent review articles; the experience with this complication at the Mayo Clinic; methods to prevent the complication; and treatment of the complication.

Nerve Injury

Physical examination of the operated upper extremity is the key to diagnosis following surgery. It is quite practical to ask the patient to perform active movement of the hand and wrist and to test for isometric contractions of the elbow flexors and the posterior portion of the deltoid muscle. This usually can be accomplished on the day of surgery; however, interscalene block is now commonly used, making it sometimes necessary to perform the neurologic examination the day following surgery. Should a nerve injury be identified, the common peripheral nerve injury classification that is defined by Seddon or Sunderland is probably useful in retrospect, but has less value in the acute setting.[59,62] Weber and coworkers developed a post-hip arthroplasty nerve palsy severity scale based on symptoms, physical examination, electromyographic findings, and the compromise of postsurgical rehabilitation,[66] and it is useful as a grading system. This scale though, as with the more standard classification scheme, is fully applicable only over time, as the nerve injury evolves, and less helpful in the acute setting. If a nerve injury is identified on the initial-screening examination, a more careful neurologic examination of the upper extremity is performed to define the lesion more precisely. Electromyographic testing may be useful after the initial 3 weeks, but as will be explained later, is probably more practical at 4 to 6 weeks, should neurologic recovery not occur in the interim.

In the 22-patient series encompassing 1,183 operated on shoulders that were reported since 1980 and defined in Table 1, seven nerve injuries (0.6%) were identified following total shoulder arthroplasty. In the 20-patient series involving 498 shoulders reported since 1980, eight nerve injuries (1.6%) were identified following hemiarthroplasty. The slightly higher frequency following hemiarthroplasty may be attributed to this surgery often occurring in the acute setting where some degree of nerve injury might complicate the initial fracture and yet not be fully defined because of the inability to perform a complete examination before surgery. Only one article has been published on neurologic complications after total shoulder arthroplasty.[43] These authors identified eight neurologic deficits reported in the literature. Of these eight injuries, five were axillary nerve palsies, only one of which completely resolved and two partially recovered. One musculocutaneous nerve palsy did not resolve. One radial nerve palsy responded completely to removal of cement that had extruded through a humeral defect during revision surgery. The final injury produced ulnar nerve dysesthesias which resolved.

Nerve injuries have received comment in review articles of shoulder arthroplasty. Miller and Bigliani mention that nerve injuries are uncommon, that they most often represent a neuropraxia, and that the axillary nerve is the most likely to be injured.[47] They are of the opinion that if the initial lesion is partial and improving, observation is indicated. If there is a suspicion that the nerve was lacerated at surgery and electromyography at 6 weeks reveals a complete lesion with no improvement at 12 weeks, exploration and surgical repair are suggested. Wirth and Rockwood were able to identify 14 reported nerve injuries following total shoulder replacement.[67] Again they felt most of the injuries represented a neuropraxia with nonoperative treatment being appropriate. Six lesions involved the axillary nerve, 3 the ulnar nerve, 2 the musclocutaneous nerve, 1 the median nerve, and 2 were a more general brachial plexus injury. Resolution was complete in 7, incomplete in 2, did not occur in 1, and in 4 the extent of recovery was not defined. Importantly, in two shoulders there was a laceration of the axillary nerve occurring in a heavily scarred operative field. Soghikian and Neviaser[61] presented a thorough discussion of complications of hemiarthroplasty, and similarly, Muldoon and Cofield[50] presented material on complications of hemiarthroplasty for proximal humeral fractures, and in neither of these reviews was nerve injury identified as a complication, other than recognition of the literature reported in Table 2.

Lynch reported the Mayo Clinic experience with neurologic complications after total shoulder arthroplasty.[43] Four hundred seventeen arthroplasties were studied. Seventeen patients with 18 operated shoulders had a neurologic deficit after surgery (4.3%). All appeared to be traction injuries; 13 involved the brachial plexus. The upper and middle trunk were involved in 6, the upper trunk in 3, the lateral cord in 2, the lower trunk in 1, and all trunks in 1. Interestingly, 3 were thought to represent the initiation of an idiopathic brachial neuritis. One patient with dysesthesias after earlier radiation therapy had an increase in the level of dysesthesias in the lower trunk and 1 patient developed median neuropathy at the wrist. The quality of recovery in the first 16 patients was graded as good in 11 and fair in 5. Time to recovery was less than 3 months in 8, 3 to 6 months in 4, 6 to 12 months in 1, and more than 12 months in 3. Numerous patient factors were studied, including diagnosis, age, sex, height, weight, use of corticosteroids, the presence of diabetes mellitus, preoperative range of motion, the presence or absence of rotator cuff disease, previous surgery and the use of interscalene block. None of these were related to a nerve injury. However, exposure through the slightly more demanding deltopectoral approach ($P=0.003$) and the use of methotrexate in patients with rheumatoid arthritis ($P<0.0001$) were statistically associated with the development of a postoperative nerve palsy. Thus, this series of a large number of shoulder arthroplasties defines that brachial plexus stretch injuries are by far the most frequently recognized neurologic deficits following prosthetic shoulder arthroplasty, that when searched for, nerve injuries are more common than has been recognized, and thankfully, that recovery is the rule—without significant compromise to the arthroplasty per se.

As identified by the foregoing information, prevention of nerve injuries at surgery is usually, but not always, possible. Certainly, locating the axillary nerve at the inferior aspect of the subscapularis and near the posterolateral aspect of the humerus is useful, and careful retraction of the conjoined group is important. Dissection on the undersurface of the superior and posterior aspects of the rotator cuff should not extend more than 1 cm medial to the glenoid rim, to avoid injury to the suprascapular nerve. Positioning of the arm in extension and abduction with external rotation should be limited in extent and time as much as possible. To facilitate all of these protective measures, it is important to have a dry operative field and to be especially cautious when there is distortion of anatomy, such as following an old fracture or fracture–dislocation.

Concerning treatment, definition of the injury by careful physical examination is important. If there is weakness of hand, wrist, or elbow function, splinting may be necessary. Swelling should be minimized by elevation and use of compressive dressings. If active motion is not possible for the hand, wrist, or elbow, passive motion should be used. Passive motion of the shoulder should be commenced during the early postoperative period (within the limits determined at surgery) with active-assisted motion initiated as the return of strength will allow.

If there is no improvement in neurologic function by 4 to 6 weeks, electromyography with nerve conduction should be performed to determine more precisely the localization and extent of the nerve injury. If the lesions are diffuse and incomplete, one would suspect a brachial plexus stretch type lesion, and conservative measures would continue. If a focal complete nerve injury is identified, such as to the axillary nerve, one would be more concerned about a significant adverse intraoperative event. Quite likely in this setting, continued observation would occur. Further examination would be performed at 3 months. If there was no apparent recovery, electromyography would be repeated at that time, and more serious consideration would be given to operative intervention to address the isolated nerve lesion. There is an important caveat, however: so few nerve lesions have occurred owing to trauma to a specific nerve it is hard to be concrete about the recommendations for surgical exploration, other than those indications that apply in general to focal peripheral nerve injuries associated with surgical intervention.

Periprosthetic Fractures

Fractures can occur both intraoperatively and postoperatively. Intraoperatively, humeral shaft fractures are most common. Fractures can also involve the proximal humeral metaphysis, the humeral tuberosities, the glenoid, and the coracoid process. Postoperatively, humeral shaft fractures are also most common. Fractures can involve other areas, including the acromion process and the coracoid process. The recognition of a fracture intraoperatively may be obvious, but sometimes undisplaced cracks develop in the bone that are detected only on subsequent radiographs. Postoperative humeral shaft fractures have been classified by Wright and Cofield.[68] Type A extends proximally from the tip of the prosthesis more than one-third of the length of the stem and may create stem loosening. A type B fracture is centered at the tip of the stem with less proximal extension, and the type C fracture involves the humeral shaft distal to the tip of the prosthesis and usually includes fracturing into the distal humeral metaphysis.

All of these fractures following total shoulder arthroplasty are relatively uncommon, as can be seen from Table 1. Intraoperative fractures occur in less than 1% of cases and postoperative fractures occur in less than one-half of 1% of cases. Following humeral head replacement (see Table 2), intraoperative fractures and postoperative fractures are even less common. However, it is not unusual for a number of arthroplasty series to report one or two humeral shaft fractures and such is the case with reports by Kelly and Foster,[40] Boyd,[11] Barrett,[4] Hawkins,[34] and Faludi.[22] The fractures occurred during varying maneuvers during surgery including exposure, humeral preparation/reaming and humeral implant insertion. Additionally, three glenoid fractures were described, one by Kelly and Foster and two by Hawkins. In a similar vein, several of these series have described the occasional postoperative fracture, including the report of one humeral shaft fracture by Barrett,[4] one humeral shaft fracture by Neer,[52] one humeral shaft fracture by Brenner,[13] three humeral shaft fractures by Post,[55] one humeral shaft fracture by McElwain,[46] and one acromial fracture by Arnst[3] and another by Thomas[64]. Thus, although fracturing is indeed uncommon, it does, in fact, occur and many of the authors reporting on shoulder arthroplasty have experienced this complication at some time.

Only a few reports have specifically addressed this problem. Boyd identified seven humeral shaft fractures after shoulder arthroplasty.[12] Treatment was complicated, and five fractures did not unite until surgery was performed. Fractures that were treated operatively healed. In 5 of the 6 patients who had union of their fracture, shoulder motion was lost compared with prefracture levels. The authors of this study identified many associated factors, including injury to the radial nerve, the high frequency of delayed or nonunion, the question of mechanical interference with fracture healing by the prosthesis or cement, the advanced age of many patients, the presence of osteopenia or systemic disease, the questionable effectiveness of immobilization, the extensive time to union, and the compromise of function of the shoulder arthroplasty. Because of the small size of the patient group, the many diverse factors that need to be considered and the variation in outcome, it was difficult for the authors to reach clear recommendations relative to fracture treatment.

Bonutti and Hawkins identified 4 patients with fracture of the shaft of the humerus.[9] They recognized the historical success with treatment of humeral shaft fractures by conservative means, but felt that aggressive treatment was needed for fracture of the shaft of the humerus associated with shoulder arthroplasty. Groh identified 11 fractures adjacent to humeral prostheses.[31] Four fractures extended from the proximal portion of the humeral shaft to beyond the distal tip of the prosthesis, and two occurred immediately proximal to the tip of the prosthesis. Three proximal fractures were managed with an orthosis. The remainder were treated with the combination of a long-stem prosthesis and cerclage wires. All fractures healed and function of the shoulder arthroplasty was maintained.

Campbell identified 16 intraoperative and 5 postoperative periprosthetic humeral fractures.[15] Fracture outcome was analyzed according to three groups: cast or brace immobilization, intramedullary fixation with a humeral stem plus cerclage wiring, and plate or screw fixation. Stable intramedullary fixation provided superior results in time to union, had less effect on rehabilitation of the shoulder, and demonstrated a trend toward fewer complications. They felt that cast or brace immobilization could be acceptable for postoperative fractures distal to a well-fixed prosthetic stem. More proximal fractures should be fixed with a stem of appropriate length and cerclage wiring.

Two reviews have been performed at the Mayo Clinic. The first reported by Wright and Cofield identified nine humeral fractures occurring following 499 shoulder arthroplasties.[68] Seven fractures were in women, and the average age was 70 years. Many occurred in patients with rheumatoid arthritis. Six fractures were centered at the tip of the prosthesis with one fracture extending proximally (type A) and five (type B) not extending proximally. The remaining three fractures involved the humeral shaft distal to the implant, extending into the distal humeral metaphysis (type C). Two of these fractures had initial unacceptable alignment and were treated operatively. Four others healed with nonoperative external support. An additional three treated with immobilization in a splint failed to heal; two eventually united after revision of the humeral prosthesis and bone grafting. Five of the patients in this group had poor shoulder function before the fracture, and 2 lost even more motion after fracture treatment. The authors feel that operative treatment should be undertaken for fractures that compromise the fixation of the humeral implant with revision to a long-stem implant and cerclage wiring in addition to autogenous bone grafting. For those other humeral shaft fractures that have acceptable skeletal alignment, nonoperative treatment may be successful, but if union is delayed, internal fixation should be undertaken in association with bone grafting.

Krakauer and Cofield reviewed both intraoperative and postoperative periprosthetic fractures in total shoulder replacement.[42] Intraoperatively, over an 18-year period, there were nine humeral shaft fractures, five greater tuberosity fractures, two proximal humeral metaphyseal fractures, four glenoid fractures, and two coracoid fractures. Of the intraoperative humeral shaft fractures, stability was achieved with a long-stem implant in six and with cerclage fixation in one. Two fractures were undisplaced and no fixation was performed; healing occurred in one but nonunion developed in the other. Three of the greater tuberosity fractures were sutured. The other two were undisplaced fractures and treated without fixation. One of the sutured greater tuberosities went on to nonunion and compromised active shoulder function. The proximal humeral metaphyseal and coracoid fractures created no adverse effect on arthroplasty outcome. The four glenoid fractures precluded placing an implant, and 2 of these patients continued to have moderate pain with their hemiarthroplasty. Postoperative humeral shaft fractures occurred in 15 shoulders. In 7 shoulders the implant was cemented and in 8 it was uncemented. Two were type A fractures, 9 type B fractures, and 4 type C fractures. Surgery was performed in 9, including internal fixation of the fracture in 5, conversion to a long-stem humeral implant in 3, and conversion to a custom humeral implant in 1. Range of motion of the shoulder arthroplasty remained the same in 10 and was decreased in 5. Of note, external support was initially attempted in 11 of these 15 cases, with union occurring in 6. The authors conclude that a trial of external support is acceptable if the implant is not loose and skeletal alignment is satisfactory, but if delayed union occurs internal fixation with a plate, screws, and cerclage wiring or conversion to a long-stem implant is desirable.

Most intraoperative fractures can be prevented. As a part of preoperative planning any stress-risers in the bone should be identified and osteopenia should be noted. One must be careful twisting the humerus during exposure, bone preparation or seating of the implant. Forces across the humerus or other bones can be diminished by appropriate release of scar and capsular contractures. For patients with extreme osteopenia, one should consider the anteromedial surgical approach with release of the deltoid origin on the clavicle and anterior acromion, rather than the deltopectoral approach. This greatly lessens the forces needed for exposure.

Even with the small experience reported by each individual author, the accumulating experience suggests that recommendations for treatment can be made. If an intraoperative humeral shaft fracture occurs, it should almost always be internally fixed; typically this would be with a long-stem humeral implant and wire cerclage. For very distal fractures, plate fixation may be preferred. Similarly, greater tuberosity fractures should almost always be sutured with heavy, nonabsorbable suture or wire. Postoperative humeral fractures should probably be considered in three categories in the manner of Wright and Cofield. For proximal fractures that involve the implant and are associated with implant loosening, revision arthroplasty with insertion of the long-stem humeral implant and cerclage fixation should be strongly considered. For those fractures centered around the tip of the implant without a great deal of proximal fracture extension, external support can be undertaken if skeletal alignment is adequate. If skeletal alignment cannot be achieved or delayed union occurs, open reduction and internal fixation with a plate, screws and cerclage would be indicated. For fractures involving the distal humerus, treatment would be dictated according to the guidelines for distal humeral fractures. This might include external support in the presence of excellent skeletal alignment or open reduction and internal fixation for displaced, unstable fractures. It is important to recognize for the first two types of fractures that include the area of bone around or near the humeral prosthesis, there is something detrimental about the fractures occurring in this situation that mutes the healing response. As such, autogenous bone graft should almost always be used as an adjunct during open fracture fixation.

Infection

Evolution in thinking about infections around the prosthetic joint arthroplasty has been directed toward four categories of infections. The first is a positive culture obtained at the time of the arthroplasty, perhaps associated with previous internal fixation. The second is an acute infection developing within 2 to 3 months following the arthroplasty. The third is an apparently acute, probably hematogenous, infection developing quite typically a year or several years following the initial arthroplasty, and the fourth is a chronic infection, sometimes associated with sinus tract formation.

The recognition of a latent, low-grade infection at the time of the arthroplasty can be somewhat difficult. The joint fluid may be slightly opaque. The synovial lining may include scattered areas of mild erythema, small foci of granulation tissue may be present on the ebernated bone surfaces, and the reactive fibrosis may be somewhat softer and slightly more pink than white. However, all these changes may be absent or, if not, quite subtle. A frozen section may show a few foci of polymorphonuclear leukocytes, or in fact, it may show a mild rather nonspecific low-grade inflammatory response with lymphocytic cells—not atypical of many patients with arthritis. Occasionally in this setting, particularly in persons who have had previous surgery and internal fixation, it may be prudent to remove the internal fixation to debride any abnormal tissue, to close the wound, and to await cultures before proceeding with the arthroplasty. Judgment in these cases can be extremely difficult, and it seems there are no clear-cut guidelines for these borderline situations.

When infection develops in the acute phase, within the first 2 to 3 months following surgery, distinction between a superficial infection and a deep infection can be difficult. The presence of a postoperative hematoma may also cloud the issue. The patient often has the symptoms and signs of an acute infection, but they may be muted. There may be some malaise of varying degree; a fever may or may not be present; the wound can be slightly more swollen than usual, particularly in the presence of a focal hematoma; or the wound may be slightly to markedly reddened. There may be drainage, or there may not be. The erythrocyte sedimentation rate will be elevated and probably will not be of much diagnostic value. Serum C-reactive protein holds some promise in identifying patients with subacute infections (developing after 3 to 6 weeks), but many physicians do not have extensive experience with the nuances of the use of this test. Similarly, the white blood cell count can be abnormal in the acute postoperative phase, but abnormalities in the subacute phase will be suggestive of the presence of an infection. Standard radiographs may show gas in the tissues, but this would be unusual. Scintigraphic techniques are probably of little value. Needle aspiration is usually indicated. In the end, debridement, with culture of the deep tissues, may be the only way to diagnose an infected shoulder arthroplasty in the immediate postoperative period.

An acute, presumably hematogenous, infection developing in a previously well-functioning arthroplasty is usually diagnosed clinically, in association with laboratory studies and joint aspiration.

Distinguishing a late, indolent, chronic infection from a mechanical problem can be easily accomplished, or it may be extraordinarily difficult. Certainly in a patient with a painful arthroplasty, infection should always be considered. The external examination may be normal; the radiographs, however, may show lucencies surrounding the components. In the humerus there may be resorption of bone, particularly in the area of the humeral calcar, laminated periosteal new bone formation, scalloping of the endosteal bone surface, or evident sinus formation through bone. The more chronic and low grade the infection the more likely the laboratory studies will be normal. Scintigraphy can be quite revealing. Usually the technetium-labeled scan will be positive throughout the arthroplasty region if infection is present. However, this can also be active in the presence of noninfectious inflammation or mechanical problems. We prefer to supplement that scan with an indium-labeled leukocyte scan. This will not always be clearly abnormal, but when it is, it is highly suggestive of infection. Joint aspiration should be performed, and arthrography should not be forgotten. Arthrography can be quite useful showing irregularities, that is hypertrophic changes within the synovium, fistula formation from the joint perhaps communicating with a pseudobursa, and dye tracking along the interface of the implant or implant and cement with the bone—in an irregular fashion. It is usually possible with the diagnostic armanentarium we have to define the presence of infection in this chronic setting even when the presentation is subtle. On the other hand, there are a few individuals who present with chronic infections and draining arthrocutaneous sinuses for whom the diagnosis is quite clean.

Referring to Table 1, infections reported in the recent total shoulder arthroplasty literature occurred in 0.4% of cases. Infections are reported somewhat more commonly following humeral head replacement. In the recent literature (see Table 2), infections are reported in 1% of cases. When we reviewed the literature specifically for complications of humeral head replacement for proximal humeral fractures, delayed wound healing or infection occurred in 6 of 203 acutely treated cases and in 3 of 100 shoulders having delayed treatment for chronic fracture-related problems.[50] Thus, the literature suggests that the infection rate is less than 1% for elective shoulder arthroplasty and may well be several times that for arthroplasty used for the treatment of complex fractures.

There is surprisingly little literature directed specifically toward infections associated with shoulder arthroplasty. Codd and coauthors reported their experience with 16 patients.[17] They recognized, as formulated earlier in this chapter, there is no single preoperative study that is consistent for the diagnosis of infection, and they suggested relying quite strongly on the operative histology. Interestingly, their group included 5 patients who had positive cultures while undergoing revision surgery, but negative intraoperative histology. These patients were treated with antibiotics and none of the patients developed infection following this treatment. Eight patients presented with infection of their arthroplasty, 4 underwent resection arthroplasty, and 4 had reimplantation of a prosthesis with antibiotic-containing bone cement. The patients undergoing reimplantation had better shoulder function. In another subgroup 5 patients apparently had earlier shoulder infection, which was treated, and then had humeral head replacement at a later date. This report typifies the information on infected shoulder arthroplasties. There is information available, but the numbers of patients are small and one hesitates to be too forceful in recommendations for treatment.

Three review articles have additional, useful information on the treatment of infection associated with shoulder arthroplasty. Wirth, in 1996, reviewed 1,615 total shoulder arthroplasties in 32 scientific reports.[67] Infection was identified as the fifth most common complication. Reported associations included host-related risk factors of diabetes mellitus, rheumatoid arthritis, systemic lupus erythematosus, previous shoulder operations, remote sites of infection, compromise of the immune system, and the speculation as to whether or not previous steroid injections predispose to infection in this circumstance. The value of preoperative laboratory testing is difficult to ascertain because of inconsistent reporting methods. Suggested treatment options include antibiotic suppression, incision and drainage, removal of the implant with reimplantation, resection arthroplasty, arthrodesis, and amputation. The specific treatment selected depends on the timing of the infection, the pathogen, and the stability of the implant. For early infections with a gram-positive organism: exploration with incision, drainage, and debridement; the use of antibiotics; and retention of the prosthesis are recommended. For late infections and those with gram-negative organisms: removal of the implant, intravenous antibiotics, and then later consideration of reimplantation are suggested. Miller in 1993 identified four infections in 1,168 reported cases.[47] He commented that the excellent vascularity and abundant soft-tissue coverage is one reason for the low rate of infection. There should always be a high suspicion of the possibility of a low-grade infection at the time of revision surgery. Preoperative evaluation should include a white blood cell count with differential, an erythrocyte sedimentation rate, consideration of use of nuclear scanning, aspiration, and certainly frozen sections. Be particularly wary of infection in an immunocompromised host. Suggested treatment for early infections included debridement, wound closure with drains, an initial broad-spectrum antibiotic with a high sensitivity to gram-positive organisms, and more specific antibiotics as the culture results become apparent. For delayed infections, removal of the implant is suggested, along with the use of intravenous antibiotics and immobilization for 3 months. If the patient is dissatisfied at 1 year, consider fusion if there is no osteomyelitis. It is possible to reinsert a hemiarthroplasty or total shoulder arthroplasty with antibiotics impregnated in the cement, but osteomyelitis should certainly not be present in this circumstance. Soghikian in 1993 reviewed complications of humeral head replacement.[61] He recommended that one be quite suspicious of infection in the presence of previous failed open reduction and internal fixation, that perioperative antibiotics be used, that hemostasis be meticulous, and that one obtain intraoperative cultures. When late infection develops the implant should be removed, there should be antibiotics for a minimum of 6 weeks, and reimplantation should be considered at that time or later.

Thirty-three patients with 34 involved shoulders were treated for an infected shoulder arthroplasty at the Mayo Clinic between 1972 and 1991. This included 19 of 1,484 primary total shoulder arthroplasties (1.3%) and 7 of 157 revision total shoulder arthroplasties (4.5%). The time to infection was quite variable. It averaged 43 months, but ranged from the first week to 14.8 years. Pain was present in almost all patients. A sinus tract had developed in slightly fewer than one-half of patients. Fever, chills, and erythema were present in approximately one-third. The sedimentation rate was elevated in 58%. The white blood count was elevated in only 7%. An indium-labeled white cell scan was performed in 9 and was positive in 7. Aspiration was performed in 18 and was positive in 14. The infection was monomicrobial in 68%, polymicrobial in 20%, and there was a negative culture with positive histology and an appropriate clinical picture in 12%. The most common organism was *Staphylococcus aureus* followed by coagulase-negative *Staphylococcus*, *Propionibacterium acnes*, and *Pseudomonas aeruginosa*. Intravenous antibiotics were used in all patients, and 13 were continued on oral antibiotics for a period of time thereafter.

Treatment was quite variable. Six underwent debridement. One debridement was performed arthroscopically in a delayed acute infection with *S. aureus*; to date there has been no reinfection, but the final result was rated as unsatisfactory because of damage to the rotator cuff during the infection and subsequent loss of active movement. Five others underwent open arthrotomy and debridement. Two remain infection-free and 3 had continuing infection or developed reinfection and later required resection arthroplasty. Twenty-three underwent a primary resection arthroplasty with only 1 having a continuation of the infection or a reinfection. Thirteen shoulders in this patient group had follow-up averaging 76 months (range 34 to 154) and underwent limited goals rehabilitation; this proved successful in 3 and unsuccessful in 10. There was no or slight pain in 8 of these patients. Average active elevation was 65 degrees with average external rotation of 38 degrees.

Two patients underwent direct exchange arthroplasty, both with chronic, but rather low-grade infections. One man with *P. aeruginosa* had direct exchange with antibiotic-impregnated cement and remains infection-free 120 months later. The second patient with coagulase-negative *Staphylococcus* and *Actinobacter* developed reinfection at 9 months with *Corynebacterium* and required resection arthroplasty. Three shoulders underwent delayed reimplantation arthroplasty with delay ranging between 2 and 15 months. The organisms were *S. aureus*, coagulase-negative *Staphylococcus*, and *Pseudomonas diminuta*. Two arthroplasties were cemented with antibiotics in the cement and one was uncemented. Current follow-up ranges between 26 and 101 months. To date there has been no reinfection. Pain state is satisfactory in all three. Average active elevation is 100 degrees with external rotation of 30 degrees. The final clinical grade is excellent in one, satisfactory in one, and unsatisfactory in one.

In summary, there are many variables involved with infections surrounding arthroplasties, including host factors, the timing and nature of the infection, and the type of organism. For the acute or delayed acute infection, arthrotomy and debridement and the use of intravenous antibiotics should be strongly considered, but this advice must be tempered, given the reinfection rate that is difficult to ascertain from the literature, but is moderate, perhaps somewhere between 30% and 60%. Resection arthroplasty has been the standard. It is successful for irradication of the infection and usually provides pain relief. Shoulder function is often unsatisfactory if rated on one of the usual shoulder rating systems. Direct exchange of the prosthesis can be considered for lower-grade infections, but the frequency of success is uncertain, because of the limited collective experience with this type of treatment in the shoulder. Delayed reimplantation has been successful for eradication of infection. It is more consistent in offering pain relief and affords better function than resection arthroplasty. The timing to reimplantation is uncertain. The suggested times extend from 6 weeks to 1 year.

Rotator Cuff Tears

Problems with rotator cuff healing or subsequent rotator cuff tearing following arthroplasty are probably substantially underreported, being identified instead as poorer outcomes and included in the lower portions of result rating scales or detailed in association with instability, rather than specifically identified as a rotator cuff stretching or tearing. Certainly, management of the rotator cuff is an important part of shoulder arthroplasty. Preexisting rotator cuff disease and tearing is common. We carefully studied 156 consecutive total shoulder arthroplasties for rotator cuff disease. Overall, 48 (27%) had tears of the rotator cuff present at surgery. Tears did vary in size being small (<1 cm in greatest length) in 10, medium (>1 to 3 cm) in 10, large (>3 to 5 cm) in 7 and massive (>5 cm) in 21. By disease category, in osteoarthritis there was no tearing in 46 shoulders, the rotator cuff was thin in 1 and torn in 6. In rheumatoid arthritis there was no tearing in 11, the rotator cuff was judged to be thin and scarred in 37, and was torn in 18. In old trauma there was no abnormality in 6, the rotator cuff was thinned and scarred in 2, was torn in 3, and in 10 there was tuberosity malunion requiring osteotomy. In rotator cuff tear arthritis the rotator cuff was torn in all 14. In other miscellaneous diagnoses there was no rotator cuff tearing in 13, the rotator cuff was thin and scarred in 2, and torn in 7. Thus, preexisting rotator cuff disease is an important consideration, may well alter the approach to shoulder arthroplasty, and certainly, if tearing is present, it would predispose the patient to having a complication related to the rotator cuff postoperatively.

The classification of rotator cuff tearing is probably no different with arthroplasty than without arthroplasty. The classification can be by location, tear size, and tear shape. Location identifies the tendon or tendons affected. Size is conveniently recorded in centimeters and is typically measured following the initial debridement before mobilization of the tendons themselves. Many cuff tears are in the impingement area or slightly posterior to this, associated with upward subluxation of the humeral head that occurs in many patients with arthritis. Occasionally, longitudinal tears occur in line with the tendon fibers, but most often, transverse tears exist. These may be essentially linear or they may include an area defect that has an oval, triangular, or trapezoidal shape, before mobilization of the tendon into the defect. Additionally, shoulder arthroplasty has made surgeons acutely aware of the possibility for interstitial tendon tearing, particularly in rheumatoid arthritis, where the tendons are quite thin and scarred, perhaps one-half to one-quarter of their normal thickness. Certainly if these tendons were examined histologically, there would be disruption of tendon fiber continuity, thus a microscopic rotator cuff tear exists in the absence of a gross full-thickness tear. The outcome of arthroplasty in these patients is strongly influenced by this compromise of rotator cuff function, although stability of the implant can usually be obtained.

The diagnosis of rotator cuff tearing following arthroplasty follows the scheme of diagnosis for rotator cuff tearing in the absence of arthroplasty. Symptomatically there is often an increase in pain, recognition of a loss of active motion, and weakness. Physical examination defines this diminution in active motion relative to passive motion and identifies weakness in the torn cuff components. Additionally, following arthroplasty, rotator cuff tearing may present most dramatically as instability, usually superiorly or anteriorly, but occasionally posteriorly (Fig. 4). Certainly when instability occurs following shoulder arthroplasty, disruption of the surgical arthrotomy or rotator cuff tearing should always be suspected. Plain radiographs may show a severe upward subluxation diagnostic of rotator cuff tearing. In the absence of this but with clinical evaluation suggesting rotator cuff tearing, an arthrogram can be performed. With a tendency for fibrosis surrounding implants, there is concern that the arthrogram may be false-negative; however, practically, this seldom seems to be an important issue, with the arthrogram typically defining the rotator cuff tear much as it would in a shoulder without prosthetic arthroplasty.

A special note relative to rotator cuff tearing in the postoperative condition relates to healing of the subscapularis. We have recognized on physical examination that a number of patients following arthroplasty have somewhat excessive external rotation and slight weakness in internal rotation. They must in fact have stretched their anterior shoulder capsule and rotator cuff repair or have disrupted it to some degree. In many of these patients there is no patient-identified adverse response with excellent pain relief and motion and maintenance of glenohumeral stability. As such, one cannot assume that disruption of the rotator cuff is the source of pain following shoulder arthroplasty. Other possible sources of pain must also be explored and identified—for apparently, rotator cuff tearing can exist following shoulder arthroplasty and, as in the nonarthroplasty state, can be minimally symptomatic or asymptomatic.

Although problems with the rotator cuff following arthroplasty are seldom at the forefront of one's thinking when considering complications of shoulder arthroplasty, if one tabulates all the complications of total shoulder arthroplasty, as defined in Table 1, rotator cuff tearing is the most common complication in this collection of reported series—having a rate of 1.9%. Following humeral head replacement, rotator cuff tearing occurs in a similar frequency (1.8%; see Table 2). Tuberosity problems also occur in fracture patients, with nonunion developing in 1.8% and tuberosity malunion in 0.4% in this 20-patient series. Interestingly, we could not identify any specific literature addressing the complication of rotator cuff tearing in the arthroplasty patient.

Neer, when discussing revision of humeral head and total shoulder arthroplasties, mentions the possibility of impingement of the rotator cuff in the postoperative state.[51] He defined that scar requires release, impingement by the anterior acromion and the coracoacromial ligament require anterior acromioplasty, and impingement by the acromioclavicular joint requires acromioclavicular arthroplasty to free the rotator cuff. Miller, in presenting the complications of total shoulder replacement, mentions a postoperative rotator cuff tear frequency of 3% to 4%.[47] He comments that repair is not always required, but recalls the admonition of Franklin's report[27] that there is an increased frequency of glenoid loosening when there are large rotator cuff tears; this might support repair of a rotator cuff tear in the postarthroplasty patient. Wirth estimates a 2% frequency of rotator cuff tearing following shoulder arthroplasty and finds that both operative and nonoperative treatment have been employed, with lack of clear definition of the benefits of one form of treatment over the other.[67]

In the Mayo series of postoperative complications of total shoulder arthroplasty, rotator cuff tearing was the second most common complication, occurring in 8% of shoulders (see Table 3). This complication occurred early in one-third and late in two-thirds of the shoulders involved (see Table 4). It was considered a minor complication in 5, a major complication affecting the outcome in 11, and a major complication requiring reoperation in 17 shoulders. As recognized in Fig. 3 there was an overlap, indeed a probable association among rotator cuff tearing, instability, and glenoid loosening.

Probably in no area is the comprehensive approach to shoulder arthroplasty more important than in the prevention of postoperative rotator cuff tearing. Balancing the joint is key to preventing large repair-threatening forces on the arthrotomy site or a repair of a preexisting rotator cuff tear. Component positioning must be carefully performed, the correct size of the component must be selected, unbalanced capsular tightness must be adjusted by appropriate releases or adjustment in component size, and impingement should be eliminated if it exists. Following implantation of the prosthetic parts, the glenohumeral joint should be stable and, in fact, will usually be stable even before the arthrotomy repair. The arthrotomy repair should then be secure. Range of motion of the shoulder should be assessed to define the limits determined by the arthrotomy repair. Sufficient postoperative limb support should be provided, as should careful pa-

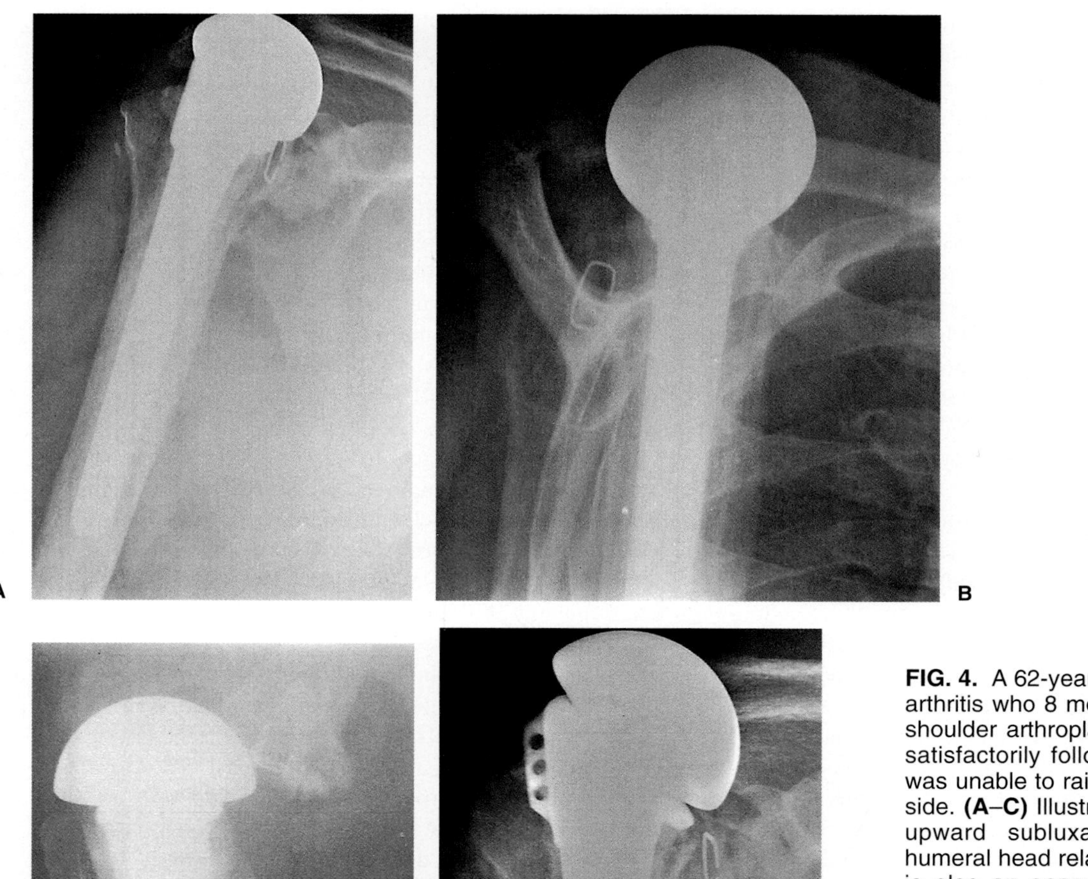

FIG. 4. A 62-year-old man with rheumatoid arthritis who 8 months previously had total shoulder arthroplasty. He never recovered satisfactorily following the procedure and was unable to raise the arm away from his side. **(A–C)** Illustrating severe forward and upward subluxation of the prosthetic humeral head relative to the glenoid. There is also an apparent high position of the humeral component within the humeral shaft. At surgery the components were tight. Tearing of the supraspinatus and infraspinatus tendons was identified and repaired. Repair was reasonably secure. However, in spite of careful postoperative support, patient instructions, and physiotherapy done passively within the limits of the tendon repair, the repair became disrupted within 1 month following surgery. The radiograph **(D)** illustrates the recurrent upward and forward subluxation of the humeral component and illustrates the difficulty in correcting this type of instability following shoulder arthroplasty.

tient instruction in protecting the limb. The physiotherapy program takes into consideration the limits of motion, as defined at the time of surgery, and the surgeon's recognition of the rate of soft-tissue healing.

There does not seem to be a yes or no answer in the recommendations for treatment of rotator cuff tearing following total shoulder arthroplasty. Certainly, there are many patients who seemingly have compromised their arthrotomy repair, yet are comfortable, have good motion, and the arthroplasty is stable. Further surgical treatment would almost certainly not be considered in these patients. Other patients express some weakness of their shoulder following arthroplasty, yet have good pain relief and fair active movement (Fig. 5). Again, in many of these older patients surgical repair of their rotator cuff stretching or tearing would not be undertaken. On the other hand, there are some patients who have been doing well with their arthroplasty who have an adverse event or an accident and have a dramatic change in shoulder function, or those who without apparent reason or following an injury develop acute instability of their arthroplasty. In these patients with a rather acute and dramatic change in their arthroplasty with substantial compromise of function, rotator cuff repair would be undertaken. Finally, there are a few patients who seem to have chronic deterioration of function in their shoulder arthroplasty. Usually, this can be attributed to other problems (such as component loosening), but occasionally it is related to a degenerative or impingement-engendered attrition and tearing of the rotator

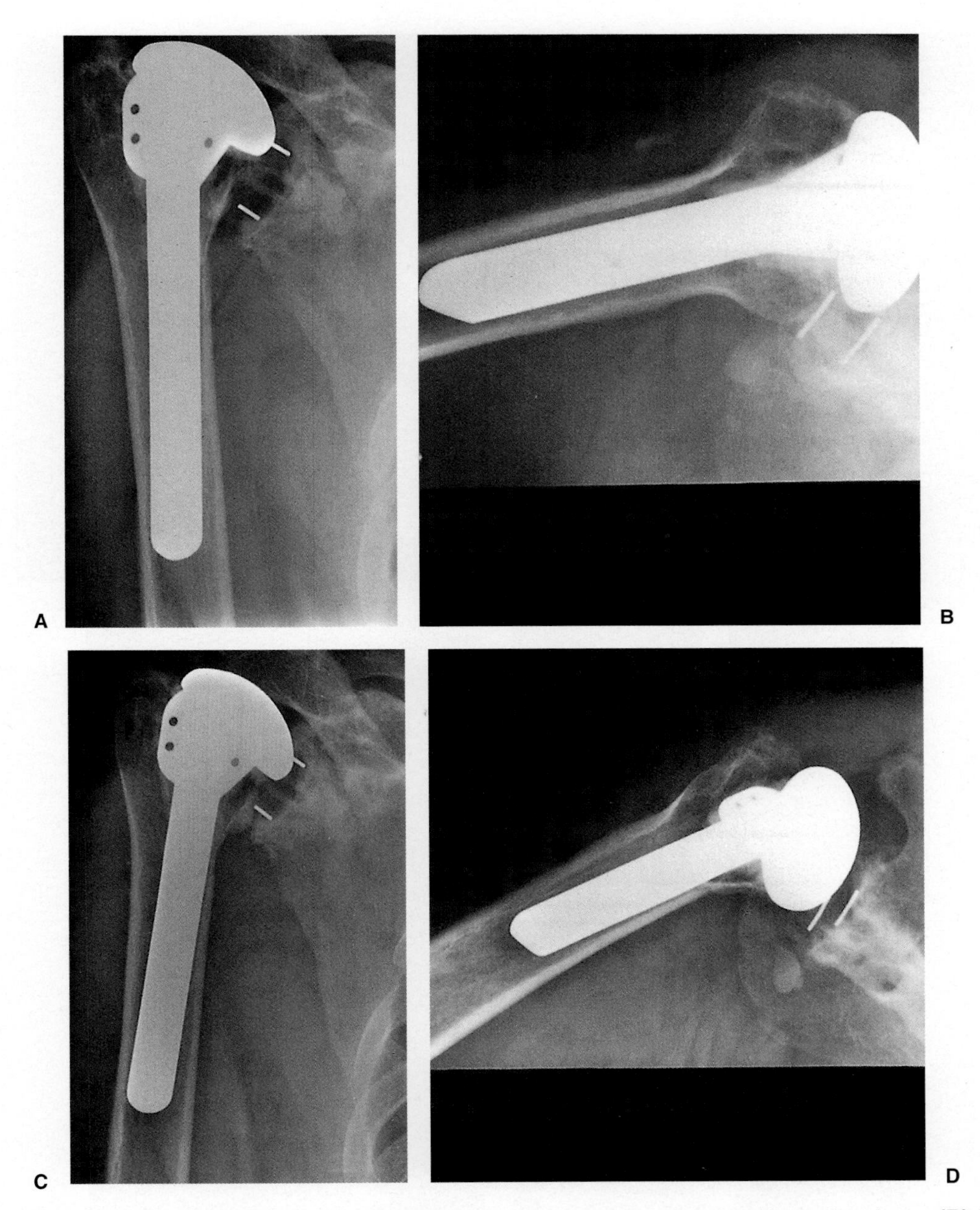

FIG. 5. (A) A 79-year-old man with osteoarthritis who underwent total shoulder arthroplasty. **(B)** Following arthroplasty and rehabilitation, he continued to have weakness and evident forward subluxation of the humeral head. In spite of rehabilitation, he did not improve. Six years later he underwent revision surgery with repair of the subscapularis tendon tearing and tearing of the anterior portion of the supraspinatus tendon. **(C,D)** Revision surgery rendered the shoulder more stable with only mild residual subluxation occurring.

cuff. In these patients, as in patients without shoulder arthroplasty, the situation should be defined and a discussion held with the patient about the benefits and limitations of rotator cuff repair. In this setting, it seems that the benefit/risk ratio is rather close, and typically, continued conservative treatment measures are recommended.

Instability

It is easiest to organize thinking about shoulder instability by using the established categorization mechanisms for shoulder instability in the absence of shoulder arthroplasty. Instability following shoulder arthroplasty does occur acutely. Chronic dislocations can occur and so do recurrent dislocations (Fig. 6). The instability can be of any degree, either mild or complete dislocation, and it can be in any direction: superiorly, anteriorly, posteriorly, or inferiorly. Perhaps the most common instability-like situation that occurs following shoulder arthroplasty is some degree of superior humeral subluxation. Boyd et al. commented on this and recognized it in 29 of 131 shoulders (22%) having a Neer prosthesis.[11] In their patient group, even in the presence of this

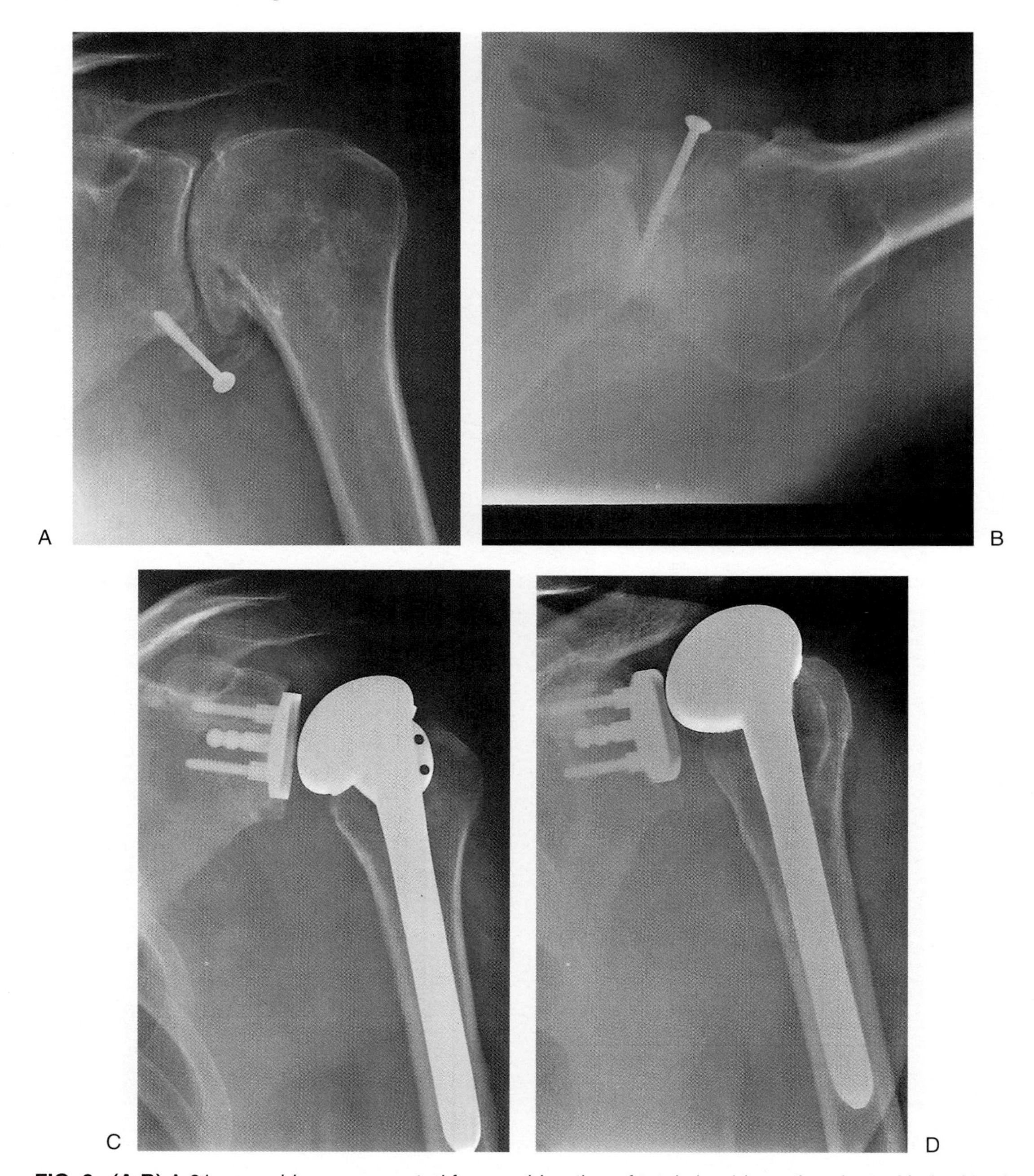

FIG. 6. (A,B) A 61-year-old man presented for consideration of total shoulder arthroplasty. He had had recurrent shoulder dislocations and had three previous anterior shoulder repairs. **(C)** He did well the first year following shoulder arthroplasty. Thereafter, he became unstable, developing both anterior and posterior subluxation of the shoulder. On one occasion he had an acute anterior dislocation that was reduced by a physician. **(D)** By 4 years following his shoulder arthroplasty, he had developed polyethylene wear, a sense of crepitus within the joint, and increased unsteadiness of the joint both anteriorly and posteriorly. Revision surgery was performed. Both the glenoid and humeral components were removed. Enough bone was lost during removal of the glenoid component that it was thought wise not to place another component. (*continued*)

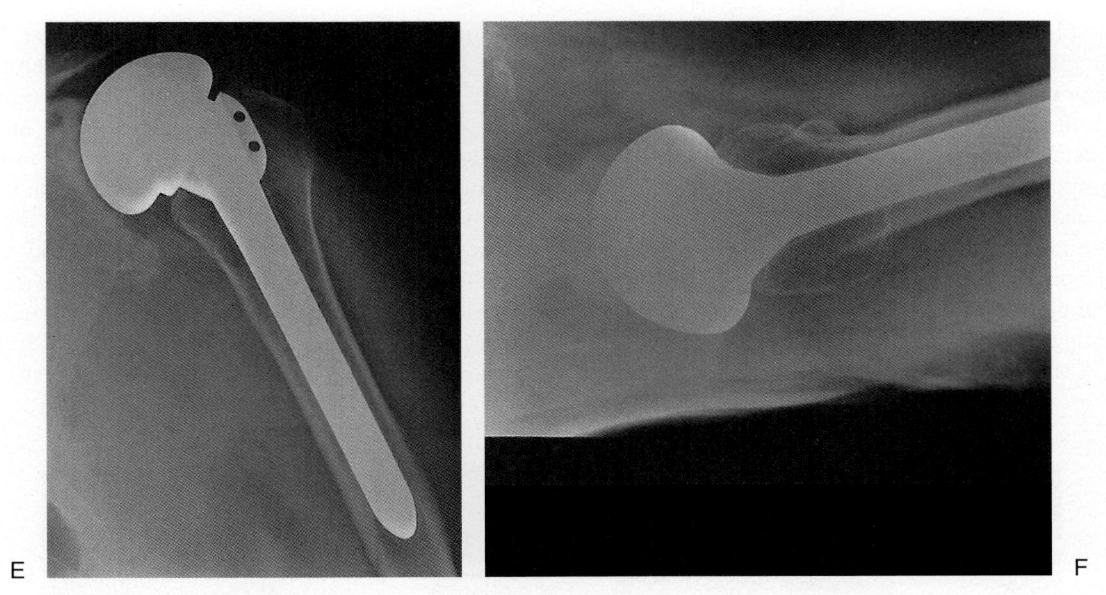

FIG. 6. *Continued* **(E,F)** The glenoid was bone grafted. A larger size humeral head was placed and the soft tissues were adjusted to have balanced tension. His inflammatory response following this revision was rather intense. By 2 years after surgery he has 95 degrees of elevation, internal rotation to L-5, and external rotation to 20 degrees. The shoulder is stable, but there is intermittent moderate pain.

situation, all patients had decreased pain compared with their preoperative state and improved range of motion. This upward subluxation seemed to be caused by a combination of factors and was not due to rotator cuff tearing alone—for they recognized major rotator cuff tears in 21% of patients with a normal glenohumeral relation and in 24% of patients with this proximal or superior subluxation.

The presence of instability is usually readily recognized by physical examination and radiography. However, there may be associated abnormalities that require more in-depth study, including the presence or absence of rotator cuff tearing, component malposition, a component size that is either too large or too small for the soft-tissue envelope, or component loosening with a change in component position.

In the literature, instability is one of the most common complications seen following total shoulder arthroplasty, occurring in 1.5% of shoulders (see Table 1). It may even be the most common complication following humeral head replacement, with 2.8% of the shoulders developing this complication in the 20 series reported since 1980.

There have been two scientific articles directly addressing postoperative instability. Moeckel et al. reported on 10 shoulders that developed instability following 236 consecutive arthroplasties.[48] The instability was anterior in seven and posterior in three (Fig. 7). They recommended correction of the soft-tissue imbalance and prosthetic revision as necessary. With particular reference to disruption of the subscapularis tendon, mobilization and repair of the tendon was recommended, but three of seven continued to have instability and required rerepair supplemented with an allograft of tendo Achilles. This latter technique proved successful in these three shoulders. Wirth reported on 18 shoulders that developed instability, 11 posterior, 6 anterior, and 1 inferior.[67] For posterior instability the treatment was directed at restoring appropriate retroversion of the humeral component, performing a posterior capsulorrhaphy and achieving appropriate position of the glenoid component or, in the absence of a glenoid component, reaming the glenoid surface to a neutral angle. For anterior instability, component version was again corrected when necessary. The anterior structures were repaired and sometimes reinforced with the pectoralis major tendon. If the coracoacromial ligament could be reconstructed, this was also done. For inferior instability, humeral length was restored.

Several review articles comment on shoulder instability. In Neer's 1982 article on revision of humeral head and total shoulder arthroplasties, he recognized loss of humeral height as extremely common following fractures or tumors and indeed that occurred in 18 or 27 failed arthroplasties in this series.[51] At revision surgery the height was restored and comment was made that bone grafting might be needed. Miller identified instability in 1% to 2% of cases.[47] He also recommended restoring humeral length, careful attention to appropriate glenoid positioning when using a glenoid component, or appropriate reaming of the glenoid surface when a glenoid component is not used. At revision surgery it would usually be necessary to correct the prosthetic's position and to perform soft-tissue reconstruction. Wirth's 1996 review of complications of total shoulder replacement noted that anterior instability was associated with dysfunction of the anterior deltoid, malrotation of the humeral component, and disruption of the subscapularis tendon.[67] This latter problem was attributed to poor tissue quality or technique, inappropriately oversized components, or aggressive physical therapy. Superior instability was associated with dynamic muscle dysfunction, attenuation of the supraspinatus muscle–tendon unit, or rotator cuff tearing. This type of instability might be associated with an increased frequency of glenoid loosening. Posterior instability was associated with a retroverted glenoid component, an excessively retroverted humeral component, and soft-tissue imbalance. If the glenoid component was not used, posterior instability was associated with posterior glenoid erosion. He recommended being aware of asymmetrical glenoid wear and to compensate for this with careful reaming or bone grafting of the glenoid. Also, the surgeon must alter the position of the humeral component to include somewhat less retrotorsion. Treatment for posterior instability would include restoring normal humeral component version, reestablishing proper glenoid component version, and addressing soft-tissue imbalance, including consideration of posterior capsulorrhaphy. Inferior instability was seemingly always associated with humeral shortening. The treatment was to reestablish humeral length. Soghikian, in reviewing the complications of humeral head replacement, identified superior subluxation as an issue and recommended careful assessment of the rotator cuff during the initial surgery and carefully positioning the height of the humeral component.[61] Adequate postoperative protection is neces-

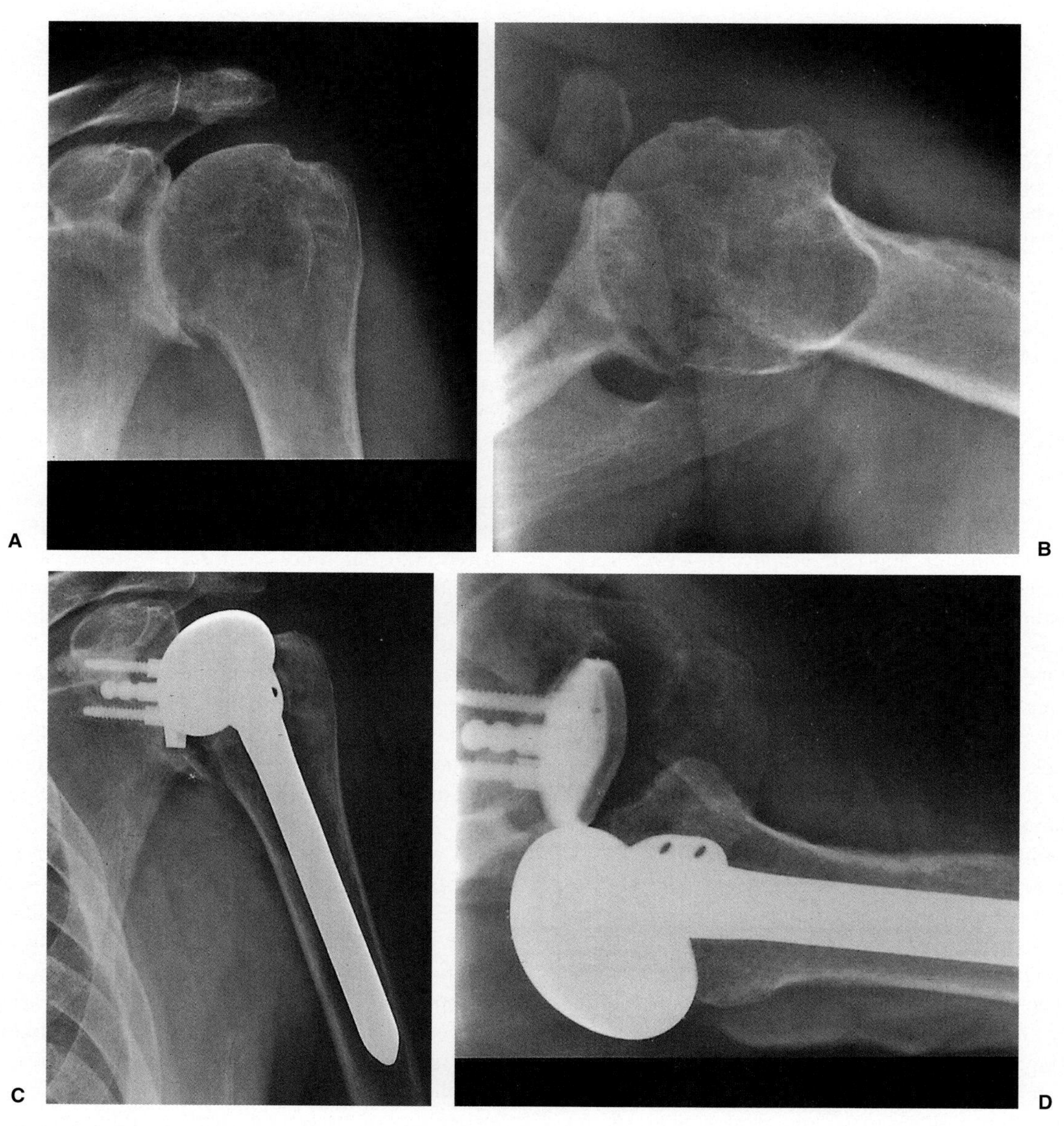

FIG. 7. (A,B) This patient with osteoarthritis and a mild cervical neuropathy underwent total shoulder arthroplasty. **(C,D)** Three years later he developed a sense that the shoulder was slipping and 31/2 years later had a posterior dislocation. At revision surgery there was minimal polyethylene wear. (*continued*)

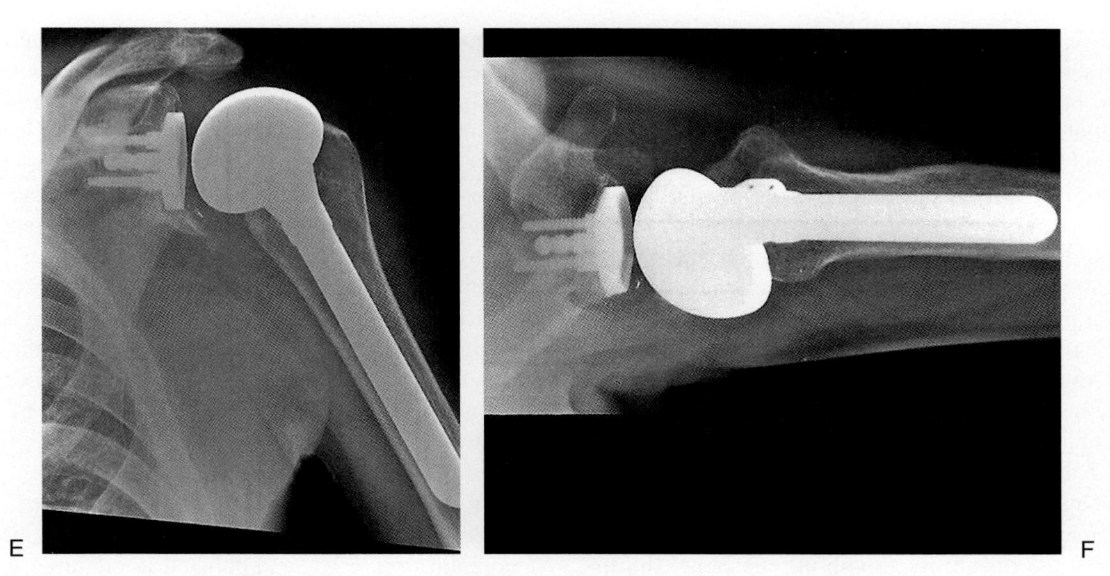

FIG. 7. *Continued* **(E,F)** The polyethylene insert was exchanged for one that was 2-mm thicker and a larger humeral head component was placed. He has remained stable following this revision surgery.

sary to allow soft-tissue healing. Should a postoperative dislocation occur, closed reduction should be performed followed by immobilization and delayed physiotherapy.

In the Mayo Clinic series analyzing postoperative surgical complications, subluxation was the most common complication identified (11%; see Table 3). This could occur early, as it did in 16 shoulders, but also developed late in 28 shoulders (see Table 4). Subluxation was usually a devastating complication (see Table 5). It was a minor complication in only 1 shoulder, it was a major complication affecting the final result in 11, and required reoperation in 32 shoulders. Because this complication was the most common one in our patients and was quite significant, a separate analysis of instability following shoulder arthroplasty was undertaken. During the time period of 1976 through 1993, 62 arthroplasties, both performed initially at our institution and referred to us from elsewhere, required revision surgery for shoulder instability. The instability was anterior in 11, posterior in 17, superior in 17, inferior in 3, and multidirectional in 2. Of the 50 shoulders with follow-up long enough to determine outcome, the primary etiologies of the instability in the anterior direction were subscapularis stretching or tearing in 11, excessive humeral component anteversion in 3, and excessive glenoid component anteversion in 1. The primary causes of the posterior instability were subscapularis tearing in 2, excessive laxity of the posterior rotator cuff and shoulder capsule in 6, detachment of the rotator cuff by the humeral osteotomy in 5, posterior glenoid erosion in 2, a malpositioned humeral component in 3, a malpositioned glenoid component in 2, and a polyethylene dissociation from the glenoid metal tray in 3. The primary causes of the superior instability were supraspinatus stretching or tearing in 15, tuberosity nonunion in 1, excessive humeral component anteversion in 1, and polyethylene dissociation in 1. The primary cause of inferior instability was a shortened humerus and humeral component position in 3. Multidirectional instability occurred in association with subscapularis tearing in 1, supraspinatus tearing in 1, and following polyethylene dissociation in 1. Thus, perhaps somewhat surprisingly, component problems, either malposition or other problems, were a primary cause of the instability in only 18 of the 50 shoulders, with the remainder of the primary causes of instability being soft-tissue abnormalities.

Average follow-up times for the five groups ranged from 32 to 88 months. Following repair of the identified abnormalities in the anterior group three remained reduced, four had moderate subluxation, and four had severe subluxation. The functional outcome rated according to the modified Neer system was satisfactory in three and unsatisfactory in eight. Following surgical treatment for instability in the posterior direction seven remained reduced, one had mild posterior subluxation, one had moderate subluxation, and eight continued to have severe subluxation. Result ratings were excellent in four, satisfactory in four, and unsatisfactory in nine. Following surgical treatment of instability in the superior direction, 4 had moderate subluxation, and 13 had severe subluxation. The result rating was satisfactory in 2 and unsatisfactory in 15. In the inferior direction two remained reduced and one had mild subluxation. All three were rated as satisfactory. In the multidirectional group one had mild subluxation and one had severe subluxation following treatment. Result ratings were excellent in one and unsatisfactory in one. When there was no change in the prosthesis but only soft tissue repair 7 of 29 or 24% had an excellent or satisfactory result rating at final follow-up. When change of prosthesis position was a component of the revision surgery 10 of 21 or 48% had an excellent or satisfactory result rating. From this experience one can conclude that subluxation following total shoulder arthroplasty that is severe enough to require revision surgery is indeed a serious complication and the chances of subsequent surgery improving the situation are only moderate.

As such, preventing subluxation and dislocation is the key. Identifiable risk factors for postoperative shoulder instability would apparently include an older patient, preexistent rotator cuff disease, subluxation or dislocation, and increased preoperative range of motion. Additional factors would include irregular, that is, asymmetrical glenoid wear—usually posterior, the use of prosthetic parts that are too small for the surrounding soft-tissue envelope, or the use of prosthetic parts that are too large, creating undue stress on the arthrotomy repair, with a potential for disruption of the repair early in the postoperative period. Component malposition should be avoided, and rotator cuff and capsule repair should be secure with appropriate postoperative external support and a carefully designed therapy program.

The treatment plan includes identification of all factors associated with the instability (involving the bone, the implants, and the soft tissues), and surgery is directed toward addressing all of these abnormalities as best one can. Postoperative support should then be ample, and the therapy program would be modified to maintain stability—recognizing that the surgical treatment we now have available is less than optimal in its effectiveness.

Component Problems

Appropriately there is significant concern in joint arthroplasty about the interface between the component–cement complex and the bone or in tissue ingrowth implants between the component and the bone. The bone is alive and can change over time because of mechanical or biologic influences. The greatest concern currently is with small–particle-induced activation of cells that resorb bone at the interface, replacing the very narrow bone to cement (or implant) or bone to fibrous tissue layer to cement interface with a softer, thicker, less mechanically stable membrane filled with histiocytes containing small particles of polyethylene, bone cement, or metal. When patients develop these changes they may be asymptomatic, or they may present having recognized a slight increase in their level of discomfort with slight reduction in limb function. Plain radiographs should be able to readily assess changes. Unfortunately, radiographs about the shoulder can be quite poor and not show the interfaces well, particularly if there is metal backing to the glenoid component, for only slight change in angle of the x-ray beam will obscure interface changes.

The 40-degree–posterior oblique view is an improvement over the standard anteroposterior view in assessing the interface between the glenoid implants and the bone of the scapula. Fluoroscopically positioned spot views are most consistent for not only evaluating the glenoid component, but also for the humeral component.[39] It is also useful to have a sequence of x-ray films, because a change in component position may be apparent with a series of films when it is not clearly demonstrated on a film taken at one point in time.

By recognizing the characteristic patient presentation and having high quality radiographs, over time it is usually possible to diagnose component loosening without needing to resort to more complex studies; however, occasionally these might be necessary and could include arthrography. Arthrography in addition to outlining the rotator cuff tendons will display synovitis, which is often present in situations during which component loosening occurs. Also dye can track between the bone–cement interface. However, the accuracy of this test for the diagnosis of component loosening has not been fully assessed. Shoulder arthroscopy has been suggested as one means to diagnose glenoid loosening, but the need for this must indeed be rare.

In the series of total shoulder arthroplasties published since 1980, glenoid loosening was the third most common complication, 1.3%, and humeral loosening was recognized to occur in 0.3%. In these series, the problem was treated with component revision slightly more than one-half the time and with removal of the loosened glenoid component, generally retaining the humeral head replacement, in slightly less than one-half the time (Fig. 8). There is little information on the treatment of loose humeral components. One of the authors in this series of reports identified two loose humeral components, but no treatment was undertaken because the patients had no pain. In another series, revision was performed because of symptomatic humeral loosening in one shoulder.

In the recent series on humeral head replacement, humeral loosening was again recognized in less than 1% of shoulders (0.6%). These cases of humeral component loosening were only recognized in a series of isoelastic prostheses and no treatment was mentioned.

Glenoid component loosening has been identified in conjunction with severe incompletely reconstructable rotator cuff tears or following the development of rotator cuff tearing in the postoperative period (Fig. 9). Franklin's seven cases occurring in this setting all exhibited large glenoid bone–cement lucent lines, often in association with a shift in component position.[27] This article was published to remind us of the importance of the rotator cuff in maintaining joint position, preventing eccentric and excessive component loading, and presumably, subsequent component loosening.

Review articles are more ample in their discussion of glenoid component loosening. Miller in 1993 reported that radiolucent lines are common, but there is apparently no direct correlation with the level of clinical symptoms.[47] He felt lucent lines may reflect the surgical technique, the quality of the glenoid bone, and changes affected by stress shielding or disuse osteoporosis. Also, he recognized that radiographic technique must be excellent to detect these lucencies in this anatomic region. He felt that loosening could be minimized by careful bone preparation at the time of surgery, fitting the implant closely to the bone, and using a minimal amount of

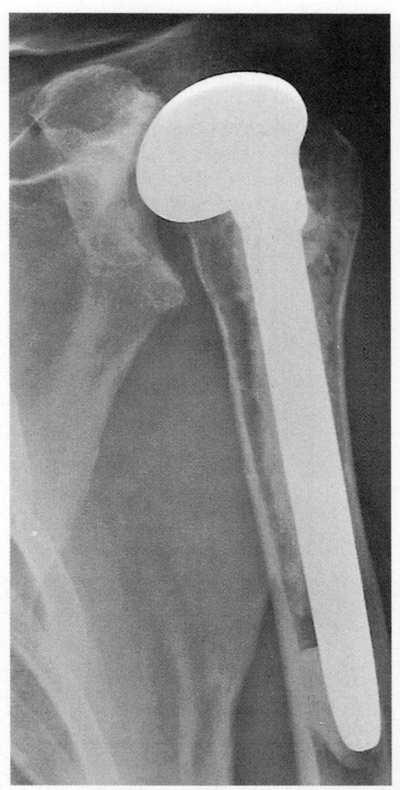

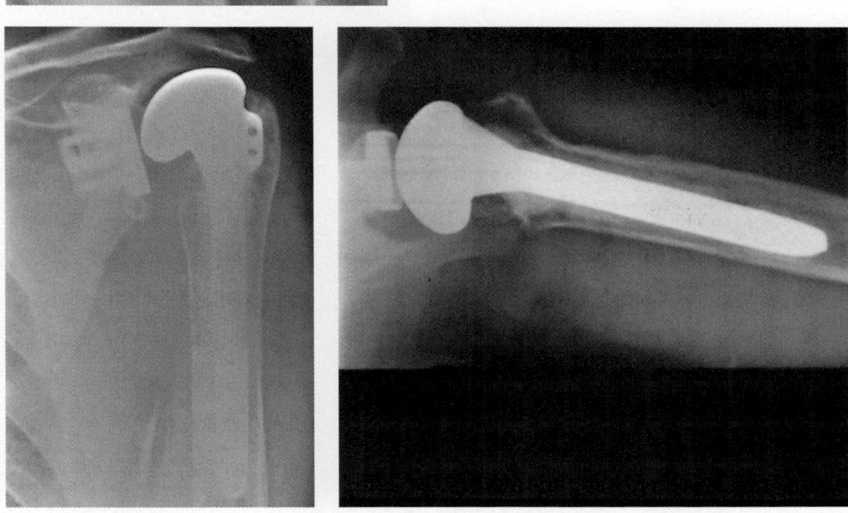

FIG. 8. This 65-year-old man with osteoarthritis underwent total shoulder arthroplasty. Five years later because of pain and loosening of the glenoid component, **(A)** he underwent revision surgery with removal of the loosened glenoid component and bone grafting. Unfortunately, he continued to have significant pain and 3 years later **(B,C)** a new glenoid component was inserted. Two years following revision surgery he is pain-free, has 140 degrees of active elevation, 70 degrees of external rotation, and internal rotation to T-7.

cement. Humeral loosening was recognized to be rare. Subsidence of the prosthesis can occur in osteoporotic bone, and the use of bone cement to fix the humeral component was suggested. Wirth and Rockwood, in reviewing 32 reports of total shoulder arthroplasty, identified that loosening represented nearly one-third of all complications and was in fact the most frequent complication reported in those studies they reviewed.[67] The authors stated that methods to enhance component fixation included concentric spherical reaming of the glenoid surface, preservation of most of the subchondral plate, a slight mismatching of the radii of the glenoid and humeral heads, and the consideration of press-fit or tissue ingrowth implants.

In the series studying postoperative complications at the Mayo Clinic, glenoid loosening was the third most common complication, occurring in 5% of shoulders. Humeral loosening occurred in 2% of shoulders. All developed late. Seventeen of the 19 shoulders diagnosed with glenoid loosening required reoperation, as did the 9 shoulders diagnosed with humeral loosening. In reviewing the complications of hemiarthroplasty for fractures, implant loosening occurred in three shoulders, the eighth most common complication.

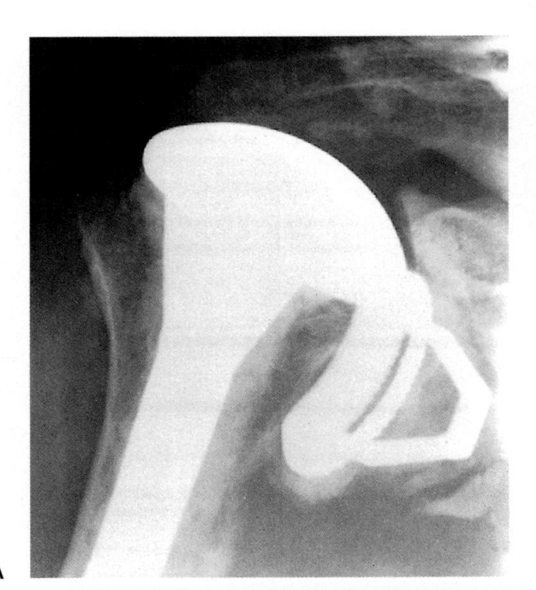

A

FIG. 9. A 71-year-old woman with rotator cuff tear arthropathy who underwent total shoulder arthroplasty. **(A)** Within several years the glenoid became loose and the shoulder became quite painful. **(B)** At revision surgery the glenoid component was replaced, recementing it into position, and the rotator cuff tear was repaired. Unfortunately, within months following revision surgery it was apparent that the rotator cuff repair had not healed or had stretched somewhat following the repair and the early healing phase. **(C)** She remains somewhat unstable superiorly and weak, but is more comfortable than during her prerevision state.

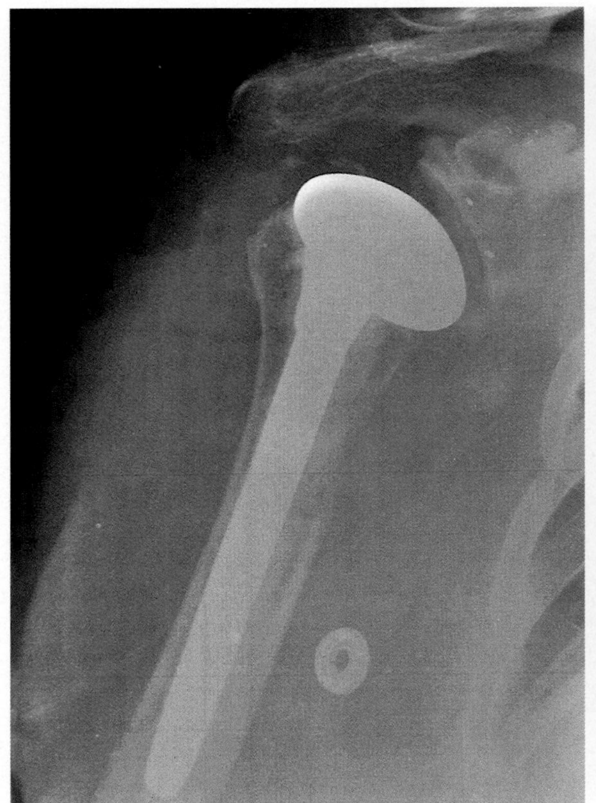

B

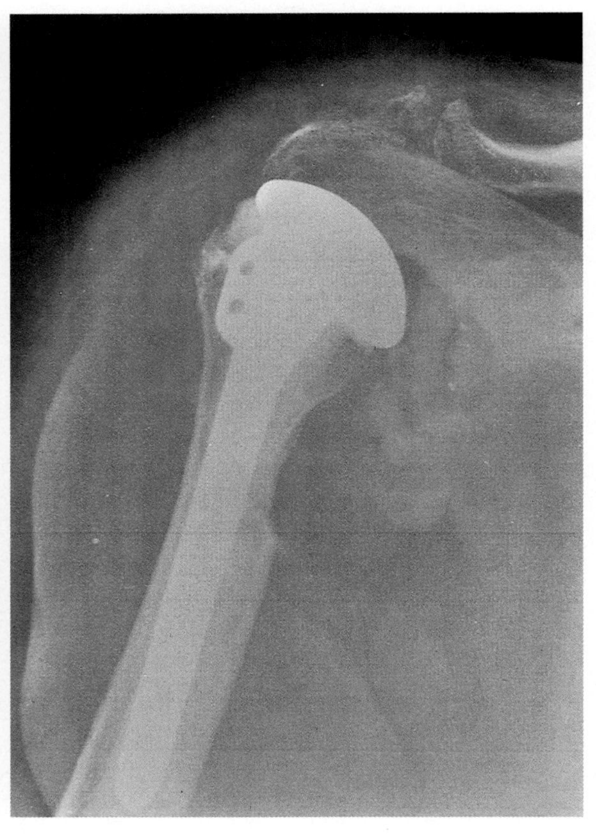

C

Longer-term follow-up of total shoulder arthroplasties and humeral head replacements is more informative concerning component loosening. Of 113 total shoulder replacements performed at the Mayo Clinic between 1975 and 1981, the probability of implant survival was 93% at 10 years, and 87% at 15 years. Seventy-nine of these patients with 89 arthroplasties were available for follow-up an average of 12.2 years following surgery, with a range of follow-up from 5 to 17 years. Seventy-five glenoid components developed bone–cement radiolucencies, and 39 glenoid components (44%) were considered to have radiographic evidence of definite glenoid loosening. This loosening was statistically associated with an increase in pain. Additionally, a change in position of the humeral component occurred in 49% of press-fitted stems, but in none of the shoulders with cemented humeral stems. Humeral component loosening was not associated with pain. In this group of patients glenoid component revision was carried out in 4, so although the radiographic frequency of glenoid loosening was quite high, the clinical need for revision surgery remained low even with long-term follow-up. Two humeral components required a revision because of loosening. One humeral component was loose at the time of revision of a loose glenoid component and was revised at that time. A second patient developed humeral component loosening in association with a humeral shaft fracture and revision was undertaken using a long-stemmed humeral component and fracture fixation.

In the series at Mayo, of 67 humeral head replacements performed for osteoarthritis or rheumatoid arthritis follow-up was possible for an average of 9.3 years. Only one of these prostheses was fixed in place with bone cement. All the remaining Neer implants were press-fitted. Six of the 35 shoulders with osteoarthritis had a lucent zone 1.5 mm or larger surrounding the humeral component and in 3 of these there was a change in humeral component position downward in the humeral canal. Three of the 32 shoulders with rheumatoid arthritis had a 1.5-mm or more lucent line surrounding most of the humeral stem. Nine of the components in rheumatoid patients had a change in component position, with the component shifting downward in the humeral canal. In these patients with substantial radiographic changes relative to the humeral component, only 1 in the osteoarthritic group had severe pain and 2 in the rheumatoid group had moderate or severe pain. Thus, there was no clear relation between the development of symptoms and the radiographic appearance of the component. However, it must be clearly noted that the frequency of radiographic changes surrounding these press-fit Neer components was quite high, which suggests that fixation with bone cement for this type of implant would be preferred.

Given the limitations of the current technology, it may be impossible to fully eliminate glenoid loosening; however, as is outlined in the foregoing series, glenoid loosening that is clinically symptomatic enough to require revision surgery is uncommon, but all attempts to reduce the incidence of component loosening will be quite worthwhile in improving the consistency of shoulder arthroplasty. The surgeon can do little if anything to address the bone quality that the individual has; however, the amount of bone in the glenoid is quite small and certainly the bone should be preserved as much as possible during insertion of an implant. This includes preserving much of the subchondral plate of the glenoid and very meticulous removal of only that quantity of bone necessary to insert the implant. Preparation of the glenoid bone requires precision instrumentation to accomplish this. Certainly, very little reaming should be performed on the glenoid surface. Only the amount of subchondral plate needed to insert the columns or keel of the component should be removed. Soft bone underlying the subchondral plate that is not mechanically sound to support a component should be removed, and by performing these steps one hopes a trial glenoid component will be stable against the glenoid even in the absence of the bone cement. Further preparation would include pulsatile water lavage, a thorough drying of the glenoid bone, mixing the bone cement to diminish porosity using a vacuum system or centrifugation, pressurization of the bone cement, and impaction of the component into position, maintaining the stability of the component against the bone until the cement hardens.

The choice of a glenoid component is somewhat controversial. Over time the radius of the glenoid component has matched the radius of the humeral head. There is anatomic and biomechanical support for a slight mismatch with the radius of the glenoid slightly greater than that of the humerus.[32,35,60] Certainly, if this difference in radius is more than a few millimeters, the theoretical stresses in the polyethylene will increase to reach the point of material failure in polyethylene.[44] There are no clinical data to support the use of either an exactly matching component or one that is slightly mismatched.

Clearly, the joint must be well balanced. Tight capsular structures should be lengthened or divided to lessen unnecessarily high compressive forces across the joint. The rotator cuff should be repaired as best possible and the humeral head should be positioned against the glenoid to eliminate subluxation, for that may create loading of the edge of the glenoid component and subsequent component loosening.

It seems that press-fitting the typical designs of humeral components that do not have surface texturing or surface ingrowth capabilities may not be wise. These components were generally designed for use with bone cement and quite likely that is the preferred mode of fixation. Loosening of a cemented humeral component is exceedingly rare. On the other hand, a cemented humeral component would be extraordinarily hard to remove should revision surgery be necessary. To attempt to address this issue, various components have been designed with texturing or ingrowth capabilities. This type of fixation will no doubt represent an improvement over press-fitting of smooth humeral stems. The security of fixation will probably not equal that of bone cement, but the frequency of clinically significant loosening of these components will probably be quite low. There is a special caveat though that the use of texturing or ingrowth surfaces on the distal portion of the humeral component will in fact also create a situation in which revision surgery will be extremely difficult or impossible, suggesting that ingrowth and textured materials should be limited to the metaphyseal area of the bone if the surgeon wishes to create better fixation in the absence of the use of bone cement, but yet retain the advantages of revisability at a later date.

It seems apparent that many glenoid components that have loosened do not require revision surgery. If a patient becomes substantially and continually symptomatic, it is important to exclude other problems as a cause of the symptoms, such as an occult low-grade infection, rotator cuff tearing, or humeral loosening. All these may occur independently or in association with glenoid loosening. Following exposure, subdeltoid and subacromial scar is lysed. The anterior arthrotomy must take into consideration the possible need for improved external rotation—typically, incising the subscapularis and shoulder capsule from the humeral neck. The inferior capsule is also incised along the humeral neck.

Synovectomy is performed as necessary following either removal of a modular humeral head component or retraction of the humeral component posteriorly. The loosened glenoid component can then be removed, samples can be taken for culture and frozen section, and any histiocytic membrane is removed from the remaining glenoid bone. Not uncommonly there is a fairly large central defect in the glenoid. If there does not appear to be enough bone remaining to offer support for a new glenoid component, one could leave the cavity and rest the humeral head against the remaining bone. Alternatively, one can use autogenous or allograft bone to fill the defect and to recontour the glenoid to a slight concavity. However, if there is enough bone remaining to support a glenoid component, it seems preferable to fix a new component in place. This can be accomplished with impaction bone grafting and the use of columns and screws to fix the tissue ingrowth component in place, cementing a component perhaps similar to the component that loosened but one with a slightly more bulky keel, or a combination of structural bone grafting and cementing a new glenoid component. It is really not clear what approach might be best. Approximately half of the cases reported have had a new glenoid replaced and half have had the loosened glenoid component removed with the glenoid either left as it is or restored with some bone graft material.

After addressing the glenoid difficulties, it is important to recall that one needs to balance the joint: to adjust humeral head size and rotator cuff tension so the shoulder seats centrally and moves smoothly through an ample arc of motion.

Humeral component loosening often includes substantial loss of the humeral metaphyseal bone and compromise of the quality of the endosteal bone surface that rested against the preceding component or component and cement. Certainly, if there is enough metaphyseal bone remaining and the canal is large enough, one could ream the canal slightly larger and put in a somewhat larger humeral stem to resecure the component. Usually this is not the case, however, and after thorough preparation of the metaphysis and endosteal surfaces, one either cements a new standard component in place or secures a component in place that is slightly longer (perhaps by 5 cm or so) than the original component. As landmarks may be distorted, it is important to pay special attention to component torsion and height.

PRINCIPLES OF REVISION SURGERY

There is a variety of complications that occur following total shoulder arthroplasty. These include not only changes in the implants and their attachments to bone, but also alterations in the soft tissues including the shoulder capsule, the rotator cuff, and the deltoid. Consideration must also be given to whether or not paresis or selective paralysis exists and whether or not there is an occult infection present. In a step-wise fashion, it is useful to understand the shoulder condition preceding the total shoulder arthroplasty or humeral head replacement, to have information about the findings at the time of the surgical procedure, and to understand what was done during that procedure. The implants are then assessed for their structural integrity, for their position relative to bone and relative to the opposing component. The deltoid is assessed for its competency and strength of contraction. The rotator cuff is evaluated considering its contributions to both glenohumeral stability and strength. The shoulder capsule is assessed for laxity or tightness. If there is question of nerve involvement, an electromyogram can be helpful. If infection is a consideration (as it often might be), laboratory assessment, indium scanning, or joint aspiration with an arthrogram may be required.

Following assessment it is useful to prepare a problem list detailing each of the abnormalities that exist. In the second column, it is helpful to prepare the alternative solutions for each one of these problems, and finally, it is helpful to realistically assess how effective each one of the treatments might be for each abnormal condition. One can then reach a conclusion about the benefits and limitations of possible revision surgery.

Finally, one must consider patient characteristics. As so much depends upon protection of the soft tissues following surgery and cautious, well planned rehabilitation, the patient must have the cooperative capacity to participate in this program. Even if the problems are recognized and the solutions are well planned and effective, if the patient is unable to cooperate in the postoperative period the revision may be for naught.

REFERENCES

1. Amstutz HC, Sew AL, Clarke IC. UCLA anatomic total shoulder arthroplasty. *Clin Orthop* 1981;155:7–20.
2. Amstutz HC, Thomas BJ, Kabo JM, Jinnah RH, Dorey FJ. The Dana total shoulder arthroplasty. *J Bone Joint Surg [Am]* 1988;70:1174–1182.
3. Arntz CT, Jackins S, Matsen III FA. Prosthetic replacement of the shoulder for the treatment of defects in the rotator cuff and the surface of the glenohumeral joint. *J Bone Joint Surg [Am]* 1993;75:485–491.
4. Barrett WP, Franklin JL, Jackins SE, Wyss GR, Matsen FA. Total shoulder arthroplasty. *J Bone Joint Surg [Am]* 1987;69:865–872.
5. Barrett WP, Thornhill TS, Thomas WH, Gebhart EM, Sledge CB. Nonconstrained total shoulder arthroplasty in patients with polyarticular rheumatoid arthritis. *J Arthroplasty* 1989;4:91–96.
6. Bell SN, Gschwend N. Clinical experience with total arthroplasty and hemiarthroplasty of the shoulder using the Neer prosthesis. *Int Orthop* 1986;10:217–222.
7. Blevins FT, Deng X, Torzilli PA, Warren RF. Dissociation of modular shoulder arthroplasty. *Orthop Trans* 1994–1995;18:977.
8. Bodey WN, Yeoman PM. Prosthetic arthroplasty of the shoulder. *Acta Orthop Scand* 1983;54:900–903.
9. Bonutti PM, Hawkins RJ. Fracture of the humeral shaft associated with total replacement of the shoulder. *J Bone Joint Surg [Am]* 1987;74:617–618.
10. Boyd AD Jr, Thomas WH, Scott RD, Sledge CB, Thornhill TS. Total shoulder arthroplasty versus hemiarthroplasty. Indications for glenoid resurfacing. *J Arthroplasty* 1990;5:329–336.
11. Boyd AD Jr, Aliabadi P, Thornhill TS. Postoperative proximal migration in total shoulder arthroplasty. *J Arthroplasty* 1991;6:31–37.
12. Boyd AD Jr, Thornhill TS, Barnes CL. Fracture adjacent to humeral prosthesis. *J Bone Joint Surg [Am]* 1992;74:1498–1504.
13. Brenner BC, Ferlic DC, Clayton ML, Dennis DA. Survivorship of unconstrained total shoulder arthroplasty. *J Bone Joint Surg [Am]* 1989;71:1289–1296.

14. Brostrom LA, Kronberg M, Wallensten R. Should the glenoid be replaced in shoulder arthroplasty with an unconstrained Dana or St. George prosthesis? *Ann Chir Gynaecol* 1992;81:54–75.
15. Campbell JT, Moore RS, Iannotti JP, Norris TR, Williams GR. Periprosthetic humeral fractures—mechanisms of fracture and treatment options. *Orthop Trans* 1996;20:59.
16. Cockx E, Claes T, Hoogmartens M, Mulier JC. The isoelastic prosthesis for the shoulder joint. *Acta Orthop Belg* 1983:49:275–285.
17. Codd TP, Yamaguchi K, Pollock RG, Flatow EL, Bigliani LU. Infected shoulder arthroplasties: treatment with staged reimplantation vs resection arthroplasty. *Orthop Trans* 1996;20:59.
18. Cofield RH. Total shoulder arthroplasty with the Neer prosthesis. *J Bone Joint Surg [Am]* 1984;66:899–906.
19. Cofield RH, Daly PJ. Total shoulder arthroplasty with a tissue-ingrowth glenoid component. *J Shoulder Elbow Surg* 1992;1:77–85.
20. Cofield RH, Frankle MA, Zuckerman JD. Humeral head replacement for glenohumeral arthritis. *Semin Arthroplasty* 1995;6:214–221.
21. Cruess RL. Corticosteroid-induced osteonecrosis of the humeral head. *Orthop Clin North Am* 1985;16:789–796.
22. Faludi II, Weiland AJ. Cementless total shoulder arthroplasty: preliminary experience with thirteen cases. *Orthopedics* 1982;321–437.
23. Fenlin JM Jr, Ramsey ML, Allardyce TJ, Frieman BG. Modular total shoulder replacement. Design rationale, indications and results. *Clin Orthop* 1994;307:37–46.
24. Figgie HED, Inglis AE, Goldberg VM, Ranawat CS, Figgie MP, Wile JM. An analysis of factors affecting the long-term results of total shoulder arthroplasty in inflammatory arthritis. *J Arthroplasty* 1988;3: 123–130.
25. Figgie MP, Inglis AE, Figgie HED, Sobel M, Burstein AH, Kraay MJ. Custom total shoulder arthroplasty in inflammatory arthritis. Preliminary results. *J Arthroplasty* 1992;7:1–6.
26. Fischer RA, Nicholson GP, McIlveen SJ, McCann PD, Flatow EL, Bigliani LU. Primary humeral head replacement for severely displaced proximal humerus fractures. *Orthop Trans* 1992;16:779.
27. Franklin JL, Barrett WP, Jackins SE, Matsen FA. Glenoid loosening in total shoulder. *J Arthroplasty* 1988;3:39–46.
28. Frich LH, Moller BN, Sneppen O. Shoulder arthroplasty with the Neer Mark-II prosthesis. *Orthop Trauma Surg* 1988;107:110–113.
29. Goldman RT, Koval KJ, Cuomo F, Gallagher MA, Zuckerman JD. Functional outcome after humeral head replacement for acute three-and four-part proximal humeral fractures. *J Shoulder Elbow Surg* 1995;4: 81–86.
30. Groh GI, Badwey TM, Rockwood CA. Treatment of cysts of the acromioclavicular joint with shoulder hemiarthroplasty. *J Bone Joint Surg [Am]* 1993;75:1790–1794.
31. Groh GI, Heckman MM, Curtis RJ, Rockwood CA. Treatment of fractures adjacent to humeral prosthesis. *Orthop Trans* 1994–1995;18: 1072.
32. Harryman DT, Sidles JA, Harris SL, Lippitt SB, Matsen FA III. The effect of articular cartilage conformity on the size of the humeral head component on laxity and motion after glenohumeral arthroplasty. *J Bone Joint Surg [Am]* 1995;77:555–563.
33. Hawkins RJ, Neer CS, Pianta RM, Mendoza FX. Locked posterior dislocation of the shoulder. *J Bone Joint Surg [Am]* 1987;69:9–18.
34. Hawkins RJ, Bell RH, Jallay B. Total shoulder arthroplasty. *Clin Orthop* 1989;242:188–194.
35. Iannotti JP, Gabriel JP, Schneck Sl, Evans BG, Missa S. The normal glenohumeral relationships. *J Bone Joint Surg [Am]* 1992;74:491–500.
36. Jonsson E, Egund N, Kelly I, Rydholm U, Lidgren L. Cup arthroplasty of the rheumatoid surgery. *Acta Orthop Scand* 1986;57:542–546.
37. Jonsson E, Brattstrom M, Lidgren L. Evaluation of the rheumatoid shoulder function after hemiarthroplasty and arthrodesis. *Scand J Rheum* 1988;17:17–26.
38. Kay SP, Amstutz HC. Shoulder hemiarthroplasty at UCLA. *Clin Orthop* 1988;228:42–48.
39. Kelleher IM, Cofield RH. Fluoroscopically positioned radiographs of total shoulder arthroplasty. *J Shoulder Elbow Surg* 1:306–311, 1992.
40. Kelly IG, Foster RS, Fisher WD. Neer total shoulder replacement in rheumatoid arthritis. *J Bone Joint Surg [Am]* 1987;69:723–726.
41. Kjaersgaard-Andersen P, Frich LH, Sojbjerg JO, Sneppen O. Heterotopic bone formation following total shoulder arthroplasty. *J Arthroplasty* 1989;4:99–104.
42. Krakauer JD, Cofield RH. Periprosthetic fractures in total shoulder replacement. *Oper Tech Orthop* 1994;4:243–252.
43. Lynch NM, Cofield RH, Silbert PL, Hermann RC. Neurologic complications after total shoulder arthroplasty. *J Shoulder Elbow Surg* 1996; 5:53–61.
44. Matsen FA III, Lippitt SB, Sedes JA, Harryman DT II. *Practical evaluation and management of the shoulder*. Philadelphia: WB Saunders, 1994.
45. McCoy SR, Warren RF, Bade HAD, Ranawat CS, Inglis AE. Total shoulder arthroplasty in rheumatoid arthritis. *J Arthroplasty* 1989;4: 99–104.
46. McElwain JP, English E. The early results of porous-coated total shoulder arthroplasty. *Clin Orthop* 1987;218:217–224.
47. Miller SR, Bigliani LU. Complications of total shoulder replacement. In: Bigliani LU, ed. *Complications of shoulder surgery*. Baltimore: Williams & Wilkins, 1993:59–72.
48. Moeckel BH, Dines DM, Warren RF, Altchek DW. Modular hemiarthroplasty for fractures of the proximal part of the humerus. *J Bone Joint Surg [Am]* 1992;74:884–889.
49. Moeckel BH, Altchek DW, Warren RF, Wickiewicz TL, Dines DM. Instability of the shoulder after arthroplasty. *J Bone Joint Surg [Am]* 1993;75:492–497.
50. Muldoon MP, Cofield RH. Complications of humeral head replacement for proximal humeral fractures. In: Springfield DS, ed, *Instructional course lectures*, 1997:15–37.
51. Neer CS, Kirby RM. Revision of humeral head and total shoulder arthroplasties. *Clin Orthop* 1982;170:189–195.
52. Neer CS, Watson KC, Stanton FJ. Recent experiences in total shoulder replacement. *J Bone Joint Surg [Am]* 1982;64:319–337.
53. Petersson CJ. Shoulder surgery in rheumatoid arthritis. *Acta Orthop Scand* 1986;57:222–226.
54. Pollock RG, Deliz ED, McIlveen SJ, Flatow EL, Bigliani LU. Prosthetic replacement in rotator cuff-deficient shoulders. *J Shoulder Elbow Surg* 1992;1:173–186.
55. Post M, Haskell SS, Jablon M. Total shoulder replacement with a constrained prosthesis. *J Bone Joint Surg [Am]* 1980;62:327–335.
56. Pritchett JW, Clark JM. Prosthetic replacement for chronic unreduced dislocations of the shoulder. *Clin Orthop* 1987;216:89–93.
57. Roper BA, Paterson JNH, Day WH. The Roper-Day total shoulder replacement. *J Bone Joint Surg [Br]* 1990;72:694–697.
58. Rutherford C, Cofield RH. Osteonecrosis of the shoulder. *Orthop Trans* 1987;11:239.
59. Seddon HJ. Three types of nerve injury. *Brain* 1943;66:237–288.
60. Severt R, Thomas BJ, Tsenter MJ, Amstutz HC, Kabo JM. The influence of conformity and constraint on translational forces and frictional torque in total shoulder arthroplasty. *Clin Orthop* 1993;292:151–158.
61. Soghikian GW, Neviaser RJ. Complications of humeral head replacement. In: Bigliani LU, ed. *Complications of shoulder surgery*. Baltimore: Williams & Wilkins, 1993:81–92.
62. Sunderland S. A classification of peripheral nerve injuries producing loss of function. *Brain* 1951;74:491–516.
63. Tanner MW, Cofield RH. Prosthetic arthroplasty for fractures and fracture-dislocations of the proximal humerus. *Clin Orthop* 1983;179: 116–128.
64. Thomas BJ, Amstutz HC, Cracchiolo A. Shoulder arthroplasty for rheumatoid arthritis. *Clin Orthop* 1991;265:125–128.
65. Vahvanen V, Hämäläinen M, Paavolainen P. The Neer II replacement for rheumatoid arthritis of the shoulder. *Int Orthop* 1989;13:57–60.
66. Weber ER, Daube JR, Coventry MB. Peripheral neuropathies associated with total hip arthroplasty. *J Bone Joint Surg [Am]* 1976;58:66–69.
67. Wirth MA, Rockwood CA. Complications of total shoulder-replacement arthroplasty. *J Bone Joint Surg [Am]* 1996;78:603–616.
68. Wright TW, Cofield RH. Humeral fractures after shoulder arthroplasty. *J Bone Joint Surg [Am]* 1995;77:1340–1346.
69. Zuckerman JD, Cofield RH. Proximal humeral prosthetic replacement in glenohumeral arthritis. *Orthop Trans* 1986;10:231–232.

PART V

Fractures

Disorders of the Shoulder: Diagnosis and Management,
edited by Joseph P. Iannotti and Gerald R. Williams, Jr.
Lippincott Williams & Wilkins, Philadelphia © 1999.

CHAPTER 23

Fractures of the Scapula: Diagnosis and Treatment

Thomas P. Goss

CLASSIFICATION AND INCIDENCE

General Considerations

Fractures of the scapula account for 1% of all fractures, 5% of shoulder fractures, and 3% of injuries to the shoulder girdle. There are two reasons for this relative infrequency: (a) the scapula lies over the posterior chest wall protected by the rib cage and thoracic cavity anteriorly and a thick layer of soft tissues posteriorly, and (b) the relative mobility of the scapula allows for considerable dissipation of traumatic forces. The vast majority of scapular fractures (90+%) are insignificantly displaced, primarily because of the strong support provided by the surrounding soft tissues, making non-

T. P. Goss: Department of Orthopaedic Surgery, University of Massachusetts Medical School, Worcester, Massachusetts 01655.

operative management the treatment of choice for most scapular fractures. As a result, these injuries have received little attention in the literature. Scapular fractures involve a major articulation, however, and when significantly displaced are capable of causing considerable morbidity. Consequently, these injuries deserve more respect and recently have received more consideration in major texts,[10,19,23,26,111,119,123,124,130,135,145,147,150,157] general and review articles,[33,42,52,53,56,75,92,107,109,110,126,127,141,144,161,170,172,180] and papers dealing with specific issues.

Scapular fractures are usually the result of high-energy (usually direct but occasionally indirect) trauma. Consequently, they have an 80% to 95% incidence of associated osseous and soft-tissue injuries (local and distant) that may

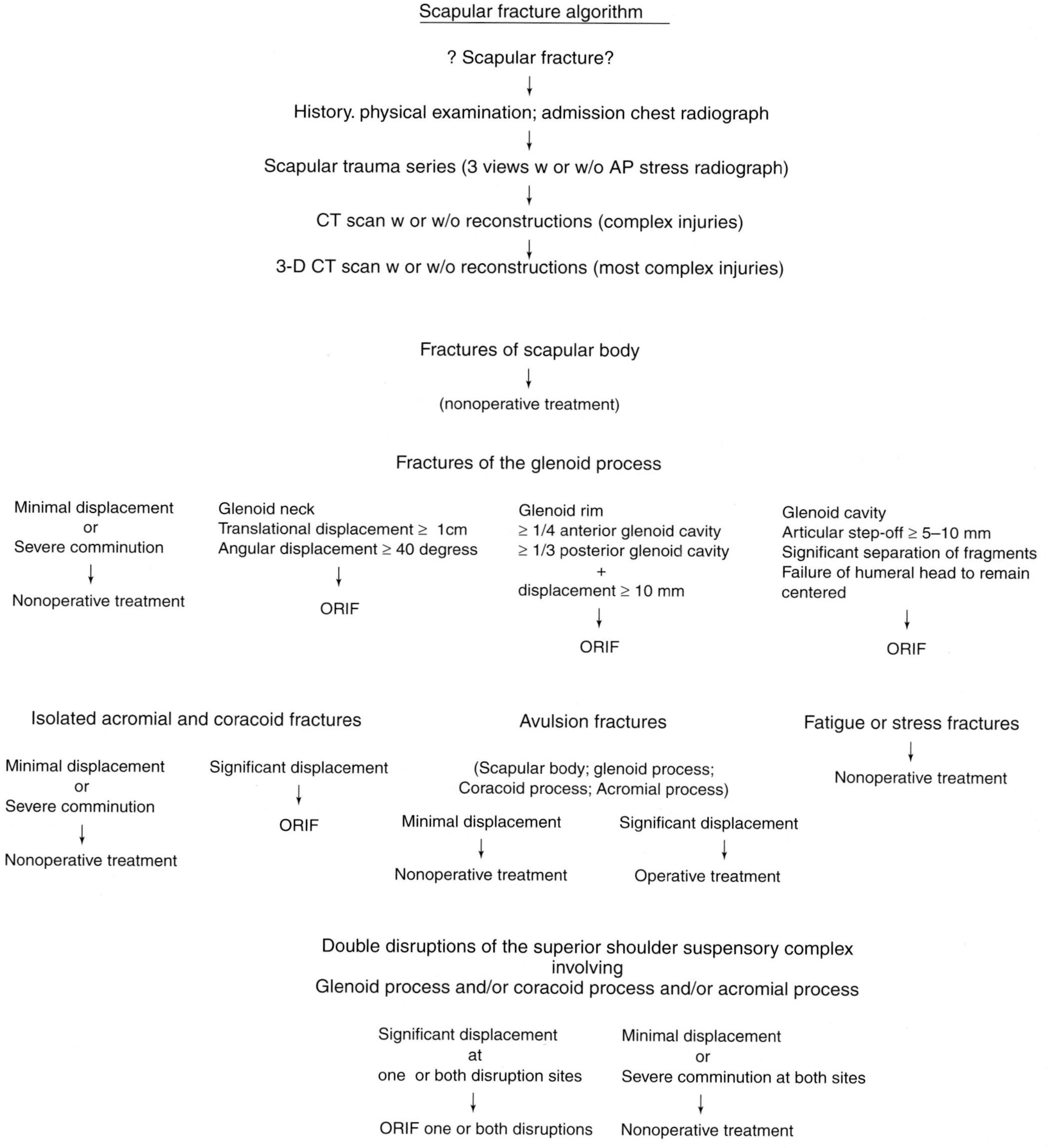

Scapular fracture algorithm

? Scapular fracture?
↓
History. physical examination; admission chest radiograph
↓
Scapular trauma series (3 views w or w/o AP stress radiograph)
↓
CT scan w or w/o reconstructions (complex injuries)
↓
3-D CT scan w or w/o reconstructions (most complex injuries)

Fractures of scapular body
↓
(nonoperative treatment)

Fractures of the glenoid process

Minimal displacement
or
Severe comminution
↓
Nonoperative treatment

Glenoid neck
Translational displacement ≥ 1cm
Angular displacement ≥ 40 degress
↓
ORIF

Glenoid rim
≥ 1/4 anterior glenoid cavity
≥ 1/3 posterior glenoid cavity
+
displacement ≥ 10 mm
↓
ORIF

Glenoid cavity
Articular step-off ≥ 5–10 mm
Significant separation of fragments
Failure of humeral head to remain centered
↓
ORIF

Isolated acromial and coracoid fractures

Minimal displacement
or
Severe comminution
↓
Nonoperative treatment

Significant displacement
↓
ORIF

Avulsion fractures

(Scapular body; glenoid process; Coracoid process; Acromial process)

Minimal displacement
↓
Nonoperative treatment

Significant displacement
↓
Operative treatment

Fatigue or stress fractures
↓
Nonoperative treatment

Double disruptions of the superior shoulder suspensory complex involving
Glenoid process and/or coracoid process and/or acromial process

Significant displacement
at
one or both disruption sites
↓
ORIF one or both disruptions

Minimal displacement
or
Severe comminution at both sites
↓
Nonoperative treatment

be major, multiple, and even life-threatening. These individuals need to be carefully evaluated when they present in the emergency room, and appropriate supportive care must be rendered (see Scapular Fracture Algorithm). As a result, scapular fractures are often diagnosed late or definitive treatment is delayed. This may compromise the patient's final functional result. In addition, if associated injuries involve the shoulder complex, the individual's "scapular fracture" recovery may be compromised still further.

Most scapular fractures involve the body and spine (approximately 50%)[109] (Fig. 1). These injuries are often rather alarming radiographically (extensive comminution and displacement are frequently present; Fig. 2); however, there is very little enthusiasm in the literature for operative treatment,[60] since bone stock for fixation is at a premium and these injuries seem to heal quite nicely with nonoperative/symptomatic treatment[63]—a good to excellent functional result can be expected. The reason for this positive prognosis probably relates to the fact that (a) the scapulothoracic interval is cushioned by a thick layer of soft tissues, and (b) the mobility of the scapulothoracic articulation compensates for most residual deformities of the scapular body. The literature does mention a fracture of the scapular body with a lateral spike entering the glenohumeral joint as an indication (albeit extremely uncommon) for surgical management.[59] On rare occasions, a scapular body malunion may result in scapulothoracic pain and crepitus requiring surgical exposure of its ventral surface and removal of the responsible bony prominence(s).[104]

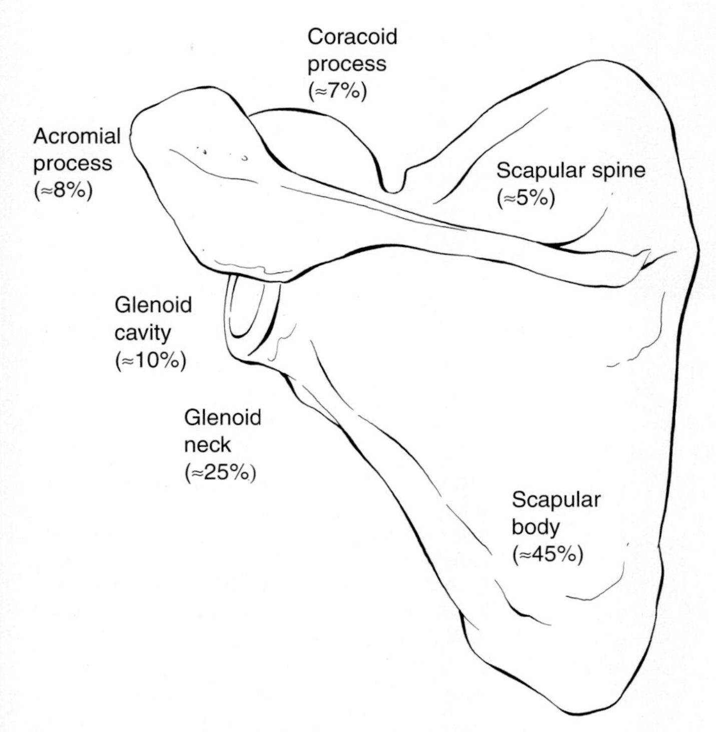

FIG. 1. Incidence of scapular fractures according to region: the scapular body (≈45%); the scapular spine (≈5%); the glenoid neck (≈25%); the glenoid cavity (≈10%), the acromial process (≈8%), and the coracoid process (≈7%). (From ref. 109, with permission.)

The remaining 50% of scapular fractures involve its three processes (see Fig. 1). Fractures of the glenoid neck constitute approximately 25% of the total, whereas fractures of the glenoid cavity (the glenoid rim and glenoid fossa) make up approximately 10%. (Fractures of the glenoid process, therefore, account for approximately 35% of all scapular fractures.) Approximately 8% of these injuries involve the acromial process, and approximately 7% involve the coracoid process.[109] (An *acromial fracture* is defined as any fracture that runs from the posterior margin of the scapular spine or acromion to the undersurface of the acromial process all the way to the deepest point of the spinoglenoid interval.)

Diagnosis

The physician's attention is initially drawn to the scapular region by the patient's complaints of pain and abnormal physical findings in the area (swelling, crepitus, ecchymosis, and such). The specific diagnosis of a scapular fracture, however, is ultimately radiographic. These injuries are often initially missed[61] or detected incidentally on the patient's admission chest radiograph (Fig. 2). A "scapula trauma series" is then indicated, including true anteroposterior (AP) and lateral views of the scapula as well as a true axillary projection of the glenohumeral joint (Fig. 3). The scapula is a complex bony structure. One must be able to visualize and evaluate the scapular body and spine as well as its three processes: the glenoid process, the acromial process, and the coracoid process. The glenoid process is composed of the glenoid neck and the glenoid cavity which, in turn, is made up of the glenoid fossa and the glenoid rim. Finally, the scapula takes part in three articulations (the acromioclavicular [AC] joint, the glenohumeral joint, and the scapulothoracic articulation), each of which must be carefully evaluated. One should look for associated shoulder girdle injuries, including those involving the clavicle, the proximal humerus, and the sternoclavicular joint.

If an injury to the linkage between the clavicle and the scapula (i.e., a disruption of the coracoclavicular and/or acromioclavicular ligaments) is suspected, a weight-bearing AP film of the shoulder should be obtained (see Fig. 3). In some situations, transthoracic lateral and oblique projections of the region may be of value. The scapula trauma series should suffice for most injuries, but if the fracture pattern appears to be complex (multiple fracture lines and significant displacement), computed tomography (CT) scanning is necessary. The superior images allow evaluation of the acromioclavicular joint and the acromial process, while the inferior images show the scapular body and spine and scapulothoracic articulation (Fig. 4). The middle images allow one to see the glenoid neck, the glenoid cavity (glenoid rim and glenoid fossa), the coracoid process, and the glenohumeral articulation (Fig. 5). In certain clinical situations, recon-

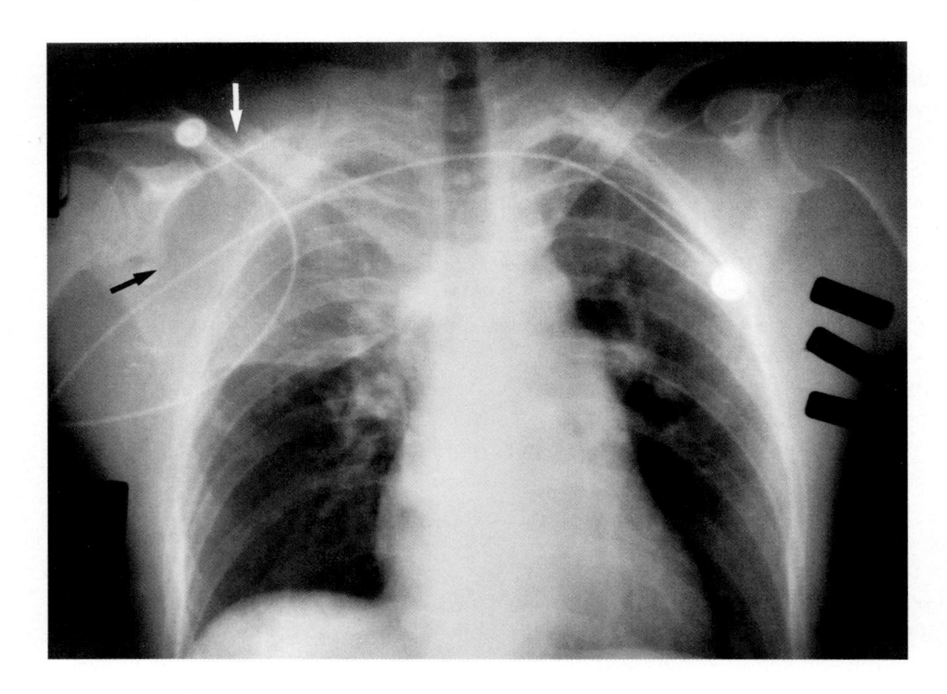

FIG. 2. An admission AP chest radiograph of a patient who sustained multiple trauma. The fractured clavicle and scapula (*arrows*) were incidental findings.

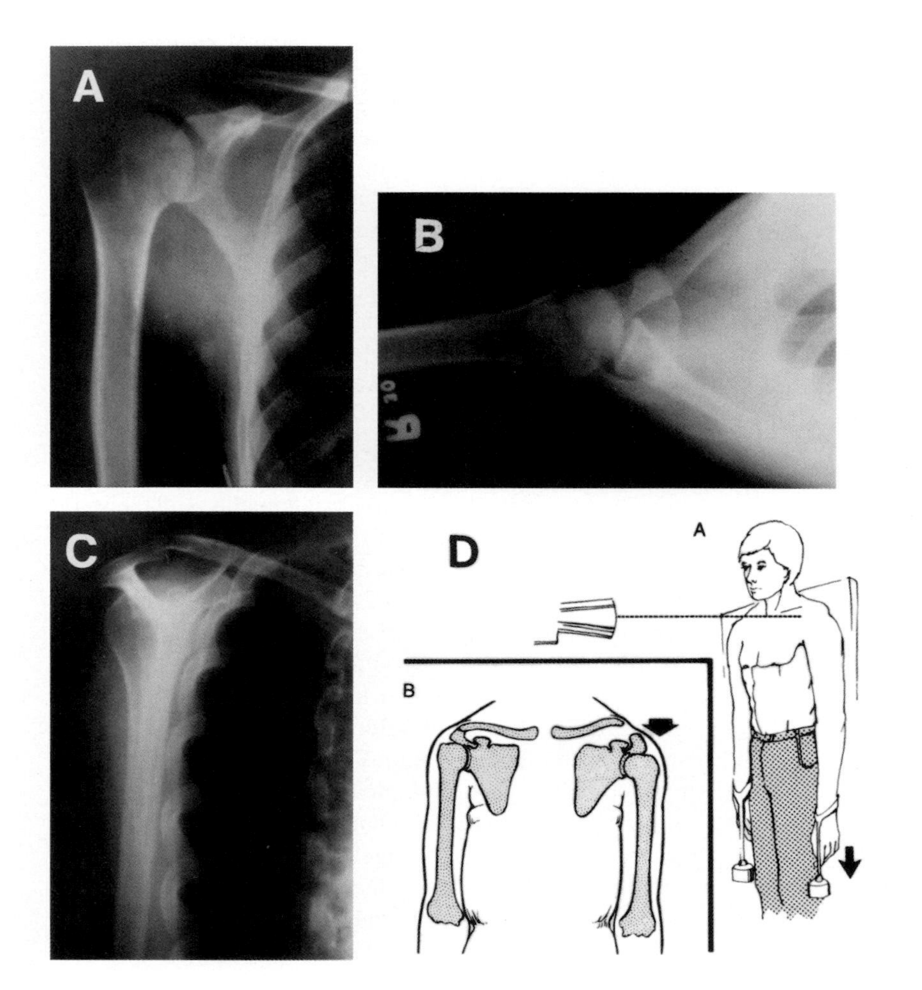

FIG. 3. The "scapular trauma series": **(A)** a true AP projection of the scapula; **(B)** a true axillary projection of the glenohumeral joint and scapula; **(C)** a true lateral projection of the scapula; and **(D)** a weight-bearing AP projection of the shoulder complex designed to evaluate the integrity of the clavicular–scapular linkage (optional and dependent on the clinical situation).(4D: From Rockwood CA. *Fractures*. Philadelphia: JB Lippincott, 1975:733, with permission.)

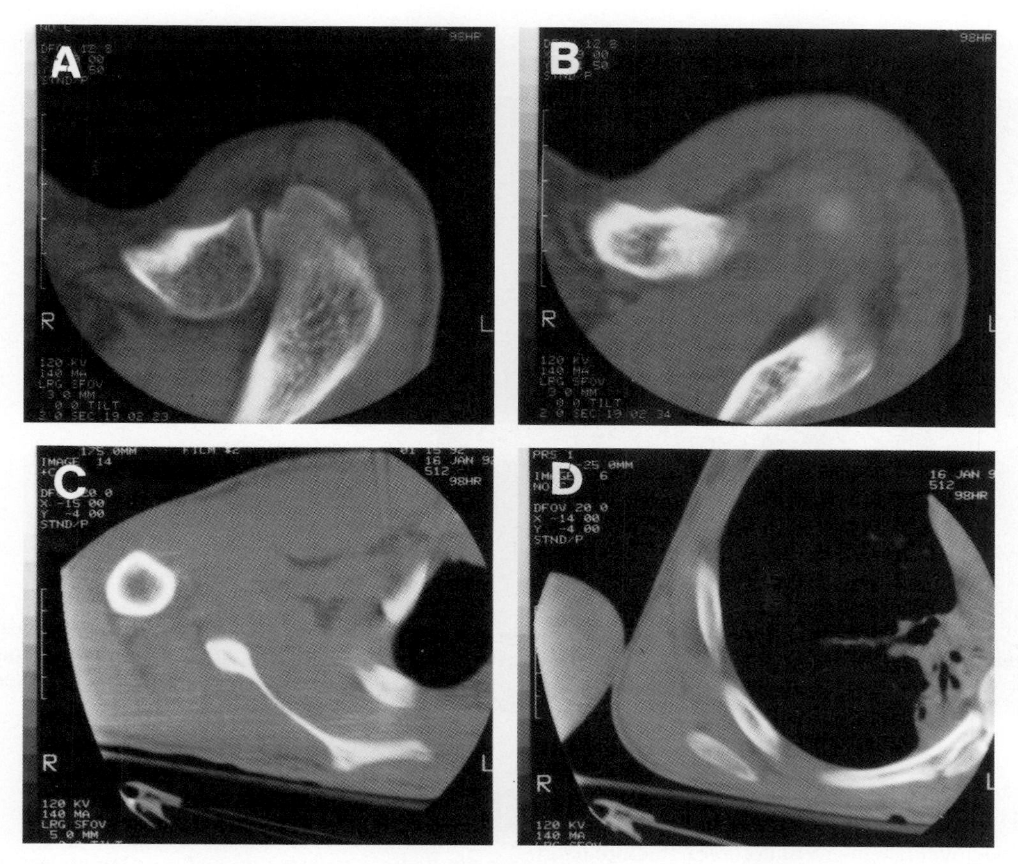

FIG. 4. Multiple axial CT images of the scapula: **(A,B)** Superior images showing the AC joint and the acromion; and **(C,D)** inferior images showing the scapular body and scapulothoracic articulation.

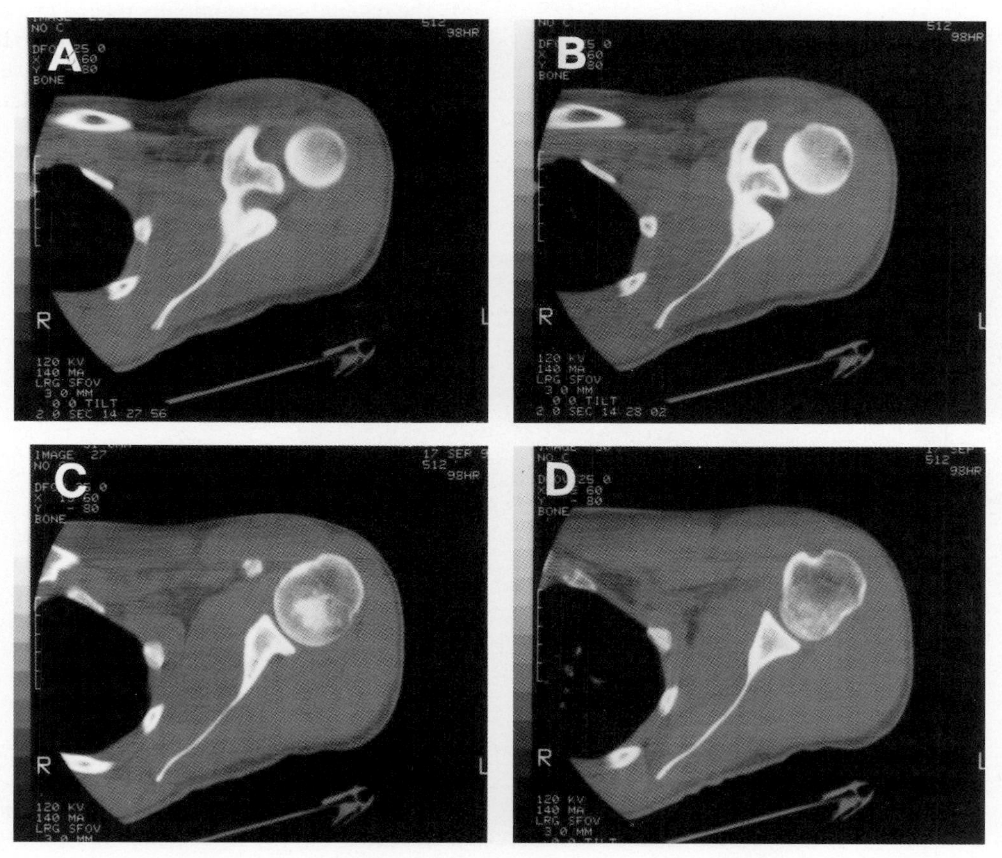

FIG. 5. Multiple axial CT images: **(A,B)** most superior; **(C,D)** most inferior, through the glenohumeral region of the scapula.

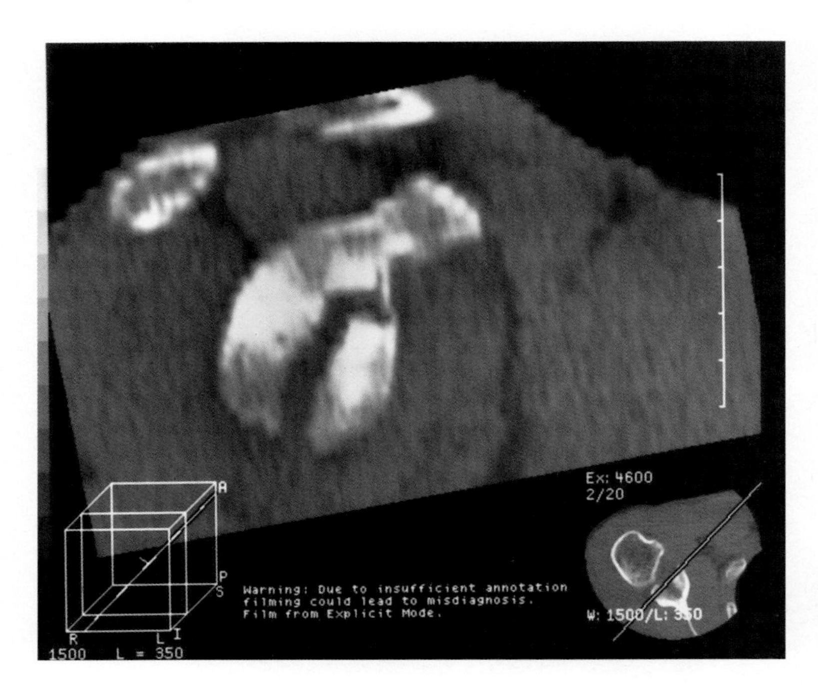

FIG. 6. A reconstructed CT image showing the glenoid cavity en face (note the large anteroinferior glenoid rim fragment with severe separation of the articular surface).

structed views can be of great value (Fig. 6). Finally, three-dimentional (3-D) scanning can be extremely helpful to the orthopedist trying to evaluate the most complex fracture patterns (Fig. 7). Images rotated at 15-degree increments in the horizontal, vertical, and oblique planes can be examined and the most useful projections printed for later reference. The proximal humerus can be eliminated for optimal visualization of the glenoid cavity and other reconstructed images are possible (see Fig. 21C). The exact role, if any, for arthroscopy (both diagnostic and therapeutic) is yet to be defined.

Nonoperative Treatment

Fractures of the scapular body and spine and insignificantly displaced fractures of the glenoid, acromial, and coracoid processes (see sections dealing specifically with injuries to these structures) are managed nonoperatively (Fig. 8). The patient's arm is initially placed in a sling and swathe immobilizer for comfort. Local ice packs to the affected area are helpful during the first 48 hours, followed by moist heat thereafter. Analgesic medications are prescribed as needed. Absolute immobilization is generally short term (48 hours), but may continue for up to 14 days, depending on the clini-

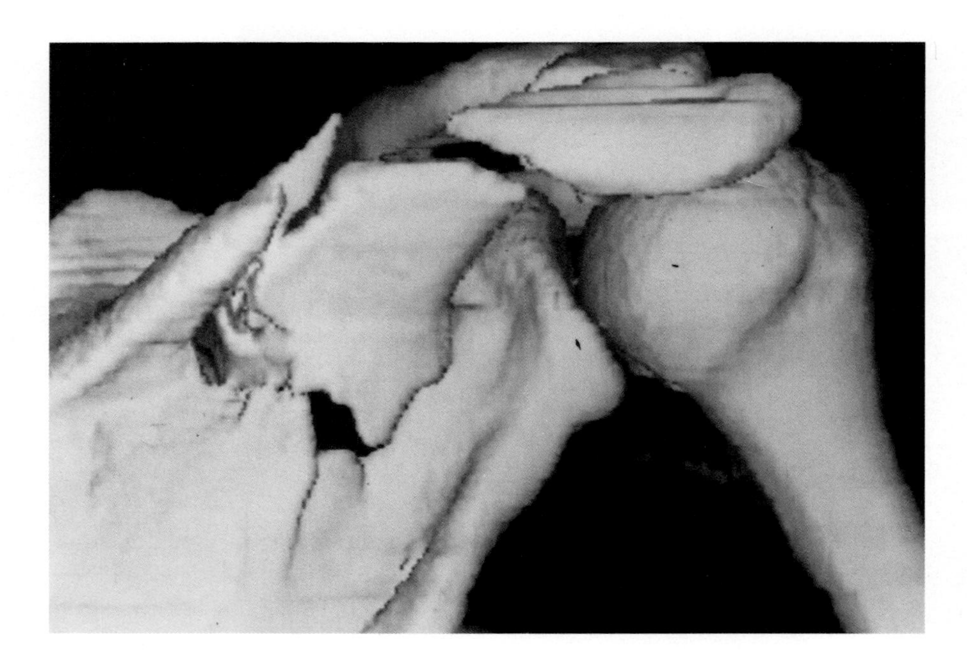

FIG. 7. A 3-D CT image of an individual who sustained a segmental fracture of the acromion (note the severely displaced intermediate segment).

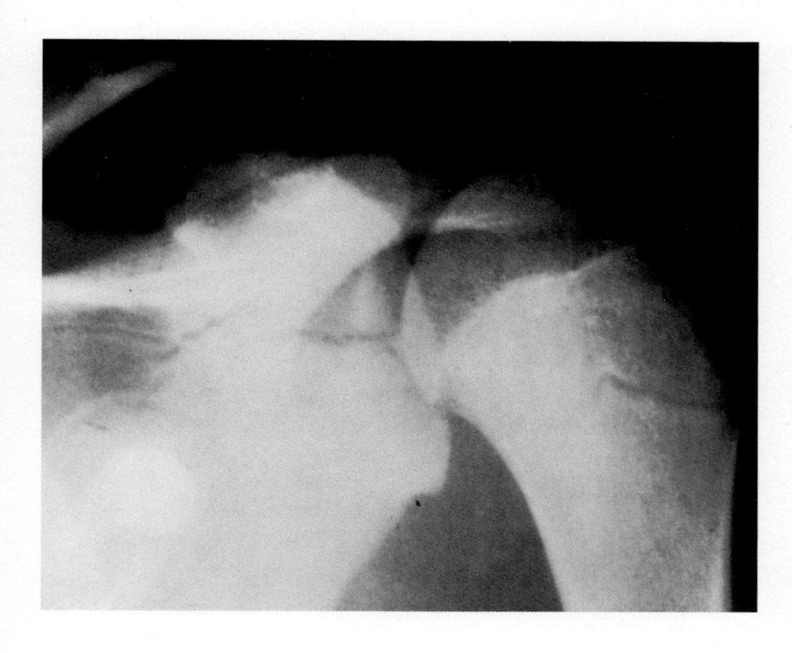

FIG. 8. An AP radiograph showing an undisplaced fracture of the scapula involving the glenoid process.

cal situation. The patient is then permitted to gradually increase the functional use of his or her upper extremity as symptoms allow and sling and swathe protection is gradually decreased until the 6-week point. Physiotherapy is prescribed during this period and focuses on maintaining and regaining shoulder range of motion. The program begins with dependent circular and pendulum movements as well as external rotation to, but not past neutral, and gradually moves on to progressive stretching techniques in all ranges. Close outpatient follow-up is necessary to monitor and guide the patient's recovery and x-ray films are obtained at 2-week intervals to ensure that unacceptable displacement does not occur at the fracture site(s). At 6 weeks, osseous union is usually sufficient to discontinue all external protection and encourage functional use of the upper extremity. The rehabilitation program continues until range of motion, strength, and overall function are maximized. Six months to 1 year may be required for full recovery, but a good to excellent result should be readily obtainable.

FRACTURES OF THE GLENOID PROCESS

The glenoid process includes the glenoid neck and the glenoid cavity which, in turn, is comprised of the glenoid rim and the glenoid fossa. Each of these areas may be fractured in a variety of ways. Most investigators agree that if significantly displaced, surgical management is indicated or should at least be considered. Several surgical principles apply.[47,49,51]

General Considerations

Surgical Approaches

Depending on the clinical situation, the glenoid process may be approached from three directions or combinations thereof.[55] The anterior approach is used for fractures of the anterior glenoid rim and some fractures of the superior aspect of the glenoid fossa. The posterior approach is used for fractures of the posterior rim, most fractures of the glenoid fossa, and fractures of the glenoid neck. The superior approach may be used for (a) fractures of the glenoid fossa with a difficult to control superior fragment (in conjunction with either a posterior or an anterior exposure), and (b) fractures of the glenoid neck with a difficult to control glenoid fragment (in conjunction with a posterior exposure).

Anterior Approach

For the anterior approach (Fig. 9), the patient is placed on the operating room table in the "beach chair" position. An anterior incision is made in Langer's lines, centered over the glenohumeral joint and running from the superior to the inferior margin of the humeral head. The deltoid muscle is exposed and split in the line of its fibers directly over the coracoid process. The conjoined tendon and pectoralis major muscle are retracted medially, whereas the deltoid muscle is retracted laterally.

The arm is externally rotated onto a sterile arm support or positioner and the subacromial bursa is removed, exposing the subscapularis tendon. (In type III glenoid cavity fractures, opening the rotator interval may allow sufficient exposure). The tendon is incised 2.5 cm medial to the medial border of the biceps groove and along its superior and inferior borders. It is then dissected off the underlying anterior glenohumeral capsule–glenoid neck periosteum and turned back medially. The anterior glenohumeral capsule is incised in the same fashion (5 mm medial to the anatomic neck) and also turned back medially. With a humeral head retractor inserted into the glenohumeral joint (the Fukuda ring retractor is especially useful[37]) and holding the humeral head out of

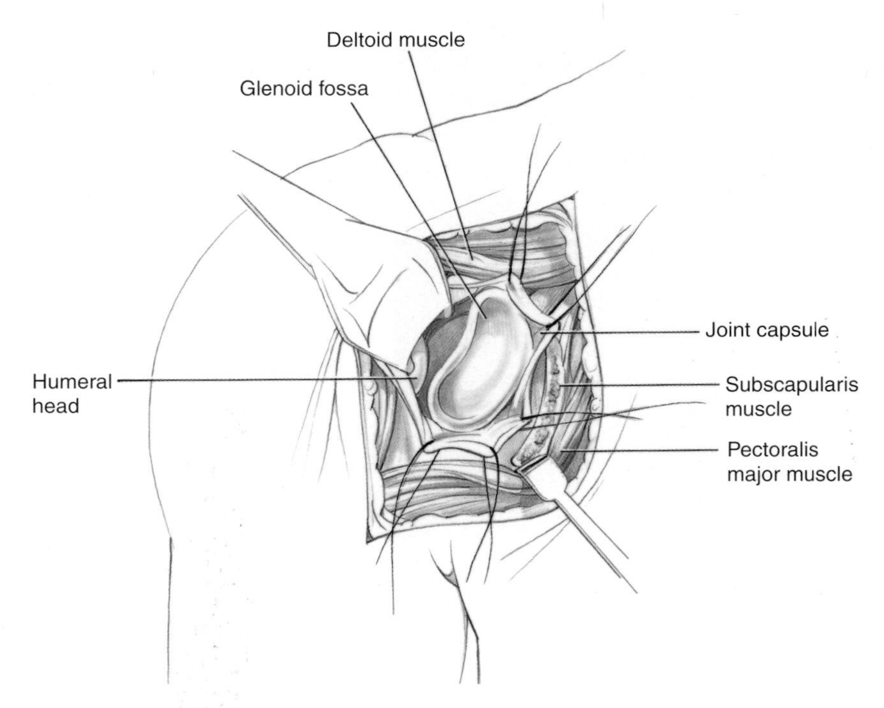

FIG. 9. Anterior surgical approach to the glenoid cavity.

the way, the entire glenoid cavity can be inspected and the surgeon has ready access to its anterior rim. One must take care to avoid injury to the nearby axillary nerve.

Posterior Approach

The patient is placed on the operating room table in the lateral decubitus position, supported by a bean bag. An incision is made over the lateral one-third of the scapular spine, along the posterior aspect of the acromion to its lateral tip and then distally in the midlateral line for a distance of 2.5 cm. Skin flaps are developed. The deltoid is dissected sharply off the scapular spine and the acromion and then split in the line of its fibers for a distance of not more than 5 cm starting at the lateral tip of the acromion. The deltoid is separated off the underlying infraspinatus and teres minor musculotendinous units and retracted down to, but not below, the inferior margin of the teres minor. (This approach allows maximal exposure; however, a more cosmetic vertical incision from the posterior axillary crease to the scapular spine with superolateral retraction of the undetached posterior deltoid muscle may suffice, especially if access to only the posteroinferior aspect of the glenoid cavity is needed; i.e., type Ib and II glenoid cavity fractures.) The infraspinatus tendon is incised 2.5 cm medial to the greater tuberosity and along its superior and inferior borders. It is then dissected off the underlying posterior glenohumeral capsule and turned back medially. The posterior glenohumeral capsule is incised in the same fashion and also turned back medially. (Depending on the particular clinical situation, one may have sufficient exposure by detaching only the lower one half of the insertion of the infraspinatus tendon and posterior glenohumeral capsule upon the humeral head, making an incision along their inferior border, and retracting the flap thereby created superiorly and medially[51]). With injuries that involve only the posteroinferior and inferior aspect of the glenoid cavity, one may be able to avoid detaching these structures completely—simply developing the infraspinatus–teres minor interval and making a linear incision in the capsule may allow adequate access.) With a Fukuda retractor inserted into the joint and holding the humeral head out of the way, the entire glenoid cavity can be inspected and the surgeon has ready access to its posterior rim as well as the glenoid neck (Fig. 10). The interval between the infraspinatus and teres minor muscles can be developed further and the long head of the triceps detached to gain access to the inferior aspect of the glenoid process and the lateral border of the scapular body (Fig. 11). One must take particular care to protect and avoid injury to the nearby suprascapular and axillary nerves.

Superior Approach

The superior approach can be added to either the anterior or the posterior exposure (Figs. 12 and 13) if a displaced, difficult-to-control or stabilize superior glenoid fragment or glenoid process fragment is present. Either incision is extended over the superior aspect of the shoulder. Soft-tissue flaps are developed and retracted, exposing the superior aspect of the distal clavicle, the AC joint, the acromion, and the trapezius muscle. In the interval between the clavicle and the acromion (posteromedial to the acromioclavicular joint), the trapezius muscle and the underlying supraspinatus tendon

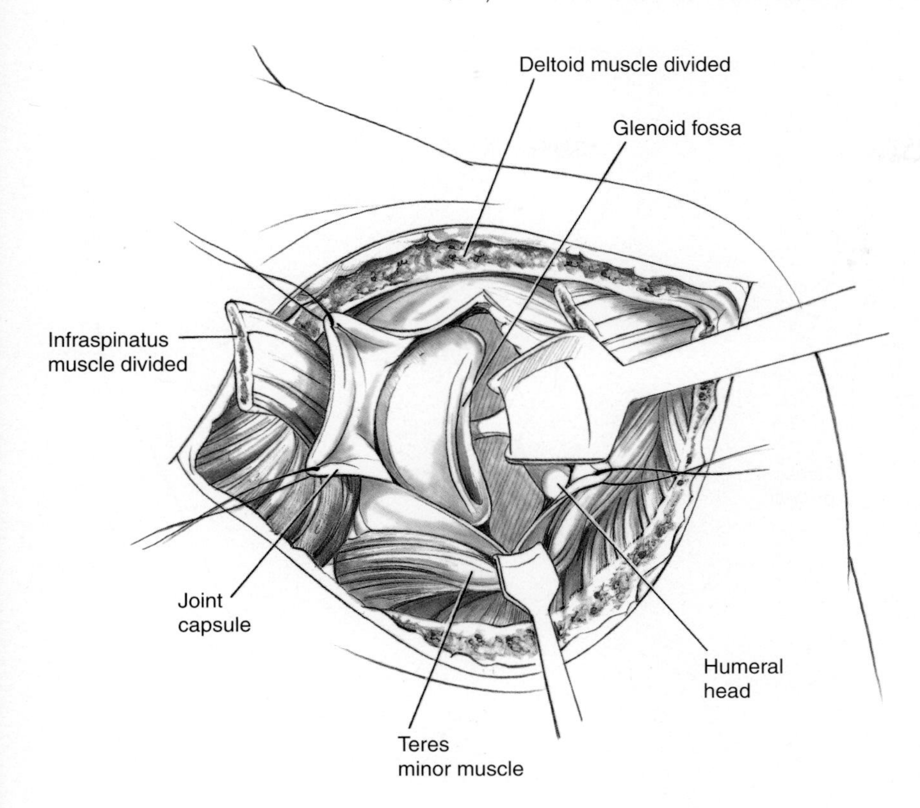

FIG. 10. Posterior surgical approach to the glenoid cavity: standard exposure.

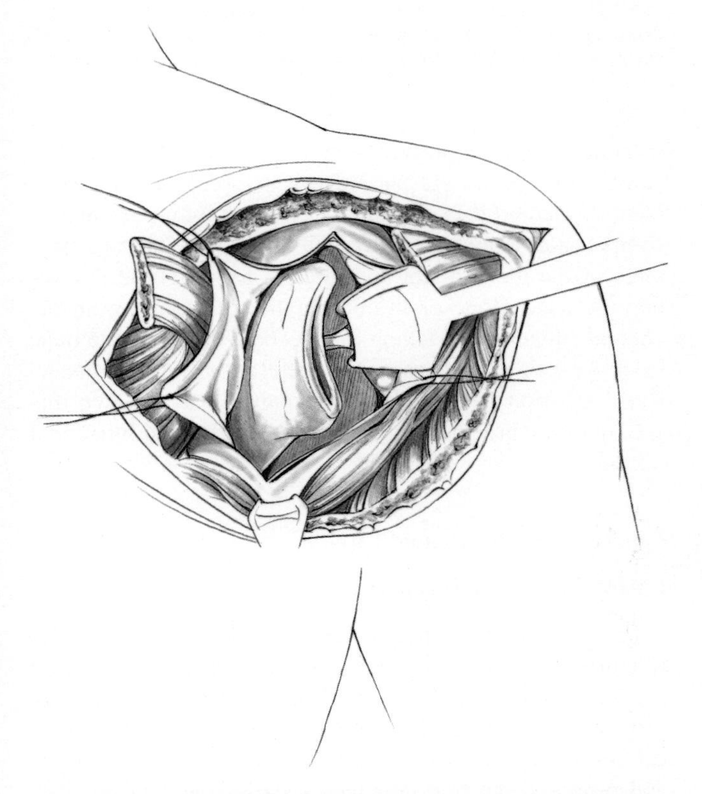

FIG. 11. Posterior surgical approach to the glenoid cavity: development of the infraspinatus–teres minor interval to expose the posteroinferior glenoid cavity and the lateral scapular border.

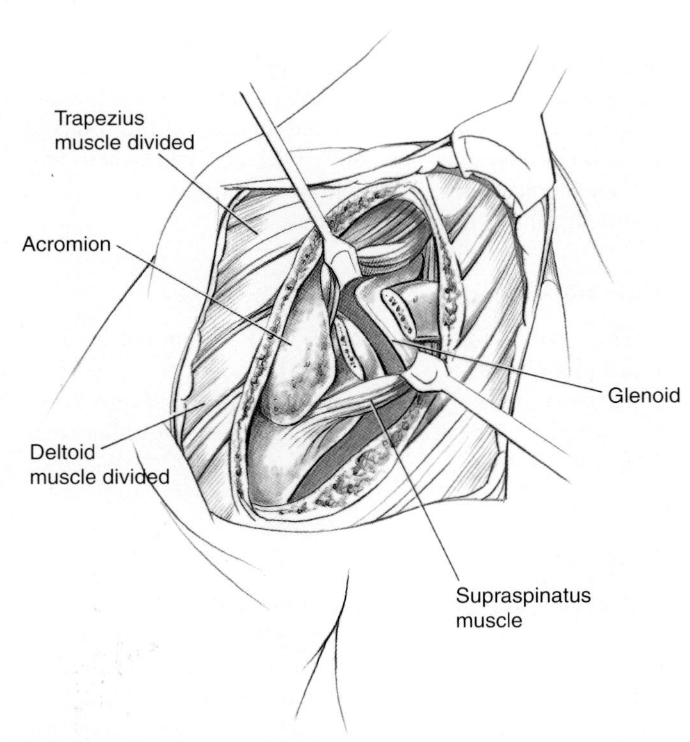

FIG. 12. Superior surgical approach to the glenoid cavity: soft-tissue and bony anatomy.

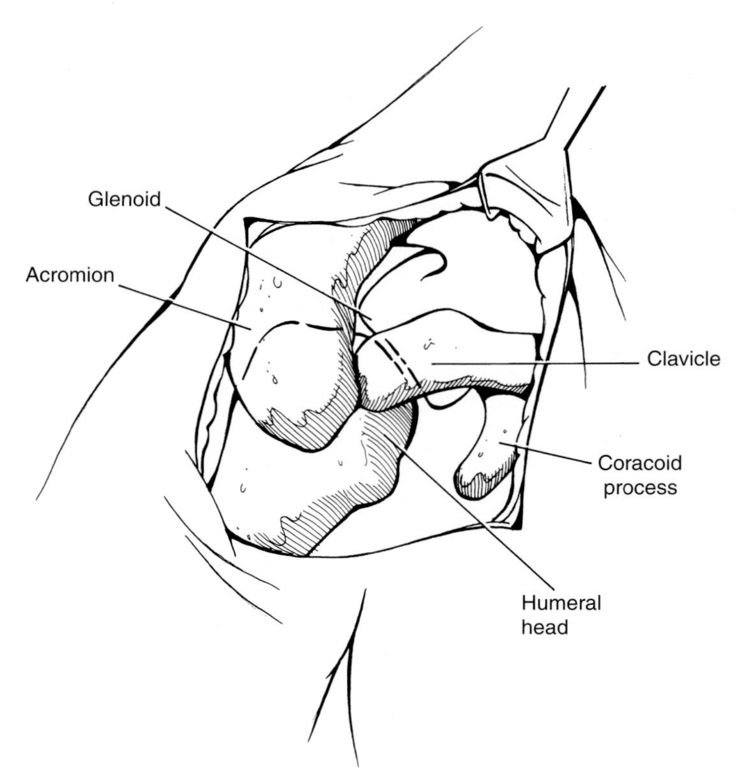

FIG. 13. Superior surgical approach to the glenoid cavity: bony anatomy.

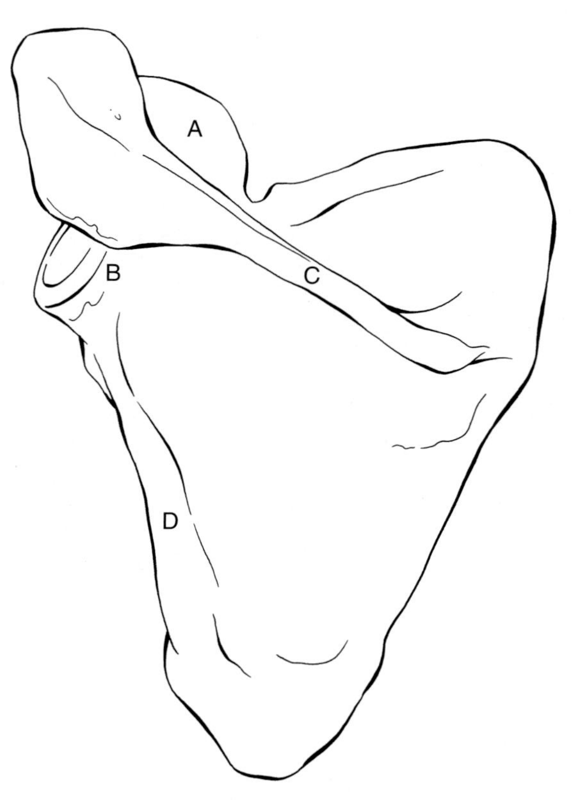

FIG. 14. Illustration depicting the scapula and areas of sufficient bone stock for internal fixation: **(A)** the coracoid process; **(B)** the glenoid process; **(C)** the scapular spine; and **(D)** the lateral scapular border. (From ref.49, with permission.)

are split in the line of their fibers bringing one down upon the superior aspect of the glenoid process (the superior glenoid rim is located posterolaterally) and the base of the coracoid process (located anteromedially). One must take care to protect and avoid injury to the suprascapular nerve and vessels that lie medial to the coracoid process.

Bone Stock

Thick, solid bone for fixation is at a premium because much of the scapula is paper-thin. There are, however, four satisfactory areas: the glenoid neck, the lateral scapular border, the base of the scapular spine, and the coracoid process (Fig. 14).

Fixation Devices

A variety of fixation devices are available (Fig. 15). The most useful, however, are K-wires, malleable reconstruction plates, and cannulated interfragmentary compression screws (Fig. 16). K-wires can be used for temporary as well as permanent fixation. The latter is the case when significantly displaced fracture fragments are too small to allow more substantial fixation, but one must be sure to bend the K-wire at its point of entry to prevent migration. 3.5 mm malleable reconstruction plates are particularly helpful in the management of glenoid neck fractures. 3.5 and 4.0-mm cannulated compression screws are especially useful in stabilizing fractures of the glenoid rim and glenoid fossa. These devices may be used alone or in combination, depending on the clinical situation and taking into account the available bone stock as well as the surgeon's preference and experience. Rigid fixation is desirable, but inability to achieve this goal does not preclude an excellent anatomic and functional result.

Fractures of the Glenoid Cavity

Classification and Incidence

Fractures of the glenoid cavity make up 10% of scapular fractures. The majority (90+%) are insignificantly displaced and managed nonoperatively. Those that are significantly displaced require surgical treatment or at least deserve surgical consideration. Ideberg reviewed over 300 such injuries and proposed the first detailed classification scheme.[72–74]. This was subsequently expanded by Goss[48](Fig. 17). Type I fractures involve the glenoid rim: type Ia, the anterior glenoid rim and type Ib, the posterior rim. Fractures of the glenoid fossa make up types II to V. Type VI fractures include all comminuted (more than two glenoid cavity fragments) injuries.

Fractures of the Glenoid Rim

Fractures of the glenoid rim occur when the humeral head strikes the periphery of the glenoid cavity with considerable violence (Fig. 18). These are true fractures, distinct from the small avulsion injuries that occur when a dislocating humeral head applies a tensile force on the periarticular soft tissues.[26] Surgical management is indicated if the fracture results in persistent subluxation of the humeral head (failure of the humeral head to lie concentrically within the glenoid cavity) or if the reduction of the fracture or humeral head is unstable. DePalma[26] stated that instability could be expected if the fracture was displaced 10 mm or more and if one-fourth or more of the glenoid cavity anteriorly or one-third or more of the glenoid cavity posteriorly was involved. Hardegger et al.[59] concurred and stated that "operative reduction and fixation of the fragment is indicated to prevent recurrent or permanent dislocation of the shoulder." Guttentag and Rechtine[56] and Butters[19] agreed with these recommendations. Several papers describing operatively managed glenoid rim fractures have also appeared in the literature.[6,90,128,152 166] A true axillary view of the glenohumeral joint, CT images (routine and reconstructive) and, if necessary, 3-D scanning allow one to determine the size and displacement of the rim fragment, whether persistent subluxation of the humeral head is present, and therefore, whether stability of the glenohumeral articulation is significantly compromised. Surgery, if necessary, is designed to restore articular stability and prevent posttraumatic degenerative

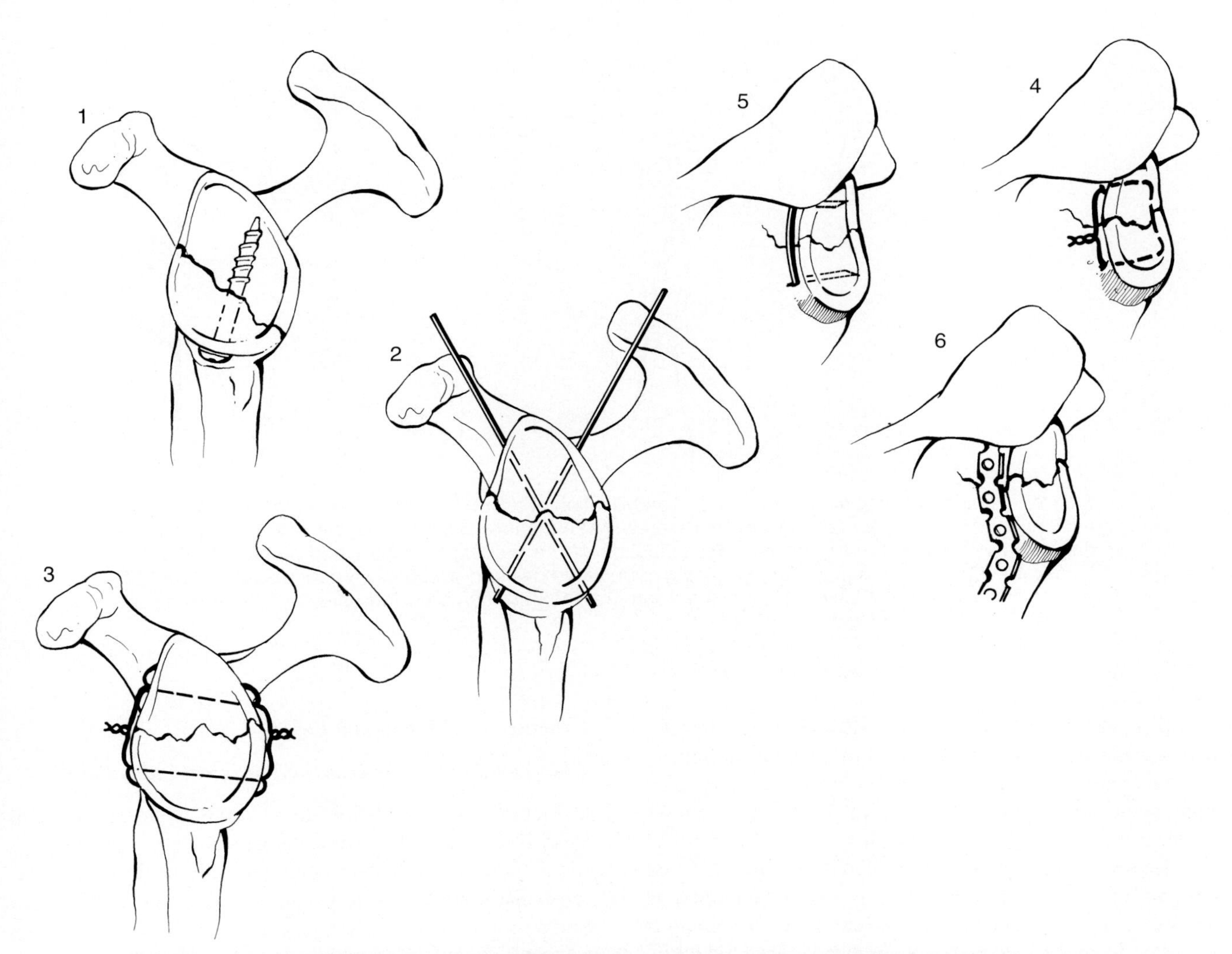

FIG. 15. Illustrations depicting fixation techniques available for stabilization of fractures of the glenoid cavity: *(1)* an interfragmentary compression screw; *(2)* Kirschner wires; *(3)* a construct using Kirschner wires and cerclage wires or Kirschner wires and cerclage sutures; *(4)* a cerclage wire or suture; *(5)* a staple; and *(6)* a 3.5 mm malleable reconstruction plate.

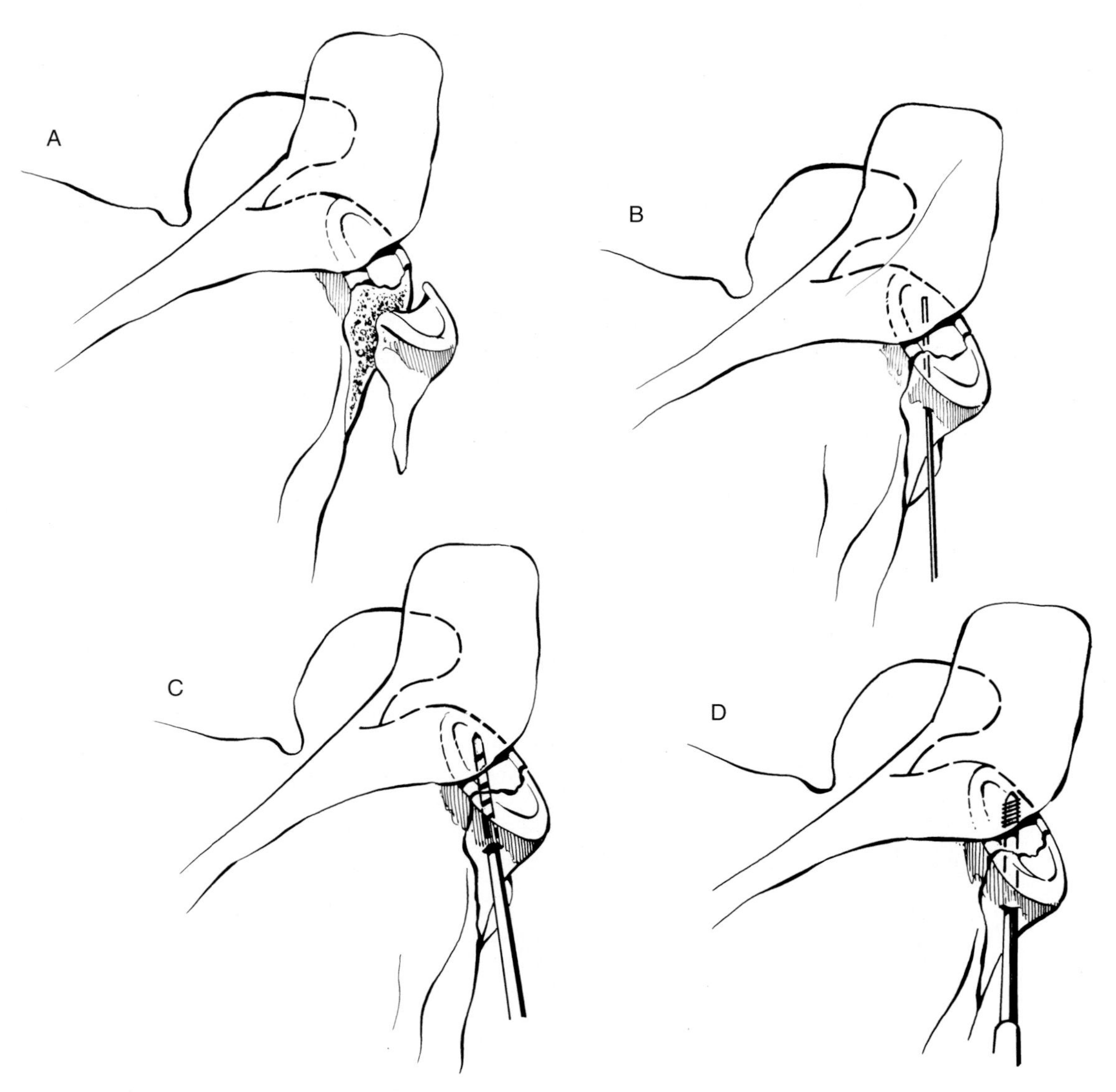

FIG. 16. Illustrations showing reduction and stabilization of a type II fracture of the glenoid cavity using a cannulated interfragmentary compression screw: **(A)** A fracture of the glenoid cavity with a significantly displaced inferior glenoid fragment; **(B)** reduction of the glenoid fragment and stabilization with a guidewire; **(C)** use of the guidewire to pass a cannulated drill and eventually a cannulated tap; and **(D)** use of the guidewire to place a cannulated interfragmentary compression screw securely fixing the glenoid fragment in position.

joint disease (Fig. 19). Type Ia (anterior rim) fractures are approached anteriorly. The displaced fragment is mobilized, reduced anatomically, and fixed in position with cannulated interfragmentary compression screws (ideally two screws are used to provide rotational stability; Fig. 20). Type Ib (posterior rim) fractures are approached posteriorly, reduced and stabilized in the same manner (Fig. 21). If the fracture is comminuted, the fragments are excised. A tricortical graft harvested from the iliac crest is then placed intraarticularly, filling the defect. A simple repair of the periarticular soft tissues to the intact glenoid cavity is an option, but restoration of rim contour is preferable.

Fractures of the Glenoid Fossa

Classification, Mechanism, and Surgical Indications

Fractures of the glenoid fossa occur when the humeral head is driven with sufficient force into the center of the glenoid concavity. The fracture generally begins as a transverse disruption (or slightly oblique) for several possible reasons: (a) the glenoid cavity is concave so forces tend to be concentrated over its central region; (b) the subchondral trabeculae are transversely oriented so fractures tend to occur in this plane; (c) the glenoid cavity is formed from two ossification centers so the central region may remain a persistently

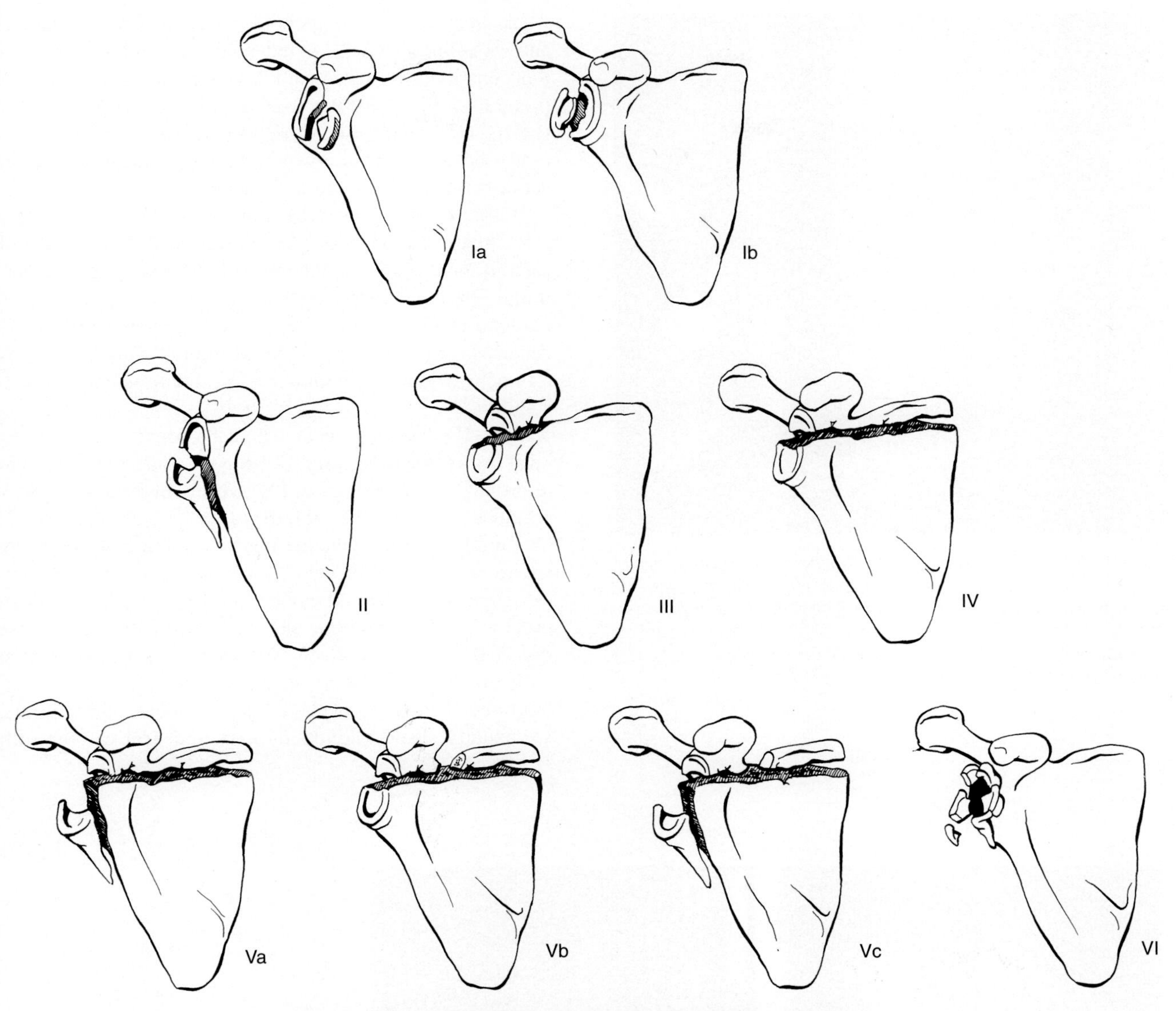

FIG. 17. Classification scheme for fractures of the glenoid cavity.

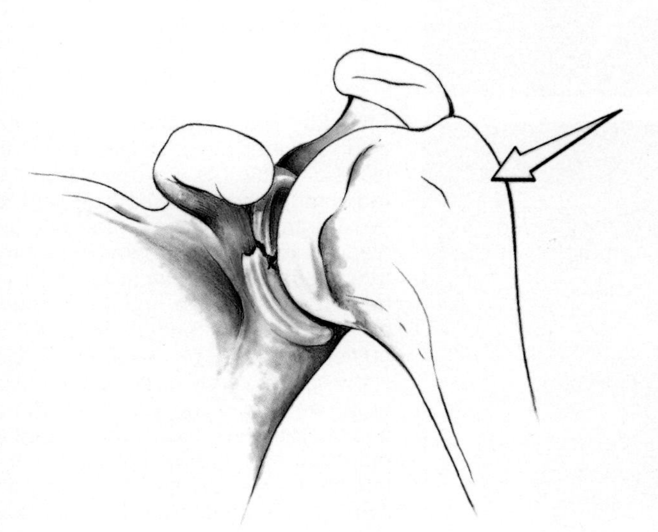

FIG. 18. Illustration depicting one mechanism of injury responsible for fractures of the glenoid rim: A force applied over the lateral aspect of the proximal humerus (a fall on an outstretched arm driving the humeral head against the periphery of the glenoid cavity with considerable violence could also cause this injury).

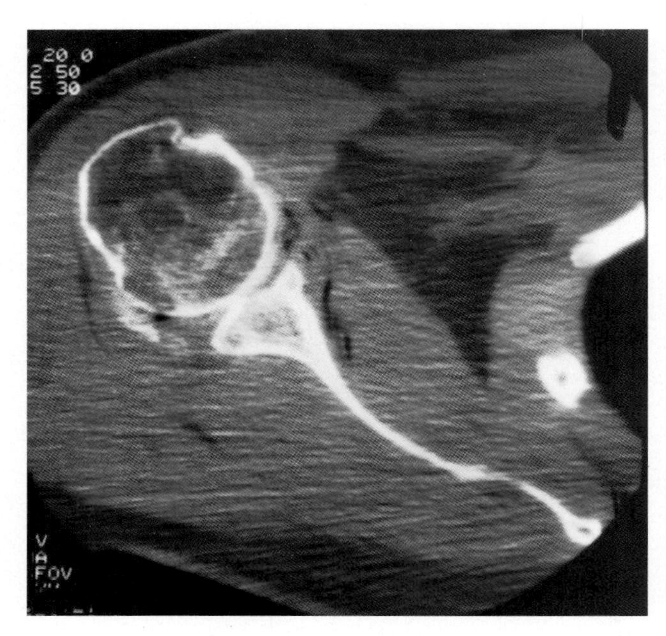

FIG. 19. An axial CT image of an individual 9 months following a traumatic event. Note the previously undiagnosed displaced type Ia fracture of the glenoid cavity with anterior subluxation of the humeral head and "bone-on-bone" contact (intraoperatively the patient had significant posttraumatic degenerative disease of the glenohumeral joint).

weak area; and (d) the glenoid cavity is narrow superiorly and wide inferiorly with an indentation along its anterior rim-this constitutes a stress riser where fractures are particularly prone to originate before coursing over to the posterior rim (Fig. 22). Once this transverse disruption occurs, the fracture may propagate in a variety of directions depending on the exact direction of the humeral head force.

With type II fractures, the humeral head is driven inferiorly, creating an inferior glenoid fragment. Surgery is indicated if there is an articular step off of 5 mm or more, and/or if the fragment displaces inferiorly carrying with it the humeral head, such that the humeral head fails to lie in the center of the glenoid cavity. These injuries can result in posttraumatic degenerative joint disease and/or glenohumeral instability.[46]

Type III fractures occur when the force of the humeral head is directed superiorly, causing the transverse disruption to propagate upward, generally exiting through the superior scapular border in the vicinity of the suprascapular notch. One might question whether this is a fracture of the glenoid cavity or a fracture of the coracoid process, since the superior third of the glenoid cavity and the base of the coracoid process are formed from the same ossification center (see Fig. 42B).[31,105] Regardless, displacement is usually minimal with the fragment lying medially. Consequently, as with fractures of the base of the coracoid process, these injuries are usually treated nonoperatively and heal uneventfully.

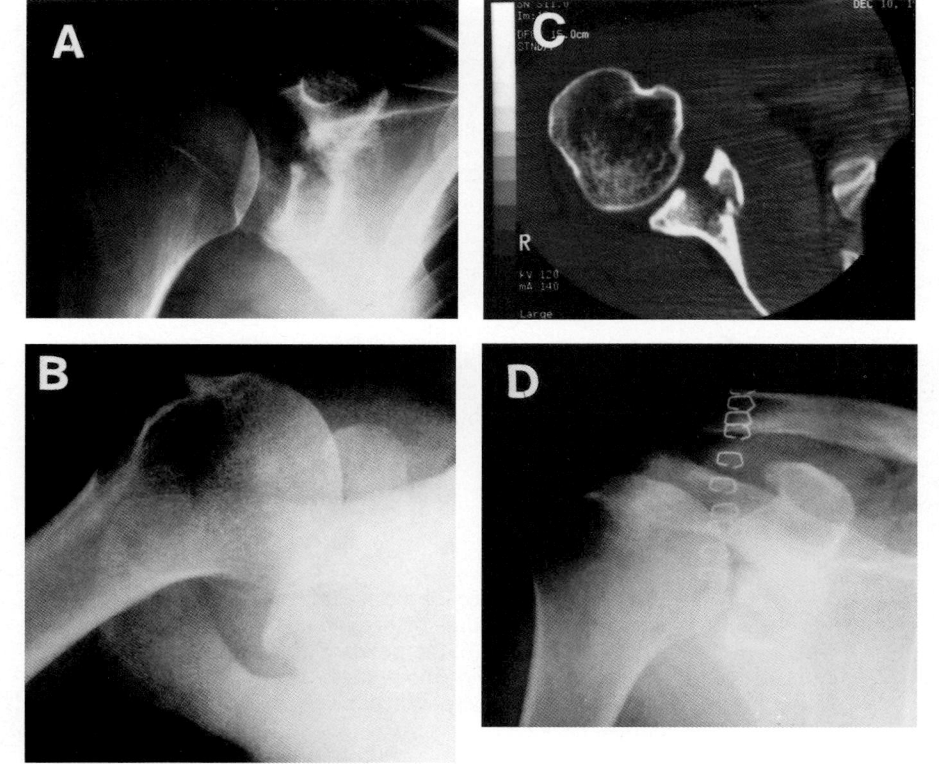

FIG. 20. Radiographs of a person who sustained a type Ia fracture of the glenoid cavity: **(A)** a preoperative AP radiograph showing what appears to be a fracture of the anteroinferior glenoid rim; **(B)** a preoperative axillary radiograph showing what appears to be a fracture of the anterior glenoid rim with anterior subluxation of the humeral head; **(C)** an axial CT image showing a severely displaced fracture of the anterior glenoid rim; and **(D)** a postoperative AP radiograph showing reduction and stabilization of the anteroinferior glenoid rim fragment with two cannulated interfragmentary screws.

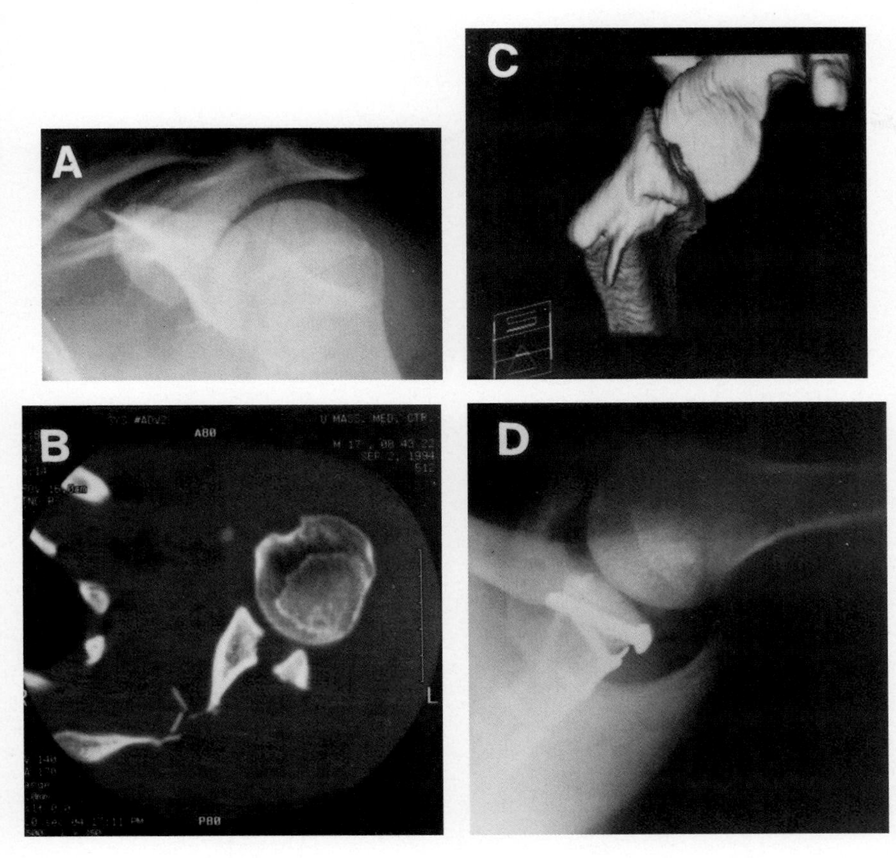

FIG. 21. Radiographs of an individual who sustained a type Ib fracture of the glenoid cavity: **(A)** A preoperative lateral scapular radiograph showing what appears to be a fracture of the glenoid cavity with significant posterior involvement; **(B)** an axial CT image showing a severely displaced fracture of the posterior glenoid rim with posterior subluxation of the humeral head; **(C)** a 3-D CT image of the glenoid cavity with the humeral head subtracted showing the severely displaced and rotated posteroinferior glenoid rim fragment; and **(D)** a postoperative axillary radiograph showing anatomic reduction and stabilization of the posterior glenoid rim fragment, with restoration of articular congruity.

Any glenoid cavity fracture may be associated with neurovascular damage owing to the proximity of the brachial plexus and axillary vessels as well as the considerable violence involved. Type III as well as type Vb, Vc, and VI injuries, however, are particularly prone, especially if there is an associated disruption of the clavicular-CC ligamentous–coracoid (C-4) linkage or the clavicular–ACJ–acromial strut. Neer considered compression of the adjacent neurovascular structures by these and fractures of the coracoid process an indication for surgery.[124] He and others also described the occurrence of suprascapular nerve paralysis resulting from fractures involving the coracoid process and glenoid neck and extending into the suprascapular notch. (An electromyogram [EMG] was essential for diagnosis, and early exploration was recommended.[23,30,31,154])

Surgical management is indicated if there is an articular step-off of 5 mm or more, with the superior fragment displaced laterally, or if there is a severe associated disruption of the superior shoulder suspensory complex[45] (the clavicular–CC ligamentous–coracoid [C-4] linkage or the clavicular–ACJ–acromial strut). These injuries can result in posttraumatic degenerative joint disease and severe functional impairment.

Type IV injuries occur when the humeral head is driven directly into the center of the glenoid fossa.[35] The fracture created courses transversely across the entire scapula, exiting along its vertebral border. If there is an articular step-off of 5 mm or more, with the superior fragment displaced laterally, or if the superior and inferior fragments are severely separated, open reduction and internal fixation is indicated to avoid symptomatic degenerative joint disease, nonunion at the fracture site (an extremely rare occurrence, but a definite concern in the case shown in Fig. 24), and/or instability of the glenohumeral joint.

Type Va, Vb, and Vc fractures are combinations of the types II, III, and IV injuries and are caused by more violent and complex forces. The same clinical concerns and operative indications detailed for the type II, III, and IV fractures apply.

Type VI fractures include all disruptions of the glenoid cavity in which more than two articular fragments are present and are caused by the most violent forces. Operative treatment is contraindicated because exposing these injuries surgically will do little more than disrupt what little soft-tissue support remains, rendering the fragments even more unstable and making a bad situation worse. An associated disruption of the superior shoulder suspensory complex may warrant operative correction, however, and this may indirectly improve glenoid articular congruity.

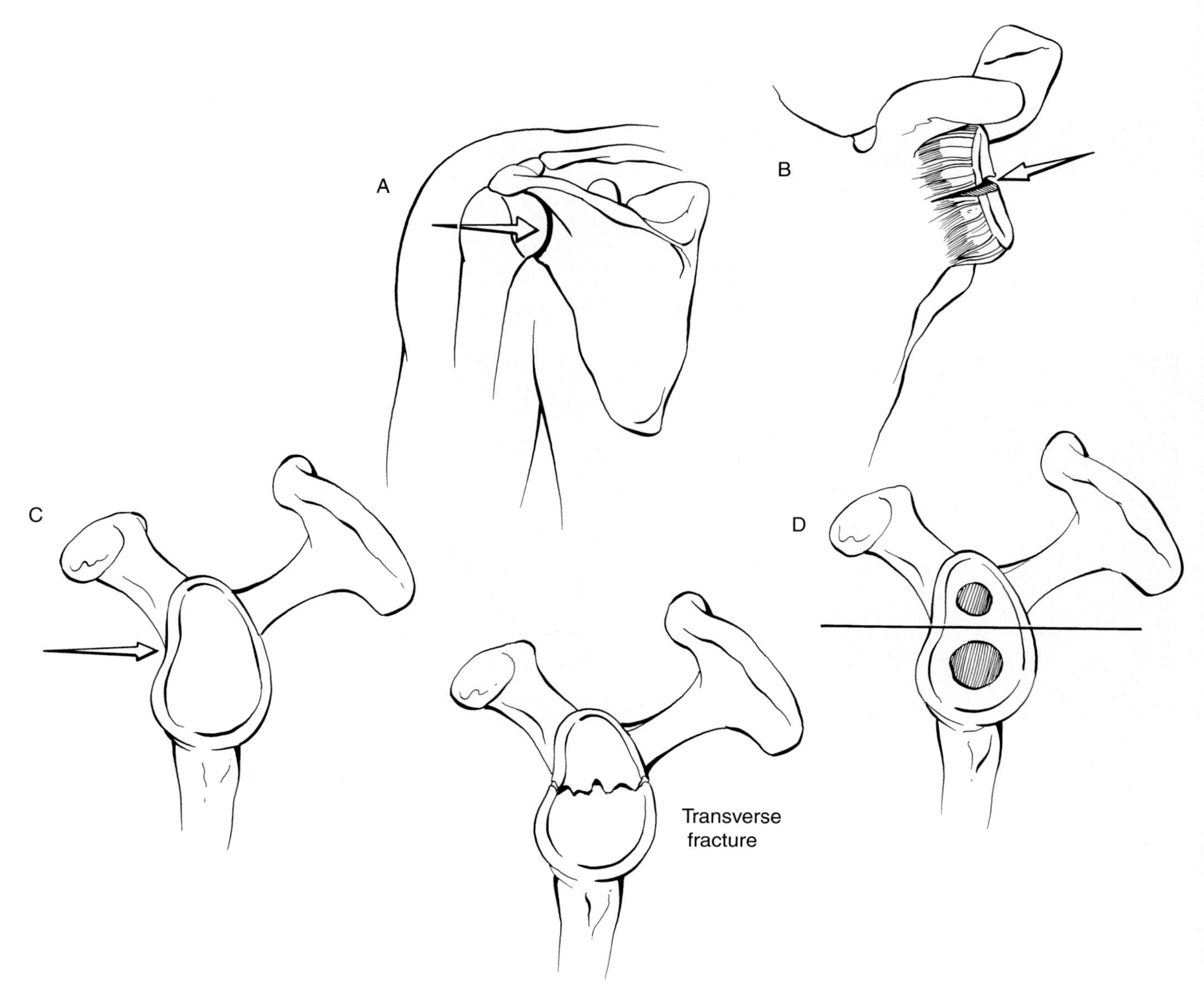

FIG. 22. Illustrations depicting a transverse disruption of the glenoid cavity and the factors responsible for this orientation: **(A)** the glenoid's concave shape concentrates forces across its central region; **(B)** the subchondral trabeculae are oriented in the transverse plane; **(C)** the "crook" along the anterior rim is a stress riser where fractures tend to originate; **(D)** formed from a superior and an inferior ossification center, the glenoid cavity may have a persistently weak central zone.

Diagnosis

A true AP projection of the glenohumeral joint, reconstructed CT images in the coronal plane, and even 3-D CT scanning may be necessary to accurately determine whether and to what degree articular incongruity and/or separation is present.

Surgical Management

Type II Fractures

These fractures are approached posteriorly. The infraspinatus–teres minor interval is developed exposing the displaced inferior glenoid fragment and the lateral scapular border. The fragment is reduced as anatomically as possible and stabilized, generally with two cannulated interfragmentary compression screws passed posteroinferiorly to anterosuperiorly or with a contoured reconstruction plate placed along the posterior aspect of the glenoid process and the lateral scapular border (Fig. 23). Excision of the fracture fragment and placement of a bone graft from the iliac crest is an option if severe comminution is present. Associated tears of the labral–capsular–ligamentous complex are repaired if possible, as they are with all fractures of the glenoid cavity. Detachments are corrected with nonabsorbable sutures passed through drill holes and intrasubstance tears are reapproximated with nonabsorbable sutures placed in a figure eight fashion.

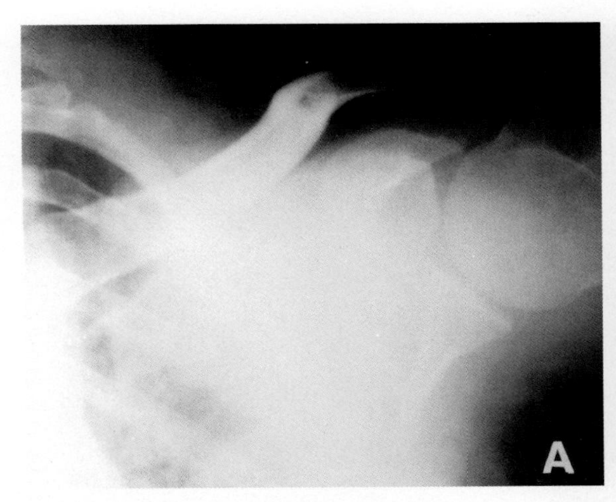

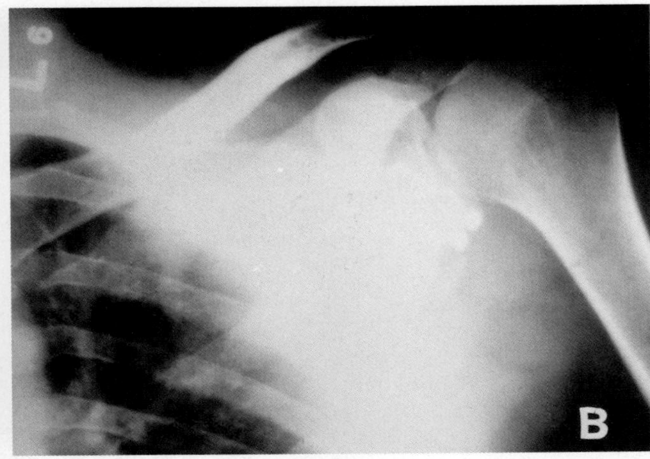

FIG. 23. Radiographs of a patient who sustained a type II fracture of the glenoid cavity: **(A)** preoperative AP radiograph showing significant displacement of the inferior glenoid fragment and a severe articular step-off; **(B)** postoperative AP radiograph showing anatomic reduction and stabilization of the inferior glenoid fragment, with restoration of articular congruity.

Type III Fractures

A posterosuperior surgical exposure (or an anterior approach through the rotator interval without taking down the subscapularis musculotendinous unit; see Fig. 41) is utilized. A K-wire can be placed into the superior glenoid fragment and then used to manipulate the fragment into satisfactory position relative to the remainder of the glenoid process, thereby restoring articular congruity. The K-wire is then driven across the fracture site and used to place a cannulated interfragmentary compression screw. When there is an associated disruption of the superior shoulder suspensory complex (SSSC), reduction and stabilization of the superior glenoid fragment may restore the integrity of this complex satisfactorily. If not, that injury may need to be addressed as well. Conversely, if the superior glenoid fragment is severely comminuted and difficult to fix, operative restoration of the associated SSSC disruption may improve glenoid articular congruity indirectly and satisfactorily.

Type IV Fractures

These fractures are approached posterosuperiorly. A K-wire is placed into the superior glenoid–scapular segment and then used to manipulate that fragment into position relative to the inferior segment while directly visualizing the reduction via the posterior exposure. The K-wire is then driven across the fracture site and used to place a cannulated interfragmentary compression screw (Fig. 24). A cerclage wire or cerclage sutures passed around the glenoid neck have also been used for fixation.

Type V Fractures

Type Va fractures are approached, reduced, and stabilized according to the principles described for significantly displaced type II fractures. The inferomedial portion of the scapula may be ignored. Type Vb injuries are approached, reduced, and stabilized according to the principles described for significantly displaced type III fractures. The superomedial portion of the scapula may be ignored. If an associated disruption of the superior shoulder suspensory complex is present, it may require operative reduction and stabilization.

Type Vc fractures are exposed by a posterosuperior approach. The superior and inferior glenoid fragments are reduced anatomically and rigidly fixed to each other. Ideally, the fixation is performed with a lag screw, which is generally easier to pass superior to inferior, or with a cerclage wire or suture that is passed through drill holes in the superior and inferior fragments. The superomedial and inferomedial portions of the scapula may be ignored. Surgical management of an associated disruption of the superior shoulder suspensory complex is dependent on the exact nature of that injury (e.g., an associated clavicle fracture may be managed with screw and plate fixation or an IM device).

Type VI Fractures: Management

The upper extremity is initially protected in a sling and swathe bandage, an abduction brace, or even overhead olecranon pin traction—whichever maximizes articular congruity as determined radiographically. Gentle passive circular and rotatory range of motion exercises performed by a therapist and the patient are initiated immediately, hoping that the movement of the humeral head will mold the articular fragments into a maximally congruous position. By 2 weeks, healing is sufficient to allow protection of all such injuries in a sling and swathe immobilizer. Exercises designed to gradually increase range of motion and progressive functional use of the shoulder out of the sling within clearly defined limits are prescribed during the subsequent 4 weeks. At 6 weeks, these fractures are sufficiently healed to allow dis-

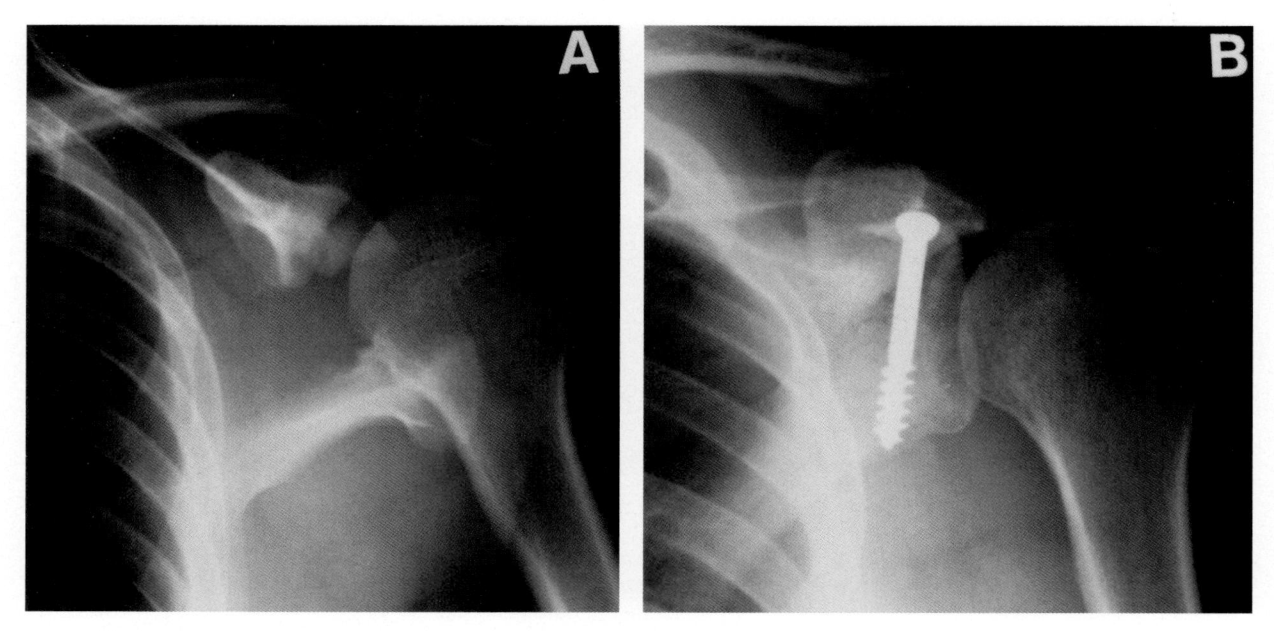

FIG. 24. Radiographs of a patient who sustained a type IV fracture of the glenoid cavity: **(A)** a preoperative AP radiograph showing severe separation of the superior and inferior portions of the glenoid fossa and scapular body; **(B)** postoperative AP radiograph showing anatomic reduction and stabilization of the superior and inferior portions of the glenoid fossa and scapular body, with restoration of articular congruity.

continuation of all external protection. Functional use of the shoulder is encouraged and physiotherapy continues until range of motion and strength are maximized. These injuries obviously have the highest potential for posttraumatic degenerative joint disease and glenohumeral instability.

Results

Bauer et al.[11] reviewed 20 patients treated surgically for significantly displaced fractures of the scapula (6.1 year average follow-up) and reported greater than 70% good or very good results based on a Constant score. They recommended early open reduction and internal fixation (ORIF) for grossly displaced fractures of the glenoid fossa as well as those of the glenoid rim, glenoid neck, and coracoid–acromial processes. Hardegger et al.[59] reported that "if there is significant displacement, conservative treatment alone cannot restore congruence" and that stiffness and pain may result. . . "For this reason, open reduction and stabilization are indicated." Kavanagh et al.[80] presented their experience at the Mayo Clinic with 10 displaced intraarticular fractures of the glenoid cavity treated with ORIF. They found ORIF to be "a useful and safe technique" that can "restore excellent function of the shoulder." In their series, the major articular fragments were displaced 4 to 8 mm. They emphasized that it remained uncertain how much incongruity of the glenoid articular surface could be accepted without risking the long-term sequelae of pain, stiffness, and/or traumatic osteoarthritis. Soslowsky et al.[155] found the maximal depth of the glenoid articular cartilage to be 5 mm. Consequently, if displacement at a glenoid fossa fracture site is 5 mm or more, subchondral bone is exposed. Case reports by Aulicino et al.[7] and Aston and Gregory[6] lend support to the role of surgery in the management of significantly displaced glenoid fossa fractures. Reudi and Chapman[147] stated that "grossly displaced intraarticular fractures of the glenoid that render the joint incongruent and unstable profit from operative reconstruction and internal fixation as incongruities will result in osteoarthritic changes." Rowe[145] has advocated surgical management of severely displaced injuries. Leung et al. reviewed 14 displaced intraarticular fractures of the glenoid treated with ORIF (30.5 month average follow-up) and reported 9 excellent and 5 good results.[98] On the basis of these reports, it seems reasonable to conclude that there is a definite role for surgery in the treatment of glenoid fossa fractures. An injury with an articular step-off of 5 mm or more should be considered for surgical intervention to restore articular congruity, and displacement of 10 mm or more is an absolute indication to avoid posttraumatic osteoarthritis.

Fractures of the Glenoid Neck

Incidence, Mechanism, and Classification

Fractures of the glenoid neck make up 25% of scapular fractures. It is somewhat surprising that these injuries are not more common, since this portion of the glenoid process is quite narrow. Fractures of the glenoid neck may be caused by (a) a direct blow over the anterior or posterior aspect of the shoulder; (b) a fall on an outstretched arm, with impaction of the humeral head against the glenoid process; or in rare cases, (c) a force applied to the superior aspect of the shoulder complex.

The glenoid neck is that portion of the glenoid process that lies between the scapular body and the glenoid cavity. The coracoid process arises from its superior aspect. Its stability is primarily osseous, specifically its junction medially with the scapular body. Secondary support is provided by its attachment superiorly to the clavicular–acromioclavicular joint–acromial strut via the clavicular–CC ligamentous–coracoid (C-4) linkage (Fig. 25) and the CA ligament. Tertiary soft-tissue support is provided anteriorly by the subscapularis muscle, superiorly by the supraspinatus muscle, and posteriorly by the infraspinatus and teres minor muscles. To be a glenoid neck fracture, the disruption must be complete—exiting along the lateral scapular border and the superior scapular margin, either just lateral or just medial to the coracoid process (Fig. 26B,C). Displacement may then occur. If in addition its secondary support is compromised (a coracoid process fracture, a coracoclavicular ligamentous disruption with or without a CA ligamentous injury, a clavicle fracture, an AC joint disruption, or an acromial fracture—i.e., a double disruption of the superior shoulder suspensory complex [SSSC]), there is the potential for severe displacement[45].

Type I fractures include all insignificantly displaced injuries and constitute 90+% of the total. Management is nonoperative, and a good to excellent functional result can be expected.

Type II fractures include all significantly displaced injuries, and *significant displacement* is defined as translational displacement of the glenoid fragment greater than or equal to 1 cm or angulatory displacement of the fragment greater than or equal to 40 degrees in either the coronal or the sagittal plane (Fig. 27).[50]

One centimeter of translational displacement was chosen by Zdravkovic and Damholt[177] and Nordquvist and Petersson,[129] and Miller and Ada[1,116] as separating major from minor injuries. Bateman[10] believed that this degree of displacement could interfere with abduction. Hardegger et al.[59] pointed out that significant translational displacement changed the normal relations between the glenohumeral articulation and the undersurface of the distal clavicle, AC joint, and acromial process, thereby altering the mechanics of nearby musculotendinous units, resulting in a functional imbalance of the shoulder complex as a whole: a "disorganization of the coracoacromial arch." Miller and Ada[1,116] believed that resultant weakness (especially abductor weakness), decreased range of motion, and pain (especially subacromial pain) were largely due to rotator cuff dysfunction. The premise that significant translational displacement of the glenoid process can lead to shoulder discomfort and dysfunction certainly makes sense intuitively—the complex bony relations in the glenohumeral region are clearly altered,

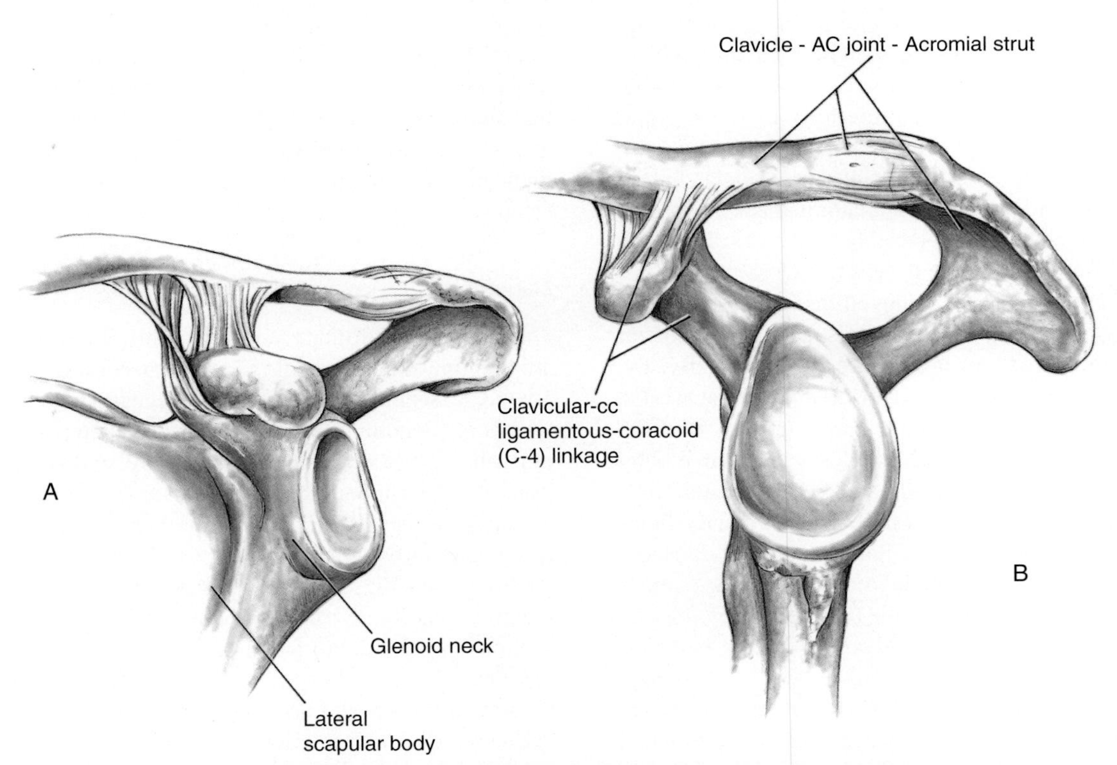

FIG. 25. Illustrations depicting structures providing stability to the glenoid process in the region of the glenoid neck: **(A)** Lateral aspect of the scapular body; and **(B)** the clavicular–AC joint–acromial strut via the clavicular–CC ligamentous–coracoid (C-4) linkage.

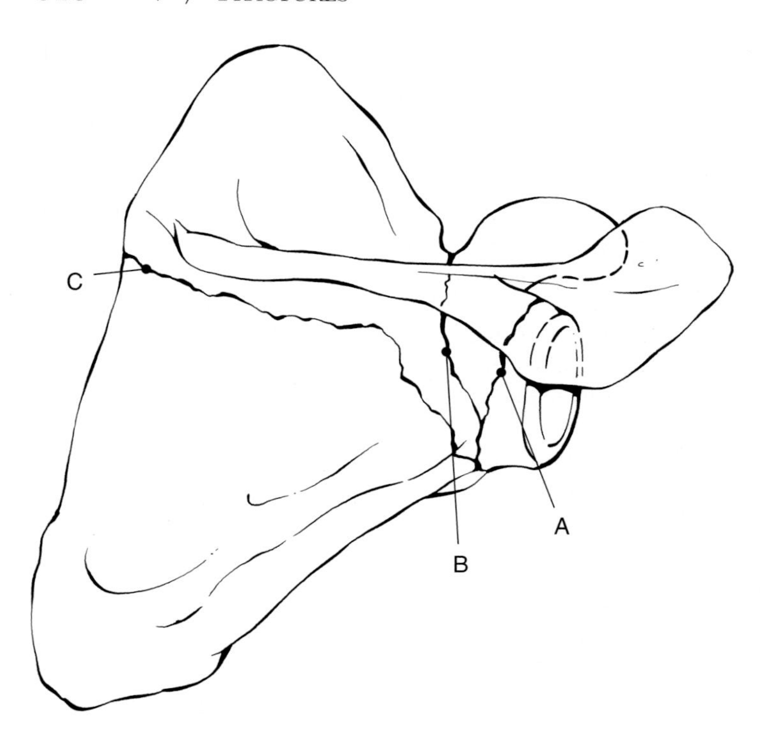

FIG. 26. Illustration depicting three basic fracture patterns involving the glenoid neck: *(A)* a fracture through the anatomic neck;[59] *(B)* a fracture through the surgical neck; and *(C)* a fracture involving the inferior glenoid neck which then courses medially to exit through the scapular body (this is managed as a scapular body fracture).

as are the mechanics of the musculotendinous structures that pass from the scapula to the proximal humerus (the deltoid muscle and the rotator cuff in particular). The fracture line usually exits the superior scapular border medial to the coracoid process (the surgical neck region). The glenoid fragment is then drawn distally by the weight of the arm and anteromedially by adjacent muscle forces or posteromedially, in which case it is usually forced inferiorly by the scapular spine (Fig. 28). (Hardegger et al.[59] described a rare case in which the fracture line exited the superior scapular border lateral to the coracoid process [the anatomic neck], allowing the glenoid fragment to be displaced laterally and distally by the pull of the long head of the triceps muscle.)

Bateman[10] and DePalma[26] believed that excessive angulation of the glenoid fragment could result in glenohumeral instability (anterior, posterior, or inferior). Normally, the glenoid cavity faces 15 degrees superiorly and is retroverted 6 degrees relative to the plane of the scapular body. With increasing angulation, the humeral head loses the normal bony support provided by the glenoid cavity (bony instability), which translates into glenohumeral discomfort and dysfunction.[1,10,26,116] Miller and Ada[1,116] felt that angular displacement greater than or equal to 40 degrees in either the coronal or transverse plane was unacceptable (Fig. 29). They felt that this degree of displacement adversely altered not only glenohumeral but also other bony relations as well as musculotendinous dynamics, particularly those of the rotator cuff, resulting in pain and overall shoulder dysfunction (diminished range of motion and loss of strength).

Miller and Ada[1,116] retrospectively reviewed 16 displaced glenoid neck fractures (greater than or equal to 1 cm of translational displacement or greater than or equal to 40 degrees of angulation in either the transverse or coronal plane) managed nonoperatively (36 month average follow-up). They found that 20% had decreased range of motion, 50% had pain (75% night pain), 40% had weakness with exertion, and 25% noted "popping." In particular, these patients frequently had shoulder abductor weakness and subacromial pain, due at least in part to rotator cuff dysfunction. They recommended open reduction and internal fixation of glenoid neck fractures with this degree of displacement.

Diagnosis

Diagnosis is ultimately radiographic. Plain radiographs are helpful, but because of the complex bony anatomy in the area, CT scanning is generally necessary to determine whether a glenoid neck fracture is indeed complete, to determine the degree of displacement, if any, and to identify injuries to adjacent bony structures and articulations. One must not confuse these injuries with the more common fractures that course through the inferior glenoid neck and the scapular body (see Fig. 26C). Computerized tomography (CT) scanning readily reveals that the latter are not complete disruptions of the glenoid process, since the superior aspect of the glenoid neck is intact. These are essentially fractures of the scapular body and do quite well with nonoperative care because the normal relations between the glenohumeral articulation and the distal clavicle–acromion are unaltered (Fig. 30).[50]

Nonoperative versus Operative Treatment

Imatini[75], McGahn et al.,[107] and Lindholm and Leven[99] recommended nonsurgical treatment for all glenoid neck fractures, but their studies give few details to justify this conclusion. A long-term follow-up study by Zdravkovic and Damholt[177] included 20 to 30 patients (it is difficult to determine the exact number from the text) with displaced glenoid neck fractures and noted that nonoperative treatment yielded satisfactory results. Nordquvist and Petersson,[129] however, evaluated 37 glenoid neck fractures treated without surgery (10 to 20 year follow-up) and found the functional result to be either fair or poor in 32%. They believed that for some fractures, early open reduction and internal fixation might have improved the result. Although somewhat ambivalent in their recommendations, three studies do mention surgical management as an option in selected cases. Armstrong and Vanderspuy[5] believed that although most of these individuals do well, more aggressive treatment including open reduction and internal fixation may be indicated in patients who are young and fit. Wilbur and Evans[170] believed that open reduction and internal fixation might be indicated if the glenoid fragment is markedly displaced or angulated, but did not believe that they had enough information or experience to warrant definitive surgical indications.

Hardegger et al.[59] reported 79% good to excellent results in five displaced glenoid neck fractures treated surgically (6.5-year follow-up). They agreed with Judet,[78] Magerl,[102] Ganz and Noesberger,[39] and Tscherne and Christ[163] that op-

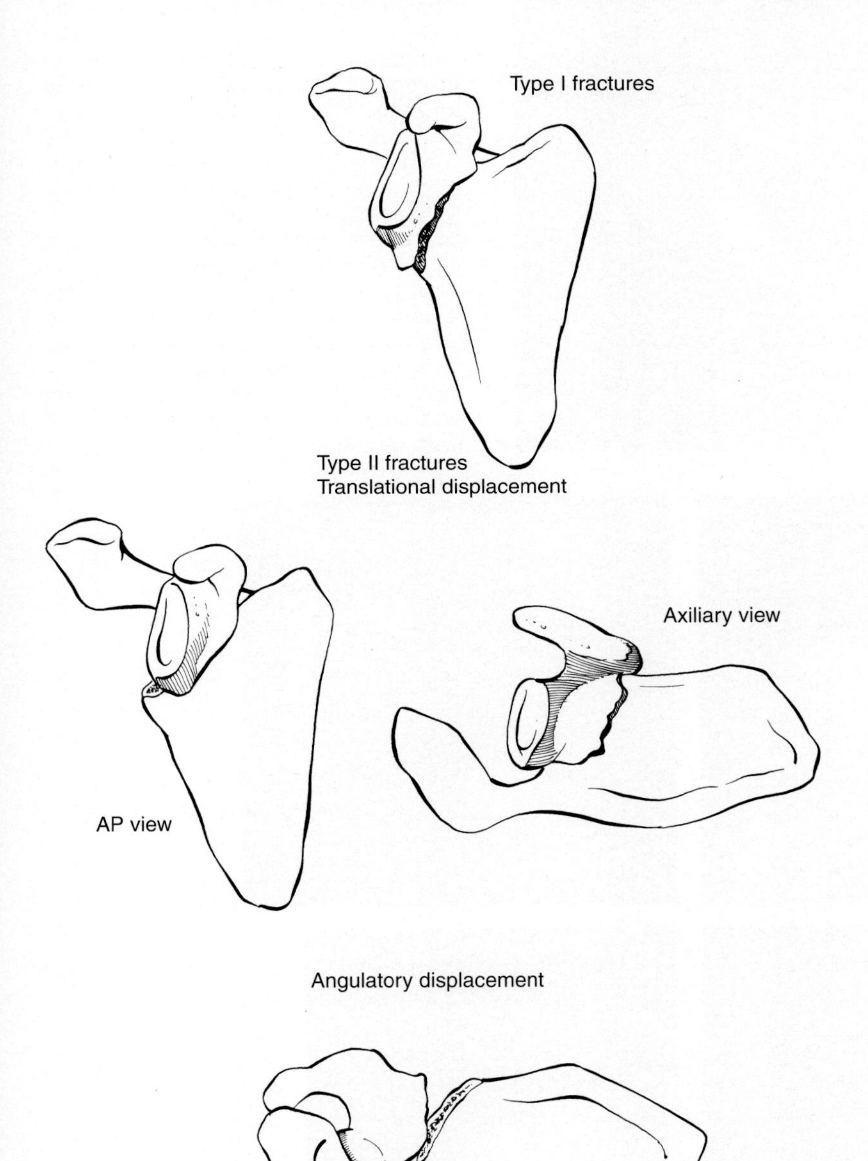

FIG. 27. Classification scheme for fractures of the glenoid neck.

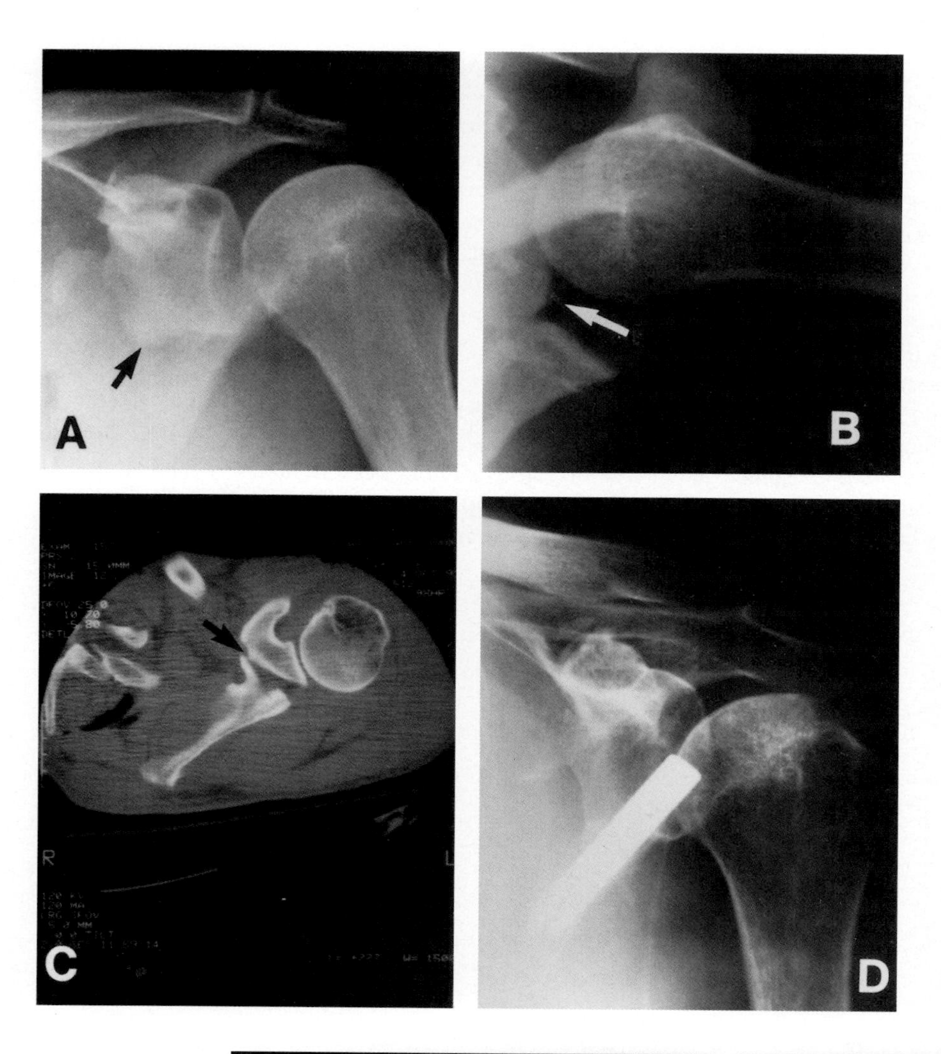

FIG. 28. Radiographs of a patient who sustained a type II fracture of the glenoid neck with significant translational displacement of the glenoid fragment: **(A)** a preoperative AP radiograph showing the glenoid neck fracture and medial translation of the glenoid fragment; **(B)** a preoperative axillary radiograph revealing that the unstable glenoid fragment is severely displaced anteromedially (the glenohumeral joint is medial to the most lateral aspect of the scapular body), probably owing to an associated disruption of the coracoclavicular ligaments (a violation of the C-4 linkage and, therefore, a double disruption of the superior shoulder suspensory complex) and possibly the coracoacromial ligament; **(C)** a preoperative axial CT image revealing the glenoid neck fracture to be complete, exiting the superior scapular border medial to the intact coracoid process (a surgical neck fracture); and **(D)** a postoperative AP radiograph showing anatomic reduction and stabilization of the glenoid neck fracture and glenoid fragment.

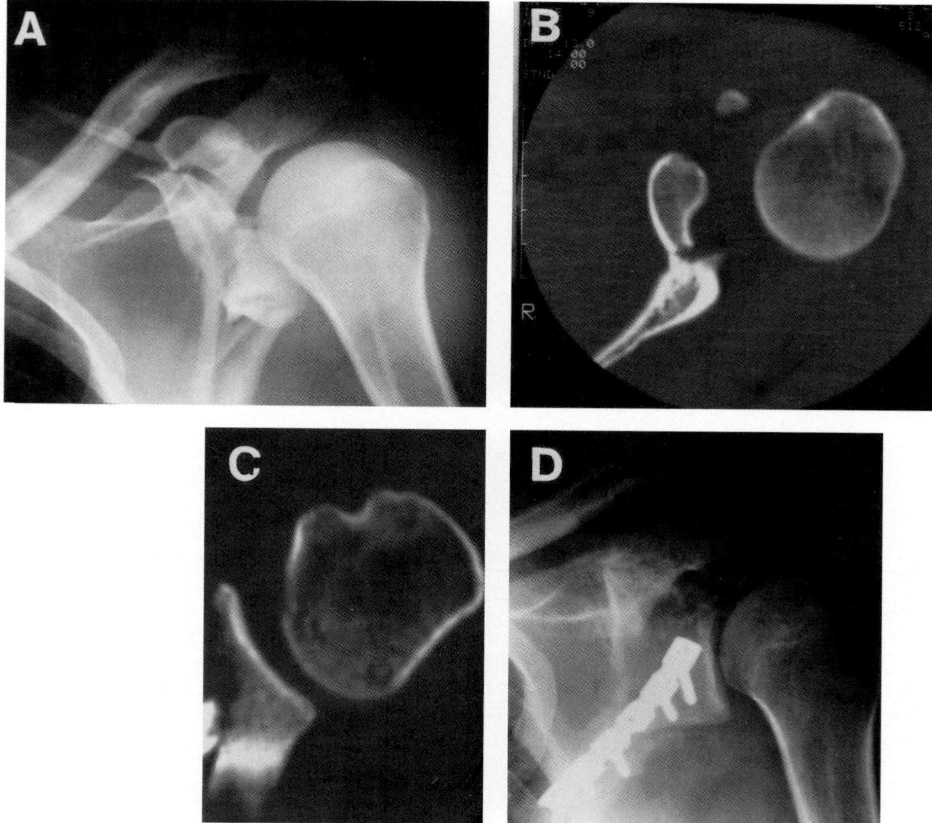

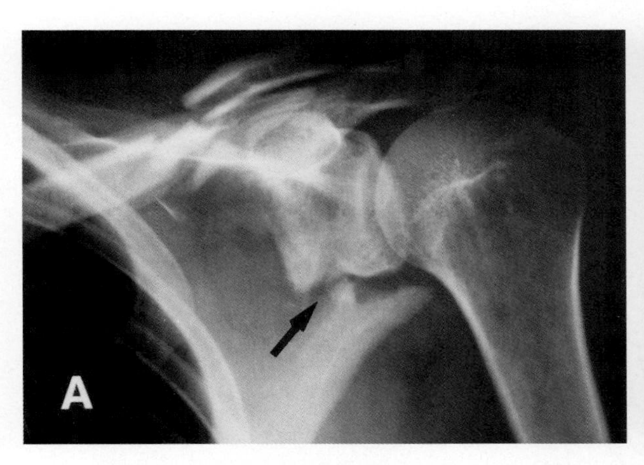

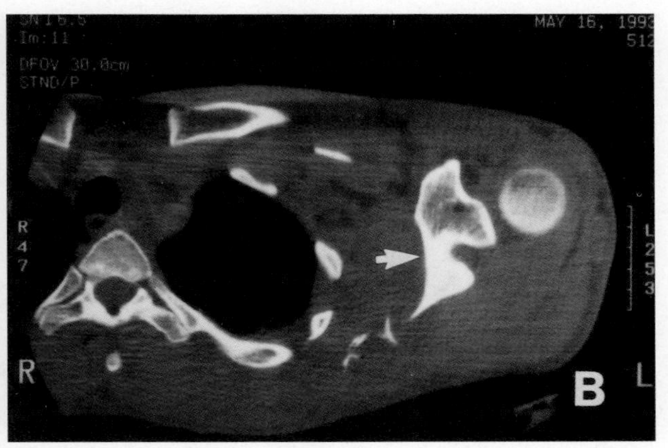

FIG. 30. Radiographs showing what appear to be a complete fracture of the glenoid neck: **(A)** An AP radiograph of the shoulder showing a fracture involving the inferior aspect of the glenoid neck and **(B)** an axial CT image showing the superior portion of the glenoid neck to be uninvolved (the fracture exited through the scapular body).

erative management of displaced glenoid neck fractures avoids late disability and yields better results. Gagney et al.[38] found a good result in only 1 of 12 displaced fractures treated nonoperatively. They believed that such injuries "could disorganize the coracoacromial arch," and recommended open reduction. Neer and Rockwood[124] and Butters[19] present the recommendations of other investigators, as does a review article by Guttentag and Rechtine.[56] Clearly, all these investigators agree that the vast majority of glenoid neck fractures can and should be treated without surgery. However, most authors believe that more aggressive treatment, including open reduction and internal fixation is at the very least a consideration, if not clearly indicated, when the glenoid fragment is severely displaced (i.e., type II injuries).

Surgical Indications and Management

Type II fractures should at the very least be considered for surgical management.

The glenoid process and fracture site are approached posteriorly. The interval between the infraspinatus and teres minor is developed to expose the posteroinferior glenoid neck and lateral scapular border. A superior approach can be added to gain control over the free glenoid fragment. Once a satisfactory reduction has been achieved, temporary fixation can be provided by placing K-wires between the glenoid fragment and the adjacent bony structures (e.g., through the glenoid fragment and into the scapular body; through the acromial process and into the glenoid fragment, and so on). Firm fixation is generally achieved by means of a contoured 3.5 mm malleable reconstruction plate applied along the lateral border of the scapula and the posterior aspect of the glenoid process. Supplemental fixation can be provided by K-wires or lag screws. K-wires providing temporary fixation can be retained or used for the placement of 3.5 mm cannulated lag screws (Fig. 31). Conceivably, comminution of the scapular body and spine may be so severe or the size of the glenoid fragment so small as to preclude plate fixation. In these cases, K-wire or lag screw fixation of the reduced glenoid fragment to adjacent intact bony structures (i.e., the acromial process, the distal clavicle, etc.) may be all that can be provided. If a disruption of the clavicular–AC joint–acromial strut is also present, fixation of that injury may indirectly reduce and stabilize the glenoid neck fracture. If significant displacement persists, however, the glenoid neck fracture must also be addressed.[50] Conversely, open reduction and internal fixation of the glenoid neck fracture may satisfactorily reduce and stabilize the second disruption. If not, that associated disruption must be addressed.[50]. A fracture of the ipsilateral glenoid neck and midshaft clavicle has been termed a "floating shoulder" (see page 30). Disruptions of the clavicular–CC ligamentous–coracoid (C-4) linkage are usually managed indirectly by reducing and stabilizing the glenoid neck fracture and any injuries compromising the

FIG. 29. A patient who sustained a type II fracture of the glenoid neck with significant angulatory displacement of the glenoid fragment: **(A)** a preoperative AP radiograph showing the glenoid neck fracture with severe angulation of the glenoid fragment and a fractured coracoid process; **(B)** a preoperative axillary CT projection showing the coracoid process fracture (a violation of the C-4 linkage) that further destabilized the glenoid fragment and allowed severe angulatory displacement (a double disruption of the superior shoulder suspensory complex); **(C)** a preoperative axillary CT projection showing the glenoid neck fracture; and **(D)** a postoperative AP radiograph showing the glenoid fragment reduced and stabilized with a contoured reconstruction plate (the coracoid process fracture was allowed to heal spontaneously).

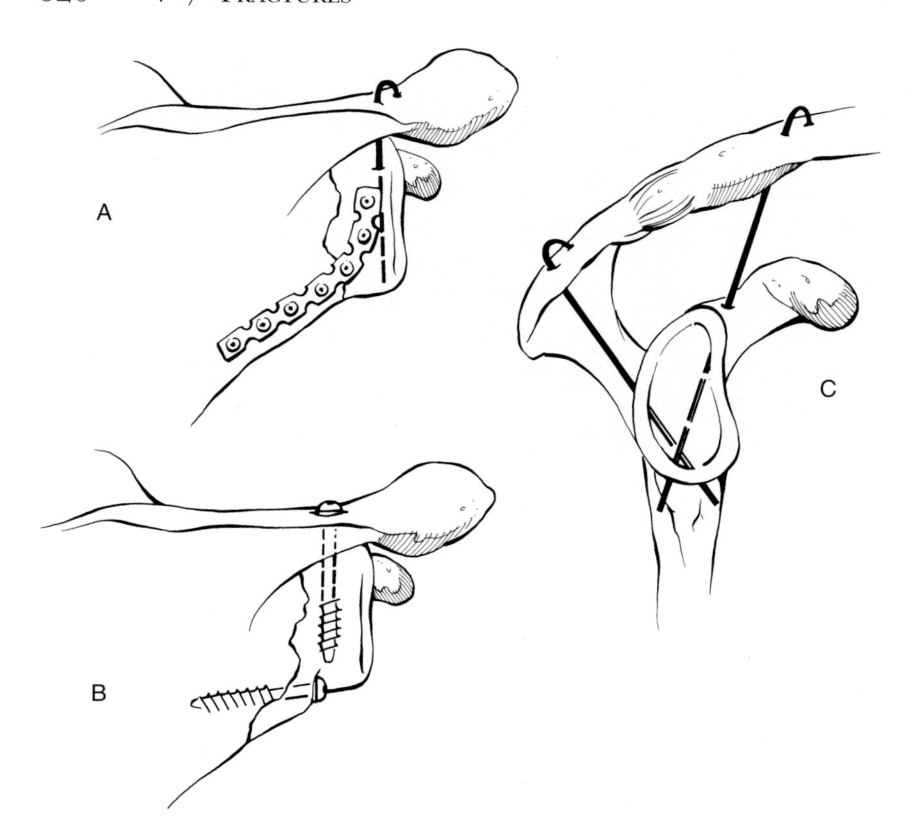

FIG. 31. Illustrations depicting fixation techniques available for stabilization of glenoid neck fractures: **(A)** stabilization with a 3.5 mm malleable reconstruction plate (note the K-wire running from the acromial process to the glenoid process that can be used for either temporary or permanent fixation); **(B)** stabilization with 3.5 mm cannulated interfragmentary screws; and **(C)** stabilization with K-wires (in this case, K-wires passed from the acromion and clavicle into the glenoid process).

integrity of the clavicular–AC joint–acromial strut. Rarely, if the scapular body–spine, acromial process, and distal clavicle are all severely comminuted, overhead olecranon pin traction must be considered or displacement of the glenoid neck fracture must be accepted and managed nonoperatively.

Postoperative Management and Prognosis

The postoperative management of glenoid process fractures depends upon the fixation–stability achieved. Immobilization in a sling and swathe bandage is prescribed during the first 24 to 48 hours following surgery. If fixation is rigid, dependent circular and pendulum movements are then initiated as well as external rotation of the shoulder to, but not past, neutral. During postoperative weeks 3 to 6, progressive range of motion exercises in all directions (especially forward flexion, internal rotation behind the back, and external rotation) are prescribed, seeking to achieve full range of motion by the end of the 6-week period. The patient is allowed to use his or her arm actively in a progressive manner within clearly defined limits (moving the weight of his upper extremity alone when sitting in a protected setting during weeks 3 and 4 and when up and about indoors during weeks 5 and 6). The patient is followed clinically and radiographically every 2 weeks to make sure displacement does not occur at the fracture site and to monitor and update the rehabilitation program. At 6 weeks, healing is sufficient so as to discontinue all external protection and encourage progressive functional use of the extremity. K-wires spanning bones that move relative to each other are removed at this time as are those passing through soft tissues [K-wires imbedded within a single osseous structure (bent at their entry site to prevent migration) may be left in place]. Physiotherapy continues to focus on regaining range of motion as progressive strengthening exercises are added. The patient's rehabilitation program continues until range of motion, strength, and overall function are maximized. Light use of the shoulder is emphasized through post-operative week 12, whereas heavy physical use of the shoulder, including athletic activities, is prohibited until the 4- to 6-month point.

If surgical fixation is less than rigid, the shoulder may need to be protected in a sling and swathe immobilizer, an abduction brace, or even overhead olecranon pin traction for 7, 10, or 14 days (dependent on the clinical situation) before the aforementioned physiotherapy program is prescribed. The patient must be encouraged to work diligently on his or her rehabilitation program because range of motion and strength can improve, and the end result is often not achieved for approximately 6 months to 1 year after injury. Hard work, perseverance, and dedication on the part of the patient, the physician, and the physical therapist are critical to an optimal functional result.

Although the literature remains somewhat deficient owing to the rarity of these injuries, interest has increased in recent years, resulting in a growing number of case reports and personal series. Although more data is needed, it is reasonable to anticipate a good to excellent functional result if: (a) surgical management restores normal or near normal glenoid anatomy articular congruity, and glenohumeral stability; (b) the fixation is secure; and (c) a well-structured, closely monitored postoperative rehabilitation program is prescribed.

DOUBLE DISRUPTIONS OF THE SUPERIOR SHOULDER SUSPENSORY COMPLEX

Biomechanics

The superior shoulder suspensory complex (SSSC) is a bony soft-tissue ring at the end of a superior and an inferior bony strut (Fig. 32). This ring is comprised of the glenoid process, the coracoid process, the coracoclavicular ligaments, the distal clavicle, the AC joint, and the acromial process. The superior strut is the middle third of the clavicle, whereas the inferior strut is the junction of the most lateral portion of the scapular body and the most medial portion of the glenoid neck. The complex can be subdivided into three units: (a) the clavicular–AC joint—acromial strut; (b) the three-process–scapular body junction; and (c) the clavicular–CC ligamentous—coracoid (C-4) linkage (Fig. 33), with secondary support provided by the C-A ligament. The SSSC is an extremely important structure as regards to the biomechanics of the shoulder complex: (a) each of its components has its own individual function(s); (b) it serves as a point of attachment for a variety of musculotendinous and ligamentous structures; (c) it allows limited, but very important motion to occur through the coracoclavicular ligaments and the AC articulation; and (d) it maintains a normal, stable relationship between the upper extremity and the axial skeleton (the clavicle is the only bony connection between the upper extremity and the axial skeleton and the scapula is "hung" or suspended from the clavicle by the coracoclavicular ligaments and the acromioclavicular articulation).

The "double disruption" concept is a principle that underlies and allows one to understand a variety of difficult-to-treat injuries to the shoulder complex, which have previously been described in isolation, but are actually united by a single biomechanical theme. This "double disruption" concept also has a certain predictive value for several injuries that are encountered only rarely.[45]

Single traumatic disruptions of the SSSC are common (e.g., a type I fracture of the distal clavicle). These are anatomically stable situations because the overall integrity of the complex is not significantly violated and nonoperative management will generally yield a good to excellent functional result.

When the complex is disrupted in two places, however (a "double disruption"), the integrity of the SSSC is clearly compromised, creating a potentially unstable anatomic situation. Significant displacement can occur at either or both sites, resulting in bony healing problems (delayed unions, malunions, and nonunions) as well as adverse long-term functional difficulties (subacromial impingement, decreased strength and muscle fatigue discomfort, neurovascular compromise due to a "drooping" shoulder, and degenerative joint disease) depending on the particular injury.

Double disruptions may take a variety of forms: two fractures of the bony–soft-tissue ring; two ligamentous disruptions of the ring; a fracture and a ligamentous disruption of the ring; fractures of both bony struts; or a fracture of one strut combined with a ring disruption (either a fracture or a ligamentous disruption; Fig. 34). Because the glenoid, acromial, and coracoid processes are all components of the superior shoulder suspensory complex, many double disruption injuries involve the scapula. Also many, if not most, significantly displaced coracoid and acromial fractures are part of a double disruption.

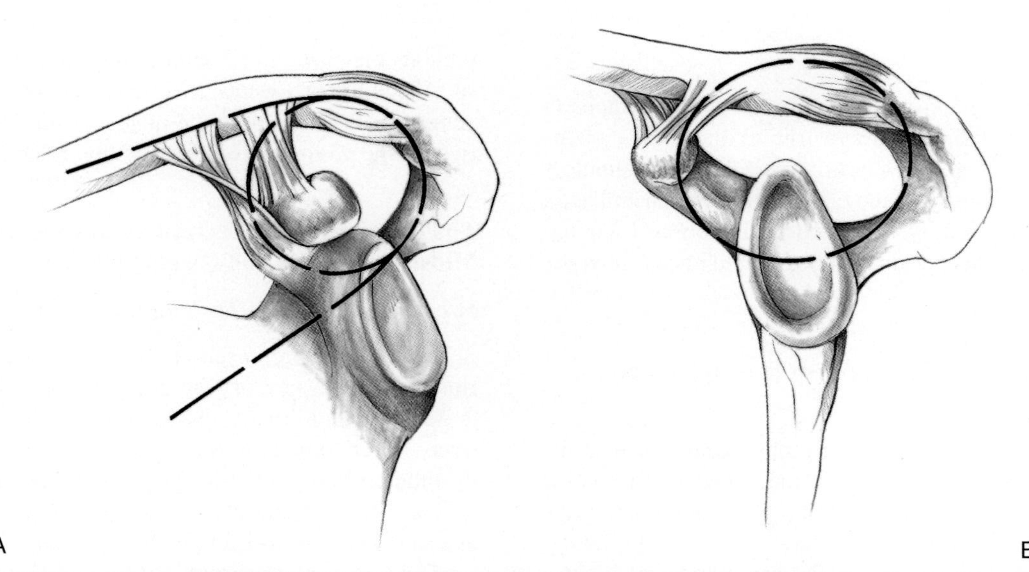

FIG. 32. Illustrations depicting the superior shoulder suspensory complex: **(A)** an anteroposterior view of the bony–soft-tissue ring and the superior and inferior bony struts and **(B)** a lateral view of the bony–soft-tissue ring.

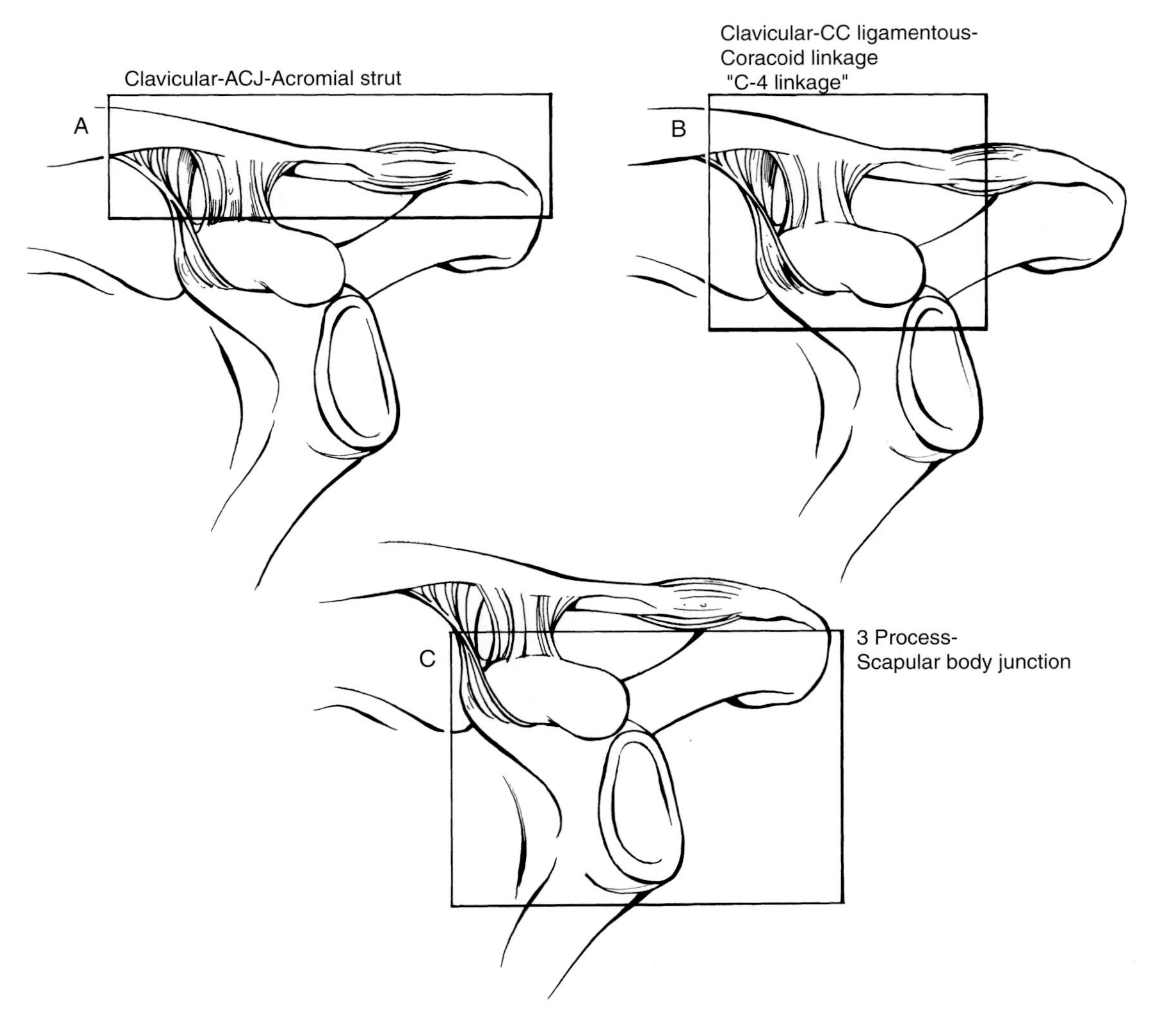

FIG. 33. The three components of the superior shoulder suspensory complex: **(A)** the clavicular–AC joint–acromial strut; **(B)** the clavicular–CC ligamentous–coracoid (C-4) linkage; and **(C)** the three process–scapular body junction.

Diagnosis

If a single disruption is noted on routine radiographs (a true AP view of the shoulder, a true axillary view of the glenohumeral joint, and a weight-bearing AP of the shoulder to evaluate the integrity of the clavicular–scapular linkage), one should look carefully for a second disruption (CT scanning is often necessary owing to the complex bony anatomy in the area).

Surgical Indications, Management Principles, and Results

If two disruptions are present, one must decide whether displacement at one or both sites is "unacceptable" (a relative term, dependent on the particular clinical situation) and if so, surgical management is generally necessary. Reducing and stabilizing one of the disruptions will frequently indirectly reduce and stabilize the other disruption satisfactorily (whichever injury is easiest to manage is chosen). If unsuccessful, both disruptions may need to be addressed (see sections dealing with specific injuries). Results, as always, are dependent on the adequacy of the reduction, the quality of the fixation, and the rigor of the postoperative rehabilitation program.

The Floating Shoulder (Ipsilateral Fractures of the Midshaft Clavicle and Glenoid Neck)

Surgical Indications, Techniques, and Results

These injuries represent a double disruption of the superior shoulder suspensory complex. In isolation, each fracture is generally minimally displaced and managed nonoperatively. In combination, however, each disruption can make the other unstable (i.e., the glenoid neck fracture often allows severe displacement to occur at the clavicular fracture site and vice versa although to a lesser degree). The situation is rendered even more unstable if an additional disruption of the clavicular–AC joint–acromial strut is present or if the C-4 linkage is violated (Fig. 35). Hardegger et al.[59] felt these

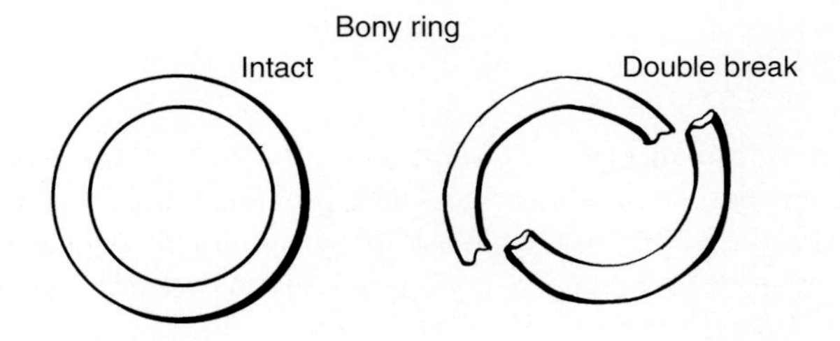

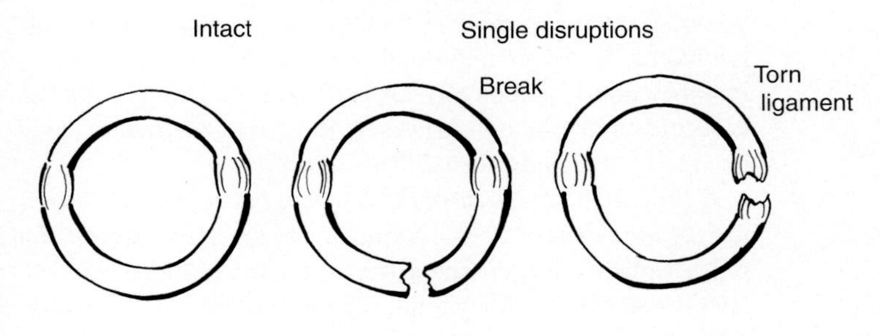

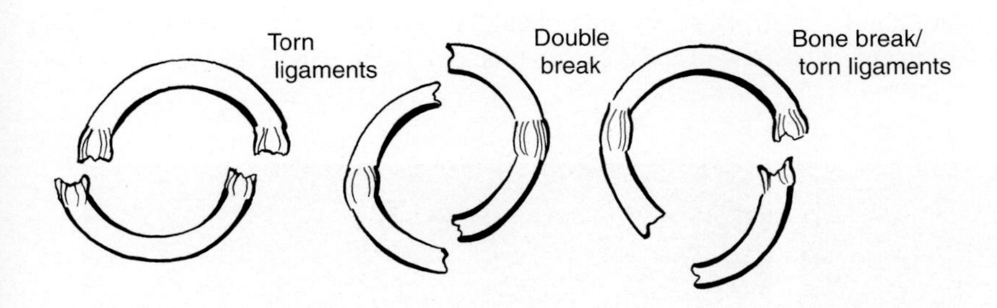

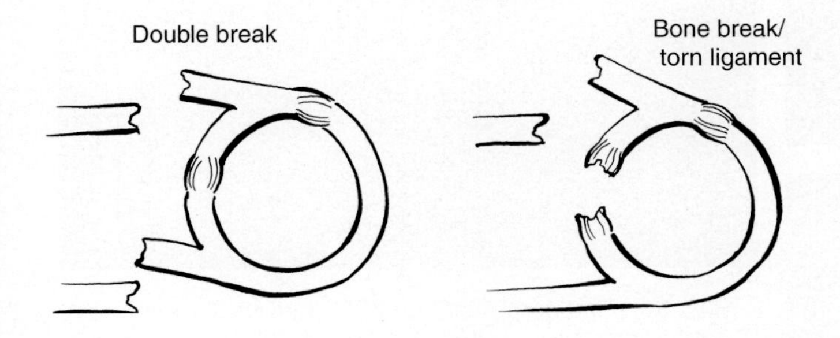

FIG. 34. Illustrations depicting the many possible traumatic ring–strut disruptions.

injuries represented a "functional imbalance" owing to the "altered glenohumeral–acromial relationships." Both he and Butters[19] recommended surgery to reduce and stabilize the injury. Surgical reduction and stabilization of the clavicular fracture site (most commonly with plate fixation) is advisable if displacement is unacceptable to avoid a nonunion, alleviate tensile forces on the brachial plexus, restore normal anatomic relationships, and ensure restoration of normal shoulder function.[66,89] The glenoid neck fracture will generally reduce and stabilize secondarily; however, if significant displacement persists, it may also require surgical management[65,96] (see *Fractures of the Glenoid Neck*). Additional injuries to the clavicular–AC joint–acromial strut may require operative treatment, whereas associated injuries of the C-4 linkage will usually heal satisfactorily if the glenoid neck and clavicular fracture sites are treated appropriately. Leung and Lam[97] reported on 15 patients treated surgically (average follow-up period 25 months). In 14 of the 15 patients, the fractures healed with a good or excellent functional result. Herscovici et al.[67] reported the results of 9 patients with ipsilateral clavicular and glenoid neck fractures (average follow-up period 48.5 months). Seven patients were treated surgically with plate fixation of the clavicular fracture and achieved excellent results. Two patients were treated without surgery and had decreased range of motion as well as "drooping" of the involved shoulder. The authors strongly recommended ORIF of the clavicle to prevent a glenoid neck malunion. Rikli et al. expanded this concept somewhat, saying that a fracture of the glenoid neck combined with either a fracture of the clavicle or a disruption of the AC joint or the SC joint results in an "unstable shoulder girdle." They reviewed 13 cases (12 patients) in which the clavicular injury was surgically stabilized and reported excellent results in nearly all.[140]

Coracoid Process Fracture as One Component of a Double Disruption of the Superior Shoulder Suspensory Complex

The coracoid process is a vital part of the SSSC serving as one of the bony components of the clavicular–CC ligamentous–coracoid (C-4) linkage that joins the scapula to the clavicular–AC joint–acromial strut. Consequently, if a coracoid process fracture is present and associated with another SSSC injury, the potential adverse consequences of a "double disruption" must be considered and treatment tailored accordingly.[45] The following are examples: *A fracture of the coracoid process and a grade III disruption of the AC joint* (see chapter 27).[14,21,31,57,68,88,95,105,118,136,153,167,178]

Fractures of the Ipsilateral Coracoid and Acromial Processes. Isolated fractures of the acromial and coracoid processes (Fig. 36) are almost always minimally displaced and, therefore, managed nonoperatively. When they occur together, however, they constitute a "double disruption" of the superior shoulder suspensory complex, a potentially unstable anatomic situation.[179] If displacement at either or both sites is unacceptable, surgical management is indicated. ORIF of the acromial fracture may be all that is required, since this will often indirectly reduce and stabilize the coracoid fracture satisfactorily and is technically less difficult than addressing the coracoid injury. If not, however, the coracoid fracture may need to be reduced and stabilized as well.

A Fracture of the Base of the Coracoid Process and a Fracture of the Glenoid Neck. A fracture of the glenoid neck can only displace if it is complete (i.e., if the fracture line exits the lateral scapular border and the superior scapular margin adjacent to the coracoid process). Even so, if continuity of the glenoid fragment with the clavicular–AC joint–acromial strut via the C-4 linkage is intact, displacement is usually minimal. If, however, this linkage is disrupted (e.g., a fracture at the base of the coracoid process), significant displacement of the

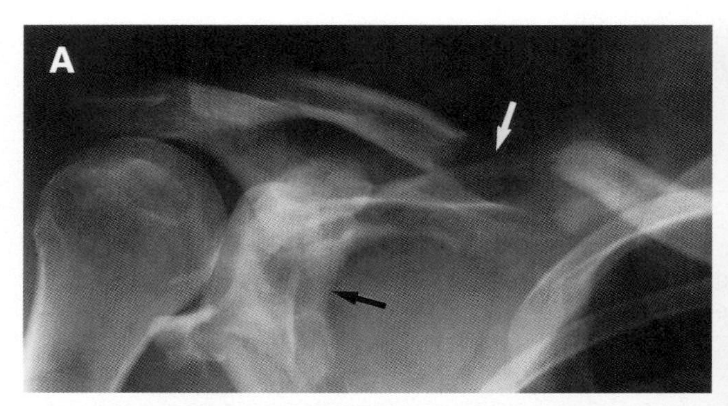

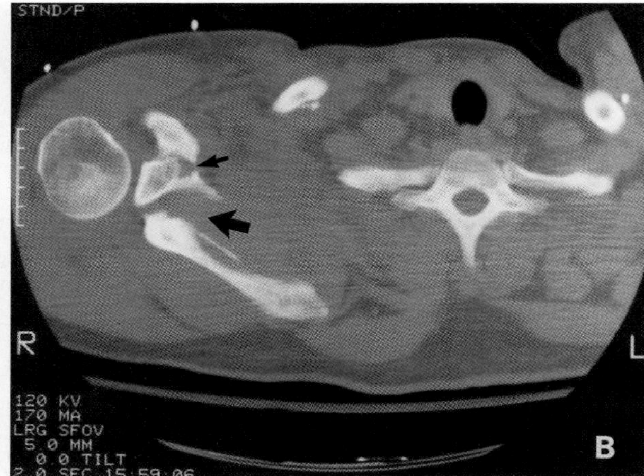

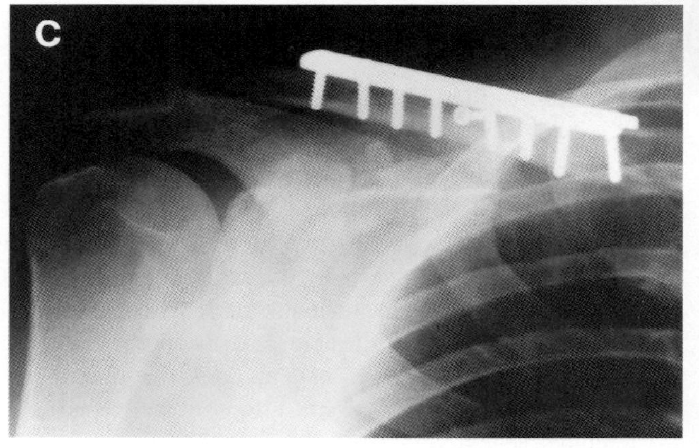

FIG. 35. Radiographs of an individual who sustained a double disruption of the superior shoulder suspensory complex resulting in a "floating shoulder": **(A)** a preoperative AP radiograph showing a fracture of the glenoid neck with medial translation and a severely displaced fracture of the middle third of the clavicle; **(B)** a preoperative axial CT image showing the glenoid neck fracture to be complete, with the glenoid fragment and the entire superior shoulder suspensory complex rendered particularly unstable by an associated fracture of the coracoid process; and **(C)** a post-operative AP radiograph showing anatomic reduction and stabilization of the clavicle fracture. The glenoid neck fracture was managed nonoperatively, although a strong case could have been made for ORIF in light of its persistent medial translational displacement (the glenoid fragment remained unstable owing to the fractured coracoid process; a double disruption of the superior shoulder suspensory complex was still present).

glenoid fragment is particularly likely (translational displacement greater than or equal to 1 cm and/or angular displacement greater than or equal to 40 degrees) and surgical management must be considered.[50] Operative treatment consists of ORIF of the glenoid neck fracture through a posterior or posterosuperior approach. The coracoid fracture will usually heal without direct intervention.

A Fracture of the Coracoid Process and a Type I Fracture of the Distal Third of the Clavicle (Fig. 37). Fractures of the distal third of the clavicle can displace unacceptably if the continuity of the coracoclavicular ligaments between the coracoid process and the proximal clavicular segment is disrupted (type II and V fractures[122,123].) The same situation can occur with type I fractures if the coracoid process is fractured. (It would probably make most sense to call all of these injuries type II fractures; i.e., situations in which the distal third of the clavicle is fractured, and the linkage between the proximal segment and the scapula [the C-4 linkage] is disrupted.) If displacement at the clavicular fracture site is of such a degree that it makes a delayed union or a nonunion likely, treatment consists of surgical reduction and stabilization of the injury (usually by means of tension band fixation). The coracoid fracture may reduce secondarily and heal uneventfully. If not, the coracoid fracture may also need to be addressed surgically.

Acromial Fracture as One Component of a Double Disruption of the Superior Shoulder Suspensory Complex

Acromial fractures that are significantly displaced are usually the result of the instability created when other fractures or ligamentous disruptions of the SSSC are present.[45] These injuries are generally the result of high-energy trauma and often require surgical intervention. The following are examples:

Ipsilateral acromial and coracoid process fractures (refer to page 623).

An Acromial Fracture and a Grade III Disruption of the Acromioclavicular Joint. This combination creates a free-

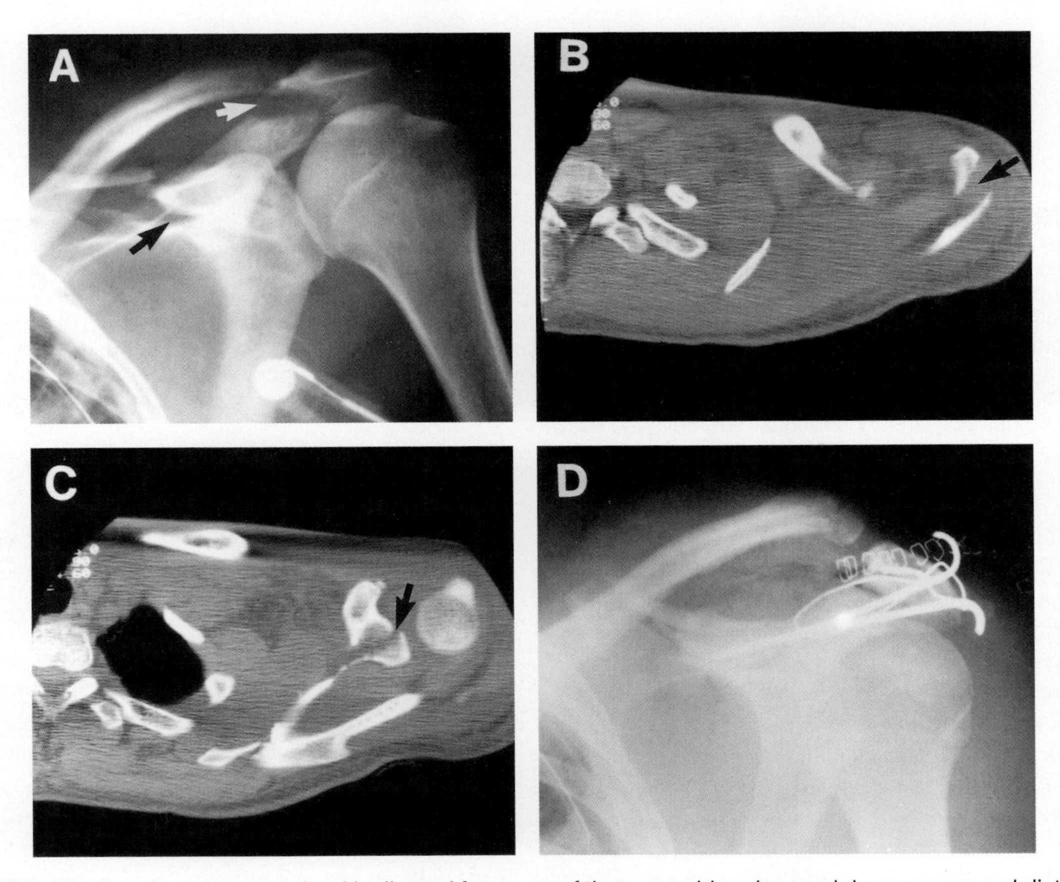

FIG. 36. A patient who sustained ipsilateral fractures of the coracoid and acromial processes and distal clavicle: **(A)** a preoperative anteroposterior (AP) radiograph of the involved area (*white arrow*, acromial fracture; *black arrow*, coracoid fracture); **(B)** a preoperative axillary CT image showing wide separation at the acromial fracture site (*arrow*) owing to the associated coracoid process fracture; **(C)** a preoperative axillary CT image showing the fractured coracoid process (*arrow*); and **(D)** a postoperative AP radiograph of the shoulder showing reduction and stabilization of the acromial fracture using a tension band construct (the coracoid process fracture and distal clavicle fracture were not addressed and healed spontaneously).

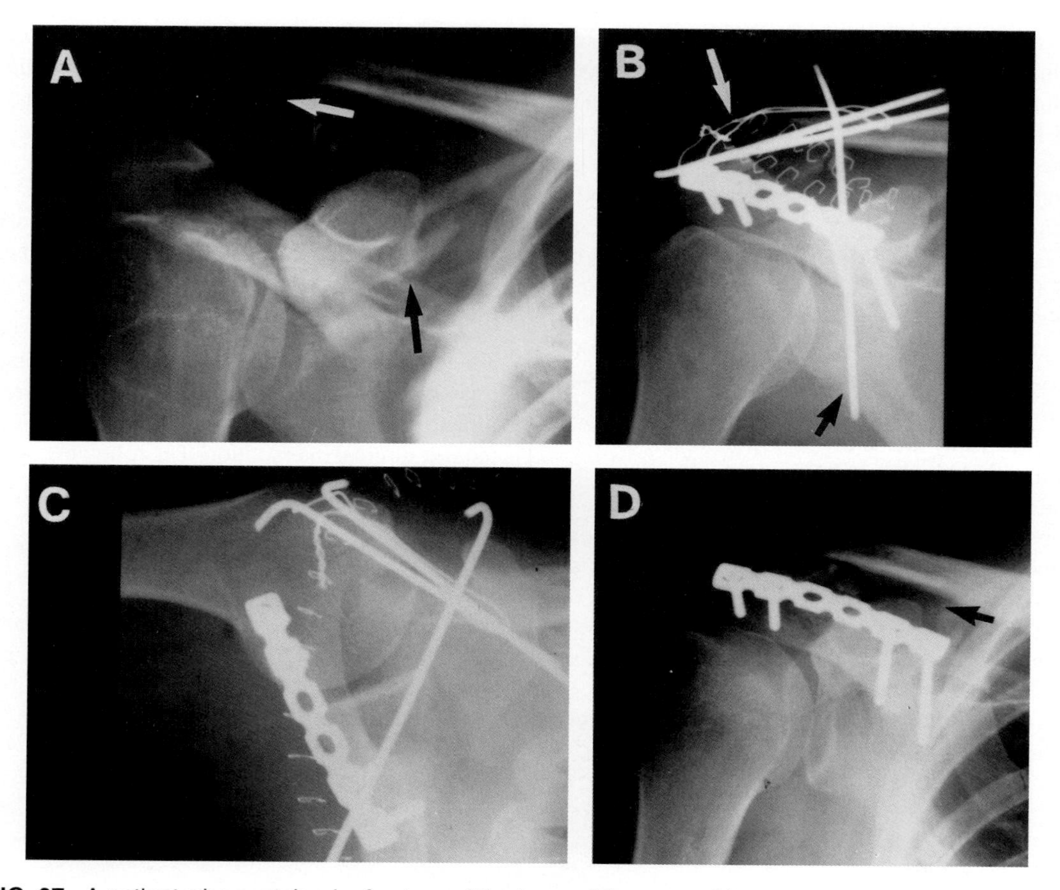

FIG. 37. A patient who sustained a fracture of the base of the coracoid process, a type I fracture of the distal clavicle, and a nondisplaced fracture of the acromion: **(A)** a preoperative AP radiograph showing severe displacement at the distal clavicular fracture site (*white arrow*) and the coracoid fracture (*black arrow*); **(B,C)** postoperative AP and axillary radiographs showing reduction and stabilization of the clavicular fracture using a tension band construct (*white arrow*) and reduction and stabilization of the coracoid process fracture by means of a transfixing K-wire passed into the glenoid process (the acromial fracture was plated; *black arrow*); and **(D)** AP radiograph taken 3 months postoperatively following removal of hardware showing the distal clavicle and coracoid fractures to be healed and the superior shoulder suspensory relations reestablished (*arrow*).

floating acromial fragment and can lead to a nonunion as well as the well-described adverse long-term functional consequences associated with AC joint disruptions. One case report describes an individual with an associated axillary nerve deficit.108 Acutely, isolated grade III AC joint disruptions are usually managed nonoperatively; however, in this situation, if displacement at the acromial fracture site is unacceptable, surgical reduction and stabilization of both injuries is indicated. Kurdy and Shah described a patient treated nonoperatively who realized a "satisfactory" outcome; however, he was 74 years old and an acromial nonunion occurred.91

A Segmental Fracture of the Acromion. As with segmental fractures of other bones, two acromial disruptions create an unstable intermediate segment. If displacement at one or both sites is unacceptable and a nonunion likely, ORIF through a posterolateral approach using plate fixation and/or a tension band construct is performed.

ISOLATED FRACTURES OF THE CORACOID PROCESS

Classification and Mechanism of Injury

The coracoid process develops from two constant ossification centers: one at its base, which also forms the upper third of the glenoid process; and one that becomes its main body. In addition, there are at least two inconstant centers: one at its angle where the coracoclavicular ligaments attach; and one at its tip where the conjoined tendon is located. The regions at which the centers finally unite are relatively weak, especially in young adults, making fractures more likely to occur when direct or indirect forces are applied.[118,136] The coracoid process has two basic functions: (a) it serves as a point of attachment for a number of musculotendinous and ligamentous structures (Fig. 38), and (b) it provides the glenohumeral joint with some anterosuperior stability. Cora-

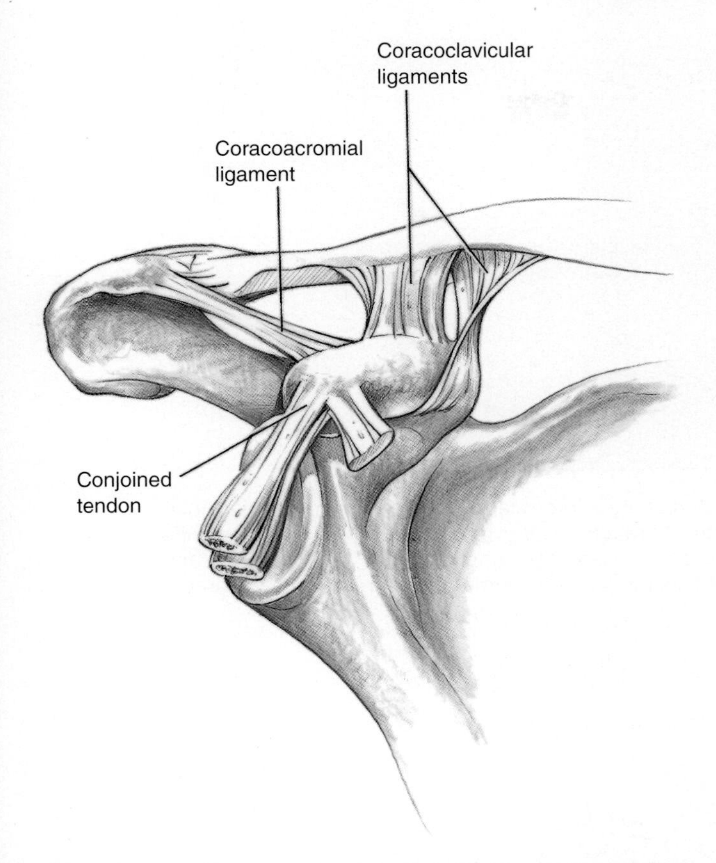

FIG. 38. Illustration showing the coracoid process as the point of attachment for, the conjoined tendon, the coracoacromial ligament and, the coracoclavicular ligaments.

coid fractures may be caused by a blow from the outside or contact by a dislocating humeral head or indirect forces applied through the musculotendinous and ligamentous structures at their attachment sites (avulsion fractures fall into this category[22,32,148]). Fatigue fractures have also been described.[17,149] Nontraumatic causes include (a) fractures associated with coracoclavicular tape fixation used in AC joint reconstructions,[117] and (b) fractures associated with massive rotator cuff tears. Despite the relative scarcity of isolated coracoid fractures, several types have been described.[31,54] These injuries can be anatomically divided into (a) fractures of the tip of the coracoid; (b) fractures between the CC and CA ligaments; and (c) fractures at the base of the coracoid process. Fractures of the coracoid tip are avulsion injuries—the result of an indirect force applied to the conjoined tendon and concentrated over its attachment to the coracoid process (see Fig. 45D). Fractures between the CC ligaments and the CA ligament may be the result of either a direct or an indirect force.[24] The distal coracoid fragment is usually significantly displaced, drawn distally by the pull of the conjoined tendon and rotated laterally by the tethering effect of the coracoacromial ligament (Fig. 39). Fractures of the base of the coracoid process are the most common coracoid fractures. They may be caused by a direct blow from the outside or a dislocating humeral head.[12] Avulsion fractures caused by strong traction forces are also possible.[103,137,143]

Diagnosis

Diagnosis is ultimately radiographic. True AP and axillary projections of the glenohumeral joint will disclose, or at least suggest, the presence of most coracoid fractures. Because of the complex bony anatomy in the area, "tilt"–oblique views,[36,43] or even CT scanning,[84] may be necessary to detect and accurately define some fractures as well as injuries to adjacent bony and articular structures. Accessory ossification centers and epiphyseal lines may complicate the evaluation. A weight-bearing AP view of the shoulder should be obtained if there is concern over the integrity of the scapular–acromial linkage.

Management

Fractures of the Coracoid Tip

Displacement may be quite marked, but nonsurgical treatment is usually in order.[175,179] Open surgical reduction and internal fixation (ORIF) has been advocated in athletes, especially those participating in sports that require optimal upper extremity function, and in persons who perform heavy, manual, physical work. Wong-Chung and Quinlan described a case in which a fractured coracoid tip prevented the closed reduction of an anterior glenohumeral dislocation.[174] Late surgical treatment may be necessary if the displaced bony fragment causes irritation of the surrounding soft tissues.[13] Surgical management (either acute or late if a symptomatic nonunion occurs[40]) takes two forms: (a) ORIF of the bony fragment if sufficiently large and noncomminuted, or (b) excision of the fragment and suture fixation of the conjoined tendon to the remaining coracoid process (Fig. 40).

Fractures Between the Coracoclavicular Ligaments and the Coracoacromial Ligament

Initial treatment may be nonsurgical or surgical, following the same reasoning described for significantly displaced avulsion fractures of the coracoid tip. Because the fragment is larger, however, symptomatic irritation of the local soft tissues is more frequent and late surgical management is more likely. The size of the fragment generally makes it amenable to interfragmentary screw fixation. Cannulated 3.5 and 4.0 mm compression screws are particularly useful. As with all coracoid process fractures managed surgically, an anterior deltoid splitting approach is used, and the rotator interval is opened as need be for optimal exposure of the fracture site (Fig. 41).

Fractures of the Base of the Coracoid Process

These injuries are generally minimally displaced owing to the stabilizing effect of the surrounding soft tissues, in par-

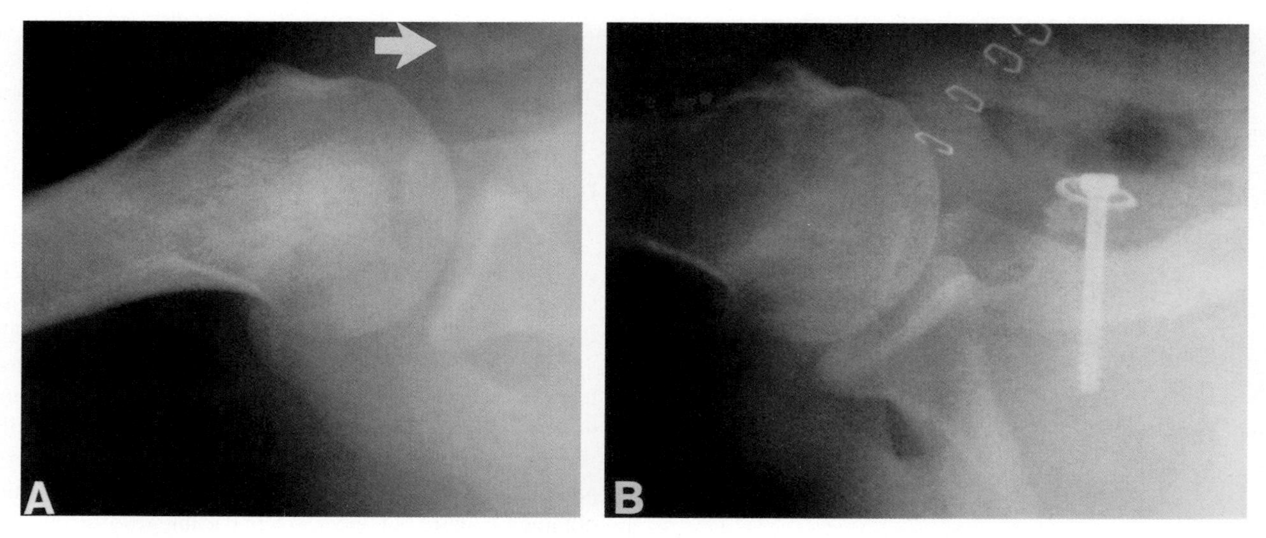

FIG. 39. A patient who sustained a fracture of the distal coracoid process between the coracoclavicular ligaments and the coracoacromial ligament: **(A)** preoperative axillary radiograph showing the significantly displaced distal portion of the coracoid process (*arrow*); and **(B)** postoperative axillary radiograph showing the bony fragment reduced and stabilized using an interfragmentary screw with a ligament washer.

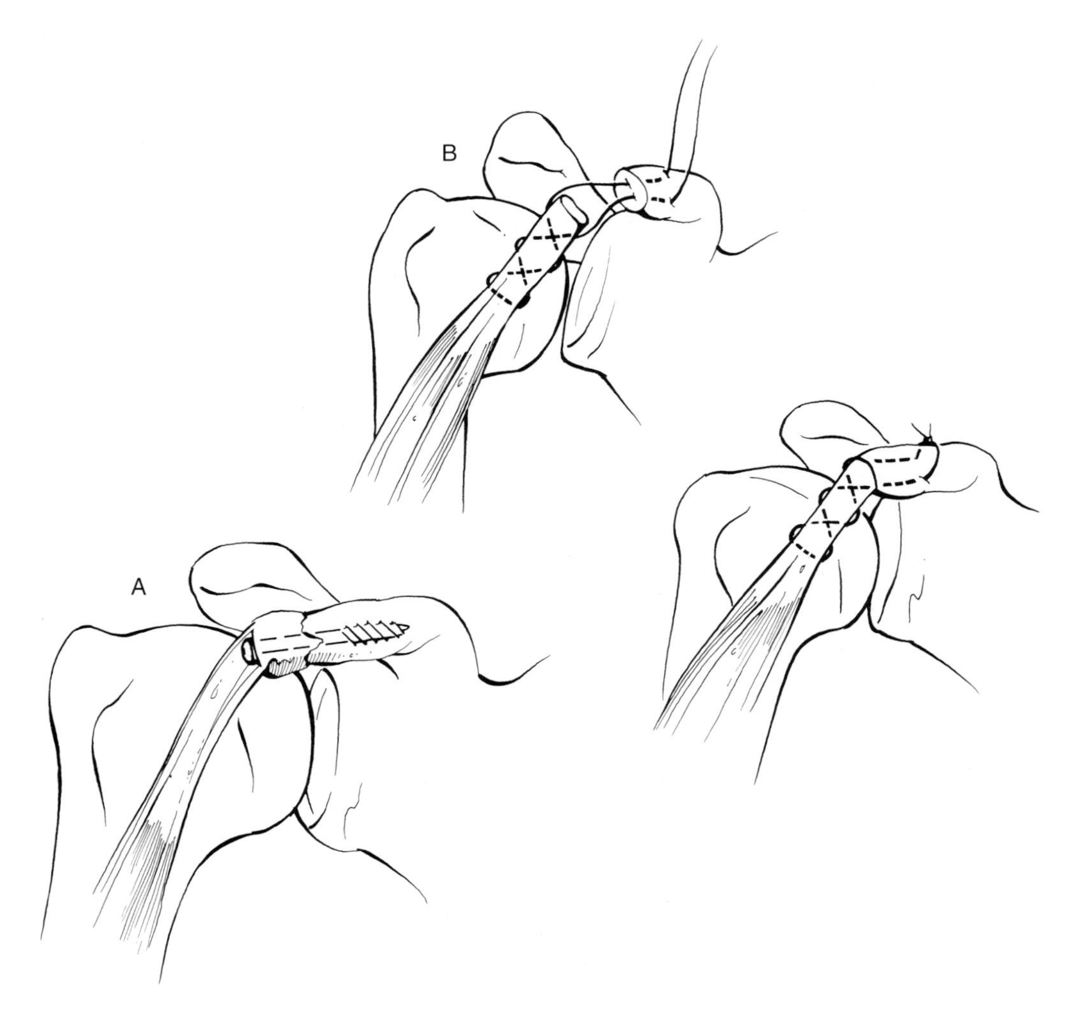

FIG. 40. Illustrations showing two surgical techniques for managing coracoid process fractures: **(A)** interfragmentary screw fixation (if the fragment is sufficiently large and noncomminuted); and **(B)** excision of the distal fragment (if small and/or comminuted) and suture fixation of the conjoined tendon to the remaining coracoid process.

ticular the coracoclavicular ligaments (Fig. 42). Symptomatic nonsurgical care is usually sufficient and union occurs within 6 weeks.[41,175,179] McLaughlin felt that fibrous union is not uncommon, but is rarely associated with discomfort.[111] If symptomatic, however, bone grafting and compression screw fixation must be considered. This is accomplished by an anterior deltoid-splitting approach, opening the rotator interval for adequate exposure.

ISOLATED FRACTURES OF THE ACROMIAL PROCESS

Classification and Mechanism of Injury

The acromial process is formed from two ossification centers: one for most of its anterior end and one for its posterolateral tip (its base is actually an extension of the scapular body and spine). The acromial process has three basic functions: (a) it provides one side of the acromioclavicular articulation; (b) it serves as a point of attachment for various musculotendinous and ligamentous structures; and (c) it lends posterosuperior stability to the glenohumeral joint.

Acromial fractures may be caused by a direct blow from the outside or a force transmitted via the humeral head. Avulsion fractures are the result of purely indirect forces. Even stress and fatigue fractures have been reported.[168] These injuries may be minimally or significantly displaced.

Kuhn et al. proposed a classification scheme that drew some discussion.[86,87,115,160] They emphasized the need for open reduction and internal fixation if an acromial fragment is displaced inferiorly by the pull of the deltoid muscle, compromising the subacromial space, thereby resulting in impingement symptoms and interfering with rotator cuff function.[85]

Diagnosis

Diagnosis is radiographic. True AP and lateral views of the scapula and a true axillary projection of the glenohumeral joint will detect most acromial fractures. The presence of an os acromionale may complicate the evaluation. On occasion, however, CT scanning may be needed to precisely define the injury and disclose involvement of adjacent bony and/or articular structures. A weight-bearing AP projection is obtained if a disruption of the scapular–acromial linkage is suspected. Arthrography to evaluate the rotator cuff should be considered if the acromial fracture is the result of traumatic superior displacement of the humeral head or chronic superior migration of the humeral head, as seen in long-standing rotator cuff disease (e.g., cuff tear arthropathy with a stress fracture of the acromion). Madhaven et al. de-

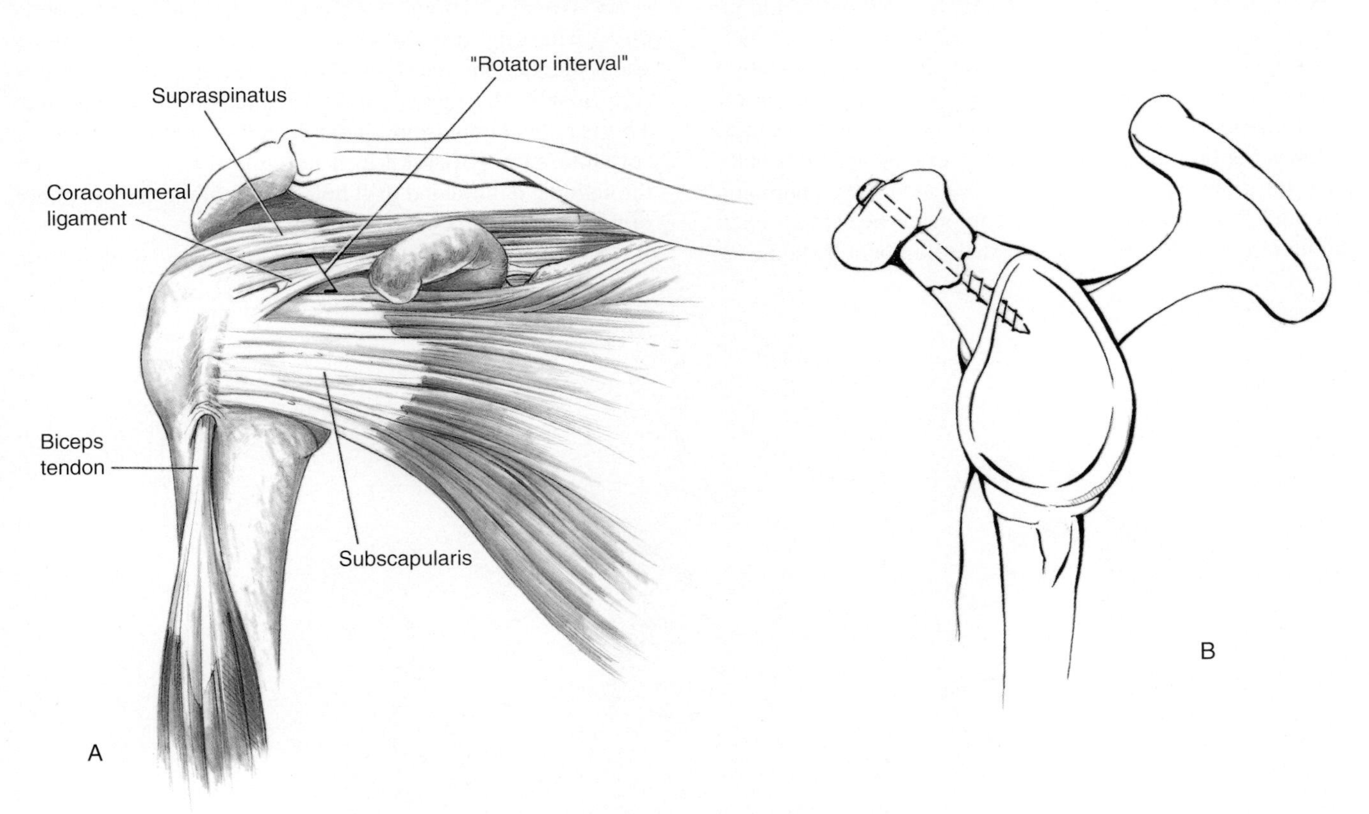

FIG. 41. Illustrations depicting **(A)** the rotator interval, which can be incised and the surrounding soft tissues retracted to expose the coracoid process including its junction with the glenoid process; and **(B)** a base of the coracoid process fracture reduced and stabilized with an interfragmentary compression screw.

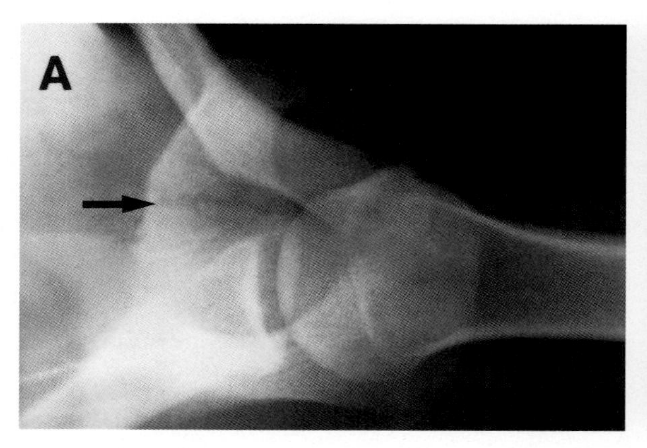

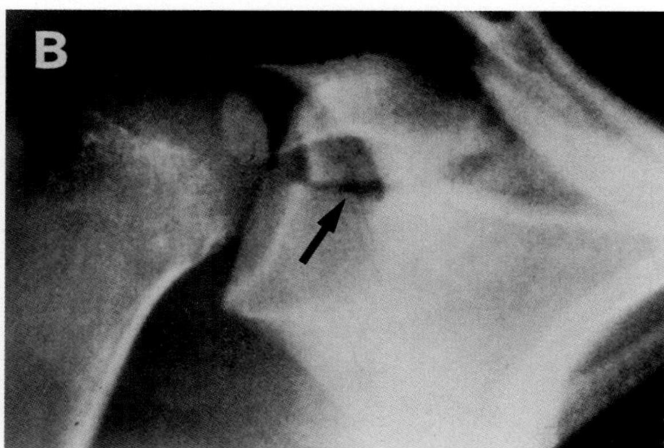

FIG. 42. Proximal coracoid fractures (two types): **(A)** an axillary radiograph showing an undisplaced fracture of the base of the coracoid process (*arrow*); and **(B)** an anteroposterior radiograph showing a type III fracture of the glenoid cavity (*arrow*) with some medial displacement (from a functional standpoint, this could be considered a very proximal coracoid process fracture).

scribed the case of an individual with an acromial fracture associated with an avulsed subscapularis tendon.[100]

Management

Although significantly displaced isolated nonavulsion acromial fractures have been described, the vast majority are nondisplaced or minimally displaced. Symptomatic, nonoperative care will reliably lead to union and a good to excellent functional result. If surgical reduction and stabilization is necessary, a tension band construct is usually chosen for distal disruptions where the acromial process is quite thin, whereas 3.5 mm malleable reconstruction plates are usually chosen for more proximal injuries (Fig. 43).[42] Symptomatic acromial nonunion although uncommon has been reported in the literature.[44] No more than a small fragment should ever be excised. The presence of a large fragment requires surgical stabilization and bone grafting.[54]

Significantly displaced avulsion fractures may occur wherever musculotendinous or ligamentous structures (the deltoid and trapezius muscles as well as the coracoacromial and acromioclavicular ligaments) attach to the acromion. Two varieties have been described in the literature.

An Avulsion Fracture of the Origin of the Deltoid Muscle.[68] The deltoid is the most important dynamic structure about the glenohumeral joint. Consequently, if a fracture is significantly displaced, surgical reattachment is indicated. This is rather simple and accomplished with multiple nonabsorbable sutures passed in a horizontal mattress fashion through the deltoid and drill holes made along the periphery of the acromial process.

An Avulsion Fracture Through the Main Body of the

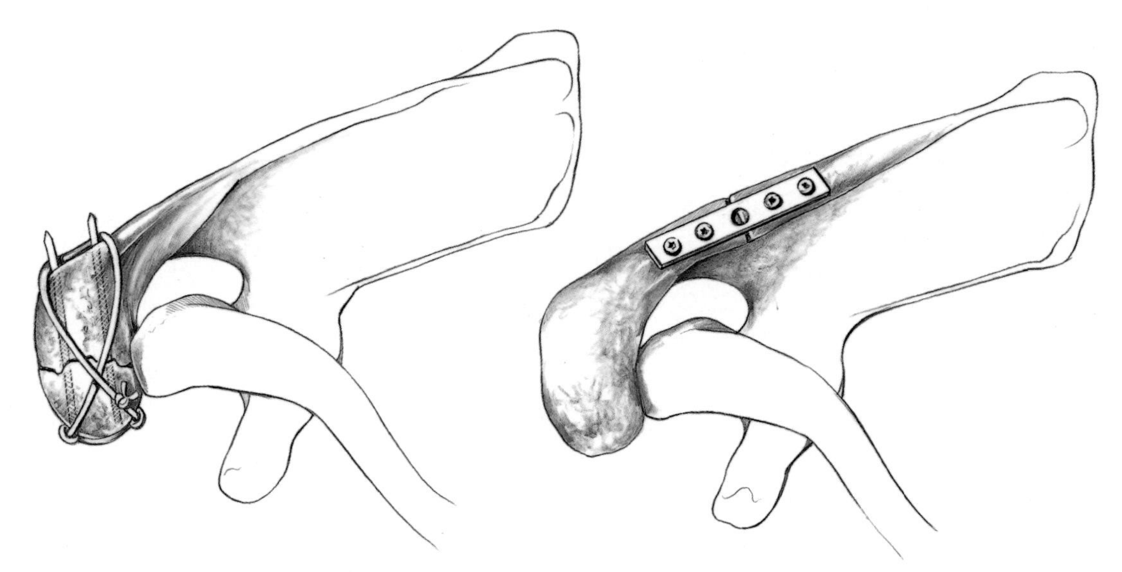

FIG. 43. Illustrations showing two surgical techniques for managing fractures of the acromial process: **(A)** a tension band construct (most appropriate for fractures through the distal portion of the acromion); and **(B)** plate–screw fixation (most appropriate for proximal fractures).

Acromion.[120,139] Two cases have been described. Both were caused by significant forces transmitted through the surrounding musculature especially the deltoid. One was treated nonsurgically, whereas the second was managed surgically. Bony union and satisfactory return of function was realized in both.

AVULSION FRACTURES OF THE SCAPULA

Classification and Mechanism of Injury

Most of the scapula is formed by intramembranous ossification, but it also has at least six or seven secondary ossification centers. The scapula has three basic functions: (a) it provides a semistable, yet fairly mobile, platform for the humeral head and the upper extremity to work against; (b) it serves as a point of attachment for a variety of soft-tissue structures (musculotendinous and ligamentous; Fig. 44), and (c) it takes part in three articulations: the glenohumeral joint, the acromioclavicular joint, and the scapulothoracic articulation. As with other scapular fractures, avulsion injuries are uncommon. By definition, they are caused by indirect forces applied to the surrounding musculotendinous and ligamentous soft tissues and concentrated at their scapular attachment sites. Three mechanisms are possible: (a) severe, uncontrolled muscular contraction caused by electroconvulsive treatment, electric shock, or epileptic seizure;[15,27,64,68,79,82,106,134,151,159,169] (b) strong indirect forces associated with a single traumatic event;[16,25,178] and (c) gradual bony failure caused by lesser but repetitive traumatic events (stress[18] or fatigue[168] fractures). The potential varieties are numerous and many have been described.

Diagnosis

True AP and lateral projections of the scapula and a true axillary view of the glenohumeral joint constitute the diagnostic trauma series. This may be supplemented as need be by CT scanning and a weight-bearing view of the shoulder complex.

Management

Treatment is by and large symptomatic/nonoperative; however, if the fracture is significantly displaced and of functional importance, surgical ORIF must be considered.[54] The following are examples of those injuries that are managed quite successfully nonoperatively.

- Avulsion fracture of the superior angle of the scapula[44](insertion of the levator scapulae; Fig. 45A).
- Avulsion fracture of the superior border of the scapula: This injury is often associated with a fracture of the base of the coracoid process and an AC joint disruption.[6,9] Some have attributed the fracture to indirect stresses applied via the omohyoid muscle,[4,76,171] whereas others have considered it an extension of the coracoid fracture.[173]

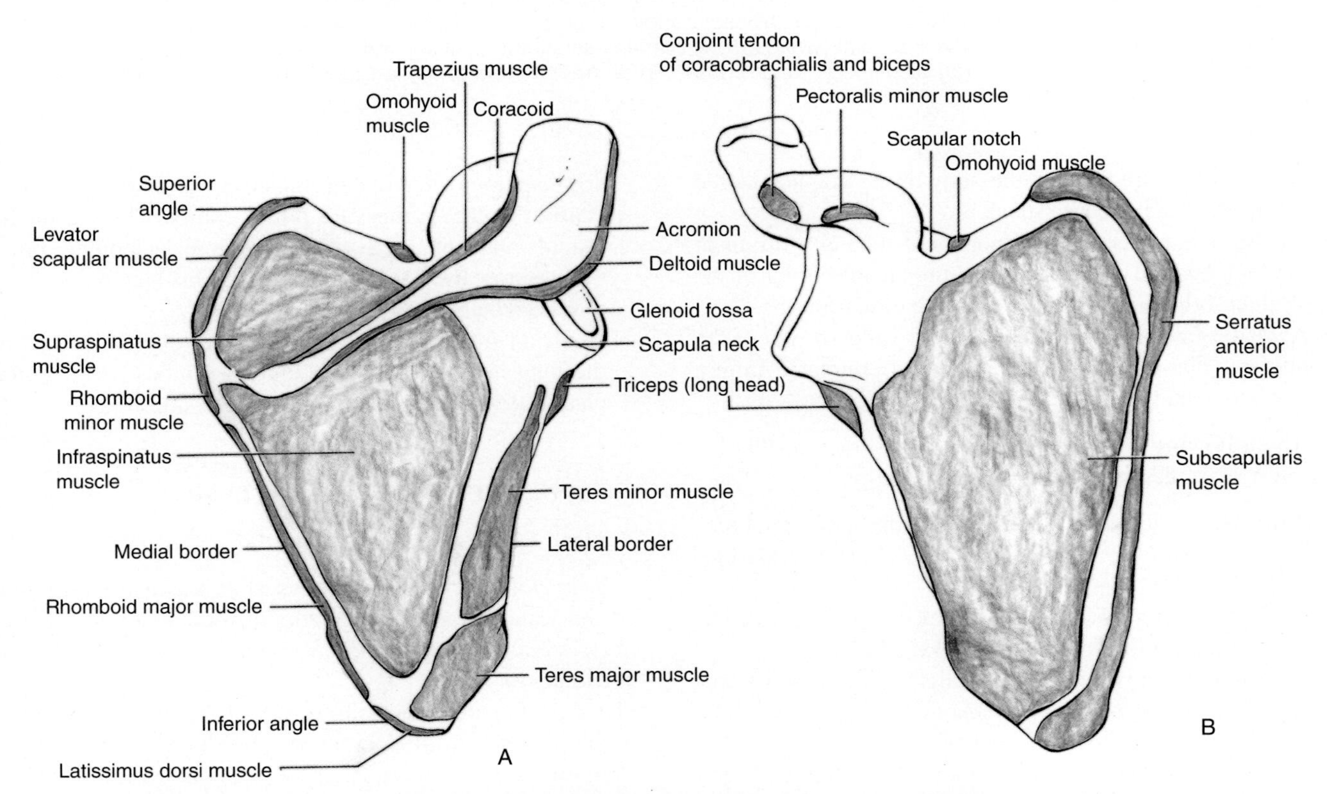

FIG. 44. Illustrations showing the many scapular musculotendinous and ligamentous attachment sites: **(A)** posterior or dorsal surface of the scapula; and **(B)** anterior or costal surface of the scapula.

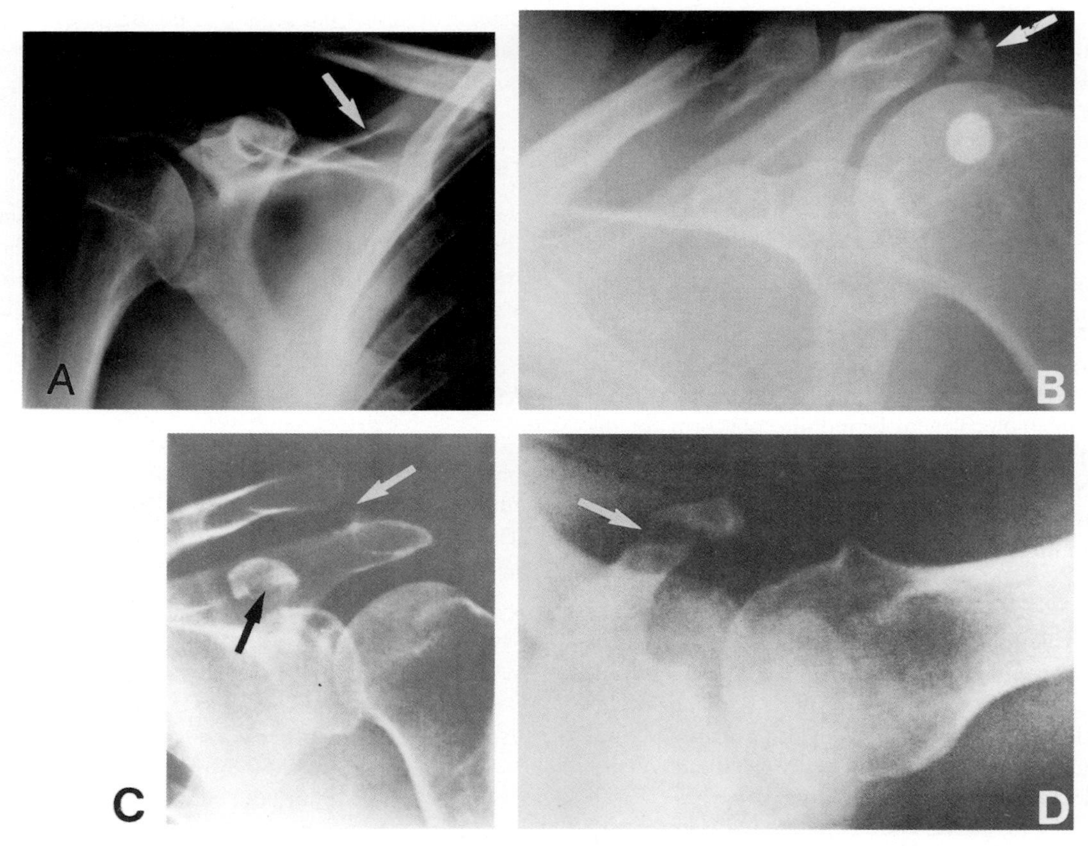

FIG. 45. Radiographs showing a variety of scapular avulsion fractures: **(A)** a minimally displaced fracture of the superior angle of the scapula (attachment of the levator scapulae; *arrow*); **(B)** a displaced fracture of the lateral margin of the acromial process (origin of the deltoid muscle; *arrow*); **(C)** a type III disruption of the acromioclavicular joint (*white arrow*) with an associated avulsion fracture at the base of the coracoid process; and **(D)** displaced fracture of the tip of the coracoid process (attachment of the conjoined tendon; *arrow*).

- Avulsion fracture through the body of the scapula caused by an accidental electric shock.[68,159]
- Avulsion fracture of the infraglenoid tubercle (origin of the long head of the triceps) and the lateral border of the scapula (origin of the teres major and minor muscles[68]).
- Avulsion fracture of the infraspinatus fossa (origin of the infraspinatus muscle[9] [this must be differentiated from a developmental anomaly[138]]).

The following are examples of avulsion fractures that, at the very least, deserve operative consideration:

- Avulsion fracture of the lateral margin of the acromial process (origin of the deltoid muscle;[68] see page 632; Fig. 45B).
- Avulsion fracture of the distal coracoid process (attachment of the conjoined tendon; see page 627).
- Avulsion fracture of the superior angle of the coracoid process (attachment of the coracoclavicular ligaments[118]) or the base of the coracoid process in association with a disruption of the acromioclavicular joint (see Chapter 27 and Fig. 45C).
- Avulsion fracture of the inferior angle of the scapula (Fig. 46; insertion of the serratus anterior muscle):[20] If significantly displaced, this rare injury causes winging of the scapula and can significantly compromise shoulder function—surgical ORIF is indicated.[62] (This may be the fracture Longbaugh described in 1924.[100])
- Avulsion fracture of the supraglenoid tubercle (origin of the long head of the biceps muscle) indicative of a displaced, possibly symptomatic SLAP lesion.[71]

SCAPULOTHORACIC DISSOCIATION

Lateral Dislocation of the Scapula

Scapulothoracic dissociation is a rare traumatic disruption of the scapulothoracic articulation caused by a severe direct force over the shoulder accompanied by traction applied to the upper extremity.[3,28,29,52,69,77,81,94,121,132,146,164] Although the skin remains intact, the scapula is torn away from the posterior chest wall, prompting some to call this injury a "closed traumatic forequarter amputation." Because of the violent forces involved, any of the three bones in the shoulder complex (the clavicle, the scapula, and the proximal

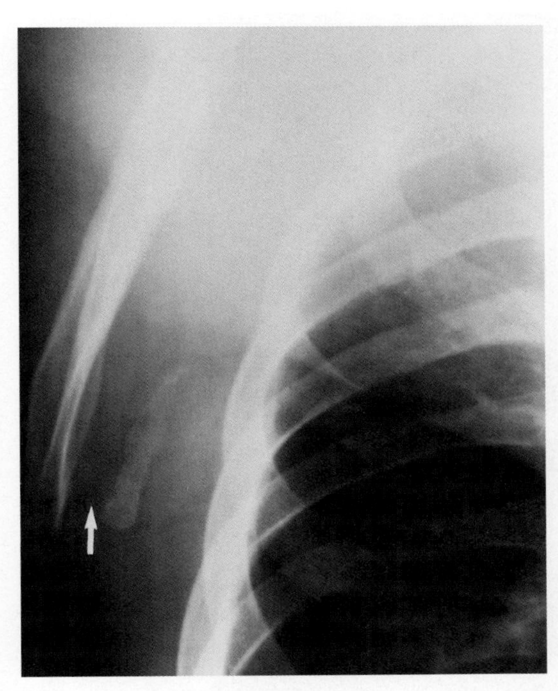

FIG. 46. A true lateral radiograph of the scapula showing a severely displaced avulsion fracture of the inferior angle (the insertion of a serratus anterior muscle).

humerus) may be fractured, and any of the remaining three articulations (the glenohumeral, AC, and sternoclavicular joints) may be disrupted. Neurovascular injury is common. Disruption of the subclavian and axillary artery (most frequently the former) and a complete or partial disruption of the brachial plexus are well described. In addition, there may be severe damage to the soft-tissue supporting structures, especially those that run from the chest wall to the scapula or the chest wall to the humerus. Complete and partial tears of the trapezius, levator scapulae, rhomboids, pectoralis minor, and latissimus dorsi, all have been reported. A presumptive diagnosis is based on a history of violent trauma in the presence of massive soft-tissue swelling over the shoulder girdle. A pulseless upper extremity, indicating a complete vascular disruption, and a complete or partial neurologic deficit, indicating injury to the brachial plexus, are quite suggestive. Significant lateral displacement of the scapula seen on a nonrotated chest radiograph confirms the diagnosis. As with all rare injuries, awareness of the clinical entity is critical to making the correct diagnosis. Treatment recommendations have focused on care of the accompanying neurovascular injury. If the vascular integrity of the extremity is in question, an emergency arteriogram is performed followed by surgical repair if necessary. The brachial plexus is explored at the same time. If a neurologic deficit is present, electromyographic testing is performed 3 weeks after injury to determine the extent of damage and to assess the degree of recovery, if any. Cervical myelography can be performed at 6 weeks. If nerve root avulsions or a complete neurologic deficit is present, the prognosis for a functional recovery is poor. Partial plexus injuries, however, have a good prognosis and most patients achieve complete recovery or regain functional use of the extremity. If some portions of the plexus are intact and others are disrupted, neurologic repair is a possibility. Late reconstructive efforts are guided by the degree of neurologic return, and musculotendinous transfers are performed as needed. Care of the surrounding soft-tissue supportive structures (musculotendinous and ligamentous) has been nonoperative, consisting of immobilization of the shoulder complex for 6 weeks to allow healing, followed by a closely monitored physical therapy program designed to restore range of motion initially, followed by strength. Magnetic resonance imaging (MRI) of the involved area now offers the ability to visualize important disruptions that may be amenable to surgical repair.

Injury to the sternal–clavicular–acromial linkage (a disruption of the sternoclavicular or AC joint or a fracture of the clavicle) is frequently, if not invariably, present for posterolateral displacement of the scapula to occur. This component of scapulothoracic dissociation has been largely ignored, both in terms of diagnosis and treatment. Of the three possible disruptions, a fracture of the clavicle seems to be the most common. This constitutes a very unstable anatomic situation—the clavicular injury allows maximal displacement of the scapula, whereas the unstable scapulothoracic articulation often leads to significant displacement at the clavicular fracture site. Consequently, surgical ORIF of the clavicle (screw plate fixation for fractures of the middle third and tension band fixation for fractures of the distal third) should be considered (a) to avoid a delayed union or a nonunion; (b) to restore as much stability as possible to the shoulder complex in order to avoid adverse long-term functional consequences; and (c) to protect the brachial plexus and subclavian and axillary vessels from further injury caused by tensile forces (Fig. 47). Uhl and Hospeder described a lesser injury characterized by progressive subluxation of the scapulothoracic articulation and a clavicle fracture (no neurovascular involvement) requiring ORIF of the latter.[165] Similar therapeutic reasoning would apply to scapulothoracic dissociations accompanied by a disruption of the AC or the sternoclavicular joint, although in the latter, metallic fixation devices must be avoided.

Intrathoracic Dislocation of the Scapula

Intrathoracic dislocation of the scapula is extremely rare. Cases associated with minimal violence and a preexisting factor (generalized laxity or locking osteochondroma) have been described.[2] The scapula becomes locked within the posterior aspect of one of the upper intercostal spaces.[125] A second type is caused by more violent trauma, either a direct blow applied over the posterior aspect of the scapula or a violent outward distractive force applied to the arm. The scapular body is displaced anterolaterally, and its inferior angle becomes lodged between the ribs. The severity of the event usually causes a fracture of the scapula and ribs as well

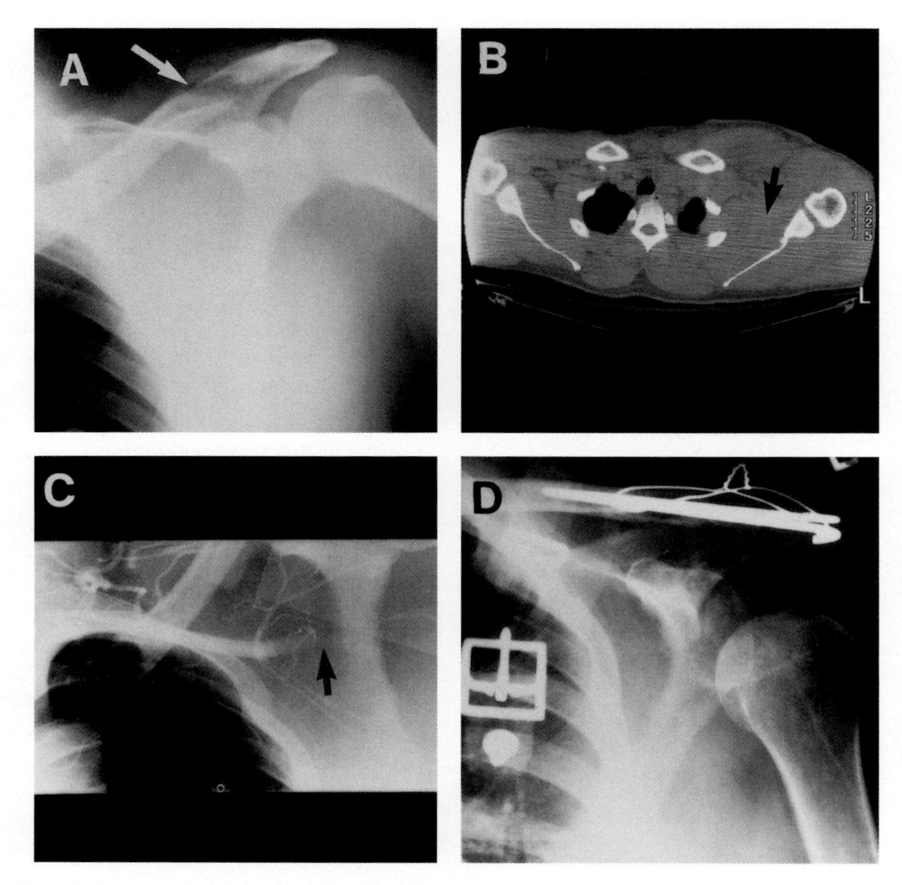

FIG. 47. A patient who sustained a left scapulothoracic dissociation. **(A)** preoperative AP radiograph showing significant lateral displacement of the scapula and a significantly displaced fracture of the distal clavicle; **(B)** CT image showing significantly increased distance between the left scapula and the rib cage as compared with the opposite (uninjured) side; **(C)** arteriogram showing disruption of the subclavian artery; **(D)** postoperative AP radiograph showing reduction and stabilization of the distal clavicle fracture (and secondarily the scapulothoracic articulation) by means of a tension band construct.

as marked disruption of the periscapular soft tissues.[83] The diagnosis may be missed initially because of associated injuries and/or inadequate radiographic projections. Displacement of the scapula may not be readily apparent on routine AP chest radiographs. Tangential views (anterior oblique or lateral scapular projections[125]) or a chest CT may be necessary to establish the diagnosis.

Acute injuries are reduced in a closed fashion under anesthesia by hyperabducting the arm and manually manipulating the scapula (rotating the scapula forward and pushing it backward[26]) while steady traction is applied to the arm. The reduction is usually stable, but securing the scapula to the chest wall with adhesive tape and immobilizing the arm in a sling and swathe are advisable for comfort and soft-tissue healing.[83] The dressing and immobilizer are changed at 7 to 10 days and discontinued 2 weeks thereafter. Unprotected and progressive functional use of the shoulder and arm is then permitted and encouraged. In long-standing cases, open reduction, with soft-tissue detachment may be necessary followed by reconstruction of the periscapular tissues to reestablish stability.[125]

COMPLICATIONS

The most significant complications associated with scapular fractures are those that result from accompanying injuries to adjacent and distant osseous and soft-tissue structures. Because of the severe traumatic forces frequently involved, these patients have an average of 3.9 additional injuries, with the most common sites being the ipsilateral shoulder girdle,[74] upper extremity, lung, and chest wall: 25% to 45% of patients have accompanying rib fractures; 15% to 40% have fractures of the clavicle; 15% to 55% have pulmonary injuries[112](hemopneumothorax, pulmonary contusion, etc.) 12% have humeral fractures; and 5% to 10% sustain injuries to the brachial plexus and peripheral nerves.[28,162] Fractures of the skull are found in approximately 25% of patients, cerebral contusions in 10% to 40%, central neurologic deficits in 5%, tibial and fibular fractures in 11%,[58,156,162] major vascular injuries in 11%, and splenic injuries that result in splenectomy in 8%; 2% of these patients die. A variety of other cardiothoracic, genitourinary, and gastrointestinal injuries have been described. Stevens et al. reviewed 173 blunt trauma patients (92 with scapular fractures and 81 controls) and concluded that scapular fractures were not a significant marker for greater mortality or neurovascular morbidity.[158]

Complications related to the scapular fractures themselves are relatively uncommon. Nonunion, although possible, is quite rare. Malunion can occur in a variety of forms, depending on the particular fracture type. Malunion of a scapular body fracture is generally well tolerated; however, painful scapulothoracic crepitus has been described on occasion. Fractures of the glenoid cavity may result in symptomatic glenohumeral degenerative joint disease. Shoulder instability can occur following significantly displaced fractures of the glenoid neck (angulatory displacement) and fractures of the glenoid rim. Fractures of the glenoid neck with significant translational displacement may give rise to glenohumeral pain and dysfunction related to altered mechanics of the surrounding soft tissues.

Various complications associated with surgical management are possible; for example, infection (both superficial and deep), intraoperative neurovascular injury, loss of fixation owing to poor surgical technique, etc. A poorly supervised postoperative physiotherapy–rehabilitation program may lead to unnecessary postoperative shoulder stiffness.

Finally, complications related to poor patient compliance may occur. Examples would include suboptimal shoulder range of motion caused by unwillingness to follow the postoperative physiotherapy program, hardware failure associated with failure to observe postoperative instructions, etc.

REFERENCES

1. Ada JR, Miller ME. Scapular fractures-analysis of 113 cases. *Clin Orthop* 1991;269:174.
2. Ainscow DA. Dislocation of the scapula. *J Coll Surg Edinb* 1982;27: 56.
3. An HS, Vonderbrink JP, Ebraheim NA, Shipple F, Jackson WT. Open scapulothoracic dissociation with intact neurovascular status in a child. *J Orthop Trauma* 1988;2:36.
4. Arenas AJ, Pampligea T. An unusual kind of fracture. *Acta Orthop Belg* 1993;59:398.
5. Armstrong CP, Vanderspuy J. The fractured scapula: importance in management based on a series of 62 patients. *Injury* 1984;15:324.
6. Aston JW Jr, Gregory CF. Dislocation of the shoulder with significant fracture of the glenoid. *J Bone Joint Surg [Am]* 1973;55:1531.
7. Aulicino PL, Reinert C, Kornberg M, et al. Displaced intraarticular glenoid fractures treated by open reduction and internal fixation. *J Trauma* 1986;26:1137.
8. Baccarani G, Porcellini G, Brunetti E. Fracture of the coracoid process associated with fracture of the clavicle: description of a rare case. *Chir Organi Mov* 1993;78:49.
9. Banerjee AK, Field S. An unusual scapular fracture caused by a water-skiing accident. *Br J Radiol* 1985;58:465.
10. Bateman JE. *The shoulder and neck*, 2nd ed. Philadelphia: WB Saunders, 1978.
11. Bauer G, Fleischmann W, DuBler E. Displaced scapular fractures: indication and long-term results of open reduction and internal fixation. *Arch Orthop Trauma Surg* 1995;114:215.
12. Benchetrit E, Friedman B. Fracture of the coracoid process associated with subglenoid dislocation of the shoulder. *J Bone Joint Surg [Am]* 1979;61:295.
13. Benton J, Nelson C. Avulsion of the coracoid process in an athlete. *J Bone Joint Surg [Am]* 1971;53:356.
14. Bernard TN, Brunet ME, Haddad RJ Jr. Fractured coracoid process in acromioclavicular dislocations. *Clin Orthop* 1983;175:227.
15. Beswick DR, Morse SD, Barnes AU. Bilateral scapular fractures from low voltage electrical injury—a case report. *Ann Emerg Med* 1982;11: 12.
16. Binazzi R, Assiso J, Vaccari V, Felli L. Avulsion fractures of the scapula: report of 8 cases. *J Trauma* 1992;33:785.
17. Boyer DW. Trap shooter's shoulder: stress fracture of the coracoid process. *J Bone Joint Surg [Am]* 1975;57:862.
18. Brower AC, Neff JR, Tillema DA. An unusual scapular stress fracture. *AJR Am J Roentgenol* 1977;129:519.
19. Butters KP. The scapula. In Rockwood CA, Matsen FA, eds. *The shoulder*. Philadelphia: WB Saunders, 1990:335.
20. Cain TE, Hamilton WP. Scapular fractures in professional football players. *Am J Sports Med* 1992;20:363.
21. Combalia A, Arandes JM, Alemany X, Romon R. Acromioclavicular dislocation with epiphyseal separation of the coracoid process: report of a case and review of the literature. *J Trauma* 1995;38:812.
22. Coues WP. Fracture of the coracoid process of the scapula. *N Engl J Med* 212:1935;727.
23. Crenshaw AH. Fractures. In: Crenshaw AH, ed. *Campbell's operative orthopaedics*, 8th ed. St Louis: CV Mosby, 1992.
24. De Rosa GP, Kettelkamp DB. Fracture of the coracoid process of the scapula: a case report. *J Bone Joint Surg [Am]* 1977;59:696.
25. Deltoff MN, Bressler HB. A typical scapular fracture—a case report. *Am J Sports Med* 1989;17:292.
26. DePalma AF. *Surgery of the shoulder*, 3rd ed. Philadelphia: JB Lippincott, 1983.
27. Dumas JL, Walker N. Bilateral scapular fractures secondary to electric shock. *Arch Orthop Trauma Surg* 1992;111:287.
28. Ebraheim NA, An S, Jackson WT, et al. Scapulothoracic dissociation. *J Bone Joint Surg [Am]* 1988;70:428.
29. Ebraheim NA, Pearlstein SR, Savolaine ER, et al. Scapulothoracic dissociation (avulsion of the scapula, subclavian artery, and brachial plexus): an early recognized variant, a new classification, and a review of the literature and treatment options. *J Orthop Trauma* 1987;1:18.
30. Edeland HG, Zachrisson HE. Fracture of the scapular notch associated with lesion of the suprascapular nerve. *Acta Orthop Scand* 1975;46: 758.
31. Eyres KS, Brooks A, Stanley D. Fractures of the coracoid process. *J Bone Joint Surg [Br]* 1995;77:425.
32. Fery A, Sommelet J. Fractures de l'apophyse coracoide. *Rev Chir Orthop* 1979;65:403.
33. Findlay RT. Fractures of the scapula and ribs. *Am J Surg* 1937;38:489.
34. Fischer RP, Flynn TC, Miller PW, et al. Scapular fractures and associated major ipsilateral upper-torso injuries. *Curr Concepts Trauma Care* 1985;1:14.
35. Fischer WR. Fracture of the scapula requiring open reduction: report of a case. *J Bone Joint Surg* 1939;21:459.
36. Froimson AI. Fracture of the coracoid process of the scapula. *J Bone Joint Surg [Am]* 1978;60:710.
37. Fukuda H, Mikasa M, Ogawa K, Isehara B. Ring retractor. *J Bone Joint Surg [Am]* 1982;64:289.
38. Gagney O, Carey JP, Mazas F. Les fractures recentes de l'omoplate a propos de 43 cas. *Rev Chir Orthop* 1984;70:443.
39. Ganz R, Noesberger B. Die behandlung der scapula-frakturen. *Hefte Unfallheilkd* 1975;126:59.
40. Garcia-Elias M, Salo JM. Non-union of a fractured coracoid process after dislocation of the shoulder. *J Bone Joint Surg [Br]* 1985;67:722.
41. Gil JF, Haydar A. Isolated injury of the coracoid process: case report. *J Trauma* 1991;31:1696.
42. Gleich JJ. The fractured scapula, a significance in prognosis. *Mo Med* 1980;77:24.
43. Goldberg RP, Vicks B. Oblique angle to view for coracoid fractures. *Skeletal Radiol* 1983;9:195.
44. Gordes W, Hessert GR. Seltene verletzungsfolgen an der spina scapulae. *Arch Orthop Unfall-Chir* 1970;68:315.
45. Goss TP. Double disruptions of the superior shoulder complex. *J Orthop Trauma* 1993;7:99.
46. Goss TP. Fractures of the glenoid cavity. *Orthop Consult* 1992;13:9.
47. Goss TP. Fractures of the glenoid cavity. Video J Orthopedics VII(6): 1992 and AAOS Physician Videotape Library.
48. Goss TP. Fractures of the glenoid cavity: current concepts review. *J Bone Joint Surg [Am]* 1992;74:299.

49. Goss TP. Fractures of the glenoid cavity (operative principles and techniques). *Tech Orthop* 1994;8(3):199.
50. Goss TP. Fractures of the glenoid neck. *J Shoulder Elbow Surg* 1994; 3:42.
51. Goss TP. Glenoid fractures—open reduction and internal fixation. In: Wiss DA, ed. *Master techniques in orthopaedic surgery: fractures* (In press).
52. Goss TP. Scapular fractures and dislocation: diagnosis and treatment. *J Am Acad Orthop Surg* 1995;3:22.
53. Goss TP. Shoulder trauma—bone. In: *Orthopaedic knowledge update 5*, American Academy of Orthopaedic Surgeons, 1996:222.
54. Goss TP. The scapula: coracoid, acromial and avulsion fractures. *Am J Orthop* 1996;25:106.
55. Goss TP, Busconi BD. Scapula fractures: Surgical Principles and Treatment. In: Fu FH, Ticker JB, Imhoff AB, eds. *An atlas of shoulder surgery*. London: Martin Funitz, 1998.
56. Guttentag IJ, Rechtine GR. Fractures of the scapula. A review of the literature. *Orthop Rev* 1988;17:147.
57. Hak DJ, Johnson EE. Avulsion fracture of the coracoid associated with acromioclavicular dissociation. *J Orthop Trauma* 1993;7:381.
58. Halpern AA, Joseph R, Page J, et al. Subclavian artery injury and fracture of the scapula. *J Am Coll Emerg Physicians* 1979;8:19.
59. Hardegger FH, Simpson LA, Weber BG. The operative treatment of scapular fractures. *J Bone Joint Surg [Br]* 1984;66:725.
60. Harmon PH, Baker DR. Fracture of the scapula with displacement. *J Bone Joint Surg* 1943;25:834.
61. Harris RD, Harris JH. The prevalence and significance of missed scapular fractures in blunt chest trauma. *Am Roent Ray Soc* 1988;151: 747.
62. Hayes J, Zehr D. Traumatic muscle avulsion causing winging of the scapula. *J Bone Joint Surg [Am]* 1981;68:495.
63. Heatly MD, Breck LW, Higinbotham NL. Bilateral fracture of the scapula. *Am J Surg* 1946;71:256.
64. Henneking K, Hofmann D, Kunze K. Skapulafrakturen nach electrounfall. *Unfallchirurgie* 1984;10:149.
65. Herscovici D. Correspondence. *J Bone Joint Surg [Am]* 1994;76: 1112.
66. Herscovici D. Fractures of the clavicle and scapular neck. Correspondence. *J Bone Joint Surg [Br]* 1993;75:509.
67. Herscovici D Jr, Fiennes AGTW, Ruedi TP. The floating shoulder: ipsilateral clavicle and scapular neck fractures. *J Orthop Trauma* 1992; 6:499.
68. Heyse-Moore GH, Stoker DJ. Avulsion fractures of the scapula. *Skeletal Radiol* 1982;9:27.
69. Hollinshead R, James KW. Scapulothoracic dislocation (locked scapula). *J Bone Joint Surg [Am]* 1979;61:1102.
70. Houghton GR. Avulsion of the cranial margin of the scapula: A report of 2 cases. *Injury* 1980;11:45.
71. Iannotti JP, Wang ED. Avulsion fracture of the supraglenoid tubercle: a variation of the SLAP lesion. *J Shoulder Elbow Surg* 1992;1:26.
72. Ideberg R. Fractures of the scapula involving the glenoid fossa. In: Bateman JE, Welsh RP, eds. *Surgery of the shoulder*. Philadelphia: BC Decker, 1984.
73. Ideberg R. Unusual glenoid fractures: a report on 92 cases [abstr]. *Acta Orthop Scand* 1987;58:191.
74. Ideberg R, Grevsten S, Larsson S. Epidemiology of scapular fractures. *Acta Orthop Scand* 1995;66:395.
75. Imatani RJ. Fractues of the scapula: a review of 53 fractures. *J Trauma* 1975;15:473.
76. Ishizuki M, Yamaura I, Isobe Y, et al. Avulsion fracture of the superior border of the scapula. A report of five cases. *J Bone Joint Surg [Am]* 1981;63:820.
77. Johnansen K, Sangeorzan B, Copass MK. Traumatic scapulothoracic dissociation: a case report. *J Trauma* 1991;31:147.
78. Judet R. Traitement chirurgical des fractures de l'omoplate. *Acta Orthop Belg* 1964;30:673.
79. Kam ACA, Kam PCA. Scapular and proximal humeral head fractures. *Anesthesia* 1994;49:1055.
80. Kavanagh BF, Bradway JK, Cofield RH. Open reduction of displaced intra-articular fractures of the glenoid fossa. *J Bone Joint Surg [Am]* 1993;75:479.
81. Kelbel JM, Hardon OM, Huurman WW. Scapulothoracic dissociation—a case report. *Clin Orthop* 1986;209:210.
82. Kelly JP. Fractures complicating electroconvulsive therapy in chronic epilepsy. *J Bone Joint Surg [Br]* 1954;36:70.
83. Key JA, Conwell HE. *The management of fractures, dislocations and sprains*. St Louis: CV Mosby, 1964.
84. Kopecky KK, Bies JR, Ellis JH. CT diagnosis of fracture of the coracoid process of the scapula. *Comput Radiol* 1984;8:325.
85. Kuhn JE, Blasier RB, Carpenter JE. Fractures of the acromion process: A proposed classification scheme. *J Orthop Trauma* 1994;8:6.
86. Kuhn JE, Blasier RB, Carpenter JE. Letters to the Editor. *J Orthop Trauma* 1994;8:14.
87. Kuhn JE, Blasier RB, Carpenter JE: Letters to the Editor. *J Orthop Trauma* 1994;8:359.
88. Kumar A. Management of coracoid process fracture with acromioclavicular joint dislocation. *Orthopedics* 1990;13:770.
89. Kumar VP, Satku K. Fractures of the clavicle and scapular neck. Correspondence. *J Bone Joint Surg [Br]* 1993;75:509.
90. Kummel BM. Fractures of the glenoid causing chronic dislocation of the shoulder. *Clin Orthop* 1970;69:189.
91. Kurdy NMG, Shah SV. Fracture of the acromion associated with acromioclavicular dislocation. *Injury* 1995;26:636.
92. Laing R, Dee R. Fracture symposium. *Orthop Rev* 1984;13:717.
93. Landi A, Schoenhuber R, Funicello R, Rasio G, Esposito M. Compartment syndrome of the scapula. *Ann Hand Upper Limb Surg* 1992; 11:383.
94. Lang RH, Noel SH. Traumatic lateral scapular displacement: an expanded spectrum of associated neurovascular injury. *J Orthop Trauma* 1993;7:361.
95. Lasda NA, Murray DG. Fracture separation of the coracoid process associated with acromioclavicular dislocation. *Clin Orthop* 1978;134: 222.
96. Leung K, Lam T. Correspondence. *J Bone Joint Surg [Am]* 1994;76: 1112.
97. Leung KS, Lam TP. Open reduction and internal fixation of ipsilateral fractures of the scapular neck and clavicle. *J Bone Joint Surg [Am]* 1993;75:1015.
98. Leung KS, Lam TB, Poon KM. Operative treatment of displaced intra-articular glenoid fractures. *Injury* 1993;24:324.
99. Lindblom A, Leven H. Prognosis and fractures of the body and neck of the scapula. *Acta Surg Chir Scand* 1994;140:33.
100. Longabaugh RI. Fracture simple, right scapula. *US Naval Med Bull* 1924;27:341.
101. Madhaven P, Buckingham R, Stableforth PG. Avulsion injury of the subscapularis tendon associated with fracture of the acromion. *Injury* 1994;25:271.
102. Magerl F. Osteosynthesen in bereich der schulter: pertuberkulare humerusfracturen. Scapulahalsfrakturen. *Helv Chir Acta* 1974;41: 225.
103. Mariani PP. Isolated fracture of the coracoid process in an athlete. *Am J Sports Med* 1980;8:129.
104. Martin SD, Weiland AJ. Missed scapular fracture after trauma. *Clin Orthop* 1994;299:259.
105. Martin-Herrero T, Rodriguez-Merchan C, Munuera-Martinez L. Fractures of the coracoid process: presentation of 7 cases and review of the literature. *J Trauma* 1990;30:1597.
106. Mathews RE, Cocke TB, D'Ambrosia RD. Scapular fractures secondary to seizures in patients with osteodystrophy. *J Bone Joint Surg [Am]* 1983;65:850.
107. McCally WC, Kelly DA. Treatment of fractures of the clavicle, ribs and scapula. *Am J Surg* 1940;50:558.
108. McGahan JP, Rab GT. Fracture of the acromion associated with axillary nerve deficit. *Clin Orthop* 1980;147:216.
109. McGahan JP, Rab GT, Dublin A. Fractures of the scapula. *J Trauma* 1980;20:880.
110. McGinnis M, Denton JR. Fractures of the scapula: a retrospective study of 40 fractured scapulae. *J Trauma* 1989;29:1488.
111. McLaughlin HL. *Trauma*. Philadelphia: WB Saunders, 1959.
112. McLellan JG, Ungersma J. Pneumothorax complicating fractures of the scapula. *J Bone Joint Surg [Am]* 1982;64:598.
113. Mencke JB. The frequency and significance of injuries to the acromion process. *Ann Surg* 1914;59:233.
114. Mick CA, Weiland AJ. Pseudarthrosis of a fracture of the acromion. *J Trauma* 1983;23:248.
115. Miller ME. Letters to the Editor. *J Orthop Trauma* 1994;8:14.
116. Miller ME, Ada JR. Injuries to the shoulder girdle. In: *Skeletal trauma*. Philadelphia: WB Saunders, 1992:1291.
117. Moneim MS, Balduini FC. Coracoid fractures—a complication of sur-

gical treatment by coraclavicular tape fixation. A case report. *Clin Orthop* 1982;168:133.
118. Montgomery SP, Loyd RD. Avulsion fracture of the coracoid epiphysis with acromioclavicular separation. *J Bone Joint Surg* 1977;59:963.
119. Moseley HF. *Shoulder lesions*, 2nd ed. New York: Paul Hoeber, 1953.
120. Mugikura S, Hirayama T, Tada H, et al. Avulsion fracture of the scapular spine: a case report. *J Shoulder Elbow Surg* 1993;2:39.
121. Nagi ON, Dhillon MS. Traumatic scapulothoracic dissociation. *Arch Orthop Trauma Surg* 1992;111:348.
122. Neer CS. Fractures of the distal third of the clavicle. *Clin Orthop* 1968;58:43.
123. Neer CS II, ed. *Shoulder reconstruction*. Philadelphia: WB Saunders, 1990.
124. Neer CS, Rockwood CA. Fractures and dislocations of the shoulder. In: Rockwood CA, Green DP, eds. *Fractures in adults*, 2nd ed. Philadelphia: JB Lippincott, 1984.
125. Nettrour LF, Krufty LE, Mueller RE, et al. Locked scapula: intrathoracic dislocation of the inferior angle. *J Bone Joint Surg [Am]* 1972;54:413.
126. Neviaser J. Traumatic lesions: injuries in and about the shoulder joint. *Am Acad Orthop Surg Instr Course Lect* 1956;13:187.
127. Newell ED. Review of over 2,000 fractures in the past seven years. *South Med J* 1927;20:644.
128. Niggebrugge AHP, van Heusden HA, Bode PJ, van Vugt AB. Dislocated intra-articular fracture of the anterior rim of glenoid treated by open reduction and internal fixation. *Injury* 1993;24:130.
129. Nordqvist A, Petersson C. Fracture of the body, neck or spine of the scapula. *Clin Orthop* 1992;283:139.
130. Norris TR. Fractures and dislocations of the glenohumeral complex. In: Chapman M, ed. *Operative orthopedics*. Philadelphia: JB Lippincott, 1988.
131. Nunley RL, Bedini SJ. Paralysis of the shoulder subsequent to comminuted fracture of the scapula: rationale and treatment methods. *Phys Ther Rev* 1960;40:442.
132. Oreck SL, Burgess A, Levine AM. Traumatic lateral displacement of the scapula: a radiologic sign of neurovascular disruption. *J Bone Joint Surg [Am]* 1984;66:758.
133. Parkes JC, Deland JB. A 3 part distal clavicle fracture. *J Trauma* 1983;23:437.
134. Peraino RA, Weinman EJ, Schloeder FX. Unusual fractures during convulsions in two patients with renal osteodystrophy. *S Med J* 1977;70:595.
135. Post M. *The shoulder: surgical and non-surgical management*, 2nd ed. Philadelphia: Lea & Febiger, 1988.
136. Protiss JJ, Stampfli FW, Osmer JC. Coracoid process fracture diagnosis in acromioclavicular separation. *Radiology* 1975;116:61.
137. Ramin JE, Veit H. Fracture of the scapula during electroshock therapy. *Am J Psychiatry* 1953;110:153.
138. Rao KG. Correspondence. *Br J Radiol* 1985;58:1057.
139. Rask MR, Steinberg LH. Fracture of the acromion caused by muscle forces. *J Bone Joint Surg [Am]* 1978;60:1146.
140. Rikli B, Regazzoni P, Renner N. The unstable shoulder girdle: early functional treatment utilizing open reduction and internal fixation. *J Orthop Trauma* 1995;9:93.
141. Rockwood CA. Management of fractures of the scapula. *J Bone Joint Surg* 1986;10:219.
142. Rockwood CA Jr, Matsen FA III. *The shoulder*. Philadelphia: WB Saunders, 1990.
143. Rounds RC. Isolated fracture of the coracoid process. *J Bone Joint Surg [Am]* 1949;31:662.
144. Rowe CR. Fractures of the scapula. *Surg Clin North Am* 1963;43:1565.
145. Rowe CR, ed. *The shoulder*. New York: Churchill Livingstone, 1988.
146. Rubenstein JD, Abraheim NA, Kellam JF. Traumatic scapulothoracic dissociation. *Radiology* 1985;157:297.
147. Ruedi T, Chapman MW. Fractures of the scapula and clavicle. In: Chapman M, ed. *Operative orthopedics*. Philadelphia: JB Lippincott, 1988.
148. Rush LV: Fracture of the coracoid process of the scapula. *Ann Surg* 1929;90:1113.
149. Sandrock AR. Another sports fatigue fracture: stress fracture of the coracoid process of the scapula. *Radiology* 1975;117:274.
150. Scudder CL, ed. *The treatment of fractures*, 4th ed. Philadelphia: WB Saunders, 1904.
151. Simon JP, VanDelm I, Fabry G. Comminuted fracture of the scapula following electric shock. A case report. *Acta Orthop Belg* 1991;57:459.
152. Sinha J, Miller AJ. Fixation of fractures of the glenoid rim. *Injury* 1992;23:418.
153. Smith DM. Coracoid fracture associated with acromioclavicular dislocation. A case report. *Clin Orthop* 1975;108:165.
154. Solheim LF, Roaas A. Compression of the suprascapular nerve after fracture of the scapular notch. *Acta Orthop Scand* 1978;49:338.
155. Soslowsky LJ, Flatow EL, Bigliani LU, Mow DC. Articular geometry of the glenohumeral joint. *Clin Orthop* 1992;285:181.
156. Stein RE, Bono J, Korn J, et al. Axillary artery injury in closed fracture of the neck of the scapula—a case report. *J Trauma* 1971;11:528.
157. Steindler A. *Traumatic deformities and disabilities of the upper extremity*. Springfield, IL: Charles C Thomas, 1946.
158. Stephens NG, Morgan AS, Corvo P, Bernstein BA. Significance of scapular fracture in the blunt trauma patient. *Ann Emerg Med* 1995;26:439.
159. Tarquinio T, Weinstein ME, Virgilio RW. Bilateral scapular fractures from accidental electric shock. *J Trauma* 1979;19:132.
160. Taylor J. Letters to the Editor. *J Orthop Trauma* 1994;8:359.
161. Thompson DA, Flynn TC, Miller PW, et al. The significance of scapular fractures. *J Trauma* 1985;25:974.
162. Tomaszek DE. Combined subclavian artery and brachial plexus injuries from blunt upper-extremity trauma. *J Trauma* 1984;24:161.
163. Tscherne H, Christ M. Konservative und operative therapie der schulterblattbruche. *Hefte Unhallheikd* 1975;126:52.
164. Tuzner S, Yanat AN, Urguden M, Ozkaynak C. Scapulothoracic dissociation: a case report. *Isr J Med Sci* 1995;32:70.
165. Uhl RL, Hospeder PP. Progressive scapulothoracic subluxation after fracture of the clavicle. *Am J Orthop* 1996;25:637.
166. Varriale PL, Adler ML. Occult fracture of the glenoid without dislocation. *J Bone Joint Surg [Am]* 1983;65:688.
167. Wang K, Hsu K, Shih C. Coracoid process fracture combined with acromioclavicular dislocation and coracoclavicular ligament rupture. *Clin Orthop* 1994;300:120.
168. Warner J, Port J. Stress fracture of the acromion. *J Shoulder Elbow Surg* 1994;3:262.
169. Wertheimer C, Mogan J. Bilateral scapular fractures during a seizure in a patient following subtotal parathyroidectomy. *Orthopedics* 1990;13:656.
170. Wilbur MC, Evans EB. Fractures of the scapula. An analysis of forty cases and a review of the literature. *J Bone Joint Surg [Am]* 1977;59:358.
171. Williamson DW, Wilson-MacDonald JW. Bilateral avulsion fractures of the cranial margin of the scapula. *J Trauma* 1988;28:713.
172. Wilson PD. *Experience in the management of fractures and dislocations (based on an analysis of 4390 cases) by the staff of the Fracture Service MGH, Boston*. Philadelphia: JB Lippincott, 1938.
173. Wolfe AW, Shoji H, Chuinard RG. Unusual fracture of the coracoid process. Case report and review of the literature. *J Bone Joint Surg [Am]* 1976;58:423.
174. Wong-Chung J, Quinlan W. Fractured coracoid process preventing closed reduction of anterior dislocation of the shoulder. *Injury* 1989;20:296.
175. Wong-Pack WK, Bobechko PE, Becker EJ. Fractured coracoid with anterior shoulder dislocation. *J Can Assoc Radiol* 1980;31:228.
176. Wyrsch RB, Spindler KP, Stricker BR. Scapular fracture in a professional boxer. *J Shoulder Elbow Surg* 1995;4:395.
177. Zdravkovic D, Damholt VV. Comminuted and severely displaced fractures of the scapula. *Acta Orthop Scand* 1974;45:60.
178. Zettas JP, Muchnic PD. Fracture of the coracoid process base and acute acromioclavicular separation. *Orthop Rev* 1976;5:77.
179. Zilberman Z, Rejovitzky R. Fracture of the coracoid process of the scapula. *Injury* 1982;13:203.
180. Zuckerman JD, Koval KJ, Cuomo F. Fractures of the scapula, In: Hedman JD, ed. *Instructional Course Lectures* 42. Rosemont, IL: American Academy of Orthopaedic Surgeons, 1993.

Disorders of the Shoulder: Diagnosis and Management,
edited by Joseph P. Iannotti and Gerald R. Williams, Jr.
Lippincott Williams & Wilkins, Philadelphia © 1999.

CHAPTER 24

Fractures of the Proximal Humerus: Diagnosis and Management

Joseph D. Zuckerman and Anthony J. Checroun

ANATOMY

Development

In the newborn infant, the spherical proximal humeral epiphysis contains the primary ossification center and the two secondary centers that will form the greater and lesser tuberosities. The primary ossification center appears within 4 to 6 months of birth, the greater tuberosity at approximately 3 years, and the lesser tuberosity by 5 years. These coalesce between 4 and 7 years and fuse to the shaft between 17 and 20 years, with earlier physeal closure in girls than in boys[1–3] (Fig. 1).

The physeal plate of the proximal humerus is concave inferiorly and almost spherical, with its apex posterior and medial to its center. This asymmetrical metaphyseal dome

J. D. Zuckerman and A. J. Checroun: New York University Hospital for Joint Diseases, 301 East 17th Street, New York, New York 10003.

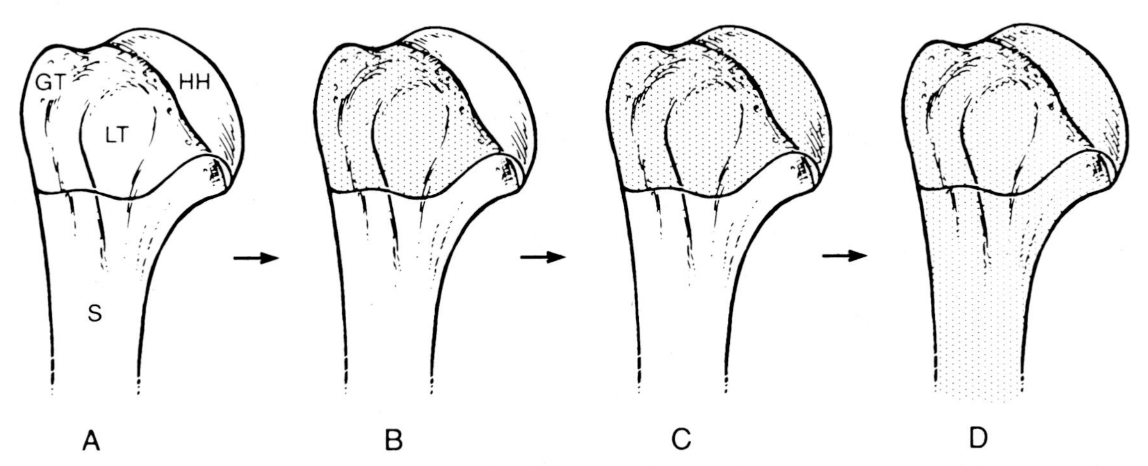

FIG. 1. (A) The humeral head (*HH*) ossification center appears at 4 to 6 months of age, the greater tuberosity (*GT*) at 1 to 3 years of age, the lesser tuberosity (*LT*) at 3 to 5 years of age. **(B)** Coalescence of the GT with the LT occurs at approximately 3 years of age; **(C)** coalescence of the primary ossification center (*HH*) with the greater tuberosity and lesser tuberosity between 4 and 7 years of age; and **(D)** fusion to the shaft between 17 and 20 years of age.

and the strong thick attachment of periosteum along the posterior surface explain why anterior, rather than posterior, displacement of the metaphysis occurs in fractures[2] (Fig. 2). Dameron et al. demonstrated, in stillborn infants, that the metaphysis could easily be displaced anteriorly at the epiphyseal plate with the humerus extended and adducted; yet posterior displacement was difficult to achieve.[2] Approximately 80% of humeral growth occurs at the proximal physis, giving this region great remodeling potential following fracture.[52]

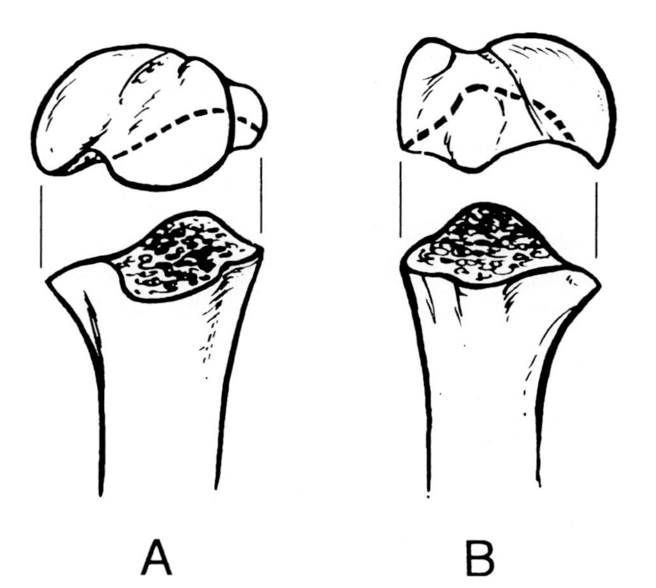

FIG. 2. (A) Lateral and **(B)** anteroposterior view of the proximal humerus, demonstrating the asymmetrical physeal plate and metaphyseal dome with an apex posterior and medial to its center.

Vascular and Neurologic Anatomy

The proximity of the nerves of the brachial plexus and vascular structures to the proximal humerus put them at risk of injury from proximal humerus fractures and dislocations, as well as during surgical approaches.

Vascular Anatomy

The rich vascular anatomy of the proximal humerus has been further delineated in the recent literature to help explain osteonecrosis of the humeral head. Laing's[4] and Gerber's[5] studies showed that the anterior lateral branch of the anterior humeral circumflex artery is the primary blood supply to the proximal humerus. The anterior humeral circumflex artery arises from the lateral side of the third division of the axillary artery approximately 1 cm distal to the inferior border of the pectoralis minor muscle (just above the teres major muscle) and courses laterally behind the coracobrachialis to reach the surgical neck of the humerus at the lower border of the subscapularis.[5–7] The anterolateral branch sends twigs to the lesser tuberosity, crosses under the biceps tendon, and then arches superiorly adjacent to the lateral side of the intertubercular groove. The vessel then penetrates bone at the cephalad portion of the transition from greater tuberosity to intertubercular groove, staying distal to the position of the old epiphysial plate. The intraosseous portion of this artery has been named the arcuate artery by Laing because of its posteromedial course after entering the humeral head. Multiple branches radiate to supply the subchondral bone of the humeral head[7](Fig. 3).

The importance of both the extra- and intraosseous arterial anastomoses has recently been described. Laing noted abundant *extraosseous* anastomoses between the anterior humeral circumflex artery and posterior humeral circumflex arteries,

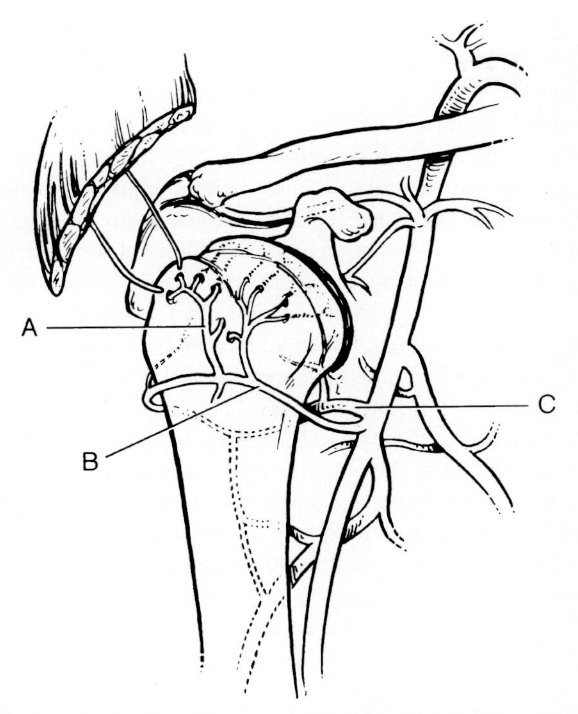

FIG. 3. The rich vascular anatomy of the proximal humerus: *(A)* The anterior lateral branch of *(B)* the anterior humeral circumflex artery is the primary blood supply. *(C)* The posterior humeral circumflex artery arises close to the anterior humeral circumflex and gives off posterior medial branches to help supply the head.

as well as with the thoracoacromial, subscapular, suprascapular, and profunda brachii arteries.[4] The anterior and posterior circumflex vessels connect with the profunda brachii artery through ascending deltoid vessels. Anastomosis of the profunda brachii artery occurs with the radial (anterior) and medial (posterior) collaterals. This rich collateral circulation about the shoulder can provide adequate circulation to maintain viability of the extremity despite axillary artery disruption after, for example, a dislocation.[8] Gerber also identified abundant extraosseous anastomoses; however, vascularization of the entire humeral head was possible only through the anterior lateral branch of the anterior humeral circumflex artery. Laing noted inconsistent contributions to the humeral head from both the lesser and greater tuberosities.[4] Gerber could not confirm that vessels of the rotator cuff directly vascularized the underlying bone.[5] The posterior humeral circumflex artery arises closely juxtaposed to the anterior humeral circumflex artery and is much larger in diameter.[6] Gerber found that the posteromedial vessels arising from the posterior humeral circumflex artery supplied the posterior portion of the greater tuberosity and a small posterior inferior part of the head. The vessels then formed an anastomosis to the arcuate artery on and within the greater tuberosity and on the joint capsule.[5] Brookes demonstrated that these posteromedial vessels pass beneath the humeral capsular attachment (which at this site extends from 1 cm onto the surgical neck), and run toward the humeral head before entering the bone just below the articular margin.[7]

The study by Brookes et al. emphasized the importance of the *intraosseous* anastomoses and, unlike Gerber's study, showed that the humeral head could be completely profused after ligation of the anterior humeral circumflex artery at its entry site into the humeral head. They found large metaphyseal arteries that passed through the fused growth plate to anastomose with the arcuate artery in six of the eight normal and control specimens. In addition, significant intraosseous anastomoses occurred between the arcuate artery and the posterior humeral circumflex artery through the posteromedial vessels described in the foregoing and the vessels of the greater and lesser tuberosities.[7]

Knowledge of the vascular anatomy may help predict osteonecrosis of the humeral head. Gerber highlighted the clinical relevance of the *intraosseous* anastomosis in a case report of a shoulder dislocation with both circumflex arteries interrupted and the extraosseous network compromised. Osteonecrosis did not develop in this patient, suggesting that the intraosseous anastomoses are important.[9] A *classic four-part* fracture will lose the blood supply to the head from disruption of the anterior humeral circumflex artery, greater and lesser tuberosities, and any metaphyseal arterial anastomosis. Thus, a high rate of osteonecrosis is expected.[10] Yet, Brookes has shown that profusion of the humeral head by the arcuate artery may continue if the head fragment includes part of the medial aspect of the upper part of the neck where the posteromedial arteries enter.[7] The so called *four-part valgus impacted fracture* with little lateral displacement of the head fragment may retain its vascularity from the posterior medial vessels, thus accounting for the lower incidence of osteonecrosis reported compared with classic four-part fractures.[11] The vascular anatomy also supports the observation that minimally displaced fractures of the anatomic neck, in which the fracture line is at the junction between the articular surface and neck, may be complicated by osteonecrosis as a result of disruption of both the extra- and intraosseous blood supply.[9]

Knowledge of the extensive collateral circulation around the shoulder helps explain the mechanism whereby the viability of the upper extremity can be maintained despite disruption of the axillary artery.

Muscles and Nerves

The proximal humerus is composed of the lesser tuberosity, which is the site of insertion of the subscapularis; the greater tuberosity, which has three facets for insertion of the supraspinatus, infraspinatus, and teres minor; the humeral head; and the shaft. The bicipital groove, a useful surgical landmark, is located between the tuberosities and contains the tendon of the long head of the biceps. The anatomic neck is at the junction of the articular margin of the humeral head and tuberosities, and the surgical neck is the area below the greater and lesser tuberosities.[6,15]

The important muscles and their innervations about the proximal humerus include the subscapularis muscle that arises from the medial two-thirds of the costal surface of the scapula. It is innervated on its costal surface by the upper and lower subscapular nerves. The supraspinatus muscle arises from the medial two-thirds of the bony walls of the supraspinatus fossa of the scapula, and from the dense fascia that covers the muscle. It is innervated from its underside by the suprascapular nerve. This nerve is relatively fixed at its origin from the superior trunk of the brachial plexus and where it passes under the superior transverse scapular ligament. Although rare, a traction injury can occur. The infraspinatus muscle takes its origin from the infraspinatus fossa of the scapula (except its lateral fourth) and from the dense overlying infraspinatus fascia. The suprascapular nerve passes through the notch of the scapular neck and under the inferior transverse scapular ligament to enter the upper part of the infraspinatus muscle.[6]

The teres minor arises from the upper two-thirds of the lateral border of the scapula and from adjacent intermuscular septa. The deltoid takes origin from the lateral third of the clavicle, the anterior and lateral border of the acromion, and the lower lip of the crest of the spine of the scapula. It inserts into the deltoid tuberosity of the humerus. Both of these muscles are supplied by the axillary nerve that arises from the posterior cord of the brachial plexus. An upper branch curves around the posterior surface of the humerus and courses from behind forward on the deep surface of the muscle, approximately 5 cm distal to the lateral border of the acromion, supplying muscular branches throughout its course. A lower branch supplies the teres minor as it ascends onto its lateral and superficial surface.[6] The axillary nerve is relatively fixed at its origin from the posterior cord and as it enters the deltoid. It also passes in close proximity to the inferior capsule, placing it at risk for a traction injury with downward motion of the proximal humerus, as in a dislocation. In fact, it is the most commonly injured nerve, especially from anterior dislocations.[26] This nerve can also be damaged with surgical approaches that split the deltoid fibers beyond 5 cm from the acromial edge or with percutaneous pins inserted from an inferior starting point.[16,147] The pectoralis major muscle has clavicular, sternocostal, and abdominal origins. It is innervated by both the lateral and medial pectoral nerves.[6]

The conjoined tendon is composed of the coracobrachialis and short head of the biceps brachii muscles, which take origin from the coracoid process. They are supplied by the musculocutaneous nerve, which is a branch of the lateral cord of the brachial plexus. This nerve enters the coracobrachialis muscle medially at a mean of 5.6 cm from the coracoid, but may be as close as 3.1 cm.[17] Therefore, retraction during anterior approaches places this nerve at risk for neuropraxia.[16]

The cords of the brachial plexus surround the axillary artery at the level of the humeral neck. Therefore, neurologic injury can result from fractures in this area. These injuries, though uncommon, are encountered more frequently than vascular injuries. Most commonly, they represent either a contusion or mild traction injury with a good prognosis for spontaneous recovery.[12] Electrophysiologic evidence of nerve injury is found in up to 45% of humeral neck fractures and primary dislocations, most commonly involving the axillary nerve, followed by the suprascapular, radial, and musculocutaneous nerves. Older patients and those with clinical evidence of hematomas have more neurologic injuries.[13] Although the neurologic injury does not have the limb-threatening potential of the vascular injury, long-term disabilities are determined by the brachial plexus injury. Although most patients with low-energy injuries recover partially or completely in less than 4 months,[13] permanent motor loss from brachial plexus injury will result in impairment of hand function. Treatment is focused on preservation of hand function, which is more important than shoulder motion.[14]

Muscle Forces

The attachment site of each muscle and the direction of pull are important determinants of fracture deformity and displacement.

The teres minor, infraspinatus, and supraspinatus muscles insert onto the greater tuberosity epiphysis, as does the subscapularis in the area of the lesser tuberosity. When the epiphysis is separated from the metaphysis as in Salter-Harris type I and II fractures, the muscular forces displace it into a position of flexion, abduction, and slight external rotation. The metaphysis often pierces the periosteum anterolateral to the biceps tendon and is pulled anteriorly and medially by the pectoralis major, which attaches to the metaphysis just below its junction with the physeal plate. It is also pulled proximally by the deltoid. The thick posterior periosteum remains intact[2,6] (Fig. 4). In the adult, Codman noted that after coalescence of the ossification centers and physeal plate, fractures tend to occur along the lines of the old epiphyseal plate scar, with patterns involving four important segments: the greater and lesser tuberosity, articular surface, and humeral shaft[18] (Fig.5).

Neer emphasized the importance of the muscular attachment sites in determining fracture deformity and displacement[19,20] (Fig. 6A). In minimally displaced fractures (one-part), the periosteum, joint capsule, and rotator cuff attachments hold the fracture fragments together.[18] In a displaced surgical neck fracture (two-part), the humeral shaft is displaced forward and medially by the pectoralis major, while the head and attached tuberosities remain in neutral rotation because the rotator cuff is intact and balanced. In displaced fractures of the greater tuberosity (two-part), the supraspinatus and external rotators (infraspinatus and teres

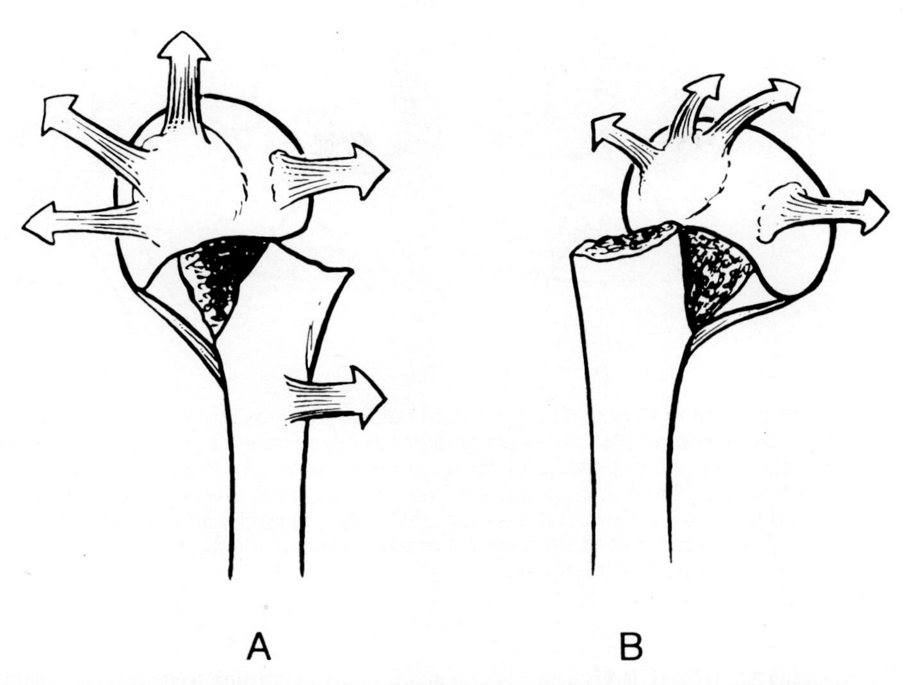

FIG. 4. **(A)** Lateral and **(B)** anteroposterior view of proximal humerus, showing the muscle forces of the rotator cuff displacing the head and tuberosities into flexion abduction and slight external rotation. The metaphysis is pulled anteriorly and medially by the pectoralis major. The thick periosteum remains intact posteromedially.

minor) actively retract fragments of the greater tuberosity superiorly and posteriorly. When a displaced surgical neck component is also present (three-part), unopposed pull of the subscapularis internally rotates the articular segment, causing the articular surface to face posteriorly. This pattern of displacement is accompanied by a longitudinal tear of the rotator cuff (Fig. 6B). Similarly, a lesser tuberosity fracture will be displaced (two-part) medially by the subscapularis muscle. When this is accompanied by a displaced surgical neck fracture (three-part), the unopposed pull of the external rotators causes the articular segment to face anteriorly (Fig. 6C). Similarly, a longitudinal rotator cuff tear also occurs.

If both tuberosities and the surgical neck are displaced (four-part), the greater tuberosity is retracted posteriorly and superiorly by the external rotators; the lesser tuberosity is retracted anteromedially by the subscapularis; and the pectoralis major retracts the shaft medially. The articular segment may be impacted on the upper shaft, displaced laterally, or dislocated anteriorly, posteriorly, or inferiorly. A longitudinal rotator cuff tear occurs between the subscapularis and supraspinatus in the rotator interval area (Fig. 6D).

In general, the deforming forces produced by the attached musculature prevent obtaining or maintaining a satisfactory closed reduction. Ultimately, this will determine fracture treatment.

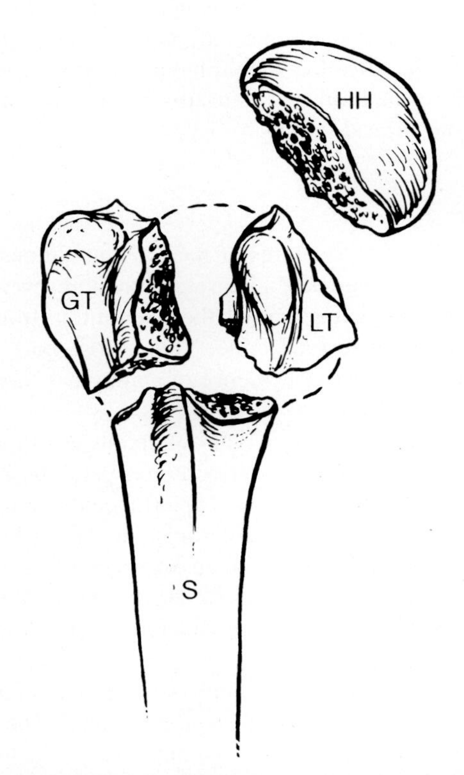

FIG. 5. Proximal humerus fractures tend to occur along the lines of the old epiphyseal plate scar. The four important segments are the greater tuberosity (*GT*), lesser tuberosity (*LT*), articular surface (*HH*), and shaft (*S*).

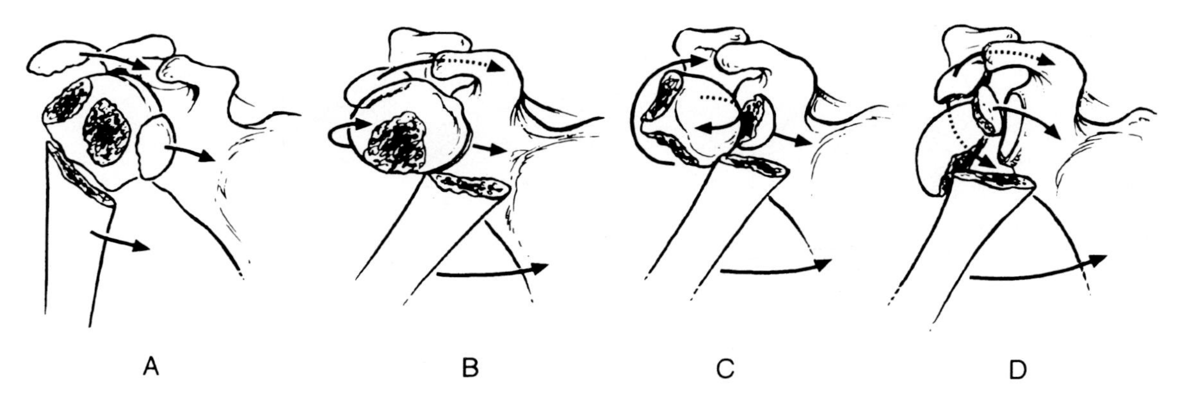

FIG. 6. **(A)** *Arrows* demonstrating muscle forces on each segment of proximal humerus that determine fracture deformity and displacement. **(B)** Three-part greater tuberosity fracture demonstrates internal rotation of the articular segment and superior and posterior displacement of the greater tuberosity. **(C)** Three-part lesser tuberosity fracture demonstrates external rotation of the articular segment such that it faces anteriorly, and medial displacement of the lesser tuberosity. **(D)** Four-part fracture demonstrating posterior and superior displacement of the greater tuberosity, anterior medial retraction of the lesser tuberosity, and medial displacement of the shaft.

CLASSIFICATION OF PROXIMAL HUMERAL FRACTURES

A classification system for proximal humerus fractures should provide a comprehensive means of describing fracture fragment displacement and position, and the presence of dislocation. It should also assist in determining treatment, in predicting long-term clinical outcomes, and in providing an acceptable level of inter- and intraobserver reliability. And finally, the classification should be based on a standard radiographic evaluation that is easily and reproducibly obtained in the clinical setting.

Pediatric

Aitken classified fractures of the proximal humerus into three types. In his series of 11 cases, all fractures were of the first type: a fracture line through the layer of transitional cartilage and newly formed bone. There were no fractures through the epiphysis or evidence of epiphyseal "crush" injuries.[21]

Salter-Harris defined five types of epiphyseal injuries on the basis of radiologic and pathoanatomic patterns. Type I is a separation through the physis. Type II includes a metaphyseal fragment that is always posteromedial. Type III is a separation through the physis, with an extension of the fracture through the epiphysis and articular surface. Type IV is an intraarticular and transmetaphyseal fracture. Type V is physeal crush injury[22] (Fig. 7).

In a more pathophysiological classification, Shapiro classified fractures of the physis as type A, B, or C. The neonatal epiphyseal separation of the proximal part of the humerus is considered a type A fracture (Salter-Harris I or Salter-Harris II), in which the separate epiphyseal and metaphyseal circulation remains intact and the longitudinal growth of the humerus is not arrested.[23] Neer and Horwitz further graded each fracture according to their initial displacement: grade I, less than 5 mm; grade II less than one-third the width of the shaft; grade III up two-thirds of the shaft width; in grade IV displacement exceeds two-thirds of the width.[3]

Adult

History

The classification of proximal humeral fractures has evolved over the last century parallel to our understanding of these injuries. Major milestones in this evolution include Kocher's[24] classification that was based upon the different anatomic levels of fracture: anatomic neck, epiphysial region, and surgical neck. The disadvantages of this simplistic system included the lack of attention to important issues, such as the presence of fractures at multiple levels, the degree of fracture displacement, the presence of dislocation, or the mechanism of injury.

Recognizing that classification systems based solely on the anatomic level of fracture did not provide information about mechanism of injury nor assist in the choice of treatment, Watson-Jones[25] proposed a different classification system. He divided proximal humeral fractures into three types: contusion "crack" fractures, impacted adduction fractures, and impacted abduction fractures. He believed that each type was caused by a specific mechanism of injury and required a specific treatment approach. A major disadvantage of this system was that changes in humeral rotation altered the radiographic appearance of the fracture; specifically, the same fracture patterns could appear as an abduction or adduction type fracture, depending on the rotational position of the humerus when the x-ray film was obtained.[19] In 1934, Codman presented a classification system based on the epiphyseal regions of the proximal humerus.[18] This system identifies four possible fracture fragments: greater tuberos-

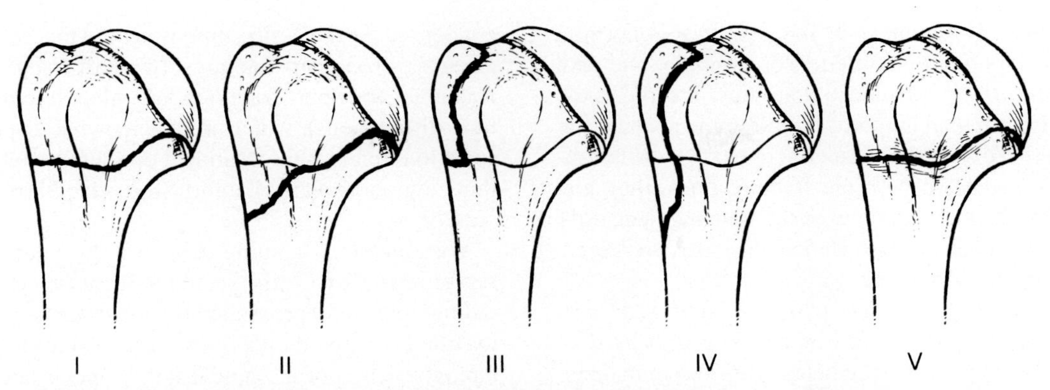

FIG. 7. The Salter-Harris classification of physeal fractures of the proximal humerus (see text).

ity, lesser tuberosity, anatomic head, and shaft. His appreciation that fractures occurred along the lines of the epiphyseal scars formed the basis for Neer's development of his classification system.

Neer Classification

Neer[10,19] proposed his classification of proximal humeral fractures in 1970, and since then it has become the most widely used system in clinical practice[26–31] (Fig. 8). This system is based on the anatomic relations of the four major anatomic segments: articular segment, greater tuberosity, lesser tuberosity, and the proximal shaft, beginning at the level of the surgical neck. Knowledge of the rotator cuff insertions and the effects of the muscular-deforming forces on the four segments is essential to understanding this classification system. Fracture types are based on the presence of displacement of one or more of the four segments. For a segment to be considered displaced, it must be either displaced more than 1 cm or angulated more than 45 degrees from its

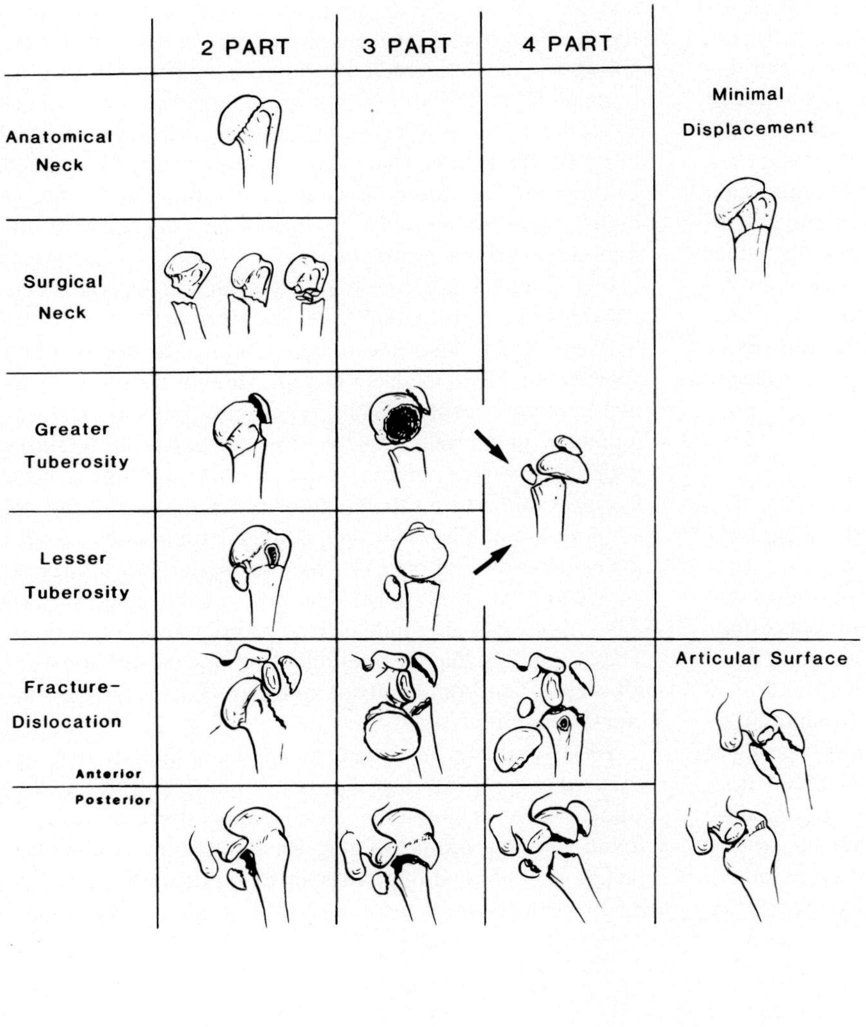

2 PART
3 PART
4 PART
Minimal Displacement
Anatomical Neck
Surgical Neck
Greater Tuberosity
Lesser Tuberosity
Fracture-Dislocation
Anterior
Posterior
Articular Surface

FIG. 8. The Neer classification of proximal humeral fractures (see text).

anatomic position. The number of fracture lines is not important in this classification system. For example, one-part fractures, or minimally displaced fractures, are the most common type of proximal humerus fractures and account for up to 85% of all proximal humerus fractures.[32–34] Although these fractures may have multiple fracture lines, they are characterized by the fact that none of the four segments fulfill the criteria for displacement. Hence, they are considered one part or minimally displaced.

Displaced fractures include two-part, three-part, and four-part fractures. A two-part fracture is characterized by displacement of one of the four segments, with the remaining three segments either not fractured or not fulfilling the criteria for displacement. Four types of two-part fractures can be encountered (greater tuberosity, lesser tuberosity, anatomic neck, and surgical neck). A three-part fracture is characterized by displacement of two of the segments from the remaining two nondisplaced segments. Two types of three-part fracture patterns are encountered. The more common pattern is characterized by displacement of the greater tuberosity and the shaft, with the lesser tuberosity remaining with the articular segment. The much less commonly encountered pattern is characterized by displacement of the lesser tuberosity and shaft, with the greater tuberosity remaining with the articular segment. A four-part fracture is characterized by displacement of all four segments.

Neer also categorized fracture–dislocations, which are displaced proximal humerus fractures: two-part, three-part, or four-part, associated with either anterior or posterior dislocation of the articular segment. Therefore, six types of these fracture dislocation patterns can occur. Neer also described articular surface fractures that were of two types: impression fractures or head-splitting fractures. Impression fractures of the articular surface most often occur in association with chronic dislocations. As such, they can be either anterior or posterior and involve variable amounts of articular surface.[26] Head-splitting fractures are usually associated with other displaced fractures of the proximal humerus in which the disruption or "splitting" of the articular surface is the most significant component.

Reliability of Neer Classification

As noted, the Neer classification is the most widely used classification system for proximal humerus fractures.[10,19,29,30] Recently, there have been several studies that have examined the reliability of the Neer classification.[31,35–40]

Among four observers of varying expertise who evaluated a series of 100 proximal humerus fractures, Kristiansen et al.[35] found a low level of interobserver reliability using a condensed Neer classification system. The level of expertise was noted to be an important factor on predicting interobserver reliability. However, this study was limited by various factors. First, a complete trauma series was not used; rather, only AP and lateral radiographs were examined. Second, a condensed Neer classification was used that consisted of five categories (one-part fractures, two-part fractures, three-part fractures, four-part fractures, all other fractures and fracture–dislocations), which were somewhat disparate with respect to fracture type, treatment options, and prognosis. And third, intraobserver reliability (reproducibility) was not assessed.

We conducted a study to assess the inter- and intraobserver reliability of the Neer classification system using the radiographs of 50 proximal humerus fractures.[31] Good quality trauma series radiographs were available for each fracture, consisting of a scapular AP, scapular lateral, and axillary view. The radiographs were reviewed by an orthopedic shoulder specialist, an orthopedic traumatologist, a skeletal radiologist, an orthopedic resident in the fifth year of training, and an orthopedic resident in the second year of training. The radiographs were reviewed on two different occasions 6 months apart. Interobserver reliability was assessed by comparing the fracture classification determined by the five observers. Intraobserver reliability was assessed by comparing the fracture classification determined by each observer for the first and second reviews. Kappa-reliability coefficients were used to adjust the observed proportion of agreement between or among observers by correcting for the proportion of agreement that could have occurred by chance.

All five observers agreed on the final classification in 32% and 30% of cases for the first and second viewings, respectively. Paired comparisons between the five observers showed a mean corrected reliability coefficient of 0.50 (range 0.37 to 0.62) for both testings, which corresponds to a "moderate" level of reliability. An excellent level of reliability (kappa greater than 0.81) was not obtained for paired evaluation. Attending physicians demonstrated slightly higher interobserver reliability than orthopedic residents. Intraobserver reliability ranged from 0.83 (shoulder specialist) to 0.50 (skeletal radiologist) with a mean of 0.65, which corresponds to a "substantial" level of agreement.

Brien et al.[37] also questioned whether the use of plain films is reliable in the Neer classification of complex proximal humerus fractures. They found only fair intraobserver reliability in a 5-year retrospective analysis of 28 fractures with kappa values ranging from 0.37 to 1.00. Surgical neck fractures faired better than tuberosity fractures. The authors admit to basing diagnosis on incomplete trauma series, with inclusion criteria of only two roentgenograms at 90-degree angles to each other (rather than the preferred three views). Also, there was no standardized radiographic procedure. They suggested that the addition of routine conventional radiographs and computed tomography (CT) scan may increase reliability.

The hypothesis that a better-imaging technique may increase the reproducibility of proximal humerus fracture classification was explored by several authors. Bernstein et al.[38] found findings similar to ours for intraobserver reliability (kappa = 0.64) and interobserver reproducibility (kappa = 0.52) when fractures were classified on the basis of radiographs alone. When CT scans were added to plain radiographs, intraobserver reliability increased slightly (kappa = 0.72), but interobserver reproducibility did not improve (kappa = 0.50). They concluded that because even the shoulder experts had difficulty agreeing on which fragments were fractured, new-imaging modalities rather than a new classification system may need to be developed.

Sjoden et al.[39] investigated 26 proximal humerus fractures with both plain radiographs and CT. Similar to Bernstein, they found that CT scan together with plain radiographs did not make fracture classification more consistent. Sallay et al.[40] conducted a study for which two groups of observers (experts and nonexperts in shoulder surgery) reviewed the plain radiographs and the three-dimensional CT scans of 12 patients with proximal humerus fractures. Both groups of observers displayed suboptimal reliability for the identification of displaced fracture fragments. The addition of three-dimensional CT scans did not improve the reliability or reproducibility. Unlike our study,[31] Sallay et al.[40] found that experience did not significantly improve the reliability of identifying specific fracture patterns. They recognized the limitations of their retrospective study and the small number of cases and a lack of standardized radiographs. They believed that it was not the classification system that was poor, but more likely the vague criteria for identifying the fractured segments and determining their displacement and angulation.

Burstein has questioned whether classification systems are useful at all.[44] Neer believes that the confusion is due to a bad use of the classification system that he believes is anatomically correct,[41] rather than to a bad classification system. Yet, Rockwood and even Neer stated that even the most experienced surgeon occasionally is in doubt and has to make the final classification at surgery.[41–44]

The classification of the fracture is critically important to the decision-making process. A fracture classified as minimally displaced by one observer and as a three-part by another may be treated differently by the two observers. Also, the results of treatment for a particular fracture in the literature may be inaccurate because of the difficulties of determining a reliable and reproducible classification.[43]

AO Classification

The AO group has modified the Neer classification, placing more emphasis on the vascular supply to the articular segment of the proximal humerus. Severity of the injury and risk of osteonecrosis forms the basis of the AO classification system (Fig. 9). In this system, it is accepted that if either tuberosity and its attached rotator cuff remain in continuity with the articular segment, the vascular supply is probably adequate. Proximal humerus fractures are separated into three types: extraarticular unifocal, extraarticular bifocal, and articular. Each of these types is further subdivided into different groups based on alignment, degree, and direction of the displacement; presence of impaction; and associated dislocation.

Type A fractures are extraarticular and involve one of the tuberosities with or without a concomitant metaphyseal fracture. Group A1 are the extraarticular unifocal tuberosity fractures; group A2 are the extraarticular unifocal fractures with an impacted metaphyseal fracture; and group A3 are the

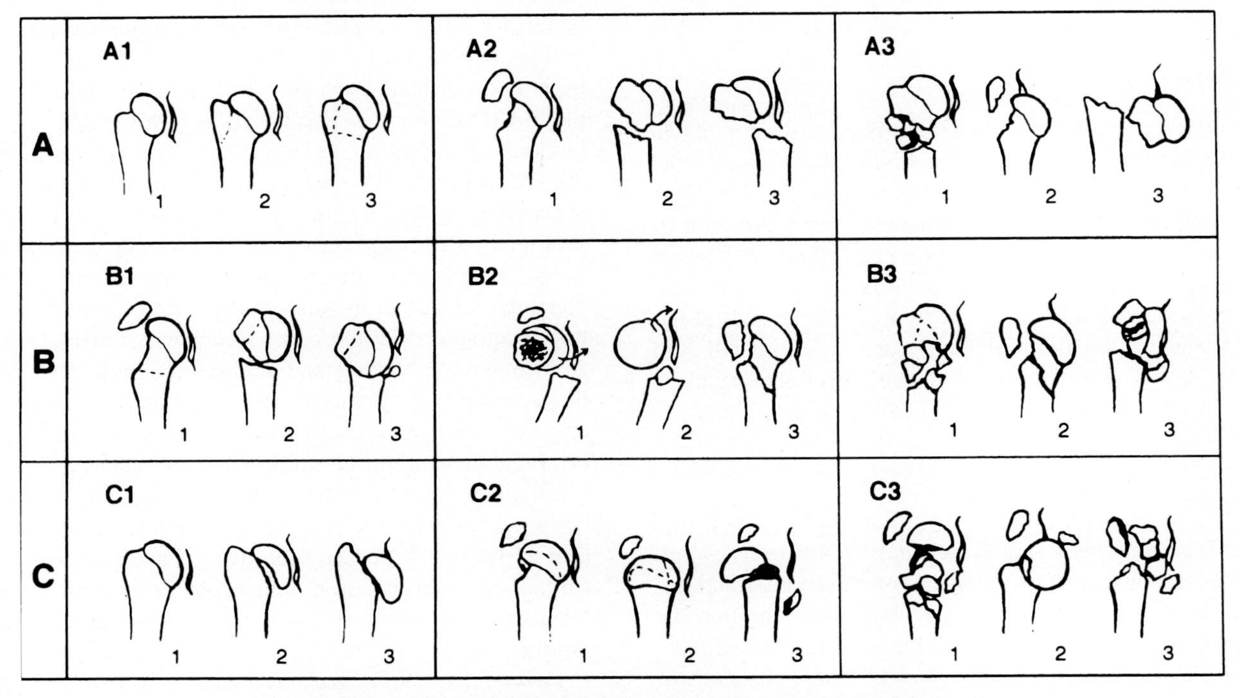

FIG. 9. The AO classification of proximal humeral fractures (see text).

extraarticular unifocal fractures with a nonimpacted metaphyseal fracture. Osteonecrosis is unlikely in type A fractures.

Type B fractures are also extraarticular, but involve both tuberosities with a concomitant metaphyseal fracture or glenohumeral dislocation. Group B1 are the extraarticular bifocal fractures associated with an impacted metaphyseal fracture; group B2 fractures are the extraarticular bifocal fractures with a nonimpacted metaphyseal fracture; and group B3 fractures are the extraarticular bifocal fractures with a glenohumeral dislocation. There is a low risk for osteonecrosis in type B fractures.

Type C fractures are extraarticular and involve vascular isolation of the articular segment. Group C1 are fractures with slight displacement; group C2 are impacted fractures with marked displacement; and group C3 fractures are associated with a glenohumeral dislocation. There is a high risk of osteonecrosis in this type.

This more complex classification system theoretically should allow development of more detailed guidelines for treatment and prognosis. However, its complexity may actually preclude attaining the widespread utilization that the Neer classification currently commands. Thus far, clinical studies using the AO classification have been quite limited. Recent assessment of its interobserver reliability has not shown it to be significantly better than the Neer system.[46] Thus far, no long-term results of treatments based on the AO classification system have been presented. Sieb and Gerber's[46] study found that when five experts in shoulder surgery evaluated 95 proximal humerus fractures using simplified versions of both the Neer and AO/ASIF classification system, there was poor interobserver reliability and acceptable intraobserver reliability for both systems.

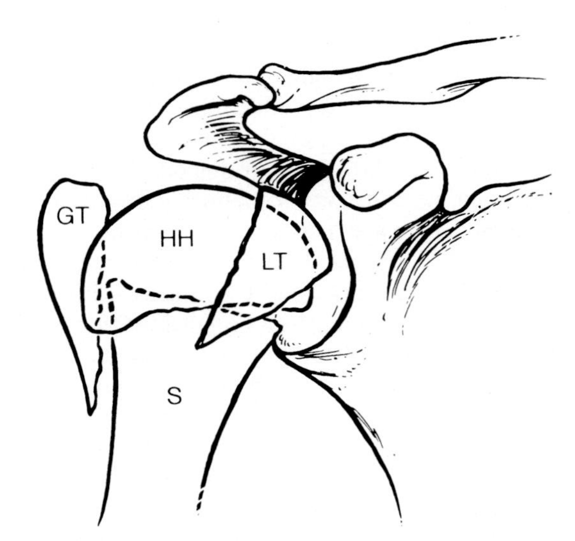

FIG. 10. Valgus-impacted four-part fracture. The articular segment (*HH*) is impacted and angulated, rather than displaced as in the classic four-part fracture. *GT*, greater tuberosity; *LT*, lesser tuberosity; *S*, the shaft.

Valgus Impacted

There is a specific type of four-part fracture described that is characterized by a valgus impaction of the humeral head and variable displacement of the tuberosities (Fig. 10). This valgus-impacted humeral head fracture pattern does not fit accurately into Neer's classification. The AO classification system classifies these fracture patterns as C2.1 and C2.2 type fractures.[47] However, because of the lower rate of osteonecrosis and the more favorable outcome compared with "classic" four-part fractures, Jakob[11] felt this fracture pattern required special consideration, as will be discussed later.

Incidence

Proximal humeral fractures account for 4% to 5% of all fractures in adults and less than 1% of children's fractures. Approximately 3% of physeal fractures occur through the proximal humerus.[15,104] Proximal humeral epiphyseal plate fractures can occur any time between birth and physeal closure at approximately 18 years of age. These are most common in adolescents between 10 and 16 years of age (owing to increased sports participation), followed by neonates who sustain birth trauma.[2,69,105,106,124] In patients younger than 17 years of age, Salter-Harris types I and II are most commonly seen with proximal humerus fractures. Salter-Harris type I injuries occur in newborn infants, whereas Salter-Harris type II injuries occur in adolescents.[2,21,48]

Salter-Harris III fractures are rare and usually occur with a dislocation in which the glenoid acts as a wedge to split the epiphysis.[50,128,209] Salter-Harris IV fractures are associated with open fractures.[48] No Salter-Harris V fractures have been reported in the literature.[2,49,118] The reason for this fracture distribution can be explained as follows. The proximal humeral epiphysial plate is very active, contributing about 80% of longitudinal humeral growth.[52] It remains open until approximately 19 years of age. The weakest area is distal to proliferating cartilage cells in the "zone of degenerative cartilage," where the cartilage is being converted to bone on the metaphyseal side of the plate.[3] Microscopic studies of fracture specimens in stillborn infants and experimental animals confirm the finding that the fracture through the plate occurs through the hypertrophied cartilage cells adjacent to the zone of provisional calcification, thus avoiding the proliferating cells and causing no harmful effects on growth.[2,22,51] The glenohumeral joint has the most mobility of any joint in the body, which limits the risk for crushing or epiphyseal splitting injuries.[3,21] Lesser tuberosity fractures occur with forced external rotation and abduction, while greater tuberosity fractures occur with dislocations, both being rare injuries.

Proximal humerus fractures account for over 75% of

humerus fractures in patients older than age 40. After age 50, women have a much higher incidence than men. An exponential increase occurs after menopause, representing the typical characteristic of an osteoporotic fracture.[33,107,203,208] In patients younger than age 50, high-energy trauma is the most common cause of proximal humerus fractures; after age 50, minimal to moderate trauma is the most common cause.[108]

Up to 85% of all proximal humerus fractures are one-part (nondisplaced or minimally displaced) fractures; 15% to 20% of all proximal humerus fractures are classified as displaced. Most two-part fractures are surgical neck fractures, with the majority of these fractures occurring in individuals older than 65 years.[109,110] Although up to 40% of proximal humerus fractures have some involvement of the greater tuberosity,[33,34] isolated two-part displaced greater tuberosity fractures are reported to comprise less than 2% of all proximal humerus fractures.[109] However, it is believed that this fracture is underdiagnosed and may be more common than the literature suggests.[43] These fractures occur in association with anterior dislocation in 5% to 33% of cases.[112, 113, 212] Two-part anatomic neck fractures have not been reported to occur in children[2] and constitute only 0.54% of proximal humerus fractures.[109] Isolated lesser tuberosity fractures comprise 0.27% of all proximal humerus fractures and 0.5% of displaced fractures. Two-part lesser tuberosity fracture–dislocations comprise 1.3% of all displaced proximal humerus fractures. Three-part fractures comprise 3% or more of displaced proximal humerus fractures.[19,109,121] Three-part lesser tuberosity fractures occur much less frequently than those of greater tuberosity displacement. Four-part fractures comprise approximately 4% of proximal humerus fractures, and articular surface fractures comprise approximately 3%.[48]

Rating System

There are many different methods currently used to assess shoulder function. Neer used a system based on 100 units: 35 units were assigned for pain, 30 units for function, 25 units for range of motion, and 10 units for anatomy. A score of 89 or higher represents an excellent result; higher than 80 units is a satisfactory result; 70 to 79 units is an unsatisfactory result, with less than 70 units representing a failure. Each assessment method places varying importance in the areas of pain, range of motion, and function. It is possible that one assessment system may indicate a good result, whereas another system may indicate a fair or poor result in the same patient. To facilitate communication between investigators, stimulate multicenter studies, and allow communication of useful and relevant outcome data to physicians, health care organizations and the general public, a standardized method of assessing shoulder function, regardless of diagnosis, was established by the American Shoulder and Elbow Surgeons (ASES) in 1994.[137]

EVALUATION

Clinical Evaluation

Newborns with an epiphyseal separation of the proximal humerus present with pseudoparalysis, with the arm held in extension, swelling at the apex of the shoulder and occasionally fever. Infection, clavicle fracture, and Erb's palsy are included in the differential diagnosis. Pain with motion of the arm points toward a fracture.[48,138]

In eliciting a history from a patient who has sustained a proximal humerus fracture, determination of the mechanism of injury can be helpful. A child usually gives a history of falling backward onto an outstretched hand with the elbow extended and the wrist dorsiflexed.[48] A loss of consciousness or a history of falls may indicate a cardiac or neurologic etiology in the older patient.[53,160] A direct mechanism can occur, such as a blow to the lateral aspect of the shoulder, in both young and older patients. However, in the elderly, the indirect mechanism is much more common and generally involves a fall onto the outstretched arm. In younger patients, this mechanism most commonly results in a dislocation. The indirect mechanism is usually associated with a greater degree of fracture displacement than the direct mechanism. Other indirect causes of proximal humerus fractures are seizures or electroconvulsive therapy without the use of muscle relaxants; both are often associated with posterior dislocations.[160]

The symptoms and signs associated with proximal humerus fractures can be quite variable. However, they most often correlate with the degree of fracture displacement and comminution. Pain, especially with any attempts at shoulder motion, is almost always present. Inspection of the shoulder usually reveals swelling and ecchymosis. The patient should be instructed that over the first 4 to 5 days following injury, the ecchymosis that develops may extend distally into the arm and forearm or even to the chest wall and breast area (Fig. 11).

Palpation of the shoulder will usually reveal tenderness about the proximal humerus. Crepitus may be evident with motion of the fracture fragments. The entire upper extremity should be examined. A fall on the outstretched arm can also result in a fracture of another area such as a distal radius fracture. The chest should also be examined, because rib fractures may also occur from a fall.[55–58]

Assessment of fracture stability is an essential part of the examination. The humeral shaft should be gently rotated internally and externally as the proximal portion of the humerus is palpated. If the proximal and distal portions move as a unit, the fracture is stable; however, motion or crepitus is consistent with an unstable or less stable fracture pattern.

Essential to the clinical evaluation of the patient with a proximal humerus fracture is a complete neurovascular examination of the involved upper extremity. Associated axillary artery and brachial plexus injuries have been reported,[12,59–62]

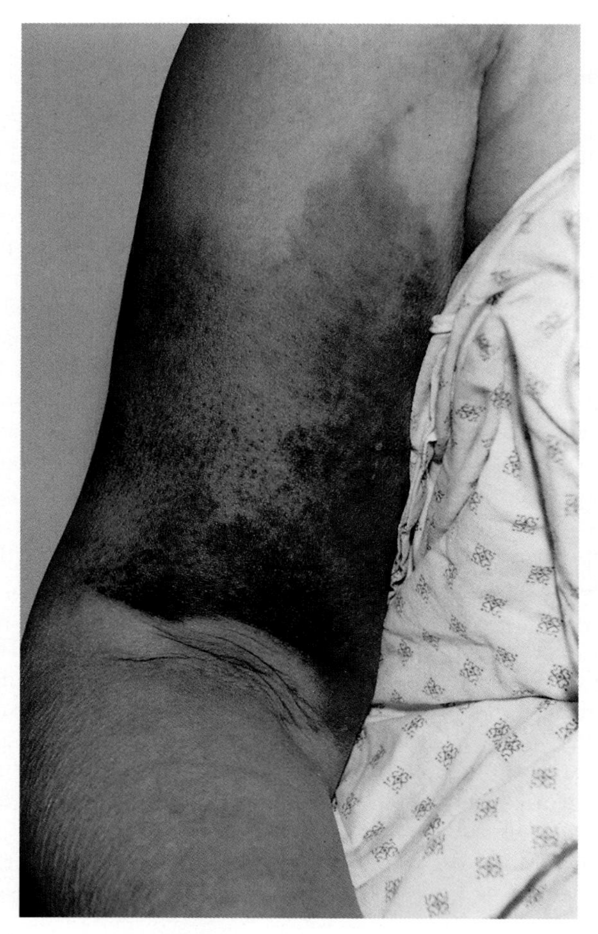

FIG. 11. A 72-year-old woman, 2 days following closed reduction of a two-part greater tuberosity fracture–dislocation; the area of ecchymosis has extended to the elbow.

especially with fracture fragments displaced medial to the coracoid process. A 45% incidence of nerve injury has recently been reported.[13] Fracture–dislocations also increase the incidence of neurovascular injury.[63] The most commonly injured peripheral nerve is the axillary nerve.[26] Both sensory and motor testing should be performed to evaluate axillary nerve function. This may be difficult in the setting of acute injury. Therefore, serial examinations should be performed.

Radiographic Evaluation

One of the most important components of the evaluation of proximal humerus fractures is the determination of the position of the fracture fragments and the degree of displacement. Thus, an adequate radiographic evaluation is mandatory.

Trauma Series

The cornerstone of the radiographic evaluation of proximal humerus fractures is the trauma series (Fig. 12). The trauma series consists of anteroposterior (AP) and lateral views of the shoulder, obtained in the plane of the scapula, and an axillary view. Fracture classification and treatment decisions are generally based on these three radiographic views. Each view contributes information obtained from three different perpendicular planes.[21,26,27,64,65]

The scapular AP view offers a general overview of the fracture and is usually evaluated first. This view should be made perpendicular to the scapular plane (as differentiated from the plane of the chest), which requires angling the x-ray beam approximately 40 degrees in a mediolateral direction. This compensates for the position of the scapula on the chest wall. It will demonstrate the glenoid in profile as well as the true glenohumeral joint space. In the undislocated shoulder, it shows the humeral head to be clearly separated from the glenoid.

At least one view obtained at 90 degrees to the scapular AP is required for assessment of proximal humerus fractures and fracture–dislocations.[66] This orthogonal view provides important information about angulation and displacement of the fracture fragments[26] and the presence of an associated dislocation.[54,67–69] Both the scapular lateral and axillary views are oriented orthogonally to the scapular AP and fulfill the criteria for a second projection. However, the trauma series generally includes all three views.

The scapular lateral, also known as the scapular "Y," can provide important information not evident on a scapular AP view.[54,69–71] This view is a true lateral of the scapula, with the x-ray beam passing parallel to the spine of the scapula. This view is taken with the patient standing. It can be obtained with the involved upper extremity immobilized in a sling and does not require any movement of the extremity and, as such, does not add to patient discomfort. The scapular lateral assists in delineating the position of the humeral head relative to the glenoid and is particularly useful in showing posteriorly displaced fragments as well as shaft displacement.

The axillary view also permits assessment of the glenohumeral relation. This is generally obtained with the patient supine. The arm must be positioned in at least 30 degrees of abduction. In the acute setting, positioning is often performed by the physician. The x-ray plate is placed above the shoulder, and the beam is directed to the plate from a caudad position. The axillary view can also be useful in identifying fractures of the glenoid rim, posterior displacement of the greater tuberosity, medial displacement of the lesser tuberosity, and humeral head articular impression fractures.[53,65,66,72,73]

The relative efficacy of these different views has not been studied extensively. Silfverskiold et al.[74] reported in their prospective study that the scapular lateral view was more sensitive than the axillary view in detecting shoulder dislocations. They did not study fractures specifically. In 92% of their 75 cases, however, the scapular lateral and axillary views resulted in the same diagnosis.

We conducted a study in which the trauma series radio-

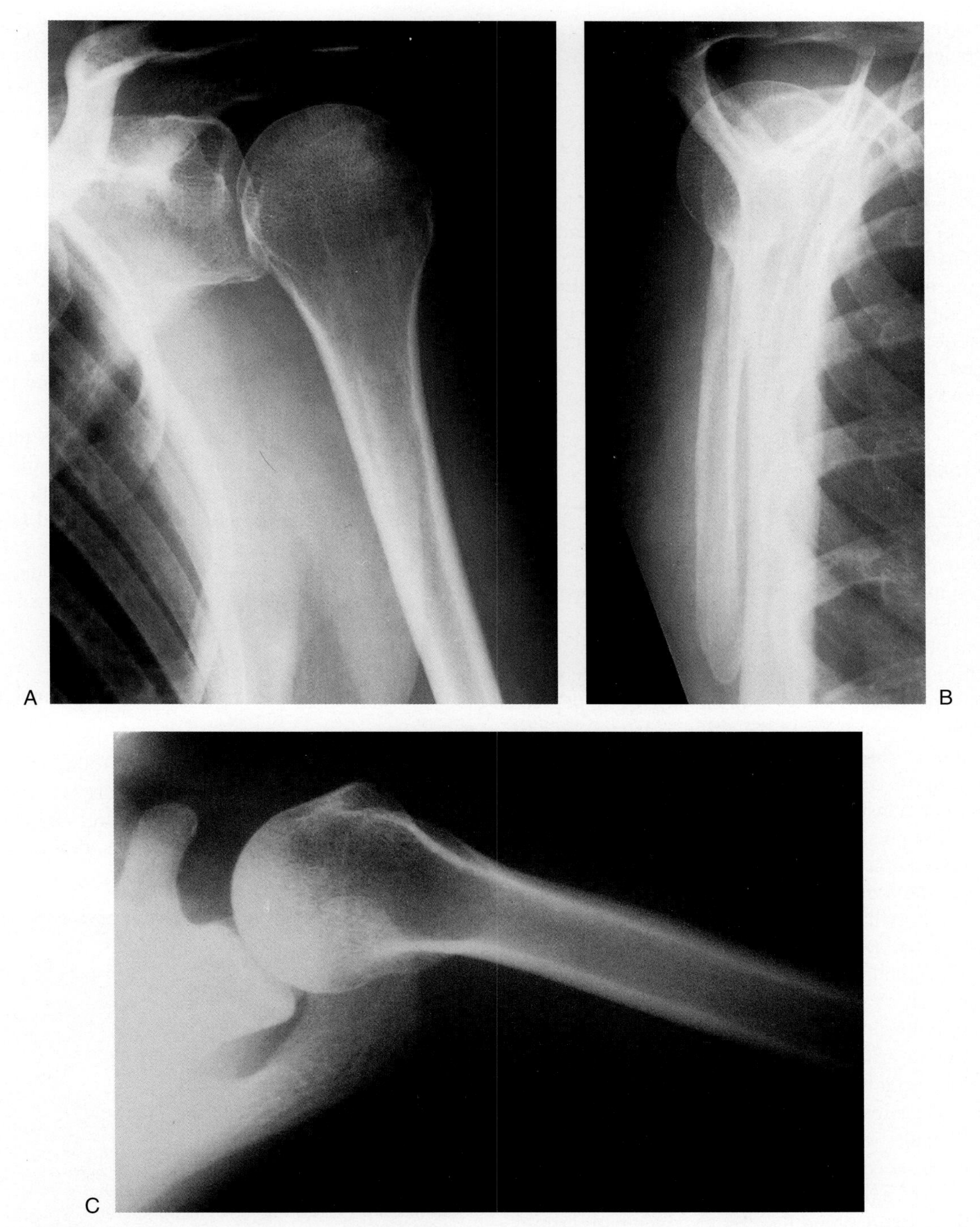

FIG. 12. The trauma series of radiographs includes an **(A)** anteroposterior view and **(B)** lateral view in the plane of the scapula, and **(C)** an axillary view.

graphs of 50 proximal humerus fractures were used to assess the relative contributions of the scapular lateral and axillary radiographs to fracture classification using the Neer system.[75] The radiographs were reviewed by five different orthopedic surgeons with varying levels of experience and expertise. In the first viewing, radiographs were reviewed and classified in the following sequence:

1. After scapular AP alone
2. After review of scapular AP and lateral views
3. After review of scapular AP, lateral, and axillary views

A second viewing of the same 50 cases was performed 6 months later in a changed sequence:

1. After scapular AP alone

2. After review of scapular AP and axillary
3. After review of scapular AP, axillary views, and scapula lateral view

For the cumulative experience of these five observers, review of the scapular AP and axillary views achieved a final classification in 99% of cases. However, after review of the scapular AP and lateral, the final classification was achieved in only 79% of cases ($P < 0.05$). These results indicate that when combined with the scapular AP radiograph, the axillary view contributes significantly more information than the scapular lateral radiograph in determining fracture classification. Posterior displacement of 1 cm of the greater tuberosity is missed 25% of the time when only AP and lateral scapular views are used alone.

Additional Radiographic Views

If any of the these three views of the trauma series is inadequate, it should be repeated. Usually, the fracture can be evaluated and treated based on this set of radiographs. Additional radiographic views may be helpful and have been advocated by others.

The apical oblique view[76] is obtained by directing the x-ray beam through the glenohumeral joint at an angle of 45 degrees to the plane of the chest wall and angled 45 degrees caudally. When compared with the scapular lateral view, it provides additional useful information in the evaluation of proximal humerus fractures and fracture–dislocations, specifically in demonstrating dislocations and posterolateral humeral head compression fractures.[77,78] However, it has not become as widely accepted as the scapular lateral view.

Modified axillary views, such as the Velpeau axillary lateral,[67] the Stripp axillary lateral,[79] and the trauma axillary lateral,[80] have been described. These views permit an axillary lateral to be obtained without removing the injured arm from the sling. The Velpeau axillary lateral is probably the most commonly used, taken with the patient leaning backward approximately 30 degrees over the x-ray table. The x-ray cassette is placed beneath the shoulder on the table, and the x-ray beam passes vertically from superior to inferior through the shoulder joint. Although this view has the benefit of avoiding the need to position the injured extremity, we prefer the standard axillary view because it offers less distortion and bony overlap and thereby provides more useful information.

Other Diagnostic Modalities.

Computed tomography scans of proximal humeral fractures and fracture dislocations may be indicated when the trauma series radiographs are indeterminate. CT scans have been recommended to evaluate the rotation of fragments, the degree of tuberosity displacement, as well as articular impression fractures, head-splitting fractures, and chronic fracture–dislocations.[26,81–85] Castagno et al. reported a small series of 17 patients in whom CT scans of acute proximal humeral fractures demonstrated important information not evident on plain radiographs.[81] Also, spiral CT with three-dimensional and multiplanar reconstructions was reported to provide additional information, compared with standard x-rays in ten patients with three- and four-part fractures. However, in this study, standard radiographs did not include an axillary view.[83]

As mentioned earlier in the classification and reliability section, CT does not seem to improve interobserver reliability and fracture classification.[39,40] In our experience, CT scans are most helpful in the evaluation of chronic fracture–dislocations, specifically to identify the size and location of humeral head impression defects and the degree of secondary glenoid changes[31] (Fig 13).

Another imaging modality to consider is magnetic resonance imaging. Magnetic resonance imaging (MRI) provides information about associated soft-tissue injuries of the rotator cuff, biceps tendon, and the glenoid labrum, which may be helpful in the management of these patients. However, cost benefits issues have to be considered carefully. Thus far, there have been no studies performed to support its routine use.

Vascular Injury and Indications for Arteriogram

The axillary artery lies just anterior and medial to the proximal humerus.[6] Vascular injury following fracture–dislocation of the humerus is uncommon; it is rare in anterior dislocation without associated fracture; and it is extremely rare in closed humeral neck fractures, despite the fracture's

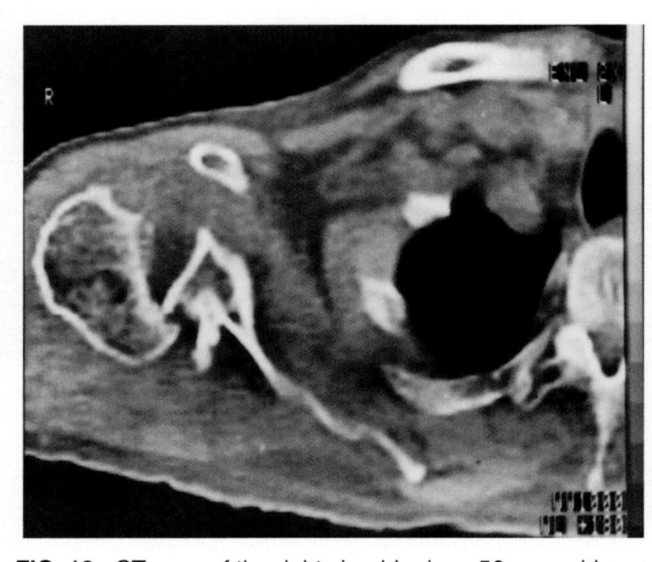

FIG. 13. CT scan of the right shoulder in a 56-year-old man with a chronic posterior dislocation of the right shoulder. The image clearly shows the impression fracture of the anteromedial portion of the humeral head, as well as the amount of the articular surface involvement. The calcification about the posterior glenoid neck provides further evidence of the chronic nature of dislocation.

proximity to the artery.[10,86–91] Morris et al. identified no vascular injuries associated with proximal humeral fractures in a series of 220 acute arterial injuries.[87] Neer reported on 117 displaced proximal humerus fractures over a 15-year period and found no vascular complications.[10] The literature documents only 16 cases of axillary artery injury from proximal humerus fractures.[12,87–92,204]

In pure anterior dislocations, the axillary artery can be damaged in its second part by avulsion of the thoracoacromial trunk or in its third part from avulsion of the subscapular and circumflex humeral vessels (with subsequent linear tears in the artery and intraluminal thrombosis). The mechanism of arterial injury in a pure dislocation is thought to be secondary to tethering of the axillary artery by the subscapular and circumflex arteries, thus accounting for the injuries primarily occurring in the third part.[93] The pectoralis minor muscle may act as a fulcrum that puts the artery on stretch and then pinches the artery with dislocation.[94] The artery may also be fixed to a scarred joint capsule from previous injury or surgery, or atherosclerotic vessels may be present. Both factors increase the risk of vascular injury. Excessive force during reduction may also cause vascular injury.[86]

Although rare, the possibility of axillary arterial injury should be considered in proximal humerus fractures with severe medial displacement of the shaft.[95] The mechanism of arterial injury may be through direct injury by sharp fracture fragments, thrombosis from vessel contusion, or damage from violent stretching or avulsion of the artery with shoulder hyperabduction, especially in fragile atheromatous vessels. Vascular spasm, although exceedingly rare, may occur from kinking.[96]

Although uncommon, when vascular complications do occur, they represent a true emergency (see Chapter 25).[97] Early recognition and treatment of vascular injuries play an important role in the eventual outcome: If an arterial repair is done in the "golden" period, within 12 hours of injury, a reasonable chance of success can be expected.[98] A careful neurologic and vascular examination is necessary at initial presentation. Axillary arterial injuries are obvious when clinical findings include an expanding hematoma, absent distal pulses in a cold, pale extremity, or the presence of a pulsatile painful mass with a bruit (in a pseudoaneurysm).[98] However, symptoms are often vague and nonspecific, particularly when ischemic changes are progressive. Because of the tremendous collateral circulation around the shoulder, peripheral pulses, initially weak, may return completely over time, despite axillary artery disruption. This may mask an injury and falsely lead the examiner to consider arterial spasm as the cause of the clinical findings. Distal pulses are reported to be palpable in 27% of patients with major arterial injuries about the shoulder.[53] Therefore, a careful assessment of peripheral pulses must be performed.[99] If a patient with a fracture or fracture–dislocation of the shoulder has no pulse, a pulse that comes and goes, or a pulse of lower volume, further investigation is necessary, even if the pulse returns to normal after manipulation or over time.[100] Any suspicion of a vascular injury requires a Doppler examination to determine both the magnitude and quality of the arterial signal. Arteriography should be performed immediately when the Doppler examination or clinical findings suggest arterial compromise.[12,99] Late signs of vascular complications, including false aneurysms and acute ischemia with gangrene, can appear weeks, months, or even years after the initial injury.[86–90,99–103] Thus, angiography is recommended when there is any clinical suspicion of a vascular injury (Fig. 14). When an arterial injury occurs in association with a proximal humeral fracture or fracture–dislocation, the fracture should be anatomically reduced and stabilized with internal fixation before vascular repair, to protect the vascular repair so that additional fracture manipulation will not be necessary after repair.[12] However, it has also been suggested that the order of treatment (reperfusion verses osteosynthesis) should be dictated by the degree of ischemia.[95]

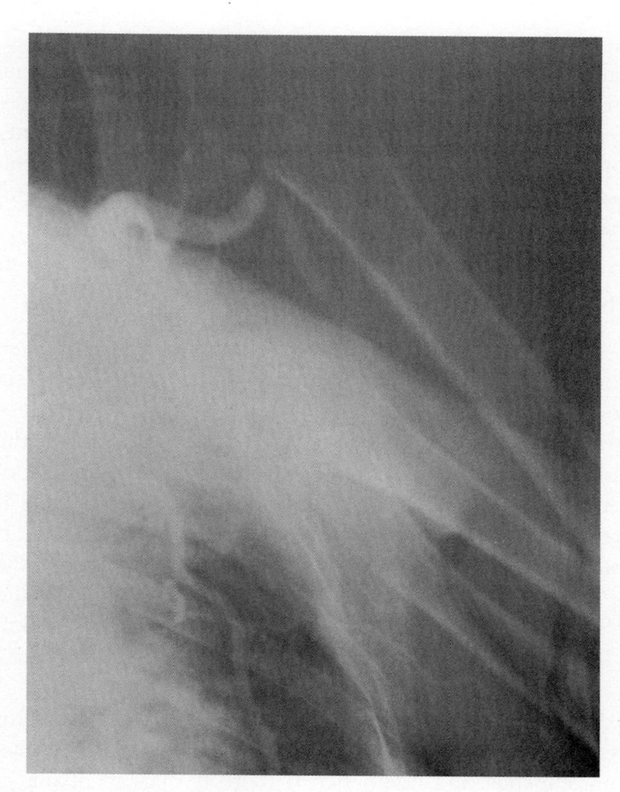

FIG. 14. Angiogram showing the humeral circumflex vessels pinched in the fracture site, with subsequent tenting of the axillary artery and obstruction of flow after closed reduction of a two-part proximal humerus fracture.

TREATMENT

The indication for operative versus nonoperative management of proximal humerus fractures is determined by numerous factors including the patient's physiologic age, arm dominance, associated injuries, the fracture type, degree of fracture displacement, and bone quality. The surgeon's knowledge and skill will greatly affect the functional outcome. He or she must also have the ability to accurately diagnose the fracture, based on an understanding of the relevant anatomy and interpretation of complete radiographs. The patient's general medical condition and ability to undergo major surgery as well as to comply with an intensive rehabilitation program are of paramount importance in developing a management plan.[53]

Physeal Fractures

Most proximal humeral physeal fractures can be treated nonoperatively, even when there is significant displacement, because of the great remodeling potential[21,207] (see algorithm 1). As a general rule, the younger the patient, the greater potential for remodeling and the greater the initial deformity that can be accepted. Neer-Horowitz grade I and II fractures do exceptionally well with sling and swath treatment without reduction, because of the remodeling potential of the proximal humeral physis. Neer-Horowitz grade III and grade IV fractures usually require reduction, but may be left with up to 3 cm of shortening or residual angulation because this is often clinically insignificant.

In newborns, most fractures are Salter-Harris type I, for the physeal plate is less resistant to trauma than the bone, joint capsule, and ligaments. If there is marked displacement, a closed reduction can be performed by applying gentle longitudinal traction with the shoulder in 135-degrees abduction, 30-degrees forward flexion, and neutral rotation, and directing a posterior force on the shaft.[114] Ultrasound can be used to evaluate the reduction. The prognosis is excellent, even if an anatomic reduction is not fully achieved. If the fracture is stable, the arm can be immobilized against the chest for 5 to 10 days, then used as tolerated. Unstable fractures should be maintained in abduction and external rotation for 3 to 4 days until callous forms.

Salter-Harris type I fractures, and less frequently Salter-Harris type II fractures, occur in children younger than age 5. Closed reduction may be necessary, but up to 70 degrees of angulation with any displacement is acceptable because of the extensive remodeling that is possible in this young age.[3] The arm is held in a sling for 4 days followed by progressive activity.

In the 5 to 11 age group, metaphyseal fractures are most common because the rapid remodeling in this area results in some degree of weakening. Closed reduction may be necessary, but bayonet apposition with 1 to 2 cm of overlap, 40 to 45 degrees of angulation, or displacement of one-half the width of the shaft are acceptable.[124] Stable fractures are immobilized in a sling and swath; a hanging arm cast is used occasionally in older children. Rarely, a spica cast is used for 2 to 3 weeks in unstable fractures to maintain the arm in the salute position. When callous is evident, the arm is slowly brought down to the side and immobilized in a sling and swath. After 3 to 4 weeks, the fracture should be healed and progressive range of motion exercises are begun. Strengthening of the rotator cuff, trapezius, and deltoid are added as range of motion progresses.[118]

From age 11 until skeletal maturity, there is less remodeling potential than in younger children, so less displacement and angulation is acceptable. The fractures encountered are

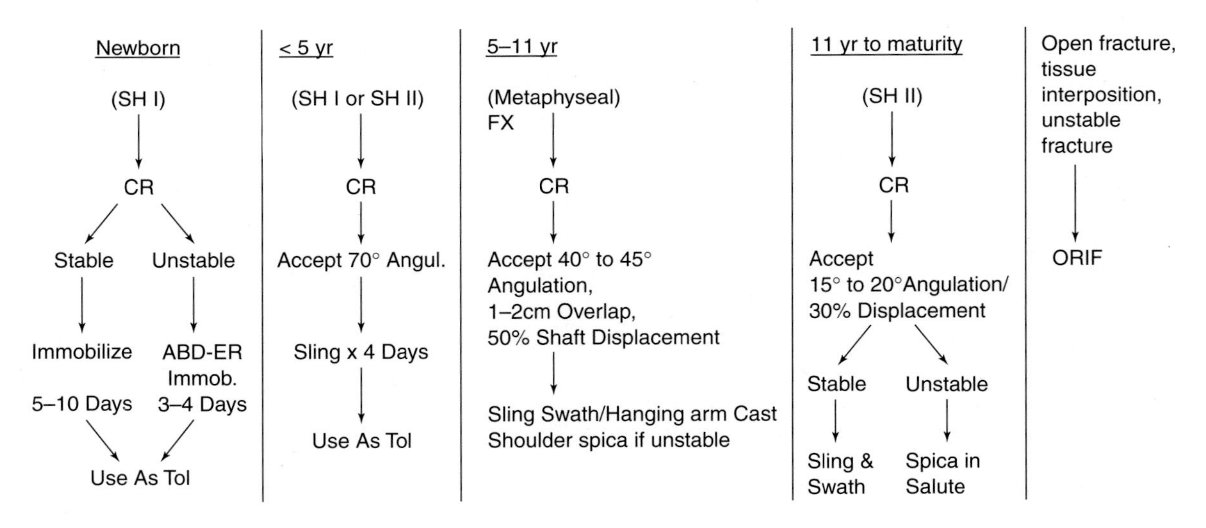

ALGORITHM

KEY: SH, Salter-Harris; CR, closed reduction; ABD, abduction; ER, external rotation; FX, fracture; ORIF, open reduction internal fixation; ROM, range of motion; AROM, active range of motion; AAROM, active assisted range of motion; PROM, passive range of motion; AVN, avascular necrosis; IR, rotator cuff tear; PP, percutaneous pinning; As Tol, as tolerated use.

more frequently Salter-Harris type II, with some Salter-Harris type I fractures. Treatment is by closed reduction with 15 to 20 degrees of angulation and less than 30% displacement considered acceptable. A stable fracture is treated with a sling and swath for 2 to 3 weeks, followed by progressive range of motion exercises; an unstable fracture may need immobilization in a shoulder spica cast with the arm in the salute position.[118]

Operative Treatment

The indications for operative treatment of physeal fractures of the proximal humerus are not well defined; many factors must be considered. Growth-remaining charts may be of benefit to determine if the patient has sufficient potential to remodel a significantly displaced fracture. The literature supports nonoperative treatment, even for markedly displaced fractures,[21] because the functional outcomes have been satisfactory even in the presence of limitation of motion and persistent deformity.[120] The literature also supports closed reduction and pinning or open reduction and internal fixation in older children with markedly displaced fractures and limited remodeling potential, in whom an acceptable reduction cannot be maintained.[123]

Open reduction and fracture fixation with smooth K-wires or Steinmann pins is indicated in open fractures to aid soft-tissue healing, in fractures with neurovascular compromise, or in multiple trauma patients to allow patient mobilization.[114] Although closed reduction is usually successful for these fractures, occasionally, the periosteum,[124] capsule,[125] biceps tendon,[127] deltoid or subscapularis[119] may be interposed between the fracture ends and block reduction. In this situation, open reduction may be needed. The shaft of the humerus may be irreducible because it is buttonholed through a capsular or periosteal tear.

The rare Salter-Harris III and Salter-Harris IV fracture–dislocations, lesser tuberosity fractures, and greater tuberosity fractures may be successfully treated by closed reduction.[128,129] If a dislocation cannot be reduced, or if the reduction is unstable, open reduction and internal fixation will be required. For acute lesser tuberosity fractures, screws or suture through drill holes, depending on fragment size, is performed to prevent future shoulder instability.[114] Displaced greater tuberosity fractures may require open reduction and repair of associated rotator cuff tears.[114]

Intramedullary fixation using smooth, flexible 2-mm nails,[122,130] inserted in a retrograde fashion from the lateral epicondyle into the head to help maintain a reduction, has been described. Rush rods[131] and a bundled wire technique[132] have also been used.

One-Part Fractures: Adult

Minimally displaced fractures account for over 80% of all proximal humerus fractures.[19] They are often referred to as "one-part" fractures, based on Neer's four-segment classification. By definition, although there may be many fracture lines, there is no significant displacement of any segment (Algorithm 2). However, it is essential to confirm the stability of the fracture. Many of these fractures are impacted and, with rotation of the humerus, the proximal humerus and shaft move together as one unit. This is a stable fracture, and an early range of motion program is appropriate. However, some minimally displaced fractures are not impacted, and rotation of the humerus indicates that the proximal segments and shaft do not move as a unit. This fracture is not stable and requires a period of immobilization until sufficient healing has occurred. Once clinical stability is present, as evidenced by movement of the head and the shaft as a unit, range of motion exercises can be initiated.

For minimally displaced stable fractures, we prefer immobilization in a simple arm sling. Padding should be placed in the axilla and around the elbow in the sling to prevent skin maceration. Elderly patients must be watched carefully for skin problems, even with use of the simple sling. Swelling and ecchymosis add to the risk of skin problems. When the humerus does not move as a unit, we prefer sling and swathe immobilization. This consists of a standard arm sling with a 6-in. elastic (Ace) bandage used as a swathe. The Ace bandage is secured to the sling with safety pins. With a sling and swathe of this type, padding should be used in the axilla and around the elbow as described. The swathe should be removed two to three times each day to check the skin about the elbow and to allow elbow, wrist, and hand range of motion. In addition, the arm can be gently abducted by gravity to check the skin and axilla.

With minimally displaced fractures that are stable, patients should be started on a range of motion program as soon as the initial discomfort subsides. Within 1 week after injury, range of motion therapy should begin, preferably under the supervision of an occupational or physical therapist. This consists of active elbow, wrist, and hand exercises in combination with assisted shoulder range of motion exercises. These are begun in the supine position for forward elevation, external rotation, and internal rotation to the chest. Therapy is supervised in one to three weekly sessions and performed three to five times daily at home by the patient. The patient's arm is maintained in a sling for 4 to 6 weeks. The sling is discontinued when clinical and early radiographic evidence of union is confirmed. At that time, an active range of motion program is begun, starting in the supine position, with gradual progression to the sitting position. Isometric deltoid and rotator cuff strengthening exercises are initiated at the same time. When a reasonable range of active shoulder motion is achieved, isotonic resistive exercises for deltoid and rotator cuff muscles are added. Gentle-stretching exercises are also added. Approximately 12 weeks after fracture, a more vigorous-stretching program is begun.

The results of treatment of minimally displaced proximal humerus fractures, using immobilization and early range of motion, have been generally reported as good to excellent.[19,29,30,32,69,133–136] In our prospective study of patients

Adult proximal humerus fracture algorithm

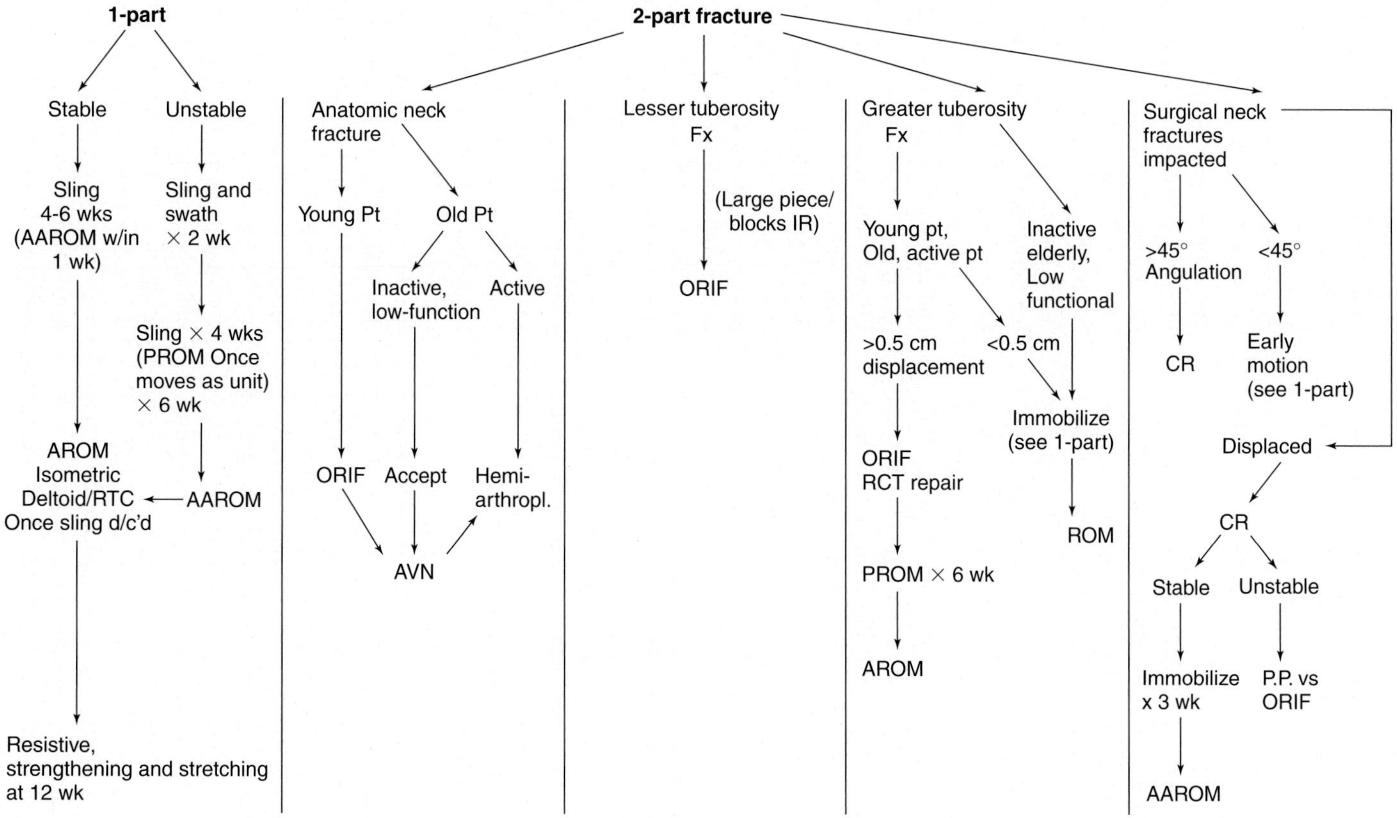

1-part

Stable
Sling
4-6 wks
(AAROM w/in
1 wk)
AROM
Isometric
Deltoid/RTC
Once sling d/c'd
Resistive,
strengthening and stretching
at 12 wk

Unstable
Sling and
swath
× 2 wk
Sling × 4 wks
(PROM Once
moves as unit)
× 6 wk
AAROM

2-part fracture

Anatomic neck
fracture
Young Pt
ORIF
Old Pt
Inactive,
low-function
Accept
Active
Hemi-
arthropl.
AVN

Lesser tuberosity
Fx
(Large piece/
blocks IR)
ORIF

Greater tuberosity
Fx
Young pt,
Old, active pt
>0.5 cm
displacement
ORIF
RCT repair
PROM × 6 wk
AROM
<0.5 cm
Inactive
elderly,
Low
functional
Immobilize
(see 1-part)
ROM

Surgical neck
fractures
impacted
>45°
Angulation
CR
<45°
Early
motion
(see 1-part)
Displaced
CR
Stable
Immobilize
x 3 wk
AAROM
Unstable
P.P. vs
ORIF

(continued)

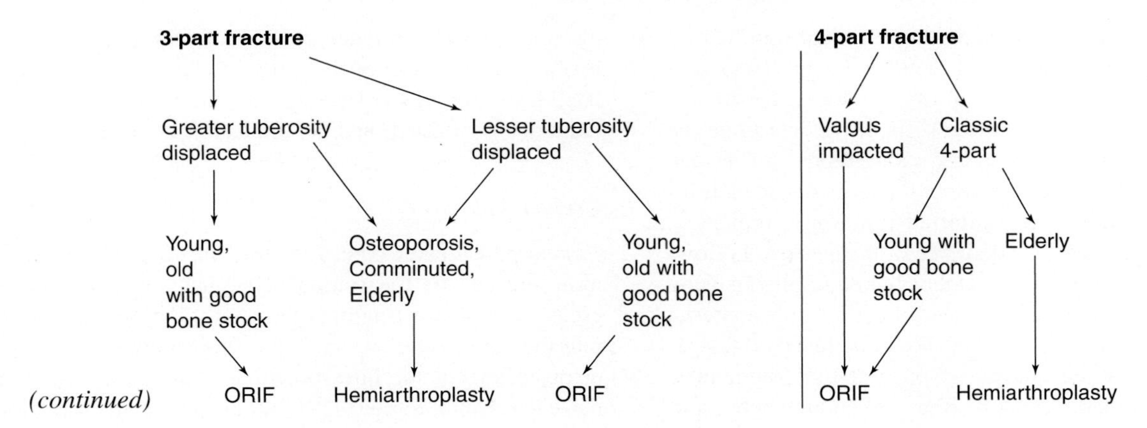

(continued)

with one-part stable proximal humerus fractures, treated with the aforementioned standardized protocol of short-term immobilization combined with an early range of motion program (mean follow-up of 22 months), recovery of range of motion was generally good. Patients regained 87% of forward elevation, 79% of external rotation, and 89% of internal rotation, compared with the opposite shoulder. However, recovery of motion did not necessarily correlate with functional outcomes. Unlike previous studies, we found a high incidence of residual shoulder pain (67%), with a significant number (27%) of patients describing the pain as moderate to severe. Moreover, almost 30% of patients required some form of medication for pain relief.

In this series, almost two-thirds (65%) of patients reported some limitation of function, with 42% reporting a significant restriction of overall function. This primarily affected activities of daily living or inability to sleep on the affected side (40%), inability to carry a package at the side (46%), and inability to use the hand over the head (51%).[139]

A similar rehabilitation program is utilized for minimally displaced fractures that do not move as a unit. The shoulder is immobilized until it moves as a unit (clinically stable). This is usually no longer than 2 to 3 weeks. Gentle passive range of motion exercises are performed until radiographic healing is evident, which is usually 6 weeks from injury. However, each day when the swathe is removed for skin checks, 5 to 10 minutes of active range of motion of the elbow, wrist, and hand should be performed. Once the fracture is stable, the swathe can be removed and only the sling portion is necessary. Range of motion regained with these fractures may be slightly less than with stable, minimally displaced fractures. However, the vast majority of patients regain a good functional range of motion.[69] Overly aggressive early passive range of motion, or active range of motion before healing, increases the risk of healing complications.[53]

Displaced Fractures: Two-Part Fractures

Two-part fractures involve displacement of one of the four segments. Therefore, four different fracture patterns are possible: anatomic neck, greater tuberosity, lesser tuberosity, and surgical neck. Even though surgical neck fractures are the most common fracture pattern, the treatment approach for all four types will be discussed.

Anatomic Neck

Displaced anatomic neck fractures in the absence of tuberosity displacement is quite rare. It may be difficult to recognize on standard radiographic views and a CT scan may be necessary. The problem with this fracture is the high risk of osteonecrosis because of disruption of the intra- and extraosseous blood supply to the humeral head. A true anatomic neck fracture occurs medial to the rotator cuff insertion and, therefore, is devoid of soft-tissue or bony attachments. As a result, these fractures are difficult to treat by closed reduction. Open reduction and internal fixation (ORIF) is preferred, with the goal of avoiding prosthetic replacement in young patients. If a displaced anatomic neck fracture occurs in an elderly patient, a choice has to be made between open reduction and internal fixation (and the risk of nonunion, malunion, and osteonecrosis) and primary hemiarthroplasty. Malunion in the absence of osteonecrosis may be compatible with a good functional outcome. However, if osteonecrosis occurs with collapse and articular incongruity resulting in significant pain, then delayed hemiarthroplasty may be necessary. We prefer primary hemiarthroplasty for the active elderly patient whose functional requirements would be better served by early prosthetic replacement and initiation of a rehabilitation program to regain range of motion. If the articular surface is comminuted, then the fracture is similar to a head-splitting fracture, and primary hemiarthroplasty is preferred. Unfortunately, these fractures are so uncommon that the reported experience is not sufficient to support broad conclusions.

Lesser Tuberosity

Two-part lesser tuberosity fractures in the absence of posterior dislocations are uncommon. When encountered, they may be found in association with nondisplaced surgical neck fractures. The fragment is displaced medially as a result of the pull of the subscapularis muscle. This invariably results in some separation of the anterior portion of the rotator cuff.

However, these fractures are of minimal clinical significance unless the fragment is large and includes a significant portion of the articular surface.[140] In this situation, internal rotation may be blocked. It is often difficult to determine the size of the fragment from standard radiographs. A CT scan may be very helpful in this situation. If a large fragment is involved, open reduction and internal fixation is indicated. This is performed through a deltopectoral approach. Following anatomic reduction, the fragment can be stabilized using tension band technique with wire or heavy suture material (no. 5 Mersilene). Screw fixation should be reserved for patients with good bone quality. If the fracture fragment is small or comminuted, it may be removed and the subscapularis tendon repaired to the fracture site. Assisted range of motion should be initiated postoperatively if secure fixation is obtained. Because of the rarity of anatomic neck and isolated lesser tuberosity fractures, no large series are available that document functional outcome after treatment.

Greater Tuberosity

Two-part greater tuberosity fractures are relatively common and can be the source of significant disability. The greater tuberosity fragment is usually displaced superiorly into the subacromial space if the supraspinatus is involved, or posteriorly if the infraspinatus or teres minor is the primary deforming force (Fig. 15). The degree and direction of displacement indicate that a longitudinal tear of the rotator

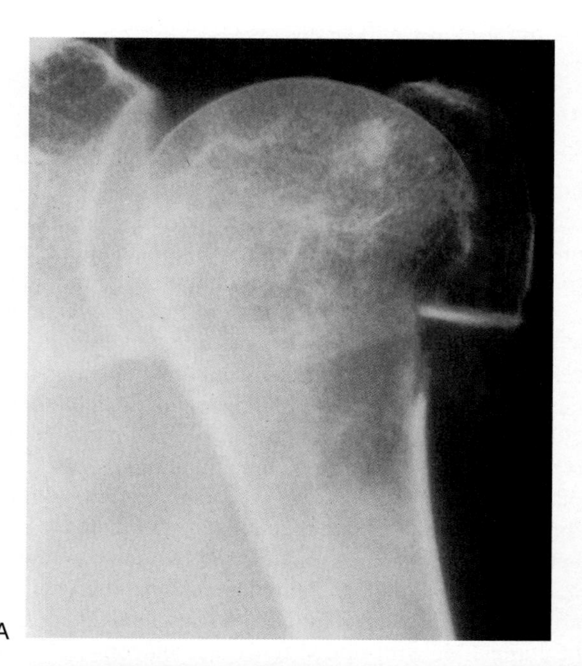

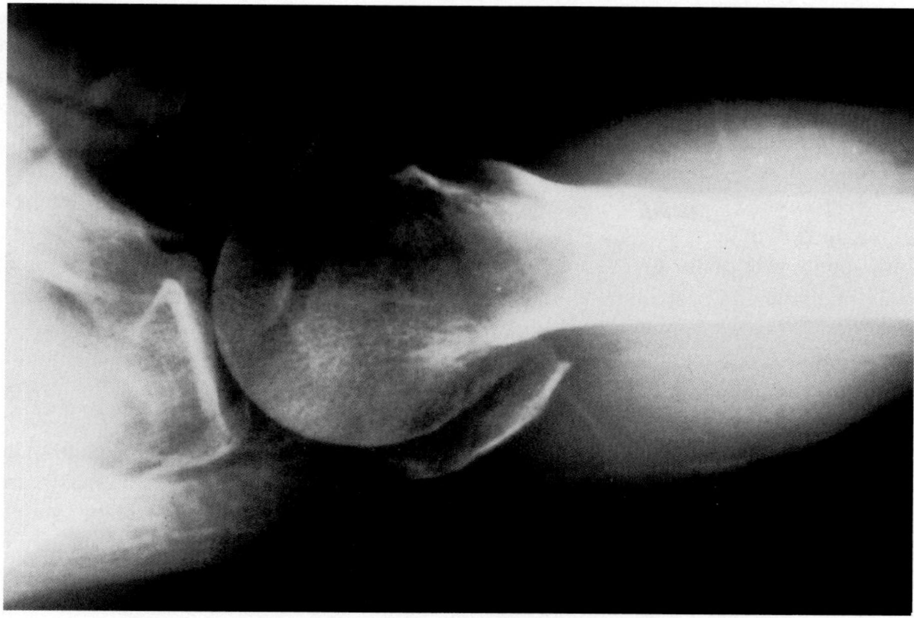

FIG. 15. (A) Anteroposterior (*AP*) and **(B)** an axillary view of a greater tuberosity fracture. Superior displacement into the subacromial space is noted on the AP view, whereas a significant amount of posterior displacement onto the articular surface of the humeral head is best seen on the axillary view.

cuff is also present. Displaced greater tuberosity fragments will often block abduction or external rotation by impinging on the underside of the acromion or posterior glenoid, respectively. Open reduction and internal fixation of the fragment and repair of the rotator cuff tear are the preferred treatment approach.[19,141,142,142a]

Although the criterion for displaced fractures is 1 cm, greater tuberosity fractures appear to be different from other proximal humerus fractures. Less than 1-cm displacement may be problematic, particularly when the displacement is superiorly into the subacromial space. Open reduction and internal fixation has been required in 20% of patients when the displacement was between 0.5 and 1 cm.[54] Concomitant subacromial spurs may exacerbate impingement, even when the tuberosity is displaced less than 1 cm. It is important to include posterior as well as superior displacement in the indication for open reduction, for posterior displacement may also lead to functional deficits, especially in external rotation. Posterior greater tuberosity displacement is best assessed on the axillary radiograph.[54,143]

Surgical repair has to be balanced against the functional demands of the patient. Active patients with significant functional demands should be treated operatively. Inactive elderly patients with low functional requirements do reasonably well with nonoperative management, consisting of acceptance of displacement and initiation of a range of motion program after a period of immobilization. In active elderly patients with greater functional demands, operative management is preferred. Techniques for repair include screw fixation alone, or in combination with tension band wire or suture, when good quality bone is present. When bone quality is compromised, tension band fixation with suture or wire is preferred. The rotator cuff tear must be repaired. We use a deltoid-splitting approach placed for optimal exposure of the fragment and its bed.

Surgical Technique: Greater Tuberosity Fracture

Preservation of the origin, innervation, and subsequent function of the deltoid is of utmost importance. The skin incision is made in Langer's lines over the anterolateral corner of the acromion and is 7 to 8 cm in length (Fig. 16A). This incision can be placed more posteriorly when the posterior portion of the greater tuberosity is involved. The skin is then undermined superiorly and inferiorly to obtain adequate exposure. The deltoid is split for 4 to 5 cm distal to the lateral aspect of the acromion. A stay suture is placed within the deltoid at the same distance, to avoid injury to the axillary nerve by preventing further splitting of the deltoid beyond the 5-cm point. A needle tip electrocautery is helpful in minimizing trauma to the deltoid during the split. The muscle is then retracted and adhesions lysed in the subdeltoid space with a blunt instrument, such as a Darrach elevator. The subacromial space is freed of bursa, scar tissue, fracture hematoma, and debris with sharp dissection and irrigation. This will now expose the fracture bed (Fig. 16B). Internal rotation and extension of the arm will aid in delivering the fracture fragment into the wound, for it is often superiorly and posteriorly displaced by the supraspinatus and infraspinatus–teres minor insertions, respectively. Control and mobilization of the greater tuberosity is then obtained with no. 5 nonabsorbable sutures placed at the bone–tendon interface at the level of the superior, middle, and inferior facets to correct both superior and posterior displacement. This incorporates the stronger rotator cuff tendon, rather than placing the suture through what is usually the osteoporotic bone of the tuberosity, where it may easily cut out. Before fracture reduction, drill holes are placed around the distal periphery of the bed for suture fixation.

Downward and forward traction on the sutures reduces the fragment into its bed. The fragment may have to be trimmed to prevent residual prominence causing impingement in abduction. These fractures are found in association with rotator cuff tears that are often either rotator interval tears or tears between the supraspinatus and infraspinatus, depending on the fracture location. Before fixation of the fragment, the sutures can be placed across the rotator cuff tear. This will facilitate the repair after fracture fixation. Repair of the rotator cuff is essential to optimize postoperative functional outcomes. The tuberosity is secured to its bed with the previously placed nonabsorbable no. 5 sutures in a figure eight fashion through the drill holes in the shaft and the bone tendon interface[143] (Fig. 16C,D). The rotator cuff sutures are then tied. The shoulder should be placed through a range of motion to assess fracture fixation. The deltoid is then closed meticulously side to side, also with nonabsorbable sutures to ensure healing.

An early passive range of motion program can be initiated, similar to that used following rotator cuff repairs. Active range of motion should not be started for 6 weeks, until the fracture and rotator cuff have healed sufficiently. This method of treatment in 12 patients with displaced greater tuberosity fractures led to 6 excellent and 6 good results.[143]

Surgical Neck

Two-part surgical neck fractures are quite common in the elderly. In these fractures, the shaft may be completely displaced and pulled medially by the deforming force of the pectoralis major, or it may be impacted and angulated at the surgical neck area. Each type of fracture pattern requires a different treatment approach. Treatment depends on fracture stability and the displacement pattern. Posterior angulation is more tolerable than varus or anterior angulation.[53] Impacted fractures with less than 45-degree angulation may be treated nonoperatively with early motion. Impacted fractures with greater than 45-degree–anterior angulation may limit forward elevation. Therefore, disimpaction, followed by reimpaction to achieve better alignment, should be considered in active patients.

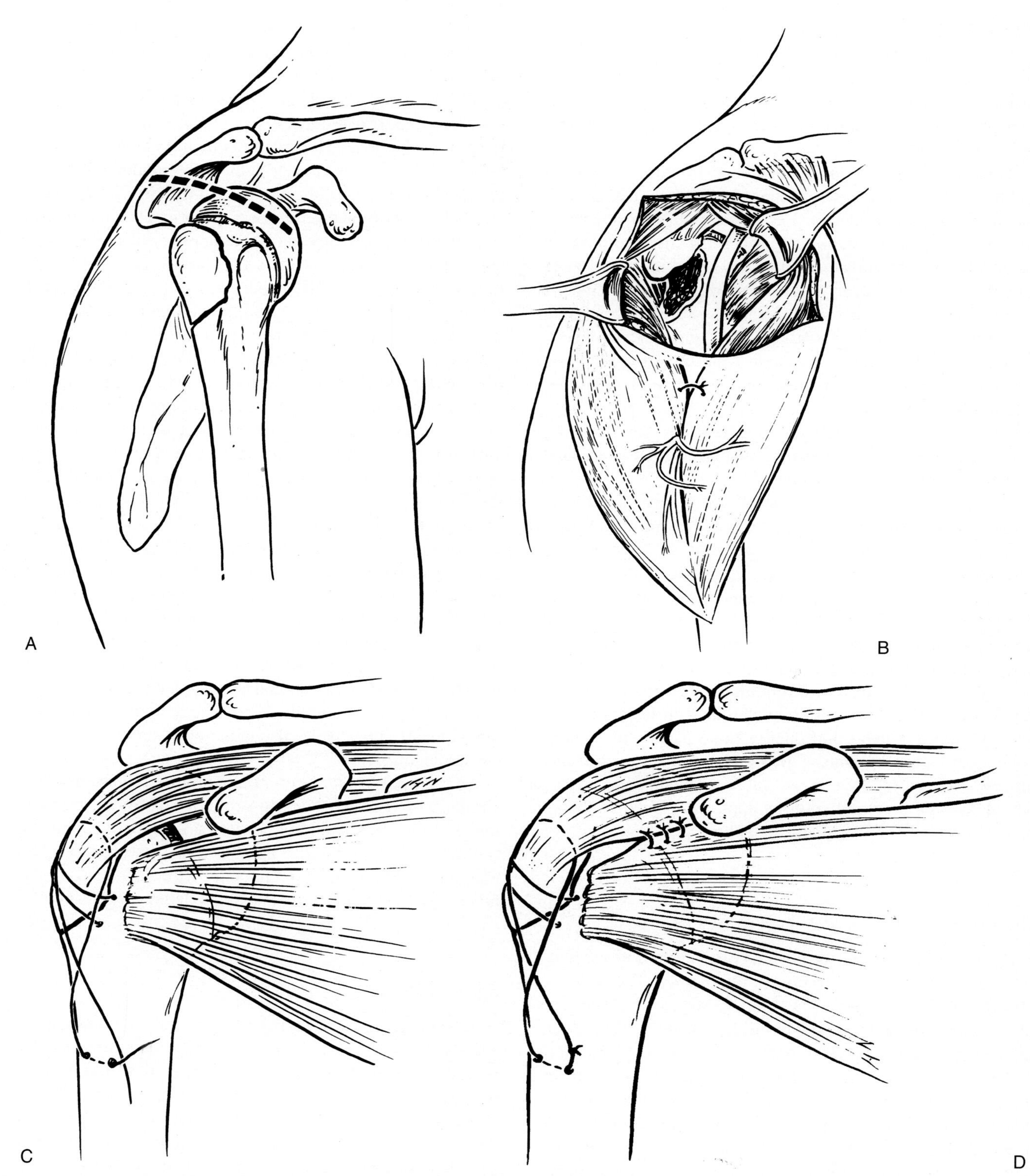

FIG. 16. Surgical technique of greater tuberosity fracture (see text): **(A)** Skin incision: the deltoid is split no more than 5 cm from the lateral aspect of the acromion. **(B)** The fracture bed is exposed. **(C)** The fracture is reduced and secured into place using no. 5 nonabsorbable sutures in figure eight fashion through drill holes in the shaft and bone tendon junction. **(D)** The rotator interval tear is closed.

Closed Reduction

When there is complete medial displacement of the shaft, achieving an acceptable functional outcome will require reduction of the fracture. We prefer to perform a closed reduction under anesthesia (regional or general) to obtain better muscle relaxation. The maneuver to achieve closed reduction requires adduction and flexion of the arm across the chest to relax the pull of the pectoralis major. The shaft is then displaced proximally for impaction into the proximal humeral fragment. In thin patients, the proximal fragment can be stabilized manually to enhance impaction. We use fluoroscopy for this maneuver, not only for the initial evaluation of the reduction but, more importantly, to evaluate the stability of the reduction. If the reduction is stable, the arm can be placed in Velpeau type immobilization (with appropriate padding) with the arm across the chest. Immobilization should be continued for approximately 3 weeks. Radiographs should be repeated during the first week to be certain displacement has not occurred. When there is radiographic evidence of healing or the fracture is stable clinically, an active assisted range of motion program can be initiated.

If the fracture can be reduced closed, but remains unstable when assessed fluoroscopically, the fracture requires fixation to maintain reduction and allow healing and initiation of range of motion. This can be accomplished in a few different ways.

Percutaneous Pinning Technique. Percutaneous pinning has been described as a useful alternative to open reduction and internal fixation for displaced proximal humerus fractures[144] that can be reduced closed, but remain unstable. Jaberg[145] reported good or excellent clinical results in 34 (70%) of 48 patients treated in this manner; 29 of these 48 patients had two-part surgical neck fractures. Before preparing and draping the patient, a closed reduction is performed to confirm that an acceptable reduction can be obtained. Before (AP and lateral) image intensification is used, the patient is positioned supine on the operating table with the arm abducted 70 to 80 degrees. To prevent loss of reduction, it has been recommended that the arm not be moved, but instead, the image intensifier repositioned to obtain acceptable axillary and AP views.[146]

Closed reduction is achieved using progressive longitudinal traction on the arm and laterally directed traction on the humeral shaft. The residual anterior angulation in the coronal plane of most fracture patterns is corrected by placing posteriorly directed pressure on the anterior aspect of the humeral shaft.[145] The slight medial displacement of the proximal fragment, relative to the shaft, permits the placement of at least one pin centrally in the humeral head. A 45-degree angle of insertion into the lateral humeral cortex is recommended, changing the angle to 30 degrees once the pin passes through the cortex. This will allow pins to pass sufficiently distal to the fracture line and obtain good purchase. The pins should enter above the insertion of the deltoid to avoid injury to the radial nerve and distal enough from the acromion to avoid injury to the axillary nerve.

Terminally threaded AO pins, 2.5 mm in diameter, inserted with a power drill without predrilling is recommended. Two pins are passed through the lateral aspect of the shaft just above the deltoid insertion across the fracture site and into subchondral bone, with the location and position confirmed with image intensification. A third pin is passed from the anterior cortex into the subchondral bone of the humeral head. The pins must be widely spaced within the humeral head to enhance fixation stability. The pins are trimmed so that they remain subcutaneous. A Velpeau dressing is applied to immobilize the arm.

Another technique has been described by Kristiansen.[148] He placed a Steinmann pin into the head for control to achieve reduction. Two half pins with continuous threads were drilled into the humeral head; two or three pins were inserted into the humeral shaft. A Hoffman external fixator neutralizing bar was applied. When the reduction was confirmed radiographically, the Steinmann pin was removed. Postoperative care includes radiographs at 10 days to evaluate for pin migration. Functional exercises start early, and active use of the arm is encouraged. All pins are removed between 4 and 6 weeks, when there is radiographic evidence of fracture healing. A more aggressive physical therapy program is then initiated.

Schanz pins and Kirschner wires can be placed percutaneously if an adequate closed reduction can be achieved. This technique provides the benefits of closed reduction and minimal soft-tissue dissection. However, placement of percutaneous pins is technically demanding and has been associated with superficial pin tract infection and migration.[145] Smooth pins and wires have a high potential to migrate and are best avoided around the shoulder.[149]

Previously, for fractures that could be reduced, but were unstable, we used percutaneous pin fixation followed by 3 weeks of immobilization. However, we have had some difficulty obtaining adequate fixation of the proximal fragment. This has led to loss of reduction. The angle of inclination for proper pin insertion often makes it difficult to obtain adequate fixation in both segments. In addition, some of our patients have complained about the pins even though they were cut off under the skin. Our experience attests to the exacting nature of this technique and the importance of the learning curve.

Open Reduction

If the closed reduction is unstable or an acceptable reduction cannot be obtained, open reduction and internal fixation is indicated. Recently, operative approaches have emphasized minimal soft-tissue dissection combined with secure fixation, with the objective to preserve the vascularity to the articular segment.[11,33,62,150–160] In young patients or in elderly patients with good bone quality, internal fixation using a T-plate and screws or a blade plate has been successfully employed. However, this requires a fairly extensive operative exposure that increases the risk of devascularization of the articular segment.[4,5] The three most common postoperative complications after plate fixation of the proximal humerus are impingement of the hardware under the acromion as a result of proximal placement of the plate, loss of fixation, and osteonecrosis of the humeral head.[161–163,170] Plate placement in a medial position may block internal rotation. If possible, one of the screws in the plate should be placed across the fracture site as a "lag screw" for additional fixation. If good stability is obtained, range of motion exercises can be started immediately.

Naidu et al. have shown that when performing percutaneous pinning of surgical neck fractures, a multiplanar pin construct optimizes torsional stiffness and the addition of tuberosity pins augments the bending stiffness.[210] Williams et al. demonstrated that the addition of intramedullary rods to figure eight interfragmentary wiring in the fixation of two-part surgical neck fractures of the proximal humerus significantly improved maximum load generated by rotational displacement.[211]

We recently performed a biomechanical cadaver study to compare the mechanical stability of ten different fixation techniques to stabilize surgical neck fractures of the proximal humerus in both osteopenic and nonosteopenic bone. T-plates and screws provided the strongest fixation in nonosteopenic bone. However, their effectiveness decreased in the presence of osteopenia. The Enders rod–tension band construct was the second strongest fixation technique, providing significantly stronger fixation than all of the remaining techniques. The strongest fixation in embalmed specimens was obtained with four Schantz pins, with one pin placed through the greater tuberosity followed by the T-plate and screws construct. Tension band fixation alone in both humeral groups provided the least effective fixation in both osteopenic and nonosteopenic bone.[164]

Surgical Technique. Open reduction and internal fixation (ORIF) of displaced surgical neck fractures is most easily performed through a deltopectoral approach (Fig.17A). When the fracture is adequately exposed, the shaft and head are mobilized and the fracture site is curetted (Fig. 17B,C). The humeral shaft is mobilized gently, and control of the humeral head is gained either by placing heavy suture at the tuberosity bone–tendon interface or with skin hooks. This will allow reduction of the head to the top of the shaft (Fig. 17D). Reduction is obtained by forward elevation of the shaft while gently pulling on the sutures controlling the head. The fracture is then impacted and the arm lowered while maintaining tension on the sutures to prevent loss of reduction.

Once adequate reduction is achieved, fixation is accomplished using a combination of tension band suture and intramedullary rods. Eighteen-gauge wire may be substituted for heavy nonabsorbable suture. Although it provides greater immediate stability, it is more difficult to handle and carries the risk of breakage and migration, which can irritate the subacromial space. Therefore, we prefer suture whenever possible. Ender nails (3.5 mm) are superior to straight rods or pins, such as Rush rods, in that they afford three-point fixation, which enhances rotational stability. The addition of the tension band configuration with intramedullary nails adds even greater longitudinal and rotational stability over that of either tension banding or intramedullary nailing alone.[164] This augmented fixation is of even greater importance when there is associated comminution of the fracture site with less inherent stability.[165]

While maintaining reduction, small longitudinal incisions are made at the insertion of the rotator cuff fibers into the greater and lesser tuberosity. These will be the sites for nail insertion. Ender nails are preferred not only for stability, as previously noted, but also for the ability to place a figure eight suture or wire through the eyelet to prevent proximal migration and impingement, which often occurs with nonfenestrated straight rods.[165,166] However, the slot of the Ender nail is long and a significant amount of metal may still protrude proximally. Therefore, the nail can be modified with placement of an additional hole above the slot. This permits deeper insertion of the nail into the humeral head, placing the tip well below the rotator cuff tendon.[165]

The site for nail insertion is dependent on the associated fractures. The goal is to insert the nail through an intact tuberosity. In the absence of tuberosity fractures, the greater tuberosity is the better choice because two nails may be used here, as opposed to the lesser tuberosity that can only accommodate one nail. Therefore, anterior and posterior longitudinal incisions are made in the supraspinatus tendon over the greater tuberosity and an awl is used to penetrate the bone. The posterior nail is best placed initially because levering on this partially inserted nail will aide in holding the reduction and preventing the humeral head from falling posteriorly (Fig. 17E). The second nail is then inserted 1.0 to 1.5 cm anteriorly. It is best to use nails of different lengths to prevent the possibility of a distal stress riser.[165] Nails between 22 and 27 cm in length are generally adequate. Before completely burying the nails, two drill holes are made in the shaft lateral to the biceps tendon for placement of the tension band suture or wire. A figure eight suture or wire (no. 5 nonabsorbable suture or 18-gauge wire) is then passed through the eyelets of the nails, passing it deep to the rotator cuff tendon between the nails to prevent proximal migration and then through the predrilled holes in the shaft. Before tying the suture or twisting both ends of the wire, the nails are impacted well below the cuff, and fracture reduction is evaluated (Fig. 17F).

Once the figure eight is secured, range of motion and fixation stability are assessed to carefully guide the postoperative rehabilitation without stressing the repair. The rotator cuff incisions and deltopectoral interval are closed, usually over suction drainage.

Use of intramedullary fixation and tension band wiring avoids the problems of intraarticular insertion that are possible with either plate and screws or percutaneous pins. Antegrade-placed Ender nails, however, may require removal if migration causes subacromial impingement during forward

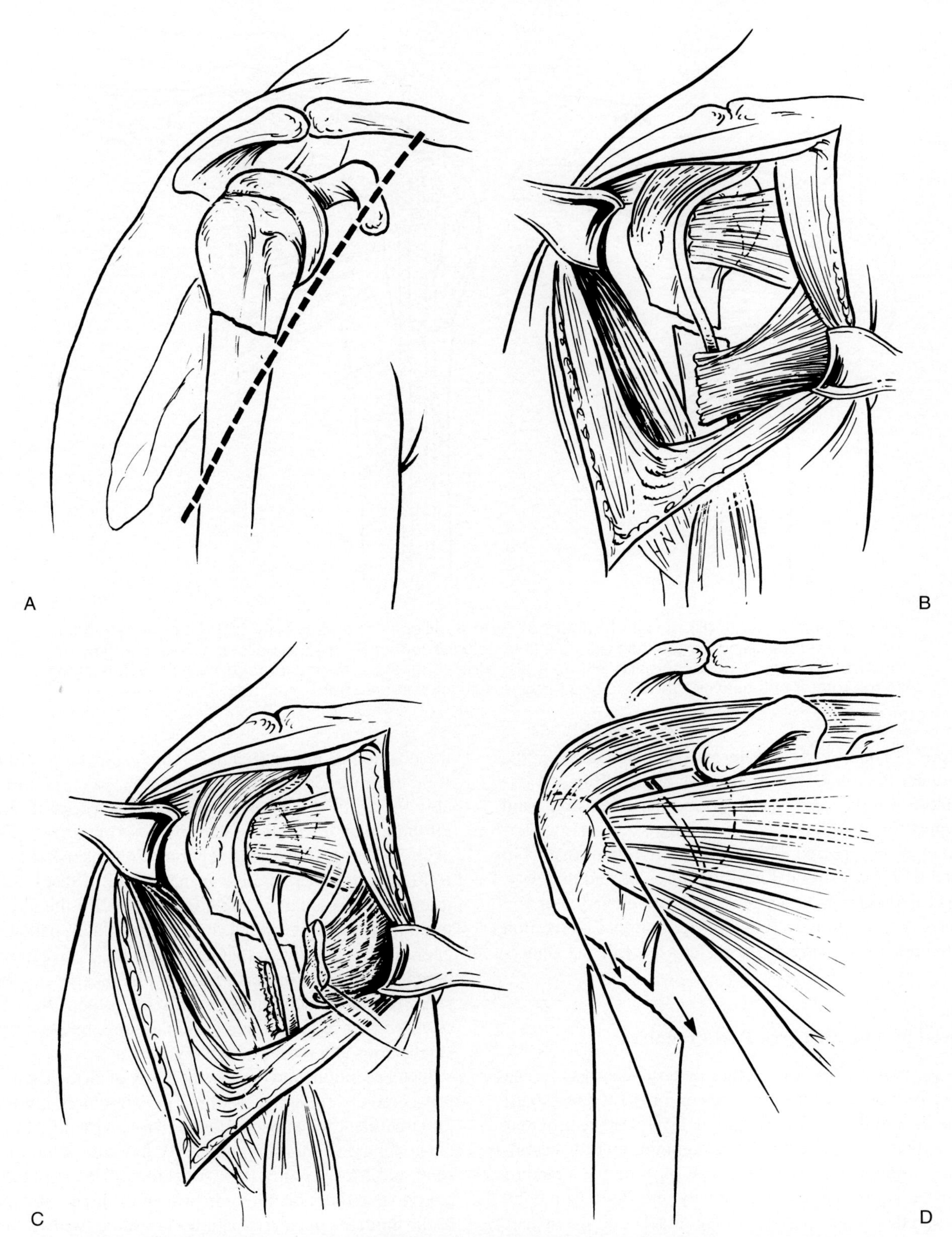

FIG. 17. Open reduction and internal fixation of surgical neck fracture (see text): **(A)** Incision for deltopectoral approach; **(B)** exposure of the fracture; **(C)** partial release of the pectoralis major tendon may help with identifying the biceps tendon and surrounding anatomy and with fracture reduction; **(D)** the fracture is reduced controlling the humeral head with skin hooks or no. 5 suture at the bone tendon interphase; *(continued)*

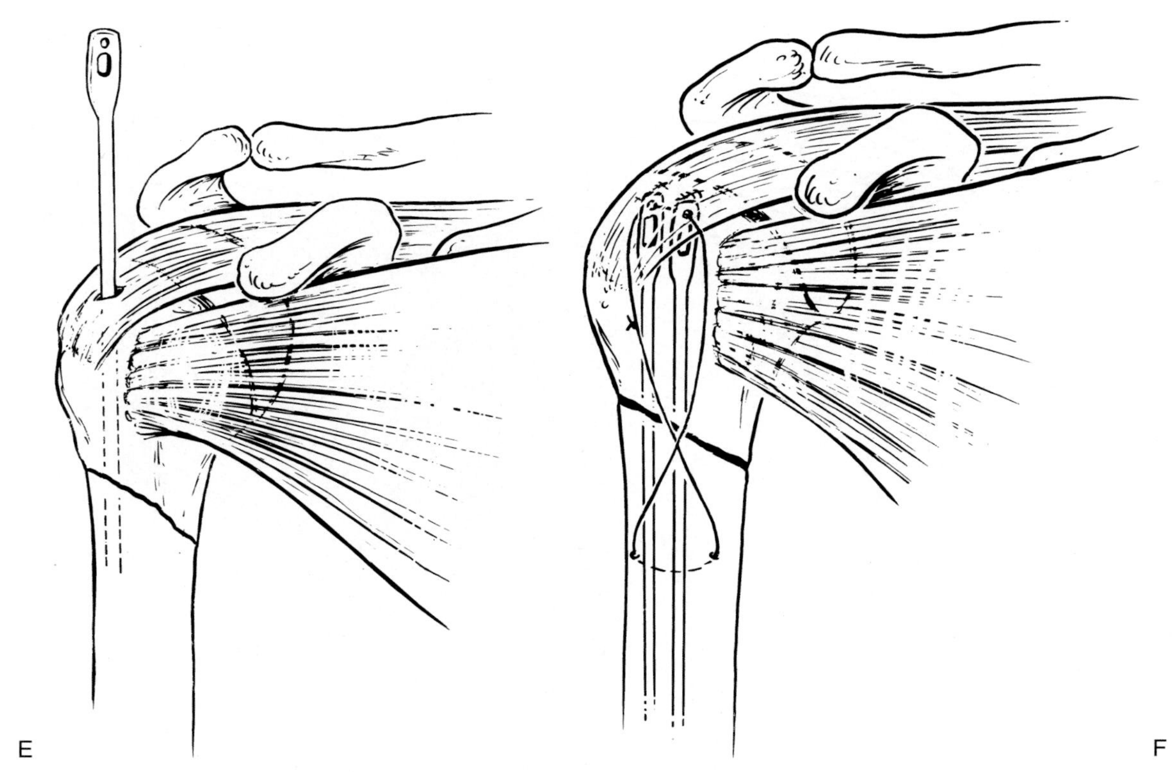

FIG. 17. *(continued).* **(E)** modified Ender nail (with additional hole above the slot) being inserted into greater tuberosity and across the fracture site to hold the reduction; **(F)** two nails of different lengths are passed, and a no. 5 nonabsorbable suture is placed in figure eight fashion through the nail eyelets, deep to the rotator cuff between the nails and through drill holes in the shaft.

elevation.[168] The modified Ender nail and placement of the suture under the rotator cuff helps avoid this problem.

Variable results have been reported using tension band techniques for surgical neck fractures.[153,167] However, Cuomo et al.[168] reported 82% good and excellent results in two- and three-part surgical neck fractures treated this way. Patients achieved an average active forward elevation of 142 degrees. Complications included one partial loss of fixation and late humeral fracture at the distal aspect of the Enders nail.

Displaced Fractures: Three-Part Fractures

Two types of three-part fracture patterns can occur. The first type is displacement of the greater tuberosity and shaft, with the lesser tuberosity remaining attached to the articular segment. This pattern occurs more commonly. The second, and less commonly, encountered type of three-part fracture is displacement of the lesser tuberosity and shaft segments, with the greater tuberosity remaining attached to the articular segment.

Treatment options for these fractures include closed reduction, open reduction and internal fixation, or prosthetic replacement. At best, an adequate closed reduction is difficult to achieve, and more difficult to maintain, because the deforming muscular forces cannot be adequately offset by the position of immobilization. The results of closed reduction for three-part fractures have been quite variable.[19,30,136,169,170,188] Neer reported no successful results in 20 three-part fractures treated by closed reduction.[19] However, Young and Wallace reported 76% acceptable results following the nonoperative management of displaced fractures.[136] Unfortunately, they did not specify the number of three-part fractures treated. Leyson treated 34 patients nonoperatively with 76% satisfactory results.[188] Because of inherent difficulties in performing a prospective randomized study for these uncommon injuries, the orthopedic literature on three-part proximal humerus fractures comprises mainly small series and retrospective reviews.

One exception, however, is the study of Zyto et al.[171] They prospectively followed 37 three-part fractures randomized into treatment with open reduction and internal fixation with tension band versus sling and early motion. Using the Constant and Murly score, they concluded that the outcome of operative and nonoperative treatment of three-part fractures of the humerus in elderly patients is similar, with more complications found in the surgically treated group. Criteria to be in the study included injuries not caused by high-energy trauma, at least 30% contact between the humeral head and shaft, and the ability of the patients to cooperate. They did not specify the methods used to classify the fracture patterns or whether interobserver selectablity issues were considered.

Currently, open reduction and internal fixation is the treatment of choice for uncomplicated three-part fractures of the proximal humerus.[26,153,168,172,173] Paavolainen et al. reported 74% satisfactory results in a series of 14 three-part fractures treated operatively with screws alone or plate and screw devices.[162] Hawkins et al. reported 87% satisfactory results using tension band wire technique in 15 patients with an average age of 61 years; postoperative forward elevation averaged 126 degrees and osteonecrosis occurred in 13% of patients.[153] Cuomo et al. reported 100% satisfactory results after open reduction and internal fixation of three-part fractures in eight patients with an average age of 45 years; forward elevation averaged 150 degrees and no osteonecrosis occurred after an average 3.3 years of follow-up.[168] Of the 31 patients with three-part fractures that Neer treated operatively, results were excellent or satisfactory in 19. He felt that most of the unsatisfactory results were secondary to inadequate fixation.[10]

Different techniques of internal fixation have been used for these fractures, including plate and screws, percutaneous pins, tension band wires, and intramedullary devices.[53,152,162,173–175,181]

Percutaneous pinning is performed as described previously for two-part fractures; if the greater tuberosity is displaced, two pins should be inserted into the greater tuberosity, with engagement of the medial cortex of the humeral shaft.[145–148] Resch recommends advancing a cannula and blunt trocar superomedially and then following the bone inferiorly with the sheath to deflect the axillary nerve and, thereby, avoid injury.[147]

The T-plate has been commonly used for three-part fractures of the proximal humerus. However, recent reports from several investigators have documented poor results with this implant.[162,170,175a,202] Complications with a T-plate include increased risk of osteonecrosis, superior placement of the plate leading to impingement, loss of plate fixation with screw loosening, malunion, and infection. Because of its relative stiffness, the AO-plate cannot be bent to exactly fit the lateral aspect of the proximal humerus, nor can the T-part of the plate be contoured to exactly fit the curve of the tuberosities. The two large cancellous screws placed through the proximal portion of the plate can cause extensive damage to the bony shell of the tuberosities before penetrating into the humeral head. For the screws to have some purchase on the tuberosities, the plate must be placed as proximal as possible, which can cause impingement. In addition, the anterior arm of the T-plate rests on the biceps tendon and any compression between the plate and the humeral head for more stable fixation will compress the tendon against the bone. Thus, the AO plate is more appropriately used for two-part surgical neck fractures, because it can be placed more distally and tuberosity fixation is not required.[162,170,175a,176]

Esser treated 26 patients (average age of 55 years), 16 with three-part fractures and 10 with four-part fractures, with a modified cloverleaf plate. All patients with three-part fractures had excellent results using the American Shoulder and Elbow Surgeons rating system. exactly fit the proximal part of the h 4.0-mm cancellous screws could be i and the tuberosities. This implant could b imal, covering the entire greater tuberosity quent impingement observed. However, Esser a demanding procedure, even for the exper geon.[177,184]

In general, the trend for three-part fractures has be ward avoidance of plate-and-screw fixation because of difficulties in obtaining adequate fixation in osteoporoti bone.[160] High incidences of postoperative pain, disability, osteonecrosis (from 12% to 34%), nonunion, malunion, and other complications have been reported with open reduction and internal fixation of three-part fractures in elderly patients with osteoporosis or extensive comminution of the fracture.[26,64,158,162,163,170,172,178–181,185,186,200] Thus, with these fracture patterns, prosthetic replacement with tuberosity reconstruction is a more reasonable treatment alternative in elderly patients.

The results with prosthetic replacement have generally been good. Neer reported 8 of 11 satisfactory results in three-part fractures of all types in his initial series.[10] Other authors have reported variable but generally satisfactory results with prosthetic replacement for three-part fractures.[64,158,182,183]

Our preferred approach for three-part fractures in the elderly is open reduction and internal fixation, using a tension band technique in combination with Enders nail. The degree of difficulty of these injuries becomes clear when operative intervention is undertaken. Attention to detail, anatomy, and fracture fixation is mandatory. If there is significant comminution or very poor bone quality, we prefer prosthetic replacement.

Surgical Technique: Three-Part Fractures

A deltopectoral approach affords the most extensive exposure. After developing this interval, the sternal head of the pectoralis may be partially released as needed. At this point, identifying the long head of the biceps tendon becomes extremely helpful in identifying the surrounding anatomy. The biceps is found directly beneath the pectoralis insertion. Once located, it is followed up to the bicipital groove and rotator interval, which is incised to the glenoid rim if the fracture displacement has not already accomplished this. Dividing the rotator interval enhances exposure and fragment mobilization. The tuberosities can be identified by their relation to the biceps tendon, with the greater being lateral and the lesser located medial to the tendon. The displaced tuberosity, greater or lesser, is then mobilized with heavy nonabsorbable suture at the tendon insertion site. The fracture site is curetted and irrigated. The head and attached tuberosity are mobilized with skin hooks and sutures at the bone–tendon interface, as previously described for two-part surgical neck fractures. If the articular surface is dislocated,

...n on the sutures

...ments is begun ...agments are re- ...sity to the head ...rbable suture ...aving one su- ...re eight fixa- ...ad and fixed ...eviously de- ...re is carried ...l tuberosity. ... are inserted; ... the lesser is the site of insertion (Fig. 18B). Four drill holes are then placed in the shaft for a figure eight fixation of both the fractured tuberosity and head. One set of holes is placed lateral to the bicipital groove and the other medial. The involved tuberosity is therefore secured both to the head and the uninvolved tuberosity, in addition to being secured to the shaft; the surgical neck fracture is fixed to the shaft with a combination of intramedullary nailing and tension band fixation. Fracture stability is then assessed, and the limits of postoperative rehabilitation are determined accordingly. The rotator interval and incisions for nail placement are repaired, as is the deltopectoral interval. The skin is closed in layers.

Passive range of motion can usually be started early in the postoperative period, depending on the security of the fixation. Active range of motion should not be started for 6 weeks until adequate fracture healing has occurred.

If secure fixation cannot be obtained by the tension band technique, either because of osteoporosis or excessive comminution of the fragments, or if the remaining soft-tissue attachments to the articular surface are tenuous, hemiarthroplasty with tuberosity reconstruction is preferred. The technique and postoperative rehabilitation for a prosthetic replacement will be discussed in the section on four-part fractures.

Displaced Fractures: Four-Part Fractures

Valgus Impacted

In "classic" four-part fractures, all four segments are displaced and the articular surface is devoid of soft-tissue attachments. This results in disruption of the blood supply to the humeral head and a high likelihood of osteonecrosis. There is great variation in the reported incidence of os-

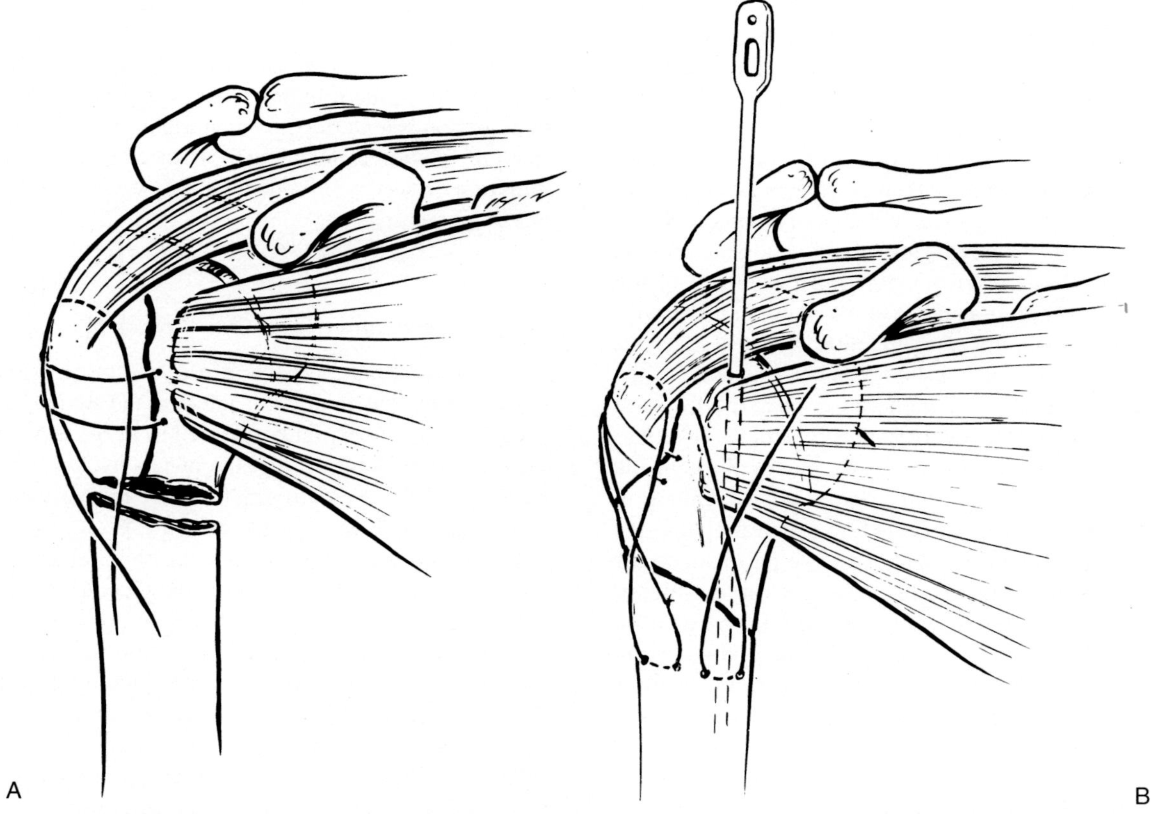

FIG. 18. Open reduction and internal fixation of three-part fracture (see text): **(A)** The three fragments are reduced to two by securing the displaced tuberosity to the head and intact tuberosity by a no. 5 nonabsorbable suture. This is then reduced to the shaft and a modified Ender nail is placed through the uninvolved tuberosity across the fracture site. **(B)** Figure eight fixation of both the fracture tuberosity and head to the shaft is done.

teonecrosis after these injuries, ranging from 21% to 75%.[10,11,163,180,187,188] Neer reported osteonecrosis in 6 of 8 patients with four-part fractures treated with open reduction and internal fixation.[10] Leyson reported osteonecrosis in 6 of 8 treated nonoperatively.[188] Lee and Hansen reported a 21% incidence.[180] The variation could be secondary to the inclusion of four-part valgus impacted fractures, which have a lower rate of osteonecrosis. In this fracture pattern type, the articular segment is impacted and angulated, rather than displaced, and may thus retain its vascularity from the posterior medial vessels traveling within the periosteum.[7,199] Theoretically, this source of blood supply can be interrupted by either a fracture line passing along the edge of the articular surface or through destruction of these vessels by lateral displacement of the articular segment relative to the main distal fragment.[189] Brookes simulated four-part fractures in cadavers and found that perfusion of the humeral head was prevented, unless the head fragment extended distally below the articular surface medially; this allowed some perfusion of the head to persist by the anastomoses of the posterior medial vessels with the arcuate artery.[7]

Reconstruction rather than replacement for the valgus impacted humeral head fracture has been extensively discussed in the recent literature, because the rate of osteonecrosis following this fracture pattern has been much lower than with the classic four-part fracture.[190] Jakob et al. reported that only 5 out of 19 (26%) valgus impacted fractures developed osteonecrosis after either treatment by closed (5 patients) or open (14 patients) reduction and minimal internal fixation with either AO screws or K-wires. They believed that replacement of the humeral head was not indicated because 74% of these patients had good results after 4 years. However, they also did not advocate nonoperative treatment because of anticipated problems with joint incongruity, impingement from the malpositioned tuberosities, and shoulder stiffness.[11]

More recently Resch et al.[189] performed an open reduction in 22 valgus impacted humeral head fractures by elevating the impacted humeral head, relocating the tuberosities, and filling the void with cancellous bone chips. Minimal osteosynthesis was used, with 1.8-mm K-wires to secure the head to the shaft and with numerous sutures anchoring the tuberosities to each other and the shaft. At minimum follow-up of 18 months, the incidence of osteonecrosis was only 9%, and a positive correlation was found between the quality of reduction achieved and the functional results. Three of 22 patients had moderate arthrosis at follow-up. The authors suggested that the low incidence of osteonecrosis and encouraging results were also related to the relatively young patient age (average 52 years) and the strict inclusion criterion for reconstruction (minimal lateral displacement of the shaft in relation to the head, which minimizes damage to the medial periosteal vascularity).[189,190]

In a small series of 8 patients (average age 66 years) of four-part valgus impacted fractures, Vandenbussche et al.[191] anatomically reconstructed the fracture by rai pacted segment of the humeral head, filling the void w tologous and tricortical iliac bone graft, and relocating tuberosities with transosseus suture fixation to each other and the shaft. No hardware was placed. On follow-up of 7 of these patients, an average of 16 months from the procedure, two results were excellent and three good or very good according to Constant criteria. Radiographic findings showed healing and incorporation of the graft in all cases. MRI results showed only one asymptomatic partial osteonecrosis (14%). This is the technique that we have employed, with the exception that we prefer to use corticocancellous allograft chips, rather than the additional procedure of iliac crest bone grafting (Fig. 19).

Classic Four-Part Fractures

The results of nonoperative treatment for classic four-part fractures have been consistently unsatisfactory as reported in the literature. Studies that appear to show acceptable results with nonoperative treatment of displaced fractures either have included no true four-part fractures or the classification of the fractures was such that an analysis of four-part fractures was not possible. Compito et al. reviewed 97 fractures from five series of true four-part fractures treated nonoperatively and showed that this resulted in a satisfactory outcome in only 5%.[192]

Open reduction and internal fixation of four-part fractures has consistently yielded poor results. Compito's analysis of the literature of true four-part fractures treated with open reduction and internal fixation showed 17 satisfactory outcomes (30%) of 56 fractures in five series.[192] Neer reported 100% unsatisfactory results in 13 cases.[10] Sturzenegger et al. reported 8 unsatisfactory results in 13 cases.[163] Mouridan reported satisfactory results in 6 out 7 four-part fractures treated with his modified Zickel nail, but 4 of the 6 developed osteonecrosis; patients were followed for only an average of 18 months.[181]

Adequate open reduction and secure internal fixation is difficult to achieve. In the elderly, the head segment is often a shell that cannot be adequately stabilized using tension band techniques. Because of problems in achieving stable internal fixation and a high risk of osteonecrosis, primary hemiarthroplasty with tuberosity reconstruction has become the treatment of choice for four-part fractures, particularly in the elderly.

In selected younger patients with good bone stock, open reduction and internal fixation may be attempted, but there is a high risk of osteonecrosis, particularly because these usually are the results of higher-energy injuries.[11,29,163] Hardware problems are commonly encountered as well.[29,162,163] There are no large series in the literature on the results of open reduction and internal fixation of four-part fractures in younger patients to help guide treatment. Primary hemiarthroplasty has been advocated by some in these young patients, because a more consistent clinical result can be ob-

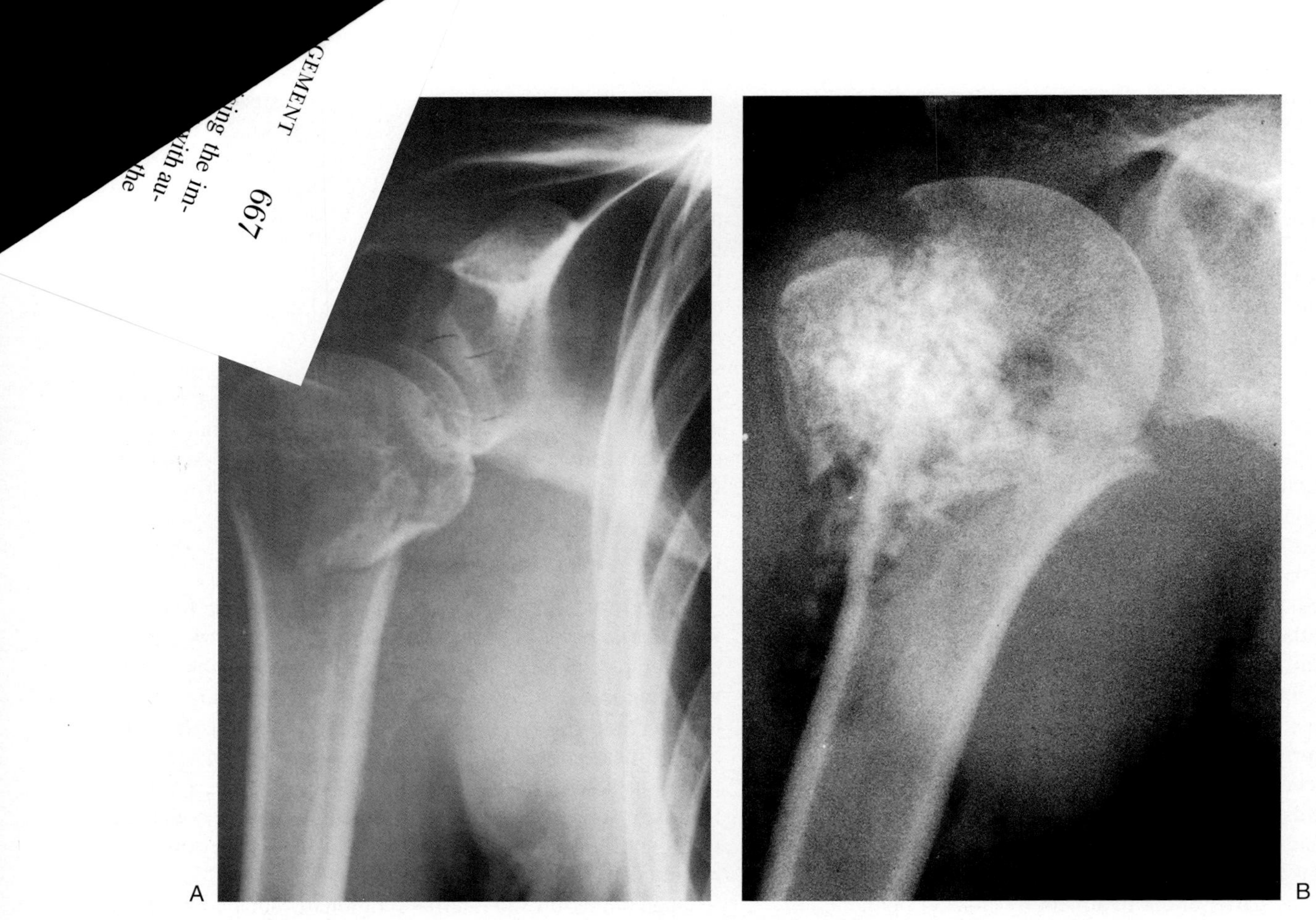

FIG. 19. **(A)** Anteroposterior view of four-part valgus impacted fracture. **(B)** Fracture fixed by raising the impacted segment of the humeral head, filling the void with cortical cancellous allograft bone chips, and relocating the tuberosities with transosseous suture fixation to each other and the shaft.

tained and poor functional outcome from complications of malunion and osteonecrosis following open reduction and internal fixation can be avoided. Also, primary hemiarthroplasty yields better results than hemiarthroplasty for revision of failed ORIF. In revision or salvage procedures, severe soft-tissue scarring and contractures, disuse osteoporosis, and tuberosity malunions are frequently encountered. Therefore, most agree the initial procedure is the best opportunity to obtain a good clinical outcome.[193]

The reported results of humeral head replacement for a four-part fracture have been variable but generally satisfactory.[19,62,158,182,183,194,195] The variability is probably related to both patient selection and the outcome criteria used. Compito et al. reviewed nine series of true four-part fractures treated with humeral head replacement and found 80% (136 of 171) satisfactory or better results.[192] Pain relief after humeral head replacement is fairly predictable in most series. Functional results can be quite variable.[196] Neer reported 100% satisfactory results in seven patients following hemiarthroplasty for four-part fractures.[19] McIlveen and Neer reported equally satisfactory results in a larger series of patients.[194] Tanner and Cofield reported satisfactory pain relief in their series of 8 patients with acute four-part fractures.[158] Stableforth prospectively studied 32 patients with four-part fractures; 16 patients treated by hemiarthroplasty made a more complete functional recovery in half the time, compared with the group treated nonoperatively. Range of motion and level of comfort were consistently better in the hemiarthroplasty group.[62] Willems and Lim reported a pain-free shoulder in 9 of 10 patients, but only 4 had satisfactory functional results.[195] Switlyk and Hawkins reported 60% fair or poor results in their series of 20 shoulders.[183] They stressed the importance of careful patient selection, meticulous surgical technique, and a supervised postoperative rehabilitation program.[183]

Green et al. studied 22 patients with humeral head replacements using the American Shoulder and Elbow Surgeons evaluation form. They found an average active forward elevation of 100 degrees, average active external rotation of 30 degrees, and average active internal rotation to the L-1 vertebra. Patients younger than 60 years had better functional range of motion than did older patients. Functional outcome was variable and appeared to depend on age and pain.[197]

Goldman et al., in a series from our institution, also found humeral head replacement for acute three- (12 fractures) and four- (14 fractures) part fractures effectively relieves pain (73%), but recovery of active motion and function were not as predictable. Active range of motion was significantly influenced by age, fracture type, and sex. Age older than 70 years, four-part fractures, and female sex correlated with a poorer recovery of active range of motion. Active forward elevation averaged 107 degrees, external rotation averaged 31 degrees, and internal rotation averaged to the L-2 vertebra. Three-part fractures averaged 31 degrees more forward elevation, 10 degrees more external rotation, and three vertebral segments more in internal rotation than four-part fractures. We also stress meticulous care in tuberosity reattachment and rotator cuff repair, soft-tissue tensioning, and an intensive supervised rehabilitation program with a well motivated patient as factors contributing to a successful outcome.[196]

Wretenberg and Ekelund evaluated the outcome of acute shoulder hemiathroplasty in 18 patients (mean follow-up of 3.5 years) following 7 displaced three-part, and 11 displaced four-part fractures in patients with a mean age of 82 years old (range 70 to 92 years old). They found their older patients recovered less motion than reported for younger patients. They believed that the tuberosity fragments, which were more osteoporotic and comminuted than in younger patients, did not allow secure reattachment; in addition, the elderly patients' inability to participate fully in the intense and prolonged rehabilitation program further compromised functional outcome.[198]

Indications and Surgical Technique of Proximal Humeral Replacement. Indications for prosthetic replacement following acute proximal humeral fractures include (a) four-part fractures and fracture–dislocations, as described; (b) three-part fractures and fracture–dislocations in elderly patients with osteoporotic bone, particularly with nondisplaced comminution; (c) head-splitting fractures; (d) anatomic neck fractures that cannot be adequately reduced and internally fixed; and (e) chronic anterior or posterior humeral head dislocations with impression fractures that involve more than 40% of the articular surface.

The basic principles of the surgical technique include (a) use of the deltopectoral approach that preserves the origin and insertion of the deltoid muscle; (b) insertion of the proximal humeral prosthesis to restore humeral length and proper retroversion; and (c) fixation of the tuberosities to the prosthesis and to each other, such that they are secure enough to optimize postoperative functional recovery.

Surgical Technique

The patient is positioned supine on the operating table in a 30-degree modified beach chair position, with a bolster placed behind the involved shoulder. A standard anterior deltopectoral approach is used. The biceps tendon is identified and provides an orientation to the greater and lesser tuberosities, the former being lateral and the latter being medial to the tendon. Each tuberosity is tagged with a no. #2 suture at the tendon insertion, which is more secure than through the tuberosity itself. The tuberosities are retracted out of the way, the articular segment is removed, and the glenoid articular surface is inspected. The axillary nerve is inspected and its continuity confirmed by the "tug test," which consists of palpation of the nerve as it comes around the humeral neck on the underside of the deltoid and as it passes inferior to the glenoid. A gentle back and forth "tugging" motion confirms its continuity.[69]

The humerus is placed in extension and the canal is prepared with a series of intramedullary broaches; a trial component is inserted. It is placed "proud" to compensate for the loss of metaphyseal bone.

Humeral length determines the tension of the deltoid muscle unit. If the prosthesis is seated too low, the deltoid function will be poor because of laxity, and inferior instability will occur. If seated too high, the shoulder will be prone to impingement and decreased range of motion.[193] A preoperative scanogram or full-length radiograph of the contralateral humerus can be helpful.[205] Also, the tension in biceps tendon can sometimes aid in establishing the proper height.[193]

To help hold the trial prosthesis in the "proud" position during a trial reduction, a surgical sponge can be wrapped around the prosthesis (Fig. 20). The desired position is 20 to 35 degrees of retroversion that is confirmed by comparing

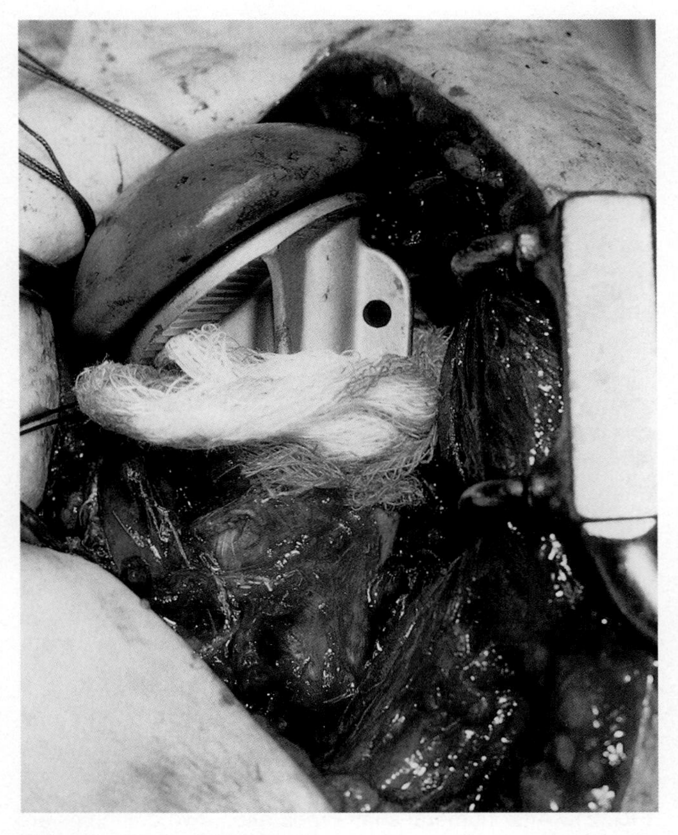

FIG. 20. A surgical sponge, making up for proximal bone loss, is wrapped around the trial implant to maintain a "proud" position of the prosthesis while testing position and stability.

the prosthesis position with the transepicondylar axis. This version should be modified if there is a preexisting chronic dislocation or fracture–dislocation. Satisfied with the position, the humeral cortex is marked near the lateral or anterior flange to reproduce positioning during cementing.

A head size equal to the removed head is used, and a trial reduction is performed. The tuberosities are pulled into position with the humeral head reduced, and anterior, posterior, and inferior stability is assessed. Up to 50% posterior translation, 50% inferior translation, and 25% anterior translation is acceptable. A larger humeral head should be used if there is excessive soft-tissue laxity; a smaller size if soft-tissue tension is excessive. When a final decision is made concerning component size and position the trial prosthesis is removed.

Two drill holes are placed 1.5 to 2.0 cm distal to the surgical neck level through the humeral cortex, with one medial and one lateral to the bicipital groove. Two or three no. 5 nonabsorbable sutures are passed through the drill holes for later tuberosity fixation (Fig. 21). The medullary canal is then irrigated and dried. A cement restrictor may be used. We use a cement restrictor to enhance cement distribution, but avoid cement pressurization to decrease the possibility of humeral shaft fracture. The canal is packed with a sponge to obtain adequate drying before cementing.

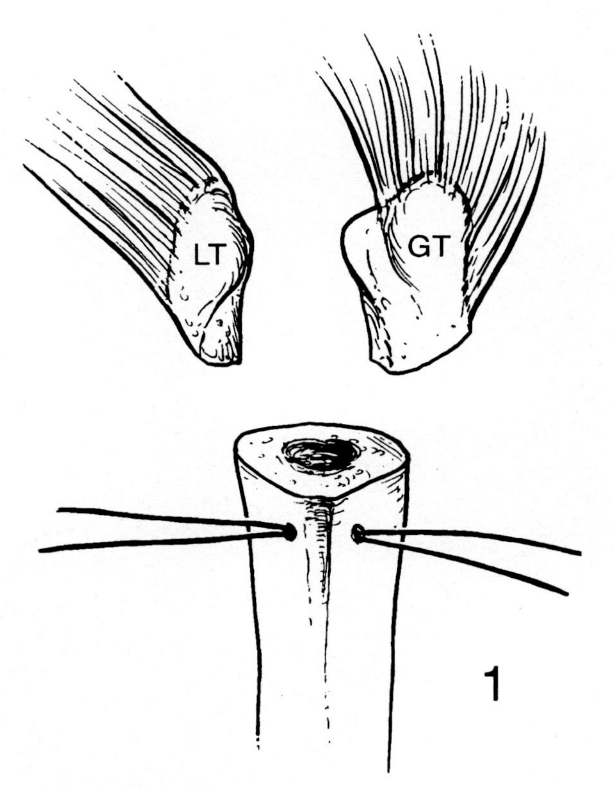

FIG. 21. After humeral shaft preparation, two drill holes are placed through the humeral cortex, one medial and one lateral to the bicipital groove. Heavy nonabsorbable sutures are passed through the drill holes.

The cement is mixed and poured into a vented 60 mL Toomey-type syringe approximately 1 minute after mixing (Fig. 22). This syringe should be vented by preparing a hole at the 20- to 30-mL level. This hole allows air to escape during insertion of the plunger so that a continuous column of cement is formed. The cement is then injected into the canal. During insertion of the prosthesis, it is essential to maintain the prosthesis in the proper proud position, as well as in the desired position of retroversion. The prosthesis should be held in position until the cement is completely set, to avoid inadvertent subsidence or rotation into an unacceptable position. When the cementing is complete, the position should be confirmed. When a modular component is used, the modular head should be impacted into place, making certain that the taper is dry and free of any debris.

Tuberosity Fixation

Fixation of the tuberosities to the prosthesis and the shaft is a critical component of this procedure. Proper reattachment and secure fixation will enhance the probability of a successful outcome in terms of range of motion and overall function. However, careful attention must be given to the technical aspects of this portion of the procedure. Heavy (no. 5) nonabsorbable sutures should be used. These sutures are generally passed through the rotator cuff tendons just at their insertion into the tuberosities. The biceps tendon is allowed to fall between the tuberosities and is incorporated into the fixation. This results in a "functional tenodesis," but probably preserves at least a portion of its humeral head depressor function.

The principles of tuberosity fixation include (a) placement of longitudinal sutures to bring the tuberosities into a position below the prosthetic articular surface and into contact with the humeral shaft; and (b) transverse suture fixation, which brings the tuberosities into contact with each other and maintains the tuberosities in the distal position obtained with the longitudinal sutures.

At this point, the two longitudinal sutures, which have already been passed through the humeral cortex, are used. The first longitudinal suture should be placed in a figure eight fashion through the supraspinatus tendon as it inserts into the greater tuberosity, and then through the upper portion of the subscapularis tendon as it inserts into the lesser tuberosity. The second longitudinal suture should be passed in similar fashion through the infraspinatus tendon as it inserts into the greater tuberosity, and through the lower portion of the subscapularis tendon as it inserts into the lesser tuberosity. These sutures are passed but not tied. The first transverse suture is then passed through the supraspinatus tendon as it inserts into the greater tuberosity, through the upper hole of the lateral or anterior flange, the prosthesis, and then through the upper portion of the subscapularis tendon as it inserts into the lesser tuberosity. The second transverse suture is passed, in similar fashion through the infraspinatus tendon, through the lower hole in the lateral or anterior flange, and through the

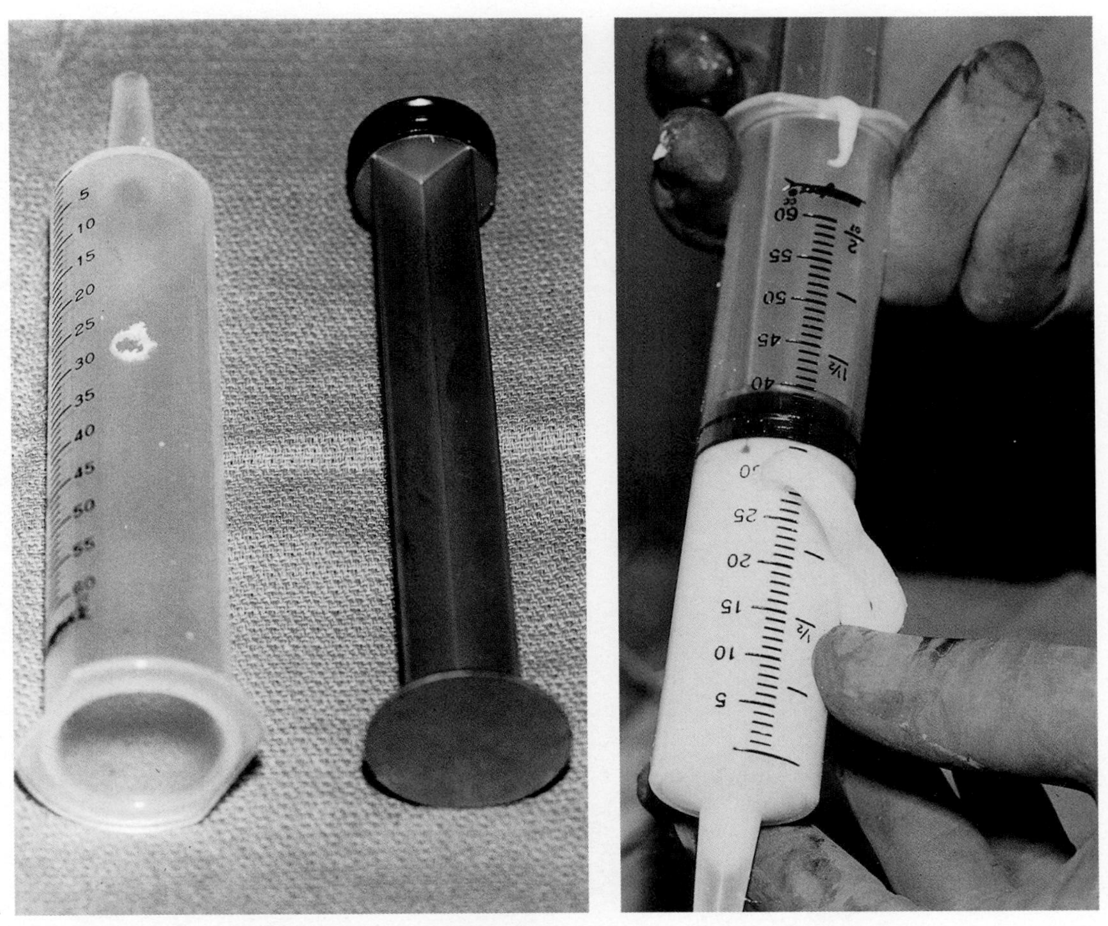

FIG. 22. (A) A hole is placed through the wall of a 60-mL Toomey-type syringe at the 30-mL level. Cement in its liquid stage is then poured into the syringe. **(B)** Air and excess cement are released through the vent hole after inserting the plunger. A column of cement can be obtained for continuous injection into the humeral canal.

lower portion of the subscapularis tendon (Fig. 23A). The suture-tying sequence is important. The first longitudinal suture should be tied first. This will advance the tuberosities distally below the articular surface of the prosthesis and into contact with the humeral cortex, which is essential to obtain bone-to-bone healing. The second longitudinal suture should then be tied for enhanced fixation (Fig. 23B). When the tuberosities are confirmed to be in proper position, the superior transverse suture is tied, followed by the inferior transverse suture. Transverse fixation brings the tuberosities into contact with each other and maintains the position obtained by the longitudinal sutures (Fig. 23C,D). Tuberosity reattachment should be performed with the arm in approximately 20 degrees of abduction, neutral flexion, and 10 to 20 degrees external rotation. When the tuberosity fixation is completed, the stability of the fixation should be carefully assessed. Range of motion in forward elevation, external rotation, internal rotation, and abduction should be performed to determine the specific limits of motion that will be allowed in the postoperative rehabilitation program. In addition, we have found that bone grafting the tuberosities can enhance healing potential. Cancellous bone from the humeral head should be placed in the area of contact between the shaft and the tuberosities, as well as between the tuberosities.

Closure includes repair of the rotator interval with no. 1 or no. 2 nonabsorbable sutures. This repair should be performed with the humerus in external rotation to decrease the possibility that rotator interval closure will restrict rotation. A closed suction drain is usually placed deep to the deltopectoral interval and brought out through the skin distally and laterally. The deltopectoral interval is repaired with absorbable suture, as is the subcutaneous tissue. This skin closure is performed with either sutures or staples. A sterile dressing is applied and the upper extremity is placed in a sling.

We feel it is very important to obtain a complete set of radiographs in the operating room. These should include an AP view of the shoulder with the humerus in internal rotation (on the chest) and maximum external rotation as defined by the intraoperative assessment. An axillary view should be

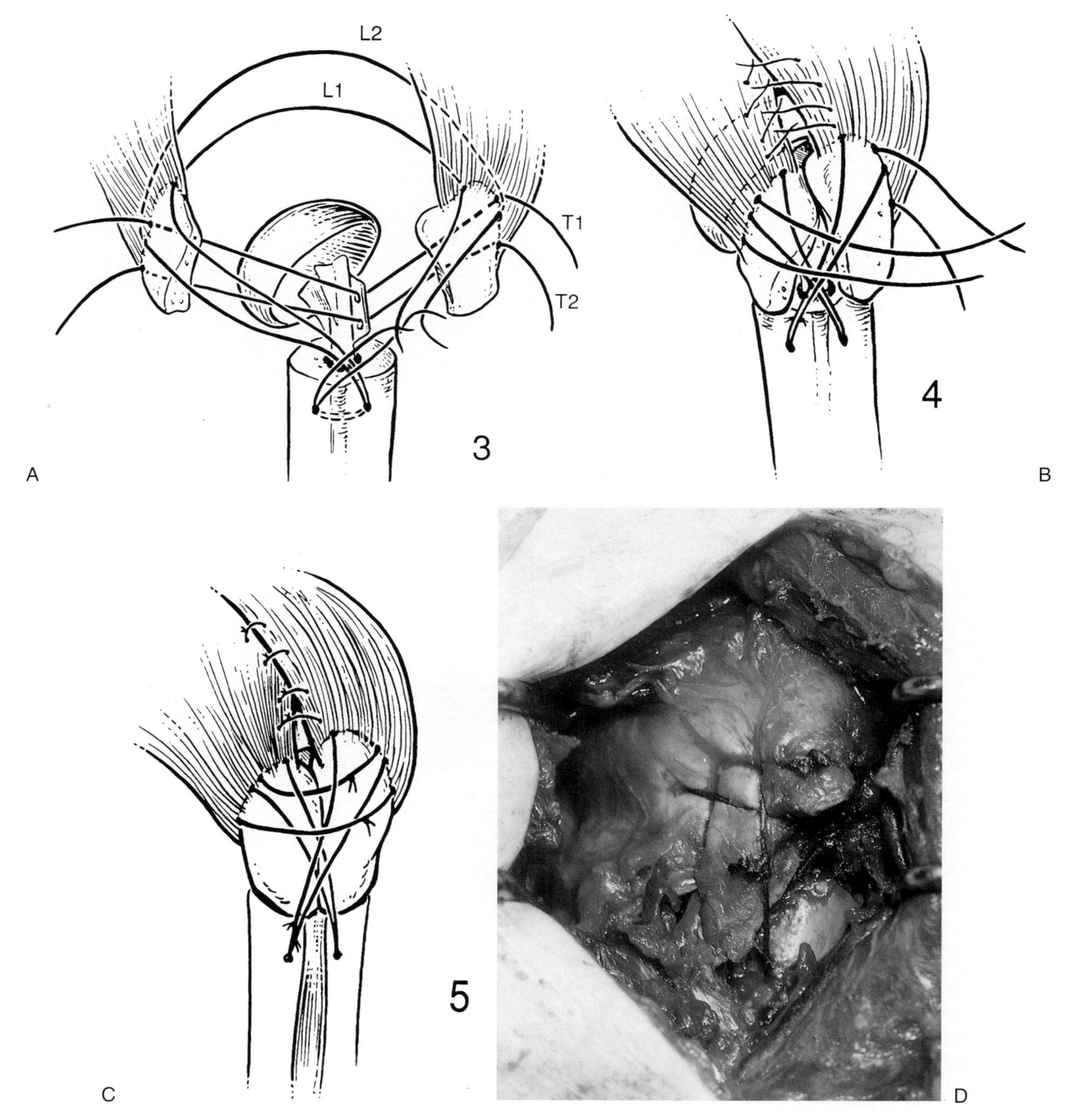

FIG. 23. The tuberosities are fixed by **(A)** placing two longitudinal sutures (*L1* and *L2*) from the humeral canal to the tuberosities, as well as two transverse sutures (*T1* and *T2*) through the tuberosities and through the lateral keel of the implant. **(B)** The longitudinal sutures are tied first, **(C,D)** followed by the transverse sutures. The rotator interval sutures are passed before completion of tuberosity attachment, but are not tied until the tuberosity repair is completed.

obtained (Fig. 24). These radiographs provide excellent visualization of the position of the prosthesis, as well as the position of the tuberosities.[69]

Postoperative Rehabilitation

On the first postoperative day, the patient is started on a rehabilitation program that consists of active range of motion of the elbow, wrist, and hand, and passive range of motion of the shoulder. External rotation should be limited, based on the intraoperative evaluation. This is important to avoid any excess stress on the tuberosity repair that could compromise healing. Internal rotation is allowed to the chest. These exercises are continued for the first 6 to 8 weeks. Radiographs are obtained approximately 2 weeks following surgery to confirm the position of the tuberosities. Additional radiographs are obtained

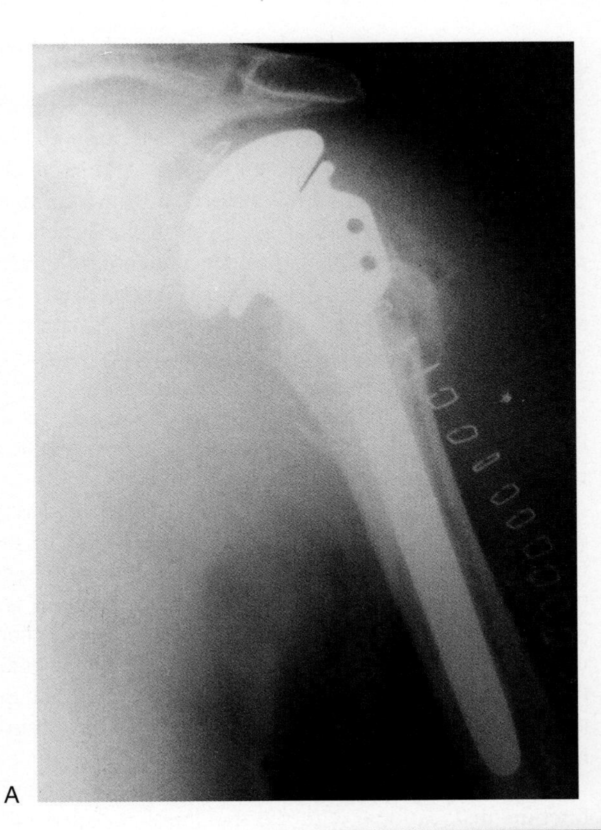

A

FIG. 24. (A) An AP view in internal and external rotation and **(B)** an axillary view should be obtained in the operating room to confirm proper prosthesis position and the position of the tuberosities adjacent to the prosthesis and in contact with the humeral shaft.

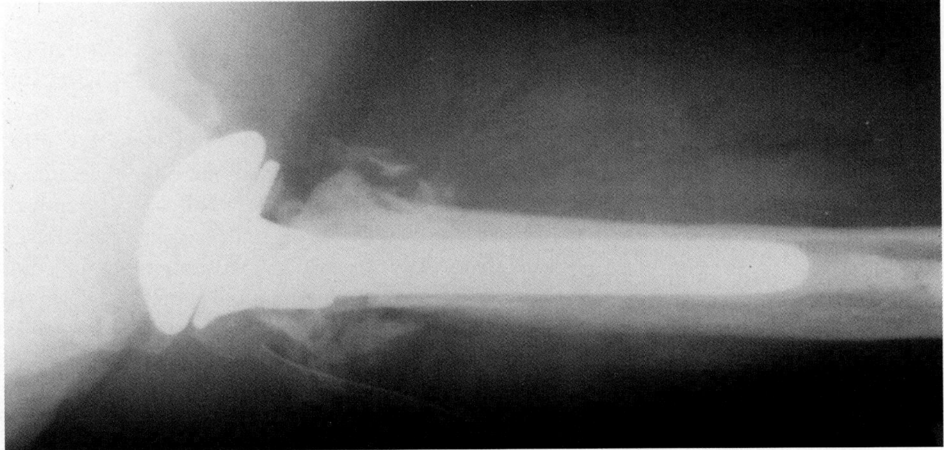

B

at 6 to 8 weeks following surgery to assess the degree of tuberosity healing. If tuberosity healing is sufficient, the sling is discontinued and an active range of motion program is begun. The patient is encouraged to use the involved upper extremity for activities of daily living. Passive range of motion is continued with gentle stretching to increase the overall range. At 8 weeks following surgery, isometric deltoid and internal and external rotator strengthening exercises are begun. Vigorous strengthening exercises are not begun until active forward elevation of at least 90 degrees is obtained. Our experience has shown that patients can expect continued recovery during the first year following surgery, although most of the recovery will occur during the first 6 months.

FRACTURE–DISLOCATIONS

Fracture–dislocations of the glenohumeral joint are characterized by a fracture of the proximal humerus in the presence of a complete loss of contact between the articular surfaces of the humeral head and glenoid. These injuries are usually associated with significant disruption of the soft tissues. Such traumatized tissues are prone to develop periarticular scarring and heterotopic bone formation. Repeated forceful attempts at closed reduction will increase the risk and severity of these problems. Therefore, although the first goal of treatment is prompt definitive reduction of the dislocation, multiple manipulations are to be avoided. Excessive force should never be used in the manipulation of fracture–dislocations, because it adds to the amount of soft-tissue injury, endangers the adjacent neurovascular structures, and risks displacing previously nondisplaced fractures.

Fracture–dislocations are classified by the direction of the dislocation (anterior versus posterior) and the type of proximal humerus fracture present. The most systematic method to categorize these injuries is the Neer classification of proximal humeral fractures, as described earlier. The category of intraarticular fractures of the humeral head includes not only "head-splitting" fractures, but also the much more common impression fractures frequently associated with dislocations. Posterolateral impression fractures occur in association with anterior dislocations, whereas anterolateral impression fractures occur in cases of posterior dislocation.

Clinical and Radiographic Evaluation

Clinical Evaluation

Fracture–dislocations of the shoulder may occur at any age and by either indirect or direct mechanisms. In general, fracture–dislocations represent higher-energy injuries than simple dislocations or fractures alone. The history may indicate as much. The most common indirect mechanism involves a simple fall onto the outstretched upper extremity. Seizures and electroconvulsive therapy are other potential indirect causes of fracture–dislocations. The direct mechanism of injury involves a direct blow to the proximal humerus, and usually is the result of a fall directly onto the shoulder. As with proximal humerus fractures, patients should be asked about the circumstances surrounding their injury. If a fall was involved, patients should be asked about any head trauma, possible loss of consciousness, other injuries to the ipsilateral upper extremity, any subjective numbness or tingling involving that extremity, or any other focal sites of pain and tenderness. Other important history facts include: patient age, occupation, hand dominance, and length of time since the injury.

Common presenting complaints include pain and swelling about the shoulder, especially with attempted motion. On examination, patients will typically exhibit crepitus and severe pain with minimal active or passive range of motion. Ecchymosis generally does not occur until 24 hours or more after the injury, but can occur sooner, usually in elderly patients. Eventually, ecchymosis may involve the entire extremity, as well as the axilla and down along the chest wall.

As with simple dislocations, there will be a change of the normal contour of the shoulder. In anterior fracture–dislocations, there is an anterior prominence in the shoulder, the lateral acromion becomes more prominent, and the coracoid more difficult to palpate. There is a flattening of the posterior aspect of the joint. Conversely, in cases of posterior fracture–dislocations, the posterior aspect of the shoulder will be full, the anterior aspect of the shoulder hollow, and the coracoid more prominent. These findings can be quite subtle in large, muscular individuals, especially if considerable swelling is present.

Most fracture–dislocations result in the affected arm being held in a very characteristic manner. If anteriorly dislocated, the arm will usually be held in a position of relative abduction and external rotation; there can be a firm, painful block to passive internal rotation as the posterior aspect of the humeral head abuts against the anterior glenoid. Conversely, in posterior dislocations, the arm may be in internal rotation, with a firm, painful block to passive external rotation as the anterior aspect of the humeral head impacts on the posterior rim of the glenoid. The primary exception to these findings occurs when a surgical neck fracture is present, in which case motion in any plane may be possible through the fracture site, rather than at the articulation.

A thorough neurovascular examination of the involved extremity is of paramount importance in cases of glenohumeral fracture–dislocation because of the increased risk of associated vascular or neurologic complications. Vascular injuries, although rare, are devastating when they occur and usually involve injury to atherosclerotic axillary vessels in the elderly. Suspicion of a vascular injury is worked up in a manner similar to that discussed with proximal humerus fractures.

Neurologic injuries are much more common sequelae of fracture–dislocations, with the incidence reported ranging from 2% to 30%.[213–218] The axillary nerve is most commonly involved, although the entire brachial plexus or any component thereof may be affected. These injuries almost always represent traction neuropraxias, and most resolve clinically within 5 months.[219,220] However, it is critical that a thorough neurologic examination of the entire extremity be documented, both before and after any attempted manipulations. In evaluation of axillary nerve function, electromyographic (EMG) studies have shown that the commonly used method of testing sensation over the lateral aspect of the shoulder is quite unreliable.[219] A much more reliable method is to test for isometric deltoid motor function, which can be performed even in the context of the acute injury.

Despite the numerous signs and symptoms described in the foregoing, glenohumeral fracture–dislocations may be difficult to diagnose and can be missed by the initial examiner, particularly those involving posterior dislocations.[221–223] It is estimated that up to 50% of these injuries are initially misdiagnosed.[224] To avoid this pitfall, it is important to maintain a high level of suspicion for these relatively uncommon injuries, and to obtain a thorough and accurate radiographic evaluation.

Radiographic Evaluation

The plane of the glenohumeral articulation lies approximately 40 degrees anterior to the sagittal plane of the body. This must be taken into account if precise radiographs of this joint are to be obtained. Misdiagnosis of shoulder injuries is often attributed to radiographs being obtained in the plane of the body, rather than in the plane of the scapula centered on the glenohumeral joint. This results in overlapping structures that can be confusing and preclude accurate assessment of the injuries.

The axillary view is essential for evaluating glenoid and humeral articular surfaces, to identify displaced tuberosities, and it is the most sensitive view for detecting glenohumeral dislocations and subluxations. This view is most easily obtained with the patient in the supine position and the affected arm gently abducted to at least 30 degrees. If possible, the arm can be supported in this position by the patient holding onto an intravenous (IV) pole. If the patient is unable to assist, the arm should be positioned by someone wearing a lead gown.

Although the axillary view is the most difficult of the three views to obtain and requires moving the patient's painful arm, if done carefully, the great majority of patients will be able to tolerate the procedure. For those few patients who are unable to do so, however, the Velpeau axillary view described earlier, is a suitable substitute that does not require removing the arm from the sling.[67]

Computed tomography is another imaging modality that can be used in the more complex or comminuted cases. This test provides unparalleled resolution for bony detail and, therefore, provides the most accurate assessment of fragment displacement, amount of articular involvement with a head-splitting or impression fracture (see Fig. 13), glenoid rim fractures, and chronic fracture–dislocations.

Although it is not as precise in assessing bony detail as a CT scan, MRI plays a very important role in evaluating traumatic shoulder injuries. It is the test of choice for evaluating soft-tissue injuries about the shoulder and so can be used in patients for whom associated glenoid labral or rotator cuff tears are suspected. It can also assess injuries involving the axillary vessels and brachial plexus, and it remains the most sensitive method to detect osteonecrosis, a potential sequela of fracture dislocations.

Associated Injuries

Rotator Cuff Tears

All fracture–dislocations in which either or both tuberosities are significantly displaced will, by necessity, have a longitudinal split in the rotator cuff—often along the rotator interval between the supraspinatus and the subscapularis. In these cases, rotator cuff repair should be performed at the time open reduction and internal fixation is performed. In patients in whom the tuberosities do not fulfill the criteria for "displacement," associated cuff tears are not uncommon as a result of the gradual deterioration that occurs with advancing age. Therefore, the elderly are particularly susceptible to this injury, because their already degenerated cuff tendons are less able to withstand the high-tensile forces generated during dislocation.

Neurologic Injuries

Injury to peripheral nerves and the brachial plexus accompany fracture–dislocations of the shoulder, with a reported incidence of between 2% and 30%. This variability partly reflects age differences of the groups studied, as well as the method of assessing neurologic deficits—physical examination versus EMG. The axillary nerve, which courses anteriorly along the anterior border of the subscapularis, is especially vulnerable to traction injury during an anterior dislocation. It is the most commonly injured nerve in shoulder fracture–dislocations,[213–218] and the likelihood of injury increases with the age of the patient, the duration of the dislocation, and the severity of the trauma producing the injury.[213,225] The vast majority of these injuries represent traction neuropraxias and usually resolve spontaneously within 5 months.[219,220] Other isolated nerve injuries to the musculocutaneous, radial, and ulnar nerves are much less common.

When a neurologic injury is suspected, the initial physical examination findings should be carefully documented. An EMG should be obtained 3 weeks following the injury for further documentation. This is a much more sensitive method of assessing a neurologic injury than the physical examination. The difficulties in assessing axillary neuropathy based on physical examinations are twofold. First, dermatomal sensory testing is very unreliable.[213] Second, the high incidence of rotator cuff tears associated with these shoulder injuries confuses the picture somewhat. Clinical findings of weak abduction can be due to rotator cuff tear, axillary neuropathy, or the acute pain associated with the injury.

Vascular Injuries

Fracture–dislocations of the shoulder can, on rare occasions, be associated with vascular injuries—usually involving the axillary artery, its branches, or the axillary vein. These injuries can occur either during the injury itself or during the reduction maneuver. Attempted reductions of chronic dislocations are particularly risky and should be discouraged. Invariably, too many attempts are made and too much force used. Vascular damage most frequently occurs in elderly patients with fragile, atherosclerotic vessels and in patients whose soft tissues (and vessels) may be adherent as a result of previous dislocations or other injuries.[226–228] When a vascular injury occurs, it is an emergency and must be addressed immediately. These injuries are associated with a mortality rate of up to 50%.

Different types of arterial damage can occur, including intimal damage followed by thrombosis, avulsion of a large arterial branch, and laceration of the artery itself. As discussed earlier, anatomic studies have shown the axillary artery to be relatively fixed at the lateral border of the pectoralis minor muscle.[230] The artery becomes taut with abduction and external rotation of the arm, and is vulnerable to injury when the humeral head dislocates anteriorly and the pectoralis minor acts as a fulcrum over which the artery is stressed. There is the further risk with fracture–dislocations that the artery can be impaled or lacerated by the fracture fragments. The clinical findings and management of axillary artery injury is as discussed previously.

Impression Fractures of the Humeral Head

All shoulder dislocations impact the humeral head against the glenoid to some extent. An anteriorly dislocated humeral head is compressed against the anterior glenoid by the concomitant muscular contraction, thereby causing an impression fracture of the posterolateral humeral head. This defect, referred to as a Hill–Sachs lesion, can be quite large, especially in cases of chronic dislocation. Posterior dislocations frequently result in impression fractures of the anteromedial portion of the humeral head, referred to as a "reverse Hill–Sachs lesion" (see Fig. 13). These impression fractures can be quite large, especially in chronic posterior dislocations. In general, the larger the size of the defect, the more difficult it is to obtain a successful closed reduction. These impression fractures play a much more prominent role in the treatment of chronic dislocations.

Treatment

Two-Part Fracture–Dislocations: Surgical Neck

Two-part surgical neck fracture–dislocations are very uncommon, but when they occur, the dislocation is almost always anterior.

In general, the approach to these injuries is to first achieve a gentle, closed reduction of the dislocation and then to determine the appropriate treatment for the fracture, based on the evaluation of the postreduction radiographs. Although conscious sedation is usually sufficient, if closed reduction is unsuccessful, general anesthesia should be used to avoid multiple attempts. Closed reduction of the anteriorly dislocated humeral head can often be accomplished with gentle fingertip mobilization of the humeral head while longitudinal traction is applied to the arm. There are a few circumstances in which open reduction is indicated:

1. Vascular injury
2. Open fracture
3. Failed or difficult closed reduction
4. Anterior or posterior dislocation associated with a nondisplaced surgical neck fracture (closed manipulation risks fracture displacement)

Following successful closed or open reduction, the operative approach is essentially the same as that used for two-part surgical neck fractures without dislocation. The deltopectoral interval is opened and the clavipectoral fascia is divided lateral to the conjoint tendon. When open reduction is necessary, the dislocated humeral head should be carefully dissected free of the glenoid rim and away from the brachial plexus. Opening the rotator interval will improve visualization of the humeral head and glenoid and facilitate mobilization of the humeral head. This should permit a gentle reduction of the humeral head into the glenoid fossa. Once this has been accomplished, ORIF of the surgical neck can be performed, using a number of the different techniques described earlier, based on bone quality, as well as the surgeon's experience and preference.

Postoperatively, the arm is protected in a sling and swath for 1 to 2 days. A simple sling can then be used for support for 4 to 6 weeks, while a rehabilitation program is initiated consisting of passive range of motion of the shoulder. Active range of motion begins at 4 to 6 weeks depending on the progress of fracture healing. Stretching and strengthening are usually begun 10 to 12 weeks following surgery.

Two-Part Fracture–Dislocations: Greater Tuberosity

Greater tuberosity fractures have been reported to occur in up to 33% of anterior shoulder dislocations.[212] This is the most common type of fracture–dislocation. The initial step in treatment of these injuries should always be gentle, closed reduction of the dislocation, followed by a complete set of postreduction radiographs. In many cases, the reduction restores the greater tuberosity fragment to near-anatomic position (Fig. 25). When this occurs, nonoperative management is preferred, consisting of sling immobilization for approximately 4 weeks. However, passive range of motion exercises should be started as soon as discomfort subsides. Frequent follow-up radiographs are essential in the postreduction period to ensure that the tuberosity has not redisplaced with the early motion program.

Management is as with greater tuberosity fractures, discussed earlier. In cases where the greater tuberosity remains displaced by more than 5 mm, operative management is indicated, unless the patient's medical condition or limited functional demands indicate otherwise.[229] Prognostically, dislocations associated with a greater tuberosity fracture rarely go on to become recurrent, because the anterior soft tissues are usually spared, and the joint stability is restored once fracture healing occurs.

Two-Part Fracture–Dislocations: Lesser Tuberosity

Posterior glenohumeral dislocations are sometimes accompanied by lesser tuberosity fractures. This represents an avulsion-type fracture as a result of the strong pull of the attached subscapularis tendon and anterior capsule. When these injuries are acute or recent (within 2 weeks), the first step in treatment should be attempted closed reduction of the dislocation. This can be accomplished with the patient supine, by application of longitudinal traction to the arm while it is held in 90 degrees of forward flexion. The arm should then be gradually adducted across the chest while maintaining traction, in an effort to unlock the head from behind the glenoid. The maneuver can sometimes be facilitated

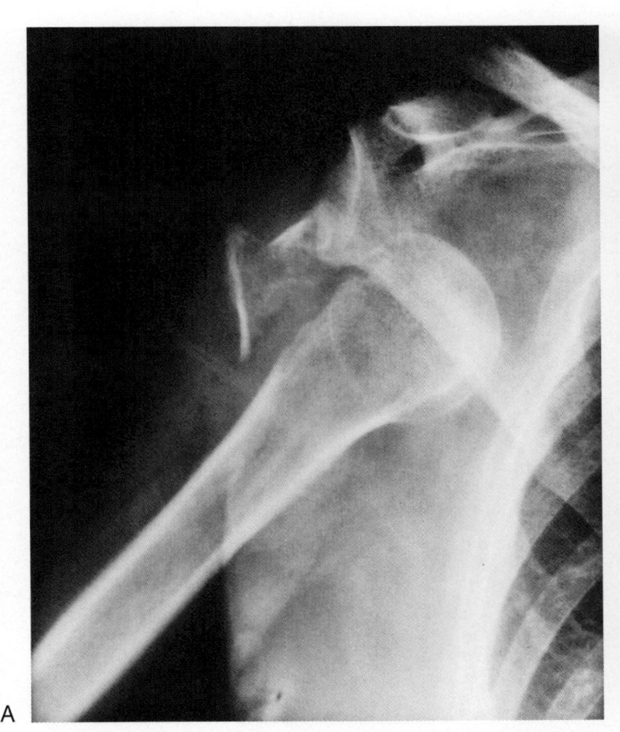
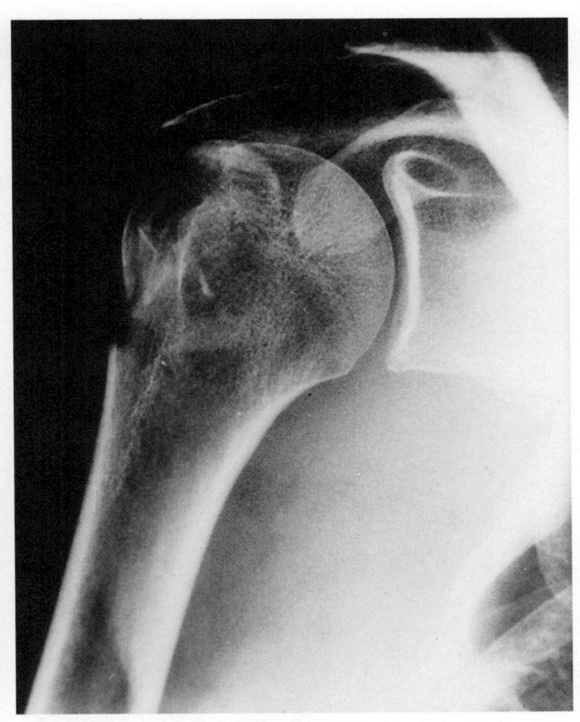

A B

FIG. 25. A 61-year-old woman who fell onto the outstretched right upper extremity sustaining **(A)** a two-part anterior greater tuberosity fracture dislocation. **(B)** Following closed reduction, there is near anatomic reduction of the greater tuberosity fragment.

by application of digital pressure on the humeral head from behind or a laterally directed force on the proximal humerus.

Postreduction radiographs should then be obtained to document reduction of the glenohumeral joint, to assess the position of the lesser tuberosity fragment, and to ensure that no other fractures have been displaced by the reduction maneuver. If the reduction is stable and residual tuberosity displacement is less than 1 cm, then the patient should undergo 4 weeks of immobilization in a modified shoulder spica cast or orthosis that maintains the arm at the side in 10- to 15-degrees external rotation, 10- to 15-degrees extension, and 10- to 15-degrees abduction. When residual instability is present, or the displacement of a large lesser tuberosity fragment exceeds 1 cm, operative management is indicated (Fig. 26). The goals of operative management are to restore stability and anatomically reduce and securely fix the lesser tuberosity fragment. However, the decision to proceed with operative management should be based on a careful assessment of all factors, not the last of which is the patient's own functional expectations.

Fixation of the lesser tuberosity can be achieved by use of transosseous sutures or cancellous screws, depending on the bone size and quality. The rotator interval should also be repaired. Postoperatively, an orthosis should be used for up to 4 weeks if there is concern about the fixation. If stability is achieved, a simple sling can be used for 4 weeks. As early as postoperative day 1, passive range of motion is begun with pendulum exercises, advancing to supine assisted overhead elevation, and pulley exercises. The patient is advanced to active exercises at approximately 6 weeks, when fracture union is insured.

Three-Part Fracture–Dislocations: Anterior

Three-part anterior fracture–dislocations consist of anterior dislocation of the humeral head with displaced fractures of the surgical neck and greater tuberosity (Figs. 27 and 28). The lesser tuberosity remains attached to the humeral head and provides some blood supply to the articular surface through the subscapularis and anterior capsule attachments. However, the arcuate artery of Laing, which carries most of the direct blood supply to the head, is at risk with this injury because it penetrates the medial portion of the greater tuberosity, with the resulting risk of osteonecrosis.[5] Open reduction of the dislocation should be performed, for it can be done much more gently, thus reducing the risk of further soft-tissue injury. Our preferred treatment for this injury consists of open reduction of the dislocation, followed by fixation of the displaced fragments. A deltopectoral approach is preferred. The biceps tendon may be used as a helpful guide to the tuberosities and the rotator interval. After reduction of the dislocation, if the remaining soft-tissue attachments to

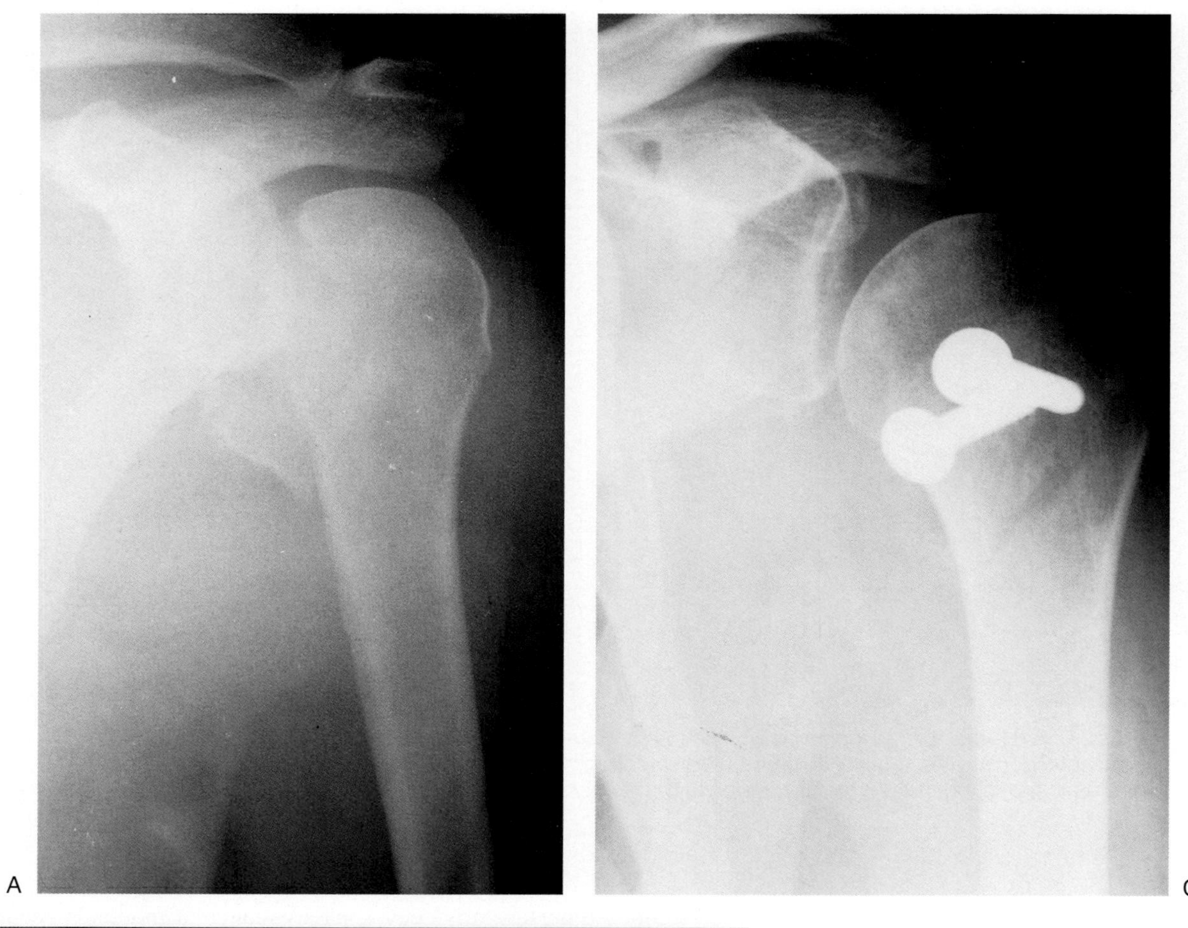

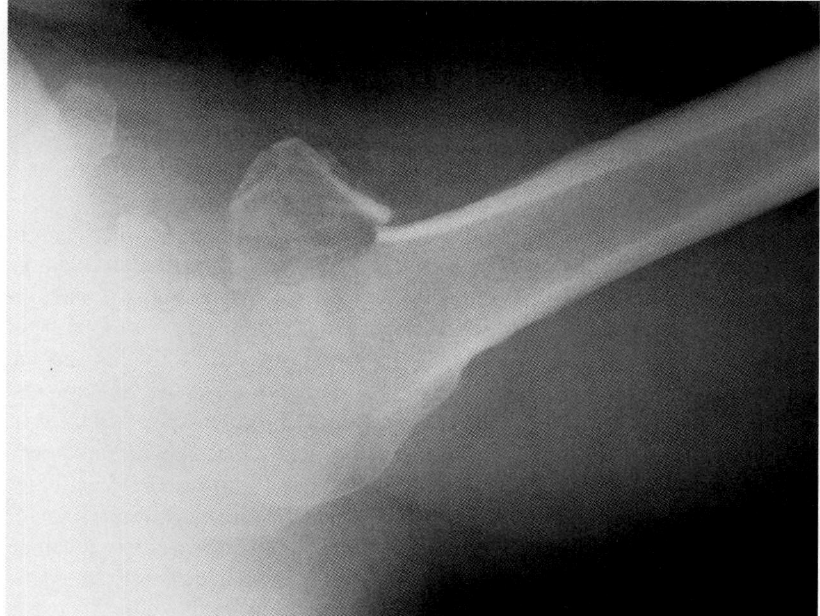

FIG. 26. A 44-year-old woman sustained **(A,B)** a left two-part lesser tuberosity posterior fracture dislocation following a seizure. With closed manipulation, the humeral head was quite unstable. **(C)** Open reduction and internal fixation with two cancellous screws was performed. The patient was maintained in a shoulder orthosis for 4 weeks following surgery.

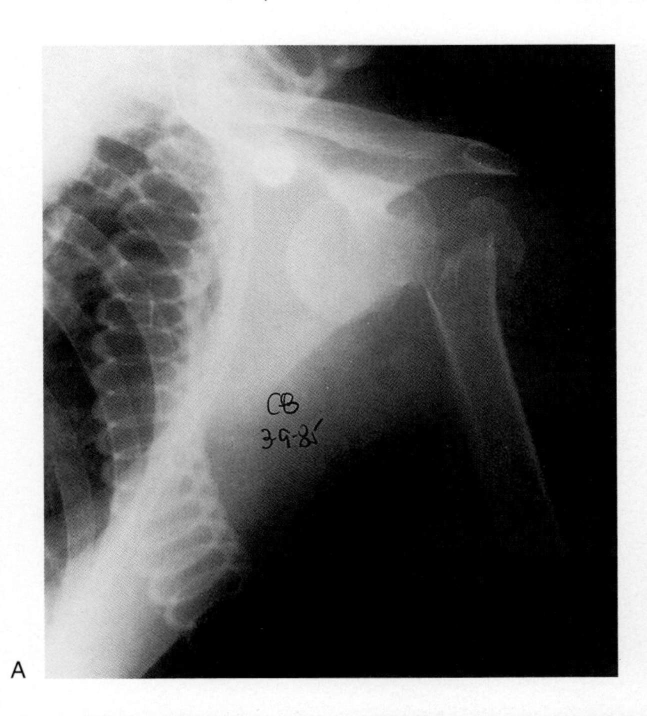

A

FIG. 27. A 32-year-old woman with **(A)** a three-part anterior fracture-dislocation of the left shoulder. This was treated by open reduction and internal fixation, using Ender rods in combination with multiple tension band sutures. **(B,C)** Postoperative x-rays films show excellent alignment and reduction of the fracture dislocation.

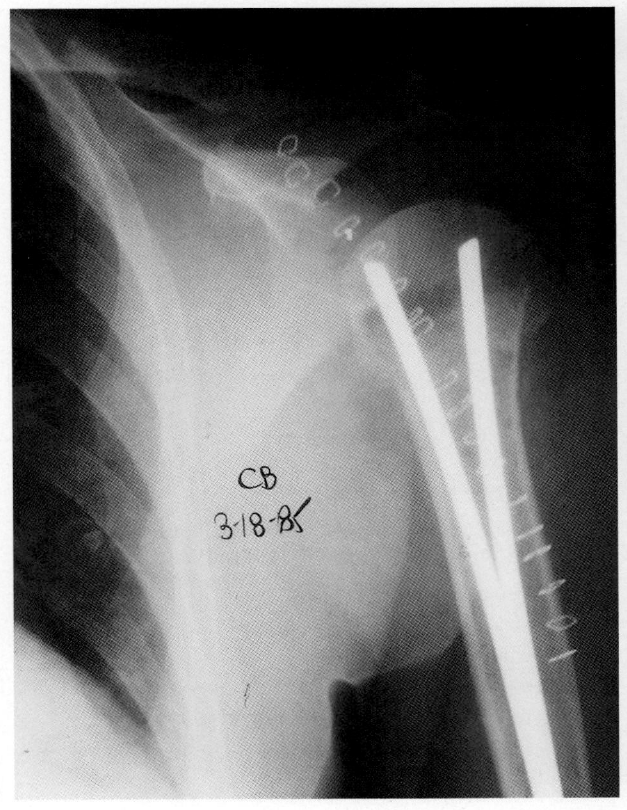

B

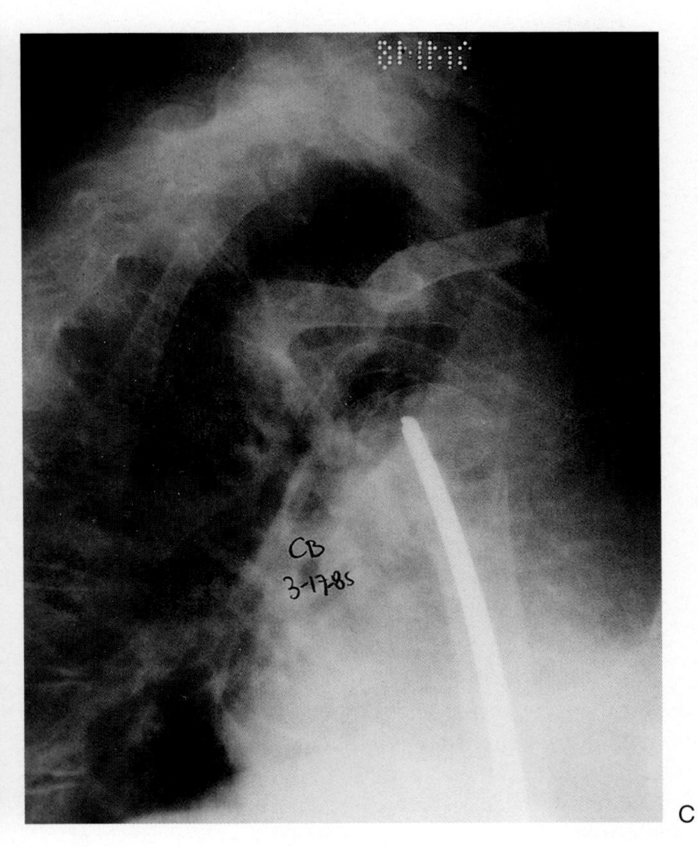

C

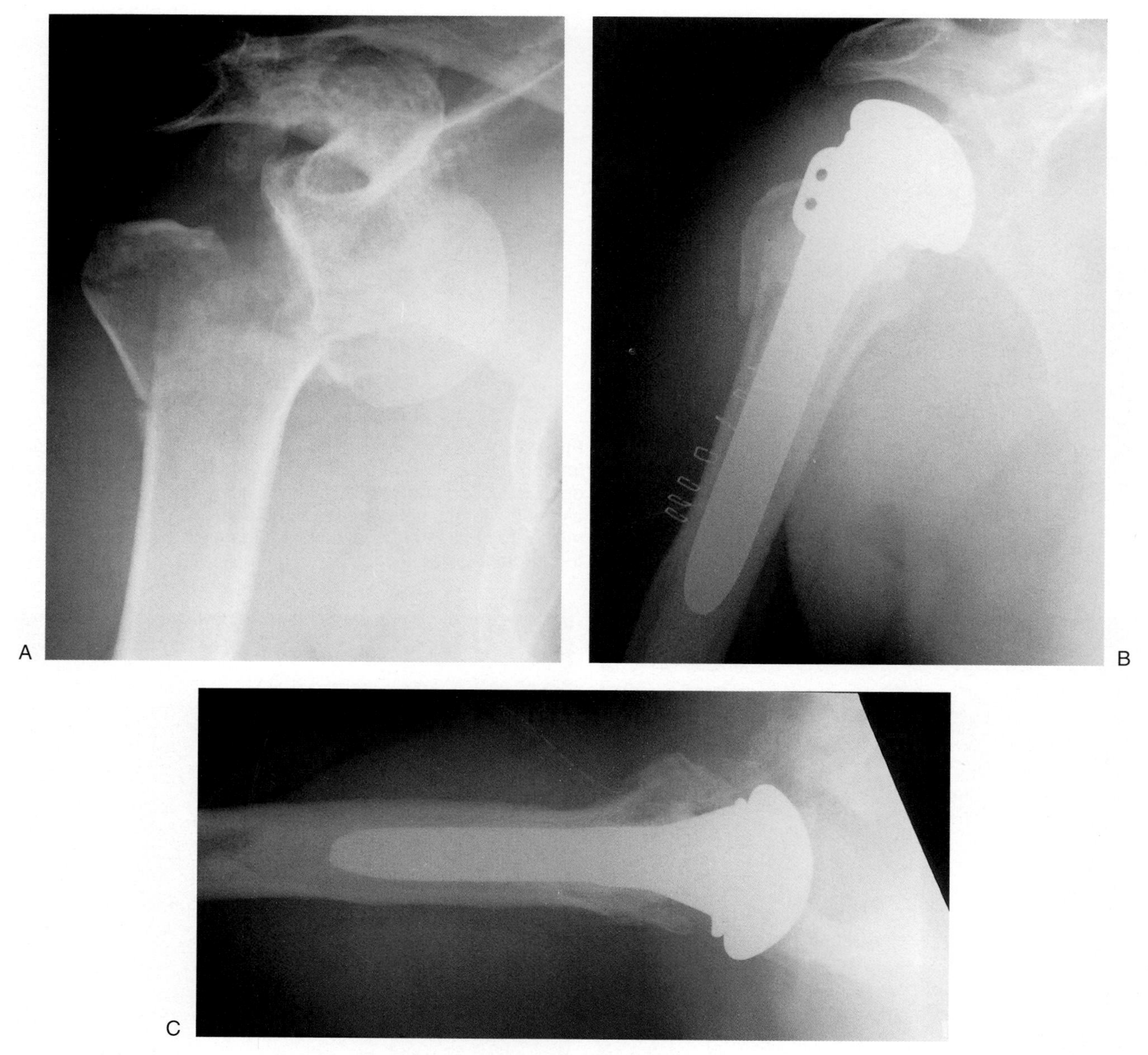

FIG. 28. A 72-year-old woman with **(A)** a three-part anterior fracture–dislocation of the right shoulder. Because of the patient's age and osteoporotic bone, **(B,C)** a proximal humeral replacement with tuberosity attachment was performed.

the head appear secure and the bone is not severely osteoporotic or comminuted, ORIF should be performed, using tension band technique alone or in combination with intramedullary device, as previously described (see Fig. 27). A repair of the rotator cuff interval should also be performed.

When osteoporotic bone or comminution preclude stable fixation, proximal humeral replacement (PHR) is preferred, in combination with reconstruction of the tuberosities (see Fig. 28). The prosthesis should be inserted with cement, with the goal of achieving proper version and humeral length, because both are critical to the function and stability of the shoulder. Aftercare and rehabilitation protocols are as described for two-part fracture dislocations.

Three-Part Fracture–Dislocations: Posterior

Three-part posterior fracture–dislocations are characterized by posterior dislocation of the humeral head, with the greater tuberosity attached, in combination with displaced fractures of the surgical neck and lesser tuberosity. Complete radiographs (trauma series) are essential to accurately assess this injury and to avoid overlooking the posterior dislocation.

As with three-part anterior dislocations, these injuries require open reduction of the dislocation performed as soon as possible after the injury. This can be performed through an anterior deltopectoral approach. The fractured lesser tuberosity should be identified and mobilized to expose the glenoid. The shaft should also be mobilized to allow visualization of the posteriorly dislocated articular segment. Gentle manipulation and a levering type retractor should be used to reduce the dislocated segment. The decision to proceed with ORIF (using the tension band technique described), or proximal humeral replacement, should be based upon bone quality, comminution, and soft—tissue integrity.

Four-Part Fracture–Dislocations

All four-part fracture–dislocations, whether anterior or posterior, are associated with significant disruption of the blood supply to the humeral head. Osteonecrosis of the articular segment is almost inevitable, and for this reason, PHR is the treatment of choice; ORIF is considered only in young patients with good bone quality. A deltopectoral approach is preferred and the articular segment is removed. The prosthesis should be cemented in place with special focus on restoring proper version and humeral length. However, proper version may not necessarily mean anatomic version. In cases of subacute fracture–dislocations, stability can be enhanced by either decreasing retroversion (for posterior dislocations) or increasing retroversion (for anterior dislocations). The tuberosities should be reconstructed such that they are securely fixed to each other, to the prosthesis, and to the shaft. It is very important that the tuberosities be brought down to a level below the articular head of the prosthesis to avoid subacromial impingement.

Rehabilitation following PHR for fracture–dislocations is the same as after PHR of proximal humerus fractures. A passive range of motion program, within the limits of the repair, should be initiated 1 or 2 days after surgery and continued for 6 to 8 weeks. After this point, tuberosity healing should be stable enough to allow an active motion program.

REFERENCES

1. Hodges PC. Development of the human skeleton. *AJR Am J Roentgenol* 1933;30:809.
2. Dameron TB, Reibel DB. Fractures involving the proximal humeral epiphyseal plate. *J Bone Joint Surg [Am]* 1969;51:289–297.
3. Neer CS II, Horwitz BS. Fractures of the proximal humeral epiphysial plate. *Clin Orthop* 1963;41:24–31.
4. Laing PG. The arterial supply to the adult humerus. *J Bone Joint Surg [Am]* 1956;38:1105–1116.
5. Gerber C, Schneeberger AG, Vinh T. The arterial vascularization of the humeral head. *J Bone Joint Surg [Am]* 1990;72:1486–1494.
6. Netter FH. Upper limb. In: *The CIBA collection of medical illustrations,* vol 8. Summit, NJ: CIBA-GEIGY, 1987:20–74.
7. Brookes CH, Revell WJ, Heatley FW. Vascularity of the humeral head after proximal humeral fractures: an anatomical cadaver study. *J Bone Joint Surg [Br]* 1993;75:132–136.
8. Fitzgerald JF, Keates J. False aneurysm as a late complication of anterior dislocation of the shoulder. *Ann Surg* 1975;181:785–786.
9. Gerber C, Lambert SM, Hoogewoud HM. Absence of avascular necrosis of the humeral head after post-traumatic rupture of the anterior and posterior humeral circumflex arteries: a case report. *J Bone Joint Surg [Am]* 1996;78:1256–1259.
10. Neer CS II. Displaced proximal humeral fractures Part II: treatment of three-part and four-part displacement. *J Bone Joint Surg [Am]* 1970; 52:1090–1103.
11. Jakob RP, Miniaci A, Anson PS, Jaberg H, Osterwalder A, Ganz R. Four-part valgus impacted fractures of the proximal humerus. *J Bone Joint Surg [Br]* 1991;73:295–298.
12. Zuckerman JD, Flugstad DL, Teitz CC, King HA. Axillary artery injury as a complication of proximal humeral fractures. *Clin Orthop* 1984;189:234–237.
13. DeLatt EAT, Visser CPJ, Coene LNJEM, Pahlplatz PVM, Tavy DLJ. Nerve lesions in primary shoulder dislocations and humeral neck fractures. *J Bone Joint Surg [Br]* 1994;76:381–383.
14. Simmen MB, Neff V, Habegger R. Subcapital humerus fracture with lesion of the axillary artery. 2 case reports and review of the literature. *Unfallchirurg* 1996;99:154–157.
15. Bigliani LU, Flatow EL, Pollock RG. Fractures of the proximal humerus. In: *Rockwood and Green's fractures in adults*, 4th ed. Philadelphia: Lippincott–Raven, 1996.
16. Hoppenfeld S, de Boer P. The shoulder. In: *Surgical exposures in orthopaedics: the anatomic approach*. Philadelphia: JB Lippincott, 1984.
17. Flatow EL, Bigliani LU, April EW. An anatomic study of the musculocutaneous nerve and its relationship to the coracoid process. *Clin Orthop* 1989;244:166–171.
18. Codman EA. *The shoulder: rupture of the supraspinatus tendon and other lesions in or about the subacromial bursa*. Boston: Thomas Todd, 1934:262–293.
19. Neer CS II. Displaced proximal humeral fractures: Part I. Classification and evaluation. *J Bone Joint Surg [Am]* 1970;52:1077–1089.
20. Neer CS II. Four-segment classification of displaced proximal humeral fractures. *AAOS: Instr Course Lect* 1975;24:160–168.
21. Aitken AP. End results of fractures of the proximal humeral epiphysis. *J Bone Joint Surg [Am]* 1936;18:1036–1041.
22. Salter RB, Harris WR. Injuries involving the epiphyseal plate. *J Bone Joint Surg [Am]* 1963;45:587–622.
23. Shapiro F. Epiphyseal disorders. *N Engl J Med* 1987;317:1702–1710.
24. Kocher T. *Bietrage zur Kenntnis einigir praktisch wichtiger Fracturen formen*. Basel: Carl Sallman Verlag, 1896.
25. Watson-Jones R. *Fractures and joint injuries*, 3rd ed. Baltimore: Williams & Wilkins, 1943:438–445.
26. Bigliani LU. Fractures of the shoulder. Part I: Fractures of the proximal humerus. In: Rockwood CA, Green DP, Bucholz RW, eds. *Fracture in adults*, 3rd ed. Philadelphia: JB Lippincott, 1991:871–927.
27. Seeman WR, Siebler G, Rupp HG. A new classification of proximal humeral fractures. *Eur J Radiol* 1986;6:163–167.
28. Habermeyer P, Schweiberer L. Frakturen des proximalen humerus. *Orthopade* 1989;18:200–227.
29. Kristiansen B, Christensen SW. Proximal humeral fractures. Late results in relation to classification and treatment. *Acta Orthop Scand* 1987;58:124–127.
30. Mills HJ, Horn G. Fractures of the proximal humerus in adults. *J Trauma* 1985;25:801–805.
31. Sidor ML, Zuckerman JD, Lyon T, Koval K, Cuomo F, Schoenberg N. The Neer classification of proximal humeral fractures: an assessment of inter-observer reliability and intraobserver reproducibility. *J Bone Joint Surg [Am]* 1993;75:1745–1750.
32. Neer CS and Rockwood CA Jr. Fractures and dislocations of the shoulder. In Rockwood CA, Green DP, eds. *Fractures in adults*, 2nd ed. Philadelphia: JB Lippincott, 1984:675–721.
33. Rose SH, Melton LJ, Morrey BF, Ilstrup DM, Riggs LB. Epidemiologic features of humeral fractures. *Clin Orthop* 1982;168:24–30.
34. Horak J, Nilsson B. Epidemiology of fractures of the upper end of the humerus. *Clin Orthop* 1975;112:250–253.
35. Kristiansen B, Andersen VLS, Olsen CA, Varmarken JE. The Neer classification of fractures of the proximal humerus. An assessment of interobserver variation. *Skeletal Radiol* 1988;17:420–422.
36. Ackerman C, Lam Q, Linder P, Kull C, Regazzoni P. Problematik der Fractur Klassification am proximalen Humerus. *Z Unfall Chir* 1986; 79:209–215.

37. Brien H, Noftall F, MacMaster S, Cumming T, Landells C, Rockwood P. Neer's classification system: a critical appraisal. *J Orthop Trauma* 1995;38:257–260.
38. Bernstein J, Adler LM, Blank JE, Dalsey RM, Williams GR, Iannotti JP. Evaluation of the Neer system of classification of proximal humeral fractures with computerized tomographic scans and plain radiographs. *J Bone Joint Surg [Am]* 1996;78:1371–1375.
39. Sjoden GOJ, Movin T, Guntner P, et al. Poor reproducibility of classification of proximal humeral fractures. Additional CT of minor value. *Acta Orthop Scand* 1997;68:239–242.
40. Sallay PI, Pedowitz RA, Mallon WJ, Vandemark RM, Dalton JD, Speer KP. Reliability and reproducibility of radiographic interpretation of proximal humeral fracture pathoanatomy. *J Shoulder Elbow Surg* 1997;6:60–69.
41. Correspondence. *J Bone Joint Surg [Am]* 1994;76:789–790.
42. Neer CS. Four-segment classification of proximal humeral fractures. In: Copeland S, ed. *Shoulder surgery*. London: WB Saunders, 1997: 321–331.
43. Cowell HR. [Editorial]: Patient care and scientific freedom. *J Bone Joint Surg* 1994;76:640–641.
44. Burstein AH. [Editorial]: Fracture classification systems: do they work and are they useful? *J Bone Joint Surg [Am]* 1993;75: 1743–1744.
45. Jakob RP, Kristiansen T, Mayo K, Ganz R, Muller ME. Classification and aspects of treatment of fractures of the proximal humerus. In: Bateman JE, Welsh RP, eds. *Surgery of the shoulder*. Philadelphia: BC Decker, 1984:330–343.
46. Siebenrock KA, Gerber C. The reproducibility of classification of fractures of the proximal end of the humerus. *J Bone Joint Surg [Am]* 1993;75:1751–1755.
47. de Anquin CE, de Anquin CA. Prosthetic replacement in the treatment of serious fractures of the proximal humerus. In: Bayley I, Kessel L, eds. *Shoulder surgery*. Berlin: Springer-Verlag, 1982:207–217.
48. Alpert SW, Ben-Yishay A, Koval KJ, Zuckerman JD. Proximal humerus. In: Green WS, ed. *Fractures and dislocations: a manual of orthopaedic trauma*. Lippincott-Raven Publishers, Philadelphia 1994:48–53.
49. Sherk HH, Probst C. Fractures of the proximal humeral epiphysis. *Orthop Clin North Am* 1975;6:401–413.
50. Wang P Jr, Koval KJ, Lemman W, Strongwater A, Grant A, Zuckerman JD. Case report: Salter-Harris type III fracture-dislocation of the proximal humerus. *J Pediatr Orthop* Part B Vol 6. No. 3, 1997 pp. 219–222.
51. Brashear HR Jr. Epiphyseal fractures. A microscopic study of the healing process in rats. *J Bone Joint Surg [Am]* 1959; 41:1055–1064.
52. Digby KM. The measurement of diaphysial growth in proximal and distal directions. *J Anat Physiol* 1916;50:187–188.
53. Cuomo F. Proximal humerus fractures in the elderly: Instructional course lecture #247. American Academy of Orthopaedic Surgeons. Annual meeting. San Francisco, CA. February 14, 1997.
54. McLaughlin HL. Posterior dislocation of the shoulder. *J Bone Joint Surg [Am]* 1952; 34:584–590.
55. Glessner JR. Intrathoracic dislocation of the humeral head. *J Bone Joint Surg [Am]* 1961;43:428–430.
56. Hardcastle PH, Fisher TH. Intrathoracic displacement of the humeral head with fracture of the surgical neck. *Injury* 1981; 12:313–315.
57. Patel MR, Parsee ML, Singerman RC. Intrathoracic dislocation of the head of the humerus. *J Bone Joint Surg [Am]* 1963; 45:1712–1714.
58. West EF. Intrathoracic dislocation of the humerus. *J Bone Joint Surg [Br]* 1949;31:61–62.
59. Hayes MJ, Van Winkle N. Axillary artery injury with minimally displaced fracture of the neck of the humerus. *J Trauma* 1983;23: 431–433.
60. Smyth EHJ. Major arterial injury in a closed fracture of the neck of the humerus: report of a case. *J Bone Joint Surg [Br]* 1969;51:508–510.
61. Lindholm TS, Elmstedt E. Bilateral posterior dislocation of the shoulder combined with fracture of the proximal humerus. *Acta Orthop Scand* 1980;51:485–488.
62. Stableforth PG. Four-part fractures of the neck of the humerus. *J Bone Joint Surg [Br]* 1984;66:104–108.
63. Pasila M, Jeroma H, Kivilnoto O, Sundholm A. Early complications of primary shoulder dislocations. *Acta Orthop Scand* 1978;49: 260–263.
64. Cofield RH. Comminuted fractures of the proximal humerus. *Clin Orthop* 1988;230:49–57.
65. Hawkins RJ, Angelo RL. Displaced proximal humeral fractures: selecting treatment, avoiding pitfalls. *Orthop Clin North Am* 1987;18: 421–431.
66. Rockwood CA, Szaleay EA, Curtis RJ, Young DC, Kay SP. X-ray evaluation of shoulder problems. In: Rockwood CA, Matsen FA, eds. *The shoulder*, vol 1. Philadelphia: WB Saunders, 1990:178–184.
67. Bloom MH, Obata WG. Diagnosis of posterior dislocation of the shoulder with use of Velpeau axillary and angle-up roentgenographic views. *J Bone Joint Surg [Am]* 1967;49:943–949.
68. Brems-Dalgaard E, Davidsen E, Sloth C. Radiographic examination of the acute shoulder. *Eur J Radiol* 1990;11:10–14.
69. Zuckerman JD, Buchalter JS. Shoulder injuries. In: Zucklermam JD, ed. *Comprehensive care of orthopaedic injuries in the elderly*. Baltimore: Urban & Schwarzenberg, 1990:307.
70. DeSmet AA. Anterior oblique projection in radiography of the traumatized shoulder. *Am J Radiol* 1980;134:515–518.
71. Rubin SA, Gray RL, Green WR. The scapular "Y": a diagnostic aid in shoulder trauma. *Radiology* 1974;110:725–726.
72. Neviaser RJ. Radiologic assessment of the shoulder: plain and arthrographic. *Orthop Clin North Am* 1987;18:343–349.
73. Whiston TB. Fractures of the surgical neck of the humerus: a study in reduction. *J Bone Joint Surg [Br]* 1954;36:423–427.
74. Silfverskiold JP, Straehley DJ, Jones WW. Roentgenographic evaluation of suspected shoulder dislocations: a prospective study comparing the axillary view and the scapular "Y" view. *Orthopedics* 1990;13: 63–69.
75. Sidor ML, Zuckerman JD, Lyon T, Koval K, Cuomo F, Schoenberg N. Classification of proximal humerus fractures: the contribution of the scapular lateral and axillary radiographs. *J Shoulder Elbow Surg* 1994;3:24–27.
76. Garth WP Jr, Slappey CE, Ochs CW. Roentgenographic demonstration of instability of the shoulder: the apical oblique projection—a technical note. *J Bone Joint Surg [Am]* 1984;66:1450–1453.
77. Korngluth PJ, Salazar AM. The apical oblique view of the shoulder: its usefulness in acute trauma. *AJR Am J Radiol* 1987;149:113—116.
78. Richardson JB, Ramay A, Davidson JK, Kelly IG. Radiographs in shoulder trauma. *J Bone Joint Surg [Br]* 1988;70:457–460.
79. Horsfield D, Jones SN. A useful projection in radiography of the shoulder. *J Bone Joint Surg [Br]* 1987;69:338.
80. Tietge RA, Cuiollo JV. C.A.M. axillary x-ray. Exhibit to the Academy meeting of the American Academy of Orthopaedic Surgeons., *Orthop Trans* 1982;6:451.
81. Castagno AA, Shuman WP, Kilcoyne RF, Haynor DR, Morris ME, Matsen FA. Complex fractures of the proximal humerus: role of CT in treatment. *Radiology* 1987;165:759–762.
82. Kilcoyne RF, Shuman WP, Matsen FA III, Morris M, Rockwood CA. The Neer classification of displaced proximal humeral fractures: spectrum of findings on plain radiographs and CT scans. *AJR Am J Radiol* 1990;154:1029–1033.
83. Jurik AG, Albrechtsen J. The use of computed tomography with two- and three dimensional reconstructions in the diagnosis of three and four-part fractures of the proximal humerus. *Clin Radiol* 1994;49: 800–804.
84. Billet FP, Schmitt WG, Gay B. Computed tomography in traumatology with special regard to the advances of three dimensional display. *Arch Orthop Trauma Surg* 1992;111:131-137.
85. Kuhlman JE, Fishman EK, Ney DR, Magid D. Complex shoulder trauma: three-dimensional CT imaging. *Orthopedics* 1988;11: 1561–1563.
86. Drury JK, Scullion JE. Vascular complications of anterior dislocation of the shoulder. *J Bone Joint Surg* 1980;67:579–581.
87. Morris GC Jr, Beall AC Jr, Roof WR, et al. Surgical experience with 220 acute arterial injuries in civilian practice. *Am J Surg* 1960;99:775.
88. Leborgne J, Le Neel JC, Mitard D, et al. Les lesions de l' artere axillaire et de ses branches consecutives a un traumatisme firme de l'epaule. A propos de 10 observations. *Ann Chir* 1973;27:587.
89. Linson Marca. Axillary artery thrombosis after fracture of the humerus. *J Bone Joint Surg [Am]* 1980;62:1214.
90. Smythe EHJ. Major arterial injury in closed fracture of the neck of the humerus. Report of a case. *J Bone Joint Surg [Br]* 1969;51:508.
91. Theodorides T, de Keizer G. Injuries of the axillary artery caused by fractures of the neck of the humerus. *Injury* 1976;8:120.
92. Marty B, Simmen HP, Neff U, Habegger R. Subcapital humerus fracture with lesion of the axillary artery. 2 case reports and review of the literature. *Unfallchirurg* 1996;99:154–157.

93. Milton GW. The circumflex nerve and dislocation of the shoulder. *Br J Phys Med* 1954;17:136–138.
94. Brown FW, Navigato WJ. Rupture of the axillary artery and brachial plexus palsy associated with anterior dislocation of the shoulder. *Clin Orthop* 1968;60:195–199.
95. Stromqvist B, Lidgren L, Norgren L, Odenbring S. Neurovascular injury complicating displaced proximal fractures of the humerus. *Injury* 1987;18:423–425.
96. McQuillan WM, Nolan B. Ischaemia complicating injury: a report of thirty-seven cases. *J Bone Joint Surg [Br]* 1968;50:482.
97. Sathyarup D, Hulgol AK, Iyer KM. Axillary artery thrombosis following a fracture of the neck of the humerus. *Injury* 1988; 19:45–47.
98. White EM, Kattapuram SV, Jupiter JB. Case report 241. *Skeletal Radiol* 1983;10:178–182.
99. Barra JA, LeSaout J, Gaultier Y. Manifestations tardives des complications vasculaires des trauma tismes fermes de l'epaule. *J Chir* 1978; 115:151–157.
100. Fitzgerald JF, Keates J. False aneurysm as a late complication of anterior dislocation of the shoulder. *Ann Surg* 1975;181:785–786.
101. Hildinsson C, Toolanen G, Hedlund T. Late vascular complication after fracture of the proximal humerus. *Arch Orthop Trauma Surg* 1996; 115:357–358.
102. Stein E. Case report 374: post-traumatic pseudoaneurysm of axillary artery. *Skeletal Radiol* 1986;15:391–393.
103. Bhamra M, Ferris BD, Paton DF. Axillary aneurysm after shoulder injury. A report of 2 cases. *Acta Orthop Scand* 1989;60:225–226.
104. Norris TR. Fractures of the proximal humerus and dislocations of the shoulder. In: Browner BD, Jupiter JB, Levine AM, Trafton PG, eds. *Skeletal trauma*. Philadelphia: WB Saunders, 1992:1201–1290.
105. Hawkins RJ, Neer CS II, Pianta RM, Mendoza FX. Locked posterior dislocation of the shoulder. *J Bone Joint Surg [Am]* 1987;69:9–18.
106. Broker FHL, Burbain T. Ultrasonic diagnosis of separation of the proximal humeral epiphysis in the newborn. *J Bone Joint Surg [Am]* 1990;72:187–191.
107. Kristiansen B, Barfod G, Bredesen J, et al. Epidemiology of proximal humeral fractures. *Acta Orthop Scand* 1987;58:75–77.
108. Jensen GF, Christiansen C, Boesen J, et al. Relationship between bone mineral content and frequency of postmenopausal fractures. *Acta Med Scand* 1983;213:61–63.
109. Jakob RP, Kristiansen T, Mayo K, et al. Classification and aspects of treatment of fractures of the proximal humerus. In: Bateman JE, Welsh RP, eds. *Surgery of the shoulder*. Philadelphia: BC Decker, 1984.
110. Wentworth ET. Fractures involving the shoulder. *NY J Med* 1940;40: 1282.
111. Roberts SM. Fractures of the upper end of the humerus: an end-result study which shows the advantage of early active motion. *JAMA* 1932; 98:367–373.
112. Schweiger G, Ludolph E. Fractures of the shoulder joint. *Unfallchirurg* 1980;6:51–56.
113. Greeley PW, Magnuson PB. Dislocation of the shoulder accompanied by fracture of the greater tuberosity and complicated by spinatus tendon injury. *JAMA* 1934;102:1835–1838.
114. Bourdillan JF. Fracture–separation of the proximal epiphysis of the humerus. *J Bone Joint Surg [Br]* 1950;32:35–37.
115. Jeffrey CC. Fracture separation of the upper humeral epiphysis. *Surg Gynecol Obstet* 1953;96:205–209.
116. Whitman RA. Treatment of epiphyseal displacement and fractures of the upper extremity of the humerus designed to assure deficit adjustment and fixation of the fragments. *Ann Surg* 1908;47:706–708.
117. Larsen CF, Kiaer T, Lindequist S. Fractures of the proximal humerus in children: 9-year follow-up of 64 unoperated on cases. *Acta Orthop Scand* 1990;61:255–257.
118. Saunders JO, Rockwood CA Jr, Curtis RJ. Fracture dislocations of the humeral shaft and shoulder. In: Rockwood CA Jr, Wilkins KE, Beaty JH, eds. *Fractures in children*, 4th ed. Philadelphia: Lippincott–Raven, 1996:905–1019
119. Smith FM. Fracture–separation of the proximal humeral epiphysis: a study of cases seen at the Presbyterian Hospital, 1929–1953. *Am J Surg* 1956;91:627–635.
120. Burgos-Flores J, Gonzalez-Herranz P, Lopez-Mondejar JA, Ocete-Guzman JG, Amay a-Alarcon S. Fractures of the proximal humeral epiphysis. *Int Orthop* 1993;17:16–19.
121. Muller ME, Allgower M, Schneider R, et al. *Manual of internal fixation. Techniques recommended by the AO-ASIF group*, 3d ed. Berlin: Springer-Verlag, 1991.
122. Sessa S, Lascombes P, Prevot J, Gagneux E, Blanquart D. Centromedullary nailing in fractures of the upper end of the humerus in children and adolescents. *Chir Pediatr* 1990;31:43–46.
123. Stewart MJ, Hundley JM. Fractures of the humerus: a comparative study in methods of treatment. *J Bone Joint Surg [Am]* 1955;37: 681–692.
124. Fraser RL, Haliburton RA, Barber JR. Displaced epiphyseal fractures of the proximal humerus. *Can J Surg* 1967;10:427–430.
125. Lentz W, Meuser P. The treatment of fractures of the proximal humerus. *Arch Orthop Trauma Surg* 1980;96:283–285.
126. Lee HG. Operative reduction of an unusual fracture of the upper epiphyseal plate of the humerus. *J Bone Joint Surg* 1944;26:401–404.
127. Visser JD, Rietberg M. Interposition of the tendon of the long head of biceps in fracture separation of the proximal humeral epiphysis. *Neth J Surg* 1980;32:12–15.
128. Cohn BT, Froimson AI. Salter 3 fracture–dislocation of glenohumeral joint in a 10-year-old. *Orthop Rev* 1986;15:403–404.
129. Ross GJ, Love MB. Isolated avulsion fracture of the lesser tuberosity of the humerus: report of 2 cases. *Radiology* 1989;172:833–834.
130. Metaizeau JP, Ligier JN. Surgical treatment of fractures of the long bones in children. Interference between osteosynthesis and the physiological processes of consolidation. Therapeutic indications. *J Chir (Paris)* 1984;121:527–537.
131. Weseley MS, Barenfeld PA, Eisenstein AL. Rush pin intramedullary fixation for fractures of the proximal humerus. *J Trauma* 1977;17: 29–37.
132. Putz P, Arias C, Bremen J, Delvaux D, Simons M. Treatment of epiphyseal fractures of the proximal humerus using Hackethal's bundled wires apropos of 136 cases. *Acta Orthop Belg* 1987;53:80–87.
133. Clifford PC. Fractures of the neck of the humerus: a review of the late results. *Injury* 1980;12:91–95.
134. Kristiansen B, Angermann P, Larsen TK. Functional results following fractures of the proximal humerus: a controlled clinical study comparing two periods of immobilization. *Arch Orthop Trauma Surg* 1989; 108:339–341.
135. Lundberg BJ, Svenungson-Hartvig E, Wikmark R. Independent exercises versus physiotherapy in nondisplaced proximal humerus fractures. *Scand J Rehabil Med* 1979;11:133–139.
136. Young TB, Wallace WA. Conservative treatment of fractures and fracture–dislocations of the upper end of the humerus. *J Bone Joint Surg [Br]* 1985;67:373–377.
137. Richards RR, Bigliani LU, Friedman RJ, et al. A standardized method for the assessment of shoulder function. *J Shoulder Elbow Surg* 1994; 3:347–352.
138. Broker FHL, Burbach T. Ultrasonic diagnosis of separation of the proximal humeral epiphysis in the newborn. *J Bone Joint Surg [Am]* 1990;72:187–191.
139. Koval KJ, Gallagher MA, Marsicano JG, Cuomo F, McShinawy A, Zuckerman JD. Functional outcome after minimally displaced fractures of the proximal part of the humerus. *J Bone Joint Surg [Am]* 1997;79:203–207.
140. Neer CS II, Craig EV, Fukuda H. Cuff tear arthropathy. *J Bone Joint Surg [Am]* 1983;65:1232–1244.
141. Bateman JE. *The shoulder and neck*. Philadelphia: WB Saunders, 1972.
142. DePalma AF. *Surgery of the shoulder*, 2nd ed. Philadelphia: JB Lippincott, 1973.
142a. Post M. *The shoulder. Surgical and nonsurgical management*, 2nd ed. Philadelphia: Lea & Febiger, 1988:535–536.
143. Flatow EL, Cuomo F, Maday MG, Miller SR, McIlveen SJ, Bigliani LU. Open reduction and internal fixation of two-part displaced fractures of the greater tuberosity of the proximal humerus. *J Bone Joint Surg [Am]* 1991;73:1213–1218.
144. Dahners LE. Internal fixation of proximal humeral fractures. *J South Orthop Assoc* 1995;4:3–8.
145. Jaberg H, Warner JJP, Jakob RP. Percutaneous stabilization of unstable fractures of the humerus. *J Bone Joint Surg [Am]* 1992;74: 508–515.
146. Ebraheim N, Wong FY, Biyani A. Percutaneous pinning of the proximal humerus. *Orthopaedics* 1996;500–501.
147. Resch H, Povacz P, Frohlich R, Wambacher M. Percutaneous fixation of three- and four-part fractures of the proximal humerus. *J Bone Joint Surg [Br]* 1997;79:295–300.
148. Kristiansen B, Kofoed H. External fixation of displaced fractures of the proximal humerus: techniques and preliminary results. *J Bone Joint Surg [Br]* 1987;69:643–646.

149. Kolialkowski A, Wallace WA. Closed percutaneous K-wire stabilization for displaced fractures of the surgical neck of the humerus. *Injury* 1990;21:209–212.
150. Angehrn F, Schultheiss HR. Percutaneous drill wire osteosynthesis of fractures of the proximal humerus. *Z Unfallchir* 1986;79:155–160.
151. Hagg O, Lundberg B. Aspects of prognostic factors in comminuted and dislocated proximal humerus fractures. In: Bateman JE, Welsh PR, eds. *Surgery of the shoulder*. Philadelphia: BC Decker, 1984: 51–59.
152. Hawkins RJ, Kiefer GN. Internal fixation techniques for proximal humeral fractures. *Clin Orthop* 1987;223:77–85.
153. Hawkins RJ, Bell RH, Gurr K. The three-part fracture of the humerus. Operative treatment. *J Bone Joint Surg [Am]* 1986; 68:1410–1414.
154. Jakob RP, Ganz R. Proximale Humerusfrakturen. *Helv Chir Acta* 1981;48:595–610
155. Kriastiansen B, Bjarne, Kofoed H. Transcutaneous reduction and external fixation of displaced fractures of the proximal humerus. *J Bone Joint Surg [Br]* 1988;70:821–824.
156. Kyle RF, Conner TN. External fixation of the proximal humerus. *Orthopedics* 1988;11:163–168.
157. Magerl F. Osteosynthesen im Bereich der Schulter. Pertuberkulare Humerusfrakturen. Skapulahalsfra kturen. *Helv Chir Acta* 1974;41: 225–232.
158. Tanner MW, Cofield RH. Prosthetic arthroplasty for fractures and fracture–dislocation of the proximal humerus. *Clin Orthop* 1983;179: 116–128.
159. Vukov V, Bumbasirevic M. Drahtosteosynthese bei Frakturen im Schulterbereich. *Beitr Orthop Traumatol* 1986;33:494–500.
160. Kristiansen B, Christensen SW. Fractures of the proximal end of the humerus caused by convulsive seizures. *Injury* 1984;16:108–109.
161. Kuner EH, Siebler G. Fracture–dislocations of the proximal humerus. *Unfallchirurgie* 1987;13:64.
162. Paavolainen P, Bjorkenheim JM, Slatis P, et al. Operative treatment of severe proximal humeral fractures. *Acta Orthop Scand* 1983;54:374.
163. Sturzenegger M, Fornaro E, Jacob RP. Results of surgical treatment of multifragmented fractures of the humeral head. *Arch Orthop Trauma Surg* 1982;100:249.
164. Koval KJ, Blair B, Takei R, Kummer FJ, Zuckerman JD. Surgical neck fractures of the proximal humerus: a laboratory evaluation of ten fixation techniques. *J Trauma* 1996;40:778–783.
165. Cuomo F, Flatow EL, Maday MG, Miller SR, McIlveen SJ, Bigliani LU. Open reduction and internal fixation of two- and three-part displaced surgical neck fractures of the proximal humerus. *J Shoulder Elbow Surg* 1992;1:287–295.
166. Contreras D, Day L, Bovill D, Appleton A. Combined Enders rods and tension banding for humeral neck fractures. Presented at the 57th Annual Meeting, American Academy of Orthopaedic Surgeons, New Orleans, February 9, 1990.
167. Koval KJ, Sanders R, Zuckerman JD, et al. Modified tension band wiring of displaced surgical neck fractures of the humerus. *J Shoulder Elbow Surg* 1993;2:85.
168. Cuomo F, Flatow EL, Maday MG, et al. Open reduction and internal fixation of two- and three-part displaced surgical neck fractures of the proximal humerus. *J Shoulder Elbow Surg* 1992; 1:287–295.
169. Clifford PC. Fractures of the neck of the humerus: a review of the late results. *Injury* 1980;12:91–95.
170. Kristiansen B, Christiensen SW. Plate fixation of proximal humeral fractures. *Acta Orthop Scand* 1986;57:320–323.
171. Zyto K, Ahrengart L, Sperber A, Tornkvist H. Treatment of displaced proximal humeral fractures in elderly patients. *J Bone Joint Surg [Br]* 1997;79:412–417.
172. Bigliani LU. Fractures of the proximal humerus. Rockwood CA, Matsen FA, eds. *The shoulder*. Philadelphia: WB Saunders, 1990: 278–334.
173. Savoie FH, Geissler WB, Vander Griend RA. Open reduction and internal fixation of three-part fractures of the proximal humerus. *Orthopaedics* 1989;12:65–70.
174. Ruedi T. The treatment of displaced metaphyseal fractures with screws and wiring systems. *Orthopaedics* 1989;12:55–59.
175. Yamano Y. Comminuted fractures of the proximal humerus treated with hook plate. *Arch Orthop Trauma Surg* 1986;105:359–363.
175a. Kuner EH, Siebler G. Luxationsfrakturen des proximalen Humerus. *Unfallchirurgie* 1987;13:64.
176. Munst P, Kuner EH. Osteosynthesen bei dislozierten Humeruskopffrakturen. *Orthopade* 1992;21:121–130.
177. Esser RD. Treatment of three- and four-part fractures of the proximal humerus with a modified clover leaf plate. *J Orthop Trauma* 1994;8:15–22.
178. Fournier P, Martini M. Post-traumatic avascular necrosis of the humeral head. *Int Orthop* 1977;1:187–190.
179. Hagg O, Lundberg B. Aspects of prognostic factors in comminuted and dislocated proximal humeral fractures. Bateman JE, Welsh RP, eds. *Surgery of the shoulder*. Philadelphia: BC Decker, 1984.
180. Lee CK, Hansen H. Post-traumatic avascular necrosis of the humeral head in displaced humeral fractures. *J Trauma* 1981;21:788–791.
181. Mouradin WH. Displaced proximal humeral fractures, seven years' experience with a modified Zickel supracondylar device. *Clin Orthop* 1986;212:209–218.
182. Kraulis J, Hunter G. The results of prosthetic replacement in fracture dislocations of the upper end of the humerus. *Injury* 1976;8:129–131.
183. Switlyk P, Hawkins RJ. Hemiarthroplasty for treatment of severe proximal humeral fractures. Presented at the American Shoulder and Elbow Surgeons' Meeting, Las Vegas, February 12, 1989.
184. Esser RD. Open reduction and internal fixation of three- and four-part fractures of the proximal humerus. *Clin Orthop* 1994;299:244–251.
185. Knight RA, Mayne JA. Comminuted fractures and fracture dislocations involving the articular surface of the humeral head. *J Bone Joint Surg [Am]* 1957;39:1343–1355.
186. Sven-Hensen H. Displaced proximal humeral fractures. *Acta Orthop Scand* 1974;45:359–364.
187. Marti R, Lim TE, Jolles CW. *On the treatment of comminuted fracture- dislocations of the proximal humerus: internal fixation or prosthetic replacement*. Berlin: Springer-Verlag 1987:135–148.
188. Leyshon RL. Closed treatment of fractures of the proximal humerus. *Acta Orthop Scand* 1984;55:48–51.
189. Resch H, Beck E, Bayley I. Reconstruction of the valgus-impacted humeral head fracture. *J Shoulder Elbow Surg* 1995;4:73–80.
190. Cuomo F. Fractures about the shoulder. *Curr Opin Orthop* 1996;7: 77–82.
191. Vandenbussche E, Peraldi P, Naouri JF, Rougereau G, Augereau B. Four-part valgus impacted fractures of the proximal humerus: graft reconstruction. Report of 8 cases. *Rev Chir Orthop* 1996;82: 658–662.
192. Compito CA, Self EB, Bigliani LU. Arthroplasty and acute shoulder trauma. *Clin Orthop* 1994;307:27–36.
193. Connor PM, D'Alessandro DF. Role of hemiarthroplasty for proximal humeral fractures. *J South Orthop Assoc* 1995;4:9–23.
194. McIlveen SJ, Neer CS. Recent results and technique of prosthetic replacement for four-part proximal humerus fractures. Presented at the annual meeting of the American Shoulder and Elbow Surgeons, Atlanta, Georgia, February 1988.
195. Willems W, Lim TE. Neer arthroplasty for humeral fracture. *Acta Orthop Scand* 1985;56:394–395.
196. Goldman RT, Koval KJ, Cuomo F, Gallagher MA, Zuckerman JD. Functional outcome after humeral head replacement for acute three- and four-part proximal humeral fractures. *J Shoulder Elbow Surg* 1995;4:81–86,
197. Green A, Barnard LW, Limbird RS. Proximal humeral replacement for acute three- and four-part fractures and fracture–dislocations. *Orthop Trans* 1992;16:335.
198. Wretenberg P, Ekelund A. Acute hemiarthroplasty after proximal humerus fracture in old patients. A retrospective evaluation of 18 patients followed for 2–7 years. *Acta Orthop Scand* 1997;68:121–123.
199. Segal W, Weiglein A. Die arterielle Blutversorgung des Oberarmkopfes und ihre prognostische Bedeutung bei Luxationen, Frakturen and Luxationsfrak turen des Oberamkopfes. *Acta Chir Austriaca Suppl 92* 1991;23:1–19.
200. Bosch U, Fremerey RW, Skutek M, Lobenhoffer P, Tscherne H. Hemiarthroplasty—a primary or secondary procedure for three- and four-part proximal humeral fractures in elderly patients? *Unfallchirurg* 1996;99:656–664.
201. Kohler A, Simmen HP, Duff C, Kach K. Trentz Osteosynthese subkapitaler humerusfrakturen mit unkonventionell. Applizierten implantaten. *Swiss Surg* 1995;2:114–117.
202. Speck M, Lang FJH, Regazzoni P. Proximale humerusmehrfragment frakturen—Misserfolgenach T-Platten Osteosynthesen. *Swiss Surg* 1996;2:51–56.
203. Baron JA, Barrett J, Malenka D, et al. Racial difference in fracture risk. *Epidemiology* 1994;5:42–47.

204. Marty B, Simmen HP, Neff U, Habegger R. Axillary artery injury after proximal humeral fractures. Two case reports and a review of the literature. *Unfallchirurg* 1996;99:154–157.
205. Dines DM, Warren RF. Modular shoulder hemiarthoplasty for acute fractures. Surgical considerations. *Clin Orthop* 1994;307:18–26.
206. Zuckerman JD, Cuomo F, Koval KJ. Proximal humeral replacement for complex fractures: indications and surgical technique. In: Springfield DS, ed. *Instructional course lectures*, vol 46. Rosemont, IL: 1997:7–14.
207. Baxter MP, Wiley JJ. Fractures of the proximal humeral epiphysis. Their influence on humeral growth. *J Bone Joint Surg [Br]* 1986;68: 570–573.
208. Nordqvist A, Petersson CJ. Incidence and causes of shoulder girdle injuries in an urban population. *J Shoulder Elbow Surg* 1995;4:107–112.
209. Wang JR, Koval KJ, Lehman W, Strongwater A, Grant A, Zuckerman JD. Salter-Harris type III fracture–dislocation of the proximal humerus. *J Pediatr Orthop B* 1997;6:219–222.
210. Naidu SH, Bixler B, Capo JT, Moulton MJR, Radin A. Percutaneous pinning of proximal humerus fractures: a biomechanical study. *Orthopedics* 1997;20:1073–1076.
211. Williams GR Jr, Copley LA, Iannotti JP, Lisser SP. The influence of intramedullary fixation on figure-of-eight wiring for surgical neck fractures of the proximal humerus: a biomechanical study. *J Shoulder Elbow Surg* 1997;6:423–428.
212. Rowe CR. Prognosis in dislocations of the shoulder. *J Bone Joint Surg [Am]* 1956;38:957.
213. Wirth MA, Rockwood CA. Complications of treatment of injuries to the shoulder. In: Epps CH, ed. *Complications in orthopaedic surgery*, vol 1. Philadelphia: JB Lippincott, 1994:229.
214. Gristina AG, Bigliani LU, Nevaiser RJ, et al. Symposium: management of displaced fractures of the proximal humerus. *Contemp Orthop* 1987;15:61.
215. De Palma AF. *Surgery of the shoulder*, 2nd ed. Philadelphia: JB Lippincott, 1973.
216. Leffert RD, Seddon H. Infraclavicular brachial plexus injuries. *J Bone Joint Surg [Br]* 1965;47:9.
217. Ferkel RD, Hedley AK, Eckhardt JJ. Anterior fracture–dislocations of the shoulder: pitfalls in treatment. *J Trauma* 1984;24:363.
218. Watson-Jones R. Dislocation of the shoulder joint. *Proc R Soc Med* 1936;29:1060.
219. Blom S, Dahlback LO. Nerve injuries in dislocations of the shoulder joint and fractures of the neck of the humerus. *Acta Chir Scand* 1970; 136:461.
220. Brown JT. Nerve injuries complicating dislocation of the shoulder. *J Bone Joint Surg [Br]* 1952;34:526.
221. Rowe CR, Zarins B. Chronic unreduced dislocations of the shoulder. *J Bone Joint Surg [Am]* 1982;64:494.
222. Wilson JC, McKeever FM. Traumatic posterior (retroglenoid) dislocation of the humerus. *J Bone Joint Surg [Am]* 1949;31:160.
223. Blasier RB, Burkus JK. Management of posterior fracture–dislocations of the shoulder. *Clin Orthop* 1988;232:197.
224. Clancy WG, Brand RL, Bergfeld JA. Upper trunk brachial plexus injuries in contact sports injuries. *Am J Sports Med* 1977;5:209.
225. Pasila M, Jaroma H, Kiviluoto O, et al. Early complications of primary shoulder dislocations. *Acta Orthop Scand* 1978;49:260.
226. Baratta JB, Lim V, Mastromonaco E, Edillon EL. Axillary artery disruption secondary to anterior dislocation of the shoulder. *J Trauma* 1983;23:1009.
227. Curr JF. Rupture of the axillary artery complicating dislocation of the shoulder: report of a case. *J Bone Joint Surg [Br]* 1970;52:313.
228. Henson GF. Vascular complications of shoulder injuries. *J Bone Joint Surg [Br]* 1956;38:528.
229. Warrren R. Symposium: management of displaced fractures of the proximal humerus. *Contemp Orthop* 1987;15:61.
230. Brown FW, Navigato WJ. Rupture of the axillary artery and brachial plexus associated with anterior dislocation of the shoulder: report of a case with successful vascular repair. *Clin Orthop* 1968;60:195.

Disorders of the Shoulder: Diagnosis and Management,
edited by Joseph P. Iannotti and Gerald R. Williams, Jr.
Lippincott Williams & Wilkins, Philadelphia © 1999.

CHAPTER 25

Complications of Proximal Humerus Fractures: Diagnosis and Management

Tom R. Norris

Complications associated with proximal humerus fractures are more frequent than commonly appreciated. The complications can be divided into those caused by the injury and those from the treatment rendered. Frequent complications include stiffness, malunion, nonunion, subacromial impingement, rotator cuff tears, and traumatic arthritis.[85] Less common complications include instability (fixed versus recurrent), osteonecrosis, infection (following an open fracture or treatment), and heterotopic ossification. Complications that are even more devastating can be those of nerve or vascular injury, either from the injury or from subsequent closed or open reductions.

In addition to the upper extremity problems to be evaluated, consideration needs to be given to the patient's medical and psychologic status.[38] Medical problems that complicate treatment include substance abuse, such as alcoholism, smoking (which interferes with bone and cuff healing); abnormal calcium metabolism, including osteoporosis; and inflammatory arthritis.[42,55,97] Preexisting neurological disorders such as Parkinson's syndrome, seizure disorder, multiple sclerosis, and myesthethenia gravis, complicate the rehabilitation as well as the healing.

T. R. Norris: Department of Orthopaedic Surgery, California-Pacific Medical Center, San Francisco, California 94115.

DIAGNOSTIC IMAGING

A major source of complication is the missed or incomplete diagnosis that can be avoided by adequate and appropriate imaging.[37,83,88,89] The standard in orthopedic trauma is to have two, preferably three, orthogonal roentgenographic views in the scapular plane. These include an anteroposterior (AP), lateral scapular, and an axial view. If there is any difficulty in obtaining the axial view, then a limited computed tomography (CT) scan will very adequately identify tuberosity fracture–displacement, status and position of the articular surface relative to the glenoid, as well as head-splitting fractures.[13] Additional imaging may include rotational AP views to evaluate tuberosity or head shaft malunion, and scanograms to compare the injured with the uninjured side for possible shortening. The goal is to restore the deltoid myofascial length for leverage and strength. Practical measurements are comparative scanograms from the top of the humeral articular surface to the capitellum[82] (Fig. 1). This allows for correction of the articular height and any shortening of the deltoid length at the time of reconstruction. In late cases, a magnetic resonance imaging (MRI) scan may define with greatest accuracy the extent of

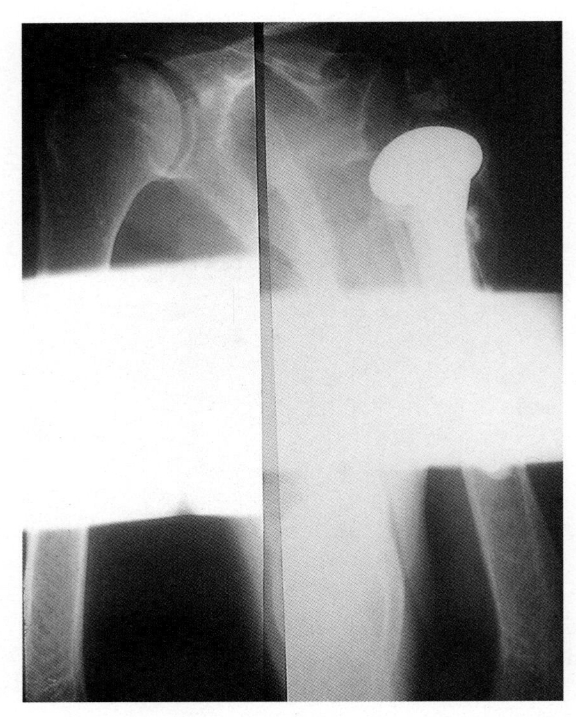

FIG. 1. Scanograms compare the two humeri for articular height discrepancies. These are measured between the top of the humeral head and the capitellum. The inferior subluxation in this patient follows a humeral head replacement for a four-part fracture. The prosthesis is low because (a) it was placed at the height of the surgical neck without accounting for the height of the tuberosities, and (b) the function of the axillary nerve was lost either with the original nerve injury or at the time of the humeral head replacement.

osteonecrosis and assist in staging the status of any rotator cuff pathology.

COMPLICATIONS OF INJURY

Neurologic Injury

With neurologic injury there are common patterns associated with certain fracture patterns. The incidence of neurologic injury is reported to be between 21% and 50%.[8,23,98] There have been numerous reports that outline the risk of temporary and permanent nerve or vascular injury with fractures and fracture–dislocations of the proximal humerus. The literature is not always clear. Some articles quote neuraprasias, without clarifying which ones have resolved spontaneously. Nerve injuries are more common than previously recognized. De Laat, Visser, and Coene et al. evaluated nerve lesions in primary shoulder dislocations and surgical neck fracture–dislocations with a prospective clinical and eltromyographic (EMG) study. Electrophysiologic evidence of nerve lesions was found in 45% of the 101 patients evaluated. The most commonly injured nerves were the axillary, suprascapular, radial, and musculocutaneous. These authors stress the importance of early diagnosis and treatment to prevent lasting impairment in those that involve more than a transient neurapraxia. In three other electrophysiologic studies of surgical neck fractures associated with glenohumeral dislocations, the axillary and other nerves were injured 20% to 30% of the time. Age was a factor; in those older than 50 years, the brachial plexus injury rate was 50%.[8,27,92]

The patient- and fracture-related factors associated with neurologic injury include the elderly and hematoma formation. Most have partial or complete recovery; 5% to 8% have persistent motor loss. The three common shoulder injuries associated with nerve injuries include the anterior shoulder dislocation, the two-part greater tuberosity fracture with an anterior dislocation, and the surgical neck fracture.[17,114] The most common single injury causing a nerve injury in the shoulder is the isolated two-part greater tuberosity fracture with an anterior dislocation.[98] The most common isolated fracture location is the surgical neck. This includes the two-part, three-part, and four-part surgical neck fractures. With a posterior fracture–dislocation, the axillary neurapraxia rate is 31% to 37% of the cases.[8,68] Following a four-part fracture, the nerve injury rate is 6.1%. Of this percentage, only one-third fully recover,[104] whereas following the three- and four-part fractures with a subsequent failed open reduction and internal fixation (ORIF), the permanent nerve injury rate rises to 17.4%, or approximately 8.7 times that of the permanent neuraprasias with the injury before treatment.[87] Thus, an ORIF as an intermediate step before arthroplasty has additional and significant risk. Worse yet, permanent loss of the axillary nerve occurs following blunt trauma in 50% of the cases.[4] Even an isolated anterior dislocation has a 10% to 20% axillary injury rate.[14,72] In summary, the risk increases with advancing patient age, the surgical neck fracture site, an associated dislocation, hematoma formation, blunt trauma, and a failed ORIF.

The diagnosis of nerve injury is more difficult with acute fractures, owing to pain, swelling, and immobilization; later, the physical examination for each motor group is more straightforward.[17,84,114] The major muscle groups to evaluate include the three divisions of the deltoid, the spinatii, the internal rotators, trapezius, serratus anterior, rhomboids, and the biceps and triceps. Within the internal rotators, the subscapularis can be isolated with the Gerber lift-off test.[32] The two external rotators, the infraspinatus and the teres minor, can be isolated by palpation and inspection before electrical confirmation.[99] These physical examination tests are unreliable with acute fractures, but can be performed after initial fracture healing.

The sensory examination, which has often been used for the evaluation of the deltoid, unfortunately, does not necessarily correlate with the motor integrity: EMG studies have documented the unreliability of sensory examination.[4,8] Specifically, the sensation can be intact in the axillary distribution, with disruption of the motor fibers. This has important implications in patient management as well as in the medical–legal exposure. If there is any question about the nerve integrity at any stage in the patient's course, EMG and nerve conduction studies may better delineate the patient's status preoperatively. This permits rational treatment plans (i.e., timing of nerve exploration, followed by decompression, primary or secondary repair or graft, or even in selected cases, muscle transfers). The shift in recent years has been to surgically explore those individuals who have complete loss without any recovery in any one motor group by 3 to 4 months.

The treatment of nerve injuries will depend on the nerves involved, the type of injury, as well as the age and health of the patient. Nerve recovery is better with younger patients and with less distance from the injury site to the motor endplate when reinnervation can occur. The prognosis for recovery from a sharp injury is better than from a blunt injury. Certainly, an early exploration and repair are justified with a penetrating injury with complete motor loss in a given motor group. The debatable area is the closed fracture with or without an accompanying dislocation and an associated brachial plexus deficit. The recent monograph *Traumatic Brachial Plexus Injuries* by Alnot and Narakas is an excellent guide for the complex cases that arise.[1,3]

Vascular Injuries

Vascular injuries are rare with proximal humeral fractures and fracture–dislocations. They are often masked by collateral circulation early on. The incidence of vascular injury is thought to be 0.3% to 3.0% with long bone fractures.[15] Conversely, in those with documented vascular injuries, 10% to 40% had long bone fractures or dislocations; 20% to 42% originally had negative physical findings.

The patient factors associated with vascular injury include the location of the fracture or dislocation, the mechanism of injury, and the age of the patient. More information is available on the association of brachial plexus injuries with vascular injuries. The vascular injuries are less frequently recognized because of the very extensive periscapular collateral circulation.[15] Traffic accidents account for 80%. Two main patterns predominate.[2] In the first and most common pattern, the shoulder is driven down and the head and cervical spine are flexed to the opposite side. This causes a traction injury to the plexus and vascular structures at the base of the neck. In the second, there is an acute narrowing of the costoclavicular space with a crush of the neurovascular structures of the thoracic outlet from a blow to the anterior shoulder girdle. The outlet is narrowed with the arm at the side, or worse when it is abducted. Associated proximal humerus fractures need not even be significantly displaced for a vascular injury to occur at the surgical neck level.[47] Fracture patterns associated with vascular injury usually involve fractures at the surgical neck of the humerus.[70,71,109] The artery at this level forms a "tethered trifurcation" where the anterior and posterior humeral circumflex vessels and subscapular trunks arise from the axillary artery (Fig. 2). The vascular injuries are associated with direct trauma, with a dislocated humeral head or a displaced upper humeral shaft. In a three-part greater tuberosity frac-

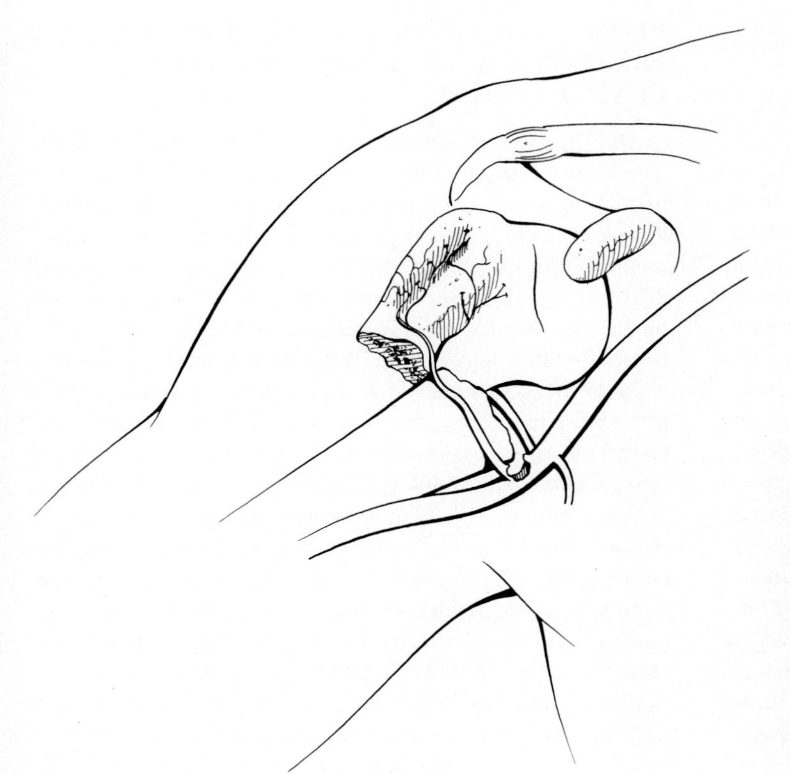

FIG. 2. Arterial tethered trifurcation: the anterior and posterior circumflex and subscapular arteries all arise from the axillary artery and diverge. These three vessels, arising from virtually the same level, tether the axillary artery. This makes it more vulnerable to tearing, rupture, or thrombosis with displaced proximal humeral fractures through the surgical neck. A simple anterior dislocation is less likely to injure these vessels, for two of the three vessels that tether the axillary artery travel with the humerus. A three- or four-part fracture–dislocation implies more trauma and more displacement. An elderly patient with more brittle atherosclerotic vessels is more likely to injure the axillary artery.

ture, the circumflex vessels can be caught in the surgical neck site. A thrombus can then develop in the axillary artery.[101] In this case report, intimal damage caused by traction injured the brachial artery and caused it to develop spasm. Thrombus removal alone was insufficient, but circulation was restorable with either a direct repair or by a vein graft. Intimal tears of the axillary artery are described in four other cases at the subscapular and circumflex branches.[49] In two, an anterior dislocation alone occurred. In two, there were three- or four-part fractures with anterior dislocations. Vessel repair restored circulation in all.

The diagnosis of vascular injury often requires a high level of suspicion when ischemia is noted. The physical findings may be subtle, for normal distal pulses may be intact in up to 27% with major arterial injuries about the shoulder. In addition to shoulder pain with the surgical neck fracture level, distal coolness and tingling develop. Palpation of the axillary artery may be precluded by pain, muscle spasm, and swelling. The brachial and radial pulses will be diminished or absent in over 70%. With time, pain on passive extension of the fingers occurs.[47] The six "Ps" to summarize vascular injury are pain, pallor, paralysis, paresthesias, poikilothermia, and pulselessness. In addition, there may be a large or expanding hematoma, pulsatile external bleeding, unexplained hypotension, or a bruit. Usually, a vascular injury accompanies a nerve injury at the same level. These signs and findings are indications for vascular investigation along with imaging. The single-injection trauma angiography is accurate in the operating room setting. If more time is available, then formal angiography can be obtained in the radiographic suite with retrograde femoral arteriogram. In addition, more sophisticated studies include digital subtraction angiography and Doppler arterial pulse volume recordings.

Most authors agree vascular injuries should be repaired. This is done immediately if there is acute ischemia. When performed on a delayed basis, it is to provide better nutrition for associated fracture and nerve healing.[2] At the time of emergency vascular repairs, the nerve repairs are best deferred until later. Then a good level of transection can be determined for the stretch injuries. The optimal time of nerve repair is 2 weeks to 3 months and may be combined with the elective vascular reconstructions. The one contraindication to a vascular repair is when the distal circulation is good through the collateral circulation and there is a complete plexus avulsion. Here, no plexus reconstruction is possible.

At the time of acute vascular repairs, the tradition has been to rigidly fix all fractures with plates and screws. More recently, the need for rigid fixation has been debated as more fractures are pinned percutaneously or with limited pin, intramedullary rod, and tension band techniques. This avoids much of the periosteal stripping.[20,21,89] In support of this transition, Sturznegger noted five times the osteonecrosis rate in treating multifragmented proximal humerus fractures with AO buttress plates as with tension band wiring.[106]

COMPLICATIONS OF MANAGEMENT

The complications of closed versus open treatment of fractures have many similarities. The advantage of closed reduction and treatment is the avoidance of an operative procedure and its inherent potential complications. Open reductions ideally permit an accurate and secure restoration of anatomy. This facilitates removal of any interposed muscle that would preclude a closed reduction,[54] the repositioning of the displaced tuberosities, rotator cuff repair, as well as any neurovascular exploration warranted. With secure fixation, earlier, safe motion may be instituted to prevent the pervasive scar and adhesions that accompany proximal humerus fractures. There are many variables to consider in determining which approaches to use. In addition,[44] many potential pitfalls complicate the treatment of proximal humerus fractures.

Stiffness is probably the ubiquitous complication. Attention has been directed to the importance of early motion in the postfracture and postoperative rehabilitation in an effort to prevent stiffness.[10,28,30,39,108,115] The etiology can be intracapsular as well as extracapsular. The intracapsular causes of stiffness include tightness at the rotator interval, loss of the inferior pouch, and articular incongruity. The last may be associated with tissue contracture on one or more sides of the joint. Extracapsular tightness derives from shortening of the coracohumeral ligament, adhesions in the subacromial and subdeltoid bursae, or bony incongruence with malunited fractures that can then act as bony blocks to motion. Although the results are thought to correlate with anatomic restoration, stiffness is the one variable not seen on the x-ray film.[57]

CLOSED VERSUS OPEN MANAGEMENT OF FRACTURES WITH THEIR POTENTIAL COMPLICATIONS

The first goal in trauma care is to ensure that the patient has stable vital signs and an adequate airway. Next, an accurate diagnosis is made with the history of injury and a physical examination. Imaging studies are the keystone to diagnosing and classifying the fracture types and associated dislocations. The options for treatment are based primarily on the fracture types with allowances for the individual's medical status, motivation, and the surgeon's familiarity with the options. Other than a pathologic fracture, nondisplaced fractures are treated with a sling for comfort, followed by early pendulum motion beginning at 2 weeks to prevent strong adhesions.[115] The goal is to treat the entire upper extremity to obtain early healing of muscle and rotator cuff attachments as well as the osseous components. This becomes more of a challenge with displaced fractures. Options include a closed reduction, percutaneous pinning, open reduction with various forms of internal fixation, and reconstruction around a humeral head replacement. Closed reduction is a good possibility for an isolated two-part surgical neck fracture; however, closed treatment has not fared well for these displaced fractures when an adequate and stable closed reduction is not achieved. The literature gives mixed reviews on the closed treatment of displaced proximal humeral fractures.[12,31,113] Svend-Hansen reported a failure in 63% of two-, three- and four-part displaced fractures of the proximal humerus.[107] Other studies have reported between 11% and 50% excellent and satisfactory results with three- and four-part fractures of the proximal humerus.[16,75] Leyshon reported 70% three-part fractures with satisfactory results, but all four-part fractures had unsatisfactory results.[69] One concern in reviewing some of the aforementioned articles is that not all fractures are considered displaced by Neer's criteria; hence, the percentage of good results is likely overreported.

The trend prevails for poor results with the rotator cuff detached, such as in three- and four-part fractures.[77] One of the main differences between closed and open treatment with displaced fractures is the lack of an anatomic reduction and a concomitant need to hold the fracture longer while waiting for early healing. Overly aggressive early passive motion, before fracture healing, has been associated with increased rates of nonunion.[77,78,91] Even with nondisplaced or minimally displaced fractures, treated nonoperatively, good to excellent functional recovery was found in only 77%. Earlier passive motion at 2 weeks was correlated with an improved result.[115] One must balance potential for adhesions and stiffness when early motion is delayed with potential scar and increased rate of nerve injury with operative treatment.[87] Other general operative complications may include inadequate open reduction; infection; dehiscence of any detached deltoid, the tuberosities, or rotator cuff; deltoid weakening from overly aggressive acromial excisions; and osteonecrosis.[48,91] The last may occur either from the fracture type or from excessive periosteal stripping when plates are used in preference to newer techniques with less invasive percutaneous pinning or tension band techniques.[53,106] Tuberosity malunion may result in subacromial impingement or blockage of motion. Hardware loosening, breakage, or joint penetration with malunions and nonunions are potential other complications. Uses of nonreamed intramedullary nails have the least favorable prognosis in Healy's series.[48]

Stiffness is the most pervasive problem in fracture care. This can occur even in one-part non- or minimally displaced fractures.[115] In a detailed functional outcome analysis on 104 nondisplaced or minimally displaced proximal humerus fractures treated nonoperatively, earlier motion at 14 days improved the results; although 94% reported functional recovery, 44% still had persistent pain. In an attempt to clarify one of the factors of stiffness, Gerber suggests that the intraarticular fractures are more prone to develop stiffness than extraarticular fractures. Thus, fractures involving a tuberosity or the articular surface will require more aggressive and early measures.

The principles include obtaining an anatomic and stable reduction, followed by a careful postoperative exercise program, in an effort to prevent stiffness. Adhesions that could arise from intraarticular joint incongruity should be addressed at the time of the original fracture, with perfect restoration of the anatomy. Later, articular incongruities may be addressed by prosthetic arthroplasty.

Another major cause of stiffness could be a fixed subluxation or dislocation; again, the imaging studies are critical. An axillary view eliminates much of the confusion over the position of the fragments (Fig. 3). If there is still any concern, a CT scan will clarify the position of the tuberosities relative to the articular surface, as well as the articular surface relative to the glenoid. Deltoid atony resulting in an inferior subluxation may be treated with upward support from a modified sling. Other significant causes for persistent inferior subluxation need to be evaluated and addressed.[112]

Later on, the treatment options, if physical therapy does not restore functional range of motion, include a manipulation under anesthesia, or a capsular release performed open or arthroscopically. Finally, for pure loss of external rotation that does not respond to a capsular release, a recession or lengthening of the subscapularis will improve external rotation.[40,82,111] Approximately 20 degrees are gained for every centimeter of subscapularis lengthening or recession of its insertion point on the lesser tuberosity closer to the articular surface (Fig. 4).

MALUNIONS

Malunions affecting function are more common than may be appreciated. They are almost assured to follow closed treatment of a displaced tuberosity fragment when the unopposed muscle pull retracts the fragment. The indications for treatment include pain, weakness, and significant stiffness. These all contribute to poor function, especially when full range of motion is needed. The goal is to restore the anatomy.

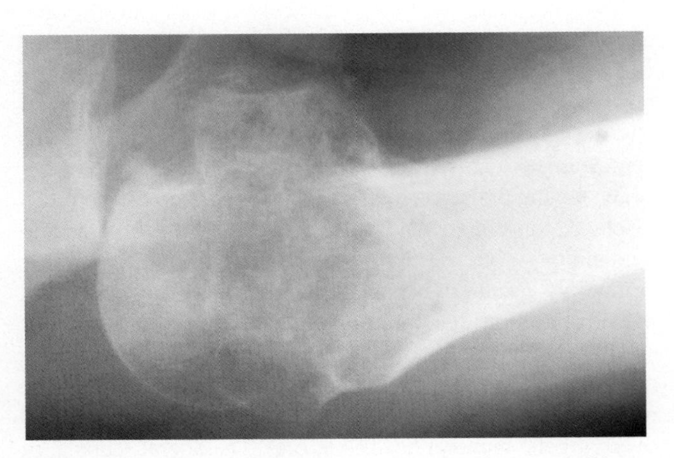

FIG. 3. Three-part malunion with a fixed posterior subluxation of the articular surface relative to the glenoid. Plans for lengthening the tight front structures and tightening the stretched posterior capsule need to be considered at the time of arthroplasty.

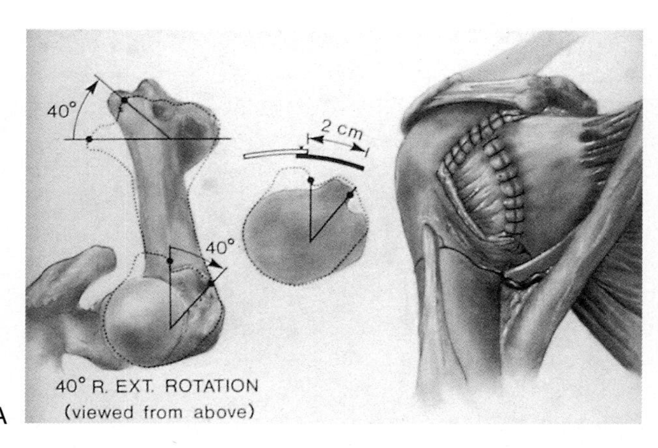

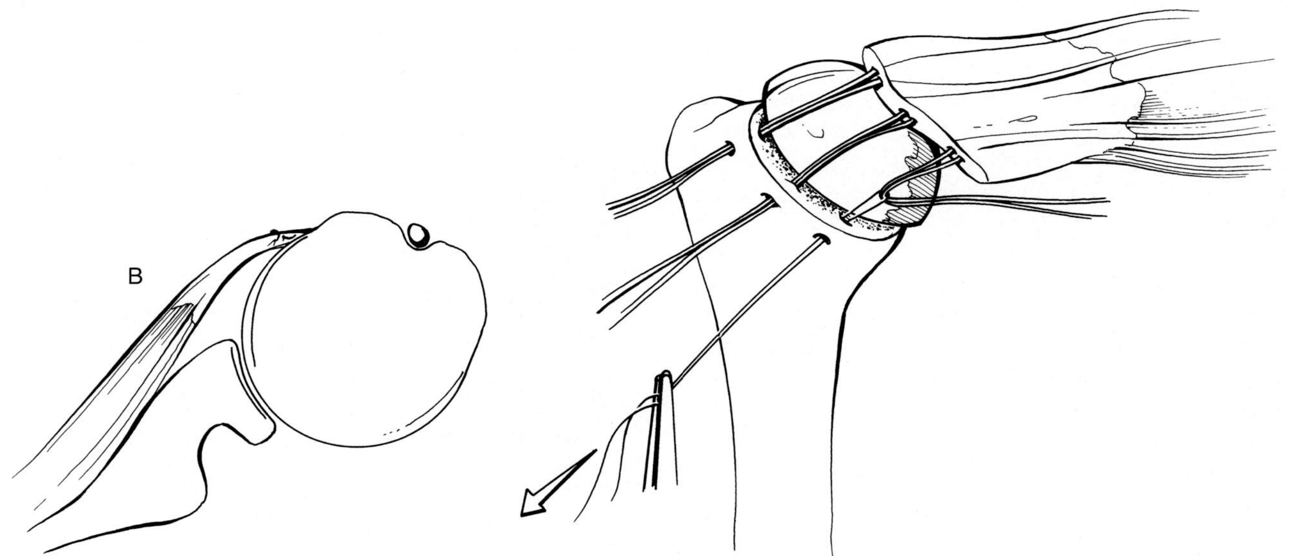

FIG. 4. Subscapularis lengthening restores 20 degrees of external rotation for every 1 cm gained. **(A)** Approximately 2 cm can be gained with subscapularis lengthening, and **(B)** 1 to 1.5 cm with a subscapularis recession.

Greater Tuberosity

The greater tuberosity malunion is likely the most troublesome. Two patterns predominate:[85] If the supraspinatus only is involved, then the displacement is superior into the subacromial space. The diagnosis is readily appreciated on an AP radiograph (Fig. 5). A significant tuberosity displacement represents a rotator cuff tear. If only a minor displacement exists, the avulsion fracture heals in situ, with an intact cuff. The supraspinatus can retract the tuberosity until it wedges between the top of the articular surface and the acromion. When displaced this far, such a displacement will probably go on to a nonunion, whereas 0.5- to 1-centimeter displacement more commonly results in a malunion. Any of the upwardly displaced malunions result in rotator cuff impingement.

The second pattern of displacement is posterior from the predominant pull of the infraspinatus. Diagnosis may be missed by an AP x-ray view alone, for the fragment may be overlying the humeral head (Fig. 6A). The lateral scapula, or better, an axial view, will demonstrate the greater tuberosity displacement (Fig. 6B). In these late cases, rotational views in the AP plane offer additional information. Here, a CT scan is indicated when plain films are inconclusive. The CT scan is the most accurate in demonstrating the fracture lines with segment displacement and any rotation of the articular surface.[13,81,83,84,89] Interobserver variations exist in the interpretation of plain films for tuberosity displacement. Castagno et al. report that the CT findings altered the treatment in 15 of 17 patients.[13] In 9, in whom significant displacement was diagnosed by plain films, the displacement was not confirmed by CT scan. Hence, the patients were treated by closed reduction. In 6 of the remaining 8, who underwent surgery, additional findings added to or altered the surgical treatment.

Implications of tuberosity malunion involve subacromial impingement, with as little as 3 to 5 mm of superior displacement. The symptoms include catching and pain. It is reasonable to anticipate that the tuberosity prominence will predispose the individual to an earlier rotator cuff tear. The posterior greater tuberosity displacement will impinge on the glenoid with attempted external rotation. Not only can there be posterior cuff weakness, but the posterior bony block will limit the range of motion for external rotation, as well as overhead elevation.

The indications and rationale for surgical treatment for these late complications are predominately pain and loss of

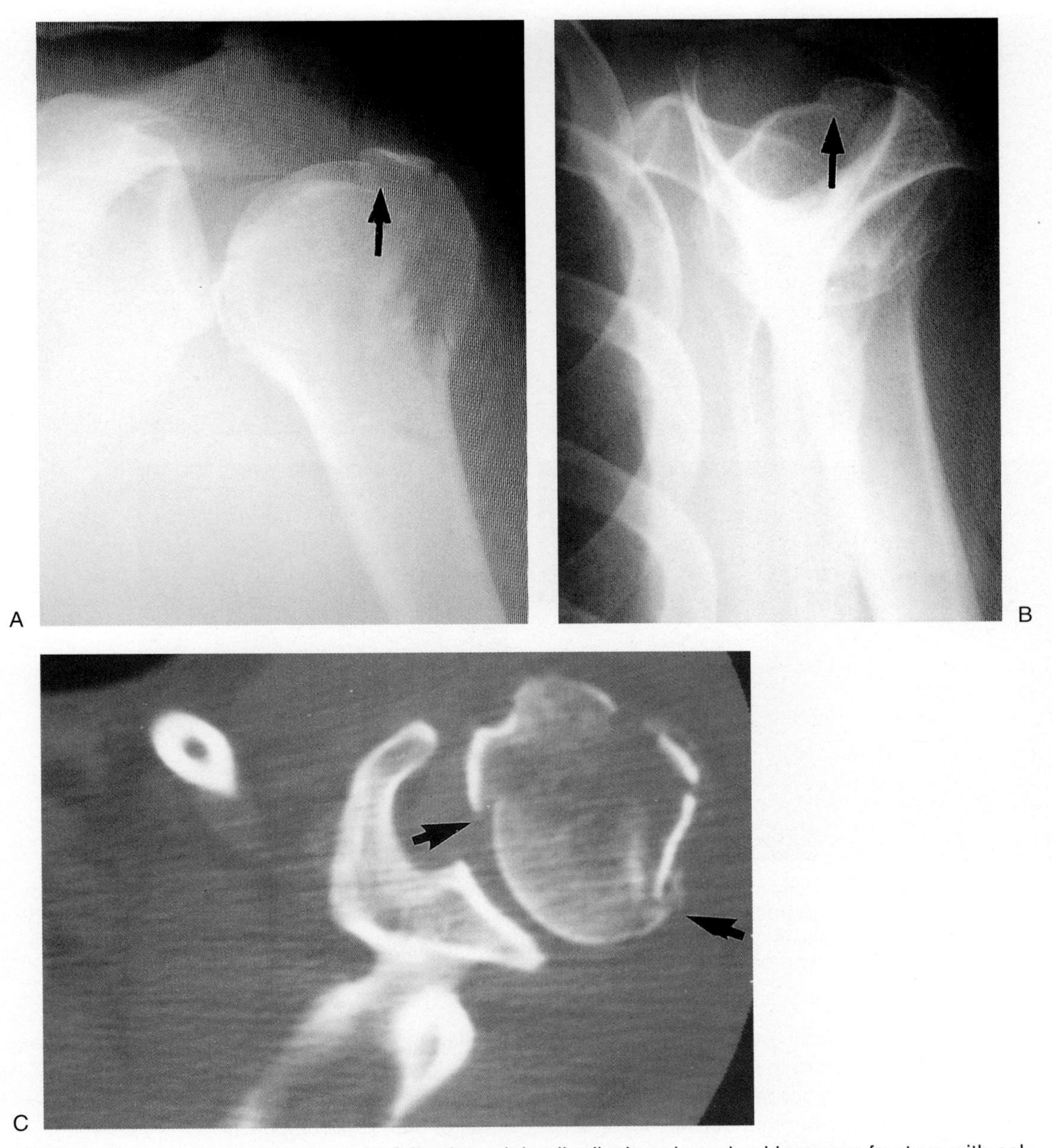

FIG. 5. Prominent greater tuberosity following minimally displaced proximal humerus fracture with collapse of the articular surface late. The greater tuberosity was prominent originally, and an early CT scan raised the possibility that this late complication could occur. **(A,B)** prominent greater tuberosity with fracture; **(C)** separate articular surface fracture.

function. The options for a superiorly displaced malunited greater tuberosity include an acromioplasty versus osteotomy and mobilization of the rotator cuff, with a more distal and anatomic repair. If the displacement is small, symptoms of impingement may be treated with an arthroscopic acromioplasty while preserving the rotator cuff attachment. If it were larger, with a posterior displacement, an acromioplasty would have little benefit. A tuberosity osteotomy and repositioning in a more anatomic position, combined with a capsular release, should permit an early range of motion (Fig. 6C,D).

Lesser Tuberosity

An isolated two-part fracture with a malunion of the lesser tuberosity is exceedingly rare. A common finding is loss of motion of both external and internal rotation because of the medial malposition over the articular surface. The diagnosis is confirmed by routine radiographs and CT scans. A trauma radiography series demonstrates an anterior displacement of the lesser tuberosity. It would not be difficult to confuse this with a greater tuberosity on an AP view alone, but the lateral scapula and axillary views confirm that it is the lesser tuberosity alone (Fig. 7). Treatment options, when substan-

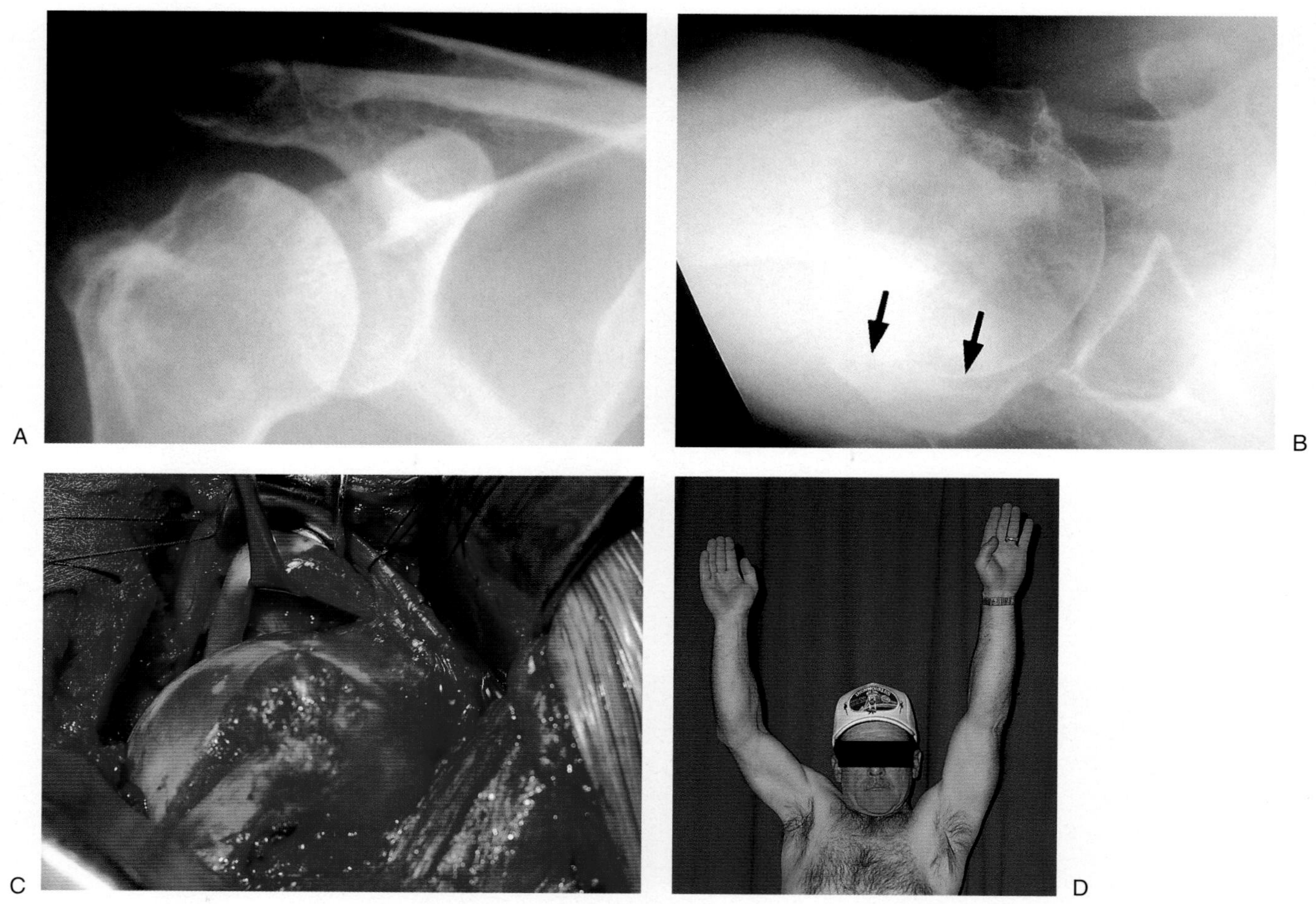

FIG. 6. Greater tuberosity malunion from the pull of the infraspinatus: **(A)** The AP view is suggestive of the "missing greater tuberosity"; **(B)** The posteriorly retracted greater tuberosity is found with the axillary view. **(C)** The tuberosity is osteotomized off of the articular surface; and **(D)** then repositioned, reestablishing the ability for overhead motion and external rotation.

tial symptoms are present, include an osteotomy of the malunited lesser tuberosity, with a return to a more anatomic position. Given that stiffness usually accompanies this fracture, a medial placement of the tuberosity may suffice, for it will approximate the normal subscapularis recession. It is preferable to keep at least a portion of the tuberosity with the subscapularis for a more secure repair, so that early motion may be instituted.

Surgical Neck

Surgical neck malunions associated with two-part fractures are often multiplanar, with an anterior angulation, internal rotation, and a varus deformity. The pectoralis displaces the shaft medialward. A significant amount of deformity can be accepted, with the understanding that for every degree of angulation, there is a concomitant degree of loss of elevation. The varus deformity positions the greater tuberosity into the subacromial space (Fig. 8). The normal lateral humeral offset is lost. If traumatic arthritis develops, the malpositioned greater tuberosity may block a prosthetic replacement. Surgical approaches to remedy this require an osteotomy either through the greater tuberosity, with repositioning it lower, or through the surgical neck, with elimination of the varus component.[102]

Plain films are usually sufficient to characterize the deformity; however, a CT scan is preferable if there is a loss of rotation and these plain films cannot be adequately positioned. One must consider carefully tackling this correction late for in order for it to be successful, an osteotomy is necessary through the deformity, with subsequent ORIF that is strong, stable, and will permit early motion to avoid stiffness. It would not be difficult to worsen a patient's condition if secure fixation were not obtained.

The long deltopectoral approach will facilitate the lysis of subacromial and subdeltoid scar and adhesions. The axillary nerve is freed from the inferior aspect of the subscapularis muscle belly back to the quadrilateral space. It is then protected at the time of an osteotomy through the malunion site. Bone grafting is indicated with bone loss or significant osteoporosis. The options for internal fixation include tension band techniques, with or without Ender rods, and blade plate

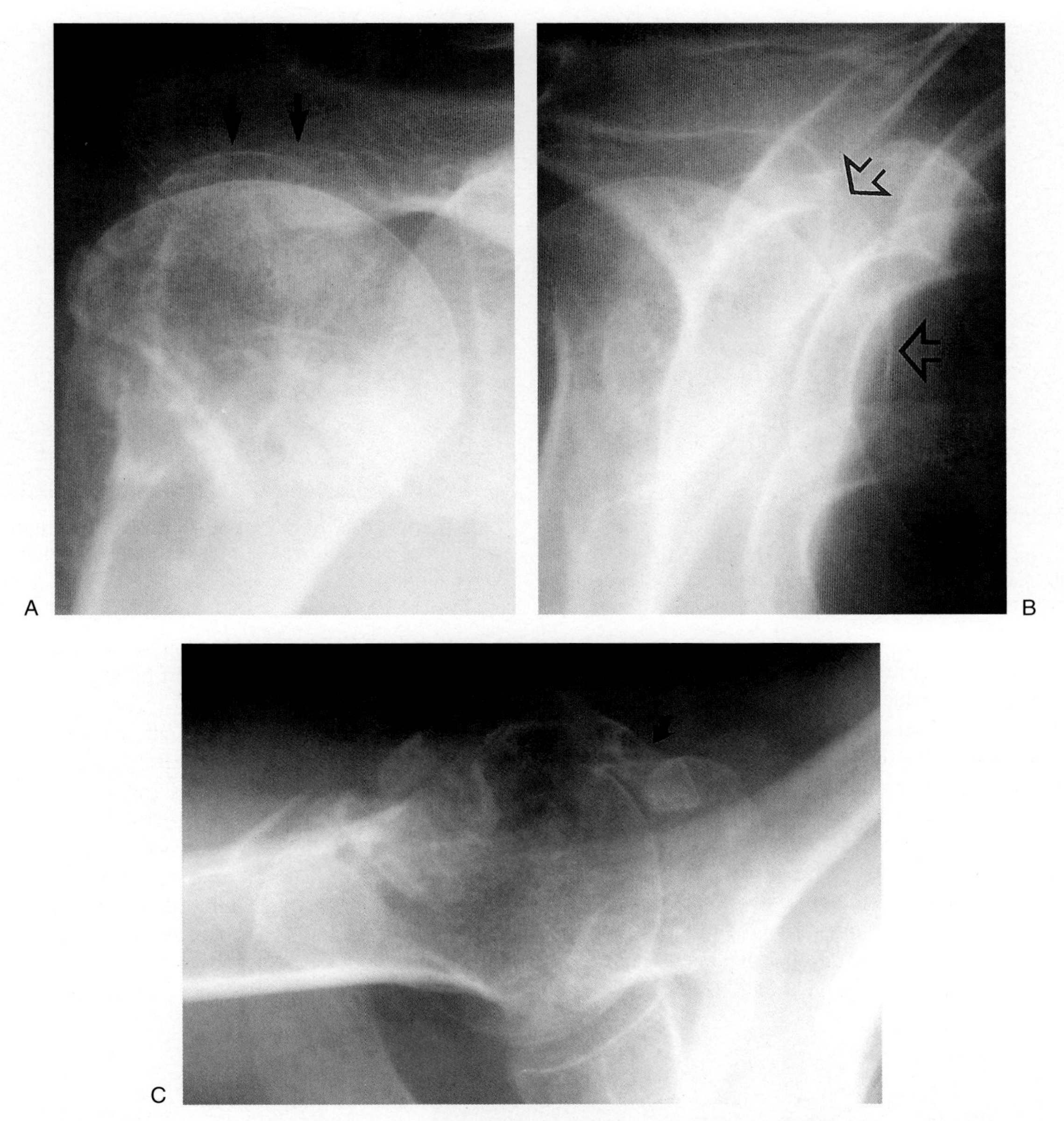

FIG. 7. Displaced lesser tuberosity malunion: **(A)** the AP demonstrates a malunion that could be confused with a greater tuberosity. In this case, **(B)** the lateral scapular and **(C)** axillary views show that the retracted tuberosity is anterior and, therefore, not the greater tuberosity.

fixation.[21,89,100] The standard plate fixation is fraught with difficulties. Often the screws will not hold in the osteoporotic humeral head, or if they do, hardware impingement has been problematic[58] (Fig. 9). Rush rods and pins may not provide adequate and anatomic fixation (Fig. 10). This may lead to malunion, nonunion, or osteonecrosis of the fragments.

COMPLEX MALUNIONS

The nature of complex malunions is multifactorial.[26] They are osseous and soft-tissue abnormalities. The osseous abnormalities include tuberosity malposition and fracture, collapse. or malalignment of the articular surface. Complex malunions are differentiated from two-part fractures with malunion in that there is usually more than one segment that is displaced or malrotated. Osteotomy for tuberosity malposition applies to these cases, similar to the two-part fractures with loss of the articular integrity, then the osseous and soft-tissue structures are reconstructed around a humeral head or total shoulder replacement. At times, malalignment of the articular surface with a fixed subluxation may be treated with contracture releases. Rotational alignment may be approached either by an osteotomy to derotate the articular surface or an arthroplasty (Fig. 11). By the time one has removed the tuberosity and performed an osteotomy to

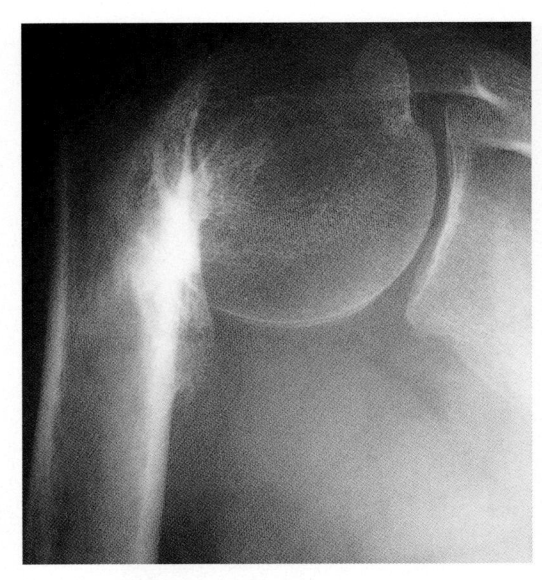

FIG. 8. Varus surgical neck malunion positioned with the greater tuberosity under the acromion restricts motion and impinges on the acromion and superior glenoid rim.

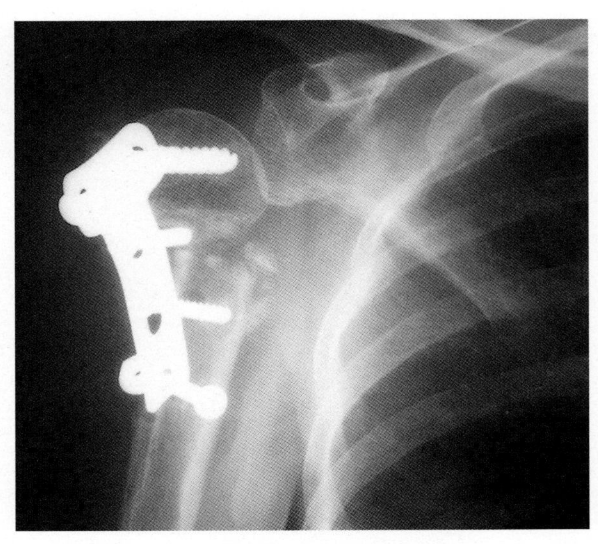

FIG. 9. An ORIF of osteoporotic proximal humerus fracture with plates and screws risks hardware pullout before the fracture heals.

derotate the articular surface, if no collapse were present, there is a significant chance that the articular surface may then go on to osteonecrosis. Prosthetic replacement increasingly becomes more attractive.[5]

Soft-tissue abnormalities include capsular and cuff contracture, neurologic deficits, and cuff deficiencies. Capsular contractures may be released by a manipulation under anesthesia. If there is a concern that a manipulation will likely disrupt the cuff or healing fractures, then an arthroscopic capsular release is preferred. An internal rotation contracture was formerly approached by a coronal plane subscapularis lengthening.[82,86] Increasingly, this has been replaced by a recession of the subscapularis insertion closer to the articular surface.[111]

Neurologic deficit, in special cases, may be treated with tendon transfers. For anterior deltoid loss, the middle deltoid and the clavicular pectoralis are moved together to fill the deficit.[82] For more widespread loss of the deltoid, many muscle transfers with only limited success have been tried during the years of treating poliomylitis. Recently, better results have been obtained by bringing the latissimus dorsi up on its neurovascular bundle to provide an anterior deltoid.[52a]

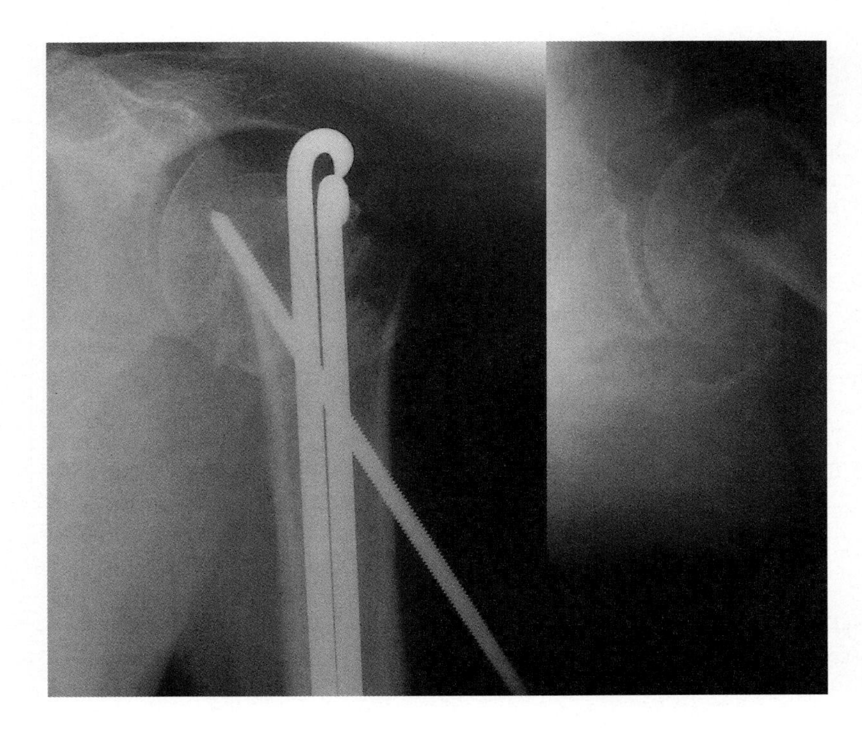

FIG. 10. A three-part proximal humerus fracture, treated with Rush rods, a Steinman pin, and inadequate reduction, which went on to a nonunion and traumatic arthritis.

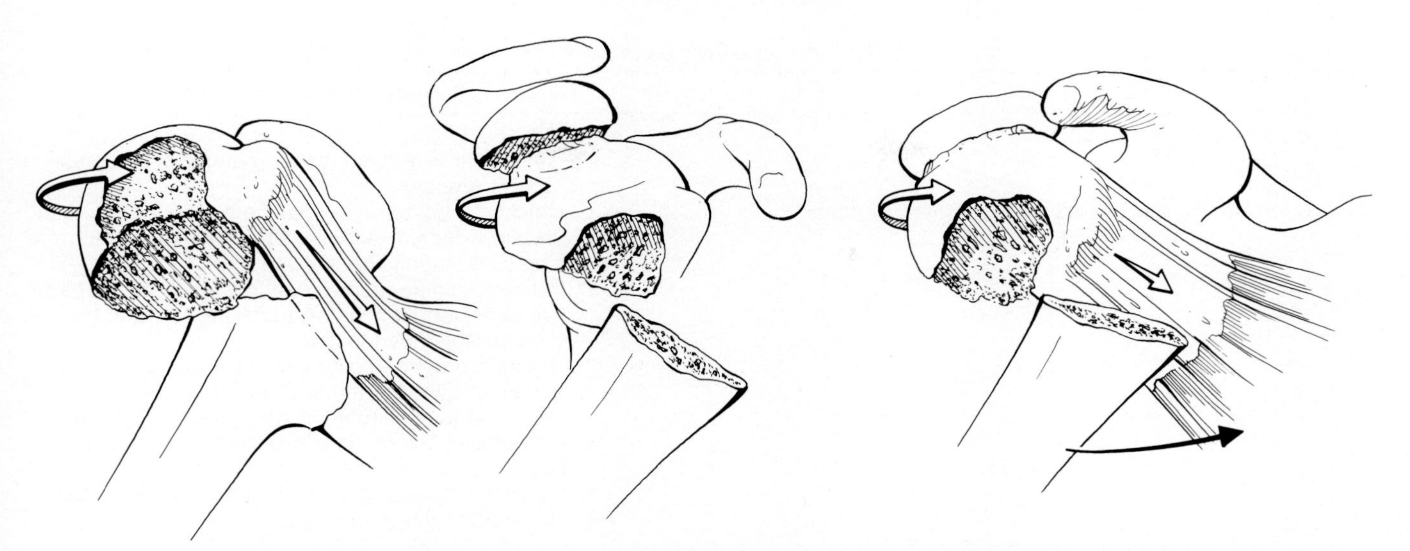

FIG. 11. Three-part malunion with posterior articular rotatory deformity and malunion of the greater tuberosity over the humeral head.

For subscapularis loss, if this is mechanical, it might then be retrieved by dissecting all the tissue off the scapular neck and bringing this tissue upward. If it is neurologic, then lateral transfer of the pectoralis has been reported to offer some success.[96] When the subscapularis is lost with total shoulder arthroplasty, an allograft, using the calcaneous, fixed to the anterior scapular neck, and the Achilles out to the humerus, serves as a tenodesis.[76] For spinatii loss, the latissimus dorsi posterior and superior transfer has been reported by Gerber.[33] Follow-up EMG studies have demonstrated that most of these transfers are active.[33]

For combined axillary and suprascapular nerve loss, the decision is between no operative treatment versus an arthrodesis. Both groups of muscles cannot be adequately replaced to warrant extensive tendon transfers.

ROTATOR CUFF DEFICIENCY

If there is a rotator cuff tear[52] that can be closed, a primary closure is preferred. Superior transposition of the subscapularis and infraspinatus for supraspinatus loss is possible to a limited degree. One must carefully weigh the advantage of detaching an intact internal or external rotator and transposing it to where, if it does not heal adequately or if it is stiff, the patient may be worse off than before surgery. If the deficit is the subscapularis, retrieval of the subscapularis is the preferred technique. Alternatively, an allograft placing the calcaneous over the anterior scapular neck and the Achilles tendon anteriorly will assist with stability for an anterior tenodesis. Any tissue that could be mobilized off the anterior scapular neck consisting of residual shortened subscapularis is sutured over this. One then might consider whether a lateral and superior transposition of the pectoralis insertion would be helpful.[96] Finally, a superior transposition of the latissimus dorsi insertion has had some mixed success.

Indications for surgical treatment of complex malunions include pain and loss of function. There should also be a reasonable chance that an improvement by these techniques can be accomplished. The surgical management involves restoration of humeral length, with or without a prosthetic replacement. The tuberosities are then repositioned anatomically. The reconstruction of three- and four-part malunions are formidable problems that usually require humeral head or total shoulder replacements. The results have usually been satisfactory for pain relief, but range of motion and overall function vary with the specific problems addressed.

NONUNION OF PROXIMAL HUMERUS FRACTURES

The incidence of nonunion of proximal humerus fractures is seldom reported. The highest incidence involves fractures of the surgical neck. Up to 23% of these may go on to nonunion.[78] These include fractures that may have started as minimally displaced, and then, unexpectedly went on to a nonunion.[19,25,66,74,78,80,83,103] Some estimate is made at the time of surgery of how secure the fixation is in determining when and what motions may be implemented. Other fracture patterns that have a higher incidence of nonunion include those with displaced tuberosities, which are treated closed, and four-part fractures which are treated either closed or open.

Factors associated with nonunion may be characterized as patient and treatment factors. The patient factors include diabetes, drug or alcohol addiction, smoking, and general noncompliance. The treatment factors involve a missed diagnosis, such as a missed tuberosity fracture from inadequate early imaging, as well as the iatrogenic factors. These include the use of a hanging arm cast, which can result in distraction at the surgical neck fracture site, inadequate internal fixation, and too early or aggressive motion before heal-

TABLE 1. *Metabolic bone workup*[85,95]

Tests	Reasons for and interpretation of tests
I. Blood tests (Screen a,b,c)	
a. CBC, sedimentation rate	a. To determine if anemia, inflammatory, or neoplastic process is present
b. SMAC-23, for overall view of metabolic state	b. 1. Calcium, phosphorus, alkaline phosphatase, total protein, albumin, globulin, albumin/globulin ratio, to assess metabolic bone state 2. BUN, creatinine, BUN/creatinine ratio, and electrolyte panel (sodium, potassium, chloride, and HCO_3 to assess kidney function 3. Serum glutamic–oxaloacetictransaminase, serum glutamic–pyruvic transanimase, alkaline phosphatase, and total bilirubin to assess liver function 4. Cholesterol and triglycerides to assess fat metabolism 5. Glucose to assess glucose metabolism for diabetes 6. Uric acid to assess for gout
c. Parathyroid screen (IRMA assay)	
d. 25-Hydroxyvitamin D screen	
e. Protein electrophoretic pattern to rule out myeloma (anemia, etc.)	
f. T_4 and T_3 by radioimmunoassay, free thyroxine index and thyroid-stimulating hormone to evaluate thyroid function	
g. Luteinizing hormone, follicle-stimulating hormone and prolactin to evaluate pituitary and gonadal function	
h. Cortisol to evaluate adrenal function	
i. Estrogen or testosterone levels to evaluate gonadal function	
j. Osteocalcin level to assess "bone turn over"	
k. Bone-specific alkaline phosphatase	a. To determine bone activity vs. liver disease
II. 24-hr urine tests	
a. Calcium	a. 1. Low a. Osteomalacia from malabsorption of calcium or lack of vitamin D b. Low bone turnover state a. 2. High a. Hypercalciuria b. High turnover state c. Hyperparathyroidism
b. Phosphorus	b. 1. Low a. Poor absorption b. Inadequate vitamin D intake c. Phosphate depletion from excessive antacid use or poor kidney function
c. Creatinine	c. Indicates appropriate specimen has been obtained and renal function is adequate; if creatinine level remains the same from one test to the next, it indicates like specimens are being compared.
d. Total hydroxyproline (Paget's disease etc.)	d. Indicates high or low turnover state because hydroxyproline is breakdown of bone matrix
e. Uric acid	e. R/O gout
III. 2-hr urinary pyridinoline cross-links	a. New test for bone resorption
IV. X-ray films	
a. AP of hands for bone resorption (if hyperparathyroidism likely)	a. Preferably on industrial film 1. Resorption of bone from radial side, especially of middle phalanges, indicative of hyperparathyroidism 2. Assesses cortical thickness of metacarpal (cortical bone loss)

TABLE 1. *Continued*

Tests	Reasons for and interpretation of tests
b. Lateral skull for hyperparathyroidism	b. 1. Determines if lamina dura present 2. Assesses size of sella turcica (posterior clinoids gone with severe demineralization) 3. Evaluates mineralization of skull; ("salt and pepper" skull in hyperparathyroidism, or in severe osteoporosis or myeloma)
c. Special scan films of involved area (CT/MRI/scanograms prn)	c. Evaluate fracture MU, NU, position and condition of articular surfaces, humeral height compared with opposite side
V. Bone scan: technetium (^{99m}TC methylene diphosphate)	a. Persistent hot spot in fusion over 1 yr old indicative of delayed fusion or pseudoarthrosis b. Bright scan of skeleton with pale kidneys indicative of osteomalacia c. Symmetric lesions indicative of pseudofractures as seen in osteomalacia d. Bright bone and kidneys: high-turnover state e. Pale scan: low-turnover rate f. Scattered or asymmetric-lesions: cancer or Paget's disease
VI. Bone densitometry	
a. Dual energy x-ray absorptiometry (DXA)	a. Evaluation of amount of mineral in spine and hip 1. Method very accurate and reproducible
b. CT scan of lumbar spine	2. CT scan method measures primarily trabecular bone and rate of bone loss
c. SXA (single energy x-ray absorptiometry) of forearm and of humerus	c. 1. Evaluation of amount of mineral in radius and humerus 2. Evaluates primarily cortical bone
c. Total body by DXA	
VII. Calcium loading	
a. Oral calcium 1,500 mg/day for 3 days. At end of second day, repeat 24-hr urine test for calcium, phosphorus, and creatinine	a. 1. Low urinary calcium level indicative of malabsorption 2. Usually no malabsorption problem if low urinary calcium normalizes 3. If urinary calcium becomes excessively high, patient is an overabsorber and overexcreter (hypercalcuric); occurs in about 10% of patients.
VIII. Bone biopsy in some cases, usually after tetracycline label (rarely done since advent of more sophisticated imagery procedures: i.e., DXA scans)	a. Usually, iliac crest undecalcified biopsy preceded by a single or double tetracycline label; most commonly done when osteomalacia is suspected, and to differentiate low turnover from high bone turnover states

ing.[48,51,83,89,91,108] Clearly the better the reduction and fixation, the earlier the rehabilitation can safely begin. This will ultimately offer the best chance to avoid stiffness. Some estimate is made at the time of surgery of how secure the fixation is in determining when and what motions may be implemented.

One major cause, often overlooked, can be attributed to advanced age and osteoporosis. Often nonunions may occur, despite adequate orthopedic treatment, owing to the patient's poor-healing potential. It is understood that the head may be osteoporotic and not hold screws well. Therefore, plate fixation can be problematic. Even with good fixation, these fractures in the elderly and debilitated patient may not heal. The roentgenographic evaluation demonstrates osteopenia, bone resorption, and a nonunion. Although this may be suspected as a possibility with an acute fracture, it is essential to consider a metabolic screening after the patient has developed a nonunion. The summary of the screening tests and their implications for the metabolic bone workup are presented in Table 1.[85,95] Unfortunately, even the best surgical techniques may fail without the cooperation of the patient's calcium metabolism.

Tuberosity Nonunion

Plain films that include three orthogonal views define the position of the tuberosity fragments that have gone on to nonunion. Those that are retracted upward in the subacromial space and preponderantly involve the supraspinatus and greater tuberosity can be diagnosed on an AP film (Fig. 12). At times, a portion of the supraspinatus is still attached to the upper part of the lesser tuberosity; hence, the axial and lateral scapula views will clarify whether the fragment is anterior or superior to the coracoid. The axial view is most useful in defining the posteriorly retracted greater tuberosity fragment. Here, the AP view would demonstrate an absent tuberosity. If stiffness or pain preclude adequate positioning, a CT scan will most clearly define the position of the articular surface and whether or not it is intact. In addition, the position of the tuberosities and any associated fractures can be clearly defined.

Indications for surgical reconstruction of tuberosity nonunion are similar to, but even more pressing, than for the malunited tuberosities. Loss of either tuberosity represents a moderate to massive rotator cuff defect. In a lesser tuberosity avulsion, the prime restraint against anterior instability is missing: 100% of patients with anterior instability after prosthetic replacement have avulsed the subscapularis.[76] This is a more important muscle than previously appreciated when it was suggested that the subscapularis could be released indiscriminately for shoulder stiffness. A greater tuberosity avulsion is similar to a large to massive rotator cuff deficiency. It may be expected that loss of the fulcrum of the head in the glenoid will be lost over time. If, at the same time, there is loss of the coracoacromial ligament, then the superior instability occurs as the head escapes the confines of the acromion and coracoacromial arch. This places the humeral head anterior and superiorly underneath the skin. With no fulcrum, any significant active elevation or abduction is impossible. With major cuff deficits, resection of the coracoacromial ligament should be avoided at all costs.

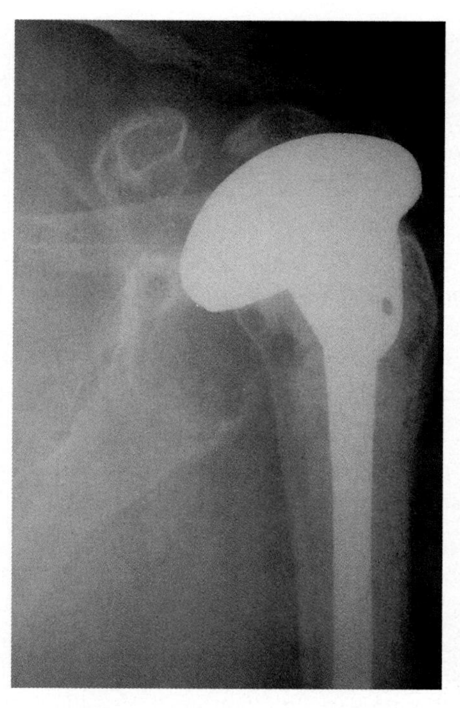

FIG. 12. Greater tuberosity nonunion following cemented humeral head arthroplasty. The supraspinatus retracts the greater tuberosity over the humeral head. This is easily appreciated on an AP roentgenograph.

Surgical techniques to manage a lesser tuberosity avulsion involve a deltopectoral approach, with release of any capsule, the lesser tuberosity, and subscapularis from the anterior scapular neck. The subscapularis is mobilized in a 360-degree manner, superficially, as well as deep, and then advanced back to the humeral shaft for secure repair. This may be done with heavy nonabsorbable suture through drill holes in bone for secure fixation.

The technique for the repair of a greater tuberosity nonunion may be carried out through a superior approach. If it is a superior fragment, then this may be done with a deltoid split. However, if this is a large posterior fragment, then removal of the anterior deltoid and the anterior half of the middle deltoid off the acromion will facilitate the exposure and mobilization. The chronic massive tuberosity avulsions that have retracted back to the level of the glenoid for more than 6 months usually cannot be adequately mobilized and successfully repaired. Even when repaired, the shortened muscle serves more as a tenodesis than an active motor. Here, an arthrodesis may be a better alternative.

Nonunions in the Surgical Neck

Surgical neck nonunions present with loss of an adequate fulcrum for elevation and no attached external rotators. The rotator cuff attached to the head does not transfer power to rotate with the humeral shaft. Crepitus is felt at the fracture site unless the deltoid or long head of the biceps is interposed. Joint fluid accumulates at the nonunion site and retards healing. These nonunions are adequately diagnosed with plain films (Fig. 13A). If some question exists over whether or not a fibrous or a nonunion is present, a CT scan will clarify this difference. The characteristic roentgenographic picture is that of osteoporosis, with bone resorption at the surgical neck site. In the extreme cases, there is cavitation of the humeral head, with little bone available to fix to the upper shaft.

Nonoperative treatment may be indicated in certain debilitated patients. These include those who would have medical difficulty with an interscalene regional block anesthesia, or those in whom motivation is highly suspect.[18] This is particularly true of the uncontrolled alcoholic.

Indications for surgical reconstruction, therefore, include those with pain and recognizable loss of function. The person should be both motivated to participate in postoperative exercise plan and have appropriate medical clearance. The operative options include ORIF, with or without a bone graft, or reconstruction around a prosthetic replacement. An open reduction and internal fixation of the nonunion is preferred if there is sufficient bone in the humeral head fragment.[48] This may be supplemented with bone graft from the iliac crest. The long deltopectoral approach facilitates removal of scar and fibrous tissue from the nonunion site. The long head of the biceps is preserved partly for orientation in restoring the correct version. The adjacent ends of the bone at the nonunion site need to be reopened to establish the intramedullary canal. Any bone that

FIG. 13. (A) Two-part surgical neck nonunion; **(B)** ORIF with tension band and Ender rods; **(C)** clinical example of tension-band Ender technique.

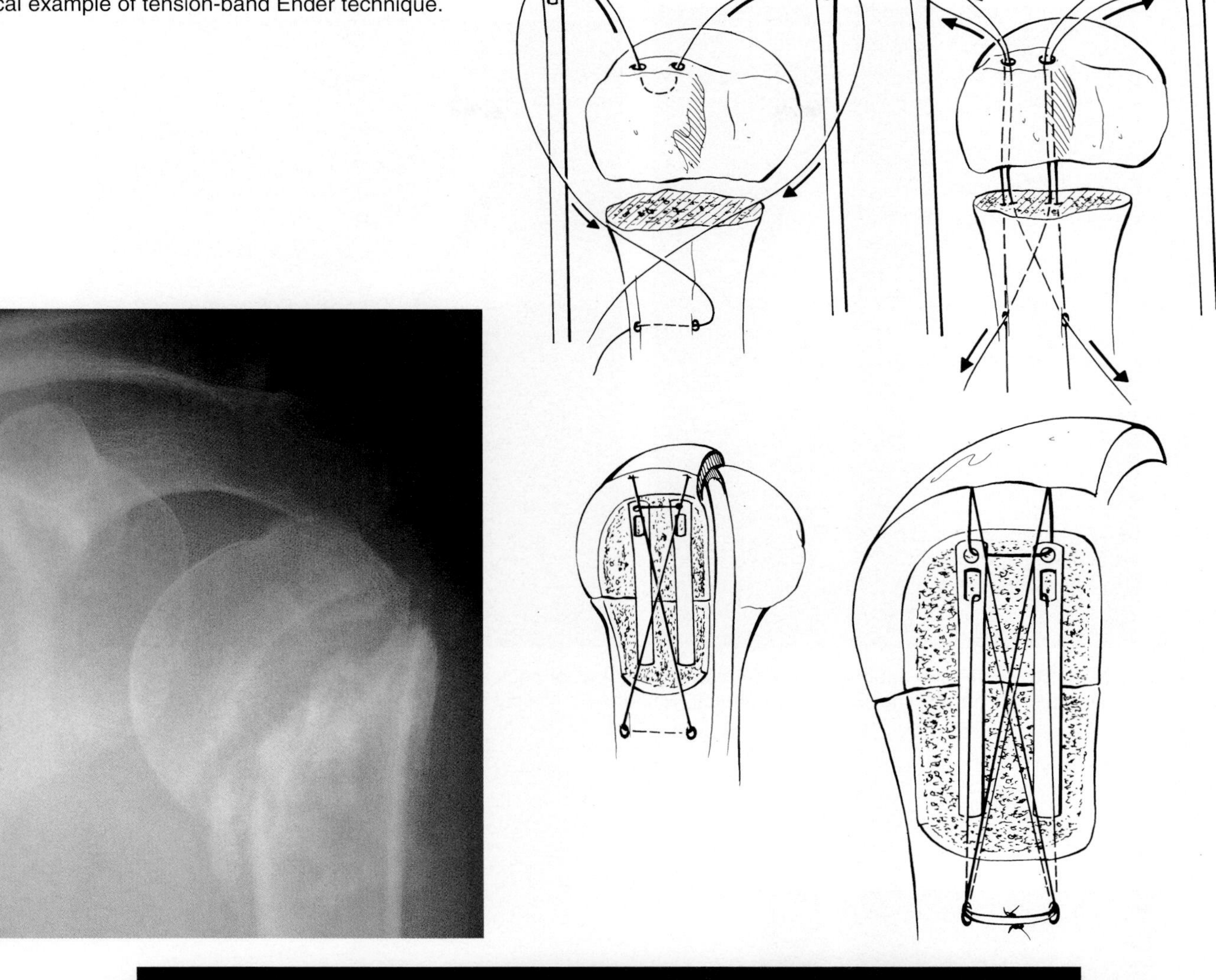

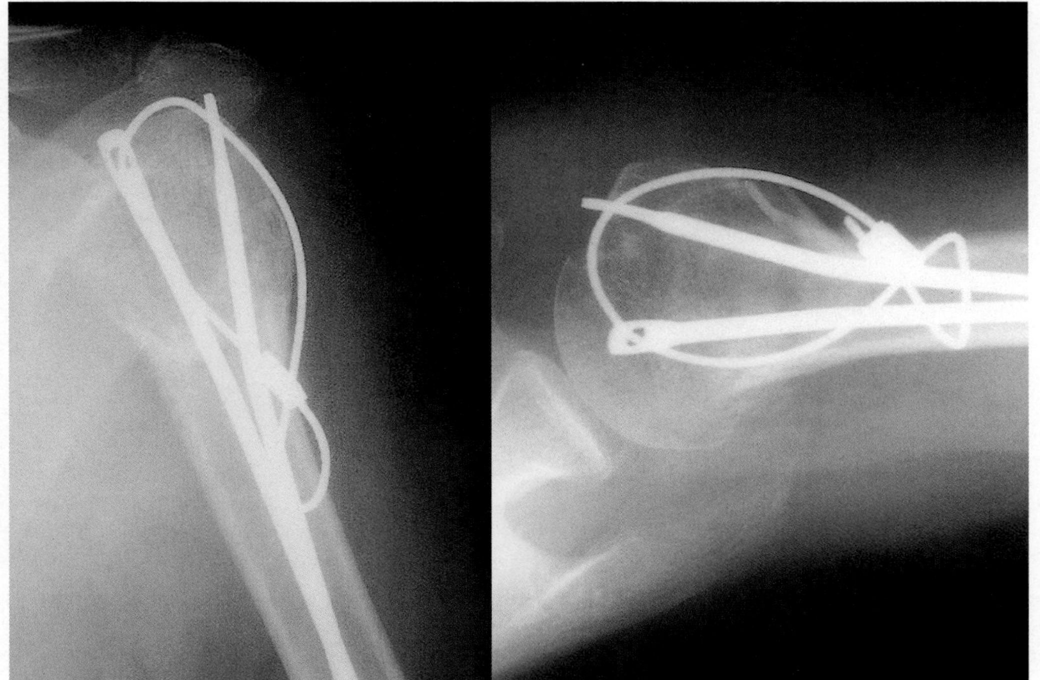

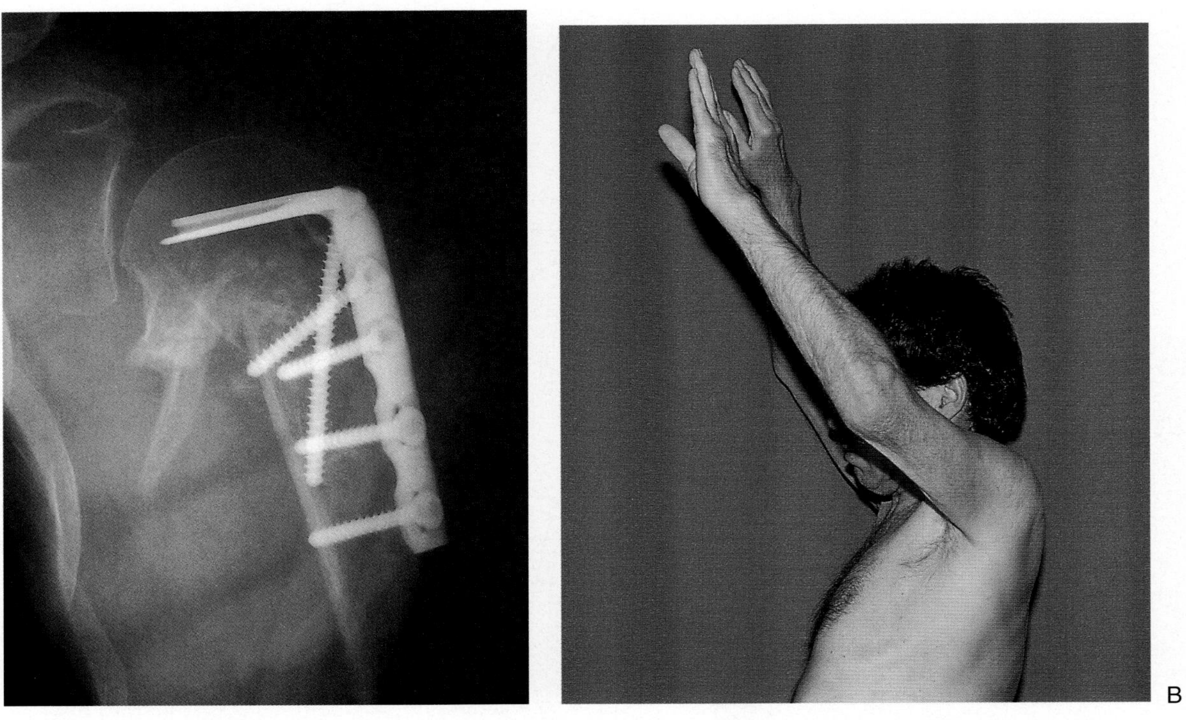

FIG. 14. ORIF with Jupiter AO blade plate for a surgical neck nonunion: **(A)** x-ray film demonstrating valgus reduction for maximal bony contact; **(B)** 2-month clinical motion.

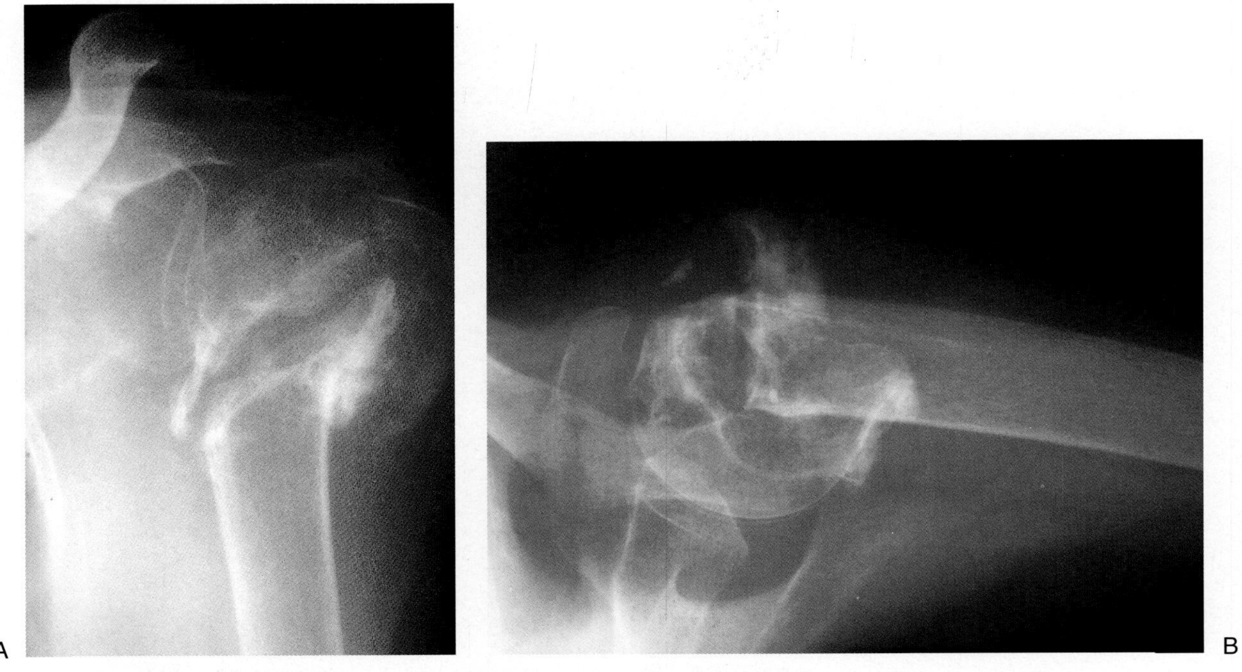

FIG. 15. **(A)** through **(D)**: Humeral head replacement for surgical neck nonunion in which little bone remains in the head fragment. A periprosthetic fracture during surgery was handled by use of a long stem humeral component and cables. (*continued*)

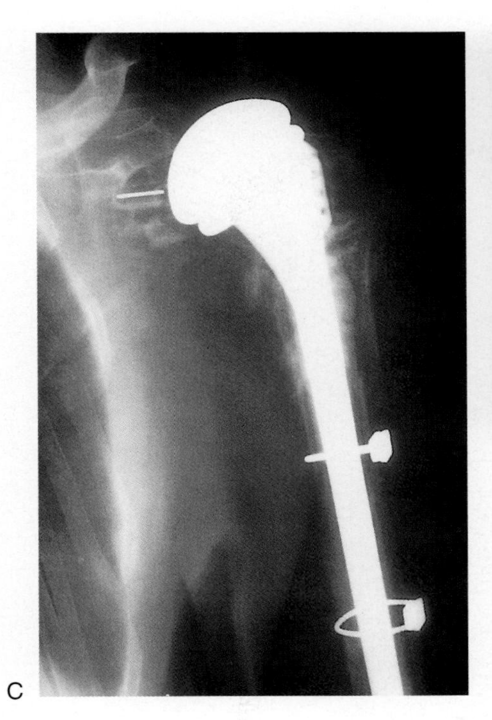
C

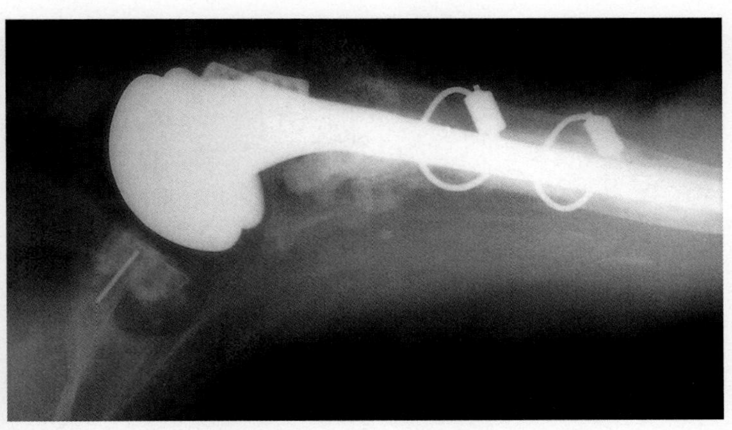
D

FIG. 15. *Continued*

is removed in reshaping this nonunion site is carefully saved on the back table for later graft material. An opening made in the rotator interval will allow direct visualization of the articular surface of the proximal humerus. Release of the coracohumeral ligament and, if necessary, the anterior capsule, will facilitate mobilization of the articular segment. Once the ends have been opened and freshened, then the shaft can be impacted into the articular surface, with care to restore its rotation and angulation. The arm at the side can be held in neutral rotation, with the articular surface facing directly back to the scapula. Aligning the long head of the biceps is another key to ensuring proper version.

The two techniques for reducing and fixing a surgical neck nonunion include a tension band or a blade plate fixation. The first is a tension band technique, with or without additional stabilization with Ender rods[89] (see Fig. 13B). The essential principles involve grasping the rotator cuff at its insertion on the tuberosity and angling it down to the shaft. Hence, the greater tuberosity is looped down to the medial shaft and the lesser tuberosity is angled down to the lateral shaft. Any harvested bone graft is packed in the discrepancy between the size of the upper shaft and the larger head fragment as these two are compressed together. When Ender rods are employed, a secondary round hole is made just above the oval slot.[21] A suture is passed into the articular surface near the cuff attachment, through the eyelet in each of two Ender rods, and then back through the articular surface near the opposite tuberosity. Thus, a figure eight tension band technique is created.[21,36,89]

With sufficient articular surface present, a blade plate will then facilitate excellent fixation without prominent hardware that one might expect with the standard AO or buttress plate[100] (Fig. 14). The same principles are used to obtain a fracture preparation and adequate reduction. An angled screw compresses the head to the shaft.

In those surgical neck nonunions with excavation of the head, a prosthetic replacement offers an opportunity to fix the nonunion with a cemented intramedullary rod; namely, a humeral head replacement[85](Fig. 15). Occasionally, the nonunion site can be freshened and the prosthesis can be inserted through the rotator interval to "shish kabob" the head to the shaft. This requires that a hole be made in the top of the articular fragment with an adjustment of the proper height and version. Somewhat more easily accomplished is the standard approach. The tuberosities are split. The scant remains of the head are excised and packed as bone graft around the upper shaft and the tuberosities as the newly created four-part fracture is reconstructed.[37] Cables provide more secure tuberosity fixation than heavy sutures and are less prone to fragmentation than monofilament wire.[22] However, the use of dissimilar metals must be avoided. As with all fractures for which a humeral head prosthesis is inserted, the height of the prosthesis is placed well above the surgical neck. Enough room is left to place the tuberosities above the surgical neck. This avoids the potential for an inferior instability if the humeral length is not restored (Fig. 16).

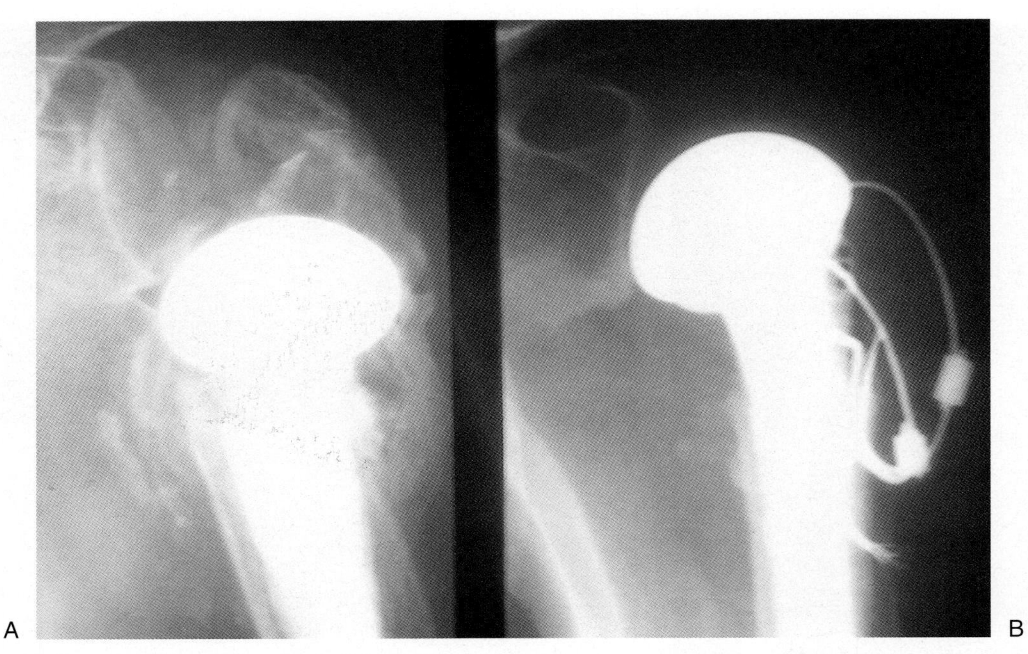

FIG. 16. (A) Inferior prosthesis placement is one cause of a fixed inferior instability. **(B)** Repositioning of the prosthesis out to length restores glenohumeral stability.

COMPLEX OR THREE- AND FOUR-PART FRACTURES

The more complex fractures, with both surgical neck and tuberosity segments displaced, are more likely to go on to nonunion with closed treatment than with open repair. Alternatively, osteonecrosis is common following ORIF of four-part fractures, with varying effects on the final pain and function.[5,41,45,59,93,105] These are more difficult to treat than an acute fracture, owing to the shortened muscles, scar, and increased osteopenia of the ununited fragments. These may have combinations of malunions, nonunions, and distortions of the articular surfaces. Fixed subluxations, dislocations, and articular splitting fractures contribute to the need for concomitant glenoid replacement. After 6 months, the glenoid cartilage may soften to the point that it peels off easily. If the rotator cuff can be reconstructed, then glenoid replacement should be considered when the cartilage is absent. An even stronger case for glenoid replacement exists when the bone is eccentrically eroded, with loss of the normal concavity.[94]

There are many studies reviewing the results of acute fracture treatment with ORIF and arthroplasty.[7,24,29,35,40,46,56,60,61,79] There are few comparative studies of the results of ORIF with or without bone grafting and prosthetic arthroplasty. For two-part surgical neck nonunions, Healy and Jupiter reported better results with ORIF than with prosthetic arthroplasty.[48] No differentiation was made between the humeral heads that still had good bone and the ones that were excavated. Neer noted satisfactory results in the acute ORIF of three-part proximal humerus fractures with only 2 out of 33 cases developing osteonecrosis.[77] In contrast, none of his four-part fractures had satisfactory results with ORIF. Prosthetic arthroplasty results were quite superior in the four-part displaced fractures. With long-standing nonunions, the tendency has been to use a prosthetic arthroplasty to reconstruct the humerus. Results are still superior to ORIF, but not as good as published results for treatment of acute fractures.[87]

COMPLICATIONS ASSOCIATED WITH INJURY OR TREATMENT

Osteonecrosis, avascular necrosis, and ischemic necrosis are terms to describe the loss of circulation to the terminal articular surface. This is followed by collapse in most cases. Although rare, it can occur after two-part and minimally displaced fractures (Fig. 17). It occasionally occurs with a three-part displaced proximal humeral fracture, but most commonly occurs after four-part fractures or fracture–dislocations. Although the amount of osteoporosis and severity of the trauma may play a role, loss of the arcuate artery of Laing in the biceps groove that provides humeral head vascularity is a major contributing factor.[34,65] This artery comes off the anterior circumflex humeral artery near the same point that the posterior circumflex humeral artery, the brachial artery, and the subscapular artery arise from the axillary artery. This point of rigid fixation is vulnerable to displacement of the shaft with fractures, and, especially, with fracture–dislocations. The more segments fractured and displaced at the time of a humeral shaft fracture, the greater the increase in the incidence of injury to this artery. If the articular surface is no longer attached to any tuberosity, the incidence significantly increases. Neer reported 2 cases of osteonecrosis out of 33

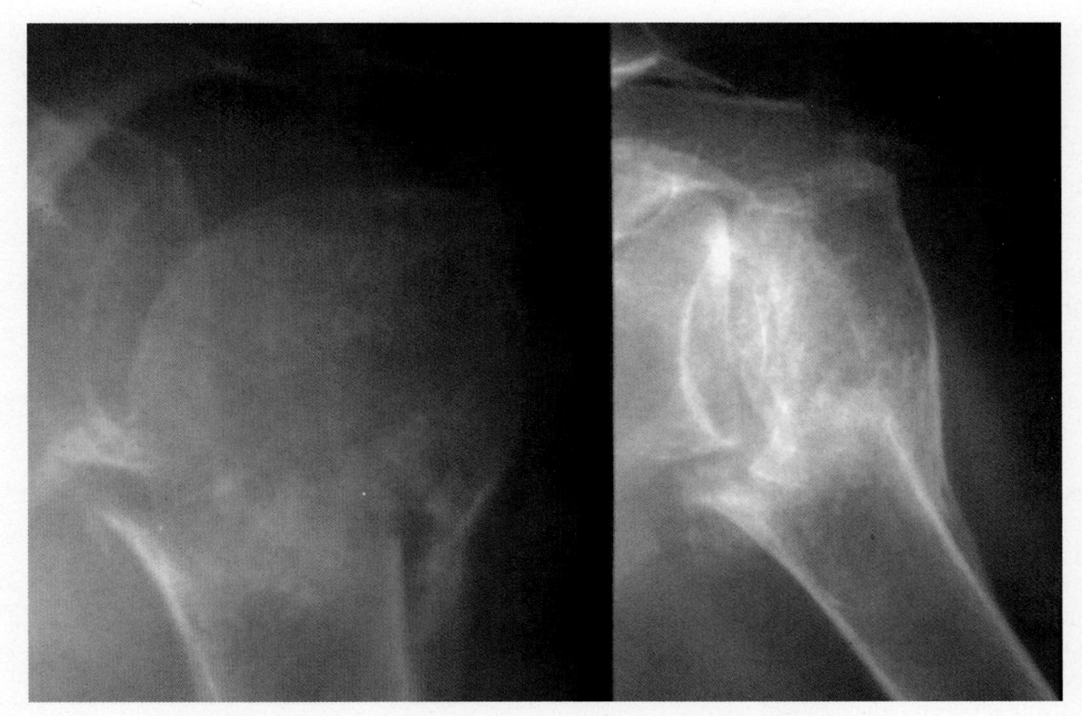

FIG. 17. Two-part fracture at the surgical neck that developed osteonecrosis 8 months after closed treatment.

ORIFs of three-part proximal humeral fractures.[77] Sturzenegger noted six times the incidence of osteonecrosis with use of plates for the proximal humerus as compared with when he used wires and pins to provide what he termed "minimal fixation."[106] Although there are isolated reports without osteonecrosis following ORIF of four-part fractures, many of these have short follow-up. For example, Lee and Hanson reported a case of a vascularization of the humeral head after ORIF of a four-part fracture at 2 years, which then went on to collapse at 3½ years.[67] In Sturzenegger's report of ORIF of three- and four-part fractures, three cases developed sympathetic dystrophy with osteonecrosis following hardware complications. Screw penetration into the joint can cause traumatic arthritis. Collapse of the joint makes the use of screws even more problematic.[73,83,106,116] The timing of replacement if this complication occurs is important. The longer one waits, the more likely it is that both sides of the joint will need to be replaced. Either use of the plate that compresses the artery, or stripping to place the plate on the fracture sites at the lateral edge of the biceps groove, contributes to the demise of the artery with subsequent osteonecrosis. Nonunion, malunion, and eventual osteonecrosis are the frequent complications associated with ORIFs of displaced four-part fractures.[5,85]

Another attempt to decrease the incidence of osteonecrosis and extend the indications for ORIF of four-part fractures is a closed pinning and external fixation.[50,62,63,64] Although this has been a successful technique in Europe, Gerber reports that when absolute anatomic reconstruction is not established, the result will be a failure. In this author's experience, there has been a significant increase in the number of nonunions, infections, and axillary nerve palsies following the closed pinning attempts. There is a steep learning curve. As with every new or resurrected technique, a set of complications also emerges.

In those patients in whom traumatic arthritis has developed, humeral head replacement may suffice. If the glenoid is destroyed, and in particular if the concavity of the glenoid is altered with bony erosion at one edge, a total shoulder is preferred.

Occasionally, when revising a malunion or nonunion, a humeral shaft fracture may occur. Long stem prostheses permit the opportunity for stable fixation and normal rehabilitation.[90]

AUTHOR'S TREATMENT ALGORITHM

Eighty percent of proximal humeral fractures are thought to be nondisplaced. A sling for early comfort followed by pendulum motion at 2 weeks may decrease the ubiquitous complication of stiffness and shorten the recovery time.[115] Approximately 77% of these patients will recover completely. More violent passive stretching is avoided until fracture healing is secure.

Treatment of displaced fractures ideally is based on the anatomy of the fracture as determined by the x-ray films and, at times, CT scan. More practically, it is also determined by the age, health, and motivation of the patient. For revision surgery, a cell saver is available. This avoids the need for additional blood transfusions.[9] Two-part surgical neck fractures can be treated with a closed reduction, if the reduction is stable. An open reduction is reserved for those that are not reducible closed, and in particular, those that have retraction of the rotator cuff. Excessive angulation at the surgical neck, if accepted, will restrict motion and function. Ideally, the decision to change the angulation will be made early, for later reconstructions are more difficult.

In general, three-part fractures of the proximal humerus can be treated with an ORIF, and a prosthetic arthroplasty is reserved for the four-part fractures.[6,11,43] In malunions, prosthetic arthroplasty becomes more frequently indicated when traumatic arthritis has developed. In disassembling a malunion, to restore normal architecture, loss of the circulation to the articular surface is more probable. If so, then a prosthetic replacement is chosen. One variable is what type of fixation might be obtained. This facilitates early motion and, potentially, better functions. A prosthetic reconstruction is preferred for a malunion, following osteotomies, with tenuous fixation and in those situations in which the head is excavated and osteoporotic. Similarly, prosthetic arthroplasty is employed in the extreme cases of a surgical neck nonunion with an excavated head. Although most three-part fractures can be treated with an open reduction and internal fixation, adequate bone needs to be present to effectively restore the rotator cuff. The longer a nonunion has existed, the more likely that both sides of the joint will be involved. In addition, if there has been a fixed subluxation, or malrotation of the articular surface, damage to the glenoid may be inevitable.

With four-part nonunions, prosthetic arthroplasty is preferred. The decision rests on whether a humeral or a total shoulder replacement is necessary. If the glenoid is not involved, then a humeral head reconstruction is appropriate. Even if the glenoid is significantly involved, if the rotator cuff cannot be adequately repaired, the glenoid should be omitted. If the cuff can be repositioned with the tuberosities around the humeral head replacement, then replacement of a damaged glenoid will more likely provide better pain relief. This offers a chance for earlier and more successful motion in a difficult rehabilitation.

REFERENCES

1. Alnot JY. Traumatic brachial plexus palsy in the adult. Retro- and infraclavicular lesions. *Clin Orthop* 1988;237:9–16.
2. Alnot JY, Banyon P. Associated nerve and vascular lesions. In: Alnot JY, Narakas A, eds. *Traumatic brachial plexus injuries*. Paris: Expansion Scientifique Francaise, 1996:110–114.
3. Alnot JY, Narakas A, eds. *Traumatic brachial plexus injuries*. Paris: Expansion Scientifique Francaise, 1996.
4. Berry H, Bril V. Axillary nerve palsy following blunt trauma to the shoulder region: a clinical and electrophysiological review. *J Neurol Neurosurg Psychiatry* 1982;45:1027–1032.
5. Bigliani LU. Malunion of four-part anterior fracture dislocation following open reduction internal fixation. *Tech Orthop* 1994;9:99–101.
6. Bigliani LU. Treatment of two and three part fractures of the proximal humerus. *Am Acad Orthop Surg Instr Course Lect* 1989;38:231–244.
7. Bigliani LU, McCluskey GM. Prosthetic replacement in acute fractures of the proximal humerus. *Semin Arthroplasty* 1990;1:29–37.
8. Blom S, Dahlback LO. Nerve injuries in dislocations of the shoulder joint and fractures of the neck of the humerus. A clinical and electromyographic study. *Acta Chir Scand* 1970;136:461.
9. Boville DF, Norris TR. The efficacy of intraoperative autologous transfusion in major shoulder surgery. *Clin Orthop* 1989;240:137–140.
10. Brostrom F. Early mobilization of fractures of the upper end of the humerus. *Arch Surg* 1943;46:614.
11. Burkhead WZ Jr. Use of porous-coated modular prosthesis in the treatment of complex fractures of the proximal humerus. *Tech Orthop* 1993;8:184–191.
12. Callahan DJ. Anatomic considerations. Closed reduction of proximal humeral fractures. *Orthop Rev* 1984;13(3):79–85.
13. Castagno AA, Shuman WP, Kilcoyne RF, et al. Complex fractures of the proximal humerus: role of CT in treatment. *Radiology* 1987;165:759–762.
14. Celli L, Rovesta C, Marongiu MC, Mingione A. Peripheral nerve lesions in anterior scapulo-humeral dislocations. In: Alnot J-Y, Narakas A, eds. *Traumatic brachial plexus injuries*. Paris: Expansion Scientifique Francaise, 1996.
15. Chervu W, Quionrs-Baldrich WJ. Vascular complications in orthopaedic surgery. *Clin Orthop* 1988;235:275–288.
16. Clifford PC. Fractures of the neck of the humerus: a review of the late results. *Injury* 1981;12:91–95.
17. Coene LN, Narakas AO. Surgical management of axillary nerve lesions, isolated or combined with other infraclavicular nerve lesions. *Periph Nerve Repair Regen* 1986;3:47–65.
18. Conn RA, Cofield RH, Byer DE, et al. Interscalene block anesthesia for shoulder surgery. *Clin Orthop* 1987;216:94–98.
19. Coventry MB, Laurnen EL. Ununited fractures of the middle and upper humerus. Special problems in treatment. *Clin Orthop* 1970;69:192–198.
20. Cuomo F. Proximal humeral fractures In: Norris TR, ed. *Orthopaedic knowledge update: shoulder and elbow*. Rosemont, IL: American Academy of Orthopaedic Surgeons, 1998:181–189.
21. Cuomo F, Flatow EL, Maday MG, et al. Open reduction and internal fixation of two- and three-part displaced surgical neck fractures of the proximal humerus. *J Shoulder Elbow Surg* 1992;1:287–295.
22. Dall-Miles Cable Grip System: Pfizer Howmedica Inc., Rutherford, NJ.
23. de Laat EA, Visser CP, Coene LN, et al. Nerve lesions in primary shoulder dislocations and humeral neck fractures: a prospective clinical and EMG study. *J Bone Joint Surg [Br]* 1994;76:381–383.
24. DesMarchais JE, Morais G. Treatment of complex fractures of the proximal humerus by Neer hemiarthroplasty. In: Bateman JE, Welsh RP, eds. *Surgery of the shoulder*. Philadelphia: BC Decker, 1984.
25. Drapanas T, Hewitt RL, Weichert RF, et al. Civilian vascular injuries. A critical appraisal of three decades of management. *Ann Surg* 1970;172:351–360.
26. Duralde XA, Rodosky MW, Pollock RG, Flatow EL, Bigliani LU. Operative treatment of malunions of the proximal humerus. *J Shoulder Elbow Surg* 1995;4:S11.
27. Ebel R. Uber die ursachen der axillaris parese bei schulterluxation. *Msche Unfallheilk* 1973;76:445–449.
28. Ekstrom T, Lagergren C, von Schreeb T. Procaine injections and early mobilization for fractures of the neck of the humerus. *Acta Chir Scand* 1965;130:18–24.
29. Frisch LH, Sojbjerg JO, Sneppen O. Shoulder arthroplasty in complex acute and chronic proximal humeral fractures. *Orthopedics* 1991;9:949–954.
30. Garceau GJ, Coglang S. Early physical therapy in the treatment of fractures of the surgical neck of the humerus. *J Indiana Med Assoc* 1941;34:293–295.
31. Geneste R, et al. Closed treatment of fracture dislocations of the shoulder joint. *Rev Chir Orthop* 1980;66:383–386.
32. Gerber C, Krushell RJ. Isolated rupture of the tendon of the subscapularis muscle: clinical features in 16 cases. *J Bone Joint Surg [Br]* 1991;73:389.
33. Gerber C. Latissimus dorsi transfer for treatment of irreparable tears of the rotator cuff. *Clin Orthop* 1992;275:152–160.
34. Gerber C, Schneeberger A, Vinh TS. The arterial vascularization of the humeral head: an anatomic study. *J Bone Joint Surg [Am]* 1990;72:1486–1494.
35. Green A, Limbird RS. Humeral head replacement for acute four-part fractures. *J Shoulder Elbow Surg* 1993;2:249–254.

36. Green A, Norris TR. Humeral head replacement for four-part fractures and fracture-dislocations. *Oper Tech Orthop* 1994;4:13–20.
37. Green A, Norris TR. Imaging techniques in glenohumeral arthritis. *Clin Orthop* 1994;307:18–26.
38. Green A, Norris TR, Becker GE, Smith RB. Failed shoulder surgery: psychological. *J Shoulder Elbow Surg* 1997;6:173.
39. Gristina AG. Symposium: Management of displaced fractures of the proximal humerus. *Contemp Orthop* 1987;15:61–93.
40. Groh GI, Rockwood CA Jr. Surgical anatomy and technique. In: Friedman RJ, ed. *Arthroplasty of the shoulder*. New York: Thieme Medical, 1994:80–98.
41. Hagg O, Lundberg BJ. Aspects of prognostic factors in comminuted and dislocated proximal humeral fractures. In: Bateman JE, Welsh RP, eds. *Surgery of the shoulder*. Philadelphia: BC Decker, 1984.
42. Hall MC, Rosser M. The structure of the upper end of the humerus with reference to osteoporotic changes in senescence leading to fracture. *Can Med Assoc J* 1963;88:290.
43. Hawkins RJ, Bell RH, Gurr K. The three-part fracture of the proximal humerus. *J Bone Joint Surg [Am]* 1986;68:1410–1414.
44. Hawkins RJ, Kiefer GN. Internal fixation techniques for proximal humeral fractures. *Clin Orthop* 1987;223:77.
45. Hawkins RJ, Angelo RL. Displaced proximal humeral fractures. Selecting treatment, avoiding pitfalls. *Orthop Clin North Am* 1987;18:421–431.
46. Hawkins RJ, Switlyk P. Acute prosthetic replacement for severe fractures of the proximal humerus. *Clin Orthop* 1993;289:156–160.
47. Hayes MJ, Van Winkle N. Axillary artery injury with minimally displaced fracture of the neck of humerus. *J Trauma* 1983;23:431–433.
48. Healy WL, Jupiter JB, Kristiansen TK, et al. Nonunion of the proximal humerus. In: Post M, Morrey BF, Hawkins RJ, eds. *Surgery of the shoulder*. St Louis: Mosby Year Book, 1990:59–62.
49. Henson GF. Vascular complications of shoulder injuries: a report of two cases. *J Bone Joint Surg [Br]* 1956;38:528–531.
50. Hinsenkamp M, Burny F, Andrianne Y, et al. External fixation of the fractures of the humerus. A review of 164 cases. *Orthopedics* 1984;7: 1309–1314.
51. Hudson RT. The use of the hanging cast in treatment of fractures of the humerus. *South Surg* 1941;10:132–134.
52. Iannotti JP. Rotator cuff impingement. Section in: Norris TR, ed. *Orthopaedic knowledge update: shoulder and elbow*. Rosemont, IL: American Academy of Orthopaedic Surgeons, 1998:123–177.
52a. Itoh Y, Sasaki T, Ishiguro T, Uchiniski K, Yabe Y, Fukuda H. Transfer of latissimus dorsi to replace a paralyzed anterior deltoid: a new technique using an inverted pedicle graft. *J Bone Joint Surg [Br]* 1987; 69:647–651.
53. Jaberg H, Warner JJ, Jacob RP. Percutaneous stabilization of unstable fractures of the proximal humerus. *J Bone Joint Surg [Am]* 1992;74: 508–515.
54. Janecki CJ, Barnett DC. Fracture–dislocation of the shoulder with biceps tendon interposition. *J Bone Joint Surg [Am]* 1979;61:142–143.
55. Jensen GF, Christiansen C, Boesen J, et al. Relationship between bone mineral content and frequency of postmenopausal fractures. *Acta Med Scand* 1983;213:61–63.
56. Jones L. Reconstructive operation for non-reducible fractures of the head of the humerus. *Ann Surg* 1933;97:217–225.
57. Keene JS, Huizenga RE, Engber WD, Rogers SC. Proximal humerus fractures: a correlation of residual deformity with long-term function. *Orthopedics* 1983;6:173–178.
58. Knight RA, Mayne JA. Comminuted fractures and fracture–dislocations involving the articular surface of the humeral head. *J Bone Joint Surg [Am]* 1957;39:1343–1355.
59. Kofoed H. Revascularization of the humeral head. A report of two cases of fracture–dislocation of the shoulder. *Clin Orthop* 1983;179: 175–178.
60. Kraulis J, Hunter G. The results of prosthetic replacement in fracture–dislocations of the upper end of the humerus. *Injury* 1976;8: 129–131.
61. Kristiansen B, Christensen SW. Plate fixation of proximal humeral fractures. *Acta Orthop Scand* 1986;57:320–333.
62. Kristiansen B, Kofoed H. External fixation of displaced fractures of the proximal humerus. *J Bone Joint Surg [Br]* 1987;9:643–646.
63. Kristiansen B, Kofoed H. Transcutaneous reduction and external fixation of displaced fractures of the proximal humerus. *J Bone Joint Surg [Br]* 1988;70:821–824.
64. Kyle RF, Conner TN. External fixation of the proximal humerus. *Orthopedics* 1988;11:163–168.
65. Laing PG. The arterial supply to the adult humerus. *J Bone Joint Surg [Am]* 1956;38:1105–1116.
66. Leach RE, Premer RF. Nonunion of the surgical neck of the humerus. Method of internal fixation. *Minn Med* 1965;45:318–322.
67. Lee CK, Hansen HR. Post-traumatic avascular necrosis of the humeral head in displaced proximal humeral fractures. *J Trauma* 1981;21: 788–791.
68. Leffert RD, Seddon H. Infraclavicular brachial plexus injuries. *J Bone Joint Surg [Br]* 1965;47:9–22.
69. Leyshon R. Closed treatment of fractures of the proximal humerus. *Acta Orthop Scand* 1984;55:48–51.
70. Lim EVA, Day LJ. Thrombosis of the axillary artery complicating proximal humeral fractures. *J Bone Joint Surg [Am]* 1987;69: 778–780.
71. Linson MA. Axillary artery thrombosis after fracture of the humerus. A case report. *J Bone Joint Surg [Am]* 1980;62:1214.
72. London PS. Treatment and aftercare for dislocation of the shoulder. *Physiotherapy* 1971;37(2):2–6.
73. Lower RF, McNiesh LM, Callahan JJ. Complications of intraarticular hardware penetration. *Complications Orthop* 1989;May/June:89–93.
74. Mauclaire M. *Bull Mem Soc Chir Paris* 1920;46:572.
75. Mills HJ, Horne G. Fractures of the proximal humerus in adults. *J Trauma* 1985;25:801–805.
76. Moeckel BH, Altchek DW, Warren RF, et al. Instability of the shoulder after arthroplasty. *J Bone Joint Surg [Am]* 1993;75:792–797.
77. Neer CS II. Displaced proximal humeral fractures. Part II. Treatment of three-part and four-part displacement. *J Bone Joint Surg [Am]* 1970;52:1090–1103.
78. Neer CS II. Nonunion of the surgical neck of the humerus. *Orthop Trans* 1983;7:389.
79. Neer CS II, McIlveen SJ. Humeral head replacement with tuberosity and cuff reconstruction for 4 part displacement. Current results and technique. *Rev Chir Orthop* 1988;74(suppl 2):31.
80. Neer CS II, Watson KC, Stanton FJ. Recent experience in total shoulder replacement. *J Bone Joint Surg [Am]* 1982;64:319–336.
81. Norris TR. Diagnostic techniques for shoulder instability. In: Stauffer ES, ed. *American Academy of Orthopaedic Surgeons instructional course lectures*, vol 34. St Louis: CV Mosby, 1985:239–257.
82. Norris TR. Unconstrained prosthetic shoulder replacement. In: Watson M, ed. *Surgical disorders of the shoulder*. London: Churchill Livingstone, 1991:473–510.
83. Norris TR. Fractures and fracture dislocations of the glenohumeral complex. In: Chapman MW, Madison M, eds. *Operative orthopaedics*, 2nd ed. Philadelphia: JB Lippincott, 1993:405–424.
84. Norris TR. History and physical examination of the shoulder. In: Nicholas JA, Hershman EB, eds. *The upper extremity in sports medicine*, 2nd ed. St Louis: CV Mosby, 1995:70–72.
85. Norris TR. Prosthetic arthroplasty in nonunions and malunions of the proximal humerus. *Semin Arthroplasty* 1997;8:304–320.
86. Norris TR, Evans J. Subscapularis lengthening for internal rotation contracture of the shoulder. *J Shoulder Elbow Surg* 1994;3:S3.
87. Norris TR, Green A, McGuigan FX. Late prosthetic shoulder arthroplasty for displaced proximal humerus fractures. *J Shoulder Elbow Surg* 1995;4:271–280.
88. Norris TR, Green A. Imaging modalities in the evaluation of shoulder disorders. In: Matsen FA III, Fu FH, Hawkins RJ, eds. *The shoulder: a balance of mobility and stability*. Rosemont, IL: American Academy of Orthopaedic Surgeons, 1993:353–357.
89. Norris TR, Green A. Proximal humerus fractures and fracture–dislocations. In: Browner BD, Jupiter JB, Levine AM, Trafton PG, eds. *Skeletal trauma*, 2nd ed. Philadelphia: WB Saunders, 1998: 1570–1638.
90. Norris TR, McElheney E. The role of long-stem humeral head prosthesis in treatment of complex humeral fractures and in revision arthroplasty. *Semin Arthroplasty* 1990;1:138–150.
91. Norris TR, Turner JA, Boville DF. Nonunion of the upper humerus: an analysis of the etiology and treatment in 28 cases. In: Post M, Hawkins RJ, Morrey BF, eds. *Surgery of the shoulder*. St Louis: CV Mosby, 1990:63–67.
92. Pasila M, Faroma H, Kiviluoto O, Sundholm A. Early complications of primary shoulder dislocations. *Acta Orthop Scand* 1978;49: 260–263.
93. Pettine KA. Open reduction and internal fixation of four-part fractures of the proximal humerus. *Contemp Orthop* 1989;19:49–54.

94. Pollock RG, Glasson JM, Djurasovic M, et al. Hemiarthroplasty for glenohumeral osteoarthritis in patients with an intact rotator cuff: results correlated to degree of glenoid wear. *J Shoulder Elbow Surg* 1997;6:177.
95. Raney F, Kolb F. The effect of metabolic bone disease on spinal fusion. In: White A, Rothman R, Ray C, eds. *Lumbar spine surgery—techniques and complications*. St Louis: CV Mosby, 1987: 246–249.
96. Resch H, Povacz P. Pectoralis major muscle transfer in case of irreparable chronic tear of the subscapularis tendon. *J Shoulder Elbow Surg* 1997;6:224.
97. Rooney PJ, Cockshott WP. Pseudarthrosis following proximal humeral fractures. A possible mechanism. *Skeletal Radiol* 1986;15:21–24.
98. Seddon HJ. Nerve lesions complicating certain closed bone injuries. *JAMA* 1947;135:11–15.
99. Seddon HJ. *Surgical disorders of the peripheral nerves*, 2nd ed. New York: Churchill Livingston, 1975:172–179.
100. Simpson NS, Jupiter JB. Reconstruction of nonunion of the proximal humerus with a custom blade plate: result of 17 consecutive cases. *J Shoulder Elbow Surg* 1997;6:182.
101. Smyth EHJ. Major arterial injury in closed fracture of the neck of the humerus: report of a case. *J Bone Joint Surg [Am]* 1969;51:508.
102. Solonen KA, Vastamaki M. Osteotomy of the neck of the humerus for traumatic varus deformity. *Acta Orthop Scand* 1985;56:79–80.
103. Sorenson KH. Pseudoathrosis of the surgical neck of the humerus. Two cases. One bilateral. *Acta Orthop Scand* 1964; 34:132–168.
104. Stableforth PG. Four-part fractures of the neck of the humerus. *J Bone Joint Surg [Br]* 1984;66:104–108.
105. Stableforth PG. Open reduction and internal fixation of displaced four-segment fractures of the proximal humerus. *Oper Tech Orthop* 1994;4:26–30.
106. Sturzenegger M, Fornaro E, Jakob RP. Results of surgical treatment of multi-fragmented fractures of the humeral head. *Arch Orthop Trauma Surg* 1982;100:249.
107. Svend-Hansen H. Displaced proximal humeral fractures. A review of 49 patients. *Acta Orthop Scand* 1974;45:359.
108. Tanner MW, Cofield RH. Prosthetic arthroplasty for fracture and fracture–dislocations of the proximal humerus. *Clin Orthop* 1982;179: 116–128.
109. Theodorides T, Dekeizer G. Injuries of the axillary artery caused by fractures of the neck of the humerus. *Injury* 1976;8:120.
110. Willems WJ, Lin TE. Neer arthroplasty for humeral fracture. *Acta Orthop Scand* 1985;56:394–395.
111. Williams GR, Iannotti JP. Total shoulder replacement—surgical technique. *Tech Orthop* 1994;9:160–170.
112. Yosipovitch Z, Tikkva P, Goldberg I. Inferior subluxation of the humeral head after injury to the shoulder. *J Bone Joint Surg [Am]* 1989;71:751–753.
113. Young TB, Wallace WA. Conservative treatment of fractures and fracture–dislocations of the upper end of the humerus. *J Bone Joint Surg [Br]* 1985;67:373–377.
114. Zuckerman JD, Flugstad DL, Teitz CC, King HA. Axillary artery injury as a complication of proximal humeral fractures. Two case reports and a review of the literature. *Clin Orthop* 1984;189: 234–237.
115. Zuckerman JD, Koval KJ, Powell SE, et al. One-part proximal humerus fractures: a prospective study. In: Vastamaki M, Jalovaara P, eds. *Surgery of the shoulder*. Amsterdam: Elsevier Science, 1995: 423–427.
116. Zuckerman JD, Matsen FA. Complications about the glenohumeral joint related to the use of the screws and staples. *J Bone Joint Surg [Am]* 1984;66:175–180.

Disorders of the Shoulder: Diagnosis and Management,
edited by Joseph P. Iannotti and Gerald R. Williams, Jr.
Lippincott Williams & Wilkins, Philadelphia © 1999.

CHAPTER 26

Fractures of the Clavicle

Jesse B. Jupiter and David Ring

INTRODUCTION

Most orthopedic surgeons consider the clavicle a relatively agreeable and cooperative bone. Fracture of the clavicle is common, and it has long been thought that its inherent reparative capacity will lead to rapid healing despite little more than symptomatic treatment.[241] Deformity has been described as merely a cosmetic concern, for function is satisfactory despite malunion.[164] It has been suggested by many that primary operative intervention is meddlesome and will only make things worse.[189,241] Despite the proximity of major vascular, nervous, and cardiopulmonary structures, associated injury is uncommon.

As this chapter will indicate, there may be reason to question some of these established beliefs. In actual fact, our understanding of clavicular fractures and clavicular function, for the most part, is based on only a modest amount of recorded data. A large percentage of clavicular fractures occur in children and heal readily with remodeling of deformity.[201,269] Failure to evaluate these fractures separately from displaced fractures in adults has clouded the issues.

J. B. Jupiter: Department of Orthopaedic Surgery, Harvard Medical School and Massachusetts General Hospital, Boston, Massachusetts 02114.

D. Ring: Department of Orthopaedic Surgery, Massachusetts General Hospital, Boston, Massachusetts 02114.

Interest in clavicular nonunions is relatively new[19] and has demonstrated that displaced fractures of the middle portion of the clavicle can in fact be troublesome injuries in adults.[120,163,288,290] Failure to unite following these injuries can lead to progressive shoulder deformity, pain, impaired function, and neurovascular compromise. Malunion may also contribute to weakness, pain, and neurovascular compromise.[74,75] Data on displaced distal clavicular fractures in adult patients have demonstrated sufficient difficulties with healing to consider primary operative treatment.[56,190–192] A recent investigation focusing on the results of the treatment of displaced midclavicular fractures in adult patients suggests that this subset of fractures may also be prone to nonunion and delayed union.[288]

ANATOMY

The clavicle is unique among long bones in many respects, among them its development, shape, structure, and anatomic relations. It is the first bone to ossify in the embryo, occurring in the fifth gestational week, and the only long bone to ossify from a mesenchymal anlage (intramembranous ossification). Although several investigations documenting the histologic evaluation of the embryonic clavicle report that ossification proceeds from two separate centers,[6,85,86,100,162] others assert that a narrow interconnection between these two centers is present from the outset, but may not be seen in any one particular histologic section and, therefore, will result in sampling error.[80,89,130] Dispute exists as to the etiology of congenital pseudoarthrosis of the clavicle, with some suggesting that it is a result of the failure of these two centers to coalesce,[129,281] whereas others believe that pressure from the subclavian artery inhibits ossification, leading to pseudoarthrosis.[155]

Growth in length initially occurs through expansion of the central ossification centers, and later by enchondral ossification of epiphyseal growth centers acquired at each end of the bone. The medial (sternal) physis accounts for approximately 80% of the longitudinal growth of the clavicle.[205] Ossification of the sternal epiphysis of the clavicle occurs in the midteenage years and is very difficult to visualize on routine radiography.[53,205] The acromial epiphysis does not ordinarily form a secondary ossification center.[274] Both the sternal and acromial physes can remain open into the third decade of life, particularly the sternal physis which typically remains open until approximately age 25 years in females and 26 in males.[116,205,274] As a result, apparent dislocations of the acromioclavicular or sternoclavicular joints are more likely to be physeal separation injuries in adolescents and young adults.[53,171,283]

The clavicle is named for its "s"-shaped curvature with an apex anteromedially and an apex posterolaterally, resembling the musical symbol, *clavicula*.[179] The larger medial curvature widens the space for passage of neurovascular structures from the neck into the upper extremity through the costoclavicular interval. The transition from medial to lateral curvature occurs at approximately two-thirds the length of the bone as measured from its sternal end, a site that roughly corresponds to both the medial limit of attachment of the coracoclavicular ligaments and the entrance point of the main nutrient artery of the clavicle.[205]

Inman has suggested that the curvature of the lateral third of the clavicle contributes to the range of motion of the shoulder girdle by allowing approximately 30 degrees of motion between the scapula and clavicle through the acromioclavicular joint.[110,111,154] According to his description, this motion occurs by inferior translation of the medial portion of the scapula, leading to abduction of the scapula through the acromioclavicular joint, a motion which might be thought impossible considering the rigid interrelation between the clavicle and scapula maintained by the stout coracoclavicular ligaments. However, the lateral curvature and 50-degree–rotational motion of the clavicle on its longitudinal axis permit inferior translation of the attachment of the coracoclavicular ligaments on to the posteriorly directed apex of the lateral clavicle along with the scapula. Inman has likened this to the action of a crankshaft[111] (Fig. 1). Others

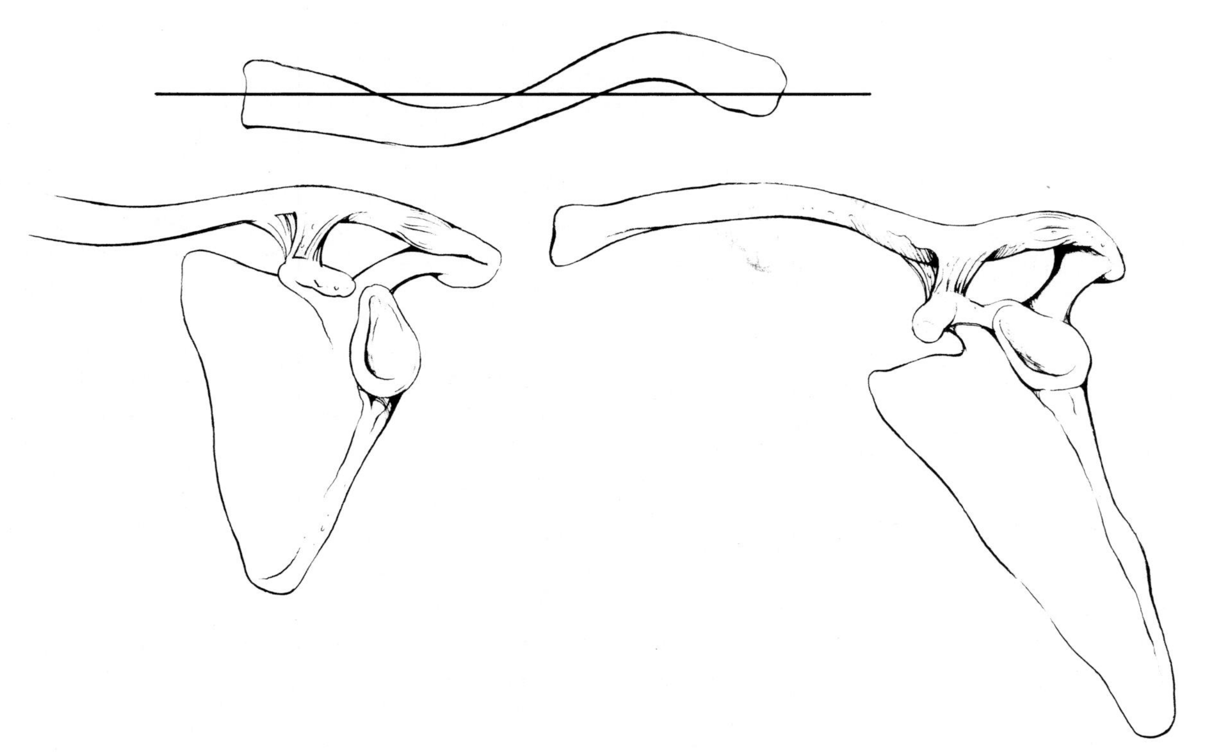

FIG. 1. There are three axes of clavicular motion: anteroposterior, superoinferior, and rotational. The 50-degree–rotational motion of the clavicle, in combination with the apex posterior curvature of the lateral clavicle, permits inferior translation of the attachment of the coracoclavicular ligaments on the lateral clavicle. This, in turn, permits the medial aspect of the scapula to translate inferiorly, with the glenoid abducting through the acromioclavicular joint. This so-called crankshaft mechanism provides 30 degrees of the total 60-degree contribution of scapulothoracic motion to shoulder abduction.

dispute this description, claiming that little motion occurs at the acromioclavicular joint and that the scapula actually rotates along with the clavicle.[42]

The clavicle is made up of very dense trabecular bone lacking a well-defined medullary canal. In cross section the clavicle transitions gradually between a flat lateral aspect, a tubular midportion, and an expanded prismatic medial end.[11,102] The peculiarities of both its curvature and cross-sectional anatomy as well as its bony structure become important when intramedullary fixation of the clavicle is considered.[241]

The clavicle is subcutaneous throughout its length and makes a prominent aesthetic contribution to the contour of the neck and upper chest. The supraclavicular nerves run obliquely across the clavicle just superior to the platysma muscle and should be identified and protected during operative exposure to offset the development of hyperesthesia or dysesthesia over the chest wall.

The articulation of the clavicle with the trunk is stabilized by the stout costoclavicular and sternoclavicular ligaments. The subclavius muscle may also contribute to stability in this region of the clavicle. The coracoclavicular and acromioclavicular ligaments stabilize the relation of the distal clavicle with the scapula. The upper portion of the insertion of the trapezius muscle and the anterior portion of the deltoid origin further stabilize the lateral clavicle through their attachments to its posterior and anterior aspects, respectively. Fractures in these regions of the clavicle tend to be relatively stable, provided that the described ligamentous and muscular relations are not disrupted in the traumatic injury.[190–192]

In displaced fractures and ununited fractures of the clavicle, the most common deformity includes mediolateral shortening, drooping, adduction, and protraction of the shoulder girdle. We find it useful to refer to this characteristic deformity as ptosis of the shoulder (Leffert RD, personal communication; Fig. 2). The forces contributing to persistence or worsening of deformity following fracture include the weight of the shoulder, as transmitted to the distal fragment of the clavicle primarily through the coracoclavicular ligaments, as well as the deforming forces of the attached muscles and ligaments. The medial fragment is elevated by the clavicular head of the sternocleidomastoid muscle, which inserts onto the posterior aspect of the medial portion of the clavicle. The pectoralis major contributes to adduction and inward rotation of the shoulder.[190–192]

The apex of clavicular deformity is typically superior. A plate placed superiorly may act as a tension band, thereby contributing to the stability of the construct, as well as promoting forces conducive to healing at the fracture site.

It is not surprising that the middle third is the most common site of clavicular fracture. The midportion is the thinnest and narrowest portion of the bone and represents a transitional region of the bone, both in curvature and cross-sectional anatomy, making it a mechanically weak area.[102] The middle third also is the only area of the clavicle that is not supported by ligamentous or muscular attachments. It is possible that this circumstance was selected during evolution because clavicular fracture protects the brachial plexus during difficult births (shoulder dystocia).

Considering the intimate relation of the clavicle to the brachial plexus, subclavian artery and vein, and the apex of the lung, it is surprising that injury to these structures in association with fracture of the clavicle is so uncommon. Brachial plexus palsy may develop weeks or years following injury owing to hypertrophic callus, with or without malalignment of the fracture fragments, leading to compromise of the costoclavicular space.[10,35,46,72,95,109,120,125,133,167,174,232,244,280,294]

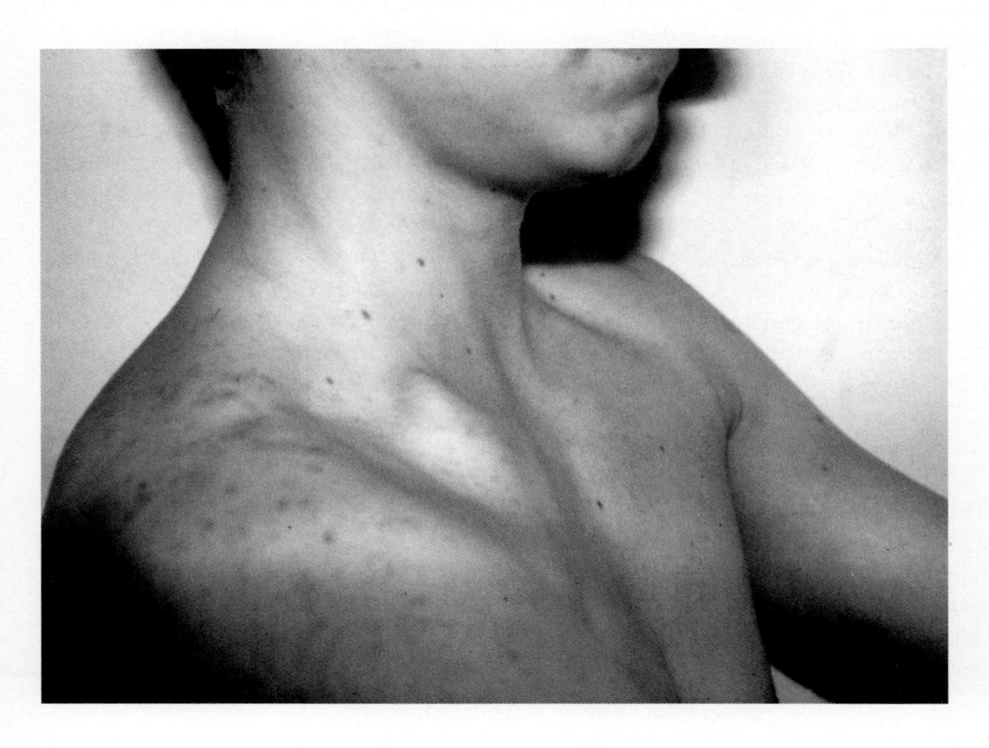

FIG. 2. Many patients with clavicular nonunion develop shortening, drooping, adduction, and protraction of the shoulder. Following Leffert (personal communication), we refer to this deformity as ptosis of the shoulder girdle. (From Browner, Jupiter, Levine and Trafton (eds). *Skeletal Trauma: Fractures, Dislocations, Ligamentous Injuries* (Second Edition). WB Saunders, Philadelphia, 1998).

Narrowing of the costoclavicular space by malunion or nonunion can also lead to a dynamic narrowing of the thoracic outlet.[9,14,25,44,77,156,180,222,264]

FUNCTION

A review of the comparative anatomy literature would support the contention that the clavicle enhances overhead activity, particularly in actions requiring power and stability, and resists those tensile forces that become so prominent in activities required by arboreal mammals in which the clavicle evolved. A clavicle was not beneficial to running and jumping quadruped mammals.[14,35,53,154,212,213] In contrast to the quadrupeds, who derive stability and strength from close association of the shoulder girdle with the trunk, the clavicle enhances upper extremity function in simians swinging through trees by holding the glenohumeral joint and the upper extremity away from the trunk in all positions. The clavicle also serves as a bony framework for muscular attachments, provides protection for the underlying neurovascular structures, transmits the forces of accessory muscles of respiration (e.g., the sternocleidomastoid) to the upper thorax, and contributes to the aesthetics of the base of the neck.[154,179]

Interestingly, children with cleidocranial dysostosis (clavicular aplasia) adapt surprisingly well to an absence of clavicles. However, limitations have been observed for overhead activities requiring strength, stability, and dexterity in patients with cleidocranial dysostosis.[51,110,111,164,271] If these congenitally aclavicular children have notable functional deficiencies in comparison with normal children, then one must be concerned about what will happen when the learned coordinated manipulation of the complex interaction of various muscle groups, ligamentous attachments, and interarticulations of the shoulder girdle is disrupted by sacrificing clavicular continuity in adult patients.[11,65] In fact, some studies have suggested that malunion alone (particularly shortening) can cause pain and inhibit function.[74,75]

Because some reports document good function following total or subtotal resection of the clavicle for infection, malignancy, or access to neurovascular structures in small series of patients,[1,49,70,78,98,111,259,291] some authors went so far as to encourage consideration of the clavicle as an expendable or surplus part of the skeleton.[97] Resection of the clavicle has been recommended in the treatment of clavicular nonunion,[31,187] as well as in the treatment of fresh clavicular fractures.[169,218]

It is certainly clear that some patients do very poorly following clavicular resection,[51,53,120,238,259] especially those with trapezial paralysis.[216,291] We therefore feel strongly that this procedure should be reserved for the unusual situation in which a salvage procedure becomes necessary. The clavicle plays an important functional role in the shoulder girdle and every effort should be made to preserve or restore normal length and alignment in the treatment of clavicular disorders.

CLASSIFICATION

Surgeons interested in clavicular fractures have long distinguished midclavicular fractures from fractures of the medial or lateral end.[16,108] Following descriptions by Allman,[4] Rowe,[241] and Neer,[190–192] the clavicle has been divided into thirds for purposes of classification. This proves somewhat arbitrary when one considers that most clavicular fractures occur at a distance from the lateral most aspect of the bone, which falls on a roughly gaussian distribution between approximately 30% and 60% of the length of the bone.[268] In the majority of reported series, separation of clavicular fractures as occurring in one of the thirds of the bone was most likely based on interpretation from standard radiographs, rather than precise measurement. This implies that separation of the large numbers of clavicular fractures occurring about the middle third–distal third junction as belonging to either the distal third or middle third group is often imprecise and may be arbitrary.

In Neer's defining work on distal clavicular fractures,[190,192] he considered fractures distal to the proximal limit of the trapezoid ligament as distal clavicular fractures and distinguished two types: type I represents a fracture in which both the trapezoid and conoid ligaments remain intact and are attached to the medial fragment, thereby providing stable reduction of the fracture; a type II fracture consists of a fracture in which the trapezoid ligament remains attached to the distal fragment while the conoid ligament is ruptured and no longer maintains reduction of the medial fragment. In type II fractures, the loss of coracoclavicular ligament restraint on the medial fragment results in wide displacement of the fracture fragments, and in Neer's experience, an increased risk of nonunion[189] (Fig. 3).

Rockwood subsequently recommended division of type II fractures of the distal clavicle into two subsets: he included fractures of the distal clavicle in which both the conoid and trapezoid ligaments remain attached to the distal fragment as type IIA and those in which medial fragment instability is a result of disruption of the coracoclavicular ligaments (Neer's original description) as type IIB.[239,240] It is unclear, however, how type IIA fractures differ from more distal midclavicular fractures, especially considering that the most common site of midclavicular fracture is at the junction of the mid- and distal thirds.[268] We believe Neer's classification to be more applicable, for it serves the role of distinguishing fractures that might potentially be stabilized by ligamentous attachments as either stable (ligaments intact) or unstable (at least partial ligamentous disruption; see Fig. 3).

In unusual instances, fractures of the distal clavicle may be unstable in the absence of ligamentous injury. This occurs when both of the coracoclavicular ligaments remain attached to an inferior fracture fragment that lacks attachment to either of the primary medial and lateral fragments.[216]

Neer noted in his initial report that fractures of the distal clavicle are occasionally associated with extension into the acromioclavicular joint[190–192] and, subsequently, distin-

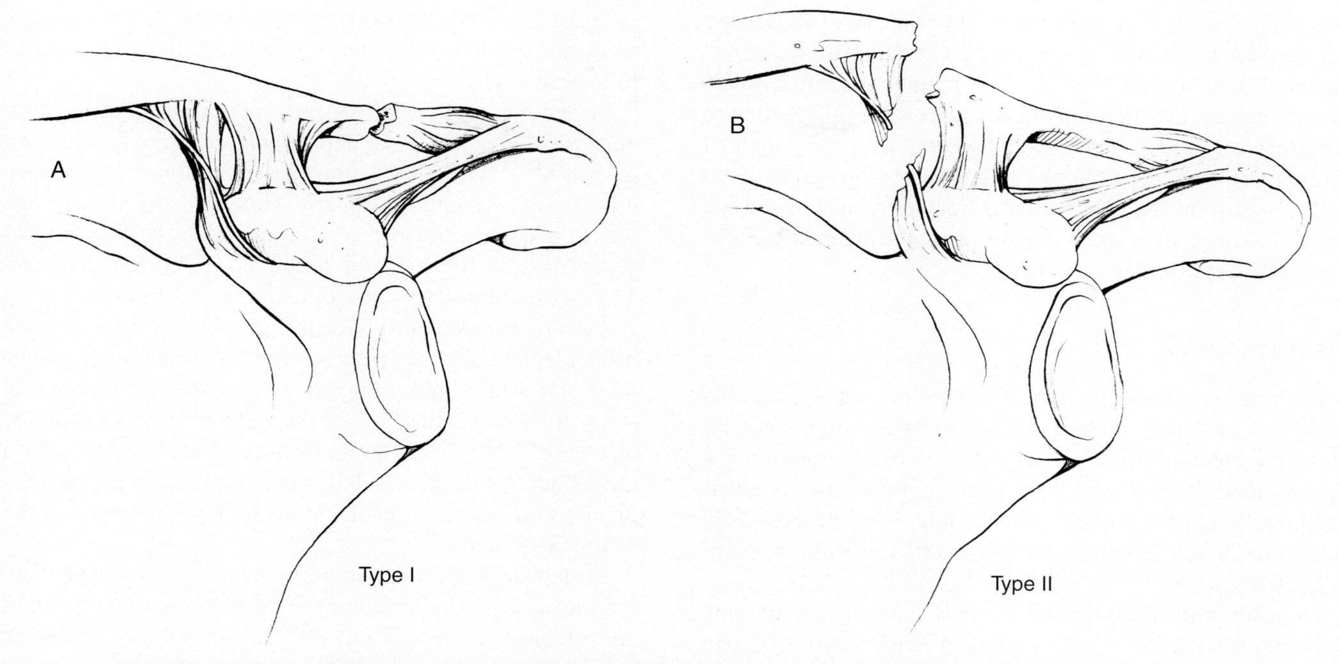

FIG. 3. When the distal end of the clavicle is fractured, the ligaments may either **(A)** remain intact and serve to maintain apposition of the fracture fragments (type I), or **(B)** rupture allowing wide displacement of the fragments (type II).

guished such fractures in his classification system as type III.[191] It has been suggested that some injuries diagnosed as type I acromioclavicular joint separation may in fact be intraarticular distal clavicular fractures and that posttraumatic osteolysis of the distal clavicle[34,114,158,230] occurs in part as a result of an undetected intraarticular fracture.[51,191]

In children and adolescents, medial and lateral clavicular injuries most frequently take the form of physeal separation injuries, although metaphyseal fractures also occur.[205,206,283] In distal clavicular physeal injuries and metaphyseal fractures (so-called pseudodislocation of the acromioclavicular joint), the proximal fragment may displace and separate from the surrounding periosteum, whereas the thin distal clavicular epiphysis, with or without an attached metaphyseal fragment, retains its anatomic relation with the acromion and the remainder of the shoulder.[78,124,206,284] The acromioclavicular and coracoclavicular ligaments are intact and remain attached to the periosteal sleeve.[206,283,289] Analogous patterns of injury occur at the sternal end of the growing clavicle.[31,121,151,226,295] Because both the medial and lateral physis typically remain open into the third decade of life,[116,205,274] it is important to realize that apparent acromioclavicular or sternoclavicular dislocations in some young adults may actually be physeal separation injuries.[31,48,121,151] As a result, these injuries can generally be expected to heal and become stable with nonoperative treatment. They may even remodel somewhat.

Fractures of the sternal end of the clavicle are uncommon and almost without exception treated symptomatically.[4,46,51,74,106,121,148,151,191,241,295] Craig has subdivided these as minimally displaced (type I), displaced (type II), intraarticular (type III), physeal separation (type IV), and comminuted (type V) fractures. Fractures in this region of the clavicle are so uncommon that the patterns of medial clavicular injury have rarely been described and studied, and it remains unclear how different fracture patterns might influence treatment or prognosis.

Fractures occurring between the medial limit of the coracoclavicular ligaments and the lateral limit of the costoclavicular ligaments represent by far the most common type of clavicular fracture, but there is no subclassification in common usage. The most important element of a midclavicular fracture is the amount of displacement or deformity. Therefore, we distinguish nondisplaced or minimally displaced fractures (including greenstick and plastic bowing[22] type fractures in children), which will heal with symptomatic treatment and little concern for either cosmesis or function, from displaced fractures, which may result in deformity, shoulder dysfunction, and an increased risk of nonunion.[273] Furthermore, it is possible that more distal midclavicular fractures are subject to increased displacement and instability as a result of muscular and ligamentous relations on a continuum with type II fractures of the distal clavicle, although there are no data to support this contention.

Pathologic fractures of the clavicle occur, although they are unusual. Rowe reported fractures through eosinophilic granuloma, pagetoid bone, and metastatic carcinoma involving the clavicle.[241] Fractures related to enchondroma[20] and arteriovenous malformation[177] have also been reported. Stress fractures of the clavicle have been described following radical neck dissection as a result of the devascularizing dissection and radiation osteitis that complicate the treatment of these tumors.[52,81,210,221,265] Fatigue fracture has also been reported in a 12-year-old boy who, while attempting to improve his grades, had apparently been carrying an inordinately large number of books under the arm on the involved side for several months.[126] Stress fracture related to the use of a Dacron graft loop for coracoclavicular ligament reconstruction has also been reported.[64]

MECHANISM

In general, clavicle fractures in all regions are typically the result of moderate- or high-energy traumatic injury in adolescents and adults, such as a fall from a height, motor vehicle accident, sports, or a blow to the point of the shoulder, and rarely a direct injury to the clavicle. In children and the elderly, clavicle fractures usually occur following low-energy trauma.[4,46,105,190–192,200,201,241,248,257,260,261,268]

It has become clear that the clavicle fails most commonly in compression.[18,82,248,261] Failure in compression is seen following falls onto the shoulder and direct blows to the point of the shoulder.[82,248,261] A direct blow to the clavicle, seen to occur in some stick-wielding sports such as Lacrosse,[257] may also fracture the clavicle. Although a fall onto the outstretched hand has traditionally been considered a common mechanism of midclavicular fracture,[4] recent observations[261] bring this into question.

Stanley et al. studied 122 of 150 consecutive patients, presenting to one of two separate hospitals in Sheffield, with a fractured clavicle providing a detailed account of their injury: 87% were the result of a fall onto the shoulder, 7% a direct blow to the point of the shoulder, and 6% a fall onto an outstretched hand.[261] A fall on the outstretched hand was the apparent mechanism of 5 of 79 (6.3%) midclavicular fractures and 2 of 34 (5.9%) distal clavicular fractures, suggesting that a direct injury to the shoulder is the most common mechanism of clavicular fracture at all sites. These authors hypothesized that even those patients who recall their injury as a fall onto the outstretched hand may have fallen secondarily onto the shoulder. This second impact may have been the injuring force, suggesting that an isolated fall onto the outstretched hand is actually an unusual mechanism of injury.[261]

Neer has stated that distal clavicular fractures tend to be the result of a high-energy, direct blow to the shoulder.[105,190] However, distal clavicular fractures have also been identified in the elderly following lower-energy injuries.[201]

EPIDEMIOLOGY

An understanding of the frequency and distribution of clavicular fractures is provided by data collected in Malmo, Sweden.[201] Four percent of all fractures occurring in Malmo in 1987 involved the clavicle. This represented 35% of all fractures in the shoulder region. The overall incidence of clavicle fractures increased from 52:100,000 persons per year in 1952 to 64: 100,000 persons per year in 1987, mostly as a result of an increase in sports-related injury and injuries following a fall.[201]

Seventy-six percent of the fractures occurred in the middle third of the clavicle, a figure that is similar to previous reports.[46,74,148,189,241] The average age overall in this subgroup was 21 years (median 13 years). However, the average age was 11 years (median 6 years) for nondisplaced fractures, 25 years (median 16 years) for simple displaced fractures, and 43 years (median 41 years) for comminuted fractures.

Twenty-one percent of fractures in Malmo involved the distal clavicle, with an average age of 47 years (median also 47 years). This is also comparable with the rate reported in some previous studies,[46,74,148] but is double the rate reported in others.[69,105,190,241] The incidences of middle and lateral third fractures of the clavicle were comparable for middle-aged adults (approximately 35 to 60 years of age) in the Malmo experience.[201]

Medial clavicular fractures represented only 3% of clavicular fractures.[201] Although many of the published studies report an incidence of 4% to 6%,[46,74,48,241] even 3% is probably an overestimate based on inclusion of many of the more medial midclavicular fractures into this group. Taylor measured the distance of 550 fractures from the lateral aspect of the clavicle and found only 0.5% in the medial third of the bone.[268] According to the data of Nordqvist et al., the average age of a person sustaining a mid-clavicular fracture was 51 years (median 59 years), with a large proportion of fractures occurring in adolescent and young adult males and the elderly. The incidence of both lateral and medial clavicular fractures rose sharply after age 75, suggesting that these areas become substantially more susceptible to fracture when osteoporotic.

EVALUATION

Clavicle fractures resulting from low- to moderate-energy traumatic injuries are easily diagnosed and are associated with few complications. The deformity and swelling associated with the fracture are usually apparent. The location of the fracture along the clavicle can usually be determined by close inspection and palpation, although distinction of fractures of the medial or lateral ends of the clavicle from dislocation of the adjacent joints can be difficult before radiographic examination. The patient typically resists all motion of the ipsilateral shoulder, is tender at the fracture site, and holds the arm against the trunk.

Open clavicular fractures are uncommon, even following high-energy traumatic injury, and are usually the result of a direct blow to the clavicle. Tenting of the skin by either one of the major fracture fragments or an intervening fragment of comminuted bone is not uncommon, but a true threat to the integrity of the skin is unusual.[231]

Neurovascular injury,[109] pneumothorax,[61,155,173,294] and hemothorax[241] have been reported in association with fracture of the clavicle, but are uncommon. In contrast to late dysfunction of the brachial plexus following clavicle fracture in which medial cord structures are typically involved, acute injury to the brachial plexus at the time of clavicle fracture usually takes the form of a traction injury to the upper cervical roots. Such root traction injuries usually occur in the setting of high-energy trauma and have a relatively poor prognosis.[13,144,253]

The prevalence of pneumothorax in association with fracture of the clavicle is often quoted as being 3%, based on Rowe's study of over 600 fractures at Massachusetts General Hospital.[241] In that study, Rowe did not distinguish between moderate- and high-energy injuries, and he did not distinguish isolated fractures from those injuries associated with ipsilateral scapular fracture or dissociation from the thorax, or ipsilateral upper rib injuries.[66,67,107,140,149,236,287] The presence of these associated injuries indicates an extremely high-energy injury mechanism. Pneumothorax and hemothorax are more common in this situation and are likely to be a result of a more generalized chest wall injury, rather than a direct injury to the apical pleura by the fractured clavicle.[107] Nonetheless, the importance of an evaluation for possible pneumothorax by both physical examination and close inspection of an upright film which includes the ipsilateral upper lung field should be emphasized.[50,160,173,294]

Vascular injuries may not always be apparent. These may consist of an intimal injury or a small puncture wound and can present from weeks to years later in the form of an aneurysm or psudoaneurysm or thrombosis of the involved vein or artery.

When a clavicle fracture occurs in the setting of a high-energy traumatic injury (such as a motor vehicle accident or a fall from a height), evaluation of life-threatening injury takes precedence and should follow the protocol promoted by the American College of Surgeons.[5] Major vascular disruption can occur in association with fracture of the clavicle, but is extremely rare.[50,58,60,62,96,109,115,166,168,188,207,219,266] Injury to the thoracic duct has also been reported.[15,28] Death following a tear of the subclavian vein with resultant pseudoaneurysm was recorded in the famous case of the death of Sir Robert Peel.[60,138] Arterial thrombosis may occur following intimal injury.[112,143,278] Fracture of the clavicle or dislocation of either the sternoclavicular or acromioclavicular joint in association with lateral scapular translation represents a scapulothoracic dissociation, an injury often associated with severe neurovascular injury.[66,67,92,140,211,242]

Evaluation of the vascular status of the upper extremity should include an assessment of relative temperature and color as compared with the uninvolved extremity. Because of the extensive collateral blood supply to the upper extremity, these factors may appear normal in spite of the presence of a major vascular injury. A difference in peripheral pulses or blood pressure between injured and uninvolved upper extremities may be the only clue that a vascular injury is present. When the limb is threatened or there is persistent unexplained hemorrhage, angiography can help detect and localize any vascular injury, thereby assisting with definitive management.

Compression[55,73,86,176,233] and even thrombosis[152,250,262] of the subclavian vein can occur in the early postinjury period. Pulmonary embolism has been reported in the setting of subclavian vein thrombosis following clavicular fracture.[262]

RADIOGRAPHIC EVALUATION

An anteroposterior (AP) view in the coronal plane of the clavicle will identify and localize most clavicular fractures, and it should differentiate displaced from nondisplaced or minimally displaced fractures. The film should be large enough to evaluate both the acromioclavicular and sternoclavicular joints, as well as the remainder of the shoulder girdle and the upper lung fields.[241] To further gauge the de-

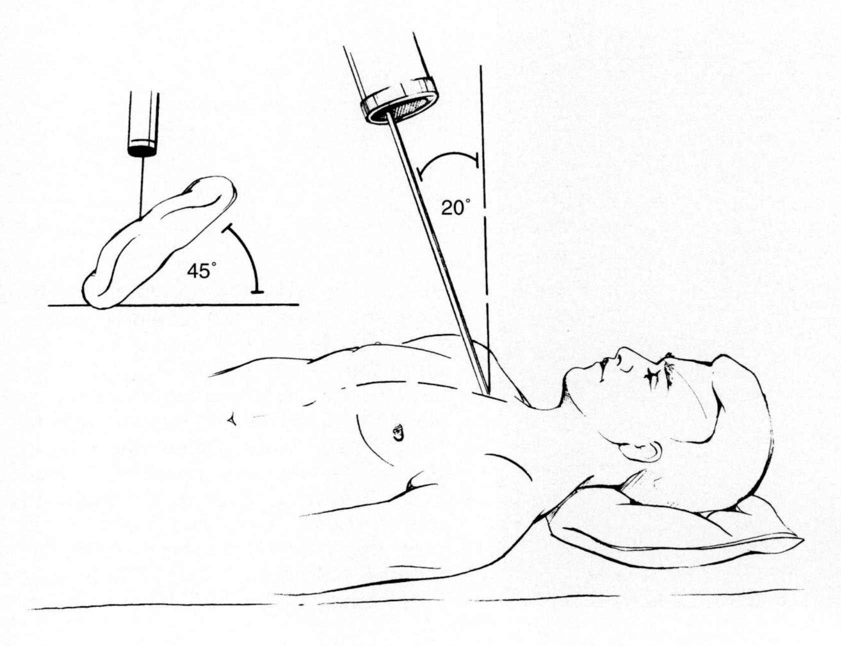

FIG. 4. The apical oblique view is taken with the involved shoulder angled 45 degrees toward the x-ray source and the x-ray source angled 20 degrees cephalad.

gree and direction of displacement of clavicular fractures, oblique views of the clavicle will be necessary.[228,241] Quesada recommended 45-degree–caudad and cephalad views, which he felt would facilitate evaluation by providing orthogonal views. In practice, a single 20- to 60-degree–cephalad tilted view provides an adequate second view, for interference with thoracic structures is minimized. Medial clavicular fractures may be difficult to characterize on this view, and computed tomography (CT) is often necessary.

Evaluation of distal clavicular fracture displacement in the anteroposterior plane requires a different set of radiographs because cephalad and caudad tilted views are hindered by overlap of the bones of the shoulder, overexposure of the distal clavicle, and frequent failure to accurately depict the degree of displacement. Neer has suggested a stress view (with 10 lb of weight in each hand) to evaluate the integrity of the coracoclavicular ligaments and 45-degree–anterior and posterior oblique views to gauge displacement.[189]

A radiograph taken with the x-ray source angled with a combination of both anteroposterior and cephalad–caudad obliquity has recently been advocated in the evaluation of midclavicular fractures.[234,286] The so-called apical oblique view (45 degree anterior [plane of the scapula], 20 degree cephalad tilt) may facilitate the diagnosis of minimally displaced fractures (e.g., birth fractures and fractures in children).[286] Ultrasound is also a very sensitive diagnostic tool in the evaluation of birth fractures[123] (Fig. 4).

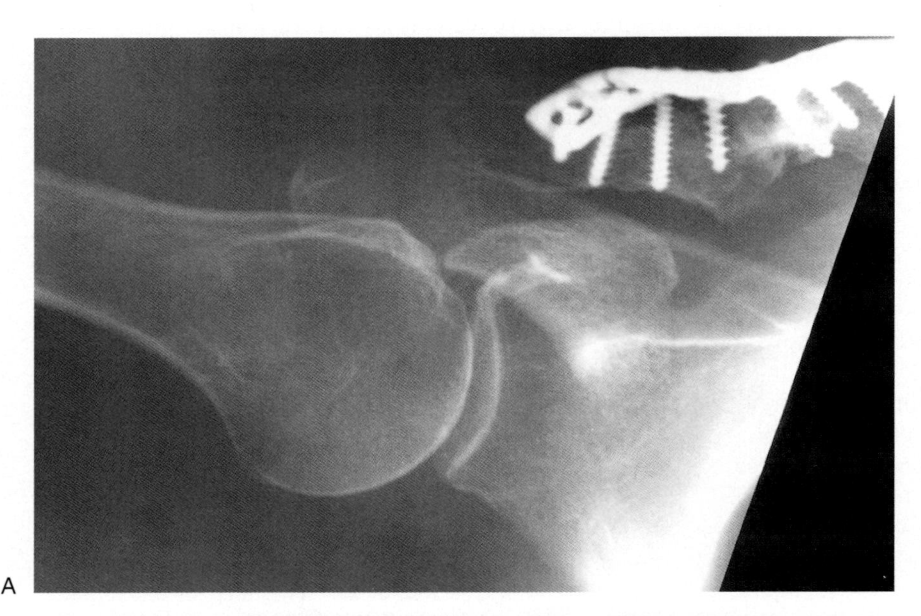

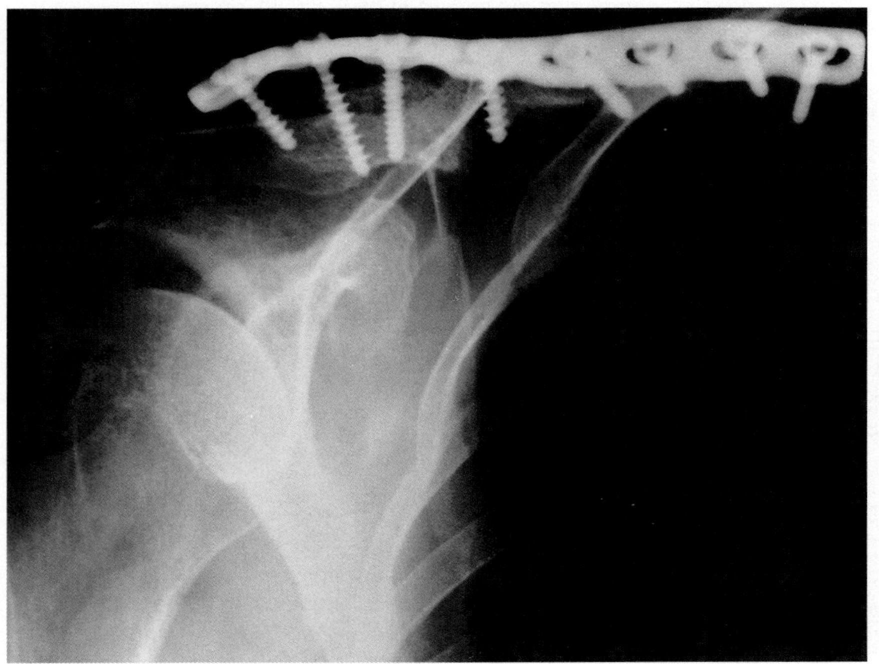

FIG. 5. The **(A)** abduction lordotic view takes advantage of the rotational motion of the clavicle with abduction of the shoulder to provide an alternative view of the clavicle. This radiographic projection is useful for visualizing the fracture site under the plate, which is often obscured in **(B)** the routine anteroposterior view. (From Browner, Jupiter, Levine and Trafton (eds). *Skeletal Trauma: Fractures, Dislocations, Ligamentous Injuries* (Second Edition). WB Saunders, Philadelphia, 1998).

The abduction–lordotic view, taken with the shoulder abducted above 135 degrees and the central ray angled 25 degrees cephalad, proves useful in evaluating the clavicle following internal fixation.[234] The abduction of the shoulder results in rotation of the clavicle on its longitudinal axis, causing the plate to rotate superiorly and thereby exposing the shaft of the clavicle and the fracture site under the plate (Fig. 5).

MANAGEMENT OF SPECIFIC INJURIES

Birth Fractures

Fracture of the clavicle is the most common traumatic birth injury.[243] Clavicle fracture must be distinguished from less common birth injuries, including brachial plexus palsy, fracture–separation of the proximal humeral epiphysis, and fracture of the humeral shaft.[243,209] High birth weight and shoulder dystocia are clearly associated with an increased risk of all types of traumatic birth injury. [32,40,43,79,91,93,118,150,159,209,237,243,254,279,282] However, upwards of 75% of neonates with clavicle fractures are the product of a normal labor and delivery and weigh less than 4,000 g.[37,40,118,237]

Shoulder dystocia results in a wide separation of the head and shoulder as passage of the shoulder through the birth canal is blocked by the symphysis pubis. This may result in a traction injury to the upper roots of the brachial plexus (Erb's palsy). Fracture of the clavicle may actually protect the brachial plexus by allowing passage of the fetus and decreasing tension on the upper roots.[209]

Identification of a clavicle fracture in a neonate who is not moving an upper extremity can be reassuring in that the fracture may explain the findings and generally will heal without long-term sequelae. However, between 1.8% and 5.3%[150,209,282] of clavicle fractures will have associated brachial plexus injury, and approximately 13% of patients with birth injury to the brachial plexus also have clavicle fractures.[93] Concurrent clavicular fracture apparently does not alter the prognosis of the brachial plexus injury.[3]

The incidence of birth fracture of the clavicle is uncertain, for many fractures are asymptomatic and may not be detected. Prospective investigations of consecutive births using either radiography or serial physical examinations have detected birth fracture of the clavicle at an incidence of 1.7%[79] and 2.9%,[118] respectively. The prospective examination of neonates demonstrated that many fractures are not detectable until callus begins to form 1 to 2 weeks following the birth injury.[118] The traditional signs of birth fracture of the clavicle—instability, motion, or crepitation at the fracture site; significant local swelling; and asymmetric Moro reflex[247]—are commonly absent.[79,118]

Most birth fractures of the clavicle occur during a vertex delivery, although they may also occur with a breech presentation or caesarean section.[209] The anterior shoulder is more commonly involved in most studies. However, in some reviews, the posterior shoulder was more commonly involved,[279] and bilateral fracture may also occur.[93,209] This suggests that both clavicles are subject to compressive forces during delivery as the widest part of the neonate (the shoulders) passes through the birth canal and that either clavicle may fracture, occasionally both.

The level of experience of the obstetrician has been implicated in some studies[43] and was unrelated in others.[32] Considering the difficulty making the diagnosis, the benign nature of the injury, and the lack of a clear association with level of experience, the incidence of birth fracture of the clavicle is probably a poor indicator of the quality of obstetric care, although it has been used as such.[32,118,203,237] It is difficult to assess the risk of forceps delivery because it is now infrequently used and may have simply been associated with more difficult deliveries in previous investigations.[32,43,150,243]

Most studies demonstrate normal apgar scores in neonates with birth fracture of the clavicle, indicating that this injury is not associated with postnatal difficulties. On the other hand, at least one study suggests that intrapartum fetal distress may be associated with an increased risk of clavicle fracture as the second stage of labor is iatrogenically shortened by a concerned obstetrician.[32]

Despite a great deal of investigative effort, no reliable risk factors have been determined that distinguish neonates at high risk of birth fracture of the clavicle, and no management recommendations can be made. Recent studies concur that birth fracture of the clavicle may be an unavoidable, and fortunately inconsequential, complication of normal birth.[32,40,237]

Isolated birth fractures of the clavicle heal quickly, remodeling any deformity. Immobilization is probably unnecessary, but is commonly used for a brief period to reassure the parents. Careful handling of the infant is the most important measure for reducing discomfort and irritability. If treatment is instituted, a simple, safe method of holding the arm at the side, such as strapping the arm to the trunk with stockinette, a gauze roll or an elastic bandage with the elbow flexed to 90 degrees and a cotton pad between the arm and trunk, should be used for about a week, after which spontaneous movement should return to the arm, indicating that interval healing has increased the stability and decreased the pain associated with the fracture.

Midclavicular Fractures

Nonoperative Treatment

Surviving writings from ancient Greece and Egypt document that for over 5,000 years humans have been concerned primarily with the deformity, rather than healing of fractures of the clavicle.[2,26] In fact, the method of closed reduction of clavicle fractures described in the Edwin Smith papyrus differs little from methods used today.[26]

To effect a closed reduction in most cases, the distal fragment must be brought upward, outward, and backward while the medial fragment is depressed. A hematoma block (10 mL of 1% lidocaine injected into the fracture site) can provide adequate anesthesia, but in some cases conscious sedation or general anesthesia may prove necessary. The reduction technique described in the Edwin Smith papyrus,[26] and still commonly used,[229] involves placing a pillow between the shoulder blades of the recumbent patient while shoulders are spread outward and upward.[26,47,229] Another method for achieving reduction is to bring the shoulders backward and upward with the patient in a sitting position while the physician's knee or clenched fist is placed between the shoulder blades to control the position of the trunk.[214,277]

Innumerable devices have been devised in an attempt to effect or maintain closed reduction and thereby minimize the deformity associated with fracture of the clavicle. Most of these were cumbersome, painful, and even dangerous.[197] Dupuytren in 1839 and Malgaigne in 1859, argued that despite these valiant attempts, deformity of the clavicle was inevitable.[63,161] They emphasized the use of the simplest and most comfortable method of treatment, which for Dupuytren consisted of placing the arm on a pillow until healing occurred.[63] It has long been suggested that excellent function can be expected despite residual deformity.[82,83,141,148,184,241,248]

Nonetheless, devices intended for the maintenance of reduction and immobilization of clavicle fractures have remained popular and commonly take the form of either the figure-of-eight bandage, with or without a sling, and only on rare occasions a figure-of-eight plaster (Billington yoke[21]) or a half shoulder spica cast.[4,214,229,241] Others have followed Dupuytren and Malgaigne in arguing that accurate reduction and immobilization of clavicular fractures is, as stated by Mullick, neither essential nor possible.[67,68,115,148,184,248] These authors advocate the use of a simple sling for comfort, forgoing any attempts at reduction.

The advantage of the figure-of-eight bandage is that the arm remains free and can be used to a limited degree. Disadvantages include increased discomfort,[6,82,68] the need for frequent readjustment and repeat office visits,[6,171] and a potential for complications, including axillary pressure sores[171,223] and other skin problems,[6] upper extremity edema and venous congestion,[6,171,184] brachial plexus palsy,[246] worsening of deformity,[82,171,184] and perhaps an increased risk of nonunion.[289]

Very few investigations have compared treatment with a figure-of-eight (or reducing) bandage with the use of a simple sling (or supporting bandage).[7,148,171,260] Although the details of patient selection and evaluation in these investigations remain unclear based upon the data published, the authors claim to have found no difference in shoulder function,[6,148,171] residual deformity,[6,171] or time to return to full range of motion and full activity.[260]

It is important to emphasize that, although the clavicle is one of the most commonly fractured bones, very little in the way of stringent, detailed analysis of clavicular fracture data has been performed. The existing literature on nonoperative treatment consists of relatively few series,[46,74,82,148,241,248,268] relatively limited studies comparing treatment modalities,[6,171,260] and some technique descriptions,[21,47,103,128,214,277] anecdotal observations,[83,74,197,229] and general reviews.[4,106,193,194,196,225]

Few reports have attempted to evaluate the relation between residual deformity and shoulder function.[74,75,208] Eskola et al. invited all 118 patients treated for fracture of the clavicle at Helsinki University Central Hospital in 1982 to return for evaluation 2 years following the injury. Among the 89 who presented for the follow-up examination, 24 (27%) had either slight pain on exercise or restricted shoulder movement, with 4 identified as having major functional problems. Primary fracture displacement and shortening of the clavicle as compared radiographically with the opposite, uninvolved side at the 2-year follow-up were used as measures of deformity. Among the 15 patients with a primary fracture displacement greater than 15 mm at the time of injury, 8 (53%) had pain with exercise, whereas only 12 of the remaining 74 patients had pain (16%), a difference found to be statistically significant using chi-squared analysis ($P=0.02$). Among 47 patients with demonstrable shortening at the final follow-up, 17 (36%) had pain with exercise, compared with 3 of 42 patients (7%) without shortening ($P=0.02$ by chi-square analysis). Given these findings, they recommend reduction of deformity associated with displaced clavicular fractures, particularly relative to shortening. One might question the authors' conclusions based on the simple fact that the more displaced fractures were those associated with higher-energy traumatic injury and might be expected to do worse regardless of residual deformity. The question of which clavicular fractures can be expected to do poorly and why remains uncertain. Even though 27% of their patients returning for 2-year follow-up reported problems with pain during exercise or restricted shoulder movement suggests that there may be room for improvement in the treatment of clavicle fractures, we must await more focused and rigidly controlled investigations for data that might alter our approach to treatment (Fig. 6).

Operative Treatment

Operative treatment of clavicular fractures has traditionally been discouraged. Early reports documented that the clavicle heals readily and predictably unless primary operative treatment is undertaken.[189,241] According to Neer, only 3 of 2,235 (0.1%) patients with midclavicular fracture treated by closed methods failed to heal, whereas 2 of 45 (4.6%) treated with immediate open reduction and fixation developed nonunion.[189] Rowe found 0.8% nonunion following closed treatment as compared with 3.7% following initial open treatment.[241] Considering the technical difficulty of operative treatment[241] and the potential for catastrophic complications associated with implant migration,[33,41,135,147,157,170,172,186,199,202,215,217,235,276] it is easy to understand why treating physicians were reluctant to operate on the clavicle primarily, reserving operative treatment for the rare case of delayed or nonunion.[189,241]

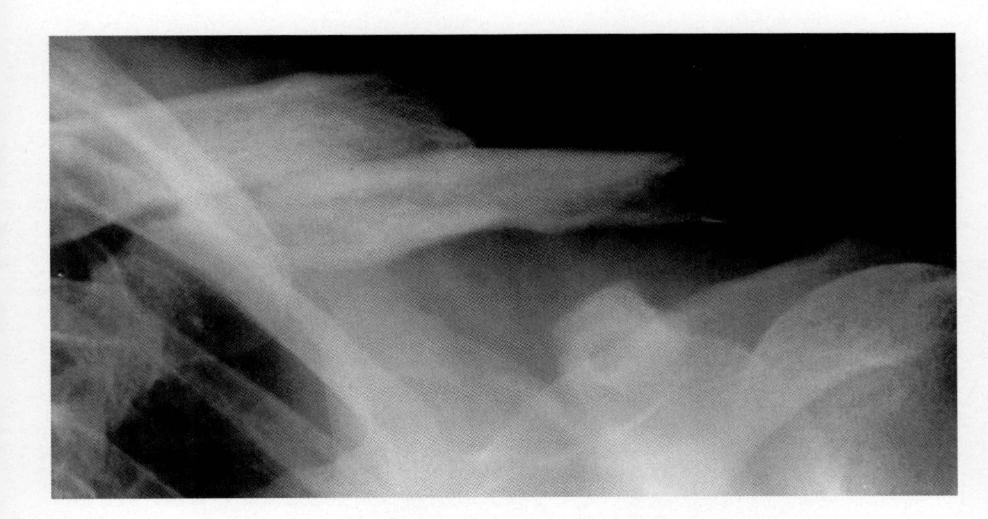

FIG. 6. Anteroposterior radiograph demonstrating healing of a clavicular fracture with 2 cm of overlap. This patient had restricted shoulder motion and required osteotomy for restoration of clavicular length. (From Browner, Jupiter, Levine and Trafton (eds). *Skeletal Trauma: Fractures, Dislocations, Ligamentous Injuries* (Second Edition). WB Saunders, Philadelphia, 1998).

Furthermore, operative fixation has been suggested to be necessary only when the fractured clavicle is widely displaced, a situation that typically occurs in the setting of high-energy trauma.[191,241] This selection bias alone toward a more severe fracture of the clavicle may be sufficient to explain the difference in union rates observed between operative and nonoperative treatment. In addition, it is now well recognized that the fixation provided by early techniques of internal fixation, as used in the studies of Neer and Rowe, is often inadequate to allow healing.

With the development of more rigid implants, there has been some interest in the use of primary operative treatment.[127,146,204,224,252,296] The good results with open reduction, internal fixation, and bone grafting of clavicular nonunion that have been documented in recent reports, also support the contention that internal fixation of the clavicle, when performed properly, should not impede healing.[22,120,163]

Zenni et al. treated operatively 25 of 800 fractures of the clavicle presenting over an 8-year period. Their indications for operative treatment included fracture of the distal third of the clavicle, with coracoclavicular ligament disruption, or severe angulation which threatened the integrity of the overlying skin, or comminution of a fracture of the middle third of the clavicle. When a threaded intramedullary wire was used for fixation, all of the fractures united after the initial operative procedure. Zenni et al. recommend as additional indications for primary operative treatment: neurovascular compromise by compression from fracture fragments, or the patient's inability to tolerate prolonged immobilization, for example, because of associated neuromuscular disorders.

Several authors have reported good results using plate fixation of clavicular fractures that are open fractures, fractures with severe angulation that could not be reduced closed, or in multiple traumatic injury, especially in the setting of ipsilateral upper extremity trauma or bilateral clavicular fracture.[30,127,136,204,224,252] In particular, scapulothoracic dissociation and the so-called floating shoulder, representing a combination of displaced clavicular and glenoid neck fractures, are felt to be important indications for open reduction and plate and screw fixation of the clavicular fracture.[66,67,92,107,140,149,236]

Khan noted no nonunions among 19 patients treated with primary plate fixation.[127] Schwartz et al. used 2.7-mm plates and reported nonunion in 3 of 36 patients, which they attributed to using a plate of inadequate length.[252] Poigenfürst has had extensive experience with plate fixation of fresh clavicular fractures and reports nonunion in 5 of 122 patients (4.1%) treated operatively.[224] He also related these failures to technical errors, including the use of a plate of inadequate length or strength, or devitalization of fracture fragments during operative exposure.

External fixation has also been used for fixation of the clavicle.[251] In a study by Schuind et al., good results were obtained in 15 fresh midclavicular fractures and in 5 delayed unions. However, considering the rarity of severe soft-tissue injury in this area, the role of external fixation remains unclear.[54]

Authors' Preferred Treatment

Nondisplaced and minimally displaced fractures of the midclavicle require little more than symptomatic treatment.[241] This is best achieved with a simple sling that can be supplemented by a swathe component if necessary for added comfort early on postinjury. Most of these nondisplaced fractures will be encountered in children who will heal quickly, and although they may not be compliant with sling wear, usually self-regulate their activity level until healing has progressed, and merely require more gentle handling during the healing period.[241] The clavicle typically heals sufficiently to discontinue immobilization within 3 to 4 weeks in young children, 4 to 6 weeks in older children, and 6 to 8 weeks in adults.[241] Limitation of activity is usually encouraged for a minimum of 8 weeks following clinical and radiographic union to reduce the risk of refracture.

The optimal treatment of displaced and comminuted fractures of the clavicle is disputed. Wide displacement and

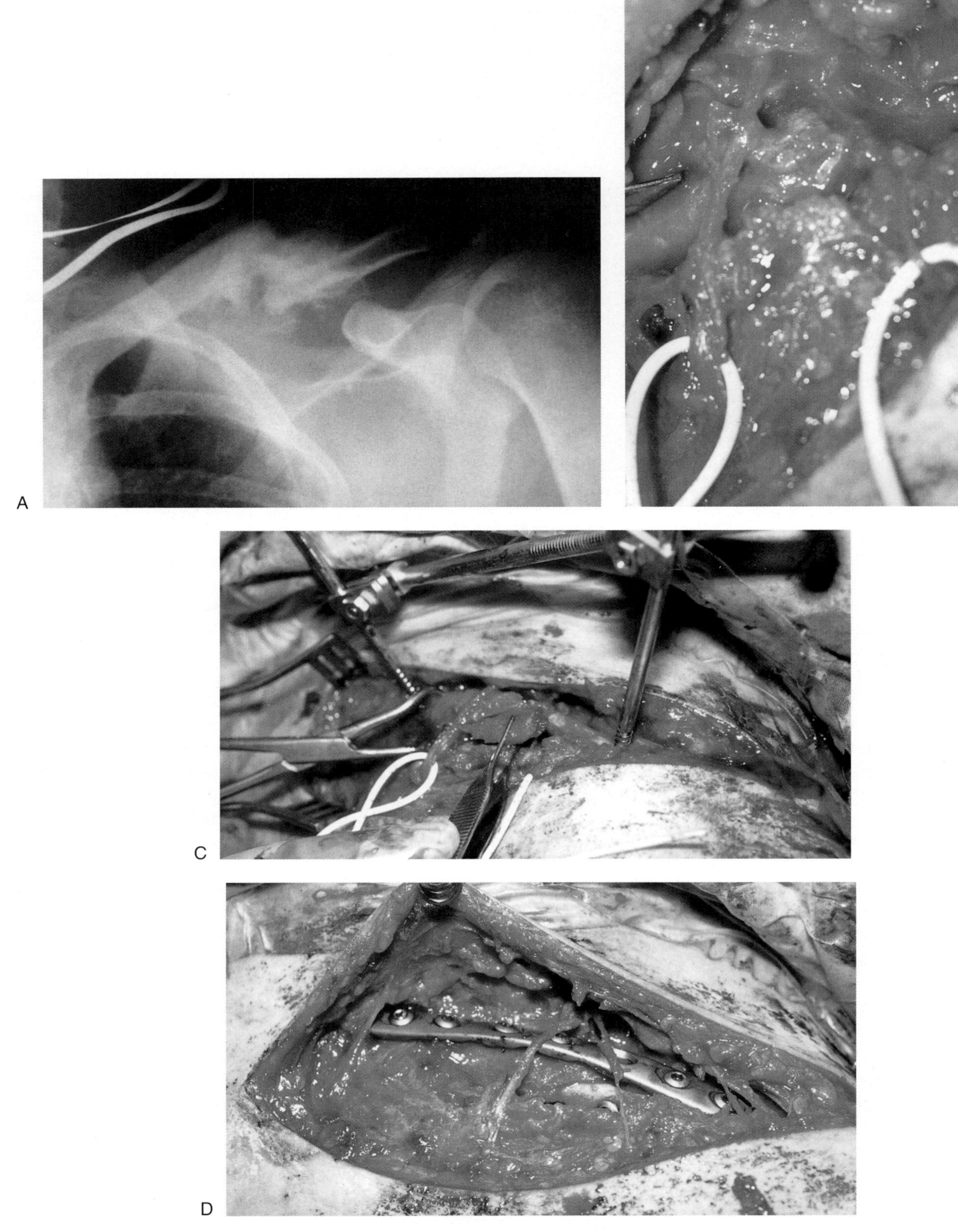

FIG. 7. A 30-year-old man presented with an ununited fracture of the clavicle associated with excessive callus formation. He had complaints of numbness and weakness in the ipsilateral upper extremity. **(A)** Anteroposterior radiograph demonstrates the nonunion and hypertrophic callous formation. **(B)** The supraclavicular nerves are preserved during exposure of the clavicle. **(C)** A distractor is used to restore clavicular length and alignment. A sculptured tricortical iliac crest graft is placed into the resulting bony defect. **(D)** The clavicle is then stabilized with a 3.5-mm limited-contact dynamic compression plate. (*continued*)

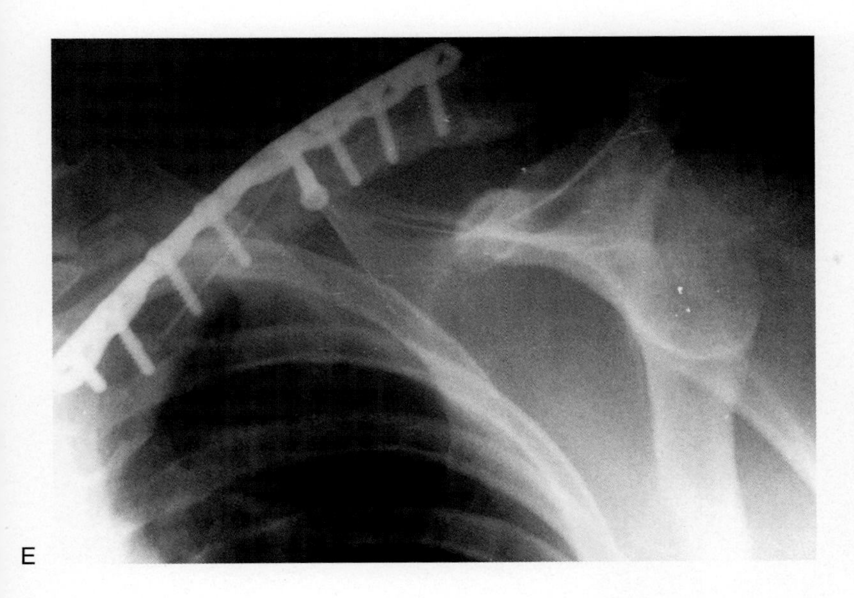

E

FIG. 7. *Continued* **(E)** Postoperative radiograph demonstrates restoration of length and alignment of the clavicle and stable plate fixation. (From Browner, Jupiter, Levine and Trafton (eds). *Skeletal Trauma: Fractures, Dislocations, Ligamentous Injuries* (Second Edition). WB Saunders, Philadelphia, 1998).

soft-tissue interposition have been implicated as risk factors for the development of nonunion,[113,120,163] and at least one study has suggested that residual deformity may alter function.[74] Open reduction and internal fixation of so-called irreducible fractures of the clavicle has been reported with good results.[30,122,127,136,204,224,252,296] However, further work is needed to determine: (a) what is the percentage of displaced midclavicular fractures that will go on to nonunion, and is it high enough to consider routine operative treatment? and (b) does the potential loss of function related to persistent deformity justify the risks of routine operative intervention?

We attempt reduction of displaced midclavicular fractures using the methods described in the foregoing and use a sling for comfort following reduction. Considering the difficulty in stabilizing clavicular reduction as well as the discomfort, encumbrance, time burden, and potential for complications associated with figure-of-eight dressings or spica casts, we no longer routinely apply these devices.

The indications for operative fixation of clavicular fractures remain uncertain. The indications that we would consider are uncommon and include open fracture, scapulothoracic dissociation,[66,67,140] so-called floating shoulder injuries,[92,106,149,236] and associated major vascular injury in which an open approach will be necessary for vascular repair. Although isolated fractures of the sternal end or middle third of the clavicle do well with nonoperative treatment, complex clavicular injuries involving dislocation or epiphyseal separation at one end of the clavicle, in combination with a fracture of the middle third, would probably benefit from open reduction and internal fixation.[71,101,139,145,271,292] Likewise, the rehabilitation of associated ipsilateral upper extremity trauma may be facilitated by operative fixation of the clavicle. In the absence of these indications, nonoperative treatment remains our preference. Operative fixation of the clavicle is most frequently performed at a time remote from the initial injury as treatment for malunion or nonunion.

It is often stated that when the skin is threatened by pressure from a prominent clavicular fracture fragment, then open reduction and internal fixation should be considered. It is extremely rare that the skin will be perforated from within.[231] However, in the head-injured patient operative stabilization may be required.

The merits of open reduction and internal fixation in the setting of neurovascular compromise are also unclear. Certainly, when an open approach for vascular repair is required, internal fixation of the clavicle should be performed, but fortunately acute neurovascular injury is rare in association with clavicular fracture.[86] The most frequent vascular disturbance encountered is venous congestion of the arm which, in the absence of deep venous thrombosis, aneurysm, or pseudoaneurysm can be treated expectantly.

Acute injury to the brachial plexus is extremely uncommon following fracture of the clavicle, and when present, is more likely to be the result of a traction injury to the upper roots of the brachial plexus.[13,109,144,253] What may prove to be an indication for operative intervention is a plexopathy which develops in relation to abundant callus in a malaligned fracture presenting at a time remote from the injury.[10,72,167,174,232,244,280] In these instances, open realignment, reduction of callus bulk, and internal fixation of the fracture should be considered (Fig. 7).

We prefer plate and screw fixation when performing open reduction and internal fixation of the clavicle. Before the advent of AO/ASIF techniques, the small, thin plates that were used gave poor results,[241] leading many to prefer intramedullary fixation with wires or screws.[27,137,142,178,185,195,220,245] Given that intramedullary fixation of the clavicle is technically very difficult owing to the curvature, high density, and poorly defined intramedullary canal of the bone,[241] it is remarkable that good results with this technique have been observed.[22,36,296]

Alterations in intramedullary devices were made, including using threaded pins, pins with a head, or bending the end of the pin in an attempt to prevent the complications associated with pin migration.[33,41,135,147,157,170,172,186,199,202,215,

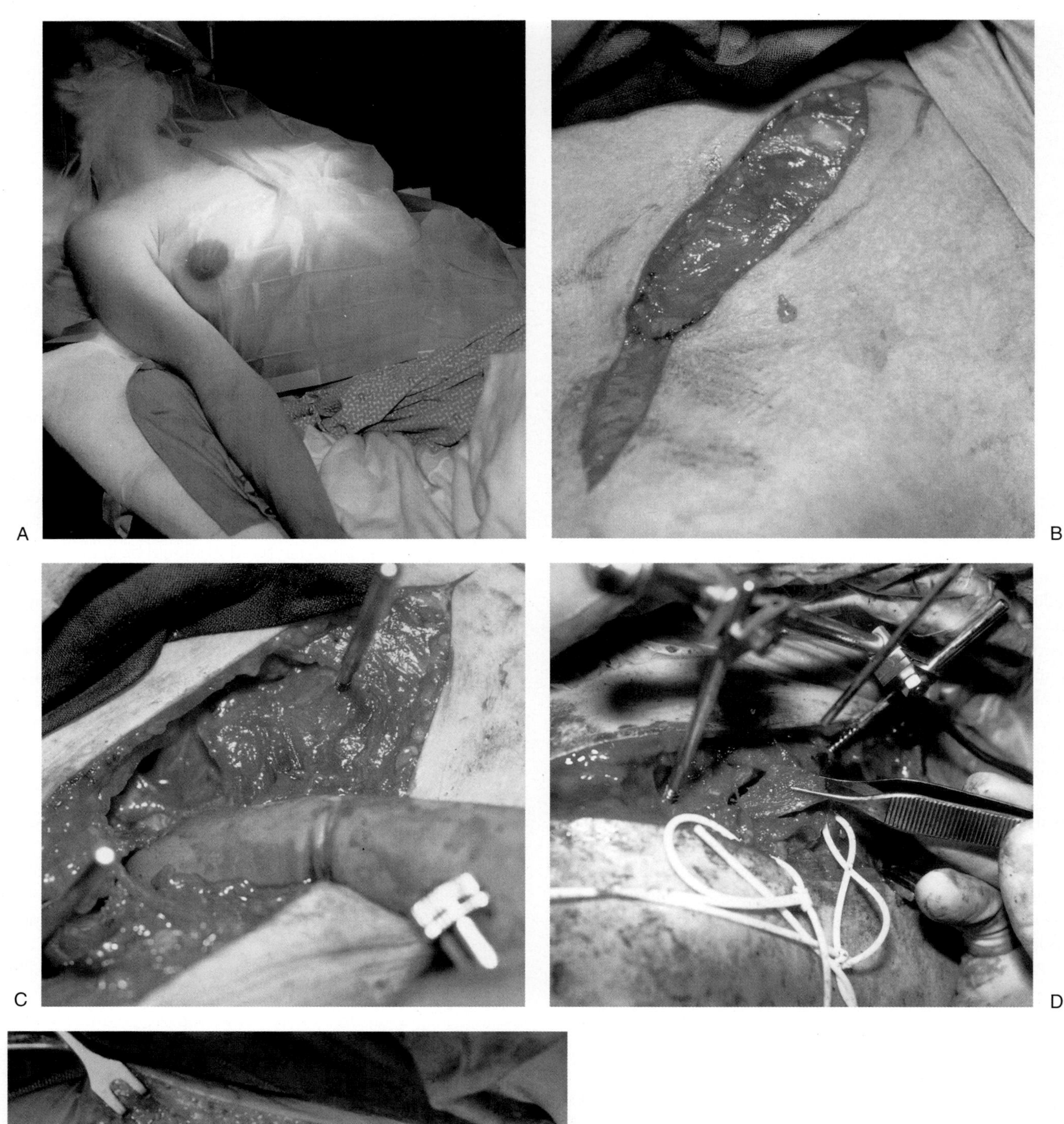

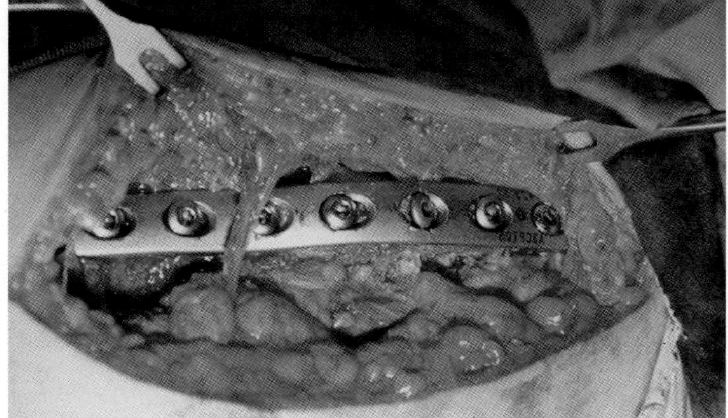

FIG. 8. Operative technique for plate fixation of the clavicle. **(A)** The patient is positioned in the beach chair position. **(B)** Incision of the skin is chosen to respect the relaxed skin tension lines. **(C)** The supraclavicular nerves are identified under loupe magnification and protected. Schantz screws are placed medial and lateral to the fracture site. **(D)** A small distractor is used to restore the length and alignment of the clavicle. When comminution results in a bony defect after anatomic reduction, an autogenous iliac crest autograft is applied. **(E)** The clavicle is stabilized using a 3.5-mm LC-DC plate. (*continued*)

F

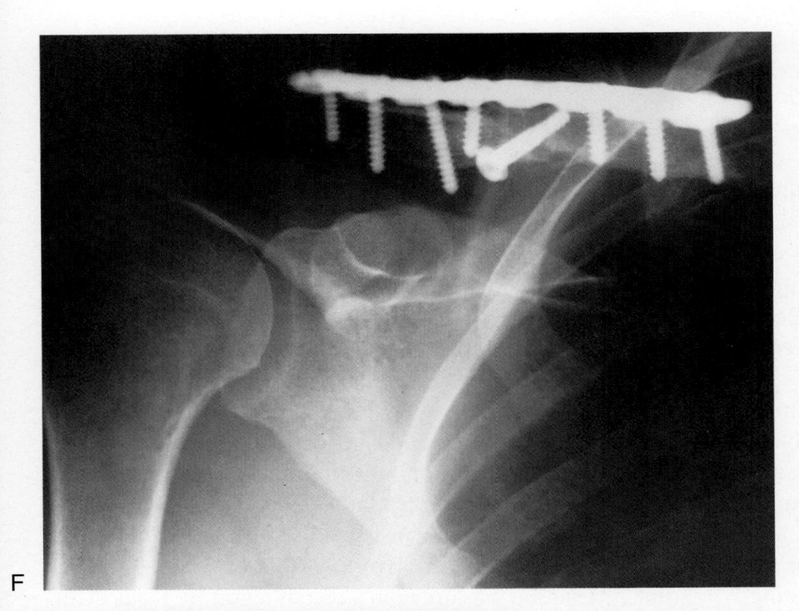

G

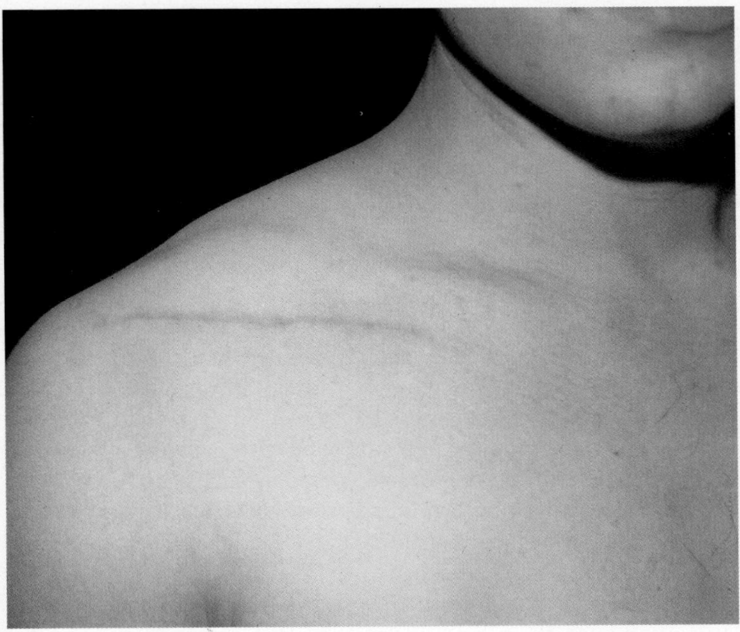

FIG. 8. *Continued* **(F)** When the fracture pattern allows, an interfragmentary lag screw is used to obtain compression between the fracture fragments. **(G)** Hypertrophy of the scar is uncommon. (From Browner, Jupiter, Levine and Trafton (eds). *Skeletal Trauma: Fractures, Dislocations, Ligamentous Injuries* (Second Edition). WB Saunders, Philadelphia, 1998).

[217,235,276] However, even threaded and bent pins can migrate, particularly if they break.[157,186,202] The potential advantage of intramedullary fixation—namely a smaller, more cosmetic scar—is disputable considering that the incision required for open reduction is not a great deal smaller than that required for plate fixation, and a second, more lateral scar is necessary for implant removal. Perhaps the greatest disadvantage of intramedullary fixation, in our view, is its inability to control the rotational forces experienced by the clavicle, making postoperative immobilization necessary in the vast majority of cases. Advocates of intramedullary fixation state that a large screw will provide sufficient rotational control to allow early postoperative mobilization, and suggest that the diminished stress shielding with this implant might lessen the risk of refracture following plate removal. Our experience with plate fixation suggests that refracture is not a problem, provided that plate removal is performed at a minimum of 18 months after the initial operation.

Our technique for internal fixation of the clavicle is as follows[153,258]: The patient is positioned in the semisitting (beach chair) position. The opposite iliac crest is routinely prepared and draped. Although an incision made parallel to Langer's lines and crossing the clavicle obliquely can be used, we prefer an incision in line with the long axis of the clavicle. The crossing supraclavicular nerves are identified under loupe magnification and preserved. The goals of alignment and apposition of the fracture fragments can often be achieved without stripping the periosteum and surrounding musculature from the bone by using a small distractor. This device can help control the fragments and aid in obtaining the desired length and alignment, while obviating the need for devascularizing and potentially dangerous circumferential clamps in many cases (Fig. 8).

We apply a 3.5-mm limited-contact dynamic compression plate (LCDC Plate; Synthes, Paoli, Pa) to the superior aspect of the clavicle.[181] A minimum of three screws should be placed in each major fragment. When the fracture pattern allows, an interfragmentary screw will greatly enhance the stability of the construct. In the presence of fracture comminution or gaps in the cortex opposite the plate, we recommend the addition of a small amount of autogenous iliac crest cancellous bone graft (see Fig. 8).

We prefer to close the wound over a suction drain, ensuring meticulous hemostasis. If the skin condition allows, wound closure is accomplished in an atraumatic fashion with a subcuticular suture. These measures will reduce the incidence of wound hematoma and promote cosmetic wound healing.

Our current practice, provided we are confident with the security of fixation, is to use a sling for patient comfort during the initial 7 to 10 postoperative days. The sling may be removed for short periods of passive shoulder pendulum and overhead elbow-flexion range of motion exercises without resistance, which are continued until fracture union has been demonstrated, which usually occurs between 6 and 8 weeks postoperatively. Thereafter, progressive strengthening exercises are permitted, and full overhead activities are gradually resumed. A return to all occupational duties and recreational pursuits is usually possible by 3 months after operative treatment.

Usually, plate removal is unnecessary; on occasion, however, hardware may cause skin problems owing to its prominence. In those instances, we remove the plate, provided a minimum of 12 to 18 months have elapsed since the injury and the cortex under the plate has reconstituted as viewed from an apical lordotic projection.

Distal Clavicular Fractures

Fractures of the distal clavicle with little or no displacement are treated symptomatically with a sling. Although some cases of nonunion following such fractures have been reported,[200] the chance of this occurrence is extremely low.

Displaced distal clavicular fractures, on the other hand, are recognized as the only general type of clavicle fracture for which routine primary operative treatment should be considered. This is based on the work of Neer[190–192] and others,[69,200] who have found that between 22% and 33% of these fractures will fail to unite following nonoperative treatment. An additional 45% to 67% will require longer than 3 months to heal the fracture.[69,190]

A number of surgeons have reported healing in 100% of operatively treated displaced lateral clavicle fractures within 6 to 10 weeks after surgery, with few associated complications.[69,90,190] The period of disability in these cases was shortened, with a relatively rapid return to full shoulder mobility and function.

Other authors have reported acceptable results with nonoperative treatment,[175,200] stating that those few nonunions that become symptomatic can be treated with a reconstructive procedure at a time remote from the injury if necessary.

Neer recommended stabilization of displaced distal clavicular fractures using two Kirschner wires to control rotation.[190–192] The wires are first passed into the distal fragment from proximal to distal through the fracture site, crossing the acromioclavicular joint, and exiting the acromion and the skin on the lateral aspect of the shoulder. The protruding part of the wires is then engaged and advanced proximally across the fracture site and into the medial fragment. The wires are then bent to decrease the risk of migration, and cut beneath the skin. Shoulder motion must be restricted to prevent pin breakage and migration. Others have used a single wire,[105,216,241] threaded wires,[105] or screws,[193–196] and some have made a point of avoiding the acromioclavicular joint.[216] Caution was urged in a recent report by Kona et al., who noted high rates of both nonunion and infection with transacromial wire techniques.[132]

Alternative techniques for operative fixation of distal clavicular fractures include coracoclavicular screw fixation[8,23,69] or transfer of the coracoid to the clavicle.[38,71,99] The AO/ASIF group has recommended using a tension band wire construct with two Kirschner wires that enter on the superior aspect of the clavicle, avoiding the acromioclavicular joint.[104] In addition, they also suggest consideration of a small plate, particularly a small "T"-shaped plate, and occasionally direct one of the screws into the coracoid.[104] A specially designed plate that is contoured so that its distal limit curves under the acromion through the acromioclavicular joint has also been used.[104]

We prefer to use a tension band wire technique. The distal clavicle and acromion are exposed through an incision in the relaxed tension lines of the skin with the development of thick flaps. Provisional fracture reduction can be held with a transacromial Kirschner wire. Definitive fixation consists of two stout smooth Kirschner wires passed through the outer edge of the acromion and crossing obliquely across the acromioclavicular joint and fracture to purchase in the solid cortex of the dorsal clavicle medial to the fracture. An 18-gauge wire is then looped through a drill hole medial to the fracture and around the tips of the wires, which are bent 180 degrees, turned downward and impacted into the acromion (Fig. 9). If a tear in either the trapezoid or conoid ligaments is identified, an attempt is made to perform a suture repair. The wound is closed over a suction drain. The postoperative managment differs from that for the midclavicular fracture in that the patient is maintained in a sling for a minimum of 4 to 6 weeks.

Medial Clavicular Fractures

Little exists in the literature about fractures of the medial clavicle.[4,31,106,121,151,226,295] These fractures are very

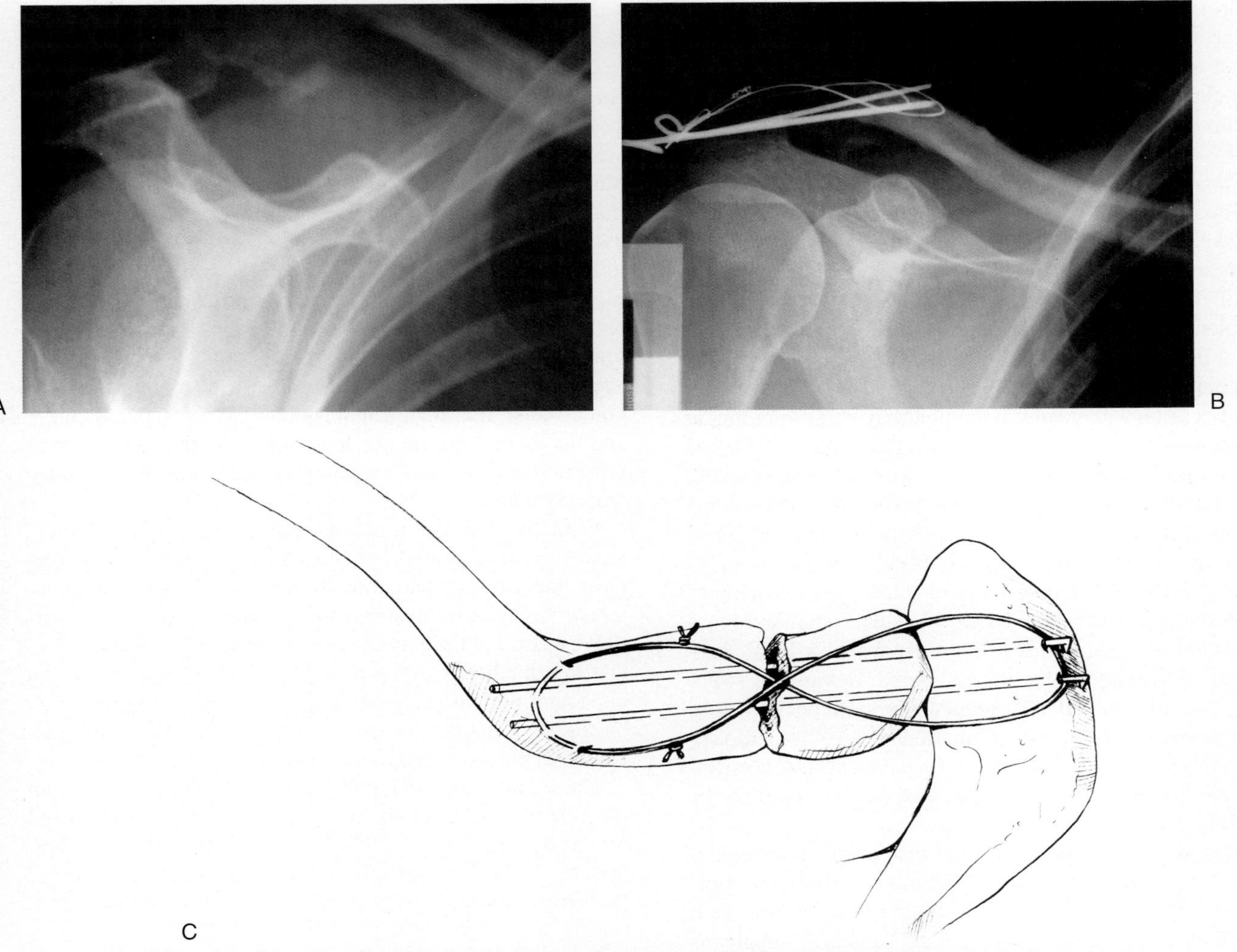

FIG. 9. **(A)** A 55-year-old woman sustained a comminuted type II fracture of the distal clavicle in a motor vehicle accident. **(B)** Fixation was achieved using two transacromial Kirschner wires exiting through the thick dorsal cortex of the medial fragment in combination with a tension band wire. (Figs. 9A & B, from Browner, Jupiter, Levine and Trafton (eds). *Skeletal Trauma: Fractures, Dislocations, Ligamentous Injuries* (Second Edition). WB Saunders, Philadelphia, 1998).

uncommon and most surgeons have limited experience with them. The literature offers little more than case reports, most of which describe medial physeal separation injuries.[31,121,151,226,295] Although some authors recommend open reduction and internal fixation,[31,226] most advocate nonoperative treatment initially, with resection of the medial clavicle if symptoms persist.[4,31,46,51,74,106,121,148,151,191,226,241,295] Considering the risks attendant with implant insertion and migration in this region, we rarely consider operative treatment. The generally good results of nonoperative treatment are related to the fact that fractures of the sternal end of the clavicle are often physeal separations that heal with stability and may even remodel somewhat. Displaced fractures must be evaluated with computed tomography scanning to be certain that posterior displacement of the fragments does not present a threat to neurovascular structures at the base of the neck.

COMPLICATIONS

Nonunion and Malunion

The percentage of nonoperatively treated clavicular fractures that fail to heal within 6 months of injury has been reported variously as 0% (of 342 patients),[248] 0.1%,[189] 0.47%,[122] 0.8%,[241] 0.9%,[268] 0.94%,[134] and 2.2%.[74,75] White et al. reported that they had encountered 8 nonunions (8%) and 18 delayed unions (16%) among 112 adult fractures of the clavicle proximal to the coracoid, most occurring as a result of a high-energy traumatic injury.[288] Proposed risk factors for nonunion, based on series of patients presenting with nonunion, include the severity of the initial trauma,[19,88,117,246,290] fracture comminution,[290] and refracture.[290] Jupiter and Leffert,[120] as well as others,[163,246,290] found that the degree of fracture fragment displacement was the most important risk factor for nonunion.[120] These risk factors often are interrelated and reflect more severe soft-tissue injury, decreased stability, and limited apposition of fracture fragments. The role of soft-tissue interposition remains unclear.[113,163]

That midclavicular nonunion is far more common than distal clavicular nonunion has been ascribed to the fact that midclavicular fractures are far more common overall.[19,88,113,117,204,290]

Primary operative treatment of fractures of the clavicle has been associated with a risk of nonunion (3.7% according to Rowe[241] and 4.6% according to Neer[189]). Although contemporary series report high union rates with internal fixation of fresh clavicular fractures,[30,69,127,136,190,204,224,252,296] they identify improper technique, including too small or too short a plate and excessive soft-tissue stripping, as reasons for operative failures[224,252] (Fig. 10).

On occasion a clavicular nonunion may be asymptomatic and discovered incidentally on a chest radiograph.[117] Before more reliable means of internal fixation were developed, some authors[117,290] recommended against operative intervention. In fact, patients presenting with an ununited clavicle are more likely than not to have specific complaints of increasing deformity that consists of adduction, shortening, and protraction of the shoulder girdle. Altered shoulder function occurs as a result of the deformity, pain, or local compression of the underlying brachial plexus or vascular structures.[120,258] Occasionally, patients will present decades after the original injury requesting treatment.[117,120,290] Unfortunately, this may be partly because these patients had been advised previously that nothing operative could or ought to be done (Fig. 11).

The neurovascular problems that may accompany a clavicular nonunion include thoracic outlet syndrome,[9,14,25,44,77,156,180,222,264] subclavian artery or vein compression[56,133] or thrombosis,[56,95,293] and brachial plexus palsy.[35,59,109,120,125] The prevalence of neurovascular dysfunction in patients presenting with clavicular nonunion has varied widely in reported series, from as few as 6% to as many as 52% of patients.[117,120,131,290]

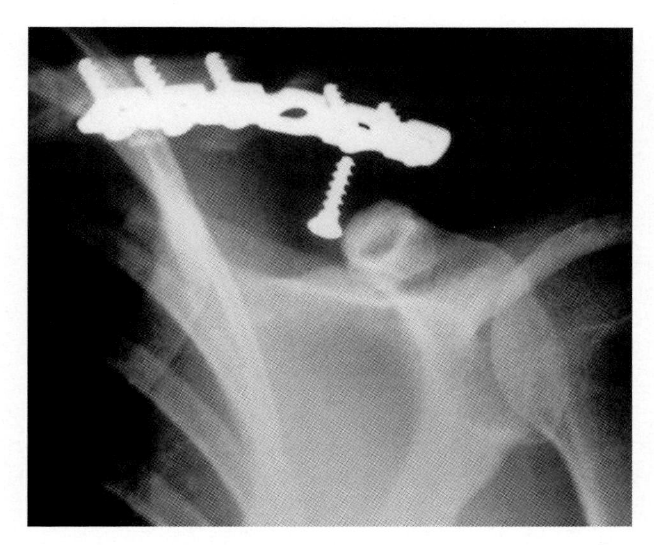

FIG. 10. Implant loosening and nonunion are typically related to inadequate plate size and length. (From Browner, Jupiter, Levine and Trafton (eds). *Skeletal Trauma: Fractures, Dislocations, Ligamentous Injuries* (Second Edition). WB Saunders, Philadelphia, 1998).

In the treatment of clavicular nonunions, we prefer to distinguish between reconstructive procedures, in which the goals of both pain relief and neurovascular compression, as well as enhanced function, are sought by restoration of the alignment and continuity of the clavicle; and salvage procedures in which the clavicle is either resected, contoured, or avoided altogether (i.e., first rib resection[55]), with the limited goal of relieving symptoms. Although treatment of clavicular nonunion with electrical stimulation has been attempted,[29,45,57,187] there are few indications for its use. Symptomatic clavicular nonunion typically has elements of both shoulder deformity and dysfunction, as well as neurovascular compromise, that are not addressed by electrical treatment,[187] and the union rates do not approach those obtained by open reduction and internal fixation with provision of an autogenous bone graft.

With the advent of improved techniques of stable fixation, the results of reconstructive procedures have improved to the point that salvage operations are now largely of historical interest.[258] The only situation in which we would consider partial resection of the clavicle is in a chronically infected clavicle in a medically compromised patient or in a very distal clavicular nonunion. A small distal clavicular fragment can be resected and the coracoclavicular ligaments securely attached to the outer end of the medial fragment.[258]

The treatment of clavicular nonunion has evolved from the screw fixation of tibial or iliac crest bone grafts used by early authors,[12,19,88,246] to intramedullary fixation,[117,165,189,267] which still has a few advocates,[22,36] to our preferred method of rigid plate and screw fixation.[68,75,94,120,122,131,163,182,208,227,258,272,275,290]

Our preference for plate fixation and our operative technique and rehabilitation protocol are described in the foregoing under Authors' Preferred Treatment. A few points on the treatment of midclavicular nonunions deserve further discussion.

In hypertrophic nonunions, the exuberant callus can be resected and saved for use as bone graft, making harvest of an iliac crest graft unnecessary in some cases. The nonunion site does not require debridement, for the fibrocartilage will progress to union following stable internal fixation. If the fracture line is oblique, it is sometimes possible to secure the fragments using an interfragmentary screw in addition to the superiorly placed plate.

Atrophic nonunions present sclerotic ends with interposed fibrous tissue, whereas pseudoarthroses will have a false synovial-lined cavity. Resection of the ends of the fracture fragments and the intervening tissue is required in both situations. In this situation, a small distractor often proves invaluable in helping to control the fragments, as well as to attain the desired length and alignment. A sculptured tricortical iliac crest bone graft will be useful to ensure restoration of length and alignment and to promote healing.

We harvest the iliac graft from the crest through an oblique incision along the midpoint of the ilium. The crest is exposed subperiosteally and a tricortical section, measuring one and one-half times the anticipated size of the final graft,

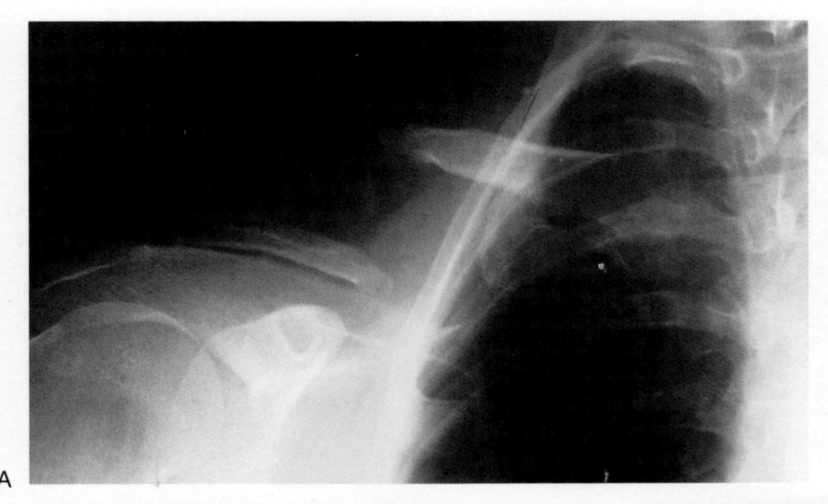
A

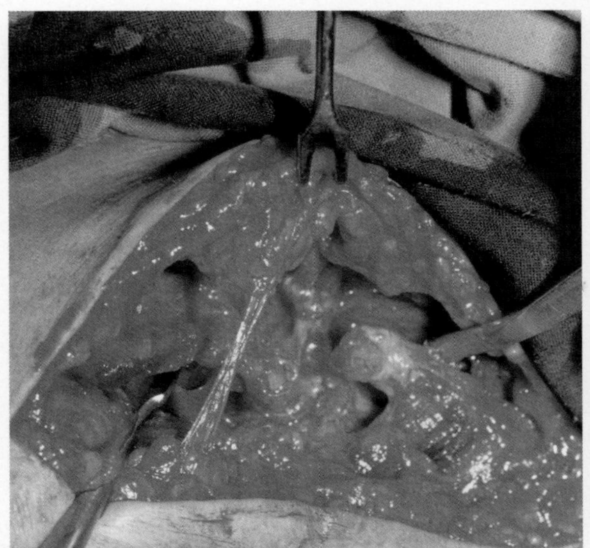
B

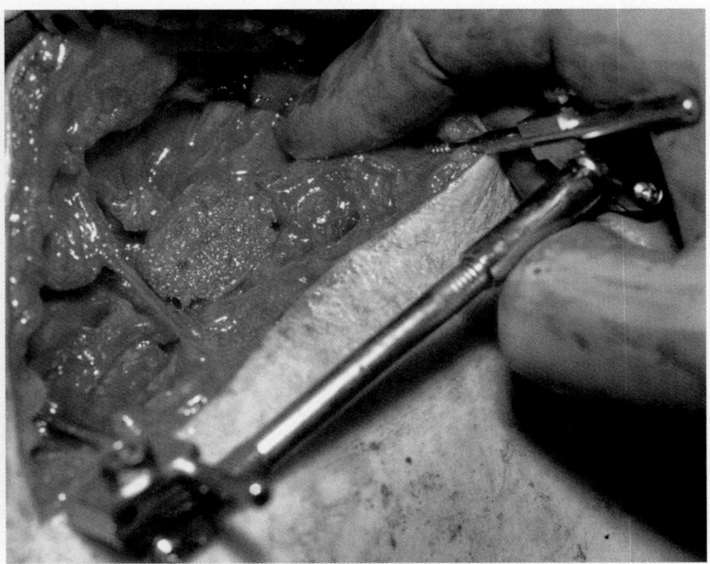
C

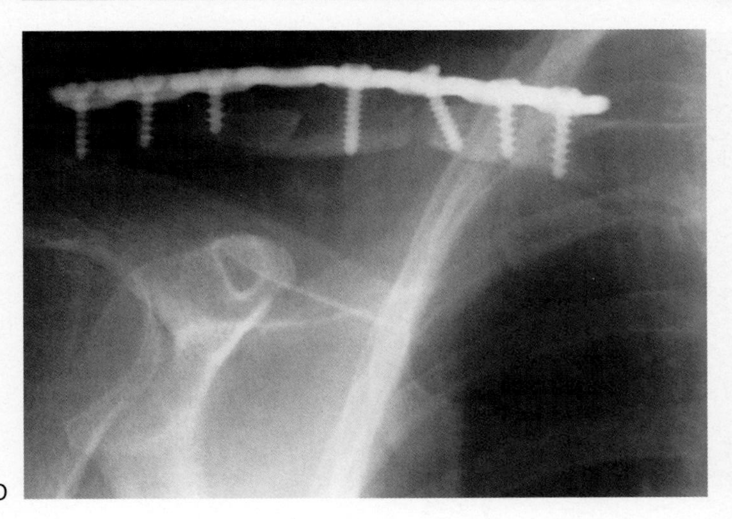
D

FIG. 11. A 56-year-old woman presented with complaints of increasing shoulder pain, stiffness, and deformity after injuring her clavicle at age 14. **(A)** An anteroposterior radiograph demonstrated an ununited fracture of the clavicle, with widely displaced, atrophic fragments. **(B)** The supraclavicular nerves were identified under loupe magnification and protected throughout the operative procedure. **(C)** A distractor was used to restore the anatomic length and alignment of the clavicle, and a tricortical bone graft from the iliac crest was used to bridge the residual bony defect. **(D)** One of the screws through the plate transfixes the bone graft. (From Browner, Jupiter, Levine and Trafton (eds). *Skeletal Trauma: Fractures, Dislocations, Ligamentous Injuries* (Second Edition). WB Saunders, Philadelphia, 1998).

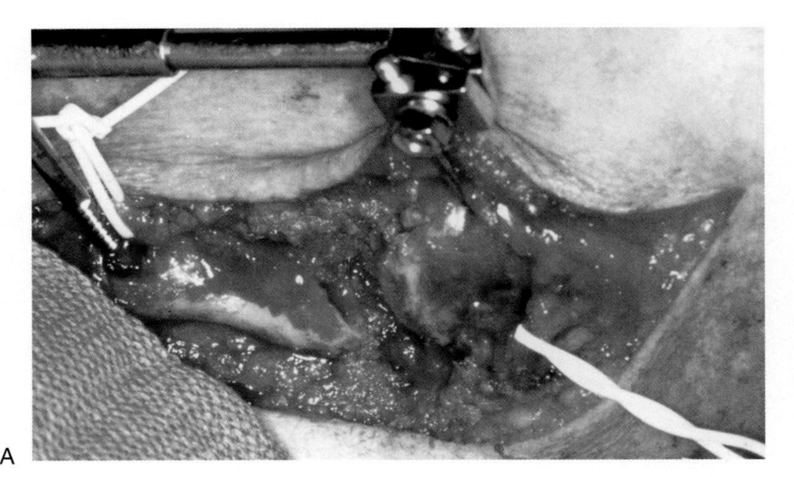

A

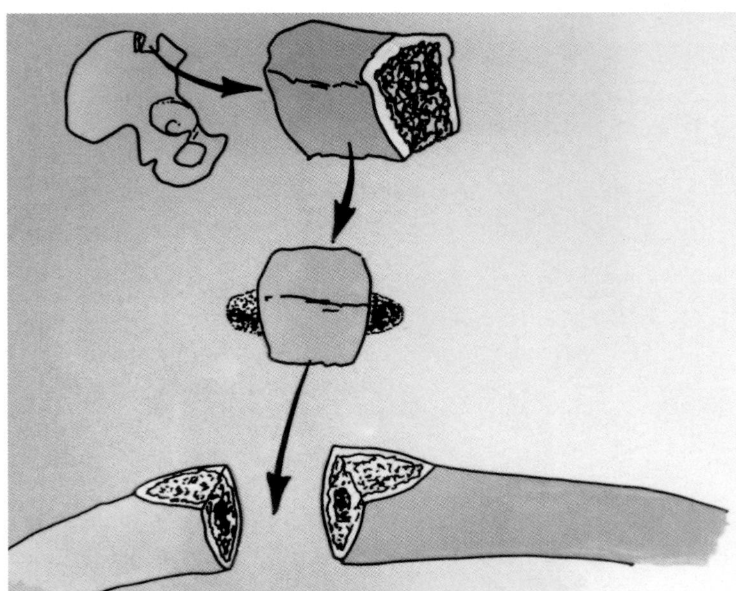

B

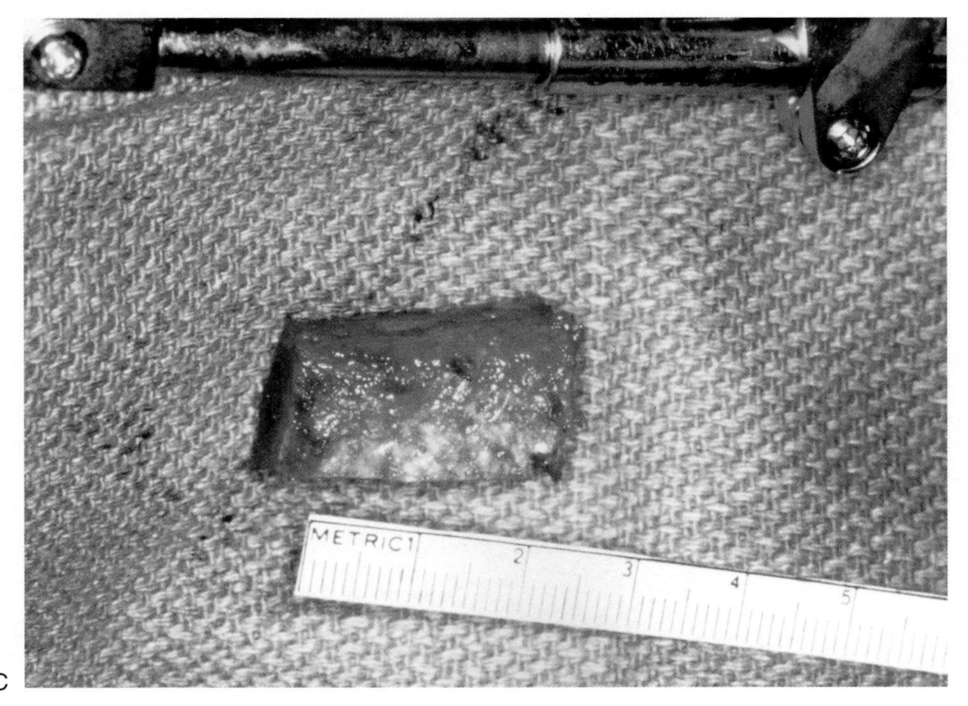

C

FIG. 12. Sculpturing of the tricortical iliac crest autograft allows interdigitation of the graft with the fracture fragments increasing the stability of the construct and enhancing healing. **(A)** Following resection of the nonunion back to viable bone and distraction of the clavicle to restore length and alignment, a substantial bony defect is common. **(B)** A tricortical graft is harvested from the iliac crest and cancellous pegs are sculptured at the medial and lateral aspects. The medullary canals of the fracture fragments are opened with a drill and the pegs interdigitate with the fragments. **(C)** The harvested iliac crest graft before sculpturing. (*continued*)

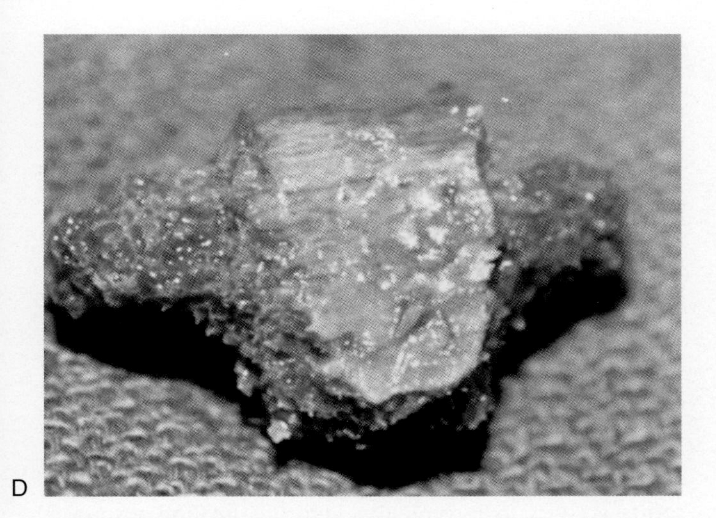

D

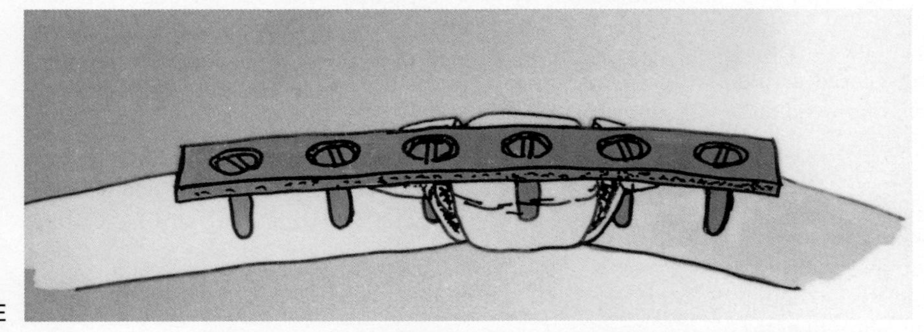

E

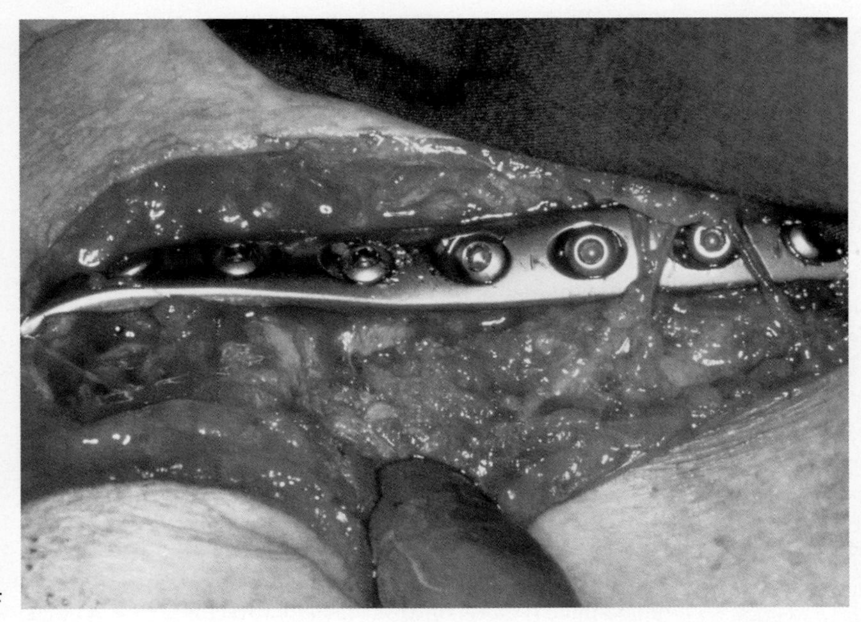

F

FIG. 12. *Continued* **(D)** The graft following sculpturing. **(E)** The interdigitation of the graft with the fracture fragments provides a measure of stability, facilitating plate fixation. One of the screws transfixes the plate. **(F)** Intraoperative photograph demonstrating plate fixation following graft interposition. (From Browner, Jupiter, Levine and Trafton (eds). *Skeletal Trauma: Fractures, Dislocations, Ligamentous Injuries* (Second Edition). WB Saunders, Philadelphia, 1998).

is removed with either osteotomes or a small oscillating saw. The graft is then sculptured to create large cancellous pegs at each end, which plug into the medullary canals of the clavicular fragments (Fig. 12). This interdigitation increases the stability of the construct and facilitates plate fixation. The graft is positioned so that the dorsal cortical margin of the iliac crest lies on the inferior surface of the clavicle, affording the advantages of better purchase of a screw as well as more resistance to bending forces at the nonunion site. Additional cancellous graft from the iliac crest is compacted into the medullary canals of each fragment before the final impaction of the corticocancellous segmental graft.

A 3.5-mm limited-contact dynamic compression plate (Synthes, Paoli, Pa) is then applied, with a minimum of three screws in each major fragment and a single screw transfixing the graft. Compression is applied to both surfaces of the graft to enhance its incorporation. The wound is closed with a subcuticular suture over suction drainage.

Malunion has traditionally been considered primarily a cosmetic concern.[197] However, it is not surprising that some reports exist of difficulties in shoulder function in patients with overriding of clavicular fragments.[74,75] In addition, compression of underlying neurovascular structures has been reported in association with malaligned clavicle fractures from narrowing of the costoclavicular space[9,14,25, 44,72,77,156,167,174,180,222,232,244,264,280] and compression of the brachial plexus, subclavian artery, or vein.[35,46,95,109,120,125,133,294] Malunited fractures typically may give rise to neurovascular symptoms weeks or months after the injury owing to proliferative callus.[9,44,72,77,232,244,280]

The senior author (JBJ) has treated 4 patients with malunited clavicular fractures for deformity associated with ipsilateral glenohumeral dysfunction either alone or in combination with scapulothoracic dysfunction (unpublished series). The malunion was osteotomized through the plane of deformity, realigned using a small distractor, and secured with a plate and screws. In each case, function was improved and the outcome deemed satisfactory (Fig. 13).

Some patients are unhappy with the appearance of their healed clavicular fractures because of a prominent bump at the apex of the deformity. These patients should be advised that an operation to smooth the contour of the deformity would essentially trade a bump for a scar. There is a risk that the scar could be hypertrophic and more unsightly than the bump. Furthermore, the removal of bone places the clavicle at an increased risk for refracture.

Neurovascular Complications

Acute neurovascular complications are rare and typically occur in association with scapulothoracic dissociation,[50,109,188] or are unrelated to the clavicular fracture (e.g., brachial plexus traction injury).[109,144] Neurovascular dysfunction as a result of narrowing of the thoracic outlet can occur within the first 2 months of injury when the fracture is malaligned, or many months or even years later as a result of hypertrophic callus in the setting of nonunion.

Further mention should be made here of thrombosis and pseudoaneurysm of the subclavian or axillary artery or subclavian vein presenting at a time remote from the injury. Cases of axillary or subclavian artery thrombosis presenting late with symptoms of atrophy and cold intolerance of the involved upper extremity, most likely represent missed acute intimal injury,[109,112,143,256,278] but may also result from compression in a narrowed costoclavicular space.[270] Cerebral embolism has been reported following subclavian artery thrombosis in this setting.[293]

True aneurysms of the subclavian artery may occur as poststenotic aneurysms when the costoclavicular space is narrowed.[58,270] Displaced clavicular fracture fragments may very rarely cause a small perforation injury of the subclavian artery. Occasionally, a psudoaneurysm develops that may present months to years later with brachial plexus dysfunction from compression.[39,50,94,99,109,188,255,263,266,294]

Subclavian vein thrombosis may also occur in relation to compression or intimal injury.[152,250,262] Pulmonary embolism may occur in this setting.[250]

Neurovascular symptoms related to compression by hypertrophic nonunion have been mistaken for sympathetically maintained pain (shoulder–hand syndrome) in the past.[222] Damage to the supraclavicular nerves can cause anterior chest wall pain.

Refracture

Repeat fracture of the clavicle usually occurs on premature resumption of full activity, in particular contact sports activity. The typically vigorous-healing response of the clavicle results in a rapid decrease in pain and return of shoulder function so that overenthusiastic patients will often ignore their physician's admonition to avoid contact sports for at least 2 to 3 months, or longer, following healing of the fracture. Refracture following plate removal is unusual if the plate remains in place a minimum of 12 to 18 months following healing of the fracture.[224,258]

Complications of Operative Treatment

Despite the proximity of important anatomic structures beneath the clavicle, intraoperative complications are rare. (Eskola et al. reported tearing of the subclavian vein, pneumothorax, air embolism, and brachial plexus palsy all in a single patient during dissection of a clavicular nonunion[75]). On the other hand, wires and pins show a remarkable ability to migrate once inserted[157] and may ultimately be found in the abdominal aorta,[186] ascending aorta,[199] the aorta and pericardium causing fatal tamponade,[41] the pulmonary artery,[147] the mediastinum,[33] the heart,[217] the lung,[170,172,215,235,276] (sometimes the opposite lung[235]) or the spinal canal.[202] A patient presenting to Kremens and Glauser[135] brought in a Steinman pin that he reported having expectorated 1 month following fixation of his medial clavicular fracture.

Poigenfurst et al. documented superficial infection in 9 (7.4%) and deep infection in 2 (1.6%) of 122 patients undergoing plate fixation of fresh clavicular fractures,[224] but other authors have had little trouble with infections following plate fixation.[30,120,127,136,163,204,224,252]

Many authors cite hypertrophic scar formation as one of the potential complications of operative treatment of clavicular fractures,[127] particularly the proponents of intramedullary fixation who advocate a more oblique incision in alignment with Langer's lines.[193–196] We have had no particular problem with cosmetically displeasing scars.

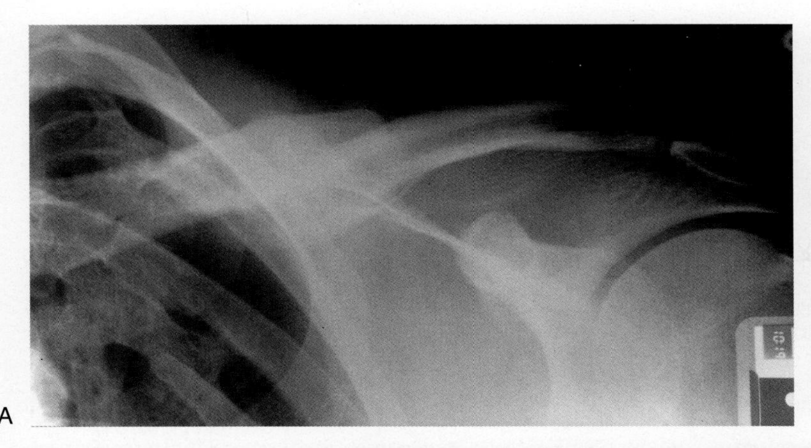
A

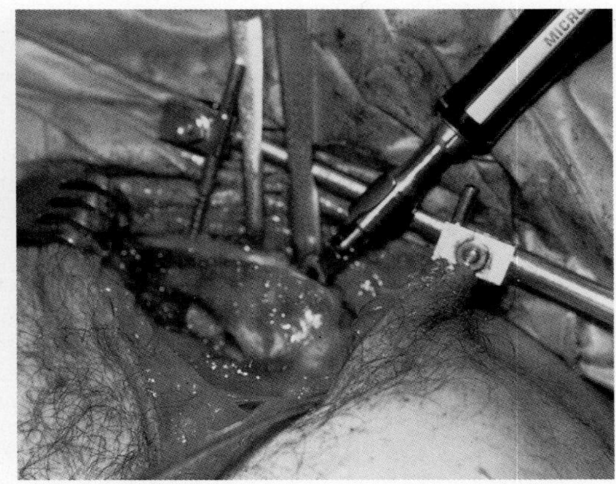
B

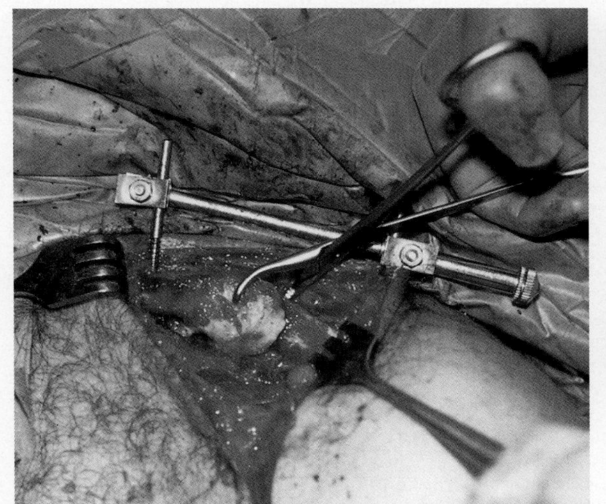
C

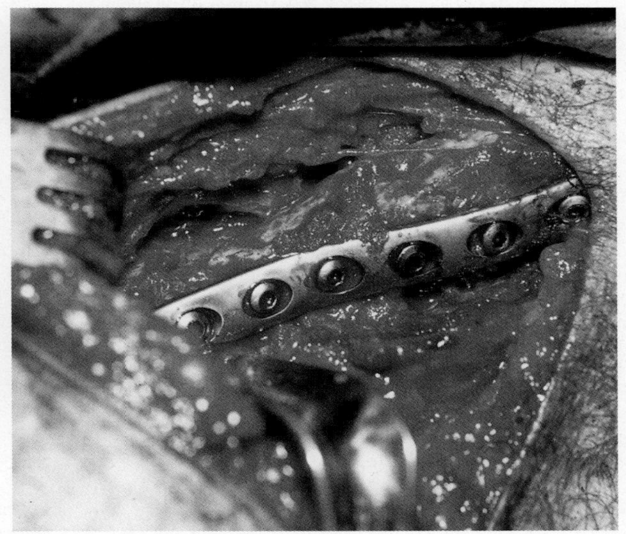
D

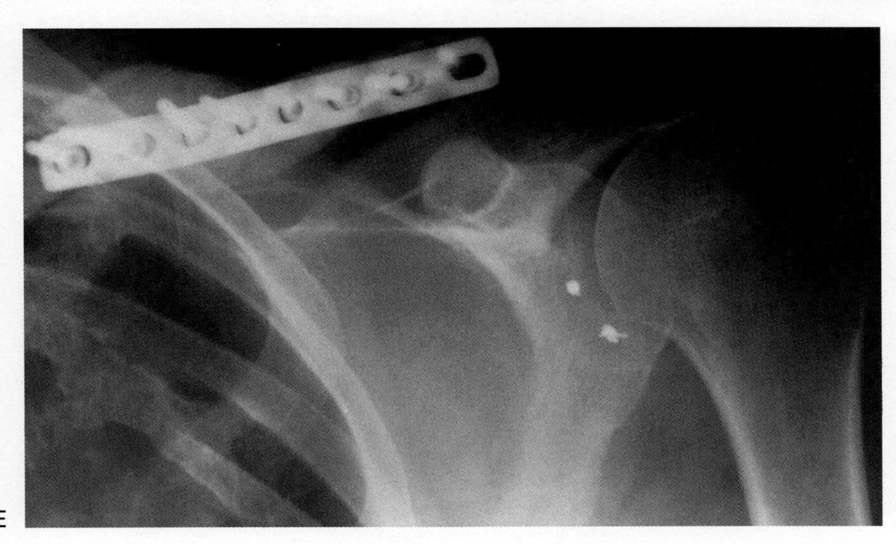
E

FIG. 13. A 35-year-old man presented with complaints of restricted shoulder motion, weakness, and discomfort after healing of his fractured clavicle with 2 cm of shortening. **(A)** Anteroposterior radiograph demonstrating malunion of the clavicle. **(B)** An oscillating saw is used to create a long oblique osteotomy of the clavicle. **(C)** A distractor is used to restore length and alignment. **(D)** Fracture reduction forceps help maintain alignment while an anterior plate incorporating an interfragmentary screw is applied. **(E)** Radiograph demonstrates stable plate fixation with restoration of clavicular length. (From Browner, Jupiter, Levine and Trafton (eds). *Skeletal Trauma: Fractures, Dislocations, Ligamentous Injuries* (Second Edition). WB Saunders, Philadelphia, 1998).

REFERENCES

1. Abbott LC, Lucas DB. The function of the clavicle: its surgical significance. *Ann Surg* 1954;140:583–599.
2. Adams CF. *The genuine works of Hippocrates*. Baltimore: Williams & Wilkins, 1939.
3. Al-Qattan MM, Clarke HM, Curtis CG. The prognostic value of concurrent clavicular fractures in newborns with obstetric brachial plexus palsy. *J Hand Surg [Br]* 1994;19:729–730.
4. Allman FL. Fractures and ligamentous injuries of the clavicle and its articulation. *J Bone Joint Surg [Am]* 1967;49:774–784.
5. American College of Surgeons Committee on Trauma. *Advanced trauma life support course*. Chicago: American College of Surgeons, 1990.
6. Andersen H. Histochemistry and development of the human shoulder and acromioclavicular joints with particular reference to the early development of the clavicle. *Acta Anat* 1963;55:124–165.
7. Anderson K, Jensen PO, Lauritzen J. Treatment of clavicular fractures. *Acta Orthop Scand* 1987;57:71–74.
8. Ballmer FT, Gerber C. Coracoclavicular screw fixation for unstable fractures of the distal clavicle. *J Bone Joint Surg [Br]* 1991;73: 291–294.
9. Bargar WL, Marcus RE, Ittleman FP. Late thoracic outlet syndrome secondary to pseudarthrosis of the clavicle. *J Trauma* 1984;24:857–859.
10. Bartosh RA, Dugdale TW, Nielsen R. Isolated musculocutaneous nerve injury complicating closed fracture of the clavicle: a case report. *Am J Sports Med* 1992;20:356–359.
11. Basmajian JV. The surgical anatomy and function of the arm–trunk mechanism. *Surg Clin North Am* 1963;43:1471–1482.
12. Basom WC, Breck LW, Herz JR. Dual grafts for non-union of the clavicle. *South Med J* 1947;40:898–899.
13. Bateman JE. Nerve injuries about the shoulder in sports. *J Bone Joint Surg [Am]* 1967;49:785–792.
14. Bateman JE. Neurovascular syndromes related to the clavicle. *Clin Orthop* 1968;58:75–82.
15. Beatty OA. Chylothorax: case report. *J Thorac Surg* 1936;6:221–225.
16. Bechtol CO. Biomechanics of the shoulder. *Clin Orthop* 1980;146: 37–41.
17. Beckman T. A case of simultaneous luxation of both ends of the clavicle. *Acta Chir Scand* 1934;56:156–163.
18. Bennett EH. The mechanism of fractures of the clavicle. *Ann Surg.* 1885;1:293–303.
19. Berkheiser EJ. Old ununited clavicular fractures in the adult. *Surg Gynecol Obstet* 1937;64:1064.
20. Bernard TN, Haddad RJ. Enchondroma of the proximal clavicle. An unusual cause of pathologic fracture dislocation of the sternoclavicular joint. *Clin Orthop* 1982;167:239–241.
21. Billington RW. A new (plaster yoke) dressing for fracture of the clavicle. *South J Med* 1931;24:667–670.
22. Boehme D, Curtis RJ, DeHann JT, Kay SP, Young DC, Rockwood CA Jr. Non-union of fractures of the mid-shaft of the clavicle. *J Bone Joint Surg [Am]* 1991;73:1219–1226.
23. Bosworth BM. Acromioclavicular separation: a new method of repair. *Surg Gynecol Obstet* 1941;73:866–871.
24. Bowen A. Plastic bowing of the clavicle in children. *J Bone Joint Surg [Am]* 1983;65:403–405.
25. Braun RM. Iatrogenic compression of the thoracic outlet. *Johns Hopkins Med J* 1979;145:94–97.
26. Breasthead JH. *The Edwin Smith surgical papyrus*: published in facsimile and hieroglyphic transliteration and commentary in two volumes, vol 1. Chicago: University of Chicago Press, 1930:596.
27. Breck LW. Partially threaded round pins with oversized threads for intramedullary fixation of the clavicle and the forearm bones. *Clin Orthop* 1958;11:227–229.
28. Brewer LA III. Surgical management of lesions of the thoracic duct. *Am J Surg* 1955;90:210–227.
29. Brighton CT, Pollack SR. Treatment of recalcitrant non-union with a capacitively coupled electrical field. *J Bone Joint Surg [Am]* 1985;67: 577–585.
30. Bronz G, Heim D, Pusterla C, et al. Die stabile clavicula-osteosynthese. *Unfallheilkunde* 1981;84:319–321.
31. Brooks AL, Henning GD. Injury to the proximal clavicular epiphysis. *J Bone Joint Surg [Am]* 1972;54:1347–1348.
32. Brown BL, Lapinski R, Berkowitz GS, Holzman I. Fractured clavicle in the neonate: a retrospective three-year review. *Am J Perinatol* 1994; 11:331–333.
33. Burman M, Grossman S, Rosenak. The migration of a fracture-transfixing pin from the humerus into the mediastinum. *AJR Am J Roentgenol* 1956;76:1061.
34. Cahill BR. Osteolysis of the distal part of the clavicle in male athletes. *J Bone Joint Surg [Am]* 1982;64:1053–1058.
35. Campbell E, Howard WP, Burklund CW. Clinical notes, suggestions and new instruments. *JAMA* 1949;139:91–92.
36. Capicotto PN, Heiple KG, Wilbur JH. Midshaft clavicle nonunions treated with intramedullary Steinman pin fixation and onlay bone graft. *J Orthop Trauma* 1994;8:88–93.
37. Carter G, Tarvin C. Clavicular fractures in neonates. *Am J Dis Child* 1991;145:251–252.
38. Caspi I, Ezra E, Oliver S, Lin E, Lotan G, Horoszowski H. Treatment of avulsed clavicle and recurrent subluxations of the ipsilateral shoulder by dynamic fixation. *J Trauma* 1986;27:94–95.
39. Cayford EH, Tees FJ. Traumatic aneurysm of the subclavian artery as a late complication of fractured clavicle. *Can Med Assoc J* 1931;25: 450–452.
40. Chez RA, Carlan SC, Greenberg SL, Spellacy WN. Fractured clavicle is an unavoidable event. *Am J Obstet Gynecol* 1994;171:797–798.
41. Clark RL, Milgram JW, Yawn DH. Fatal aortic perforation and cardiac tamponade due to a Kirschner wire migrating from the right sternoclavicular joint. *South Med J* 1974;67:316–318.
42. Codman EA. *The shoulder: rupture of the supraspinatus tendon and other lesions in or about the subacromial bursa*. Boston: Thomas Todd, 1934.
43. Cohen AW, Otto SR. Obstetric clavicular fractures: a three-year analysis. *J Reprod Med* 1980;25:119–122.
44. Connolly JF, Dehne R. Nonunion of the clavicle and thoracic outlet syndrome. *J Trauma* 1989;29:1127–1133.
45. Connolly JF. Electrical treatment of nonunions. Its use and abuse in 100 consecutive fractures. *Orthop Clin North Am* 1984;15:89–106.
46. Conwell HE. Fractures of the clavicle. A simple fixation dressing with a summary of the treatment and results attained in ninety-two cases. *JAMA* 1928;90:838–839.
47. Cook TW. Reduction and external fixation of fracture of the clavicle in recumbency. *J Bone Joint Surg [Am]* 1954;36:878–879.
48. Cope R, Riddervold HO, Shore JL, Sistrom CL. Dislocations of the sternoclavicular joint: anatomic basis, etiologies, and radiologic diagnosis. *J Orthop Trauma* 1991;5:379–384.
49. Copeland SM. Total resection of the clavicle. *Am J Surg* 1946;72: 280–281.
50. Costa MC, Robbs JV. Nonpenetrating subclavian artery trauma. *J Vasc Surg* 1988;8:72–75.
51. Craig EV. Fractures of the clavicle. In: Rockwood CA Jr, Matsen FA III, eds. *The shoulder*, vol 1. Philadelphia: WB Saunders, 1990:367–412.
52. Cummings CW, First R. Stress fracture of the clavicle after a radical neck dissection. *Plast Reconstr Surg* 1975;55:366–367.
53. Dameron TB Jr, Rockwood CW Jr. Fractures of the shaft of the clavicle. In: Rockwood CA, Wilkins KE, King RE, eds. *Fractures in children*. Philadelphia: JB Lippincott, 1984.
54. Dameron TB. Letter to the editor. *J Bone Joint Surg [Am]* 1989;71: 1272.
55. Dash UN, Handler D. A case of compression of subclavian vessels by a fractured clavicle treated by excision of the first rib. *J Bone Joint Surg [Am]* 1960;42:798–799.
56. Daskalakis E, Bouhoutsos. Subclavian and axillary vein compression of musculoskeletal origin. *Br J Surg* 1980;67:573–576.
57. Day L. Electrical stimulation in the treatment of ununited fractures. *Clin Orthop* 1981;161:54–57.
58. DeBakey ME, Beall AC, Wukasch DC. Recent developments in vascular surgery with particular reference to orthopedics. *Am J Surg* 1965;109:134–142.
59. Della Santa D, Narakas A, Bonnard C. Late lesions of the brachial plexus after fracture of the clavicle. *Ann Hand Surg* 1991;10:531–540.
60. Dickson JW. Death following fractured clavicle. *Br Med J* 1952;2: 666.
61. Dugdale TW, Fulkerson JP. Pneumothorax complicating a closed fracture of the clavicle. A case report. *Clin Orthop* 1987;221:212–214.
62. Dupuytren G. Fracture de la clavicule en plusieurs fragments par cause indirecte. *Gaz Hopitaux* 1831;4:315.
63. Dupuytren, Le Baron. *On the injuries and disease of bone, being selections from the collected edition of the clinical lectures of Baron Dupuytren*. Translated by F. G. Clark. London: Syndenham Society, 1847.

64. Dust WN, Lenczner EM. Stress fracture of the clavicle leading to nonunion secondary to coracoclavicular reconstruction with Dacron. *Am J Sports Med* 1989;17:128–129.
65. Dvir Z, Berme N. The shoulder complex in elevation of the arm: a mechanism approach. *J Biomech* 1978;11:219–225.
66. Ebraheim NA, An HS, Jackson WT, et al. Scapulothoracic dissociation. *J Bone Joint Surg [Am]* 1988;70:428–432.
67. Ebraheim NA, Peralstein SR, Savolaine ER, Gordon SL, Jackson WT, Corray T. Scapulothoracic dissociation (closed avulsion of the scapula, subclavian artery, and brachial plexus): a newly recognized variant, a new classification, and a review of the literature and treatment options. *J Orthop Trauma* 1987;1:18–23.
68. Edvardsen P, Odegard O. Treatment of posttraumatic clavicular pseudarthrosis. *Acta Orthop Scand* 1977;48:456–457.
69. Edwards DJ, Kavanagh TG, Flannery MC. Fractures of the distal clavicle: a case for fixation. *Injury* 1992;23:44–46.
70. Elkin DC, Cooper FW. Resection of the clavicle in vascular surgery. *J Bone Joint Surg [Am]* 1946;28:117–119.
71. Elliot AC. Tripartite injury of the clavicle: a case report. *S Afr Med J* 1986;70:115.
72. Enker SH, Murphy KK. Brachial plexus compression by excessive callus formation secondary to a fractured clavicle. A case report. *Mt Sinai J Med* 1972;37:678–682.
73. Erichsen J. Clinical lecture on a case of comminuted fracture of the clavicle with compression of the subclavian vein by one of the fragments. *Br Med J* 1873;1:637–638.
74. Eskola A, Vaininonpää S, Myllynen P, Pätiälä H, Rokkanen P. Outcome of clavicular fracture in 89 patients. *Arch Orthop Trauma Surg* 1986;105:337–338.
75. Eskola A, Vaininonpää S, Myllynen P, Pätiälä H, Rokkanen P. Surgery for ununited clavicular fracture. *Acta Orthop Scand* 1986;57: 366–367.
76. Fairbank HA. Cranio-cleido-dysostosis. *J Bone Joint Surg [Br]* 1949; 31:608–617.
77. Falconer MA, Weddell G. Costoclavicular compression of the subclavian artery and vein. Relation to the scalenus anticus syndrome. *Lancet* 1943;1:539–543.
78. Falstie-Jensen S, Mikkelsen P. Psuedodislocation of the acromioclavicular joint. *J Bone Joint Surg [Br]* 1982;64:368–369.
79. Farakas R, Levine S. X-ray incidence of fractured clavicle in vertex presentation. *Am J Obstet Gynecol* 1950;59:204–206.
80. Fawcett J. The development and ossification of the human clavicle. *J Anat* 1913;47:225–234.
81. Fini-Storchi O, LoRusso D, Agostini V. Psuedotumors of the clavicle subsequent to radical neck dissection. *J Larygol Otol* 1985;99:73–83.
82. Fowler AW. Fracture of the clavicle. *J Bone Joint Surg [Br]* 1962;44:440.
83. Fowler AW. Treatment of the fractured clavicle. *Lancet* 1968;1:46.
84. Freeland A. Unstable adult midclavicular fracture. *Orthopedics* 1990; 13:1279–1281.
85. Gardner E, Gray DJ. Prenatal development of the human shoulder and acromioclavicular joint. *Am J Anat* 1953;92:219–276.
86. Gardner E. The embryology of the clavicle. *Clin Orthop* 1968;58: 9–15.
87. Gearen PF, Petty W. Panclavicular dislocation. *J Bone Joint Surg [Am]* 1982;64:454–455.
88. Ghormley RK, Black JR, Cherry JH. Ununited fractures of the clavicle *Am J Surg* 1941;51:343–349.
89. Gibson DA, Carroll N. Congenital pseudarthrosis of the clavicle. *J Bone Joint Surg [Br]* 1970;52:629–643.
90. Golser K, Sperner G, Thoni H, Resch H. Fruh- und mittelfristige Ergebnisse konservativ und operativ behandelter lateraler Kalvikulafrakturen. *Akt Traumatol* 1991;21:148–152.
91. Gordon M, Rich H, Deutschberger JR, et al. The immediate and long term outcome of obstetric birth trauma: brachial plexus paralysis. *Am J Obstet Gynecol* 1973;117:51.
92. Goss TP. Double disruptions of the superior shoulder suspensory complex. *J Orthop Trauma* 1993;7:99–106.
93. Greenwald AG, Schute PC, Shiveley JL. Brachial plexus birth palsy: a 10-year report on the incidence and prognosis. *J Pedatr Orthop* 1984;4:689–692.
94. Gryska PF. Major vascular injuries: principles of managment in selected cases of arterial and venous injury. *N Engl J Med* 1962;266: 381–385.
95. Guilfoil PH, Christiansen T. An unusual vascular complication of a fractured clavicle. *JAMA* 1967;200:72–73.
96. Guillemin A. Déchirure de la veine sous-clavière par fracture fermée de la clavicule. *Bull Mém Soc Nat Chir* 1930;56:302–304.
97. Gurd FB. Surplus parts of the skeleton: a recommendation for the excision of certain portions as a means of shortening the period of disability following trauma. *Am J Surg* 1947;74:705–720.
98. Gurd FB. The treatment of complete dislocation of the outer end of the clavicle: a hitherto undescribed operation. *Ann Surg* 1941;113: 1094–1097.
99. Hansky B, Murray E, Minami K, Korfer R. Delayed brachial plexus paralysis due to subclavian psuedoaneurysm after clavicle fracture. *Eur J Cardiothorac Surg* 1993;7:497–498.
100. Hanson FB. The history of the earliest stages in the human clavicle. *Anat Rec* 1920;19:309–325.
101. Hardy JRW. Complex clavicular injury in childhood. *J Bone Joint Surg [Br]* 1992;74:154.
102. Harrington MA Jr, Keller TS, Seiler JG, Weikert DR, Moelianto E, Schwartz HS. Geometric properties and the predicted mechanical behavior of adult human clavicles. *J Biomech* 193;26:417–426.
103. Hawley GW. A method of treating fracture of the clavicle. *J Bone Joint Surg* 1937;19:232.
104. Heim U, Pfeiffer KM. *Internal fixation of small fractures. Technique recommended by the AO-ASIF group*, 3rd ed. Springer-Verlag. New York, New York: 1987.
105. Heppenstall RB. Fractures and dislocations of the distal clavicle. *Orthop Clin North Am* 1975;6:477–486.
106. Herscovici D Jr, Sanders R, Dipasquale T, Gregory P. Injuries of the shoulder girdle. *Clin Orthop* 1995;318:54–60.
107. Herscovici D Jr, Fiennes AGTW, Allgower M, Ruedi T. The floating shoulder: ipsilateral clavicle and scapular neck fractures. *J Bone Joint Surg [Br]* 1992;74:362–364.
108. Hienz WM, Misamore GW. Mid-shaft fracture of the clavicle with grade III acromioclavicular separation. *J Shoulder Elbow Surg* 1995; 4:141–142.
109. Howard FM, Shafer SJ. Injuries to the clavicle with neurovascular complications: a study of 14 cases. *J Bone Joint Surg [Am]* 1965;67: 1335–1346.
110. Inman VT, Saunders JB, De CM. Observations on the function of the shoulder joint. *J Bone Joint Surg* 1944;26:1–30.
111. Inman VT, Saunders JB. Observations on the function of the clavicle. *Calif Med* 1946;65:158–166.
112. Iqbal O. Axillary artery thrombosis associated with fracture of the clavicle. *Med J Malaya* 1971;26:68–70.
113. Jablon M, Sutker A, Post M. Irreducible fracture of the middle third of the clavicle: report of a case. *J Bone Joint Surg [Am]* 1979;61: 296–298.
114. Jacobs P. Post-traumatic osteolysis of the outer end of the clavicle. *J Bone Joint Surg [Br]* 1964;46:705–707.
115. Javid H. Vascular injuries of the neck. *Clin Orthop* 1963;28:70–78.
116. Jit I, Kulkarni M. Times of appearance and fusion of epiphysis at the medial end of the clavicle. *Indian J Med Res* 1976;64:773–781.
117. Johnson EW, Collins HR. Nonunion of the clavicle. *Arch Surg* 1963; 87:963–966.
118. Joseph PR, Rosenfeld W. Clavicular fractures in neonates. *Am J Dis Child* 1990;144:165–167.
119. Joukainen J, Karaharju E. Psuedarthrosis of the clavicle. *Acta Orthop Scand* 1977;48:550–551.
120. Jupiter JB, Leffert RD. Non-union of the clavicle. *J Bone Joint Surg [Am]* 1987;69:753–760.
121. Kanoksikarin S, Wearne WM. Fracture and retrosternal dislocation of the clavicle. *Aust N Z J Surg* 1978;48:95–96.
122. Karaharju E, Joukainen J, Peltonen J. Treatment of pseudarthrosis of the clavicle. *Injury* 1981;13:400–403.
123. Katz R, Landman J, Dulitzky F, et. al. Fracture of the clavicle in the newborn. An ultrasound diagnosis. *J Ultrasound Med* 1988;7:21–23.
124. Katznelson A, Nerubay J, Oliver S. Dynamic fixation of the avulsed clavicle. *J Trauma* 1976;16:841–844.
125. Kay SP, Eckardt JJ. Brachial plexus palsy secondary to clavicular nonunion. Case report and literature survey. *Clin Orthop* 1986;206: 219–222.
126. Kaye JJ, Nance EP Jr, Green NE. Fatigue fracture of the medial aspect of the clavicle. *Radiology* 1982;144:89–90.
127. Khan MA, Lucas HK. Plating of fractures of the middle third of the clavicle. *Injury* 1977;9:263–267.
128. Kini MG. A simple method of ambulatory treatment of fractures of the clavicle. *J Bone Joint Surg* 1941;23:795–798.

129. Kite JH. Congenital pseudarthrosis of the clavicle. *South J Med* 1968; 703–710.
130. Koch AR. Die Frühentwicklung der clavicula beim menschen. *Acta Anatomica* 1960;42:177–212.
131. Koelliker F. Behandlungsergebnisse der clavicula—psuedarthrose. *Unfallchirurg* 1989;92:164–168.
132. Kona J, Bosse MJ, Staeheli JW, Rosseau RL. Type II clavicle fractures: a retrospective review of surgical treatment. *J Orthop Trauma* 1990;4:155–120.
133. Koss SD, Goitz HT, Redler MR, Whitehill R. Nonunion of a midshaft clavicle fracture associated with subclavian vein compression. A case report. *Orthop Rev* 1989;28:431–434.
134. Kreisinger V. Sur le traitement des fractures de la clavicule. *Rev Chir* 1927;46:376.
135. Kremens V, Glauser F. Unusual sequela following pinning of medial clavicular fracture. *AJR Am J Roentgenol* 1956;76:1066–1069.
136. Kuner Eh, Schlickewei W, Mydla F. Operative therapie der clavicu-lafrakturen, indikation, technik, Ergebnisse. *Hefte Unfallheilkunde* 1982;160:76–77.
137. Lambotte A. L osteo-synthese des fractures de la clavicule. *Rev Tech Chir* 1932; 24:33.
138. Lancourt JE. Acromioclavicular dislocation with adjacent clavicular fracture in a horseback rider. *Am J Sports Med* 1990;18:321–322.
140. Lange RH, Noel SH. Traumatic lateral scapular displacement: an expanded spectrum of associated neurovascular injury. *J Orthop Trauma* 1993;7:361–366.
141. Le Vay D. Treatment of midclavicular fractures. *Lancet* 1967;1:723.
142. Lee HG. Treatment of fracture of the clavicle by internal nail fixation. *N Engl J Med* 1946;234:222–224.
143. Leese G, Belch JJF, Rickhss P, Nimmo M. Post-traumatic axillary artery thrombosis dissolution with low-dose intra-arterial streptokinase. *Injury* 1993;24:212–213.
144. Leffert RD, Seddon HJ. Infraclavicular brachial plexus injuries. *J Bone Joint Surg [Br]* 1965;47:9–22.
145. Lemire L, Rosman M. Sternoclavicular epiphyseal separation with adjacent clavicular fracture. Case report. *J Pediatr Orthop* 1984; 4: 118–120.
146. Lengua F, Nuss J-M, Lechner R, Baruthio J, Veillon F. Traitment des fractures de la clavicule par embrochage a foyer ferme de dedans en dehors sans va-et-vient. *Rev Chir Orthop* 1987;73:377–380.
147. Leonard JW, Gifford RW Jr. Migration of a Kirschner wire from the clavicle into the pulmonary artery. *Am J Cardiol* 1965;16:598–600.
148. Lester CW. The treatment of fractures of the clavicle. *Ann Surg* 1929; 89:600–606.
149. Leung KS, Lam TP. Open reduction and internal fixation of ipsilateral fractures of the scapular neck and clavicle. *J Bone Joint Surg [Am]* 1993;75:1015–1018.
150. Levine MG, Holroyde J, Woods JR Jr, Siddiqi TA, Scott M, Miodovnik M. Birth trauma: incidence and predisposing factors. *Obstet Gynecol* 1984;63:792–795.
151. Lewonowski K, Basset GS. Complete posterior sternoclavicular epiphyseal separation. A case report and review of the literature. *Clin Orthop* 1992;281:84–88.
152. Lim EVA, Day LJ. Subclavian vein thrombosis following fracture of the clavicle: a case report. *Orthopedics* 1987;10:349–351.
153. Lipton HA, Jupiter JB. Nonunion of clavicular fractures: characteristics and surgical managment. 1988: *Surg Rounds Orthop*
154. Ljunggren AE. Clavicular function. *Acta Orthop Scand* 1979;50: 261–268.
155. Lloyd-Roberts GC, Apley AG, Owen R. Reflections upon the aetiology or congenital pseudarthrosis of the clavicle. *J Bone Joint Surg [Br]* 1975;57:24–29.
156. Lusskin R, Weiss CA, Winer J. The role of the subclavius muscle in the subclavian vein syndrome (costoclavicular syndrome) following fracture of the clavicle. *Clin Orthop* 1967;54:75–83.
157. Lyons FA, Rockwood CA Jr. Migration of pins used in operations on the shoulder. *J Bone Joint Surg [Am]* 1990;72:1262–1267.
158. Madsen B. Osteolysis of the acromial end of the clavicle following trauma. *Br J Radiol* 1963;36:822–828.
159. Madsen ET. Fractures of the extremities in the newborn. *Acta Obstet Gynecol Scand* 1955;34:41.
160. Malcolm BW, Ameli FM, Simmons EH. Pneumothorax complicating a fracture of the clavicle. *Can J Surg* 1979;22:89.
161. Malgaigne JF. *A treatise on fractures* (translated by Packard JH). Philadelphia: JB Lippencott, 1859:374–401.
162. Mall FP. On ossification centers in human embyros less than one hundred days old. *Am J Anat* 1906;5:433–458.
163. Manske DJ, Szabo RM. The operative treatment of mid-shaft clavicular non-unions. *J Bone Joint Surg [Am]* 1985;67:1367–1371.
164. Marie P, Sainton P. The classic: on hereditary cleidocranial dysostosis. *Clin Orthop* 1968;58:5–7.
165. Marsh HO, Hazarian E. Pseudarthrosis of the clavicle. *J Bone Joint Surg [Br]* 1970;52:793.
166. Matry C. Fracture de la clavicule gauche au tiers interne. Blessure de la veine sous-clavière . Osteosynthese. *Bull Mém Soc Nat Chir* 1932; 58:75–78.
167. Matz SO, Welliver PS, Welliver DI. Brachial plexus neuropraxia complicating a comminuted clavicle fracture in a college football player. Case report and review of the literature. *Am J Sports Med* 1989;17:581–583.
168. Maunoury G. Fracture de la clavicule compliquée de déchirure de la veine sousclavière. Operation. Mort par hémorrhagie et entrée de l air dans les veines. *Prog Med Paris* 1881;10:302.
169. Mayer JH. Non-union of fractured clavicle. *Proc R Soc Med* 1965;58: 182.
170. Mazet R Jr. Migration of a Kirschner wire from the shoulder region into the lung: report of two cases. *J Bone Joint Surg* 1943;25: 477–483.
171. McCandless DN, Mowbray MAS. Treatment of displaced fractures of the clavicle: sling versus figure-of-eight bandage. *Practitioner* 1979; 223:266–267.
172. McCaughan JS, Miller PR. Migration of Steinmann pin from shoulder to lung. *JAMA* 1969;207:1917.
173. Meeks RJ, Riebel GD. Isolated clavicle fracture with associated pneumothorax: a case report. *Am J Emerg Med* 1991;9:555–556.
174. Miller DS, Boswick JA. Lesions of the brachial plexus associated with fractures of the clavicle. *Clin Orthop* 1969;64:144–149.
175. Miller MR, Ada JR. Injuries to the shoulder girdle. In: Browner BD, Jupiter JB, Levine AM, Trafton PG, eds. *Skeletal trauma*. Philadelphia: WB Saunders, 1991:1291–1310.
176. Mital MA, Aufranc OE. Venous occlusion following greenstick fracture of the clavicle. *JAMA* 1968;206:1301–1302.
177. Mnaymneh W, Vargas A, Kaplan J. Fractures of the clavicle caused by arteriovenous malformation. *Clin Orthop* 1980;148:256–258.
178. Moore TO. Internal pin fixation for fracture of the clavicle. *Am Surg* 1951;17:580–583.
179. Moseley HF. The clavicle: its anatomy and function. *Clin Orthop* 1968;58:17–27.
180. Mulder DS, Greenwood FAH, Brooks CE. Posttraumatic thoracic outlet syndrome. *J Trauma* 1973;13:706–715.
181. Mullaji AB, Jupiter JB. Low-contact dynamic compression plating of the clavicle. *Injury* 1994;25:41–45.
182. Muller ME, Allgower M, Willenegger H. *Technique of internal fixation of fractures*. New York: Springer Verlag, 1970.
183. Muller ME, Thomas RJ. Treatment of non-union in fractures of long bones. *Clin Orthop* 1979;138:141–152.
184. Mullick S. Treatment of mid-clavicular fractures. *Lancet* 1967;1:499.
185. Murray G. A method of fixation for fracture of the clavicle. *J Bone Joint Surg* 1940;22:616–620.
186. Naidoo P. Migration of a Kirschner wire from the clavicle into the abdominal aorta. *Arch Emerg Med* 1991;8:292–295.
187. Naidu SH, Heppenstall RB, Brighton CT, Wright DW, Esterhai JL. Clavicle non-union: results of treatment with electricity, AO dynamic compression plating and autogenous bone grafting, and excision of the nonunion in 43 patients. *Orthop Trans* 1994;18:1072.
188. Natali J, Maraval M, Kieffer E, Petrovic P. Fractures of the clavicle and injuries of the subclavian artery: report of 10 cases. *J Cardiovasc Surg*. 1975;16:541–547.
189. Neer CS II. Nonunion of the clavicle. *JAMA* 1960; 172: 1006–1011.
190. Neer CS. Fracture of the distal clavicle with detachment of the coracoclavicular ligaments in adults. *J Trauma* 1963;3:99–110.
191. Neer CS. Fractures about the shoulder. In: Rockwood CA Jr, Green DP, eds. Philadelphia: JB Lippencott, 1984:707–713.
192. Neer CS. Fractures of the distal third of the clavicle. *Clin Orthop* 1968;58:43–50.
193. Neviaser JS. Injuries of the clavicle and its articulations. *Orthop Clin North Am* 1980;11:233–237.
194. Neviaser JS. The treatment of fractures of the clavicle. *Surg Clin North Am* 1963;43:1555.

195. Neviaser RJ, Neviaser JS, Neviaser TJ, Neviaser JS. A simple technique for internal fixation of the clavicle. A long term evaluation. *Clin Orthop* 1975;109:103–107.
196. Neviaser RJ. Injuries to the clavicle and acromioclavcular joint. *Orthop Clin North Am* 1987;18:433–438.
197. Nicoll EA. Miners and mannequins. *J Bone Joint Surg [Br]* 1954;36: 171–172.
198. Nogi J, Heckman JD, Hakala M, Sweet DE. Non-union of the clavicle in a child. *Clin Orthop* 1975;110:19–21.
199. Nordback I, Markkula H. Migration of Kirschner wire from clavicle into ascending aorta. *Acta Chiropract Scand* 1985; 151:177–179.
200. Nordqvist A, Petersson C, Redlund-Johnell I. The natural course of lateral clavicle fracture. 15 (11–21) year follow-up of 110 cases. *Acta Orthop Scand* 1993;64:87–91.
201. Nordqvist A, Petersson C. The incidence of fractures of the clavicle. *Clin Orthop* 1994;300:127–132.
202. Norrell H Jr, Llewellyn RC. Migration of a threaded Steinman pin from an acromioclavicular joint into the spinal canal. *J Bone Joint Surg [Am]* 1965;47:1024–1026.
203. O'Halloran MJ. Clavicular fractures in neonates: frequency vs. significance. *Am J Dis Child* 1991;145:251.
204. O'Rourke IC, Middleton RWD. The place and managment of operative managment of fractured clavicle. *Injury* 1974;6:236–240.
205. Ogden JA, Conlongue GJ, Bronson ML. Radiology of postnatal skeletal development. III. The clavicle. *Skeletal Radiol* 1979;4:196.
206. Ogden JA. Distal clavicular physeal injury. *Clin Orthop* 1984;188: 68–73.
207. Ogle JW. Laceration of the internal jugular vein by a portion of fractured clavicle. *Br Med J* 1873;2:82–83.
208. Olsen BO, Vaesel MT, Sojbjerg JO. Treatment of midshaft clavicular nonunion with plate fixation and autologous bone grafting. *J Shoulder Elbow Surg* 1995;4:337–344.
209. Oppenheim WL, Davis A, Growdon WA, Dorey FJ, Davlin LB. Clavicle fractures in the newborn. *Clin Orthop* 1990;250:176–180.
210. Ord RA, Langon JD. Stress fracture of the clavicle. A rare late complication of radical neck dissection. *J Maxillofac Surg* 1986;14: 281–284.
211. Oreck SL, Burgess A, Levine A. Traumatic lateral displacement of the scapula: A radiographic sign of neurovascular disruption. *J Bone Joint Surg [Am]* 1984;66:758–763.
212. Oxnard CE. The architecture of the shoulder in some mammals. *J Morphol* 1968;126:249–290.
213. Oxnard CE. The functional morphology of the primate shoulder as revealed by comparative anatomical, osteometric and discrimination function techniques. *Am J Phys Anthropol* 1967;26:219–240.
214. Packer BD. Conservative treatment of fracture of the clavicle. *J Bone Joint Surg* 1944;26:770–774.
215. Pannier R, Daems J. A propos d'un cas de corps etranger intrapulmonaire apres osteosynthese de la clavicule. *Acta Tuberc Belg* 1949; 40:360–362.
216. Parkes JC, Deland JT. A three-part distal clavicle fracture. *J Trauma* 1983;23:437–438.
217. Pate JW, Whilhite JL. Migration of a foreign body from the sternoclavicular joint to the heart: a case report. *Am Surg* 1969;35: 448–449.
218. Patel CV, Adenwalla HS. Treatment of fractured clavicle by immediate partial subperiosteal resection. *J Postgrad Med* 1972;18:32–34.
219. Penn I. The vascular complications of fractures of the clavicle. *J Trauma* 1964;4:819.
220. Perry BF. An improved clavicle pin. *Am J Surg* 1966;112:143–144.
221. Pfeifle K, Rehrman A, Nwoke AL. Psuedotumors of the clavicle following neck dissection. *J Maxillofac Surg* 1974;2:14–18.
222. Pipkin G. Tardy shoulder hand syndrome following ununited fracture of clavicle. *J Mo State Med Assoc* 1951;48:643–646.
223. Piterman L. The fractured clavicle. *Aust Fam Physician* 1982;11:614.
224. Poigenfürst J, Rappold G, Fischer W. Plating of fresh clavicular fractures: results of 122 operations. *Injury* 1992; 23:237–241.
225. Post M. Current concepts in the treatment of fractures of the clavicle. *Clin Orthop* 1989;245:89–101.
226. Prime HT, Doig SG, Hooper JC. Retrosternal dislocation of the clavicle. A case report. *Am J Sports Med* 1991;19:92–93.
227. Pyper JB. Non-union of fractures of the clavicle. *Injury* 1977;9: 268–270.
228. Quesada F. Technique for the roentgen diagnosis of fractures of the clavicle. *Surg Gynecol Obstet* 1926;42:424–428.
229. Quigley TB. The management of simple fractures of the clavicle. *N Engl J Med* 1950;243:286–290.
230. Quinn SF, Glass TA. Posttraumatic osteolysis of the clavicle. *South Med J* 1983;76:307–308.
231. Redmond AD. Letter to the editor. *Injury* 1982;13:352.
232. Reichenbacher D, Siebler G. Early post-traumatic plexus lesions—a rare complication after clavicle fractures. *Unfallchirurgie* 1987;13: 91–92.
233. Reid J, Kennedy J. Direct fracture of clavicle with symptoms simulating cervical rib. *Br Med J* 1925;2:608–609.
234. Reimer BL, Butterfield SL, Daffner RH, et al. The abduction lordotic view of the clavicle: a new technique for radiographic visualization. *J Orthop Trauma* 1991;5:392–394.
235. Rey-Baltar E, Errazu D. Unusual outcome of Steinman wire: case of fractured clavicle. *Arch Surg* 1964;89:1024–1025.
236. Rikli D, Regazzoni P, Renner N. The unstable shoulder girdle: early functional treatment utilizing open reduction and internal fixation. *J Orthop Trauma* 1995;9:93–97.
237. Roberts SW, Hernandez C, Maberry MC, Adams MD, Leveno KJ, Wendel GD Jr. Obstetric clavicular fracture: the enigma of normal birth. *Obstet Gynecol* 1995;86:978–981.
238. Rockwood CA Jr, Wirth MA. Don't throw away the clavicle. *Orthop Trans* 1992;16:763.
239. Rockwood CA Jr. Fractures and dislocations of the ends of the clavicle, scapula, and glenohumeral joint. In: Rockwood CA, Wilkins KE, King RE, eds. *Fractures in children*. Philadelphia: JB Lippincott, 1984:624–681.
240. Rockwood CA Jr. Fractures of the outer clavicle in children and adults. *J Bone Joint Surg [Br]* 1982;64:642.
241. Rowe CR. An atlas of anatomy and treatment of midclavicular fractures. *Clin Orthop* 1968;58:29–42.
242. Rubenstein JD, Ebrahiem NA, Kellam JF. Traumatic scapulothoracic dissociation. *Radiology* 1985;157:297–298.
243. Rubin A. Birth injuries: incidence, mechanisms, and end results. *Obstet Gynecol* 1964;23:218–221.
244. Rumball KM, Da Silva VF, Preston DN, Carruthers CC. Brachial-plexus injury after clavicular fracture: a case report and literature review. *Can J Surg* 1991;34:264–266.
245. Rush LV, Rush HL. Technique of longitudinal pin fixation in fractures of the clavicle and jaw. *Miss Doctor* 1949;27:332–336.
246. Sakellarides H. Psuedarthrosis of the clavicle. A report of twenty cases. *J Bone Joint Surg [Am]* 1961;43:130–138.
247. Sandford HN. The Moro reflex as a diagnostic aid in fracture of the clavicle in the newborn infant. *Am J Dis Child* 1931; 41:1304–1306.
248. Sankarankutty M, Turner BW. Fractures of the clavicle. *Injury* 1975; 7:101–106.
249. Sayre LA. A simple dressing for fracture of the clavicle. *Am Pract* 1871;4:1.
250. Scarpa FJ, Levy RM. Pulmonary embolism complicating clavicle fracture. *Conn Med* 1979;43:771–773.
251. Schuind F, Pay-Pay E, Andreianne Y, Donkerwolcke M, Rasquin C, Burny F. External fixation of the clavicle for fracture or nonunion in adults. *J Bone Joint Surg [Am]* 1988;70:692–695.
252. Schwarz N, Höcker K. Osteosynthesis of irreducible fractures of the clavicle with 2.7 millimeter ASIF plates. *J Trauma* 1992;33:179–183.
253. Seddon HJ. Nerve lesions complicating certain closed bone injuries. *JAMA* 1947;135:691–694.
254. Sever JW. Obstetric paralysis: report of eleven hundred cases. *JAMA* 1925;85:1862.
255. Shih J-S, Chao E-K, Chang C-H. Subclavian psuedoaneurysm after clavicle fracture: a case report. *J Formosan Med Assoc* 1983;82: 332–335.
256. Siffre A. Thrombose post-traumatique de l'artere sous-claviere gauche. *Lyon Chir* 1956;51:479–481.
257. Silloway KA, Mclaughlin RE, Edlich RC, Edlich RF. Clavicular fractures and acromioclavicular joint injuries in Lacrosse: preventable injuries. *J Emerg Med* 1985;3:117–121.
258. Simpson NS, Jupiter JB. Clavicular nonunion and malunion: evaluation and surgical managment. *J Am Acad Orthop Surg* 19??; 4(1):1–8.
259. Spar I. Total claviculectomy for pathological fractures. *Clin Orthop* 1977;129:236–237.
260. Stanley D, Norris SH. Recovery following fractures of the clavicle treated conservatively. *Injury* 1988;19:162–164.
261. Stanley D, Trowbridge EA, Norris SH. The mechanism of clavicular fracture. *J Bone Joint Surg [Br]* 1988;70:461–464.

262. Steinberg I. Subclavian vein thrombosis associated with fractures of the clavicle: report of two cases. *N Engl J Med* 1961;264:686–688.
263. Stone PW, Lord JW Jr. The clavicle and its relation to trauma to the subclavian artery and vein. *Am J Surg* 1955;89:834–839.
264. Storen H. Old clavicular pseudarthrosis with late appearing neuralgias and vasomotoric disturbances cured by operation. *Acta Chir Scand* 1946;94:187.
265. Strauss FM, Bushey MJ, Chung C, Baum S. Fracture of the clavicle following radical neck dissection and postoperative radiotherapy: a case report and review of the literature. *Laryngoscope* 1982;92: 1304–1307.
266. Sturm JT, Strate RG, Mowlem A, Quattlebaum FW, Perry JF Jr. Blunt trauma to the subclavian artery. *Surg Gynecol Obstet* 1974;138:915–918.
267. Taylor AR. Non-union of fractures of the clavicle: a review of thirty-one cases. *J Bone Joint Surg [Br]* 1969;51:568–569.
268. Taylor AR. Some observations on fractures of the clavicle. *Proc R Soc Med* 1969;62:33–34.
269. Taylor W. Traumatic aneurysm of the left subclavian artery produced by fracture of the clavicle. *Ann Surg* 1903;38:638–651.
270. Telford ED. Pressure at the cervico-brachial junction. An operative and anatomical study. *J Bone Joint Surg [Br]* 1948;30:249–265.
271. Thomas CB, Friedman RJ. Ipsilateral sternoclavicular dislocation and clavicular fracture. *J Orthop Trauma* 1989;3:355–357.
272. Thompson AG, Batten RL. The application of rigid internal fixation to the treatment of non-union and delayed union using the AO technique. *Injury* 1976;8:188–198.
273. Thompson JS. Operative treatment of certain clavicle fractures in orthopedic controversy. *Orthop Trans* 1988;12:141.
274. Todd TW, D'Errico J Jr. The clavicular epiphysis. *Am J Anat* 1928;41: 25–50.
275. Tregonning G, Macnab I. Post-traumatic pseudarthrosis of the clavicle. *J Bone Joint Surg [Br]* 1976;58:264.
276. Tristan TA, Daughtridge TG. Migration of a metallic pin from the humerus into the lung. *N Engl J Med* 1964;270:987.
277. Trynin AH. The Bohler clavicular splint in the treatment of clavicular injuries. *J Bone Joint Surg* 1937;19:417–423.
278. Tse DHW, Slabaugh PB, Carlson PA. Injury to the axillary artery by a closed fracture of the clavicle. *J Bone Joint Surg [Am]* 1980;62: 1372–1374.
279. Turnpenny PD. Fractured clavicle of the newborn in a population with a high prevalence of grand-multiparity: analysis of 78 consecutive cases. *Br J Obstet Gynecol* 1993;100:338–341.
280. Van Vlack HG. Comminuted fracture of the clavicle with pressure on brachial plexus. *J Bone Joint Surg* 1940;22:446–447.
281. Wall JJ. Congenital pseudarthrosis of the clavicle. *J Bone Joint Surg [Am]* 1970;52:1003–1009.
282. Walle T, Hartikainen-Sorri A-L. Obstetric shoulder injury: associated risk factors, predilection and prognosis. *Acta Obstet Gynecol Scand* 1993;72:450–454.
283. Webb LX. Fractures and dislocations about the shoulder. In: Swiontkowski M, Green N, eds. *Skeletal trauma in children.* Philadelphia: WB Saunders, 1992:257–281.
284. Weber BG, Brunner C, Freuler S, eds. *Die Frankturenbehandlung bei kindern und jugendilichen.* Berlin: Springer-Verlag, 1978:87–94.
285. Weber BG, Cech O. *Psuedarthrosis.* New York; Grune & Stratton, 1976.
286. Weinberg B, Seife B, Alonso P. The apical oblique view of the clavicle: its usefulness in neonatal and childhood trauma. *Skeletal Radiol* 1991;20:201–203.
287. Weiner DS, O'Dell HW. Fractures of the first rib associated with injuries to the clavicle. *J Trauma* 1989;9:412–422.
288. White RR, Anson PS, Kristiansen T. Adult clavicle fractures: relationship between mechanism of injury and healing. *Orthop Trans* 1989;13:514–515.
289. Wilkes JA, Hoffer MM. Clavicle fractures in head-injured children. *J Orthop Trauma* 1987;1:55–58.
290. Wilkins RM, Johnston RM. Ununited fractures of the clavicle. *J Bone Joint Surg [Am]* 1983;65:773–778.
291. Wood VE: The results of total claviculectomy. *Clin Orthop* 1986;207: 186–190.
292. Wurtz LD, Lyons FA, Rockwood CA Jr. Fracture of the middle third of the clavicle and dislocation of the acromioclavicular joint. A report of four cases. *J Bone Joint Surg [Am]* 1992;74:133–137.
293. Yates AG, Guest D. Cerebral embolism due to an ununited fracture of the clavicle and subclavian thrombosis. *Lancet* 1928;2:225.
294. Yates DW. Complications of fractures of the clavicle. *Injury* 1976;7: 189–193.
295. Zaslav KR, Ray S, Neer CS. Conservative management of a displaced medial clavicular physeal injury in an adolescent male. *Am J Sports Med* 1989;17:833–836.
296. Zenni EJ, Krieg JK, Rosen MJ. Open reduction and internal fixation of clavicular fractures. *J Bone Joint Surg [Am]* 1981;63A: 147–151.

PART VI

Acromioclavicular Joint

Disorders of the Shoulder: Diagnosis and Management,
edited by Joseph P. Iannotti and Gerald R. Williams, Jr.
Lippincott Williams & Wilkins, Philadelphia © 1999.

CHAPTER 27

Disorders of the Acromioclavicular Joint: Pathophysiology, Diagnosis, and Management

Gordon W. Nuber and Mark K. Bowen

INTRODUCTION

The acromioclavicular (AC) joint is commonly involved in traumatic and degenerative conditions that affect function of the shoulder girdle. Treatment of acromioclavicular joint disorders has at times been controversial. Most injuries are related to direct trauma, such as a fall on the shoulder; or repetitive use of the shoulder girdle, as with an overhead athlete. This chapter will review the pertinent anatomy, biomechanics, and diagnosis of injuries to the acromioclavicular joint and suggest a logical approach to treatment and restoration of function.

G. W. Nuber and M. K. Bowen: Department of Orthopaedic Surgery, Northwestern University, Chicago, Illinois 60611.

ANATOMY

The acromioclavicular joint is a diarthrodial joint involving the medial facet of the acromion and the distal clavicle. Its articular surfaces are covered with hyaline cartilage. Along with the sternoclavicular joint, the acromioclavicular joint provides a bony link of the shoulder to the axial skeleton. The inclination of the joint is variable in both the sagittal and coronal planes.[68] A fibrocartilaginous disk of varying size and shape is present in the joint.[21] A complete disk is noted in less than 10% of the population. Degenerative changes of the disc increase in frequency with age. The primary stabilizers of the acromioclavicular joint are the ligaments that surround the joint. A thin capsule surrounds the joint and is stabilized by anterior and posterior as well as superior and inferior ligaments. The superior acromioclavicular ligament is the most robust of the ligaments and is reinforced by fascial attachments of the deltoid and trapezial muscles. These ligaments provide horizontal stability (anteroposterior) to the acromioclavicular joint.[72,81] The acromioclavicular ligament capsular insertion on the clavicle is approximately 1.5 cm from the joint. An acromioclavicular resection of 2 cm would potentially compromise anteroposterior stability of the distal clavicle owing to loss of capsular insertion.

Vertical stability (superoinferior) is provided by the coracoclavicular ligaments (conoid and trapezoid; Fig. 1). These ligaments pass from the inferior surface of the clavicle to the base of the coracoid process of the scapula. The trapezoid ligament is the most lateral of the two. It is a broad, thin quadrilateral-shaped ligament running obliquely from the superior surface of the coracoid process to the oblique ridge on the inferior surface of the clavicle. The conoid ligament is more conical in form, with its base directed superiorly. Its apex attaches to a rough impression at the base of the coracoid process medial to the trapezoid ligament. It attaches by its base to the coracoid tuberosity on the inferior surface of the clavicle and a line proceeding medial for 1 cm on this bone. These ligaments are the primary stabilizers of the acromioclavicular joint and constitute the primary supports by which the scapula is suspended from the clavicle. Division of the acromioclavicular ligaments and joint capsule, along with detachment of the trapezius and deltoid, allows less than 50% subluxation superiorly. Posterior dislocation, though, is possible.[81] Complete superior dislocation of the acromioclavicular joint will occur only after complete division of the coracoclavicular ligaments has also occurred.

In children, the clavicle is surrounded by a thick periosteal tube that extends all the way to the acromioclavicular joint. A secondary ossification center is present at the distal clavicle and fuses with the clavicle at about the age of 19.[19] Because of the variation in anatomy compared with adults, children are more prone to fracture and pseudodislocations than true dislocation of the acromioclavicular joint.[26,64]

An ossification center appears in the body of the coracoid at approximately 1 year of age. Another combined ossification center for the base of the coracoid and upper fourth of the glenoid occurs close to age 10.[19] These centers fuse to the scapula at about age 15. Near puberty, the acromion forms two to five ossification centers that fuse at about age 22. Failure to fuse the acromial ossification center leads to an os acromiale.

Anatomic variations in this area are infrequent. Occasionally a bony, cartilaginous or fibrous bar may form in place of the coracoclavicular ligaments, the so-called coracoclavicular bar.[73] This connection may be complete or incomplete. In 1% of the population, an actual diarthrodial joint may be present.[62] A complete bar may interfere with scapular rotation. Coracoclavicular articulations have also been linked to compression of the subclavian artery and brachial plexus, along with early degenerative changes of the acromioclavicular and sternoclavicular joints.[73,87]

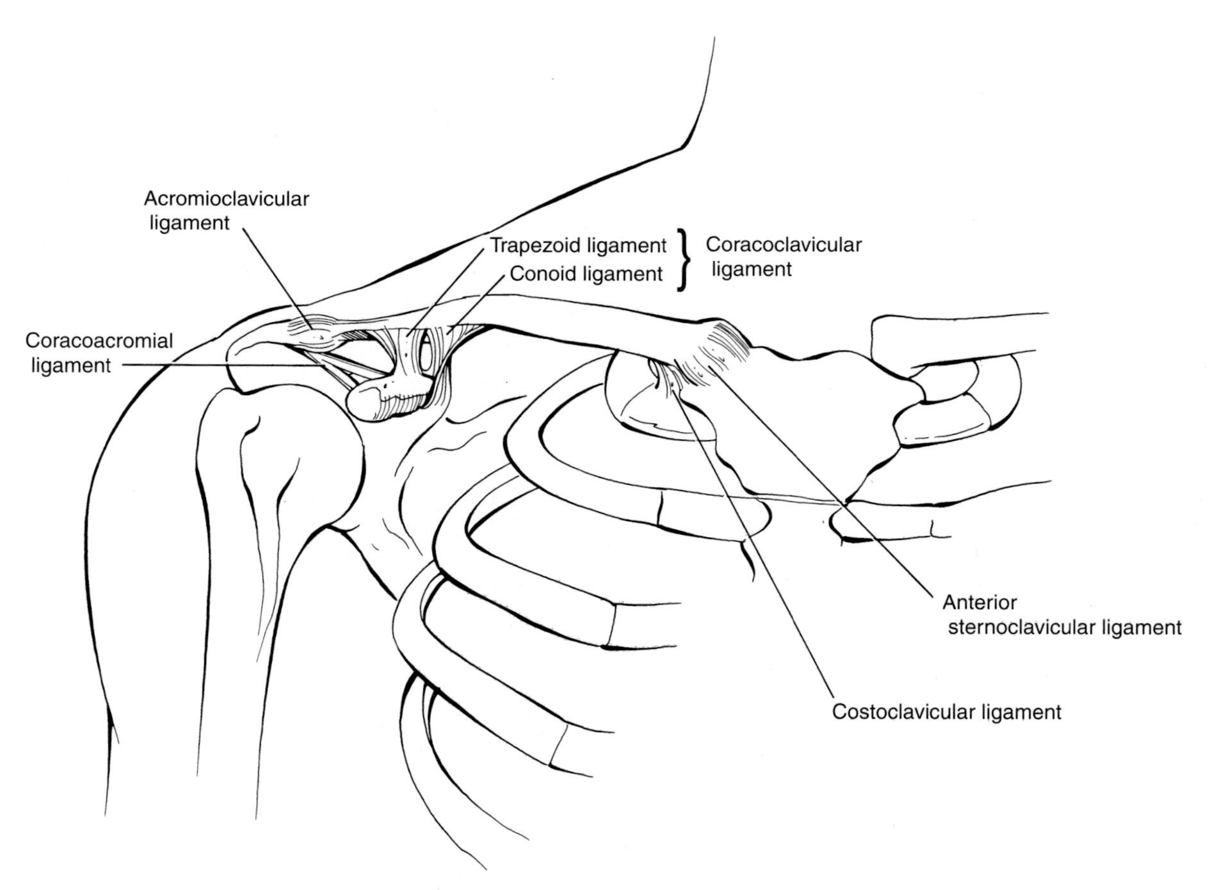

FIG. 1. Ligamentous anatomy of the acromioclavicular joint.

BIOMECHANICS

Observations by Inman et al. indicated that the clavicle rotates as the arm is elevated.[39] This was always felt to imply that motion (rotation) must be present at the acromioclavicular joint for overhead motion to be achieved. This finding was contradicted by observation by other authors who found little motion restriction after acromioclavicular joint fusions or fixations.[28,69] Rockwood, in a classic study in which percutaneous pins were implanted in volunteers, found little motion between the acromion and clavicle.[69] His findings led him to conclude that there was synchronous movement of the scapula and clavicle. As the clavicle rotates, the scapula rotates with it; thus, minimal rotation is required between the two. Hence, most scapulothoracic motion must occur at the sternoclavicular articulation. Clinically, fusions of the acromioclavicular joint will lead to minimal dysfunction.

Stability of the acromioclavicular joint is rendered by the ligamentous complex. Fukuda et al. used 12 fresh-frozen specimens and studied ligamentous contributions to joint constraint by performing load displacement tests, along with sequential cutting of the ligaments.[31] The contributions of the different ligaments to constraint changed not only with direction of loading, but also with amount of loading and displacement. With small amounts of load and induced displacement, the acromioclavicular ligament contributed more restraining force to superior displacement. With larger loads and displacement, the coracoclavicular ligaments (conoid) were major restraints. The acromioclavicular ligaments (superior and posterior) acted as the primary constraint to posterior clavicular displacement and posterior axial rotation at all loads. For axial compressive loading of the acromioclavicular joint, the trapezoid was the major restraint. This work implies that, to achieve normal physiologic function of this joint, preservation of both stabilizing groups of ligaments is important. Surgical procedures that excise the distal clavicle may not make this possible. Posterior abutment of the resected distal clavicle against the base of the acromion may be a cause of failure after open distal clavicle resection.[28] Traditionally, large amounts (1 to 2 cm) of resection were recommended. Acromioclavicular resection of 2 cm would potentially compromise anteroposterior stability of the distal clavicle by loss of capsular insertion. Resection of less bone (5 mm) along with preservation of part of the acromioclavicular ligament, either superior or inferior, will ensure that no bone-to-bone abutment occurs. This can be accomplished either through an open or arthroscopic technique.[13,30]

TRAUMATIC DISORDERS

Injuries to the acromioclavicular joint can be classified according to findings on physical examination and anteroposterior (AP) and axillary radiographs. The amount and degree of damage to the acromioclavicular and coracoclavicular ligaments, as well as the deltoid and trapezius attachments, determines the current classification.

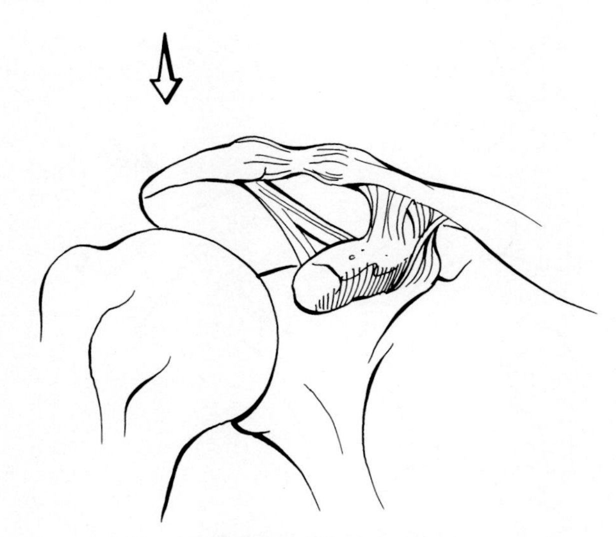

FIG. 2. Type I injury.

Classically, injuries to this joint were classified as either types I, II, or III.[3,80] Rockwood added three other types of injury to the acromioclavicular joint and expanded the classification to the current six types.[69]

Classification

Type I injury (Fig. 2)
  Sprain of the acromioclavicular ligaments only
Type II injury (Fig. 3)
  Acromioclavicular ligament and joint capsule disrupted
  Coracoclavicular ligaments intact
  Up to 50% vertical subluxation of the clavicle

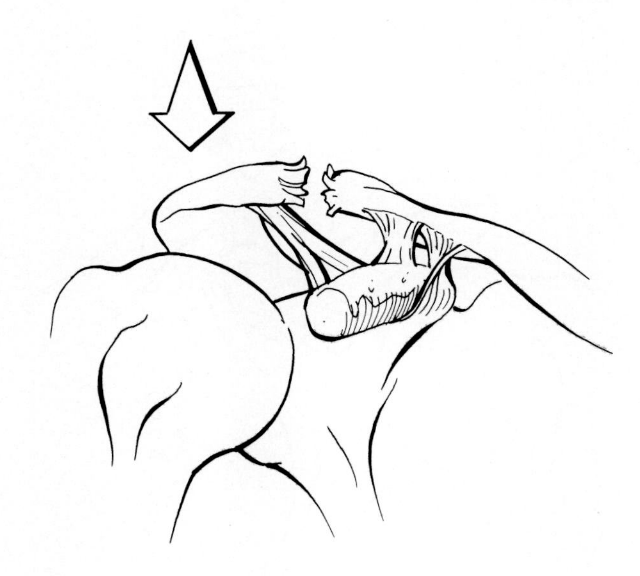

FIG. 3. Type II injury.

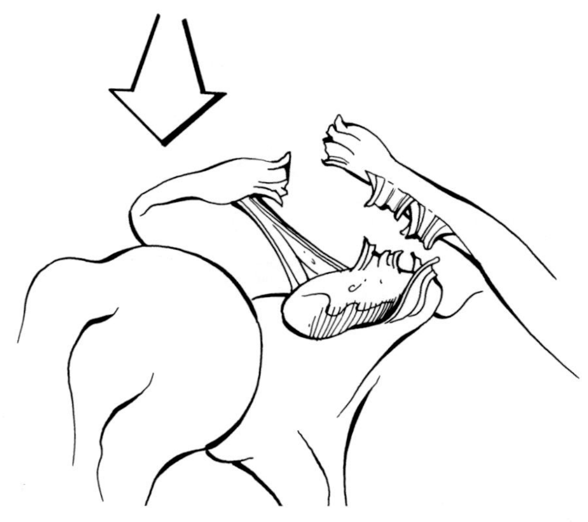

FIG. 4. Type III injury.

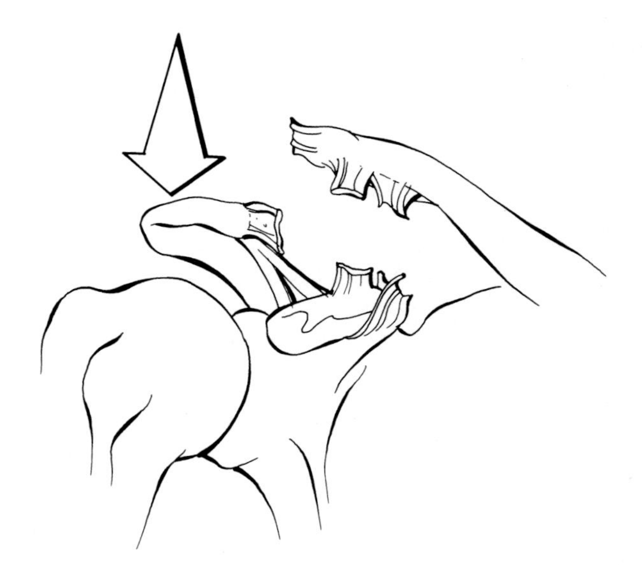

FIG. 6. Type V injury.

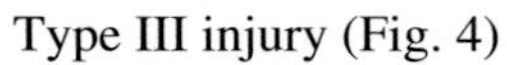

Type III injury (Fig. 4)
- Acromioclavicular ligament and capsule disrupted
- Coracoclavicular ligaments disrupted
- Dislocation of acromioclavicular joint, with the clavicle displaced superiorly, and loss of contact between the clavicle and acromion

Type IV injury (Fig. 5)
- Acromioclavicular ligament and capsule disrupted
- Coracoclavicular ligaments disrupted
- Acromioclavicular joint dislocation with clavicle displaced posteriorly into or through the trapezius muscle (posterior displacement confirmed by axillary radiograph)

Type V injury (Fig. 6)
- Acromioclavicular ligament and capsule disrupted
- Coracoclavicular ligaments disrupted
- Complete detachment of deltoid and trapezius fascia from the distal clavicle
- Acromioclavicular joint dislocated with extreme superior elevation of the clavicle (100% to 300% of normal)

Type VI injury (Fig. 7)
- Acromioclavicular ligament and capsule disrupted
- Coracoclavicular ligaments disrupted
- Acromioclavicular joint disrupted with the clavicle displaced inferior to the acromion or coracoid process

Various type III equivalent injuries have been described, primarily in children. Children younger than 15 years typically do not sustain true dislocations of the acromioclavicular joint, but rather, fractures of the distal clavicle.[19] Disruption of the periosteal sleeve of the clavicle allows the bone to displace superiorly without disruption of the coracoclavicular ligaments (Fig. 8). Thus, in children the classification of acromioclavicular injuries is based on the position of the clavicle with injury to the periosteal sleeve and intact ligaments.

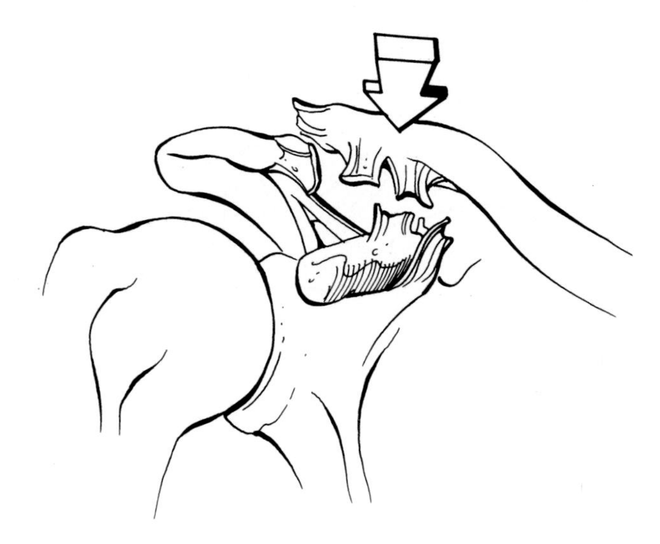

FIG. 5. Type IV injury.

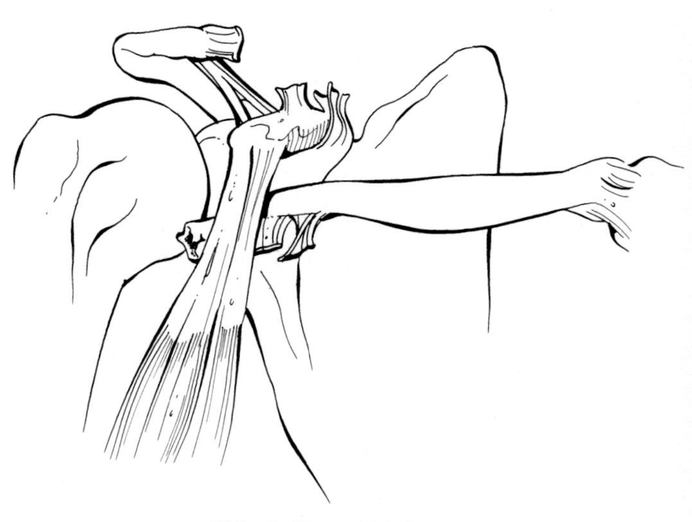

FIG. 7. Type VI injury.

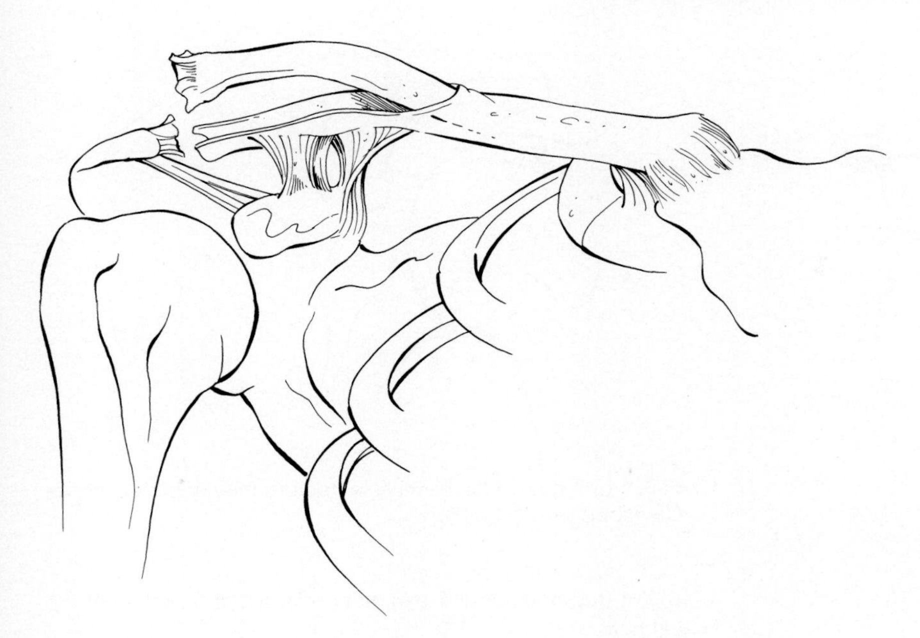

FIG. 8. Periosteal sleeve disruption of the clavicle in a child allows superior migration of the bone without disruption of the coracoclavicular ligaments.

Classification of Acromioclavicular Joint Injuries in Children

Type I injury
- Sprain of acromioclavicular ligaments
- Periosteal sleeve intact

Type II injury
- Partial disruption of periosteal sleeve
- Slight widening of acromioclavicular joint

Type III injury
- Periosteal tube disrupted with instability of the distal clavicle
- Superior displacement 25% to 100% of distal clavicle on AP radiograph

Type IV injury
- Periosteal tube disrupted
- Distal clavicle displaced posteriorly through or into trapezius viewed on axillary radiograph

Type V injury
- Periosteal tube disrupted
- Deltoid and trapezial detachment
- Clavicle displaced subcutaneously greater than 100% of normal

Type VI injury
- Inferior displacement of clavicle beneath the coracoid process

Fractures of the coracoid, if through the common growth plate with the upper glenoid fossa, may mimic an acromioclavicular injury, but the coracoclavicular interspace remains intact.[45] Fracture of the base or tip of the coracoid combined with acromioclavicular ligament disruption is an atypical form of injury to this area. An axillary view will best demonstrate a fracture of the coracoid.[9,54,78] This injury should be suspected in acromioclavicualar injuries in the first three decades of life.

Diagnosis

Injuries of the acromioclavicular joint most commonly occur as a result of direct trauma. Typically, a fall onto the superior aspect of the shoulder with the arm in adduction occurs, as with a fall off a bike or horse (Fig. 9). Another mechanism of injury is a laterally based force directed to the shoulder, as in a hockey player hitting the boards. If the upper extremity is not used to absorb the force, the area of impact is distributed across the acromioclavicular joint. Because of significant stability of the sternoclavicular joint, the energy of impact is distributed to the acromioclavicular and coracoclavicular ligaments or the clavicle itself.[7,61] The direction and magnitude of the forces determines the severity of injury and the structures injured. Typically, with an acromioclavicular injury, the force is initially distributed to the acromioclavicular ligaments. If the magnitude of force is severe, injury progresses to the coracoclavicular ligaments along with the deltoid and trapezial fascia. Fractures of the distal one-third of the clavicle occur rarely, but should be recognized (Figs. 10 and 11). These fractures may or may not be associated with coracoclavicular ligament disruption.

Injuries to the acromioclavicular joint by indirect injury have also been described. Force is typically directed superiorly by the humeral head upward into the acromion. This may occur with a fall on an elbow or outstretched arm. With this mechanism, injury is primarily to the acromioclavicular joint as the coracoclavicular ligaments are relaxed with upward movement of the scapula relative to the clavicle.

The mechanism of injury for the most severe dislocation, the type VI, is felt to be a severe force directed onto the superior surface of the distal clavicle along with abduction of the arm and retraction of the clavicle.[35,52,66]

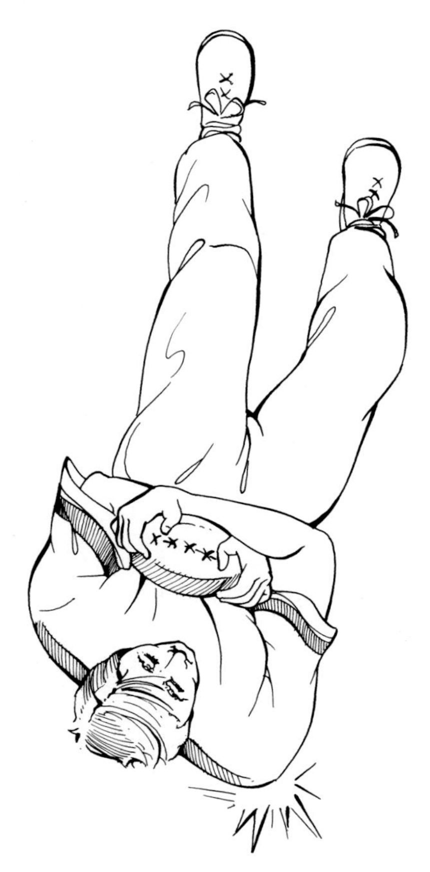

FIG. 9. Acromioclavicular joint injuries typically are the result of a fall on the superior aspect of the shoulder.

Injuries to the acromioclavicular joint should be suspected in anyone with trauma to the shoulder and a history demonstrating the typical mechanism of injury. Not infrequently, the patient will present with a significant abrasion over the superior aspect of the shoulder secondary to the fall. Inspection will also reveal swelling or prominence of the distal clavicle. It is important to remember that the prominence of the distal clavicle is actually accountable to the downward sag of the shoulder and arm, not upward displacement of the clavicle.

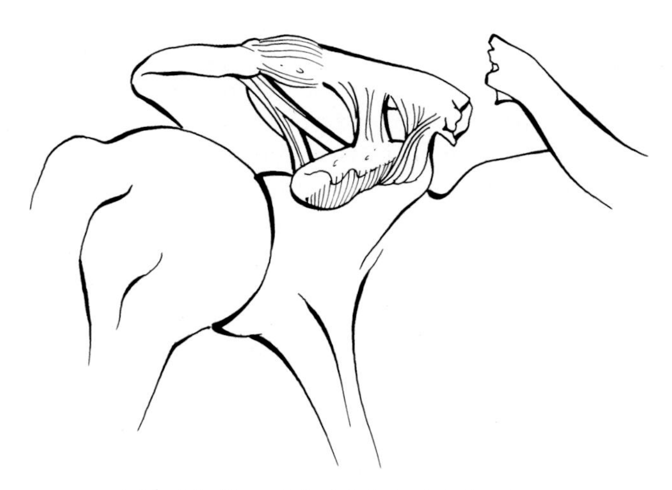

FIG. 10. Type IIA distal clavicle fracture.

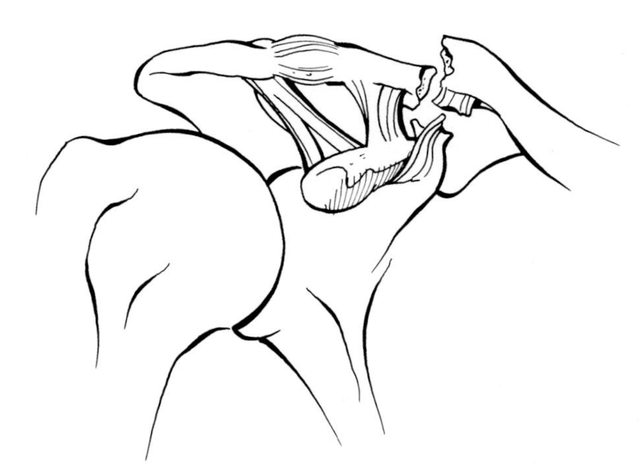

FIG. 11. Type IIB distal clavicle fracture may mimic acromioclavicular joint disruption.

Initial discomfort of the injury may cause the patient to tense his shoulder musculature or cradle his arm and make the prominence of the clavicle less noticeable. As the initial swelling subsides, the deformity and prominence of the distal clavicle become more noticeable. Palpation will typically reveal local tenderness. In type I injuries, the only finding may be localized tenderness. Direction of instability will be difficult to discern initially because of the patient's discomfort. With time, the swelling and pain will subside and make detection of the instability easier. As the patient becomes more comfortable, anteroposterior and superoinferior translation of the distal clavicle can be assessed. Depending on the severity of the injury, motion of the shoulder joint is typically restricted most in abduction or cross-body adduction. With lesser injuries (type I), pain may be produced only with resisted abduction or cross-body adduction and direct palpation of the acromioclavicular joint. Rotation of the humerus with the arm at the side is generally comfortable with these injuries and can be used to detect associated injuries of the glenohumeral joint.

Assessment of Each Type of Acromioclavicular Injury

Type I Injury

Because type I injury is the least severe of the injuries, therefore there is generally mild to moderate pain and swelling. Athletes will often continue to participate in the athletic activity that caused the injury. Arm movements typically are comfortable except for cross-body adduction. The only obvious abnormality is tenderness to palpation.

Type II Injury

The patient will display moderate to severe pain over the acromioclavicular joint. If seen before swelling occurs, slight prominence of the clavicle is noted. Anteroposterior motion of the distal clavicle can be noted when grasping the clavicle and stabilizing the shoulder. Pain may be present over the costoclavicular interspace.

Type III Injury

In type III injury (Fig. 12), moderate to significant pain is usually present. Initially the prominence of the distal clavicle may be diminished by the patient cradling the arm upward to relieve pressure and discomfort on the injured joint. Abduction of the arm or cross-body adduction increases the discomfort. With palpation, the distal clavicle feels unstable both anteroposteriorly and superoinferiorly. Typically, the patient is tender at the acromioclavicular joint as well as the coracoclavicular interspace.

Type IV Injury

Typically, the patient is in more pain than with the more common type III injury. Palpation along the clavicle will demonstrate posterior displacement of the distal clavicle through the trapezius muscle (Fig. 13). The clavicle does not have the "free floating" feel of the type III injury. Once swelling subsides, observation from above and behind the patient will demonstrate posterior displacement of the clavicle in a thin patient. Motions of the shoulder are much more painful than in the type III injury.

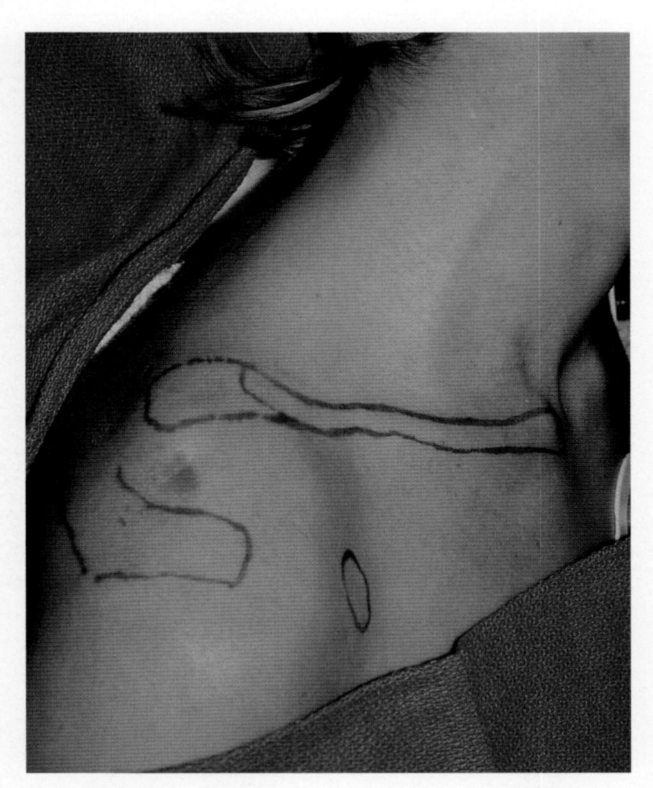

FIG. 13. Type IV injury. Clavicle and acromion outlined, with distal clavicle buttonholed through trapezius.

Type V Injury

This injury presents with findings very similar to the type III, but with more displacement of the clavicle (Fig. 14). This generally has more of the "ear tickler" presentation, owing to the more extensive injury to the deltoid and trapezial fascia. Typically, the patient is in more pain than with a type III. The skin is severely tented and it appears that the clavicle may protrude through it.

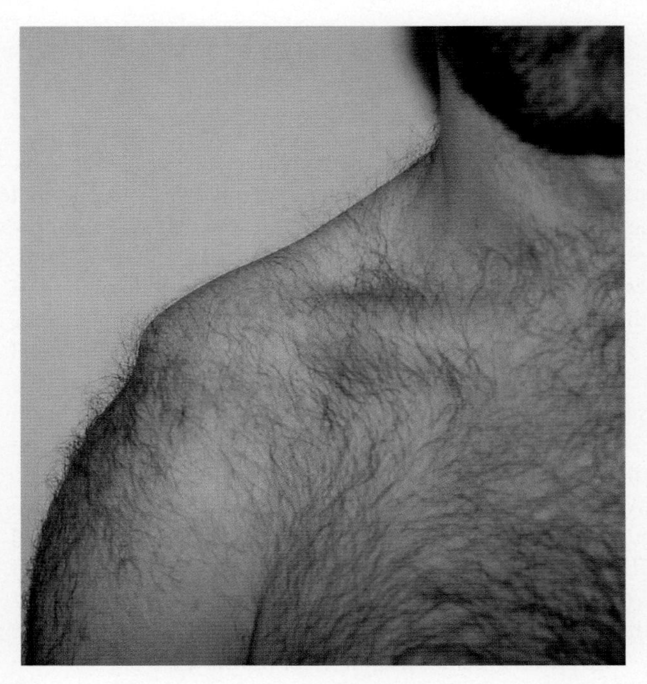

FIG. 12. Type III injury. Prominence of the distal clavicle accountable to the downward sag of the shoulder.

Type VI Injury

With this injury, the superior aspect of the shoulder appears flatter because of the downward displacement of the clavicle. The acromion is more prominent and palpable with a stepdown or depression over the distal clavicle. This rare injury may also present with neurologic changes because of proximity to the upper roots of the brachial plexus. Because of the severity of the injury, associated injuries should be suspected, including fractures of the ribs, pneumothorax, and sternoclavicular joint injuries.

Radiography

Standard anteroposterior radiography of the shoulder joint overpenetrates the acromioclavicular joint and makes interpretation difficult. An anteroposterior acromioclavicualar joint radiograph as well as a 15-degree—cephalic tilt view (Zanca) are recommended to evaluate the acromioclavicular joint.[88] The superior tilt of the Zanca view makes sure the spine of the scapula is not superimposed on the acromio-

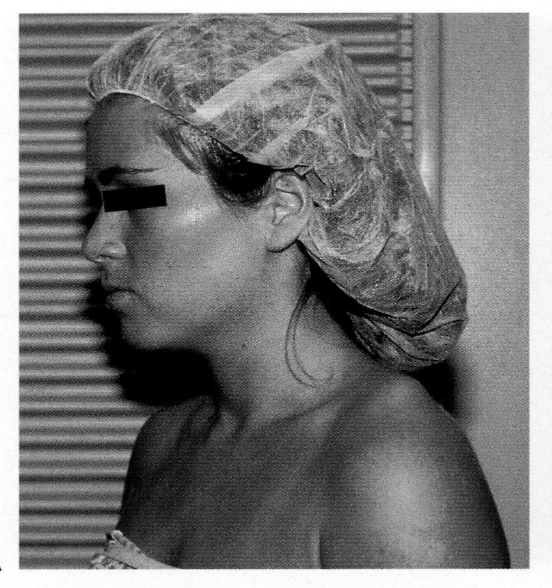
A

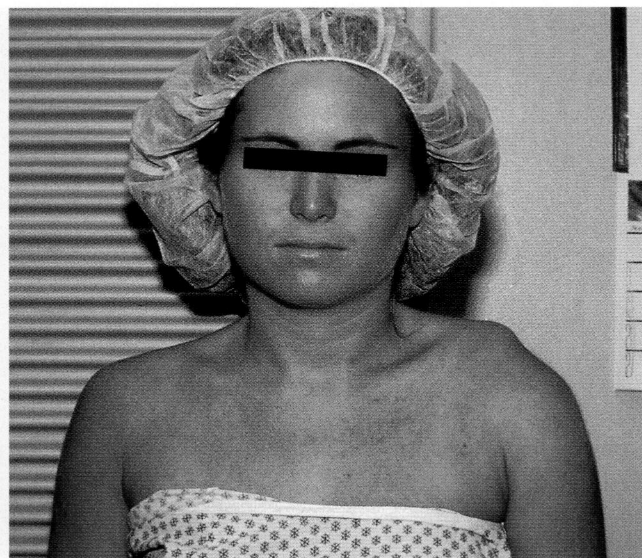
B

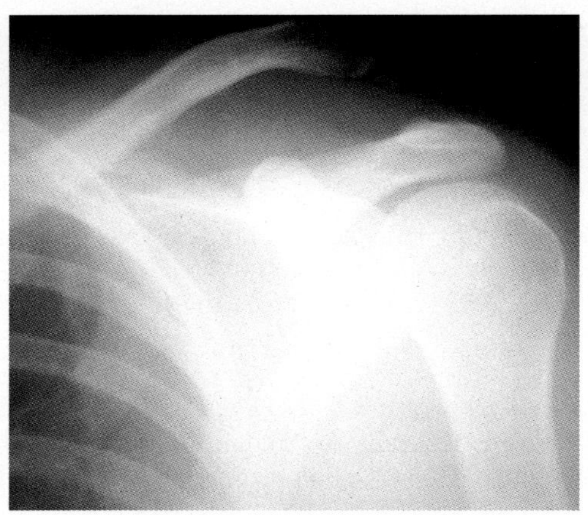
C

FIG. 14. (A,B) Clinical photograph, **(C)** and AP nonstress radiograph of the shoulder demonstrating the typical appearance of a type V acromioclavicular separation.

clavicular joint. Thus subtle fractures of the distal clavicle will not be missed. Axillary lateral view radiographs are also useful to evaluate the position of the clavicle relative to the acromion. This is particularly useful in the evaluation of type IV acromioclavicular joint injuries.

Alexander described the scapular lateral radiograph as a technique to evaluate acromioclavicular joint injuries.[1] In this view, a comparison superolateral radiograph is taken with the shoulders protracted forward. In the normal shoulder, the integrity of the acromioclavicular joint is maintained. With an acromioclavicular joint dislocation, the distal clavicle displaces superiorly to the acromion (Fig. 15).

Stress or weighted radiographs have been recommended in the past to differentiate type II from type III acromioclavicular injuries. These radiographs, with the patient seated or standing with weights (15 lb) strapped to the wrists, will accentuate the difference between the normal and injured shoulder (Fig. 16). Typically, a large 14 ×17-in. cassette is used to visualize both shoulders on the single plate. A comparison of the coracoclavicular space between the normal and injured shoulder is made. In large individuals, two separate plates may be required. A difference of 25% to 40% increase in space is felt to be significant for full disruption of the coracoclavicular ligaments.[6,69] It is important to have the patient relax or muscle forces may lift the arm superiorly and reduce the injured joint, distorting the interpretation. The same may occur if the patient is asked to hold the weights in their hands. The importance of these views is dependent on their use as a prognostic factor in treatment of these injuries. With the tendency to nonsurgical treatment of type III injuries, stress radiographic differentiation between type II and III injuries becomes clinically irrelevant. Others have noted low clinical yield as a reason to discourage use of stress radiographs.[11]

Our current recommendation for routine assessment of the acromioclavicular joint radiographically is an anteroposterior or Zanca view, along with an axillary lateral view.

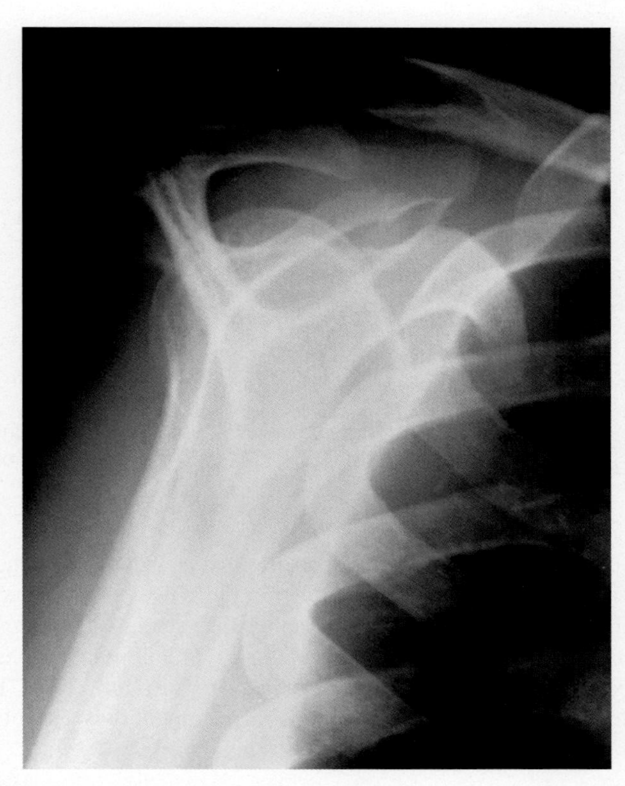

FIG. 15. Alexander scapular lateral view with complete acromioclavicular joint dislocation.

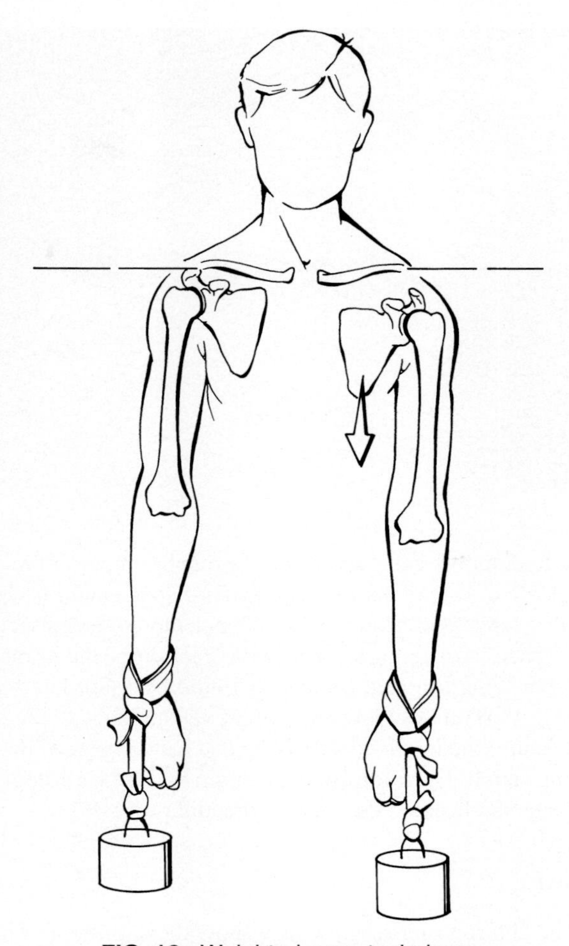

FIG. 16. Weighted x-ray technique.

Radiographic Findings

Type I

Typically these radiographs are essentially normal when compared with the uninvolved shoulder. Radiographs years later may display degenerative changes at the acromioclavicualar joint (Figs. 17 and 18).

Type II

Radiographic findings display slight widening of the acromioclavicular joint when compared with the normal side. Even with stress radiographs, the coracoclavicular space is maintained.

Type III

The joint is totally displaced on the anteroposterior radiograph compared with normal (Fig. 19). The axillary view

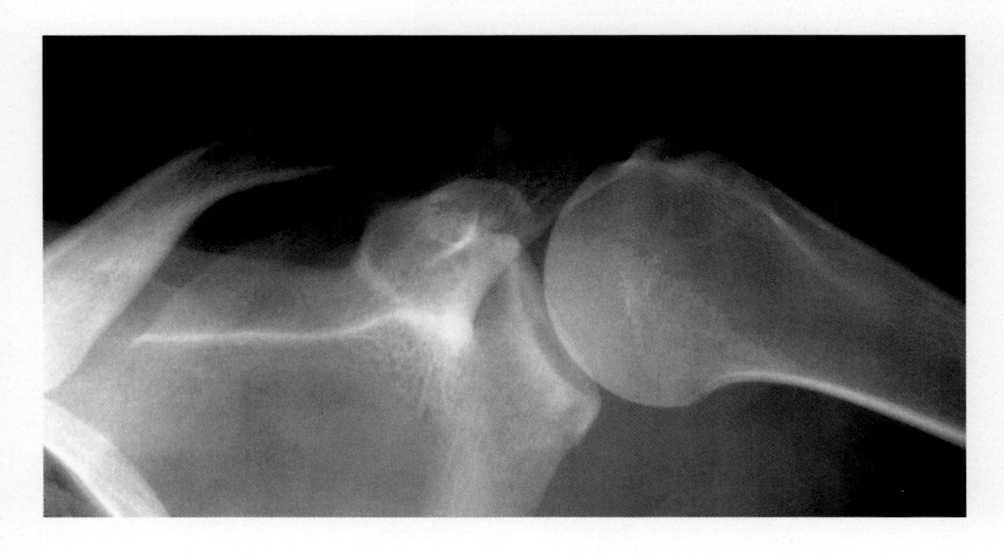

FIG. 17. Radiograph of acromioclavicular joint at time of Type I injury.

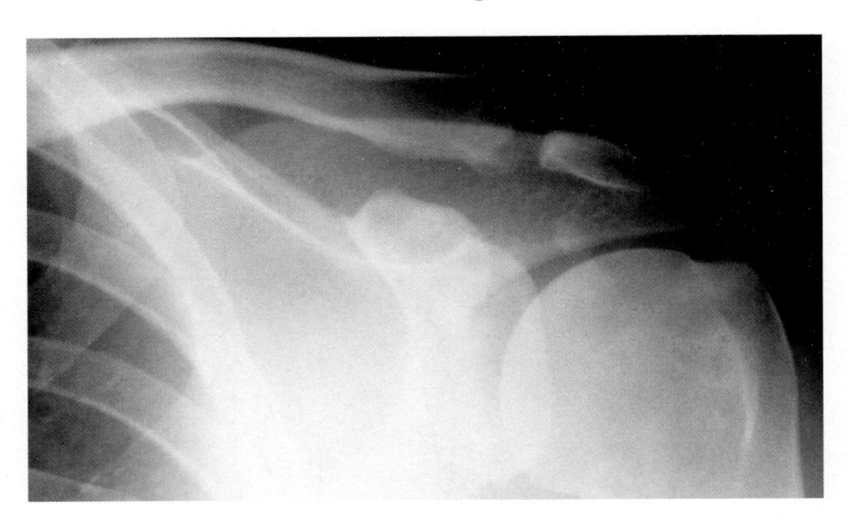

FIG. 18. Radiograph of acromioclavicular joint 10 years after Type I injury. Note irregularity of distal clavicle.

fails to demonstrate anteroposterior displacement of the distal clavicle. If total acromioclavicular displacement is noted on the anteroposterior radiograph but the coracoclavicular interspace is maintained, suspect a fracture of the coracoid process. This can best be demonstrated by a Stryker notch view.[37,70] With this view, the patient lies supine with the cassette under the involved shoulder. The hand is placed on top of the head. The radiographic beam is tilted 10 degrees cephalad and centered over the coracoid process.

Type IV

The anteroposterior view may show displacement of both the acromioclavicular joint and the coracoclavicular interspace. On the axillary view, posterior displacement of the distal clavicle in relation to the acromion is most pronounced (Fig. 20). A computed tomography (CT) scan may be warranted in heavy individuals or in those with multiple injuries that make the axillary lateral radiograph difficult. The CT scan may also be used in persons for whom there is a suspicion of associated glenoid fractures.

Type V

These injuries display gross displacement of the acromioclavicular and coracoclavicular space. The coracoclavicular space may be two to three times wider than normal (Fig. 21).

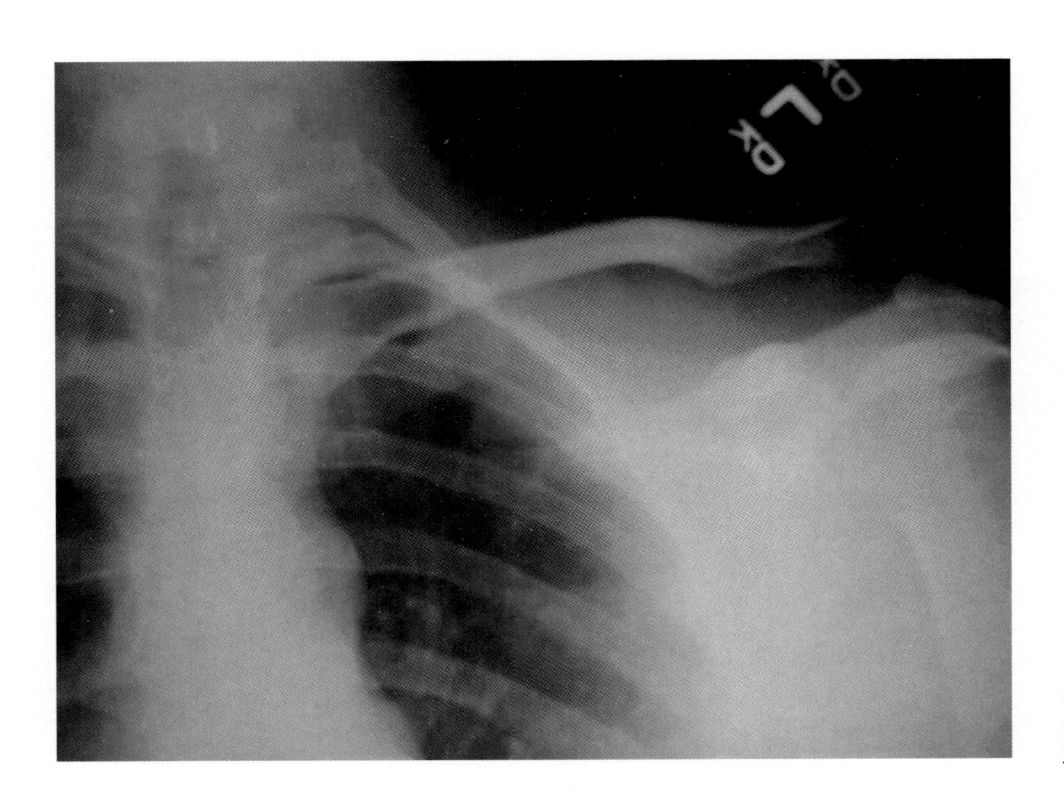

FIG. 19. Complete displacement of the acromioclavicular joint.

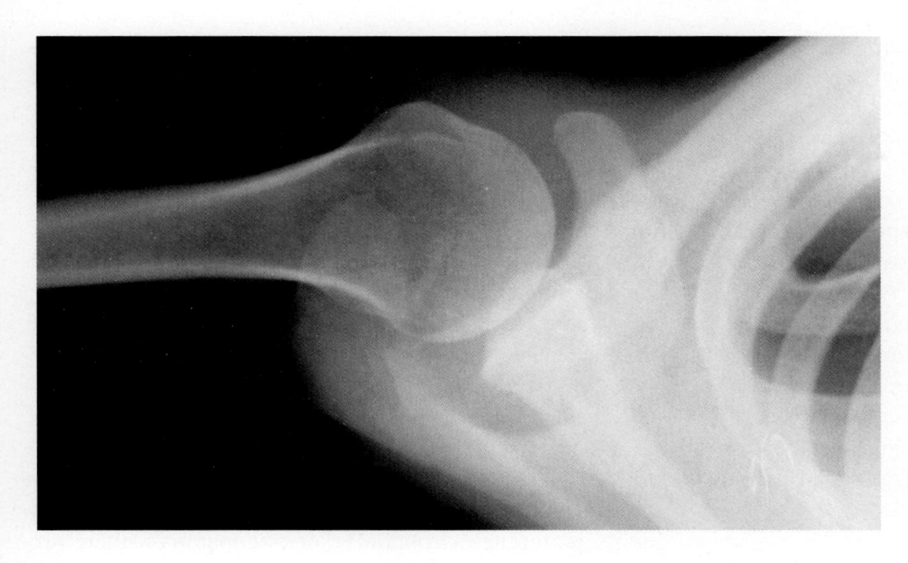

FIG. 20. Axillary radiograph demonstrating posterior displacement of the distal clavicle in relation to the acromion.

Type VI

On the anteroposterior view, the clavicle will be displaced inferior to the acromion or coracoid. Because of the magnitude of force required to produce this injury, associated fractures of the ribs or scapula should be sought.

Treatment

Although the treatment of type III acromioclavicular joint injuries remains controversial, prospective studies comparing nonoperative and surgical treatment of these injuries have yielded similar satisfactory results.[4,17,77] Thus the pendulum of care is swinging toward the initial conservative care of these patients. Not all patients, however, do well with conservative care. Guidelines for care at this time are not fixed and are frequently dictated by the patient's desires and goals as well as the surgeon's experience. Some authors who generally favor the conservative treatment of these injuries may recommend surgical repair in patients involved in heavy labor or overhead sports.[4,17,23,77,84,86] One study, though, demonstrated little effect on athletic strength or performance with acromioclavicular dislocation.[79] Questions still remain whether complete dislocation of the acromioclavicular joint affects performance of the overhead laborer or throwing athlete, or whether surgical procedures can fully restore normal anatomy and function.

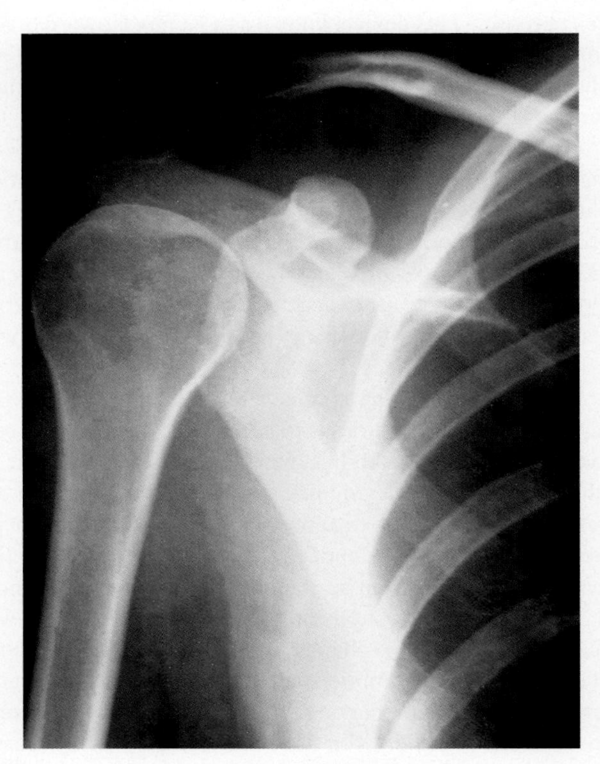

FIG. 21. Type V injury. Note gross displacement of acromioclavicular and coracoclavicular spine.

Treatment Recommendations

Type I: Acute

Type I sprains of the acromioclavicular joint are treated conservatively by all. Analgesic medications and a sling are used for the patient's comfort. Cryotherapy, for periods no longer than 15 to 20 minutes, is used to reduce swelling. Local wound care may be necessary to treat the abrasions that are frequently seen with these injuries. Early active range of motion and exercise to promote return to activity are recommended. Most active individuals, along with athletes, will return to their desired activity in 2 to 14 days. Athletes involved in contact sports, such as football, can modify their shoulder pads along with using protective cutout pads that reduce contact to the joint.

Type I: Chronic

Degenerative changes at the acromioclavicular joint in athletes are frequently the result of old type I and II acromioclavicular joint sprains.[8] Damage to the meniscus and articular cartilage with an acute injury can lead to degenerative changes later in life. Pain caused by degenerative changes at the acromioclavicular joint secondary to type I sprains can be treated with mild analgesics, nonsteroidal antiinflammatory medications, or intraarticular injections of corticosteroid preparations. Those who do not respond to conservative care may require resection of the distal clavicle to provide relief of symptoms. This can be performed with the use of an arthroscopic or open surgical approach.[29,33,34,36,56,76] The technique used depends on the surgeon's preference and experience. A potential advantage to the arthroscopic technique is the requirement for less resection of the distal clavicle (5 to 7 mm), because of the preservation of part of the capsular ligament.[29] Return to activity and athletic competition after clavicle resection is dictated by wound healing and restoration of motion, strength, and comfort.

Type II: Acute

Acute type II injuries are treated in a manner similar to the type I acute sprains: a sling, analgesic use, and icing per the patient's comfort. The potential for intraarticular damage and degenerative damage may be enhanced by the increase in sagittal plane motion of the acromioclavicular joint. Some physicians may use a sling or harness for longer periods to preclude conversion to a type III injury. Return to activity is predicted by restoration of motion, comfort, and strength.

Type II: Chronic

In patients with pain and degenerative change of the acromioclavicular joint, the treatment recommended is similar to type I injuries. Analgesic medications, nonsteroidals, and injections with corticosteroid medications seldom offer long-term relief. An evaluation of patients after isolated resection of the distal clavicle has noted some poor results attributed to abutment of the posterior clavicle on the acromion. Symptomatic type II acromioclavicular joint injuries can be treated as type III injuries, with resection of the distal clavicle along with reconstruction of the ligamentous structures. Typical reconstruction involves transferring the coracoacromial ligament to the resected distal clavicle.[83] This enhances superior-inferior stability of the joint, but provides little anteroposterior stability. Imbrication of the periosteum and deltotrapezial fascia overlying the resected clavicle may be necessary to enhance anteroposterior stability.

Type III Injuries

The trend in the treatment of these injuries is toward a more conservative approach. A distinct advantage of surgical treatment over conservative care has never been clearly demonstrated. When considering a surgical approach to treatment, the surgeon must ask himself or herself whether today's surgical options truly restore the anatomy and function of the acromioclavicular joint. We conducted an informal survey of physicians involved in the care of professional athletes involved in the sports of football, hockey, and baseball and found the majority favor a nonoperative approach for most athletes. However, these physicians would consider operative reduction for the throwing athlete's dominant extremity, particularly the baseball pitcher. Quarterbacks throw with a less specific motion and generally do not fall into the same consideration.

For those electing a surgical reconstruction, the timing of the repair may be an issue. One might consider delaying the operation to see if the patient remains symptomatic. Weinstein et al., however, noted a trend toward better results when the surgery was performed in the first 3 weeks after injury.[84] Others have found no significant difference between early and late ligamentous reconstruction.[23] Whether the surgeon's preference is operative or nonoperative, there are those who will require surgical reconstructions after the failure of conservative care.

Nonoperative care. Nonoperative care of type III acromioclavicular joint injuries is similar to that for type I and II sprains. Analgesia, icing, and a sling for comfort are also used. Because of the pain and deformity, it is unlikely the individual will return to heavy labor or athletic activity as soon as after a type I or II injury. Professional football or hockey players, though, will frequently return to their sport within a few days to weeks.

Correction of the deformity by a brace or cast has recently fallen into disfavor. Kenny Howard, a trainer at Auburn University, along with Dr. Jack Hughston, developed a brace for this purpose.[3] This device, known as a Kenny Howard brace, combines a sling with a strap over the distal clavicle that applies downward pressure on the clavicle while providing a superior force on the humerus (Fig. 22). To be effective, the brace must be worn continuously for 6 to 8 weeks while healing occurs. Any displacement of the brace during this period will lead to loss of reduction and subsequent failure. The brace can be quite cumbersome to wear and even painful. Skin maceration and breakdown is a risk, and there is even a report of an athlete who sustained an anterior interosseous nerve compression while using the sling.[63] The trend is away from using these devices.

Surgical options. Our approach to the treatment of type III acromioclavicualar injuries is to treat these injuries nonoperatively, with surgical stabilization being considered only if an athlete or laborer places significant demands on the upper extremity. If conservative treatment fails, stabilization is considered later in those who continue to note symptoms with activity. Excellent results can be obtained with late reconstruction.

Various surgical options have been described. They will be detailed later in this chapter, along with the pros and cons of each option. These options include dynamic muscle transfers, primary acromioclavicular joint fixation, primary coracoclavicular ligament fixation, and excision of the distal clavicle with or without coracoclavicular ligament reconstruction.

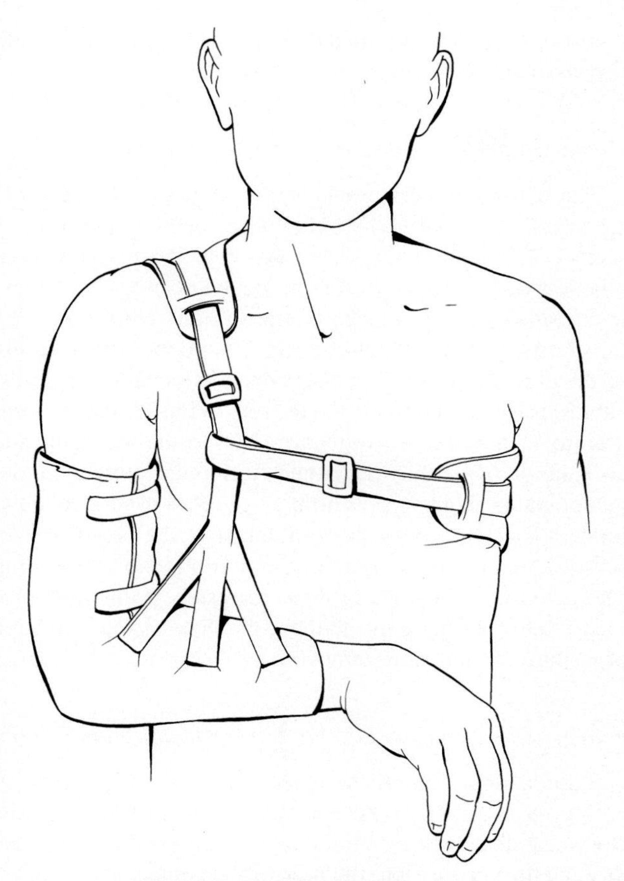

FIG. 22. Kenny Howard brace.

Type IV Injuries

We agree with most authors that posterior displacement of the clavicle through the trapezius will lead to discomfort with motion. Thus these injuries should be treated with the goal of reducing the deformity. Options include an attempt at closed reduction to displace the clavicle from its buttonholed position in the trapezius, and converting the injury to a type III and then treating it conservatively. The most common recommendation would be open reduction and fixation by one of the surgical options outlined with type III injuries. Our recommendation would be to reduce the joint operatively because the displacement involves significant stripping of the deltotrapezial fascia. Meticulous closing of the deltotrapezial fascia over the repair augments the procedure.

Type V Injuries

Type V injuries require operative reduction because of the significant stripping of deltotrapezial fascia and potential compromise of the overlying skin. Our preference is to excise the distal clavicle and reconstruct the coracoclavicular ligaments with the coracoacromial ligament. Again, meticulous repair of the deltotrapezial fascia will augment the repair. We favor excision of the distal clavicle because of the concern for later degenerative changes at the acromioclavicular joint and the potential for discomfort or rotator cuff impingement. Excision of the distal clavicle has not been shown to compromise muscle strength.[79]

Type VI Injuries

The potential for closed reduction of such an injury is remote. These are rare injuries that require open reduction and stabilization. Excision of the distal clavicle will aid in the reduction of the acromioclavicular joint.[35]

Injuries in Children

Type I, II, and III injuries in children are treated similarly to those in adults. Use of a sling, ice, and mild analgesics are all that are required. These injuries can be expected to go on and heal without sequelae.[25,38] Markedly displaced type IV, V, and VI injuries should be treated surgically. Replacement of the clavicle into its periosteal sleeve, suturing the sleeve closed, and then fixation with a coracoclavicular lag screw or transacromial fixation are generally recommended.[19,64] After 4 to 6 weeks the fixation will have to be removed before starting rehabilitation.

Type III Equivalent Injuries

A fractured coracoid along with an acromioclavicular dislocation is an exceedingly rare injury. It is easy to overlook the coracoid fracture, particularly in light of the more obvious acromioclavicular joint disruption. Most occur in the second or third decade of life. Review of the literature would indicate these injuries do well when treated conservatively or surgically. Thus we would recommend a conservative approach and avoid potential complications of surgery.[9,40]

Surgical Treatment of Acute Acromioclavicular Joint Dislocations

Indications

Mild acute acromioclavicular joint injuries (types I and II) are not associated with joint instability and have been successfully managed conservatively. Surgical management may be considered for acute acromioclavicular joint dislocations (types III, IV, V, and VI). A popular management approach to acute type III acromioclavicular joint dislocations has been to initially manage most of them nonoperatively. Surgery is discussed as a salvage for late symptoms of pain, clicking, or instability. When a type III acromioclavicular joint dislocation occurs in the dominant arm of a laborer or a throwing athlete, surgery may be considered initially. Historically, this approach has been justified, owing to concerns about shoulder girdle strength in acromioclavicular joint dislocations that are not reduced. Recent studies have not supported this theory. Typically, involved shoulder strength has been equivalent to the uninjured arm, or similar to that of patients who have undergone surgical repair.[49,79,82] Studies that have evaluated function in groups of patients treated operatively and nonoperatively have also shown little difference in outcome.[41,47,77]

A variety of surgical approaches have been described to manage these injuries and restore the anatomic relations of the acromioclavicular joint.[4,23,47,77,84] The question remains whether these techniques are effective at restoring normal functional anatomy and, therefore, offer any distinct advantage over a conservative approach.

Surgical Options

Many different operative procedures have been described to repair and stabilize acute acromioclavicular dislocations (type III, IV, V, and VI). The most popular options include dynamic muscle transfers, primary acromioclavicular joint stabilization, primary coracoclavicular and extraarticular stabilization, and excision of the distal clavicle with coracoacromial ligament reconstruction. The goal of each of these procedures is to reduce the joint and create an environment for soft-tissue healing and stabilization of the distal clavicle.

Dynamic Muscle Transfers

The clavicle may be stabilized by transfer of the tip of the coracoid process and its attached tendons of the coracobrachialis and short head of the biceps to the undersurface of the clavicle.[10,27,74] Theoretically, this transferred tendon acts as a dynamic depressor of the clavicle and holds the acromioclavicular joint reduced. Ferris et al. reviewed 20 patients managed with a dynamic transfer and found nearly half with continued aching at the acromioclavicular joint.[27] These results are most likely due to the lack of distal clavicle stability and excessive motion. Possible complications of this surgical procedure include the risks of nonunion or injury to the musculocutaneous nerve.

Primary Acromioclavicular Joint Stabilization

The dislocated acromioclavicular joint can be stabilized by transfixing it with Kirschner wires or Steinman pins or screws. This treatment typically has been performed in conjunction with repair of the acromioclavicular or coracoclavicular ligaments.[71] Technically, transfixion of this joint is demanding because of the thin acromion and the curved nature of the clavicle (Fig. 23). Other concerns include the necessity for hardware removal and the risk of pin breakage or migration.[48] In addition, surgical trauma to the meniscus and articular cartilage may occur and lead to the subsequent development of degenerative arthritis of the acromioclavicular joint.[77] There has been recent interest in the use of bioabsorbable materials to transfix the acromioclavicular joint. The potential advantage of these materials is that they provide fixation of the joint, without the necessity of a second procedure for hardware removal.

Primary Coracoclavicular and Extraarticular Stabilization

Stabilization of the distal clavicle can be achieved by securing the clavicle to the coracoid process of the scapula. Bosworth described a technique in which he placed a screw through the clavicle into the base of the coracoid (Fig. 24).[12] Initially, the screw was placed percutaneously and the acromioclavicular joint was not explored or debrided. The Bosworth screw technique is often accompanied now by joint exploration and repair of the coracoclavicular ligaments.[43,44] Repair of the deltotrapezius fascia is also accomplished during this procedure. Screw removal is typically considered between 8 and 10 weeks postoperatively. Ossifi-

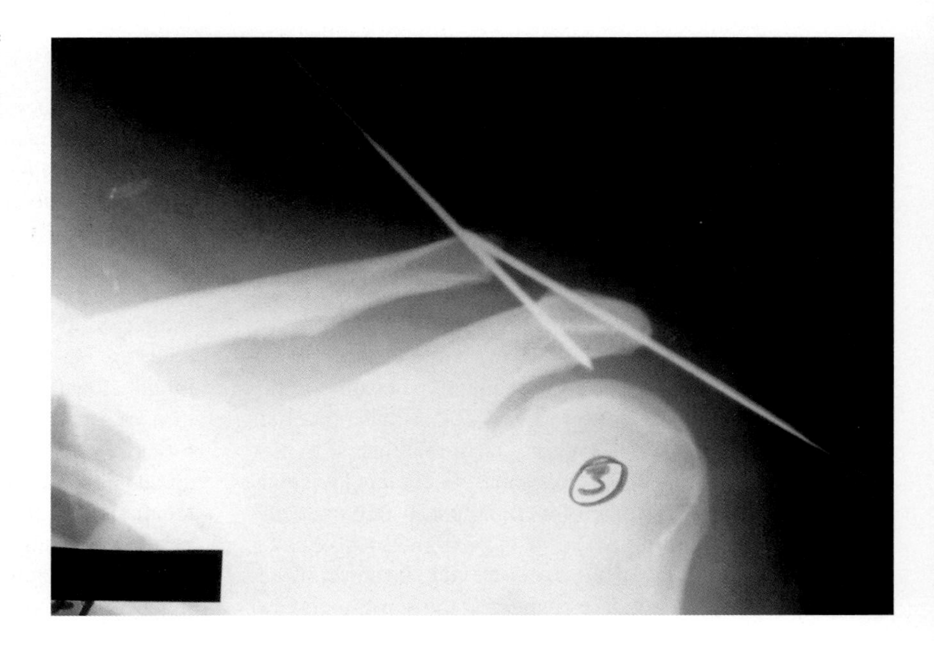

FIG. 23. Fixation failure: Transfixion of acromioclavicular joint is demanding because of the thin acromion and curvature of the clavicle.

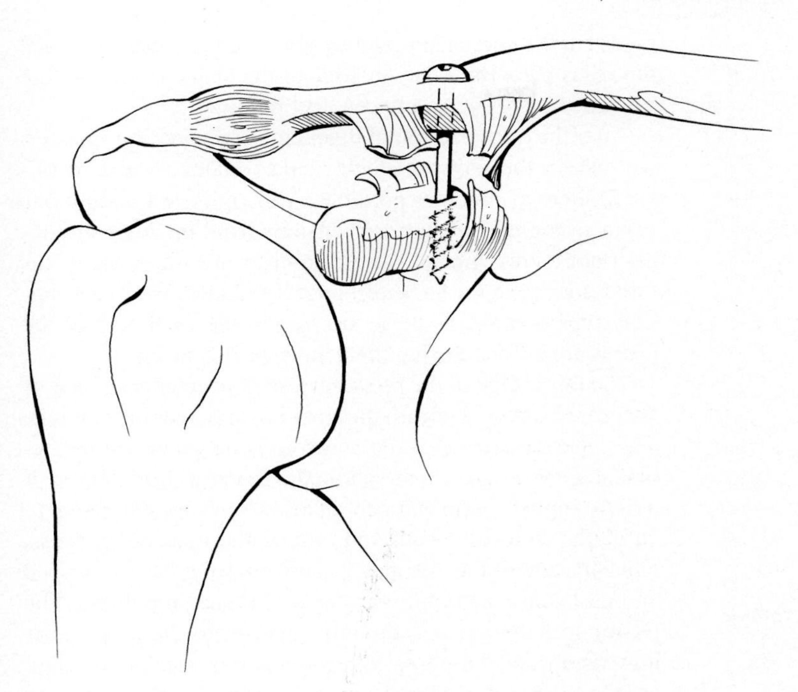

FIG. 24. Screw fixation of clavicle to base of coracoid.

cation between the coracoid and the clavicle occurs with some frequency and has not generally caused a problem with shoulder motion.[43]

Other forms of extraarticular stabilization eliminate the need for screw removal. Cerclage fixation of the clavicle to the coracoid has been accomplished using wire,[2,6] Dacron graft, or other synthetic tape,[42,58,65] and braided bioabsorbable suture. Typically, coracoclavicular fixation is accompanied by repair of the coracoclavicular ligaments, acromioclavicular joint, and deltotrapezius fascia. Use of nonabsorbable Dacron tape has been associated with erosion through the clavicle, failure of fixation,[20,32] and late infections.[61]

Accurate reduction of the acromioclavicular joint is difficult, but critical, particularly when the distal clavicle is not excised. Morrison and Lemos documented the need to accurately determine the subcoracoid and transclavicular positions of the fixation suture.[55] They determined that the loop should be placed at the base of the coracoid and then inserted through a hole at the junction of the anterior and middle third of the clavicle. They felt that if the loop is posterior or goes around the clavicle, it tends to displace the clavicle anteriorly.

Excision of the Distal Clavicle and Coracoacromial Ligament Reconstruction

In 1972, Weaver and Dunn described a technique they used to treat acute and chronic acromioclavicular joint dislocations.[83] The surgical procedure involved excision of the distal clavicle, followed by transfer of the coracoacromial ligament to the resected end of the distal clavicle. Many variations and modifications of this procedure have been used when reconstruction of the joint is performed.[14,23,84] The decision of whether to preserve or excise the distal portion of the clavicle is based on concern over the ability to completely reduce the acromioclavicular joint and the possibility for development of degenerative arthritis. In evaluating acromioclavicular joint and coracoclavicular ligament repair, Smith found no difference in symptoms, strength, or function, but did find a higher incidence of degenerative changes when the distal clavicle was not excised.[75] Symptomatic degeneration of the acromioclavicular joint has been effectively managed by excision of the distal clavicle.

Authors' Preferred Technique

Surgical management is recommended for selected type III and nearly all type IV and V acromioclavicular joint dislocations. Our preference is to stabilize the clavicle by transferring the coracoacromial ligament to the distal clavicle and supporting this repair using a braided absorbable suture over the clavicle and under the coracoid (Fig. 25). If possible, we also repair the coracoclavicular ligaments and the deltotrapezial fascia. In our opinion, the only significant surgical variable in the acute injury is deciding whether to preserve or excise the distal clavicle. We prefer its excision because of the difficulty in obtaining a perfect reduction of the acromioclavicular joint. We are concerned that the injury or incomplete reduction may lead to the development of degenerative arthritis. Pain also may occur from the degenerated joint or from inferior projecting spurs that cause mechanical impingement on the rotator cuff. No significant deficits in muscle strength were observed in athletes who have undergone excision of the distal clavicle.[79] Therefore, it may be advantageous from both a short- and long-term perspective to excise the distal clavicle as part of the reconstructive procedure.

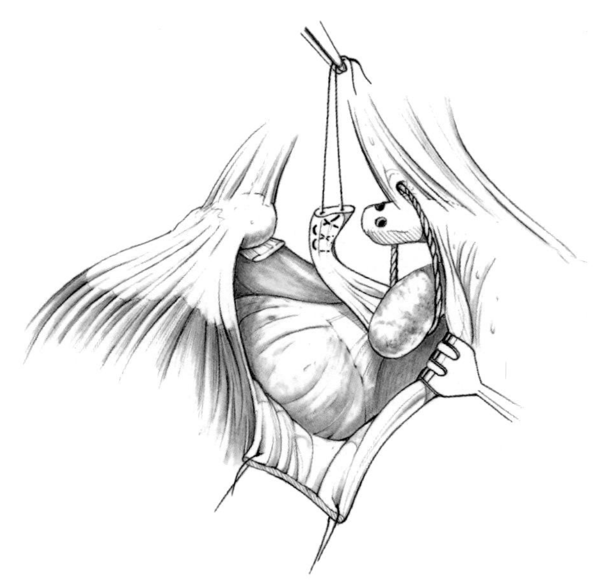

FIG. 25. Authors' preferred technique of repair of acromioclavicular joint disruption.

Patients are positioned in the beach chair position with most of the scapula and shoulder draped free. The shoulder is approached through a vertical incision from the coracoid to the posterior border of the clavicle. The incision passes approximately 2 cm medial to the acromioclavicular joint (Fig. 26A). The incision is planned and subcutaneous tissue undermined laterally so that the distal clavicle and anterior acromion can be reached. Next, the deltotrapezius fascia is incised along the clavicle using the bovie electrocautery. In type IV and V acromioclavicular joint dislocations, the deltotrapezius fascia may be disrupted, and this opening should be extended as necessary. The dissection should be performed to carefully maintain a deltoid flap for later repair (see Fig. 26B). As the incision in the fascia is carried laterally to the acromion, care is taken to dissect beneath the deltoid to expose the coracromial ligament. Once the coracoacromial ligament is completely defined, it is released from the undersurface of the acromion, with care to maximize its length. We place two independent no. 2 nonabsorbable sutures in the ligament to secure it to the distal clavicle. Typically, one suture is placed in a Bunnell fashion and the other using a Kessler-type stitch. If the coracoacromial ligament is felt to be insufficient, we add an 8- to 10-mm strip of the conjoined tendon and turn it superiorly.

At this point, the distal clavicle is exposed subperiosteally from beneath the trapezius muscle and fascia. We excise the distal 1 to 1.5 cm of the clavicle using a sagital saw. A curette is used to hollow out the intramedullary aspect of the clavicle (see Fig. 26C). A 1.6-mm–drill bit is used to create two drill holes along the superior surface of the cut end of the clavicle entering into the intramedullary canal. Looped passing sutures are then passed through each of these holes, which are used later to facilitate passage of the sutures placed in the coracoacromial ligament. Care is taken to place the holes back from the cut edge of the clavicle and provide a secure bony bridge between drill holes.

After the coracoacromial ligament is prepared for transfer, we dissect the torn coracoclavicular ligaments and reconstruct them as much as possible. Although most disruptions occur in the midsubstance, avulsions from the bone are occasionally encountered. These injuries are more easily sutured and repaired back to bone. Typically, we place tagging-type sutures, as these are tied in the final step of the procedure before closing the deltotrapezius fascia.

The third stage of the procedure involves placing a loop of absorbable suture beneath the coracoid and over the clavicle. The superior surface of the coracoid is palpated and its medial and lateral aspects are defined. We use a combination of a right-angled clamp and curved Statinsky vascular clamp to carefully dissect beneath and around the coracoid process. Once the end of the clamp is visualized, we grasp the looped end of a suture and pull it around the coracoid process. The position of the clavicle directly superior to the coracoid is now identified. This area of the clavicle is usually still covered by adherent trapezius muscle. A curved clamp is used to slip under the fascia and over the clavicle. Once exposed, a looped suture is passed around the clavicle.

The looped sutures around the clavicle and coracoid process are used to pass the suture of choice for final fixation. We have not used nonabsorbable suture or tape, owing to concerns over risks of infection and erosion through the clavicle. If available, a 5-mm tape of polydioxanonsulfate (PDS) is used; otherwise, strands of readily available no. 1 PDS are braided together. We usually braid three strands of PDS together, use two of these braids, and tie them independently (see Fig. 26D). Beginning with these coracoclavicular sutures, the three parts of this repair are secured. The knots are tied so that they end up inferior to the clavicle and do not interfere with closure of the deltotrapezius fascia. Second, the two coracoacromial ligament sutures are passed through the drill holes in the distal clavicle and tied independently. Third, the coracoclavicular ligaments are repaired as completely as possible (see Fig. 26E). Finally, the deltotrapezius fascia is carefully repaired over the clavicle. This not only covers the different parts of this reconstruction, but also reinforces and supports the repair.

Postoperatively, the arm is supported in a sling for 2 weeks. Motion exercises, including pendulums and gentle active elevation, then are begun. Progressive range of motion and strengthening exercises are not begun until 6 weeks after surgery. Heavy weight lifting, pushing, pulling, and other stressful activities are delayed until 3 months, and contact sports are allowed at 5 to 6 months.

Results

A careful review of the literature fails to demonstrate a clear choice from among the many different procedures, modifications, and combinations that have been described.

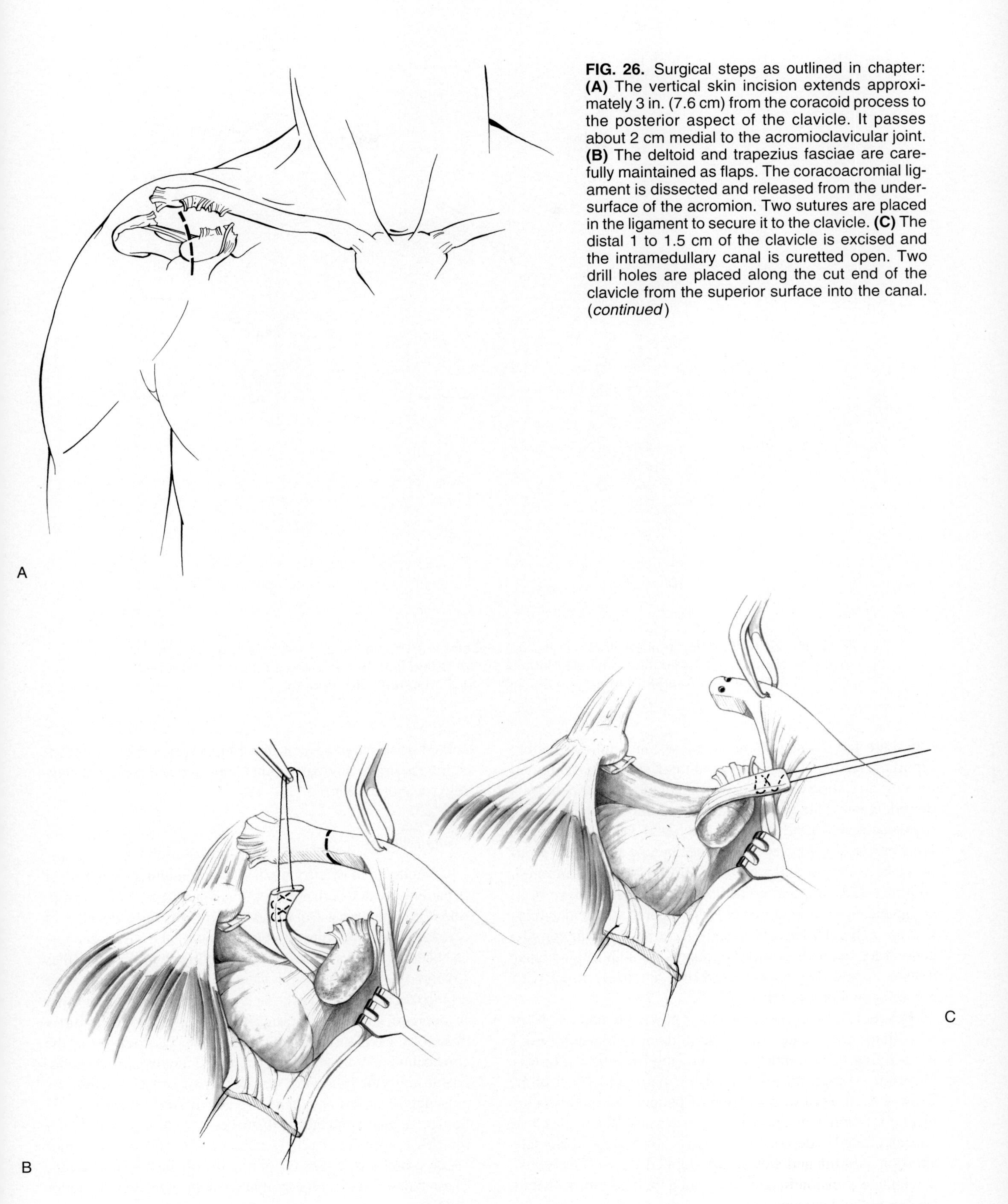

FIG. 26. Surgical steps as outlined in chapter: **(A)** The vertical skin incision extends approximately 3 in. (7.6 cm) from the coracoid process to the posterior aspect of the clavicle. It passes about 2 cm medial to the acromioclavicular joint. **(B)** The deltoid and trapezius fasciae are carefully maintained as flaps. The coracoacromial ligament is dissected and released from the undersurface of the acromion. Two sutures are placed in the ligament to secure it to the clavicle. **(C)** The distal 1 to 1.5 cm of the clavicle is excised and the intramedullary canal is curetted open. Two drill holes are placed along the cut end of the clavicle from the superior surface into the canal. (*continued*)

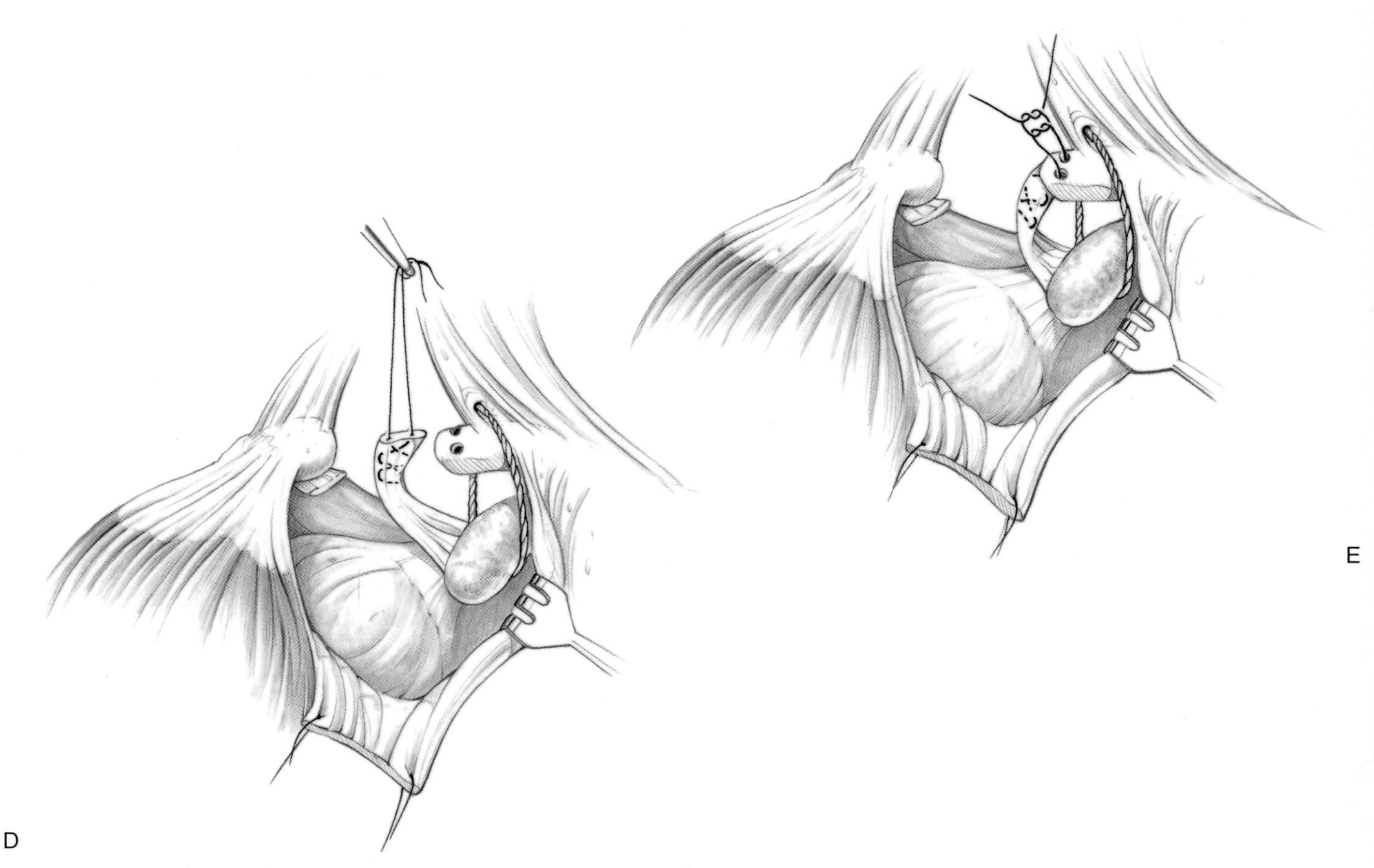

FIG. 26. *Continued* **(D)** Braided PDS sutures are placed beneath the base of the coracoid process and over the clavicle. **(E)** The coracoclavicular loop of suture is tied first. Second, the sutures from the coracoacromial ligament are tied. Finally, the coracoclavicular ligaments are repaired.

There are few comparison studies, as most authors merely report the results of a given procedure. Kennedy has reported on a modification of the Bosworth technique that includes a debridement of the acromioclavicular joint and repair of the trapezius and deltoid fascia.[44] He found that even when a bony bridge developed between the clavicle and the coracoid process, function and range of motion were maintained. Acromioclavicular and coracoclavicular fixation have been compared in several studies.[5,46,75,77] Coracoclavicular fixation has generally been favored because of its lower complication rate and overall superior results. In addition, a higher degree of late degenerative arthritis has been noted with acromioclavicular fixation.[75,77]

Weaver and Dunn described their procedure and results in 12 patients with acute type III acromioclavicular injuries.[83] Rauschning et al. reported similar good results using this procedure, based on joint stability, pain, and function.[67] Browne et al. reviewed a group of patients with coracoclavicular fixation, with and without resection of the distal clavicle, and failed to demonstrate an advantage to distal clavicle excision.[14] Smith and Stewart also looked at the effect of distal clavicle excision in patients treated with acromioclavicular fixation and coracoclavicular ligament repair.[75] They observed good results except for a higher incidence of degenerative acromioclavicular joint changes when the distal clavicle was not excised.

Complications

Complications of acromioclavicular joint injuries can occur in patients treated both nonoperatively and operatively. Symptomatic degenerative changes occur with mild degrees of acromioclavicular injury.[18] Osteolysis of the distal clavicle has been reported as a posttraumatic condition,[50,57] as well as a pathologic process seen in weight-lifting athletes who have no recollection of injury to the shoulder.[15] Pain that does not respond to conservative measures is usually successfully treated by excision of the distal clavicle. Ossification in the coracoclavicular interval may occur after coracoclavicular ligament injury or following surgical repair or stabilization. Its presence does not appear to affect outcome or results.[53,85] Some patients with chronic displaced acromioclavicular joint injuries complain of arm weakness, paresthesias, or other vague symptoms suggestive of traction on the brachial plexus. These thoracic outlet type symptoms may be related to inferior position of the shoulder girdle relative to the thorax.

The surgical treatment of these injuries is associated with a significant number of possible problems. Most common may be the persistence or recurrence of a mild prominence or deformity that is often asymptomatic. Fixation failure with complete recurrence often will require a revision procedure. The use of hardware has been associated with breakage, migration, and fixation failure.[16] Kirschner wires and Steinman pins have migrated from the acromioclavicular joint to dangerous locations, such as the lung,[24,51] spinal cord,[60] and the neck.[48] Erosion of the clavicle by wire or nonabsorbable suture used in coracoclavicular fixation has also been observed with some frequency.[42,58,65]

Chronic Acromioclavicular Dislocation

Indications

Patients with type I and II acromioclavicular joint injuries may develop degenerative changes and related pain and disability over time.[18,50,57] Conservative management involves avoidance of provocative arm positions, use of nonsteroidal medications, and steroid injections into the acromioclavicular joint. Surgery is indicated when symptoms persist. Patients who have symptoms from a chronic acromioclavicular joint dislocation (type III, IV, or V) may also consider surgery. In these acromioclavicular joint dislocations, symptoms are often related to soft-tissue pain from increased mobility of the distal clavicle.

Surgical Options

The surgical options that are considered for chronic acromioclavicular joint dislocations include distal clavicle excision and coracoclavicular stabilization. There is general agreement that excision of the distal clavicle is an effective procedure for patients with pain from a degenerated acromioclavicular joint related to prior type I and some type II injuries.[56,79] Surgical excision can be accomplished using either open or arthroscopic techniques. Some type II injuries with excision of the distal clavicle alone may remain symptomatic, owing to impingement of the resected clavicle on the posterior acromion. This is related to residual anteroposterior instability of the clavicle. These injuries require stablization of the distal clavicle to prevent these symptoms. Ideally, a procedure that addresses anteroposterior instability would suffice to eliminate these symptoms. In patients with chronic acromioclavicular dislocations (type III, IV, and V), simple excision is not sufficient to predictably eliminate symptoms. Because of the prominence and mobility of the clavicle, a coracoclavicular stabilization procedure is recommended for symptomatic patients with these injuries.

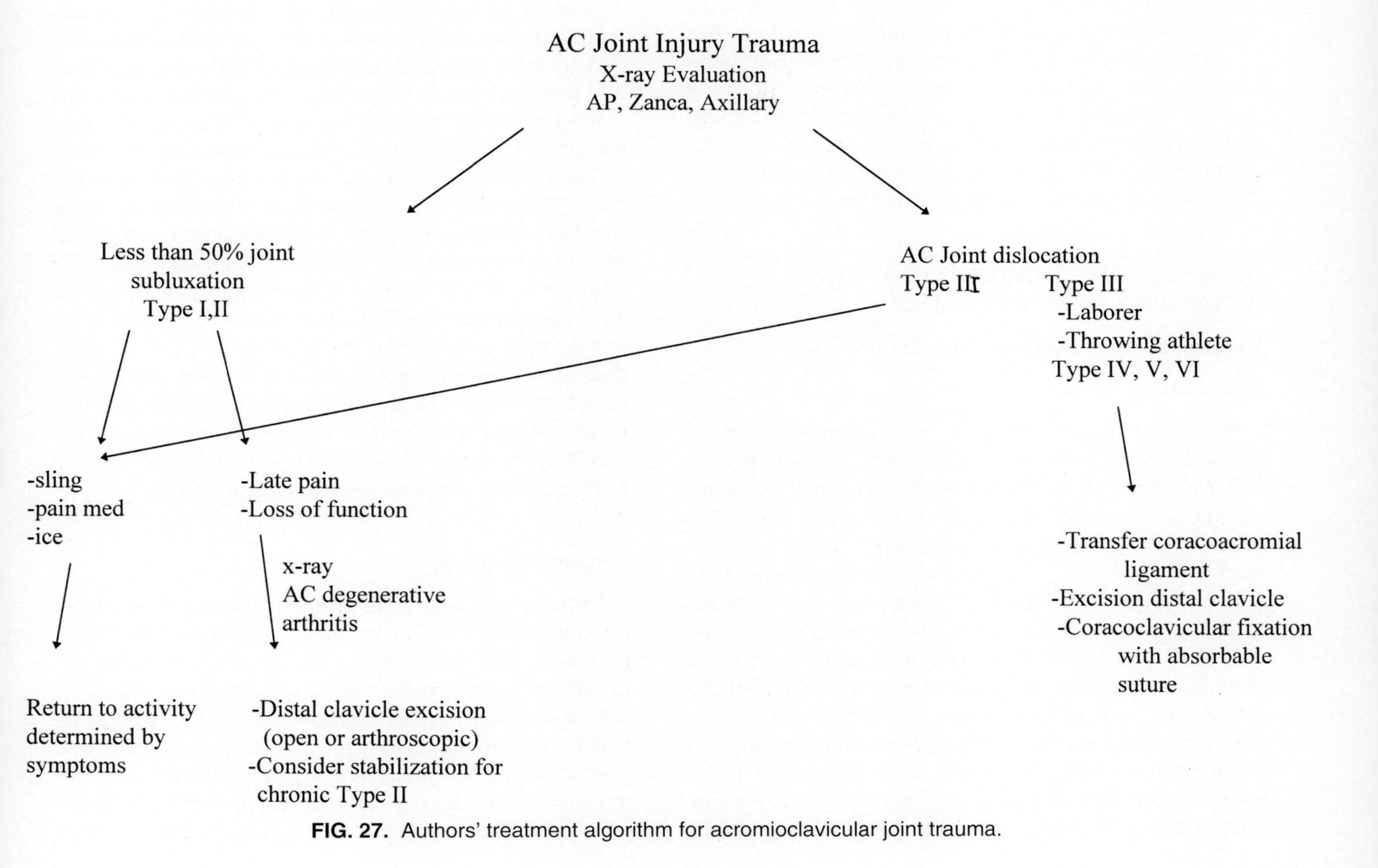

FIG. 27. Authors' treatment algorithm for acromioclavicular joint trauma.

Many of the surgical procedures discussed for acute acromioclavicular joint dislocations are also considered for chronic injuries. Transfer of the tip of the coracoid process has been used to achieve "dynamic" stability of the distal clavicle.[10,22] Weaver and Dunn initially reported their procedure, which transferred the coracoacromial ligament to the end of the clavicle for both acute and chronic acromioclavicular joint injuries.[83] Today, modifications of their original technique are among the most popular and effective surgeries for chronic acromioclavicular dislocations.[14,59,67,75] In most procedures, the coracoacromial ligament transfer is backed up with suture fixation of the coracoid to the clavicle. Other procedures combine excision of the distal clavicle and transfer of the coracoacromial ligament to the distal clavicle, which is held reduced by a coracoclavicular screw.

Authors' Preferred Technique

Excision of the distal clavicle for posttraumatic degeneration of the acromioclavicular joint can be accomplished using open or arthroscopic techniques. Details of our arthroscopic technique are described in the section on degenerative conditions of the acromioclavicular joint. Chronic acromioclavicular joint dislocations (type III, IV, and V) are usually treated by reconstruction of the coracoclavicular ligaments. Our procedure of choice is essentially the same as that described for acute acromioclavicular joint dislocations (Fig. 26). The components of the procedure include excision of the distal clavicle, transfer of the coracoacromial ligament from the acromion into the end of the distal clavicle, and temporary support for the healing ligament using absorbable suture to secure the clavicle to the coracoid process. Figure 27 outlines the authors' treatment algorithm.

DEGENERATIVE CONDITIONS OF THE ACROMIOCLAVICULAR JOINT

Degenerative and Posttraumatic Arthropathy

Presentation

Patients who have degenerative or posttraumatic arthropathy of the acromioclavicular joint most commonly present with pain. The pain may be localized to the top of the shoulder and the area of the acomioclavicular joint, but it may also be referred to the area of the upper arm. Typical impingement-type symptoms occur with abduction and overhead positions. Weight lifts, including bench press, incline press, and abduction exercises, frequently generate symptoms. Pain also occurs with crossed-body arm positions. Patients often have night pain and pain when lying on the involved side. A history of previous injury to the shoulder and the patient's diagnosis, treatment, and recovery should be elicited. Some patients notice prominence of the acromioclavicular joint and may have clicking or catching in the area. Patients with acromioclavicular joint arthropathy may be symptomatic from motion of the arthritic joint, or outlet impingement from inferior projecting spurs may cause typical rotator cuff type symptoms. A careful physical examination and radiographic evaluation are useful to determine the degree of acromioclavicular joint involvement and subacromial impingement.

Evaluation

A thorough examination is performed to evaluate the shoulder for all possible pathologies. Visual inspection may reveal asymmetry and a prominence of the acromioclavicular joint. There is asymmetrical point tenderness over the joint, which may be accentuated by horizontal crossed-body adduction. This test is sensitive, but not specific, as it may elicit pain in patients with impingement from subacromial pathology. Acromioclavicular joint stability is assessed by grasping the distal end of the clavicle between the thumb and index finger and translating the clavicle anteroposterior and superoinferior, while the other hand stabilizes the acromion. Glenohumeral stability is also evaluated with typical apprehension, relocation, and translation tests. A careful neurologic examination should determine whether there is any possible brachial plexus involvement. Selective injection of lidocaine into the acromioclavicular joint frequently helps confirm that the joint is the cause of the symptoms. Response to injection of the subacromial space may also provide useful information on the presence of rotator cuff impingement.

A complete radiographic evaluation of the acromioclavicular joint includes standard AP and coracoacromial outlet ("Y") views. The outlet view is critical to accurately asess the anatomy of the anterior acromion and the degree of outlet impingement. Because the acromioclavicular joint is frequently difficult to assess on standard AP radiographs of the shoulder owing to overpenetration, one-third less penetration is often recommended. A 15-degree–cephalic tilt (Zanca) view gives a better, unobstructed view of the acromioclavicular joint.[88] Axillary views help evaluate the anteroposterior position of the distal clavicle and the presence of an os acromion. On occasion, a bone scan may be useful to localize shoulder pathology to the acromioclavicular joint. Magnetic resonance imaging is more useful in determining the degree of acromioclavicular joint degeneration and the effect it may have impinging on the rotator cuff.

Nonoperative Treatment

Patients who have pain primarily from a degenerated acromioclavicular joint have the best chance of responding to conservative management. Those who have symptoms that appear to be secondary to the effect of narrowing of the subacromial space from acromioclavicular joint spurring may have more refractory pain. We begin all patients who have no contraindications on a regime of nonsteroidal anti-inflammatory medications and may continue them for weeks or months. They are counseled to avoid provocative activities or arm positions and instructed in range of motion and stretching exercises to minimize capsular contractures. An intraarticular injection of lidocaine and steroid into the acromioclavicular joint may provide significant and sustained symptom relief. When subacromial impingement is also apparent, we will inject the subacromial space for diagnostic and theraputic benefit. Only rarely have we used more than a total of three intraarticular acromioclavicular joint injections.

Operative Treatment

When patients have persistent pain and loss of function and activity levels despite attempts at conservative treatment, they may consider operative intervention. Excision of the distal clavicle is the procedure of choice. Similarly, patients with impingement from pathology at the acromioclavicular joint will benefit from surgical management. In these patients, excision of the distal clavicle is combined with an acromioplasty to decompress the coracoacromial outlet. Early surgical treatment may be preferred for symptomatic patients who have a complete tear of the rotator cuff.

Acromioclavicular joint resection and acromioplasty can be performed either open or by using arthroscopic techniques. The open procedure is straightforward and familiar to most surgeons. The amount of bone to be removed can be measured and predictably resected. In the absence of diagnostic errors, the results of surgery are reproducible and well documented. One disadvantage of open surgery is that it requires detachment of some portion of the deltoid from the trapezius to expose the distal clavicle. Access to the anterior acromion for an acromioplasty requires even greater dissection of the deltoid. This amount of soft-tissue trauma accounts for the fairly significant amount of early postoperative pain that is experienced with this procedure. Historically, 1 to 2 cm of distal clavicle bone has been resected. Disruption of the acromioclavicular ligaments has raised some concerns about the problem of postoperative horizontal instability of the distal clavicle. Cosmetic issues are generally of lesser concern.

Arthroscopic excision of the distal clavicle has evolved as a popular yet technically demanding procedure. It can be used for isolated acromioclavicular joint arthrosis or in conjunction with an acromioplasty when impingement anatomy

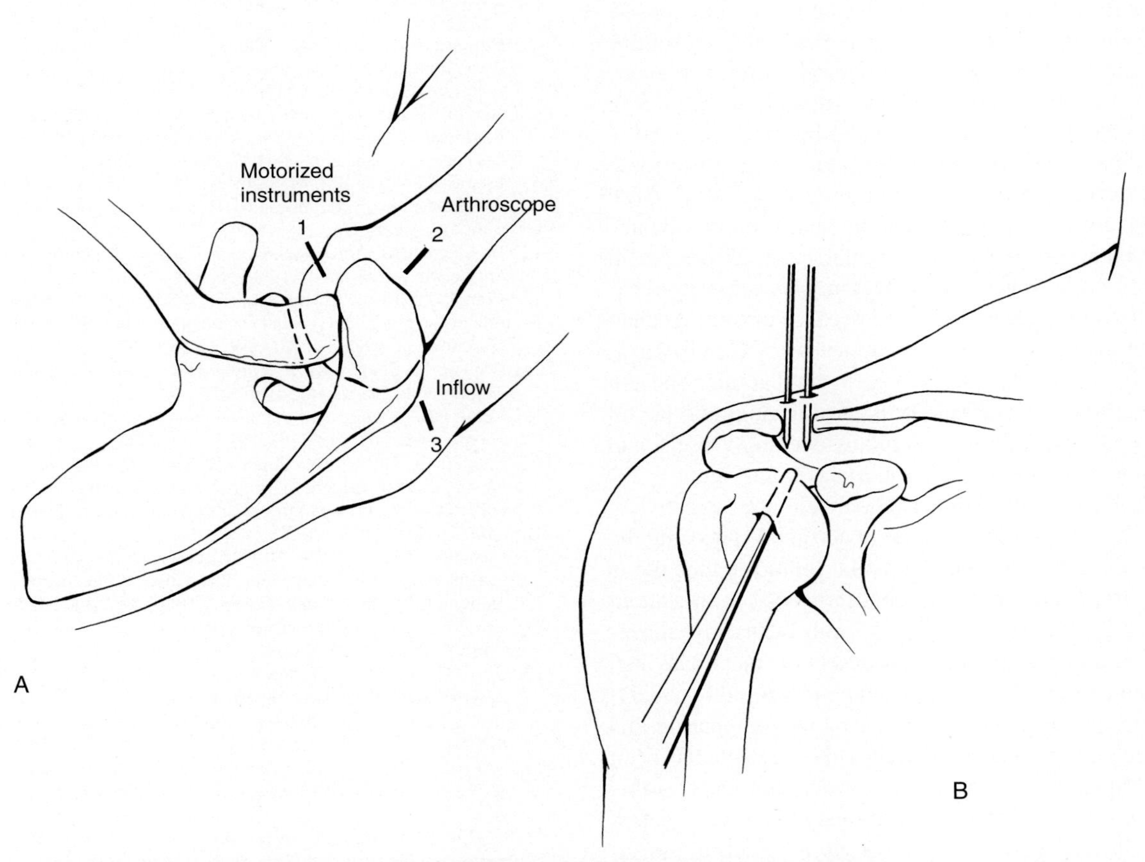

FIG. 28. Portal placement for arthroscopic distal clavicle resection: **(A)** Superior view of the shoulder demonstrating arthroscopic portal placement for subacromial decompression and excision of the distal clavicle. **(B)** Amount of clavicle resected is confirmed by placing spinal needles vertically into the resected joint at the lateral aspect of the clavicle and medial aspect of the acromion. The resection is also best viewed from the anterior portal.

is present. Other than the difficulty in obtaining precise and reproducible bone resection, arthroscopic techniques offer advantages to open surgery. There is no significant trauma to the deltoid, less postoperative pain, and minimal scarring. In addition, no protection is necessary for the deltoid postoperatively (as opposed to open surgery). The recommended amount of distal clavicle resection has been determined to be only 5 mm to 1 cm.[29,30,33] Less bone resection and preservation of the acromioclavicular ligaments should diminish concerns over horizontal instability of the distal clavicle.

Authors' Preferred Technique

We prefer arthroscopic excision of the distal clavicle because our patients experience less postoperative pain and advance more rapidly to full range of motion, strength, and function. In addition, we feel it is valuable to examine the glenohumeral joint and subacromial space as other pathologies, particularly involving the rotator cuff, are not uncommon. Pathologic, inferiorly directed spurs occur frequently on the acromial side of the acromioclavicular joint, and these are easily removed arthroscopically when excising the distal clavicle.

Patients are placed in the beach chair or lateral decubitus position, with the posterior shoulder and scapula exposed. First, the glenohumeral joint is examined through routine posterior and anterior portals. The anterior portal is planned so that it is directly in line and approximately 1 cm inferior to the acromioclavicular joint. A lateral portal is created to enter the subacromial space approximately 1 cm posterior to the anterolateral corner of the acromion (Fig. 28A). After complete examination of the glenohumeral joint, the arthroscope is advanced into the subacromial space. Debridement of the subacromial space and bursectomy is necessary to expose the distal clavicle. If indicated because of impingement anatomy of the anterior acromion or necessary for visualization, an anterior acromioplasty is performed at this time. An underwater Bovie electrocautery is used through the lateral portal to remove soft tissue, coagulate bleeding vessels, and open the undersurface of the acromioclavicular joint.

Once we have exposed the distal clavicle, we typically establish the anterior portal into the subacromial space and the inferior aspect of the acromioclavicular joint. We then move the inflow to the posterior and the arthroscope to the lateral portals (see Fig. 28B). We use a 5.5-mm full-radius shaver and a 4.0- or 5.0-mm-round burr to resect the distal clavicle. The amount of clavicle removed can be measured by resecting the anterior half of the clavicle first and comparing this with the area left untouched. Once 1 cm of clavicle has been removed, the entire distal clavicle is resected back to this level. A portion of the medial acromion is likewise resected. The most difficult part of the procedure is resecting the superior clavicle bone out of the fascia. This is particularly difficult when the distal clavicle is large and bulbous superiorly. Removal of bone is facilitated by manual downward pressure on the distal clavicle and, when necessary, viewing into the joint using a 70-degree arthroscope. Finally, we assess the resection for amount and completeness by viewing from anterior into the acromioclavicular joint. The width of the acromioclavicular joint can be approximated by placing two spinal needles vertically into the joint, one at the medial edge of the acromion and one at the lateral aspect of the clavicle (see Fig.28C). Joint width is estimated by measuring the distance between the spinal needles on the skin.

REFERENCES

1. Alexander OM. Dislocation of the acromioclavicular joint. *Radiography* 1949;15:260.
2. Alldredge RH. Surgical treatment of acromioclavicular dislocation. *Clin Orthop* 1969;63:262–63.
3. Allman FL Jr. Fractures and ligamentous injuries of the clavicle and its articulation. *J Bone Joint Surg [Am]* 1967;49:774–784.
4. Bannister GC, Wallace WA, Stableforth PG, Hutson MA. The management of acute acromioclavicular dislocation: a randomised, prospective, controlled trial. *J Bone Joint Surg [Br]* 1989;71:848–850.
5. Bargren JH, Erlanger S, Dick HM. Biomechanics and comparison of two operative methods of treatment of complete acromioclavicular separation. *Clin Orthop* 1978;130:267–272.
6. Bearden JM, Hughston JC, Whatley GS. Acromioclavicular dislocation: method of treatment. *Am J Sports Med* 1973;1:5–17.
7. Bearn JG. Direct observations on the function of the capsule of the sternoclavicular joint in clavicle support. *J Anat* 1967;101:159–170.
8. Bergfeld JA, Andrish JT, Clancy WG. Evaluation of the acromioclavicular joint following first and second-degree sprains. *Am J Sports Med* 1978;6:153–159.
9. Bernard TN, Brunet ME, Haddad RJ. Fractured coracoid process in acromioclavicular dislocations: report of four cases and review of the literature. *Clin Orthop* 1983;175:227–232.
10. Berson BL, Gilbert MS, Green S. Acromioclavicular dislocations: treatment by transfer of the conjoined tendon and distal end of the coracoid process to the clavicle. *Clin Orthop* 1978;135:157–164.
11. Bossart PJ, Joyce SM, Manaster BJ, Packer SM. Lack of efficiency of weighted radiographs in diagnosing acute acromioclavicualr separation. *Ann Emerg Med* 1988;17:47–51.
12. Bosworth BM. Acromioclavicular separation: new method of repair. *Surg Gynecol Obstet* 1941;73:866–871.
13. Branch TP, Burdette HL, Shahriari AS, Carter FM, Hutton WC. The role of the acromioclavicular ligaments and the effect of distal clavicle resection. *Am J Sports Med* 1996;24:293–297.
14. Browne JE, Stanley RF Jr, Tullow HS. Acromioclavicular joint dislocations. *Am J Sports Med* 1977;5:258–263.
15. Cahill BR. Osteolysis of the distal part of the clavicle in male athletes. *J Bone Joint Surg [Am]* 1982;64:1053–1058.
16. Cappello T, Nuber GW, Nolan KD, McCarthy WJ. Acute ischemia of the upper limb fifteen years after anterior dislocation of the glenohumeral joint and a modified Bristow procedure. *J Bone Joint Surg [Am]* 1996;78:1578–1582.
17. Carsen E, Bjerg-Nielson A, Christensen P. Conservative or surgical treatment of acromioclavicular dislocation: A prospective, controlled, randomized study. *J Bone and Joint Surg [Am]* 1986;68:552–555.
18. Cox JS. The fate of the acromioclavicular joint in athletic injuries. *Am J Sports Med* 1981;9:50–53.
19. Curtis RJ, Dameron TB, Rockwood CA. Fractures and dislocations of the shoulder in children. In: Rockwood CA, Wilkins KE, King RE, eds. *Fractures in children*. Philadelphia: JB.Lippincott, 1991: 828–919.
20. Dahl E. Follow-up after coracoclavicular ligament prosthesis for acromioclavicular joint dislocation. *Acta Chir Scand Suppl* 1981;506: 96.
21. DePalma AF. The role of the disks of the sternoclavicular and the acromioclavicular joints. *Clin Orthop* 1959;13:222–233.
22. Dewar FP, Barrington TW. The treatment of chronic acromioclavicular dislocation. *J Bone Joint Surg [Br]* 1965;47:32–35.
23. Dumontier C, Sautet A, Man M, Apoil A. Acromioclavicular dislocations: treatment by coracoacromial ligamentoplasty. *J Shoulder Elbow Surg* 1995;4:130–134.

24. Eaton R, Serletti J. Computerized axial tomography—a method of localizing Steinmann pin migration: a case report. *Orthopaedics* 1981;4: 1357–1360.
25. Eidman DK, Siff SJ, Tullos HS. Acromioclavicular lesions in children. *Am J Sports Med* 1981;9:150–154.
26. Falstie-Jensen S, Mikkelsen P. Pseudodislocation of the acromioclavicular joint. *J Bone Joint Surg [Br]* 1982;64:368–369.
27. Ferris BD, Bhamra M, Paton DF. Corcacoid process transfer for acromioclavicular dislocations. A report of 20 cases. *Clin Orthop* 1989; 242:184–187.
28. Flatow EL. The biomechanics of the acromioclavicular, sternoclavicular and scapulothoracic joints. *Instr Course Lect* 1993;42:237–245.
29. Flatow EL, Duralde XA, Nicholson GP, Pollock RG, Bigliani LU. Arthroscopic resection of the distal clavicle with a superior approach. *J Shoulder Elbow Surg* 1995;4:41–50.
30. Flatow EL, Cordasco FA, Bigliani LU. Arthroscopic resection of the outer end of the clavicle from a superior approach: a critical quantitative radiographic assessment of bone removal. *Arthroscopy* 1992;8: 55–64.
31. Fukuda K, Craig EV, An K, Cofield RH, Chao EYS. Biomechanical study of the ligamentous system of the acromioclavicular joint. *J Bone Joint Surg [Am]* 1986;68:434–440.
32. Fullerton LR Jr. Recurrent third degree acromioclavicular joint separation after failure of a Dacron ligament prosthesis. A case report. *Am J Sports Med* 1990;18:106–107.
33. Gartsman GM. Arthroscopic resection of the acromioclavicular joint. *Am J Sports Med* 1993;21:71–77.
34. Gartsman GM, Combs AH, Davis PF, Tullos HS. Arthroscopic acromioclavicular joint resection: An anatomical study. *Am J Sports Med* 1991;19:2–25.
35. Gerber C, Rockwood CA Jr. Subcoracoid dislocation of the lateral end of the clavicle: a report of three cases. *J Bone Joint Surg [Am]* 1987;69: 924–927.
36. Gund FB. The treatment of complete dislocation of the outer end of the clavicle: A hitherto undescribed operation. *Ann Surg* 1941;113: 1094–1098.
37. Hall RH, Isaac F, Booth CR. Dislocations of the shoulder with special reference to accompanying small fractures. *J Bone Joint Surg* 1956;17: 47–51.
38. Havranek P. Injuries of distal clavicular physis in children. *J Pediatr Orthop* 1989;9:213–215.
39. Inman UT, Saunders M, Abbott LC. Observations on the function of the shoulder joint. *J Bone Joint Surg* 1944;26:1–30.
40. Ishizuki M, Yamaura I, Isobe Y, Furuya K, Tanabe K, Nagatsuka Y. Avulsion fracture of the superior border of the scapula. *J Bone Joint Surg [Am]* 1981;63:820–822.
41. Jacobs B, Wade PA. Acromioclavicular joint injury: an end-result study. *J Bone Joint Surg [Am]* 1966;48:475–486.
42. Kappakas GS, McMaster JH. Repair of acromioclavicular separation using a Dacron prosthesis graft. *Clin Orthop* 1978;131:247–251.
43. Kennedy JC. Complete dislocation of the acromioclavicular joint: 14 years later. *J Trauma* 1968;8:311–318.
44. Kennedy JC, Cameron H. Complete dislocation of the acromioclavicular joint. *J Bone Joint Surg [Br]* 1954;36:202–208.
45. Kuhns LR, Sherman MP, Poznanski AK, Holt JF. Humeral head and coracoid ossification in the newborn. *Radiology* 1973; 107:145–148.
46. Lancaster S, Horowitz M, Alonso J. Complete acromioclavicular separations: a comparison of operative methods. *Clin Orthop* 1987;216:80–88.
47. Larsen E, Bjery-Nielsen A, Christensen P. Conservative or surgical treatment of acromioclavicular dislocation: a prospective, controlled, randomized study. *J Bone Joint Surg [Am]* 1986; 68:552–555.
48. Lindsey RW, Gutowski WT. The migration of a broken pin following fixation of the acromioclavicular joint: a case report and review of the literature. *Orthopaedics* 1986;9:413–416.
49. MacDonald PB, Alexander MJ, Frejuk J, Johnson GE. Comprehensive functional analysis of shoulders following complete acromioclavicular separation. *Am J Sports Med* 1988;16:475–480.
50. Madsen B. Osteolysis of the acromial end of the clavicle following trauma. *Br J Radiol* 1963;36:822.
51. Mazet RJ. Migration of a Kirschner wire from the shoulder region into the lung: report of two cases. *J Bone Joint Surg [Am]* 1943;25:477–483.
52. McPhee IB. Inferior dislocation of the outer end of the clavicle. *J Trauma* 1980;20:709–710.
53. Millbourn E. On injuries to the acromioclavicular joint: treatment and results. *Acta Orthop Scand* 1950;19:349–382.
54. Montgomery SP, Lloyd RD. Avulsion fracture of the coracoid epiphysis with acromioclavicular separation: Report of two cases in adolescents and review of the literature. *J Bone Joint Surg [Am]* 1977;59: 963–965.
55. Morrison DS, Lemos MJ. Acromioclavicular separation. Reconstruction using synthetic loop augmentation. *Am J Sports Med* 1995;23: 105–110.
56. Mumford EB. Acromioclavicular dislocation: A new operative treatment. *J Bone Joint Surg* 1941;23:799–802.
57. Murphy OB, Bellamy R, Wheeler W, Brower TD. Post-traumatic osteolysis of the distal clavicle. *Clin Orthop* 1975;109:108–114.
58. Nelson CL. Repair of acromioclavicular separations with knitted Dacron graft. *Clin Orthop* 1979;143:289.
59. Neviaser JS. Acromioclavicular dislocation treated by transference of the coracoacromial ligament: a long-term follow-up in a series of 112 cases. *Clin Orthop* 1968;58:57–68.
60. Norrell H, Llewellyn RC. Migration of a threaded Steinmann pin from an acromioclavicular joint into the spinal canal: a case report. *J Bone Joint Surg [Am]* 1965;47:1024–1026.
61. Nuber GW, Bowen MK. Injuries of the acromioclavicular joint and fractures of the distal clavicle. *J Am Acad Orthop Surg* 1997;5: 11–18.
62. Nutter, PD. Coracoclavicular articulations. *J Bone Joint Surg* 1941;23: 177.
63. O'Neill DB, Zarins B, Gelberman RH, Keating TM, Louis D. Compression of the anterior interosseous nerve after use of a sling for dislocation of the acromioclavicular joint: A report of two cases. *J Bone Joint Surg* 1990;72:1100–1102.
64. Ogden JA. Distal clavicular physical injury. *Clin Orthop* 1984;188: 68–73.
65. Park JP, Arnold JA, Coker TP, et al. Treatment of acromioclavicular separations: a retrospective study. *Am J Sports Med* 1980;8:251–256.
66. Patterson WR. Inferior dislocation of the distal end of the clavicle. *J Bone Joint Surg [Am]* 1967;45:1184–1186.
67. Rauschning W, Nordesjo LO, Nordgren B, Sahlstedt B, et al. Resection arthroplasty for repair of complete acromioclavicular separations. *Arch Orthop Traumatol Surg* 1980;97:161–164.
68. Richards RR. Acromioclavicular joint injuries. *Instrl Course Lect* 1993;42:259–269.
69. Rockwood CA Jr. Disorders of the acromioclavicular joint. In: Rockwood CA Jr, Matson FA III, eds. *The shoulder*. Philadelphia: WB Saunders, 1985:413–476.
70. Rockwood CA Jr, Sralay EA, Curtis RJ, Young OC, Kay SP. X-ray evaluation of shoulder problems. In: Rockwood CA Jr, Matsen FA III, eds. *The shoulder*. Philadelphia: WB Saunders, 1985:187.
71. Roper BA, Levack B. The surgical treatment of acromioclavicular dislocations. *J Bone Joint Surg [Br]* 1982; 64:597–599.
72. Salter EG Jr, Nasca RJ, Shelley BS. Anatomical observations on the acromioclavicular joint and supporting ligaments. *Am J Sports Med* 1987;15:199–206.
73. Samilson RL. Congenital and developmental anomalies of the shoulder girdle. *Orthop Clin North Am* 1980;11:219–231.
74. Skjeldal S, Lundblad R, Dullerud R. Coracoid process transfer for acromioclavicular dislocation. *Acta Orthop Scand* 1988; 59:180–182.
75. Smith MJ, Stewart MJ. Acute acromioclavicular separations. *Am J Sports Med.* 1979;7:62–71.
76. Snyder SJ. Arthroscopic acromioclavicular joint debridement and distal clavicle resection. *Tech Orthop* 1988;3:41–45.
77. Taft TN, Wilson FC, Oglesby JW. Dislocation of the acromioclavicular joint: an end-result study. *J Bone Joint Surg [Am]* 1987;69: 1045–1051.
78. Taga I, Yoneda M, Ono K. Epiphyseal separation of the coracoid process associated with acromioclavicular sprain: a case report and review of the literature. *Clin Orthop* 1986;207:138–141.
79. Tibone J, Sellers R, Tonino P. Strength testing after third degree acromioclavicular dislocations. *Am J Sports Med* 1992; 20:328–331.
80. Tossy JD, Mead NC, Sigmond HM. Acromioclavicular separations: Useful and practical classification for treatment. *Clin Orthop* 1963;28: 111–119.
81. Urist MR. Complete dislocations of the acromioclavicular joint: The nature of the traumatic lesion and effective methods of treatment with an analysis of forty-one cases. *J Bone Joint Surg* 1946;28:813–837.
82. Walsh WM, Peterson DA, Shelton G, Newmann RD. Shoulder strength following acromioclavicular injury. *Am J Sports Med* 1985;13: 153–158.

83. Weaver JK, Dunn HK. Treatment of acromioclavicular injuries, especially complete acromioclavicular separation. *J Bone Joint Surg* 1972; 54:1187–1194.
84. Weinstein DM, McCann PD, McIlveen SJ, Flatow EL, Bigliani LU. Surgical treatment of complete acromioclavicular dislocations. *Am J Sports Med* 1995;23:324–331.
85. Weitzman G. Treatment of acute acromioclavicular joint dislocation by a modified Bosworth method: report on twenty-four cases. *J Bone Joint Surg [Am]* 1967;49:1167–1178.
86. Wojtys EM, Nelson G. Conservative treatment of grade III acromioclavicular dislocations. *Clin Orthop* 1991;268:112–119.
87. Wood VE, Marchinski L. Congenital anomalies of the shoulder. In: Rockwood CA Jr, Matson FA III, eds. *The shoulder*. Philadelphia: WB Saunders, 1990:98–148.
88. Zanca P. Shoulder pain: involvement of the acromioclavicular joint. Analysis of 1,000 cases. *AJR Am J Roentgenol* 1971; 112:493–500.

PART VII

Sternoclavicular Joint

Disorders of the Shoulder: Diagnosis and Management,
edited by Joseph P. Iannotti and Gerald R. Williams, Jr.
Lippincott Williams & Wilkins, Philadelphia © 1999.

CHAPTER 28

Disorders of the Sternoclavicular Joint: Pathophysiology, Diagnosis, and Management

Michael A. Wirth and Charles A. Rockwood, Jr.

HISTORICAL REVIEW

Rodrigues,[155] in 1843, may have published the first case of traumatic posterior dislocation of the sternoclavicular joint in the literature, "a case of dislocation inward of the internal extremity of the clavicle." The patient's left shoulder was against a wall when the right side of the chest and thorax were compressed and rolled forward almost to the midline by a cart. Immediately, the patient experienced shortness of breath, which persisted for 3 weeks. When first seen by the physician, he appeared to be suffocating and his face was blue. The left shoulder was swollen and painful, and there was "a depression on the left side of the superior extremity of the sternum." Pressure on the depression greatly increased the sensation of suffocation. Rodrigues observed that when the outer end of the shoulder was displaced backward, the inner end of the clavicle was displaced forward, which relieved the asphyxia. Therefore, treatment consisted of binding the left shoulder backward with a cushion between the two scapulas, but only after the patient had been bled twice within the first 24 hours. Rodrigues may have seen other cases of posterior dislocation, since he stated that the patient "retained a slight depression of the internal extremity of the clavicle; such, however, is the ordinary fate of the patients who present this form of dislocation."

In the late 19th century, a number of articles appeared from England, Germany, and France; it was not until the 1930s that articles by Duggan,[48] Howard and Shafer,[91] and Lowman[114] appeared in the American literature.

M. A. Wirth and C. A. Rockwood, Jr.: Department of Orthopaedics, The University of Texas Health Science Center at San Antonio, San Antonio, Texas 78284-7774; Orthopedic Shoulder, Service, Audie Murphy Veterans Hospital, San Antonio, Texas.

SURGICAL ANATOMY AND BIOMECHANICS

The sternoclavicular joint is a diarthrodial joint and is the only true articulation between the clavicle of the upper ex-

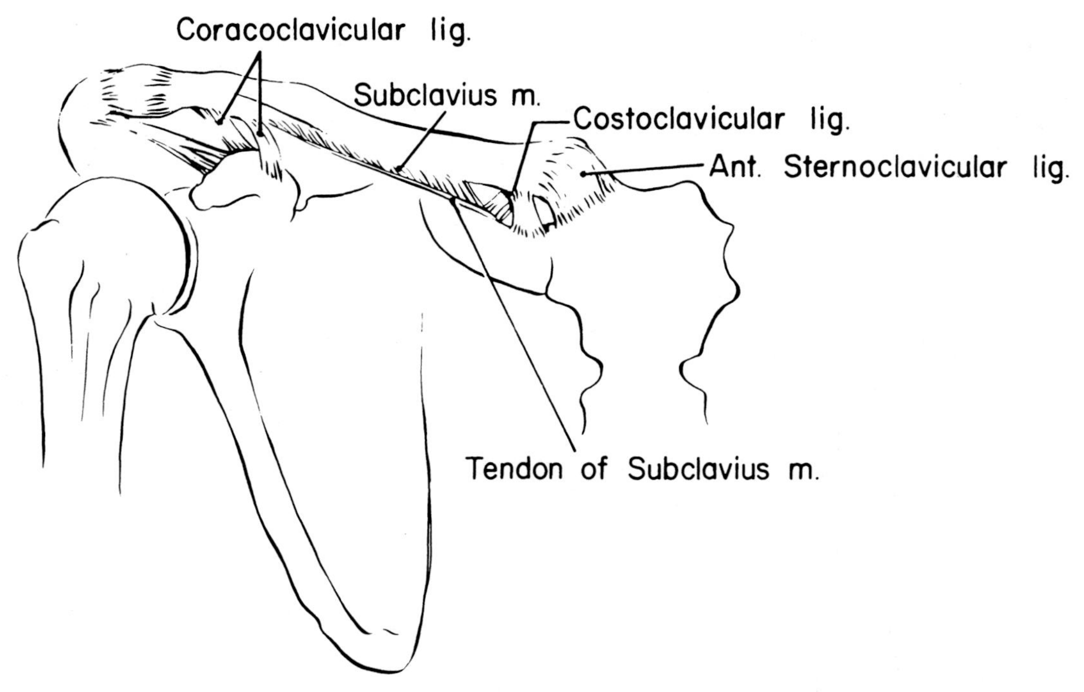

FIG. 1. Normal anatomy around the sternoclavicular and acromioclavicular joints. Note that the tendon of the subclavius muscle arises in the vicinity of the costoclavicular ligament from the first rib and has a long tendon structure.

tremity and the axial skeleton (Fig. 1). The articular surface of the clavicle is much larger than that of the sternum, and both are covered with fibrocartilage. The enlarged bulbous medial end of the clavicle is concave front to back and convex vertically, and therefore creates a saddle-type joint with the clavicular notch of the sternum.[76,77] The clavicular notch of the sternum is curved, and the joint surfaces are not congruent. Cave[27] has demonstrated that in 2.5% of patients, there is a small facet on the inferior aspect of the medial clavicle that articulates with the superior aspect of the first rib at its synchondral junction with the sternum.

Because less than half of the medial clavicle articulates with the upper angle of the sternum, the sternoclavicular joint has the distinction of having the least amount of bony stability of the major joints of the body. As Grant[76] noted, "The two (make) an ill fit." If a finger is placed in the superior sternal notch, with motion of the upper extremity one can feel that a large part of the medial clavicle is completely above the articulation with the sternum.

LIGAMENTS OF THE STERNOCLAVICULAR JOINT

There is so much joint incongruity that the integrity has to come from its surrounding ligaments: the intraarticular disk ligament, extraarticular costoclavicular ligament (rhomboid ligament), capsular ligament, and interclavicular ligament.

Intraarticular Disk Ligament

The intraarticular disk ligament is a very dense, fibrous structure that arises from the synchondral junction of the first rib to the sternum and passes through the sternoclavicular joint, which divides the joint into two separate joint spaces (Fig. 2).[76,77] The upper attachment is on the superior and posterior aspects of the medial clavicle. DePalma[45] has shown that the disk is perforated only rarely; the perforation allows a free communication between the two joint compartments. Anteriorly and posteriorly, the disk blends into the fibers of the capsular ligament. The disk acts as a checkrein against medial displacement of the inner clavicle (Fig. 2).

Costoclavicular Ligament

The costoclavicular ligament, also called the rhomboid ligament, is short and strong and consists of an anterior and a posterior fasciculus (Fig. 1).[9,27,77] Cave[27] reported that the average length is 1.3 cm, the maximum width 1.9 cm, and the average thickness 1.3 cm. Bearn[9] has shown that there is always a bursa between the two components of the ligament. Because of the two different parts of the ligament, it has a twisted appearance[77]. The costoclavicular ligament attaches below to the upper surface of the first rib and at the adjacent part of the synchondral junction with the sternum, and above to the margins of the impression on the inferior surface of the medial end of the clavicle, sometimes known as the rhomboid fossa.[76,77] Cave[27] has shown, from a study of 153 clav-

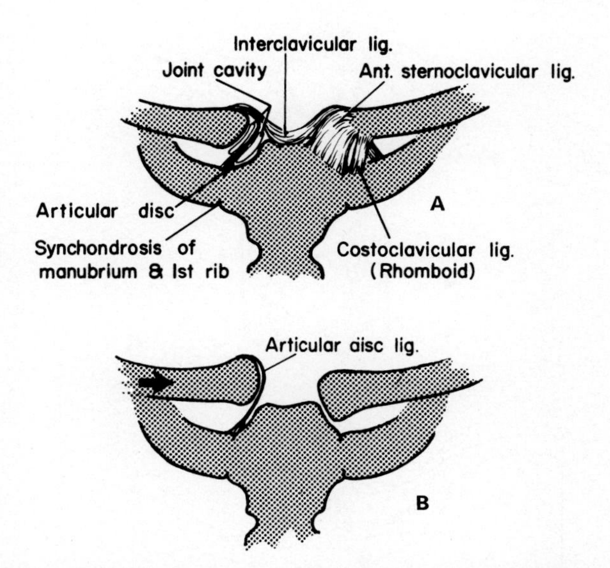

FIG. 2. (A) Normal anatomy around the sternoclavicular joint. Note that the articular disk ligament divides the sternoclavicular joint cavity into two separate spaces and inserts onto the superior and posterior aspects of the medial clavicle. **(B)** The articular disk ligament acts as a checkrein for a medial displacement of the proximal clavicle. (reprinted with permission from Rockwood CA, Matsen F III, eds. *The shoulder.* Philadelphia: WB Saunders, 1990:Fig. 13-2.)

icles, that the attachment of the costoclavicular ligament to the clavicle can be any of three types: a depression, the rhomboid fossa (30%); flat (60%); or an elevation (10%).

The fibers of the anterior fasciculus arise from the anteromedial surface of the first rib and are directed upward and laterally. The fibers of the posterior fasciculus are shorter and arise lateral to the anterior fibers on the rib and are directed upward and medially. The fibers of the anterior and posterior components cross and allow for stability of the joint during rotation and elevation of the clavicle. The two-part configuration of the costoclavicular ligament is similar to the coracoclavicular ligament on the outer end of the clavicle.

Bearn[9] has shown experimentally that the anterior fibers resist excessive upward rotation of the clavicle and that the posterior fibers resist excessive downward rotation. Specifically, the anterior fibers also resist lateral displacement, and the posterior fibers resist medial displacement.

Interclavicular Ligament

The interclavicular ligament connects the superomedial aspects of each clavicle with the capsular ligaments and the upper sternum (Fig. 2). According to Grant[76], this band may be comparable with the wishbone of birds. This ligament helps the capsular ligaments to produce "shoulder poise"; that is, to hold up the shoulder. This can be tested by putting a finger in the superior sternal notch; with elevation of the arm, the ligament is quite lax, but as soon as both arms hang at the sides, the ligament becomes tight.

Capsular Ligament

The capsular ligament covers the anterosuperior and posterior aspects of the joint and represents thickenings of the joint capsule (Figs. 1 and 2). The anterior portion of the capsular ligament is heavier and stronger than the posterior portion.

According to the original work of Bearn,[9] this may be the strongest ligament of the sternoclavicular joint, and it is the first line of defense against the upward displacement of the inner clavicle caused by a downward force on the distal end of the shoulder. The clavicular attachment of the ligament is primarily onto the epiphysis of the medial clavicle, with some secondary blending of the fibers into the metaphysis. The senior author has demonstrated this, as have Poland,[141] Denham and Dingley,[44] and Brooks and Henning.[18]

Although some investigators report that the intraarticular disk ligament greatly assists the costoclavicular ligament in preventing upward displacement of the medial clavicle, Bearn[9] has shown that the capsular ligament is the most important structure in preventing upward displacement of the medial clavicle. In experimental postmortem studies, he evaluated the strength and the role of each of the ligaments at the sternoclavicular joint to see which one would prevent a downward displacement of the outer clavicle. He attributed the lateral "poise of the shoulder" (i.e., the force that holds the shoulder up) to a locking mechanism of the ligaments of the sternoclavicular joint (Fig. 3). To accomplish his experiments, Bearn[9] dissected all the muscles attaching onto the clavicle, the sternum, and the first rib and left all the ligaments attached. He secured the sternum to a block in a vise. He then loaded the outer end of the clavicle with 10 to 20 pounds of weight and cut the ligaments of the sternoclavicular joint, one at a time and in various combinations, to determine each ligament's effect on maintaining the clavicle poise or, thinking of it in another way, which ligament would rupture first when a force was applied to the outer end of the clavicle.

He determined, after cutting the costoclavicular, intraarticular disk, and interclavicular ligaments, that they had no effect on clavicle poise. However, the division of the capsular ligament alone resulted in a downward depression on the distal end of the clavicle. He also noted that the intraarticular disk ligament tore under 5 pounds of weight, once the capsular ligament had been cut. Bearn's results have many clinical implications for the mechanisms of injury of the sternoclavicular joint.

Range of Motion of the Sternoclavicular Joint

The sternoclavicular joint is freely movable and functions almost like a ball-and-socket joint, in that the joint has motion in almost all planes, including rotation.[13,115] The clavicle, and therefore the sternoclavicular joint, in normal shoulder motion is capable of 30 to 35 degrees of upward elevation, 35 degrees of combined forward and backward movement, and 45

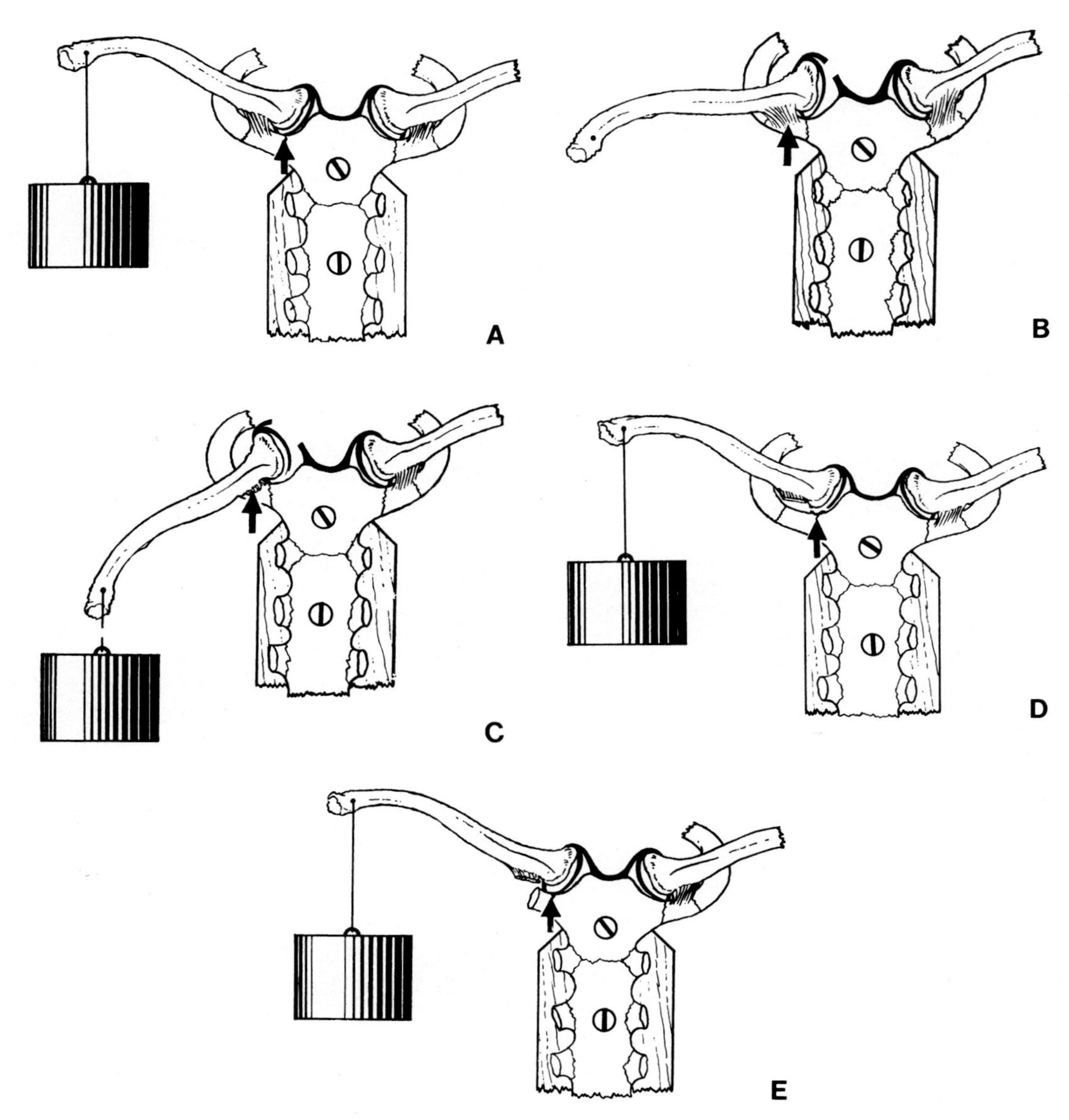

FIG. 3. The importance of the various ligaments around the sternoclavicular joint in maintaining normal shoulder poise. **A:** The lateral end of the clavicle is maintained in an elevated position through the sternoclavicular ligaments. The arrow indicates the fulcrum. **B:** When the capsule is divided completely, the lateral end of the clavicle descends under its own weight without any loading. The clavicle will seem to be supported by the intraarticular disk ligament. **C:** After division of the capsular ligament, it was determined that a weight of less than 5 pounds was enough to tear the intraarticular disk ligament from its attachment on the costal cartilage junction of the first rib. The fulcrum was transferred laterally, so that the medial end of the clavicle hinged over the first rib in the vicinity of the costoclavicular ligament. **D:** After division of the costoclavicular ligament and the intraarticular disk ligament, the lateral end of the clavicle could not be depressed as long as the capsular ligament was intact. **E:** After resection of the medial first costal cartilage, along with the costoclavicular ligament, there was no effect on the poise of the lateral end of the clavicle, as long as the capsular ligament was intact. (Reprinted with permission from Bearn JG. Direct observation on the function of the capsule of the sternoclavicular joint in clavicular support. *J Anat* 1967;101:159–170.)

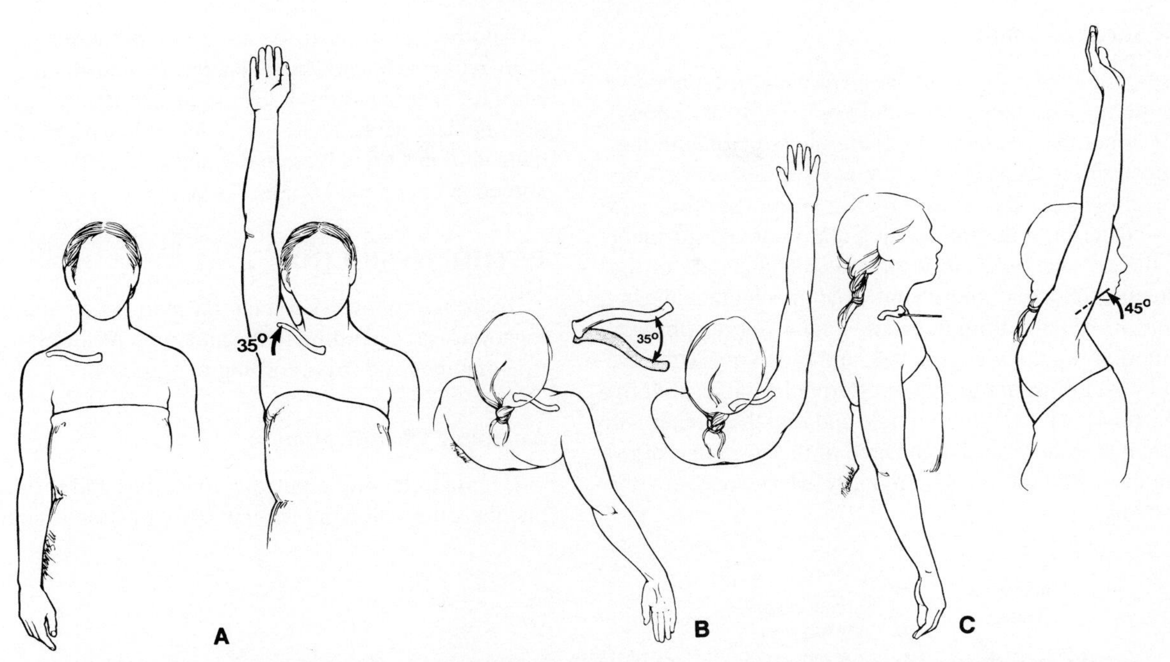

FIG. 4. Motions of the clavicle and the sternoclavicular joint. A: With full overhead elevation, the clavicle rises 35 degrees. B: With adduction and extension, the clavicle displaces anteriorly and posteriorly 35 degrees. C: The clavicle rotates on its long axis 45 degrees as the arm is elevated to the full overhead position.

to 50 degrees of rotation around its long axis (Fig. 4). It is most likely the most frequently moved joint of the long bones in the body, because almost any motion of the upper extremity is transferred proximally to the sternoclavicular joint.

Epiphysis of the Medial Clavicle

Although the clavicle is the first long bone of the body to ossify (fifth intrauterine week), the epiphysis at the medial end of the clavicle is the last of the long bones in the body to appear and the last epiphysis to close (Fig. 5). The medial clavicular epiphysis does not ossify until the 18th to 20th year of life, and it fuses with the shaft of the clavicle around the 23rd to 25th year.[76,77,141] Webb and Suchey,[186] in an extensive study of the physis of the medial clavicle in 605 males and 254 females at autopsy, reported that complete unions may not be present until 31 years of age. This knowledge of the ephipysis is important, because it is believed that many so-called sternoclavicular dislocations are actually fractures through the physeal plate.

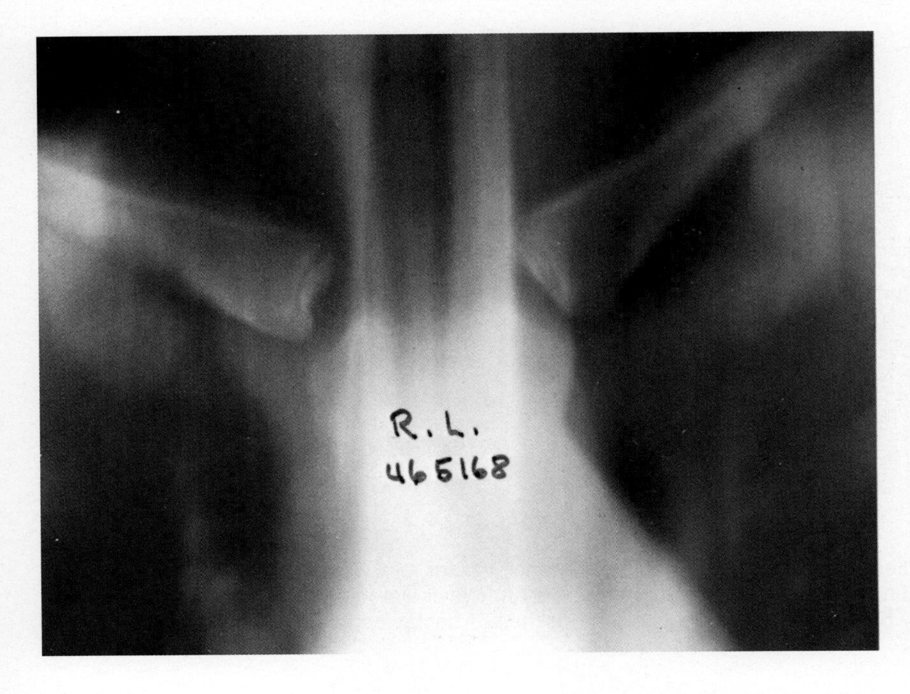

FIG. 5. Tomogram demonstrating the thin, waferlike disk of the epiphysis of the medial clavicle.

Applied Surgical Anatomy

The surgeon who is planning an operative procedure on or near the sternoclavicular joint should be completely knowledgeable about the vast array of anatomic structures immediately posterior to the sternoclavicular joint. There is a "curtain" of muscles—the sternohyoid, sternothyroid, and scaleni—posterior to the sternoclavicular joint and the inner third of the clavicle, and this curtain blocks the view of the vital structures. Some of these vital structures include the innominate artery, innominate vein, vagus nerve, phrenic nerve, internal jugular vien, trachea, and esophagus (Fig. 6). If one is considering stabilizing the sternoclavicular joint by running a pin down from the clavicle and into the sternum, it is important to remember that the arch of the aorta, the superior vena cava, and the right pulmonary artery are also very close at hand.

Another structure to be aware of is the anterior jugular vein, which is located between the clavicle and the curtain of muscles. The anatomy books state that it can be quite variable in size; we have seen it as large as 1.5 cm in diameter. This vein has no valves, and when it is nicked, it looks like someone has opened up the flood gates.

PATHOPHYSIOLOGY

There are two ways to classify sternoclavicular joint dislocations: (a) according to the anatomic position the dislocation assumes and (b) according to etiology.

Anatomic Classification

Detailed classifications are confusing and difficult to remember; the following, simple classification is suggested.

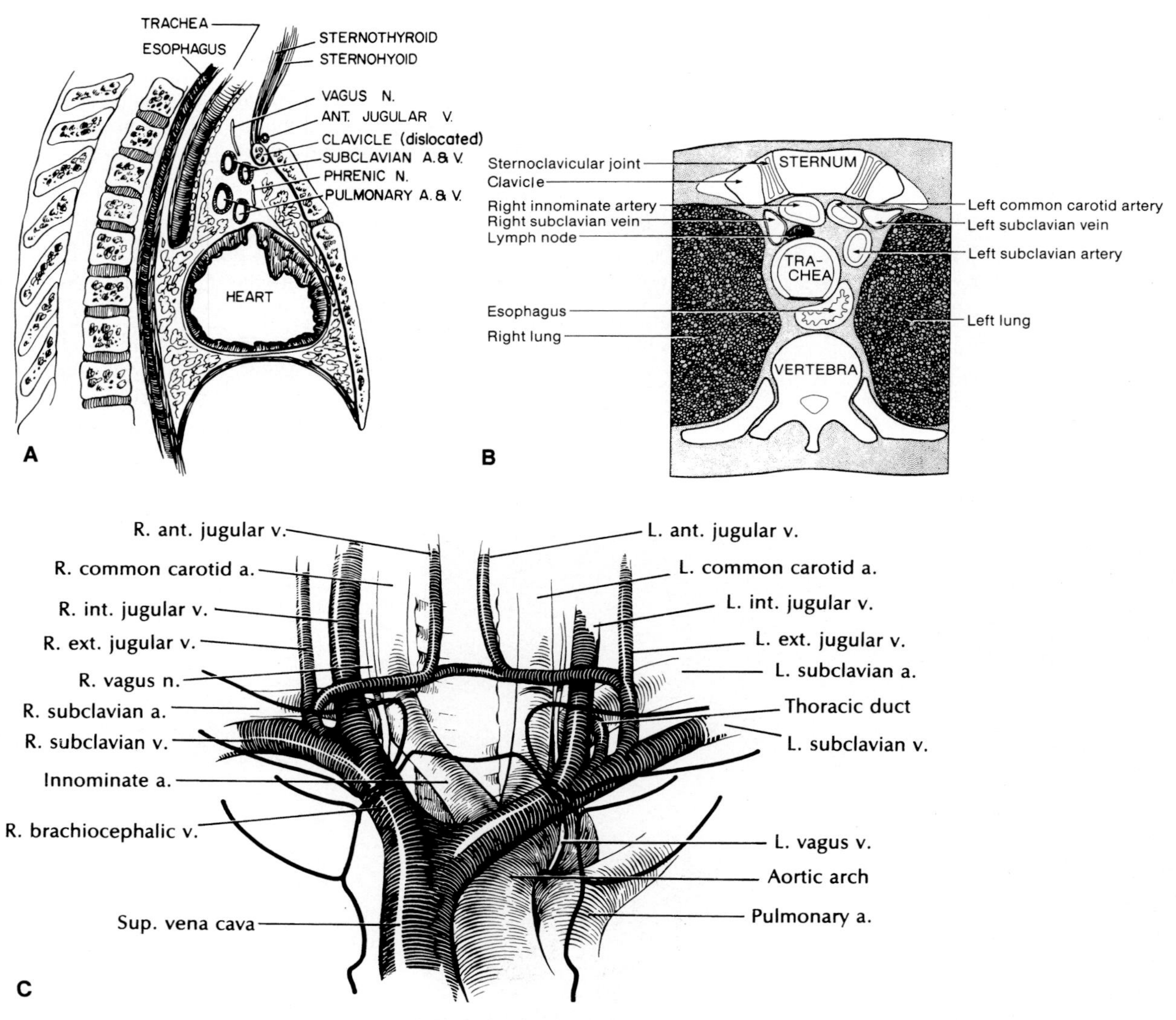

FIG. 6. Applied anatomy of the vital structures posterior to the sternoclavicular joint. **A and B:** Sagittal views in cross-section demonstrating the structures posterior to the sternoclavicular joint. **C:** A diagram demonstrating the close proximity of the major vessels posterior to the sternoclaviocular joint. *(continued)*

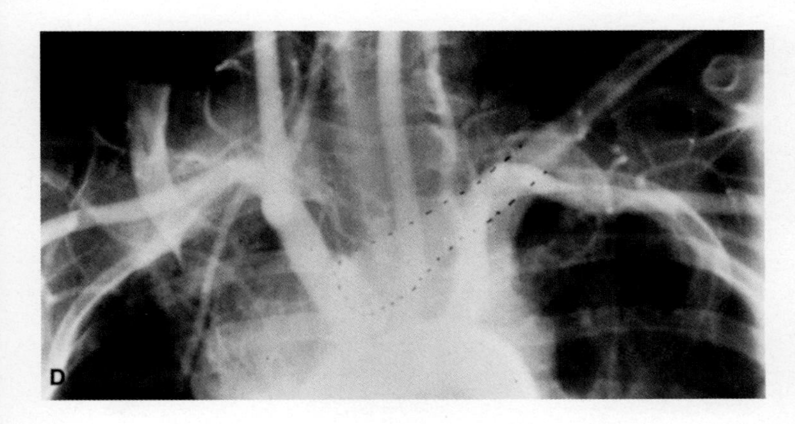

FIG. 6. *Continued.* **D:** An aortogram showing the relationship of the medial end of the clavicle to the major vessels in the mediasternum.

Anterior Dislocation

Anterior dislocations are the most common. The medial end of the clavicle is displaced anteriorly or anterosuperiorly to the anterior margin of the sternum.

Posterior Dislocation

Posterior sternoclavicular dislocation is uncommon. The medial end of the clavicle is displaced posteriorly or posterosuperiorly with respect to the posterior margin of the sternum.

Etiologic Classification

Traumatic Injuries

Sprain or Subluxation

Acute sprains to the sternoclavicular joint can be classified as mild, moderate, or severe. In a mild sprain, all the ligaments are intact and the joint is stable. In a moderate sprain, there is subluxation of the sternoclavicular joint. The capsular, intraarticular disk, and costoclavicular ligaments may be partially disrupted. The subluxation may be anterior or posterior. In a severe sprain, there is complete disruption of the sternoclavicular ligaments, and the dislocation may be anterior or posterior.

Acute Dislocation

In a dislocated sternoclavicular joint, the capsular and intraarticular ligaments are ruptured. Occasionally, the costoclavicular ligament is intact but stretched out enough to allow the dislocation.

Recurrent Dislocation

If the initial acute traumatic dislocation does not heal, mild to moderate forces may produce recurrent dislocations; this is rare.

Unreduced Dislocation

The original dislocation may go unrecognized, it may be irreducible, or the physician may decide not to reduce certain dislocations. For a variety of nontraumatic reasons, the sternoclavicular joint may subluxate or enlarge.

Spontaneous Subluxation or Dislocation

One or both of the sternoclavicular joints may spontaneously subluxate or dislocate anteriorly during overhead motion. The condition usually is not painful (Fig. 7).

Congenital or Developmental Subluxation or Dislocation

Newlin[129] reported a 25-year-old man who had bilateral congenital posterior dislocation of the medial ends of the clavicle that simulated an intrathoracic mass. Guerin[79] first reported congenital luxations of the sternoclavicular joint in 1841. Congenital defects with loss of bone substance on either side of the joint can predispose the patient to subluxation or dislocation. Cooper[34] described a patient with scoliosis so severe that the shoulder was displaced forward enough to posteriorly dislocate the clavicle behind the sternum.

Arthritis

Arthritis, with enlargement of the sternoclavicular joint, can occur secondary to osteoarthritis, arthropathies, condensing osteitis of the medial clavicle, sternocostoclavicular hyperostosis, or postmenopausal arthritis (Fig. 8).

Osteoarthritis. Osteoarthritis[82,100,101] is characterized by narrowing of the joint space, osteophytes, subchondral sclerosis, and cysts on both sides of the joint (Fig. 9). Because most of the wear occurs in the inferior part of the head of the medial clavicle, most of the degenerative changes occur in that region. The sometimes discrete degenerative changes are best seen on tomograms and computed tomography (CT) scans.[3,100] Kier and associates[100] correlated the x-ray films and the pathologic specimens of patients with osteoarthritis of the sternoclavicular joint. Sternoclavicular joint arthritus

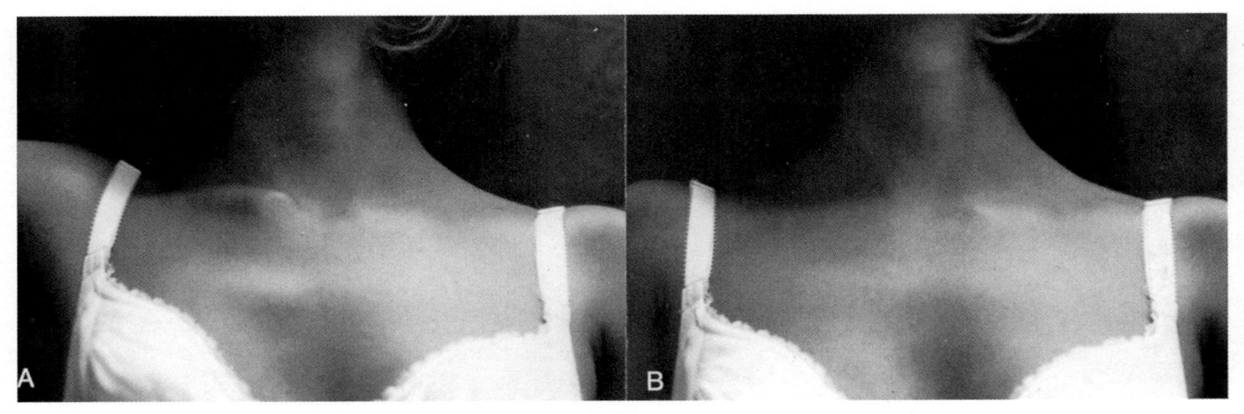

FIG. 7. Spontaneous anterior subluxation of the sternoclavicular joint. **A:** With the arms in the overhead position, the medial end of the right clavicle spontaneously subluxates anteriorly without any trauma. **B:** When the arm is lowered to the side, the medial end of the clavicle spontaneously reduces. Usually this is not associated with significant discomfort. (Reprinted with permission from Rockwood CA, Matsen F III, eds. *The shoulder.* Philadelphia: WB Saunders, 1990:Fig. 13-10.)

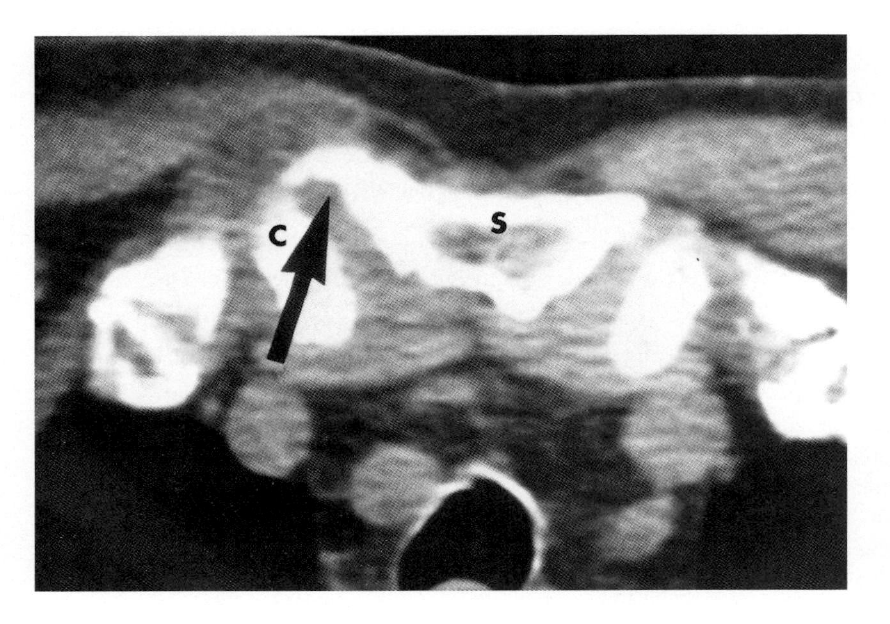

FIG. 8. CT scan of a 63-year-old right hand–dominant man who worked more than 45 years as a landscaper. Image demonstrates a hypertrophic, degenerative right sternoclavicular joint consistent with osteoarthritis (*arrow*). C, medial clavicle; S, sternum. (Reprinted with permission from Wirth MA and Rockwood CA: *Acute and Chronic Traumatic Injuries of the Sternoclavicular Joint. J Am Acad Orthop Surgeons* 1996;4:268–278 .)

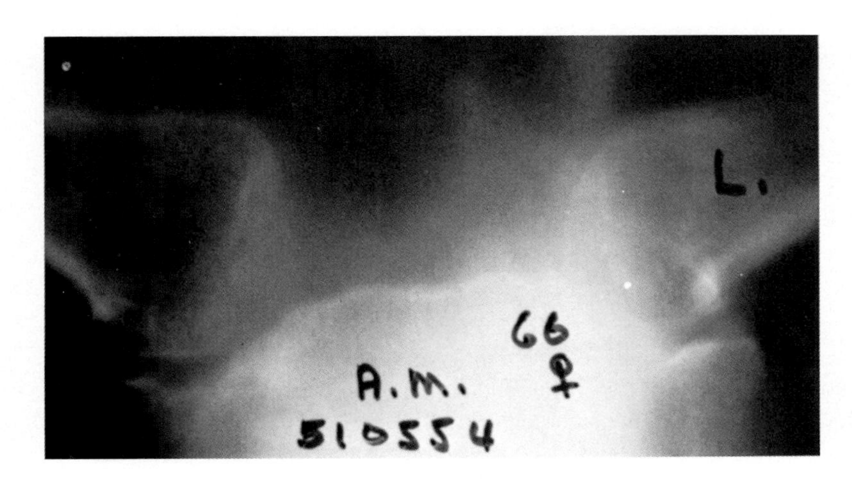

FIG. 9. Tomogram of the sternoclavicular joints in a 66-year-old patient with degenerative arthritis. (Reprinted with permission from Rockwood CA, Matsen F III, eds. *The shoulder.* Philadelphia: WB Saunders, 1990:Fig. 13-11.)

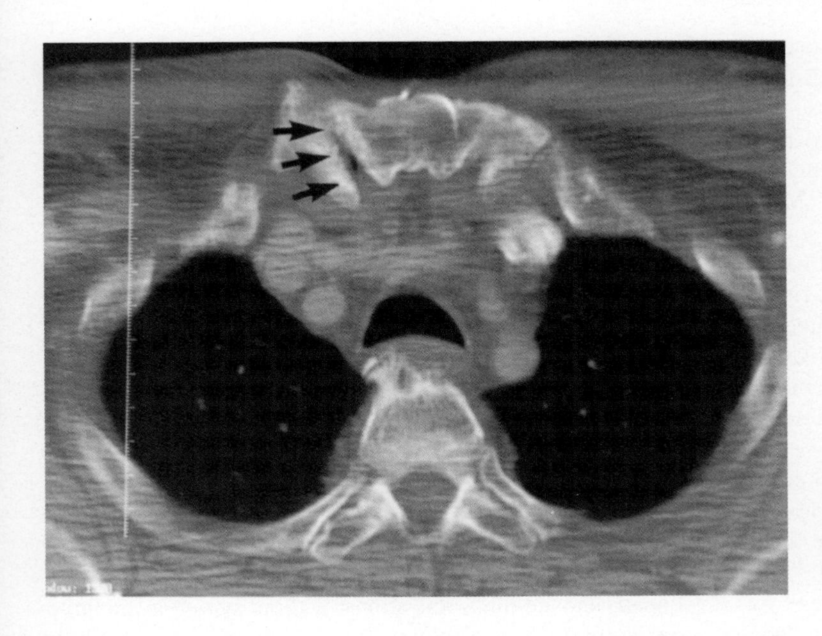

FIG. 10. CT scan of a 69-year-old patient with degenerative arthritis. The patient recalled that he injured his right sternoclavicular joint approximately 50 years earlier, while completing an obstacle course during basic training for the armed services.

and hypertrophy can develop following radical neck surgery, particularly when the spinal accessory nerve is sacrificed,[26,74,165,178] and the incidence is reported to be as high as 54%.[26] The reason for the arthritis is the downward and forward droop of the shoulder, which puts an extra stress on the sternoclavicular joint. The senior author observed one patient who had such stress on the sternoclavicular joint following a radical neck and spinal accessory nerve sacrifice that he developed a posterior dislocation of the sternoclavicular joint. The posterior displacement was so severe that the medial end of the clavicle compressed his trachea and esophagus. Baker and colleagues[3] reported that CT was useful in evaluating the pathologic changes in degenerative disease of the sternoclavicular joint (Fig. 10).

Arthropathies. Some of the disease processes that produce degenerative changes in the sternoclavicular joint are degenerative arthritis and rheumatoid arthritis (Fig. 11),[21,52,195] rheumatoid spondylitis,[146] scleroderma,[52] Reiter's syndrome,[100] psoriasis,[171] polymyalgia rheumatica,[135] secondary hyperparathyroidism,[146,179] gout,[39,118] leprosy,[131] syringomyelia,[41] metastatic carcinoma,[158] condensing osteitis,[19,165] Friedreich's disease[109] (aseptic necrosis of the medial end of the clavicle), and sternoclavicular hyperostosis.

Condensing Osteitis of the Medial Clavicle. Brower and associates[19] first described in detail the rare condition known as condensing osteitis of the medial clavicle. It usually occurs in women over the age of 40 and may occur secondary to chronic stress on the joint. The joint is swollen and tender, and radionuclide studies show an increased uptake of the isotope. Routine laboratory results are within normal limits. X-ray films show sclerosis and slight expansion of the medial third of the clavicle. The inferior portion of the sternal end of the clavicle shows sclerotic changes. Some osteophytes may be present, but the joint space is preserved. The changes of the medial clavicle are best detected via CT. The differential diagnosis includes Paget's disease, sternoclavicular hyperostosis, Friedreich's avascular necrosis of the medial clavicle epiphysis, infection, Tietze's syndrome, and osteoarthritis. More recently, Vierboom and associates[183] have described the use of magnetic resonance imaging as an adjunctive method for diagnosing this entity. The condition has been described by many authors.[32,62,96,103] Most patients do

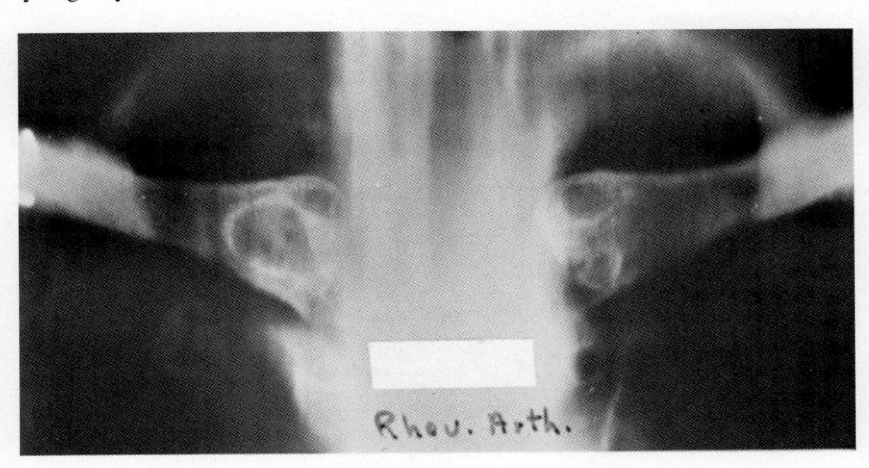

FIG. 11. Tomogram of a patient with rheumatoid arthritis with bilateral degenerative changes in the medial clavicles.

well with conservative treatment, i.e., antiinflammatory medications. Kruger and associates[103] recommend incisional or excisional biopsy in refractory cases.

Sternocostoclavicular Hyperostosis. According to most investigators,[1,30,70,73,95,105,160] sternocostoclavicular hyperostosis was first described by Sonozaki in 1974.[168–170] Many cases reported are from Japan.

This condition, usually bilateral, affects adults of both sexes between 30 and 50 years of age. The process begins at the junction of the medial clavicle, the first rib, and the sternum as an ossification in the ligaments and later involves the bones. Lagier and colleagues[105] published an excellent review of the x-ray findings and pathology from an autopsy specimen. In some cases, the hyperostosis is extensive and forms a solid block of bone of the sternum, ribs, and clavicle. Patients may have peripheral arthritis. Subperiosteal bone changes have been noted in x-ray films of other bones (i.e., humerus, pelvis, tibia, ribs, and vertebral bodies).[70] The condition has been graded into three stages by Sonozaki.[168–170] Stage I is mild ossification in the costoclavicular ligaments; stage II is characterized by an ossific mass between the clavicle and the first rib; and in stage III, a bone mass exists between the calvicle, sternum, and first rib. As might be expected with the fusion of the sternoclavicular joint, shoulder motion is severely restricted. Dohler[47] reported that as a result of the fusion of the sternoclavicular joint, his patient developed compensatory dislocation of the acromioclavicular joint.

Pustular cutaneous lesions of the palmar and plantar surfaces of skin may be seen. There is no specific laboratory test, except for an occasional elevation of the serum alkaline phosphatase.[70]

Postmenopausal Arthritis. Bremner[17] and Bonnin[12] have both reported on "postmenopausal arthritis," so named because it is most often seen in postmenopausal women. Sadr and Swann[159] reported 22 patients with this problem who were seen in a 5-year study; 20 of the cases were in women, and the majority involved the sternoclavicular joint of the dominant arm. Nonoperative treatment was recommended. The condition is the result of normal degeneration of a frequently moved joint. It is almost without symptoms; a lump develops at the sternoclavicular joint, which occasionally is accompanied by a vague ache (Fig. 12). There is no previous history of injury or disease. X-ray studies show sclerosis and

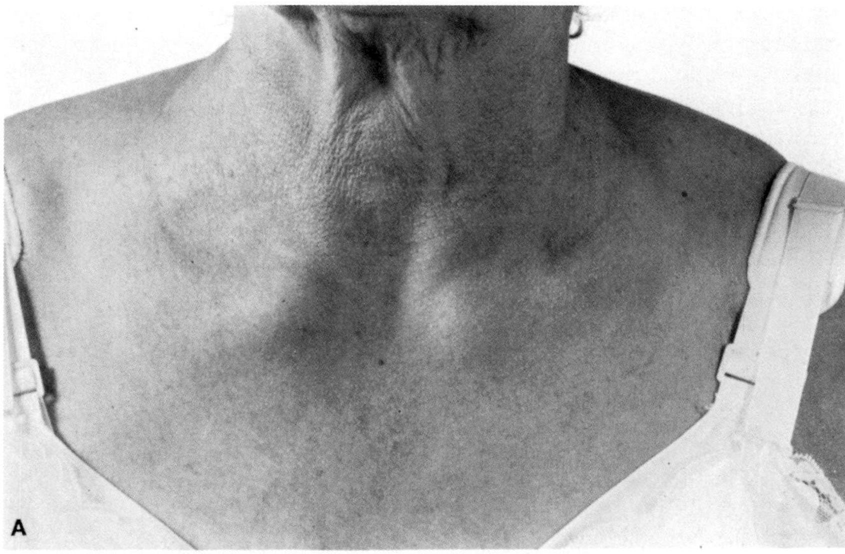

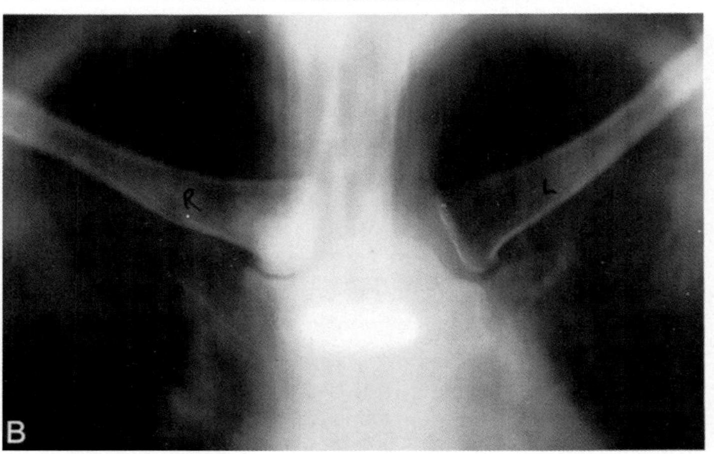

FIG. 12. A: Bilateral anterior swelling of the sternoclavicular joints in a 67-year-old woman. The right medial clavicle was more prominent because she was right handed. **B:** The tomogram demonstrates sclerosis and degenerative changes in the right sternoclavicular joint consistent with ordinary degenerative arthritis. (**B** reprinted with permission from Rockwood CA, Matsen F III, eds. *The shoulder.* Philadelphia: WB Saunders, 1990:Fig. 13-13b.)

enlargement of the medial end of the clavicle, reactive sclerosis of the sternum, and subluxation of the joint. The pathologic changes are those of degenerative arthritis.

Infection

Spontaneous swelling with the appearance of joint subluxation may be associated with acute, subacute, or chronic bacterial arthritis. Wholgethan and Newberg[192] reviewed 39 cases of infection of the sternoclavicular joint; 15 were in drug addicts. Covelli and associates[38] described 3 patients with septic arthritis of the sternoclavicular joint. Predisposing conditions included intravenous drug addiction and human immunodeficiency virus (HIV)-positive patients. Common causes of the infection in nonaddicts are bacteremia, invasion from surrounding bone, rheumatoid arthritis, alcoholism, and chronic debilitating diseases. Londsey and Leach[110] and Renoult and associates[145] reported on sternoclavicular osteomyelitis as a complication of subclavian vein catheterization, and in patients undergoing dialysis. There are many case reports of isolated infections of the sternoclavicular joint that have been caused by a variety of microorganisms, including *Staphylococcus aureus,*[40,86,111,119] *Escherichia coli,*[43,111] *Citrobacter diversus,*[64] coliform bacilli,[43] *Pasteurella multocida,*[130] *Streptococcus pyogenes,*[127] *Pseudomonas aeruginosa,*[63,175] *Brucella* species,[5,195] and *Neisseria gonorrhoeae* (Figs. 13 and 14). Blankstein and associates[11] reported a septic sternoclavicular joint that cultured *Staphylococcus aureus* secondary to bacteremia infection from a paronychia of the finger. Farrer[55] reported a 66-year-old man who had a septic sternoclavicular joint that cultured *Staphylococcus aureus.* Tabatabai and colleagues[176] reported infection of the sternoclavicular joint caused by group B *Streptococcus.* CT is useful for making an early diagnosis of a septic sternoclavicular joint (Fig. 14).

Richter and associates[148] reported 9 patients with infection of the sternoclavicular joint secondary to tuberculosis. The average time from onset of the disease until diagnosis was 1.4 years.

For some reason, intravenous drug addicts seem to have a high incidence of acute gram-negative infection of the sternoclavicular joint.[63,72] Friedman and colleagues[63] reported four cases of sternoclavicular infection in intravenous drug abusers; in three of these *Staphylocuccus aureus* was recovered, and in the fourth case *Streptococcus pneumoniae* was isolated.

Higoumenakis[87] reported that unilateral enlargement of the sternoclavicular joint is a diagnostic sign of congenital syphilis. The enlargement of the sternoclavicular joint can be mistaken for an anterior dislocation. He reported the sign to be positive in 170 of 197 cases of congenital syphilis. Glickman and Minsky[71] reported on the same condition. The enlargement is a hyperostosis of the medial clavicle, occurring in the sternoclavicular joint of the dominant extremity, which reaches its permanent stage and size at puberty. The theory of why it affects the sternoclavicular joint relates it to spirochete invasion of the sternal end of the clavicle at the time of early ossification.

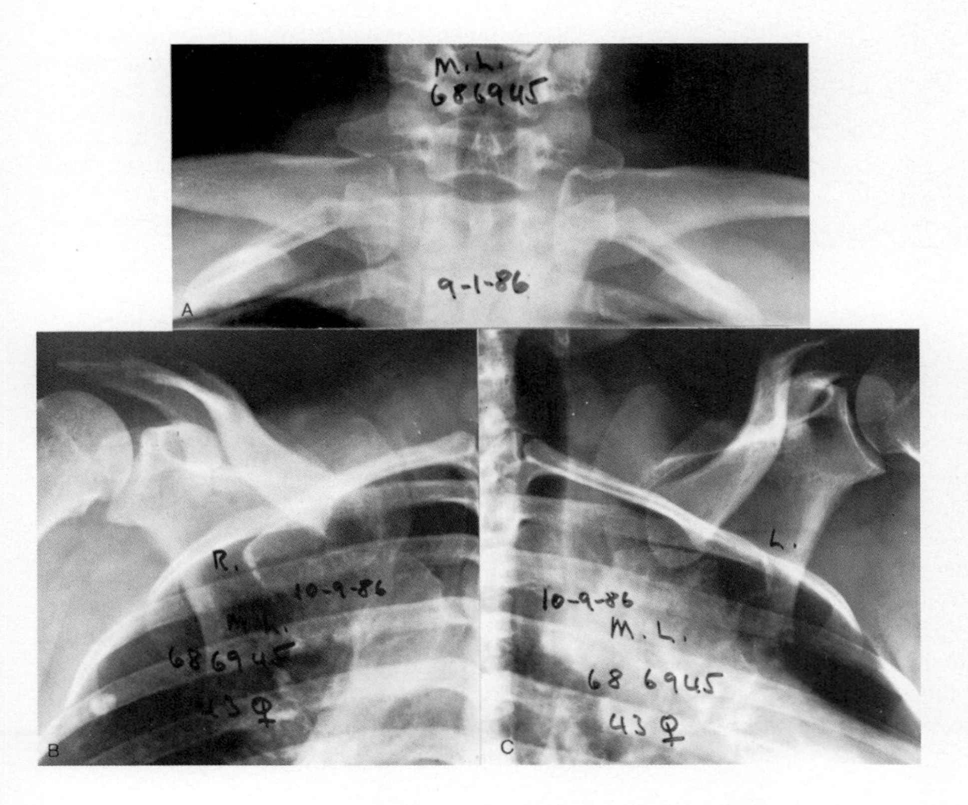

FIG. 13. Infection in the right sternoclavicular joint. **A:** On the initial x-ray, there is little difference between the right and left medial clavicles, as seen on the 30-degree cephalic tilt view. **B and C:** Thirty-eight days later, the medial end of the right clavicle is seen to be dissolving, compared with the medial end of the left clavicle. The patient had a *Staphylococcus aureus* infection in the right sternoclavicular joint, which was managed by open debridement. (Reprinted with permission from Rockwood CA, Matsen F III, eds. *The shoulder.* Philadelphia: WB Saunders, 1990:Fig. 13-14.)

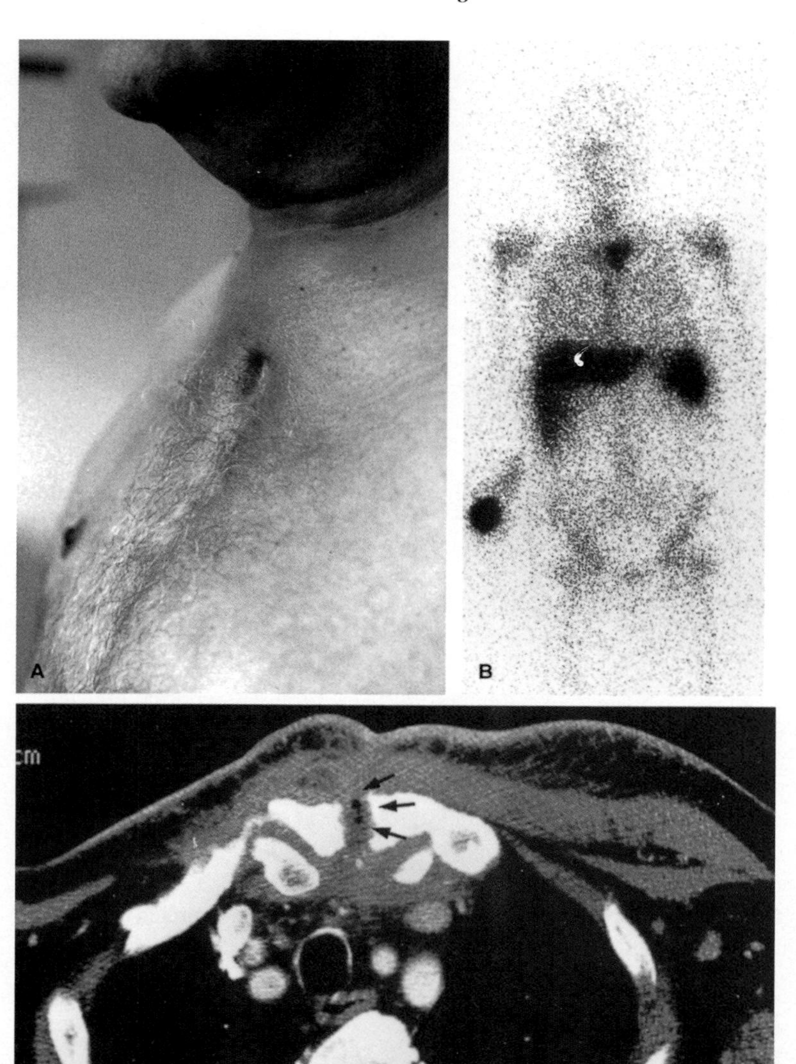

FIG. 14. A: This patient had long-standing insulin-dependent diabetes and had had a coronary artery bypass procedure that was complicated by a post-operative wound infection. **B:** Indium-enhanced white blood cell scan consistent with infection in the region of the left sternoclavicular joint. **C:** CT scan revealing significant soft-tissue swelling, interspersed locules of air within the sternal osteotomy site, and focal irregularity of the posterior aspect of the sternum consistent with an infectious process. (From Wirth MA and Rockwood CA. Injuries to the Sternoclavicular Joint In: Rockwood CA, Green DP, Bucholz RW and Hechman JD (eds.). *Fractures in Adults*, Philadelphia, JB Lippincott 1996.)

INCIDENCE OF INJURY

Sternoclavicular injuries are rare, and many of the authors apologize for reporting only three or four cases. Attesting to this rarity is the fact that some orthopedists have never treated or seen a dislocation of the sternoclavicular joint.[89,161]

The incidence of sternoclavicular dislocation, based on the series of 1,603 injuries of the shoulder girdle reported by Cave and associates,[28] is 3%. (Specific incidences in the study were: glenohumeral dislocations, 85%; acromioclavicular, 12%; and sternoclavicular, 3%). In the series by Cave and in our experience, dislocation of the sternoclavicular joint is not as rare as posterior dislocation of the glenohumeral joint.

Ratio of Anterior to Posterior Dislocation

Undoubtedly, anterior dislocations of the sternoclavicular joint are much more common than the posterior type. However, the ratio of anterior to posterior dislocations is only rarely reported. Theoretically, one could survey the literature and develop the ratio of anterior to posterior dislocations, but most of the published material on sternoclavicular dislocations is on the rare posterior dislocation. Of the references listed at the end of this chapter that address injuries of the sternoclavicular joint, more than 60% discuss only posterior dislocations and their various complications. The largest series from a single institution is reported by Nettles and Linscheid,[128] who studied 60 patients with sternoclavicular dislocations (57 anterior and 3 posterior). This gives a ratio of anterior dislocations to posterior dislocations of the sternoclavicular joint of approximately 20 to 1. Waskowitz[184] reviewed 18 cases of sternoclavicular dislocations, none of which was posterior. However, in our series of 185 traumatic sternoclavicular injuries, there have been 135 patients with anterior dislocation and 50 patients with posterior dislocation.

Bilateral Dislocations

In 1896, Hotchkiss[90] reported a bilateral traumatic dislocation of the sternoclavicular joint. A 28-year-old man was run over by a cart and suffered an anterior dislocation of the right shoulder and a posterior dislocation of the left one. The senior author has treated four cases of bilateral sternoclavicular dislocation.

Dislocations of Both Ends of the Clavicle

To our knowledge, the first reported case of dislocation of both ends of the clavicle was mentioned by Porral[142] in 1831. In 1923, Beckman[10] reported a single case and reviewed the literature on 15 cases that had been previously reported. With the exception of this patient, all patients had been treated conservatively with acceptable function. In 1 patient, a brachial plexus neuropathy developed and was treated by excision of a portion of the clavicle. Until recently, to our knowledge, only four additional cases have been reported.[33,49,68,93] In 1990, Rockwood and associates[162] reported 6 patients who had a dislocation of both ends of the clavicle (an anterior dislocation of the sternoclavicular joint) (Fig. 15). Two patients who had fewer demands on the shoulder did well with only minor symptoms after nonoperative management. The other 4 patients had persistent symptoms that were localized to the acromioclavicular joint. Each of these patients had a reconstruction of the acromioclavicular joint that resulted in a painless, full range of motion and a return to normal activity.

MECHANISMS OF INJURY

Because the sternoclavicular joint is subject to practically every motion of the upper extremity, and because the joint is so small and incongruous, one would think that it would be the most commonly dislocated joint in the body. However, the ligamentous supporting structure is so strong and so well designed that it is, in fact, one of the least commonly dislocated joints in the body. A traumatic dislocation of the sternoclavicular joint usually occurs only after tremendous forces, either direct or indirect, have been applied to the shoulder.

Direct Force

When a force is applied directly to the anteromedial aspect of the clavicle, the clavicle is pushed posteriorly behind the sternum and into the mediastinum (Fig. 16). This may occur in a variety of ways: one athlete jumps on another athlete lying on his back, and the knee of the jumper lands directly on

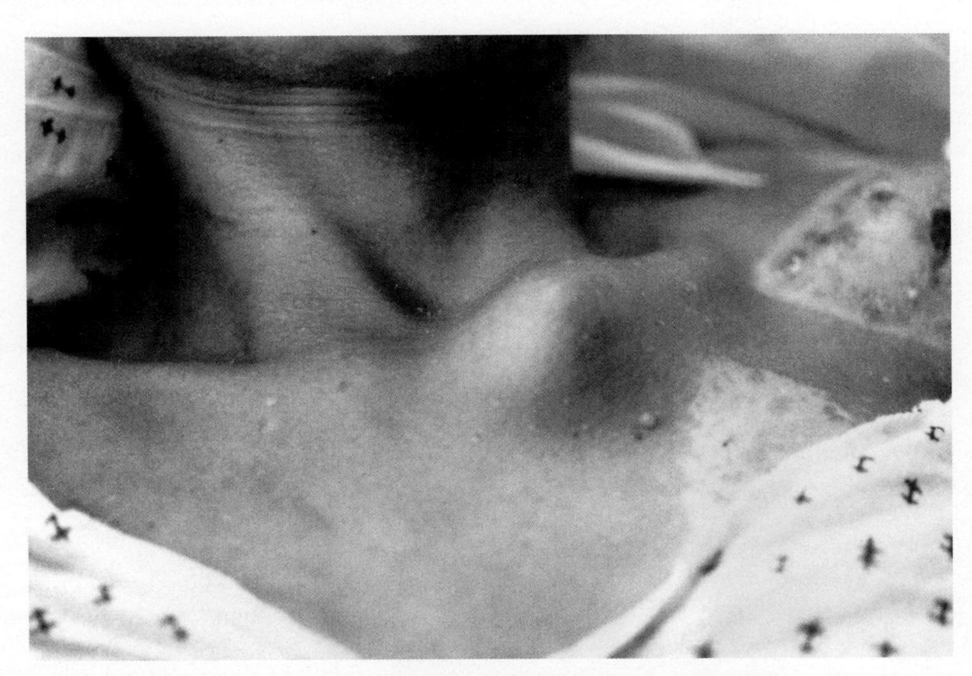

FIG. 15. Photograph of a 37-year-old woman who sustained a traumatic left anterior sternoclavicular dislocation when she was run over by a car. (Reprinted with permission from the 1996 American Academy of Orthopaedic Surgeons. Wirth MA, Rockwood CA. *J Am Acad Orthop Surgeons* 1996;4:268–278. Acute and Chronic Traumatic Injuries of the Sternoclavicular Joint.)

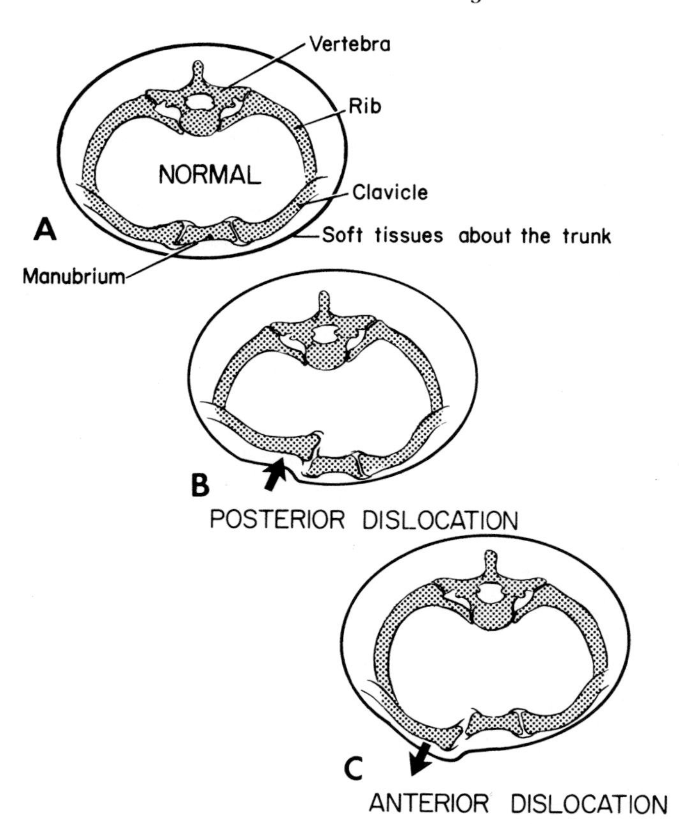

FIG. 16. Cross-sections through the thorax at the level of the sternoclavicular joint. **A:** Normal anatomic relationships. **B:** Posterior dislocation of the sternoclavicular joint. **C:** Anterior dislocation of the sternoclavicular joint.

the medial end of the clavicle; a kick is delivered to the front of the medial clavicle; a person is run over by a vehicle; or a person is pinned between a vehicle and a wall (Fig. 17). Because of our anatomy, it would be most unusual for a direct force to produce an anterior sternoclavicular dislocation.

Indirect Force

A force can be applied indirectly to the sternoclavicular joint from the anterolateral or posterolateral aspects of the shoulder. This is the most common mechanism of injury to the sternoclavicular joint. Mehta and coworkers[122] reported that three of four posterior sternoclavicular dislocations were produced by indirect force, and Heinig[85] reported that indirect force was responsible for eight of nine cases of posterior sternoclavicular dislocations. It was the most common mechanism of injury in our series of 185 patients. If the shoulder is compressed and rolled forward, an ipsilateral posterior dislocation results; if the shoulder is compressed and rolled backward, an ipsilateral anterior dislocation results (Fig. 18). One of the most common causes we have seen is a pile-on in a football game. In this instance, a player falls on the ground, landing on the lateral shoulder; before he can get out of the way, several players pile on top of his opposite shoulder, which applies significant compressive force on the clavicle down toward the sternum. If, during the compression, the shoulder is rolled forward, the force directed down the clavicle produces a posterior dislocation of the sternoclavicular joint. If the shoulder is compressed and rolled backward, the force directed down the clavicle produces an anterior dislocation of the sternoclavicular joint. Other types of indirect forces that can produce sternoclavicular dislocation are a cave-in on a ditch-digger with lateral compression of the shoulders by the falling dirt; lateral compressive forces on the shoulder when a person is pinned between a vehicle and a wall; and a person's falling on the outstretched abducted arm, which drives the shoulder medially in the same manner as a lateral compression on the shoulder.

Most Common Causes of Injury

The most common cause of dislocation of the sternoclavicular joint is vehicular accidents; the second is an injury sus-

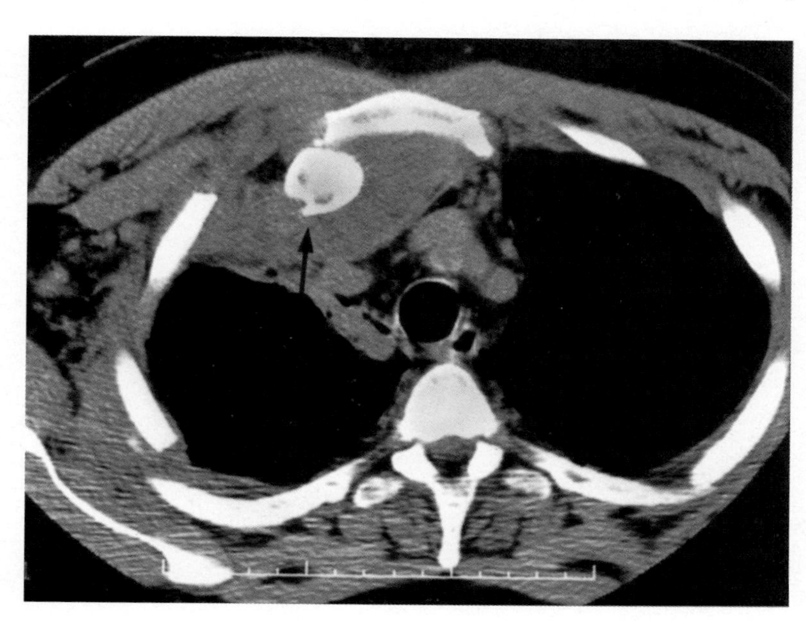

FIG. 17. Computed axial tomogram of a posterior sternoclavicular joint dislocation that occurred when the driver's chest impacted the steering wheel during a motor vehicle accident. The vehicle was totaled, and the steering wheel was fractured from the driving column. (From Wirth MA, Rockwood CA. Injuries to the Sternoclavicular Joint. In: Rockwood CA, Green DP, Bucholz RW, Hechman, JD (eds.). *Fractures in Adults*. Philadelphia. JB Lippincott, 1996.)

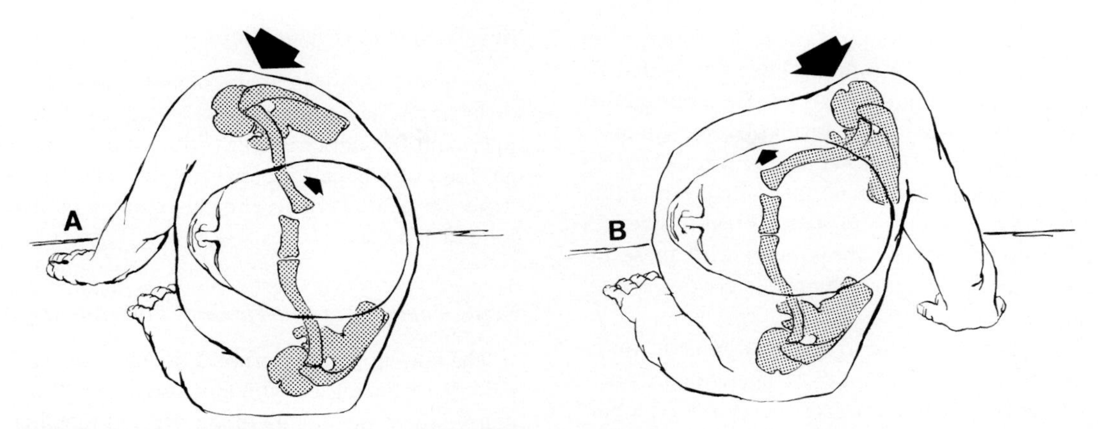

FIG. 18. Mechanisms that produce anterior or posterior dislocations of the sternoclavicular joint. **A:** If the patient is lying on the ground and a compression force is applied to the posterolateral aspect of the shoulder, the medial end of the clavicle will be displaced posteriorly. **B:** When the lateral compression force is directed from the anterior position, the medial end of the clavicle is dislocated anteriorly.

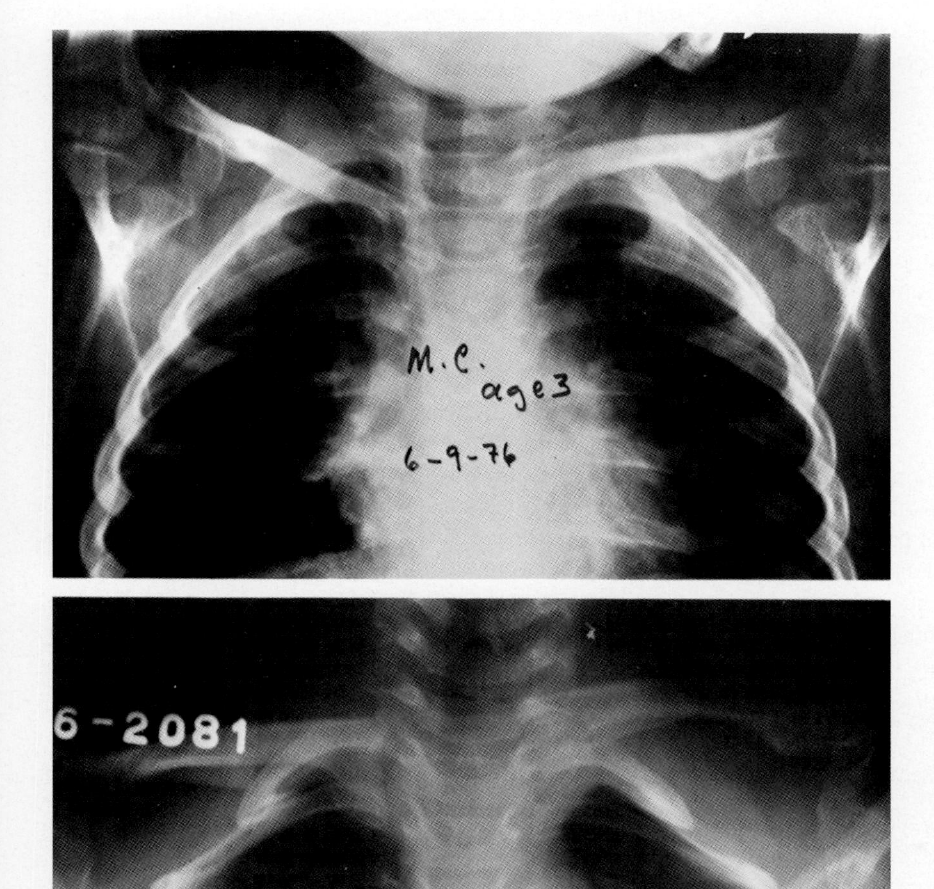

FIG. 19. X-rays of a 3-year-old child with traumatic anterior dislocation of the left sternoclavicular joint. The chest film demonstrates that the left clavicle is superior to the right, suggesting an anterior displacement of the left medial clavicle.

tained during participation in sports.[128,134,184] Omer,[134] in his review of patients from 14 military hospitals, found 82 cases of sternoclavicular joint dislocations. He reported that almost 80% of these occurred as the result of vehicular accidents (47%) and athletics (31%). We recently reviewed 19 patients with posterior sternoclavicular joint injuries that were managed at the University of Texas Health Sciences Center at San Antonio. Seventy-nine percent of these injuries were the result of a motor vehicle accident or sports-related trauma.[188]

Probably the youngest patient to have a traumatic sternoclavicular disloction was reported by Wheeler and associates.[187] They described an anterior dislocation in a 7-month-old infant. The injury occurred when she was lying on her left side and her older brother accidentally fell on her, compressing her shoulders together. The closed reduction was unstable, and the child was immobilized in a figure-of-eight bandage for 5 weeks. At 10 weeks she had full range of motion, and there was no evidence of instability. The senior author has seen an anterior injury in a 3-year-old that occurred as a result of an automobile accident (Fig. 19).

SIGNS AND SYMPTOMS

Mild Sprain

In a mild sprain, the ligaments of the joint are intact. The patient complains of a mild to moderate amount of pain, particularly with movement of the upper extremity. The joint may be slightly swollen and tender to palpation, but instability is not noted.

Moderate Sprain (Subluxation)

A moderate sprain results in a subluxation of the sternoclavicular joint. The ligaments are either partially disrupted or severely stretched. Swelling is noted and pain is marked, particularly with any movement of the arm. Anterior or posterior subluxation may be obvious to the examiner when the injured joint is compared with the normal sternoclavicular joint.

Severe Sprain (Dislocation)

A severe sprain is analogous to a joint dislocation. The dislocation may be anterior or posterior. The capsular ligament and the intraarticular disk ligament are ruptured. Regardless of whether the dislocation is anterior or posterior, there are characteristic clinical findings of sternoclavicular joint dislocation.

Signs Common to Anterior and Posterior Dislocations

The patient with a sternoclavicular dislocation has severe pain that is increased with any movement of the arm, particularly when the shoulders are pressed together by a lateral force. The patient usually supports the injured arm across the trunk with the normal arm. The affected shoulder appears to be shortened and thrust forward when compared with the normal shoulder. The head may be tilted toward the side of the dislocated joint. The discomfort increases when the patient is placed in the supine postition, at which time it will be noted that the involved shoulder will not lie back flat on the table.

Signs and Symptoms of Anterior Dislocations

With an anterior dislocation, the medial end of the clavicle is visibly prominent anterior to the sternum (Fig. 20) and can be palpated anterior to the sternum. It may be fixed anteriorly or may be quite mobile.

Signs and Symptoms of Posterior Dislocation

The patient with a posterior dislocation has more pain than does a patient with an anterior dislocation. Stankler[173] reported 2 patients with unrecognized posterior dislocations that developed venous engorgement of the ipsilateral arm. The anterosuperior fullness of the chest produced by the clavicle is less prominent and visible when compared with the normal side. The usually palpable medial end of the clavicle is displaced posteriorly. The corner of the sternum is

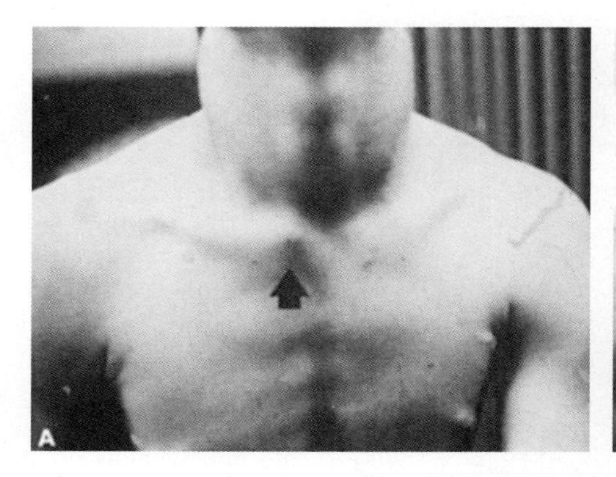

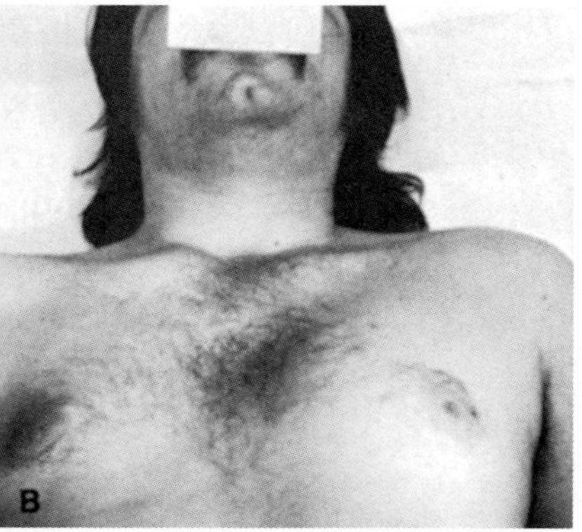

FIG. 20. **(A)** An anterior dislocation of the right sternoclavicular joint is clinically evident (*arrow*). **(B)** When the clavicles are viewed from around the level of the patient's knees, it is apparent that the right clavicle is dislocated anteriorly.

easily palpated as compared with the normal sternoclavicular joint. Venous congestion may be present in the neck or in the upper extremity. Breathing difficulties, shortness of breath, or a choking sensation may be noted. Circulation to the ipsilateral arm may be decreased. The patient may complain of difficulty in swallowing or a tight feeling in the throat, or may be in a state of complete shock or possibly have a pneumothorax.

We have seen a number of patients who clinically appeared to have an anterior dislocation of the sternoclavicular joint but on x-ray studies were shown to have complete posterior dislocation. The point is that one cannot always rely on the clinical findings of observing and palpating the joint to make a distinction between anterior and posterior dislocations.

RADIOGRAPHIC FINDINGS

Anteroposterior Views

The older literature reflects that routine x-rays of the sternoclavicular joint, regardless of the special views, are difficult to interpret. Special oblique views of the chest have been recommended, but because of the distortion of one clavicle over the other, interpretation is difficult (Fig. 21). The older literature also suggests that the diagnosis of dislocation of the sternoclavicular joint is best made from a clinical examination, not from the x-rays. However, it does indicate that tomography offers more detailed information, often showing small fractures in the vicinity of the sternoclavicular joint. Occasionally, the routine anteroposterior or posteroanterior x-rays of the chest or sternoclavicular joint suggest that something is wrong with one of the clavicles, because it appears to be displaced as compared with the normal side (Figs. 22 and 23). It would be ideal to take a view at right angles to the anteroposterior plane, but because of our anatomy, it is impossible to obtain a true 90 degree cephalic-to-caudal lateral view. Lateral x-rays of the chest are at right angles to the anteroposterior plane, but they cannot be interpreted because of the density of the chest and the overlap of the medial clavicles with the first rib and the sternum.

Regardless of a clinical impression that suggests an anterior dislocation, x-rays must be obtained to confirm one's suspicions.

Special Projected Views

Kattan[97] has recommended a special projection, as have Ritvo and Ritvo,[149] Schmitt,[164] Fedoseev,[56] Ferey and Leonard,[60] and Tricoire and coworkers.[181] Kurzbauer[104] has recommended special lateral projections. Hobbs,[88] in 1968, recommended a view that comes close to being a 90-degree cephalocaudal lateral view of the sternoclavicular joints. In the same year, Heinig[85] recommended an x-ray projection of the sternoclavicular joint that resembles a "swimmer's view" of the cervical spine.

Heinig View

With the patient in a supine position, the x-ray tube is placed approximately 30 inches from the involved sternoclavicular joint, and the central ray is directed tangential to the joint and parallel to the opposite clavicle. The cassette is placed against the opposite shoulder and centered on the manubrium (Fig. 24).

Hobbs View

In the Hobbs view, the patient is seated at the x-ray table, high enough to lean forward over the table. The cassette is on the table, and the lower anterior rib cage is against the cassette (Fig. 25). The patient leans forward, so that the nape of his or her flexed neck is almost parallel to the table. The flexed elbows straddle the cassette and support the head and neck. The x-ray source is above the nape of the neck, and the

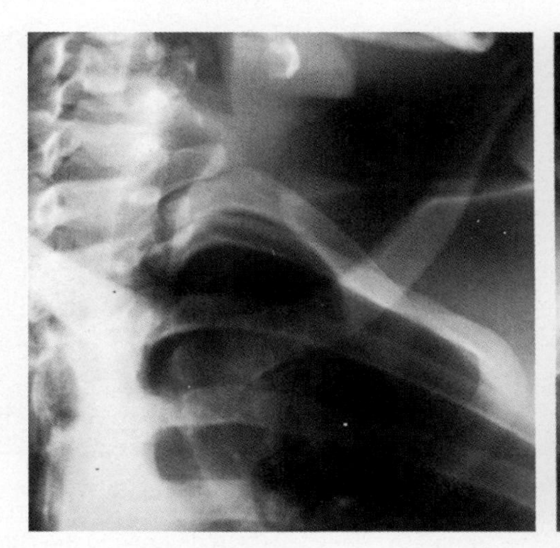

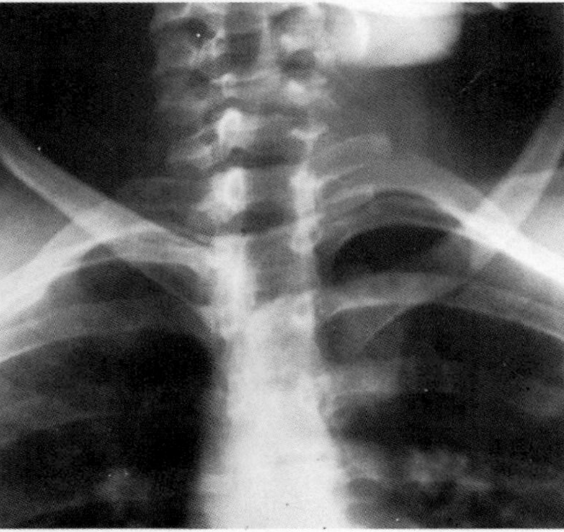

FIG. 21. Routine radiographs of the sternoclavicular joint are difficult to interpret, even with a classic posterior dislocation of the joint.

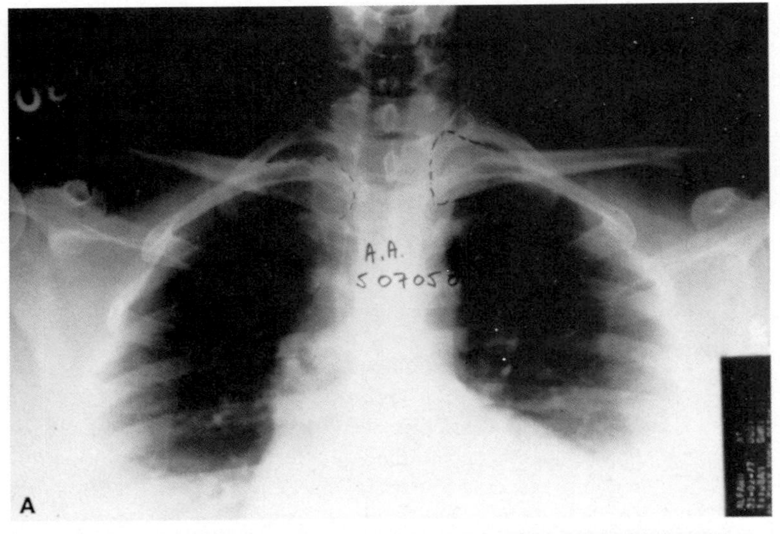

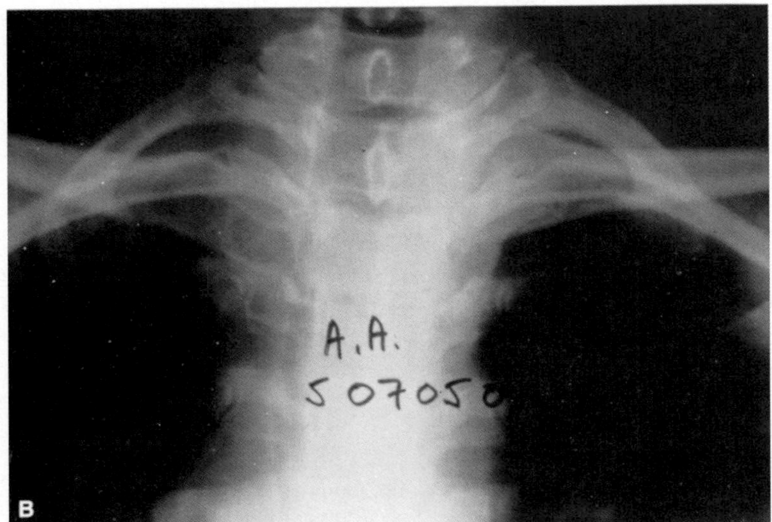

FIG. 22. Anteroposterior x-ray of the sternoclavicular joints with anterosuperior displacement of the left medial clavicle. **A:** The displacement is quite noticeable when the clavicles are outlined. **B:** However, the displacement is not so noticeable when the clavicles are not outlined.

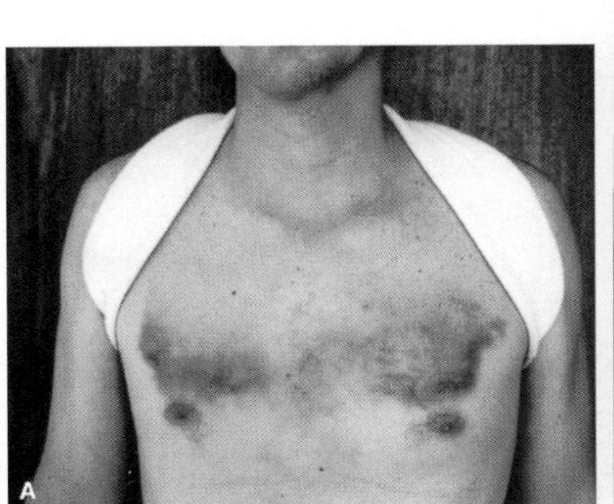

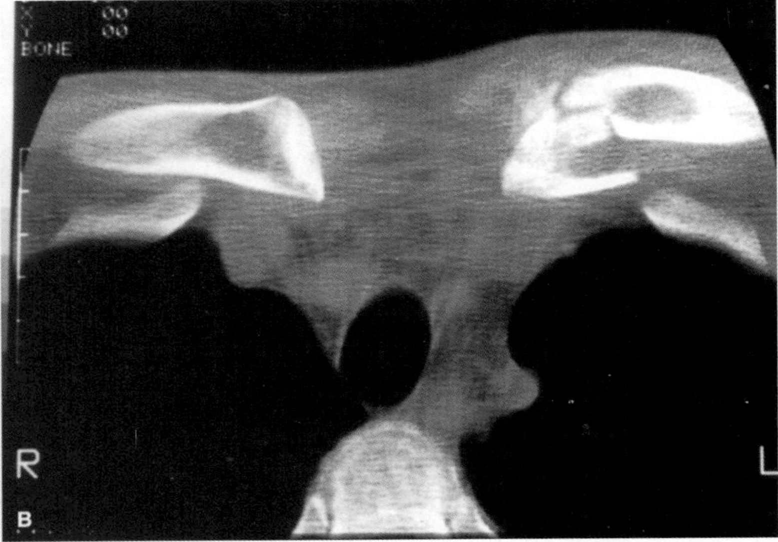

FIG. 23. A: A 34-year-old patient was involved in a motorcycle accident and sustained an anterior blow to the chest. Note the symmetric anterior chest wall ecchymosis. **B:** CT reveals a left medial clavicle fracture without disruption of the sternoclavicular joint. (From Wirth MA, Rockwood CA. Injuries to the Sternoclavicular Joint. In: Rockwood CA, Green DP, Bucholz RW, Hechman JD (eds.). *Fractures in Adults*. Philadelphia, JB Lippincott, 1996.)

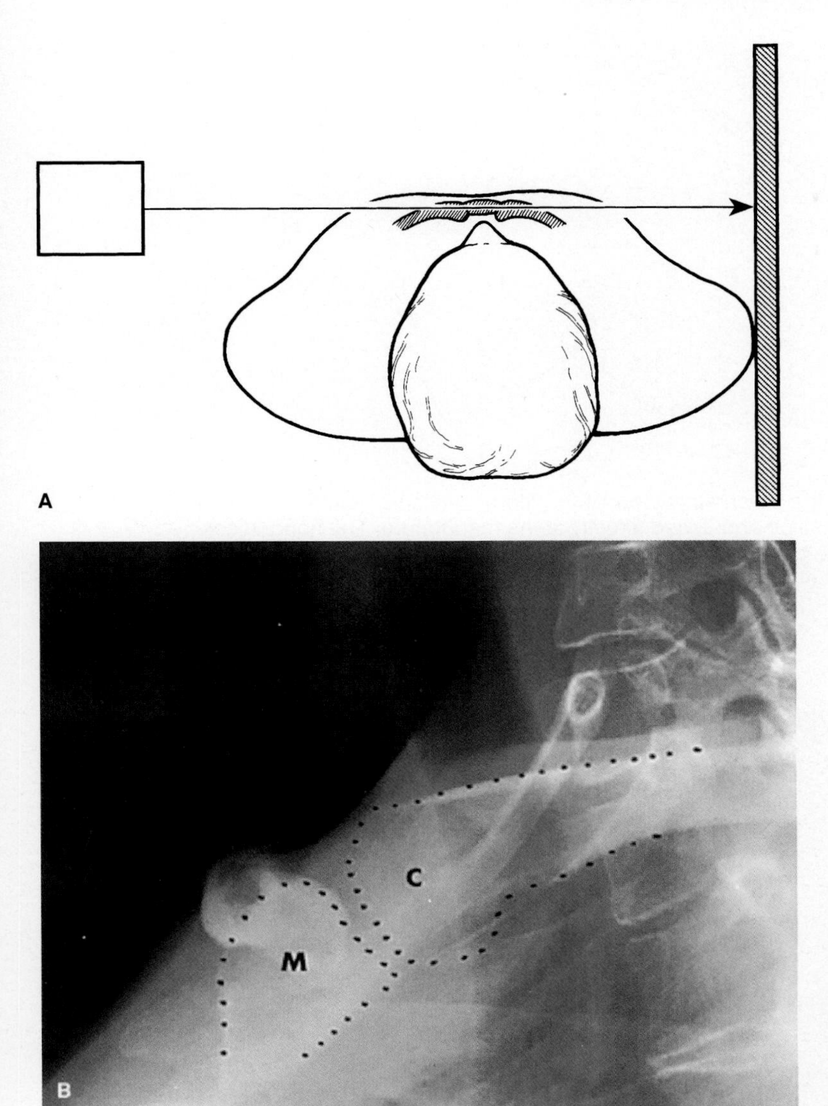

FIG. 24. **A:** Positioning of the patient for x-ray evaluation of the sternoclavicular joint, as described by Heinig. **B:** Heinig view demonstrating a normal relationship between the medial end of the clavicle (c) and the manubrium (M). (From Wirth MA, Rockwood CA. Injuries to the Sternoclavicular Joint. In: Rockwood CA, Green DP, Bucholz RW, Hechman JD (eds.). *Fractures in Adults*. Philadelphia, JB Lippincott, 1996).

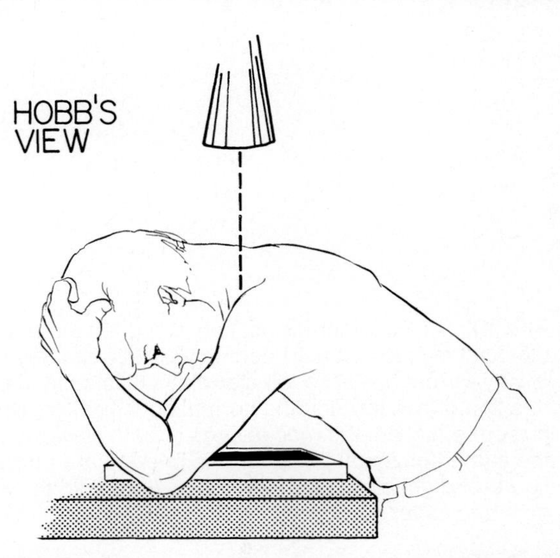

FIG. 25. Positioning of the patient for x-ray evaluation of the sternoclavicular joint, as recommended by Hobbs. (Redrawn with permission from Hobbs DW. The sternoclavicular joint: a new axial radiographic view. *Radiology* 1968;90:801.)

beam passes through the cervical spine to project the sternoclavicular joints onto the cassette.

Serendipity View

The serendipity view is rightfully named because that is the way it developed. The senior author, accidentally, noted that the next best thing to having a true cephalocaudal lateral view of the sternoclavicular joint is a 40-degree cephalic tilt view. The patient is positioned on his or her back squarely and in the center of the x-ray table. The tube is tilted at a 40-degree angle off the vertical and is centered directly on the sternum (Fig. 26). A nongrid 11 × 14-inch cassette is placed squarely on the table and under the patient's upper shoulders and neck, so that the beam aimed at the sternum will project both clavicles onto the film. The tube is adjusted so that the medial half of both clavicles is projected onto the film. It is important to note that the cassette should be placed squarely on the x-ray table (i.e., not angulated or rotated) and that the patient should be positioned squarely on top of the cassette.

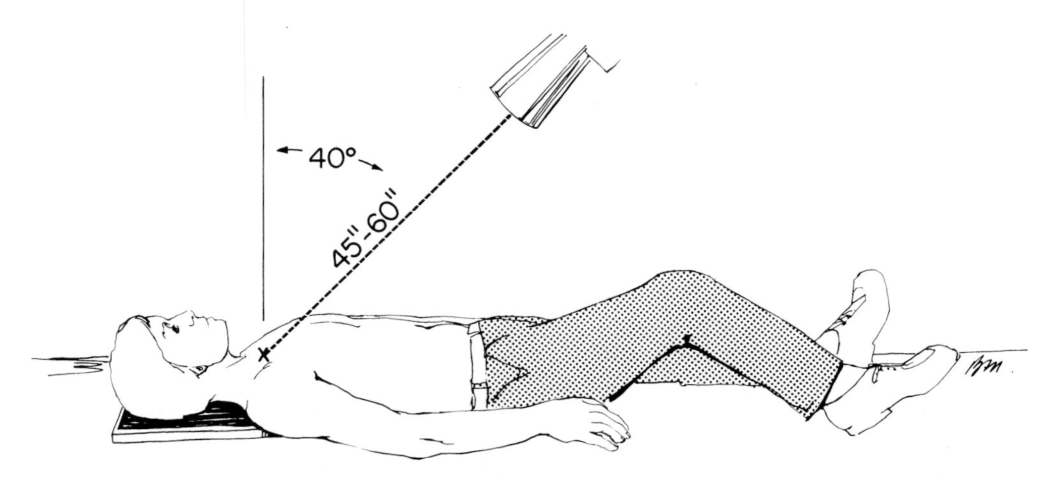

FIG. 26. Positioning of the patient to take the serendipity view of the sternoclavicular joints. The x-ray tube is tilted 40 degrees from the vertical position and aimed directly at the manubrium. The nongrid cassette should be large enough to receive the projected images of the medial halves of both clavicles. In children, the tube distance from the patient should be 45 inches; in thicker chested adults, the distance should be 60 inches.

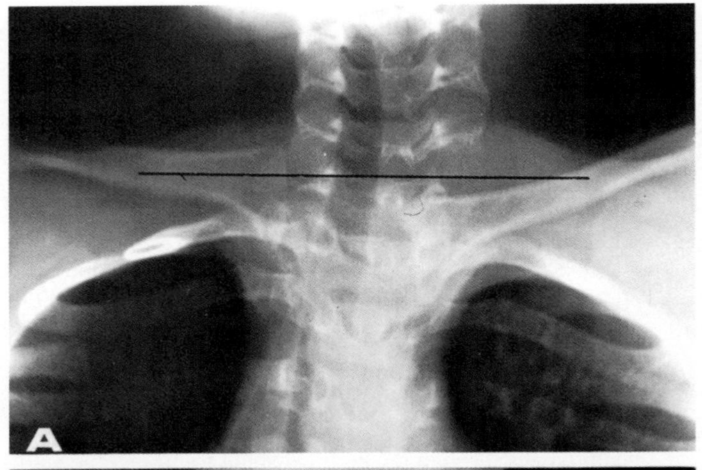

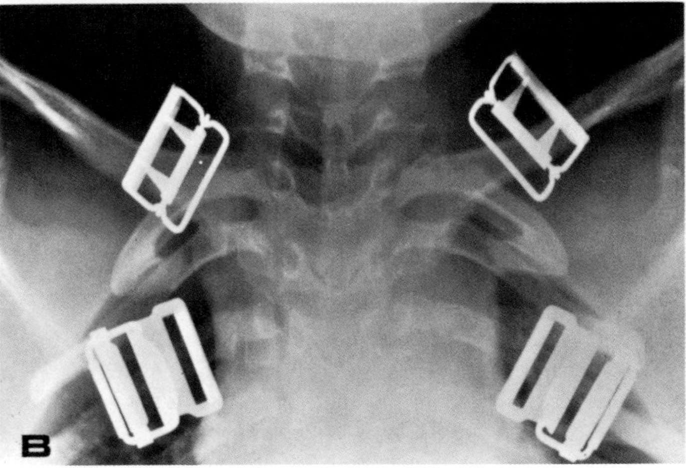

FIG. 27. A: Posterior dislocation of the left sternoclavicular joint as seen on a 40-degree caphalic tilt x-ray film of a 12-year-old boy. The left clavicle is displaced inferiorly to a line drawn through the normal right clavicle. **B:** After closed reduction, the medial ends of both clavicles are in the same horizontal position. The buckles are part of the figure-of-eight clavicular harness used to hold the shoulders back after reduction.

For children, the distance from the tube to the cassette is 45 inches; for adults, whose anteroposterior chest diameter is greater, the distance should be 60 inches. The technical setting of the machine is essentially the same as for a posteroanterior view of the chest.

To understand this view, imagine that your eyes are at the level of the patient's knees and you are looking up toward his or her clavicles at a 40-degree angle. If the right sternoclavicular joint is dislocated anteriorly, the right clavicle will appear to be displaced more anteriorly or riding higher on an imaginary horizontal line, when compared with the normal left clavicle (Fig. 20). The reverse is true if the left sternoclavicular joint is dislocated posteriorly (i.e., the left clavicle displaced inferiorly or riding lower on an imaginary horizontal plane than the normal right clavicle) (Fig. 27). The idea, then, is to take a 40-degree cephalic tilt x-ray showing both medial clavicles and compare the injured clavicle with the normal clavicle (Fig. 28).

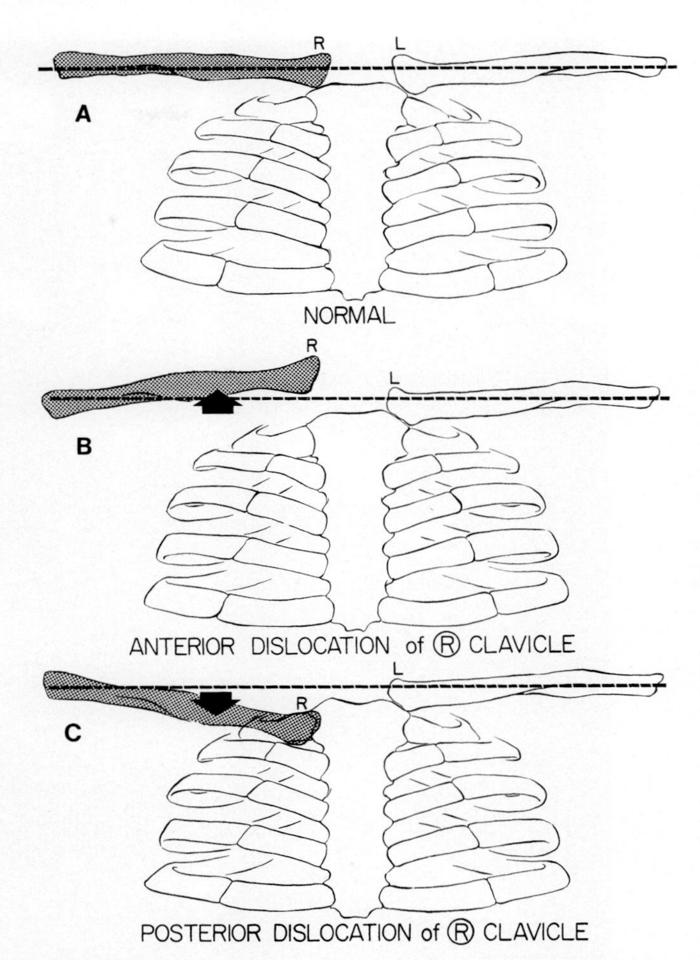

FIG. 28. Interpretation of the cephalic tilt x-ray films of the sternoclavicular joints. **A:** In the normal person, both clavicles appear on the same imaginary line drawn horizontally across the film. **B:** In a patient with anterior dislocation of the right sternoclavicular joint, the medial half of the right clavicle is projected above the imaginary line drawn through the level of the normal left clavicle. **C:** If the patient has a posterior dislocation of the right sternoclavicular joint, the medial half of the right clavicle is displaced below the imaginary line drawn through the normal left clavicle.

Special Techniques

Tomograms

Tomograms can be very helpful in distnguishing between a sternoclavicular dislocation and a fracture of the medial clavicle. They are also helpful in questionable anterior and posterior injuries of the sternoclavicular joint—to distinguish fractures from dislocations and to evaluate arthritic changes (Fig. 29).

In 1959, Baker[3] recommended the use of tomography, which was developed in the late 1920s, and said it was far more valuable than routine films and the fingertips of the examining physician. In 1975, Morag and Shahin[126] reported on the value of tomography, which they used in a series of 20 patients, and recommended that it be used routinely to evaluate problems of the sternoclavicular joint. From a study of normal sternoclavicular joints, they pointed out the variation in the x-ray appearance in different age groups.

CT Scans

Without question, the CT scan is the best technique to study problems of the sternoclavicular joint (Fig. 30). It

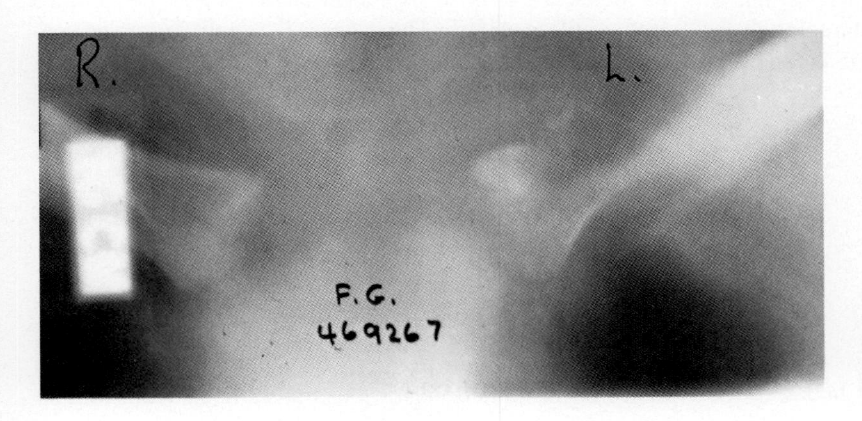

FIG. 29. Tomogram demonstrating a fracture of the left medial clavicle. The clinical diagnosis before radiography was an anterior dislocation of the left sternoclavicular joint.

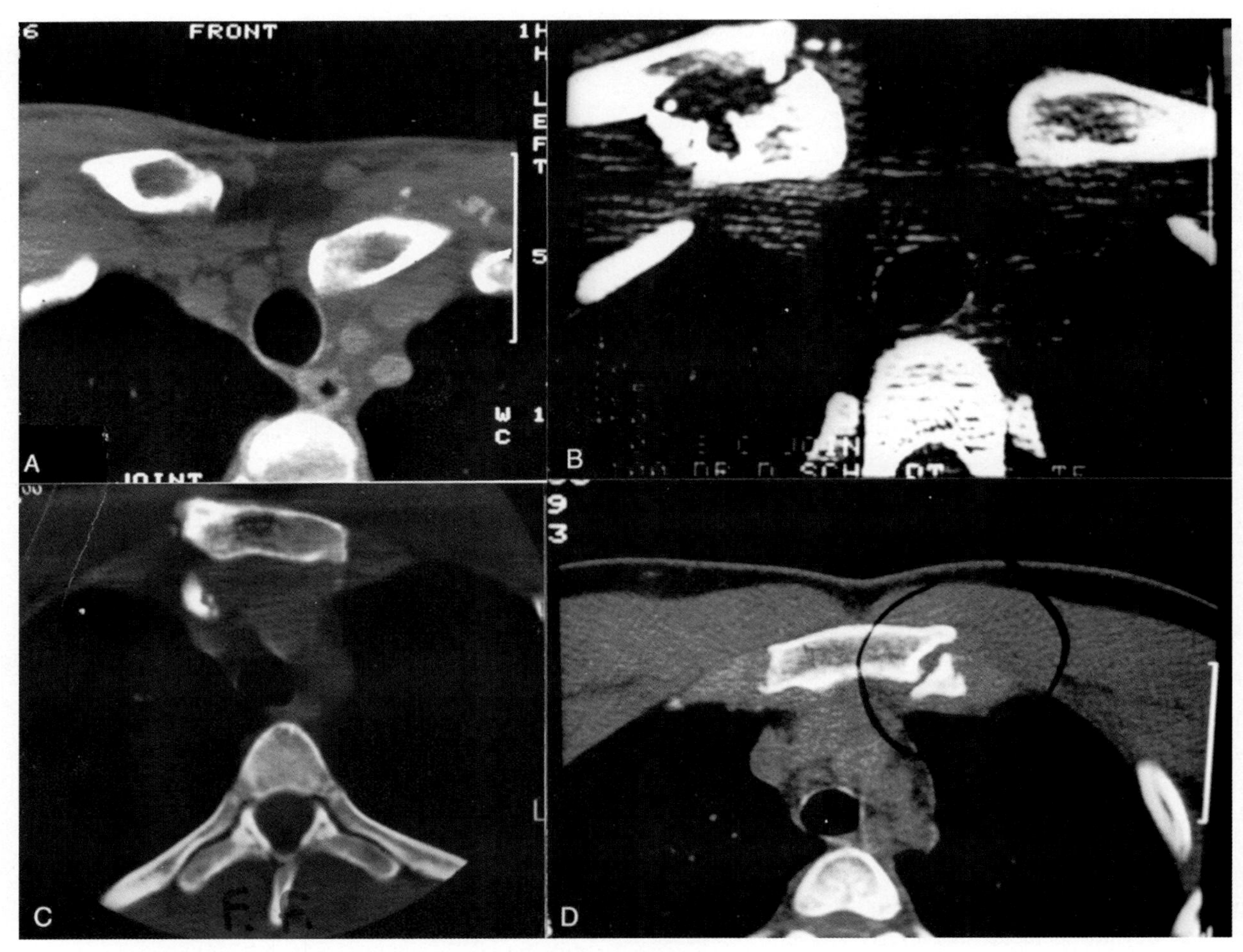

FIG. 30. CT scans of the sternoclavicular joint, demonstrating various types of injuries. **A:** Posterior dislocation of the left clavicle compressing the great vessels and producing swelling of the left arm. **B:** Fracture of the medial clavicle that does not involve that articular surface. **C:** Fragment of bone displaced posteriorly into the great vessel. **D:** Fracture of the medial clavicle into the sternoclavicular joint. (Reprinted with permission from Rockwood CA, Matsen F III, eds. *The shoulder.* Philadelphia: WB Saunders, 1990:Fig. 13-22.)

clearly distinguishes injuries of the joint from fractures of the medial clavicle and defines minor subluxations of the joint. The orthopedist must remember to ask for CT scans of both sternoclavicular joints and the medial half of both clavicles, so that the injured side can be compared with the normal side. The patient should lie flat in the supine position. If one requests a study of the right sternoclavicular joint, the x-ray technician may rotate the patient to the affected side and provide views of only the one joint.

NONOPERATIVE TREATMENT

Traumatic Injuries

Anterior Problems

Mild Sprain

The mildly sprained sternoclavicular joint is stable but painful. Application of ice for the first 12 to 24 hours, followed by heat, is helpful. The upper extremity should be immobilized in a sling for 3 to 4 days; then, gradually the patient can regain use of the arm in everyday activities. The senior author undertook a fascinating case of a young woman who, after childbirth, developed aching pain in both sternoclavicular joints. Her bra size, over a period of 4 weeks, had jumped from a 36B to a 38EE. The increase in weight depressed both shoulders and produced pain while upright in both sternoclavicular joints. The discomfort was completely relieved by pushing both elbows up, thus elevating the distal clavicles, which in turn took the strain off her sternoclavicular joints. She was requested to consult her gynecologist and surgeon to determine the quickest way to reduce the size of her breasts.

Moderate Sprain (Subluxation)

For subluxation of the sternoclavicular joint, application of ice is recommended for the first 12 hours, followed by heat for the next 24 to 48 hours. The joint may be subluxated anteriorly or posteriorly, which may be reduced by drawing the shoulders backward as if reducing and holding a fracture of the clavicle. A clavicle strap can be used to hold up the shoulder and to prevent motion of the arm. The patient should be protected from further injury for 4 to 6 weeks. De Palma[46] has suggested a plaster figure-of-eight dressing, and McLaughlin[125] has recommended the same type of treatment that would be used for fracture of the clavicle, with the addition of a sling to support the arm. Allman[2] prefers the use of a soft figure-of-eight bandage with a sling, and occasionally uses adhesive strapping over the medial end of the clavicle.

Severe Sprain (Dislocation): Anterior Dislocation

There still is some controversy regarding the treatment of acute or chronic anterior dislocation of the sternoclavicular joint. In 1990, de Jong and Sukul[42] reported long-term follow-up results in 10 patients with traumatic anterior sternoclavicular dislocations. All patients were treated nonoperatively with analgesics and immobilization. The results of treatment were good in 7 patients, fair in 2 patients, and poor in 1 patient at an average follow-up of 5 years. Most acute anterior dislocations are unstable following reduction, and many operative procedures have been described to repair or reconstruct the joint.

Method of Closed Reduction. Closed reduction of the sternoclavicular joint may be accomplished with local or general anesthesia or, in stoic patients, without anesthesia. Most investigators recommend the use of narcotics or muscle relaxants. The patient is placed supine on the table, lying on a 3- to 4-inch thick pad between the shoulders. In this position, the clavicle may reduce with direct gentle pressure over the anteriorly displaced clavicle. However, when the pressure is released, the clavicle usually dislocates again.

Occasionally, the clavicle will remain reduced. Sometimes, the physician will need to push both shoulders back onto the table while an assistant applies pressure to the anteriorly displaced clavicle. Laidlaw[106] treated an interesting case of a patient who had a dislocated clavicle. The sternoclavicular joint was dislocated anteriorly and was mildly symptomatic. The acromioclavicular joint was most symptomatic and was treated by excision of the distal clavicle. Surprisingly, the anteriorly dislocated sternoclavicular joint reduced and became pain free. More recently, Thomas and Friedman[180] reported an ipsilateral anterior sternoclavicular dislocation and clavicle shaft fracture. Unfortunately, the anterior sternoclavicular dislocation was diagnosed solely by clinical examination, without the aid of computed tomography, tomograms, or special projection views.

Postreduction Care. If, with the shoulders held back, the sternoclavicular joint remains reduced, the shoulders can be stabilized with a soft figure-of-eight dressing, a commercial clavicle strap harness, or a plaster figure-of-eight cast. Some investigators recommend a bulky pressure pad over the anteromedial clavicle that is held in place with elastic tape. A sling might be used, because it holds up the shoulder and prevents motion of the arm, Immobilization should be maintained for at least 6 weeks, and then the arm should be protected for another 2 weeks before strenuous activities are undertaken. If the sternoclavicular joint again dislocates when the reduction pressure is released, as it usually does, a figure-of-eight dressing or a sling can be used until the patient's symptoms subside. Most anterior closed reductions of the sternoclavicular joint are unstable, and even with the shoulders held back, the joint is unstable. Although some investigators have recommended operative repair of anterior dislocations of the sternoclavicular joint, we believe that the operative complications are too great and the end results are too unsatisfactory to consider an open reduction. Certainly in children, in whom many if not most of the injuries are physeal fractures, a nonoperative approach should be strongly considered.

Posterior Injuries

Posterior Dislocation

A Careful Examination of the Patient is Extremely Important. Complications are common with posterior dislocation of the sternoclavicular joint, and the patient should receive prompt attention.

A careful history and physical examination should be undertaken to rule out damage to the pulmonary and vascular systems. The sternoclavicular joint must be carefully evaluated by all available x-ray techniques, including, when indicated, combined aortogram-CT scan for potential vascular injuries (Fig. 31). If specific complications are noted, appropriate consultants should be called in before reduction is performed. Worman and Leagus[194] reported a posterior dislocation of the sternoclavicular joint, in which it was noted at surgery that the displaced clavicle had put a hole into the right pulmonary artery. The clavicle had prevented exsanguination, because the vessel was still impaled by the clavicle. Had a closed reduction been performed in the emergency department, the result could have been disastrous. Cooper and coworkers[36] reported a posterior sternoclavicular dislocation that transected the internal mammary artery and lacerated the brachiocaphalic vein. The vascular injuries were associated with fractures of the anterior ends of the first to third ribs and marked posterior instability of the medial end of the clavicle. The brachiocephallic vein was repaired, but the posteriorly displaced medical clavicle impinged on the suture line. To maintain reduction of the sternoclavicular joint, a novel method of stabilization was employed using an external fixator.

General anesthesia is usually required for reduction of a posterior dislocation of the sternoclavicular joint, because the patient has so much pain and has muscle spasms. However, for the stoic patient, some investigaotrs have performed the reduction under intravenous narcotics and muscle relaxants. Heinig[85] has successfully used local anesthesia in a posterior dislocation reduction.

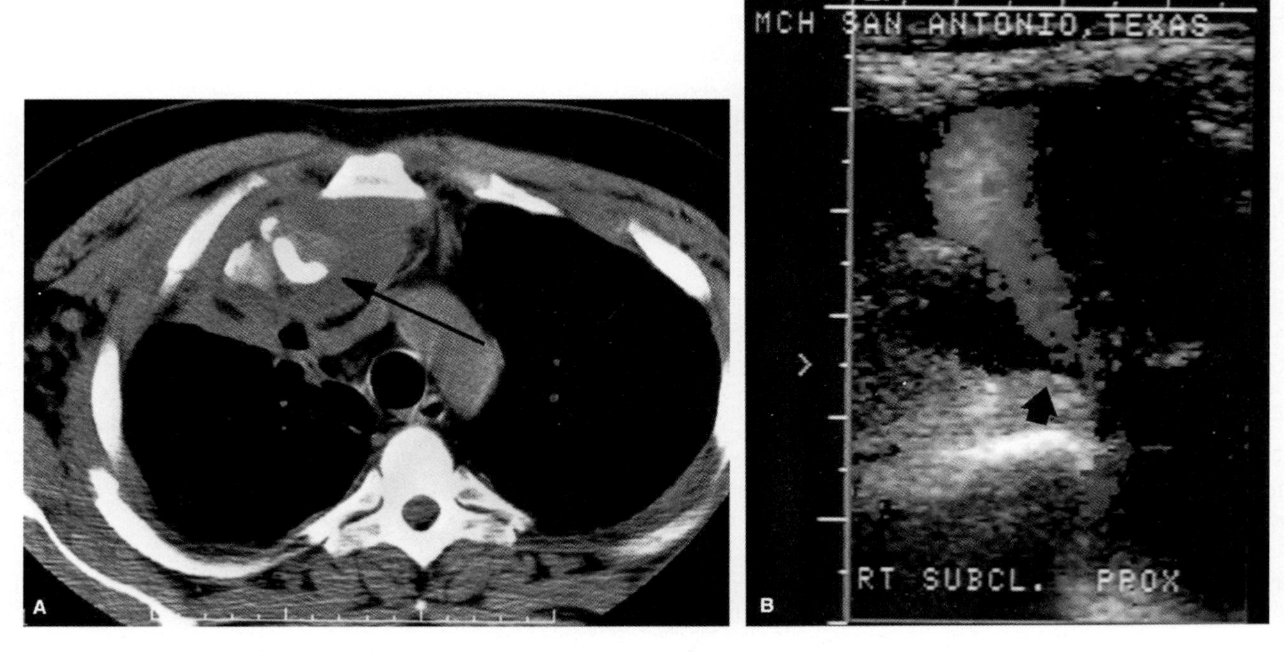

FIG. 31. A: CT scan revealing a posterior fracture–dislocation of the sternoclavicular joint with significant soft-tissue swelling and compromise of the hilar structures. **B:** Duplex ultrasound study revealing a large pseudoaneurysm of the right subclavian artery. Note the large neck of the pseudoaneurysm, which measured approximately 1 cm in diameter (*arrow*). (From Wirth MA, Rockwood CA. Injuries to the Sternoclavicular Joint. In: Rockwood CA, Green DP, Bucholz RW, Hechman JD (eds.). *Fractures in Adults.* Philadelphia, JB Lippincott, 1996).

From a review of the earlier literature, it would appear that the treatment of choice for posterior sternoclavicular dislocation was by operative procedures. However, since the 1950s, the treatment of choice has been closed reduction.[25,31,37,59,80,85,120,121,124,138,161,174] Some investigators,[138,174] who had previously performed open reductions, reported that they were amazed at how easily the dislocation reduced under direct vision, and thereafter they used closed reductions with complete success.

Methods of Closed Reduction

Many different techniques have been described for closed reduction of a posterior dislocation of the sternoclavicular joint.

Abduction Traction Technique. For the abduction traction technique,[45,59,120,124,150,161] the patient is placed on his or her back, with the dislocated shoulder near the edge of the table. A 3- to 4-inch thick sandbag is placed between the shoulders (Fig. 32). Lateral traction is applied to the abducted arm, which is then gradually brought back into extension. This may be all that is necessary to accomplish the reduction. The clavicle usually reduces with an audible snap or pop, and it is almost always stable. Too much extension can bind the anterior surface of the dislocated medial clavicle on the back of the manubrium. Occasionally, it may be necessary to grasp the medial clavicle with one's fingers to dislodge it from behind the sternum. If this fails, the skin is prepared, and a sterile towel clip is used to grasp the medial clavicle to apply lateral and anterior traction (Fig. 33).

Adduction Traction Technique. In this technique,[22] the patient is supine on the table with a 3- to 4-inch bolster between the shoulders. Traction is then applied to the arm in adducion, while a downward pressure is exerted on the shoulders. The clavicle is levered over the first rib into its normal position. Buckerfield and Castle[22] reported that this technique has succeeded when the abduction traction technique has failed. Bitterworth and Kirk[25] used a similar adducted position, except that they applied lateral traction on the upper humerus.

Other Techniques. Heinig[85] and Elting[51] have reported that they accomplished reduction by placing the patient supine on the table with three of four folded towels between the two shoulders. Forward pressure was then applied on both shoulders, which accomplished the reduction. Other investigators have put a knee between the shoulders of the seated patient and, by pulling back on both shoulders, have accomplished a reduction. Stein[174] used skin traction on the abducted and extended arm to accomplish the reduction gently and gradually. Many investigators have reported that closed reduction usually cannot be accomplished after 48 hours. However, others[22,107] have reported closed reductions as late as 4 and 5 days after the injury.

Indeed, as with other childhood fractures, the potential for remodeling is significant and may extend until the 23rd to 25th year of life. The senior author[151] has demonstrated a similar mechanism to support conservative treatment of adolescent acromioclavicular joint injuries or "pseudodislocation," in which there is a partial tear of the periosteal tube.

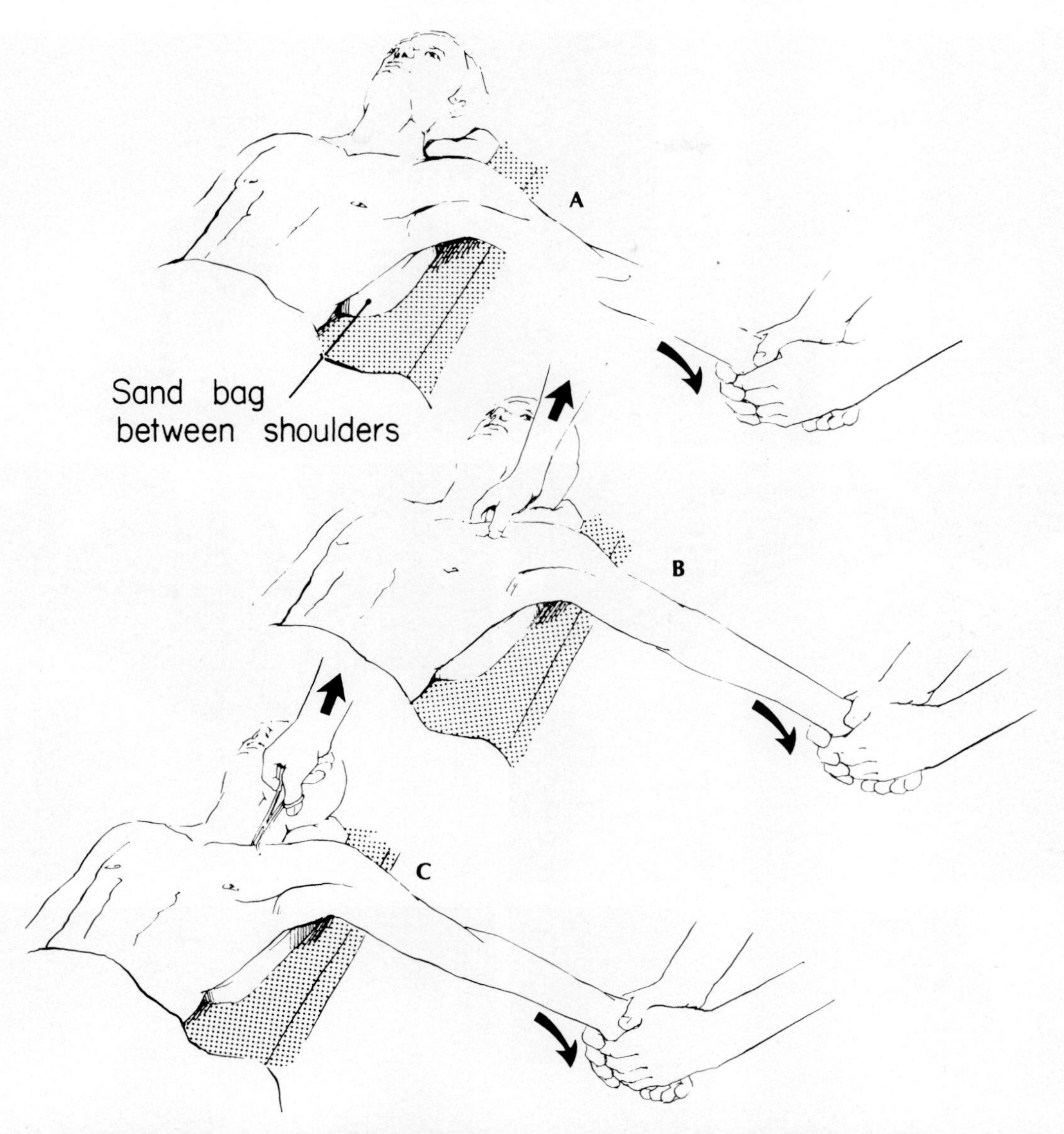

FIG. 32. Technique for closed reduction of the sternoclavicular joint. **A:** The patient is positioned supine with a sandbag placed between the two shoulders. Traction is then applied to the arm against countertraction in an abducted and slightly extended position. In anterior dislocations, direct pressure over the medial end of the clavicle may reduce the joint. **B:** In posterior dislocations, in addition to the traction, it may be necessary to manipulate the medial end of the clavicle with the fingers to dislodge the clavicle from behind the manubrium. **C:** In stubborn posterior dislocations, it may be necessary to sterilely prepare the medial end of the clavicle and use a towel clip to grasp around the medial clavicle to lift it back into position.

Because of its high osteogenic potential, spontaneous healing and remodeling to the preinjury "reduced" position occur within this periosteal conduit. Zaslav and associates[196] have reported successful treatment of a posteriorly displaced medial clavicle physeal injury in an adolescent athlete with CT documentation of remodeling, most probable within an intact periosteal tube.

Similarly, Hsu and associates[92] reported successful treatment of a posterior epiphyseal fracture dislocation of the medial end of the clavicle in a 15-year-old patient.

Postreduction Care

After reduction, to allow ligament healing, the shoulders should be held back for 4 to 6 weeks with a figure-of-eight dressing or one of the commercially available figure-of-eight straps used to treat fractures of the clavicle.

Recurrent or Unreduced Dislocation

Should closed maneuvers fail in the adult, an operative procedure should be performed, because most adult patients

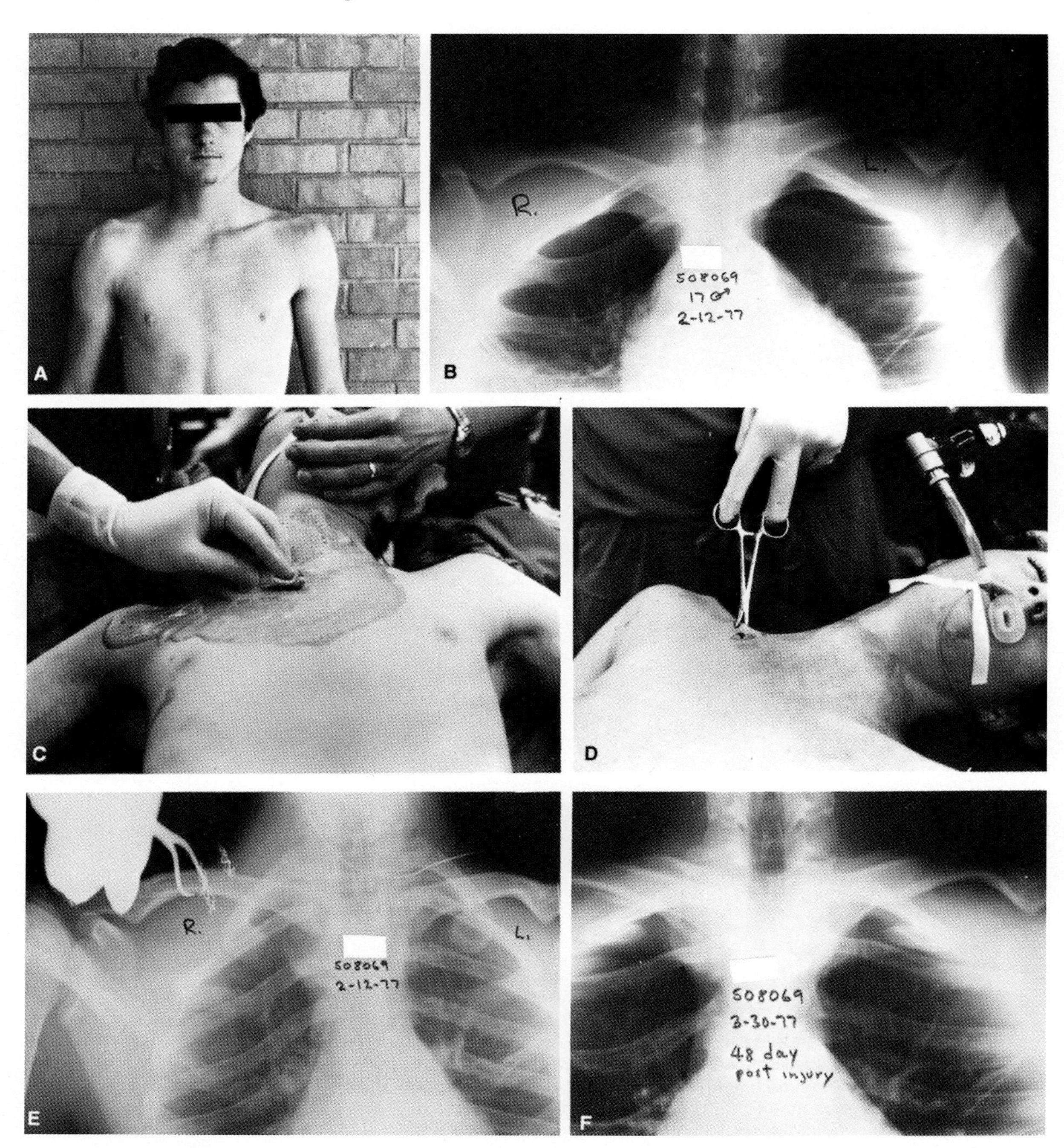

FIG. 33. Posterior dislocation of the right sternoclavicular joint. **A:** a 16-year-old boy has a 48-hour-old posterior displacement of the right medial clavicle that occurred from direct trauma to the anterior right clavicle. He noted immediate onset of difficulty in swallowing and some hoarseness in his voice. **B:** A 40-degree cephalic tilt x-ray film confirmed the posterior displacement of the right medial clavicle, as compared with the left clavicle. Because of the patient's age, this was considered most likely to be a physeal injury of the right medial clavicle. **C:** Because the injury was 48 hours old, we were unable to reduce the dislocation with simple traction on the arm. The right shoulder was surgically cleansed, so that a sterile towel clip could be used. **D:** With the towel clip securely around the clavicle and with continued lateral traction, a visible and audible reduction occurred. **E:** Postreduction x-rays showed that the medial clavicle had been restored to its normal position. The reduction was quite stable, and the patient's shoulders were held back with a figure-of-eight strap. **F:** The right clavicle has remained reduced. Note the periosteal new bone formation along the superior and inferior borders of the right clavicle. This is the result of a physeal injury, whereby the epiphysis remains adjacent to the manubrium while the clavicle is displaced out of a split in the periosteal tube.

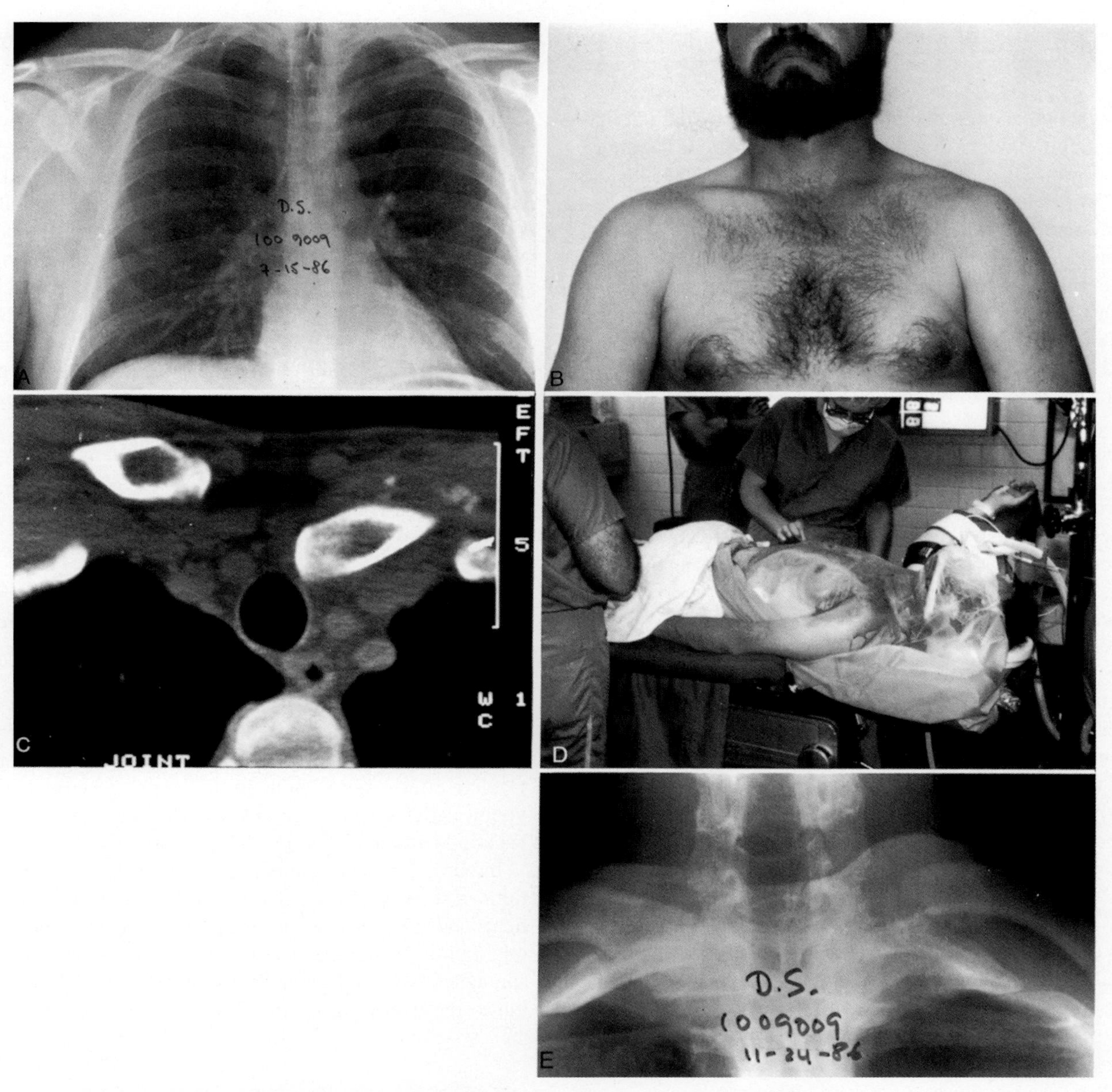

FIG. 34. Open reduction of a posterior dislocation of the left sternoclavicular joint causing compression of the great vessels in the mediastinum and resultant swelling in the patient's left arm. **A:** Chest film does not suggest any serious problem with the left medial clavicle. **B:** Clinically, the medial end of the left clavicle was depressed, as compared with the right. **C:** The CT scan reveals posterior displacement of the medial clavicle back into the mediastinum, compressing the great vessels and slightly displacing the trachea. **D:** The patient was carefully prepared for a surgical repair, in cooperation with a cardiovascular surgeon. The patient was prepared from the base of his neck down to the umbilicus, so that we could manage any type of vascular problem or complication. Open reduction was accomplished without any vascular incident. The medial end of the clavicle was totally unstable, so the medial 2 cm was resected and the remaining clavicle stabilized to the first rib. **E:** Four months after surgery, the slight anterior displacement of the clavicle was essentially asymptomatic and the remaining clavicle was stable. Reprinted with permission from Rockwood CA, Matsen F III, eds. *The shoulder.* Philadelphia: WB Saunders, 1990:Fig. 13-25.)

cannot tolerate posterior displacement of the clavicle into the mediastinum. Holmdahl,[89] Louw and Louw,[113] and Borrero[15] have reported complications following unreduced posterior dislocations. Gangahar and Flogaites[66] reported a case of late thoracic outlet syndrome following an unreduced posterior dislocation, and Borrero[15] reported late and significant vascular problems. Tircoire and colleagues[181] reported a case of respiratory compromise and dyspnea on exertion in a 65-year-old patient with a posterior sternoclavicular dislocation of 3 months' duration. The senior author was asked to evaluate a patient who, following a significant injury, complained of swelling and bluish coloration of his left arm after any type of physical activity. He did not have many local sternoclavicular joint symptoms, but by physical examination the left clavicle was displaced posteriorly. CT demonstrated a major posterior displacement of the left clavicle (Fig. 34). Because of the marked displacement and the vascular compromise, arteriography combined with CT was performed, which did not reveal any vascular leak. With the help of the chest surgeon, the clavicle was removed from the mediastinum, the medial 1.5 inches were removed, and the shaft was stabilized to the first rib. The greatest displacement we have seen was in a patient with a posteroinferior dislocation of the medial clavicle down into an intrathoracic position.

Louw and Louw[113] reported a 30-year-old patient with a T3–4 paraplegia and posterior dislocation of the left sternoclavicular joint, who had essentially no problems. He underwent an extensive rehabilitation program and could lower himself from his wheelchair to the floor and back again without assistance, and he could transfer from his wheelchair to the bed, bath, and car without difficulty.

If children and adults under 25 years of age have symptoms from the pressure of the posteriorly displaced clavicle into the mediastinum, and closed reduction is unsuccessful, an operative procedure should be performed. However, children may have no symptoms. And the physician can wait to see if the physeal plate remodeling process removes the posteriorly displaced bone.[152]

Physeal Injuries

As described earlier in this chapter, the epiphysis on the medial end of the clavicle is the last epiphysis in the body to appear on x-ray and the last one to close. The epiphysis on the medial end of the clavicle does not appear on x-rays until about the 18th year of life and does not unite with the clavicle until the 23rd to 25th year (Figs. 5 and 35).

This is important to remember, because many so-called dislocations of the sternoclavicular joint are not dislocations but physeal injuries. Most of these injuries will heal with time, without surgical intervention. In time, the remodeling process eliminates any bone deformity or displacement. Anterior physeal injuries can certainly be left alone without problem. Posterior physeal injuries should be reduced. If the posterior dislocation cannot be reduced closed and the patient is having no significant symptoms, the displacement can be observed while remodeling occurs. If the posterior displacement is symptomatic and cannot be reduced closed, the displacement must be reduced during surgery (Fig. 35).

Atraumatic Problems

Spontaneous Subluxation or Dislocation

As with classification of glenohumeral joint instability, the importance of distinguishing between traumatic and atraumatic instability of the sternoclavicular joint must be recognized, if complications are to be avoided. Rowe[157] described several patients who had undergone one or more unsuccessful attempts to stabilize the sternoclavicular joint. In all cases, the patient was able to voluntarily dislocate the clavicle after surgery. In addition, he has described several young patients who were able to "flip the calvicle out and back in" without elevation of the arms.[156]

In our experience, spontaneous subluxations and dislocations of the sternoclavicular joint are seen most often in patients under 20 years of age, and more often in females. Without significant trauma, one or both of the medial clavicles spontaneously displace anteriorly during abduction or flexion to the overhead position (Fig. 7). The clavicle reduces

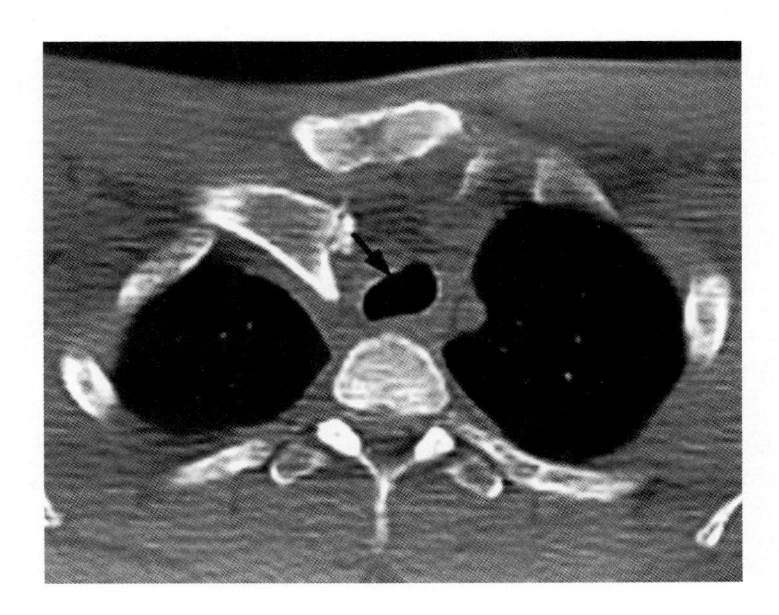

FIG. 35. CT scan of a 19-year-old patient who was involved in a motor vehicle accident and presented with complaints of chest pain and a "choking" sensation that was exacerbated by lying supine. Note the physeal injury of the medial clavicle and compression of the trachea (*arrow*). (From Wirth MA, Rockwood CA. Injuries to the Sternoclavicular Joint. In: Rockwood CA, Green DP, Bucholz RW, Hechman JD (eds.). *Fractures in Adults.* Philadelphia, JB Lippincott, 1996).

when the arm is returned to the side. This usually is associated with laxity in other joints of the extremities. Rockwood and Odor reviewed 37 cases and found it to be a self-limiting condition.[154] The conditions should not be treated with attempted surgical reconstruction, because the joint will continue to subluxate or dislocate and surgery may indeed cause more pain, discomfort, and an unsightly scar (Fig. 36). The condition should be carefully explained to the patient and the family, and they should be told that ultimately it will not be a problem and the symptoms may disappear.

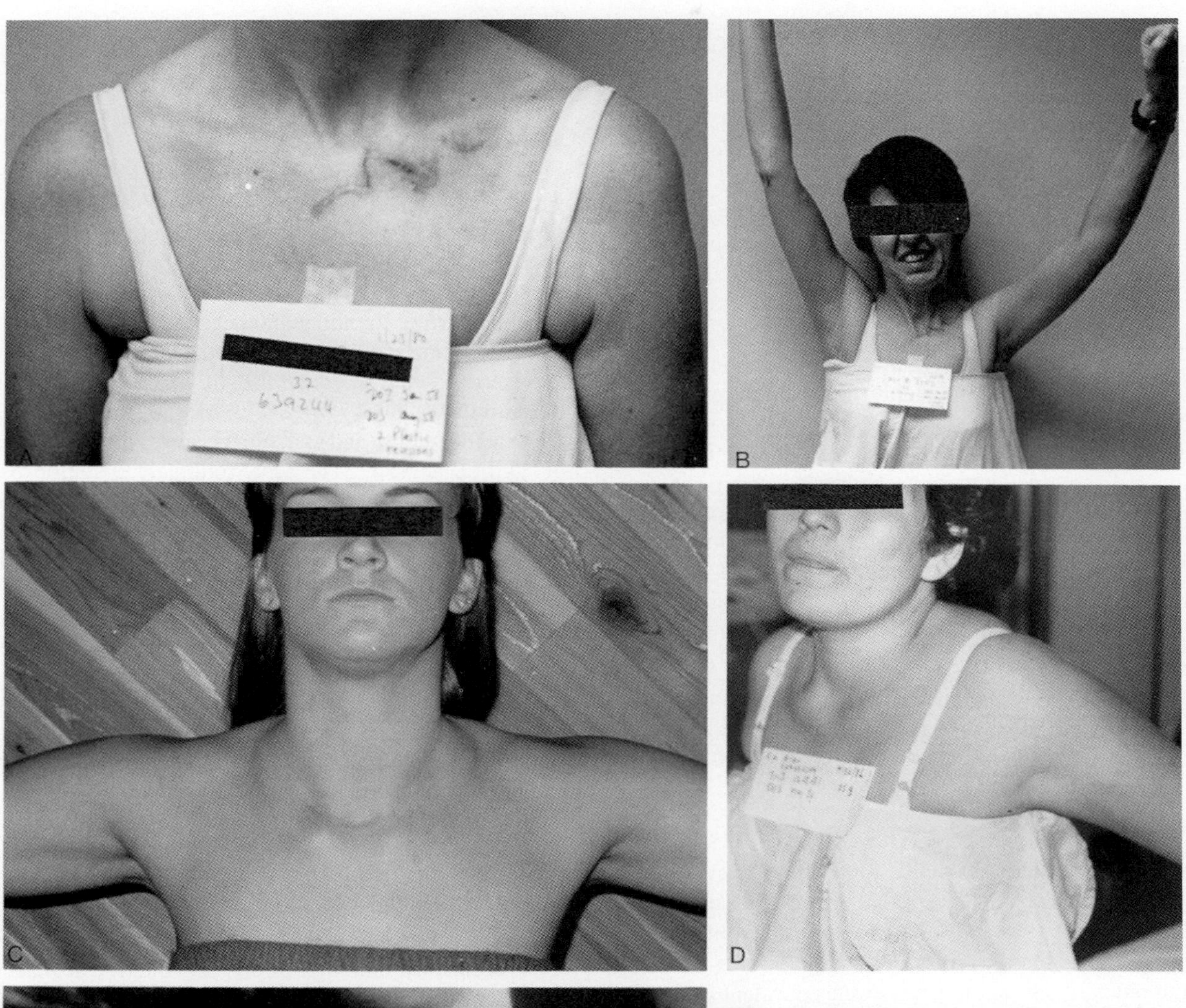

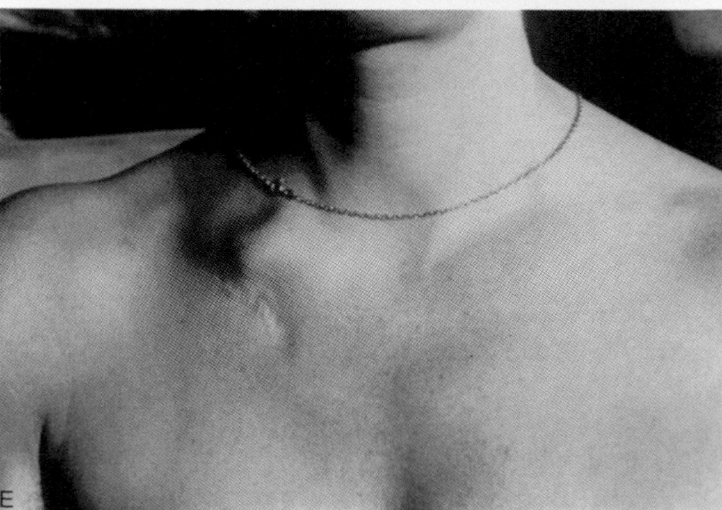

FIG. 36. Patients treated with surgery for spontaneous, atraumatic subluxation of the sternoclavicular joint had increased pain, limitation of activity, alteration of life-style, persistent instability of the joint, and a significant scar. **A and B:** Not only was the cosmetic scarring a problem, but motion and pain were worse than before the reconstruction. **C and D:** Despite surgical reconstruction, both patients shown here had persistent subluxation and pain. **E:** This patient had bilateral spontaneous, atraumatic subluxation of the sternoclavicular joints. Following reconstruction, the right shoulder continued to subluxate, was painful, and significantly altered the patient's life-style. The left shoulder had minimal subluxations and was essentially asymptomatic. (Reprinted with permission from Rockwood CA, Matsen F III, eds. *The shoulder.* Philadelphia: WB Saunders, 1990:Fig. 13-30.)

Congenital or Developmental Problems

Congenital or developmental problems (e.g., absence or partial absence of bone or muscles) can produce subluxation or dislocation of the sternoclavicular joint. Specific rehabilitation or surgical procedures are usually unnecessary.[79,129]

Arthritis

The management of patients with osteoarthritis or postmenopausal osteoarthritis can usually be accomplished via conservative nonoperative treatment (i.e., heat, antiinflammaory agents, and rest).[12,17] However, the patient must be thoroughly evaluated to rule out other conditions that mimic the changes in the sternoclavicular joint (e.g., tumor or metabolic, infectious, or collagen disorders). Patients with posttraumatic arthritic changes in the sternoclavicular joint, which follow fractures of the sternoclavicular joint and previous attempts at reconstruction, may require formal arthroplasty of the joint and careful stabilization of the remaining clavicle to the first rib.

Patients with collagen disorders, such as rheumatoid arthritis, and some patients with condensing osteitis of the medial clavicle, may require arthroplasty. Sternovostoclavicular hyperostosis is a difficult problem to manage.[1,30,70,73,95,105,160,168–170] The condition cannot be arrested with medication. Treatment is largely dependent on the amount of pain and the need for antiinflammatory medications and physical therapy. Occasionally, surgical excision of the bony mass to allow an increase in function of the upper extremity is indicated.

Infection

Infections of the sternoclavicular joint should be managed as they are in other joints, except that during aspiration and surgical drainage, great care and respect must be directed to the vital structures that lie posterior to the joint. If aspiration or a high index of suspicion demonstrates purulent material in the joint, a formal arthrotomy should be performed. This is especially important with sternoclavicular septic arthritis, due to the significant risk of abscess formation and subsequent spread of infection to the mediastinal structures. This is supported by Wohlgethan and associates' review of the literature,[192] which documented a 20% incidence of abscess formation following infections of the sternoclavicular joint. The anterior sternoclavicular ligament will need to be removed, but the posterior and interclavicular ligaments should be spared. Occasionally, the infection will arise in the medial end of the clavicle or the manubrium, which will necessitate the resection of some of the dead bone. Depending on the status of the wound following debridement, one can either close the wound loosely over a drain, or pack the wound open and close it later.

Authors' Preferred Method of Conservative Treatment

The algorithm in Fig. 37 depicts the authors' preferred treatment.

Traumatic Injuries

Anterior

Mild Sprain. For mild sprains (type I injuries), we recommend the use of cold packs for the first 12 to 24 hours and a sling to rest the joint. Ordinarily, after 5 to 7 days, the patient can use the arm for everyday activities.

Moderate Sprain (Subluxation). In addition to the cold pack, for subluxations (type II injuries) we may use a soft, padded figure-of-eight clavicle strap to gently hold the shoulders back to allow the sternoclavicular joint to rest. The harness can be removed after a week or so; then the arm is placed in a sling for about another week, or the patient is allowed to return gradually to everyday activities.

Severe Sprain (Dislocation). In general, we manage almost all dislocations (type III injuries) of the sternoclavicular joint in children and in adults via either a closed reduction or "skillful neglect." The acute traumatic posterior dislocations are reduced closed and become stable when the shoulders are held back in a figure-of-eight dressing. Most of the anterior dislocations are unstable, but we accept the deformity, because we believe it is less of a problem than the potential problems of operative repair and internal fixation.

Anterior Dislocation

Method of Reduction. In most instances, knowing that the anterior dislocation will be unstable, we still try to reduce the anterior displacement. Muscle relaxants and narcotics are administered intravenously, and the patient is placed supine on the table, with a stack of three or four towels between the shoulder blades. While an assistant gently applies downward pressure on the anterior aspect of both shoulders, the medial end of the clavicle is pushed backward where it belongs. On some occasions, although rarely, the anterior displacement may stay adjacent to the sternum. However, in most cases, either with the shoulders still held back or when they are relaxed, an anterior displacement promptly recurs. We explain to the patient that the joint is unstable and that the hazards of internal fixation are too great, and we prescribe a sling for a couple of weeks and allow the patient to begin using the arm as soon as the discomfort is gone.

Most of the anterior injuries that we have treated in patients up to 25 years of age are not dislocations of the sternoclavicular joint but type I or II physeal injuries, which heal and remodel without operative treatment. Patients over 23 to 25 years of age, with anterior dislocations of the sternoclavicular joint, do have persistent prominence of the anterior clavicle. However, this does not seem to interfere with usual activities and, in come cases, has not even interfered with heavy manual labor.

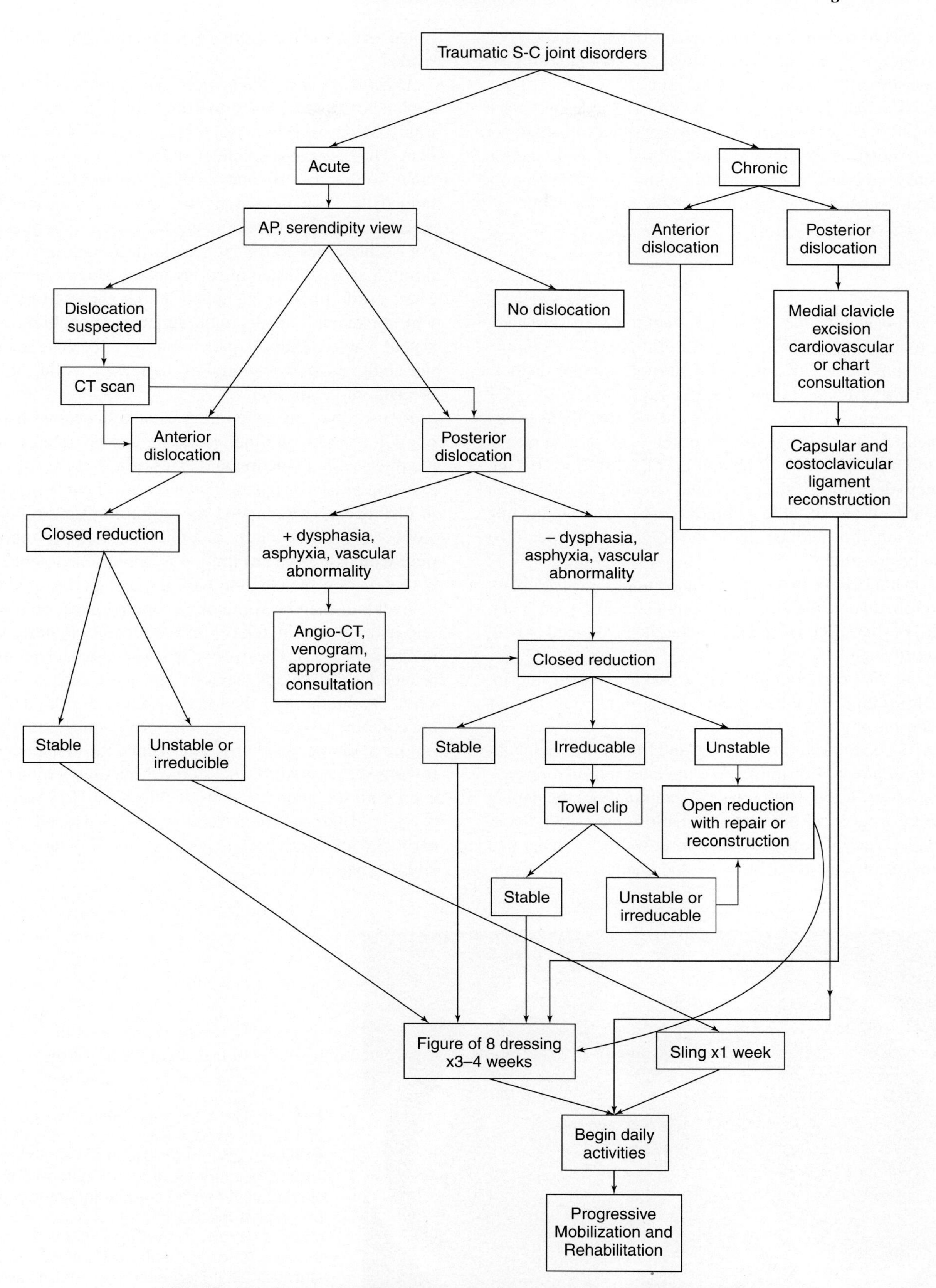

FIG. 37. Treatment algorithm for traumatic sternoclavicular joint disorders.

We wish to reemphasize that we do not recommend open reduction of the joint and would never recommend transfixing pins across the sternoclavicular joint.

Postreduction Care. If the reduction is stable, we place the patient in either a figure-of-eight dressing or in whatever device or position the clavicle is most stable. If the reduction is unstable, the arm is placed into a sling for a week or so, and then the patient can begin to use the arm for gentle everyday activities.

Posterior

Posterior Dislocation. It is important to take a very careful history and to perform a very careful physical examination in the patient with a posterior sternoclavicular dislocation. The physician should obtain x-rays, tomograms, CT scans, or angio-CT scans to document whether there is any compression of the great vessels in the neck or arm or any difficulty in swallowing or breathing (Fig. 38). It is also important to determine if the patient has a feeling of choking or hoarseness. If any of these symptoms are present, indicating pressure on the mediastinum, the appropriate specialist should be consulted.

We do not believe that operative techniques are usually required to reduce acute posterior sternoclavicular joint dislocations. Furthermore, once the joint has been reduced closed, it is usually stable (Fig. 39).

Although we used to think that the diagnosis of an anterior or posterior injury of the sternoclavicular joint could always be made on physical examination, we know now that one cannot rely on the anterior swelling and firmness as being diagnostic of an anterior injury. We have been fooled on several occasions when, from physical examination, the patient appeared to have an anterior dislocation but x-rays documented a posterior problem. Therefore, we recommend that the clinical impression always be documented with appropriate x-ray studies before a decision to treat or not to treat is made.

Method of Closed Reduction. The patient is placed in the supine position, with a 3- to 4-inch thick sandbag or three or four folded towels between the scapulas to extend the shoulders. The dislocated shoulder should be near the edge of the table, so that the arm and shoulder can be abducted and extended. If the patient is having extreme pain and muscle spasm and is quite anxious, we use general anesthesia; otherwise, narcotics, muscle relaxants, or tranquilizers are given through an established intravenous route in the normal arm. First, gentle traction is applied on the abducted arm in line with the clavicle while countertraction is applied by an assistant who steadies the patient on the table. The traction on the abducted arm is gradually increased while the arm is brought into extension.

Reduction of an acute injury usually occurs with an audible pop or snap, and the relocation can be noted visibly. If the traction in abduction and extension is not successful, an assistant grasps or pushes down on the clavicle, in an effort to dislodge it from behind the sternum. Occasionally, in a stubborn case, especially in a thick-chested person or a patient with extensive swelling, it is impossible to obtain a secure grasp on the clavicle with the assistant's fingers. The skin should then be surgically prepared and a sterile towel clip used to gain purchase on the medial clavicle percutaneously (Fig. 33). The towel clip is used to reach completely around the shaft of the clavicle. The dense cortical bone prevents the purchase of the towel clip into the clavicle. Then, the combined traction through the arm, plus the anterior lifting force on the towel clip, will reduce the dislocation. Following the reduction, the sternoclavicular joint is stable, even with the patient's arms at the sides. However, we always hold the shoulders back in a well-padded figure-of-eight clavicle strap for 3 to 4 weeks, to allow for soft-tissue and ligamentous healing.

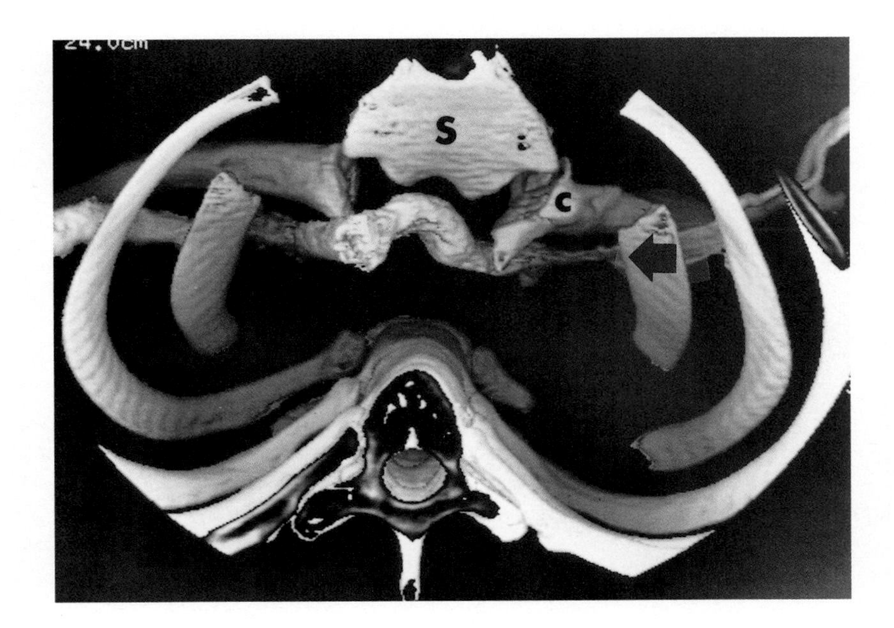

FIG. 38. Contrast material–enhanced CT scan of 16-year-old boy who presented with left arm swelling and cyanosis 14 months after a wrestling injury. A stenotic lesion of the subclavian vein can be seen adjacent to a posteriorly displaced physeal fracture of the medial clavicle (*arrow*). Note the relationship between the posteriorly displaced clavicle (C) and sternum (S). (Reprinted with permission from Wirth MA and Rockwood CA: Acute and Chronic Traumatic Injuries of the Sternoclavicular Joint. *J Am Acad Orthop Surgeons* 1996; 4:268–278.)

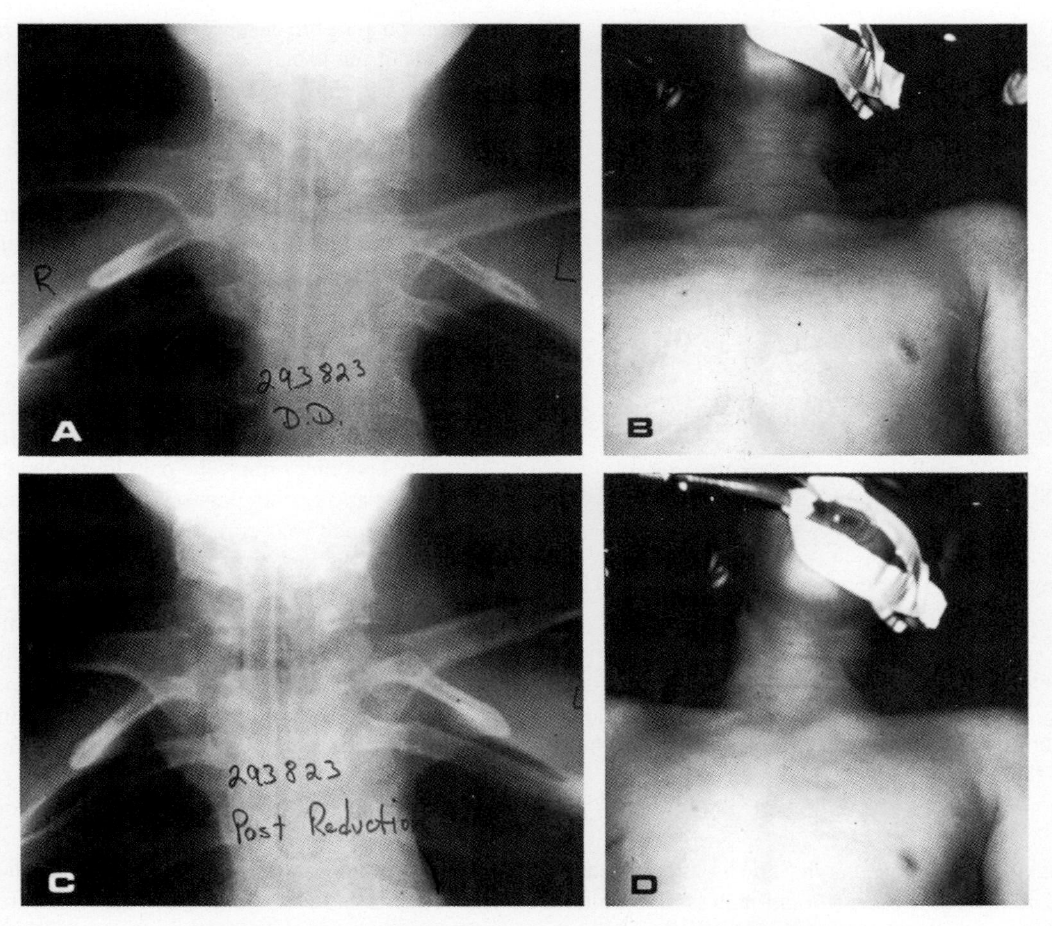

FIG. 39. Posterior dislocation or type I epiphyseal separation of the left sternoclavicular joint in a 12-year-old boy. **A:** The 40-degree cephalic tilt serendipity x-ray film reveals that the left clavicle is significantly lower on the horizintal plane than the normal right clavicle. Before reduction, the medial end of the left clavicle was displaced posteriorly, compared with the normal right clavicle. The only remaining prominence of the left sternoclavicular joint was the prominence of the superomedial corner of the manubrium. **C:** Under general anesthesia, a closed reduction was performed by traction on the arm followed by abduction and extension. The clavicle reduced with an audible pop back into position. It was restored to the same horizontal level as the normal right clavicle. **D:** Clinically, both clavicles were palpable at the same level after reduction.

Atraumatic Problems

Spontaneous Subluxation or Dislocation

We have seen 39 patients with spontaneous subluxation or dislocation of the sternoclavicular joint. They seem to have only one symptom: the medial end of the clavicle subluxates or dislocates anteriorly when they raise their arms over their head.[154] This occurs spontaneously and without any significant trauma (Fig. 40). Many of these patients have the characteristic finding of generalized ligamentous laxity (i.e., hyperextension of the elbows, knees, and fingers, as well as hypermobility of the glenohumeral joints). This problem might be considered voluntary or involuntary, because it occurs whenever the patient raises the arms to the overhead position. Some patients seen for another shoulder problem are completely unaware that with the overhead motion the medial end of the clavicle subluxates or dislocates. We have never seen a spontaneous posterior subluxation of the sternoclavicular joint. Only occasionally does the patient with atraumatic anterior displacement complain of pain during the displacement. Because it is difficult to stabilize the joint and prevent the subluxation or dislocation and end up with a pain-free range of motion, we manage the problem with skillful neglect. The anatomy of the problem is explained to the patient and the family. We explain further that surgery is of little benefit, that they should discontinue the voluntary aspect of the dislocation, and that in time either the symptoms will disappear or they will completely forget that the dislocation is a problem.

In the review by Rockwood and Odor of 37 patients with spontaneous atraumatic subluxation, 29 were managed without surgery and 8 were treated (elsewhere) with surgical reconstruction.[154] With an average follow-up of more than 8 years, all 29 nonoperated patients were doing just fine with-

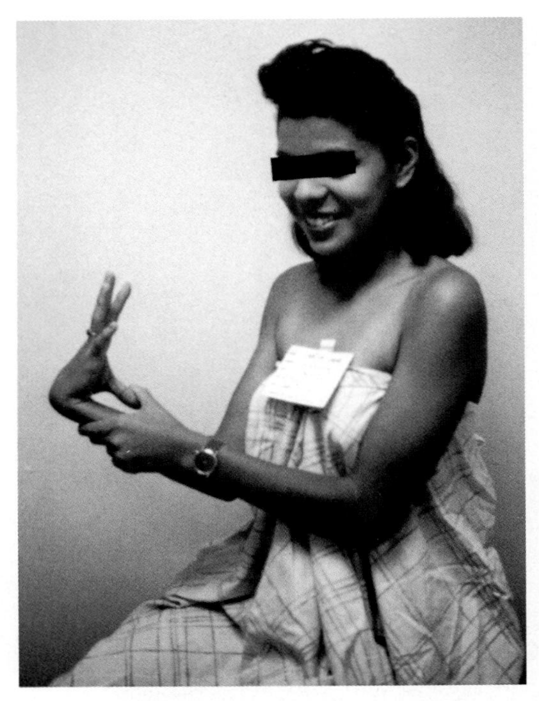

FIG. 40. This patient has developed spontaneous subluxation of her sternoclavicular joints. She also has generalized ligamentous laxity of the wrists, fingers, and elbows.

out limitations of activity or life-style. The 8 patients treated with surgery had increased pain, limitation of activity, alteration of life-style, persistent instability, and significant scars. In many instances, before reconstruction or resection, these patients had minimal discomfort, excellent range of motion, and only complained of a "bump" that slipped in and out of place with certain motions. Postoperatively, these patients still had the bump, along with scars and painful range of motion (Fig. 37).

Arthritis

Most patients with simple degenerative arthritis, or postmenopausal osteoarthritis, can be managed with rest, moist heat, and antiinflammatory medications (Figs. 11 and 12). As previously described, it is very important to do a good workup of the patient with arthritis of the sternoclavicular joint to rule out tumor, arthropathies, condensing osteitis of the medial clavicle, and sternocostoclavicular hyperostosis. Patients with posttraumatic osteoarthritis or sternocostoclavicular hyperostosis may require resection of the medial clavicle. Care must be taken to remove enough, but not too much, of the medial clavicle (Fig. 41).

Infection

We believe that pus in the sternoclavicular joint should be managed by arthrotomy and exploration. If the procedure is done soon after the onset of the infection, the arthrotomy and joint clean-out usually are sufficient. If the infection is longstanding and there is destruction of the cartilage and bone, a resection of the medial clavicle or the involved manubrium should be performed. Care should be taken to preserve the posterior, interclavicular, and costoclavicular ligaments (Fig. 13). Although some investigators report good results with nonoperative treatment of sternoclavicular joint infections, the risk of mediastinal involvement precludes us from supporting this approach.

Surgical Management

Occasionally, following conservative treatment of a type II sternoclavicular injury, the pain lingers and the symptoms of popping and grating persist. This may require joint exploration. Bateman[8] has commented on the possibility of finding a tear of the intraarticular disk, which should be excised.

Duggan[48] reported a case in which, several weeks after an injury to the sternoclavicular joint, the patient still had popping in the joint. Through a small incision, Duggan exposed the capsule and out through the capsule popped the intraarticular disk, which looked like "an avulsed fingernail." Following repair of the capsule, the patient had no more symptoms. If degenerative changes become severe in the sternoclavicular joint, excision of the medial end of the clavicle may be required.

The operative procedure should be performed in a manner that disturbs as few of the anterior ligament structures as possible. If the procedure can be performed with the anterior ligaments intact, then, with the shoulders held back in a figure-of-eight dressing, the reduction may be stable. If all the ligaments are disrupted, a significant decision has to be made to try to stabilize the sternoclavicular joint or to resect the medial 1 to 1.5 inches of the medial clavicle and stabilize the remaining clavicle to the first rib.

Some of the literature from the 1960s and 1970s recommended stabilization of the sternoclavicular joint with pins. Elting[51] used Kirschner wires to stabilize the joint and supplemented ligament repairs with a short-toe extensor tendon. Denham and Dingley[44] and Brooks and Henning[18] used Kirschner wires. DePalma[46] and Brown[20] recommended repair of the ligaments and stabilized the sternoclavicular joint with one or two Steinmann pins.

Habernek and Hertz,[81] Nutz,[133] Pfister and Weller,[140] Kennedy,[98] Tagliabue and Riva,[177] Hartman and Dunnagan,[83] Bankart,[4] Ecke,[50] and Stein[174] avoided the use of pins across the sternoclavicular joint and used loops of various types of suture wires across the joint. Burri and Neugebauer[23] recommended the use of a figure-of-eight loop of carbon fiber. Maguire,[117] Booth and Roper,[13] Barth and Hagen,[6] and Lunseth and associates[116] reconstructed the sternoclavicular joint using local tendons of the sternocleidomastoid, subclavius, or pectoralis major tendons for repair. Haug[84] reported on the use of a special plate to stabilize the joint. The complications of fixation of the sternoclavicular

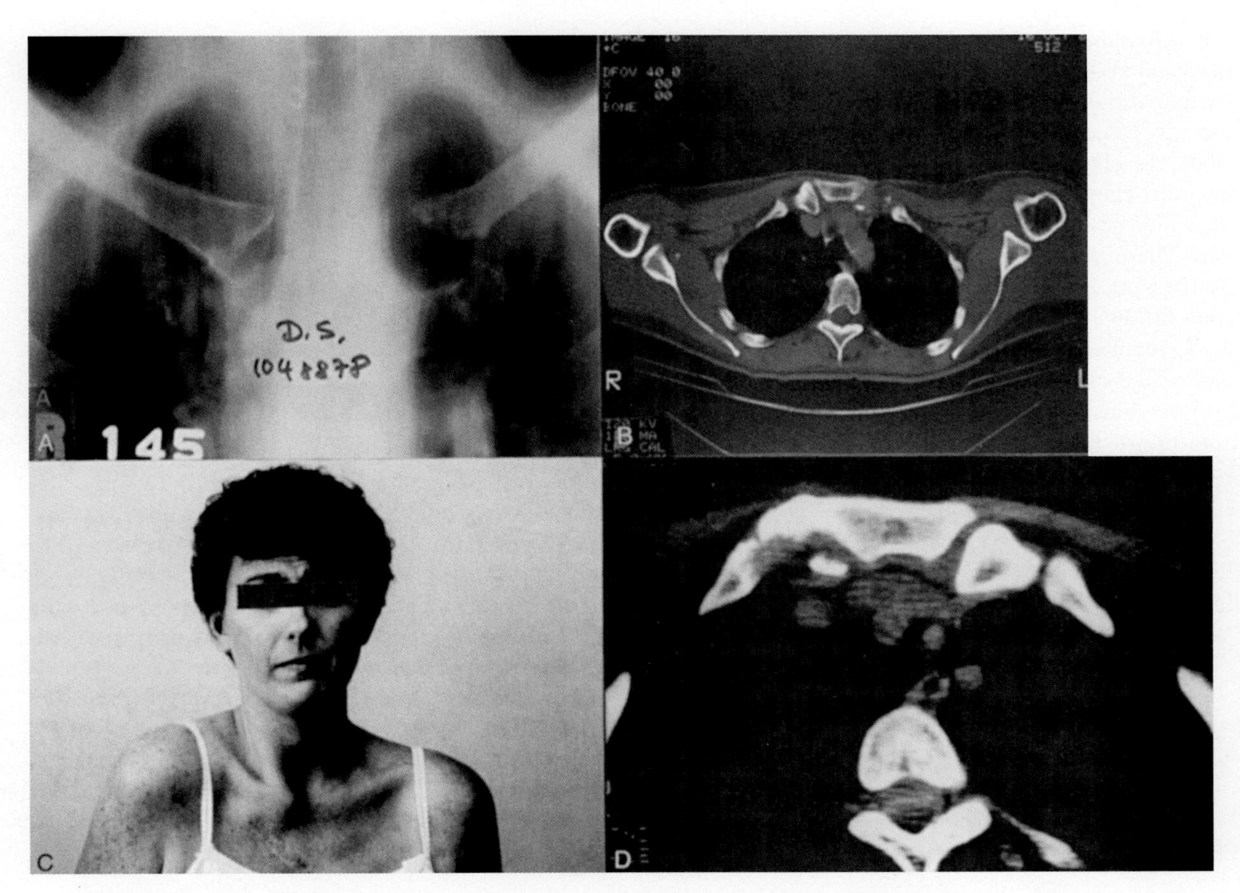

FIG. 41. In performing sternoclavicular joint arthroplasty, care must be taken to remove sufficient bone. **A and B:** After resection of the left medial clavicle, this patient continued to have pain with shoulder motion. The CT scan confirms fragments of bone in the site of the arthroplasty. **C:** After arthroplasty of the right sternoclavicular joint, the medial clavicle was still quite prominent and painful. **D:** A CT scan confirms the medial right clavicle butting into the manubrium and a loose fragment of bone in the joint. (Reprinted with permission from Rockwood CA, Matsen F III, eds. *The shoulder.* Philadelphia: WB Saunders, 1990:Fig. 13-40.)

joint with Kirschner wires or Steinmann pins are horrendous and are discussed in the section on complications.

In recent years (i.e., since 1982), various investigators have recommended open reduction and internal fixation for acute injuries, as well as for chronic problems.[53,54,58,139,140,197]

In 1982, Pfister and associates[139,140] recommended open reduction and repair of the ligaments over nonoperative treatment. In symptomatic chronic dislocation or nontraumatic cases, they recommended the use of autogenous grafts between the sternum and the first rib without placing Kirschner wires across the sternoclavicular joint. In 1988, Fery and Sommelet[61] reported 49 cases of dislocations of the sternoclavicular joint. These patients, with an average follow-up of more than 6 years, had 42% excellent results among the operative cases. Of those patients who were treated with closed reduction, 58% were satisfied. Krenzien[102] reported that a closed reduction of a posterior dislocation was difficult if not impossible and recommended an open reduction over conservative treatment. He reported that the use of Kirschner wires is not without risk and recommended that they be used only by experienced surgeons. He said use of the fascial plasties of Bunnel, Steindler, and Bankart are more suitable for fixation. Ferrandez and colleagues[58] reported 18 subluxations and dislocations of the sternoclavicular joint. Seven had moderate sprains and 11 had dislocations. Of the 3 patients with posterior dislocation, all had symptoms of dysphagia. All of the subluxations were treated nonoperatively with excellent results. The remaining 10 patients with dislocations were treated with surgery (i.e., open reduction with suture of the ligaments and Kirschner wires between the clavicle and the sternum). The wires were removed 3 to 4 weeks after surgery. At 1 to 4 years' follow-up, most of the operative cases had a slight deformity. In 2 patients, migration of the Kirschner wires was noted but was without clinical significance. Eskola and associates[53,54] strongly urged operative repair of dislocations of the sternoclavicular joint. In 1989, they reported on 12 patients treated for painful sternoclavicular joints. The average time from injury was 1.5 years, and the average follow-up after surgery was 4.7 years. In 5 patients, the sternoclavicular joint was stabilized with a tendon graft from either the palmaris tendon or the plantaris tendon between the first rib and the manubrium; in 4 patients, the medial 2.5 cm of the clavicle was resected without any type of stabilization; in 3 patients, the clavicle was fixed to the first rib with a fascia lata graft. They had four fair results and four poor results in those patients who underwent only resection of the medial clavicle. There was little discussion of the preoperative symptoms, work habits, range of motion, or degree of joint reduction following the surgery. In 1990, Tricoire and colleagues[181] reported six retrosternal dislocations of the medial end of the clavicle. They recommended reduction of these injuries secondary to the possible complications arising from protrusion of the clavicle into the thorax. Sternoclavicular capsulorrhaphy was performed in 2 patients and a subclavis tenodesis was used in the remaining 4 patients. All joints were temporarily stabilized with sternoclavicular pins for 6 weeks. Results were satisfactory in all cases at a mean follow-up of 27 months.

Surgical Reconstructions

There are several basic procedures to maintain the medial end of the clavicle in its normal articulation with the sternum. Fascia lata, suture, internal fixation across the joint, subclavius tendons, osteotomy of the medial clavicle, and resection of the medial end of the clavicle have been advocated.

Fascia Lata. Bankart[4] and Milch[123] used fascia lata between the clavicle and the sternum. Lowman[114] used a loop of fascia in and through the sternoclavicular joint, so that it acts like the ligamentum teres in the hip. Speed[172] and Key and Conwell[99] reported on the use of a fascial loop between the clavicle and the first rib. Allen[1a] used fascia lata to reconstruct a new sternoclavicular ligament.

Subclavius Tendon. Burrows[24] recommended that the subclavius tendon be used to reconstruct a new costoclavicular ligament. The origin of the subclavius muscle is from the first rib just 6 mm lateral and 1.3 mm anterior to the attachment of the costoclavicular ligament.[76,77] The insertion of the tendon is to the inferior surface of the junction of the middle third with the outer third of the clavicle, and the muscle fibers arising from the tendon insert into the inferior surface of the middle third of the clavicle (Fig. 42). The muscle fibers coming off the tendon look like feathers on a bird's wing. Burrows detaches the muscle fiber from the tendon, does not disturb the origin of the tendon, and then passes the tendon through drill holes in the anterior proximal clavicle.

In comparing his operation with the use of free strips of fascia, Burrows said that it is "safer and easier to pick up a mooring than to drop anchor; the obvious mooring is the tendon of the subclavius, separated from its muscle fiber and suitably realigned." Linseth and associates[116] have reported a modified Burrows procedure with the additional use of a threaded Steinmann pin across the joint.

Osteotomy of the Medial Clavicle. As previously described, Omer,[134] following repair or reconstruction of the ligaments, creates a step-cut osteotomy lateral to the joint and detaches the clavicular head of the sternocleidomastoid muscle from the proximal fragment.

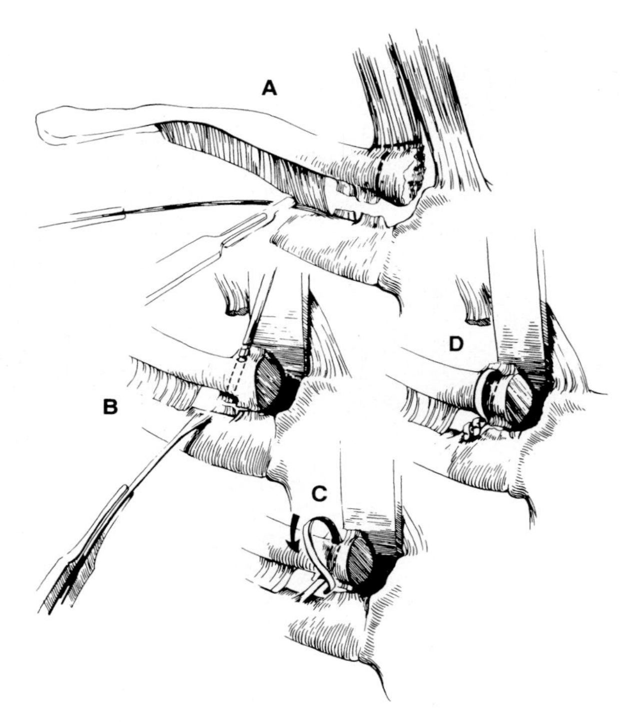

FIG. 42. The technique of Jackson Burrows, using the subclavius tendon to reconstruct the coracoclavicular ligament. (Reprinted with permission from Rockwood CA, Matsen F III, eds. *The shoulder.* Philadelphia: WB Saunders, 1990: Fig. 13-27.)

Resection of the Medial End of the Clavicle. McLaughlin,[121] Breitner and Wirth,[16] Pridie,[143] Bateman,[7,8] and Milch[123] have all recommended excision of the medial clavicle when degenerative changes are noted in the joint. If the medial end of the clavicle is to be removed because of degenerative changes, the surgeon should be careful not to damage the costoclavicular ligament.

Arthrodesis. Arthrodesis was once reported[147] in the treatment of a habitual dislocation of the sternoclavicular joint. However, this procedure should not be performed, because it prevents the previously described normal elevation, depression, and rotation of the clavicle. The end result would be a severe restriction of shoulder movement (Fig. 43).

Authors' Preferred Treatment

The complications of an unreduced posterior dislocation are numerous: thoracic outlet syndrome,[66] vascular compromise,[15] and erosion of the medial clavicle into any of the vital structures that lie posterior to the sternoclavicular joint (Fig. 37). Therefore, in adults, if closed reduction fails, an open reduction should be performed.

When operating on the sternoclavicular joint, care must be

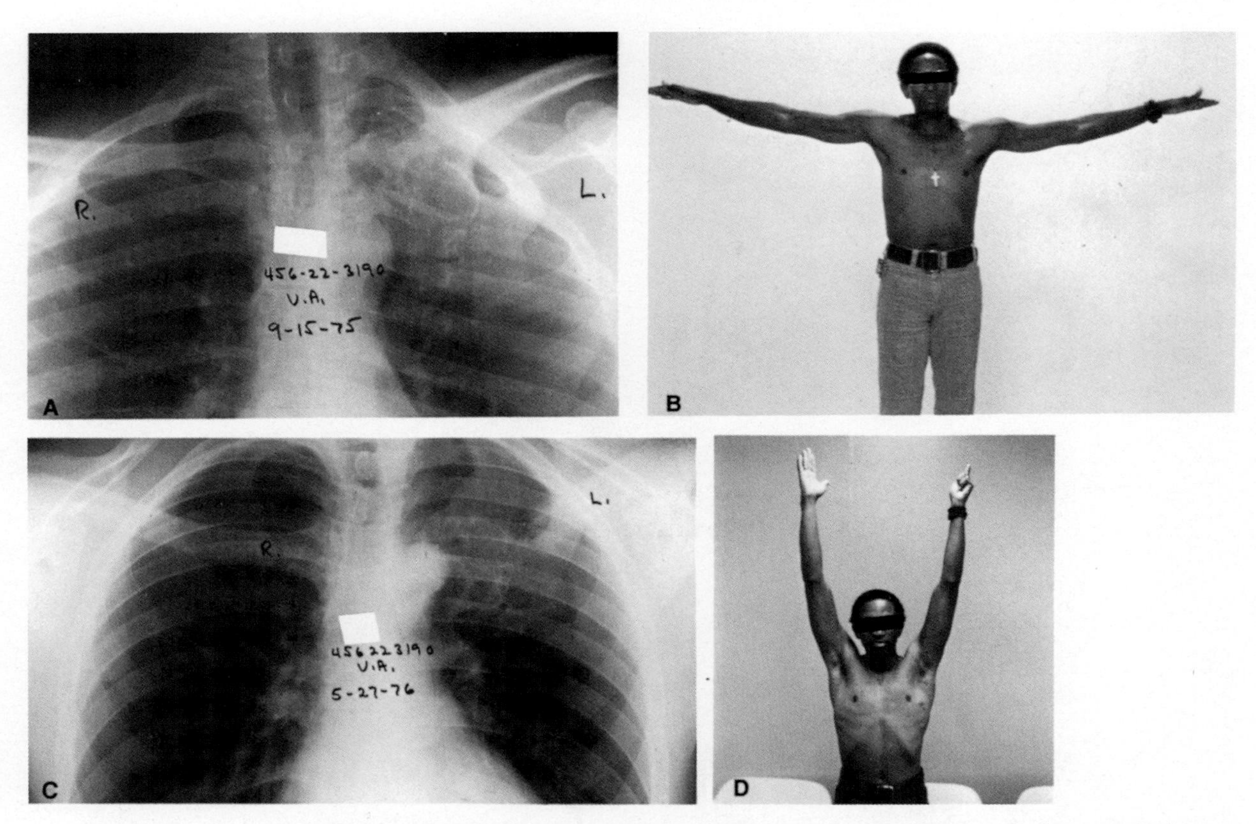

FIG. 43. The effect of an arthrodesis of the sternoclavicular joint on shoulder function. **A:** As a result of a military gunshot wound to the left sternoclavicular joint, this patient had a massive bony union of the left medial clavicle to the sternum and the upper three ribs. **B:** Shoulder motion was limited to 90 degrees flexion and abduction. **C:** Radiograph after resection of the bony mass, freeing up the medial clavicle. **D:** Function of the left shoulder was essentially normal after the elimination of the sternoclavicular arthrodesis.

taken to evaluate the residual stability of the medial clavicle. It is the same analogy as used when resecting the distal clavicle for an old acromioclavicular joint problem. If the coracoclavicular ligaments are intact, an excision of the distal clavicle is indicated. If the coracoclavicular ligaments are gone, then in addition to excision of the distal clavicle, you must reconstruct the coracoclavicular ligaments. If the costoclavicular ligaments are intact, the clavicle medial to the ligaments should be resected and beveled smooth (Fig. 44). If the ligaments are gone, the clavicle must be stabilized to the first rib. If too much clavicle is resected, or if the clavicle is not stabilized to the first rib, an increase in symptoms can occur (Fig. 45).

The patient lies supine on the table, and the three to four towels or sandbag should be left between the scapulas. The upper extremity should be draped free, so that lateral traction can be applied during the open reduction. In addition, a folded sheet around the patient's thorax should be left in place, so that it can be used for countertraction during traction on the involved extremity. An anterior incision is used that parallels the superior border of the medial 3 to 4 inches of the clavicle and then extends downward over the sternum just medial to the involved sternoclavicular joint (Fig. 46). As previously described, this should usually be done with a thoracic surgeon. The trick is to remove sufficient soft tissues to expose the joint but to leave the anterior capsular ligament intact. The reduction usually can be accomplished with traction and countertraction while lifting up anteriorly with a clamp around the medial clavicle. Along with traction and countertraction, it may be necessary to use an elevator to pry the clavicle back to its articulation with the sternum. When the reduction has been obtained, and with the shoulders held back, the reduction will be stable because the anterior capsule has been left intact. If the anterior capsule is damaged or is insufficient to prevent anterior displacement of the medial end of the clavicle, we recommend excision of the medial 1 to 1.5 inches of the clavicle and securing the residual clavicle to the first rib with 1-mm Dacron tape. The medial clavicle is exposed by careful subperiosteal dissection (Fig. 47). When possible, any remnant of the capsular or intraarticular disk ligaments should be identified and preserved, because these structures can be used to stabilize the medial clavicle. Ordinarily, the intraarticular disc ligament is a very dense, fibrous structure that arises from the synchondral junction of the first

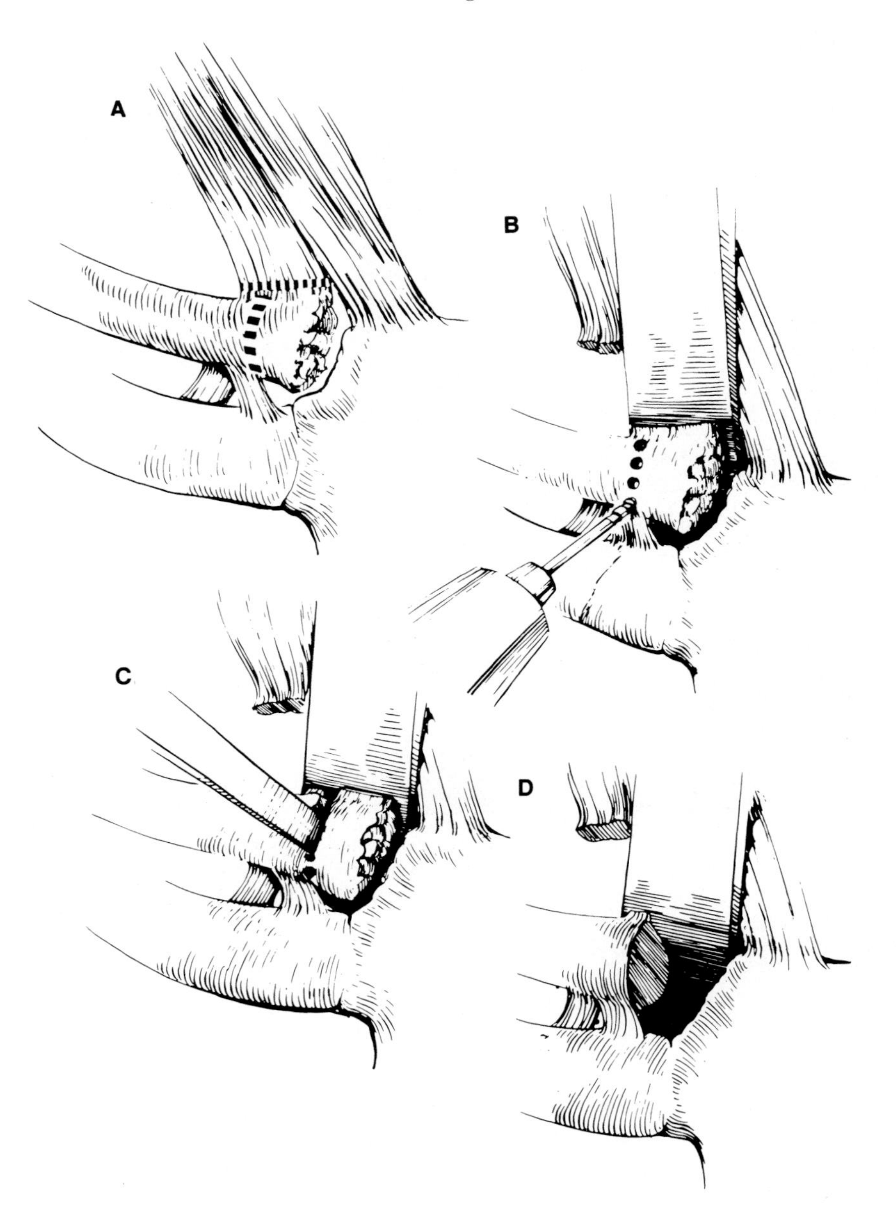

FIG. 44. Technique for resecting the medial clavicle for degenerative arthritis. **A:** Care must be taken to remove only that part of the clavicle medial to the costoclavicular (rhomboid) ligaments. There must be adequate protection for the vital structures that lie posterior to the medial end of the clavicle. **B and C:** An air drill with a side-cutting burr can be used to perform the osteotomy. **D:** When the fragment of bone has been removed, the dorsal and anterior borders of the clavicle should be smoothed, to give a better cosmetic appearance.

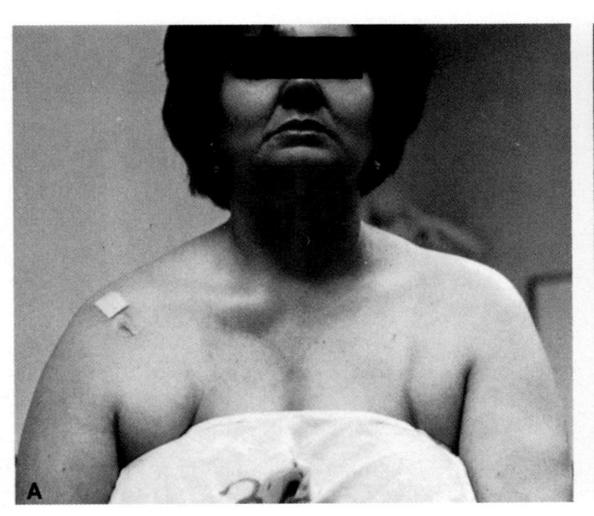

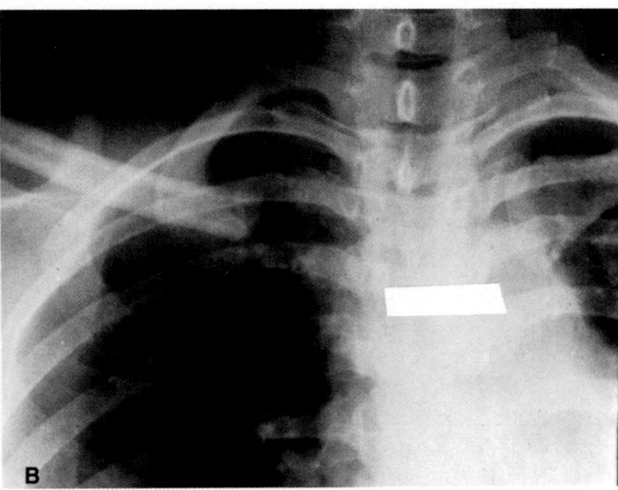

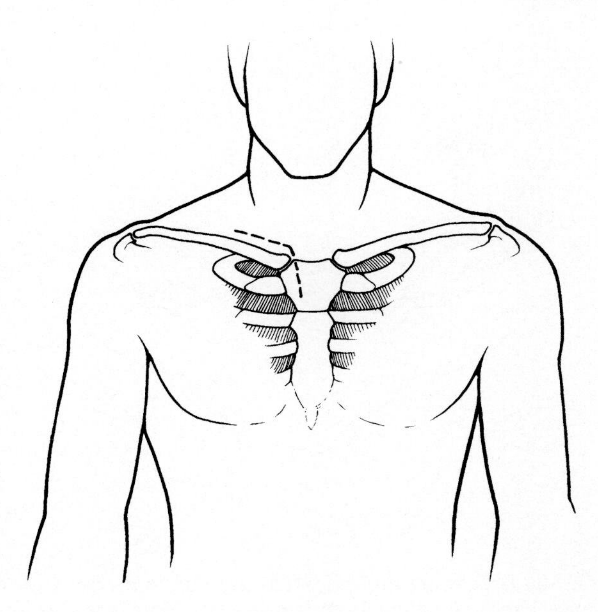

FIG. 46. Proposed skin incision for open reduction of a posterior sternoclavicular dislocation.

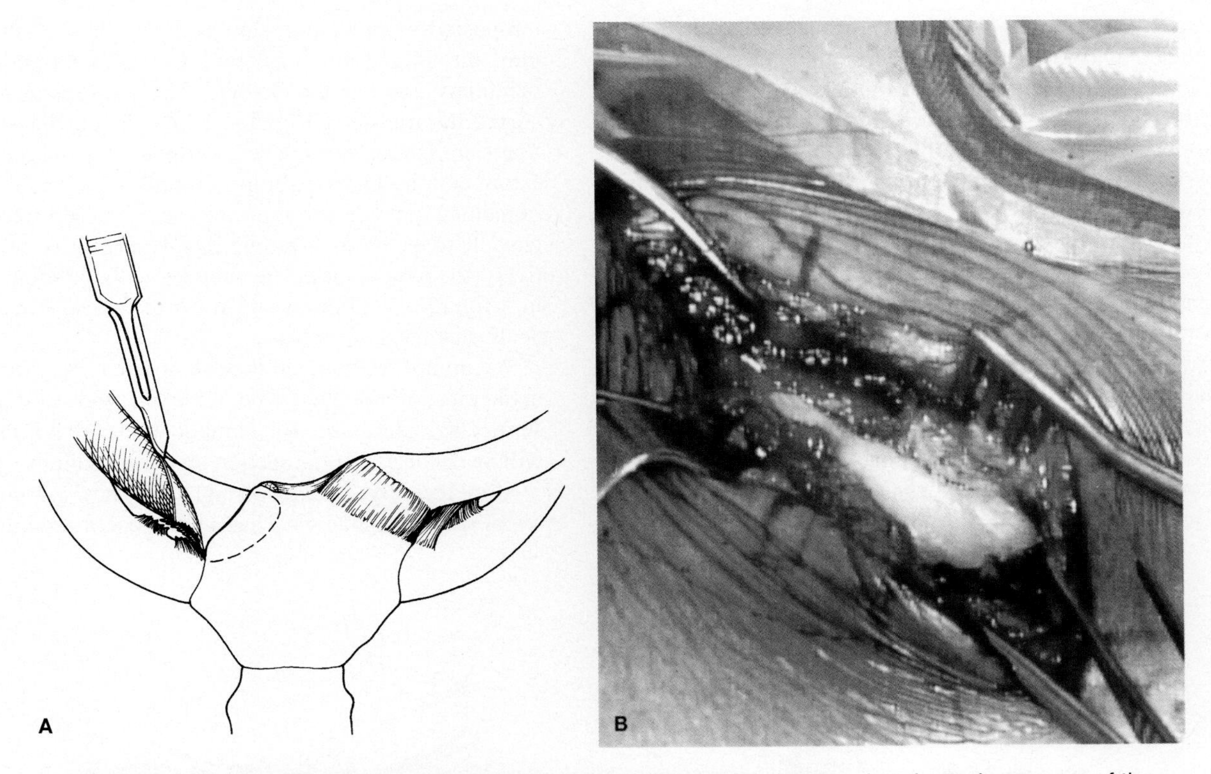

FIG. 47. Artist's depiction **(A)** and intraposterior photo **(B)** demonstratng subperiosteal exposure of the medial clavicle. Note the posteriorly displaced medial end of the clavicle. (From Wirth MA, Rockwood CA. Injuries to the Sternoclavicular Joint. In: Rockwood CA, Green DP, Bucholz RW, Hechman JD (eds.). *Fractures in Adults*. Philadelphia, JB Lippincott, 1996).

FIG. 45. A: This postmenopausal, right-handed woman had resection of the right medial clavicle, because of preoperative diagnosis of "possible tumor." The postoperative microscopic diagnosis was degenerative arthritis of the right medial clavicle. After surgery, the patient complained of pain and discomfort, marked prominence, and gross instability of the right medial clavicle. **B:** An x-ray confirmed that the excision of the medial clavicle extended lateral to the costoclavicular ligaments; hence, the patient had an unstable medial clavicle.

rib to the sternum and passes through the sternoclavicular joint, dividing the joint into two separate spaces. The capsular ligament covers the anterosuperior and posterior aspects of the joint and represents thickenings of the joint capsule. This ligament is primarily attached to the epiphysis of the medial clavicle and is usually avulsed from this structure with posterior sternoclavicular dislocation. Similarly, the intraarticular disk ligament usually is intact where it arises from the synchondral junction of the first rib and sternum and is avulsed from its attachment site on the medial clavicle.

If the sternal attachment site of these structures is intact, a nonabsorbable No. 1 cottony Dacron suture is woven back and forth through the ligament, so that the ends of the suture exit through the avulsed free end of the tissue. The medial end of the clavicle is resected, with care taken to protect the underlying structures and to not damage the costoclavicular (rhomboid) ligament or the vascular structures that are located posterior to the medial clavicle and sternoclavicular joint. These vital structures are protected by passing a curved crego or ribbon retractor around the posterior aspect of the medial clavicle, which isolates them from the operative field during the bony resection. Excision of the medial clavicle is facilitated by creating drill holes through both cortices of the clavicle at the intended site of clavicular osteotomy. Following this step, an air drill with a side-cutting burr or an osteotome is used to complete the osteotomy. The anterior and superior corners of the clavicle are beveled with an air burr for cosmetic purposes.

The medullary canal of the medial clavicle is drilled out and curetted to receive the transferred intraarticular disk ligament (Fig. 48). Two small drill holes are then placed in the superior cortex of the medial clavicle, approximately 1 cm lateral to the site of resection (Fig. 49). These holes communicate with the medullary canal and will be used to secure the suture in the transferred ligament. The free ends of the suture are passed into the medullary canal of the medial clavicle and out the two small drill holes in the superior cortex of the clavicle (Fig. 50). While the clavicle is held in a reduced anteroposterior position in relationship to the first rib and sternum, the sutures are used to pull the ligament tightly into the medullary canal of the clavicle. The suture is tied, thus securing the transferred ligament into the clavicle (Fig. 51). The stabilization procedure is completed by passing several 1-mm cottony Dacron sutures around the medial end of the remaining clavicle and securing the periosteal sleeve of the clavicle to the costoclavicular ligament (Fig. 52). Postoperatively, the patient should be wrapped with the shoulders back in a figure-of-eight dressing for 4 to 6 weeks to allow for healing of the soft tissues.

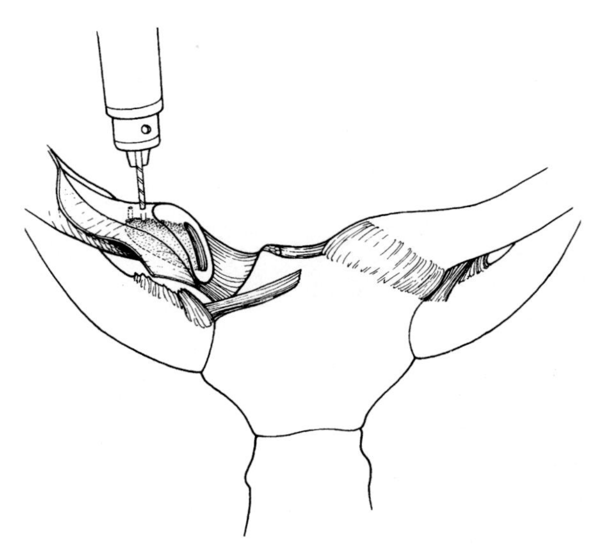

FIG. 49. Drill holes are placed in the superior cortex of the clavicle, approximately 1 cm lateral to the osteotomy site.

We do not recommend the use of Kirschner wires, Steinmann pins, or any other type of metallic pins to stabilize the sternoclavicular joint. The complications are horrendous, as will be discussed in the section on complications.

More recently, Rockwood and associates[153] reported on a series of 23 patients who had undergone a resection of the

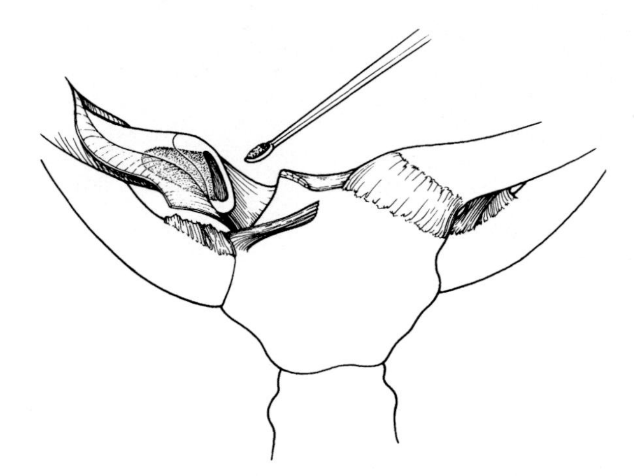

FIG. 48. The medullary canal of the medial clavicle is curretted, in preparation for receiving the transferred intraarticular ligament.

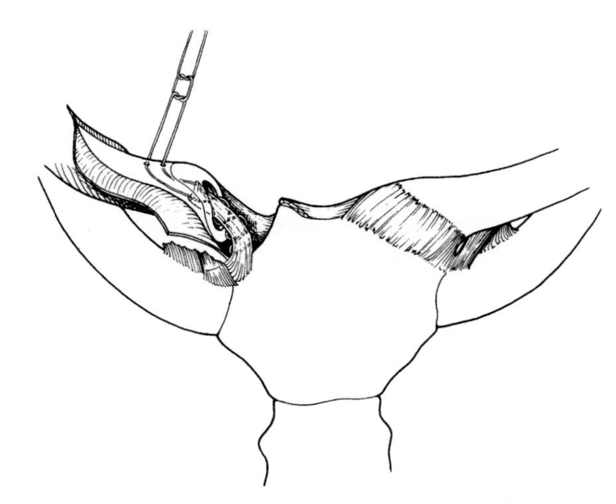

FIG. 50. The free ends of the suture are passed into the medullary canal and out the two holes in the superior cortex.

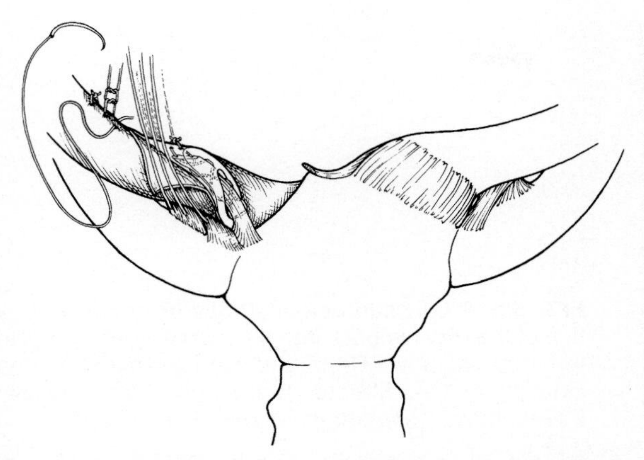

FIG. 51. The transferred ligament is secured into the medial clavicle by tying the sutures exiting from the superior cortex of the clavicle.

medial end of the clavicle. The patients were divided into two groups: group I, who underwent resection of the medial end of the clavicle with maintenance or reconstruction of the costoclavicular ligament; and group II, who had a resection without maintaining or reconstructing the costoclavicular ligament. The outcome in all but 1 of the 7 patients in group II was poor, with persistence or worsening of preoperative symptoms. The only patient of this group with a successful result experienced a posterior epiphyseal separation, in which the costoclavicular ligament remained attached to the periosteum, thus preventing instability. All of the 8 patients in group I, who underwent primary surgical resection of the medial end of the clavicle with maintenance of the costoclavicular ligaments, had an excellent result. When the operation was performed as a revision of a previous procedure with reconstruction of the costoclavicular ligaments, the results were less successful, but only 1 patient of 7 was not satisfied with the outcome of treatment.

Physeal Injuries of the Medial Clavicle

We believe that many anterior and posterior injuries of the sternoclavicular joint in patients under 25 years of age that are thought to be dislocations are, in fact, injuries to the medial physis of the clavicle. Many investigators have observed at the time of surgery that the intraarticular disk ligament stays with the sternum, and we agree with them. In addition, we submit that the unossified or ossified epiphyseal disk, depending on the age of the patient, also stays with the sternum. Anatomically, the epiphysis is lateral to the articular disk ligament, and it is held in place by the capsular ligament and can be mistaken for the intraarticular disk ligament.

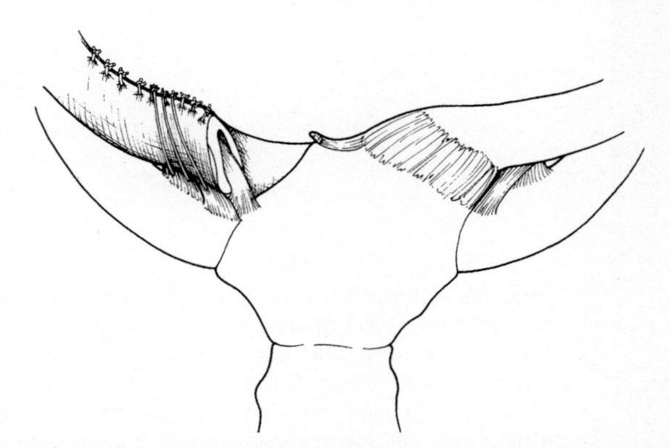

FIG. 52. Closure of the periosteal sleeve around the medial clavicle and secure fixation of these structures to the costoclavicular ligament.

Open reduction of the physeal injury is seldom indicated, except for an irreducible posterior displacement in a patient with significant symptoms of compression of the vital structures in the mediastinum. After reduction, the shoulders are held back with a figure-of-eight strap or dressing for 3 to 4 weeks.

Complications

Nonoperative. The serious complications that occur at the time of dislocation of the sternoclavicular joint are primarily limited to the posterior injuries. About the only complications that occur with the anterior dislocation of the sternoclavicular joint are a cosmetic "bump" or late degenerative changes.[189–191]

Many complications have been reported secondary to the retrosternal dislocation: pneumothorax and laceration of the superior vena cava[137]; respiratory distress[181]; venous congestion in the neck; rupture of the esophagus with abscess and osteomyelitis of the clavicle[14]; pressure on the subclavian artery in an untreated patient[91,173]; occlusion of the subclavian artery late in a patient who was not treated[173]; myocardial conduction abnormalities[181]; compression of the right common carotid artery by a fracture–dislocation of the sternoclavicular joint[91]; brachial plexus compression[120]; and hoarseness of the voice, onset of snoring, and voice changes from normal to falsetto with movement of the arm (Figs. 34 and 53).[14,98,124,161,182] Wasylenko and Busse[185] reported a posterior dislocation of the medial clavicle that caused a fatal tracheoesophageal fistula. Gangahar and Flogaites[66] reported a posterior dislocation of the clavicle that produced a severe thoracic outlet syndrome, with swelling and cyanosis of the upper extremity. Rayon[144] reported a thoracic outlet syndrome and brachial plexopathy caused by a chronic posterior sternoclavicular dislocation of 4 years' duration. The injury was presumably missed, due to an associated dislocation of the glenohumeral joint. The patient experienced paresthesias and decreased sensation, and at one time she unknowingly burned her medial forearm with a hot iron. One year following medial clavicle excision and stabilization of the remaining clavicle to the first rib, she was asymptomatic except for mild discomfort related to the glenohumeral joint. Gardner and Bidstrup[67] reported 3 patients who had severe great vessel injuries following blunt chest trauma and posterior dislocation of the sternoclavicular joint; two cases involved the innominate artery, and one involved the carotid and subclavian arteries. Gale and coworkers[65] reported a ret-

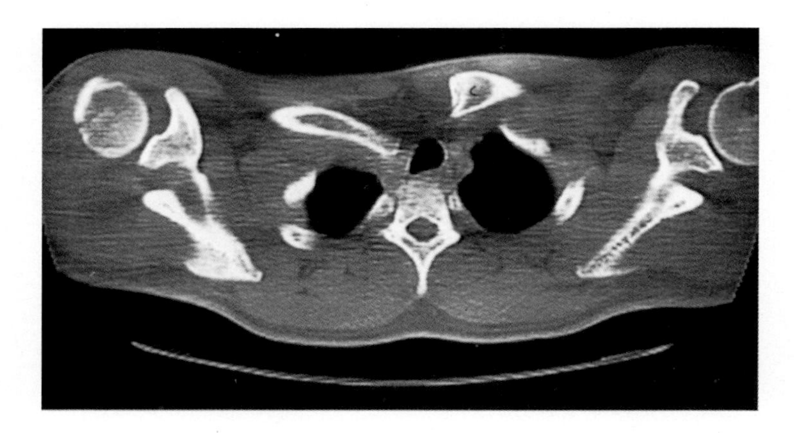

FIG. 53. A CT scan demonstrates posterior dislocation of the clavicle back into the mediastinum, displacing the trachea. (Reprinted with permission from Rockwood CA, Matsen F III, eds. *The shoulder.* Philadelphia: WB Saunders, 1990:Fig. 13-41.)

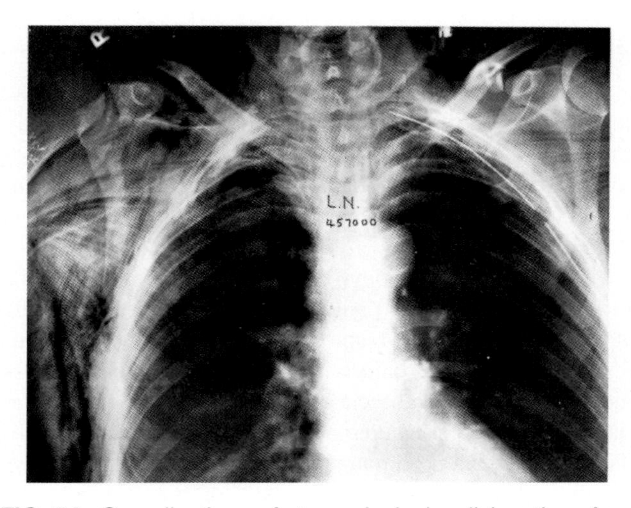

FIG. 54. Complications of sternoclavicular dislocation. As a result of posterior dislocation of the sternoclavicular joint, the patient had a lacerated trachea and developed massive subcutaneous emphysema.

rosternal dislocation of the clavicle associated with stridor and dysphagia.

Several of our patients have had unusual complications from traumatic injuries to the sternoclavicular joint. One patient, as the result of a posterior dislocation and rupture of the trachea, developed massive subcutaneous emphysema (Fig. 54). Another patient had an anterior dislocation on the right and a posterior dislocation on the left. When first seen, his blood pressure was very low. Following reduction of the posterior dislocation, his blood pressure, as recorded on his monitor, instantly returned to normal (Fig. 55). It was theorized that the posteriorly displaced clavicle was irritating some of the vital structures of the mediastinum. Another patient, who had vascular compromise, was already discussed (Fig. 34). Another patient had a traumatic injury to both sternoclavicular joints—the left was posterior and the right was anterior. Following reduction of the left posterior dislocation, the right side remained unstable. A final patient complained of dyspnea, dysphoria, and a "choking" sensation when lying in a lateral decubitus position. However, he developed a painless full range of motion (Fig. 56).

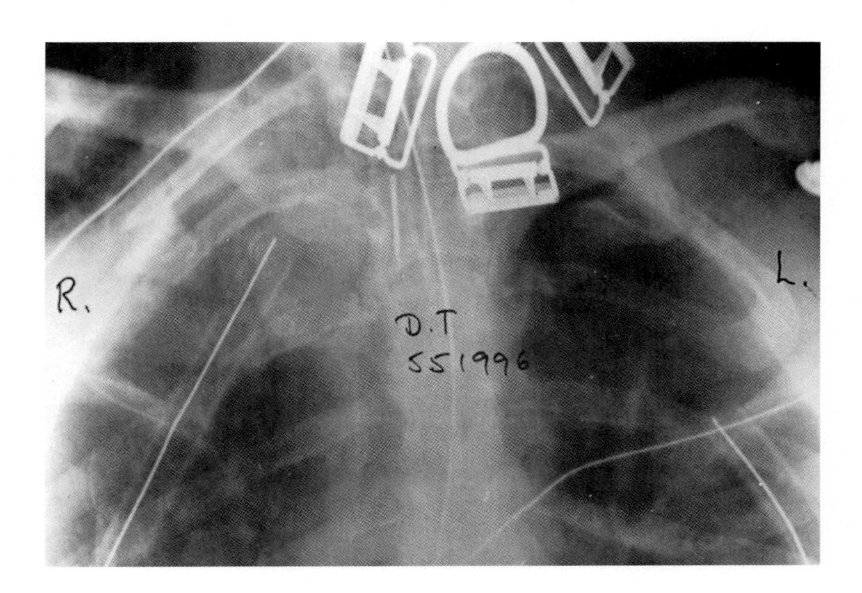

FIG. 55. Complications of sternoclavicular joint dislocation. This patient had an anterior dislocation on the right and a posterior dislocation on the left. As a result of the posterior dislocation, he had sufficient pressure on the mediastinal structures to cause significant hypotension. When the posterior dislocation was reduced, the blood pressure on the continuous monitor promptly returned to normal.

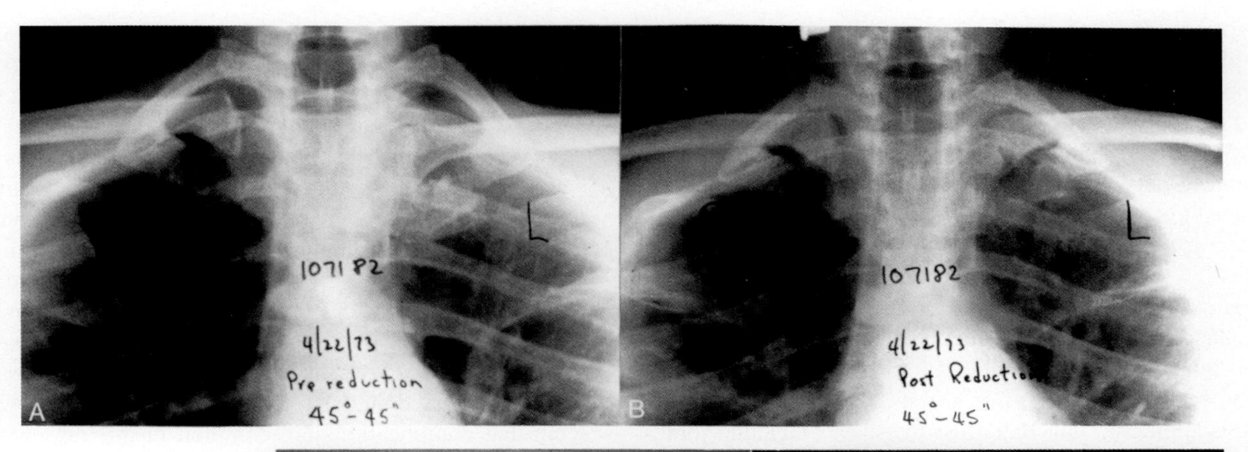

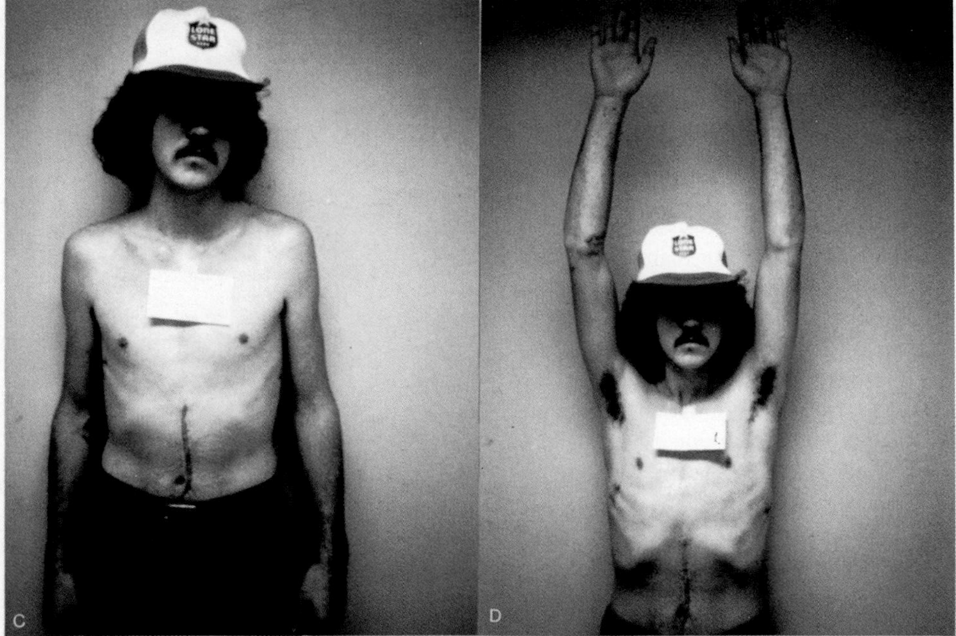

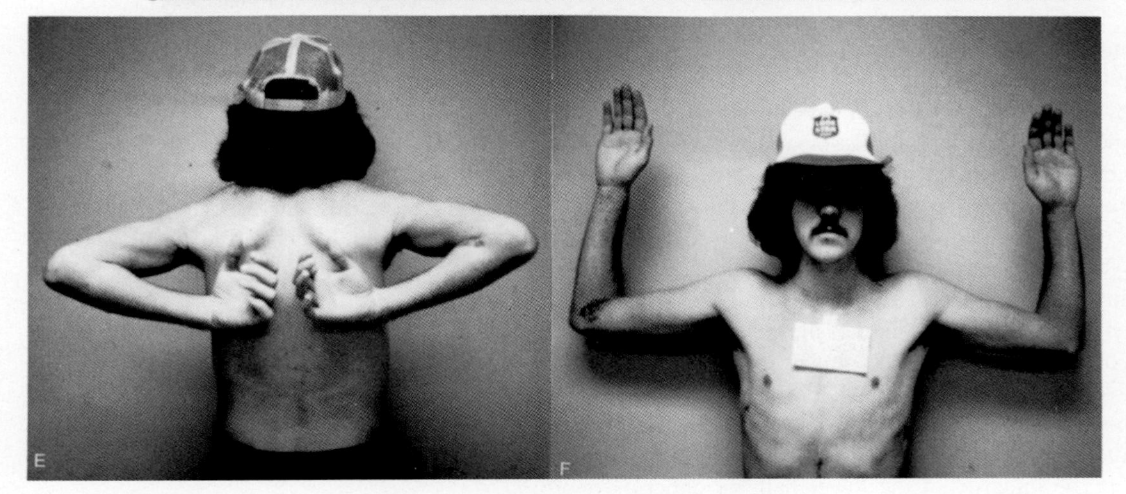

FIG. 56. A: Anterior dislocation of the right sternoclavicular joint and posterior dislocation of the left sternoclavicular joint. **B:** After reduction, the posterior dislocation was stable and the right remained slightly anteriorly displaced. **C–F:** Despite this serious injury, the patient had a full recovery and a normal range of motion of both shoulders. (Reprinted with permission from Rockwood CA, Matsen F III, eds. *The shoulder.* Philadelphia: WB Saunders, 1990:Fig. 13-44.)

Worman and Leagus,[194] in an excellent review of the complications associated with posterior dislocations of the sternoclavicular joint, reported that 16 of 60 patients had suffered complications of the trachea, esophagus, or great vessels. We should point out that even though the incidence of complications was 25%, only four deaths have been reported as a result of this injury.[78,98,141]

Operative Procedures. Through 1992, seven deaths[29,69,108,128,161,167] and three near deaths[20,136,194] from complications of transfixing the sternoclavicular joint with Kirschner wires or Steinmann pins were reported. The pins, either intact or broken, migrated into the heart, pulmonary artery, innominate artery, or aorta. Tremendous leverage force is applied to pins that cross the sternoclavicular joint, and fatigue breakage of the pins is common. Most of the deaths or near deaths were reported in the 1960s[20,108,128,136,161,194]; one each was reported in 1974[29] and 1992.[167] To our knowledge, there were no deaths reported that occurred as a result of migrating pins from the sternoclavicular joint, until the report in 1984 by Gerlach and associates[69] from West Germany. They reported two deaths from migrating nails that caused cardiac tamponade. The physicians were charged with manslaughter by negligence. We do not recommend the use of any transfixing pins—large or small, smooth or threaded, bent or straight—across the sternoclavicular joint.

Brown[20] has reported three complications in 10 operative cases: two from broken pins that had to be removed from a window in the sternum, and one a near death, in which the pin penetrated the back of the sternum and entered the right pulmonary artery. Nordback and Markkula[132] removed a pin tht migrated completely inside the aorta. Jelesijevic and associates,[94] Pate and Wilhite,[136] Rubenstein and colleagues,[166] and Schechter and Gilbert[163] reported cases where the pin migrated into the heart. Leonard and Giffors,[108] and Liu and coworkers[112] reported migration to the pulmonary artery. Sethi and Scott[166] reported migration of the pin to lacerate the subclavian artery. Ferrandez and associates[57] described two cases of Kirschner wire migration into the mediastinum. Clark and associates,[29] Gaston (in the report by Nettles and Linscheid[84)], and Salvatore[161] reported migration of pins into the aorta and resultant death. Grabski[75] reported migration of the pin to the opposite breast in a 37-year-old woman. In addition, the senior author has personally treated patients in whom the pin has migrated into the chest and up into the base of the neck.

Wolford and colleagues[193] reviewed 38 patients who had received 52 sternoclavicular grafts for reconstruction of the temporomandibular joint. The surgical technique involved osteotomy of the superior half of the medial clavicle, maintaining the integrity of the lower half for upper extremity support. Donor site morbidity included postoperative clavicle fractures in 10% of cases. Three of five clavicle fractures required open reduction and internal fixation, and two clavicle fractures healed uneventfully with expectant management.

Omer,[134] in a review of 14 military hospitals, reported 15 patients who had elective surgery for reduction and reconstruction of the sternoclavicular joint. Eight patients were followed by the same house staff for more than 6 months with the following complications: of the five patients who had internal fixation with metal, two developed osteomyelitis, two had fracture of the pin with recurrent dislocation, and one had migration of the pin into the mediastinum with recurrent dislocation. Of the three patients who had soft-tissue reconstructions, two developed recurrent dislocation (one with drainage), and the third developed arthritis and extremity weakness and was dischaarged from military service. Omer commented on this series of complications: "It would seem that complications are common in this rare surgical problem." To Omer's comment we can only add, "Amen."

REFERENCES

1. Abbott LC, and Lucas DB. The Function of the Clavicle: Its Surgical Significance. *An Surg*, 1954;140:583–599.
2. Abott LC, Saunders JB, Hagey H and Jones EW. Surgical Approaches to the Shoulder Joint. *J Bone Joint Surg*, 1949:31A:235–255.
3. Abel MS. Symmetrical Anteroposterior Projections of the Sternoclavicular Joints with Motion Studies. *Radiology*, 1979;132:757–759.
4. Aberle DR, Milos MJ, Aberle AM and Bassett LW. Case Report 407: Diagnosis: Sternocostoclavicular Hyperostosis Affecting the Sternum, Medical Ends of the Clavicles and Upper Segments of the Anteroir Ribs. *Skeletal Radiol*, 1987;16:70–73.
5. Adunsky, A, Yaretzky, A and Klajman A. Malignant Lymphoma Presenting as Sternoclavicular Joint Arthritis (letter to the editor). *Arthritis Rheum*, 1980;2:1330–1331.
6. Allen AW. Living with Suture Grafts in the Repair of Fractures and Dislocations. *Arch Surg*, 1928;16:1007–1020.
7. Allman FL. Fractures and Ligamentous Injuries of the Clavicle and Its Articulations. *J Bone Joint Surg*, 1967;49A:774–784.
8. Anderson ME. Treatment of Dislocations of the Acromioclavicular and Sternoclavicular Joints (abstract). *J Bone Joint Surg*, 1963;45A: 657–658.
9. Bachman M. Swelling of the Sternoclavicluar Joint. *Isr J Med Sci*, 17: 65–72.
10. Badgley CE. Sports Injuries of the Shoulder Girdle. *JAMA*, 1960:172: 444–448.
11. Baker EC. Tomography of the Sternoclavicular Joint. *Ohio State Med J*, 1959:55:60.
12. Baker ME, Martinez S, Kier R, and Wain S. Computed Tomography of the Cadaveric Sternoclavicular Joint: Technique, Findings, and Significance in the Degenerative Disease. Presented at the 33rd Annual Meeting of the Association of the University Radiologists, Nashville, TN, 1985.
13. Bankart ASB. An Operation for Recurrent Dislocation (Subluxation) of the Sternoclavicular Joint. *Br Surg*, 1938;26:320–323.
14. Baranda MM, Pascual JB, Gomez-Escolar IA, Abaitua LG, and Errasti CA. Sternoclavicular Septic Arthritis as First Manifestation of Brucellosis (letter to the editor). *Br J Rheumatol*, 1986;25:322.
15. Barrett J. The Clavicular Joints. *Physiotherapy*, 1971;57:268–269.
16. Barth E and Hagen R. Surgical Treatment of Dislocation of the Sternoclavicular Joint. *Acta Othop Scand*, 1983;54:746–747.
17. Basmajian JV. Joints of the Upper Limb. In: Grant, JCB (ed.): Grant s Method of Anatomy, 8th ed., pp. 158–159. Baltimore, Williams & Wilkins, 1971.
18. Bateman JE. The Shoulder and Neck. Philadelphia, W.B. Saunders, 1972.
19. Bateman JE. The Shoulder and Neck, 2nd ed. Philadelphia, W.B. Saunders, 1978.
20. Bayley I and Kesel L. Shoulder Surgery. New York, Springer Verlag, 1982.
21. Bearn JG. Direct Observations on the Function of the Capsule of the Sternoclavicular Joint in the Clavicular Support. *Anat*, 1967;101: 159–170.

22. Beckman T. A Case of Silmultaneous Luxation of Both Ends of the Clavicle. *Acta Chir Scand*, 1923;56:156–163.
23. Beller RD, Grana WA, and O'Donoghue DH. Recurrent Posterior Dislocation of the Shoulder: A Method of Reconstruction. *Orthopaedics*, 1978;384–388.
24. Berkhina FO. (Traumatic Dislocations of Clavicle.) *Orthop Traumatol*, 1935;9:11–26.
25. Bernard TN, Jr, and Haddad RJ, Jr. Enchondroma of the Proximal Clavicle: An Unusual Cause of Pathologic Fracture-Dislocation of the Sternoclavicular Joint. *Clin Orthop*, 1982;167:239–247.
26. Blankstein A, Nerubay J, Lin E, Keren G, Friedman B, and Horoszowski H. Septic Arthritis of the Sternoclavicular Joint. *Orthop Rev*, 1986;15:41–43.
27. Bloom FA. Wire Fixation in Acromioclavicular Dislocation. *J Bone Joint Surg*, 1945;27:273–276.
28. Bohle L. The Treatment of Fractures, vol. 1, pp. 540–545. New York: Grune & Stratton, 1956.
29. Bonnin, JG. Sponatneous Subluxation of the Sternoclavicular Joint. *Br Med J*, 1960;2:274–275.
30. Booth CM, and Roper BA. Chronic Dislocation of the Sternoclavicular Joint: An Operative Repair. *Clin Orthop*, 1979;140:17–20.
31. Borowiecki B, Charow A, Cook W, Rozycki D, and Thaler S. An Unusual Football Injury (Posterior Dislocation of the Sternoclavicular Joint). *Arch Otolaryngol*, 1972;95:185–187.
32. Borrero E. Traumatic Posterior Displacement of the Left Clavicular Head Causing Chronic Extrinsic Compression of the Subclavian Artery. *Physician Sports Med*, 1987;15:87–89.
33. Breitner S, and Wirth CJ. (Resection of the Acromial and Sternal Ends of the Clavicle.) *Z Orthop*, 1987;25:363–368.
34. Bremner RA. Nonarticular, Non-infective Subacute Arthritis of the Sternoclavicular Joint. *J Bone Joint Surg*, 1959;41B:749–753.
35. Brooks AL, and Henning CD. Injury to the Proximal Clavicular Epiphysis (abstract). *J Bone Joint Surg*, 1972;54A:1347–1348.
36. Brower AC, Sweet DE, and Keats TE. Condensing Osteitis of the Clavicle: A New Entity. *AJR*, 1974;121:17–21.
37. Brown JE. Anterior Sternoclavicular Dislocation: A Method of Repair. *AM J Orthop*, 1961;31:184–189.
38. Brown R. Backward and Inward Dislocation of Sternal End of Clavicle: Open Reduction. *Surg Clin North Am*, 1927;7:1263.
39. Buchmann M. Swelling of the Sternoclavicular Joint. *Acta Med Orient*, 1958;17:65–72.
40. Buckerfield CT, and Castle ME. Acute Traumatic Retrosternal Dislocation of the Clavicle. *J Bone Joint Surg*, 1984;66A:379–385.
41. Burri C, and Nuegebauer R. Carbon Fiber Replacement the Ligaments of the Shoulder Girdle and the Treatments of Lateral Instability of the Ankle Joint. *Clin Orthop*, 1985;196:112–117.
42. Burrows HJ. Tenodesis of Subclavius in the Treatment of Recurrent Dislocation of the Sternoclavicular Joint. *J Bone Joint Surg*, 1951; 33B:240–243.
43. Butterworth RD, and Kirk AA. Fracture Dislocation Sternoclavicular Joint: Case Report. *Va Med*, 1952;79:98–100.
44. Camus JP, Prier A, and Cassou B. (Sternocostoclavicular Hyperostosis.) *Rev Rhum Mal Osteoartic*, 1980;47:361–363.
45. Cantlon GE, and Gluckman JL. Sternoclavicular Joint Hypertrophy Following Radical Neck Dissection. *Head Neck Surg*, 1983;5: 218–221.
46. Cave AJE. The Nature and Morphology of the Costoclavicular Ligament. *J Anat*, 1961;95:170–179.
47. Cave EF. Fractures and Other Injuries. Chicago, Year Book Medical Publishers, 1958.
48. Cave ER, Burke JF, and Boyd RJ. Trauma Management, pp. 409–411. Chicago, Year Book Medical Publishers, 1974.
49. Christensen EE, and Dietz GW. The Supraclavicular Fossa. *Radiology*, 1976;118:37–39.
50. Clark RL, Milgram JW, and Yawn DH. Fatal Aortic Perforation and Cardiac Tamponade Due to a Kirschner Wire Migrating From the Right Sternoclavicular Joint. *South Med J*, 1974;67:316–318.
51. Codman EA. The Shoulder. Boston, Thomas Todd, 1934.
52. Colhoun EN, Hayward C and Evans KT. Inter-Sterno-Costo-Clavicular Ossification. *Clin Radiol*, 1987;38:33–38.
53. Collins JJ. Retrosternal Dislocation of the Clavicle (abstract). *J Bone Joint Surg*, 1972;54B:203.
54. Cone RO, Resnick D, Goergen TG, Robinson C, Vint V and Haghighi P. Condensing Osteitis of the Clavicle, *AJR*, 1983;141:387–388.
55. Conway AM. Movements at the Sternoclavicular and Acromioclavicular Joints. *Phys Ther Rev*, 1961;41:421–432.
55a. Cook F, and Horowitz M. Bipolar Clavicular Dislocation: A Case Report. *J Bone Joint Surg*, 1987;69A:145–147.
56. Cooper A. A Treatise on Dislocations and Fractures of the Joints, 2nd Am. ed. (From 6th London ed.). Boston, Lilly & Wait & Carter & Hendee, 1832.
57. Cooper AP. The Lectures of Sir Astley Cooper on the Principles and Practices of Surgery, p. 559. Philadelphia, E.L. Carey & A. Hart, 1935.
57a. Cooper GJ, Stubbs D, Waller DA, Eilkinson GAL, and Saleh M. Posterior Sternoclavicular Dislocation: A Novel Method of External Fixation. *Injury*, 1992;23:565–567.
58. Cope R and Riddervold HO. Posterior Dislocations of the Sternoclavicular Joint: Report on Two Cases, With Emphasis on Radiologic Management and Early Diagnosis. *Skeletal Radiol*, 1988;17:247–250.
58a. Covelli M, Lapadula G, Pipitone N, Numo R, and Pipitone V. Isolated Sternoclavicular Joint Arthritis in Heroin Addicts and/or HIV Positive Patients: A Report of Three Cases. *Clin Rheumatol*, 1993;12:422–425.
59. Currey H. Primary Gout affecting the Sternoclavicular Joint (letter to the editor). *Br Med J*, 1976;1:583–584.
60. D'Ambrosia RD. Musculoskeletal Disorders. Philadelphia. J.B. Lippincott, 1977.
61. Daffner RH, and Gehweiler JA, Jr. Case Report 236: Diagnosis: Neuropathic Arthropathy of the Sternoclavicular Joint, Secondary to Syringomyelia. *Skeletal Radiol*, 1983;10:113–116.
61a. De Jong KP, and Sukui DM. Anterior Sternoclavicular Dislocation: A Long-Term Follow-up Study. *J Orthop Trauma*, 1990;4:420–423.
62. DePalma AF. The Role of the Disks of the Sternoclavicular and the Acromioclavicular Joints. *Clin Orthop*, 1959;13:222–233.
63. DePalma AF. Surgical Anatomy of the Acromioclavicular and Sternoclavicular Joints. *Clin North Am*, 1963;43:1541–1550.
64. DePalma AF. Surgery of the Shoulder, 2nd ed., pp. 328–240. Philadelphia, J.B. Lippincott, 1973.
65. Delevette AF, and Monahan DT. Acute Arthritis of the Sternoclavicular Joint Due to Coliform Bacillus. *Conn Med*, 1970;34:629–630.
66. Deluca SA. Sternoclavicular Dislocation. *Am Fam Physician*, 1988; 37:137–138.
67. Denham RH, Jr, and Dingley AF, Jr: Epiphyseal Separation of the Medial End of the Clavicle. *J Bone Joint Surg*, 1967;49A:1179–1183.
68. Destouet JM, Gilula LA, Murphy WA and Sagel SS. Computed Tomography of the Sternoclavicular Joint and Sternum. *Radiology*, 1981;138:123–128.
69. Dohler JR. (Ankylosing Hyperostosis of the Sternoclavicular Joint.) *Dtsch Med Wochenschr*, 1987;112:304–305.
70. Duggan N. Recurrent Dislocation of Sternoclavicular Cartilage. *J Bone Joint Surg*, 1931;13:365.
71. Duthie RB, and Ferguson AB, Jr (eds.): Mercer's Orthopaedic Surgery, 7th ed., pp. 958–959. Baltimore, Williams & Wilkins, 1973.
71a. Echo BS, Domari RB, and Powell CE. Bipolar Clavicular Dislocation Treated Surgically: A Case Report. *J Bone Joint Surg*, 1988;70A: 1251–1253.
72. Ecke H. Sternoclavicular Dislocations: Personal Communication, 1984.
73. Elting JJ. Retrosternal Dislocation of the Clavicle. *Arch Surg*, 1972; 104:35–37.
74. Epps CH. Complications in Orthopaedic Surgery. Philadelphia, J.B. Lippincott, 1978.
75. Epstein BS. Sternoclavicular Arthritis in Patients with Scleroderma and Rheumatoid Arthritis. *AJR*, 1963;89:1236–1240.
76. Eskola A. Sternoclavicular Dislocations: A Plea for Open Treatment. *Acta Orthop Scand*, 1986;57:227–228.
77. Eskola A, Vainionpaa S, Vastamki M, Slatis P, and Rokkanen P. Operation of Old Sternoclavicular Dislocation: Results in 12 Cases. *J Bone Joint Surg*, 1989;71B:63–65.
78. Farrer, WE. Case Report: Sternoclavicular Pyarthrosis. J Med Soc N.J., 1985;82:735–737.
79. Fedoseev VA. (A Method of Radiographis Study of the Sternoclavicular Joint.) *Vestn Rentgenol Radiol*, 1977;3:88–91.
80. Ferrandez L, Yubero J, Usabiaga J, No L, and Martin F. Sternoclavicular Dislocation, Treatment and Complications. *Ital J Orthop Traumatol*, 1988;14:349–355.
80a. Ferrandez L, Usabiaga J, Ramos L, Yubero J, and No L. Migration of Kirschner Wires into the Mediastinum After Stabilization of Sternoclavicular Lesions: A Report of Two Cases. *Chir Organi Mov*, 1991; 76:301–304.

81. Ferry AM, Rook FW, and Masterson JH. Retrosternal Dislocation of the Clavicle. *J Bone Joint Surg*, 1957;39A:905–910.
82. Fery A and Leonard A. (Transsternal Sternoclavicular Projection: Diagnostic Value in Sternoclavicular Dislocations.) *J Radiol*, 1981;62: 167–170.
83. Fery A and Sommelet J. (Dislocation of the Sternoclavicular Joint: A Review of 49 Cases.) *Int Orthop*, 1988;12:187–195.
84. Fisk GH. Some Observation of Motion at the Shoulder Joint. *Can Med Assoc J*, 1944;50:213–216.
85. Fitchet SM. Cleidocranial Dysostosis: Hereditary and Familial. *J Bone Joint Surg*, 1929;11:838–866.
86. Foucher JTE. The Classic: Separations of the Epiphyses (1867). *Clin Orthop*, 1984;188:3–9.
87. Franquet T, Lecumberri F, Rivas A, Inaraja L and Idoate MA. Condenseing Osteitis of the Clavicle: Report of Two New Cases. *Skeletal Radiol*, 1985;14:184–187.
88. Friedman RS, Perez HD, and Goldstein IM. Septic Arthritis of the Sternoclavicular Joint Due to Gram-Postitive Microorganisms. *Am J Med Sci*, 1981;282:91–93.
89. Fuxench-Chiesa Z, Mejias E and Ramirez-Ronda CH. Septic Arthritis of the Sternoclavicular Joint due to Citrobacter diversus (letter to the editor). *J Rheumatol*, 1983;10:162–164.
89a. Gale DW, Dunn ID, McPherson S and Ini OOA: Retrosternal Dislocation of the Calvicle: The Stealth Dislocation: A Case Report. *Injury*, 1992;23:563–564.
90. Gallie WE. Dislocations. *N Engl J Med*, 1935;213:91–98.
91. Gangahar DM and Flogaites T. Retrosternal Dislocation of the Clavicle Producing Thoracic Outlet Syndrome. *J Trauma*, 1978;18: 369–372.
92. Gardner NA and Bidstrup BP. Intrathoracic Great Vessel Injury Resulting From Blunt Chest Trauma Associated With Posterior Dislocation of the Sternoclavicular Joint. *Aust NZ J Surg*, 1983;53:427–430.
93. Gartland JJ. Fundamentals in Orthopaedics, 3rd ed., pp. 249–250. Philadephia, W.B. Saunders.
94. Gazak S and Davidson SJ. Posterior Sternoclavicular Dislocations: Two Case Reports. *J Trauma*, 1984;24:80–82.
94a. Gearen PF and Petty W. Panclavicular Dislocation: A Case Report. *J Bone Joint Surg*, 1982;64A:454–455.
95. Gerlach D, Wemhoner SR and Ogbuihi S: (On Two Cases of Fatal Heart Tamponade due to Migration of Fracture Nails From the Sternoclavicular Joint.) *Z Rechtsmed*, 1984;93:53–60.
96. Gerster JC, Lagier R, and Nicod L. Case Report 311: Open-Quiz Solution. *Skeletal Radiol*, 1985;14:53–60.
97. Glickman LG, and Minsky AA. Case Reports - Enlargement of One Sternoclavicular Articulation: A Sign of Congenital Syphilis. *Radiology*, 1937;28:85–86.
98. Goldin RH, Chow AH, Edwards JE, Jr, Louie JE, and Guze LB. Sternoarticular Septic Arthritis in Heroin Users. *N Engl J Med*, 1973;289: 616–618.
99. Goossens M, Vaderstraeten CV and Claessens H. Sternoclavicular Hyperostosis: A Case Report and Review of the Literature. *Clin Orthop*, 1985;194:164–18.
100. Gorman JB, Stone RT, and Keats TE. Changes in the Sternoclavicular Joint Following Radical Neck Dissection. *AJR*, 1971;111:584–587.
101. Grabski RS. (Unusual Dislocation of a Fragment of the Kirschner Wire After Fixation of the Sternoclavicular Joint.) *Wiad Lek*, 1987;40: 630–632.
102. Grant JCB. Method of Anatomy, 7th ed., Baltimore, Williams & Wilkins, 1965.
103. Gray H. Osteology. In: Goss, CM (ed.): Anatomy of the Human Body, 28th ed., pp. 324–326. Philadelphia, Lea & Febiger, 1966.
104. Greenlee DP. Posterior Dislocation of the Sternal End of the Calvicle. *JAMA*, 1944;125:426–428.
105. Guerin J. Recherchés sur les Luxations Congenitales. *Gaz Med Paris*, 1841;9:97.
106. Gunson EF. Radiography of the Sternoclavicular Articulation. Radiog. *Clin Photog*, 1943;19:20–24.
107. Gunther WA. Posterior Dislocation of the Sternoclavicular Joint: Report of a Case. *J Bone Joint Surg*, 1949;31A:878–879.
108. Gurd FB. Surplus Parts of the Skeleton: A Recommendation for the Excision of Certain Portions as a Means of Shortening the Period of Disability Following Trauma. *Am J Surg*, 1947;74:705–720.
109. Haas, SL. The Experimental Transplantation of the Epiphysis: With Observations on the Longitudinal Growth of Bone. *JAMA*, 1915;65: 1965–1971.
110. Habernek H and Hertz, H. (Origin, Diagnosis and Treatment of Traumatic Dislocation of Sternoclavicular Joint.) *Aktuel Traumatol*, 1987; 17:25–28.
111. Haenel LC, Bradway WR, and Constantini PJ: Thrombophlebitis Complication Sternoclavicular Hyperostosis: Case Report. *Postgrad Med J*, 1980;68:113–118.
112. Hallas J and Oloesen, KP. Sterno-costo-clavicular Hyperostosis: A Case Report with Review Literature. *Acta Radiol*, 1988;58:941–945.
113. Hamilton-Wood C, Hollingsworth P, Dieppe P, Ackroyd C, and Watt, I. The Painful Swollen Sterno-clavicular Joint. *Br J Radiol*, 1985;58: 941–945.
114. Hartman, TJ, and Dunnagan, WA. Cinearthrography of the Sternoclavicular Joint. Personal communication, November, 1979.
115. Haug W. Retention Einer Seltenen Sterno-clavicular-luxationsfractur Mittels Modifizierter Y-Platte der AO. *Aktuel Traumatol*, 1986;16: 39–40.
116. Heinig CF. Retrosternal Dislocation of the Clavicle: Early Recognition, X-ray Diagnosis, and Management (abstract). *J Bone Joint Surg*, 1968;50A:830.
117. Heppenstall RB (ed.). Fracture Treatment and Healing, pp. 417–419. Philadelphia, W.B. Saunders, 1980.
118. Hermann G, Rothenberg RR, and Spiera H. The Value of Tomography in Diagnosing Infection of the Sternoclavicular Joint. *Mt Sinai J Med*, 1983;50:52–55.
119. Hernandez LA, Watson JD, and Sturrock RD. Septic Arthritis of the Sternoclavicular Joint: Complicated by Fistula Formation. *Rheumatol Rehabil*, 1976;15:292–294.
120. Higoumenakis GK. Neues Stigma der kongenitalen Lues: Die Vergrösserung des sternalen Endes des rechten Schlüsselbeins, seine Beschreibung, Deutung and Atiologie. *Dtsch Z Nervenheilkd*, 1930; 114:228.
121. Hobbs DW. Sternoclavicular Joint: A New Axial Radiographic View. *Radiology*, 1968;90:801–802.
122. Hollinshead WH. Anatomy for Surgeons, vol. 3, pp. 265–268. Philadelphia, Harper & Row, 1958.
123. Holmdahl HC. A Case of Posterior Sternoclavicular Dislocation. *Acta Othop Scand*, 1953–1954;23:218–222.
124. Hotchkiss LW. Double Dislocation of the Sternal End of the Clavicle. *Ann Surg*, 1896;23:600.
125. Howard FM, and Shafer SJ. Injuries to the Clavicle with Neurovascular Complications: A Study of Fourteen Cases. *J Bone Joint Surg*, 1965;47A:1335–1346.
126. Howard NJ. Acromioclavicular and Sternoclavicular Joint Injuries. *Am J Surg*, 1939;46:284–291.
127. Hoyt WA. Etiology of Shoulder Injuries in Athletes. *J Bone Joint Surg*, 1967;49A:755–766.
127a. Hsu HC, Wu JJ, Lo WH, Chen WM, and YU CT. Epiphyseal Fracture-Retrosternal Dislocation of the Medial End of the Clavicle: A Case Report. *Chinese Med J*, 1993;52:198–202.
128. Hynd RF, Klofkorn RW, and Wong JK. Case Report: Streptococcus anginosus-constellatus Infection of the Sternoclavicular Joint. *J Rheumatol*, 1984;11:713–715.
129. Inman VT, Saunders JB and Abbott LC. Observations on the Function of the Clavicle. *Calif Med*, 1946;65:158–166.
130. Inman VT, Saunders JB and Abbott LC. Observations on the Function of the Shoulder Joint. *J Bone Joint Surg*, 1944;26:1–30.
130a. Jain AS. Traumatic Floating Clavicle: A Case Report. *J Bone Joint Surg*, 1984;66B:560–561.
131. Jelesijevic V, Knoll D, Klinke F, Sine K, and Dittrich H. (Penetrating Injuries of the Heart and Intrapericardial Blood Vessels Caused by Migration of a Kirschner Pin After Osteosynthesis.) *Acta Chir Iugol*, 1982;29:274–276.
132. Jones R. Injuries of Joints, 2nd ed., pp. 53–55. London, Oxford University Press, 1917.
133. Jonsson G. A Method of Obtaining Structural Pictures of the Sternum. *Acta Radiol*, 1937;18:336–340.
134. Jurik AG, De Carvalho A, and Gaudal H. Sternoclavicular Hyperostosis in a Case With Psoriasis and HLA-B27 Associated Arthropathy. *Fortschr Röntgenstr*, 1985;142:345–347.
135. Jurik AG, De Carvalho A, and Graudal H. Sclerotic Changes of the Sternal End of the Clavicle. *Clin Radiol*, 1985;36:23–25.
136. Kalliomaki JL, Viitanen SM, and Virtama P. Radiological Findings of the Sternoclavicular Joints in Rheumatoid Arthritis. *Acta Rheum Scand*, 1969;14:233–240.

137. Kanoksikarin S and Wearne WM. Fracture and Retrosternal Dislocation of the Clavicle. Aust. *NZ J Surg*, 1978;48:95–96.
138. Kattan KR. Modified View for Use in Roentgen Examination of the Sternoclavicular Joints. *Radiology*, 1973;108:8.
139. Kennedy JC. Retrosternal Dislocation of the Clavicle. *J Bone Joint Surg*, 1949;31B:74–75.
140. Kessel L. Clinical Disorders of the Shoulder. London, Churchill Livingstone, 1982.
141. Key JA and Conwell HE (eds.). The Management of Fractures, Dislocations and Sprains, 5th ed., pp. 458–461. St. Louis, C.V. Mosby, 1951.
142. Kier R, Wain S, Apple J, and Martinez S. Osteoarthritis of the Sternoclavicular Loint: Radiographic Features and Pathologic Correlation. Invest. *Radiol*, 1986;21:227–33.
143. King JM, Jr, and Holmes GW. A Review of Four Hundred and Fifty Roentgen Ray Examinations of the Shoulder. *AJR*, 1927;17:214–218.
144. Kofoed H, Thomsen P, and Lindenbergs S. Serous Synovitis of the Sternoclavicular Joint: Differential Diagnostic Aspects. *Sanc J Rheumatol*, 1985;14:61–64
145. Kohler H, Uehlinger E, Kutzner J, and West TB. Sternoclavicular Hyperostosis: Painful Swelling of the Sternum, Clavicles and Upper Ribs: Report of Two Cases. *Ann Intern Med*, 1977;87:192–194.
146. Krenzien J. Acromioclavicular and Sternoclavicular Luxations. Personal Communication, July 1987.
147. Kruger GD, Rock MG, Munro TG. Condensing Osteitis of the Clavicle: A Review of the Literature and Report of Three Cases. *J Bone Joint Surg*, 1987;69A:550–557.
148. Kurzbauer R. The Lateral Projection in Roentgenography of the Sternoclavicular Articulation. *AJR*, 1946;56:104–105.
149. Lagier R, Arroyo J and Fallet GH. Sternocostoclavicular Hyperostosis: Radiological and Pathological Study of a Specimen With Ununited Clavicular Fracture. *Pathol Res Pract*, 1986;181:596–603.
150. Laidlaw JY. Treatment of Dislocated Clavicle. Personal Communication, 1985.
151. Lasher WW. Cartilage Injuries: A Clincial Study. *Am J Surg*, 1929;6: 493–500.
152. Lee HM. Sternoclavicular Dislocation: Report of a Case. *Minn Med*, 1937;20:480–482.
153. Leighton RK, Buhr AJ and Sinclairs AM. Posterior Sternoclavicular Dislocations. *Can J Surg*, 1986;29:104–106.
154. Lemire L and Rosman M. Sternoclavicular Epiphyseal Separation With Adjancent Clavicular Fracture: A Case Report. *J Pediatr Orthop*, 1984;4:118–120.
155. Leonard JW and Gifford RW. Migration of a Kirschner Wire from the Clavicle Into Pulmonary Artery. *Am J Cardiol*, 1965;16:598–600.
156. Levinsohn EM, Bunnell WP and Yaun HA. Computed Tomography in the Diagnosis of Dislocations of the Sternoclavicular Joint. *Clin Orthop*, 1979;140:12–16.
157. Levy M, Goldberg I, Fischl RE, Frisch E, and Maor P. Friedrich's Disease: Aseptic Necrosis of the Sternal End of the Clavicle. *J Bone Joint Surg*, 1981;63B:539–541.
158. Lewin KW. Rhomboid Fossa of Inflammation? (Letter to the editor). *Arch Intern Med*, 1978;138:658–659.
159. Lindesy RW, and Leach JA. Sternoclavicular Osteomyelitis and Pyoarthrosis As a Complication of Subclavian Vein Catherization: A Case Report and Review of the Literature. *Orthopaedis*, 1984;7: 1017–1021.
160. Linscheid RL, Kelly PJ, Martin WJ, and Fontana RS. Monarticular Bacterial Arthritis of the Sternoclavicular Joint. *JAMA*, 1961;178: 421–422.
160a. Liu HP, Chang CH, Lin PJ, et al. Migration of Kirschner Wire for the Right Sternoclavicular Joint into the Main Pulmonary Artery: A Case Report. *Chang Gung Med J*, 1992;15:49–53.
161. Lourie JA. Tomography in Diagnosis of Posterior Dislocations of the Sternoclavicular Joint. *Acta Orthop Scand*, 1980;51:579–580
162. Louw JA and Louw JA. Posterior Dislocation of the Sternoclavicular Joint Associated With Major Spinal Injury: A Case Report. *S Afr Med J*, 1987;71:791–792.
163. Lowman CL. Operative Correction of Old Sternoclavicular Dislocation. *J Bone Joint Surg*, 1928;10:740–741.
164. Lucas DB. Biomechanics of the Shoulder Joint. *Arch Surg*, 1973;107: 425–432.
165. Lucas GL. Retrosternal Dislocation of the Clavicle. *JAMA*, 1965;193: 850–853.
166. Lunseth PA, Chapman KW, and Frankel VH. Surgical Treatment of Chronic Dislocation of the Sternoclavicular Joint. *J Bone Joint Surg*, 1975;57B:193–196.
167. Maguire WB. Safe and Simple Method of Repair of Recurrent Dislocation of the Sternoclavicular Joint (abstract). *J Bone Joint Surg*, 1986;68B:332.
168. Marsh HO, Shellito JG, and Callahan WP, Jr. Synovial Sarcoma of the Sternoclavicular Region. *J Bone Joint Surg*, 1963;45A;151–155.
169. Martinez S, Khoury MB and Harrelson J. Imaging of Condensing Osteitis of the Clavicle: New Observations. Presented at the 33rd Annual Meeting of the Association of University Radiologists, Nashville, TN, 1985.
170. Mathews JG. Primary Gout Affecting the Sternoclavicular Joint. *Br Med J*, 1976;1:262.
171. Mazet R, Jr. Migration of a Kirschner Wire From the Shoulder Region Into the Lung: Report of Two Cases. *J Bone Joint Surg*, 1943;25A: 477–483.
172. McCarroll JR. Isolated Staphylococcal Infection of the Sternoclavicular Joint. *Clin Orthop*, 1981;16:149–150.
173. McCaughan JS, and Miller PR. Migration of Steinmann Pin from Shoulder to Lung (letter to the editor). *JAMA*, 1969;207:1917.
174. McKenzie JMM. Retrosternal Dislocation of the Clavicle: A Report of Two Cases. *J Bone Joint Surg*, 1963;45B:138–141.
175. McLaughlin H. Trauma, pp. 291–292. Philadelphia, W.B. Saunders, 1959.
176. Mehta JC, Sachdev A and Collins JJ. Retrosternal Dislocation of the Clavicle. *Injury*, 1973;5:79–83.
177. Milch H. The Rhomboid Ligament in Surgery of the Sternoclavicular Joint. *J Int Coll Surg*, 1952;17:41–51.
178. Mitchell WJ, and Cobey MC. Retrosternal Dislocation of the Clavicle. *Med Ann DC*, 1960;29:546–549.
179. Moncada R, Mantuga T, Unger E, Freeark R and Pizarro A. Migratory Traumatic Cardiovascular Foreign Bodies: Case Reports. *Circulation*, 1978;57:186–189.
180. Morag B, and Shahin N. The Value of Tomography of the Sternoclavicular Region. *Clin Radiol*, 1978;26:57–62.
181. Mosely HF. Athletic Injuries to the Shoulder Region. *Am J Surg*, 1959;98:401–422.
182. Mouchet A. Luxation Sterno-Claviculaire en Avant: Reduction Sanglante. *Rev Orthop*, 1942;28:99–100.
183. Muir SK, Kinsella PL, Trevilcock RG and Balckstone IW. Infectious Arthritis of the Sternoclavicular Joint. *Can Med Assoc J*, 1985;132: 1289–1290.
184. Nair V. Case Report - Sternoclavicular Arthritis: An Unsusual Complication of Drug Abuse. *J Med Soc NJ*, 1975;72:519–520.
185. Nettles JL, and Linscheid R. Sternoclavicular Dislocations. *J Trauma*, 1968;8:158–164.
186. Nevaiser JS. Injuries of the Clavicle and Its Articulations. Orthop. *Clin North Am*, 1980;11:233–237.
187. Newlin NS. Congenial Retrosternal Subluxationof the Clavicle Simulating an Intrathoracic Mass. *AJR*, 1978;30:1184–1185.
188. Nickel VL. Orthopaedic Rehabilitation. London, Churchill Livingstone, 1982.
189. Nitsche JF, Vaughan JH, Williams G and Curd JG. Septic Sternoclavicular Arthritis With Pasteurella multocida and Streptococcus sangius. *Arthritis Rheum*, 1982;25:467–469.
190. Nittis S. Prominence of the Right Sternoclavicular Junction in Lepers. *Urol Cutan Rev*, 1937;41:625–630.
191. Noonan TR. Sternoclavicular Dislocation. Personal Communication, July 30, 1984.
192. Nordback I and Markkula H. Migration of Kirschner Pin from Clavicle Into Ascending Aorta. *Acta Chir Scand*, 1985;151:177–179.
193. Nutz V. (Fracture Dislocation of the Sternoclavicular Joint.) *Unfallchirurg*, 1986;89:145–148.
194. O'Donoghue DH. Treatment of Injuries to Athletes, 2nd ed., Philadelphia, W.B. Saunders, 1976.
196. Ogden JA, Conlogue GJ and Bronson ML. Radiology of Postnatal Skeletal Development: III. The Clavicle. *Skeletal Radiol*, 1979;4: 196–203.
197. Omer GE. Osteotomy of the Clavicle in Surgical Reduction of Anterior Sternoclavicular Dislocation. *J Trauma*, 1967;7:584–590.
198. Orsini G, Guercio N and Paschero B. Retrosternal Dislocationof the Clavicle: Observations on Three Cases. *Ital J Orthop Traumatol*, 1984;10:533–539.
199. Paice EW, Wright FW, and Hill AGS. Sternoclavicular Erosions in Polymyalgia Rheumatice. *Ann Rheum Dis*, 1983;42:379–383.

200. Pate JW and Wilhite J. Migration of a Foreign Body From the Sternoclavicular Joint to the the Heart: A Case Report. *Am Surg*, 1969;35: 488–449.
201. Paterson DC. Retrosternal Dislocation of the Clavicle. *J Bone Joint Surg*, 1961;43B:90–92.
202. Pauleau JL and Baux S. (Sternoclavicular Dislocations: A Case Report of a Posterior Dislocation and Review of the Published Literature.) *J Chir*, 1980;117:453–456.
203. Peacock HK, Brandon JR and Jones OL. Retrosternal Dislocation of the Clavicle. *South Med J*, 1970;63:1324–1328.
204. Pendergrass EP and Hodes PJ. The Rhomboid Fossa of the Clavicle. *AJR*, 1937;38:152–155.
205. Percy EC. Sternoclavicular Dislocation (Case P55). *Can Med Assoc J*, 1971;104:1016–1017.
206. Persoons D, Copin G and Dosch J. (Retrosternal Dislocation of the Clavicle: Contribution of Computertomography in Diagnosis and Treatment - Case Report.) *Acta Orthop Belg*, 1985;51:103–109.
207. Pfister U and Ode E. Die Luxation im sterno-clavicular-gelenk. Unfallmed Arbeit October, 1983.
208. Pfister U, and Weller S. (Luxation of the Sternoclavicular Joint.) *Unfallchirugie*, 1982;8:81–87.
209. Pierce RO, Jr. Internal Derangement of the Sternoclavicular Joint. *Clin Orthop*, 1979;141:247–250.
210. Poland J. Traumatic Separation of Epiphyses of the Upper Extremity, pp. 135–143. London, Smith, Elder & Co., 1898.
210a. Porral MA. Observation d une Double Luxation de la Clavicule Droite. *J Niv Hebd Med Chir Prat*, 1831;2:78–82.
211. Post M. The Shoulder. Philadelphia, Lea & Febiger, 1978.
212. Pridie K. Dislocation of Acromio-clavicular and Sterno-clavicular Joints (abstract). *J Bone Joint Surg*, 1959;41B:429.
213. Quigley TB. Injuries to the Acromioclavicular and Sternoclavicular Joints Sustained in Athletics. *Surg Clin North Am*, 1963;43: 1551–1554.
214. Raney RB, Brashear HR and Shands AR, Jr. Shands Handbook of Orthopaedic Surgery, P.421. St. Louis, C.V. Mosby, 1971.
214a. Rayan GM. Compression Brachial Plexopathy caused by Chronic Posterior Dislocation of the Sternoclavicular Joint. *J Okla Stat Med Assoc*, 1994;87:7–9.
215. Reeves BD. Postpartum Sternoclavicular Joint Pain. *JAMA*, 1982;248: 3030–3031.
215a. Renoult E, Lataste A, Jonon B, Testevuide P and Kesler M. Sternoclavicular Joint Infection in Hemodialysis Patients. *Nephron*, 1990; 56:212–213.
216. Resnick D. Sternoclavicular Hyperostosis. *AJR*, 1980;135: 1278–1280.
217. Reuler JB, Girard DE and Nardone DA. Sternoclavicular Joint Involvement in Ankylosing Spondylitis. *South Med J*, 1978;71: 1480–1481.
218. Rice EE. Habitual Dislocation of the Sternoclavicular Articulation: Case Report. *J Okla State Med Assoc*, 1932;25:34–35.
219. Richter R, Hahn H, Nubling W and Kohler G. (Tuberculosis of the Shoulder Girdle.) *Z Rheumatol*, 1985;44:87–92.
220. Ritvo M and Ritvo M. Roentgen Study of the Sternoclavicular Region. *AJR*, 1947;53:644–650.
221. Rockwood CA, Jr. Dislocations of the Sternoclavicular Joint. Instr. *Course Lect*, 1975;24:144–159.
222. Rockwood CA, Jr. Dislocation of the Sternoclavicular Joint. In: Rockwood, CA, Jr., and Green, DP (eds.): Fractures, 1st ed. vol. 1, pp. 756–787. Philadelphia, J.B. Lippincott, 1975.
223. Rockwood CA, Jr. Injuries of the Sternoclavicular Joint (abstract). *Orthop Trans*, 1977;1:96.
224. Rockwood CA, Jr. Management of Fractures of the Clavicle and Injuries of the Sternoclavicular Joint (abstract). *Orthop Trans*, 1982;6: 422.
225. Rockwood CA, Jr. Injuries to the Sternoclavicular Joint. In: Rockwood, CA, Jr., and Green, DP (eds.): Fractures, 2nd ed. vol. 1, pp. 910–948. Philadelphia, J.B. Lippincott, 1984.
226. Rockwood CA, Jr and Odor JM. Spontaneous Atraumatic Anterior Subluxation of the Sternoclavicular Joint in Young Adults: Report of 37 Cases (abstract). *Orthop Trans*, 1988;12:557.
226a. Rockwood CA, Jr. The Shoulder: Facts, Confusions, and Myths. *Int Orthop*, 1991;15:401–405.
226b. Rockwood CA, Jr, Groh GI, Wirth MA and Grassi FA. Resection-Arthroplasty of the Sternoclavicular Joint. J Bone Joint Surg. (In press.)
227. Rodrigues H. Case of Dislocation, Inwards, of the Internal Extremity of the Clavicle. *Lancet*, 1843;1:309–310.
227a. Rowe CR. Personal Communication, June 27, 1988.
227b. Rowe CR. The Shoulder, pp. 313–327. New York, Churchill Livinstone, 1988.
228. Rozboril MB, Good AE, Zarbo RJ and Schultz DA. Sternoclavicular Joint Arthritis: An Unusual Presentation of Metastatic Carcimona. *J Rheumatol*, 1983;10:499–502.
229. Rubenstein ZR, Moray B and Itzchak Y. Percutaneous Removal of Intravascular Foreign Bodies. Cardiovasc. *Intervent Radiol*, 1982;5: 64–68.
230. Sadr B and Swann M. Spontaneous Dislocation of the Sternoclavicular Joint. *Acta Orthop Scand*, 1979;50:269–274.
231. Sala RS and Gomez JM. (Sterno-costo-clavicular Hyperostosis: Presentation of One Case and Review of Literature.) *Med Clin*, 1985;84: 483–486
232. Salvatore JE. Sternoclavicular Joint Dislocation. *Clin Orthop*, 1968; 58:51–54.
232a. Sanders JO, Lyons FA and Rockwood CA. Management of Disloations of Both Ends of the Clavicle. *J Bone Joint Surg*, 1990;72A: 399–402.
233. Santa LR. Manual of Roentgenological Technique, 9th ed., pp. 160–161. Ann Arbor, Edwards Brothers, 1942.
234. Sartoris DJ, Schreiman JS, Kerr R, Resnick CS and Resnick D. Sternocostoclavicular Hyperostosis: A Review and Report of 11 Cases. *Radiology*, 1986;158:125–128.
235. Savastano AA and Stutz SJ. Traumatic Sternoclavicular Dislocation. *Int Surg*, 1978;63:10–13.
236. Schechter DC and Gilbert L. Injuries of the Heart and Great Vessels Due to Pins and Needles. *Throrax*, 1969;24:246–253.
237. Schmitt WGH. Articulatis Sternocavicuaris: Darstellung in Einer Zweiter Ebene. *Roentgenpraxis*, 1981;34:262–267
237a. Searle AE, Gluckman R, Sanders R and Breach NM. Sternoclavicular Joint Swellings: Diagnosis and Management. *Br J Plast Surg*, 1991; 44:403–405.
238. Selesnick FH, Jablon M, Frank C and Post M. Retrosternal Dislocation of the Clavicle: Report of Four Cases. *J Bone Joint Surg*, 1984; 66A:287–291.
239. Sethi GK and Scott SM. Subclavian Artery Laceration Due to Migration of a Hagie Pin. *Surgery*, 1976;80:644–646
240. Silberberg M, Frank EL, Jarrett SR and Silberberg R. Aging and Osteoarthritis of the Human Sternoclavicular Joint. *Am J Pathol*, 1959; 35:851–865.
241. Silverman M. Sternocostoclavicular Hyperostosis (letter to the editor). *Ann Intern Med*, 87:797.
242. Simurda MA. Retrosternal Dislocation of the Clavicle: A Report of Four Cases and a Method of Repair. *Can J Surg*, 1968;11:487–490.
242a. Smolle-Juettner FM, Hofer PH, Pinter H, Friehs G and Szyskowitz R. Intracardiac Malpositioning of a Sternoclavicular Fixation Wire. *J Orthop Trauma*, 1992;6:102–105.
243. Snyder CC, Levine GA and Dingman DL. Trail of a Sternoclavicular Whole Joint Graft as a Substitute for the Temporomandibular Joint. Plast. *Reconstr Surg*, 1971;8:447–452.
244. Sokoloff, L, and Gleason, IO: The Sternoclavicular Articulation in Rheumatic Diseases. *Am J Clin Pathol*, 1954;24:406–414.
245. Sonozaki H, Azuma A, Okai K, et al. Inter-sterno-costo-clavicular Ossification With a Special Refernence to Cases of Unilateral Type. *Kanto J Orthop Traumatol*, 9:196–200.
246. Sonozaki H, Azuma A, Okai K, et al. Clinical Features of 22 Cases With Inter-sterno-costo-clavicular Ossification. *Arch Orthop Trauma Surg*, 1979;95:13–22.
247. Sonozaki H, Furusawa S, Seki H, Kurokawa T, Tateishi A and Kabata. Four Cases With Symmetrical Ossification Between Clavicles and the First Ribs of Both Sides. *Kanto Orthop Traumatol*, 1947;5:244–247.
248. Southworth SR and Merritt TR. Asymtomatic Innominate Vein Tamponade With Retromanubrial Clavicular Dislocation: A Case Report. *Orthop Rev*, 1988;17:789–791.
249. Spar I. Psoriatric Arthritis of the Sternoclavicular Joint. *Conn Med*, 1978;42:225–226.
250. Speed K. A Textbook of Fractures and Dislocations, 4th ed., pp. 282–290. Philadelphia, Lea & Febiger, 1942.
251. Stankler L. Posterior Dislocation of Clavicle: A Report of 2 Cases. *Br J Surg*, 1962;50:164–168.
252. Stapelmohr SV. Ueber die habituelle Luxation sternoclavicularis und

eine neue operative Behandlungsmethode Derselben. *Acta Orthop Scand*, 1932;3:1–42.
253. Stein AH. Retrosternal Dislocation of the Clavicle. J. *Bone Joint Surg*, 1957;39A:656–660.
254. Stimson LA. Fractures and Dislocations, pp. 588–589. Philaelphia, Lea & Febiger, 1912.
255. Streifler J, Gartz M, Rosenfeld JB, Pitlik S and Grosskopf, I. Sternoclavicular Arthritis and Osteomyelitis due to Pseudomonas aeruginosa, Not Related to Drug Abuse. *Isr J Med Sci*, 1985;21:458–259.
256. Szilasy, J Age Determination of the Sternal Articular Faces of the Clavicula. *J Human Evol*, 1980;9:609–610.
257. Tabatai MF, Sapico FL, Canawati HN and Harley HAJ. Sternoclavicular Joint Infection With Group B Streptococcus (letter to the editor). *J Rheumatol*, 1986;13:466.
258. Tagliabue D, and Riva A. Le lussazioni sterno-claveari. *Minerva Orthop*, 1985;36:876–871
258a. Takimoto T, Ishikwaw S, Tanaka S, Masuda K and Umeda R. Development of Significant Sternoclavicular Joint Hypertrophy Following Radical Neck Dissection. *ORL*, 1989;51:317–320.
259. Teplick JG, Eftekhari F, Haskin ME. Erosion of the Sternal Ends of the Clavicles: A New Sign of Primary and Secondary Hyperparathyroidism. *Radiology*, 1974;113:323–326
259a. Thomas CB, and Friedman, RJ: Ipsilateral Sternoclavicular Dislocation and Calvicle Fracture: A Case Report *J Orthop Trauma*, 1989;3: 355–357.
259b. Tricoire, JL, Colombier, JA, Choiron, P, Puget, J, and Utheza, G: Retrosternal Dislocation of the Clavicle: A Report of Six Cases. *Fr J Orthop Surg*, 1990;1:107–112.
260. Turek, SL: Orthopaedics: Principles and Their Application, 2nd ed., pp. 568–570. Philadelphia, J.B. Lippincott, 1967.
261. Tyler HDD, Sturrock WDS and Callow FM. Retrosternal Dislocation of the Clavicle. *J Bone Joint Surg*, 1963;45B:132–137.
261a. Vierboom MAC, Steinberg JDJ, Mooyaart EL and Rijswijk MHV. Condensing Osteitis of the Clavicle: Magnetic Resonance Imaging as An Adjunct Method for Differential Diagnosis. *Ann Rheum Dis*, 1992; 51:539–541.
262. Waskowitz WJ. Disruption of the Sternoclavicular Joint: An Analysis and Review. *Am J Orthop*, 1961;3:176–179.
263. Wasylenk MJ and Busse EF. Posterior Dislocation of the Calvicle Causing Fatal Tracheoescophageal Fistula *Can J Surg*, 1981;24: 626–627.
264. Watson-Jones, R. Fractures and Joint Injuries, 4th ed., vol. 2, pp. 462–463, London, E. & S. Livingstone, 1956.
265. Watson-Jones, R. Fractures and Joint Injuries, 6th ed. New York, Churchill Livingstone, 1982.
266. Webb PA and Suchey JMM. Epiphyseal Union of the Anterior Iliac Crest and Medial Clavicle in a Modern Multiracial Sample of American Males and Females. *Am J Phy Anthrpol*, 1985;68:457–466.
267. Weiner SN, Levy M, Bernstein R and Morehouse H. Condensing Osteitis of the Clavicle: A Case Report. *J Bone Joint Surg*, 1984;66A: 1484–1486.
268. Weingarten M, Tash R, Klain RM and Kearns RJ. Posterior Dislocation of the Sternoclavicular Joint. *NY State J Med*, 1985;85(5): 225–226.
269. Wheeler ME, Laaveg SJ and Sprague BL. S-C Joint Disruptions in an Infant. *Clin Orthop*, 1979;139:68–69.
270. Williams HH. Oblique Views of the Clavicle. *Radiolog Clin Photog*, 1929;5:191–194.
271. Winter J, Sterner S, Maurer D, Varecka T and Zarzycki M. Retrosternal Epiphyseal Disruption of the Medial Clavicle: Case and Review in Children. *J Emerg Med*, 1989;7:9–13.
271a. Wirth MA and Rockwood CA. Chronic Conditions of the Acromioclavicular and Sternoclavicular Joints. In Chapman, MW (ed.): Operative Orthopaedics, part XI, 2nd ed., pp. 1683–1693. Philadelphia, J.B. Lippincott, 1992.
271b. Wirth MA and Rockwood CA. Complications Following Repair of the Sternoclavicular Joint. In Bigliani, LU (ed.): Complications of the Shoulder, pp. 139–153. Baltimore, Williams & Wilkins, 1993.
271c. Wirth MA and Rockwood CA. Complications of Treatment of Injuries to the Shoulder. In Epps, CH (ed.) Complications in Orthopaedic Surgery, 3rd ed., pp. 229–253. Philadelphia, J.B. Lippincott, 1994.
271d. Wirth MA, Jensen KL and Rockwood CA: The Treatment of Traumatic Posterior Sternoclavicular Joint Injuries. Presented at the Shoulder and Elbow Surgeons 12th Open Meeting, Atlanta, February, 25, 1996.
272. Wohlgethan JR, Newberg AH. Clinical Analysis of Infection of the Sternoclavicular Joint (abstract). *Clin Res*, 1984;32:666A
272a. Wohlgetan JR, Newberg AH and Reed JL. The Risk of Abscess from Sternoclavicular Septic Arthritis: A Case Report. *J Rheumatol*, 1988; 15(8):1302–1306.
273. Wolford LM and Smith BR. Sternoclavicular Grafts for Temporomandibular Joint Reconstruction (abstract). *J Oral Maxillofac Surg*, 52:119–128.
274. Worman LW and Leagus C. Intrathoracic Injury Following Retrosternal Dislocation of the Clavicle. *J Trauma*, 1967;7:416–423.
275. Worrell J and Fernandez GN. Retrosternal Dislocation of the Clavicle: An Important Injury Easily Missed. *Arch Emerg Med*, 1986;3: 133–135.
276. Yang, SO, Cho, KJ, Kim, MJ, and Ro, IW: Assessment of Anterior Shoulder Instability by CT Anthrography. *J Korean Med Sci*, 1987;2: 167–171.
277. Yood RA and Goldenberg DL. Sternoclavicular Joint Arthritis. *Arthritis Rheum*, 1980;23:232–239.
277a. Zaslav KR, Ray S, Neer CS. Conservative Management of a Displaced Medial Clavicular Physeal Injury in an Adolescent Athlete. *Am J Sports Med*, 1989;17(6):833–836.
278. Zucman J, Robinet L, and Aubart J. (Treatment of Sternal Dislocations of the Clavicle.) *Rev Chir Orthop*, 1978;64:35–44.

PART VIII

Neuromuscular Disorders and the Scapulothoracic Articulation

Disorders of the Shoulder: Diagnosis and Management,
edited by Joseph P. Iannotti and Gerald R. Williams, Jr.
Lippincott Williams & Wilkins, Philadelphia © 1999.

CHAPTER 29

The Scapulothoracic Articulation: Anatomy, Biomechanics, Pathophysiology, and Management

John E. Kuhn

INTRODUCTION

The scapulothoracic articulation is a critical component of shoulder function; yet this region, and the disorders that affect it, have received far less attention in the medical literature than the glenohumeral joint. Disorders of the scapulothoracic articulation are frequently misunderstood and misdiagnosed. An appreciation of the anatomy of this region helps understand the pathologic conditions that may affect the scapulothoracic articulation (Fig. 1).

Surgical Anatomy and Biomechanics of the Normal Scapulothoracic Articulation

The scapula is a thin bone that serves as a site of muscle attachment for the upper extremity and the thorax. Seventeen muscles have their origin or insertion on the scapula (Table 1; Fig. 2) making it the essential link for coordinated upper extremity activity. These muscles can be divided into three major groups.

J. E. Kuhn: Department of Orthopaedic Surgery, The University of Michigan and The University of Michigan Shoulder Group, Ann Arbor, Michigan 48106-0363.

The scapulothoracic muscles coordinate scapulothoracic motion and include the rhomboideus major and minor, the levator scapulae, the serratus anterior, the trapezius, the omohyoid, and the pectoralis minor. Disorders of these muscles may manifest as scapular winging, or scapulothoracic dyskinesia. The rotator cuff muscles control activities of the glenohumeral articulation and include the supraspinatus, infraspinatus, subscapularis, and teres minor. Disorders of these muscles are common and are covered in other sections of this text. The scapulohumeral muscles provide power to the humerus and include the deltoid, the long head of the biceps, the short head of the biceps, the coracobrachialis, the long head of the triceps, and the teres major. Motion of the upper extremity occurs as a result of the coordinated activity of all of these muscles.

While at rest, the scapula is anteriorly rotated relative to the trunk approximately 30 degrees.[95,163] The medial border of the scapula is also rotated with the inferior pole diverging away from the spine approximately 3 degrees. The scapula is also tilted forward about 20 degrees in the sagittal plane when viewed from the side[95] (Fig. 3). It is thought by some that deviations in this normal alignment may contribute to glenohumeral instability.

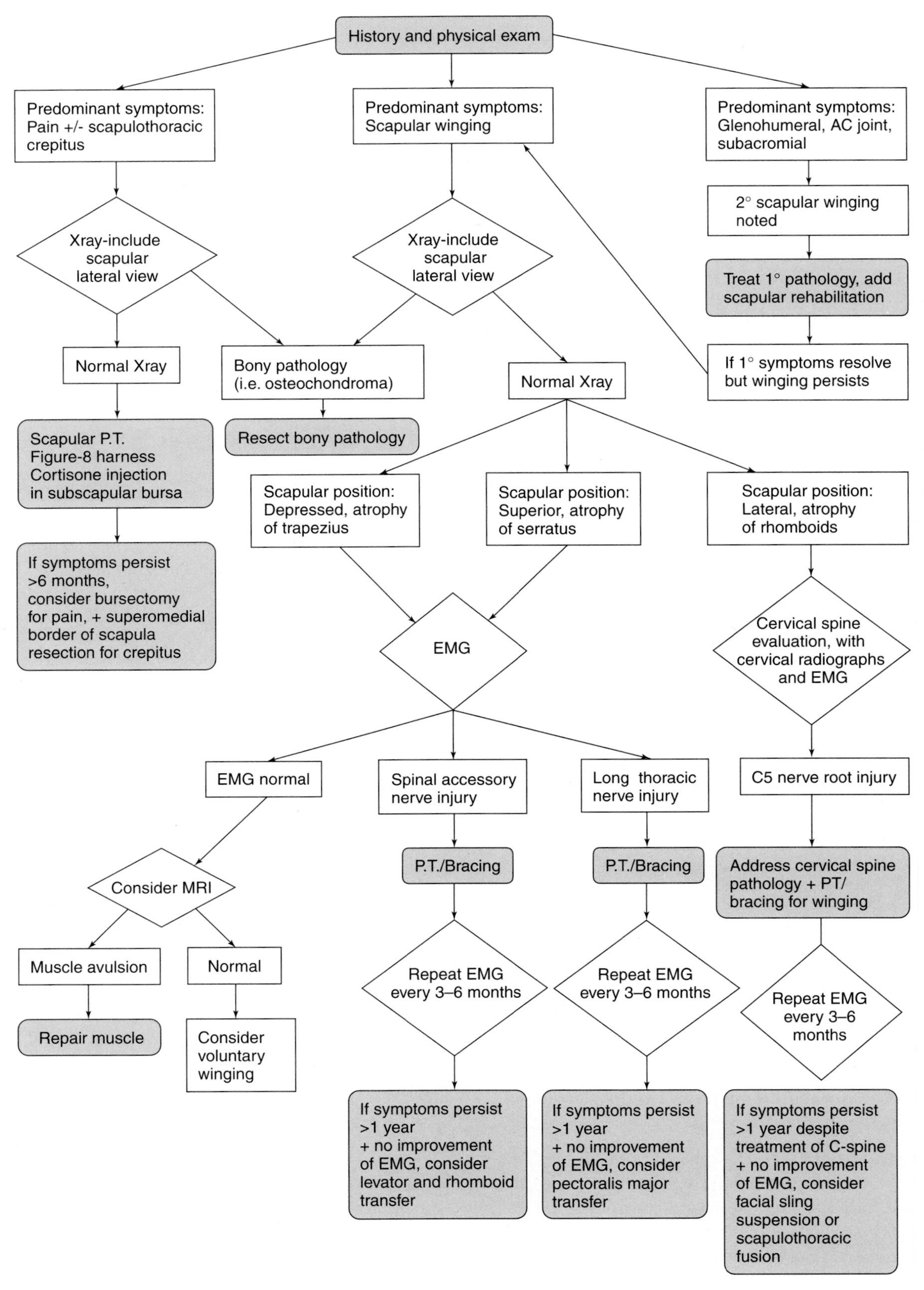

FIG. 1. An algorithm for the evaluation and treatment of scapulothoracic disorders.

TABLE 1. *Muscles of the scapula*[a]

Scapulohumeral muscles
Long head of biceps
Short head of biceps
Deltoid
Coracobrachialis
Teres major
Long head of triceps
Scapulothoracic muscles
Levator scapulae
Omohyoid
Rhomboid major
Rhomboid minor
Serratus anterior
Trapezius
Pectoralis minor
Rotator cuff muscles
Supraspinatus
Infraspinatus
Subscapularis
Teres minor

[a] Seventeen muscles attach the scapula to the neck, thorax, and humerus making it the control tower for coordinated upper extremity activity. Figure 2. displays the location of the attachments of the various muscles.

Almost every functional upper extremity movement has components of scapulothoracic and glenohumeral motion. Arm elevation has been studied extensively with efforts directed toward determining the relative contributions of scapulothoracic and scapulohumeral motion with varied and conflicting results. In general, in the first 30 degrees of elevation, most of the motion occurs at the glenohumeral joint, although this varies between individuals.[6,31,46,174] The next 60 degrees of elevation is accomplished by equal parts of scapulothoracic and glenohumeral motion. The overall effort to obtain 90 degrees of elevation requires approximately a 2:1 ratio of glenohumeral to scapulothoracic motion. During arm elevation in the scapular plane, the instant center of rotation of the scapula moves, such that from zero to 30 degrees the scapula rotates about its midportion, and from 60 degrees or more, the rotation occurs near the glenoid, resulting in a medial and upward displacement of the inferior pole of the scapula. In addition, with arm elevation, the coracoid moves superiorly, and the acromion moves superiorly, to open the impingement zone (Fig. 4).

Muscle Function about the Scapula

Cranial elevation of the scapula is accomplished by activating the upper portion of the trapezius as it inserts into the lateral spine of the scapula, acromion, and distal clavicle. This is countered by the effects of gravity and by the latissimus dorsi, which acts as the primary scapular depressor, with the lower portion of the serratus anterior, pectoralis minor, and the lower portion of the trapezius contributing.

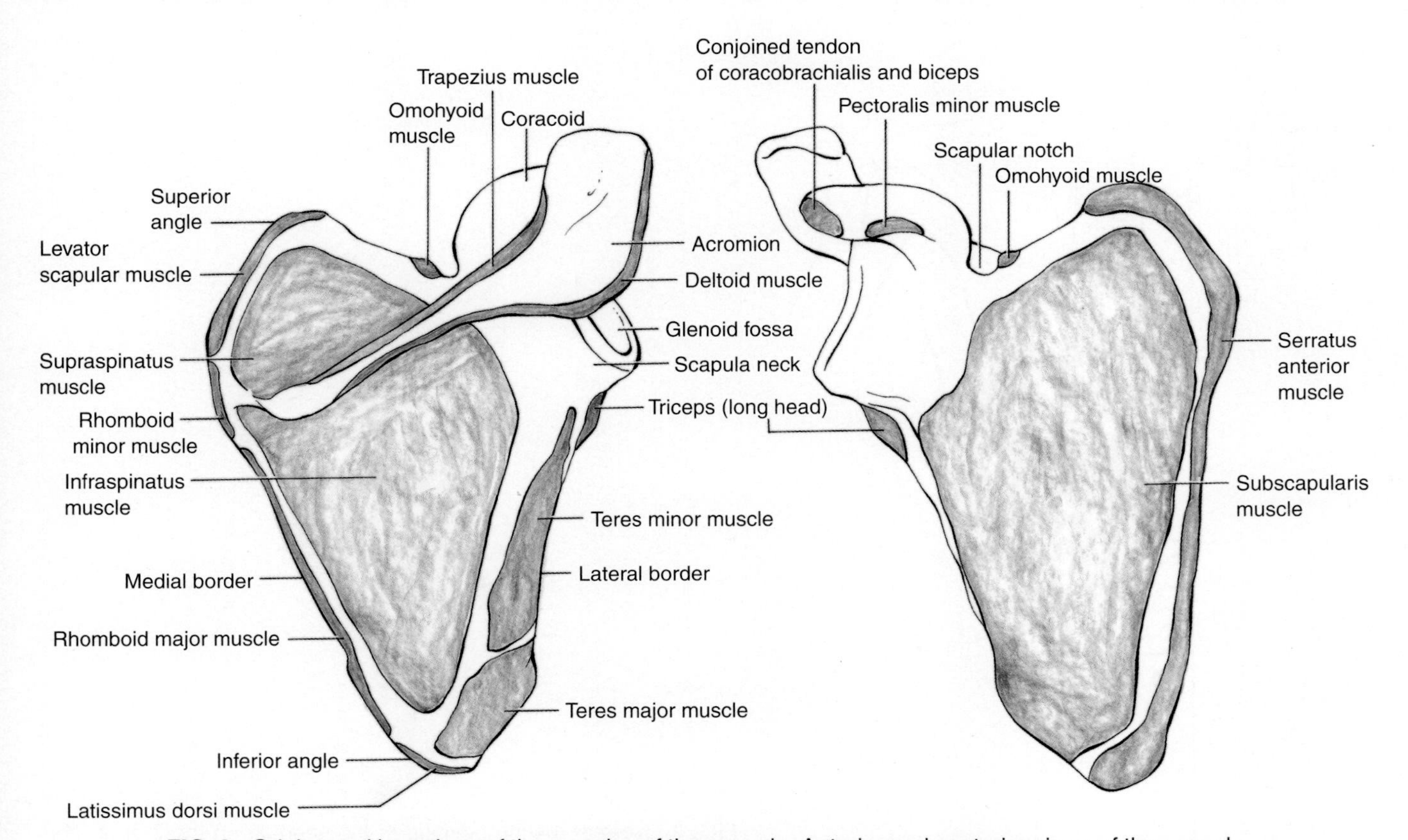

FIG. 2. Origins and insertions of the muscles of the scapula. Anterior and posterior views of the scapula demonstrate the multiple attachment sites for muscles of the scapula, making it the center for coordinated upper extremity motion.

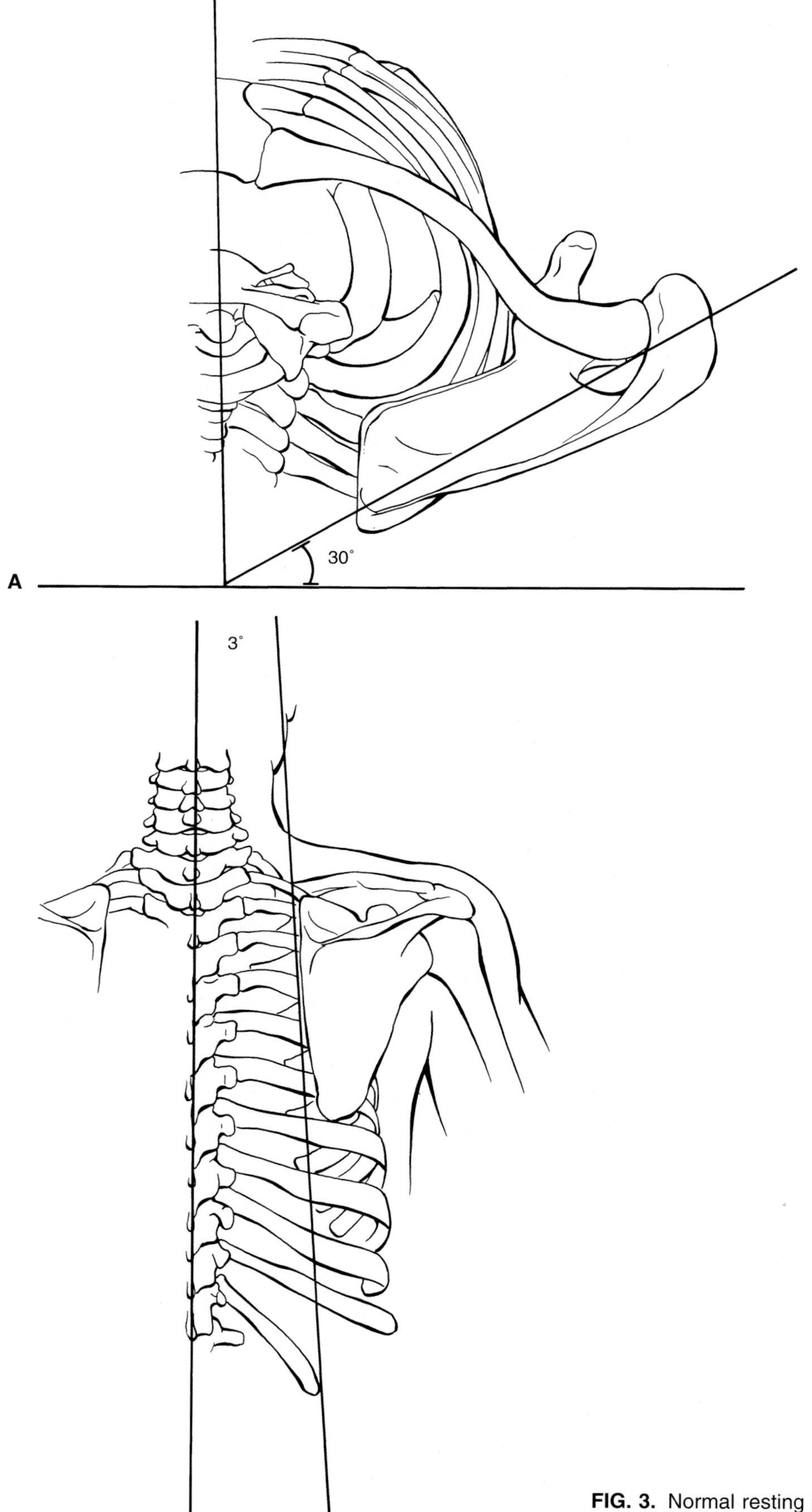

FIG. 3. Normal resting position of the scapula on the thorax. The resting scapula is 30 degrees anterior to the coronal plane, with the medial border rotated 3 degrees from the spine.

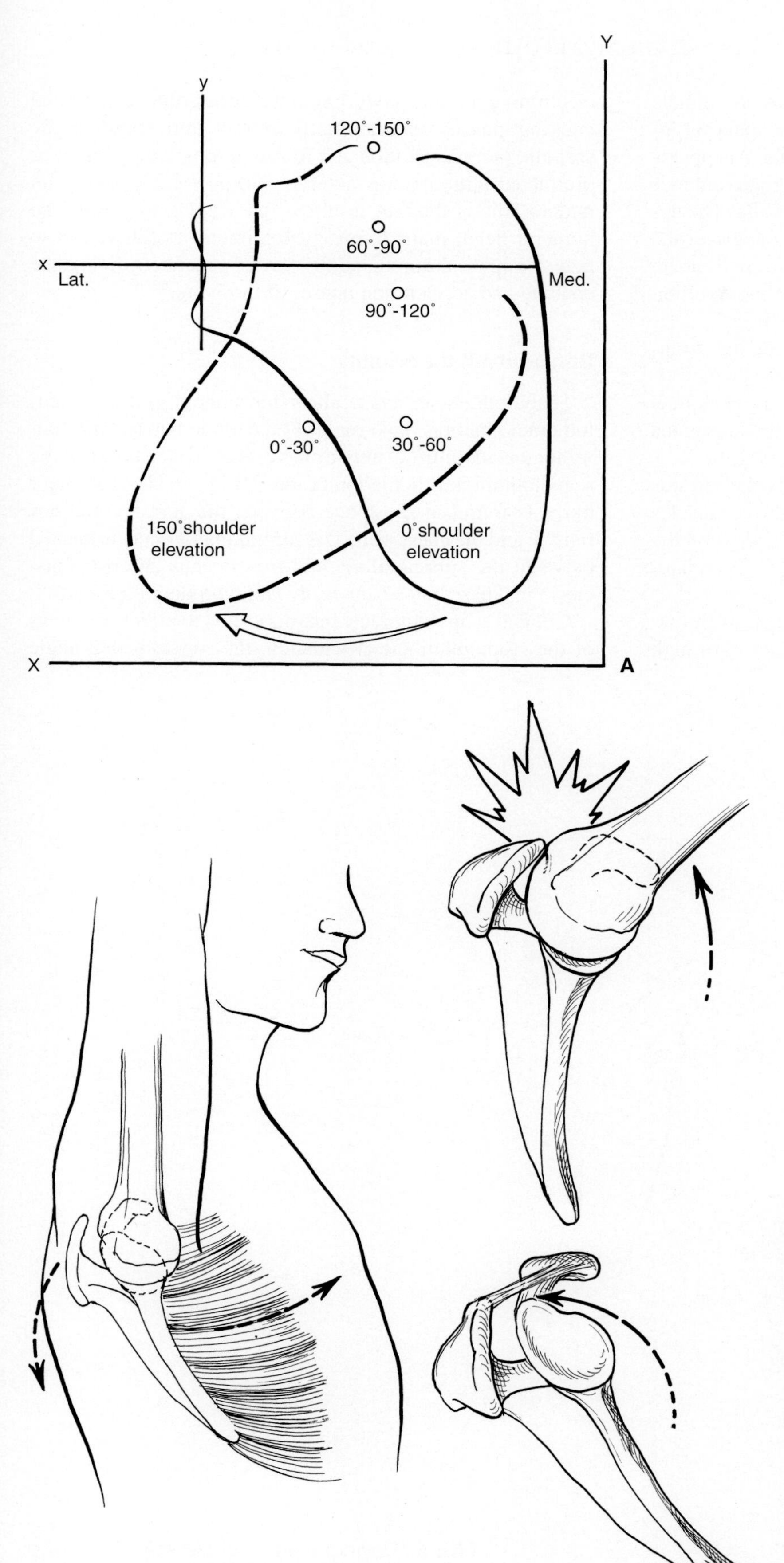

FIG. 4. Changes in the center of rotation of the scapula with arm elevations. **(A)** demonstrates that the center of rotation moves superiorly during arm elevaton, resulting in upward and medial displacement of the glenoid face, with lateral displacement of the inferior angle. (From Poppen NK, Walker PS. Normal and abnormal motion of the shoulder. *J Bone Joint Surg {Am}* 1976;58:195–201.); **(B)** The scapula rotates with arm elevation, clearing the acromion away from the impingement zone. (From Kuhn JE, Hawkins RJ. Evaluation and treatment of scapular disorders. In: Warner JP, Iannotti JP, Gerber C, eds. *Complex and revision problems in shoulder surgery*. Philadelphia: Lippincott-Raven, 1997;357–375).

Rotation of the scapula upward is initiated by the middle portion of the trapezius, which stabilizes the scapula by inserting on the medial border of the scapular spine. At approximately 45 degrees of scapular abduction, the serratus anterior acts to pull the inferior angle of the scapula laterally. The upper portion of the trapezius elevates the lateral angle of the scapula, whereas the lower portion of the trapezius pulls down on the scapula through its insertion on the medial-most portion of the scapular spine, inducing upward rotation (Fig. 5).

The downward rotators of the scapula include the rhomboideus major and minor, and the levator scapulae, which elevate the medial border of the scapula, whereas the pectoralis minor, lower portion of pectoralis major, and the latissimus dorsi depress the lateral portion of the scapula (Fig. 6).

Protraction of the scapula is accomplished by the serratus anterior and pectoralis minor and major as these muscles move the scapula lateral and forward. Retraction of the scapula relies on the middle trapezius, rhomboideus major and minor (Fig. 7).

During high-intensity shoulder activities, such as throwing, the trapezius, rhomboideus major and minor have high electromyographic (EMG) activity during the windup and cocking phases to maximally retract and stabilize the scapula. For acceleration and follow-through, the scapula is protracted with serratus anterior and pectoralis minor and major. This is thought to allow the scapula to follow the humeral head, maintaining glenohumeral stability, and to help dissipate the tremendous forces generated during the cocking and acceleration phases of throwing.[49,86]

Bursae about the Scapula

Scapulothoracic bursae allow for smooth gliding scapulothoracic motion. Two major or anatomic bursae, and four minor or adventitial bursae have been described for the scapulothoracic articulation (Table 2; Fig. 8). The first major bursa is found in the space between the serratus anterior muscle and the chest wall. The second major bursa is located between the subscapularis and the serratus anterior muscles.[18,90] These bursae are easily and reproducibly found.[90]

Clinical scapulothoracic bursitis seems to affect two areas of the scapulothoracic articulation, the superomedial angle

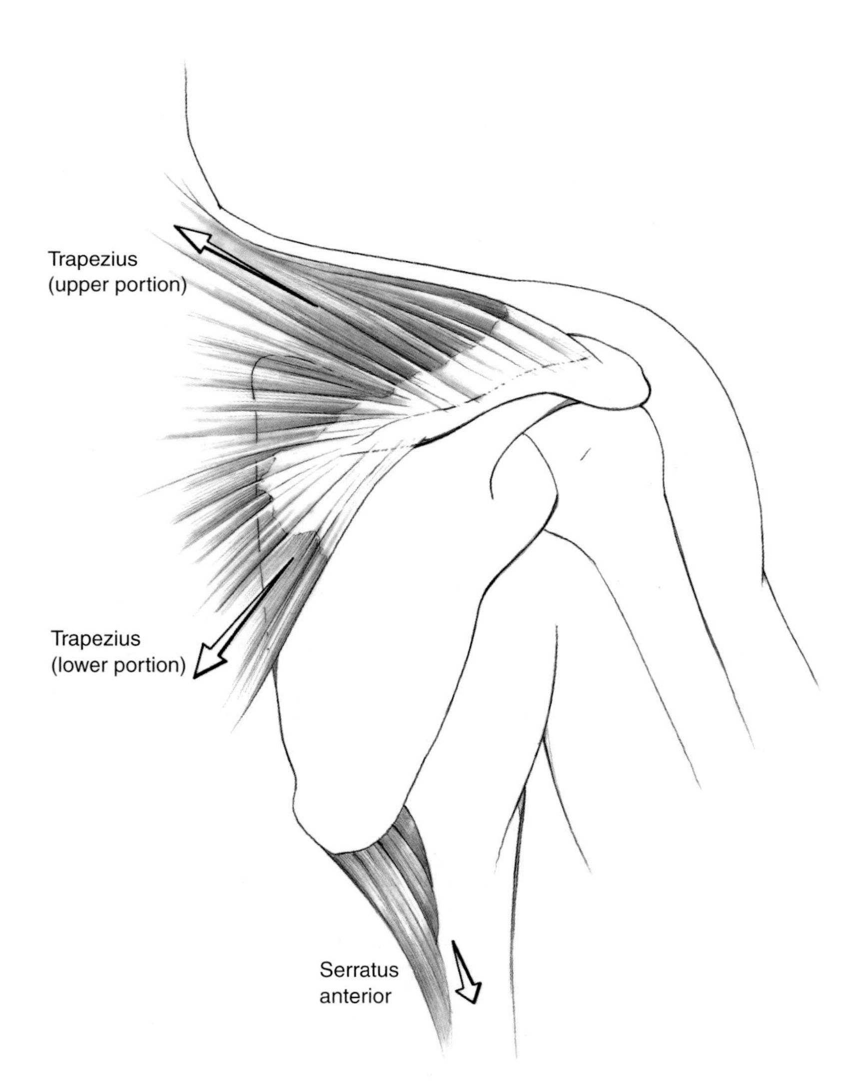

FIG. 5. Upward rotation of the scapula. As the middle trapezius stabilizes the scapula, the serratus pulls the anterior angle and the upper trapezius elevates the lateral angle.

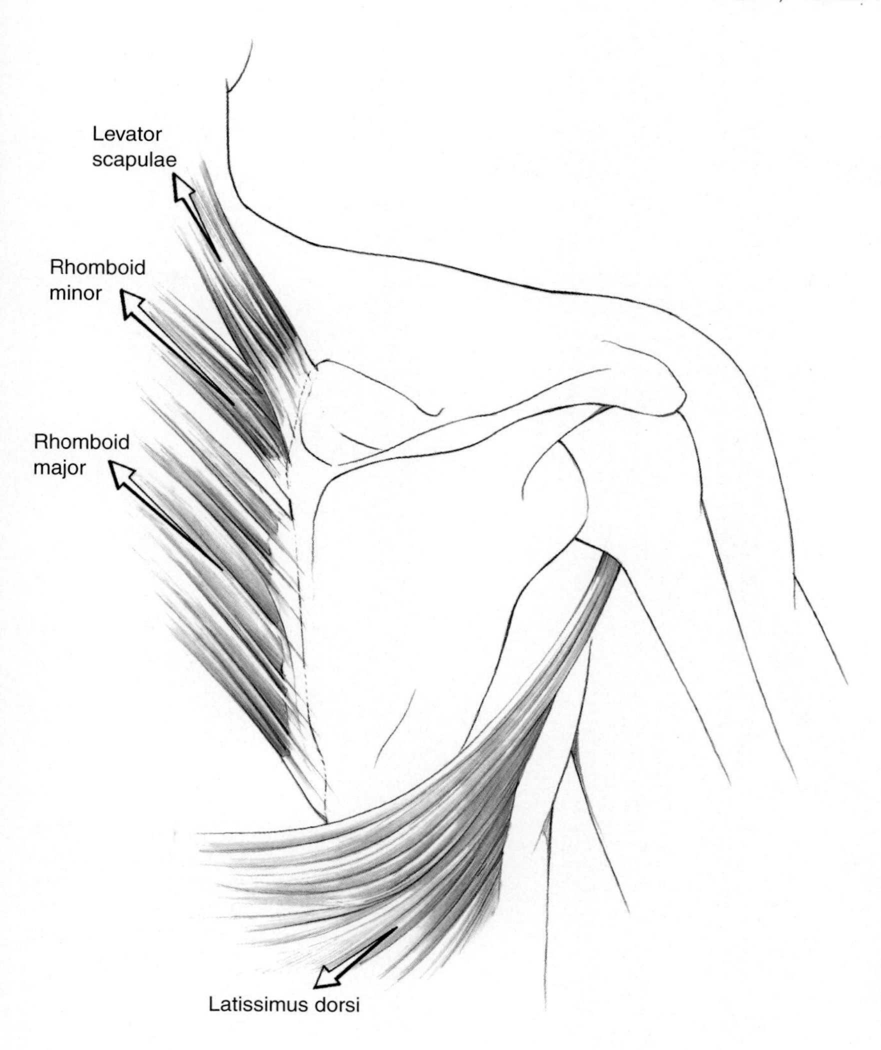

FIG. 6. Downward rotation of the scapula. The rhomboidei and levator scapulae elevate the medial border of the scapula, whereas pectoralis minor, lower pectoralis major, and latissimus dorsi depress the lateral portion of the scapula. (From ref. 107, with permission).

and the inferior angle of the scapula. When symptomatic, these areas tend to develop inflamed bursae; however, these bursae are not reliably found, and in fact, may be adventitious.[19,90,126] For inferior angle of the scapula, most authors agree that the affected bursa lies between the serratus anterior muscle and the chest wall.[20,112,153] This bursa has been given many names, including the infraserratus bursa[20] and the bursa mucosa serrata.[153,172] The second site of pathology lies at the superomedial angle of the scapula. Here, Codman[20] believed this bursa is also an infraserratus bursa, lying between the upper and anterior portion of the scapula and the back of the first three ribs. Von Gruber,[172] on the other hand, identified a bursa in this region between the subscapularis and the serratus anticus muscles, which he called the bursa mucosa angulae superioris scapulae.

A third minor or adventitial bursa, which Codman believed was the site of painful crepitus in scapulothoracic crepitus, was called the trapezoid bursa, and is found over the triangular surface at the medial base of the spine of the scapula under the trapezius muscle.[20] Some believe that these minor bursae are adventitial and develop in response to abnormal pathomechanics of the scapulothoracic articulation.[19,90,126] It would not be surprising, then, to find these bursae inconsistently or in different soft-tissue planes.

WINGING OF THE SCAPULA

Scapular winging is one of the most common abnormalities of the scapulothoracic articulation, and results from a variety of causes. Winging may be described as primary, secondary, or voluntary (Table 3). Primary scapular winging results from identifiable anatomic disorders that directly affect the scapulothoracic articulation. Secondary scapular winging usually is associated with some form of glenohumeral pathology. This type of winging will resolve as the glenohumeral pathology is addressed. Voluntary winging, which is quite rare, may have an underlying psychologic cause.

Primary Scapular Winging: Neurologic Disorders

The more common causes of primary scapular winging are attributable to neurologic disorders and include: damage to the fifth cervical nerve root, causing rhomboideus palsy; damage to the long thoracic nerve, causing serratus anterior

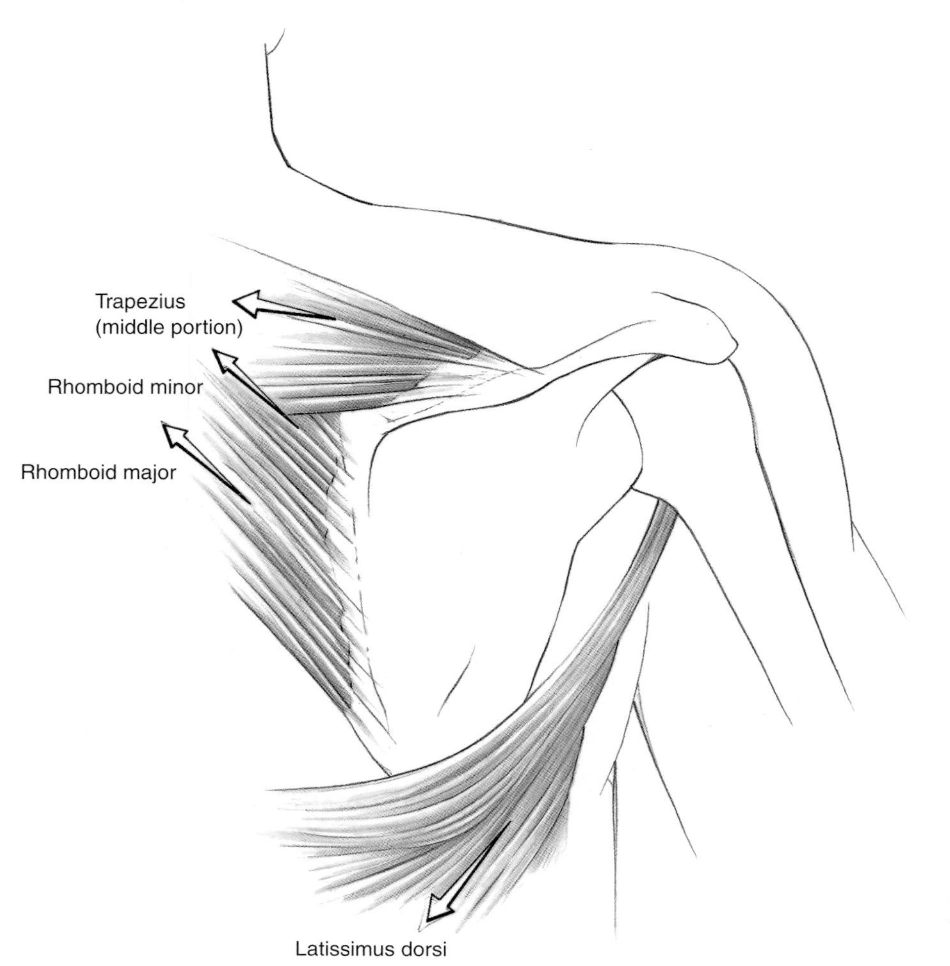

FIG. 7. Retraction of the scapula. The middle portion of the trapezius and the rhomboidei serve to counter the effect of the serratus and pectoralis and retract the scapula toward the spine. (From ref. 107, with permission).

TABLE 2. *Bursae of the scapula*[a]

Bursae of the scapula
Major/anatomic bursae
Infraserratus bursae: between the serratus anterior and chest wall
Supraserratus bursae: between the subscapularis and serratus anterior muscles
Minor/adventitial bursae
Superomedial angle of the scapula
Infraserratus bursae: between serratus anterior and chest wall
Supraserratus bursae: between supscapularis and serratus anterior
Inferior angle of the scapula
Infraserratus bursae: between serratus anterior and chest wall
Spine of scapula
Trapezoid bursae: between medial spine of scapula and trapezius

[a] The scapulothoracic articulation is associated with a number of bursae, many of which can become pathologic, causing symptomatic scapulothoracic bursitis. (From Kuhn JE, Hawkins RJ. Evaluation and treatment of scapular disorders. In: Warner JJP, Iannotti JP, Gerber C. eds. *Complex and revision problems in shoulder surgery.* Philadelphia: Lippincott–Raven Publishers, 1997:357–375.)

palsy; and damage to the spinal accessory nerve, causing trapezius palsy. Primary scapular winging may also be bony in origin, or may be due to scapulothoracic bursitis, or to disorders in periscapular musculature.

Rhomboideus Major and Minor Palsy

Pathophysiology

Weakness of the rhomboid major and rhomboid minor muscles is a rarely identified cause of scapular winging. These muscles receive innervation from the dorsal scapular nerve, which takes its origin from the C-5 nerve root. The dorsal scapular nerve passes deep to, or through the levator scapulae on its way to the rhomboids. Scapulothoracic winging may result from a C-5 radiculopathy or an injury to the dorsal scapular nerve.[142]

Evaluation

Patients with rhomboid weakness may complain of pain along the medial border of the scapula. The winging produced by rhomboideus palsy at rest is usually minimal, but

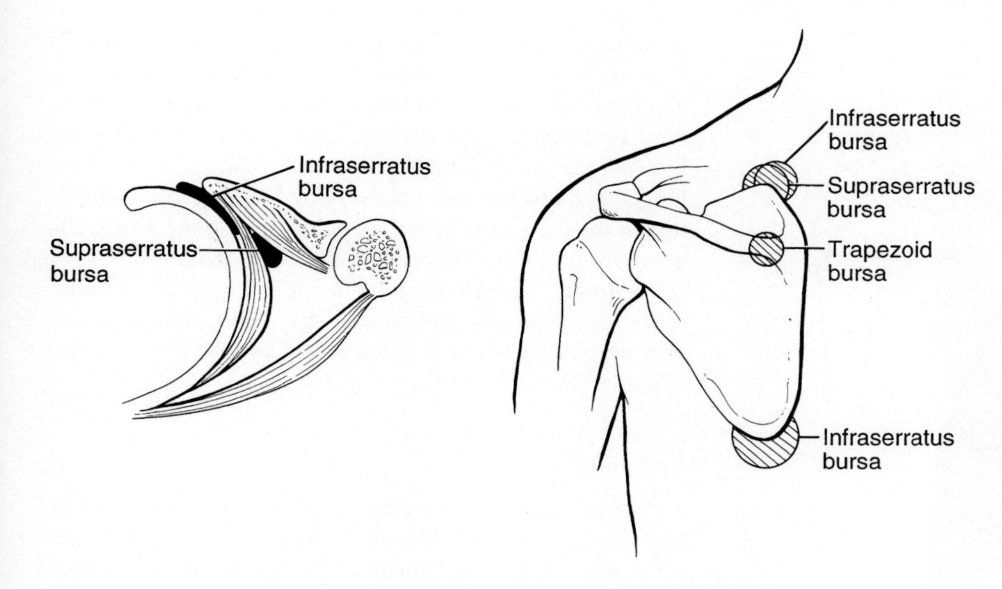

FIG. 8. Bursae of the scapula. The location of both anatomic (black) and adventitial (hatched) bursae are displayed. (From Kuhn JE, Hawkins RJ. Evaluation and treatment of scapular disorders. In: Warner JP, Iannotti JP, Gerber C, eds. *Complex and revision problems in shoulder surgery.* Philadelphia: Lippincott-Raven, 1997: 357–375.)

may appear similar to trapezius winging with the shoulder slightly depressed, the scapula laterally translated, and the inferior angle rotated laterally. In addition, atrophy along the medial border of the scapula may be evident. During arm elevation, the inferior angle of the scapula is pulled laterally and downward by the unopposed serratus anterior muscle.[27] With rhomboid weakness, the winging is accentuated by slowly lowering the arm from the forward elevated position, during which time the inferior angle of the scapula is pulled laterally and dorsally.[142] Patients will have difficulty pushing the elbows backward against resistance with the hands on the hips.[63] Electromyography and nerve conduction studies will help differentiate this type of winging from winging caused by other neurologic injury.

TABLE 3. *Winging of the scapula*[a]

I. Primary scapular winging
   A. Neurologic
      1. Long thoracic nerve: serratus anterior palsy
      2. Spinal accessory nerve: trapezius palsy
      3. Dorsal scapular nerve: rhomboideus palsy
   B. Bony
      1. Osteochondromas
      2. Fracture malunions
   C. Soft tissure
      1. Contractural winging
      2. Muscle avulsion/muscle agenesis
      3. Scapulothoracic bursitis
II. Secondary scapular winging
III. Voluntary scapular winging

[a] Primary scapular winging results from anatomic disorders of the scapulothoracic articulation. Secondary scapular winging results from glenohumeral or subacromial pathology. Voluntary scapular winging is not pathologic and may have psychologic overtones. (From Kuhn JE, Hawkins RJ. Evaluation and treatment of scapular disorders. In: Warner JJP, Iannotti JP, Gerber C. eds. *Complex and revision problems in shoulder surgery.* Philadelphia: Lippincott–Raven Publishers, 1997:357–375.)

Treatment

In patients with C-5 radiculopathies, addressing the source of the radiculopathy may provide some benefit. In general, the treatment of rhomboideus winging consists of trapezius-strengthening exercises. The patient who has significant symptoms and fails nonoperative treatment may be helped by a fascial sling operation, as described by Dickson.[27,29] In this operation, two fascia lata grafts are tubularized and used to connect the lower vertebral border of the scapula to the spinal muscles and the inferior angle of the scapula to the fibers of the latissimus dorsi. This procedure is thought to be useful in stabilizing the scapula and partially arresting the high thoracic scoliosis that may occur with rhomboid and levator scapulae paralysis.[27] There is some concern that fascial sling suspensions may elongate and fail in time.[72]

Serratus Anterior Palsy

Pathophysiology

Palsy of the serratus anterior muscle can also cause painful, disabling winging. The long thoracic nerve, which powers the serratus anterior muscle, originates from the ventral rami of the C-5, C-6, and C-7 cervical nerves and travels beneath the brachial plexus and clavicle and over the first rib. It then travels superficially along the lateral aspect of the chest wall, which makes the nerve susceptible to injury (Fig. 9). Blunt trauma or stretching of this nerve is particularly common in athletics and has been observed in tennis players, golfers, swimmers, gymnasts, soccer players, bowlers, weight lifters, ice hockey players, wrestlers, archers, basketball players, and football players.[41,55,96,170] Repetitive industrial use of the shoulder has also been implicated as a cause of serratus paralysis.[122,154] Penetrating trauma will rarely cause injury to this nerve; yet surgical procedures, such as radical mastectomy, first rib resection, and transaxillary sympathectomy, have all been identified

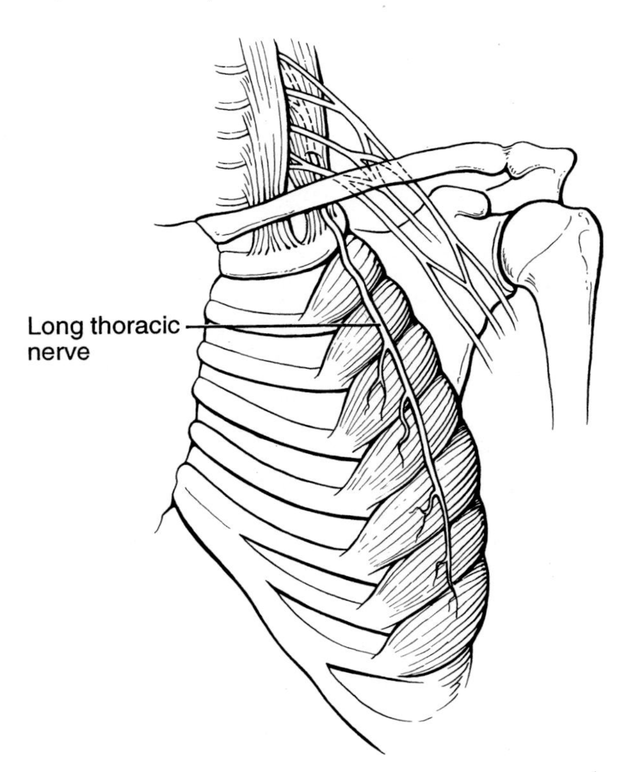

FIG. 9. Location of the long thoracic nerve. Its superficial location along the chest wall makes it susceptible to injury. (From Kuhn JE, Hawkins RJ. Evaluation and treatment of scapular disorders. In: Warner JP, Iannotti JP, Gerber C, eds. *Complex and revision problems in shoulder surgery.* Philadelphia: Lippincott-Raven, 1997:357–375).

as potential sources of injury to the long thoracic nerve.[96] This nerve can also be affected by nontraumatic events, including positioning during anesthesia,[122,154] the sequelae of viral illness,[38,133] inoculations,[4] and neuritis affecting the brachial plexus or long thoracic nerve alone.[75,76,124] Prolonged bed rest has also been reported to trigger a dysfunction of the long thoracic nerve, particularly if the arm is abducted, propping up the head to read.[98,122,131,132] Interestingly, because the long thoracic nerve has a significant C-7 component, patients with a C-7 radiculopathy may also present with serratus anterior weakness and scapular winging.[102]

Evaluation

Patients with serratus anterior palsies will complain of pain as the other periscapular muscles try to compensate. More severe pain may indicate an acute brachial plexus neuritis,[127] or Parsonage-Turner syndrome that may affect only the long thoracic nerve.[124] With an injury to the long thoracic nerve and dysfunction of the serratus anterior muscle, the scapula assumes a position of superior elevation, medial translation, and the inferior pole is rotated medially (Fig. 10). The patient will have difficulty with arm elevation above 120 degrees, which will magnify the degree of winging.[44,81] Pain may be increased with this maneuver and when the head is tilted toward the contralateral side.[127]

Electromyography is recommended to confirm the diagnosis and follow the recovery of the injured long thoracic

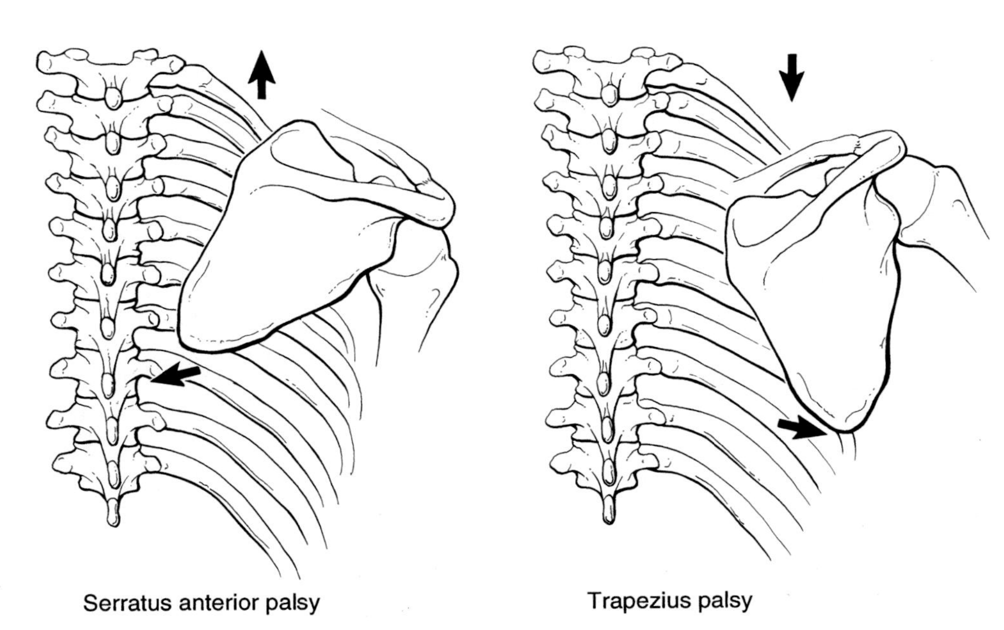

FIG. 10. Resting location of the scapula with palsy of the serratus anterior, and trapezius palsy. The unopposed muscles cause the scapula to drift into a typical position. (From Kuhn JE, Hawkins RJ. Evaluation and treatment of scapular disorders. In: Warner JP, Iannotti JP, Gerber C, eds. *Complex and revision problems in shoulder surgery.* Philadelphia: Lippincott-Raven, 1997:357–375).

nerve. When requesting an electromyographic analysis, it is important to specify an evaluation of the long thoracic nerve and serratus anterior muscle. Because most long thoracic nerve palsies will recover spontaneously, regular electromyographic examinations at 1- to 3-month intervals have been recommended to follow nerve recovery.[77,98]

Treatment

Nonoperative treatment should be implemented immediately at diagnosis and should include range of motion exercises to prevent glenohumeral stiffness. Many types of braces and orthotics have been developed, but their use is controversial.[77,107] In general, these braces attempt to hold the scapula against the chest wall, and may have some role if their cumbersome nature is overshadowed by their symptom relief.[45,81,98,180] Some have recommended bracing to limit continued traction on the nerve, in hopes of accelerating nerve regeneration. Most long thoracic nerve injuries recover spontaneously within 1 year,[7,33,40,44,45,53,55,62,75,78,81,98,122,131,132] although maximal recovery may take up to 2 years.[44,51,97]

There are scant data in the literature on the results of neurolysis, nerve grafting, or repair of an injured long thoracic nerve.[154] Nevertheless, penetrating injuries should undergo nerve exploration and early repair. Neurorrhaphy may be indicated in circumstances when the lesion can be localized.[98]

Many patients with persistent impairment of the serratus anterior are able to compensate and would not elect to have a surgical reconstruction.[98] In patients with symptomatic serratus winging that persists more than 1 year, surgical intervention may alleviate pain and improve function. Historically, the operations for serratus paralysis can be classified into three types: scapulothoracic fusions;[64] fascial sling suspensions;[29,168,177] and muscle transfers, which have utilized pectoralis minor,[17,76,134] pectoralis major,[145] the sternocostal head of pectoralis major,[103,169] the clavicular head of pectoralis major,[35] teres major,[61] the rhomboideus muscles,[67] and combinations.[161,187]

Scapulothoracic fusions as a first operation for serratus winging have been discouraged by some,[75] primarily for their inherent loss of motion. Pain relief, however, is a reasonable expectation.[64] Complications of scapulothoracic fusions are many and include nonunions and pneumothorax.[64] For these reasons, and the limited expectations for motion, scapulothoracic fusions have been generally reserved for salvage operations after failure of other techniques, or for patients with paralysis of other shoulder girdle muscles in addition to the serratus anterior.[77] Another possible indication for primary scapulothoracic fusion for serratus winging is in the laborer who places heavy demand on the shoulder.[97]

Fascial sling suspensions have had their proponents as well;[27,29,130,168,177] however, significant concern exists for potential fascial sling failure and recurrence of winging.[72]

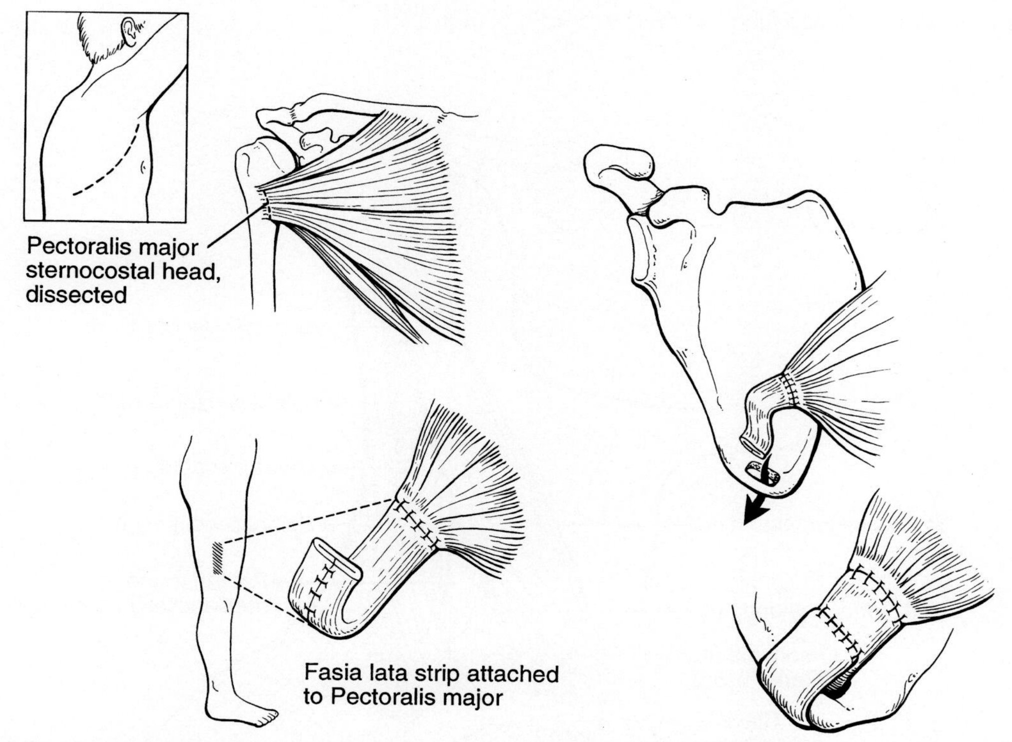

FIG. 11. Pectoralis major transfer for scapular winging. As described by Marmor and Bechtol, [103] the sternocostal head of the pectoralis major is sutured to a tubularized fascia lata graft and woven through a foramen made in the inferior angle of the scapula. (From Kuhn JE, Hawkins RJ. Evaluation and treatment of scapular disorders. In: Warner JP, Iannotti JP, Gerber C, eds. *Complex and revision problems in shoulder surgery.* Philadelphia: Lippincott-Raven, 1997:357–375).

Consequently, muscle transfers for dynamic scapular stabilization have gained wide acceptance. Although a variety of muscle transfers have been described, transferring the sternocostal head of the pectoralis major with a fascia lata graft extension[103] has become the most popular.[40,50,53,77,98,107,119,129] (Fig. 11)

In this technique,[53,103,107,129] the patient is placed in the lateral decubitus position, using a bean bag, and the involved arm and forequarter are prepared and draped. An incision is made crossing the axilla from the pectoralis major muscle anteriorly to the inferior tip of the scapula. Alternatively, two incisions can be used, with the pectoralis tendon and graft tunneled along the chest wall subcutaneously. The sternocostal head of the pectoralis major is released from its insertion on the bicipital groove of the humerus. A graft of fascia lata measuring 7 by 2 in. (18 by 5 cm) is harvested from the ipsilateral leg and sutured into a tube, 7 in. (18 cm) long. This graft is then sutured to the distal portion of the freed pectoralis tendon. After the inferior border of the scapula has been exposed, a foramen is made in the inferior angle. The graft is inserted through this defect and sutured to itself under moderate tension. It is important to position the graft such that the end of the pectoralis tendon meets the scapula, and the fascia lata graft is used as augmentation.

The wounds are closed in layers. Postoperatively, the arm is placed in a sling for comfort. Early passive motion is started immediately. Active motion is begun at 6 weeks and strengthening at 12 weeks. Although there are few large series in the literature, results using this technique have been encouraging with 70% to 91% success rates as determined by normal shoulder motion and a significant reduction in pain and winging.[53,77,96]

Surgical complications of this surgical procedure are few, but include pneumothorax, and postoperative chest radiographs should always be taken. Late complications include fracture of the inferior border of the scapula, or failure of the graft, both of which will manifest as a recurrence of winging.[129] Management of severe complications can be treated with a scapulothoracic fusion.

Trapezius Winging

Pathophysiology

The spinal accessory nerve is the only nerve supplying the vast trapezius muscle.[70,137,166] The spinal accessory nerve is superficial, lying in the subcutaneous tissue on the floor of the posterior cervical triangle. Its superficial location makes it susceptible to injury.[82,83](Fig. 12) Injury to this nerve causes significant deformity, as well as painfully disabling alterations in scapulothoracic function.[28,34,69,82,83,94,121,166, 183,185,186] This nerve can be injured in a variety of ways including blunt trauma,[8,68,186] stretching of the nerve,[186] penetrating trauma (which includes surgical biopsy of lymph nodes in the posterior cervical triangle[34,121,185,186]), and radical neck dissection.[10,137,155]

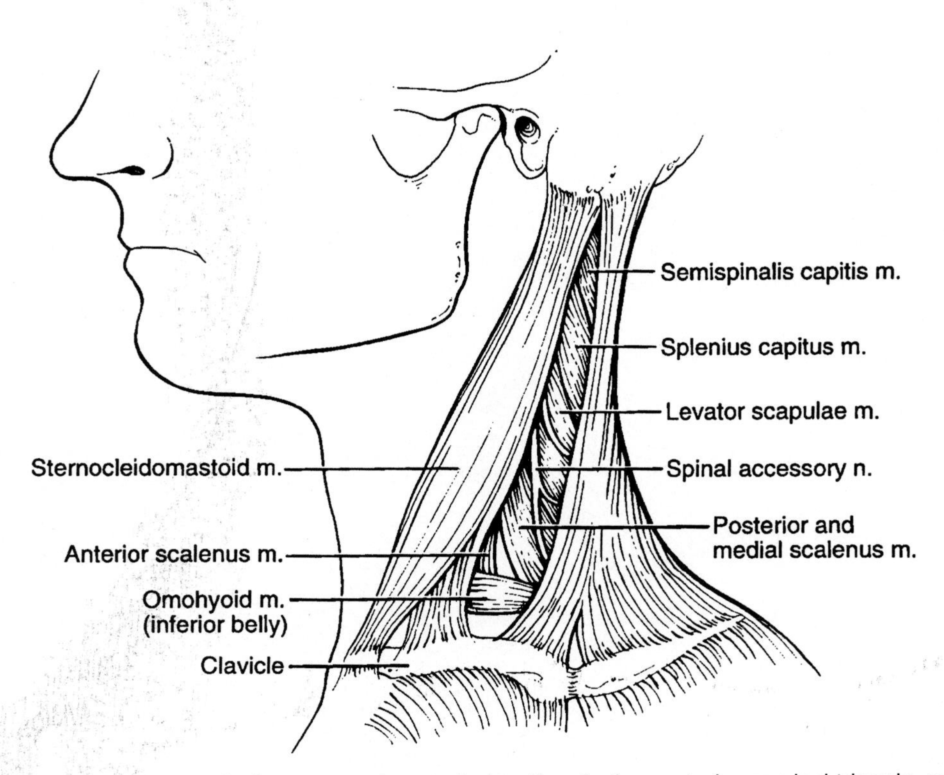

FIG. 12. Location of the spinal accessory nerve. Its location, in the posterior cervical triangle, makes it susceptible to injury during surgical procedures in this area.

Evaluation

Patients will attempt to compensate for a palsy of the trapezius by straining other muscles of the shoulder girdle including the levator scapulae and the rhomboid muscles. This strain may lead to pain and muscle spasm that can be disabling.[8] Patients can also develop pain from adhesive capsulitis, shoulder subacromial impingement, and radiculitis from traction on the brachial plexus as the shoulder girdle droops.

Upon examination, patients will have difficulty when attempting to shrug their shoulder, and will have weakness in forward elevation and abduction of the arm. The patient will assume a position with the shoulder depressed and the scapula translated laterally with the inferior angle rotated laterally (see Fig. 10). The diagnosis is confirmed by electromyography. It is important to specify an examination of the trapezius and spinal accessory nerve on the requisition, as these areas may not be routinely evaluated in a diagnostic evaluation of the shoulder.

Treatment

Treatment considerations for patients with trapezius winging depend on the duration and severity of symptoms. The initial treatment is nonoperative. The arm can be placed in a sling to rest the other periscapular muscles. Physical therapy is helpful to maintain glenohumeral motion, preventing adhesive capsulitis.[127] In cases caused by blunt trauma, serial electromyographic analysis should be performed at 4- to 6-week intervals to follow the returning function of the nerve. In cases that are due to penetrating trauma, or when there is no evidence of nerve function on electromyographic analysis, neurolysis or nerve grafting, or a combination, can be performed.[1,34,60,120,183] The results of these procedures have been variable; however, the success rate seems to be improved if the neurolysis is performed before 6 months.[8]

Patients who have had symptoms in excess of 1 year are unlikely to benefit from continued nonoperative treatment,[121,166] and surgery can be offered. Historically, a variety of procedures have been described for the treatment of trapezius winging.[28,64,72,85] These can be divided into static stabilization, including scapulothoracic fusion[64] and any of the many described operations that tether the scapula to the thoracic spine;[28,85] or dynamic stabilization that involves muscle transfers.[72]

The Dewar-Harris procedure[28] was once a popular operation for trapezius paralysis.[27,98,119,130] In this procedure the medial border of the scapula is stabilized by securing it to the T-1 and T-2 spinous processes with fascia lata strips, which attempt to compensate for the middle and lower thirds of the trapezius. In addition, the levator scapulae muscle is transferred laterally to the spine of the scapula to compensate for the upper third of the trapezius (Fig. 13). Following surgery, the arm is placed in a shoulder spica cast in 45 to 50 degrees of abduction for 6 to 8 weeks. Other operations have been described for trapezius winging that employ fascial slings as well, all with the principal effect to compensate for the three portions of the trapezius.[29,32,66,85]

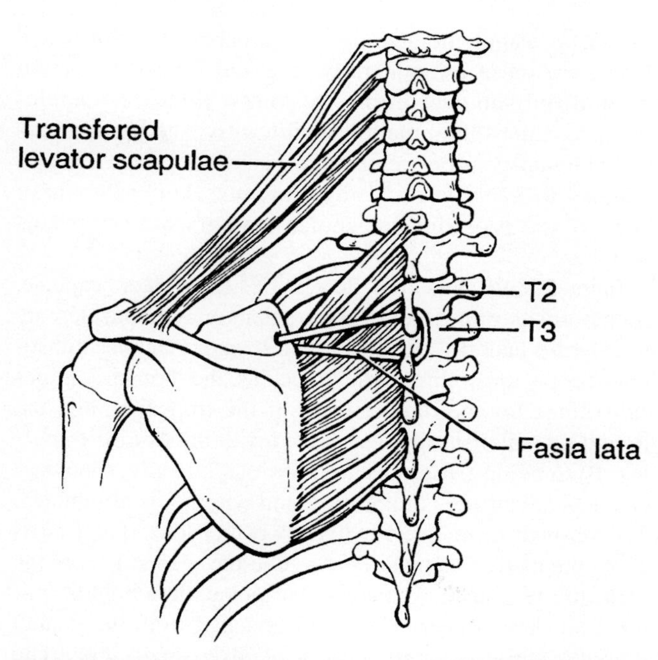

FIG. 13. Dewar-Harris operation for trapezius palsy. This procedure combines the use of fascial slings compensating for the middle and lower trapezius, and transfer of the levator scapulae to compensate for the upper trapezius.

Of historical interest, a partial fusion for trapezius winging has been described by Spira.[157] In this technique, a hole is made in the inferior angle of the scapula. The sixth rib is cut, passed through the hole, then reapproximated (Fig. 14).

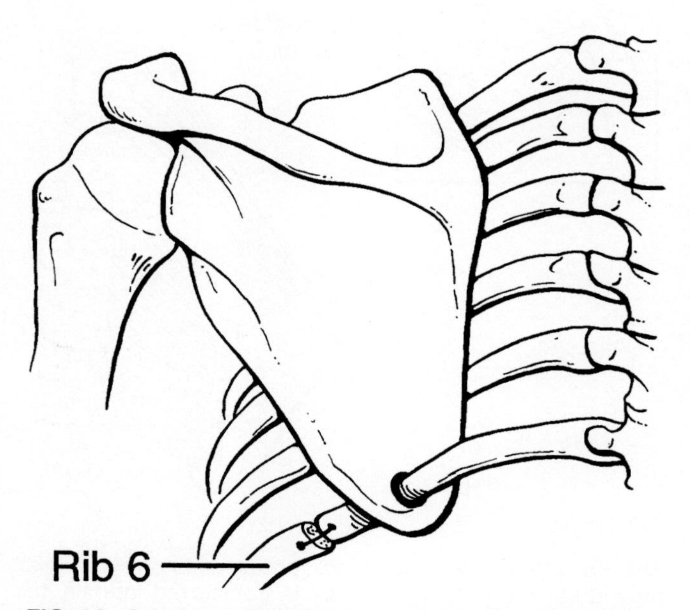

FIG. 14. Spira's partial fusion for trapezius palsy. In this procedure a hole is made in the inferior angle of the scapula, and the sixth rib is passed through the scapula, stabilizing it.

Complete scapulothoracic fusions can also be performed.[64] However, these are generally reserved for patients with generalized shoulder girdle weakness. Because scapulothoracic fusions limit motion significantly, and because fascial sling suspensions tend to fail, causing a recurrence of winging in 2 to 3 years,[8,72] dynamic muscle transfers have become the procedure of choice for persistent trapezius winging.[8,22,36,92,93,94,106]

In the Eden-Lange procedure,[36,92,93] the levator scapulae, rhomboideus minor, and rhomboideus major muscles are transferred laterally (Fig. 15). The levator scapulae substitutes for the upper third of the trapezius, the rhomboid minor substitutes for the middle third of the trapezius, and the rhomboid major substitutes for the lower third of the trapezius. By moving these muscle insertions laterally, their mechanical advantage is improved, and winging is eliminated. The surgical technique involves two incisions. The first is along the medial scapular border, and the second is over the spine of the scapula. The levator scapulae, rhomboideus minor, and rhomboideus major are detached from the medial scapula, taking a small portion of insertional bone. The rhomboideus muscles are advanced laterally under the infraspinatus and are secured with suture that is passed through drill holes placed 5 cm lateral to the medial border of the scapula. The levator scapulae is passed subcutaneously to the second incision and is sutured to the scapular spine through drill holes (see Fig. 15). Patients are kept in an abduction cast, or foam abduction pillow for 4 to 6 weeks, and then passive and active range of motion is begun. Bigliani recently reported his results using this procedure on 23 patients with trapezius scapular winging and had 87% excellent and good results.[8] Significant improvement in pain was seen in 91% of these patients and 87% had significant improvement in function.[8]

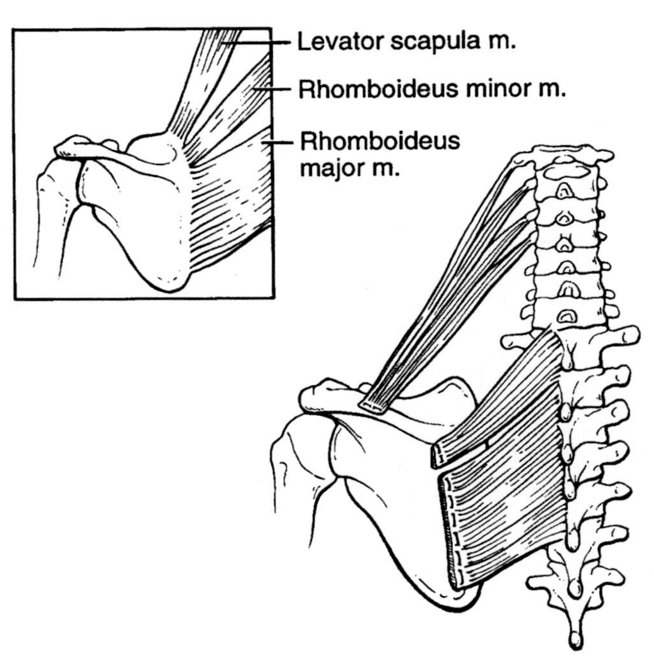

FIG. 15. Eden-Lange procedure for trapezius palsy. In this procedure, the levator scapulae is transferred laterally to function as the upper trapezius, while advancement of the rhomboid major and minor compensate for the loss of the middle and lower trapezius.

Primary Scapular Winging: Bony Abnormalities

Bone abnormalities that may present as scapular winging include osteochondromas, the most common tumor of the scapula, which can be a cause of "pseudowinging." (Fig. 16)[23,25,41,101,125] Rib osteochondromas may also cause scapular winging.[41] This type of scapular winging is structural and may be associated with scapular crepitus. Patients will have winging that may not change with varying the position of the arm. In this instance, electromyography studies will be normal, and the osteochondroma is identified by radiographs tangential to the plane of the scapula, or by com-

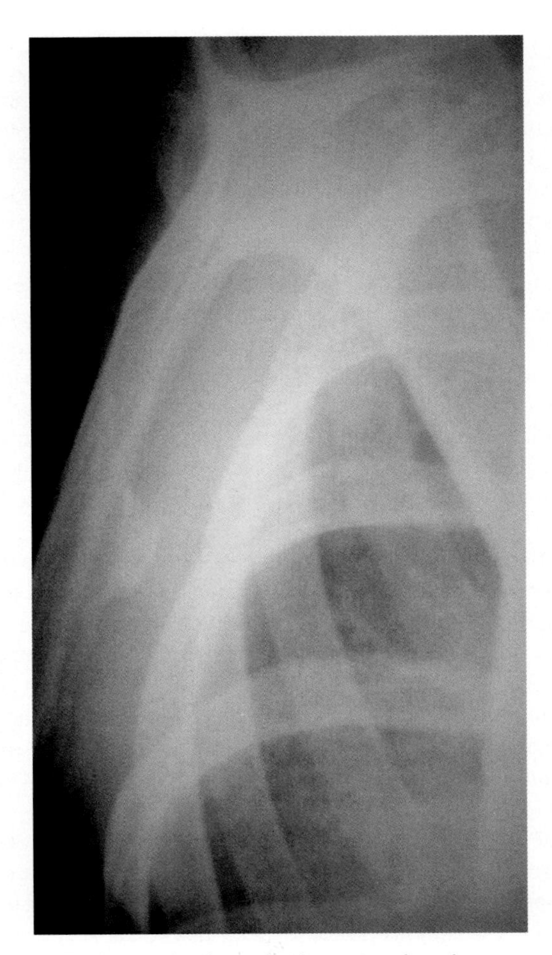

FIG. 16. Radiograph of a scapular osteochondroma causing scapular winging and crepitus. The patient's symptoms resolved completely with resection of the osteochondroma. (From Kuhn JE, Hawkins RJ. Evaluation and treatment of scapular disorders. In: Warner JP, Iannotti JP, Gerber C, eds. *Complex and revision problems in shoulder surgery.* Philadelphia: Lippincott-Raven, 1997:357–375).

puted tomography (CT). Winging is alleviated with resection of the bony pathology. Malunions of fractures of the scapula and clavicle have also been implicated as a source of primary winging of the scapula.[41,109] Because the muscle function would not be expected to be impaired, these patients may not be symptomatic.

Primary Scapular Winging: Muscle Disorders

Muscle abnormalities that cause winging have included traumatic ruptures and congenital absence of periscapular muscles. In the cases of serratus anterior muscle avulsion, significant trauma has occurred that pulls the muscle insertion from the medial border of the scapula.[43,65,110,122,176] Fiddian and King report a case of serratus anterior division during thoracotomy, which was a source of symptomatic winging.[41] In these cases, nerve conduction studies are likely to be normal and computed tomography or magnetic resonance imaging (MRI) should be considered to assist in the diagnosis. Surgical reattachment is recommended in all patients, and excellent results can be expected.[43,65,122,176] Advanced age with systemic disease may, however, be a contraindication to surgery.[110] Congenital absence of the serratus anterior,[21,100] the trapezius,[73,84,147,149] and the rhomboideus major and trapezius muscles[150] have all been reported. Patients with these congenital anomalies, however, seem to function very well without treatment.[181]

Primary Scapular Winging: Bursal Disorders

The articulation between the scapula and the thorax has bursae which in rare circumstances may become inflamed. This is one source of scapular crepitation and pain. Winging has been identified in 50% of patients with a snapping scapula and no bony abnormalities.[126] This is presumably related to the subscapular bursitis, and with treatment of the bursitis, either by nonoperative means or surgical bursectomy, the winging resolves.

Secondary Scapular Winging

Secondary scapular winging originates from disorders of the glenohumeral joint that produce abnormal scapulothoracic dynamics (Fig. 17). This phenomenon has not been thoroughly investigated in the literature. A thorough evaluation of the patient with secondary scapular winging will usually, but not always, identify the source of the glenohumeral pathology.[164] The physical examination of every patient with a shoulder condition should include looking for secondary scapular winging at rest, with dynamic forward elevation, and with resisted forward elevation. A characteristic of secondary scapular winging is a normal electromyographic examination of the long thoracic nerve and serratus anterior, the spinal accessory nerve and trapezius, and the dorsal scapular nerve and rhomboids.

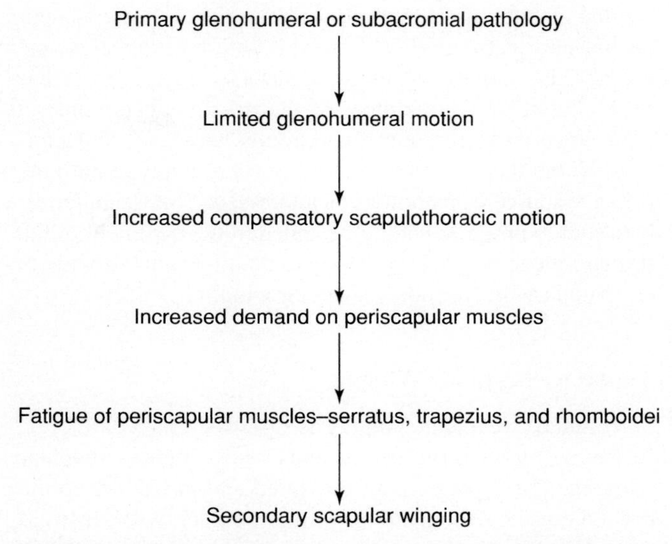

FIG. 17. Sequence of events leading to secondary scapular winging. (From Kuhn JE, Hawkins RJ. Evaluation and treatment of scapular disorders. In: Warner JP, Iannotti JP, Gerber C, eds. *Complex and revision problems in shoulder surgery*. Philadelphia: Lippincott-Raven, 1997:357–375).

Contractural winging[3] is one example in which contractures about the glenohumeral joint can produce secondary scapular winging. Patients with upper root brachial plexus injuries develop contractures owing to unbalanced muscle forces, with the humerus abducted and internally rotated relative to the scapula. When the arm is forcibly adducted to the chest wall and externally rotated, the superior corner of the scapula projects away from the chest wall, producing the "scapular sign of Putti,"[146] otherwise known as contractural winging.[3] Contractural winging can also occur with fibrosis of the deltoid muscle, in which the winging decreases with arm elevation and increases with lowering of the arm.[167] This condition is thought to be either congenital[138,179] or related to a history of injections into the deltoid muscle,[56,115] and is almost always associated with winging of the scapula.[115]

Other more common disorders involving the glenohumeral joint can be a source of secondary scapular winging. This is thought to occur by reflex muscle spasm provoked by some painful condition in the glenohumeral or subacromial areas.[167] This has been associated with rotator cuff tears,[167] nonunion of acromion fractures,[55] malunion of clavicle fractures,[41] fractures of the glenoid,[41] avascular necrosis of the humeral head,[55] acromegalic arthropathy of the shoulder,[41] acromioclavicular joint disorders,[41,164] and shoulder instability.[41,42,144,164] In our practice, we have observed secondary scapular winging in patients with adhesive capsulitis, the impingement syndrome, anterior shoulder instability, and in throwing athletes with secondary impingement caused by subtle shoulder instability. We suspect that patients with painful shoulders reflexively limit glenohumeral motion. This forces the periscapular muscles to work in excess as scapulothoracic motion must increase to compensate for the limited glenohumeral motion. With fatigue of the periscapular muscles, particularly the serratus anterior, trapezius, and rhomboids, scapular winging occurs (see Fig. 17). As has been shown,[164,167] treatment of the primary glenohumeral pathology will alleviate the scapular winging, and conversely, the scapular winging is unlikely to improve until the primary source of pathology is addressed.[164] A scapular rehabilitation program should be added to the treatment of the primary glenohumeral pathology to facilitate recovery in every patient with secondary scapular winging.[118,123]

Voluntary Scapular Winging

Voluntary scapular winging is also very rare.[41,55,140,164] Rowe has reported on four patients with voluntary scapular winging. These patients were assured and instructed on the normal muscle firing patterns of the shoulder, with "instructions not to tighten or contract their shoulder muscles when elevating the arm."[140] All four patients recovered after this coaching. Gregg et al. describe asymptomatic bilateral voluntary scapular winging in an orthopedic resident.[55] It is important to appreciate that patients with voluntary scapular winging who seek medical attention, similar to patients with voluntary subluxation of the shoulder, may have unaddressed psychologic issues complicating their care.[141]

SCAPULAR DYSKINESIA

Pathophysiology

Although static scapulothoracic abnormalities have been recognized in the past, dynamic scapulothoracic dyskinesia was an underappreciated phenomenon until recently. Recent investigations in normal and athletic patients have demonstrated significant alterations in the dynamic motion of the scapulothoracic articulation when accompanied by shoulder pathology. In their study evaluating scapulothoracic motion using Moire topographic analysis, Warner et al. found static scapulothoracic asymmetry present in 32% of patients with glenohumeral instability and 57% of patients with subacromial impingement.[175] Dynamic testing was more sensitive with asymmetrical scapulothoracic motion in 64% of patients with glenohumeral instability and all patients with impingement.[175] Furthermore, throwing athletes with anterior shoulder instability have altered scapulothoracic mechanics, with the serratus anterior demonstrating a marked reduction in activity during throwing.[49] Certainly, intrinsic shoulder pathologies, such as glenohumeral instability or subacromial impingement, may cause secondary alterations in the dynamic scapulothoracic articulation, producing scapulothoracic dyskinesia. Conversely, it has recently been appreciated that alterations in the dynamic scapulothoracic motion may be a primary cause of glenohumeral pathology.

A consistent firing pattern of the scapular-stabilizing muscles has been identified by electromyographic studies in the overhand athlete.[30,88] These studies have determined that throwing and other overhand athletic motions are dependent on synchronized, coordinated scapulothoracic motion. A coordinated firing pattern of the posterior scapular-stabilizing muscles helps stabilize the shoulder joint controlling the forces across it.[88] Alterations in this coordinated activity uncouple the force relations required for throwing and lead to decreased efficiency or an increased risk for injury. The position of the scapula during the throwing motion will determine the muscle length–tension relations and allow for maximum muscle force generation and efficiency.[86] Scapular motion also determines the location of the glenohumeral joint in space, and it is important to not only optimize glenoid placement relative to the humeral head to maintain glenohumeral joint stability, but also elevate the acromion to allow motion without impingement. Finally, periscapular muscles may be important in providing power and accepting eccentric load, as the scapula is maximally retracted during windup and cocking, and maximally protracted during acceleration and follow-through.[49,86,88] Restricted scapulothoracic retraction may limit the power stored in the windup and cocking phase of throwing. In addition, limited protraction may cause the eccentric loading to be transferred to the posterior capsule and posterior rotator cuff tendons of the glenohumeral joint during the follow-through phase of overhead throwing. These excessive repetitive stresses may lead to rotator cuff injury or glenohumeral instability. Overhand athletes often present with abnormal scapular function in the form of winging, poor retraction, poor protraction, poor positioning, or some other form of dyskinesia.

Evaluation

Kibler has described the scapular lateral slide test to evaluate patients with abnormal scapulothoracic function.[86] This test evaluates the patient's ability to stabilize the medial border of the scapula during different positions and loads. To perform this test, the arms are held in three different positions and the distance between the medial border of the scapula and the thoracic spinous processes is measured bilaterally. These positions include: (a) relative rest in neutral rotation, (b) the hands on the hips with the thumbs pointing posteriorly, and (c) the arms abducted to 90 degrees with maximal internal humeral rotation. In the asymptomatic athlete, symmetry is the general rule, with less than one centimeter side-to-side difference. In symptomatic throwers, more than 1-cm side-to-side difference in position (a) or (b) is statistically associated with pain and decreased function.[87]

The clinical implications of this abnormal lateral protraction of the scapula include increased anteversion of the glenoid, opening the anterior half of the glenohumeral articulation. This may create a situation predisposing the patient to increased instability and to glenoid labral damage.[86,143] Loss of retraction may prevent optimal energy storage during the windup and cocking phase of throwing, with reduced power. Finally, abnormal scapulothoracic dynamics may limit acromial elevation, producing rotator cuff impingement (see Fig. 4).

Treatment

When evaluating athletes with shoulder disorders, it is important to consider and treat abnormal scapulothoracic function, for the scapula is an essential component to the kinetic chain involved in overhead throwing. In treating these disorders, rehabilitation begins at the base of the kinetic chain, the legs, hips, and back, and moves distally to the shoulder when the foundation is functioning adequately.[86] Periscapular muscle-strengthening exercises then become an integral component to the complete shoulder rehabilitation program. Exercises to strengthen the rotator cuff should generally be avoided until the scapulothoracic articulation is functioning normally.

SCAPULOTHORACIC CREPITUS

Pathophysiology

Symptomatic scapulothoracic crepitus has been given a variety of names through the years, including the snapping scapula,[112] the washboard syndrome,[21] the scapulothoracic syndrome,[117] the rolling scapula,[19] the grating scapula,[119] and the scapulocostal syndrome.[152] Although Codman himself states that he was able to make his own scapula "... sound about the room without the slightest pain,"[20] Boinet[11] was the first to describe this disorder in 1867. Thirty-seven years later, Mauclaire[105] classified scapulothoracic crepitus into three groups: *froissement* was described as a gentle friction sound and was thought to be physiologic, *frottement* was a louder sound with grating and was usually pathologic, and *craquement* was a loud snapping sound and was always pathologic. These scapular noises are thought to occur from two sources, either from anatomic changes in the tissue interposed between the scapula and the chest wall, or by an incongruence in the scapulothoracic articulation (Table 4). Extrapolating from Milch,[112] *frottement* may suggest soft-tissue pathology or bursitis; whereas *craquement* may suggest bony pathology as the source of symptomatic scapulothoracic crepitus. These noises are amplified by the air-filled thoracic cavity, which acts as a resonance chamber, much like a string instrument.[5]

TABLE 4. *Causes of scapulothoracic crepitus*[a]

Interposed Tissue
Muscle
Atrophy[91,112]
Fibrosis[112,113,172]
Anatomic variation[91,160]
Bone
Rib osteochondroma[26]
Scapular osteochondroma[113,114,125]
Rib fracture[112,113]
Scapular fracture[162]
Hooked superomedial angle of scapula[112,135]
Luschka's tubercle[112,173]
Reactive bone spurs from muscle avulsion[5,165]
Other soft tissue
Bursitis[2,21,107,108]
Tuberculosis[112]
Syphilitic lues[112]
Abnormalities in scapulothoracic congruence
Scoliosis[52,172]
Thoracic kyphosis[19]

[a] A variety of structures interposed between the scapula and thorax may cause crepitus. Similarly, spinal curvatures can cause crepitus by altering the scapulothoracic congruence. (From Kuhn JE, Hawkins RJ. Evaluation and treatment of scapular disorders. In: Warner JJP, Iannotti JP, Gerber C. eds. *Complex and revision problems in shoulder surgery.* Philadelphia: Lippincott–Raven Publishers, 1997:357–375.)

There are several described abnormal structures which lie between the scapula and the chest wall that give rise to scapulothoracic crepitus. Pathologic conditions affecting muscle in the scapulothoracic articulation include atrophied muscle,[112] fibrotic muscle,[112,113,172] and anomalous muscle insertions.[160]

The most common bony pathology in the scapulothoracic space that may give rise to scapulothoracic crepitus is the osteochondroma, arising either from the ribs[26] or from the scapula[113,114,125] (see Fig. 16). Malunited fractures of the ribs or scapula are also capable of creating painful crepitus.[112,113,162] Abnormalities of the superomedial angle of the scapula, including a hooked superomedial angle[114,135] or a Luschka's tubercle (which originally was described as an osteochondroma, but has subsequently come to mean any prominence of bone at the superomedial angle[112,162,173]), have also been implicated as sources for scapulothoracic crepitus. Others[5,138,165] implicate reactive spurs of bone that are created by the microtrauma of chronic, repeated periscapular muscle avulsions.

Certainly, any bony pathology that causes scapulothoracic crepitus is capable of forming a reactive bursa around the area of pathology.[24,151] In fact, at the time of resection of bony pathology, a bursa is frequently seen. A bursa can become inflamed and painful in the absence of bony pathology, and may become an independent source of crepitus.

Other soft-tissue pathology that has been implicated in scapulothoracic crepitus includes tuberculosis lesions in the scapulothoracic region, and syphilitic lues.[112] Abnormalities in congruence of the scapulothoracic articulation are the other source of scapulothoracic crepitus. Both scoliosis[52,171] and thoracic kyphosis[19] have been implicated as sources of scapulothoracic crepitus.

Evaluation

The patient with symptomatic scapulothoracic crepitus may be able to identify the location of the crepitus. A history of overhead activity, such as sporting activities[126] or paper hanging, may be present.[19] Some suspect there is a familial tendency toward developing symptoms.[19] Patients may relate a history of trauma that precipitates symptoms,[2] and scapulothoracic crepitus may be bilateral in some patients.[18] On inspection of the scapula, fullness or winging, which may suggest a space-occupying lesion in the scapulothoracic space, may be observed. Palpation or auscultation while the shoulder goes through a range of motion may help identify the source of the periscapular crepitus.[2,18] A palpable mass, crepitus, prominence at rest, and normal scapulothoracic motion help delineate scapular winging caused by a physical mass from neurologic scapular winging. In patients with scapulothoracic crepitus, the neuromuscular examination is frequently normal. Supplemental radiographs that include tangential views of the lateral scapula and CT, or MRI scans, may be helpful in identifying anatomic pathology.

Treatment

It is important to realize that scapulothoracic crepitus is not necessarily a pathologic condition. It has been found in 35% of normal asymptomatic persons.[58] As a result of this, patients with hidden agendas or psychiatric conditions may not respond to treatment as well as other patients. However, if the scapulothoracic crepitus is truly associated with pain, winging, or other disorders of the scapulothoracic articulation, then the crepitus is considered to be pathologic.

Patients with clearly defined bony pathology, such as an osteochondroma, are unlikely to improve with conservative treatment.[112] Resection of the bony pathology is usually necessary to alleviate symptoms with a high likelihood of success.[13,116,125] Other patients should undergo a trial of conservative treatment, reserving surgery for those who fail. Conservative treatment seems to be most beneficial if soft-tissue disorders are the source of scapulothoracic crepitus.[18,112] These include postural exercises designed to prevent sloping of the shoulders.[18,111] A figure-of-eight harness may be a useful tool to remind patients to maintain upright posture. Exercises to strengthen periscapular muscles are also thought to be important.[18,112,126] Systemic nonsteroidal antiinflammatory drugs, as well as local modalities, such as heat, massage, phonophoresis, and ultrasound, and the application of ethyl chloride to trigger points may also prove useful.[18,112,126] Injections of local anesthetics and corticosteroids into the painful area have also been recommended.[13,19,107,12,126] Caution must be used, for there is a risk for creating a pneumothorax.[13] With these means, most patients are expected to improve significantly;[107,126] however, for those who fail, various operations have been described.

Muscle plasty operations include those described by Mauclaire, who reflected a flap of the rhomboids or trapezius and sutured it to the undersurface of the scapula.[105] This is thought to be inadequate, however, because the muscle flap may atrophy with time and symptoms could recur.[112] Rockwood has excised a rhomboid muscle avulsion flap, with the elimination of snapping and pain.[13] Partial scapulectomy has also been popular as a means of treating symptomatic scapulothoracic crepitus, including resection of the medial border of the scapula[14] or the superomedial angle.[2,19,91,112,135,165,181]

The surgical technique for the resection of the superomedial border of the scapula begins with the patient in the prone position (Fig. 18). An incision based over the medial spine of the scapula is made and the soft-tissue is dissected down to the spine of the scapula. The periosteum over the spine is incised, and a plane is developed between the superficial trapezius and the underlying scapula. Next, the supraspinatus, rhomboids, and levator scapulae muscles are dissected free of the scapula in a subperiosteal plane, starting at the spine of the scapula. The superomedial angle of the scapula is resected with an oscillating saw. Caution is warranted as the resection is carried laterally to avoid injury to the dorsal scapular artery or the suprascapular nerve in the suprascapular notch. After resecting the bone, the reflected muscles fall back into place, and the periosteum is reapproximated back to the spine of the scapula using suture through drill holes. Postoperatively, the patient is placed in a sling and begins passive motion immediately. Active motion is begun at 8 weeks, and resistance exercises follow at 12 weeks.

Although some authors report mixed results after partial scapulectomy for symptomatic scapulothoracic crepitus,[13] others suggest this is an excellent option.[19,91,112,135] However, most of these reports are case reports or very small series. Arntz and Matsen[2] describe their results after a resection of the superomedial border of the scapula in 14 shoulders in 12 patients with 42 months follow-up. In this relatively large series, 86% of patients obtained complete relief of pain and crepitus. Importantly, the bone resected appears normal and shows no pathology, which has prompted some to perform bursectomies and avoid a partial scapulectomy.[108,153]

Complications associated with partial scapulectomy include pneumothorax, postoperative hematoma, and in younger patients bone may form again; however, this rarely produces symptoms.

SCAPULOTHORACIC BURSITIS

Pathophysiology

Codman, in his classic text, *The Shoulder*, was clearly one of the first physicians with an interest in scapulothoracic bursitis. He described the bursa of the scapulothoracic articulation and identified and named those bursae in the superomedial border of the scapula that he thought were the cause of symptomatic scapulothoracic bursitis.[20]

Two major or anatomic bursae, and four minor or adventitial bursae have been described for the scapulothoracic articulation (see Table 2 and Fig. 8). The first major bursa is found in the space between the serratus anterior muscle and the chest wall. The second major bursa is located between the subscapularis and the serratus anterior muscles.[18,90] These bursae are easily and reproducibly found.[90]

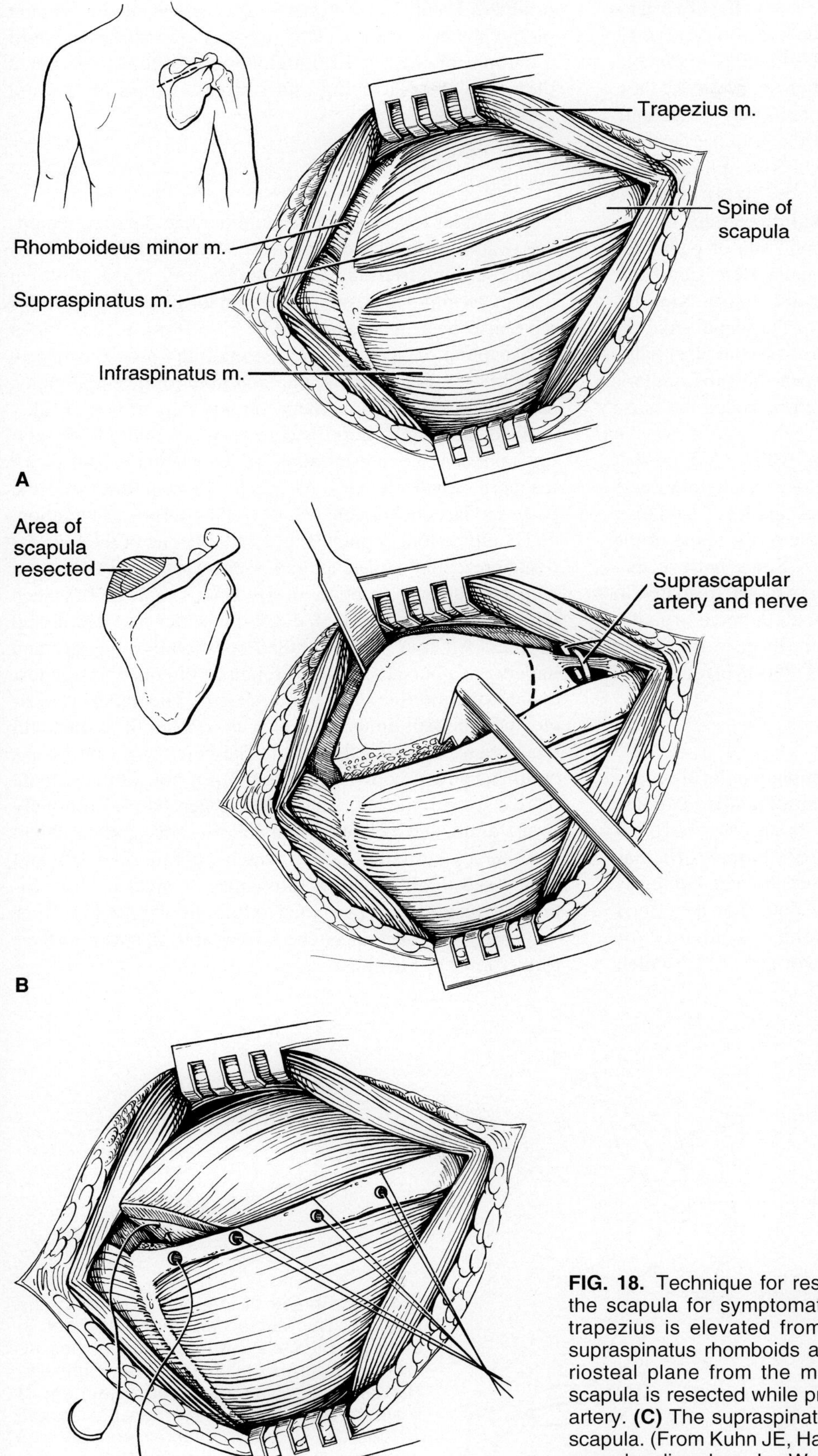

FIG. 18. Technique for resection of the superomedial border of the scapula for symptomatic scapulothoracic crepitus. **(A)** The trapezius is elevated from the spine of the scapula. **(B)** The supraspinatus rhomboids and serratus are elevated in a subperiosteal plane from the medial border, and the superomedial scapula is resected while protecting the suprascapular nerve and artery. **(C)** The supraspinatus is sutured back to the spine of the scapula. (From Kuhn JE, Hawkins RJ. Evaluation and treatment of scapular disorders. In: Warner JP, Iannotti JP, Gerber C, eds. *Complex and revision problems in shoulder surgery*. Philadelphia: Lippincott-Raven, 1997:357–375).

Clinical scapulothoracic bursitis seems to affect two areas of the scapulothoracic articulation: the superomedial angle and the inferior angle of the scapula. When symptomatic, these areas tend to develop inflamed bursae; however, these bursae are not reliably found and, in fact, may be adventitious.[19,90,126] For the inferior angle of the scapula, most authors agree that the affected bursa lies between the serratus anterior muscle and the chest wall.[20,112,153] This bursa has been given many names, including the infraserratus bursa[20] and the bursa mucosa.[112,172] The second site of pathology lies at the superomedial angle of the scapula. Here, Codman[20] believed this bursa is also an infraserratus bursa, lying between the upper and anterior portion of the scapula and the back of the first three ribs. Von Gruber,[172] on the other hand, identified a bursa in this region between the subscapularis and the serratus anticus muscles, which he called the bursa mucosa angulae superioris scapulae.

A third minor or adventitial bursa, which Codman believed was the site of painful crepitus in scapulothoracic crepitus, was called the trapezoid bursa, and it is found over the triangular surface at the medial base of the spine of the scapula under the trapezius muscle.[20] Some believe that these minor bursae are adventitial and develop in response to abnormal pathomechanics of the scapulothoracic articulation.[19,90,126] It would not be surprising, then, to find these bursae inconsistently or in different soft-tissue planes.

Evaluation

Scapulothoracic bursitis may accompany painful scapular crepitus, or it may exist as a separate entity. Patients generally complain of pain with activity and may have audible and palpable crepitus of the scapulothoracic articulation. Usually, the scapular crepitus associated with bursitis is of a much lesser quality and nature than that described with bony pathology. Patients relate a history of trauma[2,108] or overuse from sport or work,[107,108,153] which produces repetitive or constant movement of the scapula on the posterior thorax. This may irritate soft tissues until a chronic bursitis and inflammation develops. The bursa then undergoes scarring and fibrosis, with crepitus and pain to follow.

Treatment

The initial treatment of scapulothoracic bursitis, regardless of its location, is conservative, beginning with rest, analgesics, and nonsteroidal antiinflammatory drugs. Physical therapy to improve posture, heat, and local steroid injections have also been recommended.[107,153] Efforts to strengthen periscapular muscles and stretching are frequently added.[107,153] For patients who continue to have symptoms despite conservative treatment, surgery may be beneficial.

Sisto and Jobe[153] described an open procedure for resecting a bursa at the inferior angle of the scapula in four major league baseball pitchers. All pitchers had pain during the early and late cocking phases, as well as during acceleration, and could no longer pitch (Fig. 19). Only one of the four patients presented with scapulothoracic crepitus, but all had a palpable bursal sac ranging in size from 1 to 2 cm, best seen with the arm abducted to 60 degrees and elevated forward 30 degrees. All four pitchers failed conservative therapy and underwent a bursal excision through an oblique incision just distal to the inferior angle of the scapula. The trapezius muscle, then the latissimus dorsi muscle, were split in line with their fibers, exposing the bursa. The bursa was sharply excised and any osteophytes on the inferior pole of the scapula or ribs were removed. The wounds were closed routinely over a drain, and a compression dressing was applied. Physical therapy stressing motion was begun after 1 week and progressed to allow gentle throwing at 6 weeks. This progressed as symptoms permitted to full-speed throwing. After this procedure, all four pitchers were able to return to their former level of pitching.

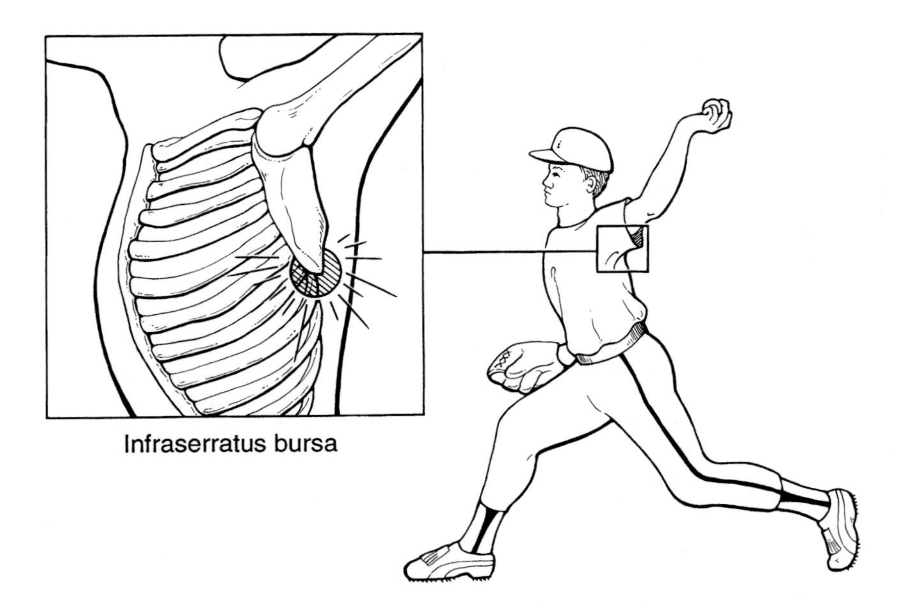

FIG. 19. Bursae of the inferior angle of the scapula. This bursa has been described in baseball pitchers, and its removal has allowed a return to pitching. (From Kuhn JE, Hawkins RJ. Evaluation and treatment of scapular disorders. In: Warner JP, Iannotti JP, Gerber C, eds. *Complex and revision problems in shoulder surgery.* Philadelphia: Lippincott-Raven, 1997:357–375).

Similarly, McCluskey and Bigliani[107,108] performed an open excision of a symptomatic superomedial scapulothoracic bursa in 9 patients, noting a thickened, abnormal bursa between the serratus anterior and the chest wall at the time of surgery. Their surgical technique involves making a vertical incision medial to the vertebral border of the scapula. The trapezius is dissected free and a subperiosteal dissection is used to free the levator scapulae and rhomboids from the medial border of the scapula. A plane is developed between the serratus anterior and the chest wall. The thickened bursa is resected, and any bony projections are removed. The medial periscapular muscles and trapezius are reapproximated to the scapula. The skin is closed in a routine fashion. The patient uses a sling for comfort and begins passive motion and pendulum exercises immediately. At 3 weeks active motion is allowed, with strengthening begun at 12 weeks. With this technique, 88% of patients with symptomatic scapulothoracic bursitis had good or excellent results. One patient with a fair result also required muscle transfers for trapezius winging.[108]

Resection of the symptomatic scapulothoracic bursa has also been performed endoscopically.[9,18,48,90,104] Ciullo and Jones[18] have the largest endoscopic series to date with 13 patients who underwent subscapular endoscopy after failing a conservative treatment program for symptomatic scapulothoracic bursitis. Debridement was performed for fibrous adhesions found in the bursa between the subscapularis and serratus muscles, as well as the bursa between the serratus and chest wall. In addition, debridement or scapuloplasty of changes at the superomedial angle or inferior angle were performed. All 13 patients returned to their preinjury activity level, except for physician-imposed restrictions in a few patients, limiting the assembly line use of vibrating tools.[18]

The technique for scapulothoracic endoscopy has been described by Matthews and colleagues.[104] Patients can be placed in the prone or lateral position; however, the lateral position is preferred because it allows arthroscopic evaluation of the glenohumeral joint and the subacromial space. In addition, if the arm is extended and maximally internally rotated, the scapula will fall away from the thorax, improving access to the bursae.

Three portals are used that are placed at least 2 cm from the medial border of the scapula in the region between the scapular spine and the inferior angle. For the middle portal, a spinal needle is inserted into the bursa between the serratus anterior and the chest wall. This needle should be inserted midway between the scapular spine and the inferior angle, at least three finger-breadths medial to the medial border of the scapula to avoid injury to the dorsal scapular artery and nerve. The bursa under the serratus anterior can be distended with fluid before a stab wound is made in the skin and the blunt obturator and endoscope are inserted. Deep penetration may traverse the serratus entering the axillary space and should be avoided.

Once this initial middle portal has been established, a superior portal placed three finger-breadths medial to the vertebral border of the scapula just below the spine will penetrate the interval between the rhomboideus major and rhomboideus minor. This portal will allow access to the superomedial angle of the scapula. Portals placed superior to the scapular spine jeopardize the dorsal scapular nerve and artery, the spinal accessory nerve, and the transverse cervical artery, and should be avoided. A third inferior portal can be made in a similar fashion at the inferior angle of the scapula.

In the bursa between the serratus anterior and chest wall, landmarks are generally absent except the ribs. A motorized shaver and electrocautery are required to perform the bursectomy and obtain hemostasis. The arthroscopic pump should be kept at low pressure throughout the procedure. After completing the bursectomy, the portals are closed in a standard fashion, and the patient is placed in a sling for comfort. Physical therapy beginning with active range of motion is initiated as tolerated by the patient.

As presented at numerous meetings, the arthroscopic techniques for performing a scapulothoracic bursectomy seem to have early promising results, and to date, no cases of injury to the long thoracic nerve, dorsal scapular artery, suprascapular nerve, axillary contents, or thoracic cavity have been reported. Despite this, no series of patients treated arthroscopically for scapulothoracic bursitis has been published in the peer-reviewed literature, and this technique still remains investigational.

SPRENGEL'S DEFORMITY

Pathophysiology

Sprengel's deformity, the most common congenital deformity of the shoulder,[128] was first described by Eulenberg in 1863, and again by Sprengel in 1891, as an apparent elevation of the scapula, [39,158] but is actually believed to occur as a result of failure of the normal caudal migration of the scapula.[15,74] Normally, at 5-weeks gestation, the fetal scapula begins differentiation opposite the fourth, fifth, and sixth vertebrae. Between the 9th and 12th week of gestation, the scapula migrates caudally to its usual thoracic position between the second and seventh ribs. Initially, the horizontal diameter of the scapula exceeds the vertical diameter, similar to a quadruped's scapula. As normal development proceeds, this orientation changes, allowing increased movement of the forelimb.[74] The arrest of this normal development explains the physical findings seen in the patient with Sprengel's deformity; however, as yet, no consensus has been reached as to the cause for this arrrested development.

Evaluation

The clinical deformity seen in the patient with an undescended scapula is a result of the arrest of the normal development (Fig. 20). The scapula is found high on the chest wall, with the inferior pole adducted and the superior angle

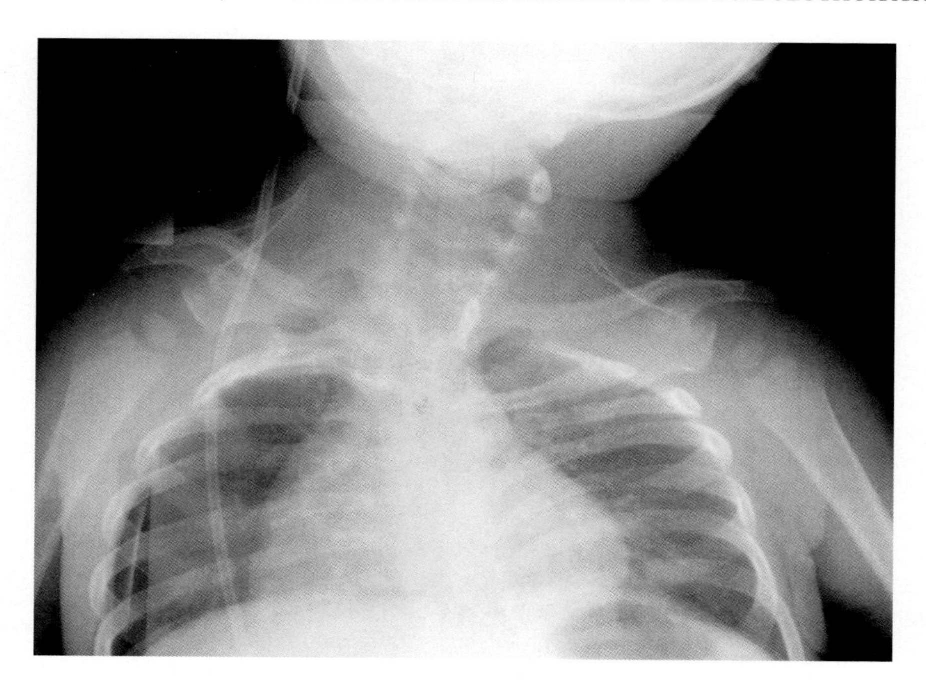

FIG. 20. Radiograph of patient with Sprengel's deformity. This infant has multiple orthopedic problems, including the failure of descent of the scapulae bilaterally. Note the relative increase in width and decrease in height of the scapula, as well as the projection of the scapula into the neck, creating an apparent webbing.

prominent in the web of the neck. The superior angle may curve anteriorly over the apex of the chest. The scapula is small with a horizontal to vertical ratio greater than normal. An omovertebral connection of fibrous tissue, cartilage, or bone connects the superior angle of the scapula to the cervical spine in up to 30% of patients,[15,16,79,80,148] which may be homologous to the suprascapular bone of the lower vertebrates.[178] These attachments severely restrict scapulothoracic motion. In addition, the scapulothoracic muscles, including the trapezius, levator scapulae, and rhomboids, are frequently hypoplastic,[16] and the serratus anterior may be weak, accentuating scapular winging.

Patients will frequently have limitation in shoulder motion, particularly in abduction as the scapula is rotated, causing the glenoid to tilt downward. Up to 40% of cases will have less than 100 degrees of abduction.[15,79,80] Flexion, rotation, and passive glenohumeral abduction may be normal. With the scapula fixed, increased stress on the glenohumeral capsule may lead to multidirectional instability.[59]

Associated anomalies are common in patients with Sprengel's deformity, affecting at least 75% of patients.[12] Spinal deformities may manifest as scoliosis, Klippel-Feil syndrome, hemivertebrae, and diastematomyelia. Patients may have fused or absent ribs. Genitourinary conditions, including solitary kidneys, pelvic kidneys, and undescended testes, are also common and patients with Sprengel's deformity should undergo abdominal ultrasound evaluations to search for these anomalies.

Treatment

Improving the cosmetic appearance of the shoulder or improving function is the usual indication for treatment. The asymmetric appearance of the neck and shoulder girdle, with severe webbing of the neck, is often the reason parents seek medical attention.[16,47] Nonoperative treatment has provided little benefit for the patient with Sprengel's deformity. Generally, surgical treatment is recommended between the ages of 3 and 6,[16,80,184] because the results seem to be better in the younger patient, and the surgery may be difficult in patients younger than age 3;[79,80] however, most series in the literature have been too small to assess outcomes in relation to patient age.

A number of different approaches have been described to treat this rare disorder. In general these approaches are all directed toward releasing the structures that tether the scapula.[57,79,156] Other procedures attempt to reposition the scapula lower on the chest wall by detaching the muscles at the scapular insertion,[54,79,89,148] or by transplanting the muscles at their midline origins.[184] Procedures in which the tethering structures alone are released are generally associated with less gain in abduction and have a higher rate of recurrence.[139] Of the procedures that relocate the scapula, the most popular are the Woodward procedure and the Green procedure.

The Green procedure (Fig. 21) consists of an extraperiosteal release of the muscles of the medial border of the scapula and a resection of the omovertebral bone and supraclavcular portion of the scapula.[54] The scapula is then relocated caudally and the muscles sutured in the new position. Piano wire that is routed through the spine of the scapula is directed through the latissimus and skin, then connected to 3 lb of traction by a spring scale molded into a body cast. The wire and cast are removed after 3 weeks. In Green's original series, he presented 16 patients with outcomes in cosmesis and function.[54] The major disadvantage was the requirement for the body cast and percutaneous traction. Recently, Leibovic[99] reviewed 18 patients with more than 3 years

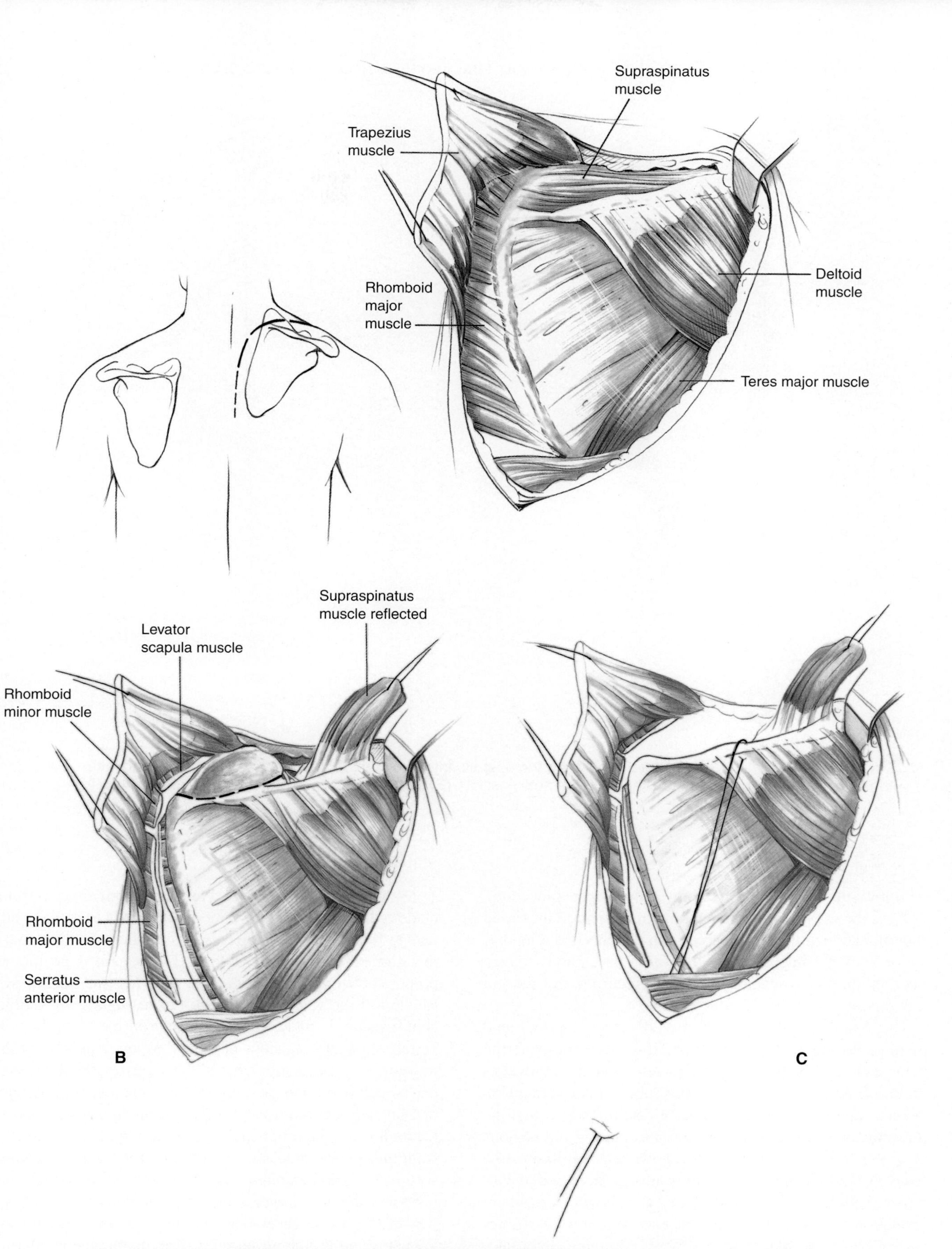

FIG. 21. Green's operation for Sprengel's deformity. **(A)** the incision is near the medial border of the scapula, and the trapezius is reflected from the spine of the scapula and retracted medially. **(B)** The rhomboid major and minor are detached from the insertion, the supraspinatus is reflected laterally in a supraperiosteal plane, and the superomedial angle is resected. **(C)** In Green's original description, wire is passed through the spine of the scapula, through the latissimus, and out of the skin for traction in a body cast. This step is frequently omitted today. (*continued*)

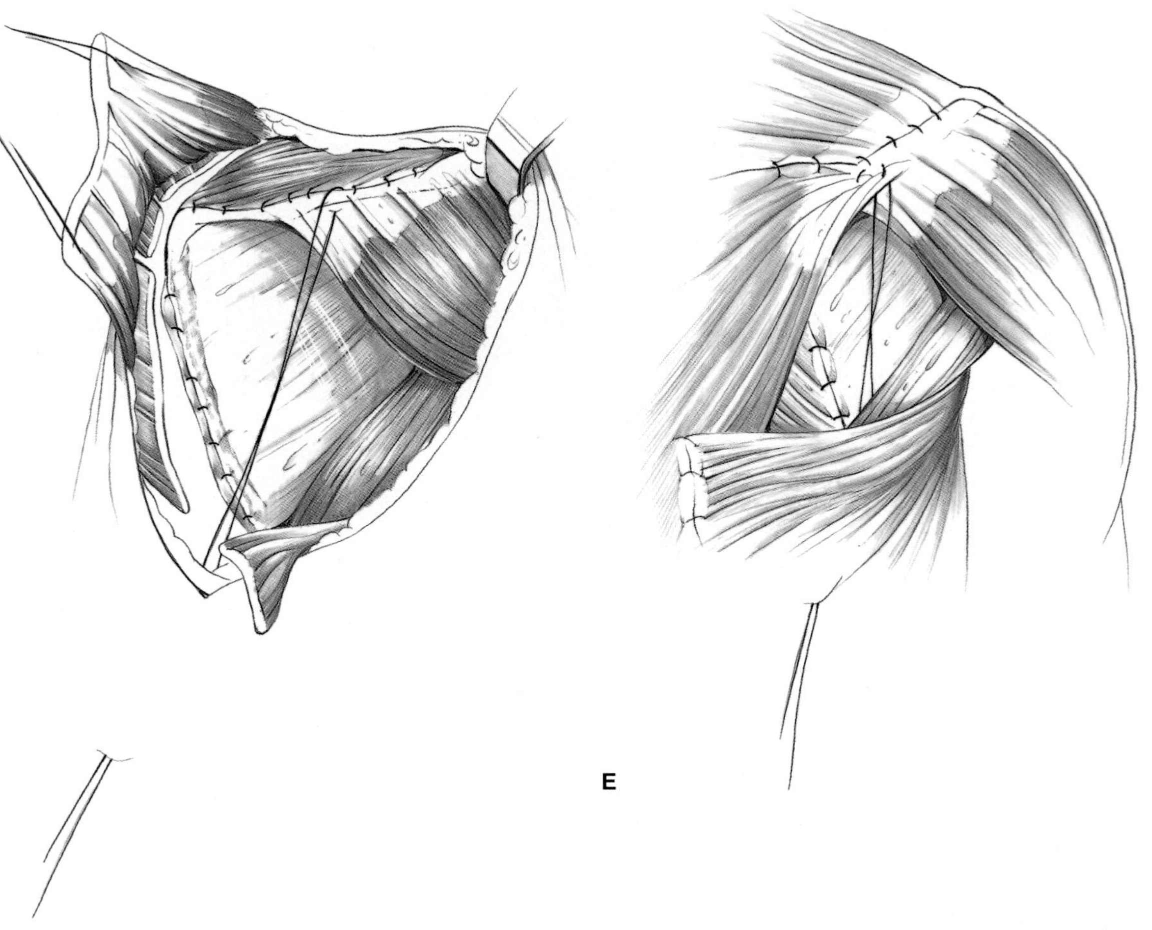

FIG. 21. *Continued* **(D)** After mobilizing the scapula inferiorly, the supraspinatus, rhomboids, and levator are reattached to the scapula in the new position. **(E)** The trapezius is reattached. (From ref. 54, with permission).

of follow-up after a modification of the Green procedure, without the use of the retaining wire, and reported increased shoulder abduction of 57 degrees. All patients had a moderate or dramatic improvement in appearance. The corrected malrotation of the scapula frequently recurred, but did not seem to influence shoulder motion.

The Woodward procedure[184] was described in 1961, and involves detaching the trapezius and rhomboid muscles from their spinous process origins, then resecting the omovertebral bone and any anterior curving supraspinatus extension of the scapula. The scapula is mobilized inferiorly, and the trapezius and rhomboids are sutured to more distal spinous processes (Fig. 22). Woodward described results in nine cases in 1961, with encouraging results in increased abduction and cosmesis.[184] Recent series have shown increases in abduction of 35 to 37 degrees, and excellent or good cosmesis in 80% to 90% of cases.[12,15,57,89,135] Although Green suggests his results are superior to those obtained by the Woodward procedure,[54] the Woodward procedure has become more popular.[57]

The Woodward procedure. Preoperative planning must include radiographs that are carefully analyzed to identify any defects in the posterior elements of the spine that might make the surgical exposure hazardous. The patient is positioned prone on the operating room table with the head resting on a Mayfield head rest, and the neck flexed slightly. A midline skin incision is made from the occiput to the tenth thoracic vertebrae. A subcutaneous plane is developed to identify the trapezius. At the inferior edge of the trapezius, the lower border is identified, and the trapezius is separated from the underlying latissimus muscle. Working from inferior to superior, the midline fascial origin of the trapezius is carefully dissected from the spinous processes with sharp dissection. As the dissection is carried cranially, the origins of the rhomboids and levator scapulae are released from the spinous processes as a part of the fascial sheet. The continuity of the origin of the trapezius and rhomboid muscles must be maintained during exposure, such that a secure caudal reattachment is possible.

After this exposure, the superomedial border of the scapula is evaluated, and any fibrous bands or omovertebral

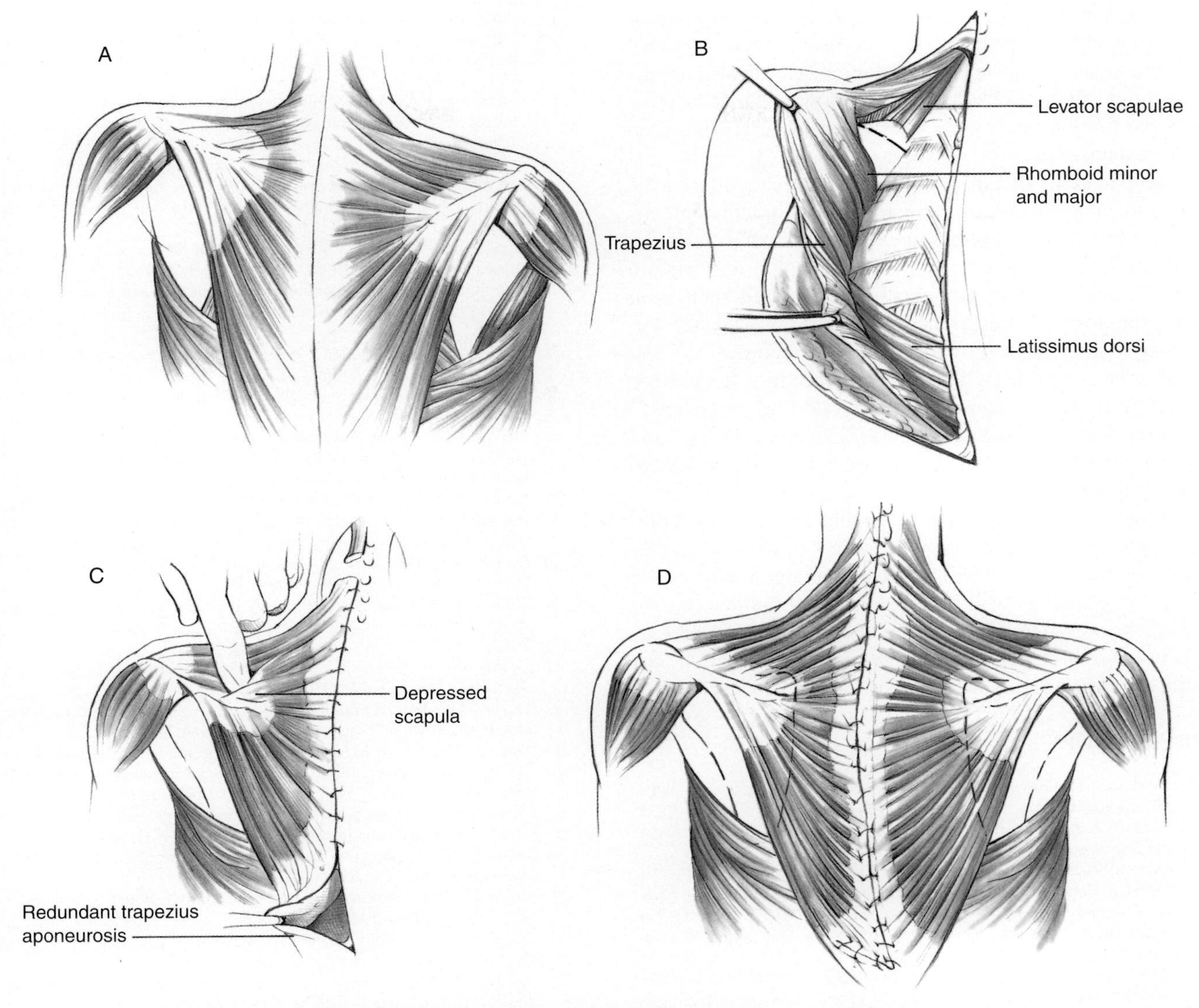

FIG. 22. Woodward procedure for Sprengel's deformity. **(A)** The trapezius origin is identified on the cervical and thoracic spine. **(B)** The trapezius, levator scapulae, and rhomboids are elevated as a flap from the cervical and thoracic spine, and bony or fibrous connections at the superomedial angle of the scapula are resected. **(C)** The scapula is mobilized distally, and the flap is sutured in its new position back to the cervical and thoracic spine. **(D)** Excess tissue is resected at the inferior margin of the flap. (From ref. 184 with permission).

bone is resected. Ideally, the omovertebral bone is resected extraperiosteally to prevent regrowth of bone. The spinal accessory nerve, which travels on the undersurface of the trapezius, must be protected. In addition, the transverse cervical artery, which passes posterior to the levator scapulae at its insertion on the superior angle of the scapula, must also be protected.

The deformed scapula is then assessed. If the superomedial border of the scapula is curved anteriorly or is enlarged, it is removed in an extraperiosteal fashion to prevent friction in the chest wall after transfer of the scapula. At this point, one may find a narrow portion of the trapezius that tethers the scapula to the spine above the fourth cervical vertebrae. This portion of the trapezius may be resected horizontally to mobilize the scapula.

After the scapula is free, it can be mobilized caudally, using traction on the aponeurosis. Because the undescended scapula is malformed, the inferior pole of the scapula is not a good reference for determining the caudal translation of the scapula. Instead, the scapular spines should be used. While the scapula is held in the desired position, the fibrous aponeurosis is sutured to the spinous processes from proximal to distal with heavy nonabsorbable suture. Distally, redundant trapezius tissue is released transversely and imbricated.

The subcutaneous tissues are closed, and then the skin is closed with a removable, nonabsorbable synthetic suture.

Because scar widening is common after the Woodward procedure, a tight subcuticular skin closure is recommended. Patients wear a Velpeau bandage for 2 weeks, then start passive range of motion of the glenohumeral joint. Active scapular motion can begin 6 weeks after surgery, with resistance exercises held for 12 weeks.

Complications of this procedure include traction on the brachial plexus creating a postoperative brachial plexus palsy, which has prompted some to recommend a clavicular osteotomy for patients with severe deformity, and when a great deal of scapular mobilization is required such as in older patients.[89,136] Recurrence of the deformity is typical in techniques that only excise the tethering structures,[12,139] and also has been reported with the Green procedure. Recurrence of deformity is very unusual in the Woodward procedure;[12] however, postoperative winging has been reported,[99,139] and as such preoperative winging may be a relative contraindication for the Woodward procedure.

Spengel's deformity, as a congenital abnormality represents one end of a spectrum of disorders of the scapulothoracic articulation. As with any other anatomic region of the body, congenital as well as acquired abnormalities can develop. As we improve in our understanding of the various conditions that affect the scapulothoracic articulation, our ability to treat patients with these disorders will improve.

REFERENCES

1. Anderson R, Flowers RS. Free grafts of the spinal accessory nerve during radical neck dissection. *Am J Surg* 1969;118:769–799.
2. Arntz CT, Matsen FA III. Partial scapulectomy for disabling scapulothoracic snapping. *Orthop Trans* 1990;14:252.
3. Aston JW. Brachial plexus birth palsy. *Orthopedics* 1979;2:594–601.
4. Ball CR. Paralysis following injection of antitetanic serum. Case report with serratus magnus involved. *US Naval Med Bull* 1939;37:305–309.
5. Bateman JE. *The shoulder and neck*, 2nd ed. Philadelphia: WB Saunders, 1978.
6. Bergmann G. Biomechanics and pathomechanics of the shoulder joint with reference to prosthetic joint replacement. In: Kibel R, et al., eds. *Shoulder replacement*. Berlin: Springer-Verlag, 1987.
7. Berkheiser EJ, Shapiro F. Alar scapula. Traumatic palsy of the serratus magnus. *JAMA* 1937;108:1790–1793.
8. Bigliani LU, Perez-Sanz JR, Wolfe IN. Treatment of trapezius paralysis. *J Bone Joint Surg [Am]* 1985;67:871–877.
9. Bizousky DT, Gillogly SD. Evaluation of the scapulothoracic articulation with arthroscopy. *Orthop Trans* 1992–1993;16:822.
10. Bocca E, Pignataro O. A conservation technique in radical neck surgery. *Ann Otol Rhinol Laryngol* 1967;76:975–978.
11. Boinet W. *Societe Imperiale de Chirurge* (2nd series) 1867;8:458.
12. Borges JLP, Shah A, Torres BC, Bowen JR. Modified Woodward procedure for Sprengel deformity of the shoulder: long-term results. *J Pediatr Orthop* 1996;16:508–513.
13. Butters KP. The scapula. In: Rockwood CA, Matsen FA, eds. *The shoulder*. Philadelphia: WB Saunders, 1990:335–366.
14. Cameron HU. Snapping scapulae. A report of three cases. *Eur J Rheumatol Inflamm* 1984;7:66–67.
15. Carson WG, Lovell WW, Whitesides TE Jr. Congential elevation of the scapula. Surgical correction by the Woodward procedure. *J Bone Joint Surg [Am]* 1981;63:1199–1207.
16. Cavendish ME. Congential elevation of the scapula. *J Bone Jont Surg [Br]* 1972:54;395–408.
17. Chavez JP. Pectoralis minor transplant for paralysis of the serratus anterior. *J Bone Joint Surg [Br]* 1951;33:228–230.
18. Ciullo JV and Jones E. Subscapular bursitis: conservative and endoscopic treatment of "snapping scapula" or "washboard syndrome." *Orthop Trans* 1992–1993;16:740.
19. Cobey MC. The rolling scapula. *Clin Orthop* 1968;60:193–194.
20. Codman EA. The anatomy of the human shoulder. In: Codman EA, ed. *The shoulder*, suppl ed. Malabar, FL: Kreiger Publishing, 1984: 1–31.
21. Cohen JA. Multiple congenital anomalies. The association of seven defects including multiple exostoses, Von Willebrand's disease, and bilateral winged scapula. *Arch Intern Med* 1972;129:972–974.
22. Compito CA, Duralde XA, Wolfe IN, Bigliani LU. Levator scapulae and rhomboid transfer for trapezius paralysis. Paper presented at the American Shoulder and Elbow Surgeons 10th open meeting, New Orleans, February 27, 1994.
23. Cooley LH, Torg JS. "Pseudowinging" of the scapula secondary to subscapular osteochondroma. *Clin Orthop* 1982;162:119–124.
24. Cuomo F, Blank K, Zuckerman JD, Present DA. Scapular osteochondroma presenting with exostosis bursata. *Bull Hosp Joint Dis* 1993;52: 55–58.
25. Danielsson LG, el-Haddad I. Winged scapula due to osteochondroma. *Acta Orthop Scand* 1989;60:728–729.
26. DeMarquay J. Exostosis of Rib. In: *Dictionaire de medicine et de chirugie pratique*, 1868.
27. DePalma AF. Shoulder-arm-hand pain of mesodermal, neurogenic, and vascular origin. In: DePalma AF, ed. *Surgery of the shoulder*, 3rd ed. Philadelphia: JB Lippincott, 1983:559–624.
28. Dewar FP, Harris RI. Restoration of function of the shoulder following paralysis of the trapezius by fascial sling fixation and transplantation of the levator scapulae. *Ann Surg* 1950; 132:1111–1115.
29. Dickson FD. Fascial transplants in paralytic and other conditions. *J Bone Joint Surg [Am]* 1937;19:405–412.
30. DiGiovine NM, Jobe FW, Pink M, Perry J. An electromyographic analysis of the upper extremity in pitching. *J Shoulder Elbow Surg* 1992;1:15–25.
31. Doddy SG, Waterland JC, Freedman L. Scapulohumeral goniomter. *Arch Phys Med Rehabil* 1970;51:711.
32. Dorling GC. Fascial slinging of the scapula and clavicle for dropped shoulder and winged scapula. *Br J Surg* 1944;32:311–315.
33. Duncan MA, Lotze MT, Gerber LH, Rosenberg SA. Incidence, recovery, and management of serratus anterior muscle palsy after axillary node dissection. *Phys Ther* 1983;63:1243–1247.
34. Dunn AW. Trapezius paralysis after minor surgical procedures in the posterior cervical triangle. *South Med J* 1974;67:312–315.
35. Durman DC. An operation for paralysis of the serratus anterior. *J Bone Joint Surg [Am]* 1945;27:380–382.
36. Eden R. Zur behandlung der trapeziuslahmung mittelst muskelplastick. *Dtsche Z Chir* 1924;184:387–389.
37. Engel D. The etiology of the undescended scapula and related syndromes. *J Bone Joint Surg [Am]* 1943;25:613–625
38. Eschner AA. Three cases of paralysis of the serratur magnus (anterior) muscle. *N Engl J Med* 1930;203:818–823.
39. Eulenberg. Beitrag zur dislocation der scapula. *Amlicht Dtsch Naturforsch Aerzte Karlsbad* 1863:37:291–294.
40. Fery A. Results of treatment of anterior serratus paralysis. In: Post M, Morrey BF, Hawkins RJ, eds. *Surgery of the shoulder*. St Louis: CV Mosby, 1990:325–329.
41. Fiddian NJ, King RJ. The winged scapula. *Clin Orthop*. 1984;185: 228–236.
42. Fishchenko PI. Paraliticheskaia scapula vara v sochetanii s zadnim podvyvikhom plecha. *Ortop Travmatol Prot* 1967;28(9):66–68.
43. Fitchet SM. Injury of the serratus magnus (anterior) muscle. *N Engl J Med* 1930;303:818–823.
44. Foo CL, Swann M. Isolated paralysis of the serratus anterior. *J Bone Joint Surg [Br]* 1983;65:552–556.
45. Foucar HO. The "clover leaf" sling in paralysis of the serratus magnus. *Br Med J* 1933;2:865–866.
46. Freedman L, Munro RH. Abduction of the arm in scapular plane: scapular and glenohumeral movements. *J Bone Joint Surg [Am]* 1966; 18:1503.
47. Galpin RD, Birch JG. Congential elevation of the scapula (Sprengel's deformity). *Orthopedics* 1987;10:965–970.
48. Gillogly SD, Bizouski DT. Arthroscopic evaluation of the scapulothoracic articulation. *Orthop Trans* 1992–1993;16:196.
49. Glousman R, Jobe FW, Tibone J, Moynes P, Antonelli D, Perry J. Dynamic electromyographic analysis of the throwing shoulder with glenohumeral instability. *J Bone Joint Surg [Am]* 1988;70:220–226.
50. Goldner JL. Tendon transfers about the shoulder for irreparable nerve injuries in children and adults. *Orthop Trans* 1977;1:115.

51. Goodman CE, Kenrick MM, Blum MV. Long thoracic nerve palsy: a follow-up study. *Arch Phys Med Rehabil* 1975;56:352–355.
52. Gorres H. Ein fall von schmerzhaften skapularkrachen durch operation geheilt. *Dtsch Med Wchnschr* 1921;472:897–898.
53. Gozna ER, Harris WR. Traumatic winging of the scapula. *J Bone Joint Surg [Am]* 1979;61:1230–1233.
54. Green WT. Sprengel's deformity: congenital elevation of the scapula. *AAOS Instr Course Lectr* 1972:11:55–72.
55. Gregg JR, Labosky D, Harty M. Serratus anterior paralysis in the young athlete. *J Bone Joint Surg [Am]* 1979;61:825–832.
56. Groves J, Goldner JL. Contracture of the deltoid muscle in the adult after intramuscular injections. *J Bone Joint Surg [Am]* 1974;56:817–820.
57. Grogan DP, Stanley EA, Bobechko WP. The congenital undescended scapula. Surgical correction by the Woodward procedure. *J Bone Joint Surg [Br]* 1983;65:598–605.
58. Grunfeld G. Beitrag zur genese des skapularkrachens und der skapulargerausche. *Arch Orthop J Unfall Chir* 1927;24:610–615.
59. Hamner DL, Hall JE. Sprengel's deformity associated with multidirectional shoulder instability. *J Pediatr Orthop* 1995; 15:641–643.
60. Harris HH, Dickey JR. Nerve grafting to restore function of the trapezius muscle after radical neck dissection. (A preliminary report). *Ann Otol Rhinol Laryngol* 1965;74:880–886.
61. Hass J. Muskelplastik bei serratuslahmung (ersatz des gelahmten musculus serratus anterior durch den muculus teres major). *Z Orthop Chir* 1931;55:617–622.
62. Hauser CU, Martin WF. Two additional causes of traumatic winged scapula occuring in the armed forces. *JAMA* 1943;121:667–668.
63. Hawkins RJ, Bokor DJ. Clinical evaluation of shoulder problems. In: Rockwood CA, Matsen FA, eds. *The shoulder*. Philadelphia: WB Saunders, 1990:149–177.
64. Hawkins RJ, Willis RB, Litchfield RB. Scapulothoracic arthrodesis for scapular winging. In: Post M, Morrey BF, Hawkins RJ, eds. *Surgery of the shoulder*. St Louis: CV Mosby, 1990:356–359.
65. Hayes JM, Zehr DJ. Traumatic muscle avulsion causing winging of the scapula. *J Bone Joint Surg [Am]* 1981;63:495–497.
66. Henry AK. An operation for slinging a dropped shoulder. *Br J Surg* 1927;15:95–98.
67. Herzmark MH. Traumatic paralysis of the serratus anterior relieved by transplantation of the rhomboidei. *J Bone Joint Surg [Am]* 1951;33: 235–238.
68. Hirasawa Y, Sakakida K. Sports and peripheral nerve injury. *Am J Sports Med* 1983;11:420–426.
69. Hoaglund FT, Duthie RB. Surgical reconstruction for shoulder pain after radical neck dissection. *Am J Surg* 1966;112:522–526.
70. Hollinshead WH. The back and limbs. In: Hollinshead WH, ed. *Anatomy for surgeons*, 3rd ed. vol 3. Philadelpia: Harper & Row, 1982.
71. Hollinshead WH. *Textbook of anatomy*. New York: Harper & Row, 1953.
72. Honey PR, Leffert RD. Operative treatment of isolated trapezius paralysis. *Orthop Trans* 1992–1993;16:761.
73. Horan FT, Bonafede RP. Bilateral absence of trapezius and sternal head of pectoralis major muscles. *J Bone Joint Surg [Am]* 1977;59:133.
74. Horowitz AE. Congential elevation of the scapula—Sprengel's deformity. *Am J Orthop Surg* 1908;6;260–311
75. Horowitz MT, Tocantins LM. An anatomic study of the role of the long thoracic nerve and the related scapular bursae in the pathogenesis of local paralysis of the serratus anterior muscle. *Anat Rec* 1938; 71:375–385.
76. Horowitz T. Isolated paralysis of the serratus anterior muscle. *Am J Orthop Surg* 1959;1:100.
77. Iceton J, Harris WR. Results of pectoralis major transfer for winged scapula. *J Bone Joint Surg [Br]* 1987;69B:108–110.
78. Ilfeld FW, Holder HG. Winged scapula: case occurring in soldier from knapsack. *JAMA* 1942;120:448–449.
79. Jeannopoulos CL. Congenital elevation of the scapula. *J Bone Joint Surg [Am]* 1952;34:883–892.
80. Jeannopoulos CL. Observations on congential elevation of the scapula. *Clin Orthop* 1961;20:132–137
81. Johnson JTH, Kendall HO. Isolated paralysis of the serratus anterior muscle. *J Bone Joint Surg [Am]* 1955;37:563–574.
82. Kauppila LI. Iatrogenic serratus anterior paralysis. Long term outcome in 26 patients. *Chest* 1996;109:31–34.
83. Kauppila LI. The long thoracic nerve: possible mechanisms of injury based on autopsy study. *J Shoulder Elbow Surg* 1993;2:244–248.
84. Kessel L. *Clinical disorders of the shoulder*. Edinburgh: Churchill Livingstone, 1982.
85. Ketenjian AY. Scapulocostal stabilization for scapular winging in fascioscapulohumeral muscular dystrophy. *J Bone Joint Surg [Am]* 1978; 60:476–480.
86. Kibler WB. Role of the scapula in the overhead throwing motion. *Contemp Orthop* 1991;22:525–532.
87. Kibler WB, Chandler TJ, Uhl T. Functional scapular instability in throwing athletes. *Orthop Trans* 1990;10:240.
88. Kibler WB, Shapiro RL, and Chandler TJ. Posterior shoulder muscle firing patterns in tennis players. AOSSM Interim Meeting, New Orleans, 1990.
89. Klisic P, Filipovic M, Uzelac O, Milinkovic Z. Relocation of congenitally elevated scapula. *J Pediatr Orthop*1981;1:43–45.
90. Kolodychuk LB, Regan WD. Visualization of the scapulothoracic articulation using an arthroscope: a proposed technique. *Orthop Trans* 1993–1994;17:1142.
91. Kouvalchouk JF. Subscapular crepitus. *Orthop Trans* 1985;9: 587–588.
92. Lange M. Die behandlung der irrepairablem trapeziuslahmung. *Langenbeks Arch Klin Chir* 1951;270:437–439.
93. Lange M. Die operative behandlung der irrepairablem tapeziuslahmung. *Tip Fakult Mecmausi* 1959;22:137–141.
94. Langenskiold A, Ryoppy S. Treatment of paralysis of the trapezius muscle by the Eden-Lange operation. *Acta Orthop Scand* 1973;44: 383–388.
95. Laumann U. Kinesiology of the shoulder joint. In: Kolbel R, et al., eds. *Shoulder replacement*. Berlin: Springer-Verlag, 1987.
96. Leffert RD. Pectoralis major transfers for serratus anterior paralysis. *Orthop Trans* 1992–1993;16:761.
97. Leffert RD. Neurological problems. In: Rockwood CA, Matsen FA, eds. *The shoulder*, vol 2. Philadelphia: WB Saunders, 1990:750–773.
98. Leffert RD. Nerve injuries about the shoulder. In: Rowe CR, ed. *The shoulder*. New York: Churchill Livingstone, 1988:435–454.
99. Leibovic SJ, Ehrlich MG, Zaleske DJ. Sprengel deformity. *J Bone Joint Surg [Am]* 1990;72:192–197.
100. Levin SE, Trummer MJ. Agenesis of the serratus anterior muscle. A cause of winged scapula. *JAMA* 1973;225:748.
101. Lynch AF, Fogarty EE, Dowling FE, Regan BF. Pseudowinging of the scapula due to osteochondroma. *J Pediatr Orthop* 1985; 5:722–724.
102. Makin GJ, Brown WF, Ebers GC. C7 radiculopathy: Importance of scapular winging in clinical diagnosis. *J Neurol Neurosurg Psychiatry* 1986;49:640–644.
103. Marmor L, Bechtol CO. Paralysis of the serratus anterior due to electrical shock relieved by transplantation of the pectoralis major muscle. A case report. *J Bone Joint Surg [Am]* 1983;45:156–160.
104. Matthews LS, Poehling GC, Hunter DM. Scapulothoracic endoscopy: anatomical and clinical considerations. In: McGinty JB, Caspari RB, Jackson RW, Poehling GG, eds. *Operative arthroscopy*, 2nd ed. Philadelphia: Lippincott-Raven 1996:813–820.
105. Mauclaire M. Craquements sous-scapulaires pathologiques traites par l'interposition musculaire interscapulo-thoracique. *Bull Mem Soc Chir Paris* 1904;30:164–168.
106. Mayer H. Trapeziuslahmung nach operativer behandlung tuberkuloser halslymphorusen. *Munch Med Woschenschr* 1953;95:170–172.
107. McCluskey GM III, Bigliani LU. Scapulothoracic disorders. In: Andrews JR, Wilk KE, eds. *The athlete's shoulder*. New York: Churchill Livingstone, 1994:305–316.
108. McCluskey GM III, Bigliani LU. Surgical management of refractory scapulothoracic bursitis. *Orthop Trans* 1991;15:801.
109. Mendoza FX, Main K. Peripheral nerve injuries of the shoulder in the athlete. *Clin Sports Med* 1990;9:331–342.
110. Meythaler JM, Reddy NM, Mitz M. Serratus anterior disruption: a complication of rheumatoid arthritis. *Arch Phys Med Rehabil* 1986; 67:770–772.
111. Michele A, Davies JJ, Krueger FJ, Lichtor JM. Scapulocostal syndrome (fatigue-postural paradox). *NY J Med* 1950;50:1353–1356.
112. Milch H. Snapping scapula. *Clin Orthop* 1961;20:139–150.
113. Milch H. Partial scapulectomy for snapping scapula. *J Bone Joint Surg [Am]* 1950;32:561–566.
114. Milch H, Burman MS. Snapping scapula and humerus varus: report of six cases. *Arch Surg* 1933;26:570–588.
115. Minami M, Yamazaki J, Minami A, Ishii S. A postoperative long-term study of the deltoid contracture in children. *J Pediatr Orthop* 1984;4: 609–613.

116. Morse BJ, Ebrahem NA, Jackson WT. Partial scapulectomy for snapping scapula syndrome. *Orthop Rev* 1993;22:1141–1144.
117. Moseley HF. *Shoulder lesions*, 2nd ed. New York: Hocher Publishing, 1933.
118. Moseley JB, Jobe FW, Pink M, Tibone J. EMG analysis of the scapular muscles during a shoulder rehabilitation program. *Am J Sports Med* 1992;20:128–134.
119. Neer CS II. Less frequent procedures. In: Neer CS II, ed. *Shoulder reconstruction*. Philadelphia: WB Saunders 1990:421–485.
120. Norden A. Peripheral injuries to the spinal accessory nerve. *Acta Chir Scand* 1946;94:515–532.
121. Olarte M, Adams D. Accessory nerve palsy. *J Neurol Neruosurg Psychiatry* 1977;40:1113–1116.
122. Overpeck DO, Ghormley RK. Paralysis of the serratus magnus muscle caused by lesions of the long thoracic nerve. *JAMA* 1940;114: 1994–1996.
123. Paine RM. The role of the scapula in the shoulder. In: Andrews JR, Wilk KE, eds. *The athlete's shoulder*. New York: Churchill Livingstone, 1994:495–512.
124. Parsonage MJ, Turner JWA. Neuralic amyotrophy. The shoulder-girdle syndrome. *Lancet* 1948;1:973–978.
125. Parsons TA. The snapping scapula and subscapular exostoses. *J Bone Joint Surg [Br]* 1973;55B:345–349.
126. Percy EL, Birbrager D, Pitt MJ. Snapping scapula: a review of the literature and presentation of 14 patients. *Can J Surg* 1988;31:248–250.
127. Pianka G, Hershman EB. Neurovascular injuries. In: Nicholas JA, Hershman EB, eds. *The upper extremity in sports medicine*. St Louis: CV Mosby, 1990:691–722.
128. Pinsky HA, Pizzutlillo PD, MacEwen GD. Congential elevation of the scapula. *Orthop Trans* 1980;4:288.
129. Post M. Pectoralis major transfer for winging of the scapula. *J Shoulder Elbow Surg* 1995;4:1–9.
130. Post M. Orthopaedic management of neuromuscular disorders. In: Post M, ed. *The shoulder, surgical and non-surgical management*. Philadelphia: Lea & Febiger, 1978:159–191.
131. Potts CS. Isolated paralysis of the serratus magnus: report of a case. *Arch Neurol Psychiatry* 1928;20:184–186.
132. Prescott MU, Zollinger RW. Alar scapula an unusual surgical complication. *Am J Surg* 1944;65:98–103.
133. Radin EL. Peripheral neuritis as a complication of infectious mononucleosis: report of a case. *J Bone Joint Surg [Am]* 1967; 59:535–538.
134. Rapp IH. Serratus anterior paralysis treated by transplantation of the pectoralis minor. *J Bone Joint Surg [Am]* 1954;36:852–854.
135. Richards RR, McKee MD. Treatment of painful scapulothoracic crepitus by resection of the superomedial angle of the scapula. *Clin Orthop* 1989;247:111–116.
136. Robinson PA, Braun RM, Mack P, Zadek R. The surgical importance of the clavicular component of Sprengel's deformity. *J Bone Joint Surg [Am]* 1967;49:1481.
137. Roy PH, Bearhs OH. Spinal accessory nerve in radical neck dissections. *Am J Surg* 1969;118:800–804.
138. Roldan R, Warren D. Abduction deformity of the shoulder secondary to fibrosis of the central portion of the deltoid muscle. In: Proceedings of the American Academy of Orthopaedic Surgeons. *J Bone Joint Surg [Am]* 1972;54:1332.
139. Ross DM, Cruess RL. The surgical correction of congenital elevation of the scapula. A review of seventy-seven cases. *Clin Orthop* 1977;125:17–23.
140. Rowe CR. Unusual shoulder conditions. In: Rowe CR, ed. *The shoulder*. New York: Churchill Livingstone, 1988:639–654.
141. Rowe CR, Pierce DS, Clark DG. Voluntary dislocation of the shoulder. *J Bone Joint Surg [Am]* 1973;55:445–460.
142. Saeed MA, Gatens PF Jr, Signh S. Winging of the scapula. *Am Fam Physician* 1981;24:139–143.
143. Saha AK. Mechanism of shoulder movements and a plea for the recognition of "zero position" of the glenohumeral joint. *Clin Orthop* 1983; 173:3–10.
144. Samilson RL Miller E. Posterior dislocation of the shoulder. *Clin Orthop* 1964;32:69–86.
145. Samter O. Sur le traitment operatoire de la paralysie du grand dentele. *J Chir* 1930;35:299.
146. Scaglietti O. The obstetrical shoulder trauma. *Surg Gynecol Obstet* 1938;66:868–877.
147. Schar W, Zweifel C. Das os acromiale und seine klinische bedeutung. *Bruns' Beitr Klin Chir* 1936;164:101–124.
148. Schrock RD. Congential elevation of the scapula. *J Bone Joint Surg* 1926;8:207–215
149. Schulze-Gocht M. Uber den trapeziusdefekt. Zugleich ein beitrag zur frage der skoliosenentstehung. *Arch Orthop Unfall Chir* 1928;26: 302–307.
150. Selden BR. Congenital absence of trapezius and rhomboideus major muscles. *J Bone Joint Surg* 1935;17:1058–1059.
151. Shogry ME and Armstrong P. Case report 630: reactive bursa formation surrounding an osteochondroma. *Skeletal Radiol* 1990;19: 465–467.
152. Shull JR. Scapulocostal syndrome: clinical aspects. *South Med J* 1969; 62:956–959.
153. Sisto DJ, Jobe FW. The operative treatment of scapulothoracic bursitis in professional pitchers. *Am J Sports Med* 1986;14:192–194.
154. Skillern PG. Serratus magnus palsy with proposal of a new operation for intractable cases. *Ann Surg* 1913;57:909–915.
155. Skolnik EM, Yee KF, Friedman M, Golden TA. The posterior triangle in radical neck surgery. *Arch Otolaryngol* 1976;102:1–4.
156. Smith AD. Congenital elevation of the scapula. *Arch Surg* 1941;42: 529–536.
157. Spira E. The treatment of the dropped shoulder. A new operative technique. *J Bone Joint Surg [Am]* 1948;30:229–233.
158. Sprengel: Die angeborne Berxhiebung des Schulterblattes nach Oben. *Arch Klin Chir* 1891 42:545
160. Ssoson-Jaroschewitsch JA. Uber skapularkrachen. *Arch Klin Chir* 1923;123:378.
161. Steindler A. Reconstruction of the poliomyelitic upper extremity. *Bull Hosp Joint Dis* 1954;15:21–26.
162. Steindler A. *Traumatic deformities and disabilities of the upper extremity*. Springfield, Il: Charles C Thomas, 1946:112–118.
163. Steindler A: *Kinesiology of the human body under normal and pathological conditions*. Springfield, IL: Charles C Thomas, 1955.
164. Steinmann SP, Higgins DL, Sewell D, Anderson C. Nonparalytic winging of the scapula. Poster presented at 61st annual AAOS meeting, New Orleans, February 25, 1994.
165. Strizak AM, Cowen MH. The snapping scapula syndrome. *J Bone Joint Surg [Am]* 1982;64A:941–942.
166. Sunderland S. *Nerves and nerve injuries*, 2nd ed. New York: Churchill-Livingstone, 1978.
167. Tamai K, Ogawa K. Intratendinous tear of the supraspinatus tendon exhibiting winging of the scapula. *Clin Orthop* 1985; 194:159–163.
168. Torok G. Scapulopexy. In: Proceedings of the Israeli Orthopaedic Society. *J Bone Joint Surg [Br]* 1963;45:806.
169. Tubby AH. A case illustrating the operative treatment of paralysis of the serratus magnus by muscle grafting. *Br Med J* 1904;2: 1159–1160.
170. Vastamaki M, Kauppila LI. Etiologic factors in isolated paralysis of the serratus anterior muscle: a report of 197 cases. *J Shoulder Elbow Surg* 1993;2:240–243.
171. Volkmann J. Uber sogenannte skapularkrachen. *Klin Wochnschr* 922; 37:1838–1839.
172. Von Gruber W. Die bursae mucosae der inneren aschselwand. *Arch Anat Physiol Wiss Med* 1864; 358–366.
173. Von Luschka H. Uber ein costo-scaplular-gelenk des menschen. Vierteljahrsschr Prakt Heilkd 1870;107:51–57.
174. Walker PS. *Human joints and their artificial replacements*. Springfield, IL: Charles C Thomas, 1977.
175. Warner JJP, Micheli LJ, Arslanian LE, Kennedy J, Kennedy R. Scapulothoracic motion in normal shoulders and shoulders with glenohumeral instability and impingement syndrome. A study using Moire topographic analysis. *Clin Orthop* 1992;285:191–199.
176. Weeks LE. Scapular winging due to serratus anterior avulsion fracture. *Orthop Trans* 1993;17:184.
177. Whitman A. A congenital elevation of scapula and paralysis of serratus magnus muscle; operation. *JAMA* 1932;99:1332–1334.
178. Willit A, Walsham WJ. An account of the dissection of the parts removed after death from the body of a woman, the subject of congenital malformation of the spinal column, bony thorax, and left scapular. *Arch Proc R Med Chir Soc Lond* 1880:8:503–506.
179. Wolbrink AJ, Hsu Z, Bianco AJ. Abduction contracture of the shoulders and hips secondary to fibrous bands. *J Bone Joint Surg [Am]* 1973;55:844–846.
180. Wolfe J. The conservative treatment of serratus palsy. *J Bone Joint Surg [Am]* 1941;23:959–961.

181. Wood VE, Marchinski L. Congenital anomalies of the shoulder. In: Rockwood CA, Matsen FA, eds. *The shoulder*. Philadelphia: WB Saunders, 1990:98–148.
182. Wood VE, Verska JM. The snapping scapula in association with the thoracic outlet syndrome. *Arch Surg* 1989;124:1335–1337.
183. Woodhall B. Trapezius paralysis following minor surgical procedures in the posterior cervical triangle. Results following cranial nerve suture. *Ann Surg* 1952;136:375–380.
184. Woodward JW. Congenital elevation of the scapula. Correction by release and transplantation of muscle origins. A preliminary report. *J Bone Joint Surg [Am]* 1961;43:219–228.
185. Wright PE and Simmons JCH. Peripheral nerve injuries. In: Edmonson AS, Crenshaw AH, eds. *Campell's operative orthopaedics*, 6th ed, vol 2. St Louis: CV Mosby, 1980:1642–1702.
186. Wright YA. Accessory spinal nerve injury. *Clin Orthop* 1975;108: 15–18.
187. Zeier FG. Treatment of winged scapula. *Clin Orthop* 1973;91: 128–133.

Disorders of the Shoulder: Diagnosis and Management,
edited by Joseph P. Iannotti and Gerald R. Williams, Jr.
Lippincott Williams & Wilkins, Philadelphia © 1999.

CHAPTER 30

Injuries of the Brachial Plexus

Scott H. Kozin

SURGICAL ANATOMY

The origin of the brachial plexus is from the fifth through eighth cervical (C5 through C8) and the first thoracic (T1) spinal nerves.[64,95] Small contributions may originate from the fourth cervical (C4) and second thoracic (T2) nerves. The dorsal and ventral rootlets (six to eight rootlets per level) exit the spinal cord, merge to form the spinal nerves, which leave the intervertebral foramina, and quickly divide into dorsal and ventral rami (Fig. 1). The small dorsal rami travel posterior to innervate the skin and muscles of the neck and upper back and are not part of the brachial plexus. The ventral rami emerge between the anterior and middle scalene muscles and are designated as the nerve roots of the brachial plexus (Fig. 2). The upper roots (C5 through C8) descend toward the first rib, whereas the lower T1 root must ascend

S. H. Kozin: Department of Orthopaedic Surgery, Temple University School of Medicine and Shriner's Hospital for Children, Philadelphia, Pennsylvania 19115.

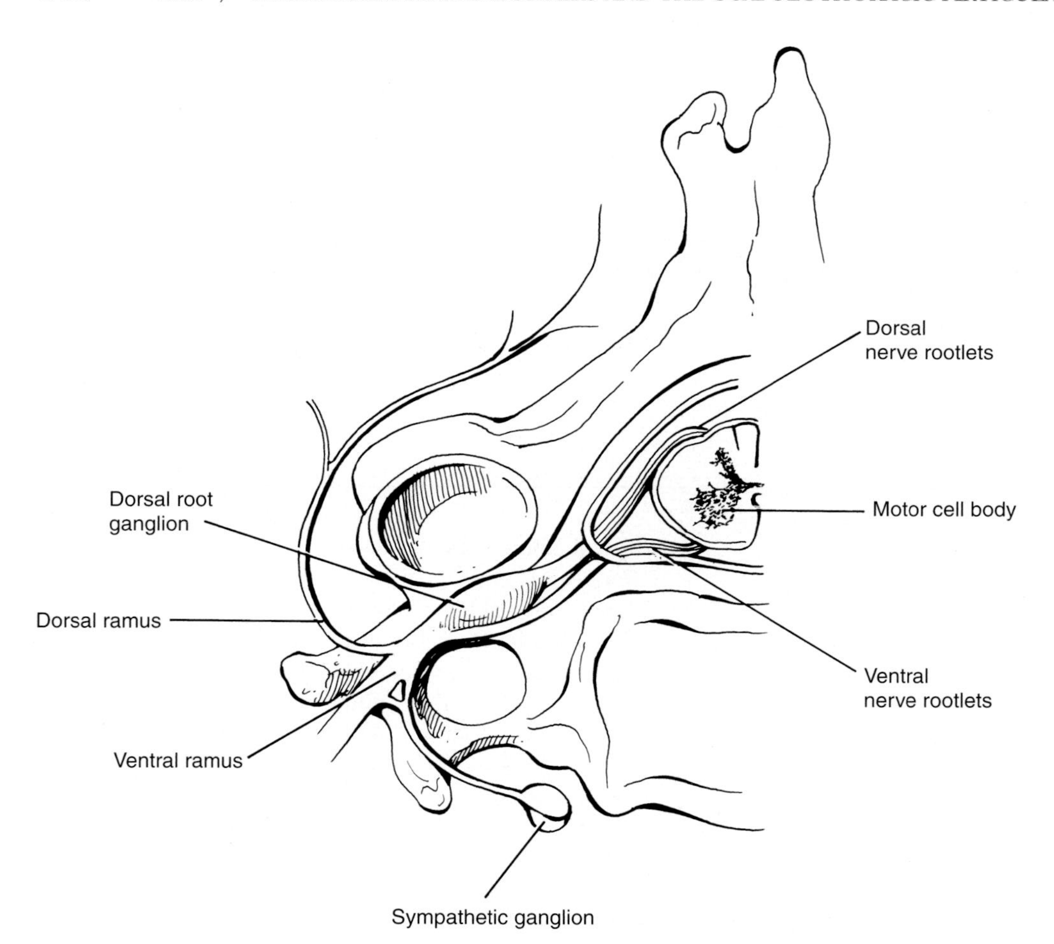

FIG. 1. Artist schematic of spinal cord with motor and sensory (dorsal root ganglion) cell bodies.

over the first rib to form the brachial plexus. Sympathetic fibers join the nerve roots as they traverse between the scalene muscles. C5 and C6 receive fibers from the middle sympathetic cervical ganglion, and C7, C8, and T1 acquire fibers from the cervicothoracic ganglion. These sympathetic fibers control blood-vessel smooth-muscle contraction (vasoconstriction) and sweat gland activity.

The motor cell bodies of the nerve roots for the brachial plexus are located within the ventral horn of the spinal cord gray matter (see Fig. 1). In contrast, the sensory cell bodies are positioned outside the spinal cord within the dorsal root ganglia. The dorsal root ganglia transfer afferent fibers to the spinal cord through the dorsal rootlets. The knowledge of the difference in anatomic location of cell bodies between motor and sensory fibers is important for the accurate diagnosis and treatment of proximal brachial plexus injuries.

The ventral rami of C5 and C6 combine to form the superior trunk, the C7 ramus continues alone as the middle trunk, and C8 and T1 unite to form the lower trunk (see Fig. 2). The trunks are located in the posterior triangle of the neck, enclosed by the posterior border of the sternocleidomastoid muscle, anterior border of the upper trapezius, and clavicle. The spinal accessory nerve (cranial nerve XI) crosses the posterior triangle to innervate the trapezius muscle. This nerve divides the posterior triangle into nearly equivalent upper and lower parts. The lower portion of the triangle contains the brachial plexus, with the upper and middle trunks superior to the omohyoid muscle and the lower trunk inferior. Each trunk divides into anterior and posterior divisions and proceeds behind the clavicle. The divisions then merge into three cords named in relation to the axillary artery. The anterior divisions of the upper and middle trunks combine to form the lateral cord. The three posterior divisions converge to form the posterior cord and the anterior division of the inferior trunk continues as the medial cord.

The cords proceed behind the pectoralis minor muscle into the axilla and divide into two terminal branches (Fig. 3). The lateral cord terminates as the musculocutaneous nerve and a branch to the median nerve. The musculocutaneous nerve perforates and supplies the coracobrachialis muscle and then becomes the principal motor nerve of the flexor compartment of the arm. The posterior cord divides into the axillary and radial nerves. At the level of the glenohumeral joint, the axillary nerve, along with the posterior humeral circumflex vessels, travels inferior to the subscapularis muscle and across the upper border of the teres major to enter the quadrangular space for innervation of the deltoid and teres minor muscles. Compression of the nerve or artery can occur at the quadrangular space from hypertrophy or anomalies of the bordering muscles. The radial nerve is the largest branch of

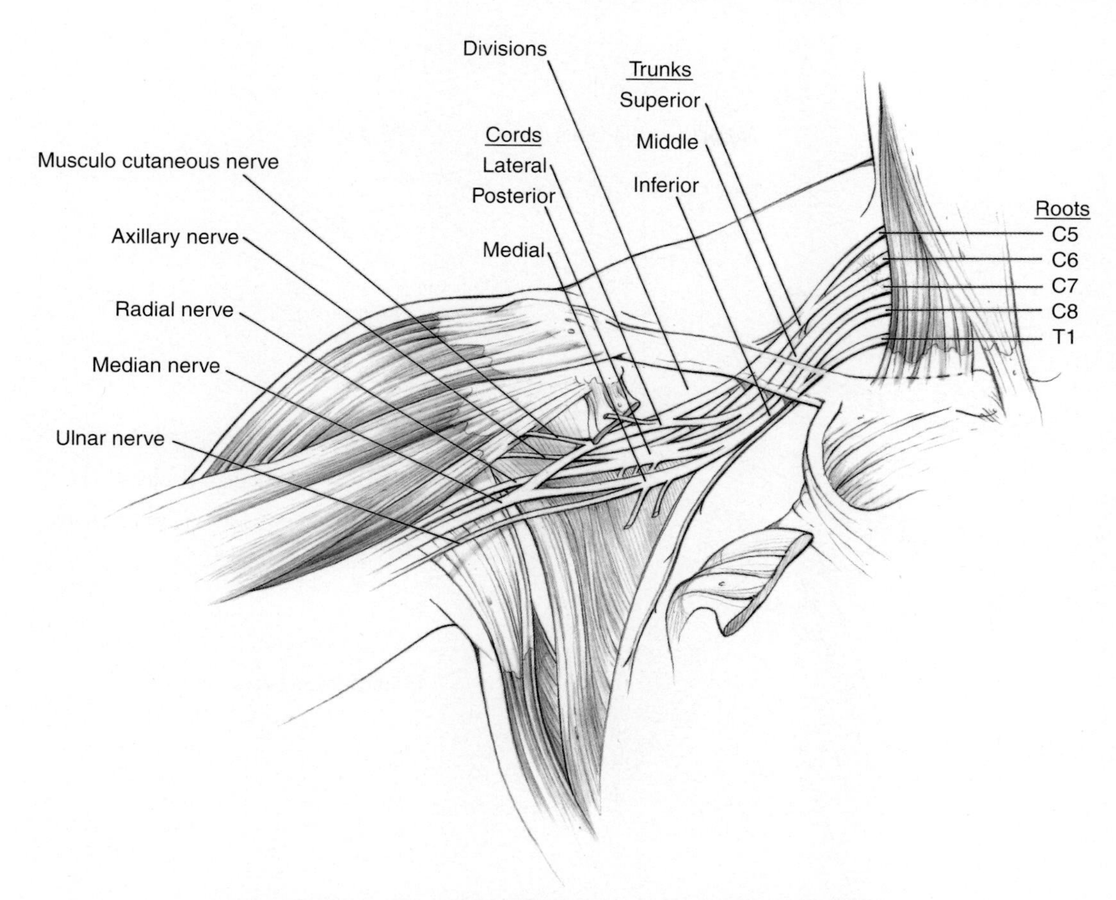

FIG. 2. Artist schematic of brachial plexus from roots to branches.

the brachial plexus and passes inferior to the teres major muscle to enter the posterior arm between the long head of the triceps and humerus. The medial cord continues as the ulnar nerve and a branch to the median nerve. The ulnar nerve travels down the arm medial to the brachial artery, pierces the medial intermuscular septum, and enters the cubital tunnel. The median nerve forms anterior to the axillary artery from the union of the medial and lateral cord branches and descends into the arm.

Several branches arise from the roots, trunks, and cords of the brachial plexus (see Fig. 2). The status of these intermediate nerves provide valuable information for the location of nerve injury and subsequent treatment algorithm. At the root level, the dorsal scapular nerve arises from C5, pierces the middle scalene to enter the posterior triangle of the neck, and innervates the levator scapulae and rhomboid muscles. The long thoracic nerve arises from C5, C6, and C7 just distal to the intervertebral foramina and travels behind the brachial plexus along the chest wall to supply the serratus anterior muscle. The phrenic nerve originates at the root level from C3, C4, and C5 and crosses the anterior scalene muscle to enter the thorax. This nerve may be injured in nerve root injuries, with subsequent hemidiaphragm paralysis.

At the trunk level, the suprascapular nerve arises from the superior trunk to travel across the posterior cervical triangle to the suprascapular notch. The suprascapular nerve advances through this notch to innervate the supraspinatus and infraspinatus muscles. The nerve to the subclavius arises from anterior surface of the upper trunk and descends anterior to the brachial plexus to innervate the subclavius muscle.

There are no branches from the plexus at the division level. At the cord level, multiple branches are present. From the lateral cord, the lateral pectoral nerve arises to pass anterior to the axillary artery, to perforate the clavipectoral fascia, and to innervate the clavicular part of the pectoralis major. The posterior cord supplies three branches: the upper subscapular, thoracodorsal, and lower subscapular nerves. The upper subscapular nerve innervates the upper portion of the subscapularis muscle, and the lower section is supplied by the lower subscapular nerve, which also innervates the teres major muscle. The thoracodorsal nerve originates between the upper and lower subscapular nerves, passes behind the axillary artery, and supplies the latissimus dorsi muscle. The medial cord provides one motor and two sensory branches. The medial pectoral nerve traverses and innervates the pectoralis minor muscle and then continues to supply the sternocostal portion of the pectoralis major muscle. The medial brachial and medial antebrachial cutaneous nerves are the only sensory branches to arise directly from the plexus and supply the arm and forearm, respectively.

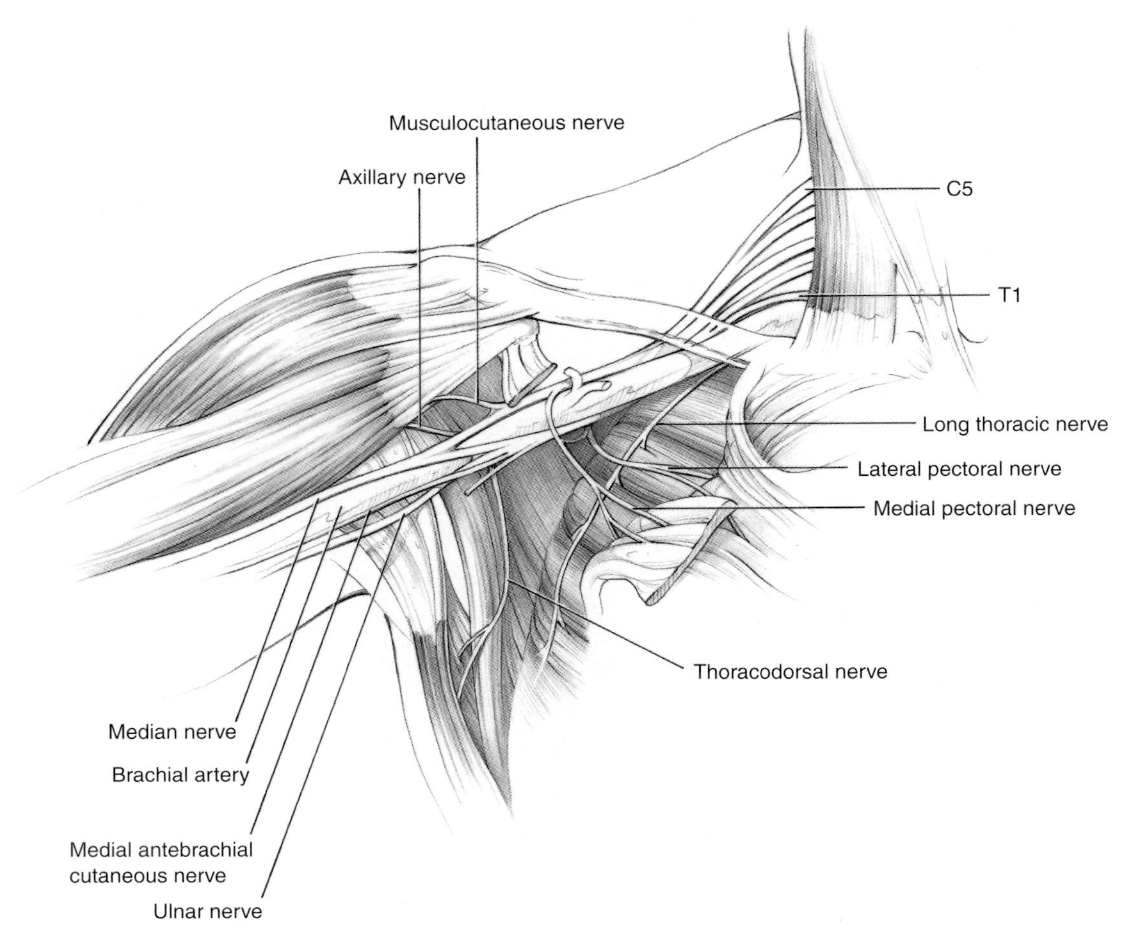

FIG. 3. Artist schematic of brachial plexus behind the clavicle pectoralis minor muscle.

The vascular anatomy of the brachial plexus centers around the subclavian and axillary vessels. The subclavian artery originates from the arch of the aorta on the left side and from the brachiocephalic artery on the right. The subclavian artery ascends over the first rib to reside between the anterior and middle scalene muscles, with the roots and trunks of the brachial plexus. In contrast, the subclavian vein is located anterior to the anterior scalene muscle. The subclavian vessels cross the first rib and become the axillary vessels with the vein medial to the artery. The axillary vessels pass behind the pectoralis minor muscle to enter the axilla. Beyond the axilla, the axillary vessels become the brachial vessels.

There is variability and asymmetry in the neural and vascular anatomy of the brachial plexus.[64,94,139] The plexus is termed *prefixed* when there is a relatively large contribution from C4 and a small allotment from T1. Similarly, a *postfixed* plexus has substantial contribution from T2 with little from C5. There are also variations in cord separation and peripheral branchings of nerves that may or may not affect segmental innervation. Branches may occasionally arise from divisions that usually originate from trunks or cords. In addition, the lateral cord may provide a branch to the ulnar nerve. The vascular relation to the plexus can be altered, with the axillary artery or vein shifted in position or even piercing a nerve.[85] The subclavian vein can travel with the artery and brachial plexus posterior to the anterior scalene muscle.[96] These anomalies should be considered when clinical, diagnostic, and surgical findings do not correspond.

Thoracic Outlet Anatomy

The thoracic outlet begins just distal to the intervertebral foramina and extends to the coracoid process. The outlet is surrounded by anatomic constraints that encompass the brachial plexus and associated vessels (subclavian and axillary). These structures include muscles (anterior and middle scalene muscles), skeleton (first rib, cervical ribs, clavicle, and coracoid), and fascia or fibrous bands. The most common sites of compression in thoracic outlet syndrome are at the superior thoracic outlet, the scalene interval or triangle, the costoclavicular space, or the subcoracoid area (Fig. 4; Table 1).[6,98,106,114] This compression can be static or dynamic with dependence on posture and activity.[74]

The superior thoracic outlet is bordered anteriorly by the sternum, laterally by the first rib, and posteriorly by the thoracic vertebrae.[147] The inferior trunk must ascend from the intervertebral foramina to navigate over the first rib. A post-

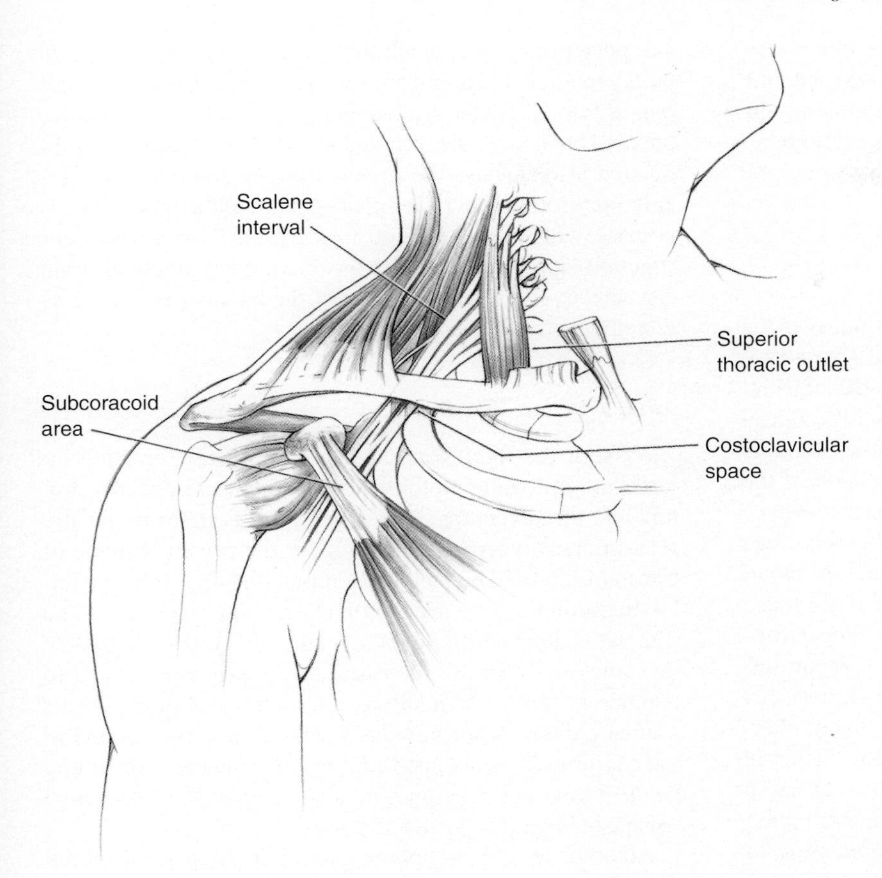

FIG. 4. Artist schematic of thoracic outlet compression sites.

fixed brachial plexus must climb even higher to exit from the thorax. The inferior trunk can be compressed or stretched over the first rib in this area.

The scalene triangle is formed by the anterior and middle scalene attachments on the first rib. These muscles originate from similar transverse processes of the upper and middle cervical vertebrae and diverge to their insertion sites. The triangle formed has a narrow base (approximately 1 to 2 cm) and elongated sides.[33, 66,106] The upper roots (C5 through C7) descend, whereas the inferior roots (C8 and T1) and subclavian artery must ascend to pass through the scalene triangle. The presence of a cervical rib or a fibrous band extending from an incomplete cervical rib to the first rib can reduce the dimensions of the triangle by elevation of its base. This forces the inferior roots and subclavian artery to further ascend to enter the scalene triangle. The incidence of cervical ribs is 0.5% to 1% of individuals, and they are present bilaterally 50% to 80% of the time.[6,74,105,127] The width of the scalene triangle can be narrowed by anterior or middle scalene muscle abnormalities, which can precipitate thoracic outlet compression.[33,60,134]

The costoclavicular interval is between the clavicle and first rib. Depression of the clavicle reduces this space and can compress the brachial plexus and subclavian or axillary vessels. A hypertrophied subclavius muscle or a clavicle with abundant callus formation can narrow the costoclavicular space. The subclavian vein is susceptible to compression between the subclavius muscle and clavicle.

The subcoracoid area can produce compression on the neurovascular structures of the brachial plexus, for the coracoid provides a fulcrum as the arm is abducted and externally rotated. Excessive arm elevation can cause a traction or compressive neuropathy along the coracoid process.[131] The pectoralis minor and conjoined (biceps brachia and coracobrachialis) tendon prevents slippage of the plexus from behind the coracoid.

TABLE 1. *Sites of compression in thoracic outlet syndrome*

Site	Principal cause
Superior thoracic outlet	First rib or cervical rib
Scalene interval or triangle	Scalene muscles or fibrous bands
Costoclavicular space	Narrow clavicle–first rib distance
Subcoracoid area	Coracoid process

PATHOPHYSIOLOGY

Brachial plexus injuries can affect a wide range of individuals from newborns to the elderly. Obstetric brachial plexus palsy can occur during passage through the birth canal, whereas adolescent and adult injury may be secondary to domestic violence, vehicular trauma, athletic endeavors, or systemic disease. The etiologies can be divided into trauma (penetrating and nonpenetrating), entrapment, and infection (Table 2). There are other less common etiologies of brachial plexopathy related to tumors, neuropathies, and iatrogenic causes.[6,53,59]

Nonpenetrating Trauma

Nonpenetrating trauma is the leading cause of injury to the brachial plexus. The mechanism of injury in almost all injuries is traction that produces tension across the brachial plexus.[131] The mechanism by which the traction is produced is variable and may be from traction to the extremity, forcible head rotation from the shoulder, or direct depression of the shoulder girdle.[131] With traction injuries, there is a stretch of the nerve beyond the physiologic limits that the nerve can withstand. There is a direct reduction of intraneural blood flow with increasing strain. A 15% elongation will reduce blood flow approximately 80% to 100%.[27,76,145] The extrinsic vascular system (longitudinal vessels in the epineurium) appears to be more susceptible to stretch than the intrinsic circulation (endoneurial vascular network).[67] Continued elongation will cause overt ischemia and disruption of nerve metabolism. Persisted traction will ultimately disrupt nerve continuity. Therefore, traction can cause nerve injury ranging from a temporary disruption in nerve fiber conduction to functional discontinuity of the nerve fibers and sheath.

Various factors affect the portion of the plexus or nerve involved and the extent of injury incurred. These determinants include the magnitude and duration of the force applied and the position of the extremity and head at time of accident.[131] The upper roots (C5 through C8) and trunks descend beneath the clavicle, whereas the lower root (T1) ascends over the first rib to form the lower trunk. The cords (medial, lateral, and posterior) pass beneath the coracoid, which can act as a pulley to direct the application of force. Therefore, the upper plexus is taut with the arm dangling at the side, and the lower plexus is taut with the arm abducted and elevated. Arm abduction also elevates the coracoid pulley and places preferential tension on the lower plexus. The middle portion (C7) is tense with lateral traction to the arm. Disruptive forces (traction) applied in line with the direction of maximal strain can selectively disrupt portions of the brachial plexus or be disseminated throughout the plexus.

TABLE 2. *Etiology of brachial plexus injuries*

Trauma
Nonpenetrating (traction)
Penetrating (knife, GSW)
Nerve entrapment
Thoracic outlet syndrome
Infection
Viral plexopathy (Parsonage-Turner syndrome)
Radiation
Fibrosis
Malignant degeneration after radiation
Tumors
Primary (schwannomas or neurofibromas)
Secondary (pulmonary apices)
Neuropathies
Iatrogenic
Axillary or scalene anesthesia
Surgical biopsy
Intraoperative positioning
Median sternotomy
Inadvertent traction

Adult Traction Injuries

Most of the significant adult brachial plexus traction injuries are following motor vehicle accidents, especially motorcycle misadventures.[92,117] The injury is more frequently seen in areas where motorcycles are the principal mode of transportation.[23] The incidence of brachial plexus injury following a motorcycle accident has been approximated to be 2%, with a prevalence in young males.[92,94] Interestingly, the incidence has recently increased and is probably related to mandatory helmet regulations and better transportation of trauma patients who previously would have succumbed to their injuries.[93] Associated injuries are common, including head trauma and fractures or dislocations of the cervical spine, shoulder, forearm, and hand.[92,117]

Automobile, bicycle, sporting, and pedestrian accidents are much less common causes of brachial plexus injuries, as are shoulder dislocations or fractures (proximal humerus, clavicle). Minor stretch injuries (burners, stingers) of the plexus are common in contact sports, especially football, because tackling drives the shoulder downward and forcibly flexes the neck toward the contralateral side.[56] The athlete experiences a burning pain and paresthesia that radiates from the supraclavicular area into the arm. Transient weakness and sensory abnormalities are present. The vast majority of burners are upper plexus traction injuries and occur without neck pain or restricted neck mobility. The symptoms and signs of these stretch injuries usually resolve spontaneously over a few minutes. However, a cervical spine fracture–dislocation or a severe brachial plexus injury can occur during impact, with subsequent quadriplegia or a permanent neurologic deficit. These injuries will have persistent weakness and limited neck motion. An extensive diagnostic evaluation similar to other nonpenetrating brachial plexus injuries is warranted in these cases.

Shoulder dislocations are often related to sporting accidents and can produce nerve injuries of the axillary, suprascapular, or musculocutaneous nerves. These are usually (80% of the time) temporary lesions that resolve over 4 to 6 months (80%).[4] However, violent high-energy trauma can cause disruption of nerve fiber integrity at the time of dislocation.

Obstetric Traction Injuries

Traction injures can occur during birth and are associated with difficult deliveries. The reported incidence has varied from 0.4 to 2.5 palsies per 1,000 live births.[29,51] Traction to the head with forceful tilting from the fixed shoulder (lateral neck flexion) during delivery can stretch the upper plexus.[45,84,126] Brachial plexus injuries have been recreated in stillborns by traction applied to a restrained shoulder.[84] Injury can also transpire during breech presentation as the lower roots are stretched during hyperabduction of the ipsilateral arm during delivery.

Penetrating Trauma

Penetrating trauma to the brachial plexus is often secondary to gunshot wounds or stabbings. Gunshot wounds occur at time of war and during domestic violence.[69,100] Bullet injuries act as projectile missiles that cause neural injury by means of a blast effect or less commonly direct nerve transection.[14,69,100] The shock wave (temporary cavity) reverberates causing a variable degree of nerve injury. The extent of blast correlates with the deformation, fragmentation, orientation, and velocity of the bullet. In contrast, stab wounds transect portions of the plexus or cause vascular injury with secondary nerve compression by expanding hematoma.[14,37] Most commonly, the upper and midplexus are involved, for the clavicle protects the lower elements.[37]

Thoracic Outlet Syndrome

The diagnosis of thoracic outlet syndrome is controversial and more common when surgeons are convinced this is a valid entity.[6,17] The etiology is presumed to be a compressive neuropathy of the brachial plexus because neurologic symptoms predominate in virtually all (94 to 97%) cases, with preferential involvement of the lower plexus. Venous and arterial thoracic outlet syndromes are much less common, appearing in 2% to 3% and 1% to 2%, respectively.[6,98] The potential sites of compression (see Table 1) are described in the preceding anatomy section. These anatomic sites are normally not problematic unless additional factors are present that initiate the compressive neuropathy. For example, shoulder muscle atrophy and loss of strength can depress the entire limb and cause the inferior trunk to be compressed or strained at the superior thoracic outlet against the first rib. Further narrowing of the costoclavicular space can occur from downward pressure on the shoulder girdle from heavy backpacks or pendulous breasts.[57,74] A preceding minor or major trauma may result in fibrosis and scarring of the thoracic outlet, which can directly compress the plexus and cause symptoms.[6,41,120] In predisposed persons, repetitive motion may play a factor, although this remains speculative.[80,118]

Irrespective of the pathologic site, intermittent compression will cause temporary alterations in nerve physiology that reverse following removal of the compression. Persistent nerve compression will cause intraneural edema and alteration of the blood supply, which results in diminished axonal transport to the pinched nerve. The initial nerve response is segmental demyelination, but prolonged ischemia will cause wallerian degeneration.[6,97,106] The degree of pathology is proportional to the intensity and duration of the entrapment pressure.

Arterial signs and symptoms can be induced by compression along the thoracic outlet. Pressure can be from the tip of a cervical rib, a fibrous band, or costoclavicular narrowing. Subclavian or axillary artery stenosis, with poststenotic dilation, can occur. This can advance to mural thrombus formation, emboli, and distal ischemia.[6]

Infection

Infection is an uncommon cause of brachial plexopathy, and the exact etiology remains enigmatic, with both viral pathogens and secondary immunologic factors proposed as possibilities. This brachial neuritis, also known as Parsonage-Turner syndrome, presents with acute onset of intense pain about the shoulder girdle without antecedent trauma.[103] Weakness of the muscles innervated by the affected nerves develops after the initial pain response. The suprascapular or long thoracic nerve is the most commonly affected (Fig. 5). Electromyographic abnormalities of the denervated muscles are apparent 3 to 4 weeks after the initial pain response, with positive sharp waves and fibrillation potentials. The treatment is conservative management with observation and serial examinations. The natural history of brachial neuritis is resolution of the pain followed by improvement in motor function. However, prolonged recovery time and persistent weakness is not uncommon years after the brachial neuritis.[56,79,90,136]

CLASSIFICATION OF BRACHIAL PLEXUS INJURY

The lesion in brachial plexus injury is classified according to the anatomic location and extent of nerve involvement. Supraclavicular lesions affect the roots, trunks, and divi-

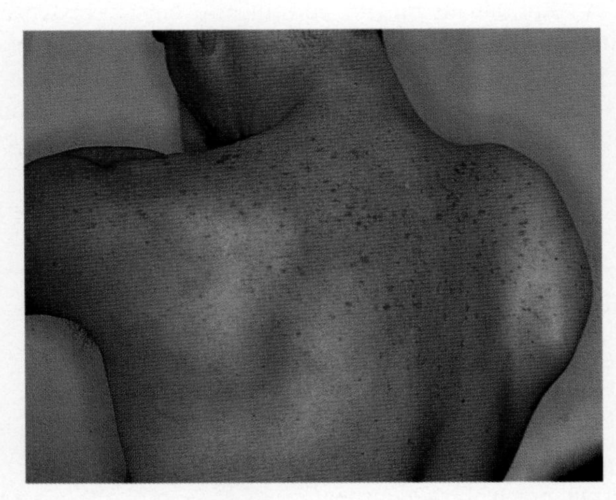

FIG. 5. A 20-year-old man who awoke with intense shoulder pain and subsequent scapula winging from isolated long thoracic nerve involvement in Parsonage-Turner syndrome.

sions, whereas infraclavicular injuries involve the cords and branches. The supraclavicular injury from traction can disrupt the rootlet connection with the spinal cord and is called an *avulsion* injury. This weak linkage along the brachial plexus is susceptible to traction injury. An avulsion separates the motor cell body in the spinal cord from its axons, but the sensory cell body located in the dorsal root ganglion remains connected to its axons (see Fig. 1). Therefore, the motor portion of the nerve undergoes wallerian degeneration, with degradation of the axons and myelin sheaths. The sensory fibers are spared from wallerian degeneration, but have been irrevocably detached from the spinal cord. The injury will cause a clinical motor and sensory loss, whereas electrodiagnostic studies will reveal abnormal motor findings with intact sensory conduction. Rarely, the rupture can effect only the motor or sensory rootlets.

The injury can also interrupt nerve continuity at the trunk level and is called a *rupture*. Ruptures of the plexus separate both motor and sensory cell bodies from their axons and wallerian degeneration occurs across all fibers. The differentiation between avulsion and rupture is a decisive element in the treatment algorithm of brachial plexus traction injuries. Discontinuity by rupture can be treated by various surgical techniques to reestablish nerve continuity, whereas avulsion injuries are irreparable. The diagnosis can be difficult, for traction can cause a combination of rupture and avulsion injuries at different levels, which will complicate accurate diagnosis.

Supraclavicular lesions account for most brachial plexus injuries (approximately 75%) and are also subdivided into groups according to the pattern of involvement (Table 3).[5,89]

The Erb-Duchenne palsy involves C5 and C6, or the upper trunk, and is characterized by loss of elbow flexion, and weakness of shoulder abduction and external rotation.[36,42] Sensory deficit is apparent in the corresponding dermatome (radial side of forearm and thumb). A C7 injury can accompany an Erb's palsy (extended upper brachial plexus lesion) and adds paralysis of elbow extension, wrist extension (extensor carpi radialis brevis), and finger extension (extensor digitorum communis and propius). The Dejerine-Klumpke palsy involves C8 and T1, or lower trunk, and is characterized by absent intrinsic hand musculature and finger flexors (flexor digitorum profundus and superficialis) with intact shoulder, elbow, and wrist function.[70] Sensory deficit is situated over the ulnar side of the forearm and hand. This isolated lower plexus palsy is uncommon in both adults and children.[45,55] The injury can include the entire plexus (C5, C6, C7, C8, and T1), which causes a flail and anesthetic arm.

TABLE 3. *Patterns of brachial plexus injuries*

Pattern	Roots involved
1. Upper brachial plexus (Erb-Duchenne)	C5 and C6
2. Extended upper brachial plexus	C5, C6, and C7
3. Lower brachial plexus (Dejerine-Klumpke)	C8 and T1
4. Total brachial plexus lesion	C5, C6, C7, C8 and T1
5. Peripheral brachial plexus lesion	Variable

Supraclavicular lesions can also be isolated to peripheral branches, such as the suprascapular or long thoracic nerve. This can be secondary to trauma, infection, surgical positioning, or iatrogenic.

Infraclavicular lesions are less common (approximately 25%) and usually represent stretch injuries from an associated shoulder dislocation or fracture.[4] These injuries represent peripheral nerve lesions of the plexus. The axillary nerve is particularly susceptible to traction because it is securely anchored as it traverses the quadrangular space. However, injury to the musculocutaneous nerve and other elements of the brachial plexus can occur after severe trauma.

Supraclavicular and infraclavicular nerve injuries can also be characterized by the degree of intraneural damage, irrespective of the location of injury and extent of plexus involvement. The gradation of nerve injury begins with neuropraxia, extends to axonotmesis, and culminates in neurotmesis.[121] A *neuropraxia* is a segmental demyelination with maintenance of intact nerve fibers and axonal sheath. A temporary conduction block follows, without axonal damage and wallerian degeneration.[17] Complete recovery occurs over the ensuing days to weeks as remyelinization is completed. An *axonotmesis* is a disruption of nerve fiber integrity with preservation of the axonal sheath and framework. Wallerian degeneration and nerve fiber regeneration are necessary for recovery. Wallerian degeneration is characterized by the proliferation of Schwann cells that phagocytose myelin and axon debris. The axons distal to the injury degrade from lack of nutrition and loss of blood supply. The regeneration rate is approximately 1 mm/day or 1 in./ month. This slow regeneration delays recovery and means that distal nerve injuries have a better prognosis because the extent of wallerian degeneration is decreased and the proximity to the motor endplates is increased. In addition, prolonged denervation of longer than 18 to 24 months results in irreversible motor endplate degradation and muscle fibrosis. In contrast, the encapsulated sensory receptors retain their capacity for reinnervation for many years. These factors make the prognosis for axonotmesis variable and guarded.

A *neurotmesis* is a disruption of the nerve fiber and axonal sheath. Transection is the classic example of this injury, but severe traction or contusion can produce a similar injury with irreversible intraneural scarring. The prognosis is bleak without surgical resection of the intervening scar and nerve coaptation by direct repair or graft interposition to allow for nerve regeneration. A severe brachial plexus injury often represents a combined lesion, with elements of neuropraxia, axonotmesis, and neurotmesis. This combination injury further complicates accurate diagnosis and predictions for recovery.

EVALUATION OF BRACHIAL PLEXUS INJURY

The clinical evaluation of the patient with a brachial plexus injury begins with a careful history and detailed examination. The examination should include the head and neck, thorax, injured extremity, and neurovascular systems. A knowledge of brachial plexus anatomy and concomitant muscle innervation is a prerequisite to accurate diagnosis. A thorough physical examination is the foundation that will dictate the treatment algorithm. Imaging studies and electrodiagnostic tests provide supplemental information to further clarify the extent of injury. The goal of this evaluation is to precisely define the location and extent of nerve injury. This information will direct treatment, which may range from continued observation to prompt surgical intervention.

Evaluation of Adult Brachial Plexus Injury

Adult brachial plexus injuries are usually not evaluated acutely, but rather referred after treatment of any life-threat-

TABLE 4. *Brachial plexus examination sheet*

Muscle tested	R	L	R	L	R	L
Trapezius (C3,C4,XI)						
Levator scapulae (C3,C4,C5)						
Rhomboids (C4,C5)						
Supraspinatous (C5,C6)						
Infraspinatous (C5,C6)						
Serratus anterior (C5,C6,C7)						
Teres major (C5,C6)						
Subscapularis (C5,C6)						
Pectoralis major clavicle (C5,C6,C7)						
Pectoralis maj. sternocostal (C6,C7,C8,T1)						
Latissimus dorsi (C6,C7,C8)						
Biceps and brachialis (C5,C6)						
Deltoid (C5,C6)						
Teres minor (C5,C6)						
Pronator quadratus (C7,C8,T1)						
Pronator teres (C6,C7)						
Flexor carpi radialis (C6,C7)						
Flexor digitorum profundus II,III (C7,C8,T1)						
Flexor digitorum superficialis (C7,C8,T1)						
Flexor pollicis longus (C7,C8,T1)						
Abductor pollicis brevis (C6,C7,C8,T1)						
Opponens pollicis (C8,T1)						
Lumbricals (C8,T1)						
Triceps (C6,C7,C8)						
Supinator (C5,C6)						
Brachioradialis (C5,C6)						
Extensor carpi radialis longus (C6,C7)						
Extensor carpi radialis brevis (C6,C7,C8)						
Extensor carpi ulnaris (C7,C8)						
Extensor digitorum communis (C7,C8)						
Extensor digiti minimi (C7,C8)						
Extensor indicis (C7,C8)						
Extensor pollicis longus (C7,C8)						
Extensor pollicis brevis (C6,C7)						
Abductor pollicis longus (C6,C7)						
Flexor carpi ulnaris (C7,C8,T1)						
Flexor digitorum prof. IV,V (C7,C8,T1)						
Abductor digiti minimi (C8,T1)						
Abductor pollicis (C8,T1)						
Opponens digiti (C8,T1)						
Interossei (C8,T1)						

Muscle grading chart

Muscle grade	Description
5, Normal	Full range of motion against gravity with full resistance
4, Good	Full range of motion against gravity with some resistance
3, Fair	Full range of motion against gravity
2, Poor	Full range of motion with gravity eliminated
1, Trace	Slight contraction without joint motion
0, Zero	No evidence of contraction

ening injuries. An inquiry into the mechanism of injury and degree of energy involved is important. The force applied (direction, magnitude, and duration), position of extremity, and concomitant injuries (fractures, dislocations, visceral damage, head trauma, and vascular disruptions) are important details. Unfortunately, the particulars of the accident are often obscured by loss of consciousness, associated injuries, or amnesia.[94] In sharp penetrating trauma, the timing of neurologic deficit is important. An instantaneous deficit implies nerve laceration, whereas a delayed onset indicates a compressive neuropathy by an expanding hematoma or false aneurysm.[14,37] Important past medical history includes overall general health before the accident, time interval from injury, hand dominance, occupation, and hobbies.

The physical examination of the adult patient begins with observation. The posture of the extremity and the manner by which the patient uses the extremity are important indicators of the segment of the brachial plexus involved. The motor and sensory deficits determined by the physical examination should be correlated with the ancillary studies to define the extent and pattern of injury to the plexus. The basis of the examination is to perform a detailed examination to determine the specific motor and sensory deficits. An inventory of the muscles innervated by the brachial plexus is imperative to accurately define the injury and provides a baseline to assess recovery. Physical findings should be recorded on a data sheet, including gradation of muscle strength according to the international muscle scoring system, and the presence or absence of sensory deficits (Table 4).[2] This documentation method eliminates inadvertent omission of important elements of the examination and allows serial examinations to be performed by different individuals.

Careful examination of the muscles innervated by the proximal branches from the brachial plexus will help define the proximity of the plexus lesion to the spinal cord (Table 5). Disruption of the dorsal rami (paraspinal muscles), dorsal scapular (rhomboids and levator scapulae), and long thoracic (serratus anterior) nerves are suggestive of an avulsion injury. The presence of a Horner's syndrome results in a drooped eyelid, constricted pupil, sunken globe, and sweating deficiency that usually implies an avulsion injury at C8 and T1 (Fig. 6). However, the false-positive response rate for a Horner's syndrome is 10% and the false-negative figure is 28%.[54] Percussion of the supra- and infraclavicular plexus is performed. A Tinel's sign is indicative of a postganglionic injury (e.g., rupture), for this sign will be absent in a preganglionic lesion (e.g., avulsion) because the link to the spinal cord and brain has been disrupted.

Postganglionic injuries are further localized by examination of the intermediate and terminal branches. The status of the suprascapular (spinati), thoracodorsal (latissimus dorsi), subscapular (subscapularis and teres major), pectoral (pectoralis major and minor) will further define the injury. Examination of the pectoralis major muscle is particularly helpful because of its dual segmental innervation from the lateral pectoral (C5, C6, C7) and medial pectoral (C8, T1) nerves from the lateral and medial cords, respectively. Selective atrophy of the clavicular head (lateral pectoral) or sternocostal head (medial pectoral) facilitates diagnosis, whereas complete atrophy implies a global injury. A peripheral vascular examination is a fundamental component of the evaluation,

TABLE 5. *Indicators of avulsion injuries and poor prognosis for recovery*

Finding	Implication
Denervation paraspinal muscles	Dorsal rami injury
Denervation rhomboid muscles	Dorsal scapular (C5) injury
Scapular winging	Long thoracic (C5,C7,C8) injury
Horner's syndrome	Cervicothoracic sympathetic injury
Absent Tinel's sign	Preganglionic separation from cord
Sensory impairment neck	Cervical plexus injury
Hemidiaphragm paralysis	Phrenic nerve injury
Cervical transverse process fx	Avulsion fracture with root injury
Pseudomeningocele	Dura and arachnoid avulsion injury
Anesthesia and intact CV	Dorsal ganglion intact, but avulsion from cord

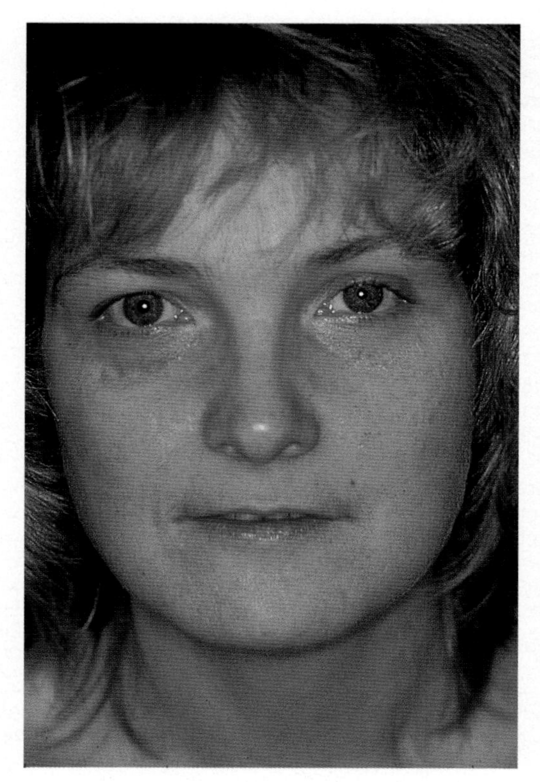

FIG. 6. A 30-year-old woman involved in a motor vehicle accident with avulsions of C8, T1 and ruptures of C5, C6, C7. Persistent subtle left Horner's syndrome years after injury.

for damage to the axillary or subclavian vessels can occur. Decreased or absent peripheral pulses, a delayed neurologic deficit (expanding hematoma), and penetrating trauma warrant arteriography.[14,37,43,132]

Evaluation of Obstetric Brachial Plexus Palsy

In obstetric brachial plexus palsy, the history is extremely important. Prenatal, postnatal, and birth information should be obtained. Risk factors for an obstetric palsy include a difficult or prolonged delivery, large birth weight, shoulder dystocia, breech presentation, and forceps or vacuum extraction.[29,42,70,45,73] Inquiry into the duration of labor, method of delivery, use of forceps or vacuum extraction, fractures of the clavicle or humerus, Horner's syndrome, postnatal position of extremity, and initial extent of involvement is required. A caesarean delivery does not negate the possibility of brachial plexus injury.[29,73] In fact, bilateral plexus injuries can occur after caesarean section.[73]

The physical examination of the newborn with obstetric brachial plexus palsy is difficult because of lack of cooperation. Observation of the affected extremity often provides valuable information of the underlying pathology. Upper root (C5, C6) or trunk injuries (Erb's palsy) present with a typical posture of shoulder adduction and internal rotation, elbow extension, forearm proration, wrist flexion, and finger flexion (Fig. 7). A completely flaccid extremity is the posture in a total plexus palsy. Isolated lower root (C8, T1) or trunk injuries (Klumpke's palsy) are rare in obstetric injuries. When present, there is normal posture of the shoulder and elbow, with paralysis of the hand's intrinsic muscles.[29,55] The presence of a Horner's syndrome (ptosis, meiosis, enophthalmos, and ipsilateral facial anhydrosis) is an important observation that implies proximal avulsion injury of the lower trunk, with disruption of the communicating branch supplying sympathetic fibers to the cervicothoracic ganglion.

Palpation of the clavicle and shoulder girdle may reveal crepitation or abundant callus formation. An acute fracture will inhibit voluntary movement and mimic brachial plexus injuries (pseudoparalysis). In addition, the passive shoulder range of motion should be assessed to exclude a posterior dislocation. A newborn with a brachial plexus injury will have full passive motion, whereas a congenital shoulder dislocation will lack passive motion.[38] Ultrasound may be required to confirm this diagnosis because the newborn humeral head is not calcified.

The assessment of motor function in the newborn or infant is a challenging task that requires patience and diligence. The initial goal is to determine the absence or presence of function, for actual grading of muscle strength is impossible. The newborn can be aroused by the startle reaction or Moro reflex. This should produce extensor tone in the legs and arms. The grasp reaction by palmar stimulation should illicit finger flexion. Absence of these primitive reflexes indicates a neurologic problem. In the infant, a collection of toys, rattles, and sweets is necessary to incite movement of the injured extremity. The effect of gravity can be altered by changing the position of the child to assess weak but functioning muscle. Gross motor function for shoulder movement, elbow motion, wrist action, and digital movement is delineated. Sensory function is also difficult to assess, for the only reaction obtained may be to painful stimuli, which will erase any chance of further cooperation.

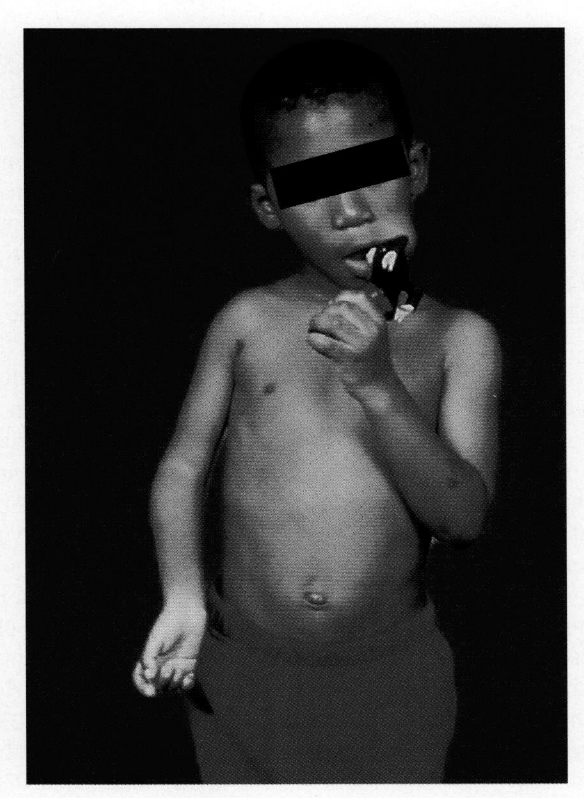

FIG. 7. A 6-year-old child, product of vaginal delivery complicated by shoulder dystocia and subsequent obstetric brachial plexus palsy. The child presents with typical posture of a residual extended upper brachial plexus injury.

Thoracic Outlet Syndrome

The clinical presentation of thoracic outlet syndrome differs drastically from an overt brachial plexus injury. The symptoms tend to be vague and the signs more subtle.[6,74,97,98] Females are more commonly effected (4:1). A thorough examination with provocative maneuvers is required for accurate diagnosis. Virtually all patients with thoracic outlet compression present with neurologic symptoms affecting the lower plexus (C8 and T1). The distribution of pain or paresthesias is often the medial side of the arm and ulnar digits. Loss of dexterity during fine manipulation is a common complaint. Vascular thoracic outlet syndrome is much less common (less than 5%) and can affect venous outflow or arterial inflow.[98] Venous thoracic outlet syndrome is more common than arterial involvement, and edema or vascular congestion may signal vascular outlet obstruction. Arterial compression may produce pain, cold intolerance (similar to Raynaud's phenomenon), and claudication. Rarely, pallor of the limb can result from arterial insufficiency.[31] The history should include inquiry about the onset of symptoms, antecedent trauma, and current activities that produce symptoms. The use of heavy backpacks and frequent maneuvers above the shoulder level are specific activities that can produce symptoms.[57,118]

The physical examination begins with an assessment of the posture of the individual. Poor posture can narrow the thoracic outlet and provoke symptoms. A careful cervical spine and peripheral nerve evaluation is critical in search of additional sites of compression that can cause a double crush neuropathy. Coexisting entrapment at the carpal or cubital tunnel can be present in thoracic outlet syndrome. The proximal thoracic compression causes the nerve to be more vulnerable to an additional distal compressive neuropathy.[6,97,143] The area of sensory abnormalities should be defined and careful manual muscle testing performed for objective signs of motor weakness that can occur in long-standing thoracic outlet syndrome. The ulnar innervated muscles of the hand are most commonly affected by neurologic thoracic outlet syndrome and should be specifically assessed for weakness. Two-point discrimination in the ulnar and median nerve distribution should be determined. Sensation may also be altered in the medial brachial and medial antebrachial nerve distribution.

The presence of edema, venous distension, or cyanosis may indicate a venous thoracic outlet syndrome, whereas pallor, splinter hemorrhages, or ischemic changes suggest arterial involvement secondary to vessel constriction or embolization.[6,120] Symmetry of the radial and ulnar pulses should be ascertained, and transient compression should be evaluated by the provocative maneuvers described in the following.

The supraclavicular region should be palpated for areas of tenderness, and percussion should be performed to illicit a Tinel's sign which indicates nerve irritation. Provocative maneuvers are instrumental in the diagnosis of thoracic outlet syndrome, but must be interpreted carefully (Fig. 8). A positive test must not only produce the expected outcome, but also reproduce the patient's symptoms to be significant. These tests attempt to narrow the anatomic constraints of the thoracic outlet and compress the neural or vascular elements. The Adson test is performed with the patient seated, placing the arm at the side, and palpating the radial pulse.[1] The patient rotates and extends the head and neck toward the affected side while taking a deep breath. This narrows the scalene triangle, and a pulse diminution or obliteration with corresponding symptoms implies thoracic outlet syndrome. The Wright hyperabduction test is performed by placing the arm in 90 degrees of abduction and external rotation.[146] The loss of a radial pulse and symptom reproduction are considered positive. The overhead exercise stress test and 3-minute stress test are similar and performed by instructing the patient to abduct and externally rotate the shoulder to place the arms above shoulder level. Active opening and closing of the hands is then executed and a positive response will reproduce symptoms such as paresthesias or fatigue.[74,113,114] The diagnostic dilemma with these provocative maneuvers is the lack of specificity for isolation of the entrapment site and the significant rate of false-positive results that occur in both asymptomatic volunteers and in other common entrapment neuropathies of the upper extremity.[98,109,146] For example, shoulder abduction and external rotation places traction across the lower plexus at the level of the first rib, narrows the costoclavicular space, and pulls the plexus around the corocoid process. This maneuver also increases the pressure within the cubital tunnel and can produce symptoms of ulnar neuropathy at the elbow.

IMAGING STUDIES

Brachial Plexus Injury

Imaging studies are an important part of the evaluation of the patient with a brachial plexus injury because they provide valuable information about the level of injury. The radiologic tests utilized are plain x-ray films, myelography, computed tomography (CT), and magnetic resonance imaging (MRI). The particular studies employed vary with the type of injury, physical examination, imaging strategy, and expertise of the radiologist.

Plain x-ray films of the cervical spine, clavicle, shoulder, and chest are obtained after an injury to the brachial plexus. Various findings are suggestive of particular levels of plexus injuries (Table 6). The bone or ligament injury often represents a failure of the supporting and protective mechanisms of the brachial plexus. For example, a transverse process fracture usually indicates an avulsion fracture with a significant traction injury to the plexus.

Hemidiaphragm paralysis from injury to the phrenic nerve may not be apparent on a static chest x-ray film and fluoroscopic evaluation during inspiration may be required. Shoulder or chest radiography may reveal the disastrous injury of scapulothoracic dissociation, with wide lateral displacement of the entire shoulder complex. This injury may cause rapid exsanguination from an avulsion of the subclavian artery and brachial plexus. If the patient survives the injury, the prognosis for return of nerve function is bleak.[39]

Angiography is indicated if there is any question of the vascular status of the extremity or integrity of the subclavian or axillary vessels. Palpable radial or ulnar pulses may be present (secondary to collateral flow) despite proximal injury.[14] Penetrating trauma or an expanding hematoma also requires angiography.[37,43,132]

Myelography is used to define the presence or absence of a pseudomeningocele, a meningeal pouch filled with cerebrospinal fluid that extends through the intervertebral foramen into the paraspinal area (Fig. 9). This represents an extraction of the dural and arachnoidal sleeve through the intervertebral foramen that often occurs during a root avulsion injury. The inability to visualize the nerve root on the

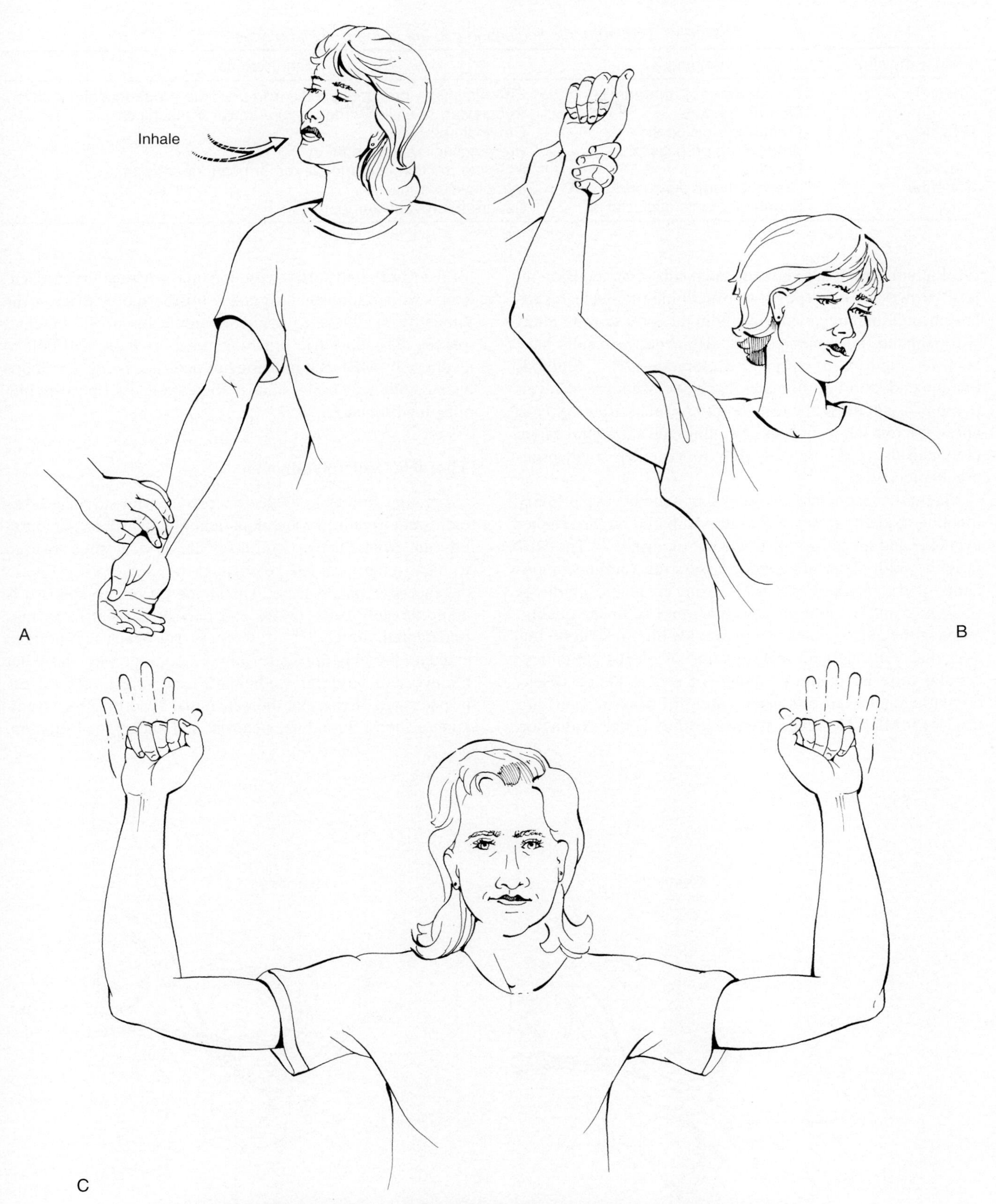

FIG. 8. Artist schematic of provocative maneuvers for thoracic outlet syndrome.

TABLE 6. *Radiographic findings in injuries to the brachial plexus*

Plain x-ray film	Findings	Significance
Chest	Elevated hemidiaphragm	Phrenic injury, proximal plexus and possible preganglionic avulsion
	First rib fracture	Subclavian or axillary artery injury, lower trunk injury
C-spine	Fracture or dislocation	Cervical spine injury
	Transverse process fx	Preganglionic avulsion injury
Clavicle	Fracture	Possible traction injury to plexus or pseudoparalysis
Shoulder	Glenohumeral dislocation	Infraclavicular injury
	Scapulothoracic dissociation	Severe neurovascular injury

myelogram further supports the diagnosis of an avulsion injury. However, false-positive psuedomeningocele results have been found in patients in whom the rootlets were intact with isolated dura rupture, and false-negative results have been reported during surgical exploration.[29,45,55] Methods recommended to improve the diagnostic accuracy of myelography are to delay the test for 4 to 6 weeks after injury to allow for resolution of local swelling and intradural blood clots and using CT myelography to visualize small pseudomeningoceles.[74,94,112]

Magnetic resonance imaging has become the primary imaging modality in some institutions, based on the scanner available and specialization of the radiologist.[99,101] The MRI provides multiplanar imaging to assess the various components of the brachial plexus.[99] Strong magnetic gradients ($\geqslant$1 tesla) and flexible surface coils improve image quality. Varying the pulse sequence will provide high-resolution images that will facilitate identification of plexus pathology. Similar criteria for the diagnosis of root avulsion (pseudomeningocele and nonvisualization of a nerve root) are used with MRI. However, the MRI offers better evaluation of the trunks and cords, with potential verification of a neuroma by an abnormal signal.[99] Furthermore, MRI is the modality of choice to evaluate neoplasms of the brachial plexus. The obstetric brachial plexus is more difficult to evaluate by MRI. But imaging protocols are being developed using adult head coils, smaller slice thickness, and variable-imaging sequences.[101]

Thoracic Outlet Syndrome

Imaging studies to evaluate a patient with suspected thoracic outlet syndrome are plain radiographic films, angiography, and MRI. Plain x-ray films of the cervical spine are used to identify cervical ribs, elongated transverse processes, or degenerative disc disease. The incidence of cervical ribs is approximately 0.5% to 1% and may be present in asymptomatic individuals.[6,105,127] A chest radiograph is routine to evaluate the lung apices for tumor. Angiography and other noninvasive vascular studies are used selectively in suspected cases of vascular thoracic outlet syndrome for visualizing a mural thrombus, stenosis, and aneurysmal dilation.

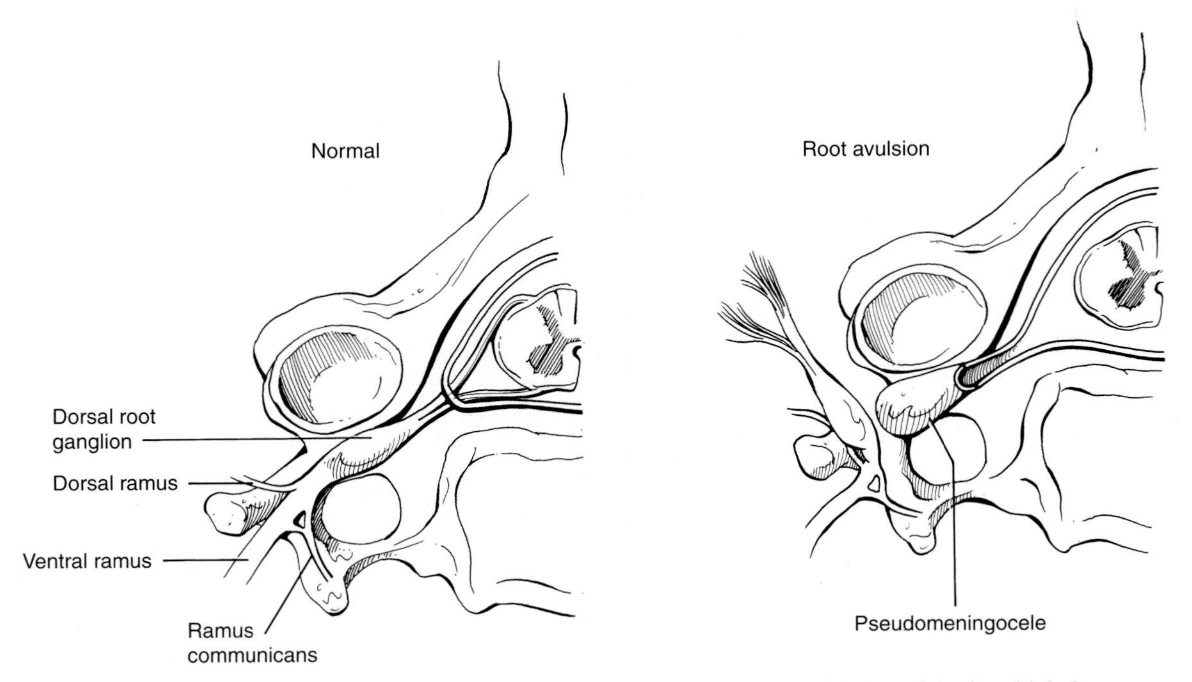

FIG. 9. Artist schematic of pseudomeningocele associated with avulsion injuries of the brachial plexus.

However, false-negative and false-positive results can occur.[6,74,138] MRI can be used to visualize the plexus anatomy and identify areas of compression and anomalous bands.[102] This study is both scanner- and radiologist-dependent and may be more applicable as imaging techniques and interpretation skills improve.

ELECTRODIAGNOSTIC STUDIES

Electrodiagnostic testing plays an integral part in the diagnosis and treatment of brachial plexus lesions.[34] The surgeon and neurophysiologist must have a dependable relationship with reciprocal communication. The results of neurophysiologic testing performed preoperatively, intraoperatively, and postoperatively may directly affect the decision-making process.[91] Methods employed to evaluate brachial plexus injuries are electromyography, nerve conduction velocity measurements, somatosensory-evoked potentials, and nerve action potentials.

Electromyography

Electromyography (EMG) records the electrical activity of muscle fibers at rest and during activation. This signal is recorded by the insertion of EMG needles into the muscle. The normal muscle is silent at rest and active during contraction with progressive recruitment of motor units. A denervated muscle will exhibit spontaneous electrical discharge (fibrillations and positive sharp wave) when the EMG needle is inserted.[17,34] These findings are not present until 2 to 4 weeks after denervation. A reinnervated muscle will begin to show reinnervation or nascent potentials (polyphasic low-amplitude recordings). These electrical changes of muscle regeneration will precede the clinical detection of muscle activity. Therefore, the EMG examination of the muscles innervated by the brachial plexus can provide valuable information about the degree of injury and early recovery.

An EMG evaluation of the more proximal branches from the brachial plexus can help differentiate an avulsion injury from a rupture (see Table 5). For example, fibrillations and positive sharp waves of the paraspinal muscles (innervated by the dorsal rami from the spinal nerve) imply an avulsion injury, whereas preservation of a normal electrical signal suggests a more distal lesion. The EMG is also useful to differentiate the degree of intraneural injury (neuropraxia, axonotmesis, and neurotmesis) and to follow the progress after injury. A neuropraxia can be differentiated from a more severe nerve injury by the absence of fibrillation potentials and positive sharp waves. These denervation changes will be present in an axonotmesis or neurotmesis. Serial EMG evaluations can distinguish an axonotmetic lesion by the spontaneous return of nascent units or reinnervation potentials that will precede clinical recovery of function. A neurotmetic injury will not exhibit EMG signs of spontaneous recovery. However, reinnervation after surgical intervention for a neurotmetic lesion can be monitored by serial EMGs.

Conduction Velocity

The integrity of the peripheral nerve is determined by the measurement of the conduction velocity. The motor or sensory latency can be measured depending on the recording of the compound motor action potential (CMAP) or the sensory nerve action potential (SNAP). The *conduction velocity* (CV) is the distance between two sites of stimulation divided by the time for the nerve action potential to travel from proximal to distal.[17] A severed nerve will lose the capability to conduct an action potential distal to the lesion as the nerve degenerates. However, the distal portion of the nerve may be able to conduct for several days after injury until degeneration occurs. Therefore, early measurement of conduction velocities can produce a false-positive result for nerve continuity, and electrodiagnostic testing should be delayed for at least 3 weeks to allow time for loss of conduction and denervation changes in muscle.

The status of the SNAP and corresponding sensory nerve conduction velocity is helpful in differentiating preganglionic avulsion injuries from postganglionic lesions. The presence of an intact sensory CV in an anesthetic part of the arm indicates a preganglionic injury, for the sensory nerve is not separated from its cell body (dorsal root ganglion). The CMAP or motor NCV is absent in both preganglionic and postganglionic injuries and is not a distinguishing factor.

Somatosensory-Evoked Potentials

Somatosensory-evoked potentials (SEPs) are electrical responses of the brain and spinal cord to stimulation of peripheral sensory fibers. Recordings of the conduction from the stimulating electrode to the central nervous system can be useful for the detection of lesions within the sensory system. This technique can be employed to assess conduction across the brachial plexus and during surgery to define irreparable nerve root avulsions. The absence of SEPs recorded over the spinal cord or contralateral sensorimotor cortex on nerve root stimulation indicates a root avulsion and is a contraindication for nerve grafting.[72,91]

Nerve Action Potentials

Nerve action potentials (NAPs) are used intraoperatively to assess lesions in continuity. Stimulating and recording of a nerve proximal and distal to a neuroma can identify the presence or absence of axonal continuity.[69] The presence of NAPs indicates propagation of an action potential along viable nerve fibers. This can help the surgeon decide between neurolysis or excision and interposition grafting.[69] This method is useful, but drawbacks include the inability to provide quantitative data and the incapacity to distinguish motor from sensory axons. Technical modifications to record the CMAP in innervated muscles or tetanic stimulation may provide better guidelines for surgical decision making.[34,69,73]

Thoracic Outlet Syndrome

Electrodiagnostic studies can be valuable in the diagnosis of thoracic outlet syndrome. Severe compression will produce denervation of the affected muscles, usually the intrinsic muscles of the hand.[46] Fibrillations and positive sharp waves will be evident upon needle insertion. However, most patients with neurologic thoracic outlet syndrome do not present with atrophy and EMG findings. A reduction of the CV across the pathologic thoracic outlet would seem to be a reliable indicator of this disorder. Unfortunately, this technique is difficult to perform, interpret, and reproduce.[74]

Dynamic recording of nerve conduction across the brachial plexus during provocative maneuvers is logical, but is also difficult to perform and to obtain consistent results.

The use of SEPs may play more of a diagnostic role in the assessment of conduction across the plexus than the standard orthodromic nerve conduction tests.[17,78] Peripheral stimulation at the wrist or forearm with recording at Erb's point, cervical spine, and sensory cortex may demonstrate changes in the pattern or timing of particular waveforms in thoracic outlet syndrome. However, the interpretation of the SEP signal remains difficult and dependent on the proficiency of the neurophysiologist.

NONOPERATIVE TREATMENT

Adult Brachial Plexus Injury

The vast majority of adult brachial plexus injuries are initially treated without surgery. Infraclavicular lesions from fracture or dislocation are treated by prompt reduction of the fracture or dislocation. The nerve injury is often an isolated peripheral lesion and treated by observation because neuropraxia and axonotmesis lesions are customary, and the prognosis for recovery is good. Exploration is reserved for those cases without spontaneous recovery.[4,94]

Supraclavicular injuries and diffuse brachial plexus injuries are often associated with other injuries that take precedence. Trauma resuscitation, with repair of visceral damage, reconstitution of vascular flow, and the stabilization of fractures, requires immediate treatment and dominates the initial postinjury period. In significant brachial plexus injuries, ipsilateral upper extremity fractures are best treated by fracture fixation because of the nonunion rate (almost 50%) and the need for early mobilization to prevent contracture, edema, and stiffness.[12] The goal of this period is to precisely define the extent of injury to the brachial plexus. This task is accomplished by a thorough examination and supplemented by the imaging studies previously described.

Following stabilization of the patient, the brachial plexus injury has certain features that require specific management (Fig. 10). Swelling and stiffness will develop in the flail limb, and physiotherapy, with range of motion exercises and antiedema measures, is required. The range of motion therapy will also maintain passive motion and supple joint structure to avoid contracture that will directly limit functional recovery. A sling is often applied to support the shoulder, to prevent any additional traction across the plexus. This sling is removed for therapy and range of motion. Electrical stimulation to diminish muscle wasting during nerve regeneration may be used, but the efficacy is unclear.

Brachial plexus pain may be a problem during this early period after injury.[15] The pain can present in both preganglionic and postganglionic injuries. Preganglionic pain can be severe and constant, with a burning or crushing sensation. In most patients, this debilitating pain gradually subsides to a tolerable level. Postganglionic pain is from afferent signals that can still travel to the central nervous system and can also be severe, but it usually dissipates over time. Pain management can be accomplished by pharmacologic treatment, transcutaneous electrical stimulation, and other analgesic measures. Unfortunately, 5% of patients will exhibit persistent intractable pain that requires valiant attempts for pain relief, including ablation of the dorsal root entry zone (DREZ) or central stimulators.[15] Even limb amputation will not necessarily relieve this pain.[141]

During this nonoperative period, serial examinations are performed to assess the initial injury and signs of early recovery indicative of a neuropraxic lesion. Radiographs of the chest, cervical spine, and shoulder girdle are evaluated for signs of brachial plexus injury (see Table 6). Incomplete recovery after 3 to 4 weeks is studied by CT myelogram or MRI to help localize the lesion. Baseline electrodiagnostic studies are also performed to assess muscle denervation and the possibility of nerve rootlet avulsions (see Table 5). Denervation of the paraspinal muscles and proximal root branches (dorsal scapular, long thoracic) and an intact sensory CV in an anesthetic limb distribution imply nerve root avulsion.

Unless a complete brachial plexus avulsion has been determined, repeat electrodiagnostic tests are performed at 3 months after injury. The presence of reinnervation potentials indicates the lesion has some potential for spontaneous recovery. At this time, the clinical information and evolution of the paralysis should be combined with the ancillary studies to define the level and extent of injury. The prognosis for recovery should be calculated. The surgeon must also decide if the lesion incurred is amenable to surgical repair or reconstruction. This observation period of 3 months is often sufficient time to adequately assess the adult brachial plexus and to decide whether spontaneous recovery will transpire. Progressive recovery that follows a sequential pattern warrants continued observation and negates the need for exploration.

In contrast, neurotmetic damage with loss of continuity (avulsion, rupture, laceration) or severe intraneural damage will not exhibit evidence of improvement at 3 months. In those reparable lesions, surgery is recommended between 3 and 6 months postinjury. This time frame for surgery is important to assure the viability of motor endplates to sprouting axons. A further delay in surgery may jeopardize the integrity of the motor endplates and prevent functional recovery, despite satisfactory nerve repair, grafting, or transfer.

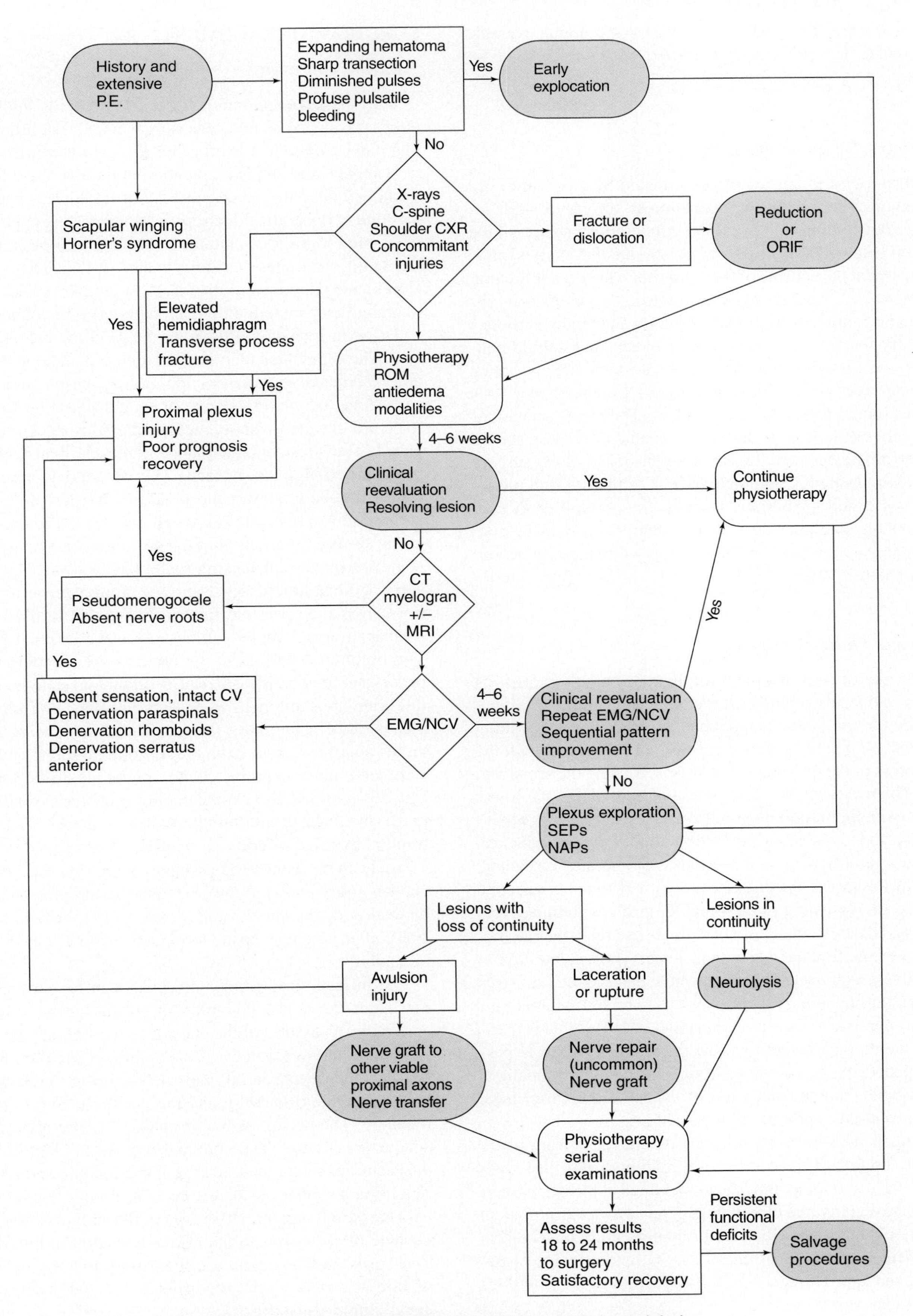

FIG. 10. Treatment algorithm for adult brachial plexus injuries.

There is a trend toward earlier surgery if a nonrecoverable and reparable lesion can be identified, to ensure endplate viability.

Obstetric Brachial Plexus Palsy

Obstetric birth palsies are also treated by a period of observation. The diagnostic evaluation is similar to adult injuries, but complicated by lack of cooperation and size of the patient (Fig. 11). Most of these palsies are mild and resolve, but permanent sequelae of these injuries can be a debilitating problem.[50,51,55] Subtle muscle deficiencies can disturb synchronous motion of the upper extremity and hinder activities of daily living. An early return of biceps and deltoid contraction is a good prognostic sign for recovery.[45,50,51,73] Lack of biceps recovery at 3 to 6 months implies a poor prognosis and warrants surgical intervention.[9,45] The reconstruction of nonrecoverable lesions that are amenable to surgery should be performed between 6 and 12 months of age. Early surgery may be indicated in complete lesions of the brachial plexus with a Horner's syndrome because the outlook is so poor without an attempt at nerve reconstruction. Also, there is always at least one root that is not avulsed that could benefit from reconstruction.[45,55]

Thoracic Outlet Syndrome

The mainstay of treatment for thoracic outlet syndrome is conservative management directed at alleviating any compression of the thoracic outlet and avoidance of aggravating factors.[74,97] There is often poor posture associated with the weakness of the parascapular muscles, causing the scapula to sag. This narrows the thoracic outlet ands drags the lower trunk over the first rib. Postural exercises and training are instituted and aimed at the correction of poor body mechanics. Activity modification and avoidance of aggravating factors is a key to success. An exercise program, directed at selective muscle strengthening of the shoulder girdle with maneuvers designed to stretch the scalene muscles and relax the first rib, is part of the treatment regimen. Supervision is required to selectively exercise and strengthen the parascapular muscles (trapezium, levator scapulae, and rhomboids) without further compression of the thoracic outlet.[6,106] The goal is to expand the thoracic outlet to allow the brachial plexus to pass unimpeded. A variety of additional therapeutic modalities (ultrasound, biofeedback, and electrical stimulation) have been proposed with ambivalent success.[6]

Women with macromastia may obtain relief from better breast support or even reduction mammaplasty in severe cases.[63,74] Ergonomic modification, aimed at the decrease of overhead activity and elimination of any downward force on the shoulder girdle, can also be beneficial. Conservative treatment is effective in improving symptoms in most patients, and approximately only 10% to 30% of these will require surgical intervention.[98,119,124]

SURGICAL MANAGEMENT

Surgical Approach

The surgical exploration for brachial plexus injuries requires a wide exposure of the supraclavicular or infraclavicular plexus, or both. The procedure is performed with the patient supine, and ample preparation of the injured extremity, neck, hemithorax, and one or both of the lower extremities for sural nerve grafts. Electrophysiologic testing apparatus is positioned for assistance during surgery, with placement of the scalp electrodes for somatosensory-evoked potentials (SEPs) and the preparation of hook or penlike probes for intraoperative stimulation to record nerve action potentials.

The skin incision varies with the required plexus exposure. The supraclavicular incision travels parallel to the posterior border of the sternocleidomastoid muscle and curves parallel to the proximal border of the clavicle (Fig. 12). Skin flaps are elevated and supraclavicular sensory nerves protected. The subcutaneous platysma muscle that covers the posterior triangle is divided. The external jugular vein, which descends across the posterior border of the sternomastoid to pierce the fascia, is identified. The spinal accessory nerve, which divides the posterior triangle in half, is identified in the cephalad portion of the exposure. The transverse cervical artery, which crosses from anterior to posterior across the operative field just cephalad to the suprascapular artery, is mobilized to expose the brachial plexus. The omohyoid muscle is the door to the supraclavicular plexus and must be identified. The omohyoid is divided at its intermediate tendon to expose the scalene muscles and plexus (upper and middle trunks). The phrenic nerve travels on the anterior scalene just anterior to the posterior triangle. This nerve must be protected throughout the dissection. The C5, C6, C7 roots and corresponding trunks are isolated between the anterior and middle scalene muscles. The lower trunk is exposed inferior to the divided omohyoid, and the T1 root can be visualized passing over the first rib. The subclavian artery and vein must be isolated and protected. The dissection of the subclavian vessels can be difficult, especially after vascular repair, for scar formation impedes mobilization.

The infraclavicular brachial plexus can be exposed primarily or the supraclavicular approach can be extended across the distal third of the clavicle to incorporate the infraclavicular nerves (see Fig. 12). The infraclavicular incision parallels the deltopectoral interval. The deeper exposure retracts the deltoid laterally and the pectoralis major muscle medially. The pectoralis major muscle may be released for adequate exposure. The coracoid process is identified and the pectoralis minor tendon tagged with a suture and divided. The infraclavicular plexus travels beneath this tendon along with the axillary artery. Dissection of the artery is often complicated by adhesions to the plexus and surrounding tissue. The cords and branches are identified and inspected. A rupture at this level can be difficult to isolate because the distal stump can retract and evade dissection. Clavicular

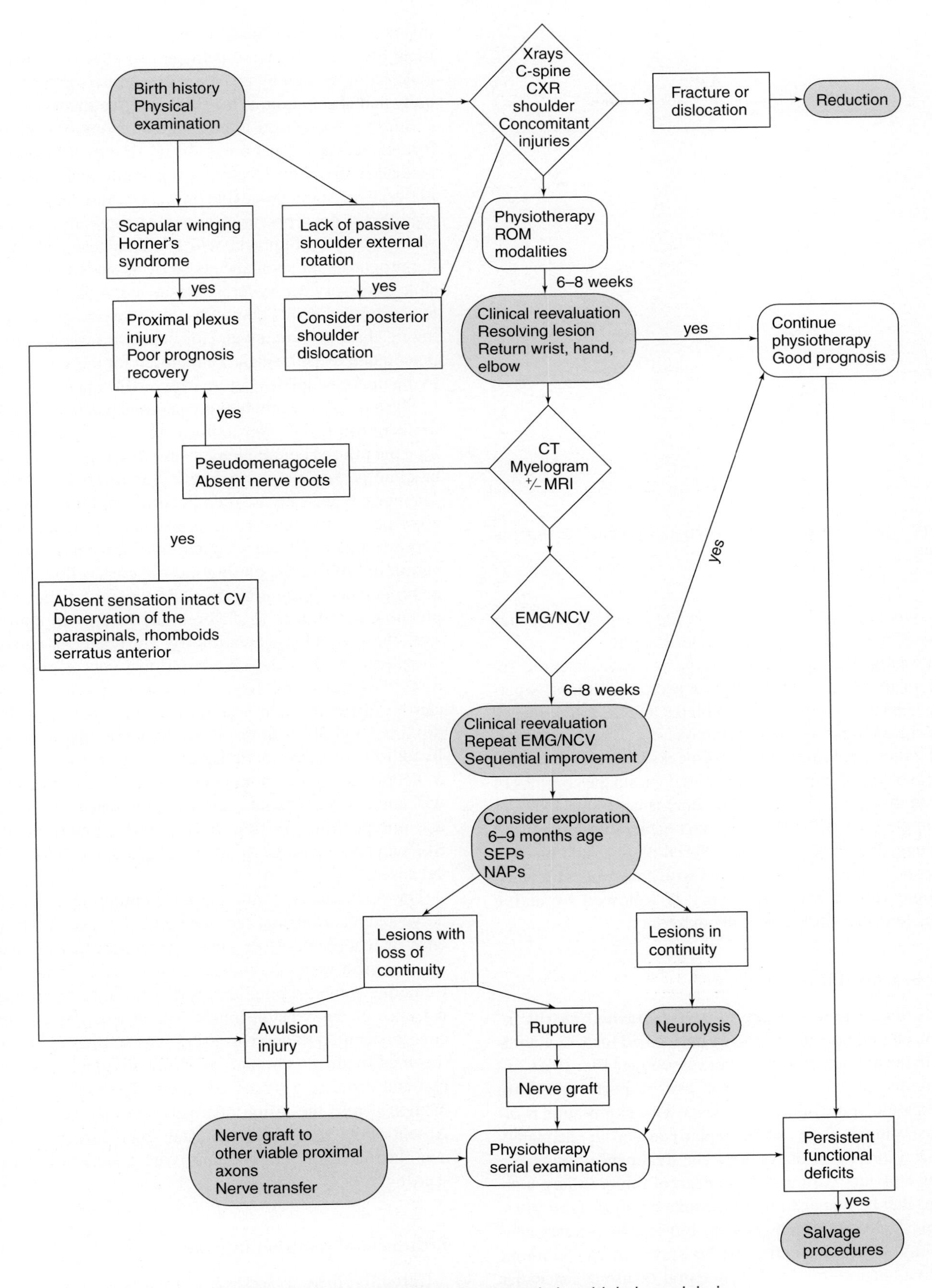

FIG. 11. Treatment algorithm for obstetric brachial plexus injuries.

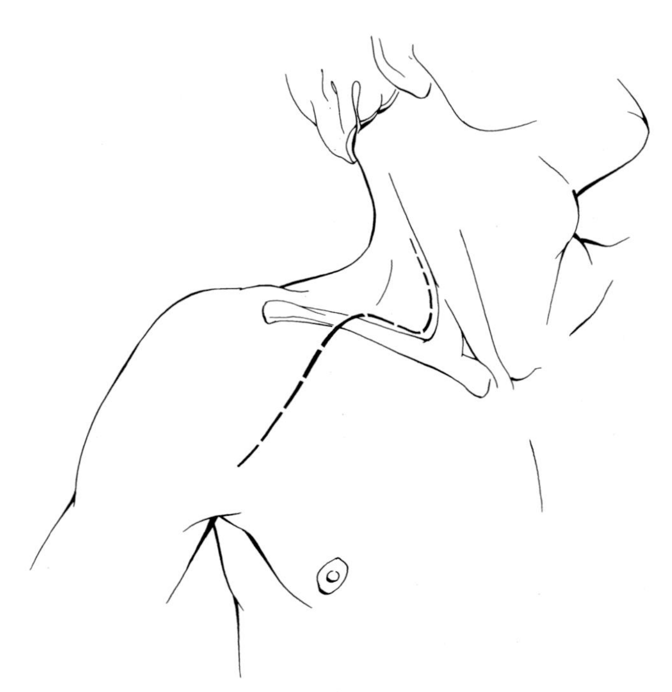

FIG. 12. Artist schematic of incision for approach to brachial plexus.

osteotomy is avoided except in unusual circumstances, such as nonunion or exuberant callus after fracture.

Following the exploration and nerve reconstruction, suturing of the divided omohyoid or pectoralis minor is performed. A layered closure is completed and the arm is placed in a Velpeau dressing. Suture removal is at 2 weeks and immobilization continued for 3 to 4 weeks. Gradual mobilization and physical therapy are instituted within the confines of nerve mobilization. Prolonged therapy is necessary to maintain supple joint structure, as nerve regeneration progresses at a sluggish rate of 1 mm/day. Serial clinical and electrodiagnostic evaluation is performed with assessment for signs of reinnervation. Motor recovery is followed by active therapy to restore function of the extremity.

Adult Brachial Plexus Surgery

Immediate surgical intervention for brachial plexus injuries is uncommon and primarily performed for vascular injuries to the axillary or subclavian vessels (see Fig. 10). Concurrent inspection of the plexus can be performed with identification of the injured segments. This exploration is often frustrating as the vascular repair can not be adequately mobilized for fear of disruption. The treatment of the nerve injuries will vary with the mechanism of injury. Sharp transections can be managed by immediate repair or graft interposition. A clean transection can be repaired by primary neurorrhaphy if the cut ends can be approximated without excessive tension.[37,87,122] An epineural or group fascicular type repair with alignment of the corresponding transected fascicles is performed. Traction or blast injuries are best treated by delayed management until one can reliably determine the extent of nerve damage and zone of injury. Most penetrating trauma by missile will not interrupt nerve continuity and observation is the preferred treatment.[14,69,100]

Surgery for closed adult plexus lesions is usually performed between 3 and 6 months postinjury. The decision to operate is based on locating a repairable lesion that would not recover spontaneously. Infraclavicular lesions usually represent a neuropraxia or axonotmesis injury and recover without surgery. Supraclavicular lesions have a less promising prognosis for spontaneous recovery and are more accessible to surgery. However, supraclavicular disruptions of the lower trunk (C8, T1) do not respond to nerve repair or grafting in adults and are not an indication for surgery. This poor outcome reflects the distance required for the axons to travel to the motor endplates before irreversible changes begin.

The surgery for brachial plexus injury is lengthy and the dissection difficult and tedious, for scar formation envelope the injured neural elements. Following exposure of the brachial plexus, the injured neural elements are identified. The normal anatomy is often distorted and basic intraoperative nerve stimulation can assist in identification of the nerve elements. Direct stimulation of the nerve and observation of any corresponding muscle contraction can assist in proper nerve identification. The focus of the brachial plexus dissection is to differentiate lesions in continuity from those with loss of continuity. The diagnosis can be uncomplicated when the dissection uncovers avulsed nerve roots or a transected nerve. However, the differentiation can be difficult when scar tissue intervenes between the proximal and distal limbs of a completely disrupted nerve. In addition, a neurotmetic lesion can occur from severe intraneural damage without overt transection, and this lesion will not recover without excision of the scarred nerve tissue and interposition grafting. Intraoperative determination of SEPs and NAP can facilitate the diagnosis in these equivocal cases.

The SEP can be evaluated by stimulating a peripheral nerve and recording the cerebral cortical response. The presence of recordable SEPs implies nerve continuity, and the absence of a response indicates nerve discontinuity. This technique can be applied to a spinal nerve to determine the presence of an avulsion injury. The absence of a SEP is a contraindication to nerve grafting. The sensory NAP can be recorded by direct stimulation of an individual nerve proximal and distal to a suspected lesion. The presence of conduction across the lesion confirms some nerve continuity. Absent nerve conduction indicates fiber discontinuity or a neurotmetic lesion in continuity with complete intraneural scarring.[68,69,88,91]

Treatment of Avulsion Injuries

Currently, there is no surgical treatment to restore nerve rootlet connection (avulsion or intraspinal injuries) with the spinal cord.[94] Experimental work is in progress to reattach the rootlets directly to the spinal cord and solve this unmanageable problem.[18,19] The current treatment options for avulsion injuries are nerve grafting to other viable proximal stumps or a nerve transfer (see Fig. 10).

Treatment of Lesions in Continuity

Neurolysis is performed for lesions in continuity and the extent of neurolysis will vary with the degree of constricting scar. Epinuerotomy may be sufficient in instances of external compression from limited fibrosis, whereas epifascicular epineurectomy may be necessary in advanced interfascicular compression from fibrosis around the fascicles.[88] If the fascicular anatomy cannot be identified during neurolysis, the injury is deemed to be a neurotmesis and resected.

Treatment of Lesions without Continuity

After the completion of this preliminary dissection and the use of intraoperative electrodiagnostic techniques, the lesions with loss of continuity have been delineated. The proximal and distal stumps available for nerve reconstruction have been defined with exclusion of any avulsed rootlets. The initial treatment is to resect the neuroma that forms at the proximal and distal nerve stumps until normal nerve consistency and fascicular anatomy is encountered. The distal stumps are now primed for coaptation with a viable inflow for regeneration of axons. The exact connection of proximal and distal stumps requires some decision making, especially in cases with loss of proximal stumps secondary to avulsion. Restoration of continuity can be accomplished by nerve grafting or nerve transfer. Nerve grafting is the placement of intercalary nerve grafts that act as scaffolding for regenerating axons. Nerve transfer is coaptation of an expendable motor nerve into the distal stump to supply axons for ingrowth.

Nerve Grafting

Nerve grafting is the preferred technique for most lesions with loss of continuity. The interposition of nerve segments link the proximal and distal axons and serve as a conduit to channel the growing axons to the periphery. The donor nerve(s) is usually the sural nerve from the lower extremity, harvested at the time of brachial plexus exploration. Other potential options are the ipsilateral medial antebrachial cutaneous and superficial radial nerves. The donor nerve graft is divided into sections that span the defect until a comparable cross-sectional area is obtained for interpositional grafting. The nerve grafts can be sutured directly between fascicular groups (interfascicular) or secured between the proximal and distal stumps (cable grafts) by epineural sutures (Fig. 13).[37,68,94] Biologic adhesives such as fibrin glue can be used to decrease operative time.[45] In general, cable grafts are used to repair the cords and trunks, and interfascicular grafts are used at the cord or branch level if corresponding proximal and distal fascicular anatomy can be identified. These nerve grafts are revascularized by vascular ingrowth from the recipient bed.[122] Therefore, numerous smaller-diameter grafts are preferable to a single large-caliber graft, to limit impermeable necrosis before revascularization begins. Tension is avoided across the proximal and distal coaptation sites because this creates an unfavorable condition for axonal sprouting.[86,88,122] Nerve grafts are best directed toward shoulder and elbow muscles for reinnervation because the distance to the branches is short and axonal regrowth can occur before there is irreversible muscle damage.[94] In addition, the plexus fascicular anatomy shifts rapidly over relatively short distances, which promotes erroneous growth of axons. Therefore, nerve-grafting strategy should attempt to preferentially direct the axons to achieve a defined function. For example, grafts that connect directly to the musculocutaneous, axillary, and suprascapular nerves have less chance of axonal dropout and misdirection compared with grafts placed imprecisely into the cords.

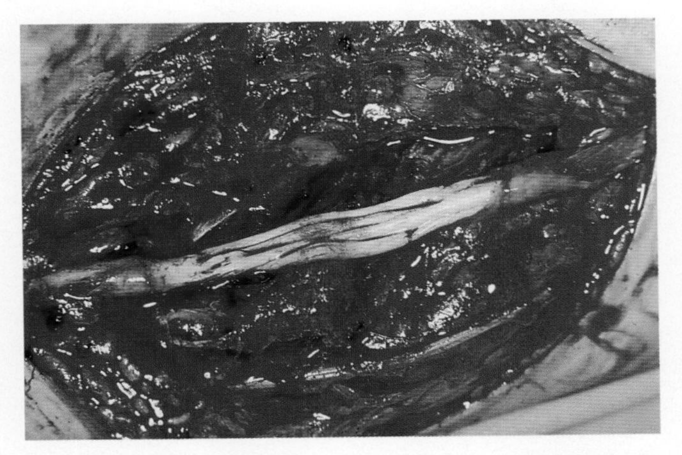

FIG. 13. A 15-year-old boy, who sustained a gunshot wound to his arm, with transection of ulnar nerve. He was treated with neuroma resection and cable graft with strands of sural nerve.

Nerve Transfer

Nerve transfer is indicated in avulsion injuries and large or extensive defects of the brachial plexus. The indications for nerve transfer increases as the number of avulsed roots multiplies. In addition, long interposition nerve grafts ($>$10 cm) are limited by available donor nerves and have less chance for recovery.[23]

This technique involves the connection of an expendable donor motor nerve to provide an axonal source for regeneration of the distal stump. The donor neurons will reinnervate the muscle, and function will require voluntary control of the transferred nerve. Similar to a tendon transfer, activation of the donor nerve to achieve function will require a period of training, and involuntary muscle activation may occur until transformation has taken place. For example, intercostal nerve transfer will initially be activated by coughing or sneezing, but reeducation will occur over time. The technique of nerve transfer can be used in tandem with nerve grafting or may be the only available option in complete avulsion injuries.

There are numerous donor nerves available for transfer, including the spinal accessory nerve, cervical plexus, phrenic, intercostal nerves, and various portions of the affected plexus (intraplexal transfer; Fig. 14).[23,24,25,52,94,122] In selected cases, branches from the opposite brachial plexus have been transferred.[23,83] The donor nerves for transfer are mobilized while maintaining their proximal connection and coapted to selected distal stumps, preferably specific peripheral nerves to achieve the desired function.

The transfer of the spinal accessory to the suprascapular nerve for spinati reinnervation and the transfer of the intercostal nerves to the musculocutaneous nerve for biceps function for avulsion injuries of C5, C6, and C7 are favored techniques.[24,71,93] The spinal accessory nerve is divided distal to the sternocleidomastoid and upper trapezius innervation to preserve some function.[24] The nerve is then coapted to the suprascapular nerve using microsurgical technique. When transferring the intercostal nerves, two to four nerves are used to provide increased motor fibers to the musculocutaneous nerve, compared with a single-nerve transfer.[22,62,71,89,93] Early reinnervation will be evident during breathing, coughing, and sneezing, which will illicit biceps activation. This involuntary reaction will subside over time as volitional activation becomes predominant.[71,89,91] Intercostal nerve transfer will have a minimal effect on pulmonary function as long as the diaphragm is functional. Diaphragmatic paralysis is a relative contraindication to intercostal nerve transfer.[71,86] In addition, combined transfer of the intercostal and phrenic nerves is not recommended.

Intercostal Nerve Transfer Technique

The intercostal transfer is performed through a transverse thoracic incision in the interspace between the third and fourth ribs, from the midaxillary line to the costochondral junction (Fig. 15).[71,89,142] The anterior surface of the ribs is exposed by separation of the pectoralis major and minor muscles. The ribs are mobilized by subperiosteal dissection, with protection of the pleura. The upper portion of the intercostal muscle is spread and the motor portion of the third intercostal nerve isolated. A portion of the rib may be resected to ease dissection.[89,142] The nerve is dissected from the costochondral junction to the midaxillary line. This length of dissection will avoid the need for an intervening nerve graft.[137] The fourth inter-

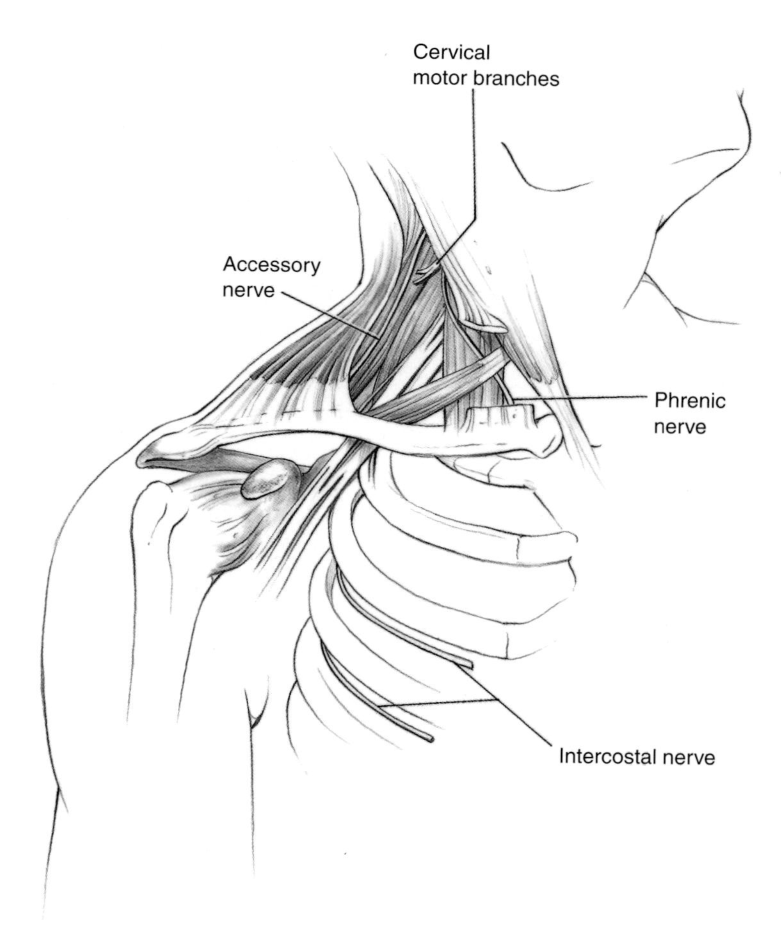

FIG. 14. Artist schematic of potential donors for nerve transfer.

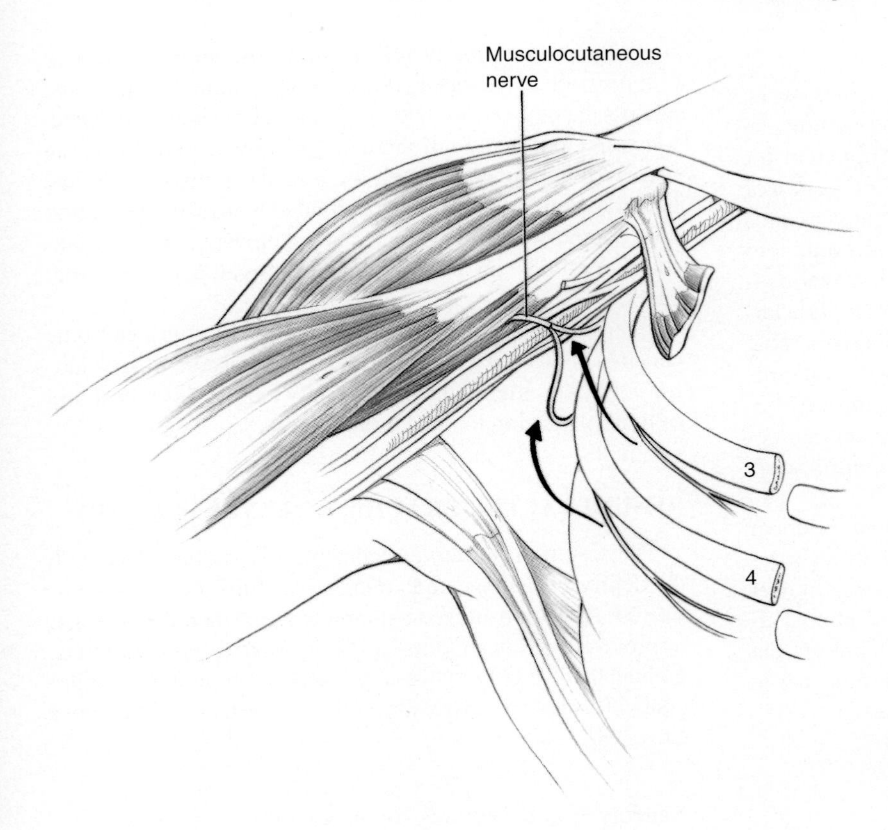

FIG. 15. Artist schematic of intercostal nerve transfer to musculocutaneous nerve for elbow flexion.

costal nerve is harvested in a similar fashion. Through a linear incision in the arm, the musculocutaneous nerve is exposed on the undersurface of the biceps brachii muscle. A subcutaneous tunnel is developed between the biceps, axilla, and the thoracic incision. The intercostal nerves are then passed to the biceps motor nerve and coapted with epineural sutures.

Additional options for nerve transfers are the cervical plexus or phrenic nerve to the suprascapular nerve, spinal accessory, or axillary nerve.[23,24,25,93] Use of the phrenic nerve does reduce pulmonary capacity, which may improve over time.[3,52,93] In infants, the use of phrenic nerve transfer is avoided because the diaphragm is not yet firmly fixed to the vertebral bodies and severe respiratory problems can occur.[24,25]

Prioritization in Severe Brachial Plexus Injuries

A priority list must be established in difficult brachial plexus injuries. This roster is based on functional importance and prognosis after nerve reconstruction. Better results are achieved from nerve reconstruction in the proximal musculature. Elbow flexion against gravity holds the highest priority in brachial plexus injuries. Restoration of elbow flexion allows the extremity to be better positioned in space and the hand flexed toward the trunk and mouth for use. Shoulder balance and stability is the next priority for reconstruction, for an unstable, dislocated, or contracted shoulder will impede use of the extremity. The triceps is next on the priority list, for nerve grafting or transfer is reliable by connection directly to the radial nerve branches that innervate the triceps. The serratus anterior muscle (long thoracic nerve) and pectoralis muscles (lateral and medial pectoral nerves) are addressed next, followed by the forearm flexors and digital sensibility (median nerve). The wrist and finger extensors are subsequently considered by linkage to the radial nerve. The ulnar innervated structures are the last priority because of the poor prognosis for recovery.[93,94] The number of axons diminish as the regenerating process moves toward the periphery and the hand has the misfortune of being last on the list. Therefore, lower trunk defects in adults are usually unsuccessful and are performed only in obstetric lesions for which reinnervation is possible.

The priority list provides guidelines for nerve reconstruction in severe cases with limited viable proximal stumps or inadequate donor nerves. The unlimited patterns of nerve lesions in brachial plexus injuries prohibit the development of specific treatment algorithms for each potential situation. The basic strategy is to precisely define the injury, perform neurolysis for lesions in continuity, and reconstruct loss of continuity (see Fig. 10). Nerve grafts are preferred for nerve reconstruction with viable proximal and distal stumps, with priority given to the elbow (musculocutaneous nerve) and shoulder (suprascapular and axillary nerves). Inadequate proximal inflow requires nerve transfer, with a priority similar to that of the elbow and shoulder function.

Obstetric Brachial Plexus Surgery

Surgery for obstetric lesions is usually performed between 6 and 12 months of age (see Fig. 11). Early intervention can be performed if a neurotmetic lesion without potential for spontaneous recovery can be accurately identified. Return of wrist, hand, and elbow flexion by 6 months almost assures near-complete recovery.[11] A diagnostic evaluation similar to that used for adult injuries is completed with serial examinations, electrodiagnostic studies, and CT myelogram. In addition, the surgical algorithm and procedures are comparable with minor modifications. There is a more aggressive attempt at nerve reconstruction for lower trunk injuries because youth favors nerve regeneration and recovery can occur.[55,122] Also, salvage procedures that include arthrodesis are avoided in the skeletally immature child.

These obstetric injuries most commonly involve the upper plexus and are usually postganglionic ruptures that can be reconstructed by interposition grafting.[55,73] In contrast, lower plexus lesions of C8 and T1 are less common and almost always avulsion injuries that require graft interposition to the upper plexus or nerve transfer. In infants, phrenic nerve transfer is avoided for fear of respiratory compromise.[24]

Thoracic Outlet Syndrome

Surgery for thoracic outlet syndrome is indicated for intractable pain, a significant neurologic deficit, vascular compromise, or when conservative measures have failed to alleviate symptoms. The surgery for thoracic outlet syndrome is not without inherent risks, and mild discomfort from inconsequential compression is better left alone. The operative procedure is directed at decompression of the thoracic outlet, with release of any anatomic constrictions. There is no consensus on the most efficacious approach or procedure to correct thoracic outlet syndrome.[98] The fundamental components to the described procedures include cervical rib resection, first rib resection, scalenotomy, scalenectomy, excision of anomalous fascial bands, claviculectomy, pectoralis minor release, or a combination of these. The procedure can be accomplished by a variety of approaches, including a supraclavicular, transclavicular, subclavicular, transaxillary, posterior, or a combined approach.

The resection of the first rib, with or without anterior scalenectomy, has become the preferred procedure for thoracic outlet syndrome in most cases.[74,98,115,116] Scalenectomy is preferred for the less common upper plexus thoracic outlet syndrome. The supraclavicular approach favors scalenectomy and upper plexus exploration, but sacrifices posterior first rib exposure. Approximately 80% to 90% of the anterior scalene muscle and 40% to 50% of the middle scalene are excised during scalenectomy.[5] The phrenic and long thoracic nerves must be identified and protected.

The first thoracic rib serves as a fulcrum for T1, an attachment site for the scalene muscles, and borders the costoclavicular space. Therefore, removal of the first rib would partially or completely relieve multiple potential sites of compression. The transaxillary route is more cosmetic and affords the best access to the first rib, but precludes scalenectomy and exploration of the upper plexus. Cervical ribs can usually be removed through the axillary approach, and the pectoralis minor tendon can be divided if suspected subcoracoid compression. A combined supraclavicular and transaxillary method can be used in complicated or recurrent cases.[95,108]

Intermittent venous or arterial thoracic outlet syndrome can also be treated by decompression. Persistent long-standing venous or arterial thrombosis may require thrombectomy or bypass grafting in recalcitrant cases.

RESULTS AFTER BRACHIAL PLEXUS SURGERY

The results from nerve reconstruction surgery vary with the degree of damage and complexity of the techniques employed. A result is judged to be successful when the outcome improves function and this usually requires a strength return greater than gravity. This antigravity strength allows independent use of the extremity without assistance of the other extremity.

Neurolysis and Primary Neurorrhaphy

Neurolysis of lesions in continuity generally produces good results with return of muscle strength against gravity in more than 90% of the cases.[30,37,69,70,100] However, the efficacy of neurolysis is difficult to prove, for spontaneous recovery may have occurred without surgery.[100] The results of nerve repair and reconstruction have paralleled the refined techniques of microneural repair.[87,88] Primary neurorrhaphy is usually not performed in brachial plexus injury.[37] However, when primary repair is indicated and performed without excessive tension, most patients regain strength to overcome gravity.[23,68,69]

Nerve Grafting

The results of nerve grafting are better with upper plexus lesions, shorter graft length, and surgery less than 9 months after injury.[23,30,37,54,123] Return of sufficient proximal muscle strength after nerve graft interposition occurs in approximately 50% to 80% of cases.[4,30,68,83,91,135] Nerve grafting for lower plexus lesions in adults is uniformly unsuccessful, but may provide some mild return of extrinsic muscle function and protective sensation.[4,14,68,69,86,122]

Nerve Transfer

The results of nerve transfer are more variable, with good results for proximal reinnervation. Better results are obtained when the transfer is performed early and placed into a peripheral nerve without an intervening graft.[23,24,71,89,91] Return of elbow flexion against gravity is achieved in 60% to 88% of cases.[23,24,52,62,86,89,135] The results for return of shoulder function are more variable when using a nerve transfer to the suprascapular nerve or axillary nerve to achieve stability and abduction. The results of transfer for suprascapular function are currently approximately 80% successful and axillary function about 40%.[25,86,88,93] The inferior results for restoration of shoulder function compared with elbow flexion are, in part, secondary to mass innervation.[94] Shoulder function is a coupled movement of scapulothoracic and glenohumeral motion to achieve abduction. Simultaneous contraction of the reinnervated shoulder muscles prevents synchronous motion and diminishes effective abduction. In contrast, elbow flexion requires a relatively uncomplicated motion. Nerve transfer for forearm and hand function is less successful, with some return of extrinsic function, but not intrinsic activity.[62]

Obstetric Brachial Plexus Reconstruction

In obstetric nerve reconstruction, the early unimpressive reports on obstetric palsy surgery tempered the eagerness for nerve surgery.[55,125] The advent of modern microsurgical techniques has renewed the interest in nerve reconstruction for obstetric brachial plexus palsy.[55] The results of surgery are more difficult to extract from the literature because complex evaluation is hampered in the child and recovery can be prolonged.[29,55] Upper plexus (C5 and C6) injuries that are reconstructed produce encouraging results, with good recovery of shoulder function in 60% to 80% and reliable return of biceps in approximately 80% to 100%.[11,45,55,73,133] As expected, better results were obtained with neurolysis than with neuroma resection and graft interposition.[73] Unfortunately, the involvement of C7 and the lower trunk diminishes outcome with a more variable recovery.[11,45,54,55] Additional functional improvement can be obtained by secondary tendon transfer surgery.[44]

Thoracic Outlet Syndrome

The results of thoracic outlet surgery are highly variable, with success rates dependent on the procedure employed and the definition of success. Isolated anterior scalenotomy has a 50% failure rate, with a significant recurrence rate.[47] The results of first-rib resection are successful (improvement of symptoms) in 37% to 92% of individuals, with lower recurrence rates.[41,75,113] Scalenectomy alone or combined with first-rib resection has reported success rates of approximately 68% to 86%.[6,119,120,108] Improvement following thoracic outlet surgery may require 2 years or longer.[6] In contrast, the initial symptomatic relief may be nullified by scar formation and cicatrization with recurrent compression and no reliable treatment. Comparison studies of first-rib resection versus scalenectomy do not reveal any appreciable difference.[120]

SALVAGE PROCEDURES

Salvage procedures are performed for residual brachial plexus injuries. These persistent deficits may result from irreparable lesions, delayed evaluation, and partial recovery after nerve reconstruction. In elderly individuals with limited capacity for nerve regeneration or if nerve reconstruction is futile, immediate salvage procedures may be recommended instead of nerve reconstruction.[94]

The goals of these secondary procedures are to improve function of the shoulder, elbow, wrist, and fingers. The specific operation performed will vary with the brachial plexus lesion and residual deficit. The timing of surgery also varies with the lesion and previous treatment performed. Early salvage procedures can be performed for irreparable injuries, whereas a delay of 18 to 24 months after nerve reconstruction is required to allow sufficient time for recovery.

The patient evaluation must consider the history of the injury and a review of previous records. The extent of the initial paralysis and subsequent neurologic recovery is a significant factor. The physical and emotional health of the patient are important components of the evaluation. The injury has altered the patient's life forever and the manner of acceptance is an important consideration in the reconstructive plan. The initial injury often overwhelms the patient's physical and social life for a time. Fear of a similar episode of dependence after reconstructive surgery is genuine, and the reconstructive plan should be formulated with minimal time away from work and activity. This strategy may require multiple procedures at a single setting.

A general assessment of shoulder, elbow, wrist, and hand function is performed. The balance of each joint complex and absence of a particular motion noted. Any joint contractures must be evaluated and may require therapy or operative release before tendon transfer. An inventory of the available muscles for transfer is recorded by completion of the brachial plexus injury sheet. A potential donor muscle must have sufficient strength against gravity because transfer will decrease strength by 1 grade.[130] The potential work capacity of a donor muscle is proportional to the cross-sectional area.[7] Reinnervated muscles often lack normal excursion and function, and ideally, they should not be used for transfer. However, often there are no other available options for donor muscles. At surgery, a slightly paler tone of a reinnervated muscle is usually evident.[94]

In general, a similar priority is based on elbow flexion to improve arm positioning and encourage hand to mouth activity. Shoulder function is addressed concurrently or following elbow flexion. Wrist extension, finger extension, and finger flexion are managed after elbow and shoulder function. In lower plexus lesions, wrist and digit motion for grasp and release assume priority.

Elbow Flexion

The restoration of elbow flexion requires a mobile joint and an available muscle for transfer. The goal of surgery is to regain a functional arc of elbow motion from 30 to 130 degrees. The potential donor muscles are the flexor–pronator group (Steindler flexorplasty), triceps, pectoralis major muscle, latissimus dorsi transfer, and free-muscle transfer.[13,20,21,26,81,128,129,130] The selection of the donor muscle varies with the strength of those available and consideration of additional tendon transfers that use similar muscles. For example, if a latissimus dorsi transfer is planned for deficient shoulder external rotation, then an alternative elbow flexorplasty should be planned. The exact choice of transfer is variable and each transfer has certain advantages and disadvantages.[8,130]

The Steindler flexorplasty transfers the flexor–pronator mass 2 in. proximal and reattaches this muscle group to the anterior humerus for elbow flexion (Fig. 16). Transfer of the flexor–pronator muscle group with a portion of the medial epicondyle and use of a compression screw provides better fixation (Fig. 17).[7] The procedure is relatively uncomplicated, but also produces weak elbow flexion.[23,65] Accordingly, this transfer has been used to augment weak elbow flexion.[23] In addition, formation of a fist and forearm pronation can occur during elbow flexion, which will compromise the functional gain of active flexion. Technical modifications to reduce the pronation and flexion contracture have been proposed.[82]

The triceps transfer sacrifices elbow extension for flexion, but is an effective flexorplasty.[20] This procedure relies on gravity for elbow extension and is contraindicated in those patients who require powerful extension for transfer or crutch ambulation. This transfer is reserved for those individuals without other options for transfer or when cocontracture of the biceps and triceps is present.[81]

The pectoralis major muscle receives innervation from throughout the plexus by the lateral (C5, C6, C7) and medial pectoral nerves (C8, T1). This muscle can be transferred by a variety of techniques, including elongation of the humeral insertion by tendon graft, transfer of the sternocostal origin to the biceps (monopolar), and transfer of the sternocostal origin to the biceps, with transfer of the humeral insertion to the acromion (bipolar).[7,13,21,28,49] The bipolar technique appears to provide the more powerful elbow flexion because the mechanical advantage is improved by transfer of the origin and insertion, and the entire mass of pectoralis major is used (increased cross-sectional area; Fig. 18).[21] However, this technique is technically demanding and cosmetically disfiguring.[81] But, the bipolar technique is the preferred technique when the pectoralis major muscle is selected for flexorplasty, for function overrides cosmesis in brachial plexus injuries.

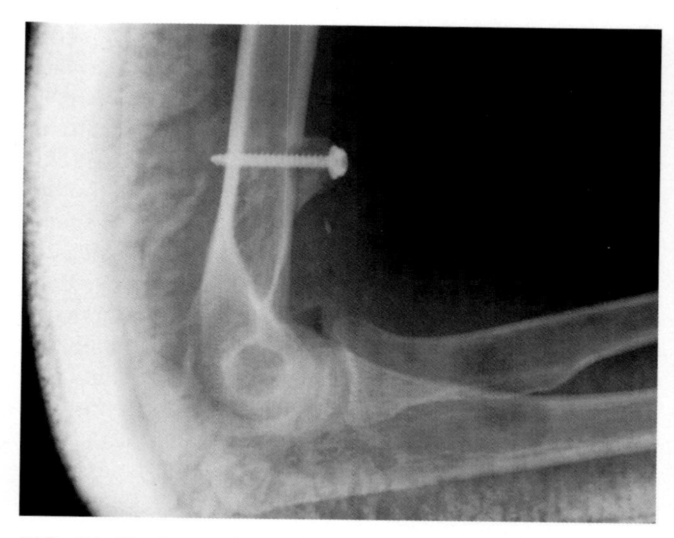

FIG. 17. Postoperative radiograph of medial epicondyle and attached flexor–pronator mass secured to the anterior humerus with a compression screw.

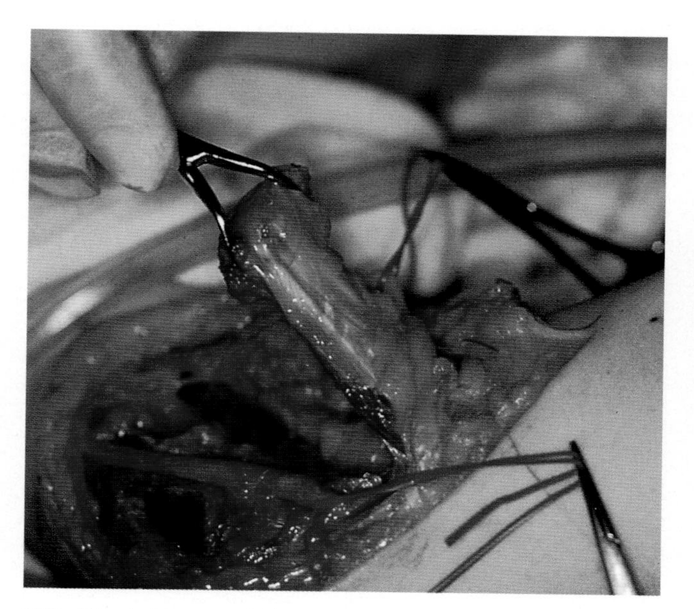

FIG. 16. A 14-year-old boy with history of C5-C6 transverse myelitis with absent elbow flexion. He was treated with proximal transfer of the medial epicondyle and flexor–pronator mass to the anterior humerus. Vessel loupes around median and ulnar nerves.

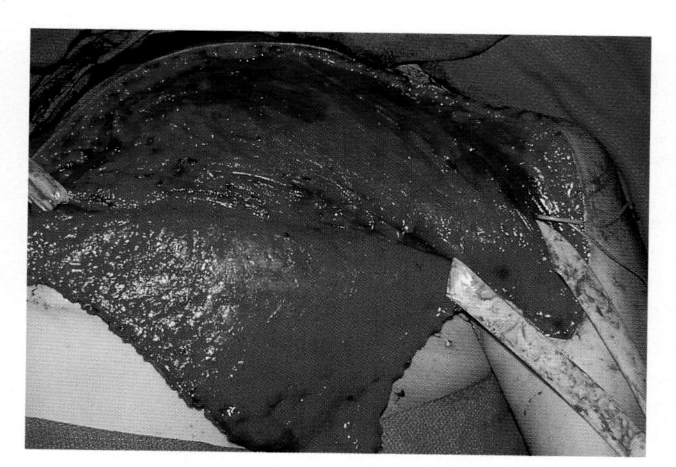

FIG. 18. A 31-year-old man, status post-brachial neuritis (Parsonage-Turner syndrome), with persistent musculocutaneous nerve palsy. He was treated with bipolar pectoralis major muscle transfer for elbow flexion.

The latissimus dorsi transfer for elbow flexion can also be accomplished by a monopolar or bipolar technique. The bipolar method transfers the origin to the biceps tendon and the humeral insertion to the coracoid process or acromion.[148] The unipolar variant does not disturb the humeral attachment. This flexorplasty has certain distinct advantages that make bipolar latissimus flexorplasty the preferred procedure for elbow flexion. The latissimus muscle can be sacrificed with minimal morbidity, provides excellent strength and excursion, and reinforces the anterior support to the shoulder, which may obviate the need for arthrodesis.[16,21] The drawbacks are related to the magnitude of the procedure and the difficult preoperative assessment of muscle grade, because bulk can overestimate strength.

Bipolar Latissimus Dorsi Transfer Technique

The bipolar latissimus dorsi transfer is performed with the patient in the sloppy lateral position. The arm and torso are prepared to the midline for adequate exposure. The ipsilateral thigh is also prepared for possible fascia lata graft. A linear incision is performed in the posterior axillary line extending proximal from the thoracodorsal origin of the latissimus dorsi muscle and distal into the axilla. A large skin flap is elevated over the posterior aspect of the latissimus to the midline. The lateral border of the muscle is identified and elevated from the underlying serratus anterior muscle. Stay sutures are placed on the surface of the muscle to record the resting length. The neurovascular pedicle is identified by palpation at the junction of the proximal and distal thirds on the undersurface of the latissimus. The muscle with some of the thoracodorsal fascia is harvested from distal to proximal from the chest wall and spinal muscles (Fig. 19). Meticulous hemostasis is attained throughout this dissection, which is performed with an electrocautery. The entire latissimus dorsi muscle is harvested on the thoracodorsal neurovascular pedicle. The vascular pedicle is mobilized to the subscapular artery, with ligation of the branch to the serratus muscle. The insertion of the latissimus tendon is tagged and divided. An anterior deltopectoral approach to the shoulder is performed and the latissimus dorsi muscle and pedicle are passed into the anterior wound (Fig. 20). Care must be taken not to kink the vessels. A large subcutaneous passage is tunneled from the deltopectoral interval to the antecubital fossa where the biceps tendon is exposed. The origin is attached to the biceps tendon by a weave technique. The addition of fascia lata interwoven into the latissimus dorsi for augmentation is necessary in certain instances. The elbow wound is closed before setting final tension at the anterior shoulder level. Final tension of the latissimus dorsi flexorplasty is determined by recreating resting length, using the previously placed stay sutures as a guideline and creating a 30-degree–tenodesis effect at the elbow. The humeral insertion is attached to either the coracoid or acromion, depending on which provides the correct tension. Suction drains are placed into the back wound and the arm immobilized to the chest for 6 weeks before active flexion. Protective extension block splinting is continued until 3 months after surgery.

The results after elbow flexorplasty are generally good, with a return of flexion against gravity (Figs. 21 and 22).[7,20,21,81,148] These transfers are often weak and lack lifting power, but there is significant improvement in function

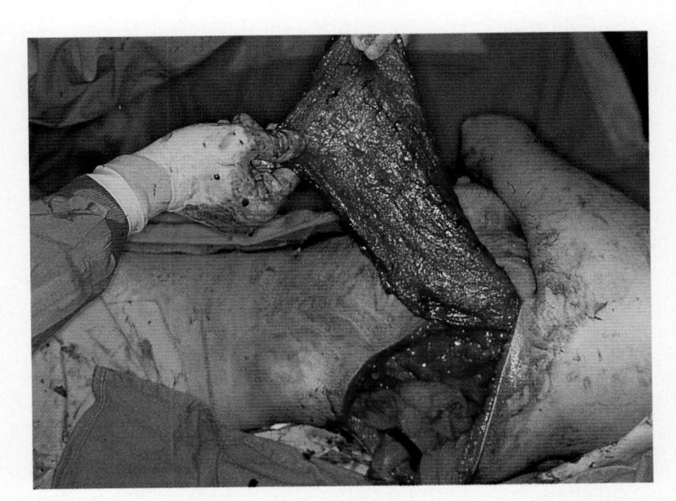

FIG. 19. A 30-year-old woman with absent elbow flexion after brachial plexus injury secondary to having her arm struck by a moving train. Latissimus dorsi muscle harvested from distal to proximal for elbow flexorplasty. Note stay sutures placed to record resting length.

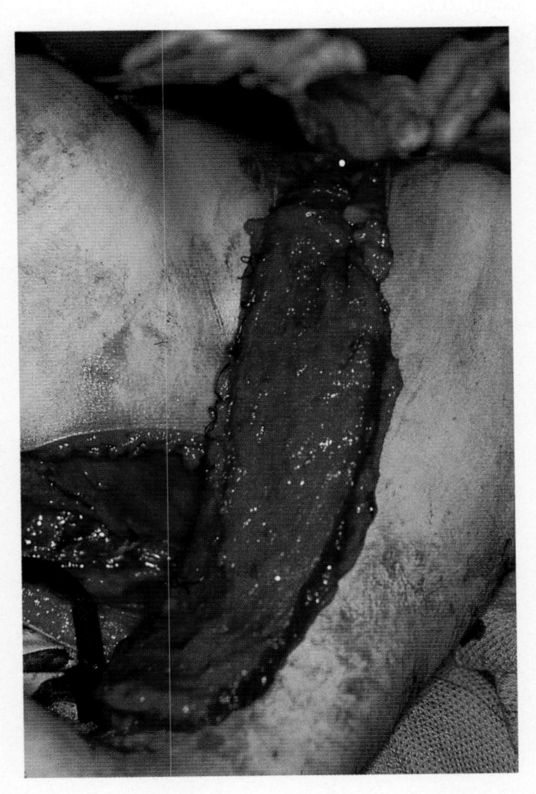

FIG. 20. Latissimus dorsi delivered into anterior wound and placed over arm in preparation for bipolar flexorplasty.

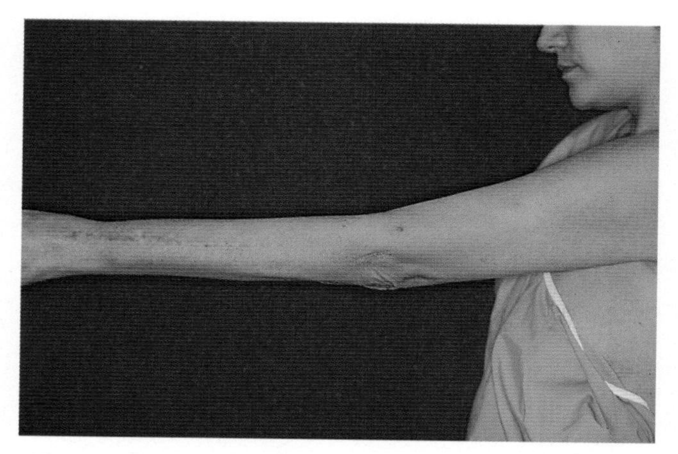

FIG. 21. Full passive elbow extension 2 years after latissimus dorsi bipolar flexorplasty.

compared with a paralyzed elbow.[7,23,93] A flexion contracture is common, but this posture also provides a mechanical advantage to initiate flexion. The presence or persistence of poor shoulder control will inhibit use of the transfer and curtail the result.[65,81,148]

Free-muscle transfer with nerve coaptation is a valiant technique to restore flexion.[26,71] This procedure involves a free microvascular muscle transfer of an expendable muscle with coaptation of a viable donor nerve to the motor nerve of the transferred muscle. This technique is indicated when other less-complicated procedures are unavailable that are most commonly used for restoration of elbow flexion. For example, long-standing denervation causes irreversible muscle atrophy with fibrosis and precludes the use of nerve grafting or nerve transfer to restore elbow flexion. The gracilis is the most common muscle used for neurovascular transfer, with the intercostal nerves coapted to the obturator motor nerve for innervation.[23,26,71] The vascular supply to the gracilis is reestablished by microsurgical anastomosis of the pedicle artery and vein to the brachial artery (end to side) and venae comitante. The muscle is attached in a similar fashion to a latissimus dorsi flexorplasty with proximal fixation to the coracoid or clavicle and distal weaving into the biceps tendon. Free-muscle transfer of the latissimus dorsi muscle to the forearm, with proximal attachment above the elbow and distal connection to the finger flexors, has been performed. Nerve transfer to the latissimus muscle has also been used to achieve combined elbow and finger flexion.[35]

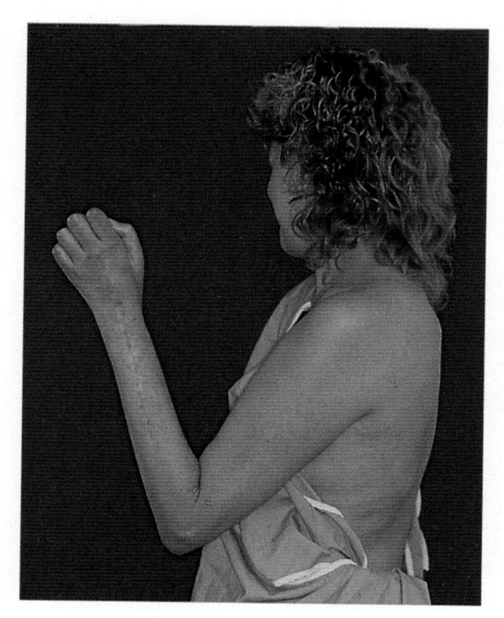

FIG. 22. Active flexion 2 years after latissimus dorsi bipolar flexorplasty which improved extremity function.

The recent results after functioning free-muscle transplantation are impressive, with elbow strength greater than gravity achieved in approximately 75% to 80% and similar results to pedicled latissimus dorsi transfer.[26,71]

Shoulder Function

Shoulder function is impaired in upper brachial plexus lesions with paralysis of the deltoid and rotator cuff muscles.[40,44] The shoulder can be completely unstable and subluxate in an inferior direction or be unbalanced by asymmetrical muscle pull. The paralysis of the infraspinatus and teres minor muscles will prevent external rotation, whereas internal rotation is preserved by the subscapularis, pectoralis major, or latissimus dorsi muscle. This creates a loss of external rotation, with a propensity for internal rotation contracture. This internal rotation posture is a disability, for hand to mouth function with the arm at the side requires some external rotation.[81,107] In addition, external rotation with active abduction promotes use of the extremity above the shoulder level. This problem is particularly relevant in patients with residual obstetric brachial plexus palsies who have had return of moderate biceps function without external rotation.[48,104] To achieve hand to mouth function, compensatory shoulder or scapulothoracic abduction is required (Fig. 23). This abduction allows the hand to be delivered to the mouth despite persistent shoulder internal rotation, but appears abnormal and is inefficient for feeding. In severe deformity, the shoulder may dislocate in a posterior direction (Fig. 24) or when the child can not obtain 80 degrees of abduction and has an internal rotation contracture greater than 45 degrees, hand to mouth function is impossible.[140]

The treatment of residual shoulder deformities is based on tendon transfer to rebalance the shoulder, humeral osteotomy to improve position, or arthrodesis to provide a stable shoulder. The most common tendon transfer used is relocation of the latissimus dorsi and teres major tendons to the infraspinatus insertion to restore external rotation.[58,104,107] This procedure is common in the residual obstetric brachial plexus population with loss of external rotation. The prerequisites for this transfer are passive external rotation and a congruent glenohumeral joint without significant dysplasia. Passive external rotation is achieved by physical therapy or surgery in recalcitrant cases. The surgery entails anterior re-

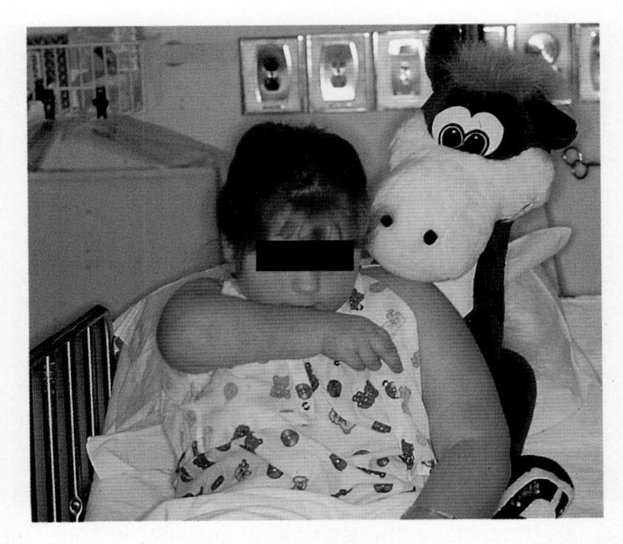

FIG. 23. An 8-year-old child with impaired hand to mouth function from residual obstetric brachial plexus palsy and lack of external rotation.

lease or lengthening of the myostatic contracture involving the pectoralis major and subscapularis muscles and is best performed at about the age of 2 to prevent potential glenohumeral dysplasia.[40,107] The anterior capsule is usually not divided for fear of instability. This procedure can be performed at the time of tendon transfer for external rotation of the shoulder, but a staged release and delayed transfer is preferred (3-month interlude) to ensure adequate passive motion. Subsequent latissimus dorsi and teres major transfer is performed between 4 and 6 years of age before development of glenohumeral dysplasia.

Older children with dysplastic glenohumeral joints diagnosed by axillary x-ray films, CT scan or MRI are treated by external rotational osteotomy of the humerus to provide ample rotation for hand to mouth function with the arm at the side.[48]

External Rotation Tendon Transfer Technique

The technique of latissimus dorsi and teres major tendon transfer is performed with the patient prone.[58,77,140] The extremity and posterior thorax are prepared for surgery. A posterior axillary incision is performed along the latissimus dorsi muscle. A skin flap is elevated and the latissimus dorsi muscle dissected to its humeral insertion. The tendons of the latissimus and teres major muscles are identified, tagged, and divided (Fig. 25). The humerus is placed in external rotation of 45 to 60 degrees and the deltoid elevated to expose the infraspinatus insertion on the tuberosity. The latissimus and teres major tendons are transferred posterior to the long head of the triceps to the greater tuberosity and sutured to the tendon–periosteum or secured through drill holes with nonabsorbable sutures. Following wound closure, a shoulder spica cast is applied with the shoulder in 30 degrees of abduction and the full external rotation. The spica cast is removed at 5 weeks and active therapy is initiated; protective splinting is continued for 3 months after surgery.

In cases of a dysplastic glenohumeral joint with inadequate external rotation for hand to mouth function, a rotational osteotomy of the humerus is performed.[48] The procedure is accomplished by an anterolateral approach to the distal humerus and mobilization of the radial nerve. Kirshner wires are placed into the humerus proximal and distal to the proposed osteotomy site to judge rotational correction. The

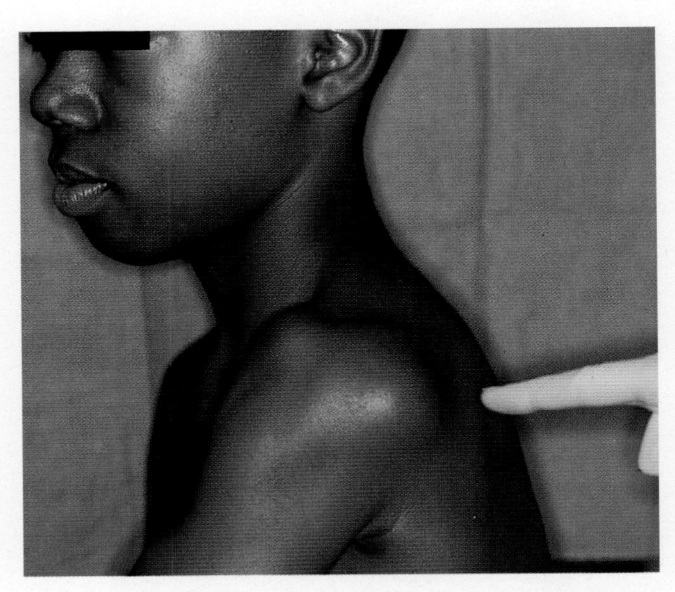

FIG. 24. A 10-year-old boy with posterior shoulder dislocation from obstetric brachial plexus injury and unbalanced muscle pull.

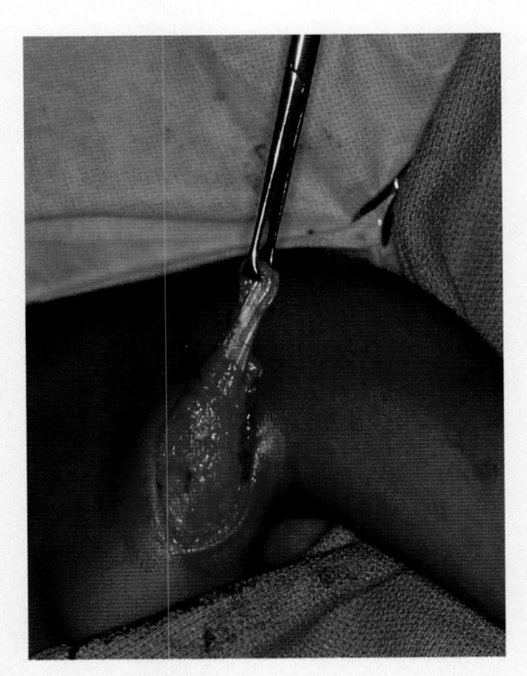

FIG. 25. A 5-year-old child with persistent lack of active external rotation after obstetric brachial plexus palsy. The latissimus dorsi muscle and tendon were harvested from the posterior approach for external rotation tendon transfer.

osteotomy is completed with a fine saw blade and external rotation of approximately 30 degrees obtained. The osteotomy is secured with dynamic plate compression to maintain alignment during the postoperative immobilization period of about 4 weeks (Fig. 26). Therapy is usually necessary to alter the preoperative pattern of combined shoulder abduction and elbow flexion for hand to mouth activity.

Another tendon transfer about the shoulder for residual brachial plexus palsy involves transfer of a muscle to restore glenohumeral abduction. Donor muscles used include the trapezius, levator scapulae, and latissimus dorsi.[40,44,61] The trapezius is transferred with a portion of the acromion to the decorticated posterolateral humerus. The levator scapulae is elongated with a fascial graft to reach the tendon of the supraspinatus, and the latissimus is transferred on a pedicle similar to the bipolar technique for flexorplasty.[40,61] Experience with these transfers is limited because obstetric palsies often regain adequate scapulothoracic abduction, and adults are treated with a bipolar elbow flexorplasty that can stabilize the shoulder. In persistent cases of shoulder instability or subluxation, arthrodesis is preferred in adult plexopathies.

Shoulder arthrodesis uses the scapulothoracic muscles for motion and predictably corrects painful glenohumeral subluxation. Absent scapular control is a contraindication for shoulder fusion. The optimal position for fusion is controversial and should allow hand to mouth function with active elbow flexion. A preferred posture is 30 degrees of abduction, internal rotation, and forward flexion.[110,111] Numerous operative techniques have been described to achieve union; rigid internal fixation is preferred, with an AO reconstruction plate across the scapular spine and onto the lateral humerus (Fig. 27). AO large cancellous screws are secured from the lateral humerus into the glenoid, and an autologous bone graft is added (Fig. 28). Postoperative immobilization varies from an abduction pillow to a shoulder spica, depending on the quality of the bone and rigidity of the fixation.

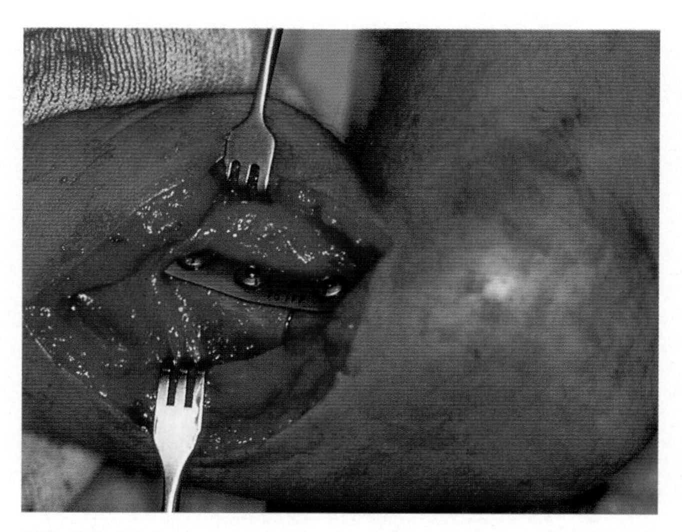

FIG. 26. Distal humeral osteotomy in a 10-year-old child with an obstetric brachial plexus palsy, lack of external rotation, and glenohumeral dysplasia.

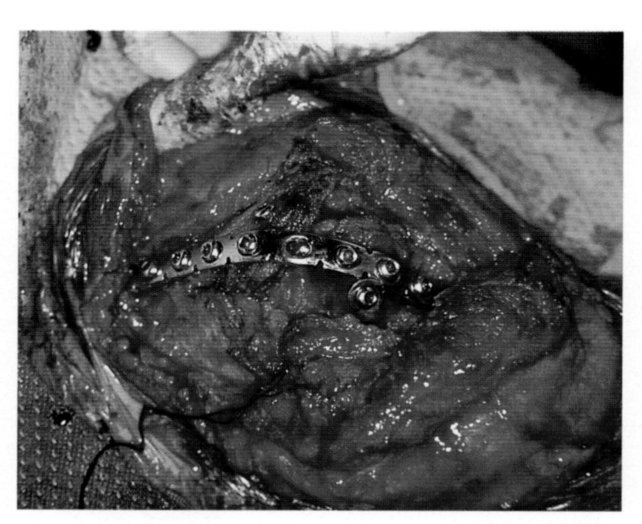

FIG. 27. Shoulder arthrodesis for an unstable, arthritic, and painful glenohumeral joint after a shoulder dislocation with persistent axillary nerve palsy.

The results for tendon transfer about the shoulder are variable. Transfers to restore shoulder abduction have limited success, although the latissimus transfer appears promising.[40,61] In contrast, the external rotation transfer has excellent success, with restoration of active abduction and the ability to achieve hand to mouth function with the arm at the side in most patients.[58,104,107,140] Restoration of external rotation by transfer rebalances the shoulder and prevents pro-

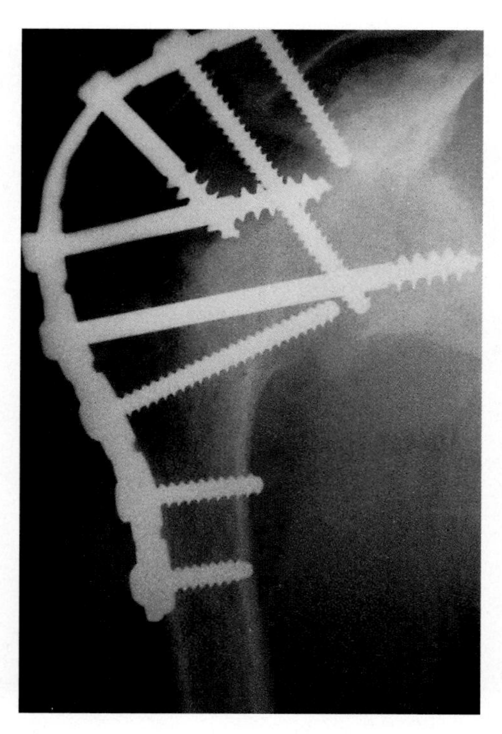

FIG. 28. Postoperative x-ray film of shoulder arthrodesis performed with reconstruction plate.

gressive deformity and possible posterior shoulder dislocation (see Fig. 24).[38,104]

Shoulder arthrodesis can reliably correct painful subluxation and provide stability to the extremity.[110,111] This proximal stability will allow better use of the extremity by scapulothoracic motion and is often combined with other tendon transfers to improve distal function. Humeral osteotomy for deficient external rotation with glenohumeral dysplasia can place the extremity in a better position for hand to mouth function, especially in the residual obstetric brachial plexus injuries (Fig. 29).[48]

Forearm, Wrist, and Hand

The forearm, wrist, and hand deformity is variable in residual brachial plexus injuries.[10] The goals are to rebalance the extremity by tendon transfer or arthrodesis. Transfer is preferred, but the limited availability of donors is a frequent problem. Wrist arthrodesis can provide a stable platform and will liberate wrist tendons as donors for transfer. The principles are to achieve grasp and release for function. The potential transfers are innumerable, but all must comply with the basic requirements and tenets of tendon transfers. The most common transfer involves restoration of wrist and digit extension with an expendable wrist or finger flexor, or both.

COMPLICATIONS OF BRACHIAL PLEXUS SURGERY

Brachial plexus surgery is a significant endeavor with potential for both minor and major complications. These problems can be mild and transient, or severe and life-threatening. The proximity of major vascular, nervous, lymphatic, and pulmonary structures, coupled with surrounding scar, increases the risk of injury (Table 7). Vascular injury can occur during the surgical approach or dissection for brachial plexus injury or thoracic outlet syndrome. The subclavian artery and vein are most susceptible to injury, especially after a previous repair or interposition grafting. A significant vascular injury can cause profuse bleeding that requires expedient measures to avert a catastrophic complication. Vascular clamps should be available to control potential bleeding .

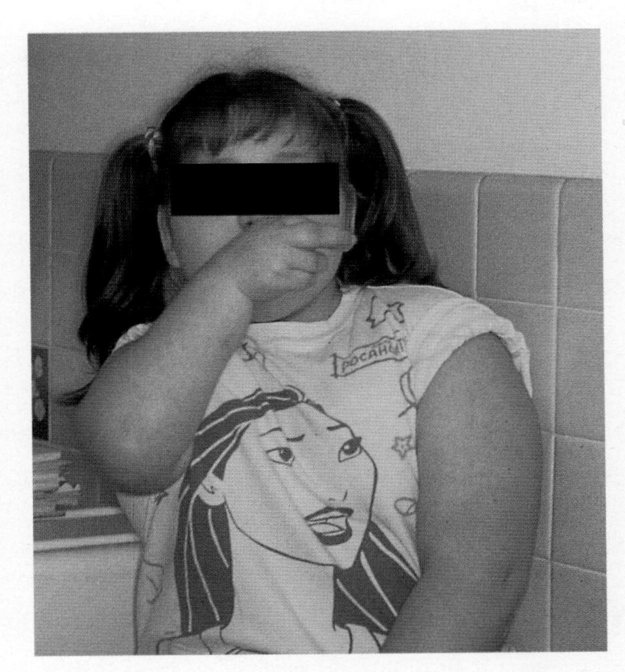

FIG. 29. Improved hand to mouth function after distal humeral rotational osteotomy in a 10-year-old with obstetric brachial plexus palsy.

Lymphatic injuries can occur during surgery on the left side of the plexus, and chylous drainage or a chylothoracic sinus may result if the injury is not recognized.[6] Pulmonary injury can occur during plexus dissection or harvesting of the intercostal nerves for transfer. During first-rib resection, pleura violation and pneumothorax are not uncommon and require chest tube placement. In addition, direct injury to the phrenic nerve during anterior scalenectomy will alter hemidiaphragm mobility during inspiration and can cause dyspnea.[6] Supraclavicular dissection can lacerate a pseudomeningocele and cause cerebrospinal fluid drainage. The pulse rate will quickly diminish and treatment requires immediate repair.[94]

Nerve injuries are the most troublesome complications and can be permanent. Inadvertent laceration, traction, and avulsion injuries can occur during surgery. The intercostal brachial cutaneous nerve is susceptible to injury during axillary dissection for first-rib resection or latissimus dorsi transfer. This nerve emanates from the third interspace and supplies sensation to the medial aspect of the arm. A neuroma or neuritis can develop that can be painful and disabling. Treatment requires localized nerve blocks or excision of the intercostal brachial cutaneous nerve. The lower plexus is particularly susceptible during first-rib resection for thoracic outlet syndrome secondary to traction from arm elevation or direct transection.[32] Intermittent arm relaxation will prevent stretching and ischemia of the lower plexus. The prognosis for recovery of a neurotmetic lower trunk lesion is poor, and residual deficits are likely. An injury at this level can also involve the sympathetic fibers, and a Horner's syndrome will

TABLE 7. *Complications of brachial plexus injuries*

System	Injury	Treatment
Vascular	Laceration	Repair
	Thrombosis	Thrombectomy
Pulmonary	Pneumothoracic pleural effusion	Tube thoracostomy
	Phrenic nerve	Avoidance
Lymphatic	Thoracic duct	Ligation
Nervous	Laceration	Repair
	Traction	Intermittent relaxation
	Dura puncture	Repair
	RSD	

result. The long thoracic nerve is also vulnerable during first-rib resection or middle scalenectomy because the nerve may travel along this muscle.[144]

REFERENCES

1. Adson AW, Coffey JR. Cervical rib: A method of anterior approach for relief of symptoms by division of the scalenus anticus. *Ann Surg* 1927;85:839–856.
2. *Aids to the investigation of of peripheral nerve injuries*, ed 2. (Medical Research Council War Memorandum, vol 7.) London: His Majesty's Stationery Office, 1943:48.
3. Allieu Y, Clauzel AM, Mekhaldi A, Triki F. Consequences sur la fonction respiratoire des paralysies du plexus brachial de l'adulte et de leur traitement chirurgical. *Rev Chir Orthop* 1986;72:455–460.
4. Alnot JY. Traumatic brachial plexus palsy in the adult. Retro- and infraclavicular lesions. *Clin Orthop* 1988;237:9–16.
5. Alnot JY. Traumatic brachial plexus lesions in the adult. Indications and results. *Hand Clin* 1995;11:623–631.
6. Atasoy E. Thoracic outlet syndrome. *Orthop Clin North Am* 1996;27: 265–303.
7. Beaton DE, Dumont A, Mackay MB, Richards RR. Steindler and pectoralis major flexorplasty: a comparative analysis. *J Hand Surg [Am]* 1995;20:747–756.
8. Berger A, Brenner P. Secondary surgery following brachial plexus injuries. *Microsurgery* 1995;16:43–47.
9. Birch R. Surgery for brachial plexus injuries. *J Bone Joint Surg [Br]* 1993;75:346–348.
10. Bonnard C, Narakas A. Restoration of hand function after brachial plexus injury. *Hand Clin* 1995;11:647–656.
11. Boome RS, Kaye JC. Obstetric traction injuries of the brachial plexus. Natural history, indications for surgical repair and results. *J Bone Joint Surg [Br]* 1988;70:571–576.
12. Brien WW, Gellman H, Becker V, Garland DE, Waters R, Wiss DA. Management of upper extremity fractures in patients with brachial plexus injuries. *J Bone Joint Surg [Am]* 1990;72:1208–1210.
13. Brooks DM, Seddon HJ. Pectoral transplantation for paralysis of the flexors of the elbow. *J Bone Joint Surg [Br]* 1959;41:36–50.
14. Brooks DM. Open wounds of the brachial plexus. *J Bone Joint Surg [Br]* 1949;31:17–33.
15. Bruxelle J, Traves V, Thiebaut JB. Occurrence and treatment of pain after brachial plexus injury. *Clin Orthop* 1988;237:87–95.
16. Brumback RJ, McBride MS, Ortolani NC. Functional evaluation of the shoulder after transfer of the vascularized latissimus dorsi muscle. *J Bone Joint Surg [Am]* 1992;74:377–382.
17. Campion D. Electrodiagnostic testing in hand surgery. *J Hand Surg [Am]* 1996;21:947–956.
18. Carlsted T, Grane P, Hallin RG, Noren G. Return of function after spinal cord implantation of avulsed spinal nerve roots. *Lancet* 1995; 346:1323–1325.
19. Carlsted T. Functional recovery after ventral root avulsion and implantation in the spinal cord. *Clin Neurol Neurosurg* 1993;95:S109–111.
20. Carroll RE, Hill NA. Triceps transfer to restore elbow flexion. A study of fifteen patients with paralytic lesions and arthrogryposis. *J Bone Joint Surg [Am]* 1970;52:239–244.
21. Carroll RE, Kleinman WB. Pectoralis major transplantation to restore elbow flexion to the paralytic limb. *J Hand Surg* 1979; 4:501–507.
22. Chuang DCC, Yeh MC, Wei FC. Intercostal nerve transfer of the musculocutaneous nerve in avulsed brachial plexus injuries. *J Hand Surg [Am]* 1992;17:822–828.
23. Chuang DCC, Epstein MD, Yeh MC, Wei FC. Functional restoration of elbow flexion in brachial plexus injuries: results in 167 patients (excluding obstetric brachial plexus injury). *J Hand Surg [Am]* 1993;18: 285–291.
24. Chuang DCC. Neurotization procedures for brachial plexus injuries. *Hand Clin* 1995;11:633–645.
25. Chuang DC, Lee GW, Hashem F, Wei FC. Restoration of shoulder abduction by nerve transfer in avulsed brachial plexus injury: evaluation of 99 patients with various nerve transfers. *Plast Reconstr Surg* 1995; 96:122–128.
26. Chuang DCC, Carver N, Wei FC. Results of functioning free muscle transplantation for elbow flexion. *J Hand Surg [Am]* 1996;21: 1071–1077.
27. Clark WL, Trumble TE, Swiontkowski MF, Tencer AF. Nerve tension and blood flow in a rat model of immediate and delayed repairs. *J Hand Surg [Am]* 1992;17:677–687.
28. Clark JMP. Reconstruction of biceps brachii by pectoral muscle transplantation. *Br J Surg* 1946;34:180–181.
29. Clarke HM, Curtis CG. An approach to obstetrical brachial plexus injuries. *Hand Clin* 1995;11:563–580.
30. Comtet JJ, Sedel L, Fredenucci JF, Herzberg G. Duchenne-Erb plasy. Experience with direct surgery. *Clin Orthop* 1988;237:17–23.
31. Cormier J, Amrane M, Ward A, Laurian C, Gigou F. Arterial complications of the thoracic outlet syndrome. *J Vasc Surg* 1989;9:778–787.
32. Dale A. Thoracic outlet compression syndrome. *Arch Surg* 1982;117: 1437–1445.
33. Daseler EH, Anson BJ. Surgical anatomy of the subclavian artery and its branches. *Surg Gynecol Obstet* 1959;108:149–174.
34. Deletis V, Morota N, Abbott IR. Electrodiagnosis in the management of brachial plexus surgery. *Hand Clin* 1995;11:555–561.
35. Doi K, Sakai K, Kuwata N, Ihara K, Kawai S. Reconstruction of finger and elbow function after complete avulsions of the brachial plexus. *J Hand Surg [Am]* 1991;16:796–803.
36. Duchenne GBA. *De l'electrisatian localisee et de son application a la pathologic et a la therapeutique*, 3rd ed. Paris: Balliere, 1872: 357–362.
37. Dunkerton MC, Boome RS. Stab wounds involving the brachial plexus. *J Bone Joint Surg [Br]* 1988;70:566–570.
38. Dunkerton MC. Posterior dislocation of the shoulder associated with obstetric brachial plexus palsy. *J Bone Joint Surg [Br]* 1989;71:764–766.
39. Ebraheim N, An HS, Jackson WT, et al. Scapulothoracic dissociation. *J Bone Joint Surg [Am]* 1988;70:428–432.
40. Egloff DV, Raffoul W, Bonnard C, Stadler J. Palliative surgical procedures to restore shoulder function in obstetrical brachial palsy. A critical analysis of Narakas' series. *Hand Clin* 1995;11:597–606.
41. Ellison DW, Wood VE. Trauma-related thoracic outlet syndrome. *J Hand Surg [Br]* 1994;19:424–426.
42. Erb W. Uber eine eigenthumliche Localisation von Lahmungen im plexus brachialis. *Naturhist-Med Ver Heidelberg* 1874;2:130–131.
43. Gallen J, Wiss D, Cantelmo N, Menzoin J. Traumatic pseudoanuerysm of the axillary artery. Report of three cases and literature review. *J Trauma* 1984;24:350–354.
44. Gilbert A, Romana C, Ayatta R. Tendon transfers for shoulder paralysis in children. *Hand Clin* 1988;4:633–642.
45. Gilbert A. Long-term evaluation of brachial plexus surgery in obstetrical palsy. *Hand Clin* 1995;11:583–594.
46. Gilliatt RW, LeQuesne PM, Logue V, Sumner AJ. Wasting of the hand associated with a cervical rib or band. *J Neurol Neurosurg Psychiatry* 1970;33:615–624.
47. Gockel M, Vastamaki M, Alaranta H. Long-term results of primary scalenotomy in the treatment of thoracic outlet syndrome. *J Hand Surg [Br]* 1994;19:229–233.
48. Goddard NJ, Fixen JA. Rotation osteotomy of the humerus for birth injuries of the brachial plexus. *J Bone Joint Surg [Br]* 1984;66B: 257–259.
49. Goldner JL. Tendon transfers for irreparable peripheral nerve injuries of the upper extremity. *Orthop Clin North Am* 1974; 5:343–375.
50. Gordon M, Rich H, Deutschberger J, Green M. The immediate and long-term outcome of obstetric birth trauma. I.Brachial plexus paralysis. *Am J Obstet Gynecol* 1973;117:51–56.
51. Greenwald AG, Schute PC, Shiveley JL. Brachial plexus palsy, a 10-year report on the incidence and prognosis. *J Pediatr Orthop* 1984;4: 689–692.
52. Gu YD, Ma MK. Use of the phrenic nerve for brachial plexus reconstruction. *Clin Orthop* 1996;323:119–121.
53. Hallikainen H, Partenen J, Mervaala E. The importance of neurophysiological evaluation of plexus bracialis injury caused by open heart surgery. *Electromyogr Clin Neurophysiol* 1993;33:67–71.
54. Hentz VR, Narakas A. The results of microneurosurgical reconstruction in complete plexus palsy. Assessing outcome and predicting results. *Orthop Clin N Am* 1988;19:107–114.
55. Hentz VR, Meyer RD. Brachial plexus microsurgery in children. *Microsurgery* 1991;12:175–185.
56. Hershman E. Brachial plexus injuries. *Clin Sports Med* 1990;9: 311–329.
57. Hirasawa Y, Sakakida M. Sports and peripheral nerve injury. *Am J Sports Med* 1983;11:420–426.

58. Hoffer MM, Wickendon R, Roper B. Brachial plexus palsies. Results of tendon transfers to the rotator cuff. *J Bone Joint Surg* 1978;69: 691–695
59. Hudson DA, Boome R, Sanpera I. Brachial plexus injury after median sternotomy. *J Hand Surg [Am]* 1993;18:282–284.
60. Huu N, Vallee B, Person H, Vu N. Anatomical bases of transaxillary resection of the first rib. *Anat Clin* 1984;5:221–233.
61. Itoh Y, Sasaki T, Ishiguro T, Uchinishi K, Yabe Y, Fukuda H. Transfer of latissimus dorsi to replace a paralyzed deltoid. A new technique using an inverted pedicle. *J Bone Joint Surg [Br]* 1987;69: 647–651.
62. Kawai H, Kawabata H, Masceda K, et al. Nerve repairs for traumatic brachial plexus with root avulsion. *Clin Orthop* 1988;237:75–86.
63. Kaye BL. Neurologic changes with excessively large breasts. *South Med J* 1972;75:177–180.
64. Kerr AT. The brachial plexus of nerves in man, the variations in its formation and branches. *Am J Anat* 1918;22:285–395.
65. Kettelkamp DB, Larson CB. Evaluation of the Steindler flexorplasty. *J Bone Joint Surg [Am]* 1963;45:513–518.
66. Kirgis HD, Reed AF. Significant anatomic relations in the syndrome of the scalene muscles. *Ann Surg* 1948;127:11
67. Kitamura T, Takagi K, Yamaga M, Morisawa K. Brachial plexus stretching injuries: microcirculation of the brachial plexus. *J Shoulder Elbow Surg* 1995;4:118–123.
68. Kline DG, Judice DJ. Operative management of selected brachial plexus lesions. *J Neurosurg* 1983;58:631–63.
69. Kline DG. Civilian gunshot wounds to the brachial plexus. *J Neurosurg* 1989;70:166–174.
70. Klumpke A. Contribution a l'etude des paralysies radicularies du plexus brachial. *Rev Med Paris* 1885;5:591–593.
71. Krakauer JD, Wood MB. Intercostal nerve transfer for brachial plexopathy. *J Hand Surg [Am]* 1994;19:829–835.
72. Landi A, Copeland SA, Wynn Parry CB, Jones SJ. The role of somatosensory evoked potentials and nerve conduction studies in the surgical management of brachial plexus injuries. *J Bone Joint Surg [Br]* 1980;62:492–496.
73. Laurent JP, Lee R, Shenaq S, Parke JT, Solis IS, Kowlik L. Neurosurgical correction of upper brachial plexus birth injuries. *J Neurosurg* 1993;79:197–203.
74. Leffert RD. Thoracic outlet syndromes. *Hand Clin* 1992;8:285–297.
75. Lepantalo M, Lindgren K-A, Leino E. Long-term outcome after resection of the first rib for thoracic outlet syndrome. *Br J Surg* 1989;76: 1255–1256.
76. Lundborg G, Rydevik B. Effects of stretching the tibial nerve of the rabbit. A preliminary study of the intraneural circulation and the barrier function of the perineurium. *J Bone Joint Surg [Br]* 1973;55: 390–401.
77. L'Episcopo JB. Tendon transplantation in obstetrical paralysis. *Am J Surg* 1934;25:122–125.
78. Machleder HI, Moll F, Nuwer M, Jordon S. Somatosensory evoked potentials in the assessment of thoracic outlet syndrome. *J Vasc Surg* 1987;6:177–184.
79. Magee KR, DeLong RN. Paralytic brachial neuritis *JAMA* 1960;174: 1258–1262.
80. Mandel S. Neurologic syndromes from repetitive trauma at work. *Postgrad Med* 1987;82:87–92.
81. Marshall RW, Williams DH, Birch R, Bonney G. Operations to restore elbow flexion after brachial plexus injuries. *J Bone Joint Surg [Br]* 1988;70:577–582.
82. Mayer L, Green W. Experiences with the Steindler flexorplasty at the elbow. *J Bone Joint Surg [Am]* 1954;36:775–789.
83. Mehta VS, Banerji AK, Tripathi RP. Surgical treatment of brachial plexus injuries. *Br J Neurosurg* 1993;7:491–500.
84. Metaizeau JP, Gayet C, Plenat F. Les lesions obstetricales du plexus brachial. *Chir Pediatr* 1979;20:159–163.
85. Miller RA. Observations upon the arrangement of the axillary artery and brachial plexus. *Am J Anat* 1939;64:143–163.
86. Millesi H. Surgical management of brachial plexus injuries. *J Hand Surg* 1977;2:367–379.
87. Millesi H. Brachial plexus injuries. Nerve grafting. *Clin Orthop* 1988; 237:36–42.
88. Millesi H. Brachial plexus injuries in adults. In: Gelberman RH, ed. *Operative nerve repair and reconstruction*. Philadelphia: JB Lipppincott, 1991:1329–1358.
89. Minami M, Ishii S. Satisfactory elbow flexion in complete (preganglionic) brachial plexus injuries: produced by suture of the third and fourth intercostal nerves to the musculocutaneous nerve. *J Hand Surg [Am]* 1987;12:1285–1301.
90. Misamore GW, Lehman DE. Parsonage-Turner syndrome (acute brachial neuritis). *J Bone Joint Surg [Am]* 1996;78:1405–1408.
91. Nagano A, Ochiai S. Restoration of elbow flexion in root lesions of brachial plexus injuries. *J Hand Surg [Am]* 1992; 17:815–821.
92. Narakas AO. The treatment of brachial plexus injuries. *Int Orthop* 1985;9:29–36.
93. Narakas AO. Neurotization in the treatment of brachial plexus injuries. In: Gelberman RH, ed. *Operative nerve repair and reconstruction*. Philadelphia: JB Lipppincott, 1991:1329–1358.
94. Narakas A. Surgical treatment of traction injuries of the brachial plexus. *Clin Orthop* 1978;133:71–90.
95. Netter FH. *The CIBA collection of medical illustrations*, vol 8, part I. West Caldwell, NJ: Ciba-Geigy, 1987:28–29.
96. Nichols H. Anatomic structures of the thoracic outlet. *Clin Orthop* 1967;51:17–25.
97. Novak CB, Mackinnon SE, Patterson GA. Evaluation of patients with thoracic outlet syndrome. *J Hand Surg [Am]* 1993;18:292–299.
98. Oates SD, Daley RA. Thoracic outlet syndrome. *Hand Clin* 1996;12: 705–718.
99. Ochi M, Ikuta Y, Watanabe M, Kimori K, Itoh K. The diagnostic value of MRI in traumatic brachial plexus injury. *J Hand Surg [Br]* 1994;19:55–59.
100. Omer GE. Injuries to nerves of the upper extremity. *J Bone Joint Surg [Am]* 1974;56:1615–1624.
101. Panasci DJ, Holliday RA, Shpizner B. Advance imaging techniques of the brachial plexus. *Hand Clin* 1995;11:545–553.
102. Panegyres PK, Moore N, Gibson R, Rushworth G, Donaghy M. Thoracic outlet syndromes and magnetic resonance imaging. *Brain* 1993; 116:823–841.
103. Parsonage MJ, Turner JWA. Neuralgic amyotrophy. The shoulder-girdle syndrome. *Lancet* 1948;1:973–978.
104. Phipps GJ, Hoffer MM. Latissimus dorsi and teres major transfer to rotator cuff for Erb's palsy. *J Shoulder Elbow Surg* 1995;4: 124–129.
105. Pollack EW. Surgical anatomy of the thoracic outlet syndrome. *Surg Gynecol Obstet* 1980;150:97–103.
106. Pratt NE. Neurovascular entrapment in the regions of the shoulder and posterior triangle of the neck. *Phys Ther* 1986; 66:1894–1900.
107. Price AE, Grossman JAI. A management approach for secondary shoulder and forearm deformities following obstetrical brachial plexus injury. *Hand Clin* 1995;11:607–617.
108. Qvarfordt PG, Ehrenfeld WK, Stony RJ. Supraclavicular radical scalenectomy and transaxillary first rib resection for the thoracic outlet syndrome. *Am J Surg* 1984;148:111–116.
109. Rayan GM, Jensen C. Thoracic outlet syndrome: Provacative examination maneuvers in a typical population. *J Shoulder Elbow Surg* 1995;4:113–117.
110. Richards RR, Sherman RMP, Hudson AR, Waddell JP. Shoulder arthrodesis using a pelvic reconstruction plate: a report of 11 cases. *J Bone Joint Surg [Am]* 1988;70:416–421.
111. Richards RR, Waddell JP, Hudson AR. Shoulder arthrodesis for the treatment of brachial plexus palsy. *Clin Orthop* 1985; 198:250–258.
112. Roger B, Travers V, Laval-Jeantet M. Imaging of postraumatic brachial plexus injury. *Clin Orthop* 1988;237:57–61.
113. Roos DB. The place for scalenectomy and first rib resection in thoracic outlet syndrome. *Surgery* 1982;92:1077–1085.
114. Roos DB. Congenital anomalies associated with thoracic outlet syndrome: anatomy, symptoms, diagnosis, and treatment. *Am J Surg* 1976;132:771–778.
115. Roos DB. The place for scalenectomy and first rib resection in thoracic outlet syndrome. *Surgery* 1982;92:1077–1085.
116. Roos DB. Transaxillary approach for first rib resection to relieve thoracic outlet syndrome. *Ann Surg* 1966;163:354–358.
117. Rosson JW. Closed traction lesions of the brachial plexus: an epidemic among young motorcyclists. *Injury* 1988;19:4–6.
118. Sallstrom J, Schmidt H. Cervicobrachial disorders in certain occupations with special reference to compression in the thoracic outlet. *Am J Ind Med* 1984;6:45–52.
119. Sanders RJ, Monsour JW, Gerber WF, Adams W, Thompson N. Scalenectomy versus first rib resection for treatment of the thoracic outlet syndrome. *Surgery* 1979;85:109–121.

120. Sanders RJ, Pearce WH. The treatment of thoracic outlet syndrome: A comparison of different operations. *J Vasc Surg* 1989;10: 626–634.
121. Seddon HJ. *Surgical disorders of peripheral nerve injuries*. 2nd ed. Edinburgh, Churchill-Livingstone, 1972.
122. Seddon HJ. Nerve grafting. *J Bone Joint Surg [Br]* 1963;45:447–461.
123. Sedel L. The results of surgical repair of brachial plexus injury. *J Bone Joint Surg [Br]* 1982;64:54–66.
124. Sellke FW, Kelly TR. Thoracic outlet syndrome. *Am J Surg* 1988;156: 54–57.
125. Sever JW. Obstetrical paralysis: report on 1100 cases. *JAMA* 1925;85: 1862.
126. Sever JW. Obstetric paralysis. Its etiology, pathology, clinical aspects and treatment, with a report of four-hundred and seventy cases. *Am J Dis Child* 1916;12:541–544.
127. Singh HK. Incidence of congenital rib anomalies. *Ind J Chest Dis* 1973;15:157–164.
128. Steindler A. Operative treatment of paralytic conditions of the upper extremity. *J Orthop Surg* 1919;1:608–624.
129. Steindler A. Tendon transplantation in the upper extremity. *Am J Surg* 1939;44:534.
130. Stern PJ, Caudle RJ. Tendon transfers for elbow flexion. *Hand Clin* 1988;4:297–307.
131. Stevens JH. The classic. Brachial plexus paralysis. *Clin Orthop* 1988; 237:4–8.
132. Sturm J, Cicero J. The clinical diagnosis of ruptured subclavian artery following blunt thoracic trauma. *Ann Emerg Med* 1983;12:17–19.
133. Terzis JK, Liberson WT, Levine R. Obstetrical brachial plexus palsy. *Hand Clin* 1986;2:773–786.
134. Thomas GI, Jones TW, Stavney LS, Manhas DR. The middle scalene muscle and its contribution to the thoracic outlet syndrome. *Am J Surg* 1983;145:589–592.
135. Tonkin MA, Eckersley JR, Gscwind CR. The surgical treatment of brachial plexus injuries. *Aust NZ J Surg* 1996;66:29–33.
136. Tsairis P, Dyck PJ, Mulder DW. Natural history of brachial plexus neuropathy. Report on 99 patients. *Arch Neurol* 1972; 27:109–117.
137. Tsuyama N, Hara T. Reconstructive surgery for traumatic brachial plexus surgery. *Clin Orthop Surg* 1968;3:675–687.
138. Vin F, Koskas F, Levy D, Goeau-Brissonniere O, Bacourt F. Thoracic outlet syndrome. Value of non-invasive arterial studies. *Presse Med* 1986;15:1709–1711.
139. Walsh JF. The anatomy of the brachial plexus. *Am J Med Sci* 1877;74: 387–399.
140. Wickstrom J. Birth palsies of the brachial plexus. Treatment of defects in the shoulder. *Clin Orthop* 1962;23:187–196.
141. Wilkinson MC, Birch R, Bonney G. Brachial plexus injury: when to amputate? *Injury* 1993;24:603–605.
142. Wood MB. Nerve repair and reconstruction. In: *Atlas of reconstructive microsurgery*. Rockville, MD: Aspen, 1990:32–34.
143. Wood VE, Biondi J. Double-crush compression in thoracic-outlet syndrome. *J Bone Joint Surg [Am]* 1990;72:85–87.
144. Wood VE, Frykman GK. Winging of the scapula as a complication of first rib resection: a report of six cases. *Clin Orthop* 1980;149: 160–163.
145. Wright TW, Glowczewskie F, Wheeler D, Miller G, Cowin D. Excursion and strain of the median nerve. *J Bone Joint Surg [Am]* 1996;78: 1897–1903.
146. Wright IS. The neurovascular syndrome produced by hyperabduction of the arms. *Am Heart J* 1945;29:1–19.
147. Young HA, Hardy DG. Thoracic outlet syndrome. *Br J Hosp Med* 1983;29:459–461.
148. Zancolli E, Mitre H. Latissimus dorsi transfer to restore elbow flexion: an appraisal of eight cases. *J Bone Joint Surg [Am]* 1973;55: 1265–1275.

PART IX

Arthroscopy and Imaging

Disorders of the Shoulder: Diagnosis and Management,
edited by Joseph P. Iannotti and Gerald R. Williams, Jr.
Lippincott Williams & Wilkins, Philadelphia © 1999.

CHAPTER 31

Shoulder Arthroscopy

Christopher M. Jobe

INTRODUCTION AND HISTORICAL OVERVIEW

Arthroscopy of any joint develops through three stages: the development of diagnostic procedures; followed by the development of ablative procedures; and finally, the development of reconstructive procedures. This pattern of development is followed because of the increasing difficulty encountered as we move from diagnosis to reconstruction. This pattern is further reproduced in the personal development of each individual arthroscopist.

Arthroscopic procedures began to develop in an attempt to recreate and possibly improve the outcomes of open procedures while doing less damage to uninvolved structures. We begin by trying to perform a procedure, such as the open procedure, without having to perform surgery on structures that are unaffected by the disease. This is accomplished with varying levels of success.

The general advantages of arthroscopy are magnification of the observed structures, better visual appreciation of color and texture, and the ability to evaluate a structure under conditions that are less disturbed than they would be in an open procedure.

There are, however, disadvantages and limitations in arthroscopy: visual distortion (Fig. 1), lack of layer-by-layer dissection, and visual inaccessibility, to name three. In visualization there is distortion inherent in the lenses. This makes it somewhat difficult to determine the flatness of a surface, especially one that the surgeon is trying to create. This dis-

C. M. Jobe: Department of Orthopaedic Surgery, Loma Linda University School of Medicine, Loma Linda, California 92354.

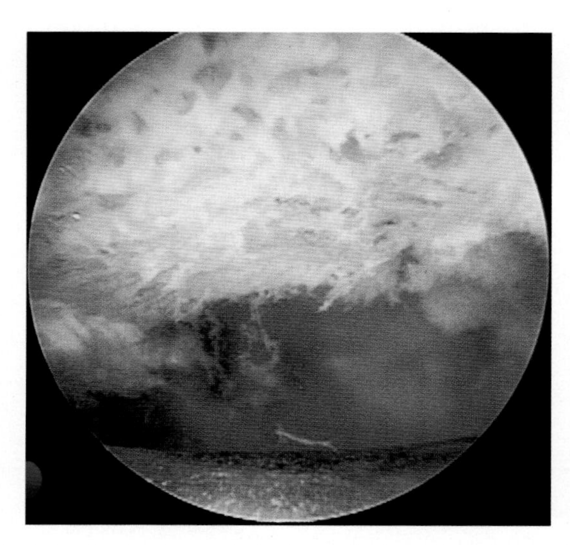

FIG. 1. Distortion through the lens. At the edge of an arthroscopic view, straight lines become concave toward the center. The shaver seen in the lower portion of this view has a straight edge. This distortion may affect a surgery where shape is important, as in judging the flatness of the undersurface of the acromion.

tortion also may lead to some disorientation early in the development of arthroscopic skills, until the surgeon becomes used to this new way of looking at things.

Arthroscopes are placed into joints with minimal disturbance to the overlying tissues. This results in less pain in the postoperative period, but takes away the advantage of a layer-by-layer dissection and, thereby, the ability to avoid injury to important but uninvolved structures, such as vessels and nerves. This inability to perform layer-by-layer dissection may preclude or delay the development of some arthroscopic portals, specifically in the shoulder, anteroinferior and posteroinferior portals. The third limitation of arthroscopy is that not all structures in a particular region of the body are contained within a space that can be filled with an arthroscopic medium. For instance, an interstitial tear of the rotator cuff will not be visible from either the joint or bursal side. Intraosseous lesions will be invisible, as well as the thoracic outlet.

In spite of these limitations, arthroscopy as a whole, and the skills of individual surgeons continue to progress.

A possible fourth stage in arthroscopic procedure development might be termed the development of the purely arthroscopic procedure. Because the arthroscope allows us to see areas and conditions of the shoulder that are not readily visible through an open procedure, new entities can be described that are seen only through the arthroscope. One of these entities, the SLAP lesion (damage to the superior labrum), is in such a location that it is also best treated through the arthroscope. In this fourth stage, the surgeon is no longer mimicking an open procedure, but has gone on to a purely arthroscopic procedure.

This developmental curve is recapitulated in the learning curve of each individual surgeon and in the indications for arthroscopic surgery. Each practitioner goes through the same process of evolution that arthroscopy of the shoulder has undergone. This process is accelerated by review of the literature, residency training, and continuing medical education courses with hands-on training, such as occurs at the AAoS Orthopaedic Learning Center. Because arthroscopy, as a whole, continues to develop, each arthroscopist is forever in a process of development. This adds an additional factor to determining the standard of care. The surgeon must be mindful to operate within his or her current level of skill. This is especially true when contemplating arthroscopic procedures for which there is an open procedure with an even higher success rate. We must remember Harold Boyd's advice that most of us should "never be the first or last" to adopt a procedure.

This final thought should be borne in mind in reading the rest of the present chapter: as we have shown that arthroscopy remains a technique in development, it is perhaps appropriate to organize the chapter along the path of procedure development. We begin with arthroscopic technique in general and the required instruments. We then discuss the procedures and indications: diagnostic, ablative, and reconstructive. We end with a discussion of complications.

SHOULDER ARTHROSCOPY TECHNIQUE

Required Spaces and Structures

In general, for arthroscopy, one needs a space fillable by a lucent medium. There are two spaces (i.e., potentially scopable spaces) in the shoulder: the glenohumeral joint and the subacromial bursa. Additional bursoscopies are reported, but are less commonly performed. The structures visible within the glenohumeral joint include the humeral and glenoid articular surfaces, the labrum of the glenoid, the long head of the biceps, the upper portion of the tendon of the subscapularis, the synovium, the subscapularis bursa, the articular surface of the rotator interval, and the thickenings of the capsule, referred to as the glenohumeral ligaments including the superior, middle, and inferior glenohumeral ligaments.

In the subacromial bursa, one can see the coracoacromial ligament, the undersurface of the acromion, the lining of the bursa, the inferior portion of the AC joint (and its contents after the inferior capsule is removed), the bursal side of the cuff and sometimes the coracohumeral ligament.

Required Instruments

The first group of instruments (Table 1) we will need are those with which we perform the diagnostic portion of the scope. One needs 30- and 70-degree lenses and various cannulae for placement of the lenses within the joint. Additional cannulae are needed, providing flow of fluids and for instrument access. These cannulae should be outfitted with blunt

TABLE 1. *Required instruments*

- A. Diagnostic equipment
  - Patient positioning
    - Beanbag for lateral position
    - Trunk stabilizer and modifiable table for beach chair position
  - Upper limb control
    - Traction device for lateral position
    - Arm rest or holder for beach chair position
  - Visualization
    - Cannulae and obturators
    - Matched endoscopes 30 degrees and 70 degrees
    - Light source and fiberoptic cable
    - Soakable television camera
    - Monitor (ergonomically positioned)
  - Fluid control and access
    - Pump with servocontrol
    - Operative cannulae
      - Side port for fluid
      - Shaped to discourage slippage
      - Transparent
  - Removal of obscuring material
    - Motorized shaver with full radius resection blades
    - Graspers
  - Testing
    - Probe
    - Biopsy forceps
- B. Ablative
  - All of the above plus
  - Bleeding control
    - Electrocautery
  - Soft material removal
    - Full selection of shaver blades for motorized shave
    - Whisker blade for synovium
    - Aggressive electrocautery
    - Laser
  - Hard material removal
    - Burrs for the motorized shaver
    - Small pituitary rongeurs
  - Tissue division
    - Scissors (various angles)
    - Basket forceps (various angles)
    - Electrocautery
- C. Reconstructive
  - All of the above plus
  - Placement of sutures
    - Suture punch
    - Suture hooks
  - Attachment to bone
    - Suture anchors and placement equipment
    - Absorbable tacks
  - Knot-tying equipment
  - Soft-tissue shrinkage
    - RF
    - Electrocautery
    - Laser

and sharp obturators. One needs an electrode for electrocautery, a motorized shaver, and a probe for palpating intraarticular structures. In addition, we need a spinal needle for portal location and a camera, monitor, and light source.

For ablative procedures, we need baskets and graspers, a set of burrs for the motorized shaver, in addition to the shaver heads, and arthroscopic knives. For reconstructive procedures, we need at least one suture punch (and probably more). We also need the appropriate reconstructive instruments, such as an absorbable tack or suture anchors, and a power drill for making holes in the bone.[1]

Anesthetic Requirements

One must be able to anesthetize the sensitive structures that are to be handled in the arthroscopy. The range, therefore, and the duration of the anesthetic required, will vary from procedure to procedure. For a diagnostic arthroscopy performed in the office with a small scope, some authors have experimented with local anesthetic. I have no experience with this, as I find visualization with the small scope inadequate. For a more extensive procedure, which will have not only intraoperative pain, but also significant postoperative pain, such as acromioplasty, an interscalene block with bupivacaine affords 12 hours of pain relief.[10] My current practice involves a mixture of interscalene anesthesia with a light general anesthetic for the extensive procedures.

Additional anesthetic issues are hypotension and paralysis. We tend not to need paralysis. Hypotension has been recommended by some authors for procedures, such as acromioplasty, during which bleeding is likely to be encountered.

Positioning Requirements

To perform the arthroscopy we need stable positioning of the patient.[19,35] This involves having control of the body and control of the upper limb. In addition, one must consider the ergonomics of the surgeon and his assistants. There are two positions for the patient for shoulder arthroscopy. By far the most popular is the lateral decubitus position. The second is the beach chair position. The lateral decubitus position is, in my opinion, the easier of the two for performing shoulder arthroscopy. There are a number of authors who insist that the beach chair position is easier. The greatest advantage of the beach chair position is that it is somewhat easier to convert to an open anterior position at the completion of the arthroscopy, without significant repositioning of the patient (Fig. 2).

To position the patient for a lateral decubitus position requires a bean bag to hold the patient, a pad to place on the thorax to take the pressure off of the contents of the axilla, and some type of arm traction device to control the limb. In placing the patient in the lateral decubitus position, we tilt the patient back about 30 degrees to place the glenoid roughly parallel to the floor. Surgeons tend to think in orthogonal planes, and placing the glenoid parallel with the floor makes orientation for the surgeon easier in addition to opening up the anterior portion of the shoulder for instrument access. Traction devices have been developed to apply

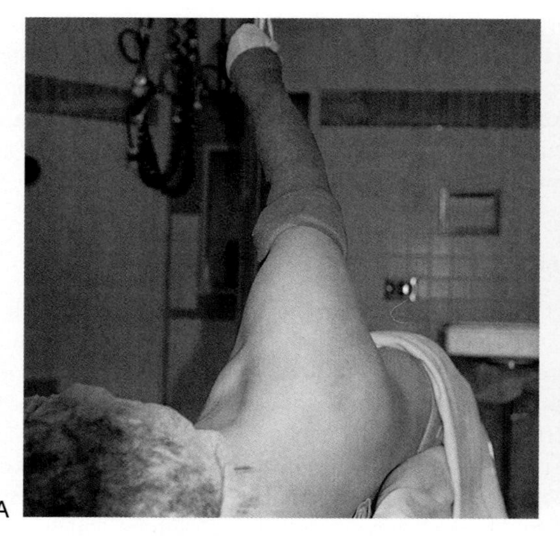

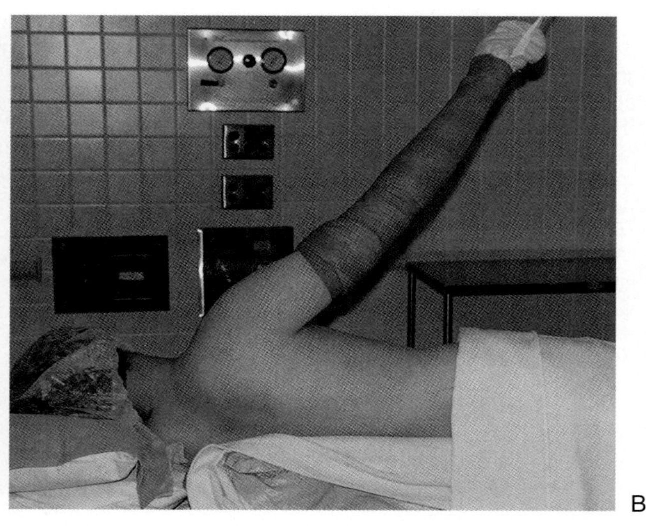

FIG. 2. **(A)** Lateral decubitus positioning and arm traction for shoulder arthroscopy, with a 30-degree–posterior tilt. This tilt places the glenoid roughly parallel with the floor and eases orientation for the surgeon. The tilt also makes the handling of instruments in the front of the shoulder easier. Note also the presence of the beanbag, which helps convert the normally round human body into a rectangular shape, so that the body will not roll anteriorly or posteriorly. **(B)** Side view of the patient in the lateral decubitus position with the arm traction. Traction is attached to a weight by pulleys, so that there is no change in the force of traction as the bed is lowered or raised. Some traction towers have an additional strap that goes on the inside of the upper arm to provide lateral traction to the glenohumeral joint.

traction in two directions, so that the humerus floats above the glenoid rather than drifting caudally.

For the beach chair position, we must also have control of the body (Fig. 3).[48] This requires an appropriate table that will allow removal of a portion of the back to leave the posterior portion of the shoulder exposed, a stable platform for the head, and some type of lateral stabilizer for the trunk so that the patient is not pulled off the table and onto the floor. After providing the stable platform for the glenoid, the arm is controlled by placing it on a Mayo stand. Some surgeons have developed arm holders that can be attached to the table to control the arm. In the beach chair position, we try to place the glenoid in the vertical position, another orthogonal plane, making orientation easier for the surgeon.

With both of these patient positions, we place the monitor directly opposite the surgeon, so that he does not have to turn his neck. We try to place it at eye level, so that he does not have to place his neck into an uncomfortable position. The height of the table for both of these positions is also adjusted for surgeon ergonomics.

Fluid and Fluid Control Requirements

A lucent medium is required for arthroscopy. Because of concerns about pneumomediastinum and pneumothorax gases, a medium such as CO_2 cannot be used. Because of concerns about osmotic cell lysis, isotonic fluids are used. These are usually normal saline or lactated Ringer solu-

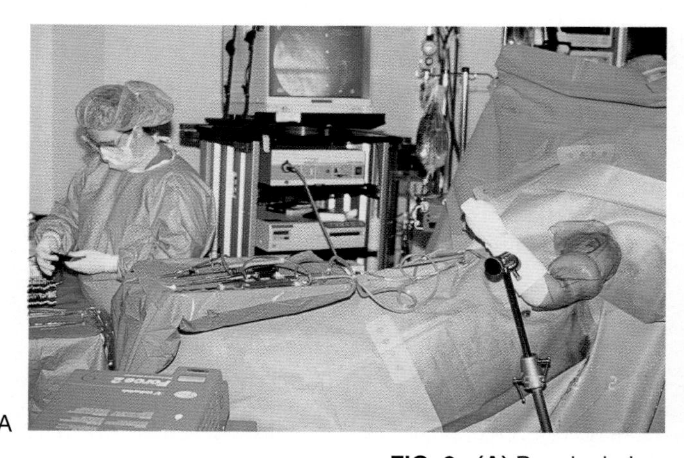

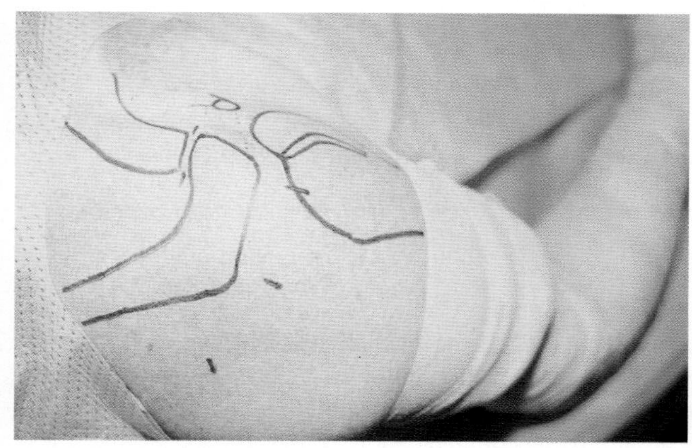

FIG. 3. **(A)** Beach chair position; **(B)** Portal placement.

tion.[7,24,25,34,35,36] For a time, nonionic isotonic solutions such as sorbitol were used when electrocautery was needed. These solutions tended to "caramelize" when the cautery was used. In addition, cautery tips were developed that made nonionic solutions unnecessary.

Control of the fluid is also important. One can err on either side of proper distension of the spaces. Underdistension provides less tamponade and allows the space to collapse. Because the boundaries of the spaces are thin, fluid extravasation into the thick muscle wall of the joint can be dramatic.

There are four handles by which the surgeon can control fluid extravasation: control of the portal, length of the procedure, fluid pressure, and rate of fluid flow. Control of the portals with cannulae allows the lining of the joint to form somewhat of a seal that slows up the extravasation of fluid into the tissues adjacent to the portal. This seal is not perfect, however, and the surgeon must continue to pay attention to the length of the procedure to decrease tissue swelling.

There are two ways to force fluid into the joint: gravity and mechanical pumps. These both allow control over the other two variables: fluid pressure and rate of flow. With gravity, fluid pressure is controlled by the height of the fluid reservoir above the shoulder. The rate of flow is controlled by the stopcocks and clamps on the line running into the shoulder. The advantage over the mechanical pump is lower cost. The disadvantage is the need to make continual manual adjustments.

Mechanical pumps also allow the surgeon to adjust pressure and flow rate. The machine is set at a prescribed pressure and flow, and from then on, it is self adjusting. The surgeon may change his settings during the surgery to meet his needs. The disadvantage here is the cost of equipment and tubing.

In any event, keeping the procedure as short as possible is the most effective control mechanism. This is an important factor in selecting which arthroscopic procedures a surgeon will attempt.

Portals and Portal Placement

Posterior Portal

The initial portal for shoulder arthroscopy is the posterior portal (Fig. 4). Our goal here is to place our lens cannula parallel to the glenoid and just slightly lateral to it to avoid an arthroscopic shadow anteriorly. The usual entry point is 2 cm medial to the posterior tip of the acromion and 2 cm inferior. With larger individuals, these distances may be a bit greater, in particular if there is a lot of exogenous obesity. This defines one point in the line of insertion. The opposite point is the palpable tip of the coracoid.[31] The posterior portion of the proposed arthroscopic path is injected with lidocaine with epinephrine. Some surgeons insufflate the joint with the needle at this time. I do not insufflate because I do not wish to scratch the articular cartilage by putting the needle into the joint. The opposing argument is that with preinsufflation

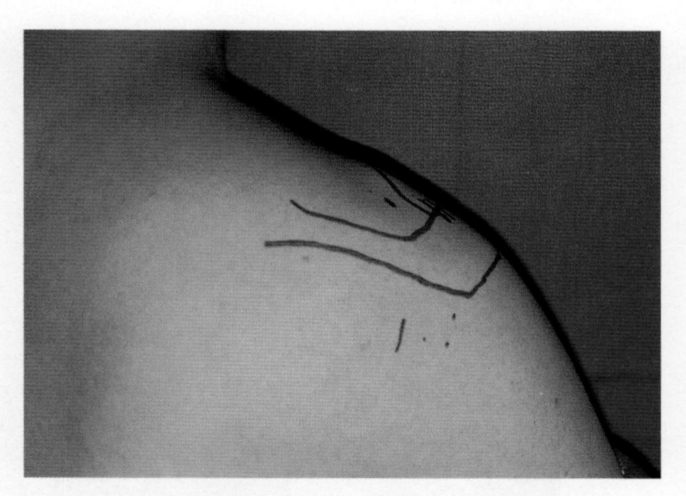

FIG. 4. A posterior view of the right shoulder showing the outline of the spine of the scapula and the back of the acromion: The position of the usual incision for the posterior portal is shown, which is roughly about 2 cm down from the posterolateral corner of the acromion and about 2 cm medial.

there is less chance of scratching the cartilage when the cannula enters the joint. The skin is incised vertically in line with the lines of skin tension. Then the cannula is advanced with a blunt obturator along the defined line of insertion, but in a slightly more inferior direction. After penetrating deltoid and infraspinatus muscles, one can palpate the posterior lip of the glenoid (Fig. 5) and determine that one is in the right position. One then punctures the capsule with the blunt obturator so as not to scratch the articular cartilage. The obturator is removed, the lens is placed, and the joint is filled with fluid. Some surgeons do an initial air arthroscopy to look at the synovium.

Superior Portal

The superior portal has been more commonly used in the past (Fig. 6).[54] The main reason for its fall from popularity has been the addition of flow portals to the other cannulae that are used for instruments, thereby obviating the need for a superior flow portal. As the superior portal is no longer needed for flow, it tends to be used only for very specific reasons: (a) the surgeon wants to keep the anterior shoulder pristine, because he is planning on following the arthroscopy with an anterior approach to the shoulder and wishes to have less anterior fluid extravasation in this region; (b) the surgeon needs to approach a specific area, such as a lesion of the superior labrum; and (c) the surgeon wants to view from above. The superior portal begins at the angle formed by the spine of the scapula with the distal clavicle. An incision is made in line with the lines of skin tension, and after predetermining the proper path with a needle, the cannula is inserted into the joint. The usual direction is about 30 degrees lateral and about 10 degrees posteriorly. This portal, because of its bony borders and the length of soft tissue it traverses,

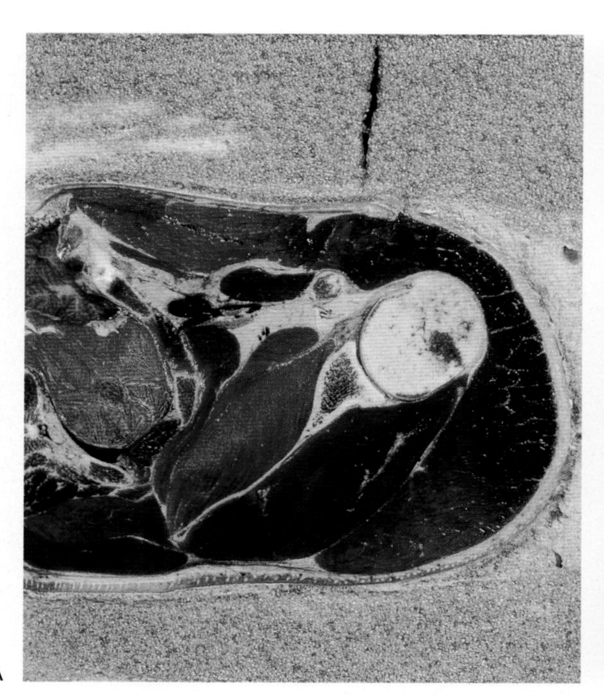

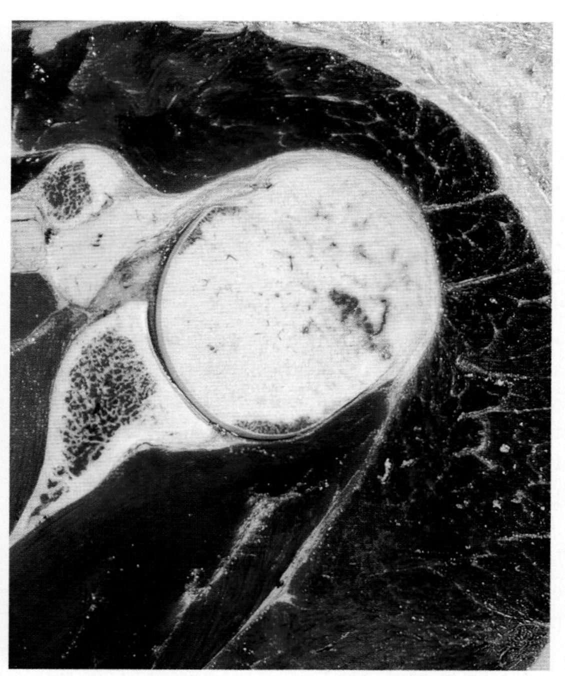

FIG. 5. (A) A cross section of the thorax and shoulder demonstrating the orientation of the scapula relative to the coronal plane of the body. Notice the tip of the coracoid anteriorly marking the line described by the plane of the glenoid. **(B)** A close-up of the same cross section. The close-up demonstrates two things: (a) that the anterior portal that is designed by placing a rod through a posterior portal will exit anteriorly either just above or just below the tip of the coracoid, (b) a laterally placed posterior portal will leave an area of anterior shoulder that cannot be observed because of the presence of the head of the humerus.

is somewhat immobile and not quite as useful for surgical procedures as the anterior and posterior portals are.

Anterior Portals

Anterior portal placement offers us a larger selection of possible portals guided by two principles: (a) complication avoidance and (b) the proposed destination of the portal (Fig. 7).[39] In choosing an anterior portal, the structure the surgeon is most likely to want to approach, based on the initial arthroscopic examination of the shoulder, determines the position of the anterior portal.

Complication Avoidance in Portal Selection

The complications avoided by proper portal technique are the anatomic complications (i.e., damage to vessel or nerve). The nerves relevant to the anterior portals are the axillary and the musculocutaneous nerves. There are abundant arteries about the shoulder, but because of abundant collaterals, no ischemic complications have yet been reported.

The anterior branch of the axillary nerve supplies the anterior two-thirds of the deltoid muscle (Fig. 8).[31] The nerve travels about 5 cm below the lateral edge of the acromion on the deep surface of the muscle. The musculocutaneous nerve comes off of the lateral cord and enters the conjoint tendon 5.5 cm below the coracoid on average. This means that at least one-half of specimens have nerves above this level. I have seen in dissection a musculocutaneous nerve that was only 1.5 cm below the coracoid.[31] There are additional branch nerves off the lateral cord to the coracobrachialis. Be-

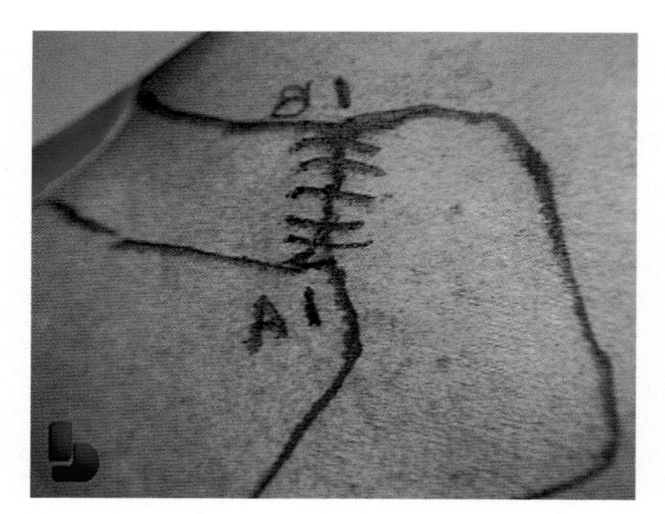

FIG. 6. A superior view of the shoulder. Portal *A* is the entry site for the superior glenohumeral portal. Incision *A* can also be used for the posterior acromioclavicular portal. Incision *B* is the anterior AC portal.

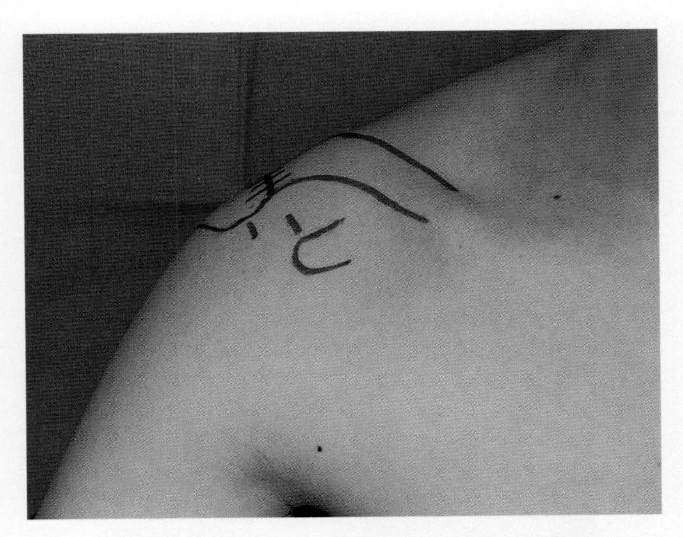

FIG. 7. Anterior view of the shoulder showing the bony landmarks of the clavicle, acromion, and coracoid, and the location of the two most frequently used anterior portals. The portal that is directly above the coracoid is the more usual portal, and this is roughly the position one would make with an inside out technique. The more superior portal is more lateral and gives the surgeon, in addition to an extra operating portal, an oblique approach to the surface of the glenoid.

cause of the position of these two nerves and of the brachial plexus, the traditional rule has been no portals below or medial to the tip of the coracoid. This rule is broken for certain specific purposes, as described later under subcoracoid portals.

There are two ways of making the anterior portal: (a) from within out (inside out), and (b) from without in (outside in). Developing the portal from inside the joint begins by using the arthroscope now located in the posterior portal to select the position of the internal orifice of our proposed anterior portal. We then place the scope on this site and replace the lens with a sharp obturator or a Wissinger rod. This is then advanced through the soft tissues out to the skin. A small cut is made in the skin and an operative cannula fed over the obturator or Wissinger rod, with the two cannulae returned together to the glenohumeral joint. In using the inside out technique, the surgeon needs to recall that the coracoid lies almost directly ahead of us in the rotator interval just above the subscapular tendon. An inferior deviation may then produce a subcoracoid portal, which is actually preferred by some surgeons for reconstructive purposes but is not necessary for diagnostic arthroscopy. The advantage of inside out technique is that it allows precise placement of the internal portal site. The disadvantage is that it provides little variation

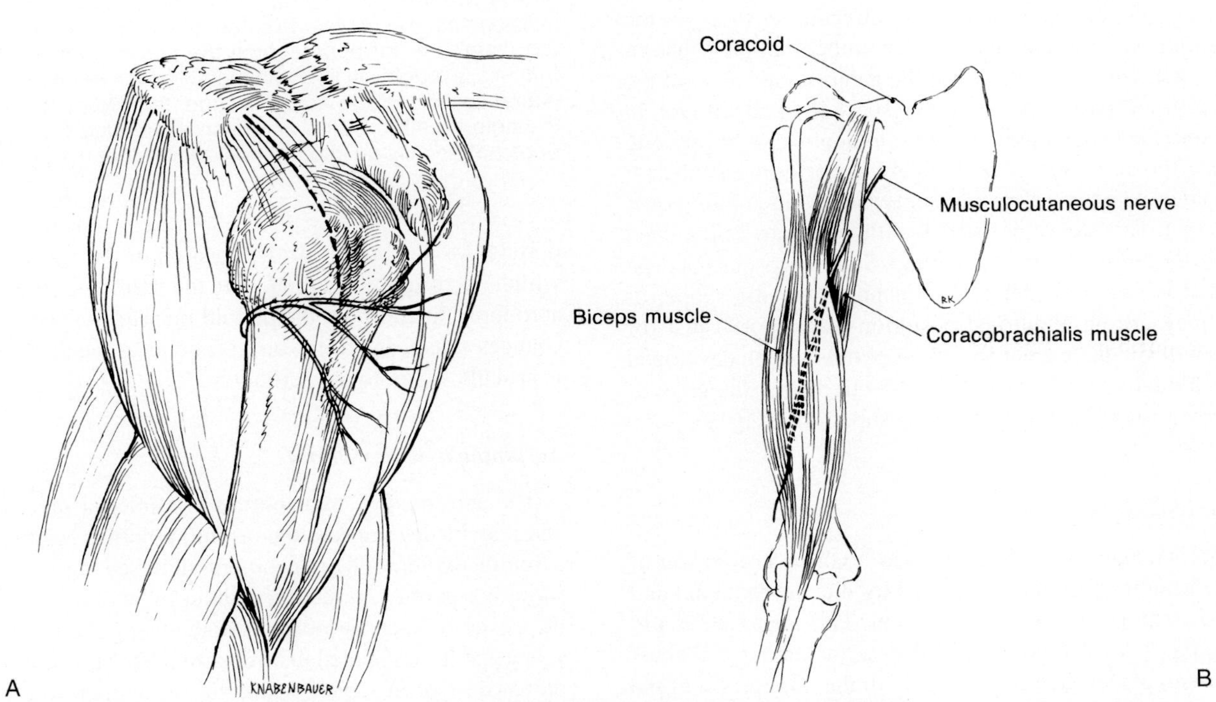

FIG. 8. Two areas that are of most concern to shoulder arthroscopists: **(A)** The axillary nerve is shown in this anterior lateral view of the deltoid. The anterior branch of the axillary nerve runs about 5.5 cm inferior to the edge of the acromion and the AC joint. Any shoulder abduction will bring the nerve closer to the acromion. **(B)** The musculocutaneous nerve shown penetrating the conjoined coracobrachialis and biceps short head about 5.5 cm below the tip of the coracoid. This penetration is highly variable, and often there is an accessory nerve to these muscles coming off of the lateral cord and entering the muscle even more proximally. (From ref. 32, with permission.)

in the angle of approach to the glenoid in the transverse plane. The angle is predetermined by the path of the posterior cannula.

The opposite technique, "outside in," allows selection not only of the internal orifice, but also of the angle of approach. In this technique, the surgeon selects what he thinks is a likely external orifice for his portal, advances a needle along the path he proposes to take, and checks this path and the internal portal with his intraarticular arthroscope. This allows a more lateral portal for anterior work.[38] The disadvantage of this technique is that it requires some experience on the part of the surgeon to be able to make an initial approximation of where the portal should lie and to place his needle appropriately without having to make multiple sticks into the shoulder. There is, therefore, a tendency for surgeons earlier in their development to use the inside-out technique and move on later to outside-in techniques.

Subacromial Portals

Inspection of the bursal side of the rotator cuff has become routine. I prefer to use my initial posterior glenohumeral portal to be the first subacromial portal. I withdraw the fluid from the glenohumeral joint and replace the lens with the blunt trochar. I withdraw the cannula until I feel it is on the outside of infraspinatus, but inside of the deltoid, and then advance the cannula along the inferior surface of the acromion. The surgeon needs to remember that the subacromial bursa only occupies about the anterior half or so of the subacromial space. The remaining space is filled with fat. In addition, the surgeon will not want to apply a lot of pressure against the acromion or he is likely to perform a subbursal dissection, leaving a sleeve of subacromial bursa lining over his scope. This sleeve of tissue will then need to be removed before the surgeon can see anything. Some surgeons make an alternative, more posterior lateral portal for the scope, or they may use an additional posterior lateral portal just for control of fluids. A great variety of portals can be developed subacromially. They start about 2.5 cm. below the edge of the acromion so that one can angle superiorly (Fig. 9).

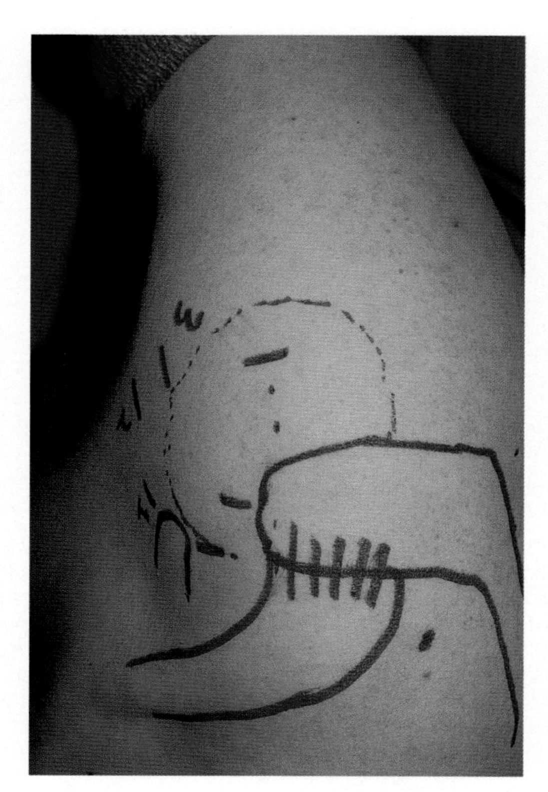

FIG. 9. A superior view of the shoulder: The *soft dotted line* shows roughly the outline of the subacromial bursa. The incision near the *midlateral* extent of the subacromial bursa is the usual one for approaching the acromion laterally. Note that this is roughly in line with the anterior medial and anterior lateral corners of the acromion and, therefore, is in line with the anterior edge of the acromion. Note also that the bursa does not usually go into the posterior half of the acromion.

Lateral Subacromial Portal

This is made 1 in. (2.5 cm) inferior to the lateral border of the acromion on a line determined by the anteromedial and anterolateral corners of the acromion. This approach would be similar to the deltoid incision that we make for rotator cuff repair and places the scope roughly in the midportion of the subacromial bursa (see Fig. 9). This portal is used most often as an instrument portal, but some surgeons have recommended using it as the observation portal for subacromial decompression, with the burr in the posterior portal. For AC joint resection, the anterolateral portal can be the viewing portal, with instruments placed in the anterior portal of the acromioclavicular (AC) joint. In all of these subacromial portals, we need to recall the position of the axillary nerve, which is roughly 5 cm below the lateral border of the acromion. In addition, the deltoid muscle is a structure that changes shape, and as the arm is abducted the axillary nerve is brought closer to the acromion.

Acromioclavicular Portals

The acromioclavicular portals are anterior and posterior and may be developed either as initial portals or after a subacromial exploration or decompression (see Fig. 6).[12] In performing a pure AC resection without subacromial disruption, the posterior superior portal is made using the wrist arthroscope and its associated instruments.[21] This is because of the narrowness of the space within the acromioclavicular joint. A straight anterior or anterosuperior portal is then developed, and through this a small shaver and burr can create a larger space within the space defined by acromioclavicular ligaments. Arthroscopic decompression of the joint is carried out without destabilizing it in the anteroposterior direction. When sufficient space has been gained, the surgeon may switch to his usual arthroscope and instruments.

Subcoracoid Portals

Additional glenohumeral portals have been developed anteriorly for reconstructive procedures (Fig. 10). These are sometimes below the level of the coracoid and are appropriate only in the hands of an experienced shoulder arthroscopist, and that surgeon will probably use these portals for only reconstructive purposes. There is usually sufficient room in the shoulder to make two of the safer anterosuperior portals, as described in the foregoing. The lower portal is in the straight-ahead position, as we described with the inside out technique, and the other lies much more superior, closer to the tendon of the supraspinatus. The surgeon will select his entry site based on which angle he wants to use to approach internal structures such as the glenoid.

One may use one of three infracoracoid approaches: the "slalom" approach, the 3:00 o'clock position approach, and the anteroinferior or 5:00 o'clock position approach.[17,19,46] The slalom approach is made directly anterior and slightly inferior. The surgeon makes a small incision for his operative cannula 3 cm below the anterior tip of the coracoid and advances his cannula with a blunt obturator until the conjoined tendon is encountered. Then the cannula and obturator are directed laterally until they encounter the humeral head and subscapularis muscle. In other words, they have gone past the lateral border of the conjoint tendon. The cannula and obturator are then swung medially and, in doing so, one pushes the conjoined tendon and musculocutaneous nerve medially. The blunt obturator is used to penetrate the fleshy part of the subscapularis muscle to give the surgeon a portal in the anteroinferior quadrant of the joint.

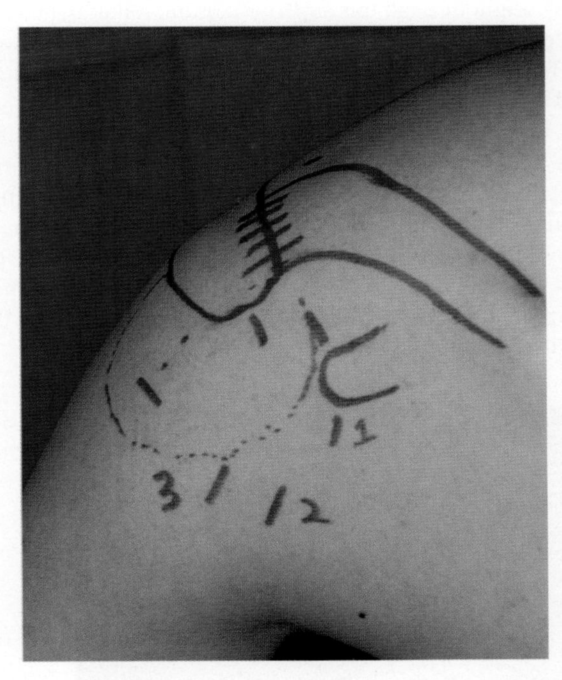

FIG. 10. Subcoracoid portals: Additional anterior operative portals located below the coracoid. Because of the increased risk involved in these portals, their use is limited to fairly specific purposes. Incision mark *1*, a subcoracoid portal, is immediately beneath the coracoid and usually made by a Wissinger rod advancing out the anterior shoulder just superior to subscapularis tendon, exiting just beneath the coracoid. Incision mark *2* is about 3 cm distal to the tip of the coracoid along the line of the conjoined tendon and is the incision made for using the slalom approach from outside to inside (see text). Incision mark *3* is a slightly more lateral portal and is achieved by an inside out technique and is the usual position for the 5:00 o'clock approach (see text).

The 3:00 o'clock position is selected in an inside out fashion. With the arthroscope, the surgeon goes directly anterior, parallel to the glenoid surface, and then uses the scope to place this cannula directly against the superior surface of the subscapularis tendon. He replaces the lens with a Wissinger rod or sharp obturator and penetrates anteriorly, ending up passing along the inferior surface of the coracoid. The anterior operating cannula is then placed over the Wissinger rod and advanced posteriorly into the joint. This portal is more inferior than the usual anterior portals, but does not allow us to go as far inferior as the slalom or 5:00 o'clock approaches.

The portal in the 5:00 o'clock position is also produced in an inside out fashion. In this technique, the arm is held in the adducted position, but with a solid pad in the axilla to distract the humeral head away from the glenoid. Adduction in this technique swings the conjointed tendon and musculocutaneous nerve medially. The Wissinger rod is advanced through the posterior cannula in an anteroinferior direction in the most lateral direction allowed by the patient's anatomy. The rod is advanced out through the soft tissues to the skin, a similar vertical incision is made, and the operative cannula admitted into the joint over the Wissinger rod.

Standard Technique for Diagnostic Arthroscopy and Relevant Anatomy

The posterior portal is the initial portal. Once the cannula and lens are within the joint, an air arthroscopy can be performed initially and then the joint distended with saline (often containing epinephrine; Fig. 11). By flushing the joint in and out through the viewing cannula, an initial visualization can be obtained. Once a semblance of clear visibility is obtained, we may use a needle to select a second portal anteriorly. Often, I do an initial quick diagnostic arthroscopy before placing the anterior portal, to determine which angle of approach to the glenoid I would like. After placement of the anterior cannula, we can use the side port on that operative cannula as our egress port and maintain clear visualization of the glenohumeral joint. Occasionally, at this early point, one might want to admit a shaver to remove some hypertrophic synovium or frayed material that is obstructing our view, but usually we move on directly to the diagnostic portion of the examination.

There are two routines that are useful for the surgeon to develop in his technique. The first is a constant orientation of the camera, and the second is a constant order of examination, so that no area is left unexamined. Orthopaedic sur-

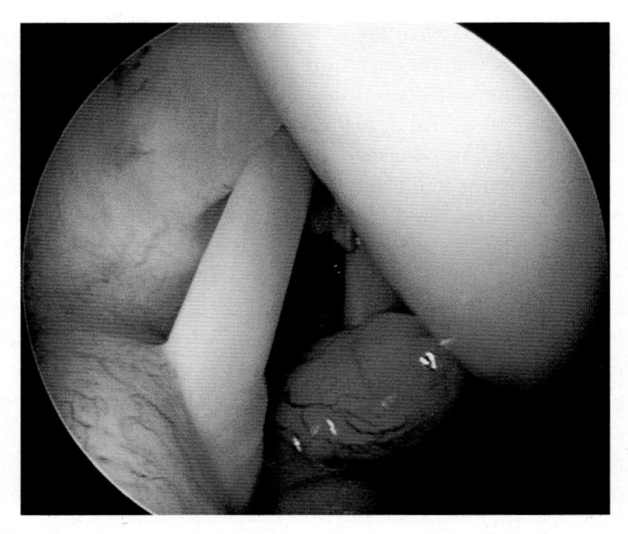

FIG. 11. Demonstration of an air arthroscopy: Note that compared with the saline medium, the air arthroscopy has less diffusion of the light, thereby better yielding delineation of shadows and sharp edges.

TABLE 2. *Author's standard order of examination*

Superior labrum with biceps origin
Anterosuperior quadrant
Anteroinferior quadrant
Posteroinferior quadrant
Posterosuperior quadrant
Biceps tendon
Bicipital groove and anterosuperior head
Superior cuff and superior head
Posterior cuff and posterior head
Center head and glenoid
Subacromial bursa

geons prefer to think in terms of lines and planes in orthogonal frames of reference. It is best to choose a position in which the glenoid is either vertical or horizontal, as seen on the monitor; otherwise, there is a tendency for the surgeon and his assistants to tilt their head one way or the other (Fig. 12).

The following is the author's routine ordered examination (Table 2). The reader will want to establish his own routine and follow it religiously. I begin by examining the superior labrum and biceps origin (Fig. 13). This is usually the area of the shoulder at which the scope is directed immediately after insertion. Compared with the inferior labrum, the superior labrum often takes an origin more medial on the glenoid. The inferior labrum comes off directly adjacent to the articular cartilage, and in many ways appears to be a continuation of the articular cartilage. In contrast, the superior labrum often takes a more medial origin, so that there is normally a gap between articular cartilage and superior labrum. In many persons, this labrum continues on to the articular surface, overhanging the articular surface in a fashion similar to the way a meniscus overlies the tibia. The biceps tendon takes its bony origin through this superior labrum, rather than having a separate insertion into the biceps tubercle. In this fashion, the biceps origin and the superior labrum usually form a unified structure.

I next evaluate the anterior superior quadrant, because this quadrant contains the largest number of normal anatomic variations (Fig. 14). The superior glenohumeral ligament takes origin off of the superior labrum and glenoid, and courses to insert into the extreme upper portion of the lesser tuberosity and often into the floor of the bicipital groove. This structure is apparent in almost 100% of shoulders.

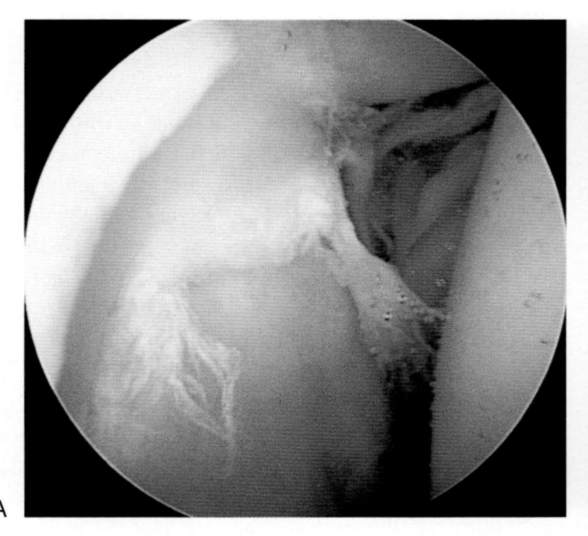

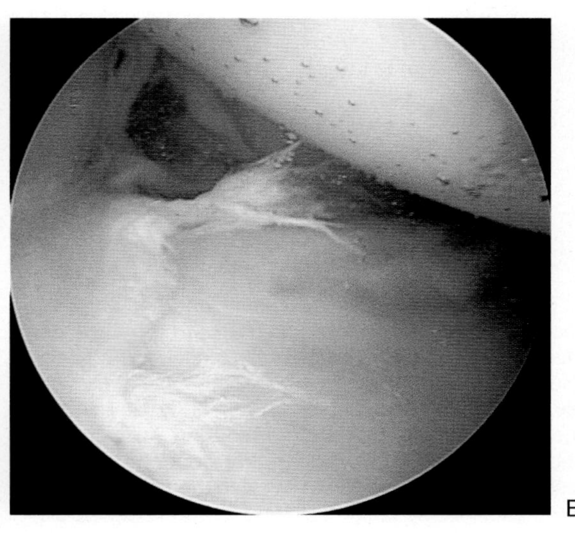

A B

FIG. 12. Desired orientations of the camera: **(A)** the vertical glenoid view and, **(B)** the horizontal glenoid view. Either of these two orientations can be used by the arthroscopist because it places the more immobile landmark, the glenoid, in one of the three orthogonal planes. This makes orientation easier for the surgeon.

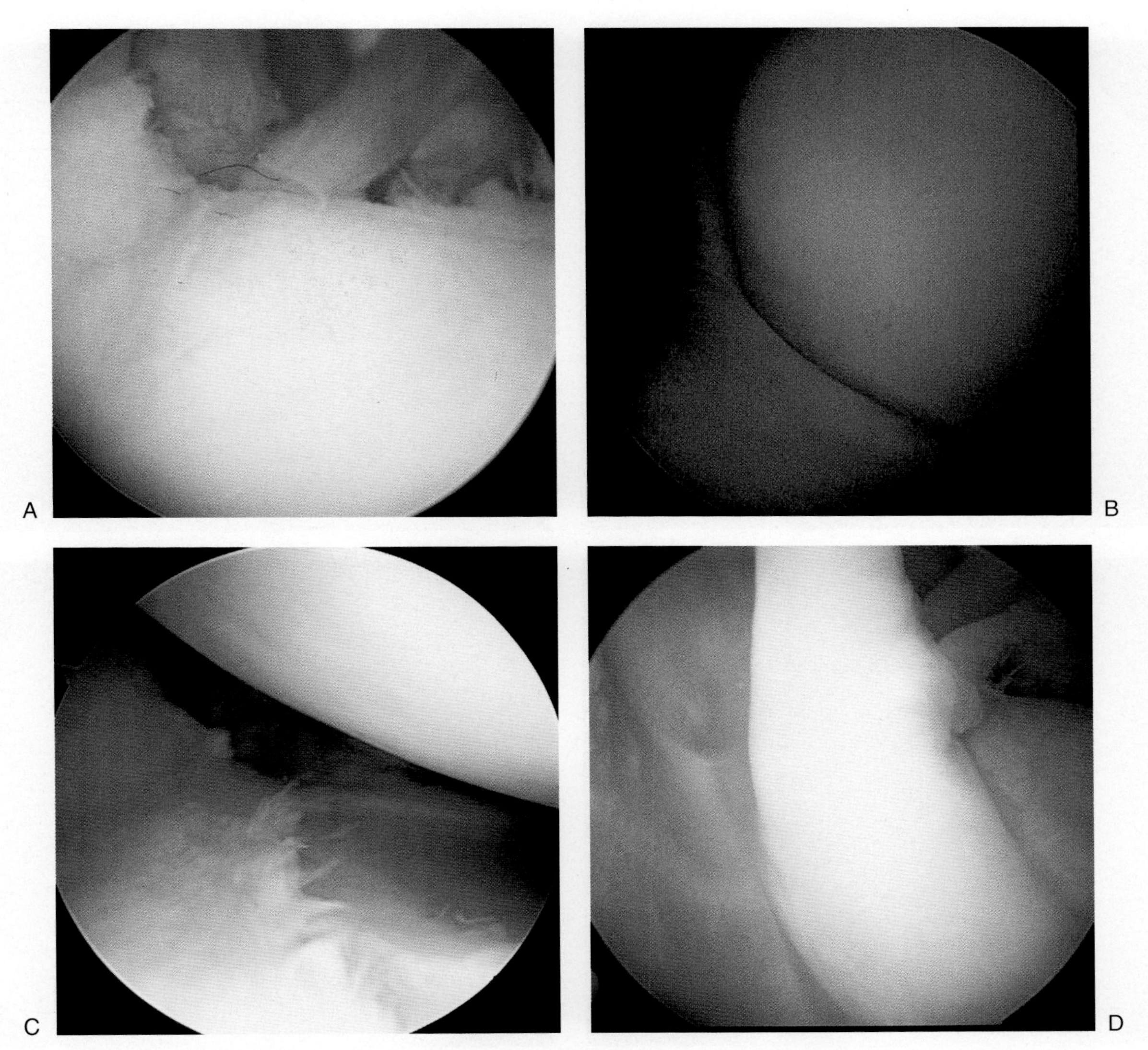

FIG. 13. Variations in the shape of the upper labrum: **(A)** In this variation, the labrum comes right off of the articular cartilage and does not have much of a medial origin, nor does it overlap the articular cartilage. **(B)** In this view, the labrum has a more medial origin on the neck, rather than coming off adjacent to the articular cartilage, but it does not heavily overlap the articular cartilage in a meniscoid fashion. **(C)** The labrum overlaps the more superior cartilage. In this variation, the labrum must be retracted with the probe to look for detachment of the biceps anchor. **(D)** Demonstrates a most important structure of the superior labrum, which is the insertion of the biceps through the labrum.

The numerous normal variants of the anterosuperior labrum lead to difficulty in differentiating the result of trauma or disease from a normal variation. Anterosuperior labrum variants arise from the actual thickness of the labrum and the mode of attachment to the bony glenoid. Up to 60% of the population has a sublabral defect. In 10% of the population, this sublabral defect will actually be complete and connect deep to the labrum with the subscapularis bursae. This presents a problem for the arthroscopist in differentiating a normal sublabral fenestration from a traumatic detachment of the anterosuperior labrum. The second form in which the anterosuperior labrum may vary is that it may be normally very small. When the middle glenohumeral ligament takes a very high origin off of the glenoid almost at the base of the biceps tendon, and this middle glenohumeral ligament has a single cordlike structure, the labrum between the origin of the middle glenohumeral ligament and the origin at the anterior band of the inferior glenohumeral ligament may appear to be so small that it is nonexistent.[63] This can be confused with a traumatic detachment of the labrum.

The middle glenohumeral ligament is the source of the largest number of variations of the glenohumeral capsule (Fig. 15). There are a number of normal specimens in which

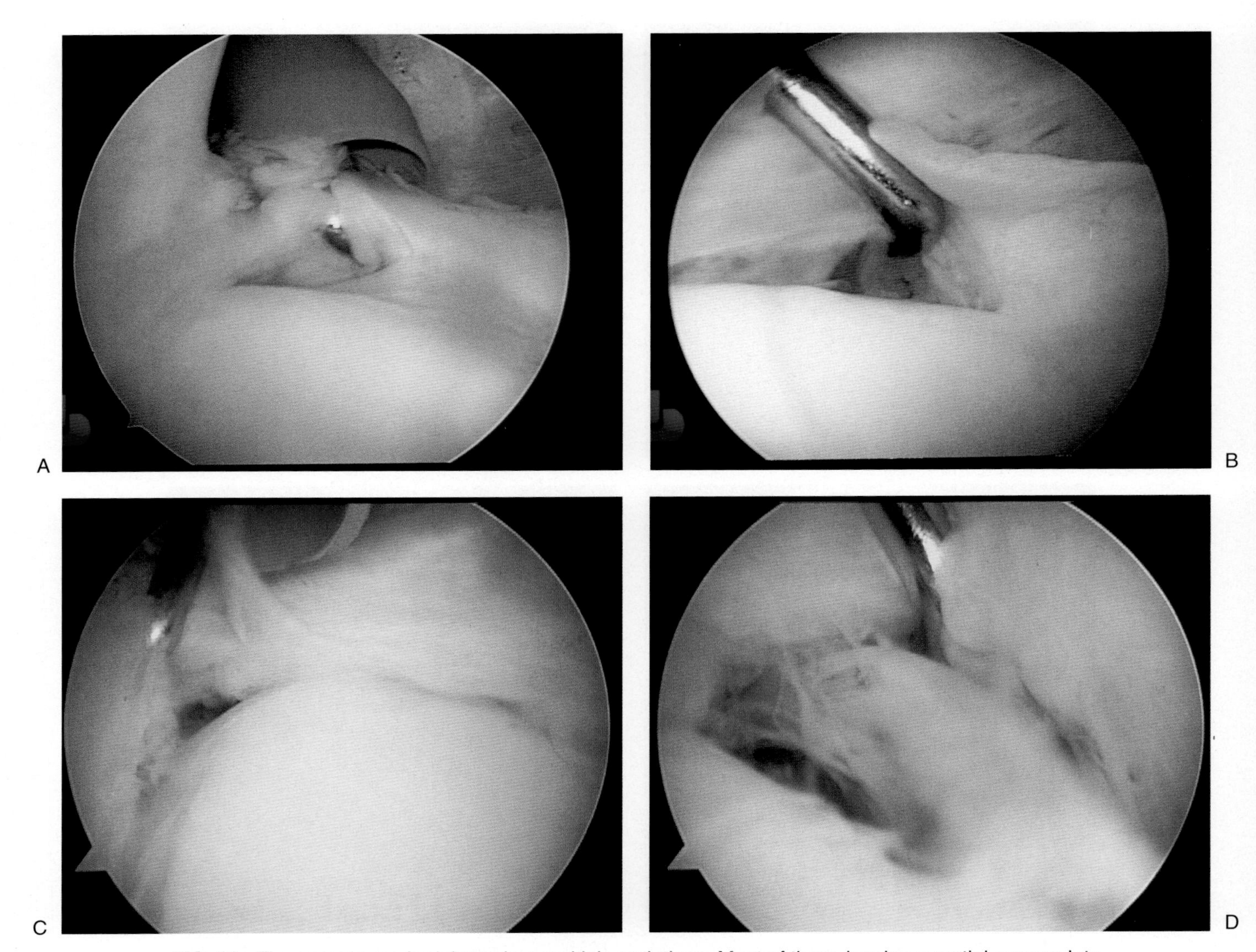

FIG. 14. The anterosuperior labrum has multiple variations. Most of these involve a partial or complete separation of the labrum off of the glenoid. **(A)** A small defect. It is the task of the surgeon to decide if this is a naturally occurring "sublabral fenestration" or a defect that has come about traumatically. **(B)** An even larger defect. The arthroscope can be passed underneath this labrum and the surgeon can see all the way to the base of the coracoid. **(C,D)** A traumatic defect, true laxity, which can be seen in D when the probe pulls radially, showing how far the labrum can be pulled away from the edge of the glenoid. Note the roughened edges of the labrum and glenoid, which point to a traumatic origin.

FIG. 15. The middle glenohumeral ligament takes variable forms: **(A)** the usual form: the middle glenohumeral ligament crossing over the vertically running subscapularis tendon and a smooth transition between middle glenohumeral ligament, running obliquely across the subscapularis and the beginning of the inferior glenohumeral ligament, which is seen more inferiorly; **(B)** sometimes the middle glenohumeral ligament is seen as a single cordlike structure with subscapularis recesses both above and below the ligament. Care must be taken to not mistake this lower entrance into the subscapularis bursa for a traumatically occurring sublabral fenestration. **(C)** Sometimes the middle glenohumeral ligament is not obvious at all and cannot be seen. **(D)** In the same individual (seen in C), if the arthroscope is moved inferiorly along the leading edge of the inferior glenohumeral ligament, a small middle glenohumeral ligament can be found further inferiorly. **(E,F)** Sometimes, however, the middle glenohumeral ligament can be missing because of the result of trauma, seen in this individual in which not only is the middle glenohumeral ligament missing, but also the upper portion of the subscapularis. On the *right-hand* side of both E and F is the remnant of capsule and a portion of the subscapularis that was not detached.

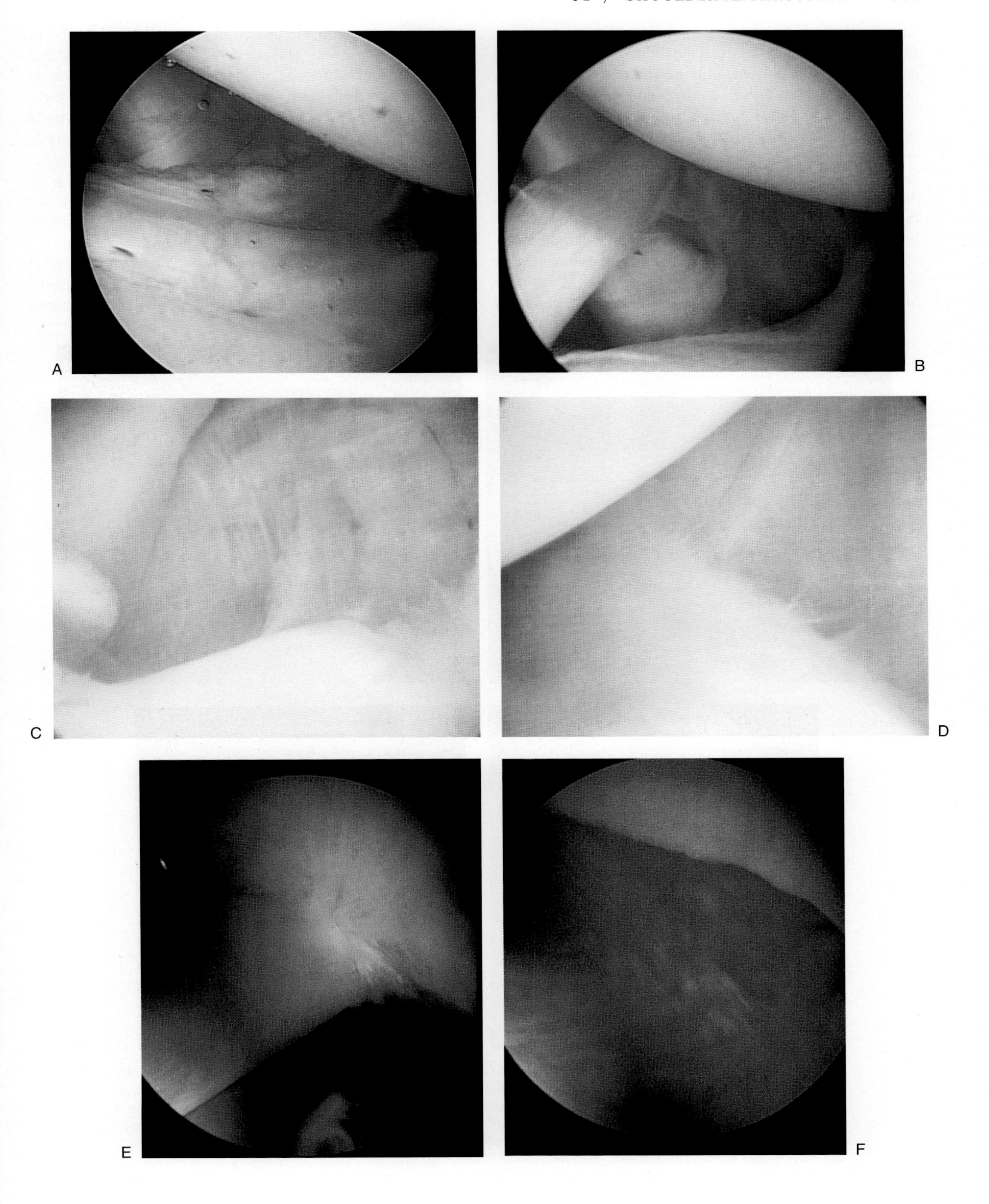
A
B
C
D
E
F

the middle glenohumeral ligament appears to be absent. Gohlke found on histology that the middle glenohumeral ligament is always present, although it is sometimes very small.[23] Gohlke also noted an inverse relation between the size of the middle glenohumeral ligament and the size of the anterior band of the inferior glenohumeral ligament.[23] This relation has been noted on arthroscopic examination of the humeral insertion site of the capsule.[23] These anatomic variants can make differentiating normal from abnormal tissues difficult, and may also result in variation in posttraumatic pathology, depending on premorbid anatomic variations.

The subscapularis bursa also is found in the anterosuperior quadrant. This bursa is a continuation of the articular surface of the rotator interval and continues as the synovium-lined structure between the upper subscapularis tendon and the neck of the glenoid. This bursa is often the site of loose bodies. The anterosuperior quadrant is often involved with inflammatory synovium associated with rheumatoid arthritis and adhesive capsulitis. The intraarticular opening to the bursa is variable. Most commonly, it appears as a single defect in the continuity of the capsule above the middle glenohumeral ligament. Alternatively, it may appear below the middle glenohumeral ligament, or above and below the middle glenohumeral ligament, or it may be so small that the anterior capsule forms a continuous layer.

The superior edge of the subscapularis tendon is also visualized on the anterosuperior quadrant. The subscapularis tendon has a uniform appearance and should be visible in all

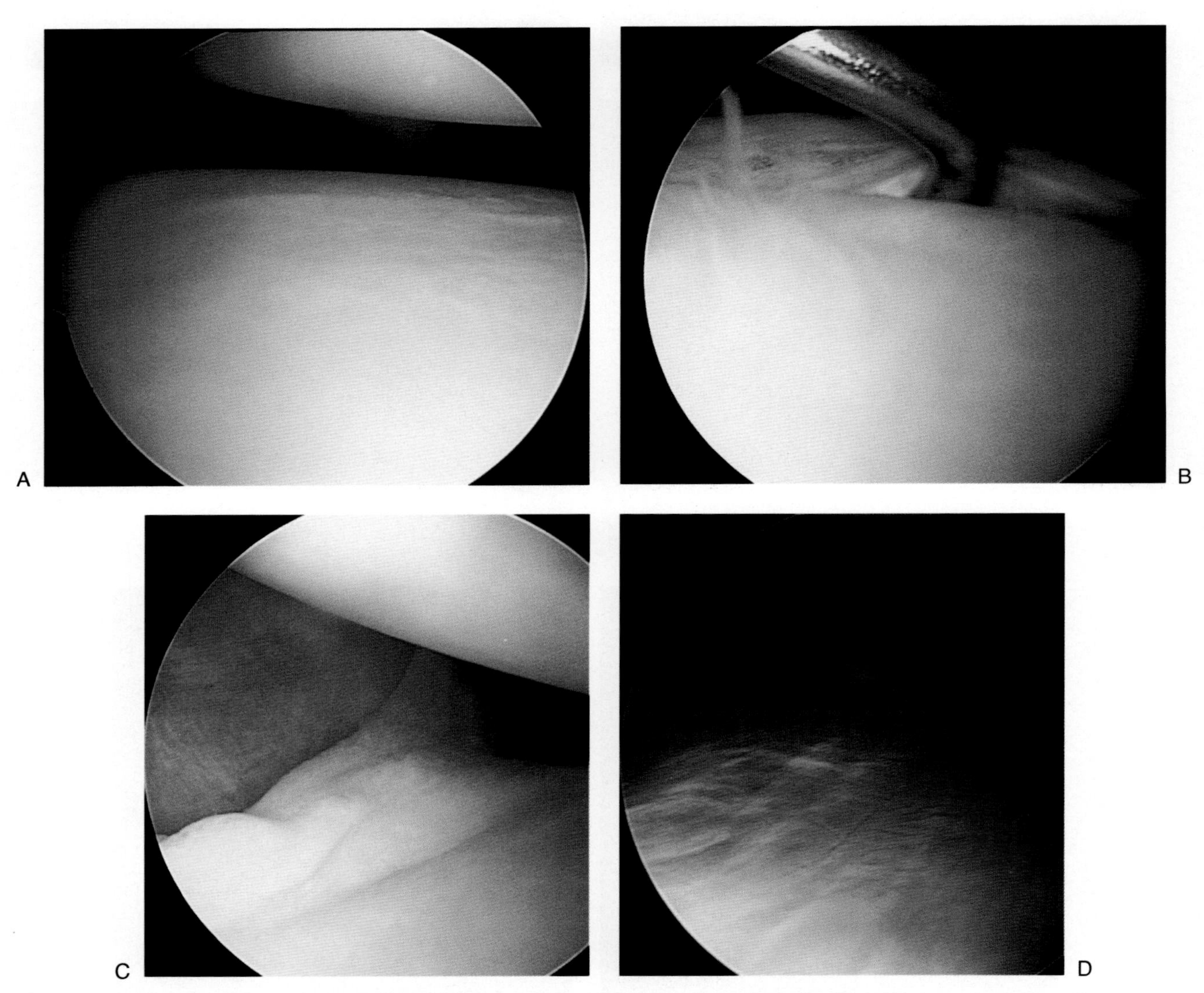

FIG. 16. Anteroinferior quadrant of the shoulder: **(A)** In the inferior joint, the labrum takes a very smooth, almost undetectable, transition between the articular cartilage and the labrum. **(B)** Any split between these structures, even if it is as subtle as in this photograph, must be considered pathologic. **(C)** Also in the anteroinferior quadrant, we can see the leading edge or anterior band of the inferior glenohumeral ligament. It is not always quite as obvious as seen in this photograph, but it can be made more obvious by having the assistant internally and externally rotate the shoulder. **(D)** The ligament can then be followed all the way to the neck of the humerus to ensure that there are no humeral detachments.

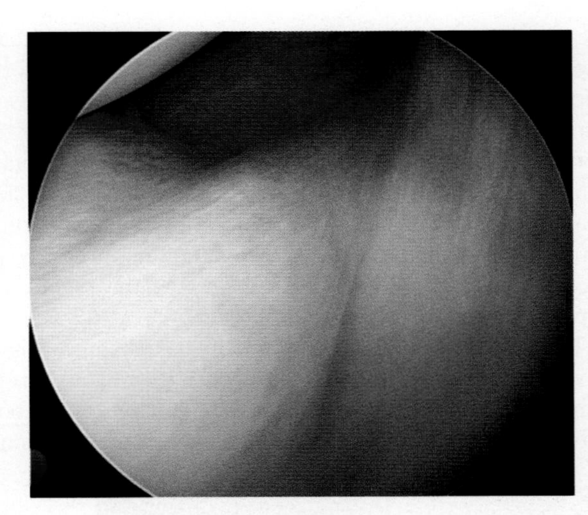

FIG. 17. Posteroinferior quadrant: In this area, one can make out the general transition between the inferior glenohumeral ligament and the more lax posterior capsule. This is sometimes referred to as the posterior band of the inferior glenohumeral ligament.

normal shoulders, so that the inability to see this structure is diagnostic either of a tear of the subscapularis tendon or of abnormal material filling the "rotator interval." This interval itself is inspected to see if it is widened.[42]

Anteroinferior Quadrant of the Shoulder

The junction between articular cartilage and labrum and the continuation of the labrum into the inferior glenohumeral ligament is normally a smooth transition and almost every incongruity, cracking, and fibrillation of this tissue suggests injury or age-related degeneration (Fig. 16). The insertion of the anteroinferior glenohumeral ligament into the humerus is difficult, if not impossible, to see from the posterior portal. Visualization through the anterior portal may be necessary to evaluate this area for a humeral attachment glenohumeral ligament (HAGL) lesion.[64] The transition between the middle glenohumeral ligament and the anterior band of the inferior glenohumeral ligament is usually a gradual transition. Rotation of the shoulder to tension these ligaments will often allow better visualization of the margins of these ligaments. This area of the joint is of primary importance to joint stability.[58]

Posteroinferior Quadrant

The inferior glenohumeral ligament complex is also seen in the posteroinferior quadrant (Fig. 17). Viewed from the posterior portal, the entire quadrant can be seen: the articular cartilage, the junction between cartilage and labrum, the labrum itself, and the inferior glenohumeral ligament. The transition between the more capacious posterior capsule and the posterior border or posterior band of the inferior glenohumeral ligament is a gradual, but distinct, transition.

Posterosuperior Quadrant

In the posterosuperior quadrant, the articular cartilage, posterosuperior labrum, and posterior capsule are evaluated for erythema on the posterosuperior labrum or deformity of that labrum (Fig. 18). This area is best evaluated later from the anterior portal. With the arm in the abducted externally rotated position, contact between the cuff and labrum can be observed.[32,33,61]

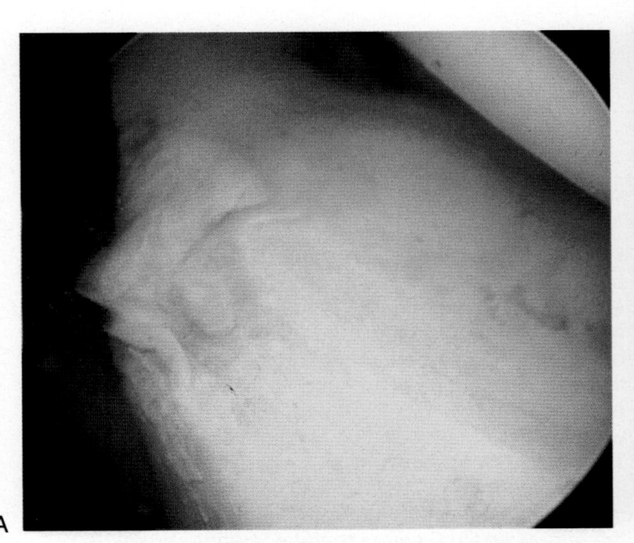

A

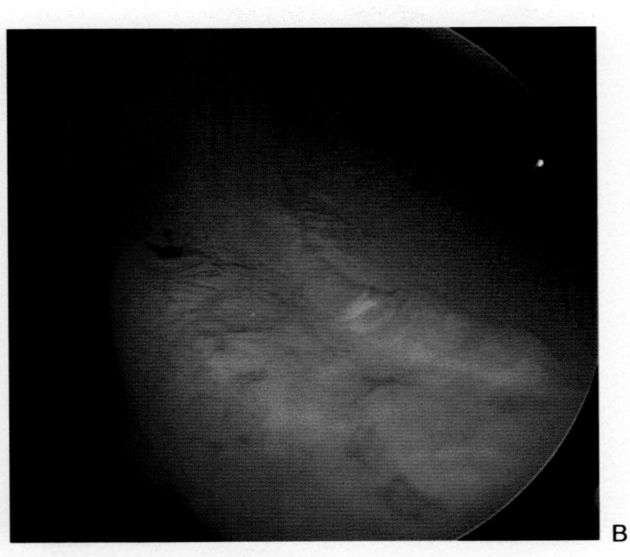

B

FIG. 18. Posterior superior quadrant: One looks for damage to articular cartilage, bone, and labrum in this area. **(A,B)** Changes may be as subtle as just a duplication of the material. A more severely affected shoulder may have erythema from contact being made in this area. Also, overt SLAP lesions can be seen.

Humeral Side of the Joint

The glenoid origin of the biceps long head origin and intraarticular portion of the long head of the biceps tendon is examined up to the bicipital groove. With a probe or Allis clamp placed into the anterior portal, 1 to 2 cm of biceps tendon can be pulled into the joint to examine the more distal aspect of the tendon and the borders of the groove. Immediately posterior to the bicipital groove, we are on the junction between articular cartilage and supraspinatus tendon (Fig. 19). The normal insertion of the supraspinatus tendon is immediately lateral to the articular cartilage; hence, there is a very sharp transition here between articular cartilage and tendon and capsule insertion. A bare area of bone between the articular cartilage and articular insertion of the supraspinatus tendon signifies a pathologic lesion and often correlates with a partial-thickness cuff tear. Also, in this superior view, we can see the more medial supraspinatus tendon and look for what Burkhart has termed the "rotator cable," or Gohlke calls the "fasciculus obliquus."[11,23] This is a group of collagen fascicles that run from the anterior insertion of the supraspinatus insertion, arching medially and then again laterally, to insert again near the junction of supraspinatus and infraspinatus.

The posterior humeral head normally has a bare area that is devoid of articular cartilage. This is the anatomic neck of the humeral head (Fig. 20). It is a gap of synovially covered bone between the edge of the articular cartilage and the insertion of

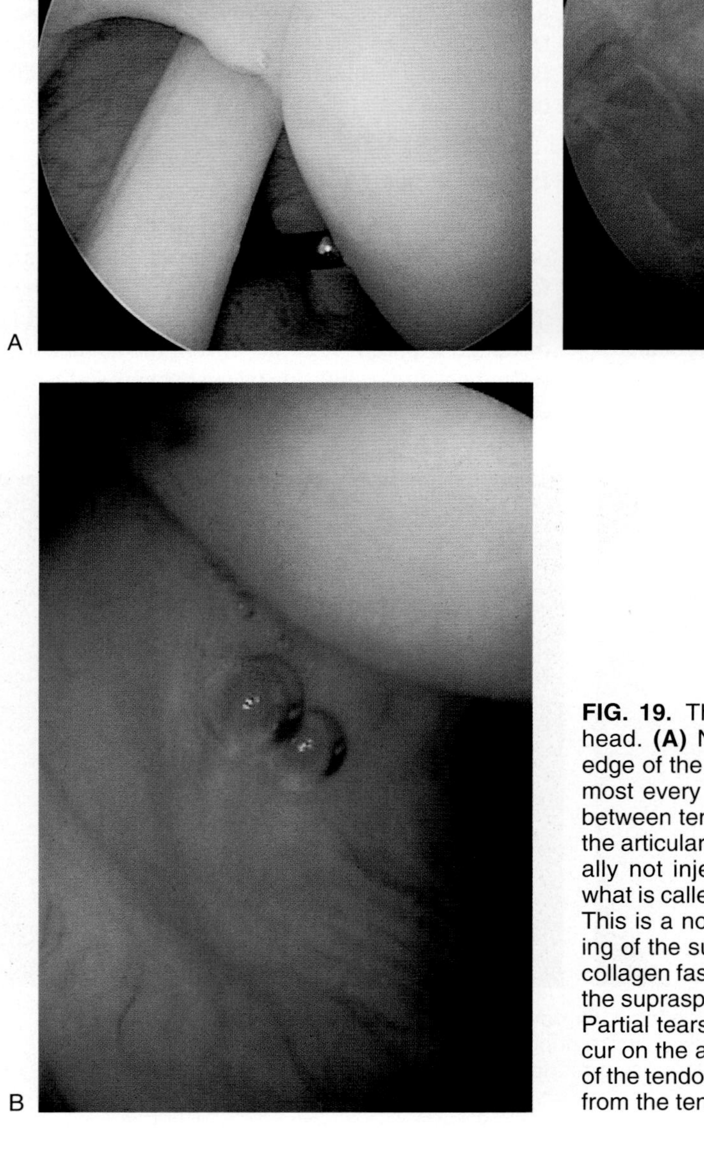

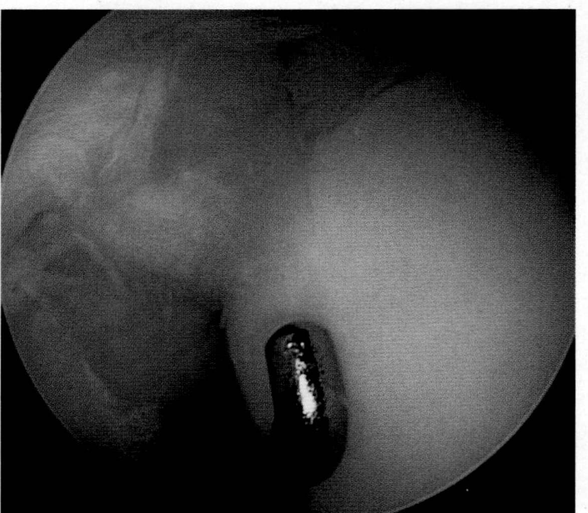

FIG. 19. The superior and anterosuperior humeral head. **(A)** Normal bicipital groove and the leading edge of the supraspinatus tendon can be seen in almost every shoulder. There is a sharp demarcation between tendon insertion and articular cartilage, and the articular surface of the tendon is smooth and usually not injected. **(B)** Further medial, one can see what is called the fasciculus obliquus or rotator cable. This is a normal structure and represents a thickening of the supraspinatus tendon created by an arc of collagen fascicles running from the anterior portion of the supraspinatus tendon to the posterior portion. **(C)** Partial tears of the rotator cuff: most partial tears occur on the articular side and appear as a roughening of the tendon and collagenous material hanging down from the tendon. *(continued)*

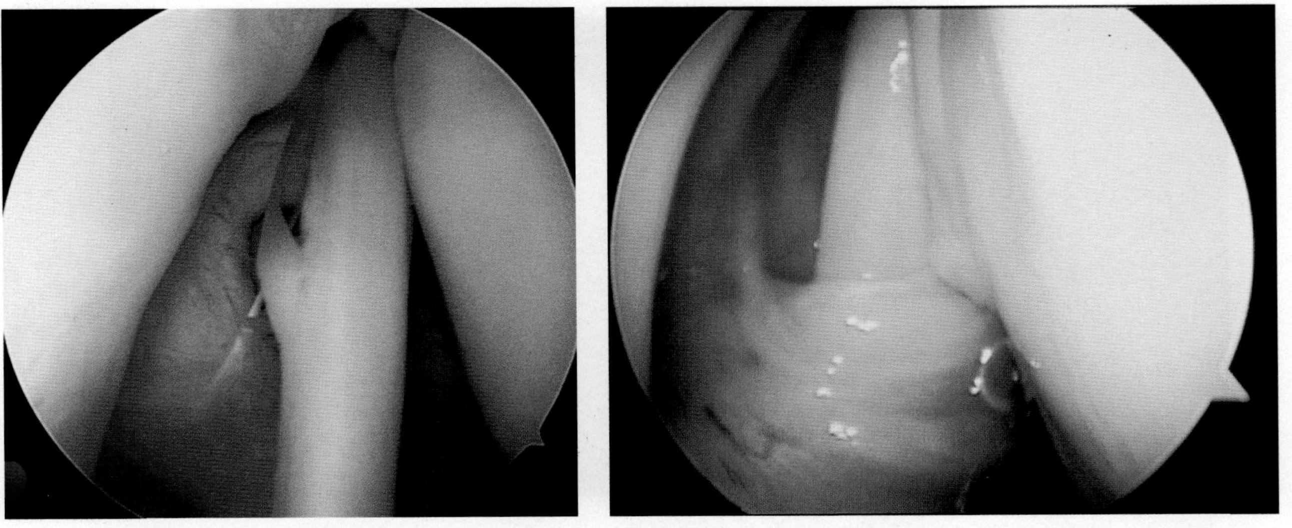

FIG. 19. *(continued)* **(D)** Also in this area, we can look for any abnormalities of the biceps tendon, which may be as subtle as the one seen here, and we can pull the biceps tendon into the joint to look for more abnormalities. **(E)** Also on the anterior portion of the humeral head, one can look for chondromalacia or actual dents in the articular cartilage that are sometimes associated with disruptions of the anterosuperior labrum or middle glenohumeral ligament complex.

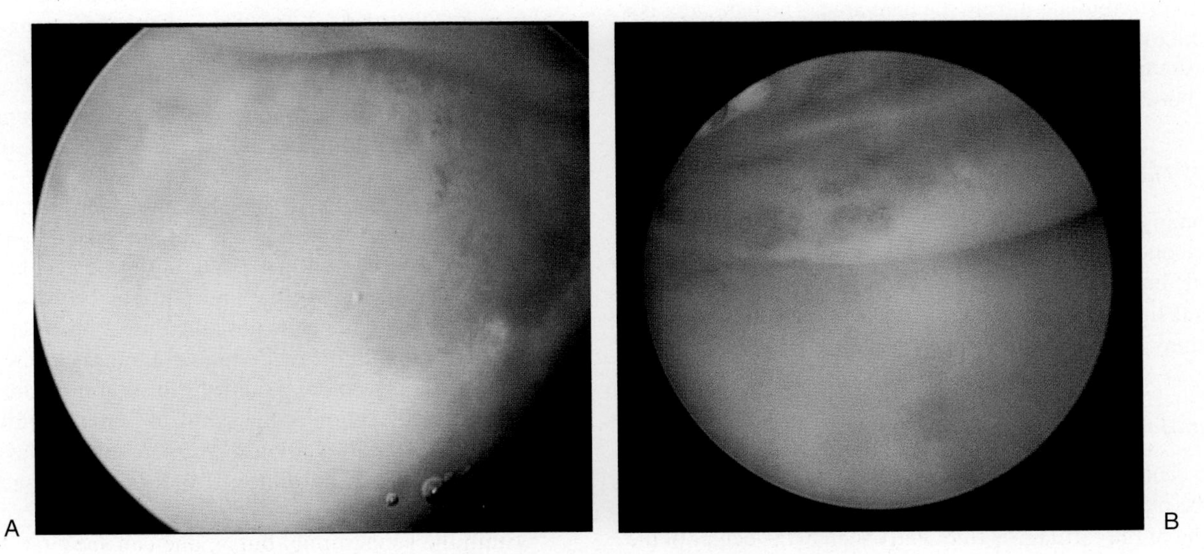

FIG. 20. The posterior humeral head usually has a bare area between articular cartilage and the insertion of the rotator cuff. In **(A)** this bare area has been continued superiorly because of some glenoid impingement. **(B)** The other abnormality is a more medial extension created by an indention fracture, as seen in this Hill–Sachs lesion.

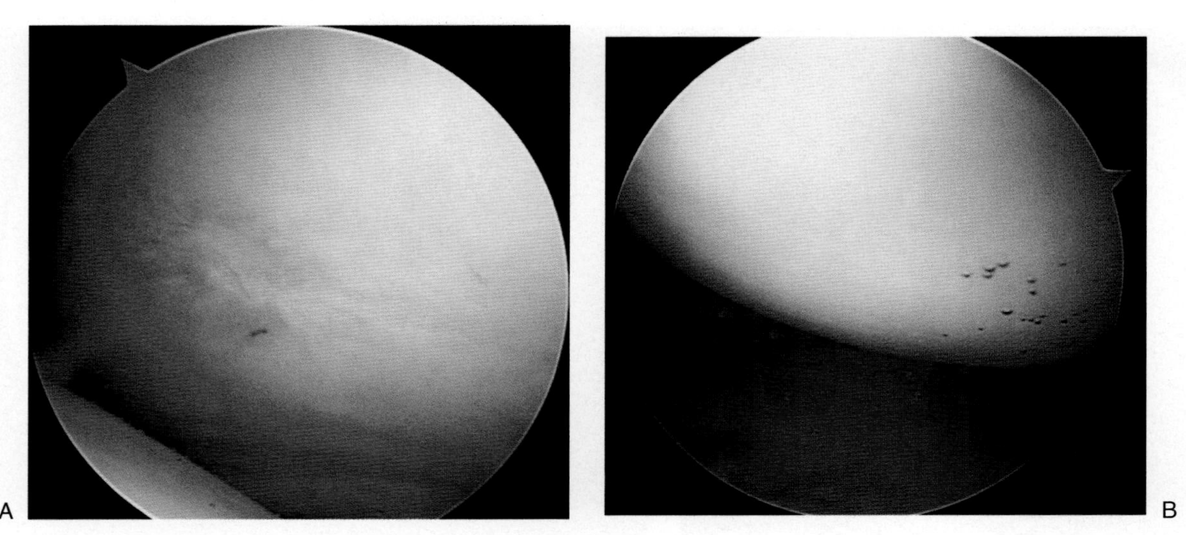

FIG. 21. Center of the joint: **(A)** the middle surface of the glenoid is seen where there is a normal thinning of the cartilage; **(B)** the normally smooth articular surface of the center of the humeral head.

the rotator cuff. This is a normal structure that needs to be differentiated from the Hermoddsen or Hill–Sachs lesion associated with glenohumeral instability.[30,32]

The Hermoddsen or Hill–Sachs lesion is an impression fracture of the articular surface of the humeral head. This helps to differentiate it from the bare area. The bare area lies adjacent to the posterior rotator cuff, while the Hill–Sachs lesion usually lies within articular cartilage and may have cartilage between it and the bare area.

Use Of The Scope Through The Anterior Portal

In many patients, the surgeon will want to place the arthroscope through the anterior cannula and examine the anterior humeral head, the insertion of the inferior glenohumeral ligament into the humeral head, and the posterior synovium in the region of the posterior portal.

Center of the Joint

The center of the joint is rarely the site of pathology, but it must be examined for articular cartilage changes. A normal thinning of the cartilage is frequently seen in the center of the glenoid (Fig. 21).

Subacromial Bursa

The final phase of diagnostic arthroscopy is viewing the subacromial bursa. My preferred technique for the subacromial bursoscopy is as follows: I replace the lens with the blunt trochar. The sheath is then withdrawn from the joint to the extraarticular surface of the infraspinatus tendon. The cannula is directed to the undersurface of the acromion, which is palpated with the tip of the blunt trochar. The cannula is then advanced below the undersurface of the acromion into the anterior aspect of the subacromial bursa.

This subacromial bursa occupies the anterior half of the subacromial space. If the bursa is not penetrated by the cannula, the arthroscope will be located in loose aveolar tissue, and clear visualization of the undersurface of the acromion and CA ligament will not be possible. Insertion of the arthroscope sheath should be gentle to avoid trauma to the undersurface of the acromion. Traumatic insertion of the sheath may result in dissection of the synovial lining, resulting in a film of subacromial synovium over the end of the arthroscope that needs to be removed before the bursa can be viewed.

Within the subacromial bursa, one can see first the synovium of the bursa on the acromial surface (Fig. 22). This

FIG. 22. Views within the subacromial bursa: **(A)** Ordinarily, the finding of a bursa is only a few cell layers thick and one can look through the bursa and see underlying blood vessels and aveolar fat. **(B)** The coracoacromial ligament ordinarily has a smooth contour and is covered by only a few cell layers of bursa. **(C)** The bursal surface of the rotator cuff is smooth, noninjected, and has no obvious defects. **(D)** An intraarticular view of what appears to be a small incomplete tear of the rotator cuff. Most rotator cuff tears appear worse from the articular side. **(E)** The bursal side view of this same tear, showing that it is actually more than 90% completed and, in effect, in terms of its mechanical effects, it is a small complete tear of the rotator cuff. **(F)** The roughening that occurs secondary to impingement in the coracoacromial ligament where it underlies the acromion. In this position, the ligament is compressed between acromion and humerus and is roughened. *(continued)*

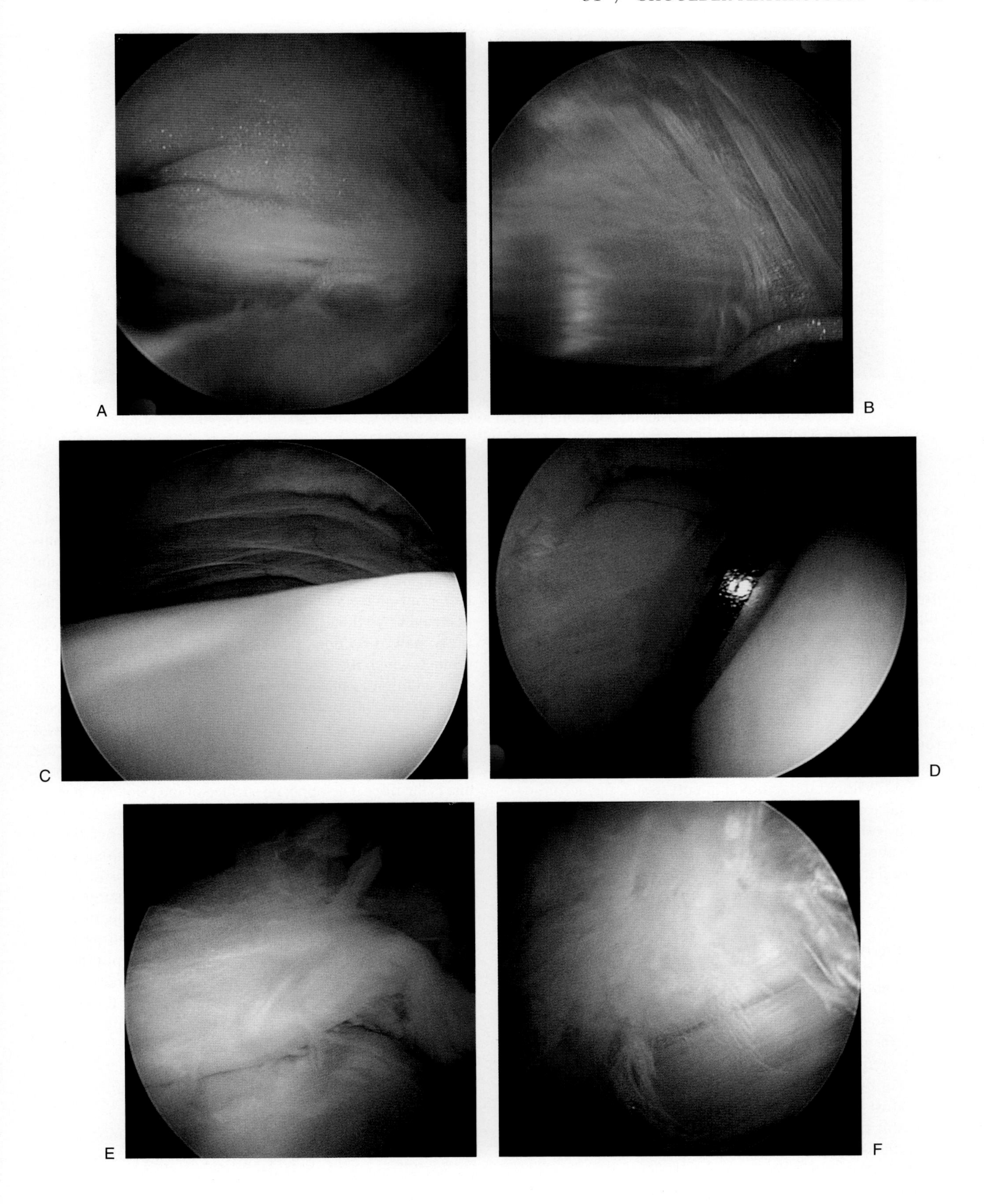
A
B
C
D
E
F

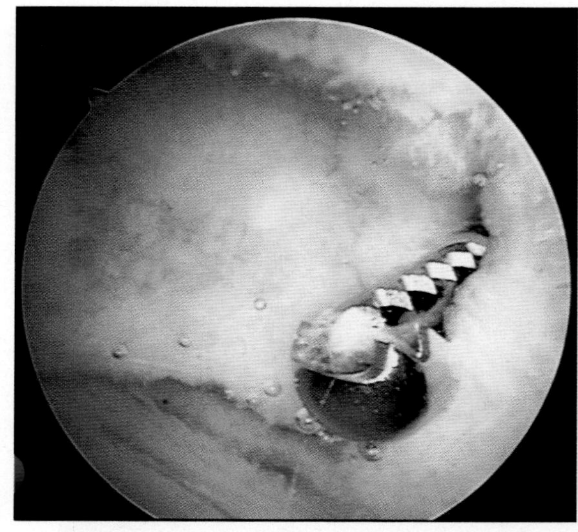

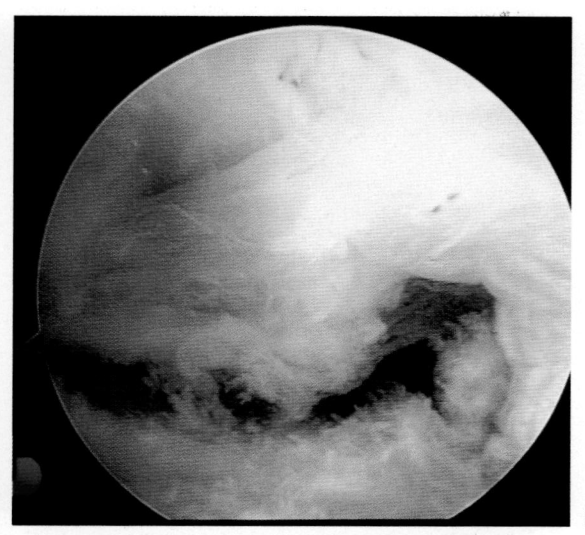

FIG. 22. *(continued)* **(G)** A view of a degenerative acromioclavicular joint after arthroscopically removing the inferior, acromioclavicular ligament. **(H)** An inflamed bursa with thickening and erythema of the lining (compare with Fig. 22A,B).

is ordinarily very thin tissue through which the acromion, the ligamentous structures, and the rotator cuff surfaces are visualized. After the synovium has been examined, the surgeon can then use a shaver through the anterolateral portal to remove tissues that are obstructing his view and complete his examination of the coracoacromial ligament. This ligament inserts on the anterior tip of the acromion and continues along the lateral border of the inferior acromion. In the normal shoulder, where the synovium is very thin, one can obtain an excellent view of this. The insertion of this ligament on the inferior surface of the acromion may continue posteriorly for a distance of up to 2 cm on the inferior surface of the acromion along the lateral edge. Without the removal of soft tissue, the acromioclavicular joint is usually not visible, for it tends to be obscured by overlying fat and synovium. Looking inferiorly, one can see the bursal surface of the rotator cuff and observe for defects here.

General Arthroscopic Technique

Arthroscope Maneuvers

There are essentially three maneuvers of the arthroscope that an arthroscopic surgeon uses in examining any joint: rotation, pistoning, and swiveling (Fig. 23). The scope is rotated often by the surgeon because there is an angle to his scope. Most commonly, he or she is using the 30-degree lens. In this fashion, without actually changing the position of the arthroscope, the surgeon can examine a much wider field of view as the scope is rotated. This rotation changes the direction of the 30-degree–angled face. By pistoning, moving the scope forward and back along a constant axis, the surgeon can change the perspective on a structure that is being viewed, moving in for a close-up visualization and moving backward to obtain some more perspective and move out of the way of the instruments. Swiveling is the maneuver by which the surgeon moves the scope in an entirely new direction, pivoting on the soft-tissue sleeve through which the scope passes.

In addition to maneuvering the scope, arthroscopists often maneuver a portion of the joint. In every joint that we arthroscope, there is one part of the joint that maintains a rather static relation with the arthroscopic portals. In the shoulder, this is the glenoid and the acromion. In the knee, this is the tibia. The opposite surface of the joint can then be maneuvered around for better observation by the surgeon. In the shoulder, the movable surface is the humerus. By detaching the arm from its traction, the assistant can move the humeral head around and show different portions of the articular cartilage and adjacent soft tissue to the surgeon, so that they can be examined for damage. In addition, there are provocative examinations that the assistant can perform, such as abduction and external rotation, that permit the surgeon to examine for anterior subluxation of the humeral head on the glenoid. The surgeon can also look for contact between the articular side of the rotator cuff with the posterosuperior labrum.

Portal Maintenance

Maintenance of the integrity of the portals is important in shoulder arthroscopy, for the large soft-tissue envelope creates a tendency for soft-tissue swelling. Repeated passages of instruments can result in tissue damage. Maintaining a

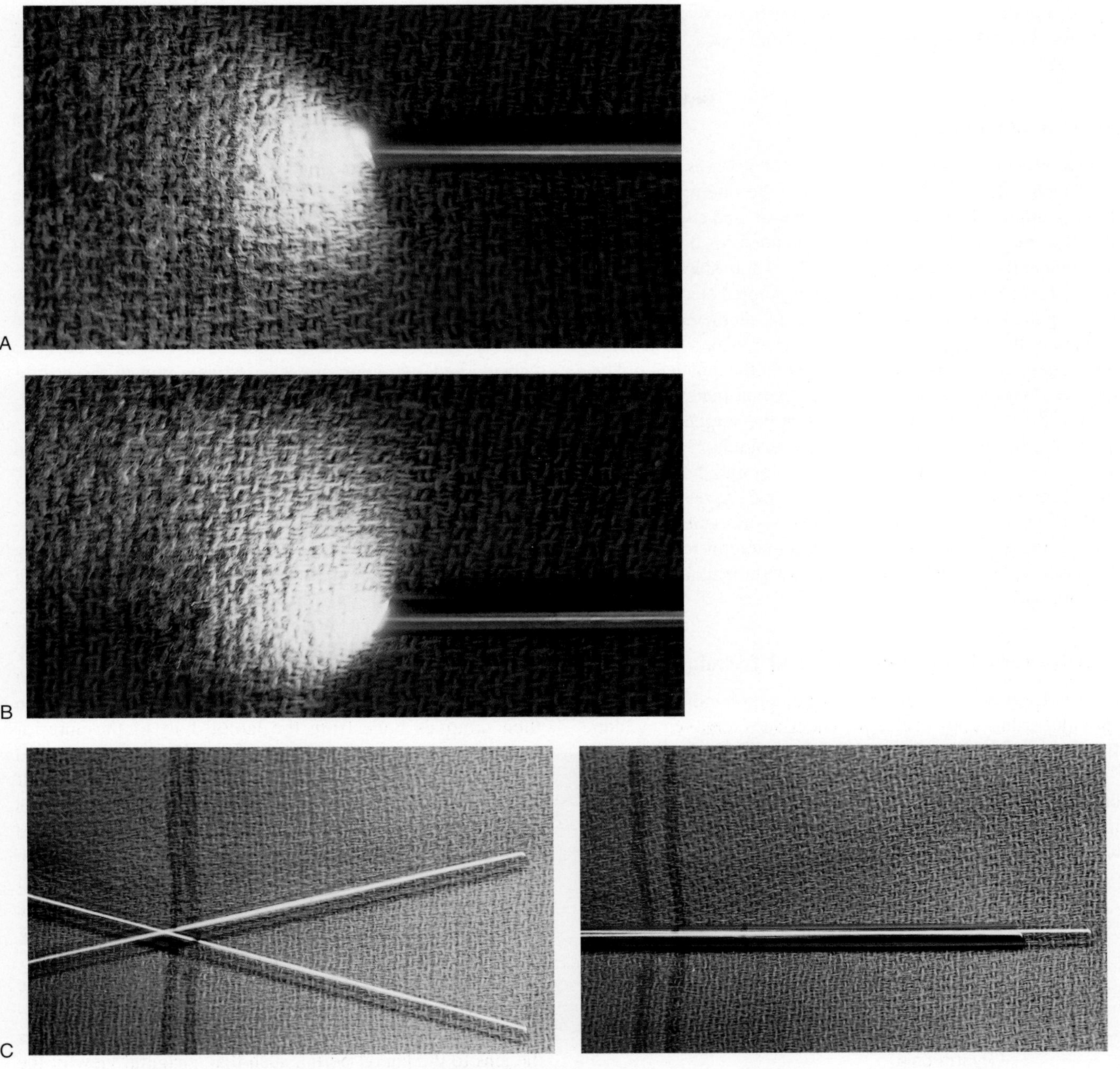

FIG. 23. Maneuvers of the scope: **(A,B)** Rotation showing the 30-degree–angled scope in two positions of rotation 180 degrees apart. The *light* demonstrates two different areas that would be viewed without any real change in the position of the scope other than rotation. **(C)** A double exposure demonstrating the swivelling maneuver by which this scope is maneuvered to a different position around the constant pivot **(D)** Pistoning, in which the scope is kept in a constant rotation and orientation and is just moved in and out of the arthroscopable space to offer the surgeon changes in perspective.

cannula in the portal tends to minimize the flow of fluid out into the soft tissues and the damage from repeat instrument passage.

Selection of Cannulae

Operative cannulae have a variety of features that influence their selection. Among these are the internal diameter of the cannula, the opacity of the material, and slippage control. The need for a certain internal diameter is based on the instrument the surgeon needs to use. A 4-mm shaver may require only a 5-mm–internal diameter. Angled electrodes and suture punches require a 7-mm–internal diameter. The first version of the Caspari suture punch required an oval cannula with a large longitudinal diameter so that the punch could be removed with the jaws open. A transparent material for the wall of the cannula is important when the surgeon wants to observe what he is doing within the cannula (e.g., arthroscopic knot tying). Most operative cannulae have ribs or threads on their external surfaces. These are to resist cannula pullout when the surgeon withdraws instruments. Because most of these cannulae have rubber diaphragms to resist water outflow, they tend to hold onto instruments as they are withdrawn.

Ablative Techniques: Indications and Techniques

Ablative procedures are the most common indications for shoulder arthroscopy (Table 3). The tissues removed include fluid, synovium, adhesion, cartilage, labrum, and bone.

Liquid materials can be easily removed from this joint or bursa, including blood or pus. In performing an arthroscopic incision and drainage, the goal is to remove all infected materials. This includes not only suction, irrigation, and the placement of a drain, but also the removal of glycocalyx or "slime" produced by the bacteria. This slime forms a lining on the joint that must be removed with a less aggressive shaver, being careful to not penetrate the capsule. In removing blood from a joint with a bleeding disorder, efforts similar to those used in the open procedures are taken to correct the bleeding diathesis.

TABLE 3. *Indications for ablative procedures*

Synovial fluid
Pyarthrosis
Hemarthrosis
Synovium
Inflammatory arthritis (RA) PVNS
Synovial chondrometaplasia
Loose bodies
Labrum
SLAP type I, III, and others
Bone
Acromioplasty
AC resection arthroplasty
Coracoplasty
Tendon
Biceps
Rotator cuff partial tear
Calcium

The tissue that is most commonly removed is synovium, although usually not as the main treatment goal. This may be done for visualization, for treatment of a specific disease such as rheumatoid arthritis, or for treatment of a source of disease as in synovial chondrometaplasia.[16,50] For those patients in whom one is concerned about removing too much synovium and getting into tissues such as capsule, there are special synovial resection blades that can be used. The capsule and synovium are released as a unit in the arthroscopic treatment of the various forms of frozen shoulder.[26,27,29,40,41,59,62]

Bone is removed most commonly in acromioplasty, and acromioplasty is the most commonly performed ablative procedure.[8,15,44,47,52,53] It is in this particular ablative technique that the shortcomings of the arthroscope in judging the flatness of a surface come to the fore. The surgeon is looking at a distorted monocular view of the undersurface of the acromion and must judge if he has created a flatter surface. One of the techniques for doing this is to measure on the preoperative x-ray film how much bone needs to be removed. Then, at the time of surgery, after removal of all of the soft tissue from the undersurface of the acromion, the surgeon then removes bone from the lateral half of the anterior acromion—the amount of bone judged to be necessary based on the preoperative x-ray films. The remaining medial half demonstrates that sufficient bone to flatten the acromion has been removed. Using the motorized burr, bone is removed from the medial half of the acromion so that it is even with the lateral half. In this fashion, the remaining medial half tells the surgeon how much bone has been resected from the lateral half. Maintaining proper camera orientation during the performance of this procedure is paramount.

The second method by which a surgeon may judge the flatness of the surface is referred to as the cutting block technique (Fig. 24). In this technique, the arthroscopist moves the lens to the lateral portal, such that a sagittal view of the undersurface of the acromion is obtained. He then uses the edge of the burr's shaft as a flat surface that can then be placed against the surface of the mid- and posterior portions of the acromion, and an attempt is made to flatten out the anterior acromion so that it resembles the flatness of the surface of the midacromion. If one attempts to make the anterior acromion parallel to the posterior acromion, one may remove too much acromion. When the arthroscopist uses the posterior acromion, but places the lever at an angle to the posterior acromion, then too much is removed. The shortcoming of the cutting block technique is that one does not obtain a good visualization of the lateral acromion. What many surgeons will do is use both of these techniques, using

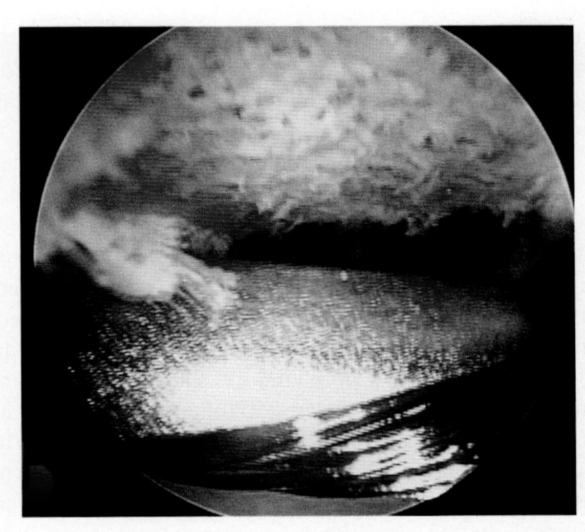

FIG. 24. Acromioplasty in progress through the lateral view: In this technique, we can use the known flat edge of an arthroscopic instrument; here, the backside of a burr, to check the flatness of the anterior acromion against the surface of the mid- and posterior acromion. In other words, we use the mid- and posterior acromion as a cutting block.

one to check the other, and in this fashion overcome the shortcomings of the monocular view of the arthroscope.

Torn glenoid labrum is sometimes removed in the shoulder in a manner similar to menisectomy.[22,45,51,57] This is done if the unstable labrum fragment is not required as a tendon or capsule anchor. Removal is done with basket forceps and graspers or by the suction motorized shaver. Damaged articular cartilage is removed and contoured in patients with degenerative changes, using the suction shaver, baskets, or graspers.

The next most commonly removed material is a loose body.[16,24] When the loose bodies are purely cartilaginous, they may be removed with the suction shaver. If they are partially ossified, they are removed using a grasper. In contrast to the knee, the shoulder arthroscopist is somewhat more wedded to maintaining his cannulae in place. For this reason, he or she is more likely to try to reduce the size of loose bodies that are being removed, so that they can be brought out through the cannula without having to remove the cannula or enlarge the portals.

Probably the least commonly resected material from the joint is tendon, such as the long head of the biceps. Some authors have reported that, in a patient with a large irreparable rotator cuff tear, resection of a very frayed biceps tendon will give pain relief, although it will not improve the performance of the patient's shoulder. In addition, following biceps tenodesis, it is a good policy to remove the intraarticular portion of the biceps. This is because as the shoulder is abducted, the intraarticular portion of the biceps will be doubled up on itself and in this fashion create a space-occupying lesion with mechanical symptoms and pain within the shoulder. Tendon removal can be accomplished by using a suture punch to place a suture in the biceps tendon and then using a knife or other cutting instrument to detach the tendon at either end of its intraarticular course. This technique avoids opening the rotator interval.

Occasionally, calcium is removed from patients in whom calcific tendinitis has failed to resolve.[2] Extraarticular cysts have also been attacked at their intraarticular end arthroscopically.[20]

Finally, man-made objects such as bullets or surgical devices can be removed.[4,5,65]

Reconstructive Techniques: Indications and Techniques

Thus far, two groups of reconstructive techniques have been described. The first of these is the reattachment of a detached structure to bone. The second is changing the dimensions of intact structures so that they more adequately perform their required function (Table 4).

The two structures that are most commonly reattached arthroscopically are the labrum with adjacent capsule and the rotator cuff. In either case, what is required is a fixation device for reattaching the structure to the bone and the ability to clean off the bone and the collagenous structure, so that they will heal to each other.[1,14,18,28,43,51,55] Removing surface debris and synovium from detached structures is easily accomplished with the suction shaver. The two most common device options in reattaching detached structures are an absorbable tack or staple and a suture anchor.

To use the absorbable tack, the surgeon has to be able to drill a hole into the bone in the appropriate angle, then place a guide wire through the detached soft-tissue structure (labrum, ligament, or tendon) into that hole, and then pass the absorbable tack over the guide pin and drive it home.[1] For the suture anchor technique, the surgeon also needs to be able to drill a hole at the appropriate angle and position, such that the suture anchor can be placed; at least one suture punch, so that he or she can then pass suture through the soft-tissue structure and be able to tie a knot in an intraarticular fashion or an intrabursal fashion. This tying of the knot is probably the most vexing part of the procedure to the surgeon. In an open procedure, the surgeon can easily tie the knot and judge its tension with his fingers. In an arthroscopic procedure, there is a learning curve and some insecurity on the part of the surgeon over knots that are tied at a relative

TABLE 4. *Indications for reconstructive procedures*

Rotator cuff tear
Instability
Traumatic
MDI
SLAP lesions
Types II, IV, and V

distance. Some practice is required before the surgeon becomes confident of his or her knot-tying ability.

The second group of reconstructive procedures is shrinkage of tissues that are lax, but are not detached from bone. The surgeon uses a heat source, either radiofrequency, laser, or electrocautery to produce changes within the collagen of the capsule, hopefully without inducing much tissue necrosis. Alternatively, suture hooks can be used to place sutures to shrink the capsule. It is hoped that some of this capsular shrinkage will be permanent and leave the patient with permanent stability in their shoulder. As to indications for this technique, the patient with a nontraumatic multidirectional instability comes to mind. In addition, there are patients who have a traumatic unidirectional dislocation, in whom there will be some residual laxity within the capsule after repair of the labrum back to the glenoid rim. There may be a place for capsular shrinking in these individuals after an arthroscopic Bankart repair.[6] This is still a technique in development. Precise ways of measuring how much capsule needs to be shortened, and how much capsule should be overshortened to compensate for postoperative capsular stretching, need to be developed.

INDICATIONS

We have described three types of procedures: diagnostic, ablative, and reconstructive. There are four groups of indications for shoulder arthroscopy: (a) the purely diagnostic, (b) a confirmatory diagnostic arthroscopy coupled with an open procedure, (c) indications for ablative procedures, and (d) indications for reconstructive procedures. As we pointed out in the Introduction, in looking over these indications, the reader needs to bear in mind two things: (a) his or her current level of arthroscopic skill, and (b) the outcomes' results reported in the literature long-term as well as short-term.

Diagnostic Indications

As these are indications for surgery for which the actual diagnosis is not known, the indication will be a complaint in combination with a set of physical findings. Considering whether there is an indication for the diagnostic arthroscopy, the surgeon needs to ask himself: does the history and physical examination in combination point to diseases for which there are pathologic findings visible within an arthroscopable space? Appropriate to this discussion is that some pathology in the shoulder is dynamic rather than static. An example of this is the discussion of laxity versus instability. In examining a large group of teenage gymnasts, a group of knowledgeable shoulder surgeons found that they were able to dislocate the shoulder in a large percentage of these gymnasts. Yet, when these same gymnasts were questioned they had no history of shoulder dislocation. They had shoulder laxity, but did not have instability symptoms during their athletic events or in their activities of daily living. The intrinsic dilemma is that instability and dynamic impingement events may occur with specific activities that cannot be accurately reproduced in the operating room. The arthroscope demonstrates anatomic pathology that is static. This static pathology may either be a cause or a result of that event. An example would be damage to the interior fibers of the rotator cuff and the fibers of the superior labrum as the result of shoulder instability (Fig. 25).

The accuracy and diagnostic value of shoulder arthroscopy in the treatment of specific disorders in an individual patient is dependent on the surgeon's ability to correctly correlate the anatomic pathology with the history and physical examination. Complaints of shoulder patients are often divided into those that involve pain, stiffness, weakness, or instability. In addition, there are accompanying physical findings of roughness, noise, or catching. Those patients who have mechanical problems with the shoulder are, in general, better candidates for arthroscopy than those whose problem is purely pain.

Confirmatory Arthroscopy Coupled with an Open Procedure

In these cases, the surgeon feels that the diagnosis is almost certain and has selected an open procedure. The surgeon must ask himself, "Is a preoperative arthroscope of benefit?" Bailey, in his Presidential Guest Lecture to the American Shoulder and Elbow Surgeons, pointed out that out of 100 arthroscopies performed before an open shoulder repair, he found additional unexpected pathology in close to 30%. Although it may not alter the overall diagnosis and treatment plan, it may modify them. This experience has been echoed by other surgeons, and it is my current practice to arthroscope the shoulder before most open shoulder surgeries, particularly for instability procedures. This allows me to examine the superior labrum and the inside of the rotator cuff and do a more thorough examination for loose bodies and articular cartilage damage.

Ablative Procedures

The ablative category comprises the largest percentage of arthroscopic surgical procedures. Acromioplasty accounts for the lion's, share of these, with distal clavicle resection also being common. The diagnosis is generally determined before surgery, and unwanted materials are removed in a fashion that causes less pain for the patient than the open procedure. Frequently, the results are as good as open surgery with less patient discomfort. This is especially true the more experienced the arthroscopic surgeon is.

Reconstructive Procedures

This remains the most rapidly changing area in shoulder arthroscopy. These are technically demanding procedures. Thus far, they consist of reattachments to bone and heat shrinkage of ligament (see foregoing section on techniques and the specific chapters).

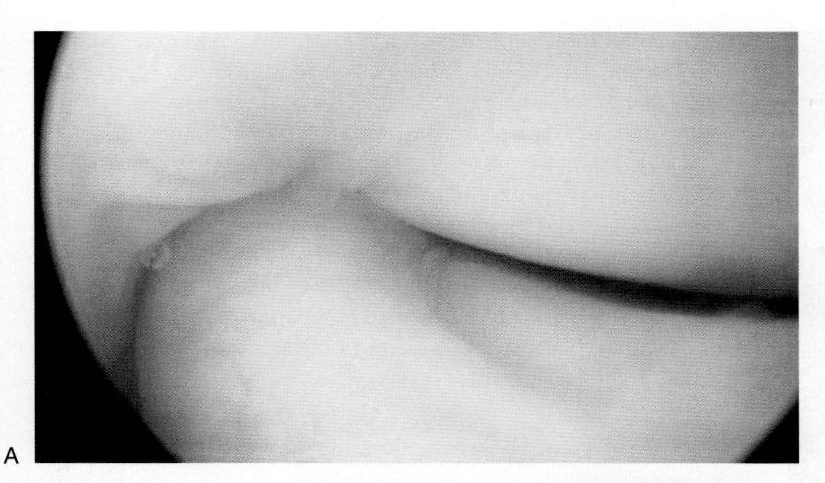

A

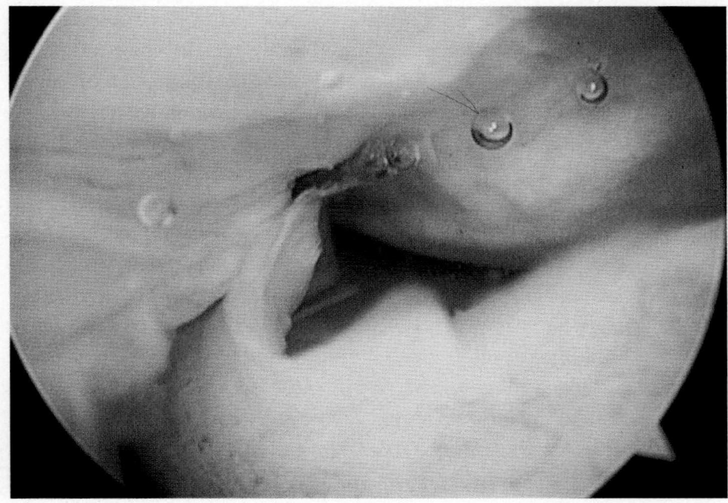

B

FIG. 25. Posterior superior impingement: **(A)** This contact can be achieved in stable shoulders that have no posterosuperior pathology. Note the smooth appearance of the posterosuperior labrum below and the rotator cuff above. In contrast, **B** shows the secondary changes in the labrum and an incomplete rotator cuff tear above. Note also that the humeral head seems to have been moved slightly anterior in comparison with the position of the humeral head in A.

COMPLICATIONS

General Complications of Shoulder Arthroscopy

The general complications of shoulder arthroscopy are relatively rare, and range from the inability to perform the arthroscopy to damage to each of the tissues about the shoulder, and continue on to the problem of saline extravasation into the soft tissues.[49] As with other arthroscopies, postoperative infection remains rare.[3] In general, the complications are least frequent in the simpler diagnostic scopes and more common for the reconstruction procedures.

The inability of the surgeon to visualize the structures that he or she wishes to visualize is usually related to one of two problems: intraspace bleeding or poor portal placement.

Bleeding into the glenohumeral joint results in poor visualization and is often handled by establishing a second portal, so that good flow of saline or lactated Ringer solution can be established. The blood is cleared, and if there is a large source of bleeding, this can be treated with electrocautery. An insulated arthroscopic meniscus electrode will allow cauterization in an isotonic medium, such as saline or lactated Ringer.

Within the subacromial space, bleeding can be more problematic because this may represent a lesion of the acromial artery. Increasing the flow within the subacromial space may not be sufficient to stop the bleeding. The acromial artery can be controlled by placing the surgeon's contralateral index and long fingers anterior to the acromion and the thumb on the spine of the scapula and pressing down, compressing the soft tissue anterior to the acromion margin. This will occlude the acromial artery and allow the surgeon to rinse out the subacromial space. Then, by establishing a flow through the scope and out through the operative portal, what bleeding occurs after the release of the surgeon's fingers disappears into the operative cannula and does not refill the subacromial space (Fig. 26). In this way, the surgeon can maintain his visualization while bringing an electrocautery to the site of bleeding.

The other visualization problem—poor portal placement—is, fortunately, usually not severe and can be remedied by using the scope through a second portal. For example, a laterally placed posterior portal may have a large area anteriorly that cannot be seen. The surgeon may compensate for this by placing the scope in the anterior portal to visual-

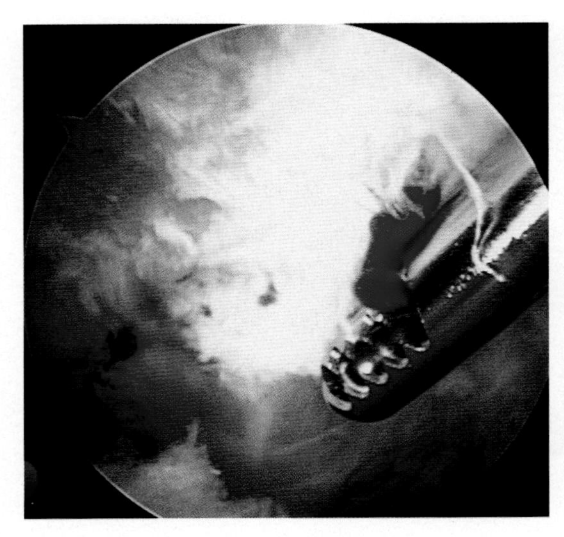

FIG. 26. Control of blood flow: When there is bleeding in a space such as the subacromial bursa, establishing an outflow through the operative cannula or in this case out through the operative instrument, can remove the blood can be removed immediately after its appearance and, thereby, the clarity of the visualization can be maintained.

ize anterior structures. In placement of the subacromial portal posteriorly, occasionally the surgeon places this between bone and synovium instead of within the bursa. In this case, the lens needs to be uncovered with a motorized shaver, taking care not to scratch the surface of the lens.

Articular Cartilage

Articular cartilage can be damaged by trochars, needles, and the use of an improper cannula with the lens. It can also be damaged chemically by some of the sterilizing chemicals that are used for soaking arthroscopic equipment. For that reason, these instruments need to be rinsed thoroughly before placement into the joint. Entering into the joint can be made less traumatic by ensuring that one uses the blunt trochar with the cannula, and one is careful about palpating the area before entering into the joint. Other than an initial joint injection, needles should be admitted to the joint only under direct arthroscopic vision. Manufacturers match their cannulae to their lenses, and if one is accidentally given the wrong lens to fit the cannula, the leading edge of the cannula may sometimes stick out beyond the lens and gouge the articular cartilage. This occasionally happens with sudden swivel type motions of the arthroscope against the articular cartilage, despite the use of the correct cannula.

Bone, Tendon, and Capsule Damage

Each of these structures can be damaged in the placement of a portal, and there is at least one publication of a rotator cuff tear that the authors felt was due to multiple arthroscopic portal placements. The portals that we have described in the foregoing all enter the joint through muscle. None of these portals enter the joint through tendon. There is a transacromial portal described that is rarely used for repair of superior labral lesions, which weakens the acromion. Excessive midacromial bone resection in acomioplasty may lead to acromial fracture. In the capsule, excessive synovectomy can damage the capsule. The capsule usually heals the defects created by the arthroscopic portals. The humeral bone in the bare space can be damaged by mistaking this indentation for the posterior glenoid at the time of initial trochar insertion. This creates a small trochar hole in the soft cancellous bone of the bare area.

Nerve Damage

Nerve damage secondary to direct injury or indirect traction injury can appear.[56] The three most worrisome nerves outside of the cutaneous nerves are the suprascapular nerve, the axillary nerve, and the musculocutaneous nerve. The suprascapular nerve is at risk in the posterior shoulder and in the supraspinatus fossa. At the upper end of the spinoglenoid notch, the suprascapular nerve may be less than 2 cm from the posterior glenoid rim.[9] In this area, a misdirected instrument might damage this nerve. As the nerve passes inferiorly it travels medially and can be damaged during transosseous suture techniques. To avoid this complication, drills and pins should be directed more medially and exit the midportion of the infraspinatus fossa. A misdirected superior portal could damage the suprascapular nerve at the suprascapular notch.

The axillary nerve may be damaged in the quadrangular space and 5 cm below the acromion within the middle and anterior thirds of the deltoid. In the quadrangular space, the axillary nerve can be injured when operating on the inferior capsule. Surgery on the inferior capsule close to the glenoid and labrum, rather than the midcapsule, helps one avoid this complication. With abduction of the arm, the axillary nerve will be brought closer to the acromion. Portals placed above the level of the coracoid for the subacromial space help prevent this injury.

The musculocutaneous nerve enters the conjoined tendon, on average, 5.5 cm below the tip of the coracoid, but it may enter closer than this average. In addition, there is frequently an additional branch from the lateral cord to the short head of the biceps and coracobrachialis muscles. When these accessory nerves are considered, about 75% of anatomic specimens have a nerve penetrating the conjoined tendon and muscles less than 5.5 cm off the tip of the coracoid. Injury to the musculocutaneous nerve or its accessory branches can occur with the 3:00 o'clock, the 5:00 o'clock, and the slalom portals. The 3:00 o'clock approach tries to avoid this complication by hugging the inferior surface of the coracoid and then exiting there. Only a rare specimen has a nerve within 1.5 cm of the tip of the coracoid. The slalom and 5:00 o'clock position portal techniques avoid damage to the musculocutaneous nerve by passing lateral to the conjoined tendon.

Indirect Damage to the Brachial Plexus

Brachial plexus traction injuries occur as a result of patient and arm position and operative time. The shorter the arthroscopic procedure, the less likely this is to occur. Klein and coworkers have shown that certain positions of the arm put more traction on the brachial plexus than others.[37] They found that the arm position of 30-degrees–forward flexion and 70-degrees abduction produced the most traction on the brachial plexus. In the more recent past, positions with less abduction have been more commonly used.

Bleeding and Blood Loss

Considering the large number of vessels about the shoulder, vessel damage is common. Abundant numbers of anastomoses make vessel damage unlikely to result in areas of ischemia. The greatest risk of vascular damage is anteriorly, where there are numerous arteries and the cephalic vein. Although there is relatively little danger of creating an area of ischemia, postoperative bleeding can be problematic. Bleeding may be difficult to detect because the portals are relatively small and there is an intervening layer of muscle. In addition, there is usually a large amount of swelling that is anticipated from leakage of the irrigant, which makes it difficult to detect hematoma postoperatively.

Fluids: Extravasation and Chemical Irritation

Fluid extravasation will usually resolve rather quickly.[13] There have been no compartment syndromes reported in the shoulder from fluid extravasation. Therefore, the surgeon must rely on failure of the swelling of the shoulder to go away and upon increased pain to be able to detect blood loss early. Some patients have bled to the point of needing a transfusion from an arthroscopic procedure.

Residual sterilization fluids remaining, or incompletely rinsed instruments, may irritate synovium or cartilage.

CONCLUSION

Shoulder arthroscopy is an essential tool for the shoulder surgeon. It remains a technique in development and each of us remains a surgeon in training. In making our patient selection and in using our arthroscope, we need not only to consider the description of the disease and the procedure and the long-term published results, but also our own current level of development of arthroscopic skill.

REFERENCES

1. Arciero RA, Taylor DC, Snyder RJ, Uhorchak JM. Arthroscopic bioabsorbable tack stabilization of initial anterior shoulder dislocations: a preliminary report. *Arthroscopy* 1995;11:410–417.
2. Ark JW, Flock TJ, Flatow EL, Bigliani LU. Arthroscopic treatment of calcific tendinitis of the shoulder. *Arthroscopy* 1992;8:183–188.
3. Armstrong RW, Bolding F, Joseph R. Septic arthritis following arthroscopy: clinical syndromes and analysis of risk factors. *Arthroscopy* 1992;8:213–223.
4. Bach BR. Arthroscopic removal of painful Bristow hardware. *Arthroscopy* 1990;6:324–326.
5. Bach BR, Novak PJ. Removal of the instrument makar shoulder staple. *Arthroscopy* 1995;11:338–339.
6. Bankart ASB. The pathology and treatment of recurrent dislocation of the shoulder-joint. *Br J Surg* 1938;26:23–29.
7. Bert JM, Posalaky Z, Snyder S, McGinley D, Chock C. Effect of various irrigating fluids on the ultrastructure of articular cartilage. *Arthroscopy* 1990;6:104–111.
8. Bigliani LU, Morrison DS, April EW. The morphology of the acromion and its relationship to rotator cuff tears. *Orthop Trans* 1986;10:228.
9. Bigliani LU, Dalsey RM, McCann PD, April EW. An anatomical study of the suprascapular nerve. *Arthroscopy* 1990;6:301–305.
10. Brown AR, Weiss R, Greenberg C, Flatow EL, Bigliani LU. Interscalene block for shoulder arthroscopy: comparison with general anesthesia. *Arthroscopy* 1993;9:295–300.
11. Burkhart SS, Esch JC, Jolson RS. The rotator crescent and rotator cable: an anatomic description of the shoulder's "suspension bridge." *Arthroscopy* 1993;9:611–616.
12. Cahill BR. Osteolysis of the distal part of the clavicle in male athletes. *J Bone Joint Surg [Am]* 1982;64:1053–1058.
13. Carr CF, Murphy JM. Deltoid and supraspinatus muscle pressures following various arthroscopic shoulder procedures. *Arthroscopy* 1995; 11:401–403.
14. Caspari R, Savoie F. Arthroscopic reconstruction of the shoulder: the Bankart repair. In: McGinty J, ed. *Operative arthroscopy*. New York: Raven Press, 1991:507–516.
15. Caspari RB, Thal R. A technique for arthroscopic subacromial decompression. *Arthroscopy* 1992;8:23–30.
16. Covall DJ, Fowble CD. Arthroscopic treatment of synovial chondromatosis of the shoulder and biceps tendon sheath. *Arthroscopy* 1993;9: 602–604.
17. Davidson PA, Tibone JE. Anterior-inferior (5 o'clock) portal for shoulder arthroscopy. *Arthroscopy* 1995;11:519–525.
18. Detrisac D. Arthroscopic staple capsulorrhaphy for traumatic anterior instability. In: McGinty J, ed. *Operative arthroscopy*. New York: Raven Press, 1991:517–528.
19. Esch JC. Shoulder arthroscopy: basic setup. In: Paulos LE, Tibone JE, eds. *Operative techniques in shoulder surgery*. Gaithersburg, MD: Aspen Publications, 1991:9–14.
20. Fehrman DA, Orwin JF, Jennings RM. Suprascapular nerve entrapment by ganglion cysts: a report of six cases with arthroscopic findings and review of the literature. *Arthroscopy* 1995;11:727–734.
21. Flatow EL, Cordasco FS, Bigliani LU. Arthroscopic resection of the outer end of the clavicle from a superior approach: a critical, quantitative, radiographic assessment of bone removal. *Arthroscopy* 1992;8: 55–64.
22. Glasgow SG, Bruce RA, Yacobucci GN, Torg JS. Arthroscopic resection of glenoid labral tears in the athlete: a report of 29 cases. *Arthroscopy* 1992;8:48–54.
23. Gohlke F, Essigkrug B, Schmitz F. The pattern of the collagen fiber bundles of the capsule of the glenohumeral joint. *J Shoulder Elbow Surg* 1994;3:111–128.
24. Gradinger R, Träger J, Klauser RJ. Influence of various irrigation fluids on articular cartilage. *Arthroscopy* 1995; 11:263–269.
25. Hamada S, Hamada M, Nishiue S, Doi T. Osteochondritis dissecans of the humeral head [case report]. *Arthroscopy* 1992; 8:132–137.
26. Harner C, Mason G, Fu FH. Cidex-induced synovitis. Presented at the Fifth Congress of the International Society of the Knee. Sydney, Australia, April 9, 1987.
27. Harryman DT. Shoulders: frozen and stiff. *Instr Course Lect* 1993;42: 247–257.
28. Harryman DT, Sidles JA, Harris SL, Matsen FA. The role of the rotator interval capsule in passive motion and stability of the shoulder. *J Bone Joint Surg [Am]* 1992;74:53–66.
29. Harryman DT, Ballmer FP, Harris SL, Sidles JA. Arthroscopic labral repair to the glenoid rim. *Arthroscopy* 1994;10:20–30.
30. Harryman DT, Sidles JA, Matsen FA. Arthroscopic management of refractory shoulder stiffness. *J Shoulder Elbow Surg* 1996;5:112.
31. Hill SA, Sachs MD. The grooved defect of the humeral head. A frequently unrecognized complication of dislocations of the shoulder joint. *Radiology* 1940;35:690–700.
32. Jobe CM. Gross anatomy of the shoulder. In: Rockwood C, Matsen F, eds. *The shoulder*. Philadelphia: WB Saunders, 1998:34–97.
33. Jobe CM. Posterior superior glenoid impingement: expanded spectrum. *Arthroscopy* 1995;11:530–536.

34. Jobe FW, Giangarra CE, Kvitne RS, Glousman RE. Anterior capsulolabral reconstruction of the shoulder in athletes in overhand sports. *Am J Sports Med* 1991;19:428–434.
35. Johnson LL, Schneider DA, Austin MD, et al. Two-percent glutaraldehyde: a disinfectant in arthroscopy and arthroscopic surgery. *J Bone Joint Surg [Am]* 1982;64:237–239.
36. Johnson LL. *Arthroscopic surgery: principles and practice*. 3rd ed. St Louis: CV Mosby, 1986.
37. Jurvelin JS, Jurvelin JA, Kiviranta I, Klauser RJ. Effects of different irrigation liquids and times on articular cartilage: an experimental, biomechanical study. *Arthroscopy* 1994;10:667–672.
38. Klein AH, France JC, Mutschler TA, et al. Measurement of brachial plexus strain in arthroscopy of the shoulder. *Arthroscopy* 1987;3: 45–52.
39. Laurencin CT, Deutsch A, O'Brien SJ, Altchek DW. The superolateral portal for arthroscopy of the shoulder. *Arthroscopy* 1994;10:255–258.
40. Matthews LS, Zarins B, Michael RH, et al. Anterior portal selection for shoulder arthroscopy. *Arthroscopy* 1985;1:33–39.
41. Neviaser JS. Adhesive capsulitis of the shoulder. A study of the pathological findings in periarthritis of the shoulder. *J Bone Joint Surg* 1945; 27:211–222.
42. Neviaser RJ, Neviaser TJ. The frozen shoulder. Diagnosis and management. *Clin Orthop* 1987;223:59–64.
43. Nobuhara K, Ikeda H. Rotator interval lesion. *Clin Orthop* 1987;223: 44–50.
44. Pagnani MJ, Speer KP, Altchek DW, Warren RF, Dines DM. Arthroscopic fixation of superior labral lesions using a biodegradable implant: a preliminary report. *Arthroscopy* 1995;11:194–198.
45. Paulos LE, Franklin JL, Harner CD. Arthroscopic subacromial decompression impingement syndrome of the shoulder: a five-year experience. In: Paulos LE, Tibone JE, eds. *Operative techniques in shoulder surgery*. Gaithersburg, MD: Aspen Publication, 1991:31–38.
46. Payne LZ, Jokl P. The results of arthroscopic debridement of glenoid labral tears based on tear location. *Arthroscopy* 1993; 9:560–565.
47. Resch H, Golser K, Sperner G. Die arthroskopische Labrumrefixation mit resorbierbaren Staples. *Arthroskopie* 1992;5:89–95.
48. Sampson TG, Nisbet JK, Glick JM. Precision acromioplasty in arthroscopic subacromial decompression of the shoulder. *Arthroscopy* 1991; 7:301–307.
49. Skyhar MJ, Altchek DW, Warren RF, Wickiewicz TL, O'Brien SJ. Shoulder arthroscopy with the patient in the beach-chair position. *Arthroscopy* 1988;4:256–259.
50. Small NC. Complications in arthroscopy: the knee and other joints. *Arthroscopy* 1986;2:253–258.
51. Smiley P, Wasilewski SA. Arthroscopic synovectomy. *Arthroscopy* 1990;6:18–23.
52. Snyder SJ, Karzel RP, Del Pizzo W, Ferkel RD, Friedman MJ. SLAP lesions of the shoulder. *Arthroscopy* 1990;6:274–279.
53. Snyder SJ. Arthroscopic acromioclavicular joint debridement and distal clavicle resection. In: Paulos LE, Tibone JE, eds. *Operative techniques in shoulder surgery*. Gaithersburg, MD: Aspen Publication, 1991:39–44.
54. Snyder SJ, Banas MP, Karzel RP. The arthroscopic Mumford procedure: an analysis of results. *Arthroscopy* 1995;11:157–164.
55. Souryal TO, Baker CL. Anatomy of the supraclavicular fossa portal in shoulder arthroscopy. *Arthroscopy* 1990;6:297–300.
56. Speer KP, Warren RF, Pagnani M, Warner JJP. An arthroscopic technique for anterior stabilization of the shoulder with a bioabsorbable tack. *J Bone Joint Surg [Am]* 1996;78:1801–1807.
57. Stanish WD, Peterson DC. Shoulder arthroscopy and nerve injury: pitfalls and prevention. *Arthroscopy* 1995;11:458–466.
58. Tomlinson RJ, Glousman RE. Arthroscopic debridement of glenoid labral tears in athletes. *Arthroscopy* 1995;11:42–51.
59. Turkel SJ, Panio MW, Marshall JL, et al. Stabilizing mechanisms preventing anterior dislocation of the glenohumeral joint. *J Bone Joint Surg [Am]* 1981;63:1208–1217.
60. Uitvlugt G, Detrisac DA, Johnson LL, Austin MD, Johnson C. Arthroscopic observations before and after manipulation of frozen shoulder. *Arthroscopy* 1993;9:181–185.
61. Walch G, Boileau P, Noel E, Donell ST. Impingement of the deep surface of the supraspinatus tendon on the posterosuperior glenoid rim: An arthroscopic study. *J Shoulder Elbow Surg* 1992;1:238–245.
62. Warner JJP, Allen A, Marks PH, Wong P. Arthroscopic release for chronic, refractory adhesive capsulitis of the shoulder. *J Bone Joint Surg [Am]* 1996;78:1808–1816.
63. Williams MM, Snyder SJ, Buford D. The Buford complex—the "cord-like" middle glenohumeral ligament and absent anterosuperior labrum complex: a normal anatomic capsulolabral variant. *Arthroscopy* 1994; 10:241–247.
64. Wolf EM, Cheng JC, Dickson K. Humeral avulsion of glenohumeral ligaments as a cause of anterior shoulder instability. *Arthroscopy* 1995; 11:600–607.
65. Zuckerman JD, Matsen FA. Complications about the glenohumeral joint related to the use of screws and staples. *J Bone Joint Surg [Am]* 1984;66:175–180.

Disorders of the Shoulder: Diagnosis and Management,
edited by Joseph P. Iannotti and Gerald R. Williams, Jr.

CHAPTER 32

Magnetic Resonance Imaging: General Principles and Techniques

J. Bruce Kneeland

Magnetic resonance imaging (MRI) has revolutionized the evaluation of disease of the musculoskeletal system in general, and the shoulder in particular. Although a profound understanding of all of the theory and physical implementation of MRI is not necessary to effectively utilize this technique as an orthopedic surgeon, an understanding of some of the basic principles, as well as an appreciation of some of the more pertinent technical considerations, can be of value.

BASIC PRINCIPLES AND TERMINOLOGY[1]

MRI is a method of forming cross-sectional images of the body that uses the magnetic properties of the hydrogen nucleus (a proton) found in water molecules that are *free* (i.e., not bound to macromolecules) and in the lightweight side chains of fatty acids.

When a subject is placed within a strong static magnetic field, the protons in the tissues will tend to align in either the direction parallel or antiparallel to the static field, with slightly more protons in the parallel direction. This gives rise to a net macroscopic magnetization. This macroscopic magnetization can be detected by irradiating the subject with a rapidly oscillating magnetic field that causes the magnetization to change its orientation (to "tip") so that all or part of it lies in a plane perpendicular to the static field. The rapidly oscillating field can change the orientation efficiently only when it is oscillating at the *resonant* frequency for the nucleus; a quantity that is determined by the strength of the static field and a constant that is unique for each nuclear species, called the *gyromagnetic ratio*. Once the magnetization has either partially or completely tipped, it will rotate around an axis that lies parallel to the static field, a type of motion called *precession*. As the magnetization precesses it emits an oscillating magnetic field, at the same resonant frequency, that can be detected by an antenna (called a *radiofrequency coil*) as a changing voltage.

Once the tipped magnetization begins precessing, two processes occur:

1. The individual protons that compose the macroscopic magnetization precess at slightly different rates, and the magnetization spreads out in the plane, decreasing its magnitude. This process is called *T2 relaxation*.
2. The macroscopic magnetization reorients itself to return to a direction parallel to the static field. This process is called *T1 relaxation*.

Typical T2 values in tissue range from as short as 10 msec to as long as 1 sec or more. Typical T1 values are much longer than T2 and range from 100 msec to 2 to 3 sec. The

J. B. Kneeland: Department of Radiology, Hospital of the University of Pennsylvania, Philadelphia, Pennsylvania 19104.

closer the tissue is to a pure liquid (e.g., urine, cerebrospinal fluid; CSF), the longer its relaxation times. Abnormal (pathologic) tissue generally has longer relaxation times than normal tissue; hence, it has the potential to be distinguished from normal tissue because of resultant differences in signal intensity.

The factors intrinsic to the tissue that predominantly control contrast in the MR image are the number of free protons in a given volume (the *proton density*) and the T1 and T2 relaxation times. The precise technique and timing used to tip the magnetization and receive the signal from the precessing protons (the *pulse sequence*) can be varied such that any one of these three parameters may become the dominant influence on the contrast of the image. In each case, the images are described as weighted by that parameter (e.g., a *T1 weighted* image), although the influence of the other two parameters can never be totally eliminated.

Normal tissues have characteristic signal intensity on differentially weighted MR images (Figs. 1 and 2). In general, on T1 weighted images (T1WI), fat is brighter than fluid, whereas on T2 weighted images (T2WI) fluid is brighter than fat. On the proton density weighted images (PDWI), fat and fluid are generally isointense. The calcified portions of the bones—namely, the cortex and trabeculae—have effectively no mobile protons and emit no signal on any sequence. They are seen as black structures on the MR image that can be identified by the surrounding higher-signal structures. Tendons and ligaments usually demonstrate uniformly low signal for the same reason, although foci of increased signal can be seen within these tissues, sometimes in characteristic locations in asymptomatic subjects. Muscle has a medium signal on the T1 and PDWI and low signal on T2WI. Both subcutaneous and marrow fat have high signal on T1 and PDWI and a moderately high signal on the T2WI. Because of this moderately high signal on T2WI, several techniques have been devised to reduce the signal from the fat on these images to increase the conspicuity of abnormal tissue (e.g., edema) located within or adjacent to the fat (see Fig. 2; with certain classes of pulse sequences, marrow fat will appear much darker than subcutaneous fat). Normal cartilage has a medium signal on T1 and PDWI, and a medium to low signal on T2WI. At higher resolution, cartilage demonstrates a laminated structure on the MR images.

The relative signal intensity of abnormal tissue depends on that of the original tissue. Abnormalities within fat generally appear lower in signal than fat on T1WI and will have a variable intensity relative to fat on T2WI. If the signal from the fat is suppressed, as mentioned in the foregoing, the abnormality will appear brighter than fat on long TE sequences. Abnormalities within tendons and ligaments generally appear slightly brighter than normal low-signal fibrous tissue on T1WI and demonstrate a variable relative signal intensity on T2WI. Abnormalities involving the cartilage are usually seen as low-signal defects within the cartilage on T1WI or high-signal defects on T2WI.

TECHNICAL CONSIDERATIONS FOR THE ORTHOPEDIC SURGEON

The selection of the technical factors used for MR imaging remains a matter of considerable controversy, even among experts in the field. These choices involve both the

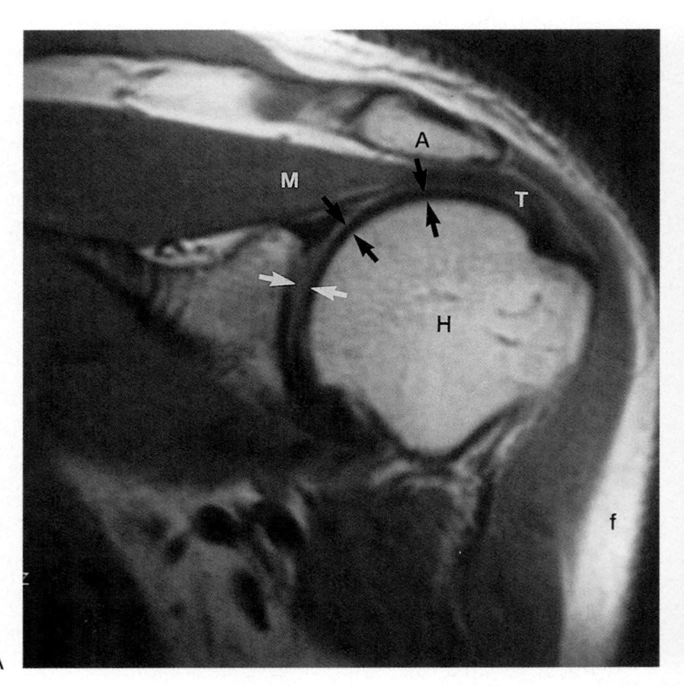

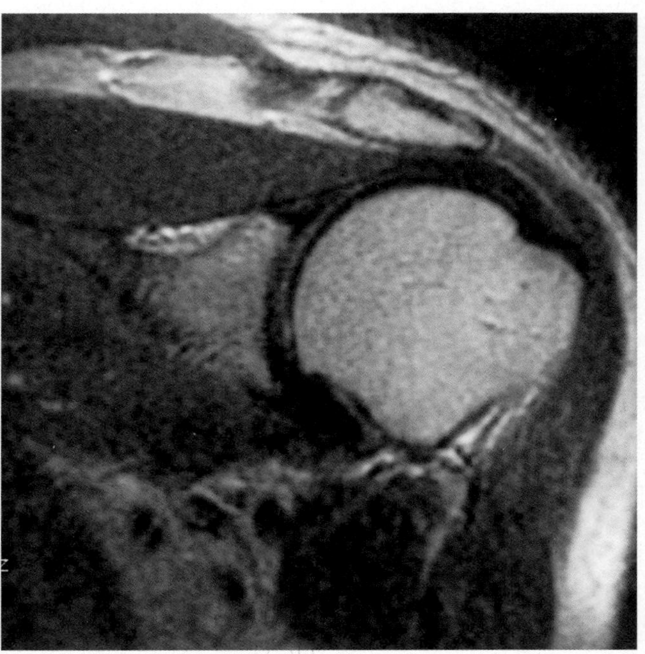

FIG. 1. **(A)** Proton density and **(B)** T2 weighted oblique coronal images of the shoulder. *M*,supraspinatus muscle; *T*, supraspinatus tendon; *H*, humeral head; *A*, acromion; *f*, subcutaneous fat. *Black arrows* outline cortical bone, *white arrows* outline articular cartilage.

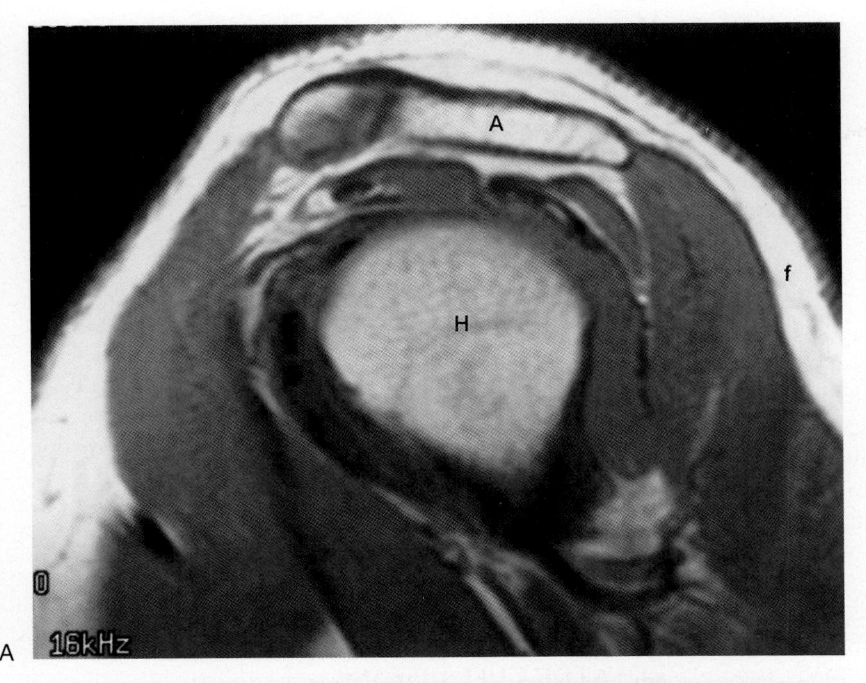

A

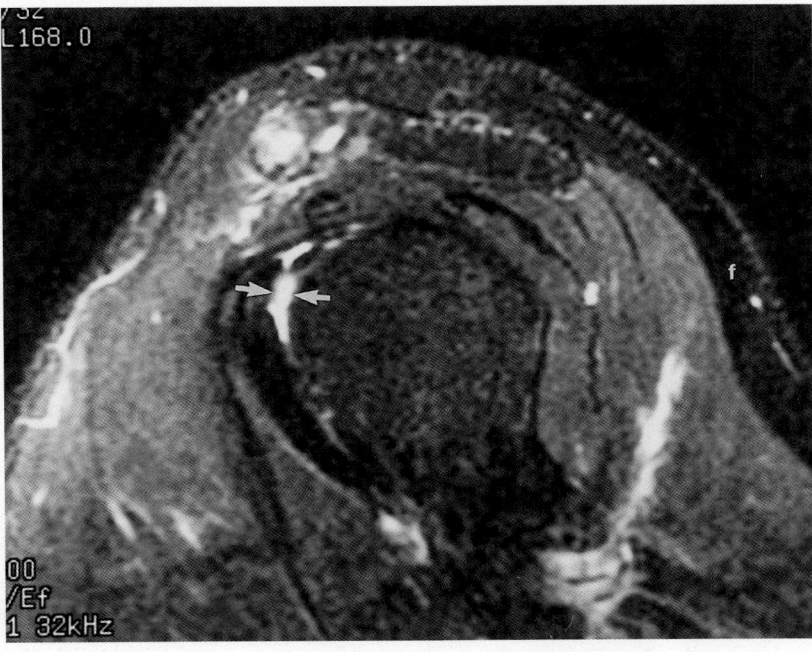

B

FIG. 2. **(A)** T1 weighted and **(B)** fat suppressed T2 weighted oblique sagittal images of the shoulder. *A*, acromion; *H*, humeral head; *f*, subcutaneous fat. Fluid in the region of the rotator interval is outlined by *white arrows.* Note the reduction in signal in the fat in 2B compared with that in 1B.

hardware, such as the magnet and radiofrequency coils, and the techniques by which the protons are excited (the pulse sequences). It is clearly not possible for the referring physician to be aware of all of these relevant factors. Moreover, there is no established best technique for the imaging of the shoulder. It is important, however, that the orthopedic surgeon study the images from different MRI facilities, decide what he finds important for patient management, and communicate this information to the radiologists at the MRI facilities. Certain factors, such as pulse sequence and associated software parameters, are often printed on the images and frequently can readily be adjusted by the radiologists. Other factors, in particular the hardware, cannot be so easily changed, although upgrades for hardware components, such as radiofrequency coils, periodically become available from the original equipment manufacturer or from smaller outside companies.

One particular technical factor of which referring physicians should become aware is the increasing use of "open" MR systems. The most commonly used types of magnets are cylindrically shaped and completely surround the patient. Open systems have magnets, the components of which are located only on top and beneath the patient, permitting much more space. The strength of the magnetic field, however, is much less (e.g., 0.3 tesla) than that of the more traditional cylindrically shaped whole-body systems (1.5 tesla). Open systems were originally designed to image claustrophobic and obese patients who cannot be readily examined within the tightly confined cylindrical magnets, as well as to permit the performance of interventional procedures under MR guidance. These systems, however, are also considerably less expensive to purchase and operate than the higher-field cylindrical systems and, in an era of increasing cost consciousness, are often being employed as a means of reducing the costs of MRI for routine cases. The lower-field strength of the open magnet systems does reduce the image quality to some extent, although just how much is arguable (Fig. 3). The orthopedist should pay particular attention to the quality of examinations from these systems to ensure that his or her patients are still receiving high-quality diagnostic examinations.

To perform an MRI examination of the shoulder, the patient is generally placed in the supine position and the shoulder is held in the neutral position. Imaging is usually performed in oblique coronal and oblique sagittal planes, obtained perpendicular and parallel to the surface of the glenoid fossa, and in the axial plane. One or two differentially weighted sequences (e.g., T1WI or PDWI and T2WI) are obtained in each of the three planes. For the MRI evaluation of posterosuperior impingement, one group of investigators has advocated placing the shoulder in abduction and external rotation (ABER position) and performing MR arthrography (see following section).[2] This view primarily improves the visualization of tears and the undersurface of the distal supraspinatus and infraspinatus tendons.

Magnetic Resonance Arthrography

Magnetic resonance arthrography refers to the performance of an MR examination after the intraarticular injection of either a dilute mixture of gadolinium chelate contrast agent in saline solution or just the saline solution.[3,4] Pulse sequences are chosen such that the solution appears brighter than the tissues. The contrast material serves both to outline the tissues and to distend the joint capsule.

The injection is usually performed under fluoroscopic guidance, with the injection of a small amount of iodinated contrast to confirm intraarticular location of the needle. The technique is straightforward to perform, although it is clearly more invasive, time-consuming, and expensive than routine noncontrast studies. In addition, it requires the coordination of efforts in both a fluoroscopic suite and an MR facility, which may be located at some distance from each other. For all of these reasons, MR arthrography is not a procedure that is performed routinely at all MRI centers.

MAGNETIC RESONANCE IMAGING OF ROTATOR CUFF DISEASE

Rotator Cuff Impingement

Magnetic resonance imaging is often used for the evaluation of the structural abnormalities that are associated with rotator cuff disease. In none of the entities, however, has it been possible to establish anatomic criteria to assess the degree of impingement or the likelihood that the anatomic impingement seen is resulting in symptoms.

Bony spurs are generally seen on MR images as marrow-filled protrusions of bone. The presence of osteoarthritis of the acromioclavicular (AC) joint with underlying spurs can

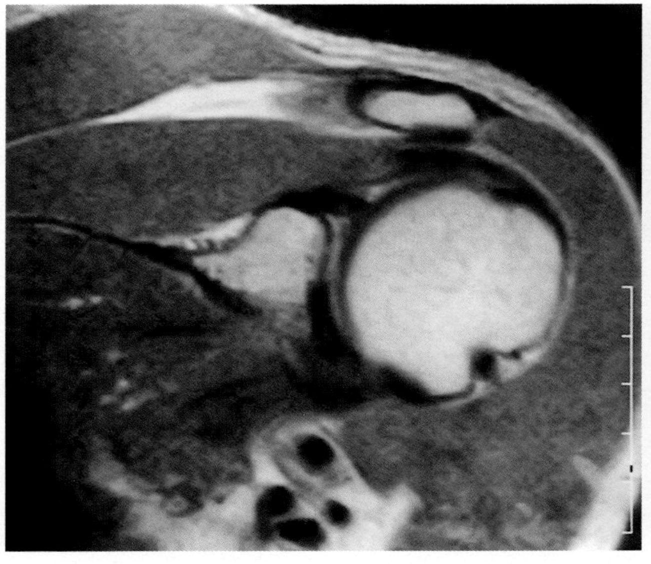

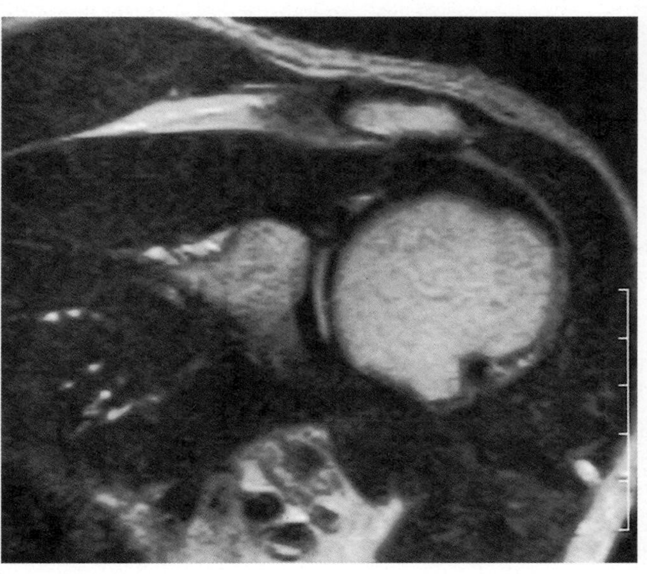

FIG. 3. PD and T2WI oblique images of the shoulder obtained on a low-field (0.3-tesla) open MR system. All of the other images in this chapter were obtained on a 1.5-tesla system. This image is probably better than most obtained on comparable systems. There is some loss of detail in this image when compared with Fig. 1.

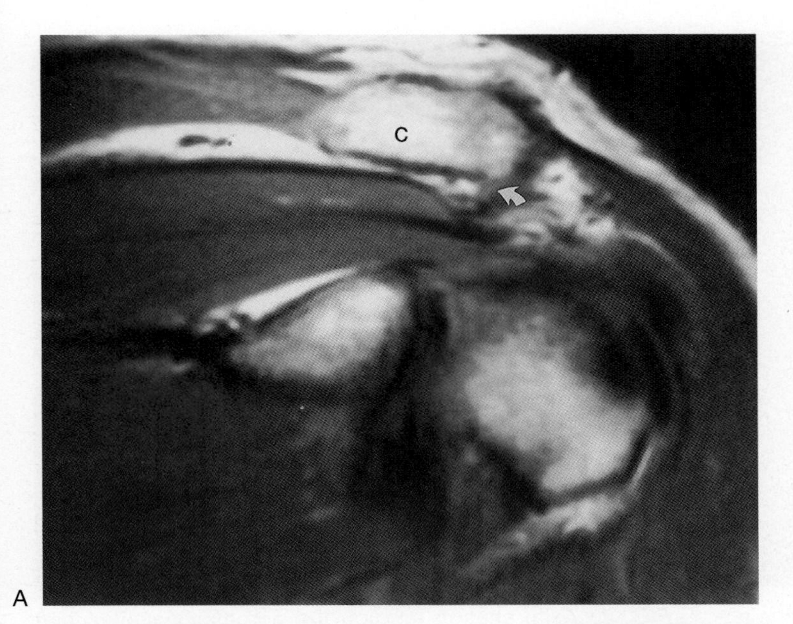

A

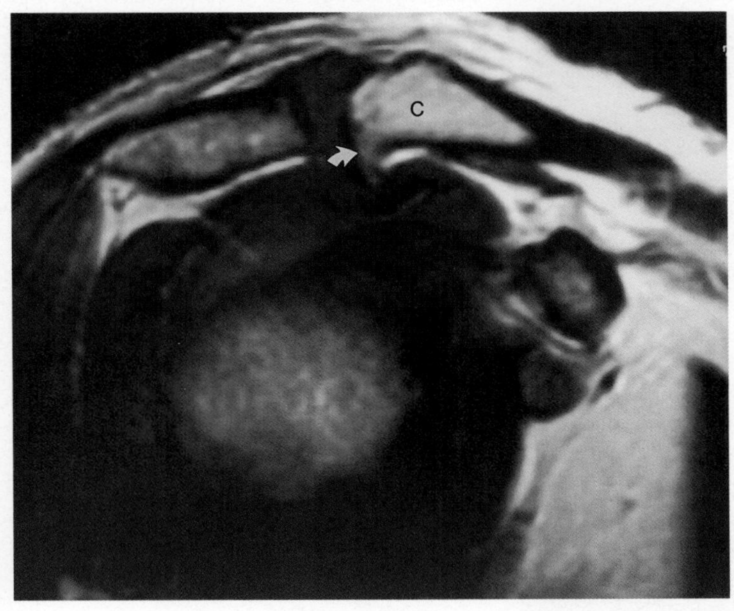

B

FIG. 4. **(A)** Oblique coronal and **(B)** oblique sagittal images of the acromioclavicular joint demonstrate a large spur (*white arrows*) on the undersurface of the distal clavicle (*C*, clavicle).

be readily detected with MR (Fig. 4). Spurs are also seen both at the insertion of the coracoacromial ligament (Fig. 5) and on the undersurface of the lateral margin of the acromion. One particular pitfall in the MRI interpretation of spurs is the presence of a low-signal wedge-shaped structure on the undersurface of the lateral margin of the acromion that, although originally believed to represent a spur, at anatomic dissections was proved to represent insertional fibers of the deltoid muscle.[5]

Acromial morphology that may be associated with rotator cuff impingement can also be readily demonstrated with MRI. This can be seen in the form of an anteriorly hooked acromion (Bigliani type III; Fig. 6), as well as a laterally or anteriorly downward-sloping acromion. A few cautionary notes in the MRI diagnoses of these acromial abnormalities are in order. First, several investigators have noted considerable interobserver disagreement in their diagnosis with MRI.[6] Second, MRI is a cross-sectional technique, whereas the Bigliani criteria were established on anatomic specimens and projection radiographs. As a result, different acromial configurations may be seen on different but contiguous MR images.

The presence of an os acromiale can also be identified with MRI as a linear focus of low signal on TIWI and variable signal on T2WI that spans the width of the acromion[7] (Fig. 7), although it can be difficult to distinguish between an os and the presence of a normally unfused apophysis up to the age of 25.

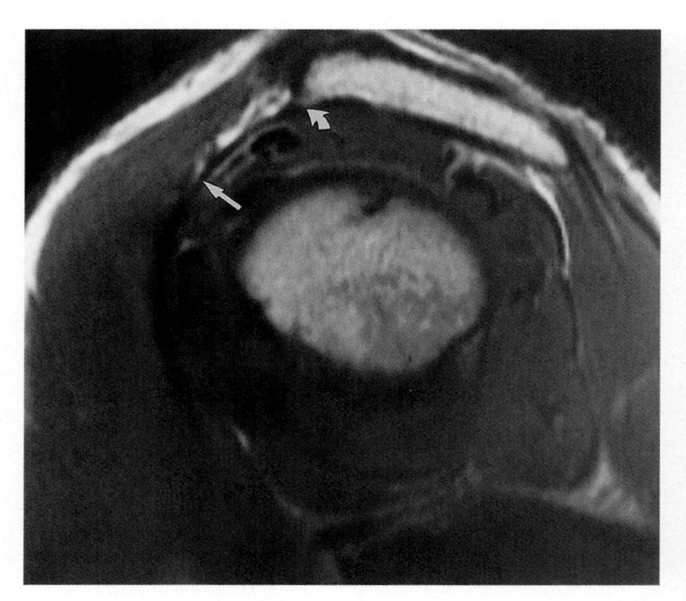

FIG. 5. Oblique sagittal image of the acromion illustrates a spur (*short, curved arrow*) at the insertion site of the coracoacromial ligament (*straight arrow*).

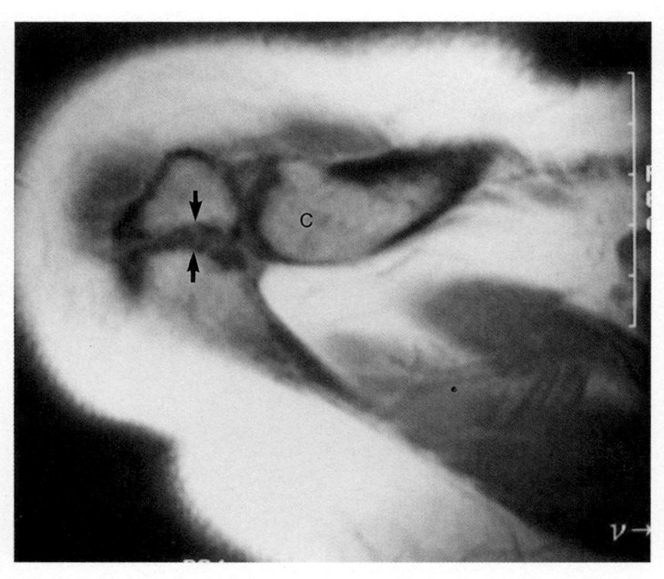

FIG. 7. Axial section through the acromioclavicular joint shows an os acromiale. The low-signal linear focus in the acromion (*arrows*) represents the site of absence of bony fusion: *C*, clavicle.

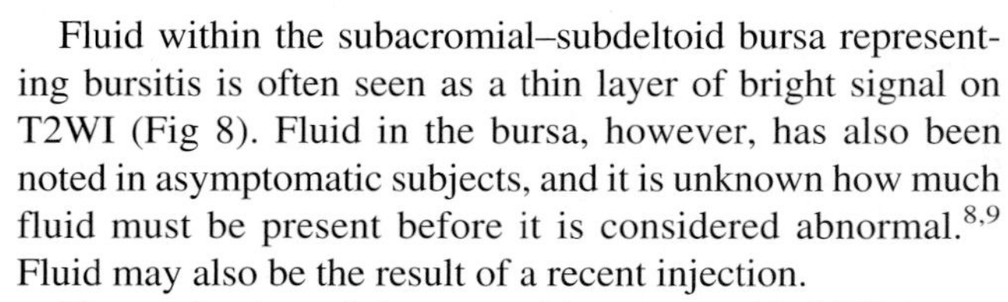

Fluid within the subacromial–subdeltoid bursa representing bursitis is often seen as a thin layer of bright signal on T2WI (Fig 8). Fluid in the bursa, however, has also been noted in asymptomatic subjects, and it is unknown how much fluid must be present before it is considered abnormal.[8,9] Fluid may also be the result of a recent injection.

The evaluation of the coracoid process with MRI in patients with suspected subcoracoid impingement has received essentially no attention in the radiology literature. No MR criteria have been developed to establish the presence of this disorder, although anecdotally, and by analogy with results from the older CT literature, there is increased lateral extension of the coracoid and a small coracohumeral distance (Fig. 9).

Rotator Cuff Tears and Tendinosis

Although the appearance of the cuff tendons was originally described as that of uniform low signal, small foci of slightly increased signal are not infrequently noted, particularly on T1 and PDWI, in asymptomatic subjects (Fig. 10). These foci have been attributed to anatomic factors, such as the interdigitation of muscle and tendon fibers,[10] the presence of subclinical degeneration, and a physicochemical phenomenon called the "magic angle effect."[11]

The earliest stages of tendon disease are marked by foci of mildly increased signal intensity that are most evident on T1 and PDWI and only faintly visible on T2WI[12] (Fig. 11). At

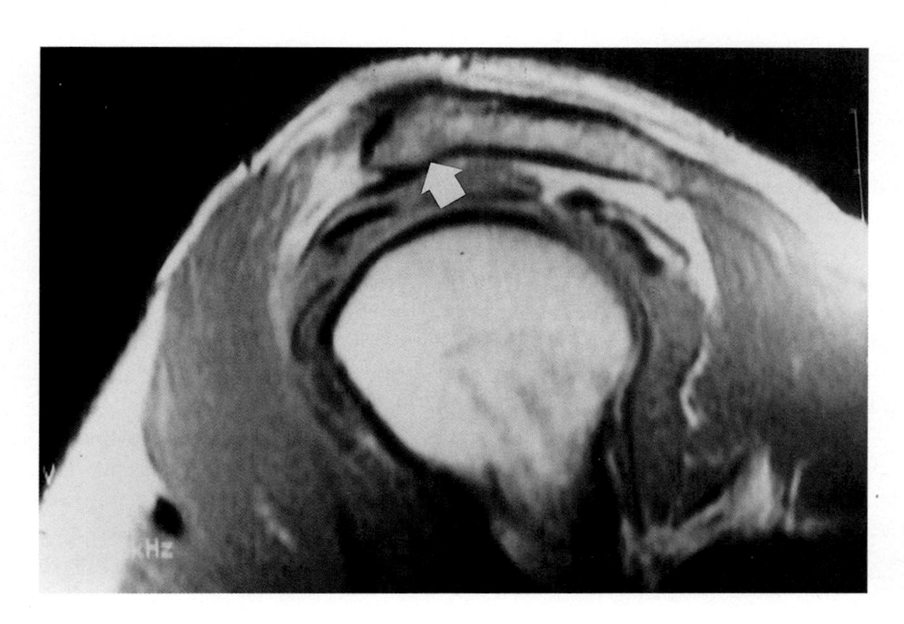

FIG. 6. Oblique sagittal image of the acromion illustrates an anterior hook (*white arrow*).

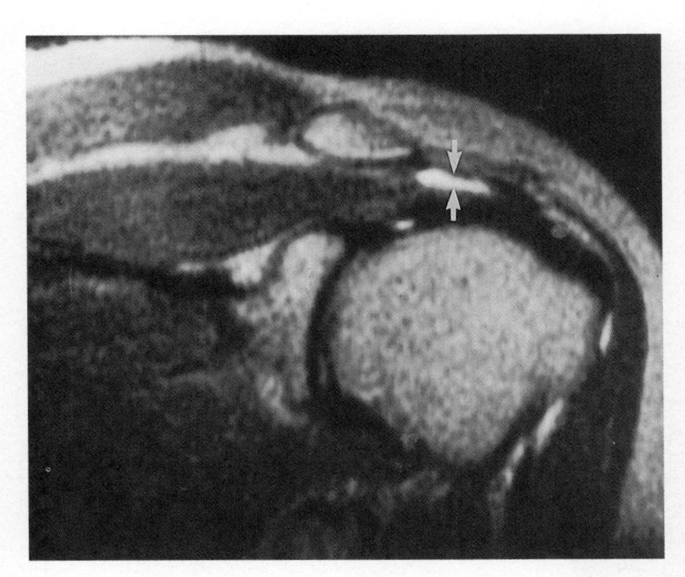

FIG. 8. T2W oblique coronal image of the shoulder demonstrates a small focus of bright signal (*arrows*) representing fluid in the subacromial bursa.

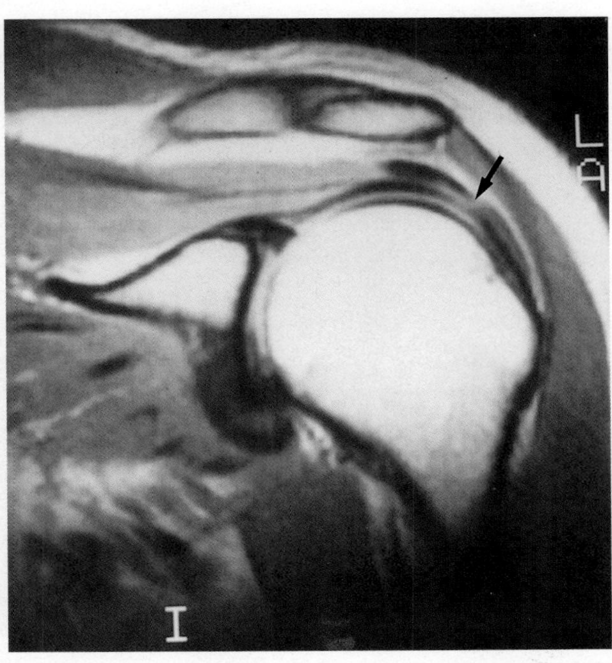

FIG. 10. PDWI demonstrates a small focus of increased signal (*arrow*) in an asymptomatic young man.

histological examination, these most typically represent degenerative rather than inflammatory changes.[13] As the tendon disease progresses, the foci of increased signal become larger, more distinct, and better seen on T2WI. In these cases, there is more likely to be inflammation, edema, and hemorrhage, although the distinction between degeneration and inflammation cannot be made with certainty.[14] The tendons may also become diffusely thickened or attenuated.

Partial thickness tears of the rotator cuff can be seen as focal areas of increased signal on all sequences that do not extend through the thickness of the cuff tendon (Fig. 12). Although they usually appear relatively brighter on the T2WI than on the T1 or PDWI, this is not always true. Partial-thickness tears can usually be classified into bursal- or articular-sided on the basis of the MR images, and the fractional thickness of the cuff involved by the tear can be estimated. It can be difficult to distinguish between focal degeneration and a partial-thickness tear in patients in whom the signal is not very bright on the T2WI. It can also be difficult to distinguish between a high-grade partial and a small full-thickness

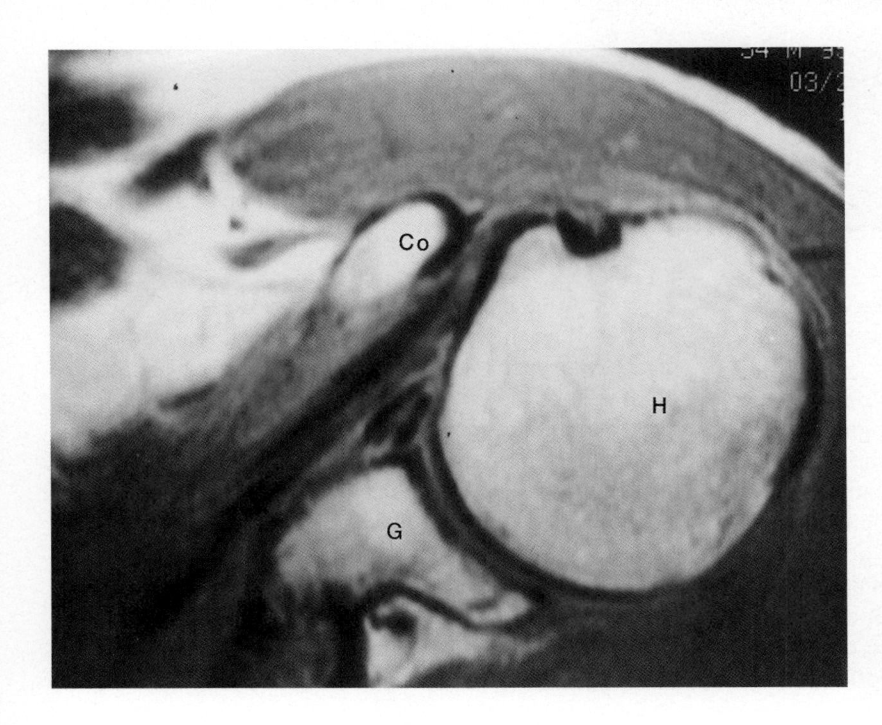

FIG. 9. Axial image through the glenohumeral joint illustrates a laterally located coracoid process (*Co*) with a small coracohumeral distance in a patient with suspected subcoracoid impingement syndrome.

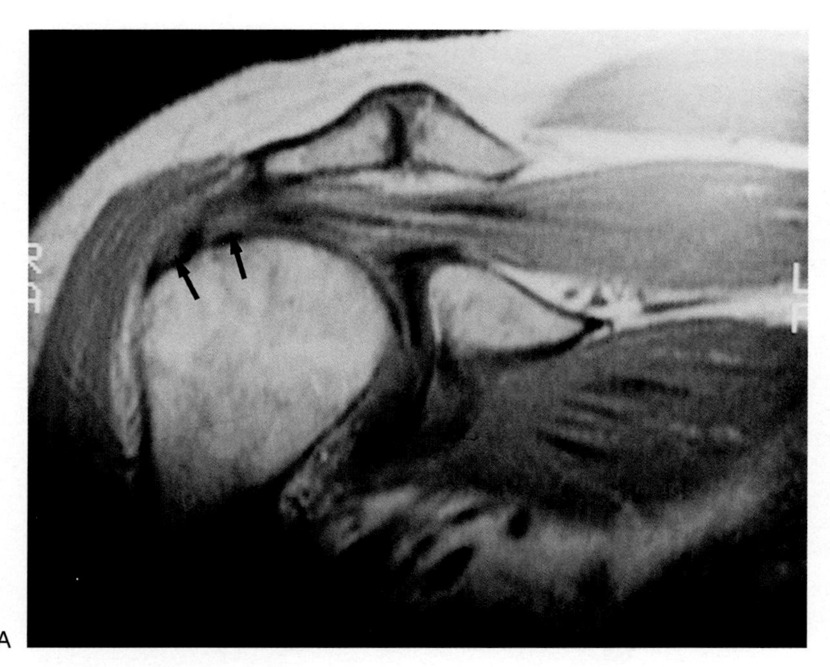

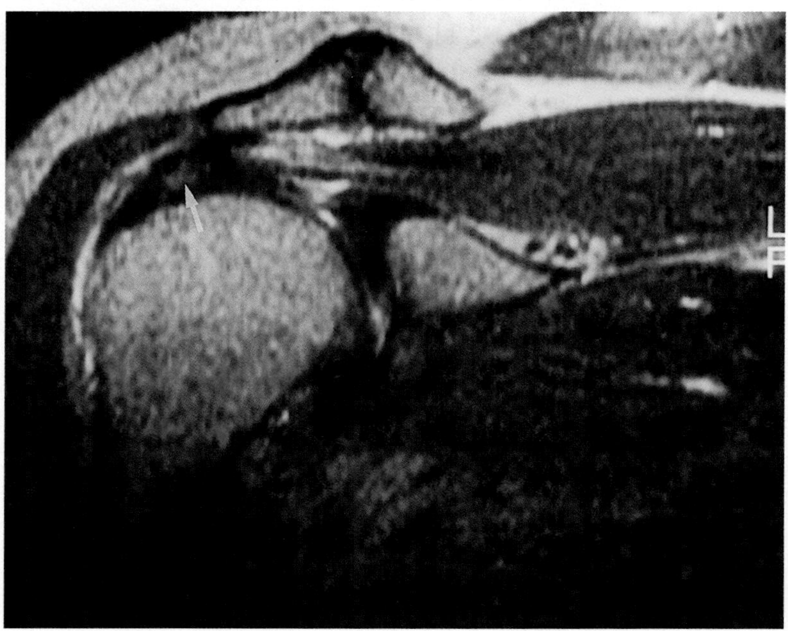

FIG. 11. (A) PDWI illustrates a diffuse focus of minimally increased signal in the supraspinatus tendon (*arrows*) that **(B)** appears smaller and less intense on the T2WI.

tear when the signal is bright on T2WI. The reported accuracy of MRI for the detection of partial-thickness tears has varied widely in the literature.[15]

Complete tears are seen as areas of increased signal intensity on T1 and PDWI that become relatively brighter on the T2WI[16,17] (Fig. 13). These foci extend through the full thickness of the cuff and represent fluid or granulation tissue. MRI has been established by numerous investigators as an accurate technique to confirm the presence of a full-thickness tear.[18] It can also provide other information that may be useful for surgical planning. The size of the cuff tear can be accurately measured with MRI, and the degree of cuff retraction can be ascertained. The quality of the cuff tendon at the margin of the tear can be assessed to some extent by studying it for fraying and increased intrasubstance signal indicating degeneration. The presence of atrophy and fatty replacement of the individual muscles of the rotator cuff can also be qualitatively assessed (Fig 14). Finally, loss of articular cartilage and underlying bony changes can occasionally be noted, although the accuracy of MRI for their diagnosis is unknown.

Post Rotator Cuff Surgery

Magnetic resonance imaging of the shoulder following rotator cuff surgery has been the subject of a small number of

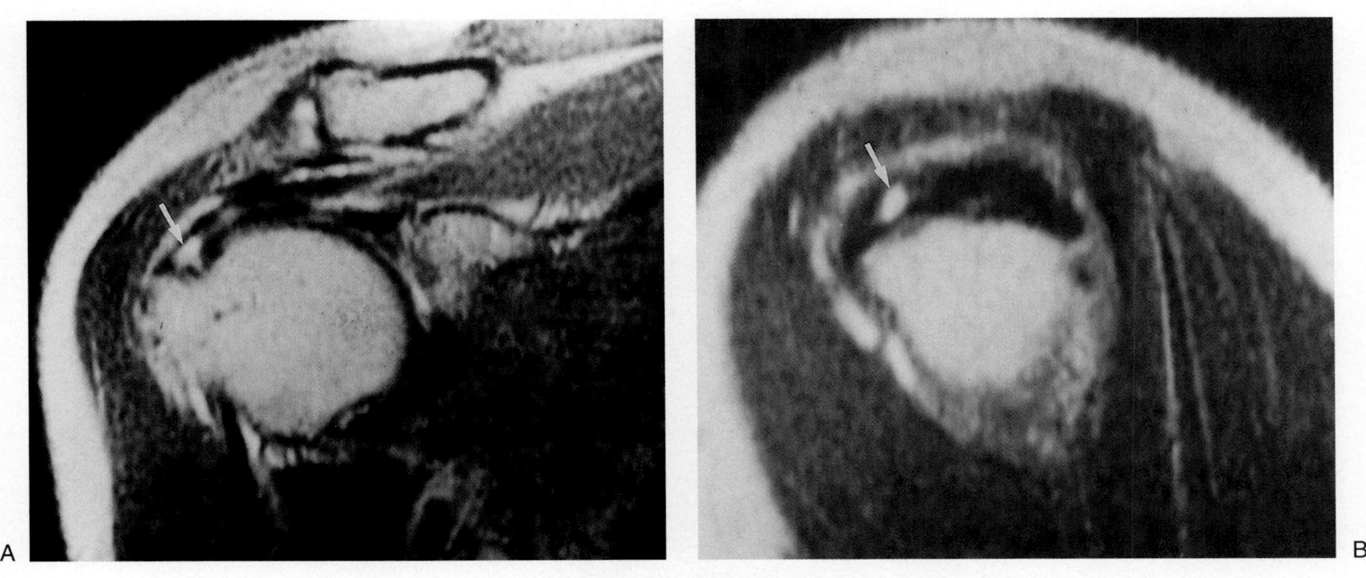

FIG. 12. (A) T2W oblique coronal and **(B)** oblique sagittal images show a small focus of bright signal within the supraspinatus tendon (*arrow*) that involves the articular surface of the tendon and extends through, most but not all, of its thickness.

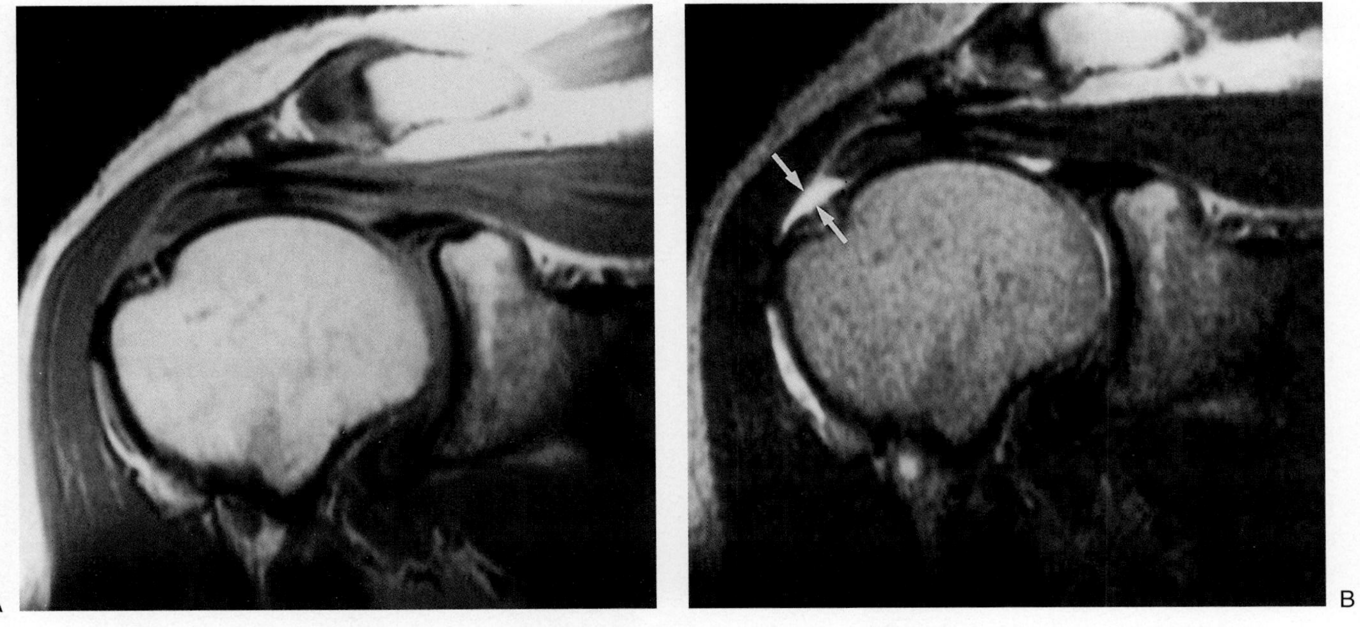

FIG. 13. (A) PD and **(B)** T2 WI demonstrate a small focus of bright signal (*arrows*) that occupies the entire thickness of the supraspinatus tendon and appears brighter on the T2WI than on the PDWI. This represents a full-thickness tear of the tendon at its insertion site on the humerus.

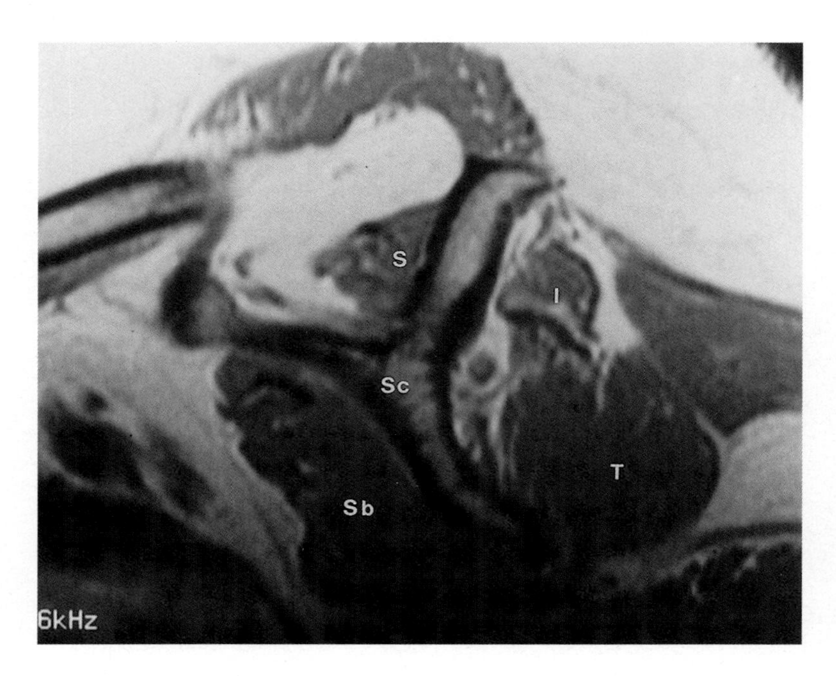

FIG. 14. Oblique sagittal image through the scapula (*Sc*) and the four muscles of the rotator cuff. Note that the supraspinatus (*S*) and infraspinatus (*I*) muscles are much smaller in their cross section than the subscapularis (*Sb*) and teres minor (*T*) muscles.

articles.[19,20] The investigators noted that ferromagnetic artifacts associated with prior surgery are generally seen, but do not as a rule limit the accuracy of the study. MRI in these small series was accurate for the detection of recurrent, full-thickness rotator cuff tears that are diagnosed using the usual MRI criteria. The diagnosis of partial-thickness tears in these patients proved somewhat more problematic. Deltoid muscle retraction and biceps tendon rupture or dislocation in conjunction with subscapularis tendon tears were also diagnosed accurately.

MAGNETIC RESONANCE IMAGING OF LABRAL DISEASE AND GLENOHUMERAL INSTABILITY

In contrast to the situation with the rotator cuff, the use of MRI for the assessment of capsulolabral complex remains controversial. Part of the controversy results from the wide variations in reported accuracy that can be found in the literature.[21,22] But there is also considerable controversy among orthopedic surgeons concerning the need for any imaging study, at least for the assessment of glenohumeral instability.

The problems associated with MRI assessment of the capsulolabral complex arise from the difficulty in visualizing the glenohumeral (GH) ligaments and the anatomic variations that can be seen in normal subjects. The labrum and glenohumeral ligaments are better visualized with MR arthrography, owing to both the outlining of soft-tissue structures with a high-contrast material and the distention of the joint capsule, with resultant separation of the structures.

The glenoid labrum most commonly demonstrates a wedge-shaped configuration (Fig. 15), but numerous shapes have been described as representing normal variants, including rounded, notched, cleaved, and flat.[23] The normal labrum typically demonstrates low signal on all sequences, with a slightly higher signal transitional zone at the junction of the labrum and glenoid. Linear, globular, and triangular foci of moderately increased signal, however, have all been described within the labrum in asymptomatic subjects, and have been found to represent a variety of histologic findings.[24] The different locations of capsular insertions on the labrum corresponding to the observations of Mosely and Overgaard[25] can also seen on MR images.[26] Other variations of capsulolabral anatomy that can be demonstrated with MRI have been described, including the relatively common sub-

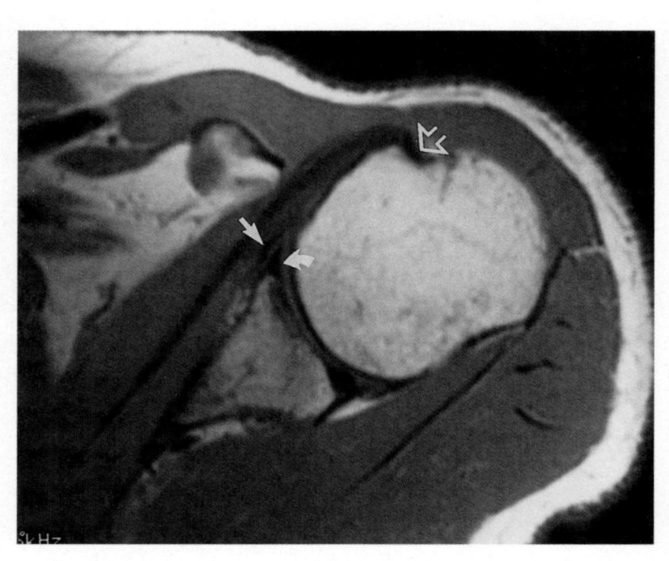

FIG. 15. Axial section through the glenohumeral joint shows the anterior labrum with a wedge-shaped cross-sectional appearance (*curved arrow*) and a linear-appearing middle glenohumeral ligament. The *dark structure* indicated by the *open arrow* is the biceps tendon.

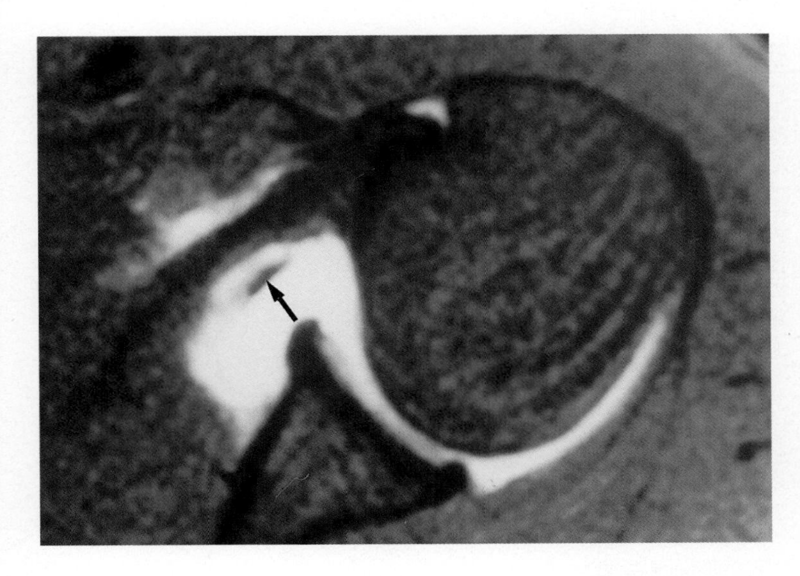

FIG. 16. Axial, fat-suppressed T1WI through the glenohumeral joint in a patient whose shoulder was just injected with a dilute solution of Gd-DTPA in saline. A short segment of the inferior glenohumeral ligament (*arrow*) is shown.

labral foramen in the anterosuperior quadrant and the much less common Buford complex that consists of a cordlike middle glenohumeral ligament (see following) and the absence of the anterosuperior segment of the labrum.[27]

The middle glenohumeral ligament is routinely seen with MRI as a low-signal linear (see Fig. 15) or, less commonly, rounded ("cordlike") structure. The superior and inferior glenohumeral ligaments are inconsistently identified as individual structures in the absence of intraarticular contrast. With intraarticular contrast, the superior and inferior glenohumeral ligaments can be consistently demonstrated as low-signal linear structures that follow a characteristic course[28] (Fig. 16).

Glenohumeral Instability

The accuracy of routine MRI for the evaluation of the anterior instability has been the subject of many investigations, with strikingly divergent results.

The most commonly observed findings on the MR images are abnormalities of the anteroinferior segment of the labrum, corresponding to a Bankart lesion. These abnormal appearances have included a high-signal linear focus in the labrum, representing a tear, with or without displacement of a labral fragment (Fig. 17); fragmentation and disruption of the labrum; and absence (Fig. 18) of the labrum.[29] The importance of identifying the GH ligaments largely lies in the importance of distinguishing between ligaments that are closely apposed to the anterior labrum and torn labral fragments. Anterior capsular abnormalities, including anterior

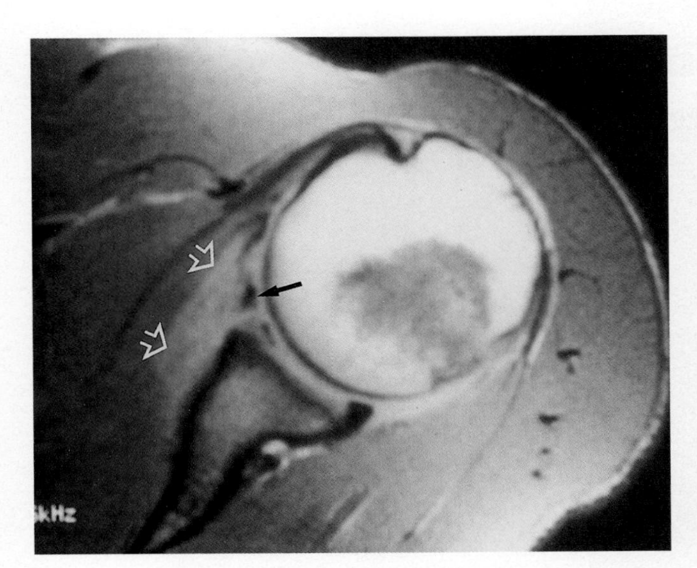

FIG. 17. Axial PDWI through the glenohumeral joint that shows an avulsed fragment of the anteroinferior labrum (*white arrow*) and anterior displacement and medial insertion of the joint capsule (*open arrows*), representing capsular stripping.

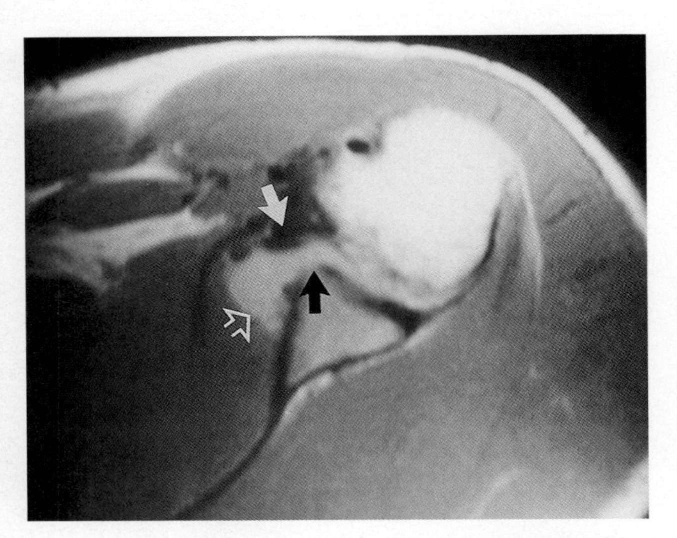

FIG. 18. Axial PDWI through the glenohumeral joint that shows the absence of the anterior labrum and the underlying bone (*black arrow*). There is also disruption (*white arrow*) and a medial insertion (*open arrow*) of the anterior capsule.

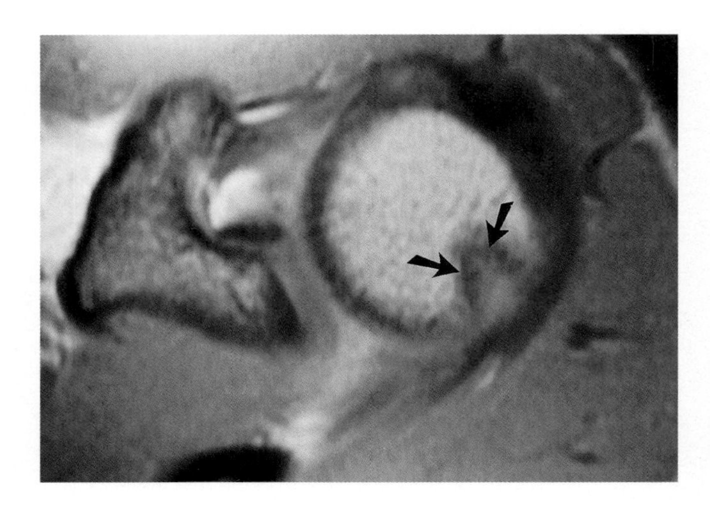

FIG. 19. Axial section through the proximal end of the humerus illustrates a Hill–Sachs defect (*arrows*) on the posterolateral margin of the humeral head.

A

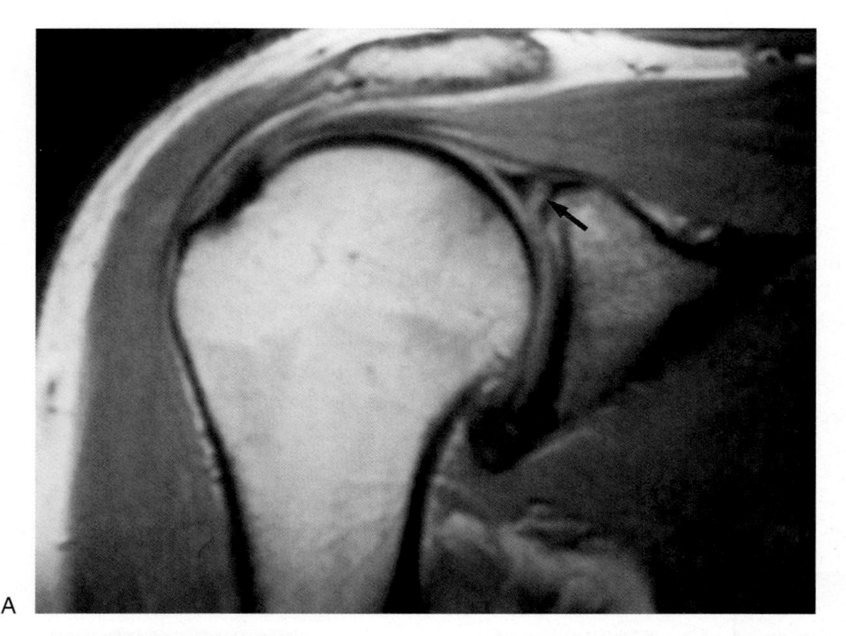

B

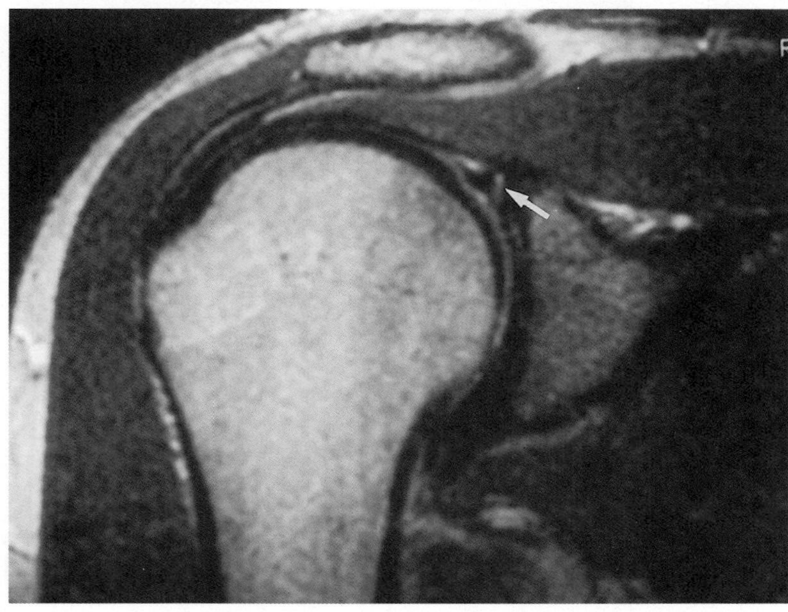

FIG. 20. (A) Oblique coronal PD and **(B)** T2WI demonstrate a high-signal–linear defect in the anterosuperior segment of the labrum (*arrow*) that represents a SLAP lesion.

displacement, disruption, and a far medial insertion, are often noted (see Figs. 17 and 18).

Magnetic resonance arthrography of the shoulder is most commonly used for the evaluation of labral tears. MR arthrography generally permits the distinction between the ligaments and labral fragments and, because of the distention of the joint, may separate torn labral fragments and make them more visible. Most investigators have concluded that the use of MR arthrography yields increased accuracy when compared to noncontrast studies.[4,30]

The MR appearance of related types of labral injuries, such as the anterior labroligamentous periosteal sleeve avulsion and glenolabral articular disruption lesions, has as yet been described only anecdotally. Similarly, the MR appearance of the rare humeral avulsion of the glenohumeral ligament type of IGL tear has only been described anecdotally.

A Hill–Sachs defect, seen as an indentation on the posterolateral margin of the humeral head, that originates within the first 7 mm of the superior margin of the humerus is commonly observed on MR images in patients with a prior anterior dislocation[31] (Fig. 19). A bright signal, presumed to represent bony edema, is often seen on T2WI in the underlying cancellous bone. It is important to distinguish between a Hill–Sachs defect and the smoother, shallower, and more distally located concavity that is often seen on the posterolateral margin of the proximal humerus of asymptomatic subjects.

The MRI appearance of posterior instability has received very little attention in the literature, reflecting its much lower incidence. In the few cases presented and that we have studied, abnormalities in the posteroinferior segment of the labrum, similar to those seen in the anteroinferior labrum, have been observed, along with the "reverse" Bankart lesion.

The MRI appearance of true multidirectional instability seen in conjunction with capsular laxity has not been described.

Superior Labral Tears

The use of MRI for the detection of tears of the superior segment of the labrum, in particular SLAP lesions, has been described in only a few articles.[32,33] Superior labral tears have most commonly been associated with the presence of a linear focus of increased signal within the labrum, similar to that seen in the anteroinferior segment of the labrum in patients with glenohumeral instability (Fig. 20). Representative examples of the MRI appearance of the different types of SLAP lesions have appeared in the literature, but the accuracy of this modality for detecting these tears or for distinguishing among the different types is unknown.

Paralabral Cysts

Paralabral cysts are readily identified by MRI as discrete, small masses with medium signal on T1WI and bright signal with T2WI. They are usually seen in conjunction with a posterior labral tear[34] (Fig. 21). Depending on their precise location, they may impinge on the nerve that innervates the infraspinatus muscle or, less commonly, on the nerve that innervates both the infraspinatus and supraspinatus muscles, leading to increased signal within the muscle(s) on T2 weighted images in the subacute stage and muscle atrophy with fatty replacement in the chronic stage.[35]

Biceps Tendon Abnormalities

The normal tendon of the long head of the biceps can be readily seen on MR images as a low-signal structure that lies within the intertubercular sulcus and extends over the superior margin of the humerus to insert at the 12:00 o'clock position on the labrum.

"Tendinitis" (actually tendinosis) of the biceps is seen as either increased intrasubstance signal, attenuation, or discontinuity of the tendon.[36] The abnormality can be located either along the intraarticular segment, usually in conjunction with rotator cuff disease, or in the intertubercular sulcus where it is generally accompanied by tendosynovitis, seen as fluid in the tendon sheath. Fluid in the tendon sheath is, however, a nonspecific finding that most commonly results from the presence of fluid in the glenohumeral joint; hence, this finding must be interpreted with caution. Proliferation of the bony structures of the sulcus can often be demonstrated.

Medial dislocation of the biceps tendon generally, but not always, occurs with readily visualized tears of the subscapularis tendon[37] (Fig. 22). Dysplastic changes of the intertubercular sulcus, such as a shallow groove, are sometimes seen and may predispose to dislocation. Spurs within the groove are also sometimes seen.

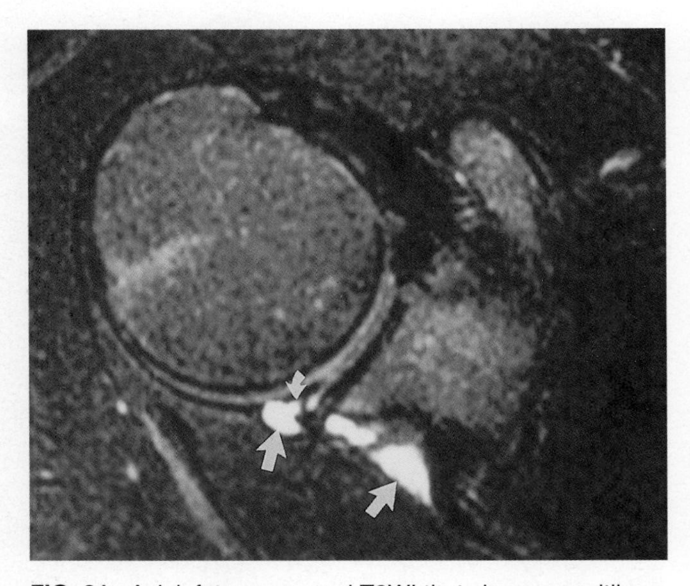

FIG. 21. Axial, fat-suppressed T2WI that shows a multiloculated, high-signal structure (*straight arrows*) that represents a paralabral cyst, originating from a tear in the posterior labrum (*curved arrow*).

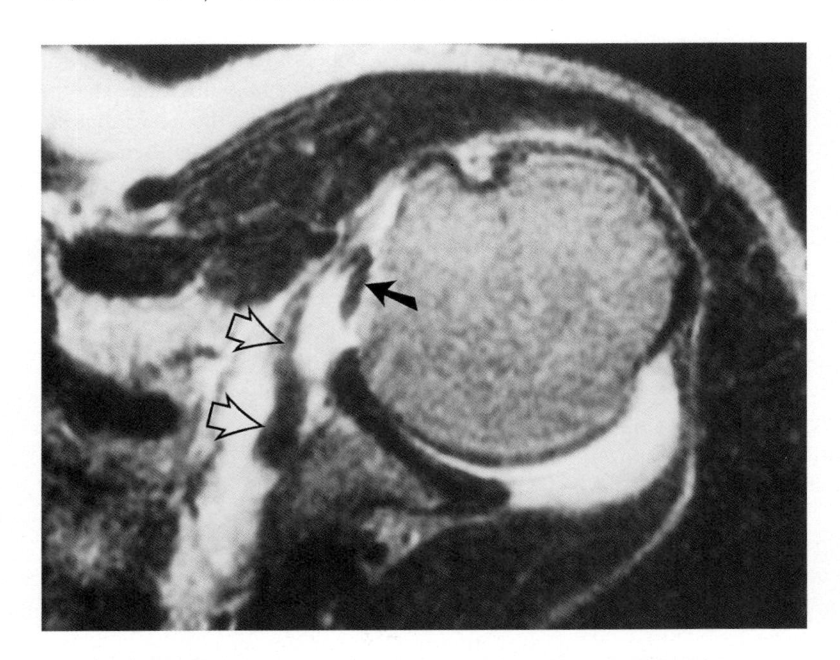

FIG. 22. Axial T2WI image illustrates a medially displaced biceps tendon (*black arrow*; compare with Fig. 15). A remnant of the torn subscapularis tendon is indicated by the *open black arrows*.

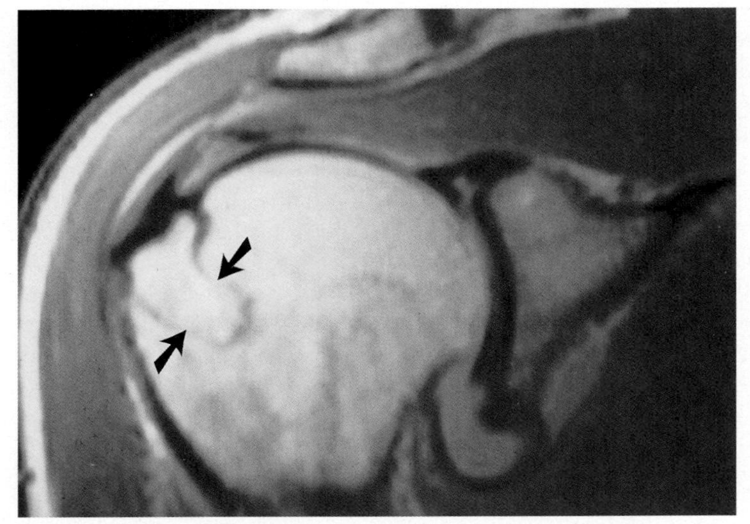

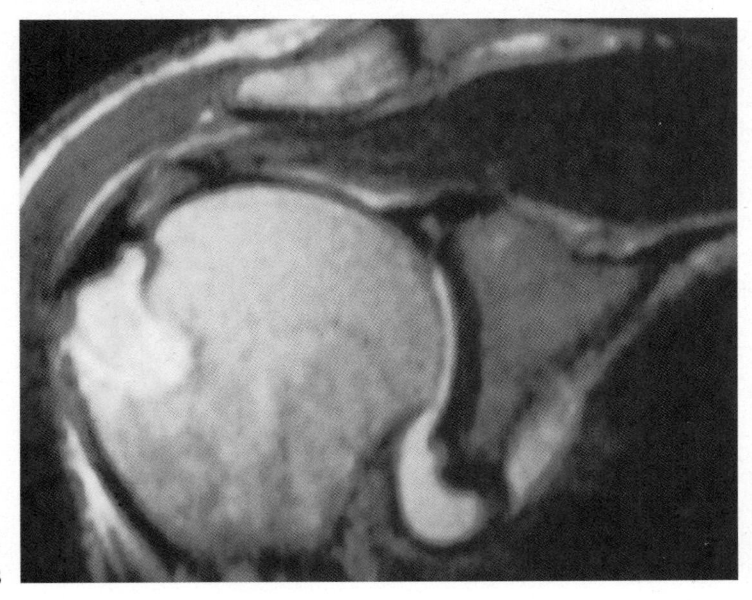

FIG. 23. (A) Oblique coronal PDWI demonstrates a low-signal curvilinear focus in the greater tuberosity of the humeral head **(B)** that turns bright on the T2WI, representing a nondisplaced fracture that was not visible on plain films.

MISCELLANEOUS ABNORMALITIES

A variety of other abnormalities about the shoulder can also be evaluated with MRI. Many of these represent disorders that occur throughout the musculoskeletal system and can involve the shoulder. These include radiographically occult fractures, such as nondisplaced fractures of the greater tuberosity (Fig. 23), primary bone and soft tissue tumors, osteonecrosis, and osteomyelitis.

REFERENCES

1. Stark DD, Bradley WG, eds. *Magnetic resonance imaging*, 2nd ed, vol 1. St Louis: Mosby Year Book, 1992:3–544.
2. Tirman PF, Bost FW, Garvin GJ, et al. Posterosuperior glenoid impingement of the shoulder: findings at MR imaging and MR arthrography with arthroscopic correlation. *Radiology* 1994; 193:431–436.
3. Palmer WE, Brown JH, Rosenthal DI. Labral–ligamentous complex of the shoulder: evaluation with MR arthrography [see comments]. *Radiology* 1994;190:645–651.
4. Palmer WE, Caslowitz PL. Anterior shoulder instability: diagnostic criteria determined from prospective analysis of 121 MR arthrograms. *Radiology* 1995;197:819–825.
5. Kaplan PA, Bryans KC, Davick JP, Otte M, Stinson WW, Dussault RG. MR imaging of the normal shoulder: variants and pitfalls. *Radiology* 1992;184:519–524.
6. Haygood TM, Langlotz CP, Kneeland JB, Iannotti JP, Williams GR Jr, Dalinka MK. Categorization of acromial shape: interobserver variability with MR imaging and conventional radiography. *AJR Am J Roentgenol* 1994;162:1377–1382.
7. Park JG, Lee JK, Phelps CT. Os acromiale associated with rotator cuff impingement: MR imaging of the shoulder. *Radiology* 1994;193: 255–257.
8. Mirowitz SA. Imaging techniques, normal variations, and diagnostic pitfalls in shoulder magnetic resonance imaging. *Magn Reson Imaging Clin North Am* 1993;1:19–36.
9. Neumann CH, Holt RG, Steinbach LS, Jahnke AH Jr, Petersen SA. MR imaging of the shoulder: appearance of the supraspinatus tendon in asymptomatic volunteers. *AJR Am J Roentgenol* 1992;158:1281–1287.
10. Vahlensieck M, Pollack M, Lang P, Grampp S, Genant HK. Two segments of the supraspinous muscle: cause of high signal intensity at MR imaging? *Radiology* 1993;186:449–454.
11. Timins ME, Erickson SJ, Estkowski LD, Carrera GF, Komorowski RA. Increased signal in the normal supraspinatus tendon on MR imaging: diagnostic pitfall caused by the magic-angle effect. *AJR Am J Roentgenol* 1995;165:109–114.
12. Zlatkin MB, Dalinka MK, Kressel HY. Magnetic resonance imaging of the shoulder. *Magn Reson Q* 1989;5:3–22.
13. Kjellin I, Ho CP, Cervilla V, et al. Alterations in the supraspinatus tendon at MR imaging: correlation with histopathologic findings in cadavers. *Radiology* 1991;181:837–841.
14. Kieft GJ, Sartoris DJ, Bloem JL, et al. Magnetic resonance imaging of glenohumeral joint diseases. *Skeletal Radiol* 1987; 16:285–290.
15. Quinn SF, Sheley RC, Demlow TA, Szumowski J. Rotator cuff tendon tears: evaluation with fat-suppressed MR imaging with arthroscopic correlation in 100 patients [see comments]. *Radiology* 1995;195: 497–500.
16. Kneeland JB, Middleton WD, Carrera GF, et al. MR imaging of the shoulder: diagnosis of rotator cuff tears. *AJR Am J Roentgenol* 1987; 149:333–337.
17. Zlatkin MB, Iannotti JP, M.C. R. Rotator cuff tears: diagnostic performance of MR imaging. *Radiology* 1989;172:223–231.
18. Iannotti JP, Zlatkin MB, Esterhai JL, Kressel HY, Dalinka MK, Spindler KP. Magnetic resonance imaging of the shoulder. Sensitivity, specificity, and predictive value. *J Bone Joint Surg [Am]* 1991;73: 17–29.
19. Gusmer PB, Potter HG, Donovan WD, O'Brien SJ. MR imaging of the shoulder after rotator cuff repair. *AJR Am J Roentgenol* 1997;168: 559–563.
20. Owen RS, Iannotti JP, Kneeland JB, Dalinka MK, Deren JA, Oleaga L. Shoulder after surgery: MR imaging with surgical validation. *Radiology* 1993;186:443–447.
21. Garneau RA, Renfrew DL, Moore TE, el-Khoury GY, Nepola JV, Lemke JH. Glenoid labrum: evaluation with MR imaging. *Radiology* 1991;179:519–222.
22. Gusmer PB, Potter HG, Schatz JA, et al. Labral injuries: accuracy of detection with unenhanced MR imaging of the shoulder. *Radiology* 1996; 200:519–524.
23. Liou JT, Wilson AJ, Totty WG, Brown JJ. The normal shoulder: common variations that simulate pathologic conditions at MR imaging. *Radiology* 1993;186:435–441.
24. Loredo R, Longo C, Salonen D, et al. Glenoid labrum: MR imaging with histologic correlation. *Radiology* 1995;196:33–41.
25. Moseley HF, Overgaard B. The anterior capsular mechanism in recurrent anterior dislocation of the shoulder. *J Bone Joint Surg [Br]* 1962; 44:913–927.
26. Neumann CH, Petersen SA, Jahnke AH. MR imaging of the labral–capsular complex: normal variations. *AJR Am J Roentgenol* 1991;157: 1015–1021.
27. Tirman PF, Feller JF, Palmer WE, Carroll KW, Steinbach LS, Cox I. The Buford complex—a variation of normal shoulder anatomy: MR arthrographic imaging features. *AJR Am J Roentgenol* 1996; 166: 869–873.
28. Palmer WE, Caslowitz PL, Chew FS. MR arthrography of the shoulder: normal intraarticular structures and common abnormalities. *AJR Am J Roentgenol* 1995;164:141–146.
29. Legan JM, Burkhard TK, Goff WB, et al. Tears of the glenoid labrum: MR imaging of 88 arthroscopically confirmed cases. *Radiology* 1991; 179:241–246.
30. Tirman PF, Stauffer AE, Crues JVD, et al. Saline magnetic resonance arthrography in the evaluation of glenohumeral instability. *Arthroscopy* 1993;9:550–559.
31. Richards RD, Sartoris DJ, Pathria MN, Resnick D. Hill–Sachs lesion and normal humeral groove: MR imaging features allowing their differentiation. *Radiology* 1994;190:665–668.
32. Cartland JP, Crues JVd, Stauffer A, Nottage W, Ryu RK. MR imaging in the evaluation of SLAP injuries of the shoulder: findings in 10 patients. *AJR Am J Roentgenol* 1992;159:787–792.
33. Monu JU, Pope TL Jr, Chabon SJ, Vanarthos WJ. MR diagnosis of superior labral anterior posterior (SLAP) injuries of the glenoid labrum: value of routine imaging without intraarticular injection of contrast material. *AJR Am J Roentgenol* 1994;163:1425–1429.
34. Tirman PF, Feller JF, Janzen DL, Peterfy CG, Bergman AG. Association of glenoid labral cysts with labral tears and glenohumeral instability: radiologic findings and clinical significance. *Radiology* 1994;190: 653–658.
35. Fritz RC, Helms CA, Steinbach LS, Genant HK. Suprascapular nerve entrapment: evaluation with MR imaging. *Radiology* 1992;182: 437–444.
36. Tuckman GA. Abnormalities of the long head of the biceps tendon of the shoulder: MR imaging findings. *AJR Am J Roentgenol* 1994;163: 1183–1188.
37. Chan TW, Dalinka MK, Kneeland JB, Chervrot A. Biceps tendon dislocation: evaluation with MR imaging. *Radiology* 1991;179:649–652.

PART X

Neoplasms

Disorders of the Shoulder: Diagnosis and Management,
edited by Joseph P. Iannotti and Gerald R. Williams, Jr.
Lippincott Williams & Wilkins, Philadelphia © 1999.

CHAPTER 33

Neoplasms of the Shoulder Girdle

Philip Z. Wirganowicz and Jeffrey J. Eckardt

INTRODUCTION

Radiographic abnormalities and bone or soft-tissue masses need to be evaluated in a well-organized and methodic fashion. An abnormal mass should not be simply attributed to a musculoskeletal strain or hematoma, and similarly, changes found on radiographs should not be ignored or assumed to be degenerative changes. The diagnostic workup and treatment of bone and soft-tissue tumors is based on principles of oncologic surgery. These should be performed promptly to improve patient survival and functional outcome. The goals in the treatment of malignant tumors about the shoulder are, first, the preservation of life, followed by preservation of limb and function. Rarely, if ever, is the sequence of these goals in primary tumors about the shoulder altered.

P. Z. Wirganowicz: Department of Orthopaedic Surgery, Hospital of the University of Pennsylvania, Philadelphia, Pennsylvania 19104.

J. J. Eckardt: Department of Orthopaedic Surgery, University of California Los Angeles, Los Angeles, California 90095-6902.

Amputation was the primary treatment for primary malignant bone tumors in the 1970s; however, sucessful limb salvage techniques have been developed for malignant and aggressive benign tumors. Improved chemotherapeutic protocols and irradiation techniques have substantially improved long-term patient survivorship and contributed to the success of limb salvage surgery for malignant tumors of the extremities. Limb-sparing surgery is considered safe and is now routine for many carefully selected patients, owing to advances in orthopedics, biomaterials, bioengineering, and radiographic imaging.

This chapter discusses the diagnosis and management of some of the more common primary benign and malignant tumors and tumorous conditions about the shoulder. There is an obvious wide range of presenting situations; therefore, clinical judgment and selection must be used in each individual case to achieve optimal outcome. Initially, a thorough patient history, a physical examination, and a basic radiologic evaluation should be performed. Once this information is known, then either patient reassurance and observation, or further workup and necessity for treatment is determined.

DIAGNOSIS

The diagnosis of bone tumors involves proceeding systematically in clinical assessment, diagnostic studies, and biopsy in selected cases.

Clinical Assessment

A thorough but directed history should document such things as how long the patient has known of any abnormality, if there is pain that awakens the patient at night, or if there has been growth of a lesion. Patients with bone tumors commonly present with complaints of pain and a noticeable mass. Some level of trauma is frequently associated with the patient's discovery of the mass; however, this is usually the factor that brings attention to the lesion, rather than the causative event. Occasionally, the lesion is discovered as an incidental finding on physical examination or on plain radiographs. Certain symptoms may be classically associated with particular lesions. For example, an osteoid osteoma frequently causes pain at night that is relieved with nonsteroidal antiinflammatory medicines, and Ewing's sarcomas may have systemic signs and symptoms, such as fevers, sweats, and elevated erythrocyte sedimentation rate. These associated factors are helpful in the diagnosis and should not be overlooked. Directed questioning is frequently needed to obtain this information, for many patients will not associate these signs with their condition. Past medical or family history is of less benefit except in cases of hereditary conditions; for example, multiple hereditary osteochondromas or multiple enchondromatosis. Previous malignancy should be ascertained to rule out metastatic disease.

With this information, a differential diagnosis is made and appropriate studies are ordered. If further workup or biopsy is performed, this information should be reported to other clinicians, such as the pathologist and radiologist. Many pathologists request to review the radiologic studies themselves to aid in a histologic diagnosis. If this information is not passed on to other clinicians, a pathologic fracture through a benign process, such as a simple bone cyst, may show an altered radiologic and microscopic appearance that leads to an incorrect diagnosis and subsequent treatment.

Diagnostic Evaluation

Plain radiographs are the most useful, cost-effective, and easily obtainable study. Radiographs are reasonably sensitive in detecting bony abnormalities, and they may show soft-tissue masses. From the clinical assessment and radiographs, a differential diagnosis is formulated, and a lesion can be more fully evaluated using other studies. Frequently, the location within the bone may suggest a diagnosis. Each tumor has a preferential location within the epiphysis, metaphysis, or diaphysis. In addition, anatomic location of the lesion may direct the clinician in making the diagnosis. For example, giant cell tumors of bone are usually lytic metaphyseal lesions located about the distal femur, proximal tibia, or distal radius. Enneking, using four parameters, has described radiographic evaluation and characterization of bone tumors.[12] First, there is anatomic location and site of the tumor, as just mentioned. Second, a determination is made concerning the effects that the lesion has on the bone. Large, destructive lesions with irregular margins or soft-tissue extensions are more often associated with malignancies; whereas smaller, well-confined lesions tend to be benign. Third, radiographs may show that the bone has a response to the lesion. Well-circumscribed lesions are usually associated with either slow-growing or benign lesions that may have sclerotic or nonsclerotic borders. A permeative or moth-eaten appearance on radiographs is characteristic of aggressive lesions. Periosteal reaction is a useful measure of lesion aggressiveness. Lesions that spread through the cortex may do so with the periosteum intact. In more slowly expanding lesions, the periosteal sleeve may remain intact and continue new bone formation during the expansion. This leads to the appearance of a Codman's triangle or lamellar periosteal reaction, typically called "onion-skinning." These periosteal reactions are frequently seen with malignant conditions; however, they are also occasionally seen with benign tumors or osteomyelitis. The periosteal reaction may be more complex, especially in rapidly growing tumors that expand beyond the periosteal sleeve. This gives the appearance of a "sunburst" reaction, typically associated with highly malignant tumors. Finally, radiographic changes may be classically associated with particular lesions. For example, an osteoid osteoma frequently has a bull's-eye appearance of the central nidus surrounded by a lucent margin.

Given the plain radiographic appearance of a lesion, a decision can be made on the need for further diagnostic workup. In the case of certain benign lesions, no further workup or treatment may be necessary. However, in cases for whom treatment is indicated, further diagnostic evaluation is usually necessary to determine the extent of tumor, either locally or distant spread, and its relation to neurovascular structures. Technetium 99m (^{99m}Tc) bone scans are helpful in determining polyostotic involvement or skip lesions. Computed tomography (CT) scans give excellent visualization of bony structures, including cortical destruction, fractures, and soft-tissue calcification. Magnetic resonance imaging (MRI) scans are useful in determining local osseous extent of tumor, soft-tissue extension, and medullary involvement, including skip lesions. Occasionally, other studies are indicated; for example, angiography, ultrasound, or other nuclear medicine studies. In cases of known malignancy or particular aggressive benign conditions, CT scans of the chest are needed to assess for metastatic disease.

Biopsy

Biopsies are indicated in cases of suspected malignancy, selected benign tumors, cases of uncertain diagnosis, or continued patient anxiety despite reassurance of a benign process. If the lesion has a classically benign radiographic appearance and location, for example a nonossifying fibroma or osteochondroma, then biopsy may be unnecessary unless the patient is symptomatic.

Biopsies can be either incisional or excisional. Incisional biopsies are often considered the procedure of choice for obtaining diagnostic tissue. By definition, incisional biopsies, including curettage, are intralesional procedures that leave either gross or microscopic residual tumor. In general, the surgeon who will perform the definitive procedure should perform the biopsy. The location of the biopsy is crucial in planning for eventual resection, especially if a limb salvage procedure is contemplated. The biopsy incision should be longitudinal along the lines of extensile exposure. A poorly placed or transverse biopsy incision may preclude adequate exposure for an en bloc resection, or eliminate the possibility for a limb-sparing surgery that necessitates amputation. The smallest size incision that provides adequate exposure is preferred. At the time of the definitive en bloc resection of the tumor, the biopsy tract and overlying skin, along with an adequate soft-tissue margin, must be excised. In obtaining the specimen, the periphery of the tumor offers the most representative tissue for diagnosis. The center of the tumor may be necrotic, and tissue obtained here is frequently nondiagnostic. The tissue biopsy should be sent for cryostat evaluation, permanent sections, and for culture. Cryostat (frozen section) evaluation ensures that there is adequate tissue for diagnosis and confirms location. The specimen is sent for multiple cultures, including aerobic, anaerobic, fungal, and acid-fast bacilli.

In performing the biopsy, meticulous hemostasis is critical to minimize the amount of hematoma. The hematoma is considered contaminated with tumor that must be resected with an adequate soft-tissue margin at the time of the definitive procedure. The biopsy site may be plugged with Gelfoam, microcrystalline collagen, or methylmethacrylate to minimize postoperative bleeding. The use of a tourniquet is not necessary, although it may be used if excessive bleeding is encountered during the biopsy. The limb may be partially exsanguinated with limb elevation before inflation of the tourniquet; however, the use of an Esmarch bandage over the site of the tumor is not recommended, for this may dislodge tumor cells into the bloodstream. If the biopsy involves bone, care should be taken to ensure that the edges of the biopsy site should be rounded and smooth, to minimize a stress concentration at this location that may lead to a pathologic fracture.

Excisonal biopsies are usually reserved for lesions smaller than 5 cm in diameter, and are usually reserved for known low-grade malignant or benign lesions. The excision is considered to be at the margin of the lesion where there is a reactive pseudocapsule. As a result, excisional biopsies are not indicated for any lesion, benign or malignant, with a propensity for recurrence or metastasis. Excisional biopsies are adequate for conditions that have little chance for local recurrence or spread; for example, simple bone cysts, osteoid osteomas, and nonossifying fibromas. Symptomatic osteochondromas can be treated with excisional biopsy if the periosteum and perichondrial sleeve is completely excised to minimize recurrence.

Needle biopsies may be performed in certain situations, especially if the tumor is easily accessible. Needle biopsies are best used for soft-tissue lesions or bone lesions with soft-tissue extension, because biopsies of bone with an intact cortex tend to be quite painful. Placement of the needle tract should be carefully planned, as in open biopsies, because this tract needs to be excised at the time of definitive procedure. The success in a needle biopsy lies in obtaining an adequate specimen. Even if an adequate amount of tissue is obtained, the tissue may not be representative of the tumor, leading to an incorrect diagnosis. The diagnostic accuracy of needle biopsies is approximately 70% to 80%. Because the diagnostic accuracy of a needle biopsy is substantially lower than an open biopsy, an open biopsy should be performed if the biopsy result is inconclusive or the diagnosis does not concur with the clinical picture. Overall, the method and accuracy of the biopsy is critical to the final outcome. Specific to the shoulder, the placement of a biopsy site must avoid contamination of the medial neurovascular structures and the intraarticular space.

Staging

Enneking promoted a standardized staging system for the evaluation of musculoskeletal tumors.[12] This system provides consistency in treatment among other surgeons, and permits the critical comparison and analysis of the treatment of the various tumors.

The staging system is based on how aggressive the tumor is, and whether it is still confined to its original compartment. The staging system was originally designed for malignant tumors; however, it has been modified to include benign conditions. In malignant tumors, the low-grade lesions are considered stage I, whereas high-grade lesions are referred to as stage II lesions. Metastatic lesions are considered to be stage III lesions, irrespective of whether the lesion is high- or low-grade. If the tumor remains intraosseous, then it is designated as A. Lesions that spread outside of the original compartment, including those that have spread outside of the overlying cortex but are still contained by the periosteum, are considered as stage B lesions. For example, a Ewing's sarcoma of the shoulder that has a large soft-tissue mass associated with the primary bone tumor and is without evidence of metastatic disease is considered a IIB lesion.

Benign bone tumors are classified in a fashion similar to that of malignant tumors. Stage 1 (Arabic numerals instead of Roman numbers for benign lesions) tumors are latent tumors that have no propensity for enlargement or spread, such as an osteochondroma after skeletal maturity. Stage 2 benign tumors are active lesions that show continued growth, but remain confined to bone. Simple bone cysts, aneurysmal bone cysts, and osteoblastomas are examples of such lesions.

Stage 3 tumors are aggressive benign tumors that have a high likelihood of local recurrence if improperly treated, may be associated with large soft-tissue masses, or may metastasize. A classic example of such a tumor is a giant cell tumor of bone.

TREATMENT

Not every tumor needs surgical intervention, or even biopsy. Lesions that have a classically benign appearance and location may be observed at regular intervals, unless the lesion is symptomatic. It is important to emphasize observation, in contrast to disregarding the lesion, because benign lesions may have a propensity for future secondary malignant change. If any doubt exists about the diagnosis of a lesion, then a biopsy needs to be performed. The surgical treatment of benign and malignant bone tumors is performed using well-established oncologic guidelines and principles. Once treatment for a bone tumor is deemed necessary, the type of treatment should be carefully considered. The type of procedure necessary is based on the patient's age, location of tumor, diagnostic studies, and tumor stage. Overall, "malignant" surgeries should be reserved for malignant diseases. Procedures for malignant tumors would include amputation or limb salvage techniques. Such surgeries are occasionally needed for benign conditions; however, they are usually not performed as initial treatment. Given the tumor stage and the biologic behavior of the tumor, an idealized treatment plan can be determined.

Oncologic Surgical Approaches to the Shoulder

Most tumors of the proximal humerus are accessed from a deltopectoral approach that is modified according to the location of the tumor (Fig. 1). Surgery is performed in either beach chair or lateral position, with the affected side up. An incision is made beginning in the deltopectoral interval and may be continued along the lateral or anterolateral arm for a more extensile approach. The incision is altered according to the extent of the resection. The biopsy should be made through the deltoid muscle itself, so that it can be widely excised at the time of definitive resection.

For resections of the proximal humerus, skin flaps are developed to allow better visualization. An interval is developed between the deltoid and pectoralis minor muscles (Fig. 2). The cephalic vein is preserved, if possible. The arm is externally rotated and adducted to protect the axillary nerve and expose the anterior circumflex vessels, which are coagulated. The subscapularis tendon is released and separated from the underlying capsule and gently retracted medially. The deltoid insertion on the humerus and the origin of the long head of the biceps is released. The shoulder capsule is

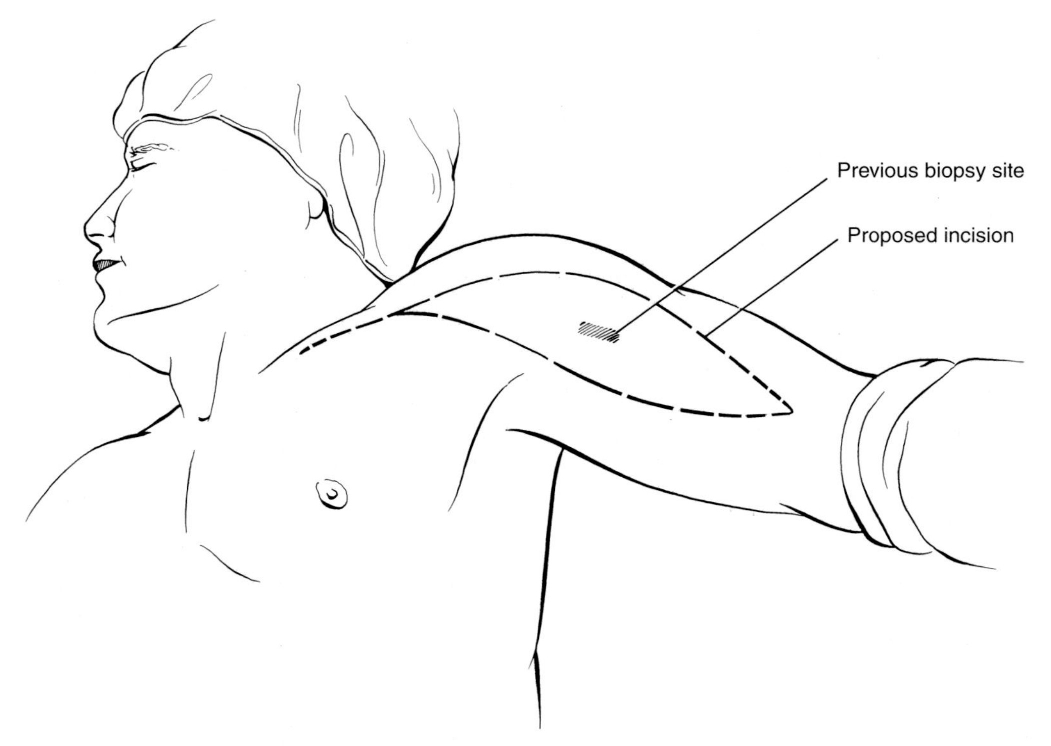

FIG. 1. The previous biopsy is performed through the deltoid muscle to minimize contamination of surrounding tissues. The biopsy site is excised at the time of definitive resection. The incision is made along the deltopectoral groove, and adjusted according to the length of resection. Skin flaps are made to increase exposure.

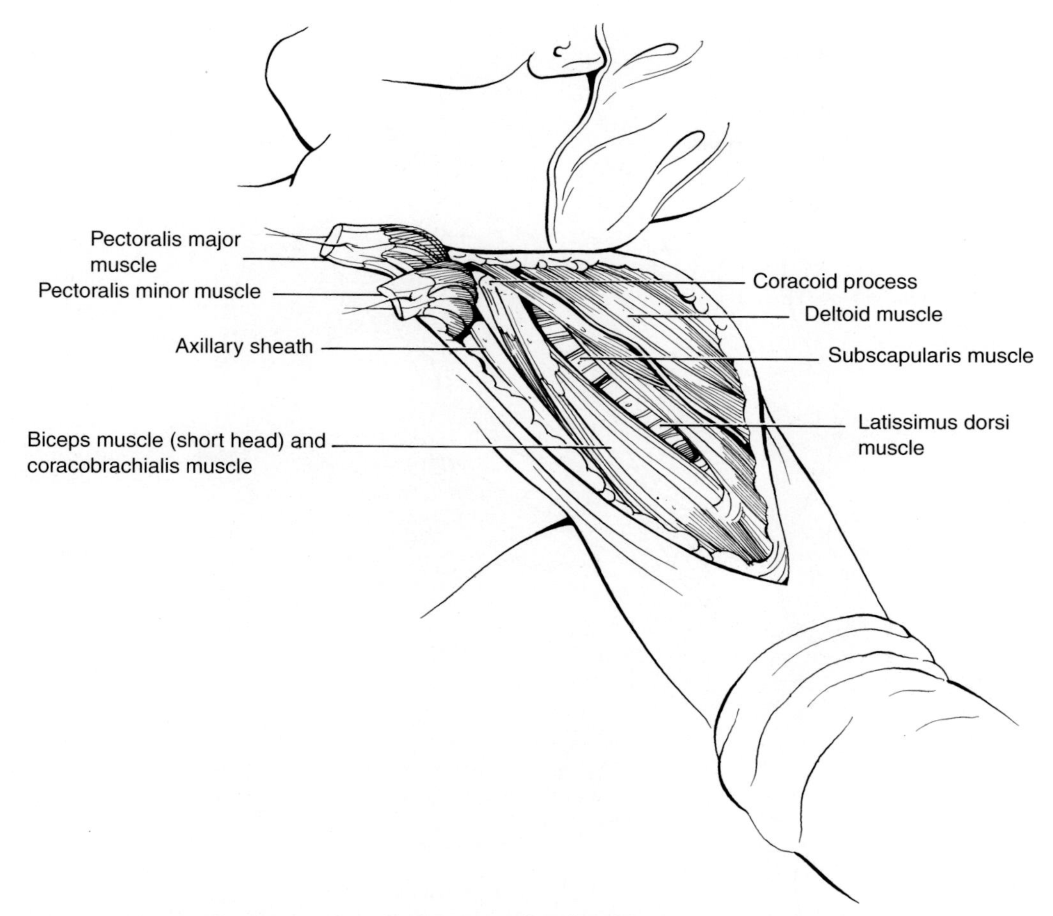

FIG. 2. The deltopectoral interval is opened and the cephalic vein is preserved, if possible. For resections of the proximal humerus, multiple muscular attachments are released. This illustrates the release of the pectoralis major and minor muscle.

divided circumferentially, and the shoulder is dislocated. A wide margin around the tumor is carried around the shaft of the humerus anteriorly, posteriorly, and medially. The neurovascular bundles are identified during dissection and retracted to prevent injury. Before performing the osteotomy, a measurement is taken from the center of the native humeral head to a location that is distal to the anticipated osteotomy. Following reconstruction, this measurement is restored to maintain proper arm lengths and soft-tissue tension. The osteotomy is performed at a level that has been determined preoperatively to be at a safe margin beyond tumor involvement, as seen on MRI. Preoperative planning is necessary to determine the level of resection that is beyond tumor and recreates equal extremity lengths following reconstruction. Once the osteotomy is performed, cryostat sampling of the distal medullary canal is performed to check for any remaining tumor at this margin. Once the margin is determined to be free of tumor, reconstruction can be performed.

Resection of the proximal humerus necessitates detachment of many soft-tissues, including the joint capsule and muscular attachments (Figs. 3 and 4). Variable amounts of soft-tissue are removed because of tumor involvement; therefore, some creativity is necessary during the reconstruction to ensure soft-tissue coverage of the prosthesis. An intact joint labrum, combined with a hemiarthroplasty component, improves overall stability of the prosthesis from dislocation. This is especially important, for the glenohumeral joint is inherently unstable, and many of the normal soft-tissue attachments to the proximal humerus, which afford some stability to the native shoulder, are no longer present. (Fig. 5). The wound is closed over suction drains, which are kept in place for several days to prevent accumulation of hematoma and serous fluid (Fig. 6). The arm is placed in a shoulder orthosis or abduction pillow for approximately 1.5 to 2 weeks before any motion at the shoulder is begun. Movement is encouraged at the fingers, wrist, and elbow to prevent stiffness. Eventually, a pseudocapsule forms around the prosthesis onto which muscles heal, allowing functional movement across the shoulder joint. The natural shoulder has a tremendous amount of motion and little inherent joint stability. After rehabilitation following oncologic reconstruction, most patients develop motion and strength neces-

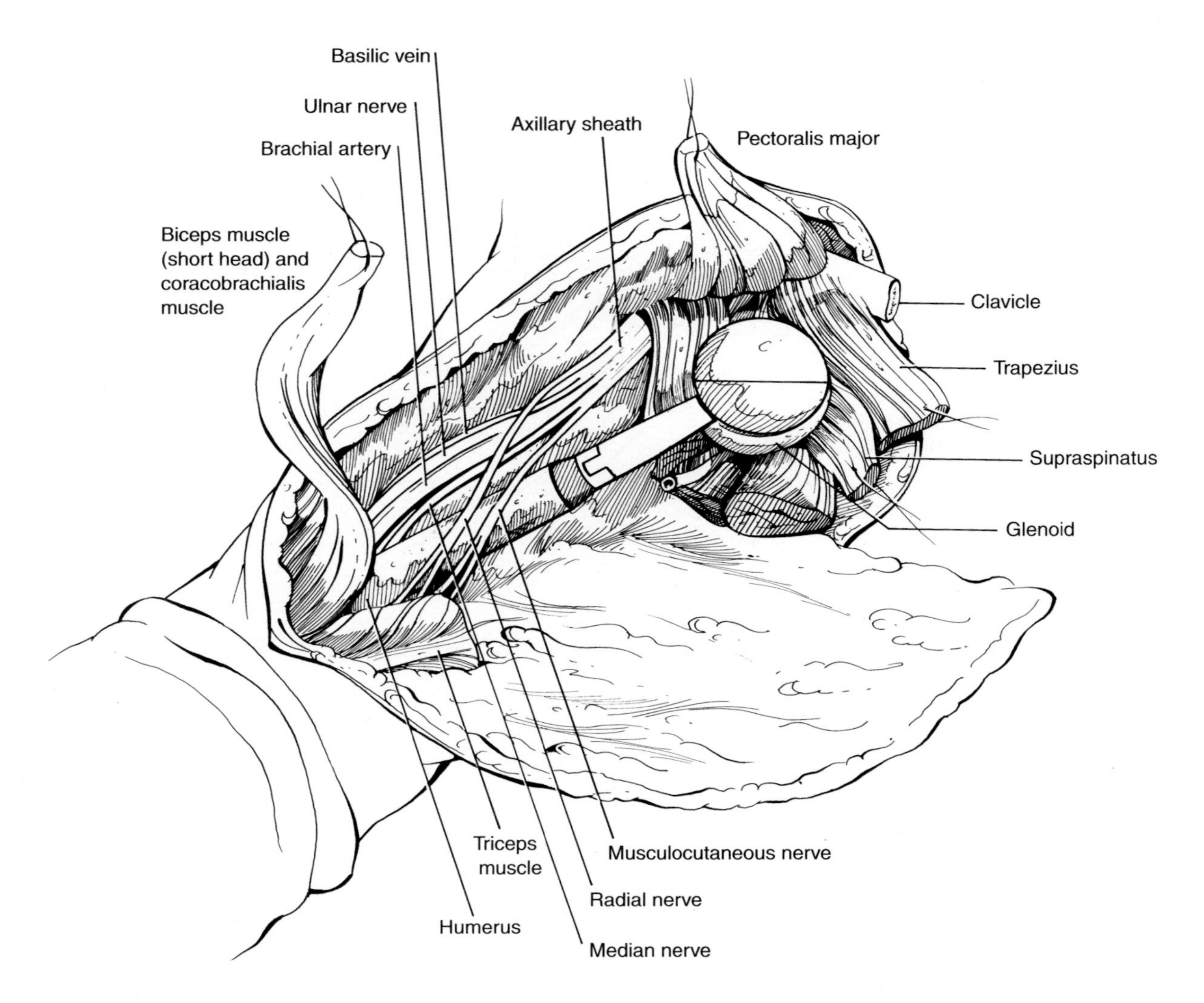

FIG. 3. Following resection, the prosthesis is cemented into the distal intramedullary canal. The length of resection is determined preoperatively by MRI to be several centimeters beyond the tumor. The detached muscles are then reapproximated to each other to secure the prosthesis into the glenoid. This is reinforced with a nonabsorbable tie, such as Mersilene tape, that is sutured to the glenoid and labrum and then wrapped around the prosthesis.

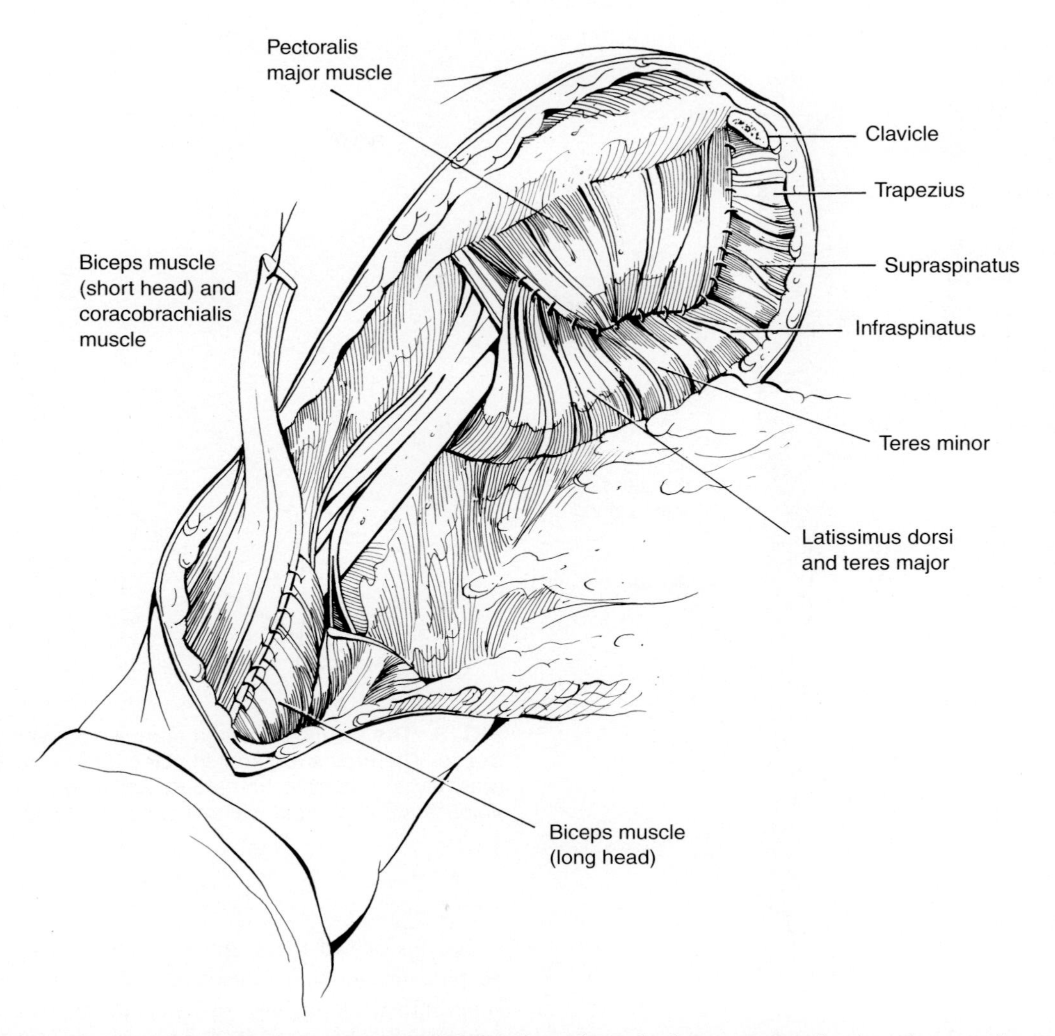

FIG. 4. To close the potential space and minimize the volume for hematoma collection, the muscles are reapproximated to each other. This also improves stability around the prosthesis against dislocation.

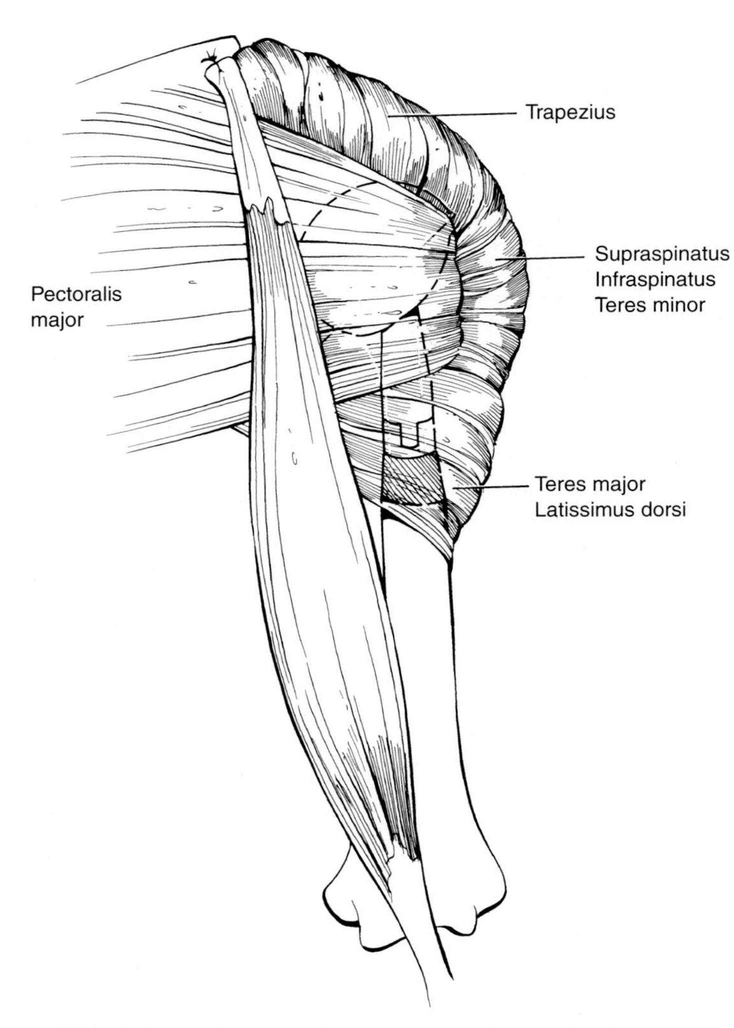

FIG. 5. The soft-tissue closure around the prosthesis: Once the muscles have healed, the myodesis created improves postoperative function and range of motion. Range of motion, particularly forward elevation and abduction, is usually limited. Movements for activities of daily living are possible, and occasionally near full range of motion is possible, if the length of resection is minimal.

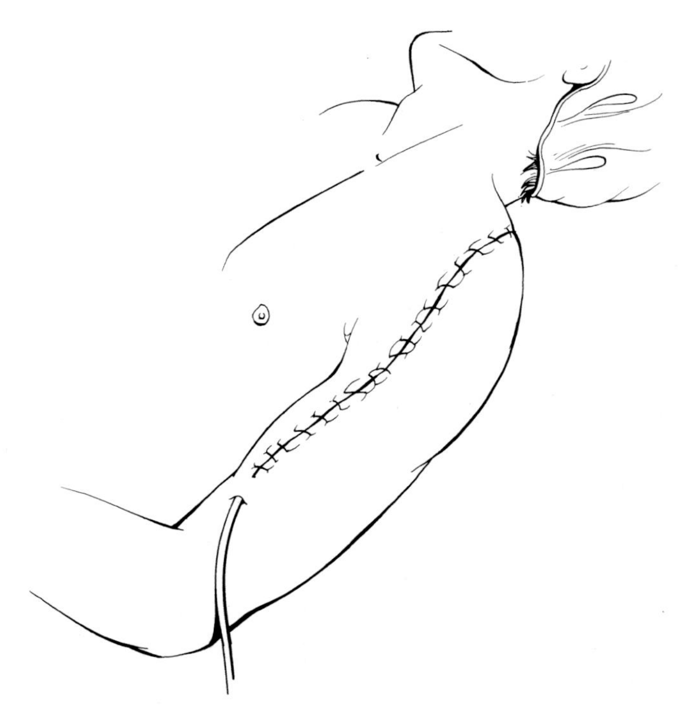

FIG. 6. The wound is closed in multiple layers over suction drains. The drains are kept in place for several days postoperatively to minimize hematoma collection. Intravenous antibiotics are continued while drains are in place.

sary for activities of daily living. Frequently, overhead activities are not possible. Postoperative dislocations are possible, and risk for this complication is minimized with meticulous soft-tissue closure around the prosthesis, which may include using a Mersilene tape wrapped around the prosthesis proximally and sutured into shoulder capsule and labrum. If the capsule or labrum is excised, a stable reconstruction is possible by use of a modified synthetic aortic graft that is secured to the circumference of the glenoid and encircles the proximal portion of the prosthesis[9] (Fig. 7). Meticulous soft-tissue closure accomplishes several goals. It decreases the amount of potential space and hematoma accumulation, improves postoperative stability, and secures muscles to allow early motion and maintains optimal muscle length (Fig. 8).

For lesions of the scapula, a posterior approach to the scapula and shoulder is used (Fig. 9). Again, this incision is longitudinal along lines of extensile exposure. The saber-type incision begins at the inferior angle of the scapula and is carried upward over the shoulder to join a deltopectoral exposure. To approach the posterior glenoid, an interval between the infraspinatus and teres minor is used. To approach other areas of the scapula, other intervals are used. Most of these approaches are purely anatomic dissections and do not use internervous planes; therefore, care must be taken not to sacrifice motor nerves or create traction neuropraxias. For complete or partial scapulectomies, there are multiple muscular attachments that must be released. Soft-tissue closure of these defects by myodesis is important for eventual postoperative function of the shoulder.

Surgical Considerations for Benign Bone Tumors

Most stage 1 or 2 benign tumors are adequately treated with curettage and filling the defect with either bone graft or methylmethacrylate bone cement. Osteochondromas may be treated with marginal excision, as long as the surrounding periosteum and perichondrial sleeve is removed. Stage 3 benign lesions may be treated with small en bloc resection or by curettage and use of adjuvant treatment, including phenol cauterization, liquid nitrogen cryosurgery, or heat cautery. In certain situations, especially in recurrent aggressive benign

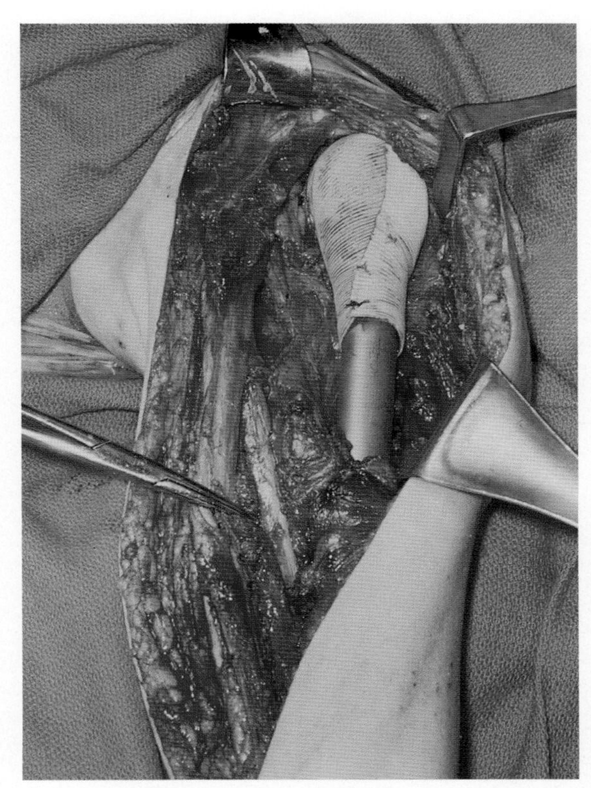

FIG. 7. After tumor resection and endoprosthetic reconstruction, the prosthesis is secured to the scapula to minimize the risk of postoperative dislocation. In patients in whom the labrum and capsule are intact, the prosthesis can be secured using nonabsorbable tape, such as Mersilene tape. In this patient, the capsule was not intact. By using a modified aortic graft attached to the glenoid, the prosthetic humeral head is encapsulated.

lesions, wide excision and reconstruction or amputation may be indicated. Other treatments are mentioned for each individual benign tumor (Table 1).

Surgical Considerations for Malignant Bone Tumors

Significant advances in adjuvant treatments, including chemotherapy and irradiation, have been made since the 1970s. As such, increasing numbers of patients who present with malignant tumors are expected to remain disease-free following amputation or limb salvage procedures. Before the advent of sophisticated adjuvant chemotherapeutic protocols, the 5-year disease-free survival of patients with osteosarcomas was approximately 15% to 20%, and approximately 5% to 10% for Ewing's sarcoma,[21] despite amputation and irradiation. With these figures in mind, it must be assumed that virtually all patients have either microscopic or macroscopic metastatic disease at the time of presentation.

Although surgery removes the primary tumor, chemotherapy is used to destroy metastatic foci of tumor. In addition, neoadjuvant chemotherapy significantly reduces tumor size, which allows limb salvage techniques to become successful.[11,35,36] Adjuvant chemotherapy is given to patients with high-grade spindle cell sarcomas, including osteosarcomas and high-grade chondrosarcomas. Many small-cell sarcomas, including Ewing's sarcomas, primitive neuroectodermal tumors, rhabdomyosarcomas, and non-Hodgkin's lymphomas are highly malignant and respond well to current multidrug chemotherapy and high-dose irradiation (Table 2).

Limb salvage techniques have dramatically improved since their introduction, and many more tumors can be successfully treated in this manner; however, there are certain contraindications to limb-sparing surgery. First, significant neurovascular involvement by tumor is the most common reason to preclude limb salvage. Limb salvage surgery may be still possible following resection of lesser nerves involved by tumor that may be treated in the long-term with either bracing or tendon transfers. Similarly, vascular in-

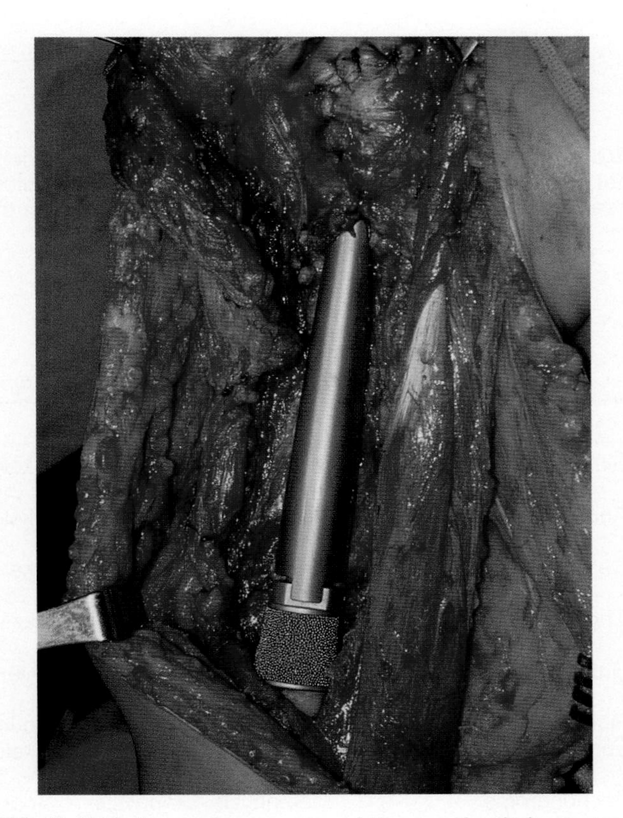

FIG. 8. Soft-tissue closure around the prosthesis is accomplished to decrease postoperative hematoma formation. The myodesis improves range of motion and function. Here, the rotator cuff, pectorals, trapezius, teres major, and latissimus dorsi muscles are imbricated to each other. Extramedullary porous ingrowth surface material is seen at the seat of the prosthesis, at the junction of prosthesis and bone. Soft-tissue ingrowth occurs at this interface that isolates the joint space and synovial fluid from the bone–cement interface. Polyethylene debris in the joint fluid is isolated from the bone–cement interface, which decreases the rate of aseptic loosening.

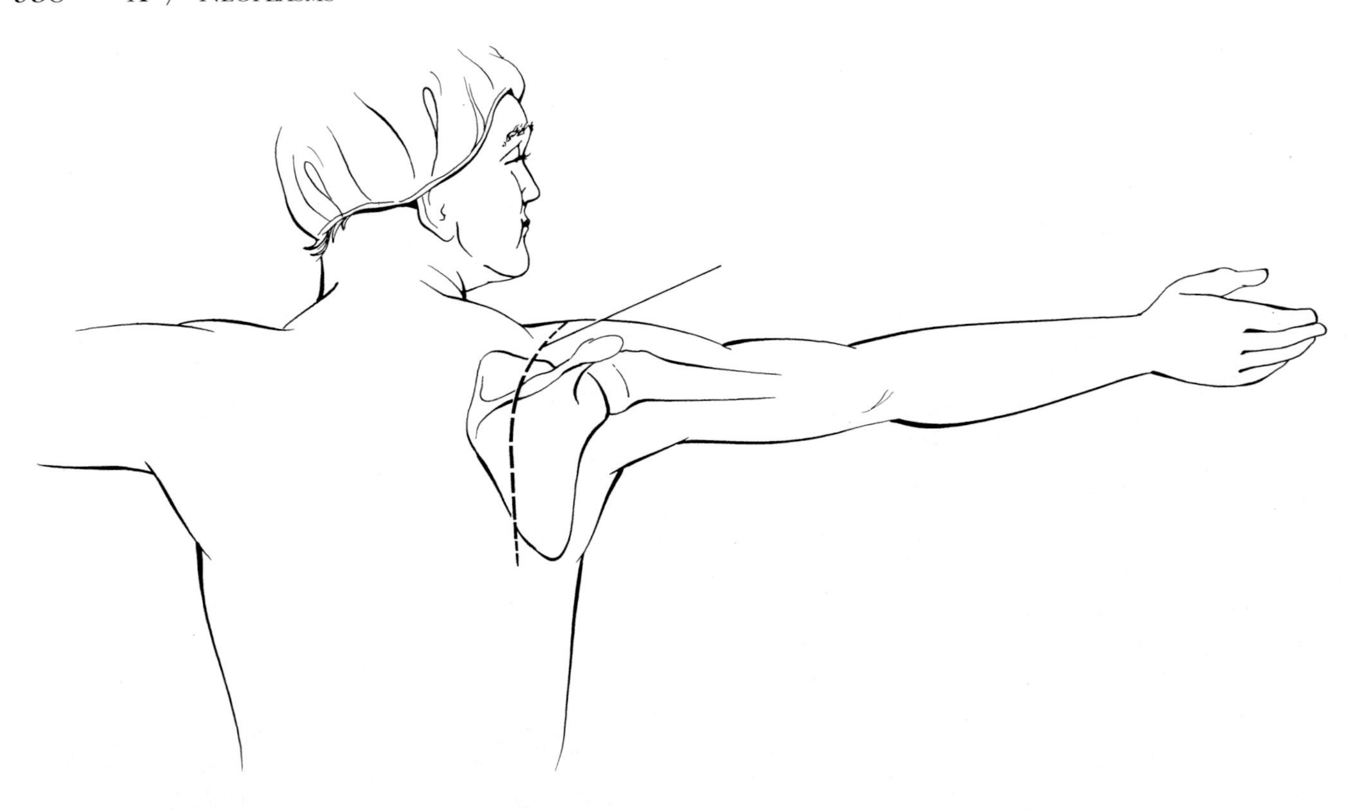

FIG. 9. The approach to the scapula and posterior shoulder employs a saber-type incision, with the patient placed in the lateral position. It may be continued over the top of the shoulder and join the deltopectoral incision, depending on the length of resection. Large full-thickness skin flaps are developed for exposure.

TABLE 1. *Common benign bone tumors and tumorous conditions of the shoulder*

Tumor	Preferred location	Age	Work-Up	Treatment*
Simple Bone Cyst	Metaphysis, Diaphysis	Skeletal Immaturity	X-rays, CT	Corticosteroid injection, Curettage/Bone Grafting
Aneurysmal Bone Cyst	Metaphysis, Diaphysis	Skeletal Immaturity	X-rays, MRI	Curettage, Adjuvant, Bone Grafting
Osteochondroma	Metaphysis, Diaphysis	Skeletal Immaturity to Adult	X-rays, MRI, CT	Excision
Chondroblastoma	Epiphysis	Skeletal Immaturity	X-rays, MRI, CT	Curettage, Adjuvant, Bone Grafting
Giant Cell Tumor	Epiphysis	Over 20 years	X-rays, MRI, CT, Bone Scan	Curettage, Adjuvant, Bone Grafting
Fibrous Dysplasia	Diaphysis	Young Adult	X-rays, CT	Curettage, Bone Grafting
Eosinophilic Granuloma	Diaphysis	Skeletal Immaturity	X-rays, MRI, CT, Bone Scan	Corticosteroid injection, Curettage/Bone Grafting
Enchondroma	Metaphysis, Diaphysis	Young Adult to Adult	X-rays, CT	Curettage, Bone Grafting
Synovial Osteochondromatosis	Intra-articular	Adult	X-rays, CT	Synovectomy
Osteoid Osteoma	Metaphysis, Diaphysis	10 to 25 Years	X-rays, CT, Bone Scan	Curettage or Excision
Osteoblastoma	Metaphysis, Diaphysis	20 to 40 Years	X-rays, CT, Bone Scan	Curettage or Wide Resection
Paget Disease of Bone	Proximal Humerus	Adult	X-rays, CT, Lab Tests	Medical Management

* General guidelines, see text for details.

TABLE 2. *Common malignant bone tumors of the shoulder*

Tumor	Preferred location	Age	Work-Up	Treatment*
Conventional Osteosarcoma	Metaphysis	Skeletal Immaturity	X-rays, MRI, CT, Bone Scan	Adjuvant Chemotherapy, Resection
Ewing's Sarcoma	Diaphysis	Skeletal Immaturity	X-rays, MRI, CT, Bone Scan	Adjuvant Chemotherapy, Resection, +/− Radiation
Chondrosarcoma	Metaphysis, Diaphysis	Adult	X-rays, MRI, CT, Bone Scan	Resection
Myeloma	Diaphysis	Over 50 Years	Skeletal Survey, Lab Tests	Chemotherapy, Radiation, Stabilization

* General guidelines, see text for details.

volvement by tumor may be treated with vascular bypass; however, this increases the risk of surgical failure and may slow recovery, especially if postoperative chemotherapy or irradiation is needed. Second, the treating surgeon must be reasonably certain that the rate of local recurrence with limb salvage surgery is no greater than with amputation and that long-term patient survival is not compromised. Local recurrence is usually associated with a fatal outcome, and limb-sparing surgery should not be considered if wide excision cannot be achieved. Third, in cases of pathologic fracture, the fracture hematoma produced allows spread of tumor along tissue planes, making a wide excision, with clear margins, a difficult prospect. Fourth, following wide tumor excision and reconstruction, there needs to be an adequate soft-tissue envelope to permit wound closure. It cannot be overemphasized that the wound must not be closed under tension because wound dehiscence may lead to deep infection, requiring a higher amputation than would have been performed primarily. Skin grafts, local muscle rotation flaps, or free tissue flaps are used occasionally; however, they may be difficult to heal in an irradiated bed. Finally, an improper biopsy may compromise future limb-sparing surgery. Improper location or orientation of the biopsy may make amputation the only alternative for complete tumor excision.

Reconstruction about the shoulder may involve the use of an endoprosthesis, allograft, allograft–prosthetic composite, or arthrodesis. Each form of reconstruction has its advantages and limitations, and as such, there are proponents for each procedure. Experience plays a large factor in the decision process for which reconstruction is suitable for different tumors. Endoprostheses were originally single-piece, custom-casted devices (Fig. 10); however, modern designs incorporate modular forged systems. These are stronger owing to the forging process, and their modularity allows for particular advantages. These include having off-the-shelf availability, intraoperative adjustment for length of reconstruction, revision surgery to replace failed hardware without having to revise the entire prosthesis, and in skeletally immature patients, the intercalated segments may be exchanged to allow for limb lengthening. Custom devices can still be ordered, although there will be a delay in surgery to allow for the manufacture of the prosthesis. Custom scapulae are available that incorporate a hooded glenoid component and a standard humeral component[9,10] Osteochondral allografts may be used; however, their use is less popular because of the long-term problems with their use, such as articular collapse. As a result, allograft–prosthetic composites are more common when allografts are used.

If limb-sparing surgery is not indicated, surgical options include amputation (shoulder disarticulation or forequarter amputation), interscapulothoracic resection and pseudoarthrosis (Tikhoff-Linberg procedure), or wide excision

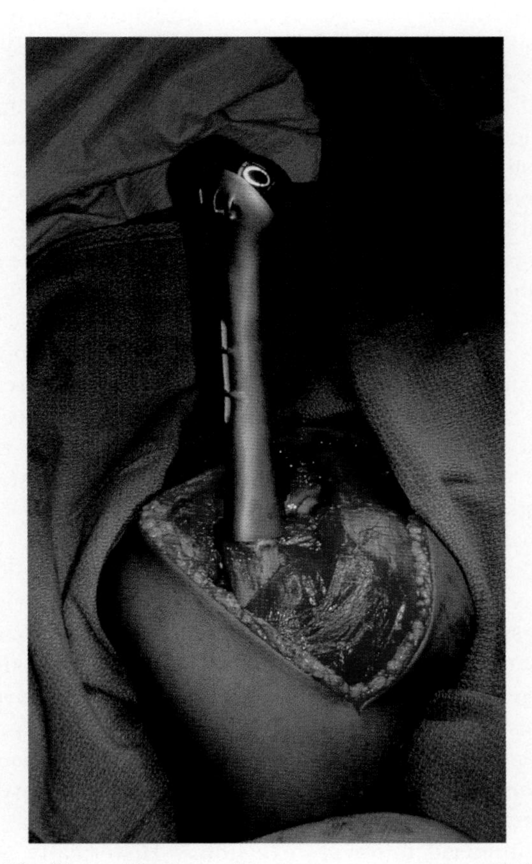

FIG. 10. The original prosthesis was a custom-casted one-piece prosthesis. Currently, modular, forged systems are available that allow the surgeon to have great flexibility for length of reconstruction and revision. The forged prosthesis is also stronger, to improve long-term durability.

and arthrodesis. Lesions that extend into the neurovascular bundles frequently require an amputation. Interscapulothoracic resection without reconstruction results in significant loss of shoulder motion, particularly with shoulder abduction. Hand and elbow function remain normal.[23] A shoulder pad prosthesis improves cosmesis and shoulder symmetry.

Arthrodesis of the shoulder following resection can be performed with use of a vascularized pedicle graft and internal fixation; however, fusion may be difficult in those patients who have received radiation or postoperative chemotherapy. In general, arthrodesis use has limited indications.

BENIGN TUMORS

Osteoid Osteoma

This lesion is characterized by a small round or oval osteoblastic mass, referred to as a nidus, surrounded by a sclerotic rim. The sclerotic rim is reactive bone to the lesion, whereas the nidus is the essential part of the tumor. In total, the lesion measures less than 1.5 cm in diameter, which distinguishes this lesion from an osteoblastoma that is histologically identical. Osteoid osteomas typically have a "bull's-eye" appearance on radiographs, especially if located in cortex. Classically, this lesion produces pain at night that is relieved with nonsteroidal antiinflammatory medicines, although many do not have such a typical presentation. The lesion may be confused with either chronic osteomyelitis (Brodie's abscess) or subacute osteomyelitis involving the epiphysis. It is extremely rare to find a patient with polyostotic osteoid osteomas. Most patients are in the 10- to 25-year-old age group.The lesion may be difficult to visualize on radiographs; therefore, either ^{99m}Tc bone scans or CT scanning are needed to identify the abnormality. The osteoid osteoma shows intense uptake activity on bone scans. With CT scans, the lesion may be easily identified as a central nidus surrounded by a sclerotic rim of bone. CT scans are routinely obtained for osteoid osteomas for preoperative localization, which may determine the operative approach.

Treatment is directed at complete removal of the lesion. The lesion may be removed in a piecemeal manner, using a high-speed burr and curettes,[3,40] or with en bloc resection. Only the nidus needs excision; the reactive sclerotic rim will resolve spontaneously once the lesion is removed. If the lesion is located in the cortex, the overlying bone may be somewhat roughened in appearance. Prophylactic stabilization with internal fixation or casting is necessary only in cases where structural integrity of the bone has been compromised following excision.[19] Historically, it has been said that osteoid osteomas may resolve spontaneously over a prolonged period of time without treatment; however, the lesion is often exquisitely painful and surgery provides consistent resolution of symptoms. In fact, many patients report dramatic improvement in pain relief on awakening from surgery in the recovery room. Recurrence of symptoms is highly suggestive of incomplete excision. Because the nidus may be difficult to identify during surgery, an intraoperative radiograph may be indicated to ensure proper location of excision.

On gross examination, the nidus appears as a discrete mass, with a deeply reddened color. The texture of the nidus is variable from being soft and granular to hard and sclerotic in cases of a mature osteoid osteoma. The nidus may be easily lifted out of its bed, analogous to a pea in a pod.

Osteoblastoma

This is also an osteoblastic lesion that is uncommon in the shoulder region. As mentioned, this lesion has histological appearance of an osteoid osteoma. By definition, these lesions are larger than 2 cm in diameter, and can be quite a large size. In contrast with osteoid osteomas, osteoblastomas generally have less sclerotic reactive bone surrounding the nidus, and they tend to cause less pain.

Computed tomography scans are generally necessary to delineate the extent of the lesion. Treatment is directed toward resection of the lesion followed by stabilization with internal fixation. There is a higher incidence of recurrence compared with osteoid osteomas,[3] and curettage alone leads to a 25% rate of recurrence. Therefore, en bloc resection is recommended whenever possible.[38]

Osteochondroma

Osteochondroma, the most common tumor of bone, may be single or multiple lesions. Multiple lesions are a hereditary condition transmitted in an autosomal dominant fashion with variable penetrance. Osteochondromas may be pedunculated on a stalk or sessile. The lesion is characterized by an outward growth of bone formed by enchondral ossification from aberrant foci of cartilage. The cortex of the exostosis is contiguous with the native cortical bone. The lesion has a cartilaginous cap that is the source of the enchondral growth. Osteochondromas develop in youth; however, the exact incidence and age group is difficult to determine, for many of the lesions are completely asymptomatic and never present to a physician. Because the lesion is a result of enchondral growth, osteochondromas continue to enlarge in size until skeletal maturity.

Osteochondromas may present with a variety of symptoms; however, many are asymptomatic. The most common complaint is that of pain. The patients may also complain of joint deformity, limited joint range of motion, nerve or vascular impingement, or cosmetic deformity.[28,33,34,39,41,42]

There is a small chance for malignant degeneration of lesions, usually to a chondrosarcoma. This degeneration usually does not occur until later in life. The exact risk for secondary malignant change in solitary exostoses is difficult to assess, owing to the uncertain incidence; however, it is estimated to be below 5% and possibly less than 1%.[39] In those patients with multiple lesions, the risk for malignancy may be as high as 30%. Two clinical features may be suggestive of malignant degeneration. When there is either a change in size of the lesion following skeletal maturity or change in symptoms without explanation, malignancy should be suspected. In addition, the cartilaginous cap rarely measures larger than 1.5 cm in thickness in benign lesions. Therefore, if there is either an enlargement in the cartilaginous cap over time or the cap measures more than 2 cm in thickness at the time of presentation, then development to a secondary chondrosarcoma should be considered.

The shoulder area is a common location of presentation for exostoses; however, treatment is less commonly indicated. Treatment is directed at symptomatic lesions or those that are suggestive of malignancy. Treatment of benign lesions consists of complete excision of the exostosis proximal to the perichondral sleeve. If the perichondrium is partially retained, recurrence is common. For lesions excised from the proximal humerus, internal stabilization or bone grafting is rarely necessary.

Enchondroma

Enchondromas are benign cartilaginous lesions that are frequently found as an incidental finding on radiographs or bone scans. These are common lesions of the proximal humerus. Although chondromas may present as a surface lesion as a periosteal chondroma, most are centrally located, giving them the name of enchondroma. The etiology of enchondromas is uncertain; however, they may be aberrant developmental cartilage rests. There is a broad age group of presentation, with a roughly even distribution throughout all decades of life. This wide distribution is primarily due to the asymptomatic nature of these lesions. Frequently, enchondromas are found during a workup for rotator cuff pathology when either radiographs or MRI reveal the lesion. Enchondromas may occur as multiple lesions in a generalized syndrome called Ollier's disease. Maffucci's disease is multiple enchondromas associated with cutaneous hemangiomas. There is a low incidence of malignant transformation of solitary enchondromas, usually to a chondrosarcoma. In multiple lesions, the incidence of secondary malignant transformation nears 25% to 30%.

The radiographic appearance of enchondromas is as a lytic lesion of the metaphysis or diaphysis. There may be stippled calcification within the lesion that occurs in 25% of all lesions. The calcification is often more radiodense than normal bone, for dystrophic calcification of cartilage produces calcium carbonate versus calcium hydroxyapatite of normal bone. The cortex overlying these lesions is frequently slightly expanded and eccentric in location. Minimal endosteal scalloping may be present. The borders may be well circumscribed. Periosteal chondromas are surface lesions that have a sharp margin, with the underlying cortex being scalloped. The cortex has a sclerotic border. Enchondromas are usually asymptomatic, unless they sustain a pathologic fracture or are undergoing malignant degeneration. Painful lesions without evidence of fracture should be highly suspect for malignant transformation.

For a classically benign-appearing enchondroma, biopsy or surgical treatment is not indicated, unless there is a possibility for pathologic fracture. Serial radiographs may follow the lesions that have a classic benign appearance. Treatment consists of complete curettage, bone grafting, and stabilization of the bone, as indicated. Some authors recommend phenol cauterization of the cavity following curettage. Treatment usually results in cure; however, recurrence of the lesion may be due to the presence of an undiagnosed chondrosarcoma, present at the time of the original surgery. Because curettage is an intralesional procedure, it may leave remaining tumor, even in the case of a benign tumor. Therefore, if there is a question of malignancy preoperatively, then an aggressive curettage with use of adjuvant therapy or wide resection should be performed.

Giant Cell Tumors of Bone

This tumor of unknown etiology is considered to be one of the more aggressive benign lesions of bone. Although named after the multinucleated giant cell seen in this lesion, the basic cell type of this tumor is the spindle-shaped stromal cell. The giant cells are a result of fusion of proliferating mononuclear cells, analogous to the osteoclast. In fact, older literature referred to this tumor as an "osteoclastoma" because of this histologic appearance. Many other lesions, both benign and malignant, have a giant cell component, leading to potential diagnostic confusion. Eighty percent of giant cell tumors occur in persons older than the age 20 years, and peak incidence occurs in the third decade of life. Most giant cell tumors are eccentrically located, epiphyseal lesions that abut the subchondral cartilage. Radiographically, they are lytic tumors, with a poorly demarcated margin adjacent to normal bone. Common symptoms include pain or limited range of motion. A palpable soft tissue mass is infrequent, although soft-tissue extension of the tumor still contained by periosteum is a common feature.

Treatment consists of an aggressive curettage, followed by adjuvant therapy with either cryosurgery or phenol cauterization, and filling of the defect. Before the advent of adjuvant therapy, the rate of local recurrence of giant cell tumors of bone was approximately 50%.[6,7,16] Phenol is a benzylic alcohol that is a surface-acting agent causing chemical cauterization. It kills tumor cells contained within the bone interstices remaining following curettage. Marcove et al.[25,27] introduced the use of liquid nitrogen in the treatment of giant cell tumors. This consisted of carefully pouring the liquid nitrogen into the cavity created by the curettage that extended the area of necrosis up to 2 cm beyond the border of the cavity. This is very effective for causing tumor necrosis; however, necrosis of the adjacent normal bone may lead to either pathologic fracture or delayed healing of bone graft, if used to fill the defect.[24] The zone of necrosis can be reduced to a few millimeters by the use of a liquid nitrogen spray. Because either phenol or surface applied liquid nitrogen have a limited zone of necrosis, it must be emphasized that the use of adjuvants is not a substitute for adequate and complete curettage. The curettage must extend to the level of normal-appearing bone, after which time adjuvants should be used. The combination of aggressive curettage and use of adjuvant therapy has reduced the rate of local recurrence for giant cell tumors to less than 5% in primary tumors treated by orthopedic oncologists.[1,5,14] The remaining bone defect usually needs to be filled with either bone graft or methylmethacrylate. Bone graft has the advantage of being a biologic reconstruction; however, the arm may require protection from full activity until there is complete incorporation of the graft. In contrast, the use of bone cement allows for early motion and use of the arm, and the heat produced by cement polymerization may have the added benefit of additional tumor kill caused by thermal necrosis.[20] A theoretical disadvantage of bone cement is less long-term durability and decreasing the amount of shock absorption if placed in a subchondral location, leading to premature arthritis. Irradiation has been used in the treatment of giant cell tumors, but owing to the increased risk of radiation associated sarcomas, its use is now reserved for lesions that are considered to be unresectable.

A CT scan of the affected area should be obtained soon after treatment as a baseline for comparison to evaluate for recurrent tumor. The median time for recurrence is 16 to 18 months, although recurrence may occur many decades following primary treatment. Local recurrence may be associated with malignant degeneration, especially if irradiation was used previously. Giant cell tumors of bone are capable of metastasis, primarily to the lung, or implantation into soft tissues at the time of surgery. Care must be taken at the time of the primary surgery to prevent tumor spillage into the soft tissues. Chest radiographs or lung CT scans should be obtained at regular intervals to assess for metastatic disease.

Chondroblastoma

Chondroblastomas are rare tumors that have radiographic and histologic similarities to giant cell tumors of bone. The basic stromal cell of a chondroblastoma appears similar to a giant cell tumor; however, these cells, which distinguish this tumor as a distinct entity, produce a chondroid matrix. The lesion is most common in the second decade of life. Chondroblastomas are epiphyseal lesions, and may occur in areas of secondary ossification. The proximal humerus is the most common location for this lesion. They are lytic lesions that may extend to the subarticular surface. They may be sharply delineated from the surrounding normal bone by a thin rim of reactive sclerosis. Thin, septated trabeculations may be seen. The lesions most commonly present with pain caused by impending or frank pathologic fracture.

Treatment consists of thorough curettage, bone grafting, and internal stabilization as indicated. This lesion is less aggressive than a giant cell tumor and recurrence is rare with proper treatment. Soft-tissue implantation has been recorded; therefore, care must be taken to prevent tumor spillage. In addition, there have been cases reported of metastasis to the lungs. As a result, regular clinical follow-up is necessary to determine any local or distant recurrence of tumor.

Eosinophilic Granuloma

This lesion is characterized by the presence of Langerhans histiocytic cells and not eosinophils as the name suggests. Histiocytosis X (Langerhans cell histiocytosis) is the generalized name for this lesion that consists of three clinical syndromes of varying severity.[22] Eosinophilic granuloma may be unifocal or polyostotic and is the most benign of these lesions. Hand-Schüller-Christian disease and Letterer-Siwe syndrome are more severe variants of histiocytosis X, of which the latter is usually fatal at an early age owing to acute, widespread dissemination of the histiocytic cells. Pain is the usual presenting complaint, and there is occasionally a palpable mass. Most lesions are radiographically lytic and well demarcated, without a sclerotic border. They tend to be diaphyseal lesions in long bones, but this lesion is most common in flat bones. Clinically, the lesion may be mistaken for a chronic bone abscess or osteomyelitis, owing to the presence of a necrotic center at the time of surgery, and histologically may appear as an abscess, owing to the presence of eosinophilic clusters. These lesions are most commonly noted in the first and second decades of life, although no treatment may have been instituted until adulthood. There is a decreased incidence with each successive decade of life.

Treatment is instituted according to severity and necessity.[4,15] These lesions may heal spontaneously, or in some cases, only injection of methylprednisolone acetate is necessary. In areas of impending pathologic fracture, curettage, bone grafting, and internal fixation may be needed. Irradiation in low doses has been curative; however, because of the risk of treatment-associated sarcoma in later life, irradiation is usually reserved for lesions that are inaccessible to injection or are difficult to approach surgically.

Synovial Osteochondromatosis

Synovial (osteo)chondromatosis is a rare condition of cartilagenous metaplasia of the subsynovial connective tissue. Multiple cartilagenous loose bodies are formed within the joint when the pedunculated metaplastic foci become detached. Patients may present with joint swelling and pain, mechanical symptoms such as locking and giving way, or a sensation of loose bodies within the joint. It is most common in middle age (40–60 years).[29]

Radiographically, multiple, small intraarticular opacities with some calcification are seen. There may be a joint effusion or soft-tissue mass in association with this condition.

Treatment is directed toward complete removal of the affected synovium with a total synovectomy. In cases of limited areas of synovial involvement, this can be performed arthroscopically; however, in most cases, including the shoulder, this excision should be performed by an open synovectomy.

If degenerative changes are seen within the joint, then a total shoulder arthroplasty can be performed. In rare cases, synovial chondromatosis can cause other problems, including shoulder joint subluxation[18] or secondary degeneration to a chondrosarcoma.[17,32]

MALIGNANT TUMORS

Osteosarcoma

Osteosarcomas are the most common primary sarcoma of bone. Only multiple myeloma occurs with greater frequency as a primary malignancy in bone. Osteosarcomas are spindle cell neoplasms that, by definition, produce osteoid. As a result, a tumor may have predominance of other elements, such as chondroid or fibromatoid tissue, but the presence of osteoid defines the lesion as an osteosarcoma. Because of this histologic variability, osteosarcomas are differentiated into chondroid, fibromatoid, or osteoid subtypes according to the predominant cellular subtype. Peak incidence is in late teens and early adulthood. Osteosarcomas usually present with pain or a palpable mass of variable duration. Radiographically, osteosarcomas are lytic, metaphyseal lesions that may be permeative (Fig. 11). There may be areas of osteoblastic activity. These lesions break through the overlying cortex and extend into the soft tissues. As they do so, there is periosteal elevation that causes the classic Codman triangle. In cases of rapid tumor growth, the soft-tissue extension may show areas of bone spicules which are perpendicular to the shaft. Most osteosarcomas present as stage IIB lesions, that is, high-grade extracompartmental tumors. Before the advent of modern chemotherapeutic regimens, there was a 15% to 20% 5-year survival rate for osteosarcomas treated with amputation. Currently, long-term survival is over 50% for all patients presenting with an osteosarcoma at treating institutions specializing in orthopedic oncology. In those patients who are without known metastatic disease (stage III) at the time of presentation, the long-term survival rate is over 75%. The proximal humerus is the third most common location for osteosarcomas, after the distal femur and proximal tibia.

Classically, osteosarcomas are considered to originate from central, medullary lesions; however, some osteosarcomas may arise from surface lesions, such periosteal and parosteal osteosarcomas. These osteosarcoma variants tend to be less aggressive. On the other hand, telangiectatic osteosarcomas are particular variants that are high-grade and have a prognosis equal to conventional osteosarcomas. These are more difficult to diagnose, owing to their different radiographic appearance, as well as their microscopic and gross histologic similarities to an aneurysmal bone cyst.

Osteosarcomas may occur as primary tumors or as a secondary malignant transformation from other preexisting lesions. Common predisposing conditions include Paget's disease and sites of previous irradiation. The incidence of treatment-associated osteosarcomas (radiation induced) is up to 20% in some studies, and the patient is at increased risk throughout the remainder of their life. The mean time interval between receiving radiation and the development of secondary osteosarcoma is approximately 15 years. Because radiation is used for a variety of conditions, both benign and malignant, long-term morbidity from its use must be considered whenever radiotherapy is contemplated. It is recommended that radiation be used in those lesions that are considered to be radiosensitive, such as Ewing's sarcoma, or

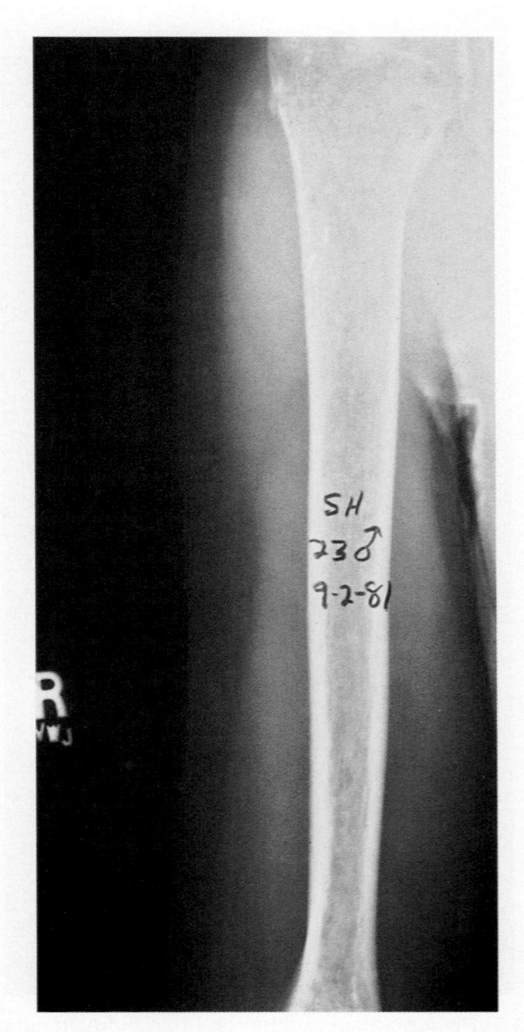

FIG. 11. Preoperative radiograph of an osteosarcoma involving the proximal humerus in a 23-year-old man. There is destruction of the humeral head, with tumor extension into the proximal diaphysis.

those lesions that are considered to be surgically unresectable. In patients with known Paget's disease, the onset of increased pain or swelling should be highly suggestive of malignant degeneration. The risk for malignant transformation in those patients with Paget's disease is 1%. The osteosarcomas that occur as secondary lesions tend to be more aggressive, with a worse prognosis than most primary osteosarcomas.

Once biopsy is performed to confirm the diagnosis, neoadjuvant chemotherapy is instituted. Preoperative studies including plain radiographs, CT scans of the extremity and lungs, MRI, and scanograms are obtained. The CT and MRI scans are used to determine the extent of tumor, soft-tissue extension, and the presence of skip lesions. These imaging studies are used to determine ability to perform a limb-salvage procedure. The scanograms are used in the design of prostheses following resection to equalize limb lengths (Fig. 12).

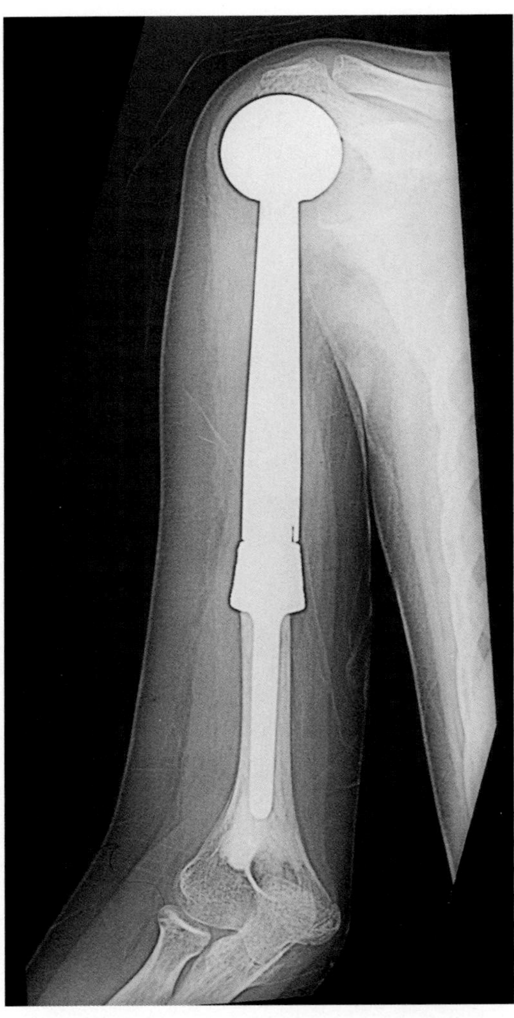

FIG. 12. Postoperative radiograph of endoprosthetic reconstruction, using a modular replacement system. Length of resection is determined preoperatively, using an MRI. The extremity is reconstructed, using a prosthesis to recreate equal limb lengths.

Chondrosarcoma

Chondrosarcomas are identified by the presence of proliferating cartilagenous cells. These tumors may also produce other stromal elements, and areas may be myxomatous, calcified, or have fibrosarcomatous cells. In contrast with osteosarcomas, chondrosarcomas tend to be less aggressive and have a slower clinical course. Metastases are less frequent and generally occur later in the disease process, although these lesions have a high propensity for local recurrence. Chondrosarcomas may develop as primary, de novo lesions; however, it is far more common for these lesions to arise as secondary chondrosarcomas from preexisting lesions.[39] Enchondromas, especially multiple enchondromas, are the most common preexisting lesion leading to secondary chondrosarcomas. Chondrosarcomas may arise from osteochondromas; however, this occurs less commonly. Chondrosarcomas develop primarily in the adult and elderly age group. Chondrosarcomas are common in the humerus and shoulder. These lesions usually present with pain, and the onset of pain in a known preexisting lesion is strongly suggestive of malignant degeneration.

Radiographically, chondrosarcomas frequently have a typical appearance of medullary destruction combined with areas of mottled calcifications. Malignant transformation may be seen as an area of lucency within a classic enchondroma. Secondary degeneration from an enchondroma is usually preceded by growth of the lesion, a change in the calcification pattern, periosteal reaction, or significant endosteal scalloping. Endosteal scalloping may be seen with chondrosarcomas; however, this finding alone is less suggestive of malignancy. Malignant degeneration of an osteochondroma should be considered when the cartilagenous cap exceeds 2 cm in thickness, or if there is a change in the thickness of the cap that occurs after skeletal maturity.

The mainstay of treatment in chondrosarcomas involves wide surgical resection of the lesion. Chondrosarcomas generally do not respond to adjuvant therapies, such as chemotherapy and radiation, except in high-grade lesions. Local spread of tumor cells or an intralesional excision of a chondrosarcoma has a high likelihood of local recurrence; therefore, particular care must be taken to not enter the tumor at the time of the resection. In addition, in those patients for whom the diagnosis is uncertain and an intralesional procedure is being performed—for example, curettage of a presumed enchondroma—the wound should be packed off to minimize tumor spillage in case the ultimate pathology indicates malignancy.

Ewing's Sarcoma

Although the exact etiology of Ewing's tumors is unclear, it is suspected that the primary cell type may be either neuroectodermal[8] or undifferentiated mesenchymal in origin. Characteristic histology shows a small, round-cell tumor that has little intervening stroma. The cells appear uniform, with little pleomorphism, anaplasia, and few mitotic figures. The humerus and scapula are frequently involved. The peak age incidence is in the second decade. Pain is the most common presenting sign, and occasionally, a mass is palpable. These tumors may also have systemic symptoms, including fevers, chills, elevated white blood cell (WBC) count and erythrocyte sedimentation rate, and anemia. The radiographs show a lytic process that is permeative with poor margination, and possible cortical expansion. There may be prominent periosteal reaction, caused by spread of tumor beyond the cortex. This typically appears as lamellations, ("onion skinning"). On MRI, a soft-tissue mass is common. Because of the systemic symptoms, the radiographic appearance, and the gross pathologic appearance of the tumor mimicking pus, Ewing's sarcomas may be mistaken for osteomyelitis.

Previously, these tumors were among the most lethal of osseous tumors. Fortunately, with newer chemotherapeutic agents in conjunction with radiation, there has been a dramatic improvement in long-term survival rates. These tumors are extremely sensitive to chemotherapy and radiation, and it is common for the entire soft-tissue extension to "melt away" and for the bone involvement to appear normal following medical treatment. As a result, an MRI should be obtained before initiating treatment to assess the medullary extent of tumor, and for possible neurovascular involvement. The medullary extent determines the proper level of resection, and neurovascular involvement with tumor before treatment may preclude limb salvage surgery. The role of surgical resection has been questioned, because of the excellent response to medical therapy in most Ewing's sarcomas; however, it is generally believed that wide resection following medical therapy is indicated.[2,31,35,41] For many Ewing's sarcomas of the proximal humerus, wide resection followed by reconstruction, using a limb salvage technique, is successful.

Myeloma

Myeloma is the most common primary malignant tumor of bone. In contrast, the orthopedic surgeon is infrequently called on to manage these tumors. This tumor is composed of a malignant proliferation of plasma cells. When the tumor is limited to one site, the tumor is called a plasmacytoma. When polyostotic involvement is present, then this lesion is called multiple myeloma. These tumors are usually seen in patients older than 50 years of age, and it is distinctly rare to see a patient with myeloma who is younger than the age of 40 years. Symptoms are usually related to increasing pain of several months' duration.[30] Fatigue, malaise, and weight loss are common. Initial presentation may be a pathologic fracture. Occasionally, other presenting symptoms occur, including neurologic compromise or polyneuropathy, renal compromise, bleeding diatheses, or fever. A soft-tissue mass may be palpable. Blood tests may show anemia, a significantly elevated erthyrocyte sedimentation rate, and hypercalcemia. When tested, Bence Jones proteins in the urine may be found in approximately 50% of patients. Immunoelectrophoresis of serum and urinary proteins provide critical information for the diagnosis. Radiographically, myelomas present with a lytic lesion of bone. There is little surrounding sclerosis and the lesions are well demarcated, giving them the appearance of a "punched-out" lesion. The cortex may be slightly expanded. Histologically, myeloma consists of uniformly packed cells, with little intervening stroma. The cells have the appearance of a plasma cell, with abundant, granular basophilic cytoplasm, and an eccentrically placed nucleus. This gives these cells the appearance of a "fried egg."

The overall prognosis is bleak for patients with myeloma. Many patients with myeloma die within 2 years of diagnosis. A plasmacytoma is considered to be the precursor for disseminated disease. Radiation is the treatment of choice for solitary lesions or patients at risk for pathologic fracture in non-weight–bearing extremities. Chemotherapy is reserved for multiple lesions. Orthopedic intervention is needed in cases of pathologic fracture, impending pathologic fracture in weight-bearing bones, and for spinal decompression in cases of neurologic compromise. The treatment of a pathologic fracture is similar to that of a metastatic carcinoma. This involves curettage and internal fixation, with supplemental cementation of the defect. Surgical resection has not been of benefit for long-term survival.

TUMORLIKE CONDITIONS OF BONE

Aneurysmal Bone Cyst

The aneurysmal bone cyst (ABC) is probably related to a reactive nonneoplastic process and is best not considered as a primary bone tumor. The exact etiology, however, is unknown. It has been suggested that ABCs occur as a result of a vascular disturbance within bone.[24] In addition, the lesion frequently regresses after incomplete excision. Aneurysmal bone cysts may occur as primary lesions, or they may be associated with other conditions, such as giant cell tumors, fibrous dysplasia, chondromyxoid fibromas, and chondroblastomas. Radiographically, they appear as lytic lesions with expansion of the overlying cortex. The cortex appears as an eggshell over the lesion. Pathologic fractures are common. On CT scans, fluid–fluid levels occur frequently. The radiographic appearance may mimic other lesions, for example, giant cell tumors; however, in nearly 80% of patients, aneurysmal bone cysts occur at ages younger than 20 years. In contrast, in over 80% of patients, giant cell tumors occur after the age of 20 years. Also, if a patient has been diagnosed with an aneurysmal bone cyst that has recurred, the diagnosis should be questioned and is more likely considered to be a giant cell tumor with an aneurysmal bone cyst component. Treatment consists of curettage, bone grafting, and internal fixation when structural integrity is compromised.[19] Some authors have advocated the use of adjuvant therapies, such as cryosurgery[24,26] or polymethylmethacrylate cement.[24] When treated appropriately, the risk of recurrence is low.

Simple Bone Cysts

Like aneurysmal bone cysts, the exact etiology of simple bone cysts is unknown. A common theory is increased intramedullary venous pressure, leading to cyst formation. The proximal humerus is the most common location for these lesions. They are usually found in children and only become symptomatic when a pathologic fracture occurs. By definition, active cysts are considered to be located within 1 cm of the growth plate, whereas latent cysts are farther away. Usually, treatment initially consists of injection of methylprednisilone acetate into the cyst; however, there is a high incidence of nonhealing with this form of therapy. Alternatively, curettage and bone grafting give more reliable healing, but must be used with caution in active cysts that are juxtaposed to the growth plate. Curettage in this area may lead to physeal arrest. In these cases, injection is warranted until the cyst grows away from the physis over time.

Fibrous Dysplasia

Fibrous dysplasia arises from an abnormality in bone development. The exact etiology, however, is unknown. As the name suggests the principal histologic feature of this lesion is the occurrence of abnormal fibrous tissue within bone. The disease develops in childhood, but usually does not become symptomatic until the second decade of life. Many cases are aymptomatic and are discovered incidentally on radiographs. When symptomatic, fibrous dysplasia presents with pain or pathologic fracture in the affected extremity or joint. There may also be bone or joint deformity, limb length discrepancy, or limited and asymmetrical range of joint motion. Rarely, a patient presents with the triad of polyostotic fibrous dysplasia, cafe-au-lait spots, and precocious puberty that is indicative of Albright's syndrome. Radiographic appearance of fibrous dysplasia shows a well-demarcated zone of slightly expanded cortex and a mildly sclerotic rim. The central portion of the lesion may have a homogeneous rarefaction, classically called "ground-glass" appearance. If the condition has been long-standing, there may be bony deformity from repeated minor pathologic fractures. Histologically, there is a proliferation of fibroblasts with an abundance of collagen matrix. There are also islands of osteoid and reactive bone formation. The trabeculae are randomly arranged, giving the appearance of scattered alphabet characters or "Chinese-letters." Osteoblasts are not present at the periphery of the trabeculae, which distinquishes fibrous dysplasia from a rare condition called osteofibrous dysplasia.

Treatment is usually conservative, unless an impending pathologic fracture necessitates stabilization. In this case, curettage and bone grafting are usually performed. Treatment may be supplemented with prophylactic internal fixation when needed.[19] If degenerative joint symptoms are present, total joint arthroplasty is indicated. The fibrous dysplasia is curetted and bone grafting is performed as needed. In the past, irradiation has been used as a form of treatment; however, benefit is questionable, and there is increased incidence of sarcomatous degeneration secondary to the radiotherapy. Therefore, irradiation is not recommended for the treatment of any fibrous dysplasia lesion.

Paget's Disease

The cause of Paget's disease is unknown, although a viral etiology is suspected. Paget's disease most commonly affects middle-aged to older individuals. Active and latent forms of the disease process are described. In the active form, bone metabolism is increased in both resorption and reparation. Early in the disease, bone resorption predominates. In the latent form of Paget's disease, the bone becomes more sclerotic and relatively less active. With progression of the disease, the bone may develop deformity; hence, the older term of osteitis deformans for Paget's disease. Histologically, broad trabeculae are present, frequently with immature lamellar bone. An increased fibrovascular stroma is present, and a prominent osteoclast activity may be seen. Paget's disease is usually treated with medical management, except in cases of secondary degenerative arthritis owing to deformity. Surgical treatment, then, is joint arthroplasty. In rare cases of Paget's disease, malignant transformation can occur, usually to an osteosarcoma. With malignant transformation, radiographically bone destruction is frequently observed, but this transformation may be difficult to diagnose, because of the underlying abnormal bone appearance. Bone scans may be difficult to interpret in the case of malignancy, because the varying stages of Paget's disease process will show different activity levels. Malignancy should be suspected in patients who have a change in the level of pain in an extremity affected by Paget's, or if there are radiographic changes, including cortical expansion or disruption and pathologic fracture.

REFERENCES

1. Aboulafia AJ, Rosenbaum DH, Sicard-Rosenbaum L, Jelinek JS, Malawer MM. Treatment of large subchondral tumors of the knee with cryosurgery and composite reconstruction. *Clin Orthop* 1994; 307: 189–199.
2. Bacci G, Toni A, Avella M, et al. Long-term results in 144 localized Ewing's sarcoma patients treated with combined therapy. *Cancer* 1989; 63:1477–1486.
3. Bettelli G, Capanna R, Van Horn JR, Ruggieri P, Biagini R, Campanacci M. Osteoid osteoma and osteoblastoma of the pelvis. *Clin Orthop* 1989;247:261–271.
4. Bollini G, Jouve JL, Gentet JC, Jacquemier M, Bouyala JM. Bone lesions in histiocytosis X. *J Pediatr Orthop* 1991;11:469–477.
5. Capanna R, Fabbri N, Bettelli G. Curettage of giant cell tumor of bone. The effect of surgical technique and adjuvants on local recurrence rate. *Chir Org Mov* 1990;75(suppl 1):206.
6. Capanna R, Sudanese A, Baldini N, Campanacci M. Phenol as an adjuvant in the control of local recurrence of benign neoplasms of bone treated by curettage. *Ital J Orthop Traumatol* 1985;11:381–388.
7. Dahlin DC, Cupps RE, Johnson EW Jr. Giant-cell tumor: a study of 195 cases. *Cancer* 1970;25:1061–1070.

8. Devaney K, Abbondanzo SL, Shekitka KM, Wolov RB, Sweet DE. MIC2 detection in tumors of bone and adjacent soft tissues. *Clin Orthop* 1995;310:176–187.
9. Eckardt JJ, Eilber FR, Jinnah RH, Mirra JM. Endoprosthetic reconstruction of the scapula including the shoulder joint, for malignant tumors: a preliminary report. In: Enneking WF, ed. *Limb salvage in musculoskeletal oncology*. New York: Churchill Livingstone, 1987.
10. Eckardt JJ, Yang RS, Ward WG, Kelly C, Eilber FR. Endoprosthetic reconstruction for malignant bone tumors and nonmalignant tumorous conditions of bone. In: *Advances in operative orthopaedics*. St Louis: Mosby Year Book, 1995:61–83.
11. Eilber F, Guiliano A, Eckardt JJ, Patterson K, Mosely S, Goodnight J. Adjuvant chemotherapy for osteosarcoma: a randomized prospective trial. *J Clin Oncol* 1987;5:21.
12. Enneking WF, Spanier SS, Goodman M. Current concepts review: surgical staging of musculoskeletal sarcoma. *J Bone Joint Surg [Am]* 1980;62:1027–1030.
13. Freedman EL, Hak DJ, Johnson EE, Eckardt JJ. Total knee replacement including a modular distal femoral component in elderly patients with acute fracture or nonunion. *J Orthop Trauma* 1995;9:231–237.
14. Gitelis S, Mallin BA, Piasecki P, Turner F. Intralesional excision compared with en bloc resection for giant-cell tumors of bone. *J Bone Joint Surg [Am]* 1993;75:1648–1655.
15. Greis PE, Hankin FM. Eosinophilic granuloma. The management of solitary lesions of bone. *Clin Orthop* 1990;257:204–211.
16. Goldenberg RR, Cambell CJ, Bonfiglio M. Giant cell tumor of bone. An analysis of two hundred and eighteen cases. *J Bone Joint Surg [Am]* 1970;52:619–664.
17. Hamilton A, Davis RI, Nixon JR. Synovial chondrosarcoma complicating synovial chondromatosis. Report of a case and review of the literature. *J Bone Joint Surg [Am]* 1987;69:1084–1088.
18. Hardacker J, Mindell ER. Synovial chondromatosis with secondary subluxation of the hip. A case report. *J Bone Joint Surg [Am]* 1991;73: 1405–1407.
19. Jaffe KA, Dunham WK. Treatment of benign lesions of the femoral head and neck. *Clin Orthop* 1990;257:134–137.
20. Leeson MC, Lippitt SB. Thermal aspects of the use of polymethylmethacrylate in large metaphyseal defects in bone. A clinical review and laboratory study. *Clin Orthop* 1993;295:239–245.
21. Li WK, Lane JM, Rose G, et al. Pelvis Ewing's sarcoma. *J Bone Joint Surg [Am]* 1983;65:738–747.
22. Lichtenstein L. Histiocytosis X: integration of eosinophilic granuloma of bone, "Letterer-Siwe" and "Schüller-Christian disease" as related manifestations of a single nosologic entity. *Arch Pathol* 1953;56: 84–102.
23. Malawer MM, Dunham W. Cryosurgery and acrylic cementation as surgical adjuncts in the treatment of aggressive (benign) bone tumors. Analysis of 25 patients below the age of 21. *Clin Orthop* 1991;262: 42–57.
24. Malawer MM. Tumors of the shoulder girdle: technique of resection and description of a surgical classification. *Orthop Clin North Am* 1991;22:7–35.
25. Marcove RC, Lyden JP, Huvos AG, Bullough PB. Giant cell tumors treated by cryosurgery. A report of twenty-five cases. *J Bone Joint Surg [Am]* 1973;55:1633–1644.
26. Marcove RC, Sheth DS, Takemoto S, Healey JH. The treatment of aneurysmal bone cyst. *Clin Orthop* 1995;311:157–163.
27. Marcove RC, Weis LD, Vaghaiwalla MR, Pearson R. Cryosurgery in the treatment of giant cell tumors of bone. A report of 52 consecutive cases. *Clin Orthop* 1978;134:275–289.
28. Masada K, Tsuyuguchi Y, Kawai H, Kawabata H, Noguchi K, Ono K. Operations for forearm deformity caused by multiple osteochondromas. *J Bone Joint Surg [Br]* 1989;71:24–29.
29. Maurice H, Crone M, Watt I. Synovial chondromatosis. *J Bone Joint Surg [Br]* 1988;70:807–811.
30. Mundy GR, Yoneda T. Facilitation and suppression of bone metastasis. *Clin Orthop* 1995;312:34–44.
31. Nesbit ME Jr, Gehan EA, Burgert EO Jr, et al. Multimodal therapy for the management of primary, nonmetastatic Ewing's sarcoma of bone: a long-term follow-up of the First Intergroup Study. *J Clin Oncol* 1990; 8:1664–1674.
32. Perry BE, McQueen DA, Lin JJ. Synovial chondromatosis with malignant degeneration to chondrosarcoma. Report of a case. *J Bone Joint Surg [Am]* 1988;70:1259–1261.
33. Peterson HA. Deformities and problems of the forearm in children with multiple hereditary osteochondromata. *J Pediatr Orthop* 1994;14: 92–100.
34. Peterson HA. Multiple hereditary osteochondromata. *Clin Orthop* 1989;239:222–230.
35. Pritchard DJ. Indications for surgical treatment of localized Ewing's sarcoma of bone. *Clin Orthop* 1980;153:39–43.
36. Rosen G, Marcove RC, Caparios B, Nirenberg A, Kosloff C, Huvos AG. Primary osteogenic sarcoma. The rationale for preoperative chemotherapy and delayed surgery. *Cancer* 1979;43:2163.
37. Rosen G, Marcove RC, Huvos AG, et al. Primary osteogenic sarcoma: eight year experience with adjuvant chemotherapy. *J Cancer Res Clin Oncol* 1983;106(suppl):55–67.
38. Schajowicz F, McGuire MH. Diagnostic difficulties in skeletal pathology. *Clin Orthop* 1989;240:281–310.
39. Schmale GA, Conrad EU III, Raskind WH. The natural history of hereditary multiple exostoses. *J Bone Joint Surg [Am]* 1994;76:986–92.
40. Ward WG, Eckardt JJ, Shayestehfar S, Mirra J, Grogan T, Oppenheim W. Osteoid osteoma diagnosis and management with low morbidity. *Clin Orthop* 1993;291:229–235.
41. Wilkins RM, Pritchard DJ, Burgert EO Jr, Unni KK. Ewing's sarcoma of bone. Experience with 140 patients. *Cancer* 1986; 58:2551–2555.
42. Wirganowicz PZ, Watts HG. Surgical risk for the elective excision of benign exostoses. *J Pediatr Orthop* 1997;

PART XI

Infection

Disorders of the Shoulder: Diagnosis and Management,
edited by Joseph P. Iannotti and Gerald R. Williams.
Lippincott Williams & Wilkins, Philadelphia © 1999.

CHAPTER 34

Sepsis of the Shoulder Girdle

Virak Tan, Matthew D. Pepe, and John L. Esterhai, Jr.

This chapter will address the issue of diagnosis and management of infections involving the shoulder. The major focus is on primary pyarthrosis of the glenohumeral joint. We will also discuss shoulder sepsis associated with osteomyelitis, septic subacromial bursitis, soft-tissue infection, infections involving the sternoclavicular and acromioclavicular joints, and postsurgical complications. No attempt has been made to specifically include Lyme disease, brachial plexus neuritis, or nonsuppurative (viral, fungal, or mycobacterial) infections, which may be part of the differential diagnoses of an infected shoulder joint. For the purpose of presentation, the topic is subdivided into pathophysiology, specific clinical entities, evaluation techniques, treatment, authors' preferred treatment, prognosis, and directions for further study.

PATHOPHYSIOLOGY

Septic arthritis of the shoulder is an inflammation of the glenohumeral joint-involving one or more foreign pathogens that cause, or are suspected of causing, the inflammation. These pathogens can be bacteria, viruses, fungi, or parasites, and can gain access to the joint through a number of different means. The defense mechanisms of the host and the properties of the invading organism play an important part in the pathophysiology of septic arthritis, as does the premorbid condition of the joint. Chronic arthritis and trauma resulting in soft-tissue damage can predispose a joint to infection.

Joint sepsis may be classified according to pathogenesis. There are three basic mechanisms: direct inoculation, con-

V. Tan, M. D. Pepe and J. L. Esterhai: Department of Orthopaedic Surgery, Hospital of the University of Pennsylvania, Philadelphia, Pennsylvania 19104.

tiguous spread from adjacent osteomyelitis, and hematogenous dissemination.

Hematogenous Septic Arthritis

Hematogenous dissemination from another organ system, such as skin breakdown, urinary system infections, or pneumonia, is the most common. In over 50% of patients with intraarticular sepsis, there is a positive blood culture.[50] Goldenberg and Cohen isolated the pathogen from a distant focus in 50% of the cases.

In the shoulder, branches of the suprascapular and subscapular arteries, along with the medial and lateral circumflex humeral arteries, form an extracapsular arterial ring, which supplies the proximal humerus. This anastamosis gives off branches, which penetrate the capsule and form an intraarticular synovial ring.[62] This has been termed the transition zone and is located between the synovium and the articular surface.[113] It is in this area that the arterioles loop acutely toward the periphery, causing a low-flow state, making the area more susceptible to receptor-specific interaction of the pathogen and the cell surface.

Spontaneous shoulder sepsis is the result of joint invasion during bacteremia. Septic arthritis has been shown to occur in experimental animals when bacteremia is created.[82] The abundance of the synovial vasculature and the absence of a basement membrane between the endothelial cells make synovial joints vulnerable to seeding by bacteria. Furthermore, most patients with hematogenous nongonococcal bacterial arthritis have at least one underlying chronic medical risk factor. These factors may be local, such as prosthetic and metallic implants, or they may be systemic, such as cancer, cirrhosis, rheumatoid arthritis, and intermittent bacteremic episodes from intravenous drug abuse or indwelling catheters[51] (Table 1).

Direct Inoculation

Direct inoculation may be traumatic or iatrogenic. Repeated corticosteroid injections[3] (Fig. 1), arthroscopy,[8] and open surgical procedures, such as rotator cuff repair and arthroplasty, have been shown to be associated with pyarthrosis of the shoulder. The incidence of infection following intraarticular steroid injection is extremely small. Hollander reported 18 infections in 250,000 injections,[68] and Gray found only two cases complicating 100,000 injections.[54] The advent of sterile disposable needles and syringes and adherence to meticulous aseptic technique helped lessen the risk. The existence of foreign bodies in or around the joint, such as nonabsorbable suture, stainless steel, cobalt chrome alloys, methylmethacrylate, and polyethylene, or devitalized bone from trauma, has provided a nidus for adhesion and colonization by bacteria.[56,60,62] This nidus allows a glycocalyx biofilm to be expressed by the bacteria, which contributes to antibiotic resistance and limits the effectiveness of the immune response of the host.

TABLE 1. *Risk factors in bacterial arthritis*

Host phagocytic defects
Complement deficiencies
Inherited disorders of chemotaxis or intracellular killing
Impaired host defense mechanism
Immunosuppressive drugs and glucocorticoids
Cancer
Chronic debilitating illness
Hypogammaglobulinemia
Direct penetration
Puncture wounds
IVDA
Joint damage
Chronic arthritis
Total or hemiarthroplasty
Other prior surgery

Septic Arthritis from Contiguous Osteomyelitis

Osteomyelitis is most often hematogenous in origin, and, in particular, is a disease of young children and the elderly. Hematogenous osteomyelitis commonly involves the metaphyseal area of rapidly growing long bones, usually occurring in the hip and knee.[94] When septic arthritis results from a contiguous infection such as osteomyelitis, it spreads from the bone to synovium, then to the joint space. This happens most often in infancy, when there is a vascular anastomosis between the epiphysis and the metaphysis. Studies conducted on the proximal femur by Trueta[128] showed a direct vascular communication between metaphyseal arterioles and the epiphyseal ossicle before 8 months of age. This allows a direct hematogenous communication between an osteomyelitis of the metaphysis and the adjacent joint synovium.[97] Between the ages of 8 and 18 months, the last vestiges of the nutrient artery system close down at the growth plate, reaching sinusoidal veins and causing a low-flow state. The open physis at this point provides an effective barrier to the spread of infection to the joint by obliterating this vascular anastomosis.[121] This situation is analogous in the proximal humerus.

At skeletal maturity, there is once again a direct osseous connection between the metaphysis and epiphysis, secondary to closing of the growth plate and reestablishment of anastomoses between the metaphyseal and epiphyseal arterioles.[4] Therefore, infection of the proximal humeral metaphysis may extend to the epiphysis and the joint through the haversian system and Volkmann canals. In addition, the proximal 10 to 12 mm of the metaphysis of the proximal humerus is intraarticular, giving the pathogens of metaphyseal osteomyelitis direct access to the synovium.

Although, in his study of the vascular supply of the proximal femur, Chung did not find direct communication between metaphyseal and epiphyseal vessels, he did demonstrate two collateral, extraosseous arterial anastomoses. One was intracapsular and subsynovial, whereas the other was extracapsular. These showed age-related changes, which he

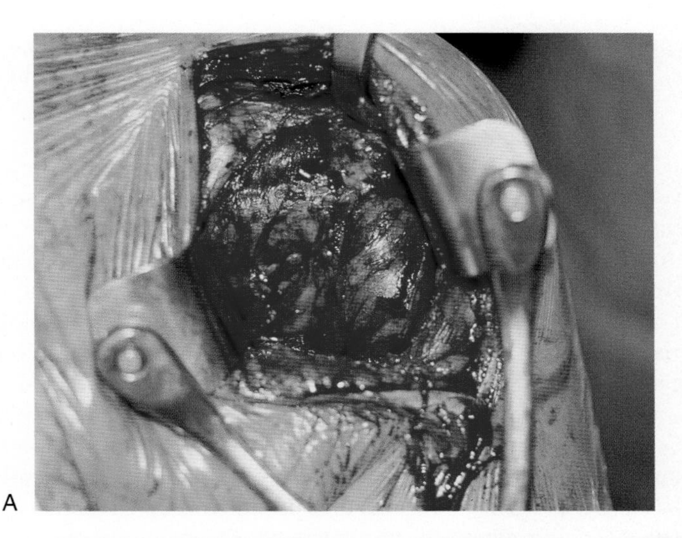
A

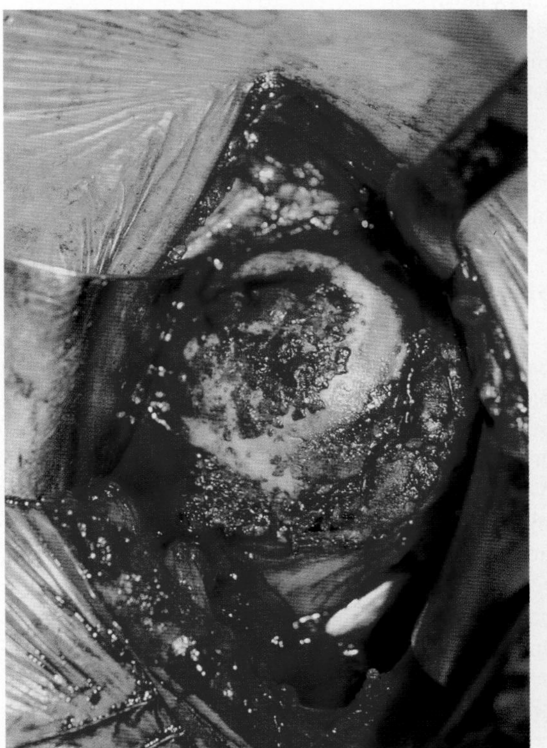
B

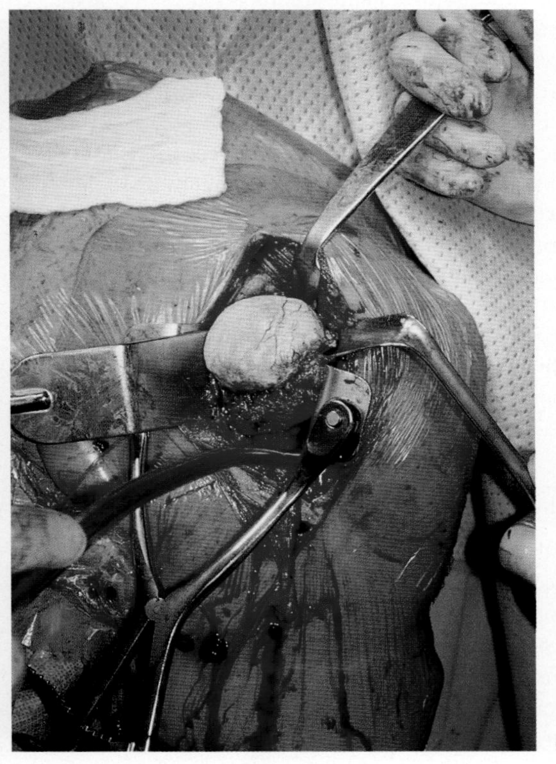
C

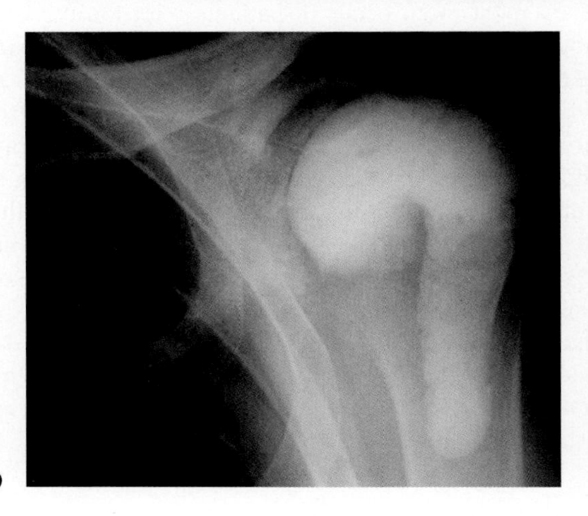
D

FIG. 1. (A and B) Acute septic shoulder from corticosteroid injection for treatment of endstage degenerative arthritis. This patient was treated with resection of the humeral head, capsulectomy, and extensive debridement of all infected tissues. **(C and D)** A tobramycin cement spacer was placed for 6 months, and the patient was given 6 weeks of intravenous antibiotics. At 6 months postdebridement, the patient was converted to a total shoulder arthroplasty (TSA) with tobramycin cement. The patient is now 12 months post-TSA treatment without signs of infection, has minimal pain, active shoulder elevation to 120 degrees, and an intact rotator cuff. (Courtesy of J.P. Iannotti, M.D., Ph.D.)

attributed to growth and changes in the position of the epiphyseal plate.[21]

Synovial Tissue and Infection

The anatomy of the shoulder joint is intricately involved in the pathogenesis of sepsis. All synovial joints contain synovial fluid, which can act as an excellent growth medium for bacteria and have a relative lack of immunologic resistance.[38] Type B synoviocytes are weakly phagocytic but in most cases are able to limit and clear a blood-borne bacterial infection.[7] Therefore, there must be an imbalance between normal synovial cell function and the invading bacteria, in order for an intraarticular infection to develop.

Synovial tissue is relatively resistant to infection.[7] Examination of joints in which experimental septic arthritis has been produced reveals infrequent colonization of the synovium.[132] Receptors for collagen have been found on several strains of *Staphylococcus aureus*. It may be a lack of ligands or a functional host resistance mechanism that helps to prevent synovial colonization.[62]

Microscopic examination of the synovium shows that it is relatively thin in the area of the transition zone, rarely being more than three or four cell layers thick. The synovial capillaries are superficial, making them more susceptible to trauma. The lack of epithelial tissue in the synovium, and thus the lack of a basement membrane, means that there is no structural barrier to the spread of bacteria from the synovium to the joint. This transient bacteremia and trauma causing intraarticular hemorrhage can play a role in the pathogenesis of septic arthritis.[62]

Bacterial Adhesion

Integral to the pathogenesis of infectious arthritis is the preferential colonization of bacteria to articular cartilage, traumatized bone, or biomaterials that are not integrated with the healthy tissues composed of living cells and extracellular matrix proteins.[60,62,116,122] Bacterial adhesion involves either very specific receptor–ligand, receptor–lectin–ligand chemical interaction, or nonspecific interaction based on charge-related, hydrophobic, and extracellular polysaccharide-based interactions.[59] *S. aureus*, has receptors for types I and II collagen,[120] fibrinogen, laminin, fibronectin, thrombospondin, bone sialoprotein, and heparin sulfate.[94] Many factors influence the adherence properties of bacteria, including (a) the surface energy and surface free energy of the bacteria and biomaterial, (b) the extracellular components of the bacteria, (c) the bacterial interaction in mixed infections, (d) the host immune system, and (e) the extracellular matrix.[38]

All natural, biologic surfaces, with the exception of teeth and articular cartilage, are protected by epithelium, endothelium, or periosteum, which decreases bacterial adhesion by desquamation or by the presence of host extracellular polysaccharide molecules. *Staphylococcus aureus* is the natural colonizer of cartilage and collagen, because it has specific surface-associated adhesins[28] for sites on collagen, not for enamel. Although the colonization of teeth by *Streptococcus mutans* is a natural symbiotic process that can be slowly destructive, the bacterial colonization of articular cartilage is unnatural and is rapidly destructive.[45,62]

Bacterial adherence is characterized by the production of an extracellular exopolysaccharide, within which the bacteria aggregate and multiply. Bacteria in aquatic environments grow predominantly in these biofilm-enclosed microcolonies adherent to surfaces.[57] Following initial colonization, the microcolonies develop coherent and continuous biofilms[40] that contain more than 99.9% of the bacteria in thick layers, within which they are protected from antibacterial agents[27,57,58] and the host immune defenses. This glycocalyx allows the bacteria to modify their local environment, limiting both the specific and the nonspecific arms of the immune response. Bacteria adherent to bone, methylmethacrylate, orthopedic devices, and surrounding tissue are harder to completely eradicate until the infected tissue and biomaterial are removed. Not infrequently, the infections are polymicrobial and difficult to culture adequately, unless special techniques are used.[50,56,58,59]

Microbiology

Patient age and host states help predict the bacterial etiology of septic arthritis. Those organisms that frequently cause bacteremia in certain age groups are usually the infecting organisms, since joint sepsis is most commonly caused by hematogenous seeding. However, certain organisms, such as *Neisseria gonorrhoeae* and *S. aureus*, seem to have an avidity for the synovium, causing septic arthritis out of proportion to their incidence of bacteremia.[121] *Staphylococcus aureus* is the most common cause of adult, nongonococcal bacterial arthritis, occurring in up to 50% of patients.[80] Ward and Goldner[134] noted 77% of infecting organisms to be gram positive, of which 46% were *S. aureus*. Joint infections with gram-negative bacilli have been increasing in incidence, ranging from 5% to 30% of all shoulder infections.[37,44,80,126] They most often occur in patients with intravenous drug abuse, malignancy, diabetes, immunosuppression, or hemoglobinopathy.[121] *Escherichia coli* and *Proteus* species are common infecting gram-negative organisms from the urinary tract, and occur in patients who are not intravenous drug abusers. Although *Pseudomonas* and *Serratia* are the common organisms in intravenous drug addicts, the incidence of *S. aureus* in this population has been increasing.[6,13,37] *Streptococcus pneumoniae* is the most common organism in patients with chronic alcoholism and hypogammaglobulinemia.[95] Polymicrobial infections of the shoulder occur in 5% to 15% of patients, often associated with an extraarticular polymicrobial infection or penetrating trauma, especially in immunocompromised patients.[107]

Incidence

The incidence of shoulder sepsis is increasing as the population ages and the prevalence of chronic, debilitating disease increases.[80,126] Currently, primary shoulder sepsis accounts for 10% to 15% of all joint infections, whereas the hip and the knee account for 20% to 25% and 40% to 50%, respectively.[37] Septic arthritis of the shoulder is a rare occurrence in the young, immunocompetent person. More frequently, it is a disease of the elderly. Most patients have chronic, systemic, immunocompromising conditions such as diabetes mellitus, blood dyscrasias, renal failure, malignancy, and malnutrition.[38,51,80,134] Local factors also play a role in some patients, such as indwelling catheters, intravenous drug use, prior joint disease (rheumatoid or osteoarthritis), trauma, bursitis, or radiation therapy.[38,51,121] Ward and Goldner reported that 74% of 27 adults with septic arthritis of the shoulder had some systemic condition causing immunocompromise or some type of local tissue abnormality. In 52% of the patients, both were present.[134]

CLINICAL ENTITIES

Natural History of Septic Arthritis

Studies conducted in animals have demonstrated that direct joint inoculation with bacteria is followed by synovial, bone, and cartilage changes within a matter of hours. Experiments have been performed on mice, rats, rabbits, chickens, and hamsters, and most have utilized direct joint inoculation. Septic arthritis caused by *S. aureus* in a rabbit model displays two processes acting simultaneously. The synovium becomes inflamed and hypertrophies within minutes of infection, with an influx of polymorphonuclear cells. This develops into an invading pannus, eroding and undermining the articular cartilage. Bacteria can be identified in and extruded by the pannus, thus maintaining the inflammatory reaction and lysosomal discharge.[106] Within 3 hours, a purulent exudate is observed, and within 24 hours multiple abscesses are seen. By day 5, synovial inflammation is so aggressive that there is extension below the cartilage interface, causing erosion and loosening in this area.

Simultaneously, by day 2, progressive loss of glycosaminoglycan occurs, as observed by a loss of safranin staining. This is most pronounced in the marginal areas near the leading edge of the pannus. The degradation of cartilage occurs through bacterial endotoxin, prostaglandins, and cytokine-mediated events that invoke a host inflammatory response and a release of destructive enzymes by synoviocytes and leukocytes.[38] Total glycosaminoglycan depletion occurs by 14 days, and the protein-polysaccharide–depleted cartilage is susteptible to degradation by collagenases released by the lysosomes.[106,135] The predominant cytokine is interleukin-1 (IL-1), which is released by synovial macrophages and circulating monocytes. IL-1 has been shown to inhibit chondrocyte proliferation and decrease expression of type II and X cartilage, making the articular cartilage more friable and susceptible to bacterial adhesion. Bremell et al., in their studies on septic arthritis in rats, noted the importance of $CD4^+$ T-lymphocytes expressing IL-2 receptors, indicating activation. Deletion of T-lymphocytes downgraded the intensity of infection, indicating a pathogenic role.[14]

If infection remains untreated for 7 to 10 days, cartilage fissuring and a decrease in height occurs, most commonly involving the weight-bearing areas. Continued infection results in joint capsule and ligament dissolution, ending in fibrous ankylosis in 5 weeks in the rabbit model.[106] Antibiotics, administered in this animal model before or at the time of inoculation, significantly reduced joint destruction.[118] Irreversible changes occurred if the joint was not sterilized within 5 days of infection.[94]

Subacromial Septic Bursitis

Pyarthrosis of the glenohumeral joint may extend into the subacromial bursa. Most commonly, the infection occurs by direct erosion through the rotator cuff (Fig. 2). However, 10% of the patients may have intact cuffs.[134]

Rarely, subacromial septic bursitis may occur in isolation, as the primary infection[125] or as a result of hematogenous seeding from a distant source of infection.[26] The diagnosis is made by aspiration of the bursa for Gram stain and culture. Aspiration is performed in an area that will likely have the highest yield, usually where there is maximal tenderness and fluctuation (Fig. 3).

Septic Arthritis of the Sternoclavicular Joint

The sternoclavicular joint is an unusual site for infection. Sternoclavicular septic arthritis usually develops in patients with an underlying medical condition or predisposing factor, such as intravenous drug abuse,[13,46,52] diabetes mellitus, rheumatoid arthritis, liver disease, alcohol abuse, renal disease, malignancy, steroid use, or infection at another site.[19,138] However, infection may occur via a hematogenous route or by direct inoculation from trauma or subclavian vein catheterization in healthy patients. Wohlgethan et al.[138] reviewed the published reports of sternoclavicular septic arthritis and found 65 cases, 19 associated with intravenous drug abuse. Approximately 20% of patients developed an abscess, regardless of the underlying condition and unrelated to the infecting organism. *Staphylococcus aureus* was the most common pathogen, responsible for infections in 37% of the cases. *Pseudomonas aeruginosa* was second, causing 23% of infections. There were associations between specific infecting organisms and predisposing conditions. *Pseudomonas* was the predominate organism in the 19 intravenous drug abusers. *Staphylococcus aureus* was responsible for infection of 8 of 10 patients with rheumatoid arthri-

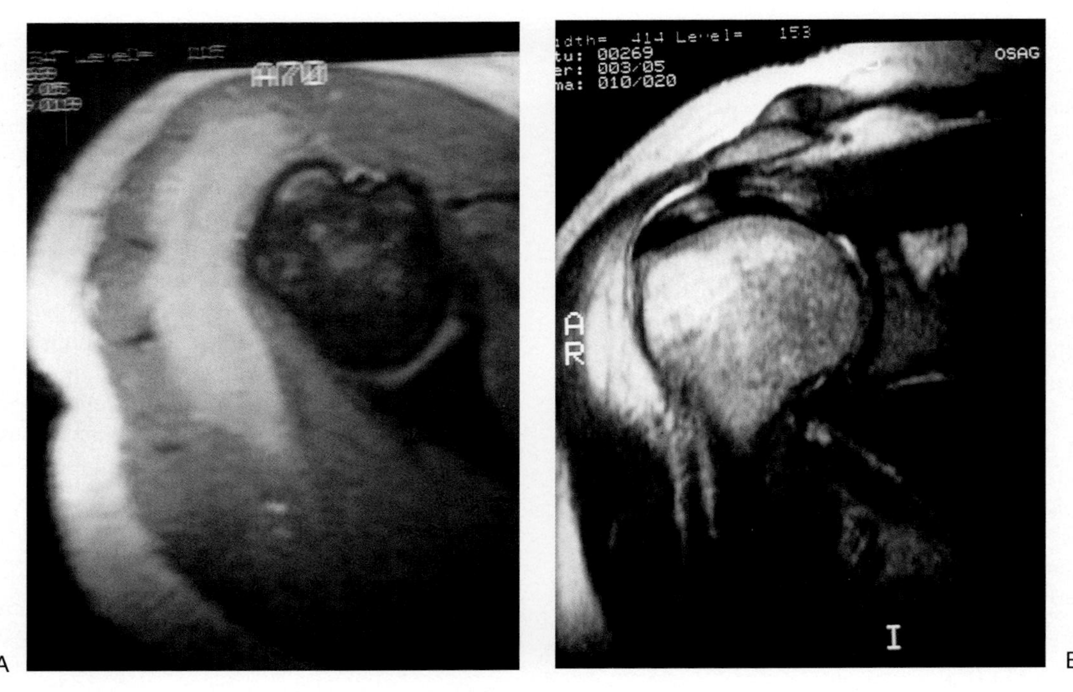

FIG. 2. (A, B) MRI of acute subacromial infection with an abscess, following open rotator cuff surgery. (Courtesy of J.P. Iannotti, M.D., Ph.D.)

tis, and 3 of 4 patients with renal failure. Of 7 patients with a history of alcohol abuse, 6 were infected with streptococci.[138]

The diagnosis of sternoclavicular septic arthritis is often difficult, and there is usually a delay between the onset of symptoms and diagnosis. Wohlgethan's review found that the duration of symptoms before diagnosis ranged from 1 day to 2 months but averaged greater than 2 weeks.[138] Symptoms most commonly involve vague pain in the anterior chest, shoulder, or neck long before other signs and symptoms occur. Fever and chills, pain on active and passive shoulder motion, swelling and tenderness over the sternoclavicular joint, and general malaise and weight loss commonly occur later.[19,42,52,138]

Infection Complicating Hemi- and Total Joint Arthroplasty

Infection of the glenohumeral joint following shoulder arthroplasty is a relatively rare, although potentially devastating, occurrence. Susceptibility is dependent on a number of host factors, such as diabetes mellitus, rheumatoid arthritis, advanced age, remote sites of infection, malnutrition, and immunosuppressive chemotherapy.[137] The reported incidence of postoperative infection from total shoulder arthroplasty ranges from 0.34% to 2.9%.[24,90] These infections can be divided into acute, subacute, or late. Acute infections are usually the result of intraoperative contamination and usually present within 3 months. Subacute infections occur

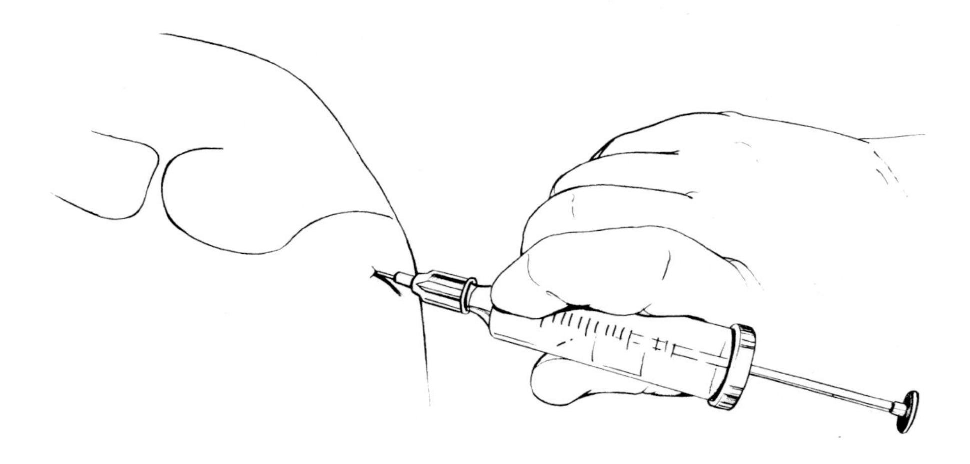

FIG. 3. Aspiration of the subacromial bursa is usually performed in an area where there is maximal tenderness and fluctuation. The needle is inserted under the acromial edge (laterally in this case) and directed slightly cephalad. This illustration also shows the outline of the acromion and acromioclavicular joint.

when there is not a routine postoperative course. An example is a case that is complicated by prolonged wound drainage or fever that spontaneously resolves. This is usually followed by evidence of infection within 12 months, with component loosening. Late infections usually represent hematogenous spread from a distant focus, but could represent a chronic infection acquired intraoperatively.[85] *Staphylococcus aureus* and *S. epidermidis* are the most common organisms involved, although *Pseudomonas* and *Candida* species have been reported in the literature.[24,83]

Antibiotic prophylaxis for the prevention of hematogenous seeding of a total joint during the transient bacteremia induced by dental or other procedures is a controversial issue. Approximately 50% of all late prosthetic joint infections are due to staphylococci. This raises the question of overemphasis being placed on infections caused by dental procedures, because *S. aureus* and *S. epidermidis* are unlikely oral pathogens.[136] Nonetheless, the consequences of prosthetic infection are so grave that bacteremic events should be avoided. In our opinion, prophylactic antibiotics should be administered in anticipation of procedures that cause bacteremia in certain instances. Animal studies have shown that the tendency toward prosthetic infection is greatest in the early postoperative period.[119] Clinical reports of infected prostheses support this finding. Over 50% of infections occur within the first 2 postoperative years.

The current recommendation is to provide prophylaxis for any patient undergoing an invasive procedure that gives the possibility of bacteremia within the first 2 years of prosthetic replacement. Regardless of the timing of the arthroplasty, a procedure performed at a distant site for an acute or chronic infectious process demands prophylaxis. Deacon et al. also believe that any patient with an immunocompromising condition, such as rheumatoid arthritis or hemophilia, should always be treated with prophylactic antibiotics.[33]

There are multiple regimens outlined in the literature, but the choice of prophylactic antibiotic depends on the normal flora of the suspected body region source.[123] The recommendations for prophylaxis during dental, head and neck, chest, and upper gastrointestinal procedures are for an oral cephalosporin, 1 g 1 hour prior to the procedure and 500 mg 4 hours after the procedure is completed.[85,123] Alternately, clindamycin and erythromycin can be used in cases of documented penicillin allergy. With high-risk biliary tract or colorectal surgery, parenteral cephalosporins should be used with clindamycin and an aminoglycoside as an alternative. Obviously, the risk of potential anaphylaxis has to be weighed against the risk of total joint infection during these procedures. Maderazo et al.[85] feel that the morbidity and possible mortality associated with a prosthetic infection warrants the small risk from the antibiotics.

Shoulder Sepsis Following Arthroscopy

Because arthroscopy of the shoulder is a sterile surgical procedure, the infection rates should be very low. They range in the literature from 0.04% to 3.4%.[8,29,74] The use of perioperative antibiotics has reduced the incidence of infection fourfold. Armstrong and Bolding, in a review of seven cases of septic arthritis following arthroscopy, noted a correlation with the use of intraarticular steroids. Four infections occurred in 101 arthroscopies during a 3-month period, and three of these involved the use of intraarticular methylprednisolone. Two of the seven infections involved the glenohumeral joint and were believed to be secondary to unsterile electrocardiogram cables contaminating the operative field. The investigators postulated that the arthroscope was inadequately disinfected between cases in the remainder of the infections. It was noted that on several occasions, the equipment was soaked for less than the 20-minute time period required for disinfection with 2% gluteraldehyde. The review by Armstrong demonstrated the importance of adequate patient, equipment, and operating room preparation.[3]

Infection Following Rotator Cuff Surgery and Open Reduction and Internal Fixation

Infection following rotator cuff repair must be diagnosed quickly and addressed expeditiously, to avoid damage to the cuff or the joint itself (Fig. 4A and B). Unfortunately, the cuff repair itself is at risk during postoperative pyarthrosis. Residual function depends on the amount and continuity of the remaining rotator cuff[101] (Fig. 4C and D). Internal fixation of fractures about the shoulder provides an environment for bacterial adhesion and glycocalyx formation, making infection more difficult to eradicate. One must also beware of the patient with postoperative drainage, slow incisional healing, and suture spitting, because occult infection following open reduction and internal fixation is one of the most common causes of infection following total shoulder arthroplasty.[63]

Septic Arthritis Superimposed on Rheumatoid Arthritis

Patients with rheumatoid arthritis are at an increased susceptibility to joint sepsis, compared with those without the disease. Their underlying chronic joint symptoms may delay the diagnosis of infection. Furthermore, the acromioclavicular joint may be involved, adding to the complexity of presentation. Gristina et al. reviewed 13 cases of septic arthritis in patients with rheumatoid arthritis and found that most presented with a sudden exacerbation of the usual arthritic pain, abrupt onset of swelling, and increased joint temperature. Only 9 of 13 were febrile. The infecting organism was *S. aureus* in 12 cases, and *E. coli* in 1 case.[61] Several factors may predispose a patient with rheumatoid arthritis to infection, including a poor overall health status with coexisting morbidities (such as diabetes), the chronic systemic administration of corticosteroids and cytotoxic drugs, and the intraarticular use of corticosteroids.[89] It also has been suggested that the synovial leukocytes of a rheumatoid may have less

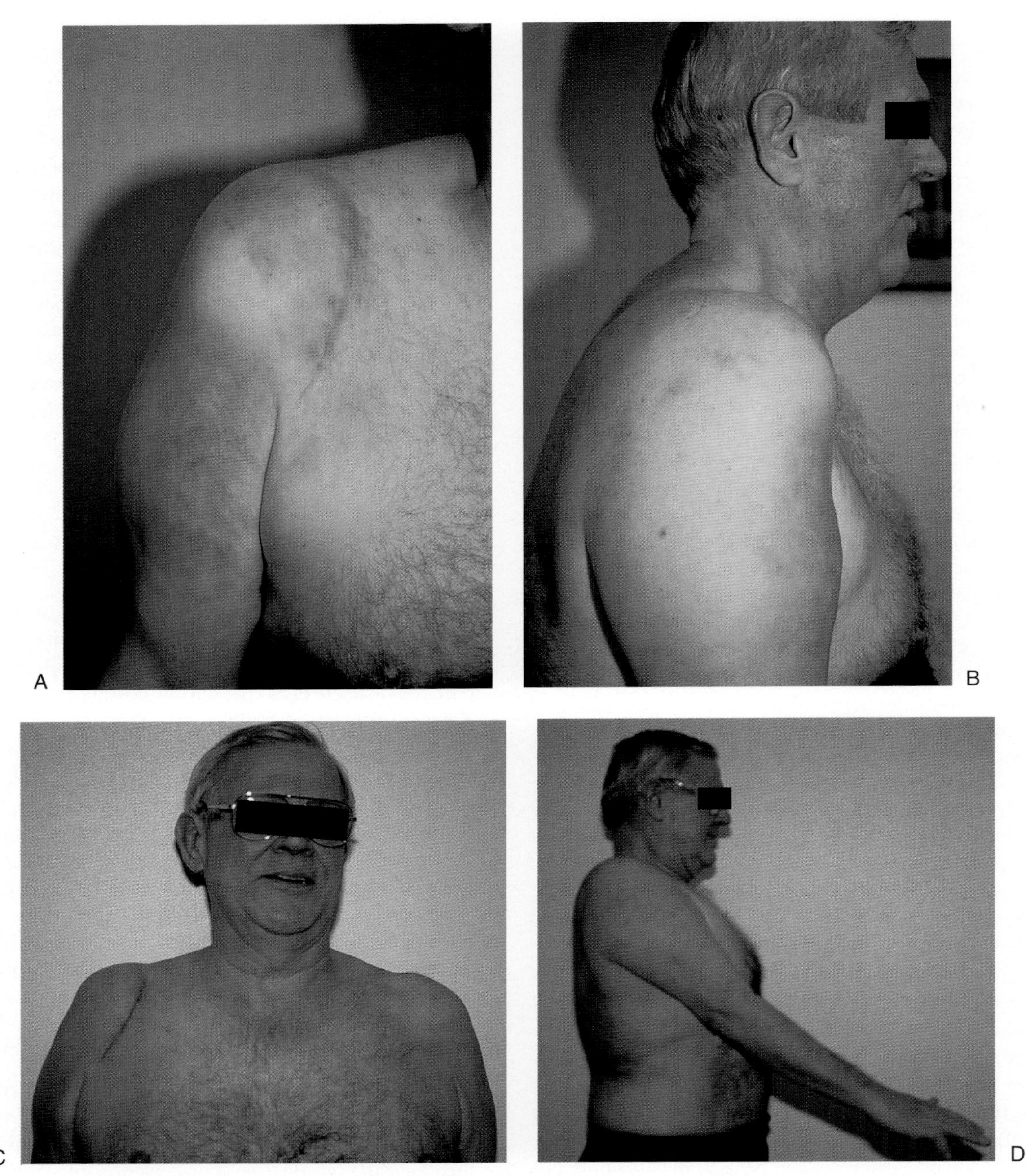

FIG. 4. (A, B) Acute infection after open rotator cuff repair. At the time of debridement of the shoulder, the cuff repair was disrupted, and the deltoid origin was detached. The shoulder was debrided, all sutures were removed. The cuff was not repaired, but the deltoid origin was repaired with absorbable suture. The patient was treated for 6 weeks with intravenous antibiotics. **(C, D)** The infection resolved with the one surgical debridement and the deltoid remained intact. Clinically, the shoulder was painless but with poor function. (Courtesy of J.P. Iannotti, M.D., Ph.D.)

phagocytic activity than normal, making their joints increasingly susceptible to sepsis.[10] The grave complication of septic arthritis should be suspected in any patient with rheumatoid arthritis when the clinical course worsens acutely, and synovial fluid should be aspirated immediately for examination. Clinical signs and symptoms are variable and inconstant, and the sedimentation rate, as well as roentgenograms, are unreliable. Upon diagnosis, prompt surgical therapy and parenteral antibiotics must be instituted, because this complication can carry a high mortality rate.

Disseminated Gonococcal Arthritis

Unlike patients with nongonoccocal shoulder sepsis, those with joint infections secondary to *N. gonorrhoeae* are generally young, healthy adults. Disseminated gonococcal infection is the most common cause of hematogenous septic arthritis of all joints. The most common clinical manifestation is a migratory polyarthralgia (70%); however, fever, tenosynovitis (67%), and dermatitis (67%) are commonly discovered on initial examination.[96] Joint aspirate yields a positive Gram stain result in only 25% of the cases, and 50% of cultures test negative.[97] Synovial fluid white cell counts are less than for nongonococcal septic arthritis, but are still greater than 50,000 white blood cells (WBC)/mm^3. Urethral, cervical, rectal, and pharyngeal cultures have a much higher yield and should be obtained from any young, sexually active patient suspected of having gonococcal arthritis. The infection shows a rapid response to ceftriaxone, and the arthritis generally resolves in 48 to 72 hours. Surgical decompression is not needed in most cases, because joint destruction is rare.

EVALUATION

Clinical Characteristics

A general workup scheme for pyarthrosis of the shoulder is outlined in Fig. 5. The typical clinical presentation of shoulder sepsis consists of complaints of pain, warmth, and swelling of the involved joint. A patient may exhibit a prodromal phase of malaise, low-grade fever, lethargy, and anorexia before the acute onset.[97] The acute phase usually consists of fevers and chills, with severe, incapacitating shoulder pain as the cardinal clinical manifestation. Physical examination reveals local signs of infection such as erythema, edema, tenderness, increased warmth, and limitation in range of motion (ROM). Previous reports have shown that fever is variably present (40% to 90% of patients), and when present may be low grade or transient.[93,107] Rosenthal noted pain in only 48 of 71 patients with septic arthritis, with limitation in ROM being the most consistent clinical sign,[121] helping to differentiate a superficial soft-tissue infection from a joint infection. Atypical presentations occur when there is chronic arthritis, immunocompromised states, extreme age, intravenous drug use, or low-grade prosthetic joint infection. Previous use of antibiotics, as well as corticosteroids or nonsteroidal antiinflammatory medication, may mask symptoms. These factors, plus the low index of suspicion for shoulder sepsis, often lead to a delay in diagnosis. Ward and Goldner, in a review of 30 patients with shoulder pyarthrosis, noted mild symptoms in the 27 adults, and a mean delay to diagnosis of 46 days.[134]

Laboratory Studies

Laboratory evaluation should consist of a peripheral WBC count with differential, erythrocyte sedimentation rate and/or C-reactive protein. The WBC count may be normal to slightly elevated and may not show a peripheral blood leukocytosis, as was demonstrated to be the case in one third of the patients with shoulder pyarthrosis described by Leslie et al.[80] Erythrocyte sedimentation rate is consistently elevated in patients with septic arthritis, but this may be elevated baseline secondary to chronic inflammatory arthritis. The C-reactive protein is an acute-phase protein produced by the liver in response to bacterial infection. It has been shown to increase more rapidly than the erythrocyte sedimentation rate, and may be of great value in the second, third, or fourth day of treatment, to evaluate recovery when the sedimentation rate is still increasing.[130] Blood cultures should be obtained from all patients with clinical signs and symptoms of systemic sepsis. In addition, cultures also should be obtained from any other possible sources of infection before antibiotics are administered.

Given the grave consequences of joint sepsis and the nonspecific clinical and laboratory findings, joint aspiration and culture are essential for making the diagnosis. The procedure must be performed with meticulous aseptic technique, preparing the skin with an iodine solution. Care must be used to enter the joint through intact, uninfected skin. An 18-gauge or larger needle should be used, so that viscous fluid can be aspirated if encountered. If difficulty accessing the joint arises, fluoroscopic guidance or contrast dye can be of assistance. Occasionally, aspirating fluid from a joint is difficult, and nonbacteriostatic saline may be injected and reaspirated, in order to obtain a sample. Joint aspiration can be painful, and appropriate analgesia and sedation (and if necessary, general anesthesia) should be used.

Synovial fluid analysis is the key to correctly diagnosing septic arthritis. The fluid should be evaluated for Gram stain, culture, cell count and differential, and polarized microscopy. Cultures should include aerobes, anaerobes, fungi, and mycobacterium. In cases where *N. gonorrhoeae* is suspected, chocolate agar or Thayer-Martin plates should be used. Ideally, the specimen is plated at the bedside; however, this will vary according to each hospital's laboratory procedures. *N. gonorrhoeae* is an extremely fastidious organism, and cultures can be negative in up to 50% of the cases. Cultures from mucosal sites should be obtained. Gram stain is only positive in 50% to 75% of patients, and the specimen should be centrifuged if a small volume is obtained.[110] Polymerase chain reaction is a technique that amplifies small amounts of bacterial DNA and provides a much higher sensitivity than culture alone. If available, it may be helpful when infection is suspected but cultures persistently remain negative.[48]

Examination of synovial fluid is an important step in the diagnosis of shoulder sepsis. Certain fluid characteristics suggest pyarthrosis, but none are absolutely specific. On gross examination, the fluid is often thick, yellow, and cloudy. Leukocyte counts are of limited use even at extreme values, because of the overlap with other types of arthritis. Values greater than 50,000 WBC/mm^3 are suggestive of bacterial arthritis, and values greater than 100,000 WBC/mm^3 are rarely from other causes. Polymorpholeukocytes are predominant, usually comprising greater than 90% of the leukocytes. Synovial fluid glucose levels may be decreased later in the process but are of limited value, unless

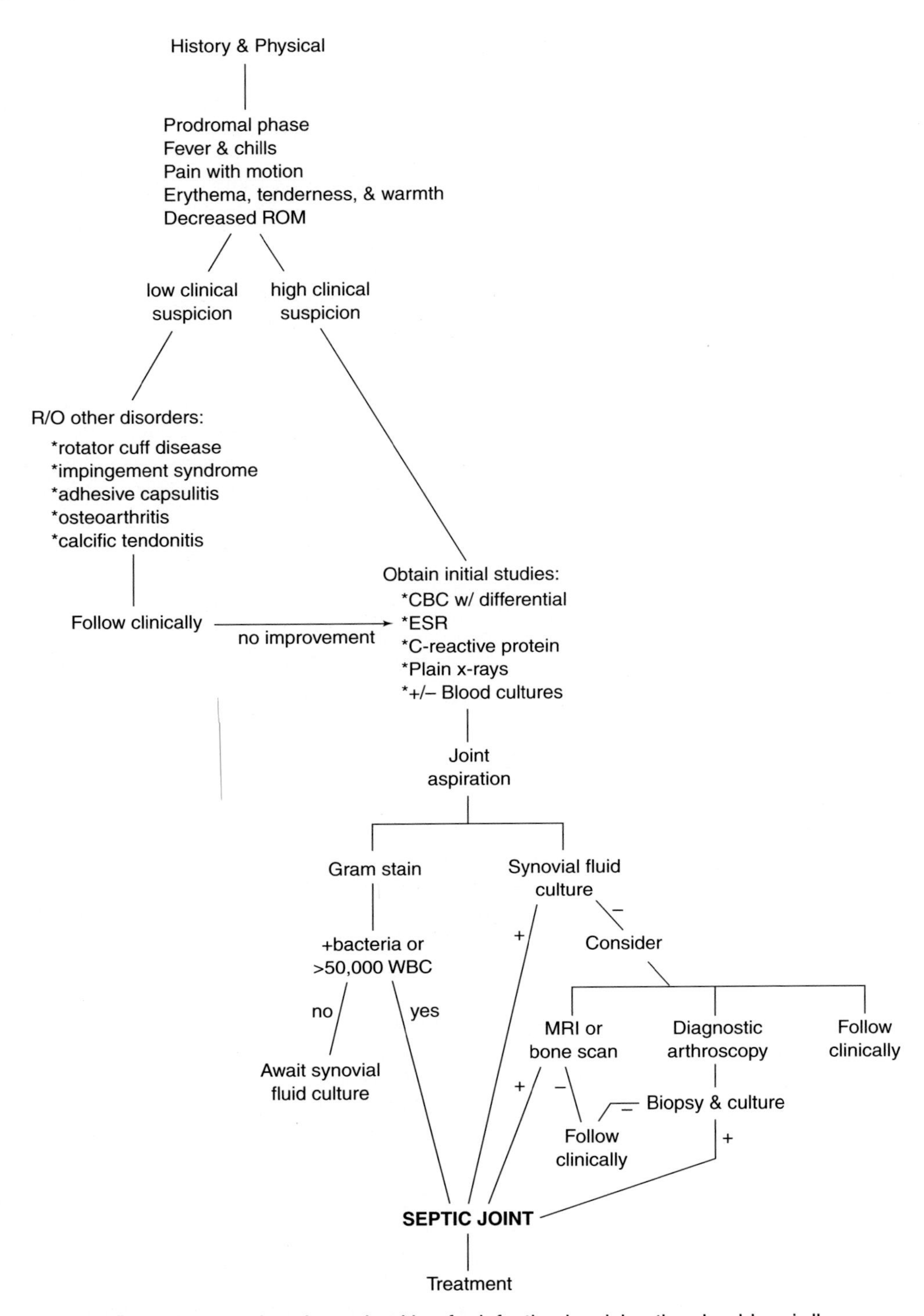

FIG. 5. A general work-up algorithm for infection involving the shoulder girdle.

serum levels are obtained at the same time and after at least 6 hours of fasting. Levels greater than 40 mg/dL below the serum level are consistent with pyarthrosis.[114] The presence of crystals in synovial fluid analysis does not rule out infection, because the two processes may coexist. Joint infection lowers the pH, occasionally causing the precipitation of urate or calcium pyrophosphate.[38] Table 2 summarizes synovial fluid findings.

Aspiration of the glenohumeral joint may be performed in one of several ways. The posterior approach (Fig. 6) may be the most commonly used route, owing to the ease of locating anatomic landmarks and the patient not being able to watch the procedure. It is performed under aseptic technique, with wide preparation of the skin with betadine. After local anesthetic is injected into the skin, muscle, and capsule, an 18-gauge spinal needle attached to a syringe is inserted 2 cm in-

TABLE 2. *Synovial fluid findings*

Synovial fluid	Normal	Noninflammatory	Inflammatory	Septic
Appearance	Clear	Clear	Opaque/translucent	Opaque, yellow/green
Viscosity	High	High	Low	Variable
WBC/mm^3	<1,000	<1,000	5,000–75,000	>50,000
Polymorphonuclear cells	<25%	<25%	>50%	>75%
Culture	Neg	Neg	Neg	Pos
Associated conditions		DJD Trauma PVNS Neuropathic SLE Acute rheumatic fever	Rheumatoid arthritis Crystal-induced arthritis Seronegative arthropathy SLE Acute rheumatic fever	Bacterial infections Immunocompromise[a]

[a] Immunocompromised patients may well not manifest an elevated synovial WBC. A normal or noninflammatory WBC does not preclude an active pyarthrosis in this patient population.

ferior and 2 cm medial to the posterolateral edge of the acromion. The needle is advanced in the direction of the coracoid process until the joint is entered. Care must be taken not to contaminate the specimen once it is obtained.

Imaging Studies

Plain radiographs should be the first study obtained when imaging septic arthritis. These are only occasionally helpful in diagnosing primary sepsis of the shoulder within the first 7 to 10 days after infection. They may show joint subluxation or soft-tissue swelling, due to either joint effusion or synovial hypertrophy.[16] Later in the infectious process, 40% of patients show abnormalities.[134] As the invading pannus erodes the articular cartilage and adjacent bone within the confines of the capsule, joint space narrowing and marginal erosions appear radiographically.[64] As the septic arthritis spreads to adjacent bone, features of osteomyelitis, such as periostitis and bone destruction, are seen.

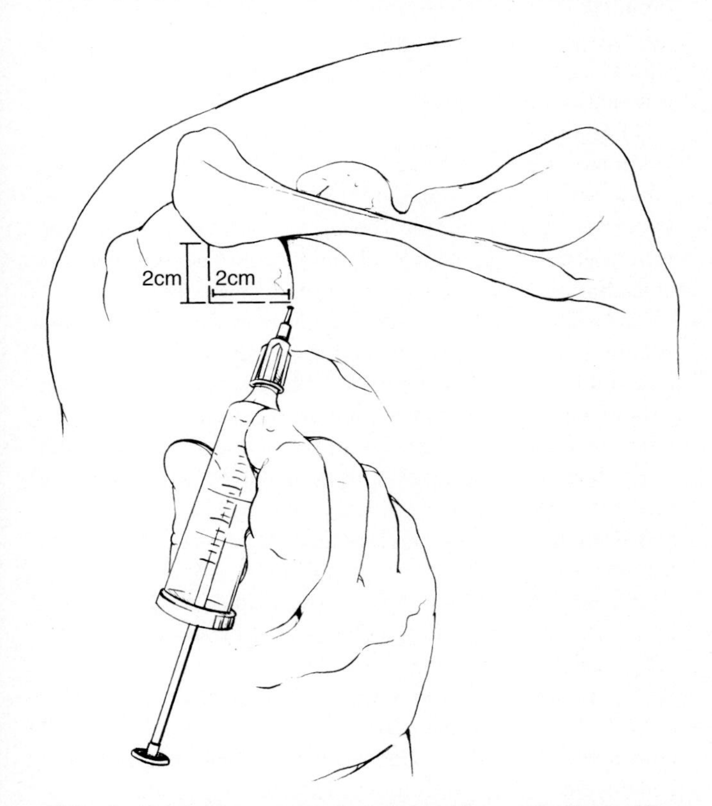

FIG. 6. Posterior approach to shoulder aspiration. After preparing the skin with betadine and injecting local anesthetic, an 18-gauge spinal needle attached to a syringe is inserted 2 cm inferior and 2 cm medial to the posterolateral edge of the acromion. The needle is advanced in the direction of the coracoid process until the joint is entered.

Plain radiographs become more important in light of postsurgical infections. They are helpful to assess the presence, condition, and location of hardware that may need removal. This is especially important for suture anchors, which may not be seen at the time of debridement surgery.

Magnetic resonance imaging (MRI) is recommended by some as the next imaging modality utilized, if the diagnosis is still in question. MRI gives excellent resolution of soft tissues and fluid collections with an extremely high sensitivity, demonstrating abnormalities within 24 hours. However, it continues to lack specificity. It cannot distinguish infected joint fluid from inflammatory, nonseptic joint fluid.[16] MRI can clearly demonstrate cartilage destruction and small joint effusions, as well as intramedullary bone destruction and marrow edema. Computed tomography (CT) can give better bony resolution than either plain radiographs or MRI, clearly depicting subtle bone destruction.

Computed tomographic scans also offer an advantage over plain x-rays in joints with complex anatomy or superimposed skeletal structures. In most cases of sternoclavicular pyarthrosis, results of plain radiography are negative, unless late bony destruction has occurred. CT is an excellent modality for diagnosis of sternoclavicular joint septic arthritis and the complication of abscess formation,[34] as well as for preoperative planning if conservative treatment has failed.[19]

Bone scintigraphy is a physiologic imaging modality and can demonstrate the presence of disease before it appears on radiography. Technetium 99m (^{99m}Tc) is the radionucleotide of choice, although new ones are being developed. A triple-phase scanning sequence should be used. The first phase is the arteriographic phase, where images are obtained every 2 seconds for 1 minute after the ^{99m}Tc bolus. The blood pool phase is obtained at 10 minutes. The third, or bone phase, is obtained 2 to 4 hours after the initial injection.

Septic arthritis manifests as an increased uptake during the first two phases, and during the third phase, there is an increased uptake at the articular ends of the affected bones.[16] This is distinguished from osteomyelitis, in that actual osteomyelitis has a more focal area of uptake. This is a very sensitive, cost-effective study, and a negative scan rules out a septic shoulder. It also may reveal additional sites of joint sepsis in a patient unable to communicate, or diagnose a septic joint in a patient with fever of unknown origin. However, it is not specific, and the findings are the same as in any inflammatory arthropathy. The specificity is increased with labeling of autogenous leukocytes with either indium 111 or ^{99m}Tc. The degree of localization depends on the mechanics of polymorpholeukocyte accumulation. This technique is more sensitive for acute inflammatory lesions. Labeling of immunoglobulin-G also has been performed with variable success in detecting joint sepsis.[129] A relatively new technique in orthopedic infection is single-photon emission computed tomography (SPECT). It is reported to have a higher sensitivity and resolution, and can differentiate the radioactivity in inflamed joints or bone from overlying normal soft-tissue activity.[129]

Role and Indications for Diagnostic Arthroscopy

Septic arthritis can be a diagnostic challenge. Patients can have negative cultures, because of prior use of antibiotics (i.e., initiation of treatment before specimen is obtained, or treatment for other infections) or because of the presence of fastidious organisms. In such cases, arthroscopy can be a helpful diagnostic, as well as therapeutic, modality. Arthroscopic examination of a septic joint usually reveals inflamed and friable synovium with fibrinous exudate. Adhesions and loculations of pus also may be present. The articular cartilage may appear normal but more often will have lost its lustrous appearance. In addition to visualization of the joint, direct synovial biopsy and culture of multiple sites can be obtained through the arthroscope.[17] The histology usually will show inflammatory cells with abundant neutrophils. Cultures of synovial tissue biopsy may have a higher yield for the fastidious organisms than the joint fluid cultures.

TREATMENT

Antibiotics

Prompt recognition, correct diagnosis, joint decompression, and an organism-specific antibiotic regimen are essential, if disabling sequelae are to be avoided.[76] Similar to infection of other parts of the body, selection of an antibiotic is ideally based on the identification of the pathogen and its susceptibility profile. However, in some patients, the organism is not isolated; therefore, an empiric treatment must be started for the most likely infecting organism in that clinical setting. This will vary with the patient's age and underlying medical conditions. Furthermore, the choice of drugs must be linked with surgical options and other supportive measures in the overall management of the disease.

Initial empiric antibiotic selection is based on information such as patient age and risk factors, including history of intravenous drug abuse, rheumatoid arthritis, chronic illness, remote sites of infection, and immune status. The treatment may be instituted after a specimen is obtained for the appropriate studies, including Gram stain, culture, and sensitivity. Usually, a penicillinase-resistant antistaphylococcal drug is the initial choice for the typical gram-positive cocci infection. In the United States, first-generation cephalosporins have been favored, because they are relatively nontoxic and inexpensive.[39] When there is a high likelihood of gram-negative bacilli or methicillin-resistant staphylococci, the initial antibiotic choice is modified to third-generation cephalosporin or vancomycin, respectively. For patients receiving immunosuppressive agents and those who have developed nosocomial infections, an aminoglycoside needs to be included for additional coverage of *P. aeruginosa*. Initial antibiotics for intravenous drug abusers should be for both *S. aureus* and *P. aeruginosa*. In the young, sexually active individual in whom the Gram stain test is negative for bacteria, gonococcal arthritis should be suspected and cefriaxone started. Table 3 summarizes the guidelines for the initial empiric antibiotic therapy.

After the microbiologic data are available, the spectrum of coverage can be narrowed, to maximize efficacy and decrease the risk of systemic toxicity. In light of the differing pathogens, their resistance profile at each hospital, and the advent of newer antimicrobial regimens, we generally obtain consultation with an infectious disease specialist.

The route of antibiotic administration is a subject of some debate. In the past, direct injection of antimicrobials into an infected joint to achieve high local levels was performed on a routine basis.[112] However, animal and human studies of intraarticular antibiotic concentrations have demonstrated that more than adequate levels can be achieved with clinically relevant parenteral doses.[81] For example, Frimodt-Moller[43] and Riegels-Nielsen[106] investigated the diffusion (after intramuscular injection) of penicillin-G, cloxacillin, clindamycin, and netilmicin into synovial fluid of infected rabbit knees and found sufficient local concentrations of all four drugs. Likewise in humans, similar studies were conducted with penicillin,[35,100] ampicillin,[5,69,92] cephalothin,[92] methicillin,[92,104] cloxacillin,[69] tetracycline,[73,100] erythromycin,[104] chloramphenicol,[73,104] lincomycin,[100] gentamicin,[87] and kanamycin.[5] All the antibiotics evaluated, with the exception of erythromycin, achieved articular concentrations in excess of the level required for bacteriostatic or bactericidal effect.[99] With the presently available agents having excellent synovial fluid penetration and the fact that there are associated risks, intraarticular antibiotic injection has fallen out of

TABLE 3. *Suggested guidelines for empiric antibiotics for septic arthritis in adults*

Clinical setting/gram stain	Likely organisms	Drug of choice	Alternative drug[a]
Gram-positive cocci	*Staphylococcus aureus*, streptococci	Nafcillin or cefazolin	Clindamycin TMP/SMX Vancomycin
Healthy, sexually active individual with gram-negative cocci (or negative stain)	*Neisseria gonorrhoeae*	Ceftriaxone	Doxycycline
Gram-negative bacilli	*Pseudomonas aeruginosa*, *Enterobacteriaceae*	Piperacillin ± gentamicin	3rd generation cephalosporins
Intravenous drug abusers	*Staph. aureus*, *P. aeruginosa*, *Serratia*	Cefazolin plus gentamicin	3rd generation cephalosporins
Patients with major underlying disease, immunocompromised, or nosocomial infection	*Staph. aureus*, *Enterobacteriaceae*, *P. aeruginosa*, streptococci	Cefazolin plus gentamicin	3rd generation cephalosporins
Patients with infected prosthesis	*Staph. epidermis*, *Staph. aureus*, *Enterobacteriaceae*, *P. aeruginosa*	Vancomycin plus gentamicin	Imipenem

[a] TMP/SMX, trimethoprim–sulfamethoxazole.

favor. Several investigators have reported chemical synovitis secondary to local tissue toxicity[2,38] and sterile abscesses[62] with the administration of intraarticular antibiotic injections. Most authorities now agree that the antibiotic regimen should almost always be given intravenously.[51]

A more controversial issue is the use of oral versus parenteral antibiotics. A number of investigators have shown good efficacy with the use of oral antibiotics to treat osteomyelitis and septic arthritis in children.[25,77,102,124] In all cases, however, the oral regimen was started only after an initial period of intravenous administration, usually 3 to 7 days. Black et al.[9] retrospectively studied this matter in 21 adults. Even though the failure rate was 14.3%, these investigators concluded that oral antibiotics are a "reasonable alternative to inpatient or outpatient parenteral therapy for treating adult patients who have bone and joint infections caused by susceptible organisms." To date, there has not been a well-designed, randomized, blinded, controlled study to determine whether oral antibiotics are as effective as parenterals in treating septic arthritis. Thus, at this time, oral antimicrobials should only be used in acute infections, after an initial period of intravenous administration. Furthermore, there should be ongoing clinical improvement as manifested by improved ROM of the joint, decreased pain, resolution of fever, as well as normalization of WBC and erythrocyte sedimentation rate.

Oral antibiotic administration has certain advantages, including cost savings, convenience, comfort, and decreased length of hospital stay. Prior to discharge, patients should be evaluated to ensure that adequate serum concentrations are being achieved. Most clinicians[91,95] have arbitrarily maintained a serum bactericidal titer (SBT) of at least 1:8. However, Prober and Yeager[102] recommend SBT peak levels of 1:16 and trough levels of 1:2. The potential risk of an oral antibiotic regimen is that patients may not take the medication as required, due to lack of compliance or difficulty obtaining the medication. Thus, the importance of a full course of therapy must be stressed, and the patients should be carefully instructed on how to take the medication(s) with regard to proper dosage and timing.

The duration of antibiotic therapy is another issue that is a subject of discussion. There are no controlled studies to document the optimal length of treatment. However, certain guidelines have been established. The total duration of antibiotic regimen varies with the pathogen isolated, the patient's underlying condition, and adjuvant medical or surgical procedures. For gonococcal septic arthritis, 7 to 10 days is generally recommended. For streptococci or *Haemophilus* species, a 2- to 3-week duration is usually adequate. In the cases in which more virulent organisms, such as *S. aureus* or gram-negative bacilli are isolated, a 4- to 6-week course of appropriate antibiotic is required. Immunocompromised patients or those with a slow clinical response will need the full 6 weeks of treatment.[115] It is generally agreed that a septic shoulder in the setting of concurrent osteomyelitis will need 6 weeks of antibiotic treatment after the last major debridement surgery.[22]

Nonsteroidal Antiinflammatory Drugs

Sterilization of the joint with antibiotics and irrigation does not completely remove all the bacterial products. These microbial fragments may persist in the joint for prolonged periods and contribute to "postinfectious synovitis."[110] Nonsteroidal antiinflammatory drugs (NSAIDs) may help to reduce this inflammatory process. In an animal model, it was shown that naproxen, when administered in combination with antibiotics, decreased the amount of glycosaminoglycan and collagen loss.[118] These results suggest that use of NSAIDs in addition to the antibiotic regimen may minimize the destruction of articular cartilage. If used, nonsteroidal drugs should not be started too early in the course of infection, because their action may mask a poor clinical response to the antibiotics. We usually start them after 4 to 5 days of antibiotic treatment.

Antibiotic-Impregnated Polymethylmethacrylate

Since described by Buchholz and Engelbrecht[18] in 1970, antibiotic-impregnated polymethylmethacrylate (PMMA) has been used in the treatment of infections of the soft tissue and joint arthroplasty, as well as osteomyelitis. The main advantage of this treatment is that it allows for a high concentration of antibiotics to be delivered locally while minimizing the risk of systemic toxicity. The antibiotic released is not absorbed systemically, therefore resulting in local concentrations five- to tenfold higher than when administered parenterally.[65] *In vitro* and *in vivo* studies have shown that this mode of therapy is safe and effective. In particular, Adams et al.[1] found that clindamycin, vancomycin, and tobramycin exhibited good elution characteristics and had consistently high concentrations in bone and granulation tissue.

Antibiotic-impregnated PMMA may be utilized in one of several ways: (a) as cement for fixation of prostheses in joint arthroplasty,[127] (b) as a spacer block (Fig. 1C and D) to maintain the soft-tissue envelope after resection arthroplasty and debridement,[11,103] or (c) as a string of beads embedded in the soft tissue or bone for chronic infection.[55] Powdered antibiotics are used in the admixture, because adding aqueous solutions of antibiotic to the cement interferes with the prepolymerization process, resulting in mechanically weakened cement.[86] When used for fixation, the fatigue strength of the cement is not significantly altered when 1.2 g of the appropriate antibiotic (usually tobramycin) is mixed per 40 g of PMMA.[31] In the form of a spacer or beads, the fatigue strength of the PMMA is less critical; therefore, a higher concentration of antibiotic may be added to the cement powder. Hofmann et al.[67] described mixing 4.8 g of powdered tobramycin in each 40-g batch of Simplex-P cement (Howmedica, Rutherford, NJ) for use as a spacer block, whereas Cierny et al.[23] reported using 4.8 to 9.6 g of tobramycin per 40 g of PMMA for making the beads.

Elution of antibiotics from the cement occurs by diffusion, in which there is a rapid initial release, followed by a sustained release that progressively diminishes over weeks to months.[41,66] Because the spherically shaped beads have a greater total surface area, more antibiotic per unit time is released when the impregnated cement is used in the form of beads than when used as a spacer block or for fixation.[66] *In vitro* studies by Marks et al.[86] demonstrated that antibiotics diffused from Palacos-R (Richards, Memphis, TN) in larger amounts and greater duration than from Simplex-P. However, these findings were not substantiated by *in vivo* studies by these same investigators. In addition, Brien et al.[15] found no statistical difference in the elution characteristics of tobramycin from these two cements.

In shoulder sepsis, antibiotic-impregnated PMMA may be a good adjunct, temporary therapy for those patients with concomitant osteomyelitis of the proximal humerus. They are placed after thorough irrigation and debridement, and the wound is closed. The cement is removed at the time of definitive surgery.

Evacuation and Decompression of the Joint

The goals of treatment of septic shoulder include sterilization and decompression of the joint with removal of all inflammatory cells, lysosomal and preoteolytic enzymes, fibrinous materials. In non–surgery-related infection; the preferred method of joint decompression remains controversial. Two schools of thought exist. One stems from the medical and rheumatologic literature, suggesting that repeated needle aspirations and appropriate antibiotics may be all that is necessary in a pyogenic arthritis of the shoulder.[51,62] The other is based on the principle that surgical debridement is the *sine qua non* of treatment for septic arthritis and osteomyelitis of the shoulder. There are studies to support both views. However, when scrutinized closely, it may be borne out that surgery offers distinct advantages.

Those who advocate repeated arthrocenteses cite extended hospitalization, wound management problems, and anesthetic risks as reasons to avoid surgical intervention. A number of retrospective studies from the 1970s and 1980s, comparing infected joints treated with needle aspirations versus surgical drainage, concluded that medically managed patients fared substantially better than patients who underwent surgery.[49,51,88,107]

Rosenthal et al.,[107] publishing in 1980, analyzed 71 nongonococcal septic joints and found that medical therapy (parenteral antibiotics and frequent aspirations) led to good result in 74%, as opposed to only 32% in the open irrigation and drainage cases. A separate study in 59 patients by Goldenberg et al.[49] showed full recovery in 67% of those treated by arthrocentesis versus only 42% of those surgically treated. Master et al.[88] reported on eight septic shoulders and concluded that needle drainage and parenteral antibiotics were all that were required for successful management.

Like other investigators,[62] we question these data. Clearly, there are weaknesses in these studies. They were all uncontrolled; therefore, the indications for the treatment modality were undefined and determined predominantly by the admitting service. Because of the lack of randomization, there were a number of biases. For example, in the Goldenberg series,[49] 47% of the surgical patients were infected with *S. aureus,* whereas only 26% of the medical patients were infected with this virulent organism (this information is not available in the Rosenthal series). Undoubtedly, infection with a more virulent organism such as *S. aureus* will result in a worse outcome.[44,80] The duration of symptoms prior to treatment (i.e., delay in treatment) will also affect the result.[2,44,49,76,] In all three series, there was a greater delay in the group of surgically treated patients who had the poor outcome. Another weakness is the outcome data. No assessment of function or follow up was reported in the study by Master.

Although the Rosenthal and Goldenberg series included ROM as part of their assessment, it is unclear how they were able to obtain the premorbid ROM because these studies were retrospective, and the patients were evaluated only after the fact. Of interest, Rosenthal pointed out that of the 6 patients who failed medical management and subsequently required surgical drainage, 3 did well. Goldenberg had 7 patients undergo surgery after medical failure but did not report follow-up.

If aspiration is the choice of therapy, it should be performed under sterile conditions with a large-bore needle. A long spinal needle may be necessary to penetrate the glenohumeral joint in an obese or muscular patient. Attempts to drain the joint completely are essential and should be repeated frequently (once or twice daily[121]) until the effusion ceases to recur.[51]

Although many internal medicine physicians view incision and drainage as an alternative form of treatment, most orthopedic surgeons believe that shoulder sepsis demands surgical treatment. Proponents of surgical drainage describe technical difficulty with shoulder aspiration, inadequate needle evacuation of purulent material secondary to loculations and adhesions, pain associated with multiple arthrocenteses, and potential iatrogenic needle inoculation of subchondral bone as reasons for surgery.[37] Again, there are only retrospective studies to support this view.

Leslie et al.[80] reviewed 18 cases of septic arthritis of the shoulder with a minimum of 1-year follow up. Ten patients were treated with arthrocenteses and 8 with surgical drainage at the outset. Of the 10 who initially had repeated aspirations, 1 died, 1 had no motion, 1 had only passive abduction and flexion to 90 degrees, and 7 required an open irrigation and drainage. Of the latter 7, 1 died, 2 had no active motion, 1 had less than 45 degrees of flexion, and 3 had greater than 90 degrees of flexion. There were no deaths in the 8 patients who underwent an operative procedure from the outset. Two had flexion of at least 90 degrees, 2 had flexion of 45 degrees or less, and 4 had no active motion. Although the sample size was too small to yield statistical significance, the investigators noted that arthrotomy resulted in a better outcome than did repeated aspirations. At Bowman Gray School of Medicine, Toby et al.[126] came to the same conclusion after reviewing 15 cases of shoulder infection. Further support for open drainage in joint infections is offered by Lane et al.,[79] who found that patients with a 3- or more day history of knee pyarthrosis and those with *S. aureus* or gram-negative bacillus infections fared better after open irrigation and drainage.

Without prospective randomized studies to provide conclusive evidence either way, the debate over medical versus surgical drainage of shoulder infections continues. However, mounting evidence is accumulating for the use of surgical arthroscopy in septic arthritis cases.[17,98] The diagnostic advantage of arthroscopy is that it allows for direct visualization of the entire joint. Visualization is essential in determining the extent of the disease and enabling tissue biopsy in atypical or challenging cases. The therapeutic advantage of arthroscopy is that the joint can be adequately drained, thoroughly debrided, and copiously irrigated. Prognostically, arthroscopic irrigation and drainage reduces hospital stay and allows for early ROM, which may be helpful in preserving joint function.[108] Recommendations for arthroscopic or open surgical drainage, as opposed to repeated arthrocenteses, are summarized in Table 4.

Early use of arthroscopy in musculoskeletal infection was entertained mostly for pyarthrosis of the knee. In 1981, Jarrett et al.[72] reported the first successful arthroscopic debridement of an infected knee in a patient who failed medical management but was too ill for general anesthesia and arthrotomy. Since then, a number of series[70,71,117] have shown good to excellent results with minimal operative morbidity. This experience with the knee has led physicians to arthroscopically treat septic arthritis of the shoulder, hip, elbow, and ankle. To date, there are only isolated case reports of the effectiveness of arthroscopic irrigation and drainage for pyarthrosis of the shoulder. The results thus far parallel those of the knee.[98]

With the advent of interventional radiology, suppurative arthritis also has been drained with percutaneous catheters placed under fluoroscopy.[105] A handful of these cases involved the shoulder.[109] Although the investigators state that septic arthritis can be successfully treated with drainage of the joint via a percutaneous catheter in combination with antibiotic therapy, the experience is relatively limited at this time. It remains to be determined whether this modality will have a future role in the treatment of joint infection.

TABLE 4. *Recommendations for arthroscopic or open surgical drainage as opposed to repeated arthrocenteses*

Duration of symptoms for 5 days or longer before the initiation of treatment
Aggressive organisms
- Methicillin-resistant *Staphylococcus aureus* (MRSA)
- Gram-negative bacilli
- Enterococcus
- Clostridia
- Glycocalyx-producing organisms

Elderly[138]
Immunocompromised host
- Immunosuppressive therapy
- Chronic debilitating illness
- Malignancy
- AIDS
- Malnutrition

Diagnostic dilemma requiring tissue biopsy
Concomitant processes
- Rheumatoid arthritis
- Osteoarthritis
- Periarticular osteomyelitis

Postsurgical infection
Failed repeated arthrocenteses
- No or little clinical improvement
- Persistent effusions after 5–7 days of treatment

Management of Sternoclavicular Joint Infection

The majority of the cases of sternoclavicular septic arthritis respond to parenteral antibiotics and repeated aspiration or simple incision and drainage. However, patients in whom the inferior part of the capsule has ruptured must be treated with more radical debridement for drainage of the intrathoracic extrapleural abscess, including excision of the medial head of the clavicle, intraarticular disc, and portions of the manubrium.[19]

Management of Postoperative Infections

The success of treatment for a postsurgical infection is dependent on obliteration of the infectious organism and the restoration of function. If the infection is superficial and limited to the subcutaneous tissue, meticulous observation, local wound care, and antibiotics are usually sufficient for successful outcome. However, for a deep postsurgical infection, a more aggressive approach is required with debridement of the glycocalyx film, avascular bone, infected sinus tract, soft tissue, and foreign material (Fig. 7).

For the infected shoulder in which foreign material is present in or about the joint, management, to be successful, must be individualized (Fig. 8). When the hardware is serving to stabilize a fracture, debridement of bone and soft tissue with adequate drainage may be attempted, while preserving the internal fixation *in situ.* If the infection persists, the hardware must be removed, in order to successfully gain control of the process. On the other hand, if the hardware is loose or not contributing to the fixation, it should be removed at the first debridement. Care must be taken to preserve cuff tissue and the tuberosities, if function of the shoulder is to be maintained.

It has been well established that suture in the wound increases the susceptibility of host tissue to infection. Elek and Conen showed that 7.5×10^6 staphylococci were required to induce an intradermal infection, whereas a bacterial inoculation count of only 300 was needed to produce a similar infection in the presence of silk suture.[36] In 1984, Chu and Williams[20] studied the attachment of bacteria to 10 different suture materials. They concluded that the number of adherent bacteria was dependent on the type of suture material, the specific bacteria, and the duration of contact. Physical configuration (monofilament versus braid multifilament) and surface area of the suture play a role in bacterial adhesion, but their chemical structure and coating may be even more important factors. These investigators also found that *S. aureus* adhered to sutures more than *E. coli*, and that the adherence is a dynamic process. Thus, in short, suture materials should be treated like any other foreign body. They may be left in place, if not grossly contaminated at the time of initial debridement, but may very well require removal to eradicate the infection.

After removal of the foreign material, several additional surgical debridements are usually needed at 2- to 5-day intervals for complete eradication of all compromised tissues. Reconstruction of the defect with bone graft and/or local or microvascular soft-tissue transfer may be performed after the wound is culture negative.

Management of Infected Arthroplasty

Fortunately, the incidence of infection after total shoulder arthroplasty is exceedingly low.[90] However, when infected arthroplasty does occur, it represents a potentially devastating complication that is often difficult to manage. Like other

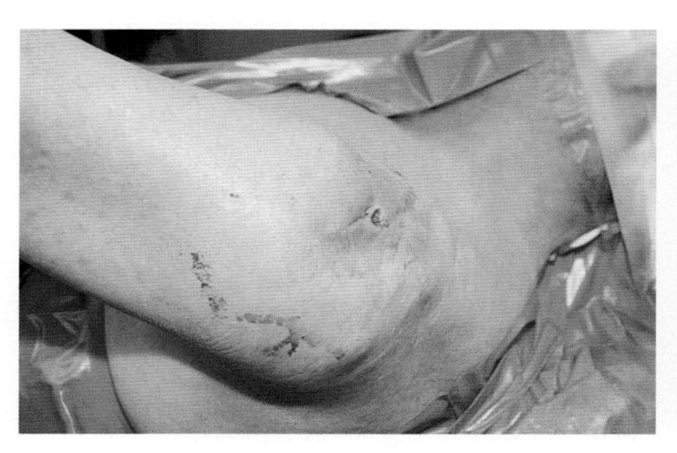
A

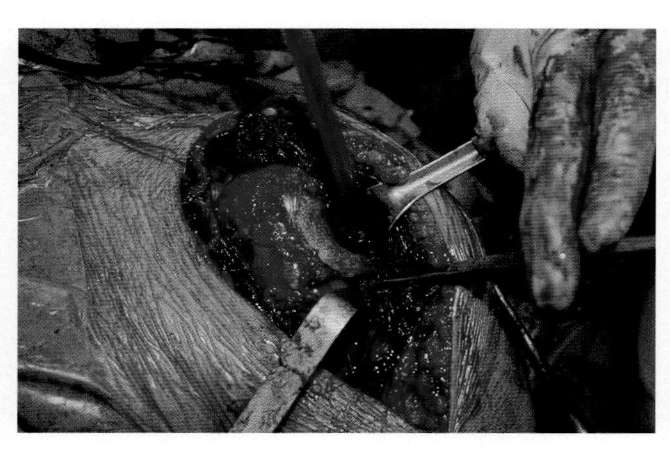
B

FIG. 7. (A and B) A 2-year chronic shoulder infection occurring after rotator cuff repair treated with multiple limited debridements. The patient presented with a chronic draining sinus and chronic osteomyelitis with a sequestrum. The patient had undergone extensive debridement of all dead bone, soft tissue, sinus tract, and suture material via both an anterior and posterior approach. The wounds were packed open and closed 3 days later, after a second irrigation and debridement. The patient had 6 weeks of antibiotics. The infection resolved without further treatment. The patient was left with a stiff but painless shoulder. (Courtesy of J.P. Iannotti, M.D., Ph.D.)

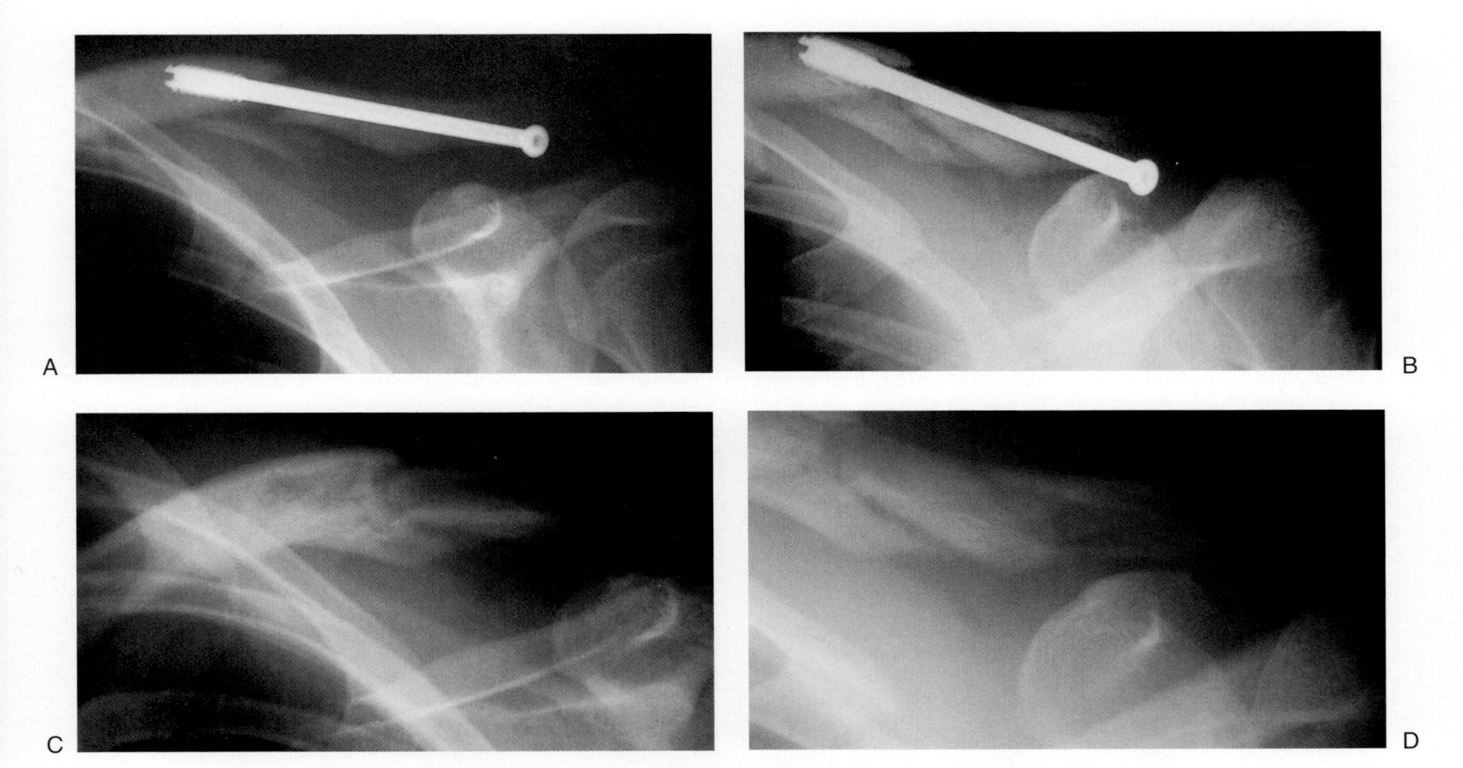

FIG. 8. (A) Immediate postoperative x-rays after open reduction and internal fixation of a comminuted, mid-shaft, clavicle fracture. **(B)** Four months postoperatively, the osteomyelitis was treated by retention of the hardware and intravenous antibiotics until the fracture healed. **(C, D)** The hardware was removed and the clavicle was debrided, which was followed by another 6 weeks of intravenous antibiotics. The patient has a healed painless clavicle with full function and no signs of infection. (Courtesy of J.P. Iannotti, M.D., Ph.D.)

joint replacement surgery, septic shoulder arthroplasty can occur early or late. Once the diagnosis is established, the treatment should follow the same principles as the larger joints. Intraoperative frozen sections may be valuable in helping to establish or confirm the diagnosis. As demonstrated by Lonner et al.[84] in revision hip and knee arthroplasties, 10 or more polymorphonuclear cells per high-power field was predictive of infection. Early infections may be managed with wound exploration, irrigation, debridement, wound closure, and antibiotics.[90,137] The implant may be left in place if the components are well fixed.[53] Wirth and Rockwood recommend that early infections with gram-negative organisms and all late infections be treated with removal of the prosthesis and all cement.[137] Thorough debridement of granulation and scar tissue is also required, combined with 6 weeks of parenteral antibiotics. Although most infected shoulder implants are treated by resection arthroplasty, other treatment options exist. Miller and Bigliani[90] have exchanged infected hemiarthroplasty for a total shoulder in several patients. They used tobramycin-impregnated cement for fixation of the components and reported acceptable short-term results. Other treatment options include antibiotic suppression, two-stage revision arthroplasty,[103] arthrodesis, and amputation.

AUTHORS' PREFERRED METHODS OF TREATMENT

Hematogenous, Isolated Subacromial Septic Bursitis

If the infection is limited to the bursa, we prefer needle aspiration of the space, organism-specific antibiotics, and careful observation. Complete evacuation of bacteria and debris is not as critical in this case, because the integrity of the articular cartilage is not in jeopardy.[78] Arthroscopic or open debridement should be performed if the process fails to clear rapidly. Patients who have a protracted course, concomitant osteomyelitis, or glenohumeral sepsis will require surgical drainage and debridement.[17] If the integrity of the rotator cuff or the involvement of the glenohumeral joint is in question, an MRI is obtained for preoperative evaluation.

Hematogenous, Isolated Pyarthrosis of the Glenohumeral Joint

In aspiration-confirmed, nongonococcal hematogenous pyarthrosis of the glenohumeral joint, we initiate appropriate intravenous antibiotic treatment and prefer surgical irrigation and debridement with the arthroscope (Table 4). After induction of anesthesia, the patient is placed in the beach-chair position. Preparation and draping are performed in the usual sterile manner for shoulder surgery. The posterior portal is made 2 cm inferior and 2 cm medial to the posterolateral edge of the acromion, in line with the posterior axillary fold. A trocar is then inserted, aiming in the direction of the coracoid. After confirming intraarticular placement by back flow of joint fluid, the arthroscope is inserted, and the joint is inspected. A second (anterior) portal is then made by first advancing a spinal needle from a location halfway between the coracoid process and the anterolateral acromion into the joint under direct arthroscopic visualization. The needle is removed, and a cannula with a trocar is inserted, following the same direction as the needle. Tissue for cultures and histology is obtained. The two portals are used for ingress and egress of irrigation fluid. After irrigation, the entire joint is once again inspected for signs of rotator cuff or articular damage and retained purulent material.

We include a limited open procedure to explore the biceps tendon, when there is tenderness along the biceps or if the infection is caused by an aggressive organism. The limited open procedure, when indicated, ensures that pockets of purulent material or soft-tissue abscesses have not developed from organisms tracking down the bicipital groove.

We recommend debridement via open arthrotomy, if the surgeon is less experienced in shoulder arthroscopy. We prefer the deltopectoral approach and opening the rotator interval. After irrigation and debridement, a closed suction drain is placed in the joint, and the interval is closed with a monofilament, absorbable suture. A second drain can be placed in the soft tissue.

Medical management with antibiotics and repeated aspirations should be reserved for less virulent infections that are diagnosed early and for patients who are medically unable to tolerate surgery. At the time of this writing, we believe that

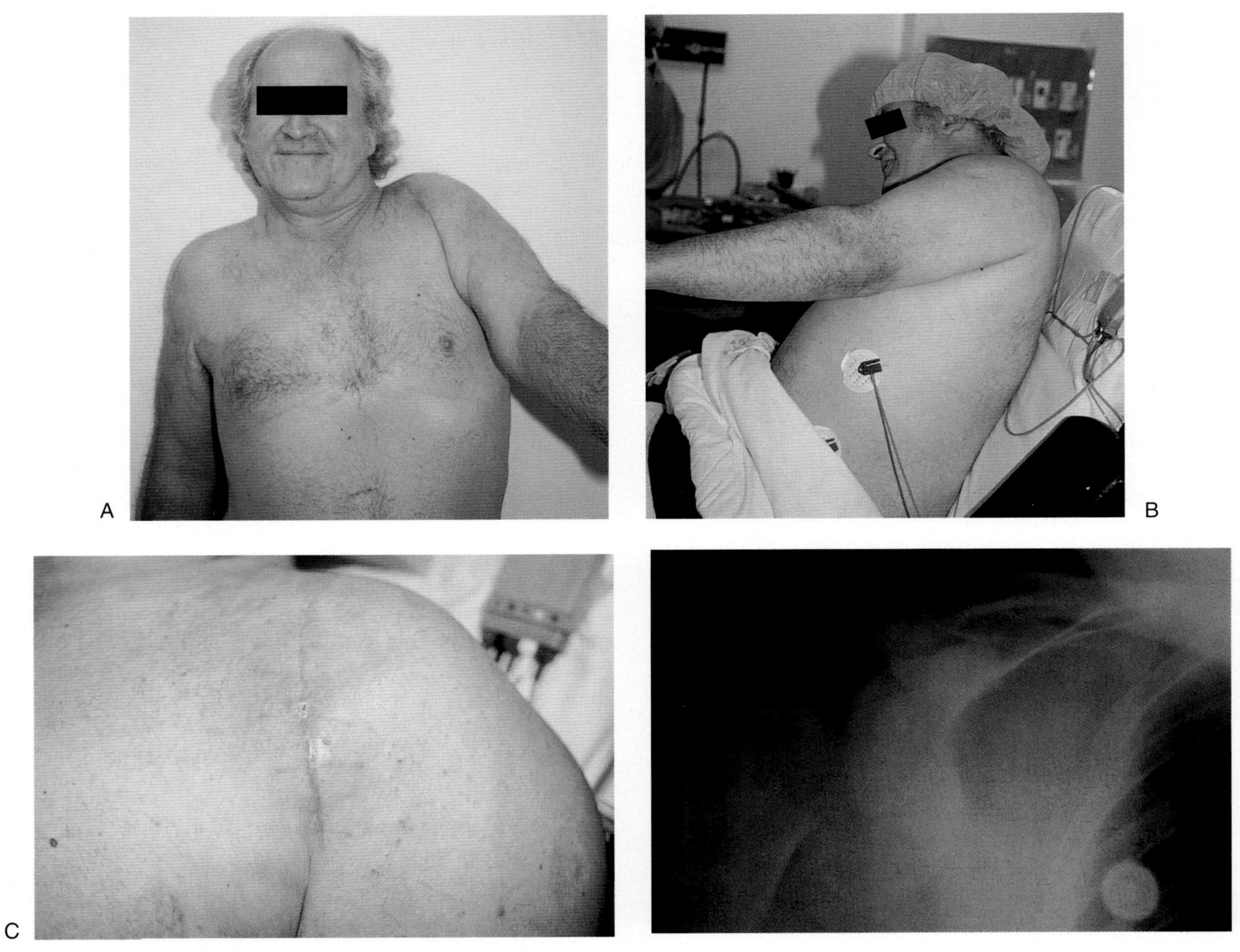

FIG. 9. (A–D) Chronic osteomyelitis after hemiarthroplasty for treatment of an acute four-part fracture. The patient had chronic wound drainage and a painful arm and was initially treated with oral antibiotics. **(E)** The postoperative x-rays showed a detached greater tuberosity and a loose cemented hemiarthroplasty.

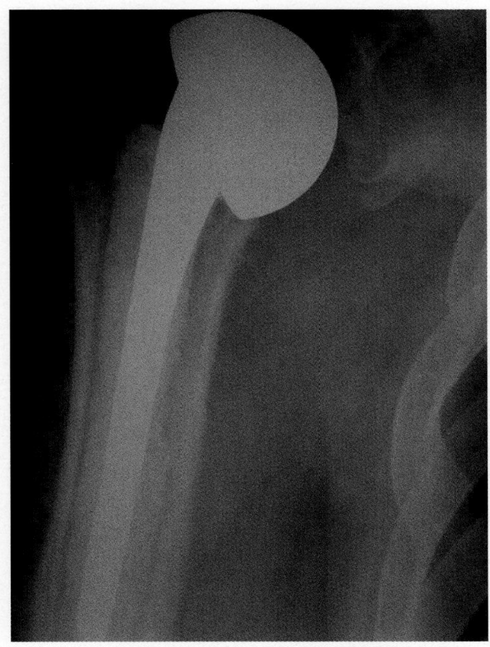

E

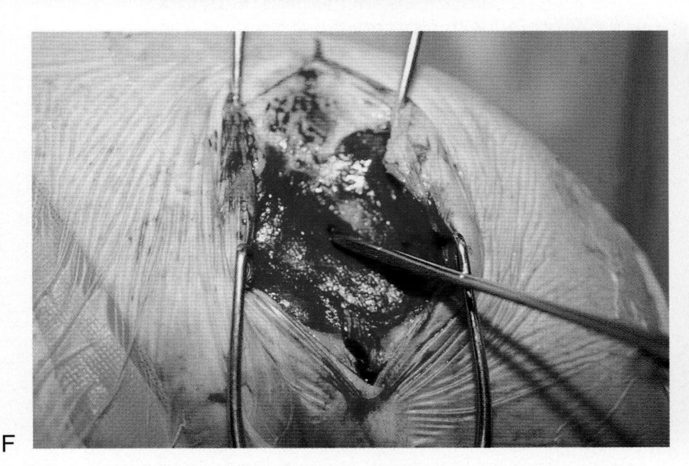

F

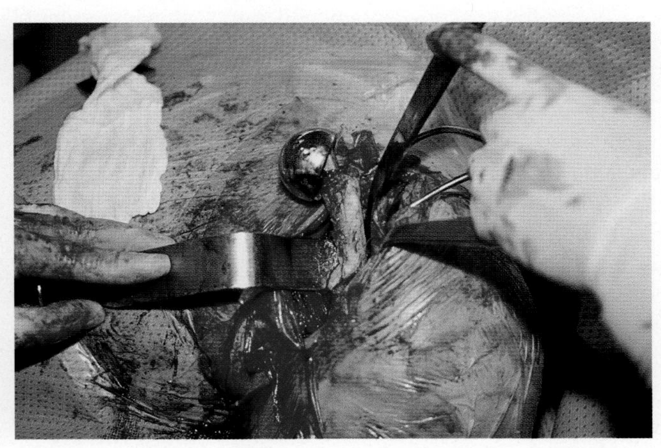

G

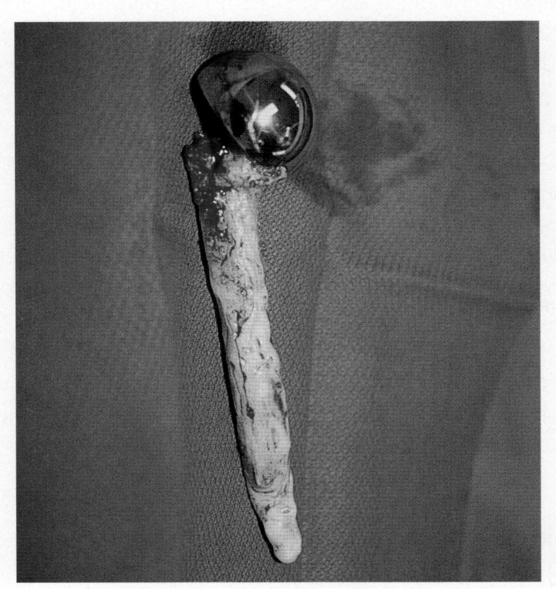

H

FIG. 9. *Continued* **(E–H)** Intraoperative photographs showing a chronic sinus tract to the prosthetic stem that was loose and easily removed with the entire cement mantle.

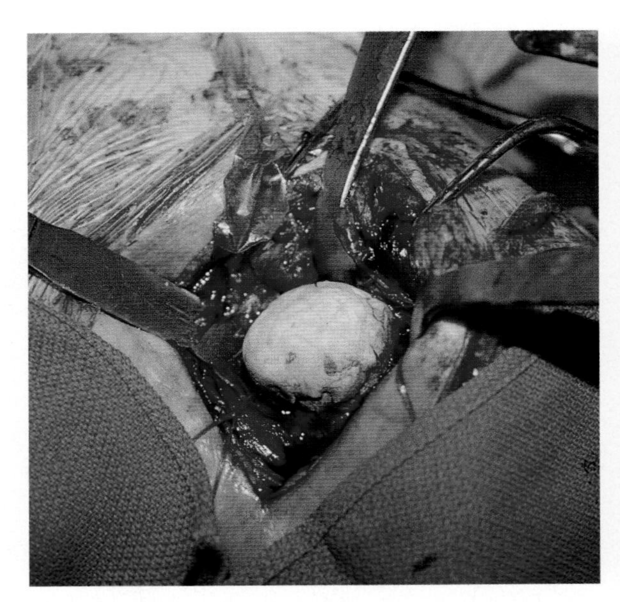

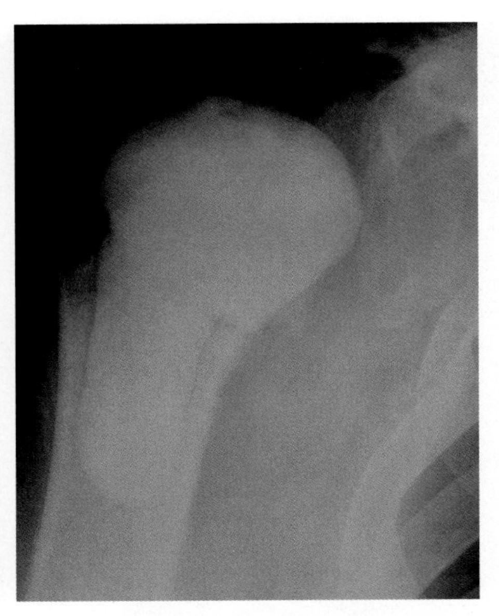

I J

FIG. 9. *Continued* **(I and J)** A tobramycin cement spacer was placed for 8 months, during which time the patient was on antibiotics. The ESR was monitored monthly. It decreased from 92 preoperatively to 20 before revision surgery, 8 months after debridement of the infected prosthesis. At the time of revision, the spacer was removed, a total shoulder arthroplasty was performed with tobramycin cement, and the tuberosity was mobilized and internally fixed to the proximal humeral shaft. (Courtesy of J.P. Iannotti, M.D., Ph.D.)

percutaneous catheter drainage is yet to be proven to offer any additional benefits.

Postoperatively, analgesics are adjusted so that the patient can participate in pendulum or passive ROM exercises within 24 hours of surgery. A sling is used for support, as needed, during ambulation. An NSAID is started after a positive clinical response to the antibiotic regimen is established, usually after 4 or 5 days.

Postoperative Wound Infection Complicating Fracture Stabilization or Rotator Cuff Repair

Although some investigators believe there is a role for arthroscopy in postoperative wound infections, we prefer an open wound debridement, including arthrotomy, as needed. The extent of debridement must be individualized for each patient. However, if the infection is caught early, at our first debridement we attempt to irrigate the wound thoroughly, debride any granulation tissue and glycocalyx, and allow the internal fixation device or cuff repair suture to remain. The patient is returned to the operating room at 2- to 3-day intervals for redebridement as needed. Closed suction drainage is used. Every attempt is made to avoid leaving the wound open or changing packing at the bed side, because of the risk of introducing a hospital-based resistant organism. Antibiotic beads are inserted, if the wound size will allow. Removal of compromised suture and fracture fixation hardware is performed as soon as it becomes obvious that the organism is not responding. We emphasize avoidance of electrocautery for dissection and meticulous soft-tissue and bone debridement, in order to have adequate host material at the time of reconstruction or definitive wound closure.

If the deltoid was taken down for exposure, care must be taken to repair it to prevent postoperative dehiscence. At the time of the definitive procedure, we suture the superficial and deep deltoid fascia directly to bone. We prefer to use monfilament, absorbable sutures in an interrupted manner for this closure.

Postoperative mobilization is restricted to pendulum exercises, depending on the stability of the cuff or fracture repair. In the case of a fracture involving the proximal humerus, fracture healing takes precedence over joint motion.

In extreme circumstances of patient noncompliance or if the soft-tissue envelope is severely damaged by the infection or multiple procedures, a shoulder spica cast is used for wound protection. Soft-tissue immobilization is maintained in the position of least tension to the repair. In our opinion, a spica cast is better immobilization than an abduction pillow, because there is less tendency for the arm to shift.

If the nonabsorbable rotator cuff suture has been allowed to remain *in situ,* parenteral, organism-specific antibiotics are delivered for 6 weeks. In the case of retained fracture fixation hardware, oral antibiotics are continued after the 6 weeks of parenteral antibiotics until the fracture is clinically and roentgenographically healed. After confirmation that healing has indeed occurred, the hardware is removed, if the infection persists.

Infection Complicating Hemi- and Total Joint Arthroplasty

Surgical wound infections that develop during or immediately after the index hospitalization are treated aggressively with debridement and irrigation, rather than expectantly, because of the underlying biomaterial.

For late deep infection, our preferred treatment is staged debridement and reimplantation, if possible. An antibiotic-impregnated cement spacer is utilized to facilitate the definitive reconstruction (Figs. 9 and 10). If a reimplantation cannot be performed, arthrodesis is the next option, if possible, because it yields better function than resection arthroplasty. However, because there is usually extensive bone loss, soft-tissue arthroplasty is performed more commonly than fusion. Deep late infection with a nonaggressive organism in an elderly patient is suppressed with antibiotics, if possible.

PROGNOSIS

The prognosis for septic arthritis of the shoulder joint is highly dependent on prompt diagnosis, the nature of the infecting organism, and the patient's immune status. Most patients will not have the typical signs and symptoms of a septic joint, and the laboratory studies may be equivocal. For

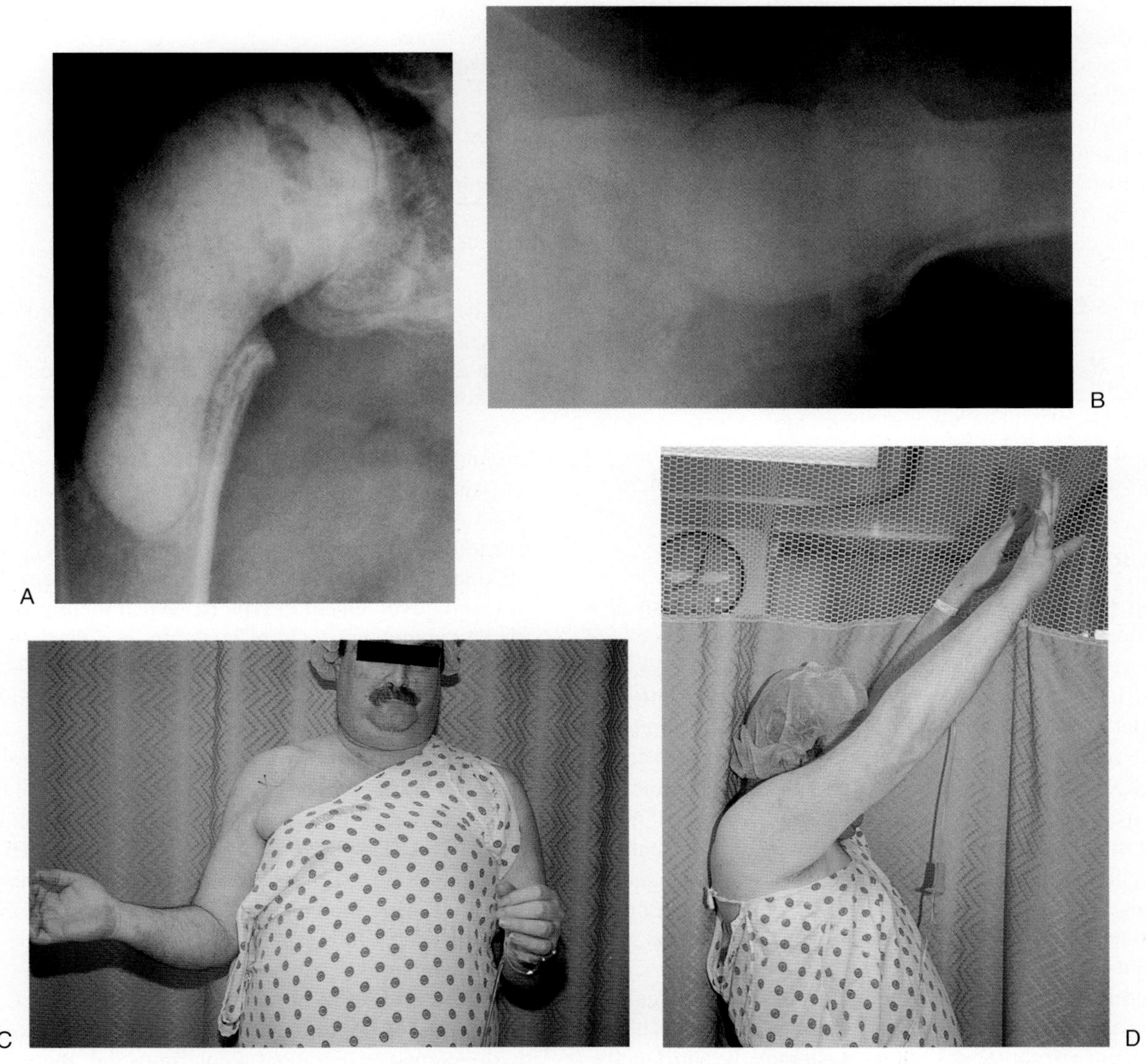

FIG. 10. (A and B) Cement spacer used on the right shoulder for treatment of a late hematogenous seeding of a hemiarthroplasty, placed 18 months prior to infection. The hemiarthroplasty was placed for arthropathy secondary to an excessively tight repair for recurrent instability of the right shoulder, 18 years before the index arthroplasty. The cement spacer maintains the soft-tissue envelope for later prosthetic conversion. In some patients, remarkable shoulder function can be maintained with a spacer in place. **(C and D)** This patient had to be called back to have the spacer replaced with a hemiarthroplasty because of progressive glenoid erosion. He maintained excellent function and minimal pain with the spacer 1 year after debridement of the infected joint. His left, uninfected shoulder had less function, due to prior shoulder surgery for treatment of recurrent dislocation 18 years previously. (Courtesy of J.P. Iannotti, M,D,, Ph.D.)

these reasons, many are initially diagnosed as having bursitis or tendonitis, and the correct diagnosis may not be made for up to 6 months.[80] It is therefore imperative that the evaluating physician have a high index of suspicion and that, if the diagnosis is entertained, the glenohumeral joint be aspirated to rule out pyarthrosis.

Gelberman et al. reported satisfactory results in 8 of 10 patients when treatment was initiated within 4 weeks of the onset of symptoms.[44] Master et al.[88] found that treatment delays of greater than 1 month resulted in therapeutic failures, with persistent infection and poor function. However, other investigators had worse outcomes in their series. Leslie et al.,[80] who defined a poor result as the death of the patient or the absence of active motion of the glenohumeral joint, found that 9 of the 10 poor results were in patients who had been diagnosed with septic shoulder within 4 weeks. Ward and Goldner[134] found that all unsuccessfully treated patients had symptoms for more than 1 week. The discrepancy between the results cited in the above series may be due to a number of factors, such as the aggressiveness of the infecting organisms or the method of treatment. However, it is clear that delay in treatment results in worse prognosis.

There is a paucity of outcome data on infected shoulder arthroplasty. There are only anecdotal reports in the literature, making it difficult to determine the prognosis for such patients. However, it is recognized that these patients generally do worse than those with primary hematogenous pyarthrosis. We have treated 3 patients with delayed exchanged arthroplasty. One patient subsequently required a resection arthroplasty. The other 2 have limited ROM.

FUTURE DIRECTIONS

Four areas deserve special attention: development of a classification system, improved prophylaxis, more accurate diagnosis, and enhanced treatment.

Part of the difficulty in reporting outcomes in infected shoulder patients is the lack of a uniform classification system for septic joints. A number of systems exist to describe osteomyelitis[23,75,133] or infection around a total joint, but none are universally accepted. The ideal system will allow for stratification of the disease, improve decision making, and facilitate outcome reporting that is suitable for meaningful comparison.[81] To our knowledge, a comprehensive classification system for septic arthritis of the shoulder, as such, does not exist at this time.

Therefore, we propose a new classification system for septic joints based on (a) the site and extent of tissue involvement; (b) the host's status, systemically and locally; and (c) the duration of symptoms and virulence of the organism (Table 5). Clearly, all three of these factors must be considered when assessing treatment results and efficacy of treatment alternatives. In this system, the infectious process is staged using four anatomic types, three host physiologic classes, and two clinical settings. Our treatment algorithm based on this classification system is outlined in Fig. 11.

TABLE 5. *Proposed classification system for septic arthritis (modified from Cierny-Mader osteomyelitis classification)*

Joint name (glenohumeral, elbow, hip, knee, etc.)
Anatomic type
- I: Periarticular soft-tissue infection without pyarthrosis
- II: Isolated septic arthritis
- III: Septic arthritis with soft-tissue extension, but no osteomyelitis
- IV: Septic arthritis with contiguous osteomyelitis

Host class
- A: Normal immune system
- B: Compromised host
  - B_L: Local tissue compromise
  - B_S: Systemic immune compromise
- C: Risk associated with aggressive treatment unwarranted

Clinical setting
- 1: Less than 5 days of symptoms and nonvirulent organism
- 2: Symptoms for 5 days or more, or a virulent organism

Clinical stage for the specific joint
- Anatomic type + host class + clinical setting = stage

The anatomic types include infection isolated to the periarticular soft tissue only, to the joint only, involvement of the joint and soft tissue, and involvement of the joint and bone. Anatomic type I is periarticular soft-tissue infection without pyarthrosis. Such a case may occur in a postsurgical deep wound infection. Isolated glenohumeral sepsis (type II) occurs when the purulent material is confined within the capsule. Anatomic type III exists when there is involvement of the joint and surrounding soft tissue, such as deep wound infection or septic bursitis, along with the joint sepsis. There is no bony involvement in type III. When there is osteomyelitis contiguous with a joint infection, it is classified as type IV. In the shoulder girdle, this usually involves the proximal humerus but may occasionally develop in the acromion, distal clavicle, or glenoid.

The host is classified into either an A, B, or C physiologic group, according to the system of Cierny and Mader.[23] An A host represents a patient with normal metabolic and immune status. The B host is compromised either locally (B_L) or systemically (B_S). Local issues include retained nonabsorbable suture or other biomaterial, local irradiation, scarring from multiple procedures, and lymphedema. Systemic compromise includes extreme age, chronic disease, or any condition causing suppression of the immune system. The C host status is reserved for those patients in whom the risks associated with aggressive treatment would outweigh the negative aspects of the infection.

The clinical setting takes into account the duration of symptoms and aggressiveness of the organism. We have grouped patients with less than 5 days of symptoms and infection with a less virulent bacterial strain into group 1. Those patients who are infected with a virulent organism or with symptoms for 5 days or greater fall into group 2. The

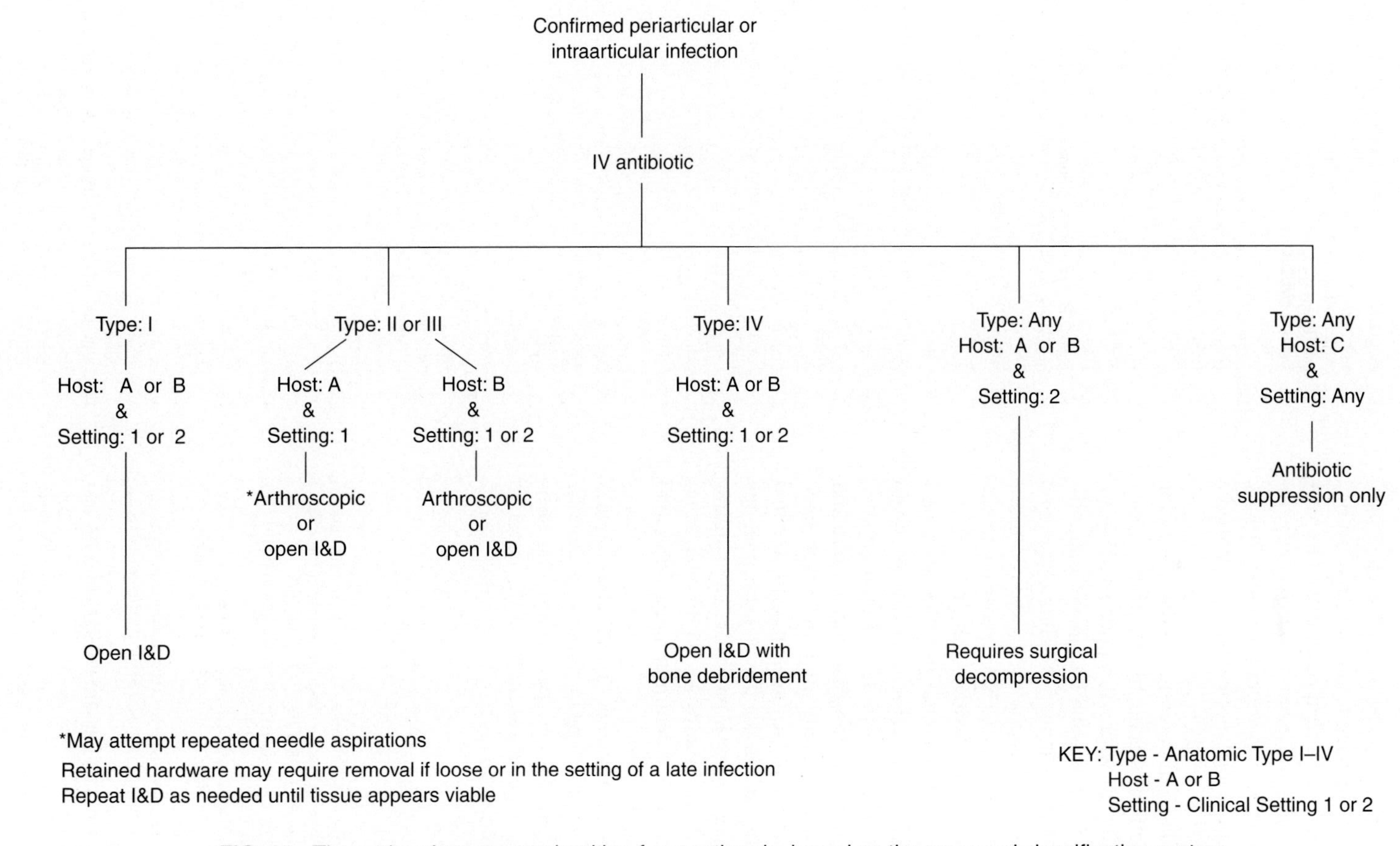

FIG. 11. The authors' treatment algorithm for pyarthrosis, based on the proposed classification system for septic arthritis (see Table 5).

cut-off was chosen at 5 days because animal studies have shown that irreversible joint damage occurs if septic arthritis persists beyond this time. The virulent organisms may vary between hospitals and geographic locations but generally include methicillin-resistant *S. aureus*, gram-negative bacilli, vancomycin-resistant enterococcal species, and clostridia (Table 4).

Exciting work is ongoing with reference to the prevention of infection associated with orthopedic biomaterials by coating fracture fixation hardware with antiseptics prior to implantation. Work in the animal model has shown a significant reduction in infection using chlorhexidrine and chloroxylenol.[30] Interestingly, Ilizarov used a sponge moistened not with saline, but rather with chlorhexedrine, to stabilize and cool transfixation pins during insertion.

Evaluation of patients with potential joint sepsis is currently imperfect at best. The application of polymerase chain reaction (PCR)[12] to synovial fluid aspiration should improve diagnostic accuracy, especially in those patients with fastidious organisms, infected arthroplasty, and those who have received partial antibiotic treatment. Presently, this method is limited by its availability and high false-positive rate, due to amplification of inactive bacterial products. The application of quantitative PCR techniques to amplify bacterial DNA and RNA shows promise in determining bacterial load and distinguishing active infection.[47]

Even after the bacteria have been destroyed, the enzymes released from the damaged tissue and by the bacteria and the host defense mechanisms can further degrade articular cartilage proteoglycan. Work is underway to blunt the negative effect of the matrix metalloproteases to diminish this postinfection degradation.

REFERENCES

1. Adams K, Couch L, Cierny G, Calhoun J, Mader JT. In vitro and in vivo evaluation of antibiotic diffusion from antibiotic-impregnated polymethylmethacrylate beads. *CORR* 1992;278:244–252.
2. Argen A, Wilson C, Wood P. Suppurative arthritis clinical features of 42 cases. *Arch Intern Med* 1966;117:661–666.
3. Armstrong R, Bolding F. Septic arthritis after arthroscopy: the contributing roles of intraarticular steroids and environmental factors. *Am J Infect Control* 1994;22:16–18.
4. Atcheson S, Ward J. Acute hematogenous osteomyelitis progressing to septic synovitis and eventual pyarthrosis. *Arthritis Rheum* 1978;21: 968–971.
5. Baciocco E, Lles R. Ampicillin and kanamicin concentrations in joint fluid. *Clin Pharmacol Ther* 1971;12:858.
6. Bayer A, Chow A, Louie J, Nies K, Guze L. Gram-negative bacillary septic arthritis: clinical, radiographic, therapeutic, and prognostic features. *Semin Arthritis Rheum* 1977;7:123–132.
7. Bhawan J, Tandon H, Roy S. Ultrastructure of synovial membrane in pyogenic arthritis. *Arch Pathol* 1973;96:155–160.
8. Bigliani L, Flatow E, Deliz E. Complications of shoulder arthroscopy. *Orthop Rev* 1991;20:743–751.
9. Black J, Hunt TL, Godley PJ, Matthew E. Oral antimicrobial therapy for adults with osteomyelitis or septic arthritis. *J Infect Dis* 1987;155: 968–972.
10. Bodel P, Hollingsworth J. Comparative morphology, respiration, and phagocytic function of leukocytes from blood and joint fluid in rheumatoid arthritis. *J Clin Invest* 1966;45:580–589.
11. Booth RE Jr, Lotke PA. The results of spacer block technique in revision of infected total knee arthroplasty. *CORR* 1989;248:57–60.
12. Booth RE Jr, Tuan RS, Gardner T, O'Rourke B, Mariani BD. Molecular genetic analysis of infection after total knee reimplantation. American Academy of Orthopaedic Surgeons 64th Annual Meeting, San Francisco, 1997.
13. Brancos MA, Peris P, Miro JM, et al. Septic arthritis in heroin addicts. *Semin Arthritis Rheum* 1991;21:81–87.
14. Bremell T, Lange S, Holmdahl R, Ryden C, Hansson G, Tarkowski A. Immunopathological features of rat *Staphylococcus aureus* arthritis. *Infect Immun* 1994;62:2334–2344.
15. Brien WW, Salvati EA, Klein R, Brause B, Stern S. Antibiotic-impregnated bone cement in total hip arthroplasty. An in vivo comparison of the elution properties of tobramycin and vancomycin. *CORR* 1993;296:242–248.
16. Brower A. Septic arthritis. *Radiol Clin North Am* 1996;34:293–309.
17. Broy SB, Stulberg S, Schmid FR. The role of arthroscopy in the diagnosis and management of the septic joint. *Clin Rheum Dis* 1986;12: 489–500.
18. Buchholz H, Engelbrecht H. Uber die depotwirkung einiger antibiotica bei vermischung mit dem kunstharz palacos. *Chirurgie* 1970;41: 411.
19. Chen W-S, Wan Y-L, Lui C-C, Lee T-Y, Wang K-C. Extrapleural abscess secondary to infection of the sternoclavicular joint. *J Bone Joint Surg [Am]* 1993;75:1835–1839.
20. Chu C-C, Williams DF. Effects of physical configuration and chemical structure of suture materials on bacterial adhesion. A possible link to wound infection. *Am J Surg* 1984;147:197–204.
21. Chung S. The arterial supply of the developing proximal end of the human femur. *J Bone Joint Surg [Am]* 1976;58:961–970.
22. Cierny G, Mader J. Adult chronic osteomyelitis. *Orthopedics* 1984;7: 1557–1564.
23. Cierny G, Mader J, Penninck J. A clinical staging system for adult osteomyelitis. *Contemp Orthop* 1985;5:17.
24. Cofield R, Edgerton B. *Total shoulder arthroplasty: complications and revision surgery*. Vol. 39. Park Ridge, IL: American Academy of Orthopaedic Surgeons, 1990:449–462.
25. Cole W, Dalziel R, Leitl S. Treatment of acute osteomyelitis in childhood. *J Bone Joint Surg [Br]* 1982;64:218–223.
26. Cooperman M. Acute hematogenous bursitis. *Ann Surg* 1938;108: 1094–1101.
27. Costerton J, Irvin R, Cheng K-J. The bacterial glycocalyx in nature and disease. *Ann Rev Microbiol* 1981;35:299–324.
28. Cunningham R, Cockayne A, Humphreys H. Clinical and molecular aspects of the pathogenesis of *Staphylococcus aureus* bone and joint infections. *J Med Microbiol* 1996;44:157–164.
29. D'Angelo G, Ogilvie-Harris D. Septic arthritis following arthroscopy, with cost/benefit analysis of antibiotic prophylaxix. *Arthroscopy* 1988;4:10–14.
30. Darouiche RO, Farmer J, Chaput C, Mansouri M, Saleh G, Landon GC. Anti-infective efficacy of antiseptic coated fracture fixation devices. *Transactions of the 43rd ORS,* 1997:306.
31. Davies JP, Harris WH. Effect of hand mixing tobramycin on the fatigue strength of Simplex P. *J Biomed Mater Res* 1991;25:1409–1414.
32. Davis JC, Heckman JD, DeLee JC, Buckwold FJ. Chronic nonhematogenous osteomyelitis treated with adjuvant hyperbaric oxygen. *J Bone Joint Surg [Am]* 1986;62:1210–1217.
33. Deacon J, Pagliaro A, Zelicof S, Horowitz H. Prophylactic use of antibiotics for procedures after total joint replacement. *J Bone Joint Surg [Am]* 1996;78:1755–1770.
34. Destouet J, Gilula L, Murphy W, Sagel S. Computed tomography of the sternoclavicular joint and sternum. *Radiology* 1981;??:123–128.
35. Drutz D, Schaffner W, Hillman J, Koenig M. The penetration of penicillin and other antimicrobials into joint fluid: three case reports with a reappraisal of the literature. *J Bone Joint Surg [Am]* 1972;49: 1415–1421.
36. Elek S, Conen P. The virulence of *S. pyogenes* for man. A study of the problems of wound infection. *Br J Exp Pathol* 1957;38:573–586.
37. Esterhai JL, Gelb I. Adult septic arthritis. *Orthop Clin North Am* 1991; 22:503–514.
38. Esterhai JL, Sawyer J, Hughes T. Shoulder infection in adults: pathogenesis and diagnosis. *Complications Orthop* 1996;??:11–15.
39. Fitzgerald RH. *Curr Concepts Antimicrob Ther* 1990;39:465–470.
40. Fletcher M, Floodgate G. An electron microscopic demonstration of an acidic polysaccharide involved in the adhesion of a marine bacterium to solid surfaces. *J Gen Microbiol* 1973;74:325–334.
41. Flick AB, Herbert JC, Goodell J, Kristiansen T. Noncommercial fab-

rication of antibiotic-impregnated polymethylmethacrylate beads. Technical note. *CORR* 1987;223:282–286.
42. Friedman R, Perez H, Goldstein I. Septic arthritis of the sternoclavicular joint due to gram positive microorganisms. *Am J Med Sci* 1981; 282:91–93.
43. Frimodt-Moller N, Riegels-Nielsen P. Antibiotic penetration into the infected knee. *Acta Orthop Scand* 1987;58:256–259.
44. Gelberman RH, Menon J, Austerlitz MS, Weisman MH. Pyogenic arthritis of the shoulder in adults. *J Bone Joint Surg [Am]* 1980;62: 550–553.
45. Gibbons R, Van Houte J. Bacterial adherence and the formation of dental plaques. In: Beachey E, ed. *Bacterial adherence: receptors and recognition,* Series B ed. Vol. 6. London: Chapman & Hall, 1980: 63–104.
46. Gifford D, Patzakis M, Ivler D, Swezey R. Septic arthritis due to *Pseudomonas* in heroin addicts. *J Bone Joint Surg [Am]* 1975;57:631–635.
47. Glaser D, Tan V, Seldes R, Williams W, Fitzgerald R Jr. Quantitative and reverse transcriptase polymerase chain reaction techniques for detection of bacterial load and active infection in total joint arthroplasty. Unpublished data, 1997.
48. Goldenberg D. Bacterial arthritis. *Curr Opin Rheumatol* 1995;7: 310–314.
49. Goldenberg DL, Brandt KD, Cathcart ES. Treatment of septic arthritis. *Arthritis Rheum* 1975;18:83–90.
50. Goldenberg DL, Cohen AS. Acute infectious arthritis. *Am J Med* 1976;60:369–377.
51. Goldenberg DL, Reed JI. Bacterial arthritis. *N Engl J Med* 1985;312: 764–771.
52. Goldin R, Chow A, Edwards J Jr, Louie J, Guze L. Sternoclavicular septic arthritis in heroin users. *N Engl J Med* 1973;289:616–618.
53. Goss TP. Shoulder infections. In: Bigliani LU, ed. *Complications of shoulder surgery.* Baltimore, MD: Williams & Wilkins, 1993: 202–213.
54. Gray R, Tenenbaum J, Gottlieb N. Local corticosteroid injection treatment in rheumatic disorders. *Semin Arthritis Rheum* 1981;10: 231–254.
55. Grieben A. Results of Septopal(R) in more than 1500 cases of bone and soft tissue infections. A review of clinical trials. *J Bone Joint Surg [Br]* 1980;62:275.
56. Gristina A, Costerton J. Bacterial adherence to biomaterials and tissue. The significance of its role in clinical sepsis. *J Bone Joint Surg [Am]* 1985;67:264–273.
57. Gristina A, Costerton J, McGanity P. Bacteria laden biofilms: a hazard to orthopedic prostheses. *Infect Surg* 1984;3:655–662.
58. Gristina A, Hobgood C, Webb L, Myrvik Q. Adhesive colonization of biomaterials and antibiotic resistance. *Biomaterials* 1987;8:423–426.
59. Gristina A, Naylor P, Webb L. Molecular mechanisms in musculoskeletal sepsis: the race for the surface. *Instruct Course Lect* 1990; 39:471–482.
60. Gristina A, Oga M, Webb L, Hobgood C. Adherent bacterial colonization in the pathogenesis of osteomyelitis. *Science* 1985;228: 990–993.
61. Gristina A, Rovere G, Shoji H. Spontaneous septic arthritis complicating rheumatoid arthritis. *J Bone Joint Surg [Am]* 1974;56: 1180–1184.
62. Gristina AG, Kammire G, Voytek A, Webb LX. *Sepsis of the shoulder: molecular mechanisms and pathogenesis.* Vol. 2. Philadelphia: WB Saunders, 1990:920–939.
63. Hawkins R, et al. The three-part fracture of the proximal part of the humerus. *J Bone Joint Surg [Am]* 1986;68:1410–1414.
64. Hendrix R, Fisher M. Imaging of septic arthritis. *Clin Rheum Dis* 1986;12:459–487.
65. Henry SL, Galloway KP. Local antibacterial therapy for the management of orthopaedic infections: pharmacokinetic considerations. *Clin Pharmacokinet* 1995;29:36–45.
66. Henry SL, Seligson D, Mangino P, Popham GJ. Antibiotic-impregnated beads. Part I: Bead implantation versus systemic therapy. *Orthop Rev* 1991;20:242–247.
67. Hofmann AA, Kane KR, Tkach TK, Plaster RL, Camargo MP. Treatment of infected total knee arthroplasty using an articulating spacer. *CORR* 1995;321:45–54.
68. Hollander J. Intrasynovial corticosteroid therapy in arthritis. *Md State Med J* 1969;19:62–66.
69. Howell A, Sutherland R, Rolinson G. Effect of protein binding on levels of ampicillin and cloxacillin in synovial fluid. *Clin Pharmacol Ther* 1972;13:724.
70. Ivey M, Clark R. Arthroscopic debridement of the knee for septic arthritis. *CORR* 1985;199:201–206.
71. Jackson RW. The septic knee—arthroscopic treatment. *Arthroscopy* 1985;1:194–197.
72. Jarrett M, Grossman L, Sadler A. Grayzel A. The role of arthroscopy in the treatment of septic arthritis. *Arthritis Rheum* 1981;24:737–739.
73. Jocson C. The diffusion of antibiotics through the synovial membrane. *J Bone Joint Surg [Am]* 1955;37:107.
74. Johnson L, Shneider D, Austin M, Goodman F, Bullock J, DeBruin J. Two percent gluteraldehyde: a disinfectant in arthroscopy and arthroscopic surgery. *J Bone Joint Surg [Am]* 1982;64:237–239.
75. Kelly J, Wilkowske C, Washington J. *Chronic osteomyelitis in the adult.* St. Louis, MO: Mosby, 1975:120–132.
76. Kelly PJ, Martin WJ, Coventry MB. Bacterial (suppurative) arthritis in the adult. *J Bone Joint Surg [Am]* 1970;52:1595–1602.
77. Kolyvas E, Ahronheim G, Marks M, Gledhill R, Owens H, Rosenthall L. Oral antibiotic therapy of skeletal infections in children. *Pediatrics* 1980;65:867–871.
78. LaCour EG, Schmid FR. Infections of bursae and tendons. In: Schlossberg, ed. *Orthopedic infection.* New York: Springer-Verlag, 1988:92.
79. Lane JG, Falahee MH, Hankin FM, Kauffer H. Pyarthrosis of the knee: treatment considerations. *CORR* 1990;252:198–204.
80. Leslie BM, Harris JM, Driscoll D. Septic arthritis of the shoulder in adults. *J Bone Joint Surg [Am]* 1989;71:1516–1522.
81. Levine S. Esterhai J, Heppenstall R, Calhoun J, Mader J. Diagnosis and staging. Osteomyelitis and joint infections. *CORR* 1993;295: 77–86.
82. Lewis G, Cluff L. Synovitis in rabbits during bacteremia and vaccination. *Bull Johns Hopkins Hosp* 1965;116:175.
83. Lichtman E. *Candida* infection of a prosthetic shoulder joint. *Skel Radiol* 1983;10:176–177.
84. Lonner JH, Desai P, Dicesare PE, Steiner G, Zuckerman JD. the reliability of analysis of intraoperative frozen sections for identifying active infection during revision hip or knee arthroplasy. *J Bone Joint Surg [Am]* 1996;78:1553–1558.
85. Maderazo E, Judson S, Pasternak H. Late infections in total joint prostheses. A review and recommendations for prevention. *Clin Orthop Rel Res* 1988;229:131–142.
86. Marks KE, Nelson CL, Lautenschlager EP. Antibiotic-impregnated acrylic bone cement. *J Bone Joint Surg [Am]* 1976;58:358–364.
87. Marsh D, Mathews E, Persellin R. Transport of gentamicin into synovial fluid. *JAMA* 1974;228:607.
88. Master R, Weisman MH, Armbuster TG, Slivka J, Resnick D, Goergen TG. Septic arthritis of the glenohumeral joint. *Arthritis Rheum* 1977;20:1500–1506.
89. Mikhail I, Alarcon G. Nongonococcal bacterial arthritis. *Rheum Dis Clin North Am* 1993;19:311–331.
90. Miller SR, Bigliani LU. Chapter 5. In: *Complications of total shoulder replacement.* Baltimore, MD: Williams & Wilkins, 1993.
91. Nade S. Acute septic arthritis in infancy and childhood. *J Bone Joint Surg [Br]* 1983;65:234–241.
92. Nelson JD. Antibiotic concentrations in septic joints. *N Engl J Med* 1971;284:349–353.
93. Newman J. Review of septic arthritis throughout the antibiotic era. *Ann Rheum Dis* 1976;35:198.
94. Norden C, Gillespie W, Nade S. *Infections in bones and joints.* Cambridge, MA: Blackwell Scientific, 1994:438.
95. Norman D, Yoshikawa T. Responding to septic arthritis. *Geriatrics* 1983;38:83–91.
96. O'Brien S, Goldenberg D, Rice P. Disseminated gonococcal infection: a prospective analysis of 49 patients and a review of the pathophysiology and immune mechanisms. *Medicine* 1983;62:395–406.
97. O'Meara P, Bartal E. Septic arthritis: process, etiology, treatment outcome. A literature review. *Orthopedics* 1988;11:623–628.
98. Parisien JS. Arthroscopic management of pyarthrosis: an overview. *Bull Hosp Joint Dis Orthop Inst* 1987;47:52–57.
99. Parker R, Schmid F. Antibacterial activity of synovial fluid during treatment of septic arthritis. *Arthritis Rheum* 1971;14:96–104.
100. Parker R, Schmidt F. Transport of antibiotics into infected joints. *Arthritis Rheum* 1968;11:503.
101. Post M. *Complications following anterior acromioplasty and rotator cuff repair.* Baltimore, MD: Williams & Wilkins, 1993:34–43.
102. Prober CG, Yeager AS. Use of the serum bactericidal titer to assess the adequacy of oral antibiotic therapy in the treatment of acute hematogenous osteomyelitis. *J Pediatr* 1979;95:131–135.

103. Ramsey M, Fenlin J Jr. Use of an antibiotic-impregnated bone cement block in the revision of an infected shoulder arthroplasty. *J Shoulder Elbow Surg* 1996;5:479–482.
104. Rapp G, Griffith R, Hebbie W. The permeability of traumatically inflamed synovial membrane to commonly used antibiotics. *J Bone Joint Surg [Am]* 1966;48:1534.
105. Renner JB, Agee MW. Treatment of suppurative arthritis by percutaneous catheter drainage. *AJR* 1990;154:135–138.
106. Riegels-Nielsen P, Frimodt-Moller N, Jensen J. Rabbit model of septic arthritis. *Acta Orthop Scand* 1987;58:14–19.
107. Rosenthal J, Giles G, Bole WDR. Acute nongonococcal infectious arthritis: evaluation of risk factors, therapy, and outcome. *Arthritis Rheum* 1980;23:889–896.
108. Salter R, Bell R, Keeley F. The protective effect of continuous passive motion in living articular cartilage in acute septic arthritis: an experimental investigation in the rabbit. *CORR* 1981;159:223–247.
109. Sanders T, Staple T. Percutaneous catheter drainage of septic shoulder joint. *Radiology* 1983;147:270–271.
110. Schmid F. Routine drug treatment of septic arthritis. *Clin Rheum Dis* 1984;10:293–311.
111. Schurman DJ, Hirshman H, Nagel DA. Antibiotic penetration of synovial fluid in infected and normal knee joints. *CORR* 1978;136: 304–310.
112. Schurman DJ, Kajiyama G. Antibiotic absorption from infected and normal joints using a rabbit knee joint model. *J Orthop Res* 1985;3: 185–188.
113. Scott J. *Copeman's textbook of rheumatic diseases,* 6th ed. Vol. 1. New York: Churchill Livingstone, 1986.
114. Sharp J. Infectious arthritis. *Arch Intern Med* 1979;139:1125.
115. Simpson ML. *Septic arthritis in adults.* Philadelphia: WB Saunders, 1989:284–287.
116. Slusher M, Myrvik Q, Lewis J, Gristina A. Extended-wear lenses, biofilm, and bacterial adhesion. *Arch Ophthalmol* 1987;105:110–115.
117. Smith MJ. ARthroscopic treatment of septic knee. *Arthroscopy* 1986; 2:30–34.
118. Smith R, Schurman D, Kajiyama G, Sarossy J. Effect of NSAID and antibiotic treatment in a rabbit model of Staph infectious arthritis. *Transactions of the 36th Annual Meeting of the ORS* 1990;15:296.
119. Southwood R, Rice J, McDonald P, Hakendorf P, Rozenbilds M. Infection in experimental hip arthroplasties. *J Bone Joint Surg [Br]* 1985;67:229–231.
120. Speziale P, Raucci G, Visai L, Switalski L, Timpl R, Hook M. Binding of collagen to *Staphylococcus aureus* Cowan 1. *J Bacteriol* 1986; 167:77–81.
121. Steigbigel N. Diagnosis and management of septic arthritis. In: Remington J, Swartz M, eds. *Current clinical topics in infectious disease.* New York: McGraw-Hill, 1983:1–29.
122. Stern G, Lubniewski A. The interaction between *Pseudomonas aeruginosa* and the corneal epithelium. *Arch Ophthalmol* 1985;103: 1221–1225.
123. Stinchfield F, Bigliani L, Neu H, Goss T, Foster C. Late hematogenous infection of total joint replacement. *J Bone Joint Surg [Am]* 1980;62:1345–1350.
124. Tetzlaff TR, McCracken GH, Nelson J. Oral antibiotic therapy for skeletal infections of children. *J Pediatr* 1978;92:485–490.
125. Thompson G, Manshady B, Weiss J. Septic bursitis. *JAMA* 1978;240: 2280–2281.
126. Toby E, Webb L, Voytek A, Gristina A. Septic arthritis of the shoulder. *Orthop Trans* 1987;11:230.
127. Trippel S. Antibiotic-impregnated cement in total joint arthroplasty. *J Bone Joint Surg [Am]* 1986;68:1297–1302.
128. Trueta J. The normal vascular anatomy of the human femoral head during growth. *J Bone Joint Surg [Br]* 1957;39:358–394.
129. Tumeh S. Scintigraphy in the evaluation of arthropathy. *Radiol Clin North Am* 1996;34:215–231.
130. Unkila-Kallio L, Kallio M, Peltola H. The usefulness of C-reactive protein levels in the identification of concurrent septic arthritis in children who have acute hematogenous osteomyelitis. *J Bone Joint Surg [Am]* 1994;76:848–853.
131. Vincent GM, Amirault D. Septic arthritis in the elderly. *CORR* 1990; 251:241–245.
132. Voytek A, Gristina A, Barth E, et al. Staphylococcal adhesion to collagen in intra-articular sepsis. *Biomaterials* 1988;9:107–110.
133. Waldvogel F, Medoff G, Swartz M. Osteomyelitis: a review of clinical features, therapeutic considerations, and unusual aspects. *N Engl J Med* 1970;282:198–206, 260–266, 316–322.
134. Ward WG, Goldner RD. Shoulder pyarthrosis: a concomitant process. *Orthopedics* 1994;12:591–595.
135. Weissman G, Spilberg I, Krakauer K. Arthritis induced in rabbits by lysates of granulocyte lysosomes. *Arthritis Rheum* 1969;12:103–116.
136. Williams D. *Antibiotic prophylaxis in bone and joint infections.* Philadelphia: WB Saunders, 1989:60–65.
137. Wirth M, Rockwood C. Complications of shoulder arthroplasty. *Clin Orthop Rel Res* 1994;307:47–69.
138. Wohlgethan J, Newberg A, Reed J. The risk of abscess from sternoclavicular septic arthritis. *J Rheumatol* 1988;15:1302–1306.

PART XII

Rehabilitation

Disorders of the Shoulder: Diagnosis and Management,
edited by Joseph P. Iannotti and Gerald R. Williams, Jr.
Lippincott Williams & Wilkins, Philadelphia © 1999.

CHAPTER 35

Shoulder Rehabilitation

Martin J. Kelley and Brian G. Leggin

Although rehabilitation of the shoulder is considered to be critical to the recovery of patients with shoulder pain, a few prospective studies demonstrate that specific techniques or protocols are effective. Controversy still exist regarding how much rehabilitation is required and whether it should be performed under a therapist's supervision or directed completely by the physician. Regardless, it is clear that the days of supervised therapy three times weekly, written as a standard order for each patient, are over. Our belief is that prudent therapy is extremely valuable if a team approach is utilized. The team is composed of the physician, the therapist, and the patient. The physician makes the diagnosis and refers the patient for therapy. The therapist further evaluates and determines the status of the patient and the level at which exercise or antiinflammatory procedures should be performed. The patient must be absolutely compliant with the program and follow through with patient education advice and exercises. The patient must interact with both the therapist and the physician to provide feedback regarding progress. Open communication between the team members is essential, particularly between the therapist and the physician, when treating the postoperative patient. The physician must provide the therapist with surgical findings, modifications, and precautions. The therapist must interact with the physician relative to the patient's progress and assist in guiding the rehabilitation. When the patient does not progress as expected, or develops complications, the therapist must make the necessary program modifications; if no changes occur, then the therapist must make appropriate recommendations to the patient and physician. If the physician, therapist, and patient are actively interacting and performing their responsibilities, the team, individually and as a whole, will be successful.

This chapter not only addresses the treatment approach to certain pathologies, but offers rationale for treatment. Unfortunately, rehabilitation is often thought of as range of motion (ROM) exercises and strengthening, but these are only components of rehabilitation.

ANATOMY AND FUNCTION

For successful shoulder rehabilitation to occur the clinician must have an excellent working knowledge of anatomy and biomechanics. Normal shoulder function is dependent on the movement harmony of the four shoulder girdle articulations: the glenohumeral joint, scapulothoracic joint, acromioclavicular joint, and sternoclavicular joint. In conjunction, appropriate movement of the spine and ribs are essential for normal shoulder girdle movement. The neuromuscular system drives the osseous structure and ensures dynamic support at the joints, whereas the capsuloligamentous structures (static stabilizers) help to maintain the appropriate orientation between the osseous structures. When the

M. J. Kelley and B. G. Leggin: University of Pennsylvania Medical Center, Penn Therapy and Fitness, Philadelphia, Pennsylvania 19104.

static and dynamic stabilizers function in synchrony, normal scapulohumeral rhythm occurs. This rhythm is classically described during arm elevation[27,31,113]; however, scapulohumeral rhythm also has been described for complex activities such as throwing and swimming. Overuse causing joint and/or soft-tissue dysfunction or injury can result in disruption of the balance between the dynamic and static stabilizers. Over time, irreversible tissue pathology may occur, requiring surgical intervention. The anatomy and biomechanics of the shoulder have been discussed in previous chapters. We will discuss specific areas of anatomy and biomechanics as they relate to pathology and rehabilitation.

Rotator Cuff

The rotator cuff is composed of four musculotendinous units—the subscapularis, supraspinatus, infraspinatus, and teres minor—that blend to form a contiguous envelope surrounding the glenohumeral joint anteriorly, superiorly, and posteriorly. These four muscles are classically described as inserting upon the lesser tuberosity (subscapularis) and the latter three upon the greater tuberosity facets, inserting superior to inferior.[36] However, the complex insertional pattern of the rotator cuff and its influence on pathology and rehabilitation is not commonly appreciated.

The rotator cuff and capsuloligamentous complex (CLC) are anatomically intimate with each other as the two become firmly integrated to surround the glenohumeral joint. Before the rotator cuff tendons actually insert to bone, the distal muscle fibers and tendons insert onto half of the CLC surface.[17,18] The tendons of the rotator cuff fuse into a contiguous structure approximately 15 mm from the humeral insertion, interdigitating anteriorly and posteriorly into the supraspinatus.[18] A triangular sheath is formed between the supraspinatus and subscapularis tendons. This sheath or space is called the rotator cuff interval and is composed primarily of the coracohumeral ligament,[18,44,76,141] superior glenohumeral ligament,[18,141] and long head of the biceps.[141] The interval appears to be a busy connective tissue intersection where multiple pathologies has been identified, including associated tears of the supraspinatus[76,141] or isolated rupture.[76] Additionally, subscapularis tears commonly are associated with medial dislocation of the long head of the biceps,[32,33,143] thereby disrupting tissues of the interval. Instability has been associated with this area, and closure has established stability.[91] Contracture of the rotator cuff interval has been found to cause significant restrictions of glenohumeral motion.[44,108] Loss of external rotation in adduction and flexion has been seen in selective imbrication of this structure.[44] A goal of rehabilitation of a patient with supraspinatus tendonitis or following surgical repair is to respect the anatomic and functional relationship between the coracohumeral ligament and supraspinatus. Stretching the arm into external rotation increases passive and dynamic tension across the coracohumeral ligament and supraspinatus. This can create painful symptoms in a person with tendonitis or can stretch a repair, particularly if performed under tension.[76]

The rotator cuff tendons eventually insert into their respective tuberosity sites. The distal 1 cm of the supraspinatus appears to be susceptible to tensile and compressive forces as well as decreased vascularity.[116,122] Histologic examination of the supraspinatus tendon–bone insertion interface reveals a protective fibrocartilage transition zone between tendon and bone.[6,18] This fibrocartilage buffer zone assists in minimizing tendon fiber separation resulting from excessive tensile, torsion, and compression forces normally encountered in high-velocity athletic activities or heavy overhead labor. Unfortunately, this natural buffer zone does not stand the test of time. Nakajima[94] compared articular and bursal sections of the supraspinatus tendon in cadavers and found the bursal side to have a sturdier connective tissue make-up and twice the tensile strength compared with the articular side. This helps to explain the high incidence of articular-sided tears. Understanding the negative effect that tension—both passive (placing the arm in adduction and performing external rotation) and dynamic (overload the cuff with too much resistance)—has on the rotator cuff is critical for the treating clinician. By modifying the position of exercise, safe and effective rehabilitation can be achieved.

The function of the rotator cuff is to stabilize the humeral head in the glenoid fossa during movement, particularly during the mid-range of motion, when the CLC is a less effective stabilizer.[80] Certainly, rotator cuff function is also paramount to glenohumeral joint stability at the end range of motion. During activities of daily living, overhead athletic use, or occupation use, the force transmitted by the supraspinatus, infraspinatus, teres minor, and subscapularis, in addition to the deltoid and biceps, provides significant joint stability. This is achieved by increasing humeral compressive forces into the glenoid[10,14,19,51,53,61,81,113,114,120,127] and by a dynamic barrier created by the contracting envelope.[127] The functional interdependency of the rotator cuff and CLC must be appreciated as the arm is moved. The rotator cuff muscles act as a primary mover of the humerus, with 50% of shoulder abduction and flexion torque output attributed to the infraspinatus and supraspinatus[50,74] and 70% of external rotation torque a result of infraspinatus function.[106] As movement occurs, the glenohumeral CLC tightens, offering assistance to joint stability.[25] At end range, stability is provided by both the rotator cuff and the now maximally taut CLC. Maximizing the rotator cuff's stabilizing function is one of the therapist's most important roles. The therapist must recognize that the dynamic stabilizers are critical to joint stability in mid-range, where the CLC is loose.

Intrinsic weakness or reflexive inhibition of the rotator cuff due to pain can cause pathologic tensile loading or secondary compression related to increased humeral head migration. This is why exercises directed toward rotator cuff strengthening—at different arcs in the range, not just with the arm at the side—are critical. To just strengthen the dynamic stabilizers with the arm at the side is accomplishing only partial rehabilitation.

Biceps

Although much of the attention in rehabilitation is directed toward the rotator cuff, the biceps is important to normal shoulder function. The biceps has been found to be an effective humeral head depressor, and activity was found to reduce strain on the inferior glenohumeral ligament (IGHL) and reduce both anterior and posterior humeral translation.[120] The long head is exposed to significant tensile load as it attempts to decelerate the elbow during the deceleration phase of throwing,[56] tennis serving,[126] or "spiking." Additionally, the biceps is susceptible to mechanical compression intraarticularly and at the biceps groove level in all overhead athletic activities.[95,99] The greater the repetition, as in swimming, the greater the mechanical stress the biceps tendon must bear.[119]

Deltoid

The last glenohumeral muscle essential to normal shoulder motion is the deltoid. Contribution of the deltoid to abduction torque is approximately 50%, equal to that provided by the supraspinatus and infraspinatus[50,74] Initial deltoid contraction produces primarily a shear force, attempting to sublux the humeral head superiorly.[114] As humeral elevation in the scapular plane increases, the direction of pull and moment arm improves, resulting in less glenohumeral joint shear force and greater compressive force.[114] Therefore, the deltoid's mechanical advantage and contribution to stability improve with elevation, as long as appropriate scapular rotation occurs. Loss of the deltoid through neurologic disruption (i.e., axillary nerve palsy) or removal can be debilitating. However, patients typically compensate well through the use of the intact musculature.[21,88] Deltoid loss in the presence of rotator cuff pathology or instability, particularly postoperatively, can be catastrophic for the patient.[39]

Capsuloligamentous Complex

The CLC is composed of the capsule, the coracohumeral ligament, and the glenohumeral ligaments—superior, middle, and inferior. This complex encases the glenohumeral joint inserting from the humerus, (superior to the lesser tuberosity and surgical and anatomic necks) to the anterior glenoid neck and glenoid rim via the labrum. The glenohumeral ligaments are distinctive collagenous capsular thickenings, the most significant is the IGHL. The IGHL is formed by an axillary pouch bordered by thickened anterior and posterior bands. The anterior band attaches between the 2 and 4 o'clock positions on the glenoid and labrum. The posterior band was found to attach between the 7 and 9 o'clock positions. This unique configuration allows this single ligament to stabilize anteriorly, posteriorly, and inferiorly.[105]

TABLE 1. *Primary restricting responsibilities of the CLC*

Ligament	Translation	Motion
Coraco-humeral	Inferior–posterior/anterior	ER (0° of abduction)
SGHL	Inferior–posterior/anterior	ER (0° of abduction)
IGHL	Inferior (in abduction)	Elevation
	Anterior (in abduction)	ER (≥90° of abduction)
	Posterior (in abduction)	IR (≥90° of abduction)

The CLC constraining function is best evident at the end range of motion, where these structures become taut. The ligament's primary role of restricting translation and motion is position dependent and summarized in Table 1. The ligaments create stabilization by (a) providing a barrier against abnormal translation,[25,139,142] (b) creating obligatory translation opposite the tightening,[43,51] and (c) increasing articular compressive forces as they tighten.[25] The extreme of this latter function is seen in the presence of capsular adhesions. In the presence of fibrotic capsuloligamentous tissue, normal glenohumeral rotation is obliterated, and articular compression is increased during elevation.

Research has demonstrated that although the isolated ligaments of the glenohumeral joint are primarily responsible for preventing directional humeral translation and restricting specific motions, they act as a functional unit as described by the circle and load-sharing concepts.[91,105,107,135,139,142,144] The circle concept refers to the global stabilizing function of the static restraints on all sides of the glenohumeral joint (i.e., the posterior capsule assists in anterior stability and *vice versa*). Load sharing refers to the shifting primary stabilizing responsibility of the isolated portions of the CLC as humeral position changes, that is, inferior translation is resisted by the coracohumeral and superior glenohumeral ligaments when the arm is positioned in adduction and by the IGHL, with the arm in abduction. Compromise of the contiguous CLC complex by trauma, Bankart lesion, or a patchulous capsule not only results in a loss of the mechanical stabilization effect, but abnormalities of proprioception. With compromise to the CLC, damage of the mechanoreceptors also may occur, resulting in inappropriate feedback to the neuromuscular system and instability.[11,40,79,78]

True understanding of the stabilizing and restricting responsibilities of the static restraints individually and as a whole guides the therapist in rehabilitation so the instability is not encouraged, the surgical reconstruction is protected and in the case of limited motion or contracture, focused stretching is emphasized.

The Dynamic–Static Complex Interdependency

Rotator cuff/CLC intimacy is more than anatomic; it results in functional interdependency. As previously discussed, rotator cuff muscle activity produces glenohumeral motion, resulting in tightening or stabilization of the static restraints. The musculotendinous units surrounding the glenohumeral joint also assist the static restraints by stabilizing at end ranges of motion but are probably the main stabilizers during movement away from the end ranges, or in mid-range. In mid-range, where the CLC is relatively lax and less effective as a barrier or in generating glenohumeral compression, the dynamic stabilizers maintain stability.

Scapulothoracic Muscles

The scapulothoracic muscles are the trapezius (upper, middle, and lower), serratus anterior (upper and lower digitations), levator scapula, rhomboids (major and minor), and pectoralis minor (Fig. 1). Scapulothoracic muscle function is classically described as force couple activity achieving lateral scapular rotation.[28,60,68]

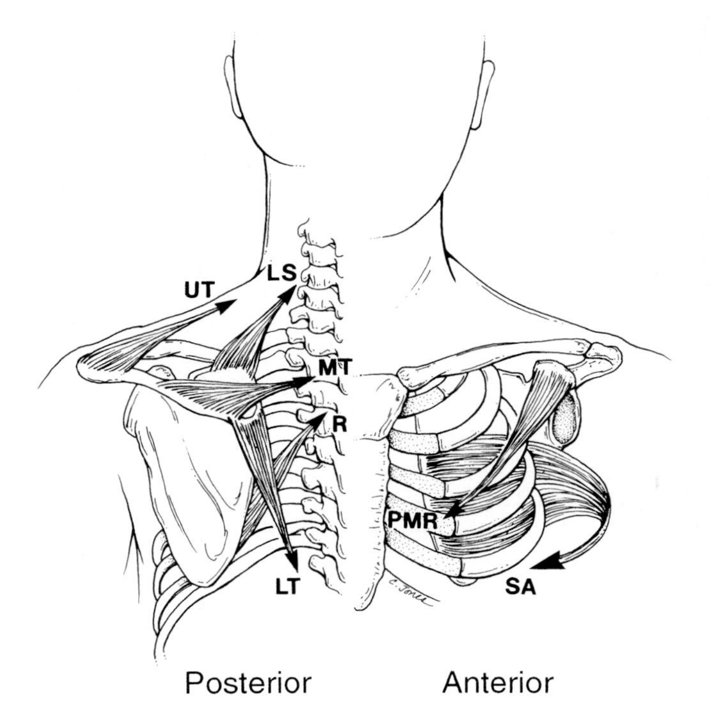

FIG. 1. Anterior and posterior view of scapular muscles.

This is a limited view of the scapular muscles' function and responsibility. We must acknowledge that the scapular muscles move the glenoid relative to the humerus and this is just as important as the glenohumeral muscles moving the humerus relative to the glenoid. The scapulothoracic muscles perform four paramount functions:

1. The muscles provide a stable base, enabling the axiohumeral and scapulohumeral muscles to move the arm against resistance. Trying to move the humerus without stabilizing scapular muscle function, particularly the trapezius and/or serratus anterior, is like to trying to push against a solid wall while standing on ice.
2. Scapular rotation results in the deltoid fibers maintaining efficient length through elevation ROM, thereby enhancing their stabilizing effect at the glenohumeral joint. Without scapular rotation, only 90 degrees of active abduction is available.[53,82]
3. The muscles prevent impingement by separating the subacromial soft tissues from the coracoacromial arch.
4. The muscles orient the scapula, maintaining the glenoid surface in an appropriate position to support the humeral head and reduce stress on the static restraints. Loss of the latter function can result in potential instability.[124] This last function is significant and requires further discussion.

Glenohumeral joint stability can be compromised when the scapular muscles function inadequately. During sagittal plane motion the serratus anterior normally translates the scapula forward (abduction) on the thoracic wall, directing the glenoid toward the sagittal plane, consistent with the position of the humerus. (Scapular abduction refers to the medial border moving away from the thoracic spine, resulting in orienting the glenoid anteriorly around the curved thorax.) However, if the glenoid remains oriented toward the coronal plane, due to poor serratus anterior strength or function, tension increases across the posterior capsule, promoting posterior instability. During coronal plane abduction, the middle trapezius, lower trapezius, and rhomboid activity increases, orienting the glenoid laterally (adducting the scapula) into optimal alignment with the humerus.[75] Attempted coronal plane abduction in the presence of weak scapular adductor muscles results in abnormal sagittal plane glenoid orientation causing increased tension across the anterior-inferior CLC, therefore jeopardizing stability. Maximizing scapular muscle strength and function to effectively position the glenoid is as important to glenohumeral stability as optimizing rotator cuff strength to centralize the humeral head.

A less appreciated aspect of scapular muscle function is the concept of scapular muscle balance. "Balance" not only refers to lateral rotation and the previously discussed movement of abduction/adduction but also scapular elevation/depression. Upon review of muscle orientation and action, it becomes clear that most of the scapulothoracic muscles have an elevation component (consider the trapezius as three separate muscles each having isolated function). Even the pectoralis minor, although considered a depressor, elevates the scapula (relative to the inferior angle) by pulling the coracoid process downward, anteriorly tilting and gliding the relatively flat scapula over the curved thorax.[64] In fact, only the middle trapezius, which acts to adduct, and lower trapezius, the only true depressor, do not elevate; however, both are significant to lateral rotation of the scapula. Although scapular elevation is important to shoulder function, overcompensation of the elevators and poor strength of the middle and lower trapezius are seen in many overhead athletes. Rarely does one evaluate any person, let alone an athlete, with a weak upper trapezius, levator scapula, rhomboid or pectoralis minor. However, athletes and nonathletes often are found to have weakness and/or poor endurance of the middle and lower trapezius. This may be related to stretch weakness, either postural[67] (chronic protracted shoulder girdle) or dynamic (due to mechanical stress during the deceleration phase). The result is excessive elevation and/or scapular anterior tilting, increased risk of impingement and instability, ineffective scapular adduction, poor eccentric control during the deceleration phase of overhead sport activities, or overdomination of the serratus during humeral coronal plane positioning.

OVERHEAD SPORT DEMANDS

Overhead activity of the shoulder(s), either unilateral or bilateral, is required during throwing, racquet sports, spiking, and swimming. These activities involve repetitive high-velocity, high-torque end range forces that test the physiologic limits of the capsuloligamentous–labral complex (CLLC) and rotator cuff. Velocities approaching 7,500 degrees/sec are experienced during the acceleration phase of pitching,[110] and thousands of strokes are endured during each swimming session.[111,118] Glenohumeral abduction and external rotation required during the late cocking and initial acceleration phase is extremely stressful to the athlete's shoulder. During the initial acceleration phase, the CLLC is tightened, creating significant articular compressive and shear forces, respectively. The rotator cuff muscles are paramount to glenohumeral joint stability in mid-range, where the capsule and ligaments are loose. Subsequently, as motion continues, and in conjunction with the static restraints, the rotator cuff assists in joint stabilization while experiencing violent torsional stresses at end range. The deceleration phase of the overhead activity (throwing, tennis serve, spike) further challenges the structural integrity of the static and dynamic restraints by distracting the joint surfaces. The rotator cuff is most vulnerable during arm deceleration because it must eccentrically contract at a high velocity. Eccentric activity is a causative factor in myotendonous strain.[11] In addition to all the forces the rotator cuff and CLC must endure, the risk of impingement constantly looms over the rotator cuff–bursal complex.

The importance of scapulothoracic muscle function is often overlooked, particularly if glenohumeral instability and/or rotator cuff pathology exist; thus, rehabilitation can be incomplete. As previously discussed, these muscles provide a fixed proximal platform for the scapulohumeral and axiohumeral muscles to create force and allow distal movement of the humerus, in addition to positioning the glenoid to maximize glenohumeral articular congruity, minimize CLLC tension, and reduce rotator cuff impingement. For example, during swimming using the free-style stroke, the scapular adductors are important in the recovery phase, directing the glenoid laterally, which results in reduced CLLC tension as the humerus elevates, horizontally abducts, and externally rotates. The serratus anterior is also important in scapular positioning in all overhead sports and was found to be significantly active during the late cocking phase of throwing and constantly active throughout all phases of the free-style stroke.[104,112] Scapular elevation domination must be identified through isolated muscle testing and evaluation of movement during shoulder muscle fatigue. Specific strengthening of the lower and middle trapezius is emphasized.

Regardless of the overhead sport, clearly the demands placed on the shoulder structures necessitate optimal flexibility, strength, and endurance.

EVALUATION

The evaluation process and goal of determining the pathology is the same for the therapist and physician, except that the therapist also attempts to focus on the reactivity of the patient's pathology. "Reactivity" is a nonspecific term that describes the irritability of the joint and/or its surrounding soft-tissue structures. The categories of reactivity are mild, moderate, and severe. Although subjective, determining a patient's reactivity defines the patient's present status and helps to guide the clinician in developing an appropriate therapeutic plan.

Because much of a therapist's training is in muscle function, subtleties of the synchronous interaction of the shoulder girdle muscles are emphasized. For example, scapular muscle destabilization can be dramatic or subtle when assessing the rotator cuff muscles with the arm at the side. One must actually look at the scapula to see if it has "locked" onto the thoracic wall. This destabilization is most evident in an individual with a spinal accessory nerve or long thoracic nerve palsy[64] (Fig. 2). Often symptoms may not be reproduced in standard positions; thus, alternative positions need to be used. For instance, a patient with subtle instability may appear to have excellent abductor and external rotation strength when tested at the side; however, when placed in a position of 120 degrees of elevation and 70 degrees of external rotation, weakness is demonstrated. This has a great deal of meaning to the therapist because this identifies the position where neuromuscular training of the dynamic stabilizers needs to be emphasized.

Therapists also tend to strongly differentiate symptoms from contractile tissue, i.e., muscle and tendon from noncontractile tissue, as well as capsule from ligament. Pain with resisted motions usually indicates that the muscle tendon unit is being provoked, and pain with passive motion indicates that noncontractile tissue is being irritated by stretching.[22] However, this is not always the case. For instance, pain with resisted abduction may occur in patients with significant glenohumeral osteoarthritis due to com-

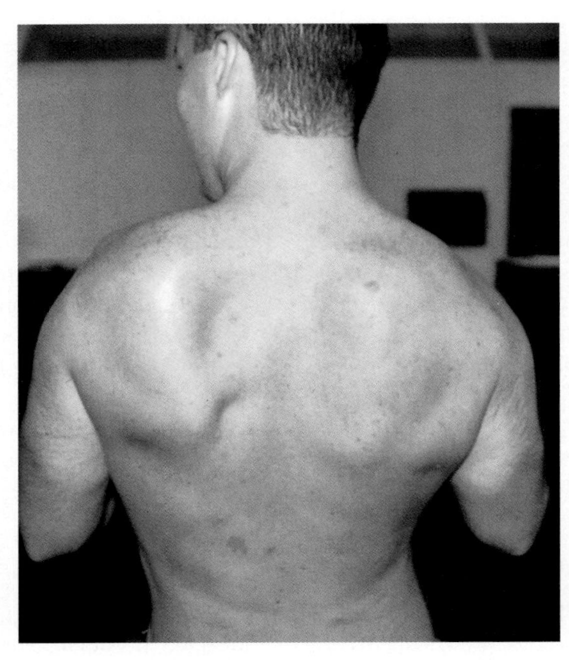

FIG. 2. Individual with left spinal accessory nerve palsy resulting in scapular destabilization. Resisting the external rotators causes the medial scapular border to flip laterally due to the loss of the middle and lower trapezius tethering function. This is not lateral ortrue medial winging.

pression of the partially denuded joint surfaces (noncontractile tissue). Pain may occur with passive functional internal rotation by placing the hand up the back, but the pain is from elongating the inflamed supraspinatus tendon (contractile tissue). Knowledge of anatomy, biomechanics, and kinesiology are extremely important in identifying the tissue status of the patient so that a safe and effective treatment plan can be established.

TREATMENT

Principles of rehabilitation remain constant regardless of whether the patient's status is postinjury or postsurgery. First, pain is always respected and rarely encouraged. The onset of pain following the introduction of a new exercise or technique probably indicates the need for reevaluation of the recent intervention. Therefore, modalities or exercises are introduced one or two at a time. Only then can the clinician identify effective treatment interventions when the patient shows progress or irritating treatment interventions when the patient regresses.

Second, performing a thorough evaluation to identify pathology, tissue reactivity, and functional deficits is critical when developing an effective treatment program. However, constant reevaluation of tissue reactivity as treatment continues is equally essential. Tissue reactivity is determined by subjective reporting and objective testing and qualifies the irritability of the involved structures. The patient's reactivity becomes the guide for program progression. An iatrogenic plateau is sometimes reached, which essentially means that further recovery is hampered by the very same process that initially allowed some degree of recovery.[65]

The plateau is characterized by stagnating mild tissue reactivity. A short but full rest from exercise, lasting 4 to 10 days, is recommended, and typically the tissue recovers as does the patients progress. Manual therapy, by resistive training and soft-tissue or joint mobilization, allows continuous reevaluation while treating. The real-time feedback gained by manual contact allows immediate modification of techniques and exercise or correction of the patient's movement patterns. Manual contact is essential in discovering subtle and sometimes blatant problems that only arise with repetitive motion or those that manifest with fatigue.

Third, exercise and techniques are advanced in motion, resistance, and movement planes based on symptoms and the functional demands of the patient. The exercise is progressed from isometrics, to short arc, to full arc. Submaximal resistance is initially used, advancing to maximal resistance. Progression of shoulder position or motion plane, during exercise, is from the nonprovocative to the provocative. Stress and safety zones are identified in Fig. 3. The plane of the scapula (POS) lies in the center of the safety zone. These nonprovocative and provocative positions and planes vary based on pathology or surgery, but most commonly the least provocative position is somewhere between 20 and 55 degrees of scapular plane abduction. Keeping the humerus below 55 degrees prevents subacromial impingement, whereas avoiding full adduction minimizes excessive tension across the supraspinatus–coracohumeral complex and/or CLC. The POS is advantageous in exercise performance for several reasons. The POS is an inherently stable position for the glenohumeral joint when working with a patient with instability because tensile and torsional stresses to the rotator cuff and CLLC are minimized during exercise.[57] Additionally, strengthening in the POS utilizes the optimal alignment of

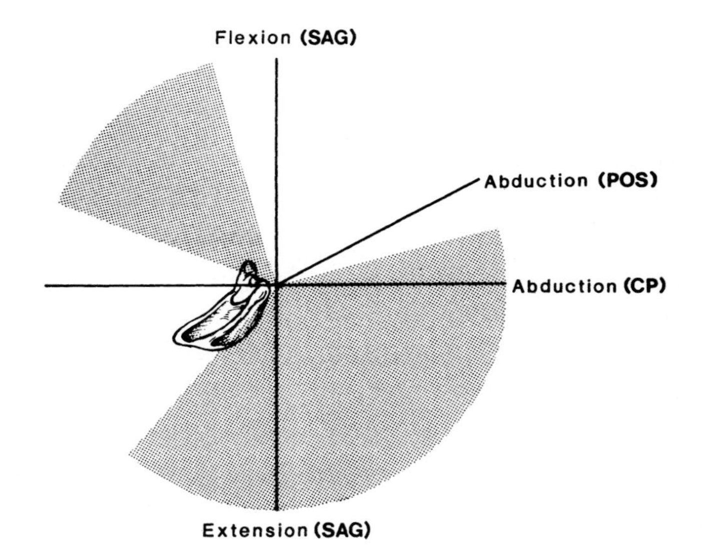

FIG. 3. Stress (*shaded*) and safety (*white*) zones.

TABLE 2. *Principles of treatment*

No pain—all gain
Constant reevaluation
Utilize the plane of the scapula
Rest when needed
Scapular muscle integration and balance
Nonprovocative → provocative
Submaximal → maximal
Short arc → full arc
Individualize program based on symptoms and functional demands

the supraspinatus and deltoid.[57] Progression to provocative positions is required, and they are typically at end ranges, where an athlete must function, particularly 90 degrees of coronal plane abduction, horizontal abduction, and full external rotation. This position not only stresses the CLLC and twists the rotator cuff but can cause supraspinatus impingement against the posterior glenoid rim.[24,54,140]

Fourth, balanced scapular muscle function is constantly integrated into all dynamic exercises from simple rotator cuff exercises to sport-specific manual resistance and isokinetics. We have found this principle to be extremely effective in returning the overhead athlete to competition.

Lastly, the patient's rehabilitation program is individualized based on reactivity, hyperelasticity/hypoelasticity, personality, goals, and surgical concerns and complications (Table 2).

Goals of Rehabilitation

The goals of rehabilitation, the problem that goal addresses, and the rationale for the goals are listed in Table 3 and will be discussed.

Patient Education

The goal and ultimate success of patient education cannot be underestimated, particularly in light of our current managed care environment. First, the patient must understand the basic concepts of their pathology so that the additional instruction about stopping irritating activities is understood. They are instructed in how to promote healing through positioning (Fig. 4) and the use of heat and ice. When appropriate, they are instructed in the proper performance of relatively pain-free exercises and, if they are to be discharged, indications for progression of the program. Without effective patient education, the rehabilitative process may be jeopardized.

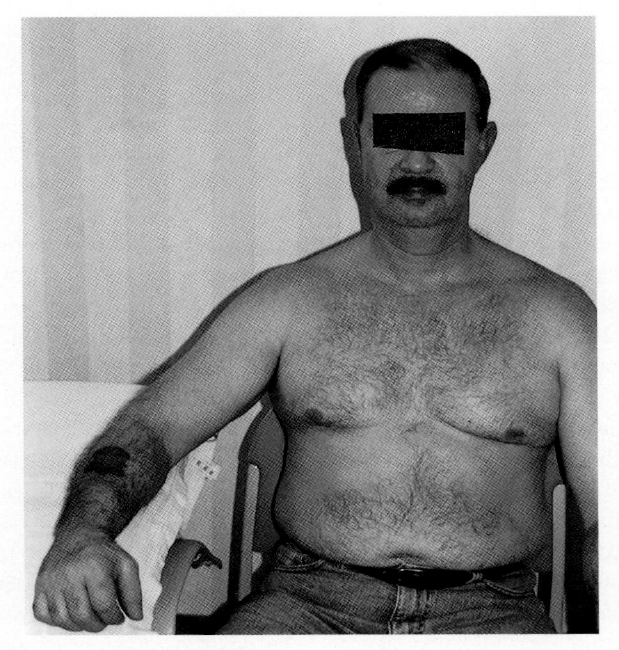

FIG. 4. Placing the patient in a supported, neutral rotation position reduces pain and discourages contracture.

Antiinflammation and Pain Reduction

In addition to terminating aggravating activities, modalities have been advocated for antiinflammation and pain reduction. Much of the evidence for their use is anecdotal or a product of questionable experimental design. A variety of modalities are used during the rehabilitation process. The four main objectives for using modalities are to (a) reduce inflammation, (b) reduce pain, (c) improve motion, and (d) promote muscle reeducation. Most modalities achieve their physiologic effect by the transfer of thermal energy. These modalities include hot packs, cold packs, ultrasonography, diathermy, and infrared. Another mode of achieving a physiologic effect is through the use of electric stimulation. Electric stimulation modalities include transcutaneous electric nerve stimulation (TENS), as well as low-voltage, high-voltage, interferential, and direct current stimulation.

TABLE 3. *Goals of rehabilitation*

Goal	Problem	Rationale
Patient education	Patient lacks knowledge	Prevent injury or reinjury
Anti-inflammation/reduce pain	Inflammation exist	Decrease prostaglandin production and reduce swelling
Facilitate collagen healing	Disruption of collagen	Gentle stress assist in collagen orientation and strength
Strengthen muscle tendon unit	Muscle weakness/dysfunction	Improve neuromuscular stabilization and control
Improve ROM	Adhesion/synovitis/contracture	Improve CLC pliability and Muscle tendon length
Optimize proprioception	Impaired mechanoreceptor input	Optimize mechanoreceptor input and sensitivity
Endurance	Fatigue	Reduce fatigue effect and vulnerability for injury

Heat therapy may be used to reduce muscle guarding and increase tissue temperature to assist with stretching.[34,77] Cold therapy may be used for pain and swelling control. Cold has been shown to be beneficial in reducing pain in the postoperative shoulder patient.[133] Phonophoresis (ultrasonography) and iontophoresis (direct current) can be used to drive antiinflammation medication, usually either hydrocortisone or dexamethasone, through the skin and into the inflamed tissue. Whether this is truly achieved is still controversial.[7,23,71] Ultrasonography does have both thermal and mechanical properties that are thought to increase vascularization and elasticity of the tissue.[34] These latter proposed effects of ultrasonography may be the most effective in conditioning the tissue for stretching and strengthening. Electric stimulation therapies also can be employed for a variety of proposed effects. There are numerous variations of electric stimulation devices based on the type of current delivered (AC or DC), the operating voltage (less than 100 V is called low voltage, versus high voltage, which operates at greater than 500 V), the available frequency (interferential utilizes 4,000 Hz), and wavelength. The desired physiologic responses for electric stimulation as a group are to reduce pain,[87,131] increase circulation,[132] increase muscle activity for reeducation or strength effects,[131] and reduce spasm (by fatigue).

Strength

Muscular strength refers to the capacity for active tension development by a muscle.[128] This is a simplistic definition of a very complex concept. Multiple factors influence muscle strength. Strength gains occur by two types of neuromuscular changes: increased motor unit recruitment and hypertrophy.[70] Significant strength gains have been shown to occur, in the absence of hypertrophy, due to improved motor unit recruitment and synchronization; in other words, the muscle learns the task. Appropriately loading a muscle will result in hypertrophy or increased muscle mass because a muscle with a larger cross-sectional area can create more tension. Although improving muscle mass may be a goal in rehabilitation, the concept of enhancing synchronization and the number of motor units recruited—neuromuscular system training—provides the rationale for why most individuals with rotator cuff tendonopathy and glenohumeral instability are placed on a rotator cuff and scapular muscle strengthening program.

The neuromuscular system is the accumulative interaction of multiple neural systems from the central nervous system (CNS) to the motor units.

1. The CNS involvement is from the motor cortex, basal ganglion, and cerebellum, where conscious and unconscious movement is initiated.
2. The brain stem is where information from the joint mechanoreceptors is relayed to maintain balance and posture.
3. The spinal cord is where reflexes are initiated from information received at the higher centers.[78,79]

The neuromuscular system continues into the afferents and efferents, which translate information back and forth from the CNS and joint, muscle, and tendon mechanoreceptors. Information is eventually processed and motor units are activated, resulting in movement or dynamic stabilization.

Proprioceptive neuromuscular facilitation (PNF) techniques such as rhythmic stabilization, alternating isometrics, and diagonal patterns are performed to enhance neuromuscular control.[134] Combining these techniques (and commonly performed isometric, isotonic, and isokinetic exercises) with our knowledge of shoulder girdle muscle and CLC anatomy, biomechanics and pathology improve our rehabilitation results.

Our ultimate objective is to teach the muscles how to work more efficiently and in an integrated manner, throughout the ROM. This brings us to some important questions:

Does submaximal strengthening of a muscle group in one position improve strength in other positions?

Does submaximal strengthening in one position result in synchronization of shoulder girdle muscle activity, i.e., rotator cuff and scapular muscles, throughout the range of movement? For example, does strengthening the external rotators with the arm placed at the side improve motor units recruitment when the arm is placed at 100 degrees of elevation with a 3-pound tool in the hand? And does performing shrugs with the arms at the side for isolation of the scapular elevators improve motor unit recruitment of these muscles when the arm is placed overhead for athletic activities?

Previous rehabilitation literature[3,63,69,145] and current research regarding proprioception and the neuromuscular mechanism[78,79] shows that rehabilitation exercise should be performed in positions of function. The point is that the commonly performed strengthening exercises for the rotator cuff–deltoid–biceps complex and scapular muscles are standardly stagnated or limited to one plane or position, unless the patient is an athlete. The concept that these exercises enhance motor learning, and thus strength and efficiency of the muscles, dictates that we also attempt to progress these exercises to elevated positions of function when or if the tissues can endure the stress. This is the basis of progressing strengthening exercises from nonprovocative to provocative positions as long as the patient remains symptom free. The provocative position for the 70-year-old sedentary woman may be placing a 16 ounce can of soup on a cabinet shelf compared with the 45-year-old plumber who must fit 95-pound pipes overhead.

To address the second question of synchronization of shoulder girdle muscle activity, we must realize that muscles do not work in isolation. Elevation of the arm requires activity of the glenohumeral muscles as well as the axiohumeral, scapulothoracic, and trunk muscles. Therefore, we need to encourage the proper sequence of motor unit synchronization of all the muscles required for a task whether it be lifting the arm overhead or throwing a baseball 100 miles per hour. Consider an individual lifting a 3-pound power drill overhead. That individual may be able to achieve the gross task of lifting the drill, but did all the necessary complex interactions of myoneural activity, soft-tissue loading, and osseous displacement occur efficiently? Did the myoneural connection happen, did the scapula rotate appropriately, did the dynamic stabilizers maintain humeral head position relative to the glenoid, did the tendon tissue accept the load without microtearing, and did the mechanoreceptors in the muscle, tendon, and capsuloligamentous tissue respond to appropriate tension to provide the necessary feedback? If all goes well, not only does the individual lift the weight, but he or she does so without injury. Now consider that person repeating the motion and driving 100 drywall screws. Can the sequence of occurrences continue without a breakdown resulting in injury. If injury does occur, is it simply a matter that the individual was not "strong" enough or has the person's neuromuscular system not efficiently learned the task or does it not have the endurance to perform it more than 50 times? Are the connective tissue properties altered so that it cannot withstand the repeated loading? The physician and therapist need to consider these questions so that a comprehensive rehabilitation program is devised that will allow the patient to recover from acute injury or following surgery and prevent recurrence of symptoms.

Exercise Versus Pathology

Many investigators have performed electromyographic (EMG) studies to evaluate muscle activity during exercise,[9,93,137] during athletic activity,[56,104,112,126] for occupational use,[58,130] and after nerve block and nerve palsy.[16,50,74] Although these studies give us useful insight regarding muscle function, the rehabilitation specialist must be careful about data interpretation and application to a patient with a pathologic condition. Townsend[137] reported on glenohumeral muscle activity during exercises used for baseball rehabilitation. They found that scaption (POS abduction) performed in internal rotation resulted in the highest muscle activity in the supraspinatus, anterior, and middle deltoid; however, the arc of motion that created peak activity was above 90 degrees (Fig. 5A). Placing an individual in this position with a reactive rotator cuff lesion will increase symptoms due to mechanical impingement. They also reported that horizontal abduction at 90 to 120 degrees of elevation combined with external rotation created maximal activity from the infraspinatus and significant activity of the middle and posterior deltoid (Fig. 5B). Blackburn[9] also advocated this position, finding maximal activity from the supraspinatus and infraspinatus in this position. Scaption with internal rotation and horizontal abduction/external rotation in elevation are two commonly performed exercises for the supraspinatus and infraspinatus, yet both of these exercises are extremely provocative to patients with reactive rotator cuff pathology or anterior glenohumeral instability. Unfortunately, we have seen overenthusiastic and uninformed rehabilitation specialists injure patients with the use of these exercises. The problem is not the research or the position, but the inappropriate use of both with the patient's pathologic condition (Table 4). Mosely et al.[93] evaluated scapular muscle function using the same exercises as Townsend[137]; however, they did not include scaption/internal rotation but only scaption/external rotation. Scaption/external rotation was found to optimally recruit six scapular muscles, but it must be noted that peak activity occurred above 120 degrees. This exercise was recommended not only for enhancing scapular muscle activity but because of the positive stabilizing effect of elevating in the POS with external rotation. Rowing was advocated due to increased trapezius (all heads), levator scapula, and rhomboid activity. Prone horizontal abduction with external rotation also increased activity of the scapular

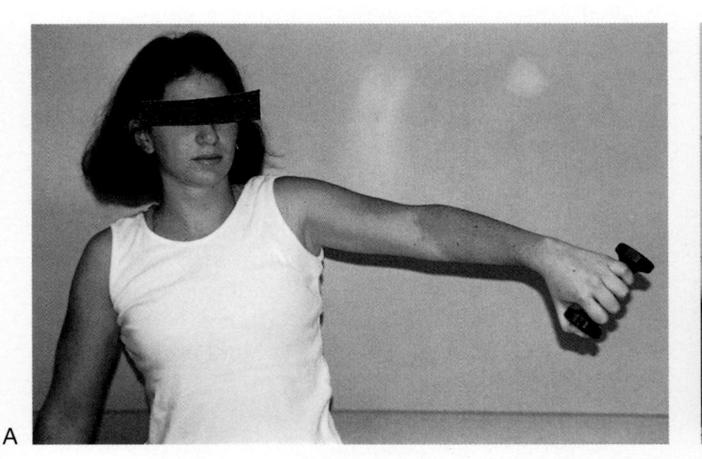
A

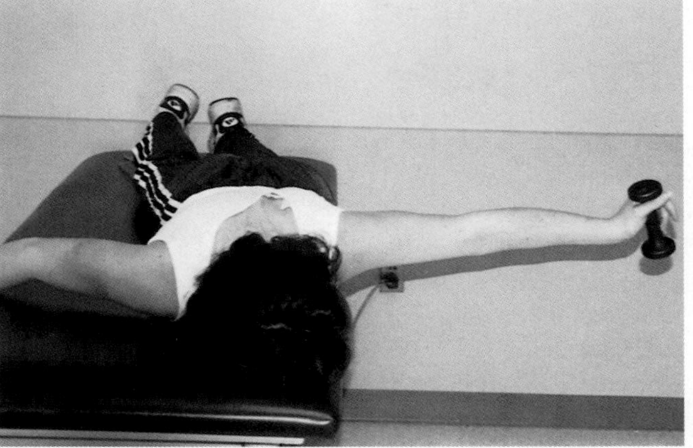
B

FIG. 5. (A) Scaption with internal rotation can create rotator cuff irritation when used in the inappropriate patient. **(B)** This exercise places the shoulder in a provocative position for patients with rotator cuff tendonopathy and anterior instability.

TABLE 4. *Problems with commonly performed strengthening exercises*

1. Nonfunctional arcs
2. Provocative positions
3. Do not integrate the scapular muscles with glenohumeral exercises

retractors, but this position must be approached with caution because it is provocative to glenohumeral soft tissues. The middle and lower fibers of the serratus anterior were found to be significantly recruited during scaption/external rotation as well as during performance of a push-up with a "plus." Again, the patient with rotator cuff tendonopathy or glenohumeral instability (particularly a primary posterior direction) must be able to safely tolerate these positions. The commonly performed exercise of lying on the involved side and internally rotating with a light weight was not found to create even 50% maximum muscle tension (level of significance) of the subscapularis. Attempting to strengthen the subscapularis with the same weight as used for the external rotators may not be effective because the cross-sectional mass of the subscapularis is significantly greater than the external rotators, and external rotator strength is typically approximately 60% of the internal rotator strength. Additionally, lying on the painful side may create symptoms. Research has shown that the commonly performed rotational exercises research do not allow for scapular muscle integration.[93] Moseley et al. found that no qualifying activity of any scapular muscles was noted when internal and external rotation strengthening exercises were performed in sidelying. The rehabilitation specialist must first consider the pathology, tissue reactivity, time from surgery, and target muscle before placing a patient into a provocative position for the potential benefit of maximizing activity of particular muscles. Only patients who have progressed to symptom-free status after adequate healing time has passed should be progressed to the most provocative positions, and with prudence.

Proprioception

Proprioception is defined as the sensation of dynamic joint motion and joint position.[79] The musculotendinous receptors are the muscle spindle and Golgi tendon organs that sense changes in muscle length and tension, respectively. These receptors provide feedback of joint motion and position while the muscle is active.[11,79] The CLC mechanoreceptors consist of the Ruffini's endings, pancinian corpuscles, and Golgi tendon organlike receptors. Nociceptive free nerve endings also mediate proprioception. Stimulation of the glenohumeral CLC mechanoreceptors is caused by tension.[79] When elongation of the CLC occurs, as in end range activity, the mechanoreceptors are stimulated by deformation and provide proprioceptive feedback or the ability to sense joint motion and position. Stimulation of the mechanoreceptors also initiates a neurologic feedback loop, causing protective stabilizing muscle function. When the CLC mechanoreceptors are injured or the CLC mechanism is disrupted, as seen in a traumatic dislocation causing a Bankart lesion, the CLC mechanoreceptors are not stimulated at end range because the normal tension developed across the CLC does not occur. This compromises the proprioceptive feedback loop, resulting in reinjury due to absent or ineffective protective muscle activity. Altered proprioception has been demonstrated in individuals who had known instability, and it was found to be restored following surgical anterior stabilization and rehabilitation.[78] Glousman[35] showed decreased activity of critical muscles during throwing in pitchers with known instability. It is difficult to say how much of a role apprehension influenced muscle activity because all subjects had a positive apprehension sign. The concept of altering mechanoreceptor input could be applied to patients with a full-thickness rotator cuff tear. This lesion also disrupts normal tensioning of the CLC because the capsule is also torn. In this case not only is the stability compromised because of a structural defect, but also because the neurologic feedback to the surrounding cuff is compromised. Consider the compromise of the neuromuscular mechanism following a total shoulder arthroplasty in which the CLC is released, the articular surfaces are replaced, and subscapularis tendon is altered by tendonotomy. Rehabilitation must address the effect of a compromised neuromuscular mechanism. These "strengthening exercises," when appropriate, must be performed at different degrees of elevation, moving toward positions of function. This enhances and retrains the neuromuscular system, proprioceptive resulting in improved function.

Range of Motion

Range of motion and stretching exercises are designed to maintain or improve soft-tissue pliability and prevent adhesions. These categories of exercises are typically passive, active assistive, and active. Passive exercise is performed when muscle activity is not wanted, as in a postoperative rotator cuff repair. Prophylactic stretching exercises to improve tissue pliability and length in the absence of pain or pathology are also considered passive. Active-assistive motions require submaximal activation of muscles to prevent disruption of surgical intervention or to reduce pain. Active motion is allowed when the repaired tissues at risk have been given adequate healing time or when the patient can move the segment without increasing symptoms. The targeted tissue and rationale for ROM exercises may be different, depending on whether the patient's status is postoperative or postinjury, whether the patient is developing a contracture or if a pre and post workout flexibility program is required.

Postoperative and postinjury ROM exercises are performed within the symptom-free or protected ROM to maintain soft-tissue mobility and prevent fibrosis. Fibrosis has been demonstrated to impair capillary circulation, which can possibly cause ischemia and further remodeling.[72] Following a rotator cuff repair, it is essential that the adhesions do not form in the subacromial space. The performance of passive ROM will maintain the proper gliding mechanism while not endangering the rotator cuff and deltoid fixation sites. Although we generally consider these exercises passive, research has shown muscle activation with passive ROM exercises.[148] Knowledge of positional effect and tissue tension is necessary for safe and effective stretching. For example, stretching into external rotation with the arm in adduction may place the cuff repair in jeopardy due to increased tension following a repair of the rotator cuff that required moderate lateral mobilization. This position has been shown to significantly increase tensile load to the repair site and rotator cuff interval.[44,151] A less stressful position that will achieve the benefits of passive rotational stretching is placing the arm at 45 degrees in the POS (Fig. 6D). In addition, gentle stress across healing tissue has been shown to enhance collagen proliferation, strength, and orientation.[70] As symptoms reduce or as the tissue heals sufficiently, activity of the involved musculature can be increased. This also improves collagen healing through an appropriate tissue stress. Active ROM is initiated when symptoms allow or are based on tissue healing parameters. This can be considered a strengthening activity in addition to achieving the previous effects on healing the soft tissues. Neer et al.[101] found that those individuals who had early passive motion, reached their motion goals for discharge much sooner than did those not involved

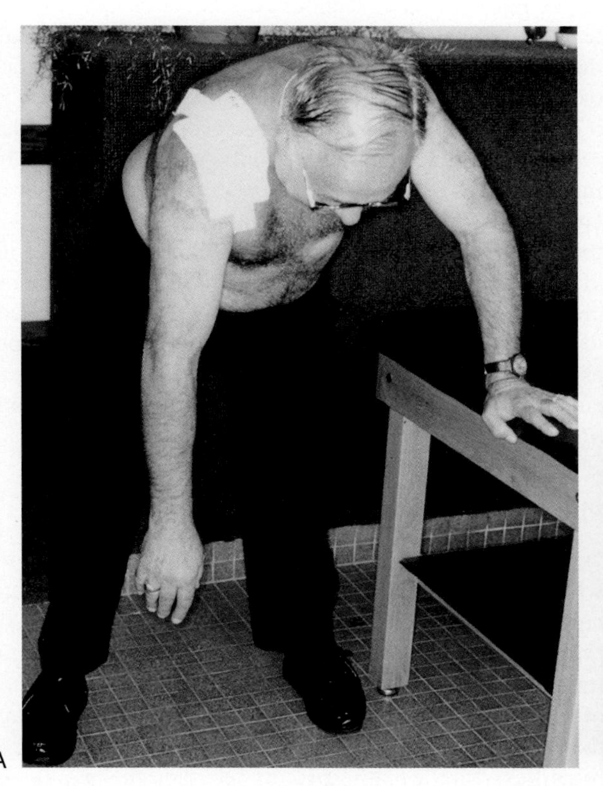

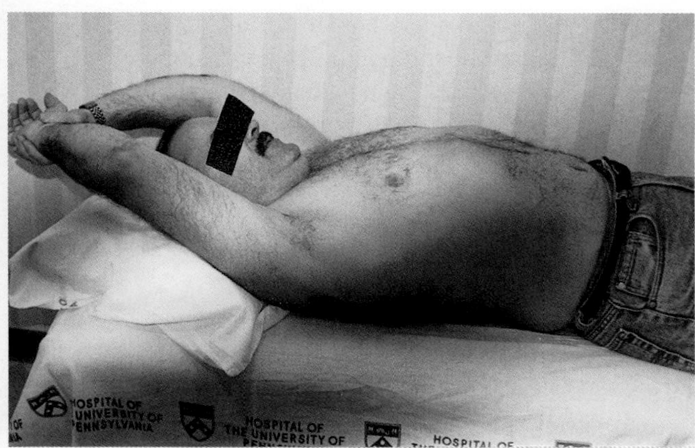

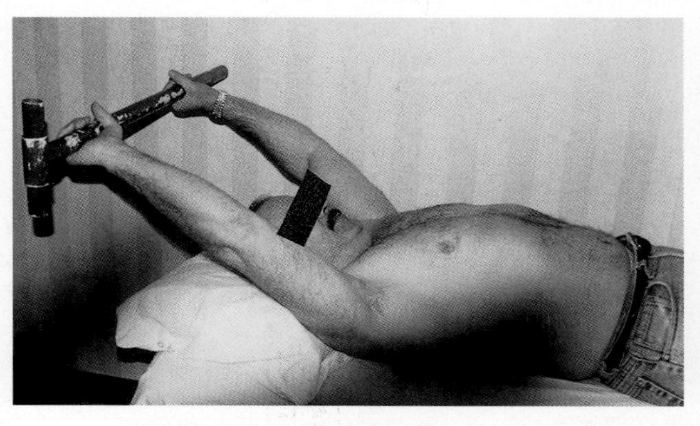

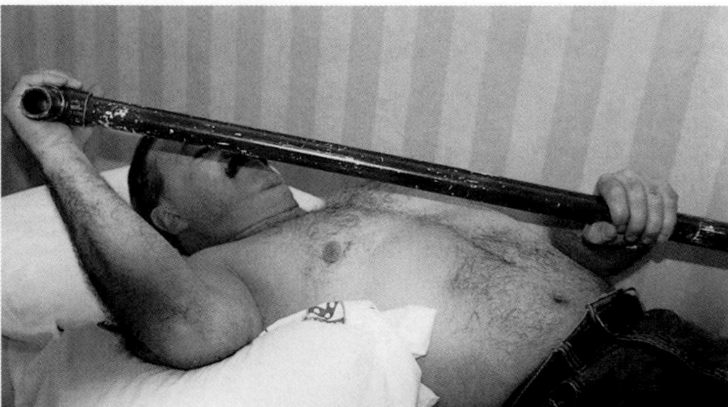

FIG. 6. Phase I ROM exercises. **(A)** Pendulum. **(B)** Passive elevation. **(C)** Active assisted elevation. **(D)** Passive external rotation in 45 degrees of elevation in the POS.

in a physical therapy program. Wingate[147] demonstrated improved function followed mastectomy when the patient was involved in a postoperative therapy program.

Stretching soft tissue in the presence of developing or established contracture is performed to mechanically elongate tissue that is in the process of losing or has lost its normal pliability. To truly mechanically deform connective tissue, it must be brought into a plastic range. Prolonged stretch is much more beneficial in causing creeping as opposed to intense short-duration stretching.[73] Unfortunately, many individuals with active inflammation either after injury or surgery cannot tolerate the required time for prolonged stretch to elongate tissue. Active inflammation, causing synovitis, is the common cause for joint contracture. Synovitis resulting in CLC fibroplasia appears to be the two stages of both primary and secondary frozen shoulders. ROM exercises performed during an active synovitis appear to minimize or prevent further loss of motion; however, one must be cautious about not being to aggressive with stretching activities because they may aggravate symptoms.

Prophylactic stretching to maintain or possibly improve pliability of the musculotendinous cuff and CLC is reasonable for recreational or competitive athletes as well as for individuals in the occupational arena. One need only evaluate the external rotation motion of a professional baseball pitcher to recognize that "abnormal" external rotation is required to generate excessive torque in order to hurl a baseball at 95 miles per hour. The occupational athletes may require a certain degree of glenohumeral/trunk mobility to perform certain tasks. Much attention has been focused on regaining elasticity by stretching the glenohumeral posterior capsule. Harryman[43] demonstrated increased anterior and slight superior humeral head translation when the posterior capsule was imbricated. Tightness of the posterior capsule has been advocated as a possible cause for secondary compressive lesions of the rotator cuff.[43,90]

Facilitate Collagen Healing

With microtearing or incomplete tearing of the CLC or muscle–tendon complex, or in the postoperative patient, collagen healing must take place. Connective tissue that is appropriately stressed promotes improved collagen tissue alignment and tensile strength.[70] This provides an aspect of the rationale for performing gentle ROM exercise and submaximal strengthening following injury or surgery. The importance of positively influencing connective tissue healing is often shadowed by the other effect of maintaining joint motion and strengthening. The performance of controlled exercises in the early phases postinjury or surgery prevents disruption of collagen tissue.

Endurance

The muscular endurance is the ability of a muscle or muscle group to repeatedly contract and sustain tension over a period of time. Strength and endurance may not always correlate well to one another because an individual may be strong but may have poor endurance. This scenario relates back to the worker who must lift a 3-pound drill gun overhead; he may certainly have the strength to do it one or 10 times, but can he do it 100 or 200 times as he may be required to do in a short time. We must not forget that a multitude of muscles from the lower extremities, trunk, and shoulder girdle contract when the arm is lifted. The weak link relative to poor endurance may be the scapular muscles or the trunk extensor and not the rotator cuff; however, the resulting injury may be demonstrated at the rotator cuff. EMG studies in the industrial population and in athletes have shown that experience and not strength may have a greater influence on fatigue. Sigholm et al.[130] found that experienced welders were able to avoid fatigue better than their less experienced counterparts. Gowan et al.[37] found that professional pitchers used all the muscles of the rotator cuff, except the subscapularis, less than amateur pitchers. Endurance therefore may relate to the efficient use of the shoulder complex through adaptation or better mechanics. Consider the difference in muscle load if our worker were to reach overhead versus using a ladder to reduce the movement required for the muscles to work. If an individual has weakness and/or poor endurance of the scapular muscles, the result may be rotator cuff tendonopathy. So the therapist must not only work on the endurance of individual muscles but in movement patterns in which the muscles work together. Certainly part of the education process is to improve mechanics and reduce potential fatigue. Another aspect of endurance that cannot be overlooked is cardiovascular endurance. One would expect that the better conditioned individual would be less prone to injury.

Phases of Rehabilitation

The speed of rehabilitation depends on the injury and whether surgery was performed. Certainly consideration needs to be given to the postsurgical patient, who should be progressed within the guidelines of safe tissue healing parameters. However, if we approach the treatment as phases of progression, based on reactivity and signs and symptoms, then a single general scheme of progression can be followed regardless of the pathology or whether the patient was treated conservatively or postoperatively. The phases will be described based on the pathology.

Pathogenesis: Rotator Cuff Tendonopathy

Rotator cuff and biceps tendon lesions are common problems affecting the shoulder. Any or all of the rotator cuff tendons may be affected, but the supraspinatus is affected most commonly due to a combination of attritional, mechanical, vascular, and traumatic factors.[102]

The anatomic position and make-up of the supraspinatus make it vulnerable to both compressive and tensile loading.[6,94] Neer classically described degenerative changes of the rotator cuff in three stages with the predominant causative factor being true mechanical impingement of the rotator cuff on the anterior acromion.[95] Biceps tendon inflammation can occur in isolation; however, pathology of this structure has been heavily correlated with rotator cuff tendonopathy.[95] Critical analysis of the rotator cuff pathogenesis reveals other causative factors. Although the morphology of the acromion is thought to cause true primary compression of the rotator cuff and bursa,[8,95] many individuals have minimal or no osseous abnormalities yet have rotator cuff tendonopathy ranging from tendonitis to full-thickness tears.

Another area of rotator cuff impingement occurs at the posterior glenoid rim.[24,54,140] At 90 degrees or slightly higher and full external rotation, the intraarticular aspect of the supraspinatus contacts the posterior labrum and glenoid. When an individual has glenohumeral instability, the humeral head may translate further, thus increasing contact of the supraspinatus and glenoid rim. This is the proposed mechanism of injury of the supraspinatus in throwing athletes who have glenohumeral instability.[24,54,140]

Other mechanisms for rotator cuff damage are from primary tensile overload, causing microtearing and inflammation of the tendon. Both compression and tensile overload can occur secondarily due to instability, scapular muscle weakness, or a tight posterior capsule.[90,92] Many individuals experience painless degenerative tears of the rotator cuff and function quite well until an event such as a fall causes an acute extension of the existing tear, resulting in pain and dysfunction.[89] Conservative treatment is usually attempted first; however, individuals with progressive loss of function and/or pain may require surgical intervention ranging from debridement, acromioplasty, and/or repair of the defect.

Tendonitis is thought to be microtearing of the tendon, which results in healing and microscarring.[89] This healing process may occur normally with appropriate rest from aggravating activity. The exercise performed during this healing phase must encourage collagen synthesis without irritation. Additionally, strength is improved. If the tissue is not given a chance to fully recover, the result will be prolonged inflammation and symptoms. Sometimes rest from exercise needs to be delayed to avoid this prolongation of symptoms. Even with adequate healing, the tendon is left slightly less tolerant of tensile loading because the residual scar tissue does not have the same tensile strength as its healthy neighboring fibers.

Rehabilitation for Rotator Cuff Tendonopathy: Conservative

Phase I. Multiple factors influence a patient's response to treatment, such as tissue reactivity, age, health status, and occupation, and it becomes difficult to place time parameters on the phases of rehabilitation. Therefore, the phases of rehabilitation for a conservatively treated patient with rotator cuff tendonopathy (Table 5) will be described and progressed based on symptom response. If the patient responds favorably to the rehabilitative intervention they can be progress to the next phase.

TABLE 5. *Rotator cuff tendonopathy—Conservative*

- Phase I
  - Goals
    1. Patient education
    2. Reduce inflammation/pain
    3. Facilitate collagen healing
    4. Improve ROM
  - Treatment
    1. Patient education
    2. Rest from painful activity
    3. Anti-inflammatory therapy
    4. Phase I and II ROM exercises (PROM, AAROM, AROM)
    5. Joint mobilization
    6. Submaximal strengthening
       - Isometrics
       - Phase I strengthening exercises
       - Scapulothoracic strengthening and integration
    7. Aerobic conditioning[a]
- Phase II
  - Goals
    1. Improve to full ROM
    2. Improve neuromuscular control and strength
  - Treatment
    1. Progress ROM
    2. Phase II strengthening exercises (submaximal → maximal)
    3. Manual
       - Multiangle isometrics
       - Short-arc excursion
       - Scapulothoracic integration and strengthening
       - Nonprovocative variable resisted exercise
    3. Aerobic conditioning
- Phase III
  - Goals
    1. Full pain-free ROM
    2. Optimize neuromuscular control
    3. Improve endurance
    4. Initiate return to functional activities
  - Treatment
    1. Prophylactic stretching
    2. Phase III strengthening/endurance exercises
       - Progress to full range
       - Emphasize eccentrics then progress to provocative positions[a]
       - Full variable and/or free-weight resistance[a]
       - Isokinetics[a]
       - Plyometrics
    3. Begin submaximal sport, occupation, or desired activities[a]
       - Interval program
       - Work-related activities
- Phase IV
  - Goals
    1. Return to sport,[a] occupation,[a] or desired activities[a]
    2. Promote concept of prevention
  - Treatment
    1. Work hardening
    2. Continue with prophylactic program

[a] Applies to athlete or laborer.

The process of rehabilitation must begin with education about rest from irritating activities, such as work activities, weight lifting, or leading with the involved arm to put on a coat. This includes terminating all painful exercises that were previously prescribed for the patient. Commonly, oral nonsteroidals are prescribed for analgesic and antiinflammatory effects. Modalities used for antiinflammatory and/or pain relief effects can be utilized. Transverse friction massage is a technique that has been advocated to improve vascularization, improve scar tissue pliability, help with appropriate orientation of the collagen, and create temporary pain relief.[22]

Anecdotally, this technique has been found to be effective in the recovery of patients with less reactive tendon lesions. The presence of a positive evaluative friction massage test indicates that the patient may respond favorably to this technique.[66]

Passive, active-assistive, or active ROM exercises are initiated in pain-free ranges to improve or maintain ROM, provide gentle stress to healing collagen tissue, and optimize the subacromial gliding mechanism. These phase I exercises include pendulums, elevation, and external rotation (Fig. 6); however, many individuals also can begin phase II ROM exercises if appropriate. These include internal rotation and horizontal adduction, extension, and combination external rotation/elevation (Fig. 7). Commonly, external rotation exercises are performed at 45 degrees of POS abduction. This position minimizes excessive tension on the superior cuff and CLC by placing them in a slackened starting position; additionally, the impingement position is avoided. Exercises are typically performed 20 times, between three to six times per day. To maximize the effect of the stretching, particularly if it is being performed in the presence of a contracture, heat should be applied to the shoulder.[72,73] Internal rotation ROM exercises performed by placing the hand behind the back must be approached with caution. This position places the supraspinatus in its most elongated state and thus may be provocative. Depending on the degree of tissue reactivity or if the patient has develop joint stiffness, grade I and II glenohumeral joint mobilization may assist in pain reduction and regaining motion limited by pain. Joint mobilization is a technique in which one joint surface (i.e., the humeral head) is directionally translated relative to the other joint surface (i.e., the glenoid)[86] (Fig. 8). Oscillations are performed at the end of the translation. Joint mobilization is usually graded from I to V, although grade V is considered a manipulation due to the high-velocity thrust performed at end range. The proposed effect of this technique is pain relief (grades I to II) and improved ROM by stretching capsuloligamentous tissue (grades III to V). Pain relief is thought to be mediated through a neurophysiologic mechanism beginning in the joint and soft-tissue mechanoreceptors and nocioreceptors.[59,86]

By translating the articular surfaces, stimulation and/or accommodation of the receptors is initiated, which results in pain reduction. If the force of the translation is significant enough, as in grades III and IV, mechanical stretching of the tight soft tissue may result.[59,86]

Pain-free submaximal isometrics and isotonic or elastic band exercises may be started either at the shoulder or elbow. Positioning of the glenohumeral joint in a slightly abducted position by using a bolster may result in less irritating passive tension of the contracting soft tissues. Isometrics can be performed in all directions, but many times resistance into abduction and flexion is painful. Therefore, the following movements are usually performed: external rotation, internal rotation, extension, elbow flexion, and elbow extension. Contractions are held for 3 to 6 seconds, and 1 to 3 sets of 10 to 15 repetitions are performed. Commonly, isometrics are reserved for the more reactive patient. Integration of the scapular muscles should be encouraged at all times. Therefore, when performing glenohumeral joint dynamic strengthening exercises, the scapular muscles should be consciously activated or "set" before the glenohumeral muscles are activated (Fig. 9). We have found that slight retraction of the shoulder girdle increases activation of the scapula adductors and balances activity with the serratus anterior. This results in better stabilization of the scapula. Because scapular muscle activity is required for normal functional shoulder movement, encouraging coactivation during glenohumeral muscles exercise, as opposed to isolated glenohumeral activity, is enormously beneficial. It allows both muscle groups to be strengthened simultaneously, reinforces synergistic firing patterns, and provides a stable base upon which the compromised rotator cuff muscles may anchor, giving them a biomechanical advantage.

Phase I strengthening exercises using free weights of 1 to 3 pounds or elastic bands are initiated. Elastic bands are easier to use, can be used in the functional erect position, and allow better integration of scapular muscles. These exercises include external rotation, internal rotation, and extension (Fig. 10). A bolster may be used between the arm and body to reduce pain; this is found to be more beneficial in patients with rotator cuff pathology. In the presence of a supraspinatus tendon lesion, placement of the arm in slight abduction slackens the tendon, thereby reducing passive irritating tendon tension. Additionally, restricting external rotation to 30 degrees past neutral rotation further minimizes passive supraspinatus tension created by the coracohumeral ligament through its intimate relationship with the supraspinatus.[44] Scapular muscle integration is emphasized but is now more challenging because the humerus is now moving compared to performing isometrics. Pain-free arcs of motion are encouraged in all exercises. Isolated strengthening of the scapulothoracic muscles also can be initiated using either elastic band/free weight resistance or manual resistance by performing scapular elevation and retraction. Cardiovascular training should be encouraged for all individuals, particularly athletes.

Phase II. As pain and inflammation resolve, modalities are discontinued, but heat may be used before exercise to precondition the soft tissues and ice may be used after exercise to assist in reducing postexercise pain and inflammation. The intensity of stretching is increased to approach the end range, but if pain persists in certain (provocative) positions, stretching is avoided. Resistive exercise using elastic bands or light free weights is continued, as is the re-

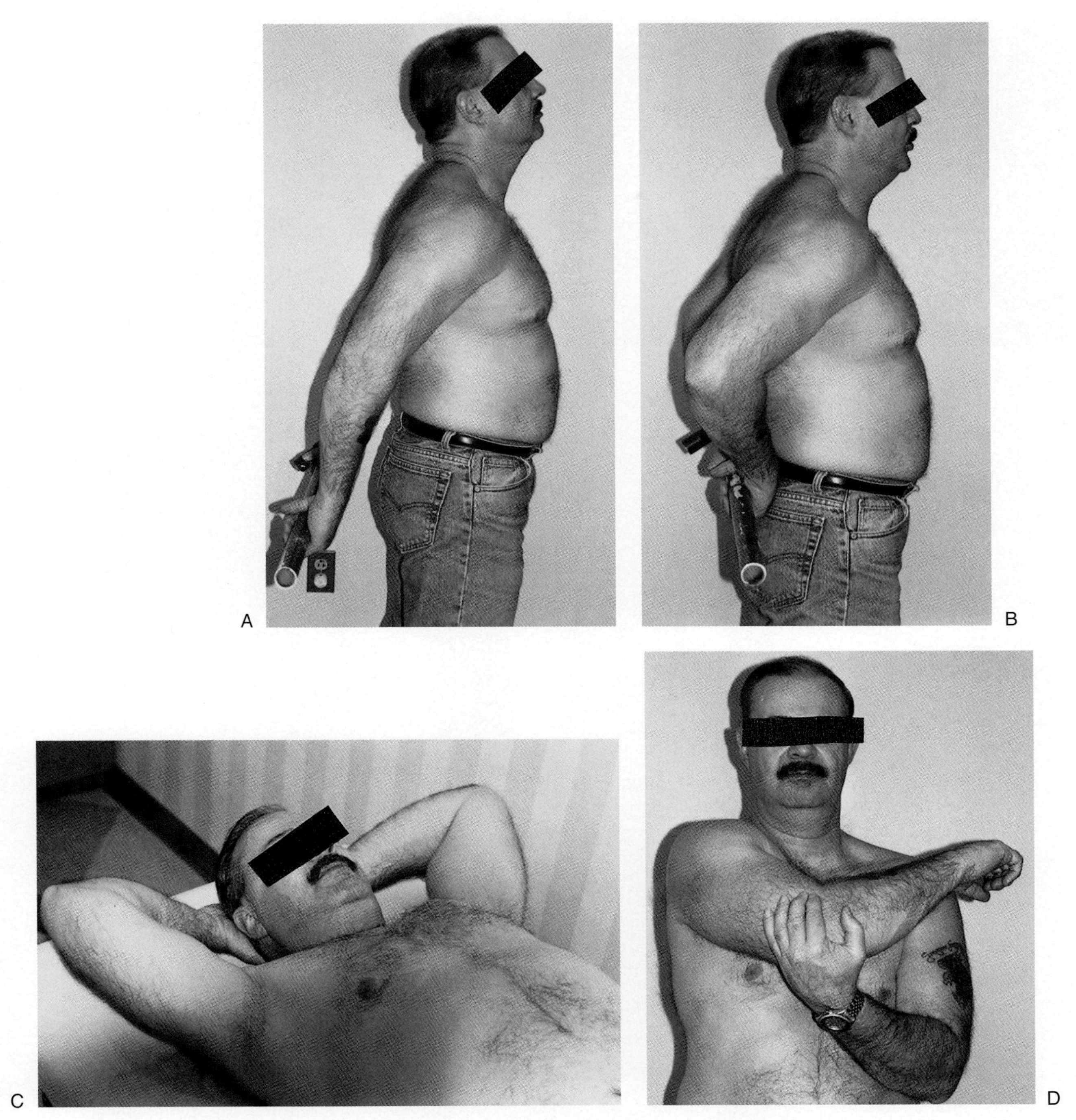

FIG. 7. Phase II ROM exercises. **(A)** Extension. **(B)** Internal rotation. **(C)** Modified elevation/external rotation. **(D)** Posterior capsule stretch.

maining part of the home and supervised rehabilitation program.

In phase II the phase I exercises for the rotator cuff–biceps–deltoid complex are continued, but the following are added: abduction (in the coronal plane limited range), scaption to 90 degrees (abduction in the POS with external rotation), flexion with "plus," elbow flexion, and extension (Fig. 11). These exercises are similar to those advocated for years, except that we integrate scapular muscles during their use. Scapular muscle integration is performed even with resisted elbow flexion and extension because the distal load can easily force proximal scapular movement, negating the stable base from which the biceps and triceps pull. The performance of a "plus" maneuver[93] (Fig. 11B) to maximize serratus anterior recruitment at the end of the shoulder flexion exercise or emphasizing scapular retraction during shoulder extension are other examples of integrating scapular muscles into commonly performed rotator cuff exercises. When performing

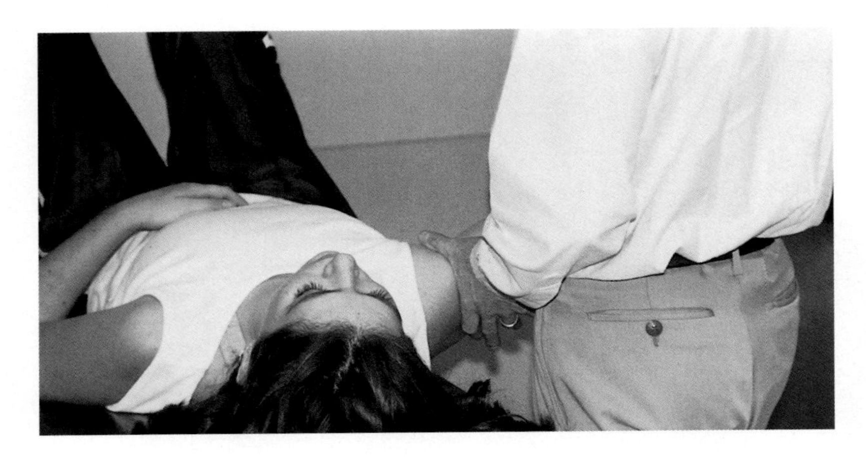

FIG. 8. Inferior glide mobilization.

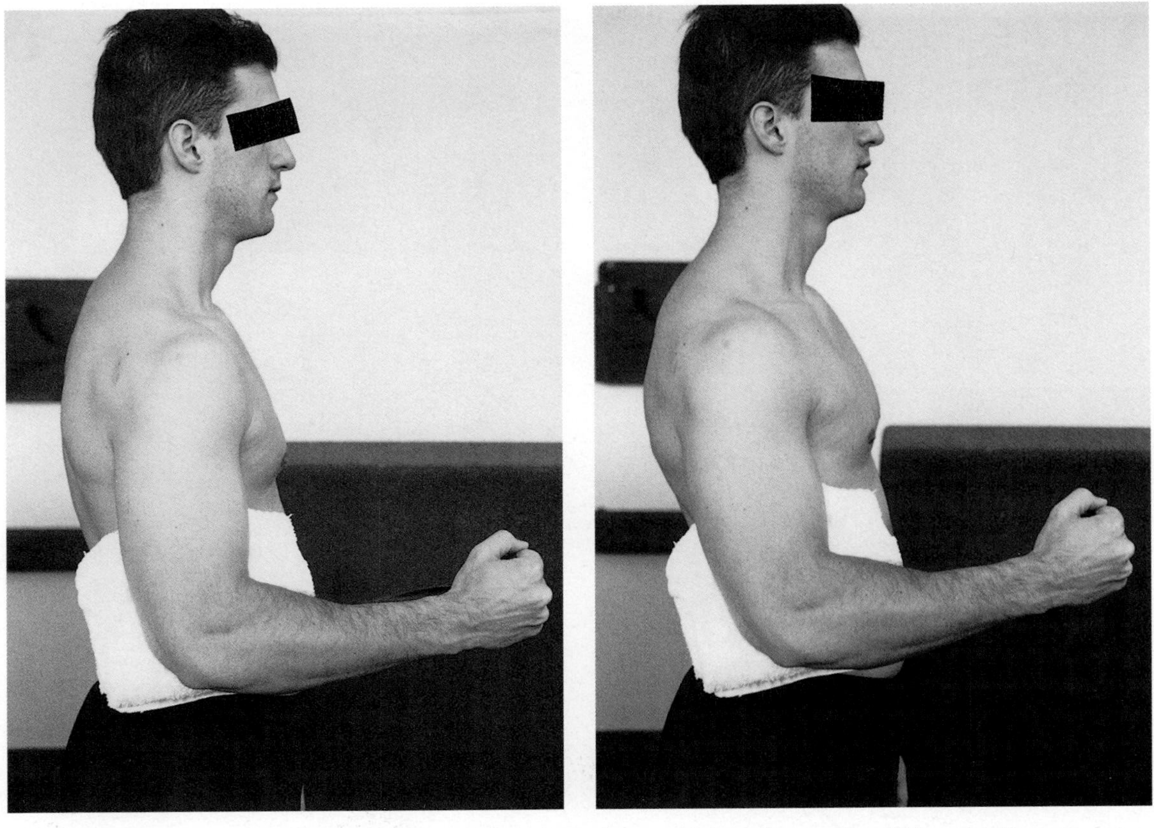

FIG. 9. External rotation strengthening with bolster. Incorrect scapular position **(A)** and with scapular muscle integration **(B)**.

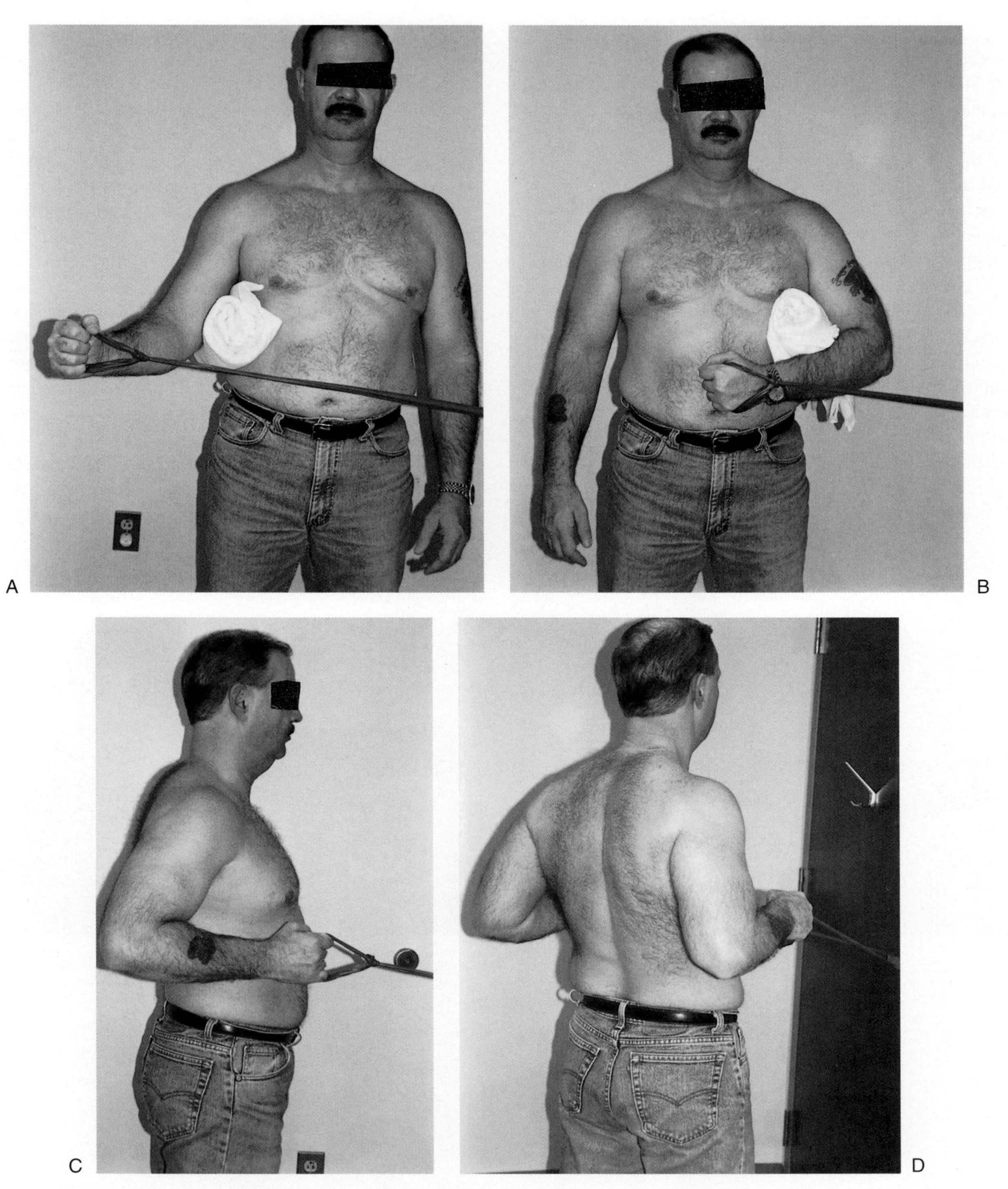

FIG. 10. Phase I strengthening exercises. **(A)** External rotation to 30 degrees. **(B)** Internal rotation. **(C)** Extension (unilateral). **(D)** Extension (bilateral) to encourage scapular adductor muscle integration.

scaption with external rotation, a free weight is typically chosen because such a long lever arm is created and the elastic can be stretched to a point of excessive resistance. External rotation as opposed to internal rotation is chosen because it is less provocative to the rotator cuff and bursal tissue. We have found that many patients have increased pain when prescribed the exercise of scaption (abduction in the POS) with internal rotation. This exercise was found to isolate the supraspinatus[55] and created the greatest muscle activity for the anterior and middle deltoid, supraspinatus, subscapularis,[137] and upper trapezius[93]; however, the higher levels of muscle activity reported were achieved above 90 degrees in all muscles tested. Performance of scaption/internal rotation above 90 degrees may be contraindicated because of potential impingement. Although this exercise may be beneficial at some stage of rehabilitation, performing it too early can result in further irritation of the rotator cuff due to increased shear forces and direct cuff compression.[46,137,143] The reader is encouraged to consult the literature on muscle activity based on EMG findings. Although these studies are valuable, direct application of study positions is not always clinically prudent because their use may be contraindicated relative to the patient's symptoms and pathology.

Commonly, exercises are performed in two to three sets of 10 to 15 repetitions, based on the patient's response and the rationale for exercise. The resistance level (elastic band thickness or free weight) is increased as the exercise becomes easier to perform. Typically we advocate that the patient move to three sets of 15 before progressing in resistance, but at some determined level the repetitions are increased to 25 to 30. We feel that increased repetition achieves all the previously stated rationale for resistive exercise in addition to improving shoulder girdle muscle endurance.

If the patient is being seen in a supervised manner, manual resistance can be performed as a form of assessment and exercise. Manual resistance is applied to isolate scapular muscles that may be weak (Fig. 12). Manual resistance in multiple directions about the shoulder (i.e., internal rotation, external rotation, and elevation) in varying positions of ele-

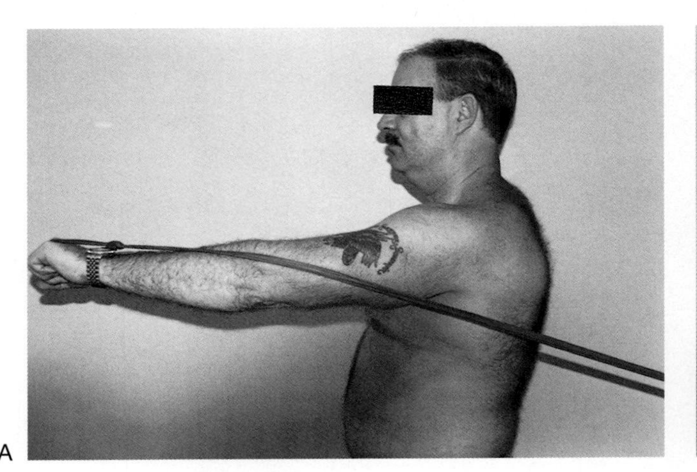

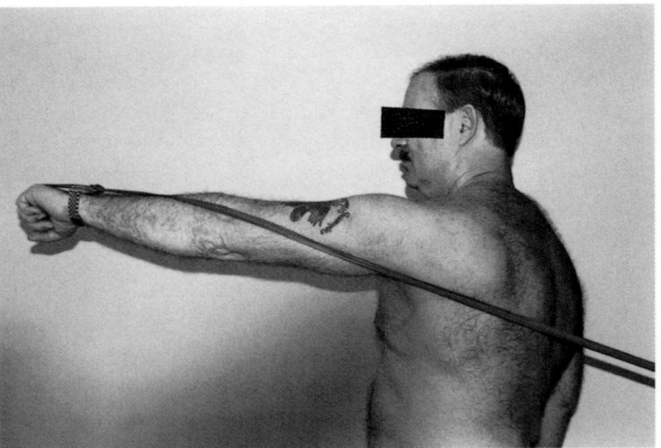

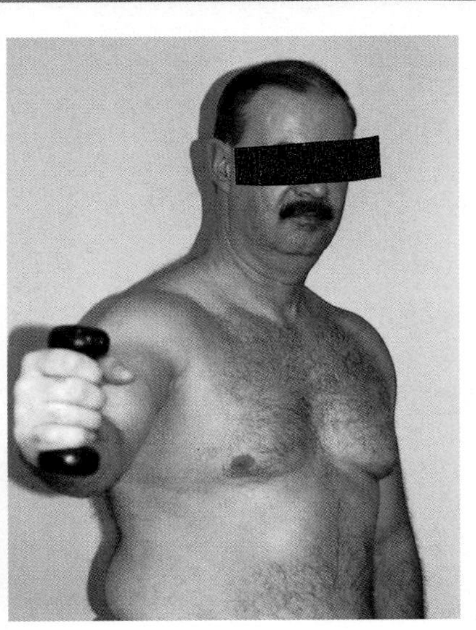

FIG. 11. Phase II strengthening exercises. **(A)** Flexion. **(B)** Flexion with "plus" to encourage serratus anterior integration. **(C)** Abduction to 45 degrees. **(D)** Abduction to 90 degrees in the POS. *(continued)*

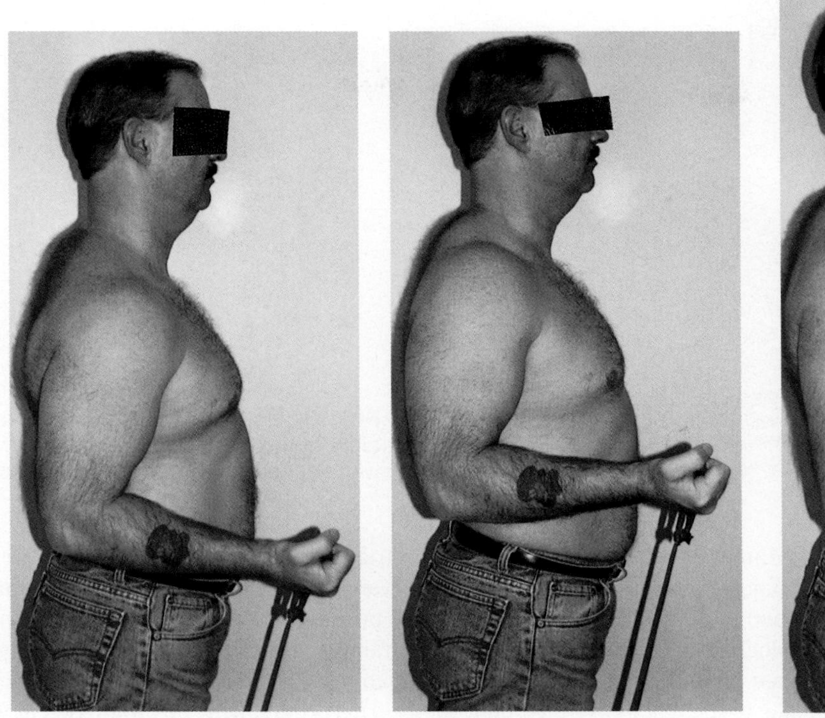
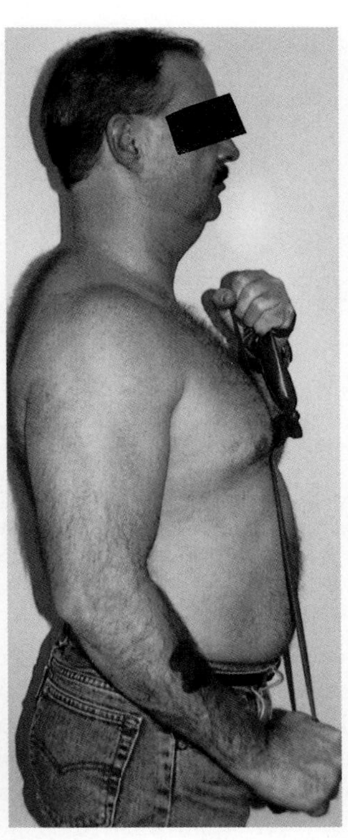

E, F G

FIG. 11. *Continued.* **(E)** Elbow flexion with incorrect scapula position. **(F)** Elbow flexion with scapular muscle integration. **(G)** Elbow extension with scapular muscle integration.

vation, to determine whether a patient is ready for resistive exercises and what positions and/or directions of resistance to choose. The typical start position is in 45 degrees of elevation in the POS (Fig. 13). If pain is felt upon appropriate submaximal resistance, the patient may refrain from resistive exercises or modifications in position are attempted. This allows some system of objectivity in determining the resistive exercise program, as opposed to placing patients on a standard protocol of resistive exercises. We have found that this reduces symptom exacerbations related to exercise. We advocate the use of manual resistance as a leading form of supervised therapy because it provides immediate feedback from the patient regarding strength, pain, integration of scapular muscles, and appropriate scapulohumeral rhythm. By systematically resisting different muscles groups (i.e., abductors/external rotation or adductors/internal rotation) in varying degrees of elevation or rotation, neuromuscular training can be enhanced and the patient's home resisted exercise program can be developed and modified.

Phase III. At this phase the patient should have relatively

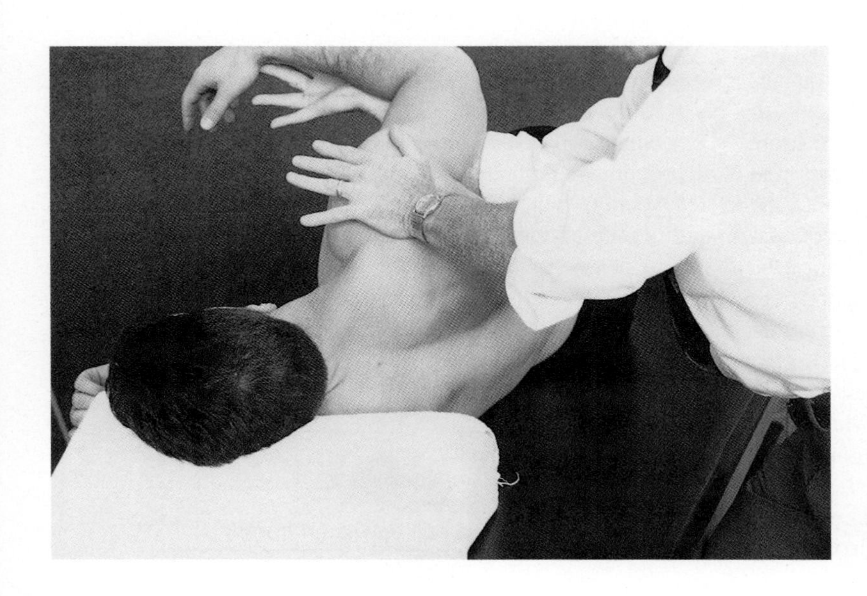

FIG. 12. Scapular adduction isolating the middle trapezius.

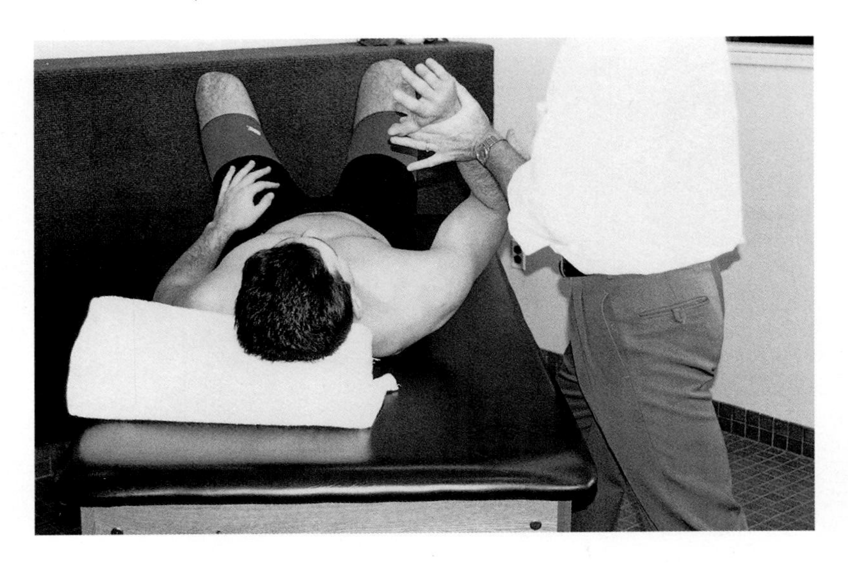

FIG. 13. Isometric manual resistance to the glenohumeral abductors and external rotators while encouraging scapular stabilization.

pain-free end range motion and is performing a full range stretching program, with emphasis on the posterior cuff and capsule. Individuals who have low demands other than activities of daily living are typically released on a home stretching and strengthening program. Their potions of exercise may be less provocative based on age, tissue reactivity, and demands. If the patient's demands are higher, we advocate that the patient, when able , be progressed to functional combination motions (Fig. 14). If a patient must repetitively function with the arm overhead, strengthening of the shoulder muscles should be progressed to that position. To maintain the patient on exercises performed at the side does not train the neuromuscular system in positions of function. Therefore, in selected patients, rotational exercise are progressed and performed at 45 degrees in the POS. This enhances neuromuscular control, joint stabilization, and strength of the shoulder complex muscles, in addition to advancing the level of difficulty for the patient. As the patient performs exercises in the elevated positions, appropriate scapulohumeral rhythm should be assessed and facilitated. Many patients who are considered to have adequate ROM and strength still demonstrated abnormal rhythm with elevation. Learned behavior appears to be the reason for the persistent abnormal rhythm and must be identified then addressed. The progression of exercises continues into more provocative positions based on the patient's response and functional requirements. The therapist must remember the rationale of exercise. Depending on the level of tendonopathy or the patient's functional requirements, the goal of the exercise may initially be to facilitate tendon healing and connective tissue alignment and to improve tensile strength. Later in the rehabilitation process, the exercises are higher and may be designed to ready the athlete or laborer, who are being seen in a supervised manner, for activity. Manual resistance exercise are progressed to full range of motion and accommodating resistance. Eccentric activity also may be emphasized. PNF techniques employing diagonal patterns, specific techniques of recruiting and sequencing isometrics, and concentric and eccentric muscle activity are performed. Resistive exercises are progressed to more functional and provocative positions based on the symptoms and need.

Weight training using variable resistive devices or barbells is started with the same nonprovocative to provocative philosophy. This program can be progressed in the clinic, or the patient can be given indications for progression of the home program (Table 6). Certain exercises that require shoulder abduction and full external rotation should be prohibited, particularly the military press, chest flies, and behind-the-neck latissimus pull-downs. These exercises may be modified to the POS.

The upper body ergometer (UBE) or rowing ergometer is used to further improve strength and endurance. This device may be used earlier in the rehabilitative process; however, care is always required when considering the patients position on the UBE. Placing the patient in a sitting position so that the machine's rotation axis is level with the glenohumeral joint requires the patient to repetitively cycle against resistance in the impingement zone. The prudent clinician initially has the patient perform the exercise in the standing position to avoid the potential rotator cuff trauma; however, the sitting position is used eventually if tolerated. Both the forward and backward direction are performed. A rowing ergometer can be used and is very effective in improving strength and endurance of the shoulder extensor and scapula retractor muscles while improving the patient's cardiovascular condition.

A device found extremely useful in rehabilitating patents with rotator cuff tendonopathy and/or glenohumeral instabil-

TABLE 6. *Phase III isotonic program*

Elbow flexors
Elbow extensors
Shoulder row
Latissimus pull downs (in front)

ity is the Bodyblade (Hymanson Inc., Playa Del Ray, CA) (Fig. 15). This device enhances strength, dynamic control, proprioception, and endurance training. Small to large oscillations of a fiberglass rod are performed in multiple positions (following the nonprovocative to provocative philosophy) and various time intervals. Oscillating the blade requires short excursion, high-speed cocontraction muscle activity of the rotator cuff–deltoid–biceps complex in addition to the scapular muscles. Therefore, dynamic stabilizing training is uniquely achieved compared with other forms of exercise. Although exercising with this device may appear easy, it can be extremely difficult and can significantly challenge the patient's shoulder muscle strength and endurance. Because the device can be used in any position, even patients in phase II can use this device. Typically the patient is placed in a slightly abducted position and oscillates the blade, primarily through elbow flexion and extension. This requires proximal stabilization at the glenohumeral and scapulothoracic joints while the distal elbow is moved. The progression of the Bodyblade is based on the rehabilitation influencing factors.

The athlete. Isokinetic exercise may be initiated for some selective patients based on their need. Typically this form of exercise is reserved for athletes or younger patients. Isokinetic dynamometers offer the unique ability of allowing maximal muscle activity at a constant speed through the ROM. The rehabilitation specialist must recognize that this requirement is usually only needed during athletic activities. Also the rotator cuff–CLC complex may not tolerate maximal tension throughout the range, particularly after injury or in the elderly. Adequate dynamic stabilization and negligible myotendinous reactivity are prerequisites to this mode of muscle strengthening. Initially speeds of 120 to 240 degrees/sec are used. Lower speeds result in increased concentric torque, greater tensile loading, and increased shear and

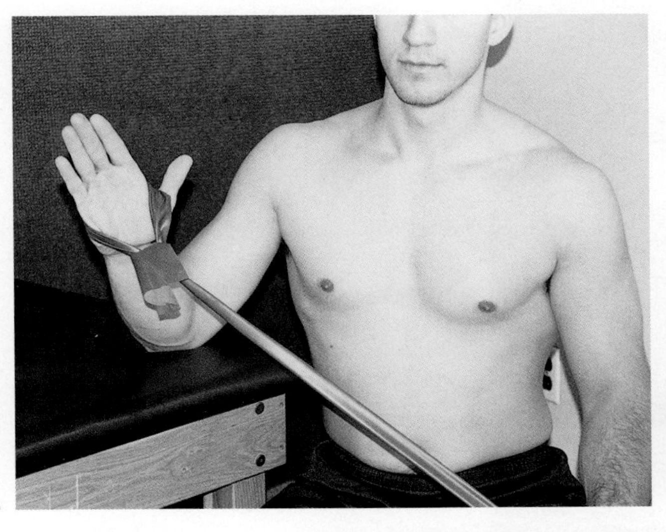

A

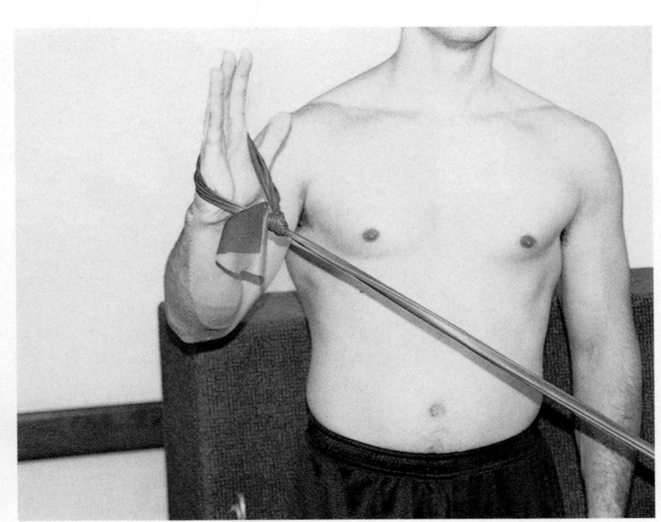

B

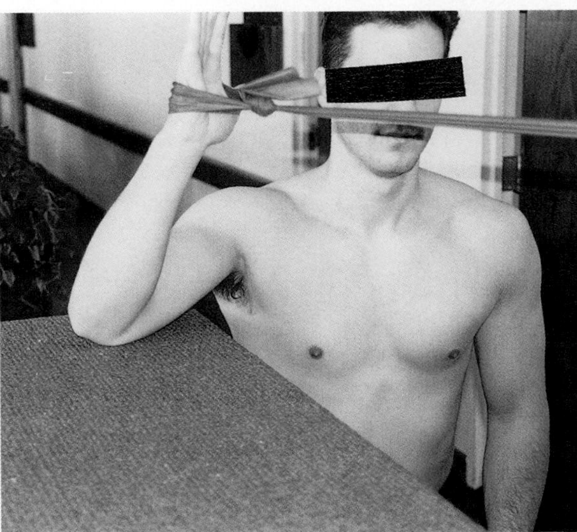

C

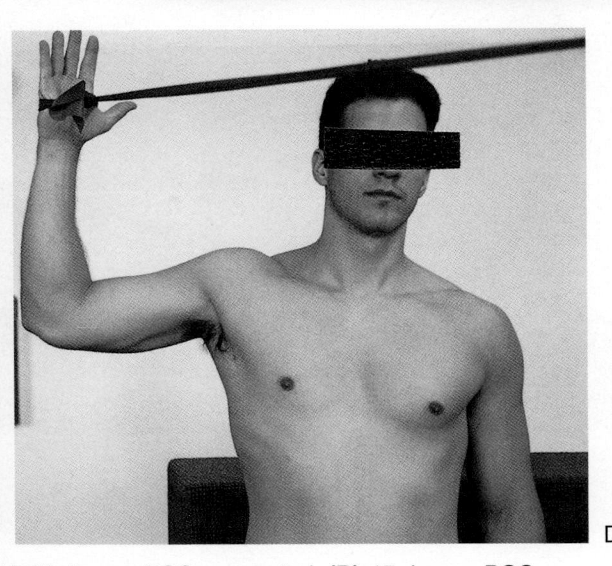

D

FIG. 14. Elastic band strengthening progression. **(A)** 45 degree POS, supported. **(B)** 45 degree POS, unsupported. **(C)** 90 degree POS, supported. **(D)** 90/90, unsupported. (Reproduced with permission from Kelly MJ. Anatomic and biomechanical rationale for rehabilitation of the athlete's shoulder. *J Sport Rehabil* 1995;4:122–154.)

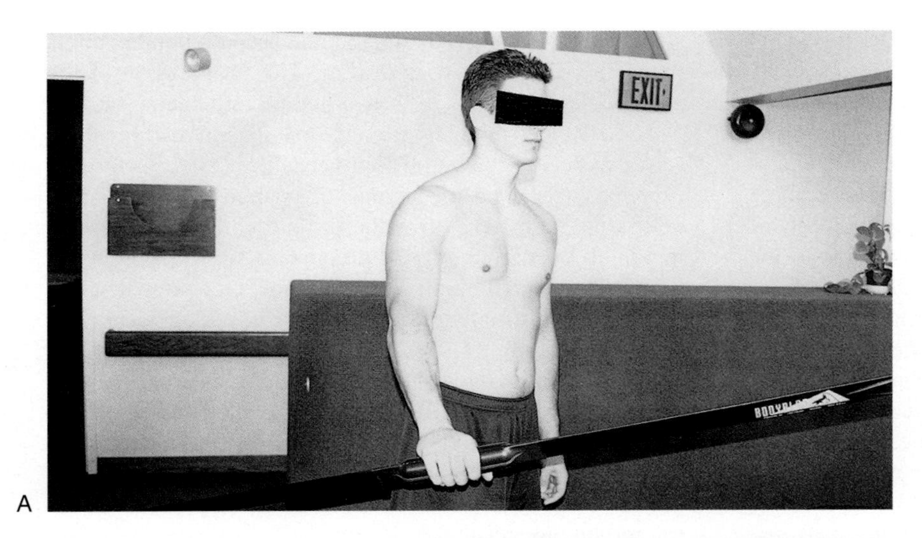

A

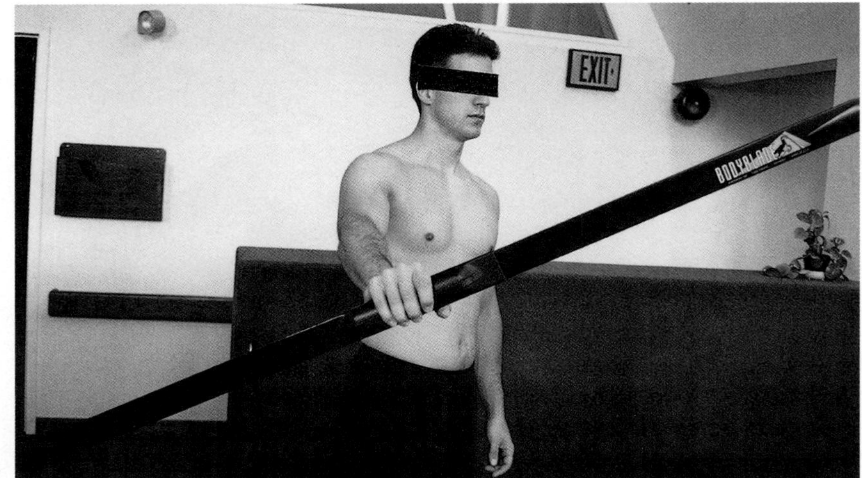

B

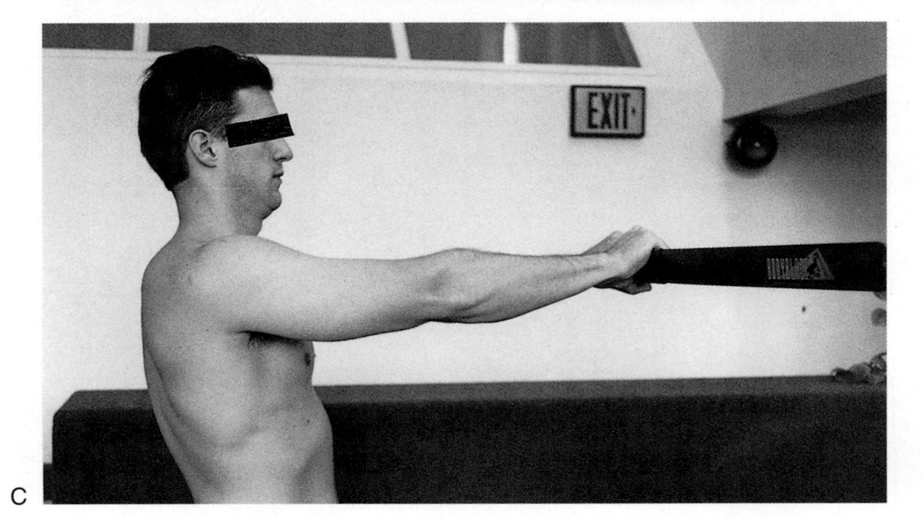

C

FIG. 15. Bodyblade progression. **(A)** 30 degrees POS. **(B)** 60 degrees POS. **(C)** 90 degrees sagittal with "plus." *(continued)*

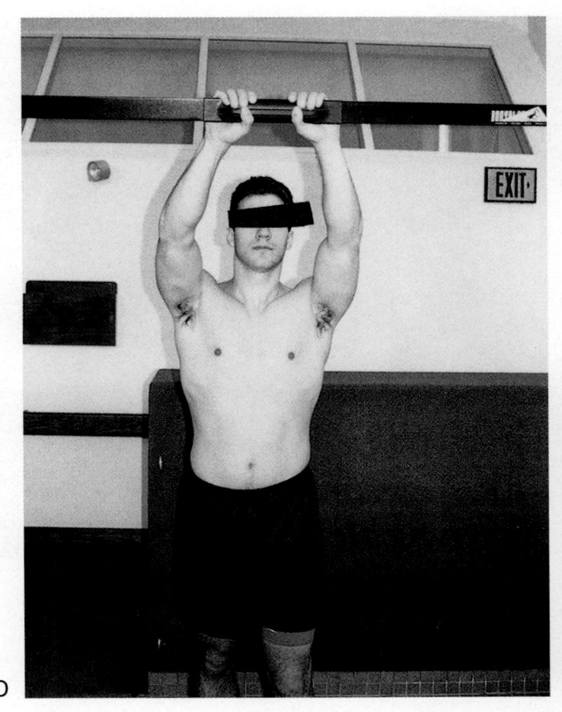

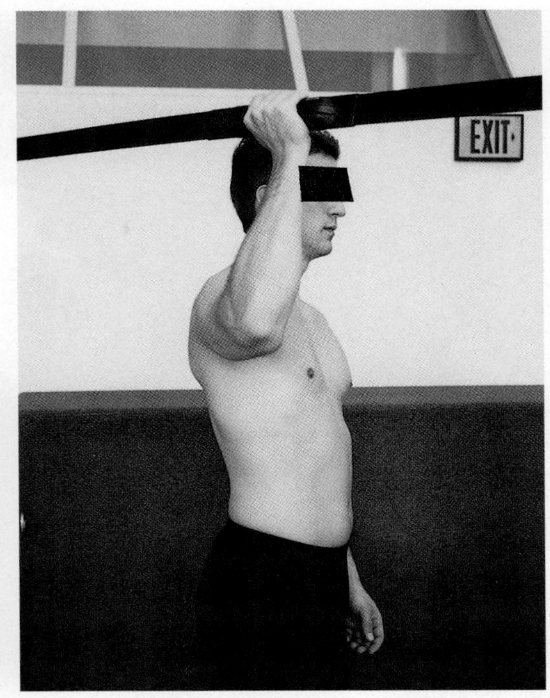

D E

FIG. 15. *Continued.* **(D)** Overhead. **(E)** 90 degrees POS. (Reproduced with permission from Kelly MJ, Anatomic and biomechanical rationale for rehabilitation of the athlete's shoulder. *J Sport Rehabil* 1995;4:122–154.)

compressive forces. Because of the potentially high torque produced, the athlete is initially placed in slight POS abduction and progressed to the provocative sport-specific positions. Eccentric training can be performed submaximally, but prudence is required when increasing resistance, particularly in provocative positions because eccentric activity is associated with myotendinous injury.[11] Caution is also required when increasing speed during isokinetic eccentric use because torque increases (as does force translated across the soft tissues) as speed increases.[32] The isokinetic dynamometers do allow other exercise modes (i.e., isometric, isotonic) that may be more suitable in the rehabilitation of the shoulder.

Plyometric training using weighted balls can be used to enhance neuromuscular control, strength, and proprioception by reproducing the physiologic stretch-shortening cycle of muscle in multiple shoulder positions. This activity can be used for any type of patient, but as with isokinetics, it is usually reserved for the younger patient or athlete. By catching and/or throwing a weighted ball (2 to 10 pounds), the adductors/internal rotators are eccentrically loaded, and thus stretched, which is followed by a concentric shortening phase. These exercises appear to enhance muscle performance by neuromuscular control. Initially concentric activity may be utilized by an activity simulating a chest pass (Fig. 16A). This places the arms into 90 degrees at ball release. The ball can then be arced to incorporate greater elevation (Fig. 16B). Sagittal plane motion may be more provocative to the athlete with posterior glenohumeral instability, and progression of difficulty should include horizontal adduction when arcing. True eccentric loading of the internal rotators is begun in the POS at 60 to 80 degrees and progressed to more provocative positions of elevation in the POS, eventually progressing to coronal plane positioning (Fig. 16C). The patient is placed upright, since this is functional and will challenge the scapular muscles better. The ball is thrown at the patient, so the velocity can be varied (varying the force of impact), yet placement of arm may be consistent or varied, which is determined by the rehabilitation specialist. Constant assessment is made of the scapular muscle to achieve balance. Typically, with repetitive throwing or catching while in humeral elevation, the patient begins to overcompensate with the scapular elevators and correction is required. Catching the ball from a vertical drop while standing or side lying is a technique to eccentrically load the posterior cuff and scapular decelerators (Fig. 17).

The laborer. The patient who must return to work is gradually progressed to work-simulated activities. This can be done by using variable resistance units that require the patient to push, pull, or lift. Specific job activities such as lifting containers can be easily reproduced in the clinic with crates filled with varying weights. Work stations are available in many rehabilitation centers that allow the patient to use tools for various tasks. The task can be elevated or lowered depending on the patient's status. Education regarding lifting, tool use, and modification and ergonomic modification should all be addressed.

Phase IV. By this time most individuals other than athletes and laborers should have returned to all necessary activities. If they still have difficulty performing some over-

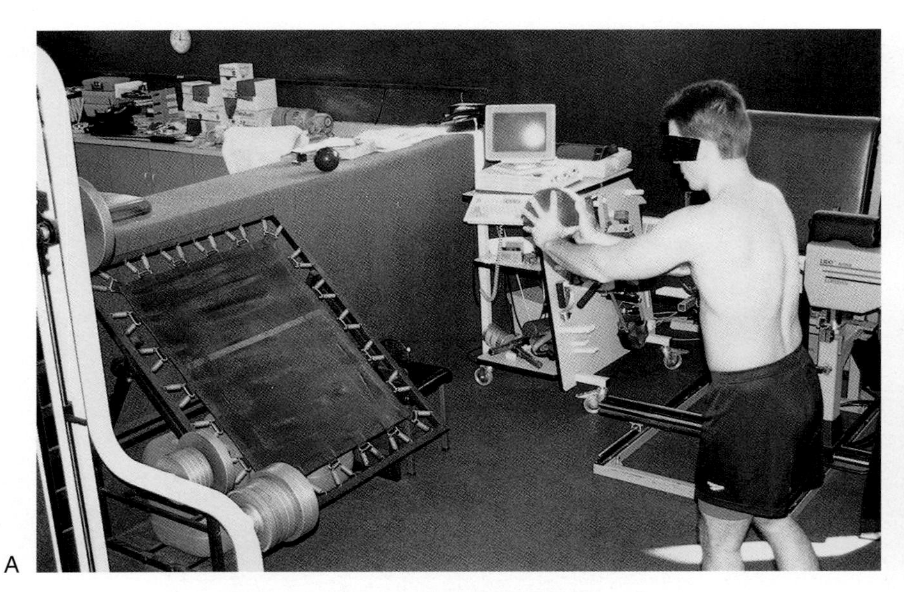
A

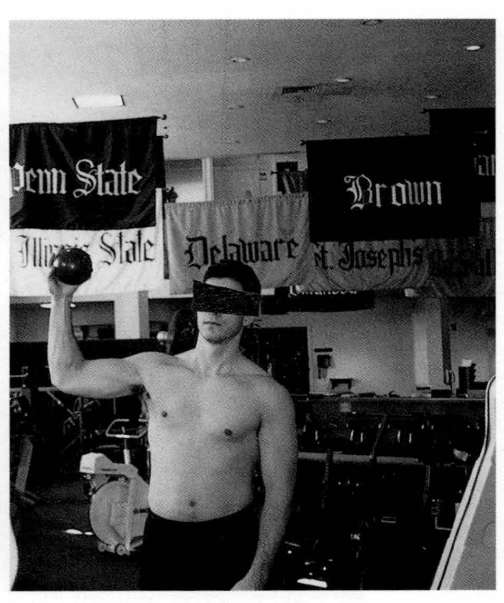

C

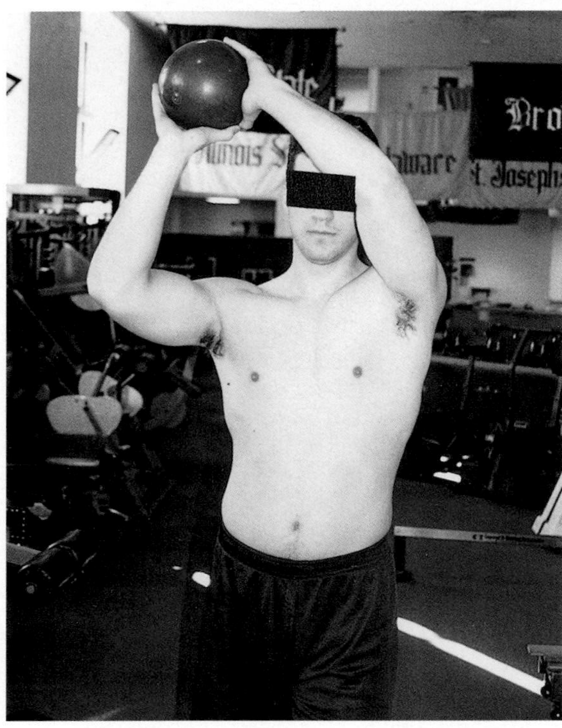
B

FIG. 16. Plyometric progression. **(A)** Chest pass. **(B)** Overhead with trunk rotation. **(C)** 90/90.

head or lifting task such as painting a ceiling or picking up a bag of leaf clippings they are taught the biomechanics of lifting to modify the task—by using a ladder, splitting the clippings, or using a wagon. In reality this is usually discussed and performed in the previous phases.

The athlete. During this phase the athlete should continue with the rotator cuff activities with a bias toward sport-specific positions. They will enter a modified off-season conditioning program. A gradual return to their sport is encouraged by allowing accommodating reentry. The pitcher will continue with an interval throwing program, and the tennis player will continue with a return to noncompetitive forehand and backhand strokes, eventually progressing to technique serving strokes. The swimmer performs low-intensity interval training. Gradually the intensity of the activity is increased.

The laborer. The laborer may be placed in a structured work-hardening program that is gradually increased in intensity. Education regarding lifting biomechanics and ergonomic modifications should be strongly emphasized during this phase. A functional capacity evaluation may help determine objective capabilities and limitations. Depending on the employer and job requirements, the patient may begin work that specifies job restrictions. This is not always possible; therefore, the patient must stay out of work until symptoms abate and/or soft-tissue healing time parameters are satisfied. Occasionally, retraining or reeducation of the individual is required due to excessive job demands.

Rehabilitation Following Rotator Cuff Repair

Rehabilitation following a rotator cuff repair may vary based on surgical technique, cuff tear size, tissue quality, patient age, patient goals, (Table 8, 9, 10) systemic disease processes, and whether it was repaired under tension. The prognosis following repair has been correlated to the cuff tear size,[42,52] presurgery atrophy,[47] presurgery ROM restrictions,[47] quality of tissue, and systemic disease processes. The goal of surgical treatment of the rotator cuff tear is to restore functional anatomy by reestablishing continuity of the rotator cuff, decrease pain, and improve function. The goals of rehabilitation are similar to those of conservative treatment, except the repair site for the rotator cuff and deltoid must be protected. The first step to ensure protection of the surgical repairs is by educating the patient about shoulder use precautions. Because the subacromial space has been surgically manipulated and bleeding occurs, emphasis is placed on preventing subacromial space scarring. Immediate passive ROM exercises are performed to maintain subacromial gliding and CLC and tendon pliability.

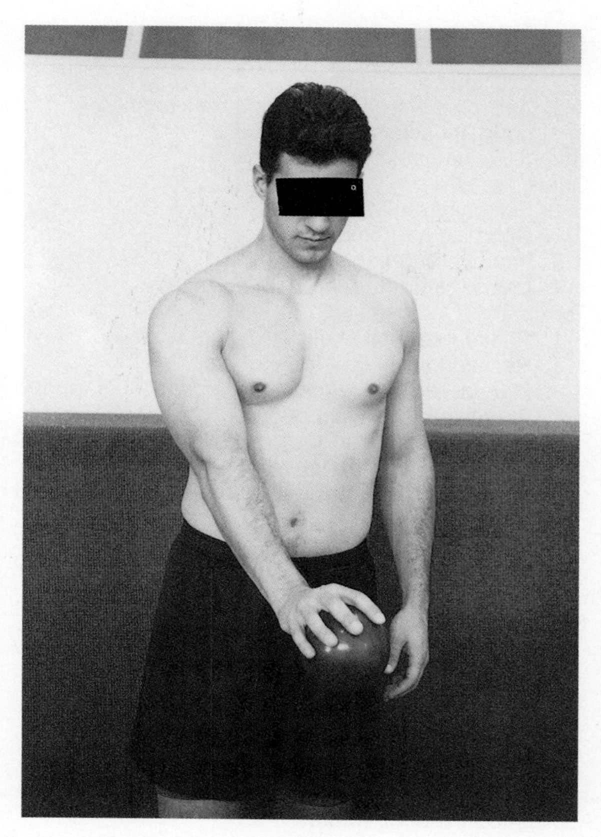

FIG. 17. Plyometrics emphasizing glenohumeral and scapular decelerators. (Reproduced with permission from Kelly MJ. Anatomic and biomechanical rationale for rehabilitation of the athlete's shoulder. *J Sport Rehabil* 1995;4:122–154.)

TABLE 7. *Influencing factors following rotator cuff repair*

Age
Quality of tissue
Size of tear
Mobilization required
Repair tension
Functional demands

As with any surgical procedure, it is essential for the rehabilitation specialist to know at least the basic surgical technique and what tissues were incised, altered, or repaired. Knowledge of the surgical intervention helps to ensure safe and educated rehabilitation by knowing what to protect. We feel it is a dangerous disservice to the patient and surgeon for the rehabilitation specialist to care for a postoperative patient without knowledge of the surgical technique. Information regarding tissue quality and presurgery ROM and strength are also valuable in guiding the rehabilitation process and predicting outcome. For example, a patient who enters surgery with a long-standing contracture restricting external rotation to 50 degrees measured at 90 degrees of abduction, can be expected to have the same limited motion, or worse, if the tight tissue is not released at the time of surgery.

Phase I. The goals of this phase are to promote patient education, control pain and inflammation, encourage healing at the repair sites, and maintain subacromial gliding and CLC and tendon pliability. This phase lasts for approximately 6 weeks and is broken down into three stages. The first stage lasts for 2 weeks and begins with patient education. Patients are instructed to use their arm for waist level activities when tolerated. They are cautioned about lifting anything, sleeping on the surgical side, leaning on the elbow, and sudden movements. They are encouraged to use ice frequently through the day. They are also instructed to place a support, such as a pillow, under the arm to position it in slight abduction and neutral rotation. Pritchett found that 10% of patients undergoing a rotator cuff repair had an inferiorly subluxed humeral head within 2 weeks after surgery.[115] Proper positioning of the shoulder helps take the weight of the extremity off the repair site and discourages an internal rotation contracture.

Active exercises are performed at the elbow, wrist, and hand. Phase I ROM exercises are initiated (Fig. 6). Pendulums are performed in tolerated ranges, as is passive shoulder flexion using the other extremity. Passive ROM into external rotation is performed with the arm at 45 degrees in the POS. The adducted position is avoided because external rotation performed with the arm adducted has been shown to increase tension across the repaired tissues.[44,151] Exercises are performed for 20 repetitions three to six times per day. Functional internal rotation is absolutely avoided because this position, shoulder extension and internal rotation, places the supraspinatus in its elongated dangerous state, endangering the integrity of the repair. For this reason, patients are warned not to tuck their shirts in behind their backs. The pa-

TABLE 8. *Acromioplasty guidelines—intact rotator cuff*

Phase I: 0–4 weeks postsurgery
- Goals
  1. Patient education
  2. Permit healing
  3. Control pain and inflammation
  4. Initiate range of motion exercises
- Treatment
  - Immediately postsurgery or postoperative day 1
    1. Immobilized in sling; use sling for comfort and public only
    2. Pendulums
    3. Hand squeezes
    4. Elbow AROM; supine PROM forward elevation (in appropriate patient)
  - 7–10 Days postsurgery
    1. Pendulums
    2. Supine PROM forward elevation and external rotation (45 degrees PO)
    3. PROM extension
    4. Heat and ice
    5. Active scapular exercises
  - 2–4 Weeks postsurgery
    1. Continue all stretches
    2. PROM internal rotation and cross body adduction
    3. PROM external rotation in abduction (below painful arc)
    4. Phase I strengthening (internal rotation, external rotation, extension)
    5. Resisted scapular exercises

Phase II: 4–6 weeks postsurgery
- Goals
  1. Improve to full ROM
  2. Improve neuromuscular control and strength
- Treatment
  1. Continue all stretches
  2. Add phase II stretches if not yet performing
  3. Progress to phase II strengthening exercises when at green for all phase I strengthening
  4. Advanced scapular strengthening
  5. Manual resistance for rotator cuff, deltoid, and PNF
  6. Body blade below 45 degrees

Phase III: 6–12 weeks postsurgery
- Goals
  1. Full pain-free ROM
  2. Optimize neuromuscular control
  3. Improve endurance
  4. Initiate return to functional activities
- Treatment
  1. Continue all stretches and strengthening, progress rotator cuff exercises into POS abduction
  2. Appropriate variable resistance and/or free-weight resistance
  3. Strengthening above 90 degrees
  4. Plyometrics[a]/body blade
  5. Work-/sport-specific exercise[a]

Phase IV: 12–16 weeks postsurgery
- Goals
  1. Return to sport,[a] occupation[a] or desired activities
  2. Promote concept of prevention
- Treatment
  1. Work hardening[a]
  2. Sport-specific training[a]

[a] Applies to athlete or laborer.

TABLE 9. *Rehabilitation guidelines for small/medium rotator cuff tears following surgical repair*

Phase I: 0–4 weeks postsurgery
- Goals
  1. Patient education
  2. Permit healing
  3. Control pain and inflammation
  4. Initiate range of motion exercises
- Treatment
- Immediately postsurgery or postoperative day 1
  1. Immobilized in sling, use sling for comfort and public only
  2. Pendulum
  3. Hand squeezes
  4. Elbow AROM, supine PROM forward elevation (in appropriate patient)
- 7–10 Days postsurgery
  1. Pendulums
  2. Supine PROM forward elevation and external rotation (45 degrees in POS)
  3. PROM extension
  4. Heat and ice
  5. Active scapular exercises
- 3–4 Weeks postsurgery
  1. Continue all stretches
  2. AAROM external rotation in abduction (below painful arc)

Phase II: 4–6 weeks postsurgery
- Goals
  1. Improve to full ROM
  2. Improve neuromuscular control and strength
  3. Emphasize normal scapulohumeral rhythm
- Treatment
  1. Continue all stretches
  2. Add phase II stretches (internal rotation and cross body abduction)

Phase III: 6–12 weeks postsurgery
- Goals
  1. Full painfree ROM
  2. Optimize neuromuscular control
  3. Improve endurance
  4. Initiate return to functional activities
- Treatment
  1. Phase I strengthening
  2. Resisted scapular strengthening
  3. Manual resistance for rotator cuff, deltoid, and PNF
  4. Bodyblade below 45 degrees
  5. Progress to phase II strengthening (abdominal and FF) when at green for all phase I exercises
  6. Appropriate variable resistance and/or free-weight resistance
  7. Strengthening above 90 degrees
  8. Body blade

Phase IV: 12 weeks to 6 months postsurgery
- Goals
  1. Return to sport, occupation, or desired activities[a]
  2. Promote concept of prevention
- Treatment
  1. Work or Sport specific exercises[a]
  2. Work hardening[a]
  3. Gradual return to sport or desired activities[a]

[a] Applies to athlete or laborer.

TABLE 10. *Rehabilitation guidelines for large/massive rotator cuff tears following surgical repair*

Phase I: 0–6 weeks postsurgery
- Goals
  1. Patient education
  2. Permit healing
  3. Control pain and inflammation
  4. Initiate range of motion exercises
- Immediately postsurgery or postoperative day 1
  1. Patients may be immobilized in sling or abduction brace
     - if sling, use for comfort and public only
     - if abduction brace, immobilized for 3–6 weeks
  2. Pendulums
  3. Hand squeezes
  4. Elbow AROM
- 7–10 Days postsurgery
  1. Pendulums
  2. Supine PROM forward elevation and external rotation above level of brace
  3. Heat and ice
  4. Active scapular exercises

Phase II: 6–10 weeks postsurgery
- Goals
  1. Improve to full ROM
  2. Improve neuromuscular control and strength
- Treatment
  1. Continue all stretches
  2. Add phase II stretches (internal rotation, CBA, extension)
  3. Rotator cuff isometrics (submaximal)
  4. Phase I strengthening (start at 6–8 weeks)
  5. Resisted scapular strengthening

Phase III: 10–16 weeks postsurgery
- Goals
  1. Full pain-free ROM
  2. Optimize neuromuscular control
  3. Improve endurance
  4. Initiate return to functional activities
- Treatment
  1. Continue all stretches and strengthening
  2. Progress to phase II strengthening when at green for all phase I exercises
  3. Manual resistance for rotator cuff, deltoid, and PNF
  4. Bodyblade in nonprovocative positions

Phase IV: 16 weeks to 6 months postsurgery
- Goals
  1. Return to work, sport, or desired activities (in appropriate patient)
  2. Promote concept of prevention
- Treatment
  1. Work hardening
  2. Gradual return to work or desired activity
  3. Progress body blade into elevated positions
  4. Work-/sport-specific exercises

tient is instructed in active scapular retraction and elevation exercises. Typically the patient returns to the surgeon in 7 to 10 days to have the sutures removed and shoulder assessed. The exercises are reinforced, as are the precautions. If the surgeons feels that the patient has excessive tightness or pain, he or she may be referred to supervised therapy. Therapy would consist of heat and/or ice, joint mobilization, and passive stretching. The home program would again be emphasized, and if the patient responded, he or she would be progressed onto a home program or intermittent supervised program.

At 4 weeks, depending on the size of the tear (less than 1 cm), some patients can start performing submaximal isometrics for the internal rotators, extensors, elbow flexors, and extensors. Passive/active-assistive ROM into external rotation can be performed at 70 to 90 degrees of POS abduction. Supine active-assistive ROM into elevation using a stick also may be initiated in this select group of patients. By the end of this phase, 70% to 80% return of passive elevation and external rotation (with the arm in 90 degrees in the POS) is expected in most patients. ROM restrictions are expected in this time frame among patients with large or massive cuff tears who required mobilization of the rotator cuff tissue and have been placed in an abduction pillow. These patients have a functionally shortened capsuloligamentous–tendonous complex that results in limited motion at the glenohumeral joint.

Phase II. This phase extends from 6 to 10 weeks and is the time when the patient will add phase II stretches (Fig. 7) and continue with phase I. Patients can begin using a stick to perform active-assistive ROM exercises in all directions; caution is required when moving into functional internal rotation. If stiffness persists, joint mobilizations and gentle, relatively pain-free manual stretching is performed. An effective stretch to improve ROM is executed by placing the hands anywhere from on the forehead to the back of the head (depending on the comfort) and letting the elbows slowly drop toward the floor (Fig. 7C). This is maintained for 10 to 20 seconds and the discomfort relieved by bringing the elbows up for 5 seconds. This sequence is repeated 10 to 20 times. If the patient had a large or massive tear, repaired restrictions are expected and respected. These patients are brought along slowly and monitored for excessive stiffness or capsulitis. Slow and gradual return of motion is allowed without attempts to instruct the patient in overstretching or iatrogenically disrupting the repair due to enthusiastic stretching by the rehabilitation therapist. The surgeon and therapist must discuss any decision to aggressively stretch any patient.

Most patients initiate resisted exercises during this phase. The decision to begin resisted exercise will be based on the rotator cuff tear size, ease of repair, and quality of tissue. If the tear was greater than 5 cm and required moderate lateral mobilization of the retracted tendon, the surgeon may want to delay resisted exercises for another week or two. We advocate that one err on the safe side when it comes to starting resisted exercises; the potential serious risk far outweighs the minimal benefits. If minimal manual resistance causes uncharacteristic pain, then resisted exercises may be delayed. The exercises performed are the same as described for conservative treatment. Care is taken to minimize excessive loading of the cuff by using a bolster when needed and choosing the appropriate resistance level. At our clinic,

Yellow Theraband®is the first band used. The patient perform the exercises in pain-free ranges. When elevation is performed, appropriate scapulohumeral rhythm is encouraged. Multi-angle isometrics are performed beginning at 45 degrees in the POS using manual resistance. Four directions of submaximal isometric resistance are performed by the patient in sequence: abduction/external rotation, adduction/internal rotation, elevation, and extension. This technique assesses the patient's resistance and pain level. This also continues the process of neuromuscular training of the glenohumeral and scapular muscles. If pain is encountered, the position is modified, resistance level changed, or the exercise is deferred until another session. The use of this manual resistance sequence helps to guide the patient's elastic band/free weight program. Depending on the patient's response to resistive exercise and time from surgery, the position of resistance is progressed toward 90 degrees in the POS. This progression continues to more provocative positions as tolerated. The rationale for this exercise philosophy has already been described, but the nuances related to a postoperative rotator cuff repair patient will be further explored.

One of the difficulties of the postoperative cuff repair patient is weakness in elevating over the shoulder level. This occurs for several reasons. One is that the anterior deltoid has been surgically repaired after detachment. The effects of this have been demonstrated in objective strength testing of patients 6 and 12 months after rotator cuff repair. These patients continued to demonstrate weakness of the abductors, external rotators, and flexors of up to 20% to 35% at 6 months and 8% to 25% at 1 year.[127,147] In both these studies the flexor group lagged behind the abductors and external rotators. Additionally, the deltoid is a one-joint muscle and is thus more susceptible to mechanical weakness because the muscle fibers shorten with elevation. Elevation also is difficult because the rotator cuff has just been reattached and many times is atrophied due to the chronicity of the tear or pain reflex inhibition. In the case of a chronic tear, it may have been 6 or 12 months since the supraspinatus translated force from its origin to insertion. This muscle is not only lacking the cross-sectional mass to translate enough force to stabilize and elevate the humerus—it forgot how. Consider a weak rotator cuff and deltoid unable to elevate the extremity because they cannot cause humeral rotation through the available range. This is analogous to a weak quadriceps not being able to elevate the tibia fully during knee extension, even though passive extension is full; this is an active extensor lag. We can describe the lack of humeral elevation or rotation as an active abduction lag. The potential problem at the shoulder is that the supraspinatus tendon is not being retracted from the subacromial space and may be painfully compressed. By providing very light resistance or assisting the arm into the elevated positions (90 to 140 degrees of POS abduction), neuromuscular training to facilitate abduction activity is achieved; the abductors can "relearn" how to contract. This cannot be achieved with strengthening exercises performed at the side. One advantage of training in this position, recognizing that the position is in the impingement zone, is that the deltoid's moment arms and line of pull are improved (relative to below 90 degrees),[114] creating stabilizing joint compressive force and less shear force. To strengthen in the elevated positions, the patient is placed supine and is first treated with heat, joint mobilization, and stretching to maximize their elevation range. Multiangle isometrics are performed at different positions of elevation to improve the muscle's ability to contract and to improve the number of motor units recruited. The patient is then placed at 90 degrees and asked to elevate through the pain-free range. Scapular shrugging is discouraged through verbal and manual cues to reinforce appropriate synergistic scapular muscle activity as the glenohumeral muscles are activated. If able, the patient is than asked to stand and place the arm on the wall and to lift the hand off the wall. This sequence has proved very effective in safely strengthening the rotator cuff–deltoid–biceps complex in functional ranges while encouraging scapular muscle integration.

In selected patients the Bodyblade may be used at 8 weeks in the nonprovocative positions (Fig. 15A and B). As the patient progresses, light free weights (5 to 10 pounds) can be used for biceps curls. Triceps isolation exercises are performed on a variable resistance unit or with Theraband® by placing the arm in a nonprovocative position. Shoulder extension exercises can usually be progressed without harm to the surgical repair. Depending on the patient's status and other influencing factors, the patient may never move beyond the initial strengthening exercises. This is a decision made by the rehabilitation team.

Phase III. The patient should have at least 80% to 90% of the ROM at this phase unless he or she had a large or massive rotator cuff repair requiring lateral mobilization of the tendon or closure of the superior defect using the subscapularis and infraspinatus. This latter group of patients are brought along slowly relative to their ROM. We expect to see limitations of external rotation when measured at the side of up to 50%; however, external rotation limitations may only be 70% to 80% when measured at 90 degrees in the POS. Functional internal rotation also may be significantly limited in this group because internal rotation requires maximal lengthening of the rotator cuff. The important finding is whether they can actively achieve pain-free end range motion. Patients should be relatively pain free at this stage and should be able to actively elevate above shoulder level with adequate scapulohumeral rhythm. Many patients may continue to shrug with elevation, and one must determine the cause of the abnormal rhythm; is it weakness, CLC tightness, pain, or learned behavior? Depending on the cause, the abnormal rhythm may be expected; however, if full PROM is present and the rotator cuff is intact with good strength, further neuromuscular control training is required to improve synchronous recruitment of the glenohumeral dynamic stabilizers and scapulothoracic muscles. If pain continues to be an issue, a subacromial or acromioclavicular joint cortisone injection may be helpful to reduce local irritation.

The patient, depending on the influencing factors, is progressed to further strengthening exercises and activity-related movements. The nonprovocative to provocative philosophy is still used with absolute respect of the rotator cuff repair and deltoid. The patient may now be advanced to isolated triceps and biceps strengthening with the arm at the side or in slight abduction: row-type pulls at chest level and progression to latissimus pull-downs (modified to the front in the POS). Both of these exercises move the patient through the impingement zone; however, they require less rotator cuff recruitment and therefore less stress. The motions are performed in pain-free arcs. The number of repetitions is progressed for their rotator cuff strengthening program. The number will vary but can approach three sets of 30 repetitions.

The laborer. The laborer will be progressed to activity-simulated movements. For example, a plumber may begin to unscrew objects (i.e., screws, light bulbs) with the arm placed at 90 degrees. This type of activity is an example of neuromuscular control training, certainly it can have an endurance affect. These types of activities can provide feedback regarding areas to focus rehabilitation, readiness to return to work, overhead function, or sport. Achievement of these activities can be very encouraging to the patient.

The athlete. The athlete will be progressed in a manner similar to that for the phase III conservative approach. The rotator cuff strengthening exercises are progressed into elevated, sport-specific positions based on signs and symptoms. Manual therapy is performed attempting to maximize neuromuscular control and integration of scapular muscles in the elevated sport-specific positions. The athlete is progressed with the Bodyblade and plyoball progression as shown in Figs. 15 to 17. Isokinetics may be used in certain select patients, but soft-tissue healing parameters must be respected and weighed against the potential injurious forces encountered during isokinetic exercise. Cardiovascular conditioning is unrestricted at this time.

Phase IV. This phase begins at 16 weeks and continues to 6 months. This is the phase in which most lower demand patients (nonathletes or laborers) continue to gradually progress their home rotator cuff strengthening program and possibly their variable resistance program. Patients are encouraged to approach overhead activities with prudence and whenever possible to use ladders or stools to raise their hand closer to the task so that the elbow can remain below shoulder level, in a less demanding position. They are again instructed in the biomechanics of lifting in efforts to reduce the incidence of rotator cuff overload. Proper lifting is strongly emphasized for patients with two and three tendon rotator cuff repairs because the literature states that these individuals are at great risk to retear their rotator cuff. [42]

The athlete and laborer will be progressed in a manner similar to what was discussed in phase IV of the conservatively treated patient. Certainly their is more consideration of soft-tissue healing parameters, and the reentry process must be slower. With advances in surgical techniques requiring less invasive procedures, the incidence to return to previous competition has improved. Athletes who require overhead use of their arm may return to their sport but may not be pain free or perform at the same level of play. Recreational athletes can temper their competitive play and have a better chance of returning to an active life-style. The laborer may need job restructuring if it is available. If it is not and they must or want to return to their previous job responsibilities, they must practice proper lifting mechanics, ergonomic modifications, and common sense.

Instability

Glenohumeral instability is defined as abnormal symptomatic translation of the humeral head relative to the glenoid. The incidence of anterior instability (80%)[15,123] far exceeds that of posterior instability; however, some believe the true incidence of posterior instability (>79%)[125] is not appreciated due to spontaneous relocation and poor diagnostics. The incidence of instability differs for those above and below 40 years of age, with a recurrence rate of more than 79% in those under 30[1,49,123] and 15% in those over 40.[122,123] The difference in recurrence rate is mostly related to activity level but also to connective tissue differences and associated pathology. One should recognize that the incidence of a rotator cuff tear in the older patient (over 40 years) who experiences a anterior dislocation is greater than 85%.[45,103] Subluxation occurs when partial dissociation of the humerus and glenoid occurs, whereas dislocation occurs when the humerus and glenoid fully separate. Instability can be classified several ways, the simplest of which are traumatic and atraumatic. Atraumatic instability can be further classified as voluntary and involuntary (Table 11). Traumatic instability can result from a high-velocity uncontrolled end range force causing a breach in the capsulolabral–bone interface or Bankart lesion. The acronym TUBS is used to describe the characteristics of the traumatic group. Commonly these individuals require surgery to repair the Bankart lesion and to remain active and without recurrence of instability. A second acronym, AMBRI, is used to describe those who suffer from atraumatic instability. These individuals have a patchulous capsule due to increased connective tissue elasticity, capsular stretching, or a combination of these two factors with dynamic stabilizer weakness. Commonly these individuals have symptomatic translation in multiple directions and are therefore described as having multidirectional instability. A strengthening program for the glenohumeral and scapulotho-

TABLE 11. *Glenohumeral instability classification*

Traumatic	Atraumatic
Unilateral	**M**ultidirectional
Bankart lesion	**B**ilateral
Surgery required	**R**ehabilitation effective
	Inferior capsular shift required

racic muscles may be beneficial to this group,[13] but if they do not respond, a capsular shift may be required.

Conservative Treatment

Following a glenohumeral dislocation, the patient may be immobilized followed by a general progressive ROM and strengthening program (Table 12). The motion is advanced as tolerated while the patient is performing the phase I and II ROM exercises (Figs. 6 and 7). The range of motion should be full by 8 weeks postinjury with minimal pain at end range. Some sense of apprehension may still be felt at the provocative end range. Strengthening should be progressed through phases I, II, and III as discussed in the rotator cuff section, moving from nonprovocative to provocative. The evidence that proprioception has been compromised reinforces the concept of strengthening toward the position of dislocation. In addition to optimizing proprioceptive input, neuromuscular training is enhanced in positions where the injured static stabilizer is less effective at end range. This type of program is rarely performed in a supervised manner for more than several visits unless dealing with an athlete who is returning to competition. Several investigators have reported excellent results in preventing recurrence of dislocation in individuals experiencing traumatic instability.[2,149] Others feel that if an individual is to participate in high-velocity end range activities (i.e., throwing, spiking, or contact sports), the likelihood of recurrence is significant regardless of the rehabilitation.

Postoperative Rehabilitation

Rehabilitation following a Bankart procedure will vary depending on whether it was performed using an arthroscopic technique or an open procedure (Table 13). Typically rehabilitation following the arthroscopic technique will lag behind that following the open repair because greater fixation is typically achieved during the latter. Respect must be shown for the subscapularis repair during the open procedure. Greis[38] reported on several cases of subscapularis rup-

TABLE 12. *Instability—conservative treatment guidelines*

Phase I: 0–4 weeks
1. Immobilize in sling to allow healing
2. Begin gentle phase I stretching at 2–3 weeks
3. Phase I strengthening

Phase II: 4–6 weeks
1. Continue phase I stretching
2. Add phase II stretching
3. Manual resistance
    - Multiangle isometrics
    - Short arc
    - Scapulothoracic integration strengthening
4. Scapular strengthening
5. Progress to phase II strengthening

Phase III: 6–12 weeks
1. Prophylactic stretching
2. Phase III strengthening (progress to more provocative positions)
3. Submaximal occupation, sport, or desired activities

Phase IV: 16 weeks
1. Work hardening
2. Gradual return to sport

TABLE 13. *Rehabilitation guidelines following Bankart procedure*

Phase I: 0–4 weeks—exercise four to six times per day
- Goals
  1. Patient education
  2. Permit capsuloligamentous-labral healing
  3. Control pain and inflammation
  4. Initiate range of motion exercises
- Treatment
- Postoperative day 1
  1. Educate patient on precautions.
  2. Pendulum exercises
  3. Elbow AROM, hand squeeze exercises
  4. Ice (instruct patient on use of ice at home)
- Postoperative days 7–10
  1. Continue with pendulum exercises.
  2. Phase I stretching
      - Forward elevation
      - External rotation at 45 degrees in POS (limit range to 30 degrees)

Phase II: 4–6 weeks
- Goals
  1. Decreased pain and inflammation
  2. Normal arthrokinematics of glenohumeral and scapulothoracic joints
  3. Improve strength
- Treatment
  1. Continue with above treatment
  2. Phase II stretching
  3. Manual resistance for glenohumeral and scapulothoracic stabilization
  4. Phase I strengthening (at 5–6 weeks)
  5. Add shoulder shrugs and scapular retraction
  6. Bodyblade in nonprovocative positions (5–6 weeks)

Phase III: 6–12 weeks
- Goals
  1. Increase strength of rotator cuff and deltoid
  2. Increase strength of scapular muscles
  3. Increase total arm strength (biceps, triceps, forearms, etc.)
  4. Initiate strengthening in provocative positions
- Treatment
  1. Continue with above (decrease frequency of stretching exercises)
  2. Add phase II strengthening when at green for phase I strengthening; progress strengthening to more provocative positions
  3. Variable resistance and/or free-weight resistance
  4. Bodyblade in functional positions
  5. Plyoball progression (begin with chest pass)

Phase IV: 12–16 weeks
- Goals: Initiate return to sport or occupational activity[a]
- Treatment
  1. Bodyblade in overhead positions
  2. Plyoball throwing
  3. Work-/sport-specific activities[a]

[a] Applies to athlete or laborer.

ture within the first 4 weeks following surgery. The mechanism of subscapularis rupture appears to be related to a fall or inappropriate use of the arm by the patient. Occasionally excessive stiffness will be seen following anterior reconstruction.[62,84,136] This has been attributed to overtightening, excessive scar tissue formation, and allergic reaction to the fixation device. If tightness persists, particularly if excessive pain is a symptom, reexploration of the joint may be required.[62,84]

Phase I. Patient education is important in the early phases following surgery. Patients are instructed to use their arm for waist level activities when tolerated. They are cautioned about lifting anything, particularly by pushing the hands together (internal rotation), sleeping on the surgical side, leaning on the elbow, and making sudden movements. They are encouraged to use ice frequently throughout the day. When sitting, the patient is encouraged to position the arm on a pillow or arm rest in slight abduction and the arm in neutral rotation. This helps to prevent prolonged internal rotation contractures.

The patient will be shown pendulum exercises the day of surgery and is to perform them four to six times per day. Hand and wrist exercises are also encouraged. The patient will typically remain in the sling until his or her return to the surgeons office. At 1 to 2 weeks the patient is examined at the surgeons office and begun on the other phase I exercises of passive external rotation with the arm at 45 degrees in the POS. External rotation is not to exceed 30 degrees (Fig. 6D). Active-assistive ROM using a stick held in both hands is also started, limiting the motion to 90 degrees. At 3 weeks the patient can begin the stretch into further elevation limited only by discomfort. Active-assistive ROM wand exercises for extension and internal rotation can be started at 3 weeks. Submaximal isometrics may be started for the external rotators, flexors, extensors, elbow flexors, and elbow extensors. Internal rotation is not performed due to the subscapularis repair. Assessment of generalized hyperelasticity and hypoelasticity should be performed and will guide the progression of ROM exercise. If a hyperelastic patient presents with 150 degrees of elevation and 45 degrees of external rotation 3 weeks following surgery, ROM exercises will be discouraged. However, if a hypoelastic patient presents with significant restriction at 3 weeks postsurgery, the progressiveness of stretching will be accelerated.

Phase II. Depending on the status of the patient and quality of repair, the patient will be progressed to phase I and II strengthening exercises at 4 to 6 weeks (Figs. 10 and 11). Either an elastic band or free weights (0.5 to 2 pounds) can be used. Stretching is continued in all directions. If the patient is being followed in a supervised manner, manual resistance starting at 45 degrees in the POS can be initiated using alternating isometrics (Fig. 13). Scapular muscle integration and appropriate scapulohumeral rhythm is encouraged in all strengthening exercises. The UBE may be used with motion performed in each direction. The Bodyblade may be used in nonprovocative positions (Fig. 15A and B). If excessive stiffness is demonstrated, more progressive stretching is performed and joint mobilization techniques can be utilized. Rotational strengthening exercises may be progressed to 45 degrees of elevation.

Phase III. At this time the patient can be progressed to light-weight isotonics, using free weights or variable resistance units. Many times these exercises can be initiated in the latter part of phase II. Strengthening of the biceps and triceps can be initiated. The shoulder should remain in a protected position (less than 20 degrees of elevation) and the scapula "fixed" to integrate scapular muscle function into the exercise. A rowing exercise also can be performed with the same type of resistive equipment. Elastic band or free weight strengthening is progressed in resistance, repetition, and position of elevation. Diagonal patterns (D2 and D1) can be incorporated into the program. The patient can progress to latissimus pull-downs performed in front of the body. The Bodyblade exercises are progressed to functional positions and increased time intervals of up to 60 seconds (Fig. 15). The plyoball progression may be used, particularly if the patient is a competitive or recreational athlete or laborer (Figs. 16 and 17). Stretching should continue in this phase until full elevation is achieved and external rotation stretching is progressed to 90 degrees of abduction (90/90 position). External rotation at neutral still may be lacking up to 20 degrees, but external rotation at 90 degrees of elevation should be within 10 degrees of the other side. One must remember that collagen tissue continues to remodel for up to 12 months; therefore, further gains will be achieved over time.

The athlete. The throwing athlete will be progressed at an accelerated pace relative to external rotation stretching in phase II since this motion is critical to performance; however, stability cannot be sacrificed. In phase III the throwing or swimming athlete will be advanced to the provocative positions for their glenohumeral dynamic stabilizer exercises. Specific manual techniques may be emphasized for the glenohumeral dynamic stabilizers and scapular muscles. Cardiovascular exercise is strongly encouraged in the group.

Phase IV. Patient will be progressed to phase IV at 12 weeks and can begin to participate in their particular activities. The swimmer is encouraged to perform slow strokes. The basketball player can begin shooting. The thrower can begin light throwing of a tennis ball; the patient then moves back into an interval program over weeks 14 to 20. The patient can progress their variable resistance for a free program. Bench pressing can be initiated after 14 weeks; however, the degree of horizontal abduction may be limited and weight will be added gradually.

Rehabilitation Following Anterior Capsulorrhaphy (Table 14)

Anterior capsulorrhaphy is performed to reduce the volume within a redundant CLC. The degree of CLC redundancy can vary significantly. Thus, one may encounter a throwing athlete with minimal redundancy and "stiff" con-

TABLE 14. *Rehabilitation guidelines following anterior capsulorrhaphy*

- Phase I: 0–4 weeks
  - Goals
    1. Patient independent with precautions and home exercise program prior to discharge from hospital (typical inpatient hospital stay = 1 day)
    2. Permit capsular healing
    3. Control pain and inflammation
    4. Range of motion exercises will be initiated depending on surgeon's preference
  - Postoperative day 1
    1. Educate patient on precautions
    2. Pendulum exercises (25 times in each direction), depending on surgeon
    3. Elbow AROM, hand squeeze exercises
    4. Ice (instruct patient on use of ice at home)
- Phase II: 4–6 weeks
  - Goals
    1. Decreased pain and inflammation
    2. Normal arthrokinematics of glenohumeral and scapulothoracic joints
    3. Improve strength
  - Treatment
    1. Continue with above treatment
    2. Add phase I stretching, limit external rotation to 45 degrees
    3. Add phase II stretching
    4. Manual resistance for glenohumeral and scapulothoracic stabilization
    5. Add phase I strengthening
    6. Add shoulder shrugs and scapular retraction
- Phase III: 6–12 weeks
  - Goals
    1. Increase strength of rotator cuff and deltoid
    2. Increase strength of scapular muscles
    3. Increase total arm strength (biceps, triceps, forearms, etc.)
    4. Initiate strengthening in provocative positions
  - Treatment
    1. Continue with above (decrease frequency of stretching exercises)
    2. Add phase II strengthening, progress to strengthening to more provocative positions
    3. Variable resistance and/or free-weight resistance
    4. Body blade in nonprovocative progressing to functional positions
    5. Plyoball progression (begin with chest pass)
- Phase IV: 12–16 weeks
  - Goal: Initiate return to sport or occupational activity[a]
  - Treatment
    1. Body blade in overhead positions
    2. Plyoball throwing
    3. Work-/sport-specific activities[a]

[a] Applies to athlete or laborer.

nective tissue as opposed to an individual with a very patchulous CLC and "loose" connective tissue who has undergone unsuccessful stabilization procedures or has true multidirectional instability. These two types of athletes would be progressed very differently, but with the ultimate goal of allowing CLC healing and optimizing neuromuscular control. In the throwing athlete, near normal ROM would be encouraged, whereas in the individual with failed previous surgeries, ROM restrictions of 10 to 20 degrees may be encouraged. Phase I may be slightly more protracted after capsulorrhaphy as compared with phase I after an open Bankart procedure.

Phase I. Patient education is emphasized and is identical to that of the postoperative Bankart patient. The patient's arm is placed in a sling following surgery. The initiation of pendulum exercises varies based on the patient's connective tissue elasticity and the surgeon's preference. Pendulum exercises typically are started within the first 4 weeks. Some patients may not begin any type of ROM exercises until 6 weeks.

Phase II. After 4 weeks the patient has started passive external rotation with the arm placed in 45 degrees POS. Rotation is limited to neutral. Active-assistive ROM of up to 90 degrees elevation using the other arm is begun. The patient begins isometric exercises with the arm placed at the side for internal rotators, external rotators, extensors, flexors, and adductors. Resisted elbow/flexion and extension also is performed. The patient is advanced to phase I strengthening exercises using elastic band and/or free weights (0.5 to 2 pounds) (Fig. 13). Elevation exercises are continued, moving toward full range. External rotation stretching may be limited to no more than 45 degrees in the POS. Phase II stretches are initiated. External rotation at 90 degrees in the POS is checked and should not progress beyond 70 degrees. The goal is for this patient to have some degree of tightness by the end of 12 weeks. Approximately 10 to 20 degrees of limited motion in all planes is desired at 12 weeks because continued collagen remodeling will occur over time. This may vary depending on the extent of the capsulorrhaphy and if the patient has hyperelastic tissue. Manual strengthening techniques using alternating isometrics in the mid-range are strongly emphasized. Although the capsule has been tightened, it is critical that the glenohumeral dynamic stabilizer function be optimized. Short arc manual resistive exercises and/or the use of free weights are utilized in efforts to maximize these muscles in their stabilization function across the glenohumeral joint. Scapular muscle integration is again strongly emphasized. Use of the UBE may begin, again performed in both directions. The Bodyblade can be started toward the end of 7 weeks, starting in the nonprovocative position (Fig. 15).

Phase III. The patient follows the same regimen as described for that following the Bankart procedure. Again, strong emphasis is placed in mid-range function with strengthening being performed and progressed toward the end range. The use of the plyoball will be determined by the surgeon based on the functional demands of the patient. If the patient is an athlete or laborer and therefore requires use of the arm in provocative positions, then plyometrics will be utilized in phase III. Various resistance exercises are also performed (Table 6).

Phase IV. The patient is progressed to activities of phase IV at approximately 16 weeks. If the patient is a throwing athlete, an interval program is initiated. For a swimming athlete, progression will be slow, with initially work on stroke and technique and finally distance. The patient will not be encouraged to aggressively stretch as many swimmers tend to do because such an action may stretch out the reconstruction. A gradual return of ROM will be encouraged in the next 6 to 9 months.

Posterior Capsulorrhaphy

Rehabilitation following posterior capsulorrhaphy is typically much slower than that following the Bankart reconstruction or individual having multidirectional instability and anterior capsulorrhaphy. The patient is commonly placed in a brace with the arm in 10 to 20 degrees of external rotation for at least 6 weeks. No exercise is performed during this time, but patient education regarding donning and doffing the brace is essential. Precautions are also reviewed.

Phase II. Starting at 4 to 6 weeks, the patient is encouraged to utilize the arm for daily activities. Phase I and II stretches are started. Passive ROM is progressed to active ROM. Stretching into internal rotation will begin somewhere around 8 weeks. Horizontal adduction also is initiated. Flexion is progressed gradually from 90 to 150 degrees. Isometrics are performed, initially using some caution when resisting external rotators. At approximately 8 weeks the patient is progressed to phase I and II strengthening exercises using elastic band and/or free weight exercises for the dynamic glenohumeral and scapulothoracic stabilizers. Manual resistance is emphasized for this group of patients, and strengthening in the mid-range is encouraged.

Phase III. In Phase III, strengthening is progressed toward the end range of motion. The patient is moved onto variable resistive exercises with the arm in protected positions. By weeks 14 to 18, the patient should be fully progressed in their strengthening exercise and stretching and are allowed to return to some limited activity such as swimming.

Phase IV. Phase IV begins at weeks 18 to 28, and the patient may be returned to throwing activities utilizing a progressive interval program. Strength training is encouraged as the exercise for the glenohumeral dynamic stabilizers. Bench pressing is executed cautiously if at all because this activity can significantly stress the posterior capsule.

Frozen Shoulder

The frozen shoulder is a common problem in orthopaedic medicine; however, the nomenclature has made it difficult to understand. Recently, a classification system of frozen shoulder was developed by Zuckerman.[150] Frozen shoulder is classified into either primary or secondary frozen shoulder. Primary frozen shoulder is characterized by idiopathic, systemic, and extrinsic features. Patients with idiopathic primary frozen shoulder develop a painful and stiff shoulder without incident or related pathology. Patients with systemic primary frozen shoulders are concomitantly affected by factors such as diabetes; patients with extrinsic primary frozen shoulder develop stiffness and pain secondary to cardiovascular incident or cerebrovascular accident. Individuals with idiopathic primary frozen shoulder are commonly said to have "adhesive capsulitis." Adhesive capsulitis is a separate entity, and this diagnosis should be reserved for individuals with the onset of a stiff and painful shoulder without incident.

Secondary frozen shoulder is seen in individuals affected by trauma. This would also include individuals with rotator cuff tendonopathy, fracture, post surgery. The incidence of frozen shoulder in the general population has been reported as approximately 2%[12,83] and has been reported as high as 19%[109] in individuals with diabetes. The etiology of primary frozen shoulder is still difficult to determine. A great deal of research has been directed toward this problem, and possible etiologies include autoimmune response,[85] biceps tenosynovitis,[26] and trigger point of subscapularis.[138]

The pathology of frozen shoulder does need clarification. Essentially, what occurs is a very significant synovitis followed by capsular and ligamentous fibroplasia. Three phases of frozen shoulder have been described: freezing, frozen, and thawing.[117] The freezing phase is characterized by an aggressive synovitis and pain. This is followed by a frozen phase in which synovitis is still active and significant fibroplasia occurs. The thawing phase is characterized by significant reduction and abatement of synovitis; however, capsular contraction remains.[41] Over time, in the thawing phase, ROM does return. Shaffer[129] performed a study in which he had up to a 15-year follow-up and found that individuals, although asymptomatic, continued to have limitations in ROM, particularly external rotation.

Rehabilitation following frozen shoulder must absolutely include patient education. Often patients do not understand the cause of their significant pain and loss of function. They may believe that they have a catastrophic disease process such as cancer. This is why patient education regarding the pathology is absolutely essential. Many of these patients cannot sleep at night and commonly are extremely fatigued and not themselves. If the pathology and natural history of frozen shoulder has not been explained to them, it is the physician's and therapist's duty to educate them as to the natural history and eventual recovery of ROM and function. Patients typically respond favorably to the information that the pain will at some point resolve and that ROM will return.

If the patient is felt to have little stiffness and pain, he or she may be treated with only a home program. The patient is instructed to use heat before and/or during stretch followed by ice afterward. Commonly, phase I or II stretching (Figs. 6 and 7) is initiated, but patients are warned not to be too aggressive with stretching, particularly if they are in the freezing or early frozen phase. Aggressive stretching can increase symptoms due to the aggravation of synovitis. They are encouraged to take their range to the onset of discomfort and to maintain that position for 5 to 10 seconds. If reactivity is not too significant, patients are also instructed in standing extension and internal rotation exercises. Commonly, resistive exercises are not performed because strength is rarely affected. If the patient does have strength deficits, resistive exercises will be added once pain and stiffness begin to decrease. Patients may be examined after 1 to 2 weeks to assess their progress. Patients who do not demonstrate progress may continue therapy under supervision, including heat and prolonged stretch, along with joint mobilization.

Joint mobilization using grade I or II or possibly grade III mobilization is performed in efforts to decrease pain. The mechanism by which joint mobilization relieves pain is not completely understood, but oscillations appear to have some neurophysiologic effect in shutting down the nociceptors of the synovium. Mobilization can reduce the pain and somewhat "kick start" the recovery process. The main objective is to reduce pain, the recovery of motion will depend on how aggressive the fibroplasia process has been. Initial treatment may result in less pain, but significant contracture may still be present. Typically, the patient is not treated for more than 4 weeks, utilizing joint mobilization and stretching. If the patient's pain decreases, he or she can move within the functional range (activities of daily living can be performed with much less pain).

If the patient remains unresponsive to treatment, an intraarticular injection is advocated. This will hopefully address the reactive synovitis and reduce the patient's pain. It is important to remember that the initial goal of treatment is to reduce the patient's pain if fibroplasia is established, ROM will return slowly. Occasionally, a patient can be caught early in the freezing phase and will demonstrate a fairly quick response in ROM return. Often individuals with primary rotator cuff tendinopathy and secondary capsulitis respond more quickly with the return of ROM because the capsulitis appears to be less aggressive than that seen in patients with the idiopathic or diabetic variety. Over time, the ROM exercises may be progressed to elevated positions with rotation or more provocative positions. The progression is based on symptoms, and the length of time spent in each stretch position is increased in efforts to improve the mechanical effect and hopeful deformation of the connective tissue. Patients may be examined every 2 months to reevaluate their progress. If the patient does not show any reduction of pain or improvement in ROM over approximately a 3-month period, and if several injections have been given, the patient may be treated with either manipulation or arthroscopic capsular release. With either of these surgical approaches, the same treatment course is followed with active assisted and passive ROM exercises, which are started in the recovery room and continued once a day for 4 to 6 weeks. Joint mobilization also is performed to reduce postoperative pain. Heat and ice are utilized as required. The patient typically is progressed in a supervised manner following manipulation or surgical release.

GLENOHUMERAL ARTHRITIS

Several diseases affect the osteoarticular surface of the glenohumeral joint and can result in the need for surgical intervention. The most common among these disorders include degenerative osteoarthritis, traumatic arthritis, osteonecrosis, arthritis of glenohumeral instability, rheumatoid arthritis, rotator cuff arthropathy, and crystal-induced arthritis.[4,20,98,146] Other less common disorders include hemophilic arthropathy, Paget's disease, psoriasis, and ochronosis.[146] Arthritic conditions can cause deformity of the normal articulating surfaces, loss of the articular cartilage, and synovitis associated with generalized joint inflammation.[146] As a result, the patient may experience joint pain, instability, limited active and passive ranges of motion, and decreased strength, which limits the patient's daily, recreational, and work activities.[146] The primary indication for prosthetic arthroplasty is pain that limits functional activity and is not improved with conservative management.[146] Limited ROM in the absence of pain is not an indication for surgery.[98]

Prosthetic joint replacement can include total shoulder arthroplasty or hemiarthroplasty (proximal humeral replacement). Indications for hemiarthroplasty include conditions in which the glenoid is intact, such as acute proximal humerus fractures, avascular necrosis, and younger patients.[29,30,98,146] Another indication for hemiarthroplasty is patients who have massive, irreparable deficiencies of the rotator cuff such as those with cuff tear arthropathy, crystal-induced arthritis, and rheumatoid arthritis.[29,30,100,146] Patients with massive rotator cuff deficiency have a higher incidence of glenoid component loosening than patient's with the same disease process but an intact rotator cuff.[30] Therefore, hemiarthroplasty is the preferred procedure for these patients.[146] Total shoulder arthroplasty in patients with an intact rotator cuff and significant glenoid degeneration will result in improved shoulder mechanics and postoperative pain level (Table 15).[20,98,146]

Postoperative Rehabilitation

Good communication between the rehabilitation specialist and orthopaedic surgeon is critical to successful outcome after shoulder arthroplasty. Rehabilitation after shoulder arthroplasty depends on the underlying diagnosis, integrity of the rotator cuff, and variations in surgical technique. The rehabilitation specialist should know the amount of external rotation and forward elevation achieved by the surgeon at the time of wound closure.[146] The kind of joint stability and quality of the subscapular repair should be determined. The patient's goals and motivation to participate in the rehabilitation process are also significant factors affecting outcome. Neer recommended classifying patients into standard goals

PROXIMAL HUMERUS FRACTURES

Fractures of the proximal humerus can produce as many as four major fracture fragments.[19] These include the head, the greater tuberosity, the lesser tuberosity, and the shaft of the proximal humerus. Neer introduced a four-part classification system based on the anatomic and biomechanical forces that contribute to the displacement of the fracture fragments.[5,97] Displacement is defined as greater than or equal to 1 cm of translation or 45 degrees of angulation from the fragment's normal anatomic position as seen on radiographs.[97] A proximal humerus fracture in which none of the major fragments is displaced is a one-part or nondisplaced proximal humerus fracture.

Management of proximal humerus fractures varies depending on the type and amount of displacement. A majority of proximal humerus fractures are nondisplaced and do not require surgery.[48,96,97,121] In these cases, the patient's arm is placed in a sling with the arm at the side. In some two-, three-, and four-part proximal humerus fractures, surgery is indicated. The preferred methods include closed reduction, open reduction and internal fixation, and prosthetic arthroplasty.[146] The type of fracture present as well as the medical and functional status of the patient determine the type of procedure to be performed.[146]

Rehabilitation of Proximal Humerus Fractures

Communication between the therapist, surgeon, and patient is essential to successful rehabilitation following proximal humerus fracture (Table 17).[5] The rate of exercise advancement is coordinated with the surgeon and depends on the severity of the fracture, stability of reduction, and formation of callus.[5] In most cases, the patient has never had a previous shoulder injury. Therefore, the patient should be educated on the importance of performing a home exercise program, techniques for pain relief, the length of the rehabilitation process, and expected outcome. Several factors affect outcome, including patient age and compliance with the home exercise program, complexity of the fracture, type of reduction, and soft-tissue involvement.[5]

A detailed history should be obtained from the patient and should include mechanism of injury, presence of additional injuries, prior functional status, and patient's goals. If the physician has not provided a detailed description of the type and stability of the fracture, the therapist should obtain this information prior to initiating movement of the extremity. The therapist should also perform a good neurovascular examination of the distal extremity.

Phase I

The rehabilitation process may begin when the surgeon is confident that adequate stabilization of the fracture has been achieved. This can be as early as the first postoperative day in many cases. In those cases in which surgery has not been performed or less than ideal fixation has been achieved, the rehabilitation program may require modification.

The importance of performing the home exercise program 4 to 6 times per day should be emphasized to the patient. Pain is a major consideration in this population and should always be respected. Many patients with proximal humerus fractures have never had shoulder pain similar to the magnitude they now experience; therefore, it is occasionally more difficult to motivate them to perform their home exercise program. Initial exercises include pendulums, supine passive forward elevation with the opposite hand, and supine passive

TABLE 17. *Rehabilitation guidelines following surgery for proximal humerus fractures with stable fixation*

Phase I: 0–4 weeks
- Goals
  1. Patient education
  2. Reduce/control pain
  3. Initiate range of motion exercises
- Treatment
  1. Patient education
  2. Modalities for pain relief
  3. Pendulums and phase I stretching
  4. Progress to phase II stretching

Phase II: 4–8 weeks
- Goals
  1. Decrease pain
  2. Improve to full ROM
  3. Improve neuromuscular control and strength
  4. Increase ADL activity
- Treatment
  1. Continue all stretches
  2. Manual resistance for glenohumeral and scapulothoracic stabilization
  3. Phase I strengthening (at 6–8 weeks if x-rays show healing fracture)
  4. Scapula muscle strengthening

Phase III: 8–12 weeks
- Goals
  1. Optimize PROM
  2. Increase strength of rotator cuff and deltoid
  3. Increase strength of scapular muscles
  4. Increase total arm strength (biceps, triceps, forearms, etc.)
  5. Initiate strengthening in provocative positions
- Treatment
  1. Phase II strengthening (if x-rays show healing fracture)
  2. Progress scapular muscle exercises
  3. Total arm strengthening
  4. Manual resistance in unsupported positions
  5. Body blade/plyoball exercises
  6. Prepare for return to work or sport

Phase IV: 12–16 weeks
- Goals
  1. Full functional activities
  2. Return to work or sport[a]
- Treatment
  1. Work- or sport-specific training[a]
  2. Suggest modifications to work, sport, or functional activities[a]

[a] Applies to athlete or laborer.

external rotation with a stick. Patients are slowly advanced to passive extension, internal rotation, and cross-body adduction at approximately 3 to 6 weeks postfixation. Special consideration is given to those patients with greater tuberosity fractures because these exercises provide tension to the rotator cuff and its attachment. If excessive tightness is determined, joint mobilization is implemented to facilitate the return of motion.

Phase II

The patient should achieve near full passive ROM at 4 to 6 weeks postfixation. Rotator cuff strengthening with isometrics and/or Theraband can begin at this time. In addition, scapular strengthening exercises also may be initiated. If the patient is being followed in supervised therapy, manual isometrics at 45 degrees in the POS can be introduced.

Phase III

Approximately 8 to 12 weeks postfixation, the patient should have full passive ROM and good rotator cuff strength. Phase II strengthening exercises with the elastic band can begin at this time. These exercises include abduction to 45 degrees, forward elevation, and external rotation at 45 degrees (Fig. 14). Progression of resistance for shoulder shrugs, scapular retraction, biceps curls, and triceps extension is also accomplished. For patients who are being followed in supervised therapy, manual resistance in unsupported positions can be progressed utilizing alternating isometrics and PNF diagonals.

SUMMARY

Proper rehabilitation of the shoulder is essential to the recovery of patients treated both conservatively and postoperatively. Successful rehabilitation is dependent on effective communication and interaction between the physician, therapist, and patient. Each of these team members has a defined role in the rehabilitation process and must fulfill their responsibilities in order for the desired outcome to be achieved.

This chapter presented principles and rationale for rehabilitation of various shoulder pathologies. In addition, guidelines for instruction and exercise progression were illustrated. Whether the patient will be followed in regular supervised therapy or seen in the office at specific intervals, extensive patient education is essential to successful rehabilitation. The patient must understand the pathology and rationale for each phase of the rehabilitation process. Constant reevaluation by the physician and therapist is important to make necessary program modifications if the patient is not achieving preset goals.

The common goals of the rehabilitation process include reduction of pain and inflammation, facilitation of collagen healing, improvement in ROM and strength, and optimization of proprioception and endurance. This is achieved by gradually increasing the program from nonprovocative to provocative positions. It is the rehabilitation specialists' and surgeons responsibility to identify when to implement the appropriate modalities or exercises in order to improve the impairment and thereby increase the patient's function.

Prospective studies that demonstrate rehabilitation of impairments and functional limitations associated with various shoulder pathologies are needed in the literature. Once these studies exist, a dialogue between physicians and therapists can be further developed. The end result will be more efficient and successful rehabilitation for the most important member of the team, the patient.

REFERENCES

1. Arciero RA, et al. Arthroscopic Bankart repair versus nonoperative treatment for acute, initial anterior shoulder dislocations. *Am J Sports Med* 1994;22:589–94.
2. Aronen JG, RK. Decreasing the incidence of recurrence of first time anterior shoulder dislocations with rehabilitation [Abstract]. *Am J Sports Med* 1988;74:283–291.
3. Arrigo CA, Wilk KE. Shoulder exercises: a criteria-based approach to rehabilitation. In: Kelley MJ, Clark WA, ed. *Orthopaedic therapy of the shoulder*. Philadelphia: JB Lippincott, 1995:337–370.
4. Barrett WP, et al. Total shoulder arthroplasty. *J Bone Joint Surg [Am]* 1987;69:865–872.
5. Basti JJ, Dionysian E, Sherman PW, Bigliani LU. Managment of proximal humerus fractures. *J Hand Ther* 1994:111–121.
6. Benjamin M, et al. The structure of the insertions of the tendons of biceps brachii, triceps and brachialis in elderly dissecting room cadavers. *J Anat* 1992;180:327–332.
7. Benson HAE, McElnay JC. Transmission of ultrasound energy through topical pharmaceutical products. *Physiotherapy* 1988;74:587.
8. Bigliani LU, Morrison D, April EW. The morphology of the acromion and its relationship to rotator cuff tears. *Orthop Trans* 1986;1:228.
9. Blackburn TA, McLeod WD, White B, Wofford L. Analysis of posterior rotator cuff exercises. *Athletic Training* 1990;25:40.
10. Blasier RB, Guldberg RE, Rothman ED. Anterior shoulder stability: contributions of rotator cuff forces and the capsular ligaments in a cadaver model. *J Shoulder Elbow Surg* 1992;1:140–150.
11. Borsa PA, LS, Kocher MS, Lephart SP. Functional assessment and rehabilitation of shoulder proprioception for glenohumeral instability. *J Sport Rehabil* 1994;3:84–104.
12. Bridgman J. Periarthritis of the shoulder and diabetes mellitus. *Ann Rheum Dis* 1972;31:69–71.
13. Burkhead W, Ca R. Treatment of instability of the shoulder with an exercise program. *J Bone Joint Surg [Am]* 1992;74:890–896.
14. Cain PR, et al. Anterior stability of the glenohumeral joint: a dynamic model. *Am J Sports Med* 1987;15:144–148.
15. Cave EF, Burke JR, Boyd RJ. *Trauma management*. Chicago: Year Book Medical, 1974.
16. Celli L, et al. Some new aspects of the functional anatomy of the shoulder. *Ital J Orthop Traumatol* 1985;11:83–91.
17. Clark J, Sidles JA, Matsen FA III. The relationship of the glenohumeral joint capsule to the rotator cuff. *Clin Orthop Rel Res* 1990; 254:29–34.
18. Clark JM, Harryman DT II. Tendons, ligaments, and capsule of the rotator cuff. *J Bone Joint Surg [Am]* 1992;74:713–725.
19. Codman EA. The shoulder: rupture of the supraspinatus tendon and other lesions in or about the subacromial bursa. *The shoulder.* Boston: Thomas Todd, 1934:262.
20. Cofield RH. Total shoulder arthroplasty with the Neer prosthesis. *J Bone Joint Surg [Am]* 1984;66:899–906.
21. Colachis SC, Strohm BR. Effect of supraspinatus and axillary nerve blocks on muscle force in upper extremity. *Arch Phys Med Rehabil* 1971;52:22.
22. Cyriax J. Diagnosis of soft tissue lesions. In: *Textbook of orthopaedic medicine,* 8th ed. Vol. 1. Baltimore: Williams & Wilkins, 1970.

23. Davick JP, Martin RK, Albright JP. Distribution and deposition of tritiated cortisol using phonophoresis. *Phys Ther* 1988;68:1672–1675.
24. Davidson PA, et al. Rotator cuff and posterior-superior glenoid labrum injury associated with increased glenohumeral motion: a new site of impingement. *J Shoulder Elbow Surg* 1995;4:384–390.
25. Dempster WT. Mechanisms of shoulder movement. *Arch Phys Med Rehabil* 1965;46:49–70.
26. DePalma AF. Surgery of the Shoulder. Philadelphia: JB Lippincott, 1973.
27. Doody SG, Freedman L, Waterland JC. Shoulder movements during abduction in the scapular plane. *Arch Phys Med Rehabil* 1970;51: 595–604.
28. Dvir Z, Berme N. The shoulder complex in elevation of the arm: a mechanism approach. *J Biomechanics* 1978;11:219–225.
29. Figgie HE, et al. An analysis of factors affecting the long-term results of total shoulder arthroplasty in inflammatory arthritis. *J Arthroplasty* 1988;3:123–130.
30. Franklin JL, et al. Glenoid loosening in total shoulder arthroplasty. *J Arthroplasty* 1988;3:39–46.
31. Freedman L, Munro RR. Abduction of the arm in the scapular plane: scapular and glenohumeral movements. *J Bone Joint Surg [Am]* 1966; 48:1503–1510.
32. Gerber C, Hersche O, Farron A. Isolated rupture of the subscapularis tendon. *J Bone Joint Surg [Am]* 1996;78:1015–1023.
33. Gerber C, Krushell RJ. Isolated rupture of the tendon of the subscapularis muscle. *J Bone Joint Surg [Br]* 1991;73:389–394.
34. Gersten JW. Effect of ultrasound on tendon extensibility. *Am J Phys Med* 1955;34:362–369.
35. Glousman R, et al. Dynamic electromyographic analysis of the throwing shoulder with glenohumeral instability. *J Bone Joint Surg [Am]* 1988;70:220–226.
36. Goss CM, ed. *Anatomy of the human body (Gray's anatomy).* Philadelphia: Lea & Febiger, 1973.
37. Gowan ID, Jobe FW, Tibone TJ. A comparative electromyographicc analysis of the shoulder during pitching: professional versus amateur pitchers. *Am J Sports Med* 1987;15:586–590.
38. Greis PE, Dean M, Hawkins RJ. Subscapularis tendon disruption after Bankart reconstruction for anterior instability. *J Shoulder Elbow Surg* 1996;5:219–222.
39. Groh G, et al. Loss of the deltoid after shoulder operations: an operative disaster. *J Shoulder Elbow Surg* 1994;3:243–253.
40. Guanche C, et al. The synergistic action of the capsule and the shoulder muscles. *Am J Sports Med* 1995;23:301–306.
41. Hannafin J, DiCarlo EF, Wickiewicz TL. Adhesive capsulitis: capsular fibroplasia of the glenohumeral joint [Abstract]. *J Shoulder Elbow Surg* 1994;3:s5.
42. Harryman DT, et al. Repairs of the rotator cuff: correlation of functional results with integrity of the cuff. J Bone Joint Surg [Am] 1991; 73:982–989.
43. Harryman DT II, et al. Translation of the humeral head on the glenoid with passive glenohumeral motion. *J Bone Joint Surg [Am]* 1990;72: 1334–1343.
44. Harryman DT II, et al. The role of the rotator interval capsule in passive motion and stability of the shoulder. *J Bone Joint Surg [Am]* 1992;74:53–66.
45. Hawkins RJ, et al. Anterior dislocation of the shoulder in the older patient. *Clin Orthop* 1986;206:192.
46. Hawkins RJ, Kennedy JC. Impingement syndrome in athletes. Am J Sports Med 1980;8:151–158.
47. Hawkins RJ, Misamore GW, Hobeika PE. Surgery for full thickness rotator cuff tears. *J Bone Joint Surg [Am]* 1985;67:1349–1355.
48. Horak J, Nilsson B. Epidemiology of fractures of the upper end of the humerus. *Clin Orthop* 1975;112:250.
49. Hovelius L, et al. Recurrences after initial dislocation of the shoulder. *J Bone Joint Surg [Am]* 1983;65:343–349.
50. Howell SM, et al. Clarification of the role of the supraspinatus muscle in shoulder function. *J Bone Joint Surg [Am]* 1986;68:398–404.
51. Howell SM, Kraft TA. The role of the supraspinatus and infraspinatus muscles in glenohumeral kinematics of anterior shoulder instability. *Clin Orthop Rel Res* 1991;263:128–134.
52. Iannotti JP, et al. Postoperative assessment of shoulder function: a prospective study of full-thickness rotator cuff tears. *J Shoulder Elbow Surg* 1996;5:449–457.
53. Inman VT, Saunders M, Abbott LC. Observations on the function of the shoulder joint. *J Bone Joint Surg* 1944;26:1–30.
54. Jobe CM. Superior glenoid impingement. *Orthop Clin North Am* 1997;28:137–143.
55. Jobe FW, Moynes DR. Deliniation of diagnostic criteria and a rehabilitation program for rotator cuff injuries. *Am J Sports Med* 1982;10: 336–339.
56. Jobe FW, Moynes DR, Tibone JE, Perry J. An EMG analysis of the shoulder in pitching. A second report. *Am J Sports Med* 1984;12: 218–220.
57. Johnston TB. The movements of the shoulder-joint: a plea for the use of the "plane of the scapula" as the plane of reference for movements occurring at the humero-scapular joint. *Br J Surg* 1937;25:252–260.
58. Kadefors R, Petersen I, Herberts P. Muscular reaction to welding work: an electromyographic investigation. *Ergonomics* 1976;19:543.
59. Kaltenborn FM. *Mobilization of the extremity joints: examination and basic treatment techniques.* Oslo: Olaf Bokhandel, 1980.
60. Kapandji IA. *The physiology of the joints.* Vol. 1. Baltimore: Williams & Wilkins, 1970.
61. Kelkar R, et al. A stereophotogrammetric method to determine the kinematics of the glenohumeral joint. *Adv Bioeng* 1992:143–146.
62. Kelley M. The zero-zero sign: a postoperative finding following anterior capsular reconstruction surgery. Presented at the American Society of Shoulder and Elbow Therapists Annual Meeting, Newport, RI, 1997.
63. Kelley MJ. Anatomic and biomechanical rationale for rehabilitation of the athlete's shoulder. *J Sport Rehabil* 1995;4:122–154.
64. Kelley MJ. Biomechanics of the shoulder. In: Kelley MJC, ed. *Orthopedic therapy of the shoulder.* Philadelphia: JB Lippincott, 1995: 64–103.
65. Kelley MJ. Case studies of the shoulder. In: Kelley MJC, ed. *Orthopedic therapy of the shoulder.* Philadelphia: JB Lippincott, 1995: 424–442.
66. Kelley MJ. Evaluation of the shoulder. In: Kelley MJC, ed. *Orthopedic therapy of the shoulder.* Philadelphia: JB Lippincott, 1995: 225–268.
67. Kendall FP, McCreary EK. *Muscle testing and function*, 3rd ed. Baltimore: Williams & Wilkins, 1982.
68. Kent B. Functional anatomy of the shoulder complex. *Phys Ther* 1971;51:867–889.
69. Kibler WB, Livingston B, Chandler TJ. Shoulder rehabilitation: clinical application, evaluation, and rehabilitation protocols. *Instruct Course Lect* 1997;46:43–51.
70. Kisner C, et al. *Therapeutic exercise: foundations and techniques.* Philadelphia: FA Davis, 1985.
71. Kleinkort JA, Wood F. Phonophoresis with 1 percent vs. 10 percent hydrocortisone. *Phys Ther* 1975;55:1320.
72. Kottke FJ. Therapeutic exercise to maintain mobility. In: KFL JF, ed. *Krusens handbook of physical medicine and rehabilitation,* 4th ed. Philadelphia: WB Saunders, 1990.
73. Kottke FJ, Pauley DL, Ptak RA. The rationale for prolonged stretching for correction of shortening of connective tissue. *Arch Phys Med Rehabil* 1966;47:345–352.
74. Kuhlman J, et al. Isokinetic and isometric measurement of strength of external rotation and abduction of the shoulder. *J Bone Joint Surg [Am]* 1992;74:1320–1333.
75. Laumann U. Kinesiology of the joints. In: Kolbel REA, ed. *Shoulder replacement.* Berlin: Springer-Verlag, 1987.
76. Le Huec JC, Shauerbeke T, Moinard M, Kind M, Diard F, Dehais J, Le Rebeller A. Traumatic tear of the rotator interval. *J Shoulder Elbow Surg* 1996;5:41–46.
77. Lehman JF, Masock AJ, Warren CG, Koblanski JN. Effect of therapeutic temperatures on tendon extensibility. *Arch Phys Med Rehabil* 1970;51:481–487.
78. Lephart SM, Pincivero DM, Giraldo JL, Fu FH. The role of proprioception in the management and rehabilitation of athletic injuries. *Am J Sports Med* 1997;25:130–137.
79. Lephart SM, Warner JP, Borsa PA, Fu FH. Proprioception of the shoulder in healthy, unstable and surgically repaired shoulders. *J Shoulder Elbow Surg* 1994;3:371–380.
80. Lippitt S, Matsen F. Mechanisms of glenohumeral joint stability. Clin Orthop Rel Res 1993;291:20–28.
81. Lippitt SB, et al. Glenohumeral stability from concavity-compression: a quantitative analysis. *J Shoulder Elbow Surg* 1993;2:27–35.

82. Lucas DB. Biomechanics of the shoulder joint. *Arch Surg* 1973;107: 425–432.
83. Lundberg J. The frozen shoulder: clinical and radiographical observations: the effect of manipulation under general anesthesia: structure and glysosaminoglycans content of the joint capsule. *Acta Orthop Scand* 1969;119:1–59.
84. Lusardi DA, Wurtz D, Rockwood CA. Loss of external rotation following anterior capsulorrhaphy of the shoulder. *J Bone Joint Surg [Am]* 1993;75:1185–1192.
85. Macnab I. The painful shoulder due to rotator cuff tendonitis. *R I Med J* 1971;54:367–374.
86. Maitland GD. *Peripheral manipulation*, 3rd ed. London: Butterworth, 1991.
87. Mannheimer JS, Lampe GN. *Clinical transcutaneous electrical nerve stimulation.* Philadelphia: FA Davis, 1984:249.
88. Markhede G, Monastyrski J, Stener B. Shoulder function after deltoid muscle removal. *Acta Orthop Scand* 1985;56:242.
89. Matsen FA, Arntz CT. Rotator cuff tendon failure. In: *The shoulder.* Matsen RA, ed. Philadelphia: WB Saunders, 1990:647–677.
90. Matsen FA, Artnz GTI. Subacromial impingement. In: Matsen RA, ed. *The shoulder.* Philadelphia: WB Saunders, 1990:623–648.
91. Matsen FA III, Thomas SC, Rockwood CA Jr. Glenohumeral instability. In: Rockwood CA Jr, Matsen FA III, eds. *The shoulder.* Philadelphia: WB Saunders, 1990:526–622.
92. Meister K, Andrews JA. Classification and treatment of rotator cuff injuries in the overhead athlete. *J Orthop Sports Phys Ther* 1993;18: 413–421.
93. Moseley JB, Jobe FW, Pink MS, Perry J, Tibone J. EMG analysis of the scapular muscles during a shoulder rehabilitation program. *Am J Sports Med* 1992;20:128–135.
94. Nakajima T, Rokuuma N, Hamada K, Tomatsu T, Fukuda H. Histologic and biomechanical characteristics of the supraspinatus tendon: reference to rotator cuff tearing. *J Should Elbow Surg* 1994;3:79–87.
95. Neer C. Impingement lesions. *Clin Orthop* 1983;173:71–77.
96. Neer CS. Displaced proximal humeral fractures. Treatment of three-part and four-part displacement. *J Bone Joint Surg* 1970;52: 1090–1103.
97. Neer CS. Displaced proximal humerus fractures. Part I. Classification and evaluation. *J Bone Joint Surg [Am]* 1970;52:1077–1089.
98. Neer CS II, Watson KC, Stanton FJ. Recent experience in total shoulder replacement. *J Bone Joint Surg [Am]* 1982;64:319–337.
99. Neer CSI. Impingement lesions. *Clin Orthop* 1973;173:70–77.
100. Neer CSI, Craig EV, Fukuda H. Cuff tear arthropathy. *J Bone Joint Surg [Am]* 1983;65:1232–1244.
101. Neer CSI, et al. Earlier passive motion following shoulder arthroplasty and rotator cuff repair. A prospective study. *Orthop Trans* 1987;2: 231.
102. Neviaser RJ. Ruptures of the rotator cuff. *Orthop Clin North Am* 1987; 18:387–394.
103. Neviaser RJ, Neviaser TJ. Recurrent instability of the shoulder after age 40. *J Shoulder Elbow Surg* 1995;4:416–418.
104. Nuber GW, Jobe FW, Perry JP, et al. Fine wire EMG analysis of the shoulder during swimming. *Am J Sports Med* 1986;14:7–11.
105. O'Brien SJ, et al. The anatomy and histology of the inferior glenohumeral ligament complex of the shoulder. *Am J Sports Med* 1990;18: 449–456.
106. Otis JC, et al. Contribution of the infraspinatus muscle to shoulder abduction and external rotation torques. Presented at the 1989 Biomechanics Symposium, La Jolla, CA.
107. Ovesen J, Nielsen S. Anterior and posterior shoulder instability: a cadaver study. *Acta Orthop Scand* 1986;57:324–327.
108. Ozaki J, et al. Recalcitrant chronic adhesive capsulitis of the shoulder. Role of contracture of the coracohumeral ligament and rotator interval in pathogenesis and treatment. *J Bone Joint Surg [Am]* 1989;71: 1511–1515.
109. Pal B, Anderson D, Dick WC, Griffiths ID. Limitation of joint mobility and shoulder capsulitis in insulin and non-insulin dependent diabetes mellitus. *Br J Rheumatol* 1986;25:147–151.
110. Pappas AM, Zawacki RM, Sullivan TJ. Biomechanics of baseball pitching. *Am J Sports Med* 1985;13:216–222.
111. Perry J. Anatomy and biomechanics of the shoulder in throwing, swimming, gymnastics, and tennis. *Clin Sports Med* 1983;2:247–270.
112. Pink M, et al. The normal shoulder during freestyle swimming. An electromyographic and cinematographic analysis of twelve muscles. *Am J Sports Med* 1991;19:569–576.
113. Poppen NK, Walker PS. Normal and abnormal motion of the shoulder. J Bone Joint Surg [Am] 1976;58:195–201.
114. Poppen NK, Walker PS. Forces at the glenohumeral joint in abduction. *Clin Orthop Rel Res* 1978;135:165–170.
115. Pritchett J. Inferior subluxation of the humeral head after trauma or surgery. *Shoulder Elbow Surg* 1997;6:356–359.
116. Rathbun JB, Macnab I. The microvascular pattern of the rotator cuff. *J Bone Joint Surg [Br]* 1970;52:540–553.
117. Reeves B. The natural history of the frozen shoulder syndrome. *Scand J Rheumatol* 1975;4:193.
118. Richardson AB, The mechanics of swimming: the shoulder and the knee. *Clin Sports Med* 1986;5:10.
119. Richardson AB, Jobe FW, Collins HR. The shoulder in competitive swimming. *Am J Sports Med* 1980;8:159–163.
120. Rodosky MW, et al. Significance of a superior labral lesion of the shoulder: a biomechanical study. *Trans Orthop Res Soc* 1990;15:276.
121. Rose SH, et al. Epidemiologic features of humeral fractures. *Clin Orthop Rel Res* 1982;168:24–30.
122. Rothman RH, Parke WW. The vascular anatomy of the rotator cuff. *Clin Orthop Rel Res* 1965;41:176–186.
123. Rowe CR. Acute and recurrent anterior dislocations of the shoulder. *Orthop Clin North Am* 1980;11:253–270.
124. Rowe CR, Sakellarides HT. Factors related to recurrences of anterior dislocations of the shoulder. *Clin Orthop* 1961;20:41.
125. Rowe CR, Zarins B. Chronic unreduced dislocations of the shoulder. *J Bone Joint Surg [Am]* 1982;64:494–505.
126. Ryu RK, McCormick J, Jobe FW, Moynes DR, Antonelli DJ. An electromyographic analysis of shoulder function in tennis players. *Am J Sports Med* 1988;16:481–485.
127. Saha AK. Dynamic stability of the glenohumeral joint. *Acta Orthop Scand* 1971;42:491–505.
128. Sapega AA, Kelley MJ. Strength testing about the shoulder. *J Shoulder Elbow Surg* 1994;3:327–345.
129. Shaffer B, Tibone JE, Kerlan RK. Frozen shoulder. *J Bone Joint Surg [Am]* 1992;74:738–746.
130. Sigholm G, et al. Electromyographic analysis of shoulder muscle load. *J Orthop Res* 1984;1:379–386.
131. Snyder-Mackler L. Electrical stimulation for pain modulation. In: Snyder-Mackler L, Robinson AJ, eds. *Clinical electrophysiology, electrotherapy and electrophysiologic testing.* Baltimore: Williams & Wilkins, 1989:203–228.
132. Snyder-Mackler L. Electrical stimulation for tissue repair. In: Snyder-Mackler L, Robinson AJ, eds. *Clinical electrophysiology, electrotherapy, and electrophysiologic testing.* Baltimore: Williams & Wilkins, 1989:229–244.
133. Speer KP, Warren RF, Horowitz L. The efficacy of cryotherapy in the postoperative shoulder. *J Shoulder Elbow Surg* 1996;5:62–68.
134. Sullivan PE, Markos PA, Minor MD. *An integrated approach to therapeutic exercise, theory and clinical application.* Reston, VA: Reston Publishing, 1982.
135. Terry GC, et al. The stabilizing function of passive shoulder restraints. *Am J Sports Med* 1991;19:26–34.
136. Torg JS, et al. A modified Bristow-Helfet-May procedure for recurrent dislocation and subluxation of the shoulder. *J Bone Joint Surg [Am]* 1987;69:904–912.
137. Townsend H, et al. Electromyographic analysis of the glenohumeral muscles during a baseball rehabilitation program. *Am J Sports Med* 1991;19:264–272.
138. Travell J, Simmons DG. *Myofascial pain and dysfunction: trigger point manual.* Baltimore: Williams & Wilkins, 1983:410–424.
139. Turkel SJ, et al. Stabilizing mechanisms preventing anterior dislocation of the glenohumeral joint. *J Bone Joint Surg [Am]* 1981;63: 1208–1217.
140. Walch G, Boileau P, Noel E, Donell T. Impingement of the deep surface of the supraspinatus tendon on the posterior glenoid rim: an arthroscopic study. *J Shoulder Elbow Surg* 1992;1:239–245.
141. Walch G, Nove-Josserand L, Levigne C and Renaud E. Tears of the supraspinatus tendon associated with "hidden" lesions of the rotator interval. *J Shoulder Elbow Surg* 1994;3:353–360.
142. Warner JJP, et al. Dynamic capsuloligamentous anatomy of the glenohumeral joint. *J Shoulder Elbow Surg* 1993;2:115–133.
143. Warner JP, Answorth AA and Gerber C. Diagnosis and management of subscapularis tendon tears. *Tech Orthop* 1994;9:116–125.
144. Warren RF, Kornblatt IB, Marchand R. Static factors affecting posterior shoulder stability. *Orthop Trans* 1984;8:89.

145. Wilk KE, Arrigo CA. Current concepts in rehabilitation of the athletic shoulder. *J Orthop Sports Phys Ther* 1993;18:365–378.
146. Williams GR, Iannotti JP. Diagnostic tests and surgical techniques. In: Kelley MJ, Clark WA, eds. *Orthopedic therapy of the shoulder*. Philadelphia: JB Lippincott, 1994:158–224.
147. Wingate L. Efficacy of physical therapy for patients who have undergone mastectomies. *Phys Ther* 1985;65:896–900.
148. Wooten ME, Kadaba MP, McCann PD. Electromyographic and kinematic analysis of shoulder rehabilitation exercises. *Trans ORS* 1989;14:569.
149. Yoneda B, Welsh RP, MacIntosh DL. Conservative treatment of shoulder dislocation in young males. *J Bone Joint Surg [Br]* 1982;64: 254–255.
150. Zuckerman J, Cuomo F. Frozen shoulder. In: Matsen F, Fu FH, Hawkins RJ, eds. *The shoulder: a balance of mobility and stability.* Rosemont, IL: American Academy of Orthopaedic Surgeons, 1993: 253–267.
151. Zuckerman JD, et al. The effect of arm position and capsular release on rotator cuff repair: a biomechanical study. *J Bone Joint Surg [Br]* 1991;73:402–405.

PART XIII

Outcome Measurement

Disorders of the Shoulder: Diagnosis and Management,
edited by Joseph P. Iannotti and Gerald R. Williams, Jr.
Lippincott Williams & Wilkins, Philadelphia © 1999.

CHAPTER 36

Shoulder Outcome Measurement

Brian G. Leggin and Joseph P. Iannotti

Documenting outcome of medical and therapeutic treatment is receiving increased emphasis from patients, administrators, and third-party payors. In order to survive in today's health-care environment, providers must document quality of treatment, compare results of different forms of treatment, and compare results reported by other clinicians. Keller has stated that the quality of medical care is based on a combination of the "efficacy" of a procedure or technology as proven in laboratory studies, the "effectiveness" of that procedure when used in the community, and the "appropriateness" of the procedure when applied to a given patient.[68]

Patient-oriented outcomes research focuses on the effectiveness and appropriateness of a treatment. Until recently, the orthopedic literature has consisted of efficacy research. Although reports such as these may be related to the success of the procedure, they do not tell us what effect the procedure had on the patient. Because there is little evidence of patient outcome, treatment recommendations have been left to the personal experience of a limited number of surgeons who most often have a special interest or expertise in the area being reported. It cannot be assumed, then, that patients with similar pathologies from different geographic locations are being treated with the same procedure, let alone achieve the same outcome.

B. G. Leggin: Penn Therapy and Fitness, University of Pennsylvania Medical Center, Philadelphia, Pennsylvania 19104.
J. P. Iannotti: Department of Orthopaedic Surgery, Hospital of the University of Pennsylvania, Philadelphia, Pennsylvania 19104.

In order for proper outcome reporting to be feasible, a standardized and widely used system must be available.[44] Before such a system can be used, it must first satisfy the needs of those using it, as well as satisfy criteria set forth for the validation of outcome tools. Various evaluation tools and scoring systems have been developed and used to document outcome of treatment of shoulder pathologies. However, evidence of proper psychometric testing of these instruments is limited. As a result, no one tool has been widely used and accepted. In order for this to occur, common guidelines and terminology must be agreed upon. This chapter will present (a) a brief history of outcome reporting, (b) the concept of disablement, (c) criteria for validation of outcome measures, (d) a review of existing shoulder scales, (e) a new scale developed by the authors, and (f) make suggestions for the future of outcome reporting.

HISTORY

The concept of reporting outcome was first conceived at the turn of the century by Dr. Ernest Amory Codman.[23] Codman's End Result Idea "was merely the common-sense notion that every hospital should follow every patient it treats, long enough to determine whether the treatment was successful and to inquire 'if not, why not' with a view to preventing similar failures in the future."[23] In his own practice, Codman found that by routinely following even the uninteresting cases, he was able to learn more about the management of his patients.

This idea was introduced to the Philadelphia County Medical Society on May 14, 1913, in an address titled "The Product of a Hospital."[23] Codman urged hospitals to make it their responsibility to know the "actual result" of the patient's treatment, the competence of the doctors on their staff, and the efficiency of their hospital. The following year, Codman highlighted many deficiencies in the medical profession with a paper titled "Study of Hospital Efficiency." It was not until a third report was published in 1916 that his idea was adopted, at least in part, by other surgeons and hospitals.

Although Codman set the groundwork for reporting outcomes over 80 years ago, there is still much work to be done in this area.

DISABLEMENT

Before we discuss measurement tools, it will be helpful to classify outcomes through the use of a disablement scheme. "Disablement" is a global term that reflects all the diverse consequences that disease, injury, or congenital abnormalities may have on human functioning at many different levels.[62] Saad Nagi introduced the first disablement scheme in 1965 (Fig. 1).[93,94] The World Health Organization followed with the International Classification of Impairments, Disabilities, and Handicaps in 1980.[53,57] The goal of these schemes is to describe the pathway from active pathology to various consequences. For simplification, we will only discuss the Nagi scheme.

Nagi describes active pathology as the interruption or interference of normal processes and the efforts of the organism to regain a normal state.[93,94] Active pathology can result from degenerative disease processes, infection, trauma, or other etiology. Attempts have been made to accurately describe pathologies, such as classification of fractures, size of rotator cuff tear, shape and size of acromion, and degree of instability. Follow-up typically consists of x-rays to document fracture healing, arthroplasty position, or acromial shape; and magnetic resonance imaging for size of rotator cuff tear or degree of healing of rotator cuff repair. Again, this tells us about the efficacy of the treatment, but nothing about its affect on the patient.

Active pathology typically leads to an impairment of some kind. Impairment is an anatomic or physiologic abnormality or loss that can be a direct result (e.g., decreased active range of motion [ROM] due to a frozen shoulder) or secondary result (e.g., decreased strength secondary to disuse) of the pathology. Much of the clinical orthopedic literature has focused on impairment data such as pain, ROM, strength, and stability as an outcome.

Pain is one of the most commonly measured impairments in shoulder literature. Pain has been measured and reported in various ways, including visual analog scales (VAS), numeric rating scales, descriptive scales, and the amount and type of pain medication. The visual analog scale has been reported to be reliable and valid.[105,112] The typical VAS consists of a 10-cm horizontal or vertical line with anchor points such as "no pain" and "worst possible pain" at either end of the line. The patient is asked to place a mark on the line indicating the amount of pain he or she is experiencing. Pain is then calculated by measuring the distance of the mark from one of the anchor points. A disadvantage of measuring pain in this way is that it can be very time consuming for the clinician, because every scale must be individually measured. It should also be noted that the 10-cm line will decrease with each photocopy, so printed forms should be used.[54] Another method used to record pain is a numeric rating scale. Much like the VAS, a numeric rating scale also uses anchor points. However, rather than using a line, numbers are typically arranged from 0 to 10. The patient is asked to circle the number that best correlates to his or her level of pain. Ferraz found the numeric rating scale to be the most reliable among both literate and illiterate subjects.[39] Good correlation of numeric rating scales to VAS has been reported.[128] Williams also favored numeric rating scales for telephone administration and longer term follow-up.[128] A descriptive pain scale typically provides the patient with verbal descriptors such as none, mild, moderate, and severe.[25,26,54,55] "Moderate" is most often chosen, even in patients who rate pain as mild or severe by other methods.[54,55] Another concern is that there are not enough options for patients to accurately record pain in the same rank order.[89] Quantifying pain by the amount and type of pain medication, such as over-the-counter, nonsteroidal antiinflammatories, or narcotics, also has been used.[35,101] Although this is useful information to have on hand, the accuracy of this type of pain scale must be questioned, because various psychological and psychosocial issues may taint the results. Pain scales that include descriptors as well as amount of medication in a single item should be regarded with caution, because multiple variables can be confusing for patients.[35]

Shoulder ROM is an important outcome of shoulder surgery. Goniometric measurement of ROM has been reported to be reliable.[14,41,86,102] However, because of the multiplanar motion of the shoulder, it can be difficult to reproduce and compare results reported by other clinicians.[102] In response to the need to standardize measurements, the American Shoulder and Elbow Surgeons (ASES) recommends that four functionally important ranges of motion be documented: forward elevation, external rotation with the arm at the side, external rotation in the 90 degree abducted position, and internal rotation.[16] Forward elevation is defined as the maximum angle the arm makes with the trunk when the patient is asked to raise his or her arm above the head with the elbow held straight. It should be noted that this

Active Pathology ⟶ **Impairment** ⟶ **Functional Limitation** ⟶ **Disability**

FIG. 1. Nagi disablement scheme.

plane of motion is not considered to be true flexion or abduction. Experience tells us that most patients will raise their arm somewhere between true flexion and the plane of the scapula. The angle that the arm makes with the thorax is measured in the upright position for active motion, whereas passive measurement is made in the supine position.

External rotation with the arm at the side is measured with the elbow flexed to 90 degrees and the forearm in the sagittal plane. External rotation at 90 degrees abduction is measured by asking the patient to begin with the arm in the same position as for external rotation at the side. The patient is then asked to abduct the arm to 90 degrees. Once at 90 degrees abduction, the patient is asked to externally rotate the shoulder. Active motion is measured with the patient upright, whereas passive motion is measured with the patient supine. Internal rotation is measured by the position reached by the outstretched hitchhiking thumb up the back, in reference to the posterior anatomy.

Common reference points include the greater trochanter, buttock, sacrum, waist line, and spinous processes of the lumbar and thoracic vertebrae.

Strength assessment is another commonly reported impairment to document effectiveness of surgical or therapeutic intervention. As with ROM testing, it is important to have standardized testing protocols for reproducibility in a clinical setting. A variety of methods for quantifying muscle performance have been available, including manual muscle testing (MMT), handheld isometric dynamometry, and isokinetic dynamometry.

Manual muscle testing is the most widely used method of clinical evaluation of muscle strength.[87] Some investigators have recommended using MMT when documenting shoulder outcomes.[35,101] This technique, however, has been criticized for its subjectivity and lack of reliability within the good and normal ranges.[5,15]

In an attempt to quantify the results of MMT procedures, handheld dynamometry was introduced in 1949.[87] Although several investigators have demonstrated handheld dynamometry to be reliable in both patient and nonpatient populations, problems include an upper limit to recording muscle force, difficulty in maintaining the device perpendicular to the limb segment, and dependency on the strength of the tester.[1,7–12,18,22,23,33,73,82,87,97,104,125,127]

Several isokinetic devices have become available for use in the clinic, including those that have the capability of measuring concentric, eccentric, and isometric strength. The reliability of these dynamometers has been well documented.[20,27,34,37,59,70,73,80,99,113] However, these devices are nonportable, relatively expensive, and require elaborate setup and stabilization procedures. Therefore, use in the clinic is time consuming and impractical.

The Isobex 2.1 (Curor Ag, Niederwanten, Switzerland) is a more recently developed isometric dynamometer that is lightweight and portable. Fixation to a wall is attained by suction cups. A cable mechanically measures force output. Reliability of this device for measuring shoulder strength is comparable with or better than isokinetic and handheld dynamometry.[73]

In order to accurately compare results of strength measurements, standardization of such variables as test position, dynamometer, stabilization, and protocol must be established. Several studies have advocated testing shoulder strength in the plane of the scapula and 15 to 45 degrees of abduction. Proponents of this test position argue that it avoids the impingement arc, avoids the apprehension position, and reduces passive tension on the rotator cuff.[111] However, positioning the arm in the scapular plane at 45 degrees for rotational testing would require appropriate stabilization of the limb, which may make reproducibility and efficiency in the clinic difficult. Testing elevation at 45 degrees in the plane of the scapula would not require stabilization. A recent study by the authors demonstrated that measuring isometric shoulder strength for internal and external rotation with the arm at the side in neutral rotation is highly reliable. In addition, elevation tested at 45 degrees in the plane of the scapula is also reliable.[73]

Interpreting strength testing data has typically consisted of comparison with the uninvolved extremity and comparison with normative data.[111] It is difficult to compare results with the normative data available in the literature because test position and dynamometer vary for each study. Although we prefer comparing ROM and strength data to the opposite uninvolved side, this method is not without controversy. The influence of hand dominance in both athletic and nonathletic populations has been debated in the literature.[20,99,111] In patients who have bilateral shoulder involvement, age-, gender-, and hand dominance–matched normative values would be ideal.

Instability is also an impairment commonly reported. The ASES recommends grading the amount of instability of the glenohumeral joint in the following way: 0 = no translation, 1 = mild (0 to 1 cm translation), 2 = moderate (1 to 2 cm translation or translates to the glenoid rim), and 3 = severe (greater than 2 cm translation or over the glenoid rim).[101] This should be noted for anterior, posterior, and inferior translation. In addition, the presence of apprehension or a positive relocation test should be noted. The ASES also recommends having the patient rate his or her level of shoulder instability on a VAS.[101]

Although knowledge of these parameters is important to the overall understanding of a pathology, they do not describe the total effect of the pathology on the person. Nagi uses the term "functional limitations" to describe limitations in performance at the level of the whole person. Physical functioning involves the patient's ability to perform activities of daily living (ADLs), dress, reach, push, pull, lift, carry, and work. Although social functioning is the person's ability to interact socially, perform usual social roles, and participate in social activities,[48,49] not all impairments lead to functional limitations. For example, a patient with limited shoulder ROM may not be able to reach the back of his opposite shoulder. However, this may not be a functional loss, because the patient may use a long-handled scrub brush to wash the axilla and back of the opposite shoulder.

Disability is the limitation in performance of socially defined roles and tasks within a sociocultural and physical environment.[62] A patient who is unable to perform or participate in usual work, school, leisure, and personal care activities can be considered disabled. It is important to note that not all impairments and functional limitations lead to disability. Disability largely depends on the patient's desired activity level. For example, a limitation in the ability to raise the arm above shoulder level may not be a disability for a computer programmer who works below shoulder level. However, this functional limitation would be a devastating disability for a painter or professional tennis player. We also can illustrate disability through the use of shoulder scoring systems. The computer programmer with a shoulder score of 90 on a 100-point scale can have no perceived disability. However, moderate disability can be perceived by the painter or tennis player with the same 90-point score.[26,56]

The disablement process can be halted at each step by appropriate surgical or therapeutic intervention. In addition, the process can be expedited or slowed by several factors, including age, gender, life-style, education, social support, motivation, and environment.[61] It is important to determine which of these factors weigh most heavily on patient outcome after shoulder surgery.

DEVELOPMENT OF SCORES

Several instruments have been reported to document outcome with little regard for the process of selecting and constructing the scale. This has caused confusion as to the best way to construct and validate outcome measurement tools for use in the clinic.[69] Clinicians should choose an outcome tool that will best suit the purpose of its use.[69] Kirshner and Guyatt classify outcome assessment tools as either discriminative, predictive, or evaluative.[69] A discriminative index is used when no "gold standard" is available to validate the measure. Items in this type of measure must be important to patients and performed by almost all of the patients to be studied. The most appropriate number of response options in this type of scale is two. Either the patient can or cannot perform the activity. This type of instrument allows comparison among different groups. However, a dichotomous scale such as this cannot detect small changes in a patient's status over time.

A predictive index is used to determine whether a patient has a specific condition or is likely to develop that condition. The patient can then be classified into a specific category. Based on a comparison of other patients in that category, one can predict the outcome the patient will achieve. However, this type of index will not measure outcome.

An evaluative index is used to quantify the amount of change the treatment intervention has provided. An evaluative index must be able to measure all clinically important effects of treatment.[69] These scales must be able to be responsive to change over time.

Increasing response options on a scale increases responsiveness. It is this type of scale that we are most interested in to document within person change over time.

Several investigators have outlined requirements for the development of new outcome measures.[13,46,50,51,63,65,66,68,69,123] In order for an index to be considered useful in the clinic, the following steps must be demonstrated: item selection, item scaling, item reduction, determination of reliability, determination of validity, and determination of responsiveness.[69]

The first step in constructing an evaluative instrument is to select a set of items that are relevant to the overall function of the type of patient to be evaluated. This can be accomplished through literature review, personal experience, consultation with colleagues, review of existing instruments, and interview with patients.[50,51,69,117] The likelihood that patient response to a particular item will change with medical or therapeutic intervention is an important consideration.[69] In addition, all clinically important treatment effects most be included in the tool.[69]

Once the items of the instrument are established, the response options or range that patients have for responding to each item must be determined. Each item must be sensitive to clinically important changes in status. Typical response options include a VAS or a Likert scale with multiple options. The optimal number of response options for a Likert scale has not been reported. However, increasing response options will increase item responsiveness. The typical Likert scale includes five to nine options. For a tool designed to discriminate between patients who can or cannot perform an activity, a simple "yes" or "no" is all that is necessary. These response options are fine for tools designed to detect between-person differences, but not small changes in an individual patient's status. Therefore, it is recommended that either a Likert scale or a VAS be used with an evaluative tool.

Because we are interested in measuring change over time, it would be counterproductive to include items in the scale that do not change after a particular intervention. This stage of scale development is item reduction. A method of reducing the items of a scale is to administer the scale to a group of patients before and after an intervention that produces change in a patient's status. Items that are unresponsive to change are then deleted from the questionnaire.

Once the questionnaire is in its final format, it is ready for reliability testing. Reliability is the extent to which a measurement is consistent and free from error.[50,51,69,100,108,123] Reliability is tested by administering the questionnaire to the same subject at two points in time. Although there may be small changes in within-person measures, they may be statistically and clinically insignificant.[69] Intrarater reliability refers to the stability of data recorded by one individual across two or more trials.[100,108] Interrater reliability is variation between two or more raters who measure the same group of subjects.[100,108] Test–retest reliability means that a measure will remain stable over repeated measures in time, provided that no change in status has taken place.[108] The extent to which the items of a scale reflect the same dimension is known as internal consistency.

Validity concerns the extent to which an instrument measures what it is intended to measure. Validating a new instrument is an ongoing process. In a shoulder score, we want to know if it can evaluate change in the magnitude or quality of a variable from one time to another. There are several types of measurement validity.

Face validity is the simplest and weakest form of validity. If the items of an index appear to make sense to the person using it, then the scale has face validity. A more formal way of measuring validity of an index is to demonstrate that the results of the new scale correlate to an external "gold standard." This is also known as criterion validity. Content validity is satisfied when it is proven that the scale measures all important aspects of the condition to be examined. Construct validity in an evaluative index is determined when within-patient change of the score over time is correlated to changes in impairment measures or a global rating of change by the patient, a relative, and/or the clinician.[50,51,69]

Before we can declare an evaluative index useful in the clinic, it must be able to detect improvement, regression, or stability of a condition over time.[120] Sensitivity to change or responsiveness can be considered an additional component of validity.[2,31,79,120] There are several methods for assessing responsiveness.[69] Stratford has discussed several study designs that can be used to determine responsiveness of an index.[120] The simplest design compares an initial score with a follow-up score after treatment intervention. More sophisticated designs compare the outcome of a group who received a treatment of known efficacy with that of a placebo group. Another design involves comparing the clinician's and patient's global ratings of change with the change in score. Whichever design is chosen, an adequate sample size must be selected.

CRITICAL REVIEW OF SHOULDER SCORES

Several tools have been developed and used to document outcome of surgical and therapeutic treatment of shoulder pathology. These include generic quality-of-life or health status measures, condition-specific tools, and tools that are applicable to all conditions of the shoulder.[21,71] Although many of these tools have been used in various reports, many have not satisfied the necessary criteria.

The SF-36 has been gaining popularity as a generic health status measure. This index consists of 36 items derived by Ware and colleagues from the Medical Outcomes Survey.[121,126] It measures eight health concepts, including physical functioning (10 items), social functioning (two items), role limitations due to physical problems (four items), role limitations due to emotional problems (three items), mental health (five items), energy/fatigue (four items), bodily pain (two items), and general health perception (five items). Using a generic health status measure in patients with shoulder pathology provides the clinician with a way of comparing the health status of various shoulder conditions. In addition, the health status of patients with shoulder pathologies can be compared to patients with other medical conditions. However, the SF-36 may not be sensitive enough to document change over time in patients with shoulder pathology. Mossberg and McFarland found lower physical functioning scores in patients with lower quarter involvement than in those with upper quarter involvement.[92] They were not surprised by this finding, given that nearly all items in the physical functioning scale are in some way associated with the use of the lower extremities. Beaton and Richards found lower correlations of five shoulder-specific questionnaires with the SF-36 than with each other.[6] They also found the scores on the physical function section of the SF-36 to be higher than the scores on the shoulder-specific measures in the same patients.

In order to capture more sensitivity to change over time, some investigators have advocated the use of condition-specific assessment tools.[71] Rowe has attempted to accomplish this with his Rating Sheet for Bankart Repair.[110] This 100-point scoring system awards 50 points to the patient who reports no recurrence of dislocation, subluxation, or apprehension. The remaining 50 points are derived from ROM and function. There have not been any reliability or validity studies on this scoring system. Several investigators have used the Rowe system to report outcome of surgical and nonsurgical treatment of shoulder instability.[19,32,38,80,81,89,90,91,109,115,129,130] These studies report only posttreatment scores, with no evidence of responsiveness to change. Although this scoring system appears well suited for the patient with shoulder instability, it would not be useful for a patient who has a comorbid shoulder disorder. Leung recently reported outcome of fixation of scapular neck and clavicular fractures using the Rowe scale.[74] One must question the validity of an outcome report on fractures when the scale used is intended for patients with instability. Using condition-specific tools makes it difficult to compare the functional limitations and disability associated with different shoulder conditions.

Therefore, it seems more practical to use assessment tools that are applicable to any condition of the shoulder. A number of these tools are available. Although they have been used extensively in the literature, evidence of the psychometric properties of many of these scales is lacking. Each of these scales will be examined for content, use in the literature, reliability, and validity.

NEER RATING SHEET

Neer published the first system to document outcome in 1972, when he discussed his results of anterior acromioplasty.[96] In 1982, he discussed results of total shoulder replacement, using the same system.[95] Although the Neer rating sheet is not a cumulative scoring system, it does take into account the important aspects of pain, motion, strength, function, and patient satisfaction. Neer graded his results as excellent, satisfactory, or unsatisfactory, depending on a combination of these parameters. In addition, x-ray findings, postoperative complications, patient's compliance with physical therapy, and patient's general physical condition were documented at each follow-up visit. Although no reliability or validity data are available, this early method of tracking shoulder outcomes has formed the basis from which more recent outcome scoring systems have been derived.

CONSTANT SHOULDER SCORE

The Constant Shoulder Score (Fig. 2) was described in 1987 by Constant and Murley.[25,26] It is a 100-point scoring system in which 35 points are derived from the patient's report of pain and function. The remaining 65 points are allocated for objective assessment of ROM and strength. A significant contribution of Constant's work is age- and gender-matched normative data based on a study of 900 individuals with no known shoulder dysfunction. The Constant Shoulder Score has been used internationally for reporting outcome of various shoulder conditions.[29,42,43,47,58,60,67,77,98,103,107,114,116,131] This may be why investigators at the 1992 International Shoulder Surgeons' meeting were required to present clinical data using the Constant Shoulder Score.[106] The European Shoulder and Elbow Society also requires results of clinical data to be reported using the Constant Shoulder Score.[71]

The content of the score appears to include all relevant aspects of shoulder outcome, with the exception of whether or not the patient is satisfied with his or her shoulder. However, each item of the scale requires a significant degree of interpretation by the patient. There is only one pain scale in which the patient is asked to rate the most severe pain experienced at rest, sleep, or with various activities. Clinical experience tells us that patients experience varying degrees of pain with different activities. One pain scale appears to be inadequate to gain a true picture of the patient's pain. There is also concern that report of function is not specific to any particular activity and therefore is left to interpretation by the patient.

The objective assessment of external rotation is also questionable.[44] The patient is awarded 4 points for placing the hand behind the head with the elbow held back, whereas 8 points is awarded for hand placement on top of the head with the elbow held back. The difference of shoulder external rotation between these two hand positions seems negligible.

The method of measuring strength has not been standardized. Constant advocates testing isometric abduction strength with a spring balance at 90 degrees abduction. He

A. Subjective Assessment:

Pain during functional use:

15 14 13 12 11 10 9 8 7 6 5 4 3 2 1 0
None Mild Moderate Severe

Daily work: (work without restriction = 4 points, 75% of normal work = 3 points, 50% of normal work = 2 points, ...etc.; undisturbed sleep = 2 points, interrupted sleep = 1 point, no sleep = 0 points)

Work	Recreation	Sleep
0	0	0
1	1	1
2	2	2
3	3	
4	4	

Ability to work at the level of:

2	the waist
4	the xiphoid process
6	the neck
8	the head
10	above the head

FIG. 2. Constant Shoulder Score.[25,26] (Adapted with permission from Constant CR, Murley AHG. A clinical method of functional assessment of the shoulder. *Clin Orthop Rel Res* 1987;214:160–164.)

Constant Shoulder Score
(continued)

B. Objective Assessment:

Flexion:	Abduction:
0 = 0 – 30º	0 = 0 – 30º
2 = 31 – 60º	2 = 31 – 60º
4 = 61 – 90º	4 = 61 – 90º
6 = 91 – 120º	6 = 91 – 120º
8 = 121 – 150º	8 = 121 – 150º
10 = > 150º	10 = > 150º

External Rotation:

2 = Hand behind head, elbow held forward

4 = Hand behind head, elbow held back

6 = Hand on top of head, elbow forward

8 = Hand on top of head, elbow back

10 = Full elevation from top of head

Internal Rotation:

0 = Hand to lateral thigh

2 = Dorsum of hand to buttock

4 = Hand to lumbosacral junction

6 = Dorsum of hand to waist (LV 3)

8 = Dorsum of hand to TV 12

10 = Dorsum of hand to interscapular region (TV 7)

Strength of abduction: (90º abduction or highest level patient can achieve)

Trial 1: ____

Trial 2: ____

Trial 3: ____

Total = ____ / 3 = ____

FIG. 2. *Continued.*

also states that testing can be performed at the highest level achieved by patients, if they are unable to achieve 90 degrees abduction. This inconsistency makes reproduction of results difficult. Furthermore, Conboy recently questioned the validity of measuring shoulder power in a single arc of movement.[24]

Although the procedures and statistical analysis for determining reliability are not reported, the investigators report an average observer error of 3% among three different observers testing 100 abnormal shoulders.[25] Conboy and colleagues recently examined the reliability of the Constant Shoulder Score in 25 patients with either arthritis, dislocation, or impingement.[24]

They found an interobserver standard deviation of 8.86 with a 95% confidence limit that the measurement of a single observer would be within 17.7 points of the true score.[24]

Therefore, studies examining pre- and post-intervention measures using the Constant Shoulder Score should be examined with caution. Another concern is that because such a large portion of the Constant Shoulder Score is derived from objective impairment measures; patients who are unable to return to the clinic will be lost to follow-up, which may lead to incomplete outcome studies.

THE ASES STANDARDIZED SHOULDER ASSESSMENT FORM AND SHOULDER SCORE INDEX

The ASES Standardized Shoulder Assessment Form (Fig. 3) was developed by the Research Committee of the ASES and published by Richards and colleagues in 1994.[101] The instrument consists of a patient self-assessment section and a clinician assessment. The patient is asked to indicate whether they are having pain in the shoulder and to record the location on a diagram. Additional questions include whether there is pain at night, type of pain medication, and number of pills taken on average each day. The patient is also asked to rate degree of pain and instability, if present, on a VAS. Ten ADLs are assessed on a 4-point Likert scale. The clinician assessment includes ROM measurements of forward elevation, external rotation with the arm at the side and at 90 degrees abduction, internal rotation up the back, and cross-body adduction. Signs of tenderness, impingement, and crepitus are also assessed. Manual muscle strength testing of forward elevation, abduction, and external and internal rotation at the side are assessed as recommended by the Medical Research Council. In addition, translation in the anterior, posterior, and inferior directions is noted on a scale of 0 (if absent) to 3 (if severe instability is noted). Questions pertaining to apprehension, voluntary instability, relocation test, and generalized laxity are recorded. The Shoulder Score Index is a 100-point scoring system in which 50 points are derived from the patient's report of pain on the VAS. The cumulative score of the 10 ADLs on the 4-point ordinal scale accounts for the remaining 50 points. To date, reliability and sensitivity to change of this index have not been established.

Although the index does include the important aspects of pain and function, it does not include the patient's satisfaction with his or her shoulder. In addition, only one pain scale is not specific to activity or time of day. The ADL section includes three items that may not be normal ADLs for some patients. This can present a problem, because there are only 10 items in this section.

The advantage of this scale is its ease of administration. It can be completed by the patient independent of an examiner or by phone interview. The clinician assessment portion provides a standardized method for clinicians to follow. Because this scale is relatively new, it has not been used extensively in the literature.

Pain:

How bad is your pain today?

0 1 2 3 4 5 6 7 8 9 10

No pain at all — Pain as bad as it can be

Activity of daily living: (Circle the number in the box that indicates your ability to do the following activities
0 = unable to do; 1 = very difficult to do; 2 = somewhat difficult to do; 3 = not difficult)

Activity	Right Arm	Left Arm
1. Put on a coat	0 1 2 3	0 1 2 3
2. Sleep on your painful or affected side	0 1 2 3	0 1 2 3
3. Wash back/do up bra in back	0 1 2 3	0 1 2 3
4. Manage toileting	0 1 2 3	0 1 2 3
5. Comb hair	0 1 2 3	0 1 2 3
6. Reach a high shelf	0 1 2 3	0 1 2 3
7. Lift 10 lbs. above shoulder	0 1 2 3	0 1 2 3
8. Throw a ball overhand	0 1 2 3	0 1 2 3
9. Do usual work - List: ______	0 1 2 3	0 1 2 3
10. Do usual sport - List: ______	0 1 2 3	0 1 2 3

FIG. 3. ASES Standardized Shoulder Assessment Form.[101] (Adapted with permission from Richards RR, An K, Bigliani LU, et al. A standardized method for the assessment of shoulder function. *J Shoulder Elbow Surg* 1994;3:347–352.)

SHOULDER PAIN AND DISABILITY INDEX

The Shoulder Pain and Disability Index (SPADI; Fig. 4) was described by Roach and colleagues in 1991.[105] This 100-point system incorporates a VAS for all items. There are five items for pain and eight for functional limitations/disability. Scoring is based on the severity of pain and disability reported. The higher the score, the more severe the disability.

The items of this scale relate mostly to self-care and dressing. Therefore, it may not be sensitive enough for higher level patients. The investigators report fair reliability with high internal consistency of the scale. They also report sensitivity to change and good correlation to objective measures of ROM. Williams and colleagues recognized the difficulties posed when using a VAS in the clinic or for telephone administration.[128] They changed the format to a numeric rating scale and studied the correlation to the original version of the

PAIN SCALE

A. How severe is your pain:

				Score
1. At its worst?....................	No pain	______________________	Worst pain Imaginable	_____
2. When lying on involved side?.................	No pain	______________________	Worst pain Imaginable	_____
3. When reaching for something on a high shelf?..............	No pain	______________________	Worst pain Imaginable	_____
4. Touching the back of your neck?......................	No pain	______________________	Worst pain Imaginable	_____
5. Pushing with the involved arm?................	No pain	______________________	Worst pain Imaginable	_____

DISABILITY SCALE

A. How much difficulty did you have:

1. Washing your hair?.........	No difficulty	______________________	So difficult required help	_____
2. Washing your back?.......	No difficulty	______________________	So difficult required help	_____
3. Putting on an undershirt or pullover sweater?.........................	No difficulty	______________________	So difficult required help	_____
4. Putting on a shirt that buttons down the front?.............................	No difficulty	______________________	So difficult required help	_____
5. Putting on your pants?....	No difficulty	______________________	So difficult required help	_____
6. Placing an object on a high shelf?..................	No difficulty	______________________	So difficult required help	_____
7. Carrying a heavy object of 10 pounds or more?...	No difficulty	______________________	So difficult required help	_____
8. Removing something from your back pocket?..........................	No difficulty	______________________	So difficult required help	_____

FIG. 4. Shoulder Pain and Disability Index.[105] (Adapted with permission from Roach KE, Budiman-Mak E, Norwarat S, Lertratanakul Y. Development of a shoulder pain and disability index. *Arthritis Care Res* 1991;4:143–149.)

SPADI and assessed its responsiveness to change over various time periods. The investigators found good correlation between the VAS and numeric scaled SPADI. They also found significant changes at each time period that correlated with the patient's global status rating. This study is fairly recent, and, as such, there are minimal clinical outcome studies using either version of the SPADI.

UCLA END-RESULT SCORE

The UCLA End-Result Score (Fig. 5) was first used by Ellman and colleagues in 1986.[35] This is a 35-point scale. The items measured include pain (10 points), function (10 points), active forward flexion (5 points), strength of forward flexion (5 points), and patient satisfaction (5 points). A score of 34 to 35 is considered an excellent result and a score of 29 to 33 a good result. Any score less than 28 is considered a poor result.

This scale appears to include all aspects relevant to rating the shoulder. However, the UCLA score uses descriptive items for pain and function. Each item contains multiple descriptions that may make it difficult for the patient to understand. The report of patient satisfaction is also questionable. The patient has two choices for this item. Five points are awarded if he or she is "satisfied and better," whereas 0 points are awarded for "not satisfied and worse." There is no option in between. The wording of these options may mislead patients into rating that although they may not be "better," they may be "satisfied" with their treatment. This method of measuring patient satisfaction also makes it difficult to use this scale prior to treatment, because many patients are typically not satisfied and worse when seeking medical attention.[44] Strength of forward flexion is assessed with manual muscle testing. We have already discussed the problems associated with this method of strength testing. In addition, the position of this measurement is not standardized. Reliability and re-

	Points
Pain:	
Present all of the time and unbearable; strong medication frequently	1
Present all of the time but bearable; strong medication occasionally	2
None or little at rest, present during light activities; salicylates frequently	4
Present during heavy or particular activities only; salicylates occasionally	6
Occasional and slight	8
None	10
Function:	
Unable to use limb	1
Only light activities possible	2
Able to do light housework or most activities of daily living	4
Most housework, shopping, and driving possible; able to do hair and dress and undress, including fastening brassiere	6
Slight restriction only; able to work above shoulder level	10
Normal activities	
Active forward flexion:	
150º or more	5
120º to 150º	4
90º to120º	3
45º to 90º	2
30º to 45º	1
Less than 30º	0
Strength of forward flexion (manual muscle testing):	
Grade 5 (normal)	5
Grade 4 (good)	4
Grade 3 (fair)	3
Grade 2 (poor)	2
Grade 1 (muscle contraction)	1
Grade 0 (nothing)	0
Satisfaction of the patient:	
Satisfied and better	5
Not satisfied and worse	0

FIG. 5. UCLA End Result Score.[35] (Adapted with permission from Ellman H, Hanker G, Bayer M. Repair of the rotator cuff: end-result study of factors influencing reconstruction. *J Bone Joint Surg [Am]* 1986;68:1136–1144.)

sponsiveness of this scale have not been established. Most likely due to its ease of administration, the UCLA score has been used frequently in the literature for both retrospective and prospective studies.[2,3,17,35,36,52,76,78,118,119] Burkart reported pre- and postoperative values for the UCLA score in a study of 14 patients who received partial repair of a massive rotator cuff defect.[17] All but one of these patients was satisfied with his or her result. However, the average postoperative score was 27.6. This is considered a poor result under the guidelines set forth by the original investigators. Therefore, it would seem more practical to only report numeric results of the UCLA score and omit using terms such as "excellent" or "good."[44]

SIMPLE SHOULDER TEST

The Simple Shoulder Test (SST) (Fig. 6) was developed by the shoulder service at the University of Washington.[4,75,83–85] The questionnaire consists of 12 functional items, derived from a review of other scales and the most frequent complaints of patients seen in their practice. The SST does not directly assess pain, ROM, or strength. Instead, these parameters are evaluated indirectly through each of the items on the questionnaire.[71] Two of the questions relate to pain, seven to function, and three to ROM.[6] Response to each item requires a simple "yes" or "no." The goal of the developers was to provide an assessment tool that does not require a clinician, elaborate equipment, or computer for calculation. Not surprisingly, investigators report excellent reliability of this scale. Beaton and Richards reported good correlation of the SST to other shoulder instruments.[6]

A dichotomous scale such as the SST provides excellent reliability and discriminates between patients who can and cannot perform a particular activity.[69] However, this type of scale would not perform well as an evaluative index. For example, a patient who had mild pain at night that occasionally disrupted sleep would answer the same as a patient who had severe pain at night that prevented sleep on a regular basis. There is no provision for the patient to assess satisfaction with the function of the shoulder.

ATHLETIC SHOULDER OUTCOME RATING SCALE

The expectations and goals of the athletic shoulder are typically far greater than those expected by the general population. Therefore, a good result for a nonathletic patient may be a poor result for a high-level athlete. Recognizing that the available shoulder outcome scales were targeted to the general population and, as such, were not sensitive enough for high-level athletes, Tibone and Bradley have proposed the Athletic Shoulder Outcome Rating Scale (Fig. 7).[122] This

Answer each question below by circling "yes" or "no" (please do not leave questions unanswered)

1. Is your shoulder comfortable with your arm at rest by your side?	**Yes**	**No**
2. Does your shoulder allow you to sleep comfortably?	**Yes**	**No**
3. Can you reach the small of your back to tuck in your shirt with your hand?	**Yes**	**No**
4. Can you place your hand behind your head with the elbow straight out to the side?	**Yes**	**No**
5. Can you place a coin on a shelf at the level of your shoulder without bending your elbow?	**Yes**	**No**
	Yes	**No**
6. Can you lift one pound (a full pint container) to the level of your shoulder without bending your elbow?	**Yes**	**No**
7. Can you lift eight pounds (a full gallon container) to the level of your shoulder without bending your elbow?	**Yes**	**No**
	Yes	**No**
8. Can you carry twenty pounds at your side with the affected extremity?	**Yes**	**No**
9. Do you think you can toss a softball underhand ten yards with the affected extremity?	**Yes**	**No**
10. Do you think you can toss a softball overhand ten yards with the affected extremity?	**Yes**	**No**
11. Can you wash the back of your opposite shoulder with the affected extremity?	**Yes**	**No**
12. Would your shoulder allow you to work full-time at your regular job?	**Yes**	**No**

FIG. 6. Simple Shoulder Test.[75] (Adapted from Lippitt S, Harryman DT, Matsen FA. A practical tool for evaluating function: The simple shoulder test. In: Matsen FA, Fu FH, Hawkins RJ, eds. *The shoulder: a balance of mobility and stability.* Park Ridge, Illinois. American Academy of Orthopaedic Surgeons, 1993.)

SUBJECTIVE (90 Points)

	Points
I. PAIN	
-No pain with competition	10
-Pain after competing only	8
-Pain while competing	6
-Pain preventing competing	4
-Pain with ADL's	2
-Pain at rest	0
II. STRENGTH/ENDURANCE	
-No weakness, normal competition fatigue	10
-Weakness after competition, early competition fatigue	8
-Weakness during competition, abnormal competition fatigue	6
-Weakness or fatigue preventing competition	4
-Weakness or fatigue with ADL's	2
-Weakness or fatigue preventing ADL's	0
III. STABILITY	
-No loosenes during competition	10
-Recurrent subluxations while competing	8
-Dead-arm syndrome while competing	6
-Recurrent subluxations prevent competition	4
-Recurrent subluxations during ADL's	2
-Dislocation	0
IV. INTENSITY	
-Preinjury versus postinjury hours of competition (100%)	10
-Preinjury versus postinjury hours of competition (less than 75%)	8
-Preinjury versus postinjury hours of competition (less than 50%)	6
-Preinjury versus postinjury hours of competition (less than 25%)	4
-Preinjury and postinjury hours of ADL's (100%)	2
-Preinjury and postinjury hours of ADL's (less than 50%)	0
V. PERFORMANCE	
-At the same level, same proficiency	50
-At the same level, decreased proficiency	40
-At the same level, decreased proficiency, not acceptable to athlete	30
-Decreased level with acceptable proficiency at that level	20
-Decreased level, unacceptable proficiency	10
-Cannot compete, had to switch sport	0
OBJECTIVE	
Range of Motion	
-Normal external rotation 90º–90º position; normal elevation	10
-Less than 5º loss of external rotation; normal elevation	8
-Less than 10º loss of external rotation; normal elevation	6
-Less than 15º loss of external rotation; normal elevation	4
-Less than 20º loss of external rotation; normal elevation	2
-Greater than 20º loss of external rotation, or any loss of elevation	0

FIG. 7. Athletic Shoulder Rating Scale.[122] (Adapted with permission from Tibone JE, Bradley JP. Evaluation of treatment outcomes for athletes[7] shoulders. In: Matsen FA, Fu FH, Hawkins RJ, eds. *The shoulder: a balance of mobility and stability.* Park Ridge, Illinois. American Academy of Orthopaedic Surgeons, 1993.)

scale includes the patient's assessment of pain, strength/endurance, stability, intensity, and performance, as well as objective measurement of elevation and external rotation ROM.

Although this scale includes parameters relevant to the athlete, the wording of each item poses the same problem as that of the UCLA score. Many of the response options have more than one variable, which can be confusing for the patient. In addition, the investigators do not specify position for testing ROM. Nor do they specify the requirement for normal ROM.

The concept of an outcome scale specifically designed for the athlete is excellent. Further refinement of this scale, and proper psychometric testing, would make this a valuable tool for clinicians.

UNIVERSITY OF PENNSYLVANIA SHOULDER SCORE

In light of the deficiencies of available shoulder scoring systems, the investigators have developed two 100-point shoulder scoring systems. The self-assessment 100-point scoring system is based on scoring of the patient's report of pain, satisfaction, and function (Figs. 8 and 9).[72] The 100-point impairment score consists of objective measures of ROM and strength (Figs. 10 and 11).[72] The items of the score were chosen from a review of the literature and consensus of a panel, consisting of orthopedic surgeons and physical therapists, with extensive experience treating shoulder disorders and knowledgeable in scale development and statistics.

Most patients with shoulder pathology typically have pain that varies, depending on the demands placed on the shoulder. Therefore, the University of Pennsylvania Shoulder Score includes three pain items that address pain with the arm at rest by the side, pain with normal activities, and pain with strenuous activities (Fig. 8). All are based on a 10-point numeric rating scale with end points of "no pain" and "worst possible pain." Ten points can be awarded for each item by subtracting the number circled from 10. Therefore, a patient can be awarded 30 points for absence of pain.

The patient's satisfaction with the function of the shoulder is also assessed with a numeric rating scale (Fig. 8). The end points chosen were "not satisfied" and "very satisfied." Scoring is based on the number circled by the patient. Therefore, the patient can achieve 10 points for this section.

Self-assessment of function is based on a 20-item questionnaire with a four-category Likert scale for responses (Fig. 9). Scoring for this section is calculated in the following way: 3 points are awarded if the patient "can perform the activity without difficulty," 2 points for "some difficulty," 1 point for "much difficulty," and 0 for "cannot do at all." Therefore, the patient can achieve 60 points if he or she can perform every item without difficulty. Because some items may not be applicable to all patients, the response option "did not do before injury" is included. When the patient chooses this response option or leaves an item blank, an av-

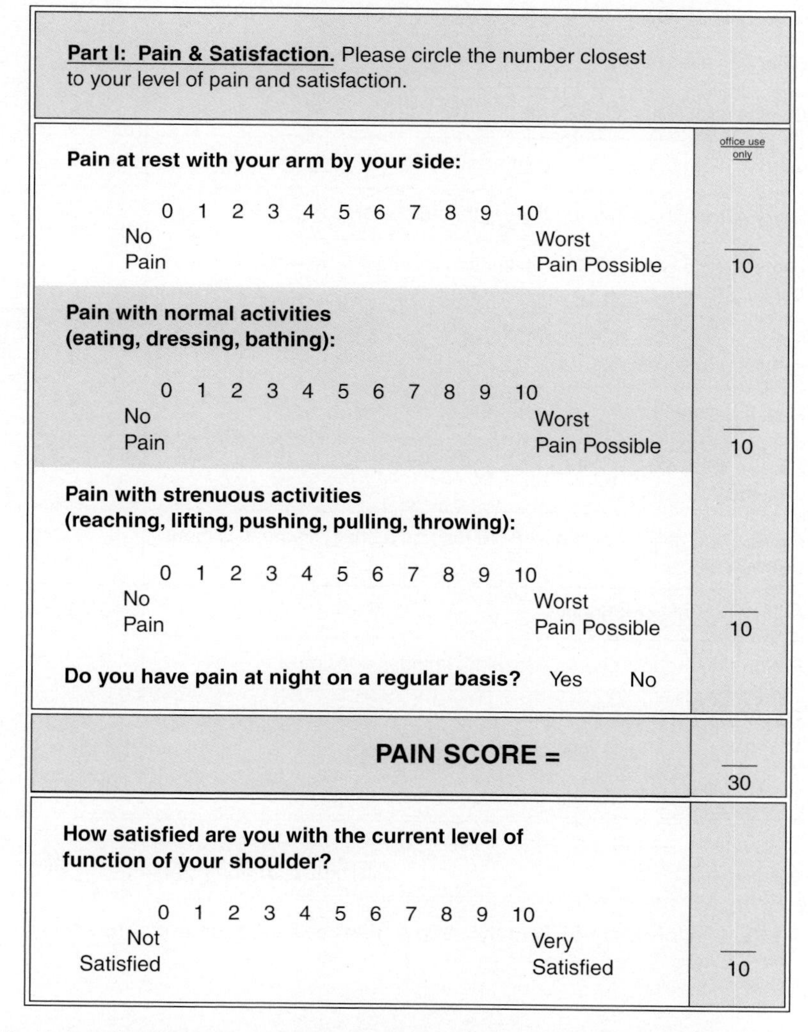
Part I: Pain & Satisfaction. Please circle the number closest to your level of pain and satisfaction.

office use only

Pain at rest with your arm by your side:

0 1 2 3 4 5 6 7 8 9 10
No Pain — Worst Pain Possible
___ /10

Pain with normal activities (eating, dressing, bathing):

0 1 2 3 4 5 6 7 8 9 10
No Pain — Worst Pain Possible
___ /10

Pain with strenuous activities (reaching, lifting, pushing, pulling, throwing):

0 1 2 3 4 5 6 7 8 9 10
No Pain — Worst Pain Possible
___ /10

Do you have pain at night on a regular basis? Yes No

PAIN SCORE = ___ /30

How satisfied are you with the current level of function of your shoulder?

0 1 2 3 4 5 6 7 8 9 10
Not Satisfied — Very Satisfied
___ /10

FIG. 8. University of Pennsylvania patient self-assessment of pain and satisfaction.[72]

Part II: Function

Please circle the number that best describes the level of difficulty you might have performing each activity.

3 = no difficulty
2 = some difficulty
1 = much difficulty
0 = can't do at all
x = did not do before injury

1. Reach the small of your back to tuck in your shirt with your hand.	3	2	1	0	x
2. Wash middle of your back/hook bra.	3	2	1	0	x
3. Perform necessary toileting activities.	3	2	1	0	x
4. Wash the back of opposite shoulder.	3	2	1	0	x
5. Comb hair.	3	2	1	0	x
6. Place hand behind head with elbow held straight out to the side.	3	2	1	0	x
7. Dress self (including put on coat and pull shirt off overhead).	3	2	1	0	x
8. Sleep on affected side.	3	2	1	0	x
9. Open a door with affected side.	3	2	1	0	x
10. Carry a bag of groceries with affected arm.	3	2	1	0	x
11. Carry a briefcase/small suitcase with affected arm.	3	2	1	0	x
12. Place a soup can (1–2 lbs.) on shelf at shoulder level without bending elbow.	3	2	1	0	x
13. Place a one gallon container (3–10 lbs.) on a shelf at shoulder level without bending elbow.	3	2	1	0	x
14. Reach a shelf above your head without bending elbow.	3	2	1	0	x
15. Place a soup can (1–2 lbs.) on a shelf above your head without bending your elbow.	3	2	1	0	x
16. Place a one gallon container (8–10 lbs.) on a shelf overhead without bending elbow.	3	2	1	0	x
17. Perform usual sport/hobby.	3	2	1	0	x
18. Perform household chores (cleaning, laundry, cooking).	3	2	1	0	x
19. Throw overhand/swim/overhead racquet sports (Circle all that apply to you).	3	2	1	0	x
20. Work full-time at your regular job.	3	2	1	0	x

TOTAL FUNCTION = ____ 60

FIG. 9. University of Pennsylvania patient self-assessment of function.[72]

Part III: ACTIVE RANGE OF MOTION						
Points are based on a % of INV/UNINV shoulder AROM	AROM		PROM		% UNINV	PTS
	INV	UNINV	INV	UNINV		
Forward elevation					%	
External rotation at 0º abduction					%	
External rotation at 90º abduction					%	
Internal rotation (level of hitchhiking thumb)					%	
TOTAL POINTS =						/40

Forward elevation & External rotation AROM scoring	Internal rotation AROM scoring
96 – 100% = 10 points 85 – 95% = 9 points 75 – 84% = 8 points 65 – 74% = 7 points 55 – 64% = 6 points 45 – 54% = 5 points 35 – 44% = 4 points 25 – 34% = 3 points 15 – 24% = 2 points 5 – 14% = 1 point 0 – 4% = 0 points	< 2 Spinal levels = 10 pts 3 – 5 Spinal levels = 8 pts 6 – 12 Spinal levels = 6 pts Sacrum = 4 pts Buttock = 2 pts Side of thigh = 0 pts

FIG. 10. University of Pennsylvania AROM scoring.[72]

Part IV: STRENGTH:				
Device: ____________(kg lbs. ft/lbs) (circle one)	INV	UNINV	% Uninv	PTS
External rotation at side			%	
Internal rotation at side			%	
Elevation at 45º in POS			%	
TOTAL POINTS =				/60

Strength Scoring
>90% = 20 points
80 – 89% = 18 points
70 – 79% = 16 points
60 – 69% = 14 points
51 – 59% = 12 points
40 – 49% = 10 points
30 – 39% = 8 points
20 – 29% = 6 points
10 – 19% = 4 points
1 – 9% = 2 points
0% = 0 points

FIG. 11. University of Pennsylvania strength scoring.[72]

erage of the items that were responded to is multiplied by 3 (maximum score for each item), to yield the maximum possible score achievable by that patient. The score for each relevant item is then added, and this total raw score is divided by the total achievable maximum score for all relevant items, to yield a percentage of the points assigned to this category. This percentage is multiplied by 60 points, to yield the final functional score.

Shoulder active range of motion (AROM) is recorded as recommended by the ASES and includes forward elevation, external rotation with the arm at the side, external rotation at 90 degrees abduction, and internal rotation.[16] All motions are measured in the seated position, with the exception of internal rotation, which is measured while standing.

Figure 10 demonstrates the scoring for each of the ROM parameters. Scoring for forward elevation and external rotation is based on a percentage of the opposite uninvolved side. Internal rotation scoring is based on the level that the hitchhiking thumb can reach, until the patient is able to reach the lumbar or thoracic spinous processes. Scoring then is based on a comparison of the spinal level achieved by the opposite uninvolved extremity. Ten points can be awarded for each ROM parameter for a total of 40 points for this section.

Strength testing should be performed with an isometric dynamometer. Internal and external rotation are measured with the arm at the side and in neutral rotation. Elevation is measured at 45 degrees in the plane of the scapula. Scoring is based on a percentage of the opposite normal side and is shown in Fig. 11. Ten points can be awarded for each position for a maximum of 30 points for this section. Excellent reliability of the self-assessment and impairment total scores were found in a study of 37 patients.[72] The subsections of each of the scales were also highly reliable, with good correlation of these total scores to the Constant and ASES shoulder scores. Responsiveness to change of these scores requires further study.

SUMMARY

The necessity of documenting outcome of surgical and therapeutic intervention of shoulder disorders is receiving increased emphasis in health care today. More importantly, clinicians must be able to compare results of different forms of treatment, compare results reported by other clinicians, and learn the confounding factors that may affect outcome. In order to accomplish this, standardized methods must be universally accepted. Available outcome scoring systems must meet the necessary criteria before they can be used. Once these systems are in place, the most effective treatments will be offered for the least cost.

Improving the patient's pain, function, and satisfaction should be the goal of any treatment intervention. Knowledge of the factors that contribute to that improvement are important in determining their relationship to the overall patient outcome. A patient self-assessment tool that measures outcome for the general population of shoulder patients should be used, in conjunction with a scale designed for the athletic population. In addition, the level of improvement in impairments such as ROM and strength should be compared with the patient's assessment of outcome. Use of a generic health status measure provides data as to the affect a shoulder problem has on the patient's overall function. Integrating these data will help to guide treatment and predict outcome, thereby improving the efficiency of our health-care system.

REFERENCES

1. Agre JC, Magness JL, Hall SZ, et al. Strength testing with a portable dynamometer: reliability for upper and lower extremities. *Arch Phys Med Rehabil* 1987;68:454–457.
2. Amstutz HC, Sew Hoy AL, Clark IC. UCLA anatomic total shoulder arthroplasty. *Clin Orthop* 1981;155:7–20.
3. Bain GI, Sandow MJ, Howie DW. Treatment of humeral shaft fractures with the Seidel intramedullary nail. *Aust N Z J Surg* 1996;66:156–158.
4. Barret WP, Franklin JL, Jackins SE, et al. Total shoulder arthroplasty. *J Bone Joint Surg [Am]* 1987;69:865–872.
5. Beasley WC. Quantitative muscle testing: principles and applications to research and clinical services. *Arch Phys Med Rehabil* 1961;42: 398–425.
6. Beaton DE, Richards RR. Measuring function of the shoulder. A cross-sectional comparison of five questionnaires. *J Bone Joint Surg [Am]* 1996;78(6):882–890.
7. Bohannon RW. Comparability of force measurements obtained with different strain gauge hand-held dynamometer. *Arch Phys Med Rehabil* 1991;72:911–914.
8. Bohannon RW, Lusardi MS. Modified sphygmomanometer versus strain gauge hand-dynamometer. *Arch Phys Med Rehabil* 1991;72: 911–914.
9. Bohannon RW. Hand-held compared with isokinetic dynamometry for measurement of static knee extension torque (parallel reliability of dynamometers). *Clin Phys Physiol Meas* 1990;11:217–222.
10. Bohannon RW. Make tests and break tests of elbow flexion muscle strength. *Phys Ther* 1988;68:193–194.
11. Bohannon RW, Andrews AW. Interrater reliability of hand-held dynamometry. *Phys Ther* 1987;67:931–933.
12. Bohannon RW. Test-retest reliability of hand-held dynamometry during a single session of strength assessment. *Phys Ther* 1986;66: 206–209.
13. Bombardier C, Tugwell P. Methodological considerations in functional assessment. *J Rheumatol* 1987;14(suppl 15):6–10.
14. Boone DC, Azen SP, Lin CM, Spence C, Baron C, Lee L. Reliability of goniometric measurements. *Phys Ther* 1978;58:1355–1360.
15. Bordon R, Colachis SC. Quantitative measurement of the good and normal ranges in muscle testing. *Phys Ther* 1968;48:839–843.
16. Boublik M, Hawkins RJ. Clinical examination of the shoulder complex. *J Orthop Sports Phys Ther* 1993;18:379–385.
17. Burkhart SS, Nottage WM, Ogilvie-Harris DJ, Kohn HS, Pachelli A. Partial repair of irreparable rotator cuff tears. *Arthroscopy* 1994;10: 363–370.
18. Byl N, Richards S, Asturias J. Intrarater and interrater reliability of strength measurements of the biceps and deltoid using a hand-held dynamometer. *J Orthop Sports Phys Ther* 1988;9:399–405.
19. Cai TD, Guo BF. Recurrent anterior dislocation of shoulder joint. *Chin Med* 1990;103:604–605.
20. Cahalan TD, Johnson ME, Chao EYS. Shoulder strength analysis using the cybex II isokinetic dynamometer. *Clin Orthop Rel Res* 1991; 271:249–257.
21. Ciepiela MD, Burkhead WZ. The end result: functional assessment of rotator cuff repair. In: Burkhead WZ, ed., *Rotator cuff disorders*. Baltimore, MD: Williams & Wilkins, 1996.
22. Clarke HH. Comparison of instruments for recording muscle strength. *Res Q* 1954;25:399–411.
23. Codman EA. *The shoulder: rupture of the supraspinatus tendon and other lesions in or about the subacromial bursa.* Malabar, FL: Robert E. Krieger Publishing, 1934.
24. Conboy VB, Morris RW, Kiss J, Carr AJ. An evaluation of the Constant-Murley shoulder assessment. *J Bone Joint Surg [Br]* 1996;78: 229–232.

25. Constant CR, Murley AHG. A clinical method of functional assessment of the shoulder. *Clin Orthop Rel Res* 1987;214:160–164.
26. Constant CR. Age related recovery of shoulder function after injury [Thesis]. University College, Cork, Ireland, 1986.
27. Cook EE, Gray VL, Sairnar-Nogue E, Mederos J. Shoulder antagonistic strength ratios: a comparison between college level baseball pitchers and nonpitchers. *J Orthop Sports Phys Ther* 1987;8:451–461.
28. Dawson J, Fitzpatrick R, Carr A. Questionnaire on the perceptions of patients about shoulder surgery. *J Bone Joint Surg [Br]* 1996;78: 593–600.
29. DeSimoni C, Ledermann T, Imhoff AB. Holmium-YAG laser in outlet impingement of the shoulder. Mid-term results. *Orthopade* 1996; 25:84–90.
30. Deyo RA, Inui TS. Toward clinical application of health status measures: sensitivity of scales to clinically important changes. *Health Ser Res* 1984;19:275–289.
31. Deyo RA, Centor RM. Assessing the responsiveness of functional scales to clinical change: an analogy to diagnostic test performance. *J Chron Dis* 1986;39:897–906.
32. Duncan R, Savoie FH. Arthroscopic inferior capsular shift for multidirectional instability for the shoulder: a preliminary report. *Arthroscopy* 1993;9:24–27.
33. Effgen SK, Brown DA. Long-term stability of hand-held dynamometers measurements in children who have myelomeningocele. *Phys Ther* 1992;72:458–465.
34. Ellenbecker TS, Daires GJ, Rouinski MJ. Concentric versus eccentric isokinetic strengthening of the rotator cuff: objective data versus functional test. *Am J Sports Med* 1988;16:64–69.
35. Ellman H, Hnaker G, Bayer M. Repair of the rotator cuff: end-result study of factors influencing reconstruction. *J Bone Joint Surg [Am]* 1986;68:1136–1144.
36. Esch JC, Ozerkis LR, Helgager JA, Kane N, Lilliott N. Arthroscopic subacromial decompression: results according to the degree of rotator cuff tear. *Arthroscopy* 1988;4:241–249.
37. Feiring DC, Ellenbecker TS, Derscheid GL. Test-retest reliability of the biodex isokinetic dynamometer. *J Orthop Sports Phys Ther* 1990; 11:298–300.
38. Field LD, Warren RF, O'Brien SJ, Altchek DW, Wickiewicz TL. Isolated closure of rotator interval defects for shoulder instability. *Am J Sports Med* 1995;23:557–563.
39. Ferraz MB, Quaresma MR, Aquino LRL, et al. Reliability of pain scales in the assessment of literate and illiterate patients with rheumatoid arthritis. *J Rheum* 1990;17:1022–1024.
40. Gartsman GM. Arthroscopic acromioplasty for lesions of the rotator cuff. *J Bone Joint Surg* 1990;72:169–180.
41. Gajdosik RL, Bohannon RW. Clinical measurement of range of motion. Review of goniometry emphasizing reliability and validity. *Phys Ther* 1987;67:1867–1872.
42. Gazielly DF, Gleyze P, Montagnon C, Bruyere G, Prallet B. Functional and anatomical results after surgical treatment of ruptures of the rotator cuff. 1. Preoperative functional and anatomical evaluation of ruptures of the rotator cuff. *Rev Chir Orthop Repar Appareil Moteur* 1995;81:8–16.
43. Gerber C, Hersche O, Farron A. Isolated rupture of the subscapularis tendon. Results of operative repair. *J Bone Joint Surg [Am]* 1996;78: 1015–1023.
44. Gerber C. Integrated scoring systems for the functional assessment of the shoulder. In: Matsen FA, Fu FH, Hawkins RJ, eds. *The shoulder: a balance of mobility and stability*. American Academy of Orthopaedic Surgeons, Park Ridge, IL 1993.
45. Gerber C, Krushell RJ. Isolated rupture of the tendon of the subscapularis muscle. Clinical features in 16 cases. *J Bone Joint Surg [Br]* 1991;73:389–394.
46. Gresham GE. Traditional approaches to functional assessment arthritis. *J Rheumatol* 1987;14(suppl 15):11–14.
47. Gshwend N, Bloch HR, Bischof A. Long-term results of surgical management of rotator cuff rupture. *Orthopade* 1991;20:255–261.
48. Guccione AA. Physical therapy diagnosis and the relationship between impairments and function. *Phys Ther* 1991;71:499–504.
49. Guccione AA. Arthritis and the process of disablement. *Phys Ther* 1994;74:408–413.
50. Guyatt GH, Bombardier C, Tugwell PX. Measuring disease-specific quality of life in clinical trials. *Can Med Assoc J* 1986;134:889–895.
51. Guyatt G, Walter S, Norman G. Measuring change over time: assessing the usefulness of evaluative instruments. *J Chron Dis* 1987;40: 171–178.
52. Habernek H, Weinstabl R, Schabus R, Schmid L. A new approach to the subacromial space. Technique and 2-year results in 28 rotator-cuff repair cases. *Acta Orthop Scand* 1993;64:92–94.
53. Heerkens YF, Brandsma JW, Lakeweld-Heyl K, Dorine van Ravensberg C. Impairments and disabilities—the difference: proposal for adjustment of the international classification of impairments, disabilities, and handicaps. *Phys Ther* 1994;74:430–441.
54. Huskisson EC. Measurement of pain. *J Rheumatol* 1982;9:768–769.
55. Huskisson EC. Measurement of pain. *Lancet* 1974;2:1127–1131.
56. Iannotti JP, Bernot MP, Kuhlman JR, Kelley MJ, Williams GR. Postoperative assessment of shoulder function: a prospective study of full-thickness rotator cuff tears. *J Shoulder Elbow Surg* 1996;5:449–457.
57. International Classification of Impairments, Disabilities and Handicaps. Geneva, Switzerland: World Health Organization, 1980.
58. Imhoff A, Ledermann T. Arthroscopic subacromial decompression with and without the Homium:YAG-laser. A prospective comparative study. *Arthroscopy* 1995;11:549–556.
59. Ivey FM, Calhoun JH, Rusche K, Brerschenk J. Isokinetic testing of shoulder strength: normal values. *Arch Phys Med Rehabil* 1985;66: 384–386.
60. Jaffe M, Frank A, Beaufils P. Endoscopic acromioplasty in total rupture of the rotator cuff. *Rev Chir Orthop Repar Appareil Moteur* 1994; 80:369–378.
61. Jette AM. Outcomes research: shifting the dominant research paradigm in physical therapy. *Phys Ther* 1995;75:965–970.
62. Jette AM. Physical disablement concepts for physical therapy research and practice. *Phys Ther* 1994;74:380–386.
63. Jette AM. The functional status index: reliability and validity of a self-report functional disability measure. *J Rheumatol* 1987;14(suppl 15): 15–19.
64. Jette AM. Diagnosis and classification by physical therapists: a special communication. *Phys Ther* 1989;69:967–969.
65. Jette AM, Davies AR, Cleary PD, et al. The functional status questionnaire: reliability and validity when used in primary care. *J Gen Intern Med* 1986;1:143–149.
66. Kane RL. Looking for physical therapy outcomes. *Phys Ther* 1994;74: 425–429.
67. Kasperczyk WJ, Engel M. Tscherne H. 4-fragment fracture of the proximal upper arm. *Unfallchirurgie* 1993;96:422–426.
68. Keller RB. How outcomes research should be done. In: Hawkins RJ, Fu FH, Matsen FA, eds. *The shoulder: a balance of mobility and stability*. American Academy of Orthopaedic Surgeons, Park Ridge, IL 1993.
69. Kirshner B, Guyatt GH. A methodological framework for assessing health indices. *J Chron Dis* 1985;38:27–36.
70. Kuhlman JR, Iannotti JP, Kelly MJ, Riegler FX, Gevaert ML, Ergin TM. Isokinetic and isometric measurement of strength of external rotation and abduction of the shoulder. *J Bone Joint Surg [Am]* 1993;74: 1320–1333.
71. Kuhn JE, Blasier RB. Measuring outcomes in shoulder arthroplasty. *Semin Arthroplasty* 1995;6:245–264.
72. Leggin BG, Shaffer MA, Neuman RM, Iannotti JP, Williams GR, Brenneman SK. Reliability of a shoulder outcome scoring system. *Am J Sports Med*, 1998 (submitted for publication).
73. Leggin BG, Neuman RM, Iannotti JP, Williams GR, Thompson ET. Intrarater and interrater reliability of three isometric dynamometers in assessing shoulder strength. *J Shoulder Elbow Surg* 1996;6:18–24.
74. Leung KS, Lam TP. Open reduction and internal fixation of ipsilateral fractures of the scapular neck and clavicle. *J Bone Joint Surg [Am]* 1993;75:1015–1018.
75. Lippitt S, Harryman DT, Matsen FA. A practical tool for evaluating function: the simple shoulder test. In: Matsen FA, Fu FH, Hawkins RJ, eds. *The shoulder: a balance of mobility and stability.* American Academy of Orthopaedic Surgeons, Park Ridge, IL 1993.
76. Lirette R, Morin F, Kinnard P. The difficulties in assessment of results of anterior acromioplasty. *Clin Orthop Rel Res* 1992;278:14–16.
77. Loew M, Jurgowski W, Mau HC, Thomsen M. Treatment of calcifying tendinitis of rotator cuff by extracorporeal shock waves: a preliminary report. *J Shoulder Elbow Surg* 1995;4:101–106.
78. Lozman PR, Hechtman KS, Uribe JW. Combined arthroscopic management of impingement syndrome and acromioclavicular joint arthritis. *J South Orthop Assoc* 1995;4:177–181.
79. MacKenzie CR, Charlson ME, DiGioia D, Kellog K. Can the sickness impact profile measure change? An example of scale assessment. *J Chron Dis* 1986;6:429–438.

80. Malebra JL, Adam ML, Harris BA, Krebs DE. Reliability of dynamic and isometric testing of shoulder external and internal rotators. *J Orthop Sports Phys Ther* 1993;18:543–552.
81. Marcacci M, Zafagnini S, Petitto A, Neri MP, Iacono F, Visani A. Arthroscopic management of recurrent anterior dislocation of the shoulder: analysis of technical modifications on the Caspari procedure. *Arthroscopy* 1996;12:144–149.
82. Marino, M, Nicholas JA, Glein GW, Rosenthal P, Nicholas SJ. The efficacy of manual assessment of muscle strength using a new device. *Am J Sports Med* 1982;10:360–364.
83. Matsen FA III, Ziegler DW, DeBartolo SE. Patient self-assessment of health status and function in glenohumeral degenerative joint disease. *J Shoulder Elbow Surg* 1995;4:345–351.
84. Matsen FA III, Lippitt SB, Sidles JA, Harryman DT II. *Practical evaluation and management of the shoulder*. Philadelphia: WB Saunders, 1994
85. Matsen FA III, Fu FH, Hawkins RJ, eds. *The shoulder: a balance of mobility and stability*. Rosemont, IL: American Academy of Orthopedic Surgeons, 1993.
86. Mayerson NH, Milano RA. Goniometric reliability in physical medicine. *Arch Phys Med Rehabil* 1984;65:92–94.
87. Mayhew T, Rothstein J. Measurement of muscle performance with instruments. In: Rothstein J, ed. *Measurement in physical therapy: clinics in physical therapy*. New York: Churchill Livingstone, 1985: 57–102.
88. Meenan RF. The AIMS approach to health status measurement: conceptual background and measurement properties. *J Rheumatol* 1982; 9:785–788.
89. Melzack R, Torgerson WS. On the language of pain. *Anesthesiology* 1971;34:50–59.
90. Mologne TS, Lapoint JM, Morin WD, Zilberfarb J, O'Brien TJ. Arthroscopic anterior labral reconstruction using a transglenoid suture technique. Results in active-duty military patients. *Am J Sports Med* 1996;24:268–274.
91. Montgomery WH III, Jobe FW. Functional outcomes in athletes after modified anterior capsulolabral reconstruction. *Am J Sports Med* 1994;22:352–358.
92. Mossberg KA, McFarland C. Initial health status of patients at outpatient physical therapy clinics. *Phys Ther* 1995;75:1043–1053.
93. Nagi S. Disability concepts revisited: implications for prevention. In: Pope A, Tarlov A, eds. *Disability in America: toward a national agenda for prevention*. Washington, DC: National Academy Press, 1991:309–327.
94. Nagi S. Some conceptual issues in disability and rehabilitation. In: Sussman M, ed. *Sociology and rehabilitation*. Washington, DC: American Sociological Association, 1965:100–113.
95. Neer CS, Watson KC, Stanton FJ. Recent experience in total shoulder replacement. *J Bone Joint Surg [Am]* 1982;64:319–336.
96. Neer CS. Anterior acromioplasty for the chronic impingement syndrome in the shoulder. A preliminary report. *J Bone Joint Surg [Am]* 1972;54:41–50.
97. Nicholas JA, Sapega A, Kraus H, Webb JN. Factors influencing manual muscle tests in physical therapy. *J Bone Joint Surg [Am]* 1978:60: 186–190.
98. Olsen BS, Vaesel MT, Sojbjerg JO. Treatment of midshaft clavicular nonunion with plate fixation and autologous bone grafting. *J Shoulder Elbow Surg* 1995;4:337–344.
99. Otis JC, Warren RF, Backus SI, Santnen TJ, Malbrey JD. Torque production in the shoulder of the normal young adult male. The interaction of function dominance, joint angle, and angular velocity. *Am J Sports Med* 1990;18:119–123.
100. Portney LG, Watkins MP. *Foundations of clinical research: applications to practice*. East Norwalk, CT: Appleton & Lange, 1993.
101. Richards RR, An KN, Bigliani LU, et al. A standardized method for the assessment of shoulder function. *J Shoulder Elbow Surg* 1994;3: 347–352.
102. Riddle DL, Rothstein JM, Lamb RL. Goniometric reliability in a clinical setting. Shoulder measurements. *Phys Ther* 1987;67:668–673.
103. Rikli D, Regazzoni P, Renner N. The unstable shoulder girdle: early functional treatment utilizing open reduction and internal fixation. *J Orthop Trauma* 1995;9:23–27.
104. Rheault W, Beal JL, Kubik KR, Nowak TA, Shepley JA. Intertester reliability of the hand-held dynamometer for wrist flexion and extension. *Arch Phys Med Rehabil* 1989;70:907–910.
105. Roach KE, Budimen-Mak E, Songsiridej N, Lertratanakul Y. Development of a shoulder pain and disability index. *Arthritis Care Res* 1991;4:143–149.
106. Romeo AA, Bach BR, O'Halloran KL. Scoring systems for shoulder conditions. *Am J Sports Med* 1996;24:472–476.
107. Rompe JD, Rumler F, Hopf C, Nafe C, Heine J. Extracorporal shock wave therapy for calcifying tendinitis of the shoulder. *Clin Orthop Rel Res* 1995;321:196–201.
108. Rothstein JM, Echternach JL. *Primer on measurement: an introductory guide to measurement issues*. American Physical Therapy Association, Alexandria, VA 1993:59–95.
109. Rothstein JM, Miller PJ, Roettiger RF. Goniometric reliability in a clinical setting. Elbow and knee measurements. *Phys Ther* 1983;63: 1611–1615.
110. Rowe CR, Patel D, Southmayd WW. The Bankart procedure: a long term end-result study. *J Bone Joint Surg [Am]* 1978;60:1–16.
111. Sapega A, Kelley MJ. Strength testing of the shoulder. *J Shoulder Elbow Surg* 1994;3:327–345.
112. Scott J, Huskisson EC. Vertical or horizontal visual analogue scales. *Ann Rheum Dis* 1979;38:560.
113. Seger JY, Westing SH, Hanson M, Karlson E, Elblom B. A new dynamometer measuring concentric and eccentric muscle strength in accelerated, decelerated, and isokinetic movements validity and reproducibility. *Eur J Appl Physiol* 1988;57:526–530.
114. Segmuller HE, Taylor DE, Hogan CS, Saies AD, Hayes MG. Arthroscopic treatment of adhesive capsulitis. *J Shoulder Elbow Surg* 1995; 4:403–408.
115. Shepard KF. Qualitative and quantitative research in clinical practice. *Phys Ther* 1987;67:1891–1894.
116. Singer GC, Kirkland PM, Emery RJH. Coracoid transposition for recurrent anterior instability of the shoulder. A 20-year follow-up study. *J Bone Joint Surg [Br]* 1995;77:73–76.
117. Smythe HA, Helewa A, Goldsmith CH. Selection and combination of outcome measures. *J Rheumatol* 1982;9:770–774.
118. Snyder SJ, Banas MP, Karzel RP. The arthroscopic Mumford procedure: an analysis of results. *Arthroscopy* 1995;11:157–164.
119. Speer KP, Lohnes J, Garrett WE. Arthroscopic subacromial decompression: results in advanced impingement syndrome. *Arthroscopy* 1991;7:291–296.
120. Stratford PW, Binkley JM, Riddle DL. Health status measures: strategies and analytic methods for assessing change scores. *Phys Ther* 1996;76:1109–1123.
121. Tarlov AR, Ware JE, Greenfield S, et al. The Medical Outcomes Study: an application of methods for monitoring the results of medical care. *JAMA* 1989;262:925–930.
122. Tibone JE, Bradley JP. Evaluation of treatment outcomes for athletes' shoulders. In: Matsen FA, Fu FH, Hawkins RJ, eds. *The shoulder: a balance of mobility and stability*. American Academy of Orthopaedic Surgeons, Park Ridge, IL 1993.
123. Tugwell P, Bombardier C. A methodological framework for developing and selecting endpoints in clinical trials. *J Rheumatol* 1982;9: 758–762.
124. Verbrugge L, Jette A. The disablement process. *Soc Sci Med* 1994;38: 1–14.
125. Wadsworth CT, Krishnan R, Sear M, Harrold J, Nielson DH. Intrarater reliability of manual muscle testing and hand-held dynametric muscle testing. *Phys Ther* 1987;67:1342–1347.
126. Ware JE, Sherbourne CD. The MOS 36-item short-form health survey (SF-36). *Med Care* 1992;30:473–483.
127. Wikholm JB, Bohannon RW. Handheld dynamometer measurements: tester strength makes a difference. *J Orthop Sports Phys Ther* 1991; 13:191–198.
128. Williams JW, Holleman DR, Simel DL. Measuring shoulder function with the Shoulder Pain and Disability Index. *J Rheumatol* 1995;22: 727–732.
129. Wirth MA, Blatter G, Rockwood CA. Ther capsular imbrication procedure for recurrent anterior instability of the shoulder. *J Bone Joint Surg* 1996;78:246–259.
130. Youssef JA, Carr CF, Walther CE, Murphy JM. Arthroscopic Bankart suture repair for recurrent traumatic unidirectional anterior shoulder dislocations. *Arthroscopy* 1995;11:561–563.
131. Zyto K, Kronberg M, Brostrom LA. Shoulder function after displaced fractures of the proximal humerus. *J Shoulder Elbow Surg* 1995;4: 331–336.

PART XIV

Pain Management

Disorders of the Shoulder: Diagnosis and Management,
edited by Joseph P. Iannotti and Gerald R. Williams, Jr.
Lippincott Williams & Wilkins, Philadelphia © 1999.

CHAPTER 37

Medical Management of Chronic Shoulder Pain

F. Michael Ferrante

Before any discussion of the management of chronic pain of the shoulder is possible, it is necessary that we define pain as an entity, as well as give some background information on its temporal characteristics and the different types of pain. The International Association for the Study of Pain (IASP) defines pain as an unpleasant sensory and emotional experience associated with actual or potential tissue damage or described in terms of such damage.[104] If we examine this definition, pain is by its innate nature a physiologic process composed of neural pathways and neurotransmitters but also a subjective and emotional experience. Juxtaposition of these phenomena cannot be dichotomized. Pain implies perception of a multitude of biochemical and physiologic processes. Without perception and a concomitant emotional experience, we do not have pain but only a series of complex physiologic and biochemical mechanisms.

Moreover, pain may serve a protective function (i.e., potential tissue damage in the IASP definition). Withdrawal reflexes, immobilization of an injured limb, and avoidance of subsequent encounters with potentially painful stimuli serve to prevent damage to tissues. The potentially protective function of pain is vividly demonstrated by individuals with the rare condition of congenital insensitivity to pain. Such patients lack a number of the normal neural structures for perception of noxious stimuli and repetitively injure themselves by failing to avoid threatening thermal, mechanical, and chemical stimuli.[40]

Acute pain signifies the presence of a noxious stimulus that is producing actual tissue damage or that possesses the potential to do so. The presence of acute pain implies a properly working nervous system (i.e., the teleologically protective mechanism is functional). There is autonomic hyperactivity: hypertension, tachycardia, sweating, vasoconstriction, etc. Temporally, acute pain is short lived.[62]

Chronic pain implies the absence of a threat of tissue damage, but the patient describes the experience in terms of such damage. The normal function of the nervous system becomes reorganized (neuroplasticity) with the potential for spontaneous and atopic nerve excitation. Autonomic hyperactivity is absent. Pain is deemed to be chronic when it persists beyond 3 to 6 months.[62]

There are two types of pain: nociceptive and neuropathic pain. Nociceptive pain implies activation and/or sensitization of nociceptors in the periphery. Nociceptors are nerves that transduce noxious stimuli into electrochemical impulses, which are subsequently transmitted to the spinal cord and more rostral centers of the central nervous system. Nociceptive pain can be further subdivided into two types: somatic pain and visceral pain. Somatic pain results from excitation and sensitization of nociceptors in tissues such as bone, periarticular soft tissue, joints, and muscles. Visceral pain is mediated by discrete nociceptors in the cardiovascular, respiratory, gastrointestinal, and genitourinary systems. The shoulder has little relevance to visceral pain, except as a

F. M. Ferrante: Department of Anesthesia, Hospital of the University of Pennsylvania, Philadelphia, Pennsylvania 19104.

referral site. Several examples of visceral pain phenomena that are typically referred to the shoulder include angina, esophageal dysmotility, various pulmonary diseases, mediastinal tumors, and processes irritating the pleural or peritoneal surface of the diaphragm (e.g., pleural effusion and subdiaphragmatic abscess).

Neuropathic pain results from injury to neural structures within the peripheral or central nervous systems. Such injury promotes spontaneous and atopic firing of nerves, as well as reorganization of the nervous system.

Chronic pain of the shoulder is usually due to somatic and/or neuropathic pain. Before we can begin any discussion of the pathophysiology of conditions of the shoulder that give rise to both somatic and/or neuropathic types of pain, it is necessary to review the underlying anatomy of the brachial plexus and its neural ramifications.

ANATOMY OF THE BRACHIAL PLEXUS

The brachial plexus is formed from the union of the ventral rami of C5–T1 (Fig. 1). The neural structures of the brachial plexus are sequentially divided into roots, trunks, divisions, cords, and subsequent individual terminal nerve branches. The ventral rami of C5 and C6 nerve roots fuse to form the upper trunk of the brachial plexus. Similarly, the ventral rami of C8 and T1 fuse to form the lower trunk. The middle trunk is formed as a continuation of the ventral root of C7.

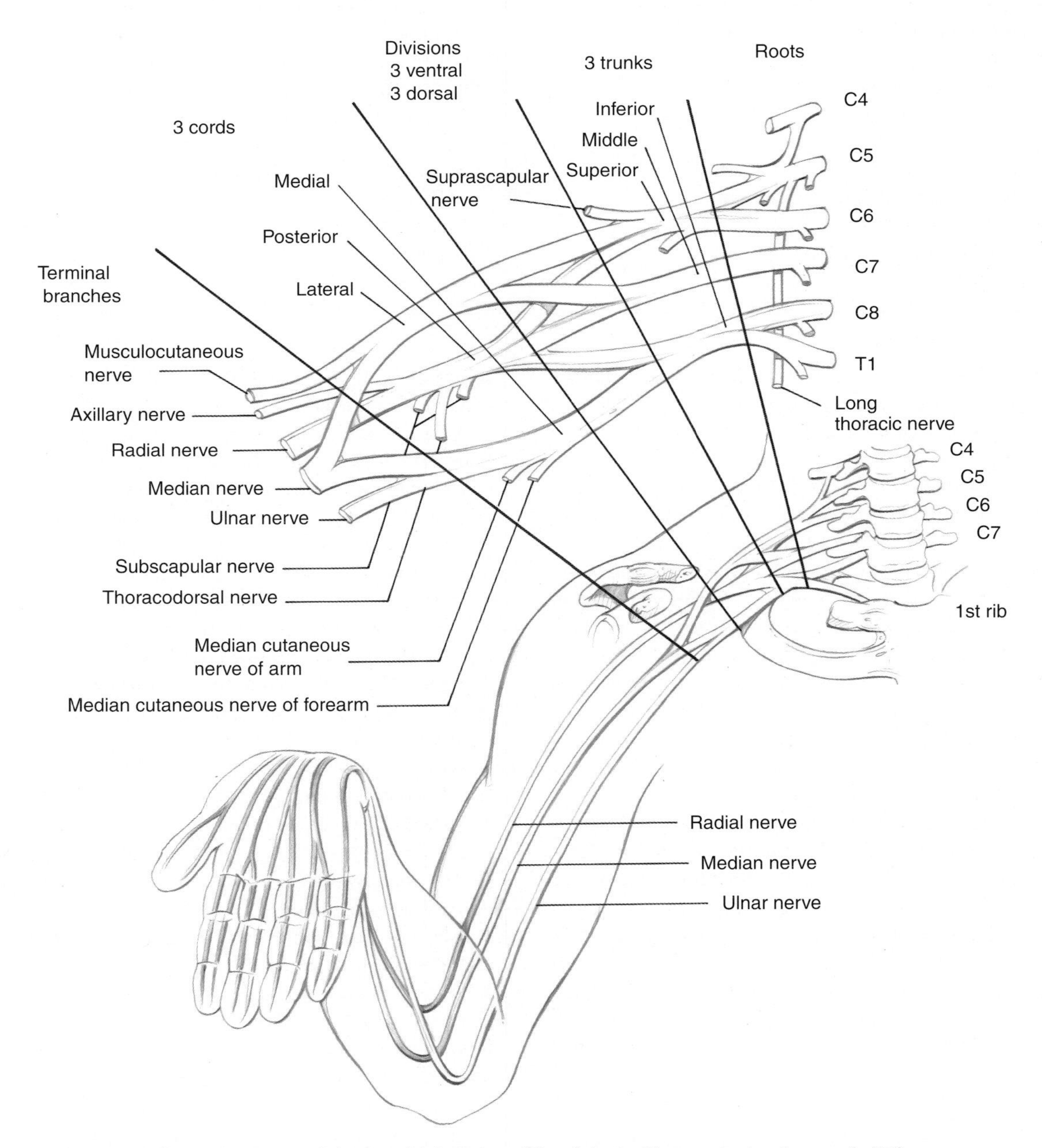

FIG. 1. Anatomy of the brachial plexus. (Reprinted with permission from ref. 17.)

In their passage from the cervical transverse processes to the first rib, the roots and subsequently the trunks can be considered to be sandwiched between the anterior and middle scalene muscles. The neural structures are invested by the fasciae of these muscles. The plexus emerges from behind the lower end of the sternocleidomastoid muscle and passes under the clavicle. The divisions are found surrounding the subclavian artery behind the clavicle. The divisions then reorganize to form the cords that pass into the axilla.

The radial nerve is a direct continuation of the posterior cord and is composed of fibers from C5 to C8. The ulnar nerve (C8–T1) is derived from the medial cord of the plexus. The median nerve receives nerve fibers from both the lateral and medial cords. Muscles supplied by the median nerve can be divided into two groups. Some are innervated from C5 to C7 (lateral portion of the median nerve: pronator teres and flexor carpi radialis). Most muscles are supplied by the C8 and T1 nerve roots, however (medial portion of the median nerve: flexors and median-innervated hand muscles).

A number of nerves arise from the brachial plexus prior to its ramifications into the radial, ulnar, and median nerves of the arm. Knowledge of the anatomy of these nerves is important for accurate localization of brachial plexus injuries (Fig. 1 and Table 1). The dorsal scapular nerve arises from the C5 ventral ramus before joining with that of C6 and innervates the rhomboid muscles. The long thoracic nerve supplies the serratus anterior muscle and is derived from the ventral rami of C5–7. The supraspinatus and infraspinatus muscles are innervated by the suprascapular nerve (C5–6), which branches off the upper trunk of the brachial plexus. The lateral pectoral nerve (C5–7) innervates the pectoralis major muscle and is derived from the upper trunk of the brachial plexus. The thoracodorsal nerve (C6–8) and the axillary nerve (C5–6) are derived from the posterior cord and supply, respectively, the latissimus dorsi and the deltoid muscles. The medial pectoral nerve and the medial cutaneous nerves (both C8 and T1) are derived from the medial cord of the brachial plexus.

Of course, the bony anatomy of the shoulder is also important in the genesis of chronic painful conditions. However, the bony anatomy of the shoulder has been exhaustively reviewed elsewhere in this text. Thus, we refer the reader to the previous excellent discussions of the bony anatomy of the shoulder in reference to any discussions of somatic pain.

PATHOPHYSIOLOGY

Somatic pain involves pathology of periarticular soft tissue, the shoulder joint itself, as well as the bones comprising the shoulder girdle (Table 2).

Somatic (Nociceptive) Pain

Somatic pain is characterized as being well localized topographically, intermittent or constant, and is described as aching, gnawing, throbbing, or cramping.

Between the site of tissue damage and the perception of pain is a complex series of electrochemical processes and mechanisms. Four physiologic processes are involved: (a) transduction, (b) transmission, (c) modulation, and (d) perception (Fig. 2).[49,72]

Transduction is the process wherein noxious stimuli in the periphery (periarticular soft tissue, joint, bone and/or mus-

TABLE 1. *Patterns of muscle weakness resulting from brachial plexus lesions*

Brachial plexus	Nerve branch	Muscles
Trunks		
Upper	Suprascapular (C5–6)	Supraspinatus, infraspinatus
	Lateral pectoral (C5–7)	Clavicular portion of the pectoralis major
	Musculocutaneous (C5–7)	Biceps
	Lateral portion median (C5–7)	Pronator teres, flexor carpi radialis
	Radial (C5–6)	Brachioradialis
	Axillary (C5–6)	Deltoid
Middle	Thoracodorsal (C6–8)	Latissimus dorsi
	Subscapular (C5–6)	Teres major
	Radial (C7)	All radial innervated muscles (except brachioradialis)
	Lateral portion median (C5–7)	Pronator teres, flexor carpi radialis
Lower	Medial pectoral (C8–T1)	Sternal portion of pectoralis major
	Ulnar (C8–T1)	All ulnar innervated muscles
	Medial portion median (C8–T1)	Flexors of hand, median innervated intrinsic muscles of hand
Cords		
Lateral	Musculocutaneous (C5–7)	Biceps
	Lateral portion median (C5–7)	Pronator teres, flexor carpi radialis
Posterior	Thoracodorsal (C6–8)	Latissimus dorsi
	Subscapular (C5–6)	Teres major
	Axillary (C5–6)	Deltoid
	Radial (C5–T1)	All radial innervated muscles
Medial	Ulnar (C8–T1)	All ulnar innervated muscles
	Medial portion median (C8–T1)	Flexors of hand, median innervated intrinsic muscles of hand

TABLE 2. *Differential diagnosis of painful pathologies of the shoulder*

Somatic pain	Neuropathic pain
Periarticular soft tissue	Spinal cord lesions
Impingement syndromes	Cervical pathology
Rotator cuff tear (partial and complete)	Spondylosis
Bicipital tendinitis	Degenerative disc disease
Bicipital tendon tear	Herniated nucleus pulposus
Calcific tendinitis	Radiculopathy
Adhesive capsulitis/frozen shoulder	Spinal nerve lesions
Glenohumeral instability	Brachial plexopathy
Joints	Stretch, compression, trauma
Osteoarthritis of glenohumeral joint	Avulsion
Primary (rare)	Stingers and burners
Secondary (after fracture, recurrent dislocation, etc.)	Intraoperative injuries
Osteoarthritis of acromioclavicular joint (traumatic)	Brachial plexus neuritis
Septic arthritis	Tumors
Rheumatoid arthritis	Radiation neuritis
Gout and pseudogout	Thoracic outlet syndrome (TOS)
Osteonecrosis (steroids, alcohol, SLE, etc.)	Neurologic TOS
Subluxation (acromioclavicular or sternoclavicular)	Vascular TOS
Bone	TOS of pain and sensory symptoms
Fracture	Entrapment syndromes
Osteomyelitis	Suprascapular nerve
Tumor	Long thoracic nerve
Muscles	Axillary nerve
Myofascial pain syndrome	Sympathetically maintained pain (RSD)
Fibromyalgia	CRPS I (reflex sympathetic dystrophy)
	CRPS II (causalgia)

cle) excite and sensitize nociceptors. Nociceptors are afferent neurons whose peripheral terminals encode chemical, thermal, or mechanical noxious stimuli into neural impulses (primary afferent nociceptors), or they are neurons that transmit impulses from noxious stimuli (nociceptive transmission) to higher order neurons (secondary order, tertiary order, etc., nociceptors). A number of chemical mediators (substance P, potassium, histamine, acetylcholine, serotonin, bradykinin, prostaglandins, leukotrienes, etc.) mediate transduction in the periphery via processes whose exact mechanisms remain obscure.

Transmission refers to the propagation of impulses to higher rostral centers. There are four neural components to the transmission pathways:

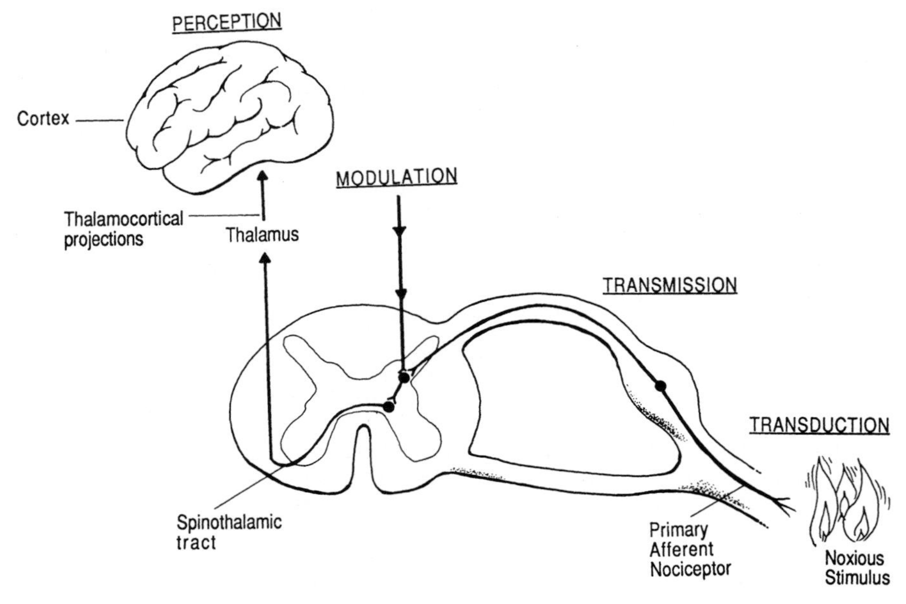

FIG. 2. Nociception is composed of four physiologic processes: transduction, transmission, modulation, and perception. (Reprinted with permission from ref. 72.)

1. Primary afferent nociceptors (Aδ and C fibers), which carry nociceptive transmission to the dorsal horn of the spinal cord. Primary nociceptors synapse in Rexed's laminae I, II, and V within the dorsal horn of the spinal cord.
2. Dorsal horn neurons that receive primary afferent input and their respective interneuronal connections with the dorsal horn. The cell bodies within the dorsal horn in turn receive input from a series of excitatory (e.g., glutamate, substance P) and inhibitory (e.g., enkephalin, serotonin, norepinephrine) neurotransmitters.
3. A series of ascending relay neurons between the spinal cord, brainstem, and thalamus (spinothalamic tract).
4. The thalamocortical projections.[49,72]

Modulation refers to the process controlling the quantity of nociceptive transmission propagated from the periphery to higher rostral centers. Endogenous analgesic substances (serotonin, norepinephrine, opioids) are produced in diffuse areas throughout the central nervous system. Axons from these diffuse locations coalesce into a pathway called the dorsolateral funiculus. The dorsolateral funiculus synapses in exactly the same areas of the dorsal horn receiving nociceptive transmission from primary nociceptors (Rexed's laminae I, II, and V). Thus, nociceptive transmission can be selectively inhibited at the level of the dorsal horn of the spinal cord.[49,72]

Because pain is, by definition, a subjective and emotional experience, perception must occur. Unfortunately, the mechanisms and processes underlying perception remain obscure. To reiterate, the individual physiologic processes comprise what we refer to as nociception. The processes of nociception in conjunction with perception (eliciting a subjective and emotional experience) are what we refer to as pain.

The Gate Control Theory of Pain

The physiologic processes of nociception all converge and impact upon the firing patterns of dorsal horn neurons within laminae I, II, and V of the spinal cord. Thus, the dorsal horn can be viewed as the focal point or gate for the integration and modulation of nociception (Fig. 3).[102,103] Processes that enhance nociceptive transmission through the dorsal horn open the gate. Administration of analgesics that mimic the endogenous analgesic substances subserving modulation, or processes that enhance modulation will close the gate.[102,103] Thus, the neural pathways and neurotransmitters subserving nociception should not be conceptualized as mere cables or telephone wires. Nociception is a dynamic and fluid process.

Neuropathic Pain

As previously stated, neuropathic pain is derived from injury to a peripheral or central neural structure. Neuropathic pain is typically described as sharp or burning. There are three subsets of neuropathic pain. Peripherally generated neuropathic pain involves such entities as cervical radiculopathy, spinal nerve lesions, brachial plexus injuries, thoracic outlet syndrome, and entrapment neuropathies. Centrally generated pain involves injury to the central nervous system at the level of the spinal cord or above. This type of pain is usually relatively unimportant with respect to shoulder pain. Sympathetically maintained pain may be generated peripherally or centrally and is characterized by localized autonomic dysregulation in the affected area with vasomotor and/or pilomotor changes, edema and sweating, and atrophic changes. It is referred to as reflex sympathetic dystrophy (RSD), causalgia, or more recently, complex regional pain syndrome. Sympathetically maintained pain is extremely important as a disease entity involving the shoulder.

Chronic Somatic Painful Conditions

A differential diagnosis of the somatic and neuropathic pathologies that can generate acute and chronic shoulder pain is listed in Table 2. Of course, a rigorous discussion of the various tendonidites, arthritides, fractures, infections, and tumors that can generate chronic somatic pain are beyond the scope of this chapter. However, myofascial pain involving the muscles of the shoulder is quite common. Therefore, it would be worthwhile to discuss this entity in detail.

Regional Myofascial Pain Syndrome

Irrespective of our focus and emphasis on the shoulder, myofascial pain represents one of the most common causes of chronic pain in general. Regional myofascial pain syndrome[151] must be distinguished from fibromyalgia[171] (which will be discussed later). The hallmark characteristics of regional myofascial pain are: (a) localization within a circumscribed muscle or group of muscles in a particular area of the body and (b) the presence of trigger points. Trigger points are hyperirritable nodules that feel like cords of rope within the body of a skeletal muscle or surrounding fascia. Trigger points can develop after different types of trauma, many of which are seemingly insignificant. Quite often, trigger points are the result of repetitive injury (e.g., trigger points with the body of trapezius in a typist).

On physical examination, the trigger point can produce a localized involuntary twitch response to palpation. This involuntary twitch response represents a brief contraction of muscle fibers within an involved muscle. At the same time, a patient also may have a voluntary response to palpation of a trigger point. This voluntary response is most commonly manifested as patient movement or vocalization and has been called the jump sign. Trigger points within specific muscles have well-described, characteristic referral patterns to other areas of the body.[171] These patterns of radiation may not seemingly follow normal anatomic radiation patterns, i.e., radiation along the course of peripheral nerves or dermatomes. However, the somewhat atypical and unusual patterns of trigger point radiation are well described and reproducible.[171]

Trigger points may be characterized as either active or

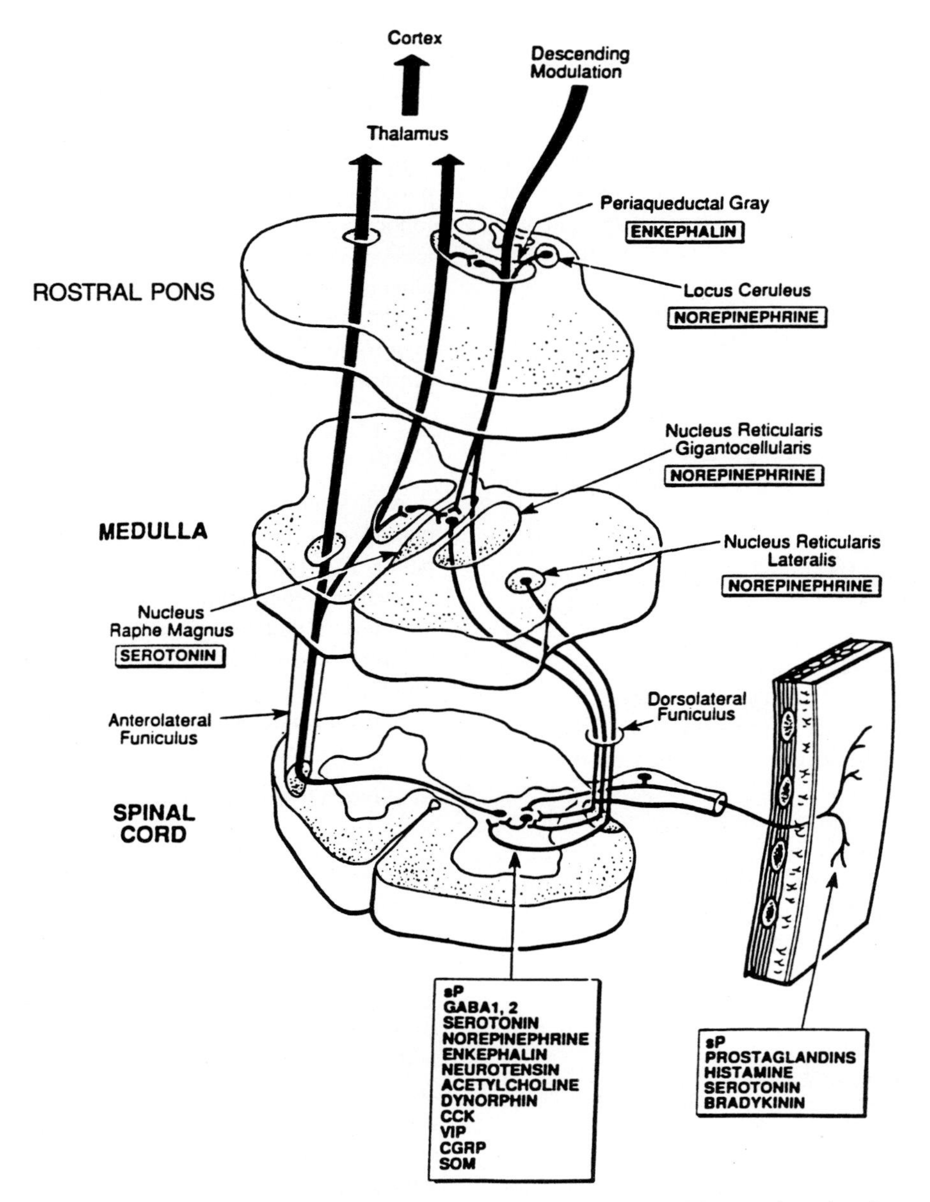

FIG. 3. The gate control theory of pain. The physiologic processes underlying nociception (transduction, transmission, and modulation). All converge on and impact on the discharge of dorsal horn neurons in Rexed's laminae I, II, and V. Thus, the dorsal horn of the spinal cord is the focal point or gate for integration of the processes of nociception. (Reprinted with permission from ref. 32.)

passive. Active trigger points are a present source of pain and elicit the characteristic responses outlined above. A passive or latent trigger point is not a present source of pain to the patient. However, passive or latent trigger points can cause pain when sufficient pressure is applied during palpation.

The pathogenesis of trigger points is unclear. Injured muscles that do not heal and progress to chronic pain appear to develop problems within the sarcomere early in the natural history of the process. Uncontrolled contraction of the sarcomere may lead to development of a trigger point.[152] On a molecular basis, inability to physiologically utilize calcium may cause actin and myosin to function improperly. Thus, a muscle fibril becomes, in essence, paralyzed and unable to relax.[150]

Histologic findings of muscle biopsies have shown a number of different abnormalities. These include disruption of myofibrillar structure, increased amounts of mucopolysaccharides, multifocal loss of oxidative enzymes, and potential mitochondrial damage.[8] In keeping with theories regarding abnormal calcium homeostasis, one study has shown a decreased level of high-energy phosphates in muscle biopsy samples from the trapezius muscle, suggesting an abnormality of actin and myosin physiology.[80]

Treatment of regional myofascial pain involves medical, invasive, and physical therapeutic modalities. Nonsteroidal antiinflammatory medications (NSAIDs) and tricyclic antidepressants (TCAs; unlike the serotonin-specific reuptake inhibitors [SSRIs]) have been shown to provide effective analgesia.[23,145] Muscle relaxants have been widely used in the treatment of myofascial pain, despite the fact that they have not been rigorously studied to the same extent as NSAIDs and antidepressants. However, some patients will anecdotally report great benefit from the use of muscle relaxants. Membrane-stabilizing drugs have not been shown to produce significant analgesia in regional myofascial pain.

Injection of active trigger points has been advocated by some investigators, although scientific studies have been inconclusive regarding their long-term effects.[132,145] Trigger point injections have utilized saline, local anesthetics, corticosteroids, or combinations of these as the injectate, or injections have been given without medications (dry needling).

Physical medicine modalities are the most important treatment for regional myofascial pain. Historically, stretch and spray exercises have been used. These techniques involve use of vapocoolant sprays (ethyl chloride, fluorimethane), with stretching of the affected muscle. More recently, specific myofascial release physical therapeutic techniques have been developed and have gained great success in the rehabilitation of patients with regional myofascial pain.

Fibromyalgia

Fibromyalgia is a musculoskeletal disorder with marked similarity to regional myofascial pain.[58,97] The prevalence of fibromyalgia in the population is approximately 0.7% to 3.2%.[69] The high prevalence of disability among patients with fibromyalgia represents a significant cost to society in health-care dollars.[88]

Although regional myofascial pain and fibromyalgia share many characteristics, they are distinct clinical entities (Table 3). Myofascial pain is topographically discrete and localized, whereas fibromyalgia is diffuse and widespread. The American College of Rheumatology has developed criteria for the diagnosis of fibromyalgia.[182] When 11 of 18 tender points elicit pain by palpation (in nine paired anatomically defined sites) with concomitant widespread muscular aching, a sensitivity of 88.4% and a specificity of 81.1% is achieved for the diagnosis of fibromyalgia.[182] Trigger points are deemed to be specific for regional myofascial pain syndrome. Trigger points elicit pain upon palpation of the muscle belly, whereas tender points occur at the muscle–tendon junction. Moreover, trigger points have reproducible patterns of radiation, whereas tender points do not radiate. No data are available on the prevalence of trigger points in fibromyalgia.

TABLE 3. *Characteristics of regional myofascial pain and fibromyalgia*

	Regional myofascial pain	Fibromyalgia
Gender	2 female:1 male	10 female:1 male
Pain	Local and referred	Local
Distribution of		
Tender or trigger points	Regional	Widespread
Tender/trigger point anatomy	Muscle belly (trigger point)	Muscle–tendon junction (tender point)
Stiffness	Regional	Widespread
Treatment	Drugs, local injection, stretch, and spray	Drugs
Prognosis	Excellent	Chronic pain

Regional myofascial pain syndrome is the result of trauma, microtrauma, or repetitive injury to muscle. On the other hand, fibromyalgia presents without a history of trauma or even an inciting event.

Fatigue and sleep disturbance are found in fibromyalgia but not regional myofascial pain.[183] The sleep disturbance is characterized by a nonrestorative pattern. The patient awakens each morning unrefreshed. These symptoms may be the result of an α-δ sleep abnormality.[98]

Fibromyalgia has been reported in conjunction with connective tissue disorders.[191] The prevalence of regional myofascial pain is not increased in rheumatologic disorders in comparison with the general population.

Two of the anatomically defined sites for the diagnosis of fibromyalgia by the American College of Rheumatology[182] lie within the musculature of the shoulder. Thus, pain in the shoulder musculature as a presenting feature of fibromyalgia is not unusual. The orthopedic surgeon must have a clear working knowledge of the distinction between regional myofascial pain and fibromyalgia. Patients with either clinical entity should be referred to a pain center for appropriate therapy.

The treatment of fibromyalgia should involve interdisciplinary expertise. The cornerstone of therapy is pharmacologic management with NSAIDs and TCAs.[23,145] Use of trigger point injections has been uniformly disappointing in patients with fibromyalgia, because of the diffuse nature of the disease. Physical therapy is paramount in the treatment of fibromyalgia, but many patients reject it because of the painful nature of the disease process. However, all physical therapeutic efforts should be formulated within the framework of a strengthening and conditioning program. Many patients with fibromyalgia lack insight into their disease, as well as coping strategies, and may appear depressed and anxious.[6] Many patients may benefit from psychological intervention, as well as psychotropic medication where appropriate.

Chronic Neuropathic Painful Conditions

The remainder of our discussions of pathophysiologic entities of the shoulder will involve neuropathic pain states.

Cervical Pathology

Cervical spondylosis involves osteoarthritic degenerative changes of the joints of the cervical spine: the disc itself, the facet, and the uncovertebral joints. Osteophytes may form at all of the aforementioned joints and encroach upon the nerve root foramina. Changes in the cervical discs themselves consist of chronic degeneration and dessication. The discs can flatten and bulge outward with promotion of osteophyte formation.

Disc herniation consists of protrusion of the nucleus pulposus through a tear in the annulus fibrosus. The nerve root may be compressed within its foramen when the herniation occurs in a lateral or dorsolateral direction, thereby potentially generating a cervical radiculopathy. Disc herniation may occur in conjunction with chronic spondylotic changes in the cervical spine.[160]

Cervical radiculopathy and myelopathy may be generated by acute, subacute, or insidious (with the possibility of spinal cord compression) disc herniation. Acute cervical disc herniation is much less common than in the lumbar area. Pain is the predominant symptom of acute cervical radiculopathy. The pain is often widely distributed over the shoulder, scapula, upper chest, and arm, and may be appreciated deep within certain muscles. Radicular pain (paresthesia) is present in a dermatomal pattern. Muscle weakness is usually mild but can be severe. The dermatomal distribution of the radicular pain, as well as weakness within certain muscles (Table 1), may be diagnostic aids in determination of the involved root.[181]

Subacute cervical radiculopathy is much more common than acute radiculopathy and results from disc herniation occurring in conjunction with chronic spondylotic changes. Pain and paresthesias are present, as in the acute form. Unlike acute radiculopathy, mild sensory loss or hyperesthesia, along with moderate weakness, is common. The most commonly involved discs are C5–6 and C6–7.[181]

Radicular myelopathy may result from compression of the spinal cord. Cervical degenerative discs, spondylosis of the facet and/or uncovertebral joints, and posterior vertebral osteophytes may be involved in the compressive mechanism. Furthermore, a hypertrophied and inelastic ligamentum flavum may compress the cord with neck extension.[162] The result of these chronic spondylotic changes with spinal cord compression is a myelopathic constellation of symptoms affecting both the arm and legs. In contradistinction to acute and subacute radiculopathy, pain and sensory changes are usually minimal with respect to upper limb symptoms. On the other hand, muscle weakness and wasting may be severe. Abnormalities in the legs include spastic weakness and variable sensory loss (with vibratory sense being most affected). Deep tendon reflexes in the legs are hyperreflexic, whereas those in the arms are hyporeflexic.[160]

As can be seen from our liberal use of radiologic images to illustrate various aspects of cervical pathology, computed tomography (CT), myelography, CT myelography, and magnetic resonance imaging (MRI) are essential for the evaluation and diagnosis of mechanical and radicular cervical spine pain. An exhaustive discussion of the indications for each ra-

TABLE 4. *Radiologic imaging techniques in the evaluation of degenerative disc disease*

Technique	Advantages	Disadvantages
Computed tomography	Visualizes location, size, migration and sequestration of herniation Evaluates status of bony canal and epidural space	More or less adequate demonstration of disc herniation Exam limited to two to three levels Tissue less well visualized than bone Difficult with scoliosis Inferior to MRI for evaluation of cervical pathology Nondynamic (flexion and extension not allowed)
Myelography	Visualizes entire subarachnoid space, cord, and roots Better visualization of disc and nerve root abnormalities Dynamic (flexion and extension permissible)	Invasive Possible side effects from subarachnoid contrast No visualization of extradural segment of roots and epidural space Poor visualization of spinal cord or nerve roots above a block
CT myelography	Combines advantages of CT with myelography Lower volume and concentration of contrast with fewer side effects Better sensitivity with block Better visualization of neural structures at or above the level of a block	Invasive Possible side effects from subarachnoid contrast
MRI	Excellent for soft-tissue visualization Survey of spine possible Multiplanar capacity Less shoulder artifact Higher contrast resolution Direct visualization of cord and discs	Contraindicated in patients with metallic hardware and prostheses Spatial resolution less than CT myelography Inferior to CT and CT myelography for study of bony pathology

diologic technique is beyond the scope of this chapter. However, some relative guidelines for use and the respective advantages and disadvantages of each technique are listed in Table 4.

Treatment of the pain of spondylosis itself may be amenable to NSAIDs. Acute and subacute radiculopathy may be ameliorated by NSAIDs and cervical epidural steroid injections (CESIs),[25,27,48,139,177] with rehabilitation facilitated by physical therapy. Judicious surgical intervention may guard against the devastating effects of radiculomyelopathy.

Cervical Epidural Steroid Injection

The utility of CESI for the treatment of cervical radiculopathy has recently been a topic of great interest.[25,27,48,139,177] A clinical classification scheme (Table 5) and an algorithm (Fig. 4) for the rational use of epidural steroid injections was recently developed by Ferrante et al.[48] In general, patients with radicular symptoms and signs have the best potential for benefit after CESI, in contradistinction to patients with axial neck pain.[48]

Cervical epidural steroid injection is performed at the interspace appropriate for the dermatomal distribution of pain[48,139,177] or at the C7–T1 interspace in all patients,[25,27,139] depending on the respective investigator and study. Patients are placed either in the sitting position with the neck flexed and resting on a pillow, or are placed in a decubitus position with the painful side most dependent. Both loss of resistance techniques and hanging-drop techniques have been used. Because of the loss of tactile strength of the ligamentum flavum as it progresses from the lumbar to the cervical area, loss of resistance may be difficult to appreciate in certain individuals when performing cervical epidural injections. Because of the large negative pressure in the cervical epidural space in the sitting position, the hanging-drop technique has a readily appreciable end point and is easier to perform.

Methylprednisolone acetate or triamcinolone diacetate is usually employed as the steroid preparation in the cervical epidural space. Certain investigators also have included morphine, although the long-term utility of morphine in the treatment of cervical pathology is unconfirmed.[25] The steroid should be mixed with local anesthetic and saline, and several treatment protocols have been described.[25,27,48,139,177] In general, a lower volume of injectate should be used as compared with the lumbar area. Saline should be used to flush the epidural needle as it is being withdrawn, in order to prevent the possible development of a tract.

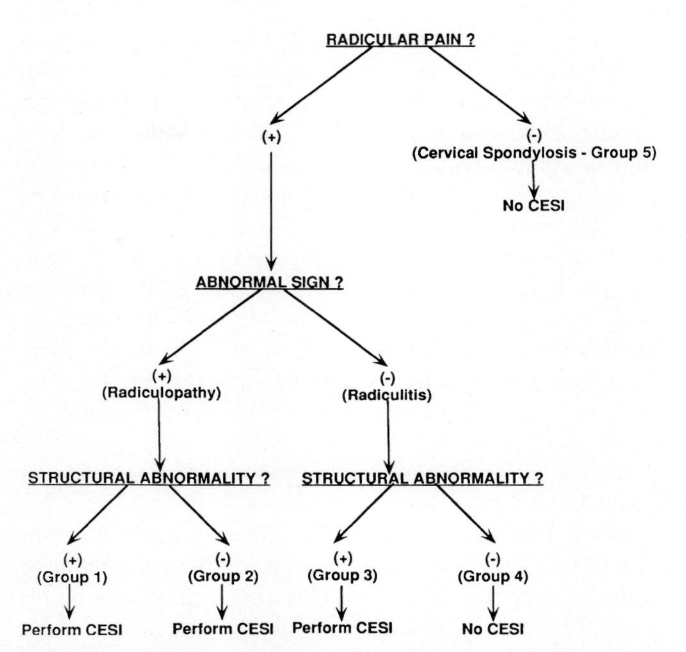

FIG. 4. An algorithm for the effective use of CESI in the treatment of cervical radiculopathy and neck pain. Group numbers refer to the clinical groups within the classification scheme from Table 5. (Reprinted with permission from ref. 48.)

Brachial Plexopathies

Stretch (Traction), Compression, and Other Traumatic Injury

Because of its superficial location, the mobility of the shoulder and the neck, and its close proximity to many bony structures, the brachial plexus is particularly susceptible to

TABLE 5. *Clinical classification schema for outcome after CESI*

Pathology	Figure 4 algorithm outcome group	Symptom	Sign	Structure[a]
Radiculopathy with structural abnormality	Group 1	+	+	+
Radiculopathy without structural abnormality	Group 2	+	+	
Radiculitis with structural abnormality	Group 3	+	−	+
Radiculitis without structural abnormality	Group 4	+	−	−
Cervical spondylosis	Group 5	−	−	−

Radiculopathy is characterized by a positive sign (hypesthesia, hyporeflexia, motor weakness, or positive electromyography) only if the sign is correlated with the nerve root responsible for pain. Radiculitis is characterized by pain in a specific dermatome without a correlating positive sign.

[a] Refers to the presence of a structural abnormality elicited by roentgenography, CT scan, MRI, or myelography if the structure correlates with the painful dermatome.

traumatic injury. Stretch (traction) injuries are particularly common after falls and motorcycle accidents, when the head and neck are moved in one direction and the shoulder is moved in the opposite direction. The brachial plexus also may be compressed or crushed between the clavicle and underlying ribs, or damaged by bony fragments, displaced muscles, hematomas, or missiles.[160]

Fractures and dislocations of the shoulder frequently damage the brachial plexus.[83,99] Dislocations of the shoulder without a concomitant fracture more frequently injure the axillary nerve than the brachial plexus itself, however. Bony fragments or hematoma associated with fractures of the clavicle can damage the plexus and cause brachial plexopathy.[187] Even after healing of a clavicular fracture, callus formation at the site of the fracture can cause chronic compression of the brachial plexus.[45]

When damage to the brachial plexus does occur, it is usually diffuse, with varying degrees of injury associated with different parts of the plexus. However, injury may be restricted to just one trunk or cord. Complicating matters, there are usually other neural injuries associated with the brachial plexopathy: (a) cervical nerve root avulsion, (b) injury to the spinal cord, and (c) damage to individual nerves which arise from the plexus.

Nerve Root Avulsion

Avulsion of spinal nerve roots involves tearing of the dorsal and ventral roots of one or more spinal nerves from the spinal cord. Of course, avulsion is a particularly serious result of stretch injuries to the brachial plexus. The lower cervical roots (including T1) are most often involved.

Neuropathic pain is almost uniformly produced after traumatic root avulsion.[111] The topographic distribution of pain conforms to the dermatome of the avulsed root(s). (Hand and forearm pain occurs after C6, C7, C8, or T1 root avulsions. Shoulder pain occurs after C5 root avulsion.) Hot, burning, electric shock, or pressure sensations form a continuous background of severe pain. Superimposed upon this background are paroxysms of pain of unbearable intensity that radiate from the hand to the shoulder and are described as sharp, shooting, or lightning-like. More typical paresthesias following normal dermatomal distributions also occur. Of note, individuals may often be aware of a phantom limb with sensations of movement when an effort is made to use any of the paralyzed musculature.[111]

Careful physical examination (Table 1) is essential in localization of the injury to a specific area of the plexus. In conjunction with physical examination, radiographic studies and electrophysiologic studies are essential in the diagnosis of root avulsion.

CT myelography[109] and myelography[115,188] are useful in the diagnosis of cervical nerve root avulsion. Root avulsions can be well demonstrated on CT myelography or myelography, because when a root is avulsed, the meninges are pulled away from the spinal cord into and through the nerve root foramen. The meninges form a small pseudomeningocele that can fill with contrast medium.[188] Experience with imaging nerve root avulsions with MRI is limited and inconclusive.[128]

Irrespective of the radiographic technique employed, the most optimal assessment of nerve root avulsion and plexus injury combines radiographic visualization with electrophysiologic testing. Electromyography (EMG) can assist in the assessment of nerve root avulsion, because it permits evaluation of the paraspinal muscles (which cannot be evaluated clinically) and because it may indicate the severity of damage. In nerve root avulsion, EMG of paraspinal muscles is abnormal, because damage to the roots is proximal to the dorsal rami.[19] Sensory action potentials recorded from the arm are normal in nerve root avulsion because distal sensory fibers are still viable, because they are not separated from their cell bodies. Sensory action potentials may be normal, even in the face of dense anesthesia in the distribution of the avulsed root(s).[178] In contrast, sensory action potentials are reduced or absent in brachial plexus lesions, because damage to nerve fibers is distal to the dorsal root ganglion.

Somatosensory evoked potentials (SSEPs) also have been used in the evaluation of brachial plexopathies.[189] However, they do not seem to be more accurate than EMG in localization of lesions.

During the first 3-4 months after avulsion, spontaneous recovery from neuropraxia can occur. During this time period, neuropathic pain should be treated with TCAs and membrane-stabilizing agents. Aggressive physiotherapy is important to prevent contractures and joint ankylosis.[105]

If no nerve regeneration is present after 4 months and if electrophysiologic studies show evidence of severe axonal degeneration, the brachial plexus should be surgically explored.[105] Surgical repair of the brachial plexus can restore function and reduce pain.[105,108] More recently, bypass coaptation procedures have resulted in significant return of neurologic function after cervical nerve root avulsion.[185,186] Complete or partial return of sensory and motor function has been achieved.[185,186] Although experience with this procedure is limited, bypass coaptation should be performed as soon as possible after the cervical nerve root avulsion, unlike older surgical procedures.[185,186]

Ablative procedures should not be entertained until the possibility of *de novo* nerve regeneration or functional recovery from bypass coaptation procedures has waned. Amputation should not be considered, because it will not relieve the pain of root avulsion. Ablation of the dorsal root entry zone (DREZ lesion) can greatly reduce the pain of nerve root avulsion.[169]

Stingers and Burners

Stingers and burners are synonymous terms for a common syndrome that is seen after a head, neck, or shoulder blow in players of contact sports. Immediately after the injury, the individual appreciates a sharp pain in the shoulder radiating into the arm and hand and often into the thumb. This may be accompanied by weakness of the biceps or the musculature of the shoulder girdle. Stingers are a transient phenomenon that can last only a few minutes but may at times persist for hours or even weeks. Permanent neurologic sequelae are uncommon. The exact nature and localization of the injury are obscure. The syndrome probably results from transient nerve damage in several locations: the cervical spinal cord, nerve roots, ventral rami, and upper trunk of the brachial plexus.[37,94]

Intraoperative Brachial Plexus Injuries

Damage to the brachial plexus also may occur during general anesthesia. Such injuries are due to hyperabduction of the arm and stretch of the plexus because of poor positioning of the patient.[95] Intraoperative brachial plexus injury is particularly common after procedures involving median sternotomy and has been estimated to occur in 5% of all such patients.[81] The lower trunk or medial cord is most commonly involved, although any part of the plexus can be damaged.

Brachial Plexus Neuritis

Acute brachial plexus neuritis can develop at any age for reasons that are obscure. The pain is of great intensity and does not follow a radicular or peripheral nerve distribution. Sensory abnormalities are usually of less intensity than the pain and ensuing muscle weakness. The serratus anterior, deltoid, infraspinatus, and supraspinatus muscles are most commonly involved, although involvement of individual muscles or muscle groups is highly variable. Weakness of the musculature may indicate involvement of a single nerve, two nerves, or a discrete part of the plexus, usually the upper trunk. Acute brachial plexus neuritis is asymmetric in only about one third of cases and is most commonly found as a bilateral condition.[173]

A number of antecedent infectious, traumatic, or surgical events have been suggested as the key factors in the pathogenesis of brachial plexus neuritis.[160] Because of the many different infections that are implicated (as well as the occasional occurrence of epidemics), a viral etiology has been suggested as the origin of the pathogenesis of acute brachial plexus neuritis.[184] A causal relationship has not been proven.[7] An immune complex vasculitis also has been hypothesized as the pathogenic mechanism. No cause-and-effect relationship has been definitively demonstrated.[160]

Malignant Invasion and Radiation Neuritis

Tumors invading the brachial plexus include cancer of the breast (most common) and Pancoast's tumor. In cancer of the breast, brachial plexus invasion occurs via spread from lymph nodes or bone metastases. The predominant symptom is shoulder pain that radiates down the medial aspect of the arm and forearm into the lateral two (ulnar) fingers. Paresthesias and weakness develop later in the natural history. Malignant invasion of the brachial plexus is rarely an early manifestation of breast cancer.

In contradistinction, brachial plexopathy presents as an early manifestation of Pancoast's tumor.[82] Pancoast's tumor (superior pulmonary sulcus tumor) is almost always caused by invasion of the lower trunk of the brachial plexus by carcinoma of the lung at the apex. The presenting symptom is usually pain radiating along the inner aspect of the arm. Weakness and sensory changes are usually localized to the lower trunk of the brachial plexus. Almost two thirds of patients will develop Horner's syndrome, due to infiltration of the inferior cervical sympathetic ganglion.[66]

If a patient has received radiation to the upper chest wall and supraclavicular area for the treatment of malignant disease, radiation-induced brachial plexopathy with fibrosis of the brachial plexus may occur. Radiation damage to the brachial plexus is dose dependent. Onset of plexopathy may be years after irradiation. Radiation-induced brachial plexopathy can occur without any sign of radiation damage to the overlying skin. The presence of non-neurologic signs (e.g., lymphedema and induration) may be found in both radiation neuritis and malignant invasion of the brachial plexus.[170]

Thoracic Outlet Syndromes

Numerous anatomic variations are found at the cervicothoracic junction. Some of these anatomic variations can compress vascular or neural structures to generate a variety of thoracic outlet syndromes. Usually, in discussion of thoracic outlet syndromes, a laundry list of these anatomic structures is presented and discussed. It is perhaps wiser to conceptualize the thoracic outlet syndromes pathophysiologically than anatomically.

The thoracic outlet syndromes comprise three different clinical pathophysiologic entities.[160] Neurologic thoracic outlet syndrome consists of weakness and sensory loss in the arm and hand and results from stretch and/or compression of the lower trunk of the brachial plexus. The presence of an accessory cervical rib with or without a fibrous band, an abnormal first rib, hypertrophy of the anterior scalene muscle (scalenus anticus syndrome), and hyperabduction syndrome are some of the anatomic variations that may be responsible for neurologic syndromes. Vascular thoracic outlet syndrome consists of narrowing of the subclavian artery as it angles over the first rib in patients with a well-developed cervical rib. There may be intermittent blanching of the fingers or the entire hand. There may be signs of ischemia and even gangrene. However, there are usually no neurologic symptoms. The third and most common type of thoracic outlet syndrome presents without neurologic or vascular abnormalities but with symptomatology of pain and/or paresthesias in the arms. It has been suggested that symptomatology results from compression of the brachial plexus between the clavicle and a normal first rib (costoclavicular syndrome). However, the anatomic and pathophysiologic bases, diagnostic criteria, and treatment for this third type of thoracic outlet syndrome are uncertain and controversial.

Neurologic Thoracic Outlet Syndrome

Neurologic thoracic outlet syndrome is found mainly in women. It begins to manifest itself as pain along the medial aspect of the arm and forearm. Paresthesias are found extending into the ulnar border of the hand. Muscle weakness and atrophy occur later. Muscle atrophy is selective for the abductor pollicis brevis and the opponens muscles of the thenar eminence. Wasting of all the intrinsic muscles of the hand is possible with progression of the condition. There are no vascular symptoms. Sensory abnormalities are referrable to the lower trunk of the brachial plexus.[56]

A well-developed cervical or rudimentary cervical rib with a fibrous band extending to the upper surface of the first rib may impinge on the lower trunk of the brachial plexus (Fig. 5).[14,56,57,85] Similarly, anatomic abnormalities of the first rib may stretch and angulate the lower trunk of the brachial plexus. The scalenus anticus syndrome involves hypertrophy of the anterior scalene muscle and compression of the brachial plexus as it passes through the interscalene groove between the anterior and middle scalene muscles (Fig. 6). Hyperabduction syndrome or subcoracoid-pectoralis minor syndrome involves compression of the brachial plexus with lateral abduction of the arm to an elevated position. In this position, the brachial plexus and vasculature are compressed by tension of the pectoralis minor muscle and, to a lesser extent, the coracoid process.[85]

Physical examination, roentgenographs, and electrophysiologic studies should be employed in determination of the diagnosis of neurologic thoracic outlet syndrome. Roentgenographs will almost uniformly show the characteristic bony abnormality responsible for the neurologic symptomotology. If a bony abnormality is not seen, then consideration must be given to the presence of fibrous bands,[14] scalenus anticus syndrome or hyperabduction syndrome. Electrophysiologic studies can differentiate neurologic thoracic outlet syndrome from carpal tunnel syndrome and ulnar neuropathy.[57] SSEPs, following stimulation of the ulnar nerve at the wrist, may actually be a more useful technique.[190]

Supraclavicular exploration with release of the compressive anatomy is the most satisfactory treatment for neurologic thoracic outlet syndrome. Patients experience immediate relief of pain. Unfortunately, muscle weakness and atrophy do not usually improve.[56]

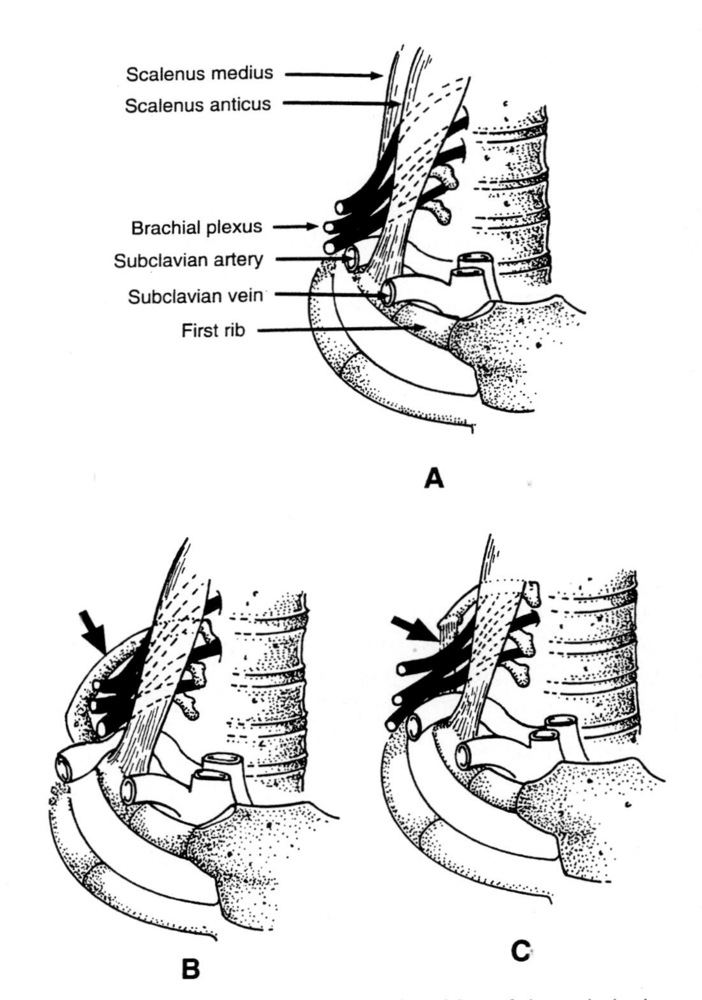

FIG. 5. (A) Normal anatomic relationships of the subclavian artery and the brachial plexus at the cervicothoracic junction. **(B)** Vascular thoracic outlet syndrome. The subclavian artery is angulated over a well-developed cervical rib. The subclavian artery is also sandwiched between the cervical rib and the anterior scalene muscle. Both these anatomic relationships cause stenosis of the subclavian artery and poststenotic dilation of the artery. **(C)** Neurologic thoracic outlet syndrome. The normal anatomic relationships of the first rib, lower trunk, medial cord of the brachial plexus, subclavian artery, and anterior scalene muscle are shown on the right. On the left, a small cervical rib and a fibrous band are depicted. The lower trunk of the brachial plexus is angulated over this band, and this anatomic relationship can generate neurologic thoracic outlet syndrome. (Reprinted with permission from ref. 160.)

Vascular Thoracic Outlet Syndrome

In patients with a well-developed first rib, the subclavian artery may be angulated over the cervical rib and wedged between the anterior scalene muscle and the cervical rib (Fig. 5). The subclavian artery will become narrowed and will develop an area of poststenotic dilation. Thrombus may accumulate in the poststenotic dilation, fragment, and embolize to the hand. This produces vascular symptomotology with intermittent blanching of the hands and fingers. Pulses may be diminished or absent. A bruit can sometimes be auscultated in the supraclavicular and/or axillary areas. The vascular thoracic outlet syndrome consists only of vascular symptomotology without neurologic abnormalities. Angiography will confirm the diagnosis. Surgical excision of the cervical rib effectively treats vascular thoracic outlet syndrome.[41]

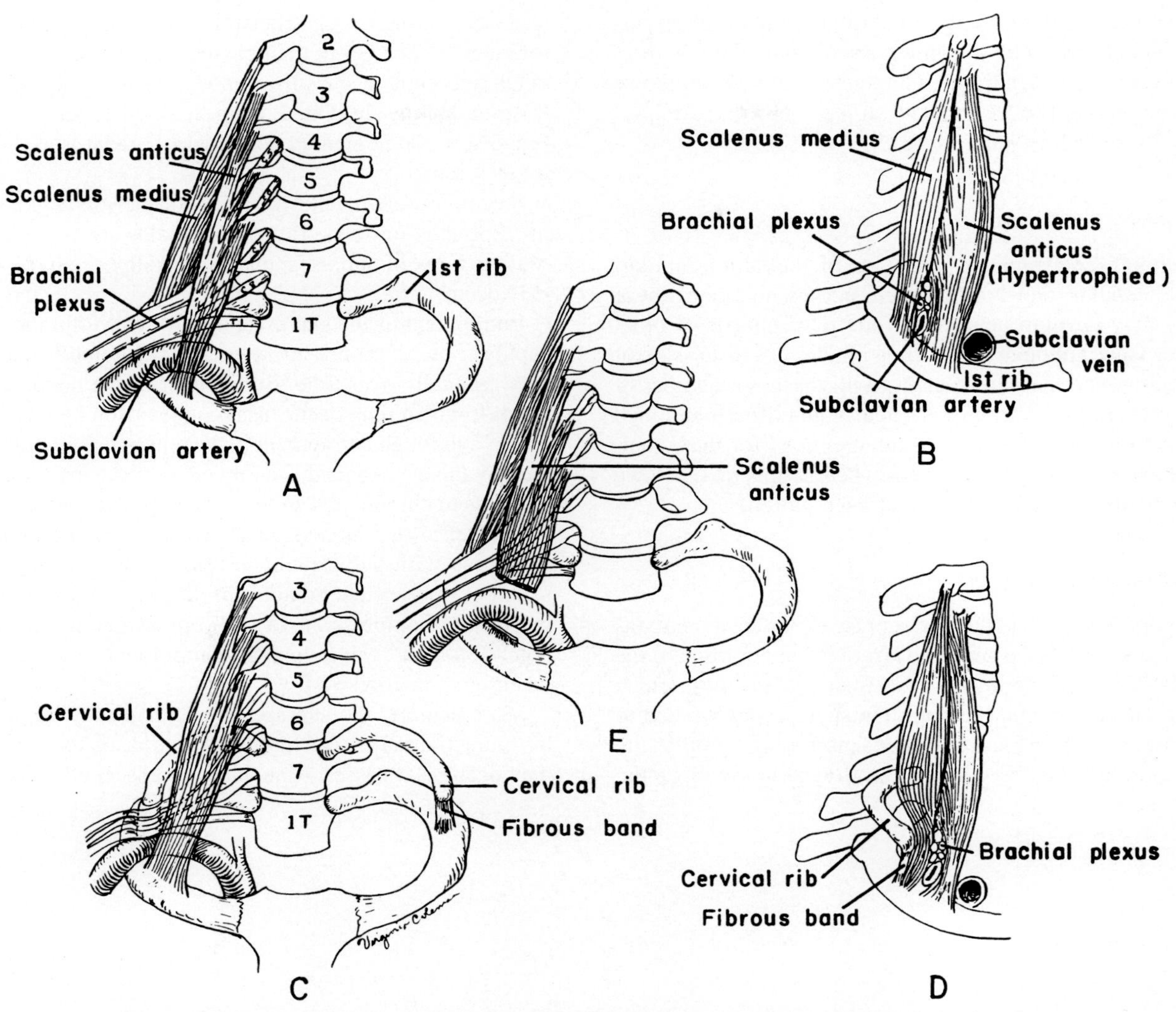

FIG. 6. Anatomic relationships generating scalenus anticus syndrome in the presence and absence of a cervical rib. **(A)** Normal. **(B)** Hypertrophied anterior scalene muscle compresses the brachial plexus and the subclavian artery. **(C and D)** Compression of the brachial plexus by a cervical rib. **(E)** Relief of compression by scalenostomy. (Reprinted with permission from ref. 85.)

Thoracic Outlet Syndrome of Pain and Sensory Symptoms

The largest group of patients with thoracic outlet syndrome will present with less clearly defined symptomotology than the aforementioned two rare, but well defined, thoracic outlet syndromes. Such patients will usually present with a diffuse nagging ache and numbness in the arm. The pain in the arm will be made worse by carrying heavy objects or holding the arm in particular positions. Paresthesias may occur concomitantly with the pain or may be temporally distinct. Paresthesias are usually appreciated in the medial aspect of the arm and forearm and sometimes in the hand.

The exact pathophysiology underlying the aforementioned symptomotology is obscure. Various proposed mechanisms include: (a) compression of the subclavian artery and/or brachial plexus between the lower end of the anterior scalene muscle and the first rib[56]; (b) vascular factors (i.e., venous rather than arterial compression[135]); and (c) costoclavicular syndrome. The costoclavicular syndrome[46,47] suggests that the subclavian artery and/or the brachial plexus are intermittently compressed between the clavicle and a normal first rib. Patients believed to have costoclavicular syndrome are women with long necks and drooping shoulders. Symptomotology has been hypothesized to result from chronic stretching of the brachial plexus.[164]

Investigations to confirm this more common but obscure form of thoracic outlet syndrome are usually unrewarding. Roentgenographs, EMG, nerve conduction studies, SSEPs, and arteriography are usually normal and of limited value.

Because costoclavicular syndrome has been hypothesized to result from chronic stretching of the brachial plexus in women with drooping shoulders, exercises to counteract and strengthen drooping shoulders have been proposed as a possible treatment. Symptomotology is believed to be reduced or relieved in 40% to 85% of patients,[164] although all studies do not report similar findings. First rib resection is often performed in patients with this more obscure but common form of thoracic outlet syndrome. Complete relief of symptoms has been reported in 55% to 85% of patients with partial relief in 7% to 35% of patients.[141]

Entrapment Syndromes

Although entrapment syndromes of the suprascapular, dorsal scapular, and long thoracic nerves do occur, these nerves may develop neuropathy due to a number of other factors. Thus, although the heading alludes to a discussion of only entrapment neuropathies, we will discuss a number of the disorders that may affect each of the aforementioned nerves. Moreover, the surgical interventions for these maladies have been fully covered elsewhere in this text, and we will only discuss their nonsurgical intervention.

Suprascapular Nerve

As previously discussed, the suprascapular nerve contains fibers from C5 and C6 and arises from the upper trunk of the brachial plexus. Coursing underneath the trapezius muscle, it passes onto the scapula through the suprascapular notch to the supraspinatus fossa of the scapula, to supply the supraspinatus muscle (Fig. 7). A ligament overlies the suprascapular notch and transforms the notch into an actual foramen.[131] The nerve then passes around the spinoglenoid notch and ends in the infraspinous fossa, to supply the infraspinatus muscle. Once again, a small ligament may be found at the spinoglenoid notch, which transforms the notch into a foramen.[2]

Selective wasting and weakness of the supraspinatus and infraspinatus muscles, rather than pain, are the usual presenting signs of suprascapular neuropathy. Pain, of course, may occur.

Entrapment of the suprascapular nerve within the suprascapular notch/foramen or spinoglenoid notch/foramen occurs gradually over time. Entrapment of the nerve in either notch/foramen may occur from compression by a tight ligament,[54] although entrapment in the spinoglenoid notch/foramen by this mechanism is a rare event.[24] A small notch predisposes to entrapment. In the suprascapular notch/foramen, the presence of a bone spur also may cause entrapment.[54] Fractures with subsequent development of callus[154] and shoulder injuries that do not cause a fracture also may result in chronic compression of the suprascapular nerve in its notch/foramen.[131] Entrapment compression may occur as a result of a ganglion cyst.

More acutely, the suprascapular nerve may be damaged by blunt trauma or fractures.[43] Traction of the nerve also may occur as it passes through the suprascapular notch after

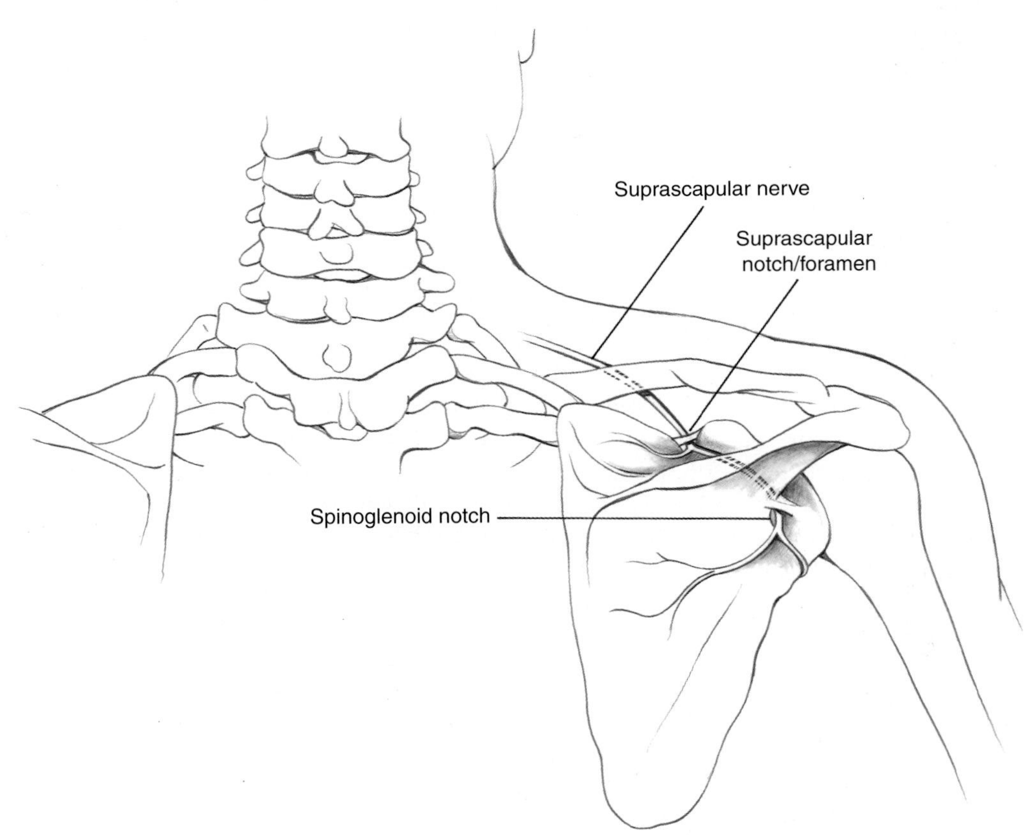

FIG. 7. Suprascapular nerve entrapment. Posterior view of the left shoulder showing the course of the suprascapular nerve and potential areas of entrapment in the suprascapular notch/foramen and the spinoglenoid notch/foramen. (Reprinted with permission from ref. 65.)

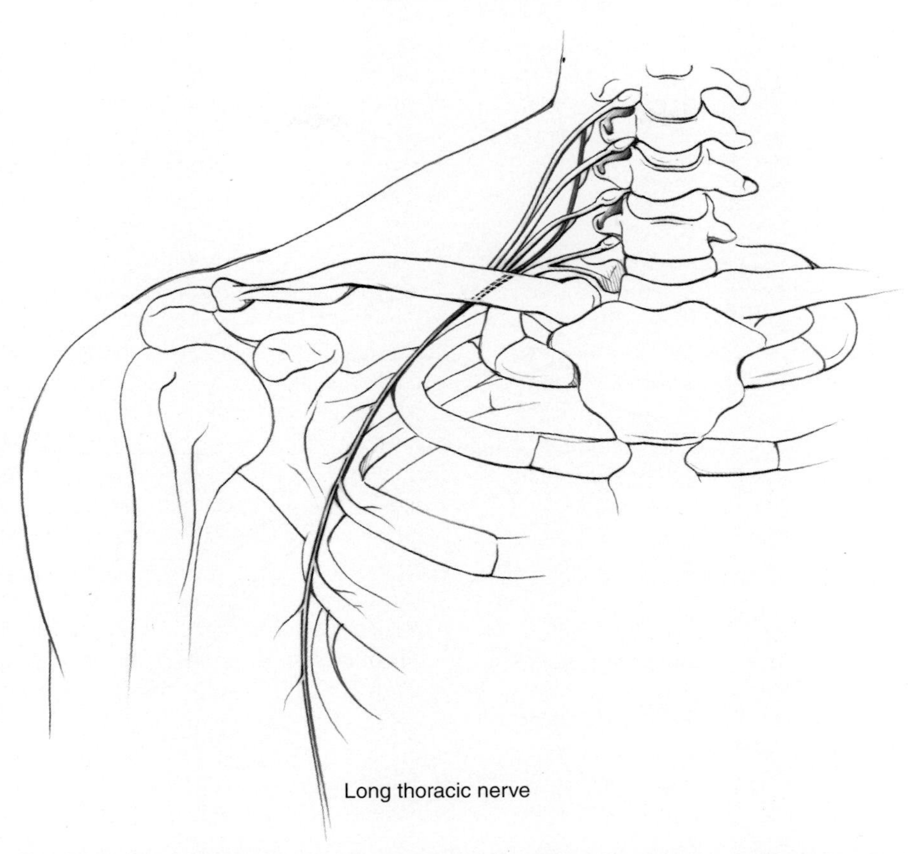

FIG. 8. Long thoracic nerve entrapment. Anterior view of the right chest and shoulder showing the course of the long thoracic nerve. (Modified with permission from ref. 65.)

forceful forward rotation of the scapula around the chest wall, due to trauma.[28]

Treatment should be based on severity of the neuropathy. In the presence of a mild focal neuropathy, injections of local anesthetic and corticosteroid may be helpful.[154] For a complete discussion of the surgical interventions for suprascapular nerve entrapment, please see the preceding chapters.

Long Thoracic Nerve

The long thoracic nerve arises from the ventral rami of C5–6 and sometimes C7. After leaving the brachial plexus, it travels down the internal aspect of the chest wall supplying the serratus anterior muscle (Fig. 8).

Patients with a neuropathy of the long thoracic nerve complain of a dull ache around the shoulder girdle at rest or upon abduction of the arm. However, motor dysfunction of the serratus anterior and its sequelae are more prominent features. As the serratus anterior stabilizes the scapula against the chest wall, weakness and difficulty in using the shoulder are the primary symptoms of long thoracic neuropathy.

Because of the formation of the long thoracic nerve from the roots of C5–7 prior to the development of the trunks, long thoracic neuropathy will seldom occur in brachial plexus injuries. Long thoracic neuropathies most often occur in the face of blunt trauma to the shoulder or the anterolateral thoracic wall.[70] The long thoracic nerve also may be injured after a number of common surgeries, including thoracotomy and radical mastectomy.[65,114] Repetitive or extreme exertional shoulder movement also has been implicated in long thoracic neuropathy. Activity such as chopping wood, golf, tennis, and jumping rope have been described as potential factors in the genesis of the neuropathy.[114] The pathogenesis of the exercise-induced neuropathy has been hypothesized to be excessive stretch or compression of the nerve, due to an underlying anatomic abnormality of the nerve itself or adjacent soft tissue and bony structures.

If the injury to the long thoracic nerve is due to excessive or repetitive use of the shoulder, cessation of activity usually results in full recovery. Physical therapy is the primary modality for management of long thoracic neuropathy after acute blunt trauma or surgical injury. Unfortunately, prognosis is poor.[59] Shoulder braces also may be of value.[172]

Axillary Nerve

The axillary nerve arises from the posterior cord of the brachial plexus. It lies lateral to the radial nerve and passes below the shoulder joint into the quadrilateral space (Fig. 9). The boundaries of the quadrilateral space are the neck of the

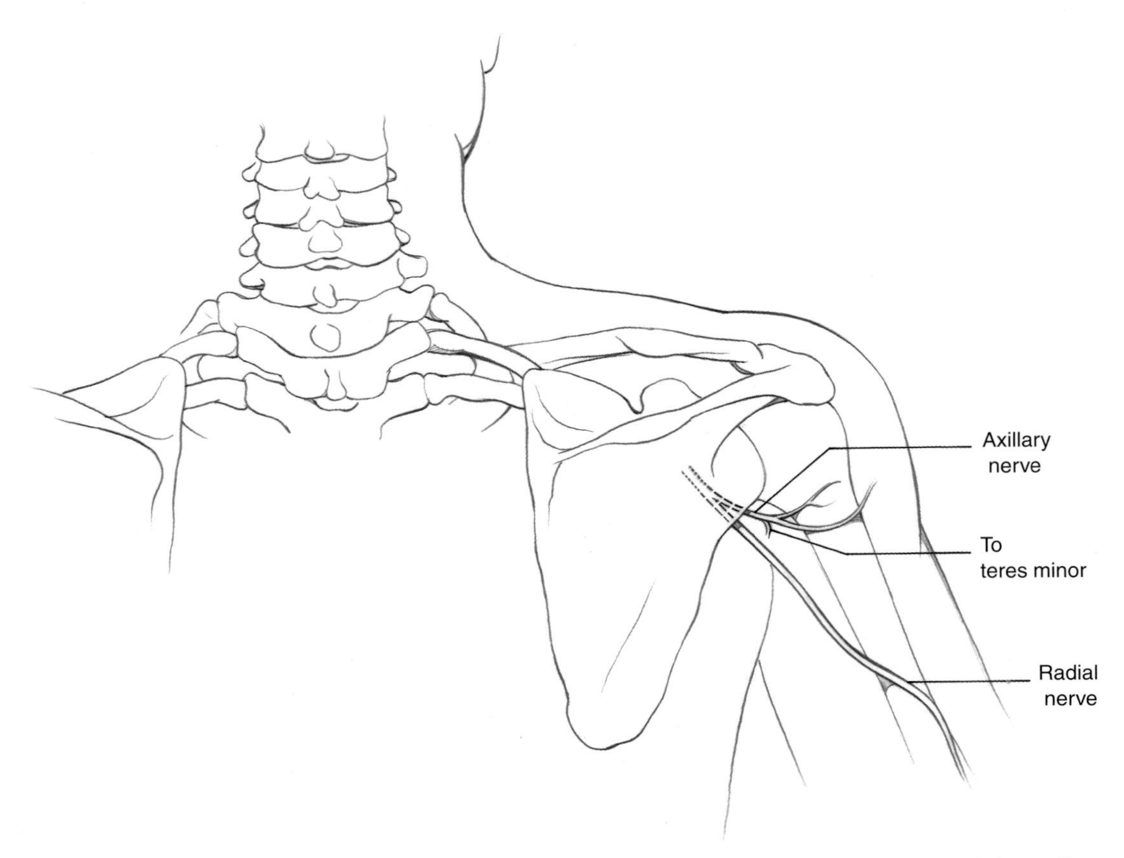

FIG. 9. Axillary nerve entrapment. Posterior view of the shoulder showing the course of the axillary nerve. (Modified with permission from ref. 65.)

humerus, the long head of the triceps, the teres major, and teres minor muscles. The axillary nerve courses along the posterior and lateral surfaces of the humerus and divides into terminal branches supplying the deltoid muscle.

As in other entrapment neuropathies, sensory aberrations can be minimal in axillary nerve entrapment. Any sensory loss is appreciated in a small area overlying the deltoid muscle near its insertion.[9] Wasting and weakness of the deltoid muscle, with marked impairment in shoulder abduction, are the chief clinical presentations of axillary neuropathy.

Shoulder dislocation or fracture of the surgical neck of the humerus are the most common causes of axillary neuropathy.[11] The axillary nerve is usually not injured in isolation, and there may be concomitant trauma to the radial, suprascapular, or musculocutaneous nerves or the brachial plexus itself.[84] Other causes of injury to the axillary nerve include blunt trauma to the shoulder without fracture or dislocation,[9] as well as intramuscular injections and bullet wounds.[146]

With respect to treatment, if traumatic damage to the axillary nerve is incomplete, no specific therapy is required. If the lesion is complete, some degree of recovery should be expected in several months. If recovery does not occur, surgical exploration and nerve grafting may be considered. Please see preceding chapters for a complete discussion of the surgical interventions for axillary nerve entrapment.

Sympathetically Maintained Pain (Reflex Sympathetic Dystrophy)

The nomenclature of pain syndromes with involvement of the sympathetic nervous system as a pathogenic mechanism is confusing, to say the least. A vast terminology has been used to describe these pathophysiologic states: causalgia, shoulder-hand syndrome, Sudek's atrophy, sympathetic overdrive, posttraumatic spreading neuralgia, etc.[157] The unifying feature of all such terminology is that pain is dependent on sympathetic efferent innervation of the affected area, i.e., the pain is sympathetically maintained.[134] Generically, these sympathetically maintained syndromes have been referred to as reflex sympathetic dystrophy in the past. Similarly, in common parlance and in a less generic sense, if an injury occurred to a minor nerve and/or the precipitating event was unknown, the terminology of RSD was employed. Causalgia referred to a similar constellation of autonomic, motor, and trophic disturbances with known injury to a major nerve trunk. In an attempt to reduce the current level of confusion with respect to taxonomy, a consensus work group was held in Orlando, FL, from October 31 to November 3, 1993. The term that was chosen for the group of disorders was "complex regional pain syndromes" (CRPS). The CRPS were divided into two types: CRPS type 1 (RSD) and CRPS type 2 (causalgia). For the purposes of our discussion, we will use the term "sympathetically maintained pain."

Irrespective of difficulties with taxonomy, the symptoms of sympathetically maintained pain represent a constellation of autonomic, motor, and sensory disturbances.[22] Sympathetically maintained pain can be defined by: (a) the appearance of pain disproportionate to that expected from the initiating injury, (b) variably expressed sympathetic dysfunction, (c) dystrophic changes, and (d) a delay in functional recovery. Clinical characteristics typically include: (a) sustained and diffusely burning pain, (b) allodynia (pain upon light touch), (c) hyperalgesia (exaggerated response to a normally painful stimulus), (d) vasomotor and pseudomotor disturbances, (e) skeletal muscle hypotonia, and (f) variable onset. Manifestations of sympathetically maintained pain are most commonly seen in the distal region of an affected extremity after an injury. Symptoms can become generalized and may not be limited to a single extremity. Moreover, they may bear little relation to the topographic localization or the severity of the initiating injury. (For example, sympathetically maintained pain may occur after minor injuries such as sprains, bruises, and needle sticks, and may spread to the contralateral limb.)

Autonomic Disturbances

Edema will frequently present in the distal portion of the affected extremity. The skin is quite often erythematous, mottled, slightly bluish, or frankly cyanotic. There will be a demonstrable difference in skin temperature between contralateral extremities.

Sympathetically maintained pain occurs spontaneously without provocation. Patients often state that it is worse at night. Pain may be exacerbated by placing the limb in a dependent position, and by movement of the joints. Dysesthesia is common, and the skin may be either hyperesthetic, hyperalgesic, or hypesthetic. Mechanical allodynia is often absent at the onset of the process but develops later in the natural history.[143,156]

Motor Disturbances

Dystonia of the distal extremity may be present. Nonphysiologic tremor of the affected extremity also may be exhibited. Motor strength may be reduced or entirely lost.[144]

Trophic Changes

A number of trophic disturbances can be seen with sympathetically maintained pain states. These include grooving of the nails, hair growth, hair loss, skin texture changes, loss of subcutaneous tissue, and osteoporosis. Characteristic bony and periarticular changes have been described with sympathetically maintained pain.[50,163] Initially, a patchy osteoporosis appears in juxtaarticular bone of the metacarpophalangeal or metatarsophalangeal joints, or the shoulder of the affected limb. A more generalized osteoporosis and erosion of the subchondral bone will subsequently develop.[75–77] Such changes may be elucidated by scintigraphy.[75,77] Today, three-phase scintigraphy is a standard diagnostic technique for defining the presence of sympathetically maintained pain.[90]

Clinical Stages of Sympathetically Maintained Pain

Autonomic, sensory, motor, and trophic disturbances occur at various times in the natural history of sympathetically maintained pain. Such a progression to trophic disturbances from autonomic, sensory, and motor changes has allowed definition of clinical stages.

Stage I: Acute Phase. Within days or weeks of an initiating event, pain occurs. It is most often described as burning and is localized to the area of injury. Because there is incident (movement-related) pain, the injured individual will attempt to maintain the affected limb in a protected stance. The limb may be warm, erythematous, and dry, or cool and pale. Edema may be present and tenderness may be exhibited over the distal joints of the limb. Radiographic examination may show spotty osteoporosis in periarticular areas of the bones of the hands or feet.[156]

Stage II: Dystrophic Phase. As the natural history of sympathetically maintained pain progresses, pain intensity may remain static, increase, or decrease. At the beginning of the dystrophic phase (which usually occurs anywhere from 3 to 6 months after the initiating event), hyperesthesia, paresthesia and allodynia may be present. The edema becomes more generalized within the limb, and joints begin to stiffen. Muscle wasting may begin to occur, and myofascial pain can involve ipsilateral as well as contralateral limb girdles. The skin is cold and pale, or cyanotic and moist. Hair and nails on the affected limb may become thickened and course. Osteoporosis may become more generalized. Technetium uptake by scintigraphy is seen in the dystrophic phase.[156]

Stage III: Atrophic Phase. This is the final stage of sympathetically maintained pain. It is characterized by severe and permanent trophic disturbances that are resistant to therapy. Pain intensity may be variable but is most often increased. Allodynia and dysesthesia are usually present. Exposure of the limb to air may exacerbate the pain. The limb is characteristically immobile with ankylosis of joints and atrophy and contracture of muscles. Edema has resolved and subcutaneous tissue is atrophied. The skin is smooth, shiny, cold and damp. Osteoporosis is diffuse.[156]

The Shoulder in Sympathetically Maintained Pain

Many patients with sympathetically maintained pain localized in the hand or the wrist also have complaints of pain in the shoulder. Such coexistence of pain symptomatology is often called the shoulder-hand syndrome[158,159] or the shoulder-hand-finger syndrome.[106] Patients complain of pain, stiffness, and/or a limited range of motion in the shoulder, with swelling and vasomotor disturbances in the hand. This limited range of shoulder motion may be passive or active because of pain. Frozen shoulder may occur in severe cases.[137,176] Many of the characteristic autonomic disturbances of sympathetically maintained pain in the hand have not been described in the shoulder.[176] Intriguingly, the joint interposed between the shoulder and the wrist (i.e., the elbow) is entirely free of symptomatology. Why this should occur is not completely understood.

The pathophysiologic mechanisms underlying shoulder-hand syndrome remain largely unknown. However, the pain complaints in the shoulder can be attributed to tendonitis of one or both tendons of the biceps muscle in a majority of patients.[176]

Although primary therapy should be directed toward resolution of the sympathetically maintained pain in the hand, injections of bupivacaine and methylprednisolone can be both diagnostically and therapeutically beneficial for the shoulder.[176] Injections should not be administered into the affected tendon or the shoulder joint, but into soft tissue surrounding the painful tendon or into the tendon sheath. Oral corticosteroids also have been beneficial in the treatment of shoulder-hand syndrome.[107]

Evaluation and Diagnostic Testing

The clinical signs and symptoms of sympathetically maintained pain states are extremely variable. Therefore, it is important to differentiate sympathetically maintained pain from other medical diagnoses. Moreover, sympathetically maintained pain may develop as a consequence of other disorders or exist alongside other medical conditions.

In order to entertain a diagnosis of sympathetically maintained pain, certain characteristic symptoms and signs must be present. As discussed previously, these may or may not include the following items (depending on the stage of the disease): burning pain, hyperpathia, allodynia, vasomotor phenomenon, edema, and hair and/or nail trophic changes.

A number of laboratory tests have been used to diagnose sympathetically maintained pain. Thermography is a method of measuring body surface temperature via infrared radiation. The thermogram can demonstrate dysfunction in the microcirculation resulting from autonomic responses to disease. The finding of temperature asymmetry can be helpful in establishing a diagnosis of sympathetically maintained pain. Moreover, temperature observations before and after sympathetic block are particularly helpful.[44] Although it is a useful adjunct in the diagnosis of sympathetically maintained pain, thermography lacks sufficient specificity and sensitivity to make a diagnosis of sympathetically maintained pain as a solitary diagnostic test.

With respect to radiologic modalities, standard roentgenograms may be useful in demonstrating patchy juxtaarticular osteoporosis. Bilaterality of these findings may be useful in suggesting the diagnosis of sympathetically maintained pain.[75,76] Similarly, three-phase scintigraphy with technetium diphosphonate has been suggested as having a 60% sensitivity and 86% specificity in the diagnosis of sympathetically maintained pain.[35] However, all radiologic tests should be viewed as representing adjunctive objective criteria in the diagnosis of sympathetically maintained pain. Unfortunately, a negative result does not necessarily rule out the presence of sympathetically maintained pain.

Although older qualitative tests such as the ninhydrin sweat test,[36] the cobalt blue filler paper sweat test,[86] and the sympathogalvanic response[86] are poor measures of sympathetic activity, the quantitative sweat test has gained popularity as a useful adjunctive modality for the diagnosis of sympathetically maintained pain.[89] This test involves measurement of the humidity exchanged with a small known volume of air that passes through a microenvironment between a capsule placed on the skin over a known time. Because sweating is under sympathetic cholinergic control, the iontophoresis of acetylcholine into the skin can be used as a measurement of the output of sweat. The stimulated sweat output is higher and temporally more protracted with sympathetic hyperactivity. Once again, this test is purely adjunctive, and used alone, it lacks sufficient specificity and sensitivity to make a diagnosis of sympathetically maintained pain.

Several lines of evidence suggest that α-adrenergic receptors may play a critical role in the genesis of sympathetically maintained pain.[5,55,125,126] Oral administration of the α-adrenergic antagonists phenoxybenzamine[55] and prazosin[1] have been therapeutically used to treat sympathetically maintained pain. Intravenous administration of the short-acting α-adrenergic blocking agent phentolamine has been developed as a test for sympathetically maintained pain.[5,125–127] Moreover, this test has been shown to be predictive as to which patients will respond to sympatholytic treatment.[5]

Despite all the aforementioned qualitative tests and despite the development of an intravenous diagnostic test with some degree of pharmacologic specificity, sympathetic effector blockade utilizing sympathetic blocks is still the most beneficial of all confirmatory diagnostic modalities, because sympatholysis is an integral part of therapy.[87]

Treatment

The treatment of sympathetically maintained pain must be multidisciplinary. Treatment protocols must utilize sympathetic blockade, prescription of appropriate medications, physical therapy, and psychologic support. Sympatholysis forms the basis for all successful treatment regimens (Table 6).

Although sympatholysis and analgesia are important, they form only one part of a comprehensive program. It is critical that patients be rapidly evaluated and diagnosed, because early intervention results in better prognosis. Once sympatholysis is initiated, aggressive physical and occupational therapy should be utilized to prevent joint and limb dysfunc-

TABLE 6. *Sympatholytic and analgesic therapies for the treatment of sympathetically maintained pain*

Neural blockade
Sympathetic nerve blocks (13)
Lumbar sympathetic
Stellate ganglion
Neurolytic (39)
Radiofrequency sympatholysis (180)
Peripheral nerve blocks
Intravenous regional block
Local anesthetic (67)
Guanethidine (10)
Bretyllium (67)
α-Receptor blockade
Oral prazocin (1)
Oral phenoxybenzamine (55)
Intravenous phentolamine (5,125–127)
α_2-Agonism
Topical clonidine (33)
Epidural clonidine (129)
Other
Surgical sympathectomy (92)
Membrane-stabilizing agents: tegretol, gabapentin (101)
Antidepressants
Nonsteroidal anti-inflammatory drugs (NSAIDs)
Opioids
Spinal cord stimulation

tion, or to minimize dysfunction if it is already present and irreversible. These physical medicine programs should include both passive and active range of motion, desensitization, coordination activities, aerobic and strength activities, and treatment of myofascial pain. Ultimately, once pain is under control and the patient is on the way to recovery, work hardening should be utilized to maximize functional return to work.

EVALUATION

Appropriate Referral

Patients are referred to practitioners of pain medicine by a vast array of physicians and health-care practitioners. These colleagues naturally vary in their expectations as to what pain medicine can achieve. Similarly, these expectations are passed on to their patients, even on a subliminal level. Sometimes referrals are a desperate attempt to get help for a distressed patient whose care has completely exasperated the referring physician. Sometimes referrals are made by physicians as a means of disposing of problem patients who will not respond to therapy as expected. Sometimes patients are referred to practitioners of pain medicine because the referring physician feels that the patient's problem is all in his or her mind, because a medical cause for symptomatology cannot be found. Sometimes patients are referred to practitioners of pain medicine because of fears of referring physicians regarding the prescription of controlled substances on a protracted basis.

Any discussion of what constitutes an appropriate versus inappropriate referral must be based on the pain medicine specialist's vision as to his or her own role, as well as a legitimate assessment of the services that can be provided. Some pain medicine specialists view themselves in the role of the primary care physician, acting as a diagnostician and utilizing all therapies (whether invasive or noninvasive) to assuage the patient's pain. Other pain medicine specialists view themselves purely in the interventional role and prefer to deal only with nerve blocks, radiofrequency ablation, and implantation of devices, etc. Such a dichotomy of vision translates itself into a disparity in the availability of services provided under the aegis of each respective physician.

An appropriate referral to a pain medicine specialist must be based on an understanding by the referring physician that suffering and pain behavior cannot be separated from patients' perception of pain and the actual nociceptive or neuropathic stimulus (Fig. 10). Any time a referring physician makes a referral to a pain medicine specialist and does not view the patient in the totality of their personhood (Fig. 10), it is an inappropriate referral. Thus, viewing patients' symp-

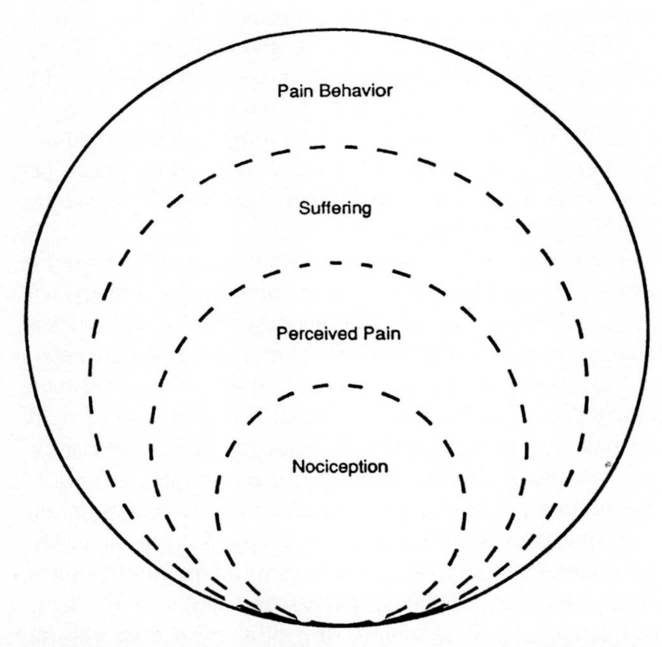

FIG. 10. Chronic pain must be viewed as a complex and dynamic interaction between a noxious stimulus (nociceptive or neuropathic), perceived pain, emotional suffering, and pain behavior. Traditional medical practice attempts to treat or remove the noxious stimulus but fails to account for patient perceptions, their suffering, and the genesis of pain behaviors. Perceived pain by the patient may be greater (e.g., somatic preoccupation) or less (e.g., distraction) than that which is commensurate with the noxious stimulus. Suffering revolves around the meaning or interpretation that an individual gives to a painful experience. The teaching of adaptations to pain, and therefore controlling suffering, forms the basis for cognitive-behavioral therapy. Pain behavior refers to actions related to the experience of pain and signal discomfort. It is maladaptive pain behaviors that make the chronic pain patient difficult at times. (Reprinted with permission from ref. 51.)

toms as purely psychosomatic, viewing patients' pain complaints as purely drug-seeking, and viewing patients' symptoms as unreal or imagined are inappropriate reasons for referral. On the other hand, any desire for assistance in dealing with the sometimes complex and distressing issues surrounding suffering, illness behavior, and the potential for drug-seeking behavior are appropriate reasons for referring patients to pain medicine specialists. Of course, referrals should be tempered by the availability of services. An interventionalist will be unable to assist with difficult diagnostic issues or potential psychological issues.

History and Physical Examination

Any history of pain must contain these descriptors in order to be complete: (a) temporal relationships, (b) spatial relationships, (c) the presence or absence of a radicular component, (d) the quality of the pain, (e) factors that palliate, and (f) factors that provoke or exacerbate the pain. The temporal characteristics of the pain are important. Continuous pain is much easier to treat than episodic pain. Similarly, acute pain is easier to treat than chronic pain.

With respect to the shoulder, spatial relationships are extremely important. If the pain is localized, it may be referable to joints, muscles, or bone. If the pain is segmental, it may be referable to nervous structures. If it follows dermatomal distributions, it may be referable to nerve roots. If the pain is peripheral in its distribution, the pain may be referable to the brachial plexus or its branches.

The quality of the pain in relation to its natural history is extremely important. What was the description of the pain at its onset? What is the description of the pain now? Duration, quality, intensity, and associated symptoms should be noted.

Various descriptors of the quality of the pain may provide diagnostic clues. If the pain is described as sharp or bright, the pain may be neuropathic. If the pain is described as burning, vascular pathology must also be entertained. Of course, a vascular etiology for pain would usually have a more diffuse spatial distribution than a neuropathic pain state. Description of pain as a deep ache is most referable to muscles, bones, and joints. Radicular pain is described as brief, sharp, and lancinating. Descriptions of continuous diffuse burning with hyperalgesia and hyperesthesia are referable to sympathetically maintained pain.

Descriptions of stiffness also can be diagnostic. Morning pain and stiffness may be attributable to myofascial disorders. Pain and stiffness that is worse late in the day after work may have a musculoskeletal etiology. Pain and stiffness that is worse at night may be referable to bony pathology.

Naturally, ameliorating or exacerbating factors are important to denote, particularly in regard to motion or position of the shoulder.

With respect to physical examination, inspection should be made for atrophy of particular muscles and muscle groups. Palpation of individual muscles, joints, and periarticular soft tissue should denote the presence of pain and tenderness. Patterns of radiation should also be noted. In any examination, the presence of trigger points and tender spots should be denoted. Range of motion of the shoulder should be assessed. This should be done for both active and passive motion, as well as against resistance for abduction, adduction, flexion, extension, external rotation, and internal rotation of the shoulder joint.

Careful neurologic examination of the neck, shoulder, and limb is extremely important in defining pathology. All flexors and extensors of the brachium, antebrachium, and hand should be evaluated. Motor examination of the shoulder has been previously mentioned. Sensory examination should be performed to determine the presence of hypesthesia, hyperesthesia, and allodynia in dermatomal patterns or in the distributions of particular peripheral nerves. Examination should be made of the deep tendon reflexes. The extremity and shoulder should be visualized for vasomotor phenomena.

The cervical examination is extremely important in differentiating pathology of the nerves supplying the shoulder. Neck range of motion should be performed with respect to flexion, extension, lateral flexion, and rotation. Peripheral palpation of the trapezius and scalene muscles should be performed, looking for trigger points and tender points.

Once a proper history and physical examination have been obtained, the clinician should avail himself or herself of both electrophysiologic and radiologic testing. The benefits of EMG, roentgenography, CT, MRI, and myelography for each specific pathophysiology of the shoulder have been previously discussed.

THERAPEUTIC ARMAMENTARIUM

Various classes of medications, as well as types of injections, can be used in the treatment of the different painful disease states affecting the shoulder. We will briefly review the pharmacology of medications that can be used to treat somatic and/or neuropathic pain. This will be followed by a discussion of injection therapy.

Nonsteroidal Antiinflammatory Medications

Nonsteroidal antiinflammatory drugs are the most commonly used group of medications for the treatment of pain of orthopedic origin. Those in common usage in the United States can be divided into three families of compounds: carboxylic acids, pyrazoles, and oxicams (Table 7). The overwhelming majority of NSAIDs are derivatives of carboxylic acid and can be divided into four groups: salicylic acids, acetic acids, propionic acids, and anthranilic acids (Table 7).

Mechanism of Action

Classically, the analgesic properties of NSAIDs were believed to be due solely to peripheral mechanisms. More re-

TABLE 7. *Pharmacologic classification of the NSAIDs*

Carboxylic acids
Salicylic acids
Acetylsalicylic acid (aspirin)
Nonacetylated salicylates
Choline magnesium trisalicylate (Trilisate)
Salicyl salicylate (Disalcid)
Diflunisal (Dolobid)
Acetic acids
Indoles
Indomethacin (Indocin)
Sulindac (Clinoril)
Etodolac (Lodine)
Pyrolle acetic acids
Tolmetin (Tolectin)
Ketorolac (Toradol)
Phenyl acetic acids
Diclofenac (Voltaren)
Naphthyl acetic acid
Nabumetone (Relafen)
Anthranilic acids
Fenamates
Meclofenamic acid (Meclomen)
Mefenamic acid (Ponstel)
Propionic acids
Phenylpropionic acids
Ibuprofen (Motrin)
Fenoprofen (Nalfon)
Flurbiprofen (Ansaid)
Ketoprofen (Orudis)
Naphthylpropionic acids
Naproxen (Naprosyn, Anaprox)
Oxicams
Piroxicam (Feldene)
Pyrazoles
Phenylbutazone (Butazolidin)

cently, a central analgesic mechanism has been proposed for NSAIDs.[91,165] For the purposes of our discussion, we will deal solely with the peripheral mechanism of analgesic action of the NSAIDs.

Nonsteroidal antiinflammatory drugs inhibit the enzyme cyclooxygenase (prostaglandin synthetase).[175] With initiation of the inflammatory response, cell membrane phospholipids are released (Fig. 11). Phospholipase catalyzes the conversion of these phospholipids into arachidonic acid intermediates. Cyclooxygenase catalyzes the conversion of arachidonic acid to cyclic endoperoxide intermediates. These cyclic endoperoxides are the precursors of the clinically relevant prostaglandins: prostacyclin (PGI_2), thromboxane (TxA_2), and prostaglandins (PGE_2, $PGF_{2}\alpha$). When NSAIDs inhibit the enzyme cyclooxygenase, the tissue levels of prostaglandins are reduced.

Because prostaglandins are algesic mediators, a reduction in their quantity causes analgesia. Prostaglandins contribute to the process of transduction wherein a noxious stimulus is converted in the periphery to a series of electrochemical events that are then transmitted to the spinal cord and higher rostral centers. In conjunction with a number of other chemical mediators (e.g., histamine, serotonin, bradykinin), prostaglandins are known to sensitize the ability of a nerve to generate action potentials. (A number of the other chemical algesic mediators also can excite neurons to fire.) Thus, a reduction in the synthesis of prostaglandins would be translated into a decrease in the ability of a noxious stimulus to be transduced into nerve action potentials.

Nonsteroidal antiinflammatory drugs do not typically inhibit the enzyme lipoxygenase (Fig. 11). NSAIDs do not, therefore, inhibit the eicosanoid pathway. However, the activity of the lipoxygenase pathway may be preferentially

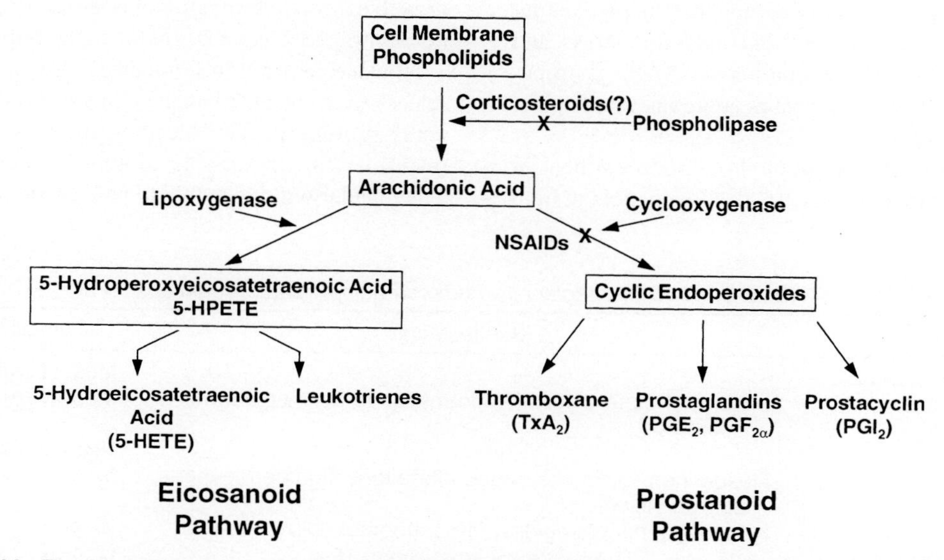

FIG. 11. The prostanoid and eicosanoid pathway for the genesis of prostaglandins and leukotrienes.

heightened by administration of NSAIDs. By blocking the conversion of arachidonic acid to cyclic endoperoxides, arachidonic acid may be shunted into the eicosanoid pathway, making more arachidonic intermediates available for conversion by lipoxygenase. Enhanced activity in the eicosanoid pathway generates leukotrienes. Such a mechanism underlies the genesis of asthma and allergic reactions with the administration of NSAIDs.[68] Meclofenamic acid (Meclomen) Myla Pharmaceuticals, is unique among the NSAIDs, because it inhibits both cyclooxygenase and lipoxygenase.[12,31] Therefore, it is the drug of choice in asthmatic patients who should receive an NSAID.

Side Effects

The side effects of NSAIDs can be divided into prostaglandin-mediated and non–prostaglandin-mediated effects. The prostaglandin-mediated effects are gastropathy, disorders of hemostasis, and nephrotoxicity. The non–prostaglandin-mediated reactions (sometimes called idiosyncratic reactions) have been attributed to cell-mediated phenomena such as inhibition of neutrophil migration and lymphocyte responsiveness. Non–prostaglandin-mediated effects also may contribute to the antiinflammatory and analgesic properties of the NSAIDs. Non–prostaglandin-mediated effects of the NSAIDs are listed in Table 8.

Gastropathy

Prostaglandins (PGE_1, PGE_2, etc.) act as autocoids within the body of the stomach. (Autocoids are locally produced hormones that act at the site of secretion.) Prostaglandins are involved in gastric mucosal cytoprotection and inhibition of ulcerogenesis.[15] Therefore, inhibition of prostaglandin synthesis by NSAIDs will enhance ulcerogenesis.

A number of factors that predispose to ulcerogenesis with NSAID administration have been identified. These include gender (greater incidence in females than males), preexisting peptic ulcer disease, use of alcohol and cigarettes, stress, and certain dietary factors.[15] The symptoms of NSAID gastropathy include dyspepsia, epigastric pain, anorexia, esophagitis, constipation, and diarrhea.

The issues surrounding the prophylaxis and treatment of NSAID gastropathy are complex.[15,64,155] In a patient at high risk for the development of gastropathy as well as ulcerogenesis, alcohol consumption and smoking should be eliminated. The use of multiple NSAIDs in the same individual has no therapeutic benefit. Such practice will only increase the risk of development of gastropathy or ulcer. A reduced risk for the development of gastropathy or ulcer has been associated with the use of nonacetylated salicylates.[30,74]

All NSAIDs undergo rapid absorption from the gut[16] and are highly protein bound.[148] Most NSAIDs undergo hepatic metabolism and excretion of inactive metabolites via the urine. The exceptions include sulindac (Clinoril) Merck & Co., nabumetone (Relafen) Beecham Pharmaceuticals, and salicyl salicylate (Disalcid) 3M Pharmaceuticals. These compounds are inactive prodrugs that must be converted to active metabolites by hepatic transformation, and they are relatively gastric sparing.[16,149]

With respect to pharmacologic therapy, consideration should be given to the use of H_2-antagonists and/or misoprostol in high-risk patients. Misoprostol is an analog of prostaglandin and causes gastric mucosal cytoprotection, inhibiting gastric and duodenal ulceration.[60,147]

If gastrointestinal symptoms do occur, patients should be treated with H_2-antagonists, antacids, or sucralfate. If ulceration develops, NSAIDs should be discontinued. If this is not possible, the NSAID dosage should be minimized as far as practicable, and treatment should be instituted with misoprostol or H_2-antagonists.[15]

Disorders of Hemostatis

Dyscrasias of the individual cell lines of the blood may occur. However, they occur with much, much less frequency than drug interactions and platelet dysfunction due to NSAID administration. Both coumadin and NSAIDs are avidly bound by plasma proteins. Competition between coumadin and NSAIDs may lead to an increase in free coumadin in the plasma, potentially causing bleeding problems. Although the concomitant use of NSAIDs and anticoagulants is not contraindicated, caution must certainly be advised.

Nonsteroidal antiinflammatory drugs affect the platelet release reaction and platelet aggregation. Thus, they will typically prolong platelet bleeding time. Acetyl salicylic acid (aspirin) will irreversibly inhibit platelet cyclooxygenase. The platelet will be unable to participate in the release reac-

TABLE 8. *Non–prostaglandin-mediated (idiosyncratic) reactions*

Reaction	Manifestation	Implicated NSAIDs
Asymptomatic transaminasemia		Most NSAIDs
Dermatologic reactions	Minor rashes to exfoliative dermatitis to toxic epidermal necrolysis	Most NSAIDs
Hepatitis		Sulindac, diclofenac
CNS symptoms	Headaches, dizziness, mood alterations, lightheadedness, blurred vision	Indomethacin
Aseptic meningitis	Headache, nuchal rigidity, fever, photophobia	Ibuprofen, sulindac, tolmetin
Bilateral pulmonary nodules		Naproxen

tion and aggregation for its lifetime. Thus, the bleeding time is prolonged for 6 to 10 days (the entire lifetime of platelets) after a single administration of one aspirin.[20] All other NSAIDs will competitively inhibit platelet cyclooxygenase.[3] Platelets will return to normal function after the NSAID is cleared from the plasma (five half-lives).

Nephrotoxicity

Under normal circumstances, renal blood flow and glomerular filtration are not prostaglandin dependent. However, in the clinical scenarios of dehydration, hepatic cirrhosis, or congestive heart failure, renal blood flow and glomerular filtration do become prostaglandin dependent. In these clinical scenarios, there is activation of the renin-angiotensin-aldosterone and sympathetic nervous systems. Prostaglandins are important as a protective mechanism against renal ischemia. Administration of an NSAID may inhibit prostaglandin synthesis, thereby leading to decreased renal perfusion and glomerular filtration.[29,112] Although the use of NSAIDs is not absolutely contraindicated in dehydration, hepatic cirrhosis, or congestive heart failure, caution must be used, and vigilance should be exercised to determine any deterioration in renal function. At that time, NSAIDs must be immediately discontinued.

In the normally functioning individual, prostaglandins inhibit tubular reabsorption of sodium and water and the secretion of renin from the juxtaglomerular apparatus. Thus, by inhibition of prostaglandin synthesis, NSAIDs can lead to fluid retention, impaired responsiveness to diuretics, and hyperkalemia in the presence of dehydration, hepatic cirrhosis, and/or congestive heart failure.[29,112]

Opioid Therapy for Chronic Nonmalignant Pain

It is beyond the scope of this chapter to present a full discussion of the pharmacology of the opioids. However, it is wise to briefly discuss the issues surrounding the protracted use of opioids for chronic pain.

Traditionally, long-term opioid administration has been viewed as ineffective and unsafe. However, a number of surveys of long-term opioid administration have suggested that administration can be effective and safe without genesis of addiction or abuse in a subpopulation of patients with chronic pain.[52,73,117,119,166–168,174,192] This evolution in the philosophy of opioid administration is actually derived from the analgesic experience with cancer. Seventy to ninety percent of patients with cancer can obtain long-term analgesia and improved quality of life without the development of analgesic tolerance, physical dependence, or addiction.[118,142]

The critical issues surrounding the use of opioids for chronic nonmalignant pain revolve around their therapeutic efficacy, the potential for adverse pharmacologic outcomes, the potential for physical dependence, and the risk of opioid addiction and abuse. Although we have dealt somewhat with therapeutic efficacy, it is important to denote that no data exist to support the conclusion that nonmalignant pain (in general), or any patient subgroup, or any particular diagnosis is inherently unresponsive to opioids. Neuropathic pain offers a useful illustration. Although the common wisdom is that neuropathic pain is generally more refractory to opioid therapy and its use is fraught with the possibility of an unfavorable response,[4,79] in the individual patient there clearly can be a gratifying response.[26,116,117,174] Thus, the diagnosis of neuropathic pain, or any other pain state, does not justify a decision to withhold opioids on a presumption of inefficacy.

Long-term opioid therapy has not been associated with major organ toxicity in large studies of cancer patients. Moreover, persistent side effects such as somnolence, confusion, nausea, or cognitive impairment do not appear to be of significance.[78,120]

Physical dependence is defined as a physiologic phenomenon that is, in essence, an abstinence syndrome induced by abrupt discontinuation of an opioid.[133] The prerequisite period of drug ingestion that is necessary in order to develop physical dependence is unknown. It should be assumed that the administration of opioids even for several days may necessitate a gradual taper of a drug, rather than abrupt withdrawal. Nevertheless, physical dependence is a physiologic phenomenon. It does not imply addiction, and it is phenomenologically distinct from addiction. Every individual placed on an opioid can develop physical dependence. It is not a behavior but a physiologic phenomenon.

Addiction is characterized by a loss of control over drug use, compulsive use of that drug, and continued use despite harm to the patient.[120] Unlike physical dependence, addiction is not a physiologic phenomenon but a behavioral phenomenon. Moreover, it is uniformly a behavior that we would hope not to induce iatrogenically.

What is the risk of addiction with the use of opioids for nonmalignant pain? Three studies give us some idea of the incidence of iatrogenically inducing addiction. The Boston Collaborative Drug Surveillance Project identified only four cases of addiction among 11,882 patients with no history of substance abuse.[121] In a survey of 10,000 patients treated for burn pain, no cases of addiction could be identified.[113] Only 3 patients developed problematic, drug-related behavior among 2,369 patients at a large headache center who had protracted access to opioids.[100]

These data are compelling when compared with the incidence of addiction within the United States. The prevalence of alcoholism in the general United States population is 3% to 16%.[130] The incidence of other forms of substance abuse in the general U.S. population is 5% to 6%.[130] Thus, from the data presently available, the incidence of iatrogenically inducing addiction with protracted opioid use is much, much smaller than the prevalence of addiction to alcohol or other drugs within the general population.

How should one proceed when an individual is possibly a candidate for this therapy? The indication for opioids for chronic nonmalignant pain is certainly a valid reason for referral to a pain center. The pain center will be able to adjust medications, as well as provide psychometric testing and psychological evaluation to determine whether the patient is a valid candidate. Once the patient is on a stable dose of opioids, it is appropriate for the patient to be referred back to their primary physician for long-term care at stable doses of opioids. Of course, increasing pain and/or escalating dosages can prompt re-referral to the pain center.

Medications for the Treatment of Neuropathic Pain

The three major classes of medications used in the treatment of neuropathic pain include antidepressants, membrane-stabilizing agents (anticonvulsants), and neuroleptic agents. Because there is considerable controversy regarding the use of neuroleptic agents, we will not discuss them further. Opioids and NSAIDs may be effective in the treatment of neuropathic pain in their role as nonspecific analgesics. However, the antidepressants and membrane-stabilizing agents truly represent the primary pharmacologic agents for treatment of neuropathic pain.

Antidepressants

The antidepressants consist of five groups of agents: (a) the tricyclics, (b) the heterocyclics, (c) the SSRIs, (d) the monoamine oxidase inhibitors, and (e) lithium (Table 9).

Certain drugs of this class are referred to as tricyclic antidepressants because they have three rings with substitution on the middle ring (Table 9). Similar to the tricyclics, maprotiline and trazodone are old antidepressants (although they do not possess three rings). Maprotiline and trazodone are sometimes referred to as heterocyclics. As a group, the analgesic, as well as antidepressant effects, of the tricyclics and heterocyclics are believed to be due to blockade of presynaptic uptake of serotonin and norepinephrine. With respect to the provision of analgesia, the TCAs are the most clinically useful of all the antidepressants and the best studied.[110] Because we are interested in the treatment of neuropathic pain, we will confine the majority of our discussion of the antidepressants to the tricyclics.

TABLE 9. *Antidepressants*

Tertiary amines
Amitriptyline (Elavil)
Clomipramine (Anafranil)
Doxepin (Sinequan)
Imipramine (Tofranil)
Trimipramine (Surmontil)
Secondary amines
Amoxapine (Asendin)
Serotonin-specific reuptake inhibitors
Paroxetine (Paxil)
Fluoxetine (Prozac)
Sertraline (Zoloft)
Fluvoxamine (Luvox)
Venlafaxine (Effexor)
Monoamine oxidase inhibitors
Lithium
Nortriptyline (Pamelor)
Maprotiline (Ludiomil)
Protriptyline (Vivactil)
Desipramine (Norpramin)

Certain of the antidepressants solely block the reuptake of serotonin and are therefore referred to as serotonin-specific reuptake inhibitors (Table 9). The SSRIs are relatively new agents. The SSRIs, while excellent antidepressants, appear to have less utility as analgesics in the treatment of neuropathic pain.[96] The exception to this may be venlafaxine. More research is necessary to fully establish venlafaxine's analgesic utility. Similar to the vast majority of the SSRIs, monoamine oxidase inhibitors have not been demonstrated to have any analgesic effect. Lithium is useful in the treatment of migraine but has limited utility for other types of pain.

Tricyclic antidepressants exist as tertiary or secondary amines. The tertiary amines are metabolized to secondary amines. These secondary amines have less of the side effects associated with their tertiary precursors. Amitriptyline is metabolized to nortriptyline. Similarly, imipramine is metabolized to desipramine.[63]

As previously stated, the mechanism of analgesia of the TCAs (and heterocyclics) is believed to be the presynaptic blockade of the amine pump with failure of reuptake of serotonin and norepinephrine. No antidepressant effects are seen for 1 to 4 weeks after initiation of therapy. However, analgesic effects are almost immediate, which allows for more rapid titration of drugs in the treatment of neuropathic pain.[63]

All TCAs are well absorbed after oral administration and undergo a significant first-pass effect.[53] The TCAs are highly lipophilic, and their elimination half-lives are long (1 to 4 days).[63] These antidepressants generally undergo metabolism in the hepatic microsomal system and are conjugated with glucuronic acid and excreted in the urine and the feces.

There is marked variability in serum or blood levels of TCAs after oral ingestion, because of idiosyncratic variations in clearance among patients.[53] Therapeutic ranges for the treatment of affective disorders have been established. However, TCA serum or blood levels bear no relationship to the production of significant analgesia in the treatment of neuropathic pain.[140] Serum or blood levels should not be used to determine the presence of therapeutic levels in the treatment of neuropathic pain; serum or blood levels should only be relied upon in the assessment of potential toxicity.

The propensity for the production of side effects complicates the clinical utility of the TCAs. The common side effects associated with use of TCAs are: (a) anticholinergic effects, (b) antihistaminic effects, (c) α_1-adrenergic blockade, and (d) miscellaneous side effects.

The anticholinergic effects of the TCAs are due to their muscarinic actions at the acetylcholine receptor. These may include dry mouth (common), visual accommodation difficulties, constipation (common), urinary retention, and delayed gastric emptying.[63] Fortunately, many people will accommodate to the presence of dry mouth if forewarned. However, care is always advised with the use of antidepressants in the face of benign prostatic hypertrophy, because of the possible exacerbation of any urinary retention. TCAs are contraindicated in patients with narrow-angle glaucoma.

Sedation is commonly seen with the initial use of TCAs. Sedation is due to blockade of H_1-receptors. Once again, patients may accomodate to its presence if forewarned. Orthostatic hypotension is a rare side effect and is caused by α_1-adrenergic receptor blockade. Miscellaneous problems with the use of TCAs include photosensitivity reactions, jaundice, and weight gain.[63]

Membrane-Stabilizing Agents

Besides the TCAs, membrane-stabilizing agents are the other commonly used group of drugs for the treatment of neuropathic pain. Drugs in common usage include phenytoin, carbamazepine, valproic acid, clonazepam, and gabapentin. These agents also have anticonvulsant properties. Similar to the TCAs, serum levels are not useful in establishing analgesia.[63] Abrupt withdrawal of these agents can precipitate seizures in patients without a prior history of epilepsy. Thus, these agents must be tapered if they are to be discontinued.

The mechanism of action of phenytoin is stabilization of excitable membranes by altering sodium, calcium, and potassium flux.[63] The side effects of phenytoin are significant. Phenytoin is associated with hirsutism, ataxia, diplopia, confusion, epigastric pain, nausea, and vomiting.[63] Fibrocyte stimulation by phenytoin may cause gingival hyperplasia.[161] Both the anemia and neuropathy of folic acid deficiency and vitamin K and D deficiencies may occur with phenytoin therapy.[21] Phenytoin also may inhibit insulin secretion and cause hyperglycemia.[63]

Carbamazepine alters sodium and potassium flux, in order to stabilize membranes. Structurally, carbamazepine is similar to imipramine. Analgesia with carbamazepine usually does not occur until a daily dose in the range of 1.0 to 1.5 g is achieved. The need for slow titration of carbamazepine dosage limits the utility of carbamazepine. Side effects of carbamazepine include a propensity for production of hematologic abnormalities (thrombocytopenia, agranulocytosis, anemia, and pancytopenia). Hepatic dysfunction also may occur. Prior to institution of therapy, it is important to determine blood counts as well as liver enzyme levels. These laboratory tests should be repeated on a regular basis while the patient is on carbamazepine therapy, in order to monitor the respective cell counts and enzyme levels. Ataxia, rash, sedation, diplopia, and nausea are also seen with carbamazepine therapy.[63]

The mechanism of action of analgesia of valproic acid appears to be inhibition of gamma-amino-butyric-acid (GABA) transaminase.[18] The most common side effects of valproic acid are gastrointestinal symptoms. However, these may ameliorate over time. Sedation, ataxia, tremor, rash, and alopecia also may be precipitated by use of valproic acid. The most devastating effect of valproic acid therapy is the production of hepatic failure in the rare individual.[63]

Clonazepam is unique among the membrane-stabilizing agents because it is a benzodiazepine. Therefore, blockade of the receptor-linked chloride channel to enhance GABA binding or activity is its mechanism of action.[153] Clonazepam is a useful agent because its analgesic effects for neuropathic pain states can be rapidly appreciated. Side effects are similar to other benzodiazepines: possible disinhibition during use and the precipitation of abstinence syndrome with abrupt withdrawal.

Gabapentin is the newest of the membrane-stabilizing agents and has tremendous potential for the treatment of neuropathic pain, at least anecdotally. The mechanism of action of gabapentin is unknown. It does bind to a specific receptor in the brain, inhibits voltage-dependent sodium currents, and may enhance the release or enhance the actions of GABA.[38] Gabapentin is unusual because it is excreted intact by the kidneys, and plasma protein binding is negligible. Thus, the dosage of gabapentin should be reduced in patients with renal impairment, and the propensity for drug interactions are few.[123] Gabapentin is also notable for its improved side effect profile in comparison with other membrane-stabilizing agents. Sedation, fatigue, ataxia, dizziness, and gastrointestinal symptoms may still occur, however.[34]

Neural Blockade

The most common neural blockade techniques utilized for treatment of various neck and shoulder conditions include suprascapular nerve block, stellate ganglion block, and CESIs (see earlier section on CESIs).

Suprascapular Nerve Block

The suprascapular nerve block may be useful as part of a comprehensive rehabilitative program for the management of chronic[136,138,179] and acute[42] shoulder pain. Although useful as an aid to physical reconditioning, too little data exist in the literature to determine the effectiveness of the block when used alone in the treatment of shoulder conditions. Similarly, few data exist as to the optimal frequency for repetition of suprascapular nerve block.

The block is easy to perform. Complications are rare and mainly involve production of pneumothorax (incidence less than 1%) by advancement of the needle deeper than recommended.

With the patient in the sitting position, the suprascapular notch can be located by identifying the tip of the acromion process and the medial border of the scapula at the level of the scapular spine. These two points can be marked and a line drawn between them overlying the spine of the scapula (Fig. 12). Another line can be drawn that bisects this line. Needle entry point is determined by making an X 1 inch lat-

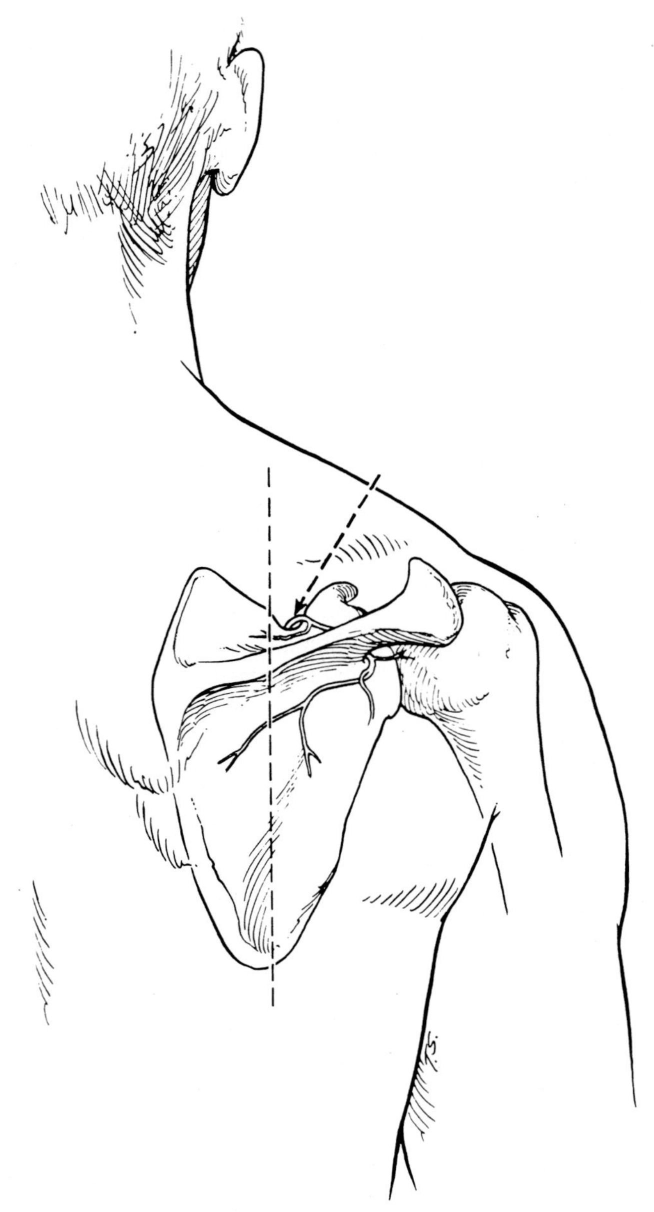

FIG. 12. Anatomic landmarks for neural blockade of the suprascapular nerve. (Reprinted with permission from ref. 124.)

erally along the scapular spine from the bisection of the two lines and 1 inch above this point, along a line parallel to the vertebral spine. After appropriate cleansing, a skin wheal with local anesthetic is made. A 7-cm, 22-gauge spinal needle with stylet is then introduced through the skin perpendicular to all planes until bone is contacted. This needle can be withdrawn to the subcutaneous tissue, redirected 15° laterally and 15° cephalad and introduced toward the suprascapular notch to a final depth of approximately 1.5 cm from the skin. At this junction, 6 to 7 ml of local anesthetic can be administered.[138] Alternatively, the block may be performed with use of nerve stimulation (although this is not mandatory).

Stellate Ganglion Block

The term "stellate ganglion block" is incorrect, because the stellate ganglion is only found in approximately 80% of people. The stellate ganglion results from fusion of the lowest ganglion of the cervical sympathetic chain with the first thoracic ganglion. Actually, the injection is a cervicothoracic sympathetic block, with spread of local anesthetic to achieve blockade of both the cervical and thoracic sympathetic chain over multiple segments. Moreover, the stellate ganglion overlies the neck of the first rib. The procedure usually is performed paratracheally at C6, and the stellate ganglion is not contacted by the needle at all.

Typically, Horner's syndrome is produced as a normal physiologic sequalae of successful blockade. Horner's syndrome consists of: (a) ipsilateral nasal stuffiness secondary to vasodilation, (b) anhidrosis in the affected area, (c) miosis of the pupil on the appropriate side, (d) ptosis, and (e) enophthalmos. Moreover, as the superior laryngeal nerve lies in close approximation to the area of injection, the patient may experience some degree of hoarseness after the block. It is always advisable to warn a patient of the production of Horner's syndrome and possible hoarseness prior to performance of the block. Actual complications (not side effects) of stellate ganglion block include intravascular injection into the vertebral artery and pneumothorax.

The technique of stellate ganglion block is easy to perform. The trachea and carotid pulse are gently palpated between the sternocleidomastoid muscle and the trachea at the level of C6 (Fig. 13). The level of C6 can be ascertained by palpation of the cricoid cartilage. A skin wheal is made for patient comfort. Using the fingers as a hook, the sternocleidomastoid muscle is then retracted laterally. The injection should not be made until the carotid pulse is appreciated lateral to the palpating fingers. A 22-gauge short-bevel needle attached to a 20-ml syringe may then be inserted as paratracheally as possible and perpendicular to the plane of the skin until it hits bone. This is the anterior tubercle of C6 or Chassaignac's tubercle. At this point, aspiration is performed. A small amount of local anesthetic can be given as an injection. If aspiration and test dose are negative, the remainder of the local anesthetic may be administered with frequent aspiration to look for the presence of blood. Aspiration and test dose are necessary because the vertebral artery lies in close approximation to the area of injection, encased within bone in the foramen transversarium.[71]

Stellate ganglion block is most useful for treatment of sympathetically maintained pain but also may be used for treatment of Raynaud's disease, scleroderma, occlusive vascular disease, herpes zoster, and other pathologies of the head, neck, and arm wherein sympathetic blockade may be therapeutic.

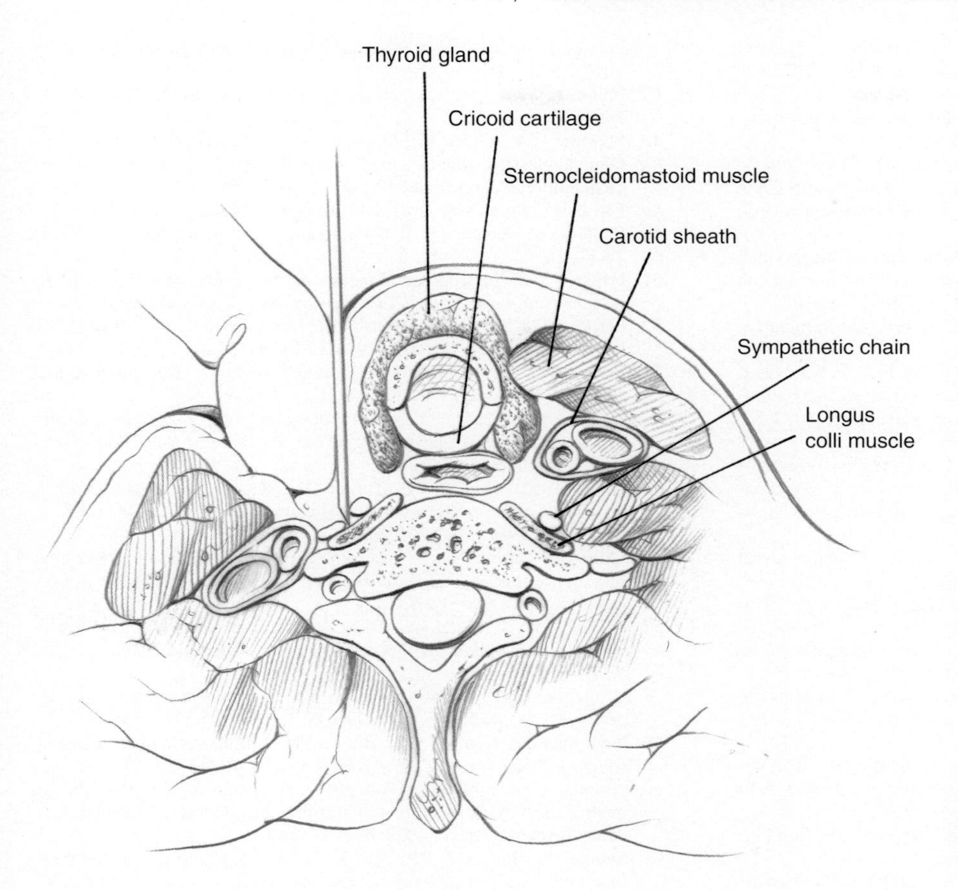

FIG. 13. Stellate ganglion block: anatomy and technique. (Reprinted with permission from ref. 17.)

CONCLUSION

This chapter has described types of pain, as well as various pathologies that may give rise to painful conditions of the shoulder. Clinicians should avail themselves of medication therapy, as well as neural blockade to the extent of their abilities. At that time, referral of patients with painful conditions of the shoulder to a practitioner of pain medicine may be advisable.

REFERENCES

1. Abram SE, Lightfoot R. Treatment of longstanding causalgia with prazocin. *Reg Anesth* 1981;6:79–81.
2. Aiello I, Serra G, Traina GC, Tugnoli V. Entrapment of the suprascapular nerve at the spinoglenoid notch. *Ann Neurol* 1982;12: 314–316.
3. Ali M, McDonald JW. Reversible and irreversible inhibition of platelet cyclooxygenase and serotonin release by nonsteroidal anti-inflammatory drugs. *Throm Res* 1978;13:1057–1065.
4. Arnér S, Meyerson BA. Lack of analgesic effect of opioids on neuropathic and idiopathic forms of pain. *Pain* 1988;33:11–23.
5. Arnér S. Intravenous phentolamine test: diagnostic and prognostic use in reflex sympathetic dystrophy. *Pain* 1991;46:17–22.
6. Baumstark KE, Buckelew SP, Sher KJ, et al. Pain behavior predictors among fibromyalgia patients. *Pain* 1993;55:339–346.
7. Beghi E, Kurland LT, Mulder DW, Nicolosi A. Brachial plexus neuropathy in the population of Rochester, Minnesota. 1970–1981. *Ann Neurol* 1985;18:320–323.
8. Bennett RM. Myofascial pain syndromes and fibromyalgia pain syndrome: a comparative analysis. In: Friction JR, Awad EA, eds. *Advances in pain research and therapy*. Vol 17. New York: Raven, 1990: 43–65.
9. Berry H, Bril V. Axillary nerve palsy following blunt trauma to the shoulder region: a clinical and electrophysiological review. *J Neurol Neurosurg Psychiatry* 1982;45:1027–1032.
10. Blanchard J, Ramamurthy S, Walsh N. Intravenous regional sympatholysis: a double-blind comparison of guanethidine, reserpine and normal saline. *J Pain Symptom Manage* 1990;5:357–361.
11. Blom S, Dahlbäck LO. Nerve injuries in dislocations of the shoulder joint and fractures of the neck of the humerus. *Acta Chir Scand* 1970; 136:461–466.
12. Boctor AM, Eickholt M, Pugsley TA. Meclofenamate sodium is an inhibitor of both the 5-lipoxygenase and cyclooxygenase pathways of the arachidonic acid cascade in vitro. *Protaglandins Leukotrienes Med* 1986;23:229–238.
13. Bonica JJ. Causalgia and other reflex sympathetic dystrophies. In: Bonica JJ, Loeser JD, Chapman CR, Fordyce WE, eds. *The management of pain*. 2nd ed. Vol. 1. Philadelphia: Lea & Febiger, 1990: 220–243.
14. Bonney G. The scalenus medius band: a contribution to the study of the thoracic outlet syndrome. *J Bone Joint Surg [Br]* 1965;47: 268–272.
15. Borda IT. The spectrum of adverse gastrointestinal effects associated with nonsteroidal anti-inflammatory drugs. In: Borda IT, Koff RS, eds. *NSAIDs: a profile of adverse effects*. Philadelphia: Hanley & Belfus, 1992:25–80.
16. Brooks PM, Day RO. Nonsteroidal anti-inflammatory drugs—differences and similarities. *N Engl J Med* 1991;324:1716–1725.
17. Brown DL. *Atlas of regional anesthesia*. Philadelphia: WB Saunders, 1992.
18. Bruni J, Wilder BJ. Valproic acid: review of a new drug. *Arch Neurol* 1979;36:393–398.
19. Bufalini C, Pescatori G. Posterior cervical electromyography in the diagnosis and prognosis of brachial plexus injuries. *J Bone Joint Surg [Br]* 1969;51:627–631.

20. Burch JW, Sanford N, Majerus PW. Inhibition of platelet prostaglandin synthetase by oral aspirin. *J Clin Invest* 1978;61:314–319.
21. Burchiel KJ. Carbamazepine inhibits spontaneous activity in experimental neuromas. *Exp Neurol* 1988;102:249–253.
22. Campbell JN, Raja SN, Meyer RA. Painful sequelae of nerve injury. In: Dubner R, Gebhart GE, Bond RF, eds. *Proceedings of the Vth world congress on pain, pain research and clinical management*. Vol. 3. Amsterdam: Elsevier, 1988:135–143.
23. Carette S, Bell MJ, Reynolds WJ, et al. Comparison of amitriptyline, cyclobenbenzaprine, and placebo in the treatment of fibromyalgia. A randomized, double-blind trial. *Arthritis Rheum* 1994;37:32–40.
24. Carlson JA, Baruah JK. Suprascapular nerve entrapment at spinoglenoid notch. *Neurology* 1985;35:78.
25. Castagnera L, Maurette P, Pointillart V, Vital JM, Erny P, Sénégas J. Long-term results of cervical epidural steroid injection with and without morphine in chronic cervical radicular pain. *Pain* 1994;58:239–243.
26. Cherny NI, Thaler HT, Friedlander-Klar H. Opioid responsiveness of cancer pain syndromes caused by neuropathic or nociceptive mechanisms: a combined analysis of controlled, single-dose studies. *Neurology* 1994;44:857–861.
27. Cicala RS, Thoni K, Angel JJ. Long-term results of cervical epidural steroid injections. *Clin J Pain* 1989;5:143–145.
28. Clein LJ. Suprascapular entrapment neuropathy. *J Neurosurg* 1975;43:337–342.
29. Clive DM, Stoff JS. Renal syndromes associated with nonsteroidal anti-inflammatory drugs. *N Engl J Med* 1984;310:563–572.
30. Cohen A, Garber HE. Comparison of choline magnesium trisalicylate and acetylsalicylic acid in relation to fecal blood loss. *Curr Ther Res* 1978;28:187–191.
31. Conroy MC, Randinitis EJ, Turner JL. Pharmacology, pharmacokinetics, and therapeutic use of meclofenamate sodium. *Clin J Pain* 1991;7(suppl 1):44–48.
32. Cousins MJ, Phillips GD, eds. *Acute pain management*. London: Churchill Livingstone, 1986.
33. David KD, Treede RD, Raja SN, Meyer RA, Campbell JN. Topical application of clonidine relieves hyperalgesia in patients with sympathetically maintained pain. *Pain* 1991;47:309–317.
34. de Jong RH. Neurontin: pie in the sky or pie on the plate? [Editorial]. *Pain Dig* 1996;6:143–144.
35. Demangeat JL, Constantinesco A, Brunot B, Foucher G, Farcot JM. Three phase bone scanning in reflex sympathetic dystrophy of the hand. *J Nucl Med* 1988;29:26–32.
36. Dhuner KG, Edshage S, Wilhelm A. Ninhydrin test-objective method for testing local anaesthetic drugs. *Acta Anaesthesiol Scand* 1960;4:189–193.
37. DiBenedetto M, Markey K. Electrodiagnostic localization of traumatic upper trunk brachial plexopathy. *Arch Phys Med Rehabil* 1984;65:15–17.
38. Dichter MA, Brodie MJ. New antiepileptic drugs. *N Engl J Med* 1996;334:1583–1590.
39. Dondelinger R, Kurdziel JC. Percutaneous phenol neurolysis of the lumbar sympathetic chain with computed tomograph control. *Ann Radiol* 1984;27:376–379.
40. Dyck PJ, Mellinger JF, Reagan TJ, et al. Not indifference to pain but varieties of hereditary sensory and autonomic neuropathy. *Brain* 1983;106:373–390.
41. Eastcott HHG. Reconstruction of the suclavian artery for complications of cervical-rib and thoracic-outlet syndrome. *Lancet* 1962;2:1243–1246.
42. Edeland HG, Stefanson T. Block of the suprascapular nerve in reduction of acute anterior shoulder dislocation. *Acta Anaesth Scand* 1973;17:46–49.
43. Edeland HG, Zachrisson BE. Fracture of the scapular notch associated with lesion of the suprascapular nerve. *Acta Orthop Scand* 1975;46:758–763.
44. Edwards BE, Hobbins WB. Pain management and thermography. In: Raj PP, ed. *Practical management of pain*. St. Louis: Mosby-Year Book, 1992:168–184.
45. Enker SH, Murthy KK. Brachial plexus compression by excessive callus formation secondary to a fractured clavicle: a case report. *Mt Sinai J Med* 1970;37:678–682.
46. Falconer MA, Weddell G. Costoclavicular compression of the subclavian artery and veins: relation to scalenus anticus syndrome. *Lancet* 1943:2:539–543.
47. Falconer MA. The costoclavicular syndrome. *Br Med J* 1947;2:539–543.
48. Ferrante FM, Wilson SP, Iacobo C, Orav EJ, Rocco AG, Lipson S. Clinical classification as a predictor of therapeutic outcome after cervical epidural steroid injection. *Spine* 1993;18:730–736.
49. Fields HL. *Pain*. New York: McGraw-Hill, 1987.
50. Fontaine R, Hurrmann L. Posttraumatic osteoporosis. *Ann Surg* 1933;26:17–26.
51. Fordyce WE. Environmental factors on the genesis of low back pain. *Advances in pain research and therapy*. New York: Raven, 1979.
52. France RD, Urban BJ, Keefe FJ. Long-term use of narcotic analgesics in chronic pain. *Soc Sci Med* 1984;19:1379–1382.
53. Friedman H, Greenblatt DJ. Rational therapeutic drug monitoring. *JAMA* 1986;256:2227–2233.
54. Garcia G, McQueen D. Bilateral suprascapular-nerve entrapment syndrome: case report and review of the literature. *J Bone Joint Surg [Am]* 1981;63:491–492.
55. Ghostine SY, Comair YG, Turner DM, Kassel NF, Azar CG. Phenoxybenzamine in the treatment of causalgia. Report of 40 cases. *J Neurosurg* 1984;60:1263–1268.
56. Gilliatt R. Thoracic outlet syndromes. In: Dyck PJ, Thomas PK, Lambert EH, eds. *Peripheral neuropathy*, 2nd ed. Vol. 2. Philadelphia: WB Saunders, 1984:1409–1424.
57. Gilliatt RW, Willison RG, Dietz V, Williams IR. Peripheral nerve conduction in patients with a cervical rib and hand. *Ann Neurol* 1978;4:124–129.
58. Goldenberg DL. Fibromyalgia, chronic fatigue syndrome, and myofascial pain syndrome. *Curr Opin Rheum* 1994;6:223–233.
59. Goodman CE, Kenrick MM, Blum MV. Long thoracic nerve palsy: a follow-up study. *Arch Phys Med Rehabil* 1975;65:352–355.
60. Graham DY, Agrawal N, Roth SH. Prevention of NSAID-induced gastric ulcer with misoprostol: multicentre, double-blind, placebo-controlled trial. *Lancet* 1988;2:1277–1280.
61. Grenier N, Baulny D, Sénégas J, Caillé JM. Lumbar intervertebral disc and facet joints. Normal and pathological. In: Manelfe C, ed. *Imaging of the spine and spinal cord*. New York: Raven, 1992:257–268.
62. Grichnik KP, Ferrante FM. The difference between acute and chronic pain. *Mt Sinai J Med* 1991;58:217–220.
63. Haddox JD. Neuropsychiatric drug use in pain management. In: Raj PP, ed. *Practical management of pain*, 2nd ed. St. Louis: Mosby-Year Book, 1992:636–659.
64. Hawkey CJ. Non-steroidal anti-inflammatory drugs and peptic ulcers. *Br Med J* 1990;300:278–284.
65. Haymaker W, Woodhall B. *Peripheral nerve injuries—principles of diagnosis*. Philadelphia: WB Saunders, 1953.
66. Hepper NGG, Herskovic T, Witten DM, Mulder DW, Woolner LB. Thoracic inlet tumors. *Ann Intern Med* 1966;64:979–989.
67. Hord AH, Rooks MD, Stephens BO, Rogers HG, Fleming U. Intravenous regional bretylium and lidocaine for treatment of reflex sympathetic dystrophy: a randomized, double-blind study. *Anesth Analg* 1992;74:818–821.
68. Izzo V, Pagnoni B, Rigoli M. Recent acquisitions in pain therapy: meclofenamic acid. *Clin J Pain* 1991;7(suppl 1):49–53.
69. Jaconsen B, Bredkaer SR. The prevalence of fibromyalgia and widespread chronic musculoskeletal pain in the general population. *Scand J Rheumatol* 1992;21:261–262.
70. Kaplan PE. Electrodiagnostic confirmation of long thoracic nerve palsy. *J Neurol Neurosurg Psychiatry* 1980;43:50–52.
71. Katz J, Renck H. *Handbook of thoraco-abdominal nerve block*. Orlando, FL: Grune & Stratton, 1987.
72. Katz N, Ferrante FM. Nociception. In: Ferrante FM, VadeBoncouer TR, eds. *Postoperative pain management*. New York: Churchill Livingstone, 1993:17–67.
73. Kell MJ, Musselman DL. Methadone prophylaxis of intractable headaches: pain control and serum opioid levels. *Am J Prev Med* 1993;3:7–14.
74. Kilander A, Dotevall G. Endoscopic evaluation of the comparative effects of acetylsalicylic acid and choline magnesium trisalicylate on human gastric and duodenal mucosa. *Br J Rheumatol* 1983;22:36–40.
75. Kozin F, Genant HK, Bekerman C, McCarty DJ. The reflex sympathetic dystrophy syndrome. II. Roentgenographic and scintigraphic

evidence of bilaterality and of periarticular accentuation. *Am J Med* 1976;60:332–338.
76. Kozin F, McCarty DJ, Sims J, Genant H. The reflex sympathetic dystrophy syndrome. I. Clinical and histologic studies: evidence for bilaterality, response to corticosteroids and articular involvement. *Am J Med* 1976;60:321–331.
77. Kozin F, Ryan LM, Carerra GF, Wortmann RL. The reflex sympathetic dystrophy syndrome (RSDS). III. Sctinigraphic studies, further evidence for therapeutic efficacy of systemic corticosteroids, and proposed diagnostic criteria. *Am J Med* 1981;70:23–30.
78. Kreek MJ. Medical complications in methadone patients. *Ann NY Acad Sci* 1978;311:110–134.
79. Kupers RC, Konings H, Adriaensen H, Gybels JM. Morphine differentially affects the sensory and affective pain ratings in neuropathic and idiopathic forms of pain. *Pain* 1991;47:5–12.
80. Larsson SE, Bengtsson A, Bodegaerd L, Henriksson KG, Larsson J. Muscle changes in work-related chronic myalgia. *Acta Orthop Scand* 1989;59:552–556.
81. Lederman RJ, Brever AC, Hanson MR, et al. Peripheral nervous system complications of coronary artery bypass graft surgery. *Ann Neurol* 1982;12:297–301.
82. Lederman RJ, Wilbourn AJ. Brachial plexopathy: recurrent cancer or radiation? *Neurology* 1984;34:1331–1335.
83. Leffert RD. Brachial-plexus injuries. *N Engl J Med* 1974;291: 1059–1067.
84. Liveson JA. Nerve lesions associated with shoulder dislocation: an electrodiagnostic study of 11 cases. *J Neurol Neurosurg Psychiatry* 1984;47:742–744.
85. Loeser JD. Cervicobrachial neuralgia. In: Bonica JJ, Loeser JD, Chapman CR, Fordyce WE, eds. *The management of pain*, 2nd ed. Vol. 1. Philadelphia: Lea & Febiger, 1990:868–881.
86. Löfström JB, Cousins MJ. Sympathetic neural blockade of upper and lower extremity. In: Cousins MJ, Bridenbaugh PO, eds. *Neural blockade in clinical anesthesia and management of pain*, 2nd ed. Philadelphia: JB Lippincott, 1988:461–500.
87. Loh L, Nathan PW. Painful peripheral nerve states and sympathetic blocks. *J Neurol Neurosurg Psychiatry* 1978;41:664–671.
88. Lorenzen L. Fibromyalgia: a clinical challenge. *J Intern Med* 1994; 235:199–203.
89. Low PA, Caskey PE, Tuck RR, Fealey RD, Dyck PJ. Quantitative sudomotor axon reflex test in normal and neuropathic subject. *Ann Neurol* 1983;14:573–580.
90. Mailis A, Meindok H, Papagapiou M, Pham D. Alterations of the three-phase bone scan after sympathectomy. *Clin J Pain* 1994;10:146–155.
91. Malmburg AB, Yaksh TL. Pharmacology of spinal action of ketorolac, morphine, ST-91, V50488H, and L-PIA on the formalin test and isobolographic analysis of the NSAID interaction. *Anesthesiology* 1993;79:270–281.
92. Manart JD, Sadler RT, Schmitt EA, Rainer WG. Upper dorsal sympathectomy. *Am J Surg* 1985;150:762–766.
93. Manelfe C, Chevrot A, Arrvé P, Mark AS. Disc herniations. In: Manelfe C, ed. *Imaging of the spine and spinal cord*. New York: Raven, 1992:269–331.
94. Maroon JC. Burning hand in football spinal cord injuries. *JAMA* 1977; 238:2049–2051.
95. Martin JT. *Positioning in anesthesia and surgery*. Philadelphia: WB Saunders, 1987.
96. Max MB, Lynch SA, Muir J, Shoat SE, Smoller B, Dubner R. Effects of desipramine, amitriptyline, and fluoxetine on pain in diabetic neuropathy. *N Engl J Med* 1992;326:1250–1256.
97. McCain GA, Scudds RA. The concept of primary fibromyalgia (fibrositis): clinical value, relation and significance to other chronic musculoskeletal pain syndromes. *Pain* 1988;33:273–287.
98. McGain GA. Fibromyalgia and myofascial pain syndromes. In: Wall PD, Melzack R, eds. *Textbook of pain*, 3rd ed. Edinburgh: Churchill Livingstone, 1994:475–493.
99. McManus F. Brachial plexus lesions complicating anterior fracture–dislocation of the shoulder joint. *Injury* 1976;8:63–66.
100. Medina JL, Diamond S. Drug dependency in patients with chronic headache. *Headache* 1977;17:12–14.
101. Mellick GA, Mellick LB. Gabapentin in the management of RSD [Letter}. *J Pain Symptom Manage* 1995;10:265–266.
102. Melzack R, Wall PD. Pain mechanisms. A new theory. *Science* 1965; 150:971–978.
103. Melzack R, Wall PD. *The challenge of pain*. New York: Basic Books, 1982.
104. Merskey H, Bogduk N, eds. *Classification of chronic pain. Description of chronic pain syndromes and definition of pain terms*, 2nd ed. Seattle: IASP Press, 1994.
105. Millesi H. Trauma involving the brachial plexus. In: Omer GE, Spinner M, eds. *Management of peripheral nerve problems*. Philadelphia: WB Saunders, 1980.
106. Moberg E. The shoulder-hand-finger syndrome. *Surg Clin North Am* 1960;40:367–373.
107. Mowat AG. Treatment of the shoulder-hand syndrome with corticosteroids. *Ann Rheum Dis* 1974;33:120–123.
108. Narakas AO. The effects of one pain of reconstructive neurosurgery in 160 patients with traction and/or crush injury to the brachial plexus. In: Siegfried J, Zimmermann M, eds. *Phantom and stump pain*. New York: Springer-Verlag, 1981:126–147.
109. Olsen WL, Chakeres DW, Berry I, Richard J. Spine and spinal cord trauma. In: Manelfe C, ed. *Imaging of the spine and spinal cord*. New York: Raven, 1992:407–444.
110. Onghena P, Van Houdenhove B. Antidepressant-induced analgesia in chronic nonmalignant pain: a meta-analysis of 39 placebo-controlled studies. *Pain* 1992;49:205–219.
111. Parry CBW. Pain in avulsion lesions of the brachial plexus. *Pain* 1980;9:41–53.
112. Patrono C, Dunn MJ. The clinical significance of inhibition of renal prostaglandin synthesis. *Kidney Int* 1987;32:1–12.
113. Perry S, Heidrich G. Management of pain during debridement: a survey of US burn units. *Pain* 1982;13:267–280.
114. Petrera JE, Trojaborg W. Conduction studies of the long thoracic nerve in serratus anterior palsy of different etiology. *Neurology* 1984; 34:1033–1037.
115. Piatt JH, Hudson AR, Hoffman HJ. Preliminary experiences with brachial plexus exploration in children: birth injury and ventricular trauma. *Neurosurgery* 1988;22:715–723.
116. Portenoy RK, Foley KM, Inturrisi CE. The nature of opioid responsiveness and its implications for neuropathic pain: new hypotheses derived from studies of opioid infusions. *Pain* 1990;43:273–286.
117. Portenoy RK, Foley KM. Chronic use of opioid analgesics in non-malignant pain: report of 38 cases. *Pain* 1986;25:171–186.
118. Portenoy RK. Cancer pain: epidemiology and syndromes. *Cancer* 1989;63:2298–2307.
119. Portenoy RK. Chronic opioid therapy for nonmalignant pain: from models to practice. *APS J* 1992;1:285–288.
120. Portenoy RK. Opioid therapy for chronic nonmalignant pain: a review of critical issues. *J Pain Symptom Manage* 1996;11:203–217.
121. Porter J, Jick H. Addiction rare in patients treated with narcotics. *N Engl J Med* 1980;302:123.
122. Prère J, Manelfe C, Salvolini U. Pathology of the neural arch, spinal stenoses, and spondylolisthesis. In: Manelfe C, ed. *Imaging of the spine and spinal cord*. New York: Raven, 1992;333–385.
123. Radulovic LL, Türck D, von Hodenberg A, et al. Disposition of gabapentin (Neurontin) in mice, rats, dogs and monkeys. *Drug Metab Dispos* 1995;23:441–448.
124. Raj PP, Johnson KS, Murphy TM, et al. Nerve blocks. In: Raj PP, ed. *Practical management of pain*, 1st ed. Chicago: Year Book, 1986: 578–681.
125. Raja SA, Treede RD, Davis KD, Campbell JN. Systemic alpha-adrenergic blockade with phentolamine. A diagnostic test for sympathetically maintained pain. *Anesthesiology* 1991;74:691–698.
126. Raja SN, Davis KD, Campbell JN. The adrenergic pharmacology of sympathetically maintained pain. *J Reconstr Microsurg* 1992;8: 63–69.
127. Raja SN, Turnquist JL, Meleka S, Campbell JN. Monitoring of adequacy of α-adrenoreceptor blockade following systemic phentolamine administration. *Pain* 1996;64:197–204.
128. Rapoport S, Blair DM, McCarthy SM, Desser TS, Hammers LW, Sostman HD. Brachial plexus: correlation of MR imaging with CT and pathologic findings. *Radiology* 1988;167:161–165.
129. Rauck RL, Eisenach JC, Jackson K, Young LD, Southern J. Epidural clonidine treatment for refractory reflex sympathetic dystrophy. *Anesthesiology* 1993;79:1163–1169.
130. Regier DA, Meyers JK, Kramer M, et al. The NIMH epidemiologic catchment area program. *Arch Gen Psychiatry* 1984;41:934–958.
131. Rengachary SS, Burr D, Lucas S, Hassanein KM, Mohn MP, Matzke

H. Suprascapular entrapment neuropathy: a clinical, anatomical, and comparative study. Part 2: anatomical study. *Neurosurgery* 1979;5: 447–451.
132. Reynolds AD. Myofascial trigger point syndromes in the practice of rheumatology. *Arch Phys Med Rehabil* 1981;62:111–114.
133. Rinaldi RC, Steindler EM, Wilford BB, Goodwin D. Clarification and standardization of substance abuse terminology. *JAMA* 1988;259: 555–557.
134. Roberts WJ. A hypothesis on the physiological basis for causalgia and related pains. *Pain* 1986;24:297–311.
135. Roos DB. Congenital anomalies associated with thoracic outlet syndrome: anatomy, symptoms, diagnosis and treatment. *Am J Surg* 1976;132:771–778.
136. Rose DL, Kelly CR. Suprascapular nerve block in shoulder pain. *J Kan Med Soc* 1964;70:135–136.
137. Rosen PS, Graham W. The shoulder-hand syndrome: historical review with observations on 73 patients. *Can Med Assoc J* 1957;77:86–91.
138. Rowlingson JC, Arasi R. The use of suprascapular nerve blocks in the management of shoulder pain. *Reg Anesth* 1986;11:156–159.
139. Rowlingson JC, Kirschenbaum LP. Epidural analgesic techniques in the management of cervical pain. *Anesth Analg* 1986;65:938–942.
140. Rubin EH, Biggs JT, Preskorn SH. Nortriptyline pharmacokinetics and plasma levels: implications for clinical practice. *J Clin Psychiatry* 1985;46:418–424.
141. Ruckley CV. Thoracic outlet syndrome. *Br Med J* 1983;2:447–448.
142. Schug SA, Zech D, Grond S, Jung H, Meurser T, Stobble B. A long-term survey of morphine in cancer pain patients. *J Pain Symptom Manage* 1992;7:259–266.
143. Schwartzman RD, McLellan TL. Reflex sympathetic dystrophy. A review. *Arch Neurol* 1987;44:555–561.
144. Schwartzman RJ, Kerrigan J. The movement disorder of reflex sympathetic dystrophy. *Neurology* 1990;40:57–61.
145. Scudds RA, McCain GA, Rollman GB, Harth M. Improvements in pain responsiveness in patients with fibrositis after successful treatment with amitriptyline. *J Rheum* 1989;16(suppl 19):98–103.
146. Seddon H. *Surgical disorder of peripheral nerves*, 2nd ed. Edinburgh: Churchill Livingstone, 1975.
147. Silverstein FE, Graham DY, Senior JR, et al. Misoprostol reduces serious gastrointestinal complications in patients with rheumatoid arthritis receiving nonsteroidal anti-inflammatory drugs. A randomized, double-blind, placebo-controlled trial. *Ann Intern Med* 1995;123: 241–249.
148. Simon LS, Mills JA. Nonsteroidal anti-inflammatory drugs (first of two parts). *N Engl J Med* 1980;302:1179–1185.
149. Simon LS, Mills JA. Nonsteroidal anti-inflammatory drugs (second of two parts). *N Engl J Med* 1980;302:1237–1243.
150. Simons DG, Travell JG. Myofascial trigger points, a possible explanation. *Pain* 1981;10:106–109.
151. Simons DG. Muscular pain syndromes. In: Friction JR, Awad EA, eds. *Advances in pain research and therapy*. Vol. 17. New York: Raven, 1990:1–41.
152. Sinald M, Merritt JL, Stillwell GK. Tension myalgia of the pelvic floor. *Mayo Clin Proc* 1971;52:717–722.
153. Snyder SH. Drug and neurotransmitter receptors. *JAMA* 1989;261: 3126–3129.
154. Solheim LF, Roaas A. Compression of the suprascapular nerve after fracture of the scapular notch. *Acta Orthop Scand* 1978;49:338–340.
155. Soll AH. Pathogenesis of peptic ulcer and implications for therapy. *N Engl J Med* 1990;322:909–916.
156. Stanton-Hicks M, Jänig W, Boas RA, eds. *Reflex sympathetic dystrophy*. Boston: Kluwer Academic, 1990.
157. Stanton-Hicks M, Jänig W, Hassenbusch S, Haddox JD, Wilson P. Reflex sympathetic dystrophy: changing concepts and taxonomy. *Pain* 1995;63:127–133.
158. Steinbrocker O, Spitzer N, Friedman HH. The shoulder-hand syndrome in reflex dystrophy of the upper extremity. *Ann Intern Med* 1948;29:22–52.
159. Steinbrocker O. The shoulder-hand syndrome. Associated painful homolateral disability of the shoulder and hand with swelling and atrophy of the hand. *Am J Med* 1947;3:402–407.
160. Stewart JD. *Focal peripheral neuropathies*, 2nd ed. New York: Elsevier, 1993.
161. Stinnett E, Rodu B, Grizzle WE. New developments in understanding phenytoin-induced gingival hyperplasia. *J Am Dent Assoc* 1987;114: 814–816.
162. Stoltmann HF, Blackwood H. The role of the ligamenta flava in the pathogenesis of myelopathy in cervical spondylosis. *Brain* 1964;87: 45–51.
163. Sudeck P. Ueber die acute enzundliche knochenatropie. *Arch Klin Chir* 1900;62:147–158.
164. Swift TR, Nichols FT. The droopy shoulder syndrome. *Neurology* 1984;34:212–215.
165. Taiwo YO, Levine JD. Prostaglandins inhibit endogenous pain control mechanisms by blocking transmission at spinal noradrenergic synapses. *J Neurosci* 1988;8:1346–1349.
166. Taub A. Opioid analgesics in the treatment of chronic intractable pain of non-neoplastic origin. In: Kitahata LM, Collins D, eds. *Narcotic analgesics in anesthesiology*. Baltimore: Williams & Wilkins, 1982: 199–208.
167. Tennant FS, Robinson D, Saherian A, Seecof R. Chronic opioid treatment of intractable nonmalignant pain. *Pain Manage* 1988;Jan/Feb: 18–36.
168. Tennant FS, Uelman GF. Narcotic maintenance for chronic pain: medical and legal guidelines. *Postgrad Med* 1983;73:81–94.
169. Thomas DGT, Jones SJ. Dorsal root entry zone lesions (Nashold's syndrome) in brachial plexus avulsion. *Neurosurgery* 1984;15: 966–968.
170. Thomas JE, Colby MY. Radiation-induced or metastatic brachial plexopahty? A diagnostic dilemma. *JAMA* 1972;222:1392–1395.
171. Travell JG, Simons DG. *Myofascial pain and dysfunction: the trigger point manual*. Baltimore: Williams & Wilkins, 1983.
172. Truong XT, Rippel DV. Orthotic devices for serratus anterior palsy: some biomechanical considerations. *Arch Phys Med Rehabil* 1979;60: 66–69.
173. Tsairis P, Dyck PJ, Mulder DW. Natural history of brachial plexus neuropathy: report on 99 patients. *Arch Neurol* 1972;27:109–117.
174. Urban BJ, France RD, Steinberger DL, Scott DL, Maltbie AA. Long-term use of narcotic-depressant medication in the management of phantom limb pain. *Pain* 1986;24:191–197.
175. Vane JR. Inhibition of prostaglandin synthesis as a mechanism of action for the aspirin-like drugs. *Nature New Biol* 1971;231:232–235.
176. Vedman AJM, Goris JA. Shoulder complaints in patients with reflex sympathetic dystrophy of the upper extremity. *Arch Phys Med Rehabil* 1995;76:239–242.
177. Waldman SD. Complications of cervical epidural nerve blocks with steroids: a prospective study of 790 consecutive blocks. *Reg Anesth* 1989;14:149–151.
178. Warren J, Gutmann L, Figueroa JR, AF, Bloor BM. Electromyographic changes of brachial plexus root avulsions. *J Neurosurg* 1969; 31:137–140.
179. Wassef MR. Suprascapular nerve block. A new approach for the management of frozen shoulder. *Anaesthesia* 1992;47:120–124.
180. Wilkinson AA. Radiofrequency percutaneous upper thoracic sympathectomy: technique and review of indications. *N Engl J Med* 1984; 311:34–36.
181. Wilkinson M. *Cervical spondylosis: its early diagnosis and treatment*, 2nd ed., London: William Heinemann, 1971.
182. Wolfe F, Smythe HA, Yunus MB, et al. The American College of Rheumatology 1990 criteria for the classification of fibromyalgia. Report of the multicenter criteria committee. *Arthritis Rheum* 1990;33: 160–172.
183. Wolfe F. Fibromyalgia. The clinical syndrome. *Rheumatic Dis Clin North Am* 1989;15:1–18.
184. Wyburn-Mason R. Brachial neuritis occurring in epidemic form. *Lancet* 1941;2:662–663.
185. Yamada S, Lonser RR, Iacono RP, Morenski JD, Bailey L. Bypass coaptation procedures for cervical nerve root avulsion. *Neurosurgery* 1996;38:1145–1152.
186. Yamada S, Peterson GW, Soloniuk DS, Will D. Coaptation of the anterior rami of C-3 and C-4 to the upper trunk of the brachial plexus for cervical nerve root avulsion. *J Neurosurg* 1991;74:171–177.
187. Yates DW. Complications of fractures of the clavicle. *Injury* 1976;7: 189–193.
188. Yeoman PM. Cervical myelography in traction injuries of the brachial plexus. *J Bone Joint Surg [Br]* 1959;41:4–35.
189. Yiannikas C, Shahani BT, Young RR. The investigation of traumatic

lesions of the brachial plexus by electromyography and short latency somatosensory potentials evoked by stimulation of multiple peripheral nerves. *J Neurol Neurosurg Psychiatry* 1983;46:1014–1022.
190. Yiannikas C, Walsh JC. Somatosensory evoked responses in the diagnosis of thoracic outlet syndrome. *J Neurol Neurosurg Psychiatry* 1983;46:234–240.
191. Yunus MB, Hussey FX, Aldag JC. Antinuclear antibodies and connective tissue disease features in fibromyalgia syndrome: a controlled study. *J Rheumatol* 1993;20:1557–1560.
192. Zenz M, Strumpf M, Tryba M. Long-term opioid therapy in patients with chronic nonmalignant pain. *J Pain Symptom Manage* 1992;7: 69–77.

Disorders of the Shoulder: Diagnosis and Management,
edited by Joseph P. Iannotti and Gerald R. Williams, Jr.
Lippincott Williams & Wilkins, Philadelphia © 1999.

CHAPTER 38

Anesthesia for Shoulder Surgery

Anthony R. Brown

Patients present for shoulder surgery with a variety of conditions. These include sports injuries, trauma, and age-related arthritic conditions. The anesthesiologist is therefore presented with patients of varying ages and levels of medical fitness who are scheduled for a wide range of procedures, varying from manipulation under anesthesia, to arthroscopic or open shoulder surgery, to total shoulder arthroplasty. The objectives of this chapter are to describe the preoperative evaluation of these patients and their anesthetic options; to provide a detailed description of the use of regional anesthesia for shoulder surgery; and, to discuss the control of postoperative pain.

PREOPERATIVE EVALUATION

The preoperative evaluation is important in establishing the patient's fitness for anesthesia and surgery. Ideally, the patient should be assessed prior to the day of surgery in a preoperative clinic or preadmission unit by a member of the anesthesia care team.[136] A registered nurse (RN) or physicians, assistant (PA) may perform the preoperative assessment on patients classified as American Society of Anesthesiologists physical status I and II (ASA I and II, Table 1). Patients requiring more detailed medical evaluation are referred to a physician member of the team. In teaching institutions, the preoperative evaluations are traditionally performed by an anesthesiologist or anesthesia resident. For ASA I and ASA II patients, the patient can be evaluated on the day of surgery. However, this negates some of the objectives of preoperative evaluation described below. Patients not evaluated prior to the day of surgery are seen by the anesthesiologist immediately prior to the surgical procedure.

The objectives of the preoperative consultation are outlined below:

I. Establishment of the patient's fitness for anesthesia and surgery. A healthy patient is examined to rule out an undiagnosed underlying condition, such as hypertension. In the case of patients with known systemic diseases, the goals are:
   A. to establish that the condition is adequately controlled (e.g., hypertension, asthma, diabetes). If the medical condition is poorly controlled, an elective surgical procedure should be postponed until the patient is medically fit to minimize the risk from the underlying condition.
   B. to evaluate multiple system involvement associated with certain medical conditions. Rheumatoid arthritis, for example, may be associated with limited cervical spine and temperomandibular joint range of motion, resulting in difficulty with intubation. In addition, these patients may suffer from

A. R. Brown: Department of Anesthesiology, College of Physicians & Surgeons, Columbia-Presbyterian Medical Center New York, New York 10032-3784.

TABLE 1. *The American Society of Anesthesiologists' Physical Status Classification*

ASA Class 1	A healthy patient (no organic, physiologic, biochemical, or psychiatric disturbance)
ASA Class 2	A patient with mild to moderate systemic disease Examples: essential hypertension, diabetes mellitus, chronic bronchitis
ASA Class 3	A patient with severe systemic disease that limits activity but is not incapacitating Examples: heart disease that limits activity, poorly controlled hypertension, diabetes mellitus with vascular complications, angina pectoris
ASA Class 4	A patient with incapacitating systemic disease that is a constant threat to life Examples: congestive heart failure, advanced renal, pulmonary, or hepatic dysfunction
ASA Class 5	A moribund patient who is not expected to survive for 24 hours with or without an operation Examples: Pulmonary embolus, cerebral trauma, ruptured abdominal aneurysm. In the event of an emergency operation, the number is preceded with an E.

cardiac, pulmonary, renal, hematologic, and neurologic dysfunction.[95,158]

C. to document medication the patient may be receiving. Medication may influence the choice of anesthetic, because certain medications may result in dangerous drug interactions with commonly used anesthetic agents (e.g., monoamine oxidase inhibitors)[164,191] or may influence the choice of anesthetic (e.g., anticoagulants and central neuraxis blocks).[155,165]

II. Review of appropriate preoperative tests. The medical condition of the patient will determine the necessity of specific preoperative tests. In the case of a healthy patient, the tests performed will depend on the guidelines laid down by the individual institution (Table 2).[136]

III. Discussion of such issues as risks and benefits of regional versus general anesthesia; expectations in the operating room (monitor placement and initiation of anesthesia); and postoperative pain management options. Previous anesthetic experience should be discussed, because it may impact on the patient's attitude toward regional versus general anesthesia. The importance of establishing rapport with the patient cannot be overemphasized, because premedication is seldom a viable option in this era of ambulatory and same-day surgery. The goal is to decrease the patient's fears and anxieties related to the perioperative experience.

IV. Examination of the patient's upper airway, cardiovascular, and respiratory systems. Preexisting neurologic deficits should be assessed and documented. This is of particular importance if regional anesthesia is being considered.

V. Discussion of anesthetic options, including relative risks and benefits.

VI. Obtaining anesthesia consent.

In a well-run preadmission unit, the patient is seen in a pleasant setting, the waiting period is minimal, preoperative testing is performed in an efficient manner, and a well-in-

TABLE 2. *Summary of preoperative test recommendations*

Asymptomatic individuals			Individuals not receiving general or major conduction anesthesia	
Age	Men	Women	Sedative hypnotics for intravenous monitored anesthesia	Peripheral or nerve block
6 mo to <40 yr	None	Hct ? Pregnancy test	None	None
40 to <50 yr	EKG	Hct ? Pregnancy test	None	None
50 to 64 yr	EKG	Hct ? Pregnancy test EKG	Hct (within 6/12)	None
65 to 74 yr	Hb/Hct EKG BUN Glucose	Hb/Hct EKG BUN Glucose	Hct (within 6/12) EKG (within 1 yr)	Hct (within 6/12)
>74 yr	Hb/Hct EKG BUN Glucose ? CXR	Hb/Hct EKG BUN Glucose ? CXR	Hct (within 6/12) EKG (within 1 yr) BUN (within 6/12) Glucose (within 6/12)	Hct (within 6/12) EKG (within 1 yr)

Reprinted with permission from ref. 136.

formed patient leaves the unit knowing what to expect on the day of surgery and comfortable with the knowledge that management of preoperative anxieties, intraoperative course, and postoperative pain will be of utmost importance to the anesthesia care team.[85]

An additional benefit of the preadmission visit is the positive influence a well-functioning unit may have on operating room efficiency and utilization. Lack of a preoperative history and physical examination and incomplete preoperative testing are common causes of operating room delays, whereas poorly controlled systemic disease may result in cancellation of a patient's surgery. Delays in initiation or cancellation of cases can wreak havoc with operating room efficiency. Although these problems cannot be totally eliminated, they can be significantly reduced by encouraging patients to attend the preadmission unit.[31,136]

ANESTHETIC OPTIONS

General Versus Regional Anesthesia

Shoulder surgery can be successfully performed under general anesthesia, regional anesthesia (interscalene brachial plexus block), or a combination of the two. The goals are to utilize an anesthetic technique that is safe and pleasant for the patient, to provide optimal operating conditions for the surgeon, and to reduce morbidity to a minimum. The final choice will depend on the planned surgical procedure, medical condition of the patient, patient preferences, and the skill and experience of the anesthesiologist. The majority of anesthesiologists are comfortable administering general anesthesia. The technique is familiar, control of the patient's airway under circumstances of limited patient access is guaranteed, and the perceived disadvantages of regional anesthesia (time to perform the block, complications, and failure of the block) are nonissues (Table 3). However, regional anesthesia offers a number of significant advantages, when administered by an individual experienced in these techniques (Table 4).

The most significant advantage of regional anesthesia in shoulder surgery is the perioperative pain control achieved by an interscalene brachial plexus block. The concept of preemptive analgesia is currently under intensive investigation.[116,141,153] It is based on the theory that peripheral tissue injury results in modification of nociceptive processing at both the peripheral and central nervous system levels. Prevention of the surgical stimulus by means of a local anesthetic block results in a decrease in the hypersensitivity of peripheral nerve endings, as well as the hyperreflexia that occurs at the spinal cord level. This results in a decrease in the overall pain experienced postoperatively by the patient, not only while the block is in effect, but also when the block has worn off. As a result, the patient's postoperative pain may be controlled with minor oral analgesics rather than with systemic opioids. The latter are associated with significantly more side effects, particularly nausea, vomiting, and sedation. These side effects may result in delayed discharge from the ambulatory surgery center (occasionally an unscheduled overnight admission may become necessary) and a decrease in patient satisfaction.[192] Inpatients experience the same opioid side effects, resulting in delayed ambulation, recovery, and hospital discharge.

Numerous muscle groups stabilize the shoulder joint. Intraoperative muscle relaxation is therefore an essential element of successful shoulder anesthesia. This can be achieved with either regional or general anesthesia. The effect of regional anesthesia is limited to the operative limb, thus obviating the necessity for endotracheal intubation and ventilation of the patient. In addition, the quality of muscle relaxation achieved with an interscalene block may be superior to that achieved with muscle relaxants. A local anesthetic of appropriate concentration and duration (e.g., mepivacaine 1.5% or bupivacaine 0.5%) will achieve a complete motor block of consistent intensity. Muscle relaxation under general anesthesia is achieved with muscle relaxants of vary-

TABLE 3. *General anesthesia—advantages and disadvantages*

Advantages	Disadvantages
Familiar technique Control of the airway ? Improved efficiency	Side effects associated with general anesthesia (e.g., postoperative nausea and vomiting, sore throat) Postoperative pain Side effects of postoperative pain medication Less patient satisfaction Increased recovery room (PACU) length of stay

TABLE 4. *Regional anesthesia—advantages and disadvantages*

Advantages	Disadvantages
Preemptive, intraoperative, and enhanced postoperative pain control	Complications (and failure) may occur, particularly in inexperienced hands
Muscle relaxation limited to the operative limb	Requires additional injections
Less intraoperative bleeding	Control of a sedated patient's airway
Improved operating room efficiency	Risks associated with an anesthetized limb
Reduced requirements for postoperative pain medication, resulting in a reduction in their associated side effects (nausea and vomiting, sedation)	
Reduced nursing care	
Shorter recovery room and/or hospital stay	
Significant patient satisfaction	
Cost benefit of regional anesthesia	

ing duration. Unless the anesthesiologist is vigilant in maintaining an adequate and consistent level of motor block, the degree of relaxation will vary, resulting in operating conditions that are not consistent.

Compared with general anesthesia, an interscalene block may result in a decrease in intraoperative bleeding.[34,101,170] Numerous mechanisms have been proposed to explain this observation:

1. Ventilation of a patient under general anesthesia results in an increase in mean intrathoracic pressure, mean venous pressure, and, as a result, venous bleeding. These conditions do not exist in a spontaneously ventilating patient under regional anesthesia.
2. An interscalene block causes a sympathectomy of the ipsilateral upper arm, resulting in dilatation of the capacitance vessels. As a result, blood tends to drain away from the surgical site.[170] Positioning the patient in the beach-chair position further reduces the venous pressure at the operative site.
3. Patients under regional anesthesia have greater hemodynamic stability, with lower average blood pressures.[34] Decreased bleeding should improve the operating conditions for the surgeon, and may therefore decrease operating time. Although requirement for blood transfusion is uncommon in patients undergoing shoulder surgery, the reduction in blood loss associated with regional anesthesia would further reduce the necessity for, and hence risks associated with, the use of blood transfusions.

Additional advantages of regional anesthesia include avoidance of the major physiologic trespass associated with induction of general anesthesia, avoidance of airway instrumentation, decrease in postoperative medical complications, reduction in unplanned hospital admissions, decreased requirement for postoperative nursing care, and shorter recovery room post anesthesia care unit (PACU) stays.[19,30,34,82,101,170,186] Regional anesthesia also may result in an increase in operating room efficiency,[19,34,96] and has been shown to be more cost effective than general anesthesia.[66] Regional techniques allow communication with the patient,which can be important under certain circumstances, e.g., symptoms of hypoglycemia could be conveyed by a diabetic patient. In the rare event of an emergency shoulder procedure, regional anesthesia will minimize the risk of aspiration of gastric contents. These benefits, coupled with the safety and efficacy of the block in experienced hands and extremely high patient satisfaction ratings,[19,169] suggest that an interscalene block should be the anesthetic technique of choice for most shoulder surgical procedures. However, it should be stated that a healthy patient receiving anesthesia from an individual inexperienced in the performance of an interscalene block may be better served receiving general anesthesia.[86]

Arguments may be made against the use of regional anesthesia. First, regional anesthesia is associated with numerous complications, a high failure rate, taking too long to perform and, as a result, delay in the start of surgery. The greater the experience of the individual performing the block, the less valid (and less vociferous) are the arguments against regional anesthesia. The failure rate, time to perform the block, and complication rate are indirectly proportional to the experience of the individual performing the block.[3,19,30,34,180] In experienced hands, the time to perform the block is not significantly different from that required to induce general anesthesia. This is true even in academic institutions, provided the instructors are skilled regional anesthesiologists. The efficiency of regional anesthesia may be further increased by the use of a regional anesthesia induction area.[19]

Second, patient's fear the additional, painful needle stick. This fear may be allayed by patient education, i.e., preoperative explanation of the technique used with particular emphasis placed on steps taken to minimize patient discomfort.

Third, some anesthesiologists (and surgeons) experience discomfort managing an awake as opposed to an anesthetized patient. In addition, care of an awake or sedated patient may be more labor intensive than an anesthetized patient. It is the author's opinion that the benefits of regional anesthesia far outweigh any inconvenience of caring for a patient under regional anesthesia.

General considerations

A number of considerations apply to all patients undergoing shoulder surgery, whether they receive regional or general anesthesia.

The minimum requirements for intraoperative monitoring include an electrocardiograph (EKG), an automatic noninvasive blood pressure monitor, and a pulse oximeter. The position of the EKG limb lead that is usually placed in the vicinity of the operative shoulder must be altered to avoid the surgical field. Although not mandatory with regional anesthesia, continuous monitoring of expired carbon dioxide is routinely used at the author's institution as a sensitive indicator of ventilation. A split nasal cannula, or a small catheter positioned alongside a regular nasal cannula, provides a continuous recording of expired carbon dioxide. Ventilation also can be monitored with a precordial stethoscope or by simple observation of the patient. Monitoring of ventilation in patients receiving regional anesthesia supplemented with sedation is essential, if potentially disastrous outcomes are to be avoided.[25,67] Use of the pulse oximeter alone for this purpose is not entirely adequate, because desaturation may be a late sign of inadequate ventilation. In addition to the above, temperature monitoring is regarded as standard care for patients undergoing general anesthesia.

Invasive monitoring (arterial line, central venous pressure, pulmonary artery pressure) is not usually indicated for patients undergoing shoulder surgery. The need for these monitors is determined by the medical condition of the patient, as well as by those situations in which the risk of rapid and extensive blood loss may exist. Attention should be directed toward the placement of the arterial line transducer (and, for that matter, blood pressure cuff) in a patient in the beach-chair position. Zeroing the arterial transducer at the arm level overreads the pressure perfusing the cerebral cortex. This is of particular importance in patients suffering from peripheral vascular disease. A more accurate recording is obtained by zeroing the transducer at the ear level.

All patients must have a functioning intravenous line (in the arm opposite to the surgical site) prior to the induction of general or regional anesthesia. Placement of the intravenous line in the antecubital fossa should be avoided, if possible, because this will limit the use of the patient's only functional upper extremity. Fluid replacement is not usually a major concern in shoulder surgery, because most procedures are of limited duration and significant blood loss is uncommon. During total shoulder replacement, blood loss occurs predominantly during reaming of the humerus in preparation for insertion of the humeral prosthesis. Average blood loss during an uncomplicated total shoulder replacement should be less than 500 ml. However, there are procedures in which blood loss can be substantial (e.g., revision total shoulder arthroplasty, open reduction and internal fixation of a fractured humerus). In these situations, adequate intravenous access should be established. In elective procedures, the patient may wish to predonate his or her own blood (autologous blood) for perioperative use.

Shoulder surgery may be performed in the beach-chair or lateral decubitus position. The majority of shoulder procedures are performed at the author's institution with the patient in the beach-chair position (Figs. 1 and 2). Benefits attributed to this position include ease of setup, lack of brachial plexus strain, excellent arthroscopic intraarticular visualization, and ease of conversion to the open approach.[159] In this position, the table is flexed at the hips and

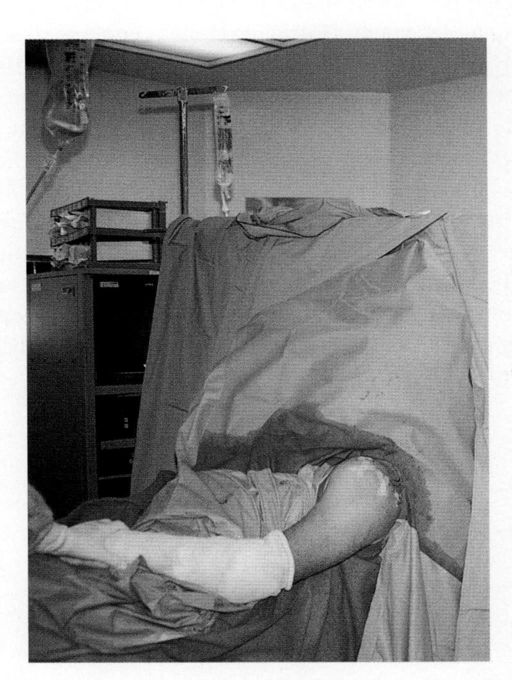

FIG. 1. Fully draped patient in the beach-chair position with the operative arm exposed.

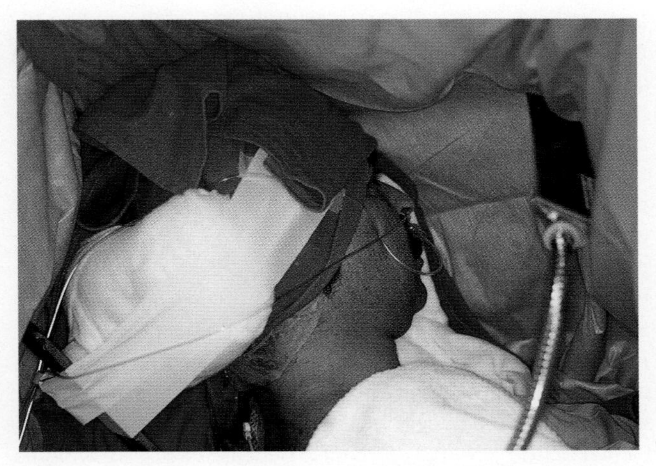

FIG. 2. Fully draped patient in the beach-chair position, demonstrating the head taped in position, free access to the face, oxygen delivery via a nasal cannula, and expired carbon dioxide monitoring via a nasal catheter.

the knees. An attempt should be made to maintain the lower extremities close to the heart level to minimize peripheral venous pooling. The patient's operative shoulder is shifted laterally off the table, so that it is free of the mattress. The patient's head is placed in a padded head rest in the neutral position and secured with tape. Turning the head away from the operative shoulder should be avoided, because this can cause traction on the operative side brachial plexus, particularly when traction is applied to the arm. A strap should be placed across the patient's hips to secure the patient and prevent further lateral movement off the table. A folded sheet is placed behind the medial border of the ipsilateral scapula to bring the operative shoulder forward and free of the mattress. In a nonintubated patient, care should be taken to optimize the patient's airway prior to securing the head in the headrest. Special consideration may need to be given to a subgroup of shoulder patients suffering from degenerative joint diseases, who may or may not have undergone multiple previous orthopedic procedures. These patients should be positioned in a way that affords them the greatest degree of comfort. This can be easily achieved in an awake patient who can not only cooperate, but also guide the operating room team in optimizing his or her position following insertion of the nerve block.

The nonoperative arm should be protected and may be placed alongside the patient. The author prefers to secure the nonoperative arm on a well-padded armboard placed at a 75 to 85 degree angle to the operating table. This facilitates intraoperative access to the patient's intravenous line and pulse oximeter.

The beach-chair position may pose a problem in the event of an emergency intubation. Although this should be a rare event, occasionally, particularly in inexperienced hands, an urgent intubation is required. Causes include failure to establish that a block is inadequate prior to surgical incision, inability to adequately sedate a patient, and excessive sedation of a patient. The surgical drapes will need to be adjusted and the back of the operating table lowered. The head may not be favorably positioned for intubation, particularly when a nonadjustable headrest is used. A headrest that can be easily and rapidly adjusted for both height and angle is a safer choice.

At the author's institution, a posterior approach to the shoulder (e.g., instability repair) is performed, using a combined technique (regional and general anesthesia) with the patient in the lateral decubitus position (Fig. 3). In this position, all pressure points should be carefully padded. Both the superior and dependent limbs are at risk for brachial plexus injury. Any extreme position of the superior limb can cause traction and subsequent ischemia to the brachial plexus. A traction pulley device with 5 pounds of weight may be attached to the operative extremity. Because excessive weights can cause traction injury to the brachial plexus, somatosensory evoked potential (SSEP) monitoring may be used intraoperatively to detect injury that may be developing. Under these circumstances, a narcotic, nitrous oxide/oxygen, relaxant anesthetic technique is recommended.[9] The dependent brachial plexus and blood vessels may be compressed between the rib cage and the head of the humerus. Neurologic and/or vascular damage can be prevented by the placement of an axillary role, to keep the weight of the patient's thorax off the head of the humerus. Adequate perfusion can be detected by monitoring the wave form of the pulse oximeter, or clinically by observing venous engorgement or poor capillary refill. Continuous monitoring is essential, because the patient's position may change during the procedure.

Hynson et al.[74] reported a case of complete airway obstruction during arthroscopic shoulder surgery in the lateral decubitus position in an awake patient under regional anesthesia. The anesthesiologist should be alert to the possibility of fluid dissection into the upper torso and neck when irrigation pumps are used. Because the lateral position may contribute to the accumulation of fluid in the soft tissues of the neck, the sitting (beach-chair) position may be preferable to reduce fluid migration and airway edema. Clinicians should maintain a high level of awareness during shoulder arthroscopy, particularly when the procedure is prolonged and involves extensive debridement or extracapsular maneuvers. Periodic evaluation of the neck for swelling, particularly in the lateral decubitus position, should be performed.

Besides fluid, extravasation of air also has been reported during or immediately after shoulder arthroscopy. This has resulted in subcutaneous emphysema, pneumomediastinum, and potentially life-threatening pneumothorax.[91,92] Early diagnosis, followed by immediate termination of the procedure, along with appropriate treatment (chest tube in the case of a tension pneumothorax), can be life-saving.

Ichai et al.[75] report a death due to cerebral edema as a result of intravascular absorption of glycine irrigating solution during shoulder arthroscopy. The patient's emergence from general anesthesia was noted to be slow. Following extubation, the patient complained of nausea and was noted to be slightly sleepy. Seven and a half hours postoperatively, the patient was found to have severe bradypnea, a Glascow Coma Scale score of 3, and fixed, dilated pupils. Glycine is absorbed intravascularly during shoulder arthroscopy; therefore, if glycine is used, patients should be closely observed in the postoperative period.

Venous air embolism is a potential problem that may be associated with the beach-chair position, because the operative site is above the level of the heart. From a practical standpoint this has not proven to be a problem. However, it might be prudent to take precautions by monitoring for the occurrence of venous air embolism in patients with a known right-to-left shunt.[52]

Total shoulder replacement involves removal of the humeral head and replacement with a prosthesis that is inserted into the shaft of the humerus. In addition, a prosthetic component may be placed into the glenoid cavity. Methylmethacrylate is used to cement the implant into the humeral shaft. The cement consists of granular methylmethacrylate, to which a liquid monomer is added immediately prior to use. Its use has been associated with hemodynamic instability (including cardiac arrest) and pulmonary changes during total hip replacement. Huffnagle et al.[73] reported no adverse hemodynamic events or increased pulmonary shunting associated with the use of methylmethacrylate in a group of patients undergoing total shoulder surgery. Despite these findings, precautions should be taken to minimize the possibility of adverse events related to embolization and/or the use of methylmethacrylate by maintaining an adequate fluid volume status and ensuring normal oxygen saturation throughout the procedure. The surgical technique should include elimination of reamed intramedullary contents and venting of the medullary cavity during insertion of the bone cement.

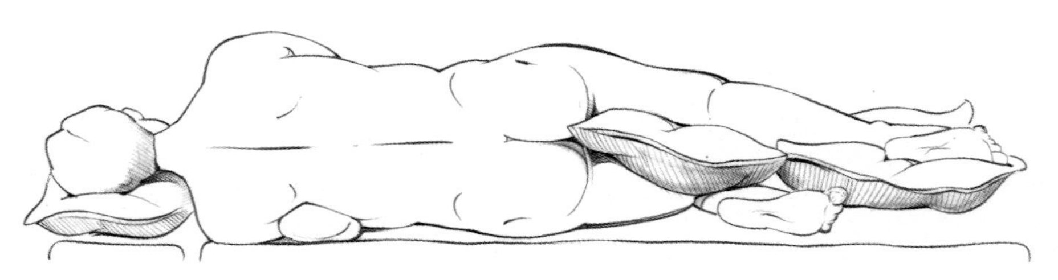

FIG. 3. Patient in the right lateral decubitus position, demonstrating the appropriate padding over bony prominences, chest roll to protect the axilla, and proper alignment of the cervical spine.

General Anesthesia

Shoulder surgery performed under general anesthesia usually requires the use of an endotracheal tube. This is due to the proximity of the surgical site to the face. The exception is the patient undergoing manipulation under anesthesia, in whom mask general anesthesia may be used. In the latter case, it is essential that an adequate depth of anesthesia is achieved to avoid laryngospasm that could result from vigorous manipulation of a painful, stiff shoulder.

In a subgroup of shoulder patients, intubation may be difficult, due to associated pathology affecting the cervical spine and/or the temperomandibular joints (e.g., rheumatoid arthritis). Under these circumstances, specialized techniques and equipment (e.g. fiberoptic intubation) will be required.

The endotracheal tube needs to be well secured on the side opposite to that of the surgery, because movement of the shoulder during the procedure may result in dislodgment of a casually secured tube.

The beach-chair position and the elaborate surgical draping required to maintain a sterile field limit the anesthesiologist's access to the patient. As a result, in addition to the endotracheal tube, all monitors, as well as the temperature probe and orogastric tube, should be well secured. The face (particularly the eyes) should be protected against accidental injury from surgeons leaning on or placing objects on the drapes overlying the face (surgeons may need to be reminded of the proximity of the face to the operative site). An ether screen or a gooseneck-shaped adjustable metal bar may be useful in preventing the drapes from covering the patient's face.

Patients undergoing shoulder surgery, particularly those with degenerative joint disease, often have other joint involvement; thus, extra care needs to be taken in positioning and protecting these patients.

The majority of open shoulder procedures are completed within 2 to 3 hours, with the possible exception of a revision total shoulder arthroplasty and an open reduction and internal fixation/hemiarthroplasty of a shoulder fracture. Under these circumstances, in which surgery may be prolonged and blood loss significant, catheterization of the bladder to monitor urinary output as a sensitive indicator of fluid volume status is prudent.

At the author's institution, where regional anesthesia is the technique of choice for shoulder surgery, the following situations are regarded as indications for combining regional with general anesthesia:

1. Anticipation of a long surgical procedure (e.g., revision total shoulder arthroplasty).
2. A patient with a potentially difficult airway, requesting more than minimal sedation.
3. The existence of an absolute contraindication to regional anesthesia (e.g., patient refusal, sepsis at the block site). A number of relative contraindications to regional anesthesia exist, e.g., preexisting nerve damage. The decision to perform an interscalene block under these circumstances will depend on the risk/benefit ratio to the patient and will vary not only with the patient's condition, but also with the experience of the anesthesiologist making the decision.
4. The anesthesiologist is inexperienced or uncomfortable utilizing an interscalene block supplemented by sedation for shoulder surgery. Numerous advantages can be attributed to regional over general anesthesia for shoulder surgery. However, as mentioned above, the success rate and complication rate are largely dependent on the experience of the anesthesiologist. Patient safety should be the prime concern of the physicians taking care of the patient. Therefore, although some of the benefits of regional over general anesthesia may be lost with the use of a combined technique, the overall comfort of the patient (and the anesthesiologist) may be best served by the use of a combined technique.
5. The inclusion of an iliac crest bone graft as part of the surgical procedure. Occasionally, an iliac crest bone graft may be required to complete a surgical procedure. A number of anesthetic options, including the use of a combined technique, have been described. Alternatively, anesthesia may be achieved by combining an interscalene block with local infiltration at the site of the iliac crest donor site. Additional sedation may be required during the removal of the bone graft. Another option is the use of a lumbar epidural catheter, placed prior to the start of surgery. Postoperatively, the donor site may cause more discomfort to the patient than the operative site. A continuous infusion of local anesthetic by means of a catheter, placed prior to closure of the donor site, has proven to be a successful form of treatment.[21]

REGIONAL ANESTHESIA

The author believes that unless contraindicated, regional anesthesia is the technique of choice for most patients undergoing shoulder surgery. Under certain circumstances (as described above), a combined technique is indicated. In these situations, the interscalene block is performed prior to the induction of general anesthesia.[114] This decision is based on the fact that permanent nerve damage (a rare complication of regional anesthesia), if directly attributable to the nerve block, is caused either by direct needle trauma to the nerve, a direct intraneural injection, or a combination of the two.[104,146,148–150] Because direct needle trauma may cause painful paresthesias, and a direct intraneural injection causes severe pain on injection, an awake (albeit mildly sedated) patient can immediately alert the anesthesiologist to the potential danger associated with initiating or continuing the injection. In this way, further nerve damage can avoided. Under general anesthesia, these warning signs cannot be relayed to the anesthesiologist, thus decreasing the safety of the technique. An exception to this rule is the young child or agitated adult who cannot be appropriately sedated. Under these circumstances, the anesthesiologist may be presented with a moving target that may increase the likelihood of complications and decrease the success rate. In this situation, it may be safer to anesthetize the patient prior to performing the block.

The benefits of regional anesthesia over general anesthesia have been described above. It should, however, be stressed that a successful nerve block does not necessarily result in successful regional anesthesia. In the author's opinion, an unsedated patient who is left in an acutely anxious state during the operative procedure, despite a perfectly functioning peripheral nerve block, should be classified as a failed regional anesthetic. De Andres et al.[39] evaluated the factors that influence patient satisfaction with regional anesthesia. They concluded that in addition to utilizing the correct anesthetic procedure, adequate sedation may favor patient acceptance of regional anesthesia. Careful patient preparation and attention to detail will improve patient acceptance and satisfaction.[160] For regional anesthesia to be classified as completely successful, the following goals should be met:

1. A successful, uncomplicated nerve block.
2. A comfortable patient.
3. Optimal operating conditions.
4. An uncomplicated postoperative period.

Successful Block

The requirements for a successful nerve block are many, and include its appropriateness for the surgery. The anatomic limitations and variations of the specific block and how this may impact on the planned surgical procedure must be taken into account. Although an interscalene block will provide complete anesthesia of the shoulder joint and surrounding muscles, the variable cutaneous innervation to the skin of the anterior/upper axillary area, as well as the posterior aspect of the shoulder (i.e., T2–3), needs to be taken into account when the surgical approach involves these dermatomes (Figs. 4 and 5). A paravertebral or intercostal block of T2 has been recommended as a solution to this problem.[44,127] Peterson[120] performed upper thoracic paravertebral blockade of T1–3 for complete anesthesia of the shoulder. This involved a large volume (dose) of local anesthetic and multiple injections. A simpler and effective technique is subcutaneous infiltration of the arthroscopic portals (particularly the posterior portal) or planned skin incision (e.g., the lower end of an anterior-inferior capsular shift skin incision that extends toward the axilla). Sedation may be required during an anterior-inferior capsular shift procedure, as retractors are deeply placed in the wound.

Also relevant is a block of adequate duration for the surgery. A nerve block that wears off before the end of surgery is a failed block. If the duration of surgery is unpredictable, a long-acting local anesthetic agent (prolonged postoperative analgesia is usually greatly appreciated by the patient) or a continuous catheter technique should be used.

Adequate muscle relaxation must also be considered. Shoulder surgery is facilitated by optimal muscle relaxation. In the author's experience, mepivacaine and bupivacaine provide excellent muscle relaxation when used in concentrations of 1.5% and 0.5%, respectively. However, the adequacy of muscle relaxation with bupivacaine has been questioned.[17] Bupivacaine exhibits the property of sensory-motor dissociation. At a bupivacaine concentration of 0.5%, sen-

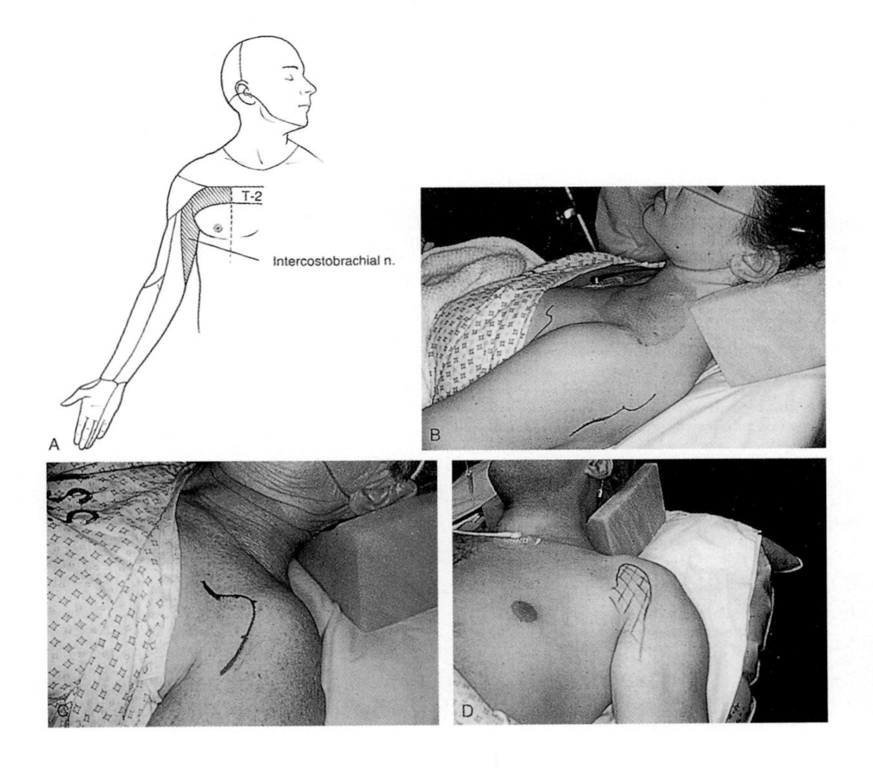

FIG. 4. (A) Sensory innervation and course of the intercostobrachial nerve (T2). Three photographs show the real sensory distribution in patients. **(B)** No tongue. **(C)** Small tongue. **(D)** Large tongue. (Reprinted with permission from ref. 181.)

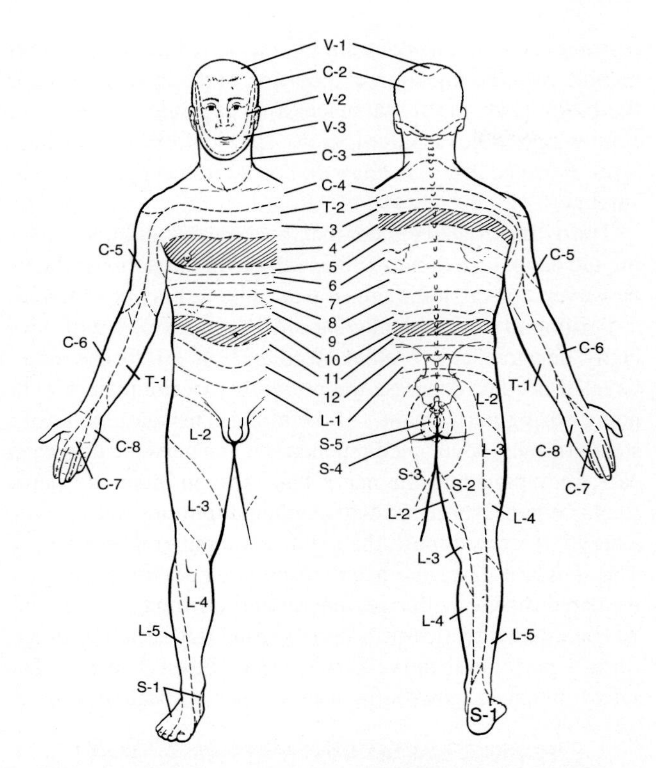

FIG. 5. Posterior cutaneous innervation of the shoulder.

sory, as well as motor blockade, is achieved. Reducing the concentration to 0.25% while still providing an adequate sensory block will result in a motor block of variable intensity that may not be adequate for surgery. At still lower concentrations, the motor block is lost, while the sensory block may still be adequate to produce analgesia.[42]

Comfortable Patient

This is one of the most important requirements of successful regional anesthesia, yet one of the most neglected. The concept encompasses the preoperative visit/assessment, the immediate preblock period, as well as the intra- and postoperative course. Communication with the patient during this entire period is essential.

Preoperatively, most patients have similar fears, anxieties, and questions they would like answered. These questions should be answered in a manner that is reassuring to the patient, so that trust and confidence between the patient and physician can be established. One frequently raised issue is the fear that the block will be painful. It should be stressed that insertion of the block is no more painful than insertion of an intravenous cannula. In fact, the patient may experience less discomfort during performance of the block, due to preblock administration of sedatives and analgesics and skin infiltration with a fine-gauge needle prior to insertion of the block. The addition of 0.1 ml of bicarbonate to 1 ml of lidocaine may further reduce any discomfort produced by an intradermal injection.[99] Unless paresthesia is unintentionally elicited, the patient may not be aware that the block is being performed.

Another fear expressed by the patient is that he or she might see, feel, or hear something, or that he or she might be left alone. The patient should be reassured that a member of the anesthesia team will be present at all times, that he or she can be sedated to a level of comfort, and that the surgery will not commence until success of the block is confirmed.

The surgical team needs to be aware that surgery is being performed under regional and not general anesthesia. This may necessitate modification both in their behavior and surgical technique.

Optimal Operating Conditions

Skilled anesthesia includes safe, effective, and efficient anesthesia. In addition, the surgeon's expectations and desires are important, as long as they are not at the expense of patient safety. Thus, quality anesthesia includes ideal operating conditions for the surgeon.

The common misconception that regional anesthesia delays the start of surgery has been disproved in a number of studies. Brown et al.[19] reported no significant difference in the anesthesia preparation time (patient in operating room to anesthesia ready i.e., patient ready for the surgical team) between regional and general anesthesia. Positioning, preparing, and draping while the block is setting helps to minimize the waiting period. At the end of the procedure, the patient is wide awake, can assist in placement of the braces and special dressings, and can leave the operating room as soon as the dressings are complete. This is in contrast to the scenario of a patient under general anesthesia, where delays can occur due to a slow awakening patient, including delayed reversal of muscle relaxants and delayed extubation.

The efficiency of regional anesthesia may be improved further by inserting the block outside the operating room in a designated holding area. This designated area should be fully equipped to monitor the patient and to treat any complications that may occur. In addition, the patient should not be left alone once the block has been inserted.

Some surgeons are uncomfortable operating on awake patients. This needs to be taken into account when discussing the anesthetic plan with the patient. Patient safety is of prime importance. A patient with a questionable airway should receive minimal, if any, sedation. If this is not acceptable, the patient's airway should be secured with either a laryngeal mask airway or an endotracheal tube.

Uncomplicated Postoperative Course

An explanation of the expected duration of the block should be given to the patient. This will allay patient fears of permanent nerve damage following a long-acting block. It is not uncommon for the duration of a bupivacaine block to exceed 24 hours before complete resolution. The benefit of prolonged postoperative analgesia, provided by a long-acting local anesthetic agent, should be emphasized to the patient.

Analgesics (systemic or oral) should be administered at the earliest signs of the block wearing off. This will allow the analgesic to take effect before the block wears off completely, resulting in a smoother transition from one form of analgesia to another. Early treatment of pain is associated with greater ease of control and reduced analgesic requirements, with a resultant reduction in associated side effects. This is particularly important in the outpatient setting, where oral analgesics are more likely to be administered.

Finally, it should be the responsibility of all individuals involved in the care of these patients to confirm that the anesthetized limb is well protected. The symptoms of excessive pressure or poor positioning of the anesthetized limb cannot be reported by the patient. Care and vigilance are therefore key components in preventing postoperative neurologic and vascular complications in an anesthetized limb following shoulder surgery.

The management of a patient undergoing shoulder surgery under regional anesthesia can be divided into three stages:

1. Preoperative preparation
2. Insertion of the block and intraoperative care
3. Postoperative management

PREOPERATIVE PREPARATION

Preoperative preparation includes the availability of appropriate equipment and supplies, as well as the preparation of the patient.

Equipment and Supplies

The area where the block is inserted should be fully equipped to monitor and, if necessary, resuscitate the patient. In addition, the operating room should be set up to provide general anesthesia. Conversion from regional to general anesthesia may be necessary for a number of reasons. First, the block may fail. Success rates vary with the experience of the individual performing the block. A success rate of 91% to 97% has been reported in experienced hands.[19,34,170,180] Following a failed block, the available options include repeating the block[46,54] or converting to general anesthesia.

Second, the patient may develop a toxic reaction to the local anesthesia agent. This should be a rare occurrence,[20] and when associated with peripheral nerve blocks, it is usually the result of a direct intravascular injection. Vigilance and early diagnosis should prevent the administration of a large intravascular dose of local anesthetic. Cessation of further administration, the avoidance of hypoxia, hypercarbia, and acidosis, and treatment of central nervous system excitability with centrally acting hypnosedatives (midazolam, thiopentone, propofol, or diazepam) are usually successful solutions.[20] Once the patient has been stabilized, the surgery may proceed either under the interscalene block (if, despite an intravascular injection of a portion of the local anesthetic, the block turns out to be successful) or general anesthesia. Following cardiovascular toxicity (particularly if associated with bupivacaine), it may be prudent to postpone the surgery.

Third, the sedated patient may become disinhibited. Altering the depth of sedation will usually overcome this problem. However, conversion to general anesthesia may be required.

Peripheral nerve blocks should be performed with specially designed nerve block needles (Fig. 6). These short-beveled needles decrease the possibility of traumatizing the nerve during performance of the block. The sharp point of a standard long-bevel needle penetrates the nerve with greater ease, may penetrate the nerve fascicles, and may cut nerve fibers. When a short-beveled needle comes into contact with a nerve, it tends to push the nerve aside rather than cut it.[151] The standard 22-gauge needle used need not necessarily be insulated for use with a peripheral nerve stimulator.[6,56,102]

The characteristics of a nerve stimulator suitable to perform a peripheral nerve block are listed in Table 5. The safety and success with the use of a nerve stimulator,[122,133]

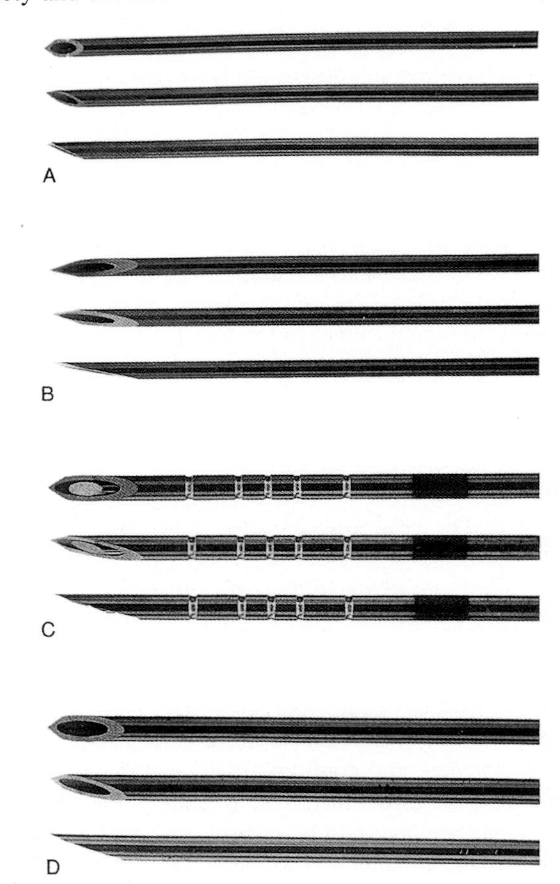

FIG. 6. Frontal, oblique, and lateral views of regional block needles. **(A)** Blunt-beveled, 25-guage axillary block needle. **(B)** Long-beveled, 25-guage (hypodermic) block needle. **(C)** Ultrasound "imaging" needle. **(D)** Short-beveled, 22-guage regional block needle. (Reprinted with permission from ref. 109.)

TABLE 5. *Characteristics of a nerve stimulator suitable for peripheral nerve block*

Constant current output
Clear meter reading to 0.1 mAmps (preferably digital)
Variable output control
Linear output
Clearly marked polarity
Short pulse width
Pulse of 1 Hz
Battery indicator
High and low output (clearly marked)
High-quality alligator-type clips

Reprinted with permission from ref. 122.

compared with eliciting paresthesia to confirm proximity of the needle tip to the nerve, is a controversial issue.[97,104,131,147] There does not appear to be any clear-cut advantage of one technique over the other. The success rate and the lack of severe complications are similar in experienced hands. The author favors the use of the nerve stimulator for two reasons. First, paresthesia requires a fully cooperative patient who needs to inform the anesthesiologist when paresthesia occurs as well as the distribution of the paresthesia. The nerve stimulator technique is dependent on a more objective muscle twitch that requires no communication or cooperation from the patient. This facilitates the performance of a block in patients in whom there is a language barrier, young patients, as well as excessively anxious patients who need to be appropriately sedated.

Second, some patients have an extremely low pain tolerance, particularly in the anxiety-provoking scenario of an operating room. Under these circumstances, paresthesia can be an unpleasant or painful experience for the unsedated patient.

Preparation of the Patient

The practice of regional anesthesia involves significant interaction with an awake patient. This requires interpersonal skills and an additional commitment to the well-being of the patient. Not only is it essential to gain the patient's confidence, but also to "sell" the block to the patient, i.e., point out the advantages of regional over general anesthesia in his or her specific case. For example, the author stresses the excellent intra- and postoperative analgesia (the potential postoperative benefit of preemptive analgesia is explained in detail) achieved with regional anesthesia, avoidance of the risks and side effects of general anesthesia, and the increased likelihood of a smooth postoperative course and shortened hospital stay.[19,34,170] The positive psychological impact on the attitude of the patient toward his or her perioperative experience cannot be overemphasized.

The patient should be given a detailed explanation of the procedure from the time he or she enters the operating room until discharge from the postanesthesia care unit. This includes the performance of the block as well as the intraoperative care of the patient. He or she should be informed that in the unlikely event of an inadequate block, supplementation with an additional block or conversion to general anesthesia will be implemented. It should be stressed that the adequacy of the block will be established prior to the start of surgery and that the patient's comfort will be of prime concern at all times.

Inadequate sedation is the only major complaint reported following successful interscalene block anesthesia for shoulder surgery.[19,169] If a relative contraindication to sedation exists (e.g., potentially difficult intubation), this should be discussed with the patient and a decision made as to whether the procedure could be performed under regional anesthesia without any sedation. If this is not possible, the airway should be protected with a laryngeal mask airway or endotracheal tube following insertion of the block. The patient may then be safely sedated and/or lightly anesthetized.

INSERTION OF THE BLOCK AND INTRAOPERATIVE CARE

An interscalene approach to the brachial plexus is regarded by many as the anesthetic technique of choice for shoulder surgery[19,30,34,170] and will therefore be discussed in detail. This approach was conceptualized by Etienne in 1925 and popularized by Winnie.[199] The brachial plexus is enclosed by a fascial sheath that extends from the cervical spine to the distal axilla. This permits local anesthetic blockade of the nerves supplying the upper limb to be performed by means of a single injection (Fig. 7). The interscalene approach to the brachial plexus is recommended for shoulder surgery. It is performed at the nerve root level, specifically at the level of C6. If an adequate volume of local anesthetic is injected, the anesthetic will diffuse upward (cephalad) to block C5 to C3, and occasionally the C2 nerve root. The local anesthetic will also spread downward (caudad) and outward (laterally) to block C6 and C7 (or the superior and middle trunks).[90] Nerve roots C8 and T1 (the inferior trunk) are blocked on a less consistent basis. The shoulder joint is supplied by C5–7 (brachial plexus), whereas the cutaneous innervation of the shoulder is predominantly derived from C4 and/or C3 (superficial cervical plexus). As a result, with a few exceptions (Figs. 4 and 5), an interscalene block will be effective in the majority of surgical approaches to the shoulder. The cutaneous innervation of the posterior (dorsal) aspect of the shoulder, as well as the lower anterior (ventral) aspect (extending caudad into the axilla), is provided by T2 and T3. Supplementary blocks of T2 and T3 (or subcutaneous infiltration of local anesthetic), when appropriate, will provide complete shoulder anesthesia. Surgical approaches in which supplementary blocks are indicated include an anterior inferior capsular shift/instability repair (if the incision extends into the axilla), a posterior instability repair, and occasionally the posterior and/or anterior arthroscopic portals (Fig. 4). The superior and deltopectoral approaches are

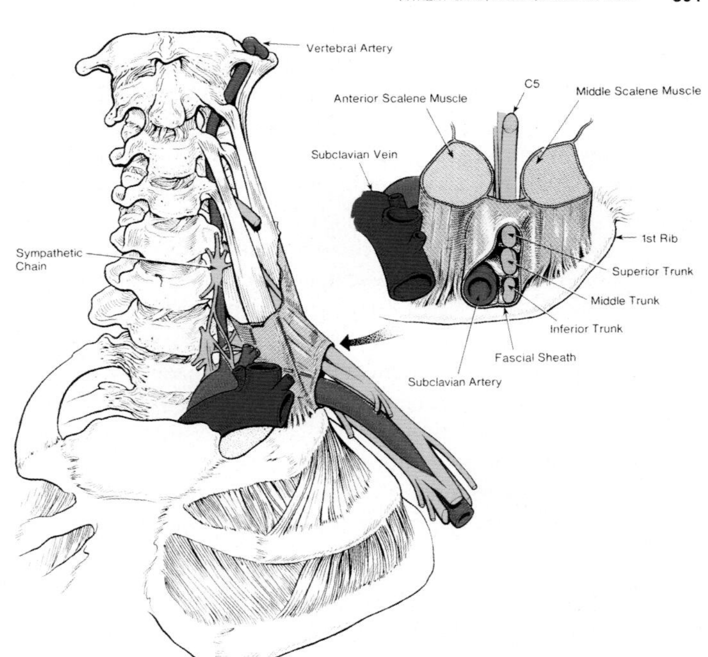

FIG. 7. Brachial plexus sheath and scalene muscles. Note brachial plexus sandwiched between the anterior and middle scalene muscles, prevertebral fascia splitting to enclose scalenes and then forming a fascial sheath around the brachial plexus. Note also the relationships to the vertebral artery, subclavian artery, and sympathetic chain. (Reprinted with permission from ref. 15.)

within the dermatomes anesthetized with an interscalene block.

The block is performed with the patient in the supine position on the operating room table. The cricoid cartilage is identified anteriorly, because this indicates the approximate level of the transverse process of C6. The head is then turned to the side opposite that to be blocked, and the shoulder is lowered as far as possible. The patient is instructed to raise his or her head slightly off the table to bring the two heads of the sternocleidomastoid muscle into prominence (sternal head medially, clavicular head laterally). It is essential that both heads are identified, because in a small percentage of cases, the clavicular head may be absent or may exist as an ill-defined broad band rather than a distinct entity. As a result, the lateral border of the sternal head may be mistakenly identified as the lateral border of the clavicular head and will result in misidentification of an interscalene groove that is medial to the true interscalene groove. The anesthesiologist's fingers are placed against the lateral border of the clavicular head and the patient is instructed to lower his or her head to the pillow and to relax the neck muscles. The operator's fingers will come to rest on the scalenus anterior muscle, which is immediately lateral and deep to the lateral border of the clavicular head. By walking or rolling the fingers laterally, a groove will be encountered that exists between the scalenus anterior and scalenus medius muscles (the interscalene groove). The point of needle insertion is where a line drawn horizontally from the cricoid cartilage crosses the interscalene groove. Some investigators have recommended that firm pressure be applied in the interscalene groove at the level of C6, to confirm the correct point of insertion. This is an unnecessary maneuver and is unpleasant if not painful for the patient. If uncertainty exists, the following aids to the identification of the interscalene groove have been described:

1. The external jugular vein often crosses the interscalene groove at the level of C6.
2. The 3.0 cm line. In a morbidly obese patient, the interscalene groove may be difficult to identify. However, the belly of the sternocleidomastoid muscle is usually palpable. A line drawn horizontally at the level of C6 from the lateral border of the main belly of the sternocleidomastoid muscle (not the lateral border of the clavicular head) and extended laterally for 3.0 cm will indicate the approximate, if not exact, point of insertion.[18]
3. A slow deep inspiration will result in contraction of the scalene muscles; this will facilitate location of the interscalene groove.[156]
4. Palpation of the subclavian artery will indicate the lower end of the groove. The subclavian artery crosses the first rib between the insertions of scalenus anterior and scalenus medius (Fig. 8). The interscalene groove extends upward (cephalad) and slightly medially from this point.

Following skin preparation, the needle is advanced at right angles to the skin, i.e., mesiad, slightly caudad and dorsad, with the bevel of the needle facing the sheath. This increases the likelihood that a click or pop through the sheath will be elicited (author's personal experience), although this is not always obvious, because the brachial plexus sheath is at its thinnest in the interscalene area. The needle is gently advanced until a paresthesia in the upper limb below the oper-

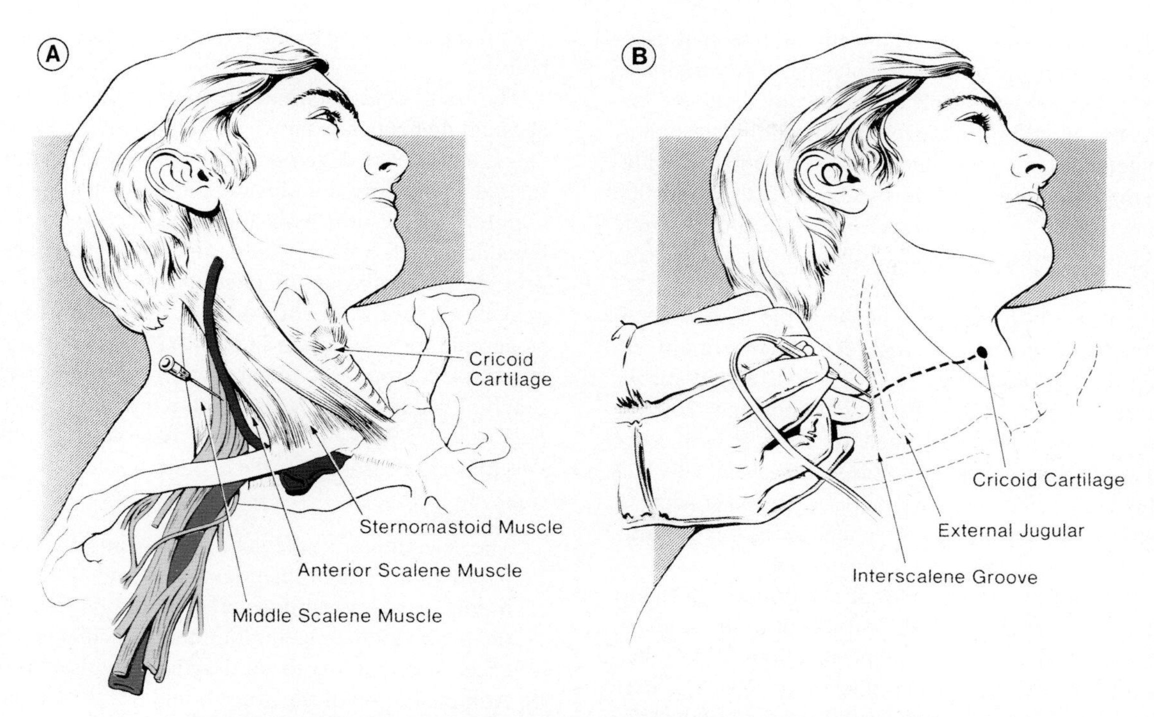

FIG. 8. Interscalene block: anatomic landmarks. (Reprinted with permission from ref. 15.)

ative shoulder is elicited. Roch et al. have suggested that a paresthesia at the level of the shoulder may be equally successful in indicating correct positioning of the needle.[135] A biceps and/or deltoid twitch at or below 0.3 mAmps is associated with a high success rate using a nerve stimulator technique (Table 6).[10]

Once the correct position of the needle (within the brachial plexus sheath) has been confirmed, the local anesthetic is injected in fractionated doses, with frequent aspiration to avoid an intravascular injection of a large dose of local anesthetic.

A variety of local anesthetic agents have been used to perform an interscalene block.[170,195] The ultimate choice will be determined by the desired duration of action of the local anesthetic and the personal preference of the anesthesiologist. Mepivacaine is commonly used for arthroscopic surgery, because it provides 2 to 3 hours of anesthesia. Longer acting agents are required for lengthy open shoulder procedures and to provide prolonged postoperative analgesia. Bupivacaine and supercaine (a mixture containing mepivacaine, tetracaine, and epinephrine)[200] provide long-acting blocks and postoperative analgesia that may exceed 24 hours in duration. Ropivacaine is a recently introduced long-acting local anesthetic that is similar in action to bupivacaine with less cardiotoxic potential.[98]

TABLE 6. *Rate of successful interscalene block as a function of the stimulating current*

Current output (mAmps)	Successful blocks (%)
0.6–1.0	36
0.5	82
0.4	84
0.3	93

Reprinted with permission from ref. 10.

Concerns have been expressed regarding the dose of local anesthetic used to perform an interscalene block, particularly when a block is repeated. These concerns are based on the maximum recommended doses of local anesthetics that appear in the literature. Although these doses of local anesthetic agents appear to offer a useful guide, particularly to the inexperienced regional anesthesiologist, the current recommendations appear illogical and without scientific foundation.[145] Moore et al., in reviewing 9,287 regional blocks, reported that the occurrence of systemic toxic reactions in adults does not correlate with the dosages and/or physical status of the patient when 400 mg or less of bupivacaine, 450 mg or less of etidocaine, or 500 mg or less of mepivacaine is used. The authors question the maximum dosages established for certain local anesthetic drugs, as well as the method by which such dosages were established.[103] Support is lent to these arguments by the following observations. First, the systemic toxic effects are dependent on the blood concentration of the specific local anesthetic agent. This is determined by the rate of vascular absorption, tissue redistribution, metabolism, and excretion. The site of injection is one of the primary factors that influences the rate of absorption.[41] Thus, the rate of absorption and maximum plasma concentration from an intercostal nerve block, epidural, or caudal anesthesia is significantly greater than that seen after a peripheral nerve blockade (i.e., interscalene block), which in turn is greater than the plasma concentration seen after local infiltration. If one assumes that a plasma concentration of 5 μg/ml of lidocaine will result in the development of toxic symptoms, this would be achieved by the administration of approximately 300 mg in the intercostal area, 500 mg epidurally, 600 mg in the region of the brachial plexus, and 1,000 mg subcutaneously.[176] Thus, recommendation of a single maximum dose without regard to the site of injection is meaningless.[145]

Second, there is a discrepancy between the United Kingdom and the United States with respect to the maximum recommended dose of lidocaine. In the United Kingdom, the maximum recommended dose for plain lidocaine is 200 mg, compared with 300 mg in the United States.[145] In both countries, 500 mg is recommended if epinephrine is added. This implies that epinephrine reduces the peak plasma concentration by 60%; however, there is no evidence for this assumption.

Third, the most common cause of acute local anesthetic toxicity is accidental intravascular injection. In the study by Moore et al., all nine systemic toxic reactions (0.1% incidence) resulted from intravascular injections. None occurred as a result of absorption.[103] The knowledge of maximum recommended doses is obviously of no value under these circumstances, because signs of toxicity will occur at significantly lower doses.

Who decides on the maximum recommended dose and how it is determined? The validity of extrapolating data obtained from research in laboratory animals to humans has been questioned.[103] With regard to lidocaine, it is not certain when or how the maximum recommended dose was determined. The 200 mg recommended currently in the United Kingdom appeared in the *Scandinavian Pharmacopoeia* around 1957.[145] Once such doses have been accepted by a government regulatory agency, they are difficult to change, even if proven wrong by animal research, human research, or both.

The traditional maximum recommended doses for local anesthetic agents are shown in Table 7. DiFazio stated that "local anesthetics develop a peak blood level that is directly related to the dose administered at a given site. In general, doubling of the dose will approximately double the blood level achieved; however, administration of a given dose of drug at different sites of injection will result in different peak blood levels."[48] For example, lidocaine 1 mg/kg given as an epidural will result in approximately a 1 μg/kg peak blood concentration, compared with 0.5 μg/kg following a brachial plexus block (less vascular area) with the same dose, and 1.5 μg/kg after an intercostal nerve block (highly vascular area). Based on these data, the following suggestions are advanced:

1. The selection of a safe dose of local anesthetic should be based on the site of injection. As a general rule, the maximum drug dose administered should be selected so that the peak blood concentration that is achieved should not exceed one half to one third of the convulsant blood level.
2. Administration of the drug should occur in a manner that will identify an unintended intravascular injection. This is achieved by adhering to the practice of fractionating the dose of local anesthetic, frequent gentle aspiration during the injection, and maintaining verbal contact with the patient.[48]
3. Revisions should be made to the standard recommendations regarding maximum recommended doses (Table 8).

The importance of the publication and acceptance of these modified maximum recommended doses cannot be overemphasized, because medicolegal problems may arise if the maximum recommended dose is exceeded and an unexpected reaction occurs (which may have little or no relation-

TABLE 7. *Traditional recommended doses of local anesthetic drugs*[a]

Drug	Plain (total mg)	Plain (mg/kg)	With epidural (total mg)	With epidural (mg/kg)	Other[b] (total mg)
Tetracaine (Amethocaine, Pontocaine)	100	1.5	200		
Lidocaine (Lignocaine, Xylocaine)	300	4.5	500	7	500
Mepivacaine (Carbocaine, Polocaine)	400		550	7	500
Prilocaine (Citanest)		10	500		500
Bupivacaine (Marcaine, Sensorcaine)	175	1–2	225	3	250
Etidocaine (Duranest)	300	4	400	6	250
Ropivacaine	150	2–3 (tentative)			

[a] Manufacturer-suggested dose limits for perineural (extravascular and extrathecal) use. This table in no way implies that these doses are either safe or the absolute maximum. Systemic reactions can be encountered with much smaller doses, whereas much larger doses, used judiciously, have been administered without ill effect (40,103).

[b] Simplified maximum doses recommended by Mulroy (107).

TABLE 8. *Comparable safe doses of local anesthetics (mg/kg)[a]*

Drugs	Peripheral blocks with epidural[b]	Central blocks[b]		Intercostal blocks with epidural[b]
		Plain	With epidural[b]	
Lidocaine	20	7	9	6
Mepivacaine	20	7	9	6
Bupivacaine	5	2	2	2
Tetracaine	—	2	2	—

[a] Estimated to produce peak plasma levels that are less than half the plasma levels at which seizures could occur.

[b] Peripheral nerve blocks represent areas of low vascularity, central neuraxis blocks (epidurals and caudals) represent areas of moderate vascularity, and intercostal nerve blocks represent areas of high vascularity (48).

ship to the local anesthetic drug itself).[145] "Unfortunately, all too often, when a systemic toxic reaction occurs, attention is focused on the dosage of the local anesthetic drug, rather than on the ability of the physician employing the drug."[103]

Numerous adjuvants have been added to local anesthetics with varying success. The addition of bicarbonate to the local anesthetic immediately prior to injection may shorten the onset of the block by increasing the percentage of unionized (lipid soluble) local anesthetic, compared with ionized (non–lipid-soluble/water-soluble) local anesthetic that is present in the commercial preparation. As a result, the passage of local anesthetic across the nerve cell membrane is facilitated.[7,70,172] The onset of a mepivacaine interscalene block was significantly faster, and the quality of motor blockade was improved without affecting the duration of the block.[171,172] These benefits apply to peripheral nerve blocks performed with lidocaine but do not apply to bupivacaine.[26] The addition of a short-acting to a long-acting local anesthetic (e.g., supercaine) also has been used to shorten the onset of the long-acting agent. This technique is safe and effective,[69] albeit at the expense of the long-acting agent.[40]

Epinephrine is added to reduce peak systemic blood concentrations, reduce absorption, and prolong the duration of short and intermediate-acting local anesthetic agents. It does not prolong the duration of long-acting agents.[121] Epinephrine (in the dilution of 1:200,000 to 1:400,000) should be added to the local anesthetic mixture immediately prior to performance of the block. The pH of commercially available premixed solutions of epinephrine and local anesthetics is substantially lower than that of plain local anesthetic solutions, with the result that a greater percentage of local anesthetic is present in the ionized (non–lipid-soluble) form. This prolongs (slows down) the onset of the block. In certain situations, the addition of epinephrine is relatively contraindicated, e.g., in patients with ischemic heart disease.

Various opioids (morphine, fentanyl, meperidine, and buprenorphine) have been added to local anesthetics in an attempt to increase the intensity and prolong the duration of peripheral nerve blocks. Although results are conflicting, it does not appear that their addition confers any significant benefit.[12,55,105,126,187] The addition of clonidine (an alpha-2 agonist) to prolong the duration of a peripheral nerve block may be of some benefit.[23,51,58,157]

Assessing the success of peripheral nerve block is a critical step in the practice of regional anesthesia. The success of an interscalene block may be tested as described below:

1. The deltoid sign describes the patient's inability to elevate his or her arm.[194] The time to develop the deltoid sign varies with the local anesthetic used and is shortened by the addition of bicarbonate to the local anesthetic solution. The onset also may be influenced by the technique used (paresthesia or nerve stimulator) and the patient's body habitat. The anesthesiologist should be familiar with the expected time frame, so that a questionable block can be recognized as soon as possible to avoid an unacceptable delay in the operating room.
2. The patient loses sensation over the anterolateral border of the upper arm in the distribution of C5 and C6. Loss of sensation over the shoulder area is not sought as an early indication of a successful block. The local anesthetic may have been injected outside the interscalene sheath, thus blocking the supraclavicular nerves at a peripheral rather than at a nerve root level (C3 and C4). Under these circumstances, the patient will report an early loss of sensation over the shoulder area, yet the interscalene block will fail.
3. The "money sign," i.e., the patient involuntarily rubs his or her thumb against the index and middle finger as he or she becomes aware of the onset of numbness or pins and needles.[17]
4. The patient experiences a decrease in handgrip strength, which is usually accompanied by unintentional pronation of the forearm.[181]

Once the success of the block has been established, the degree of sedation and overall comfort of the patient is of paramount importance in achieving a successful outcome following regional anesthesia. Herein lies a major component of the art of regional anesthesia.

Care of the patient during the procedure involves monitoring the patient's vital signs and ensuring that the patient remain comfortable. Careful positioning with appropriate padding is important, particularly in obese, thin, and elderly patients. Excessive fluid administration should be avoided, particularly in patients under regional anesthesia, because excessive bladder distention can sabotage a perfectly executed nerve block. Sedation should be tailored to the patient's needs and may vary from little to no sedation, to twilight sleep, to deep sedation.

Interscalene block anesthesia for shoulder surgery can be the most challenging of all forms of regional anesthesia, due to the proximity of the surgical site to the face; the position of the surgical drapes can result in a claustrophobic environment being presented to the patient and the limited access the anesthesiologist has to the patient. In addition, the frequently used beach-chair position further limits access and challenges the ability of the anesthesiologist to perform a rapid intubation, should this become necessary. Care should therefore be exercised to avoid sedating the patient beyond a sedation scale score of 3, because the airway may become compromised (Table 9).[188]

Opinions vary regarding the appropriate level of sedation. The patient's preference should be taken into account. Some prefer to be wide awake to observe arthroscopic surgery (or to avoid loss of autonomy), others prefer light sedation (so-called twilight sleep), while others insist on heavy sedation ("I don't want to see, feel, or hear anything"). It is important that the patient's wishes be taken into account, provided patient safety is not jeopardized.

A number of options are available to keep the patient asleep during surgery (Table 10). The simplest technique is to administer intravenous sedatives, alone or supplemented with an analgesic agent. These agents can be administered by intermittent boluses and/or continuous infusion, until the desired level of sedation is achieved. Should there be concern regarding maintenance of the patient's airway during the procedure, a number of options to circumvent this problem are available. First, a nasal airway may be utilized. This is not the author's technique of choice, because unexpected nasal bleeding may occur that, if difficult to control, may necessitate endotracheal intubation to protect the airway of a sedated patient. A laryngeal mask airway (LMA) is an excellent method of maintaining a potentially difficult airway in a sedated patient.[8,161] It provides a hands-free airway and, when compared with an endotracheal tube, has the advantage of reduced anesthetic requirements, lower incidence of postoperative sore throat, decreased acute hemodynamic changes during induction and emergence, reduced work of breathing, and avoidance of muscle relaxants and reversal agents.[192] The patient does not need to receive general anesthetic agents via the LMA, because the interscalene block provides complete anesthesia and the level of sedation may be maintained with intravenous agents. Thus, oxygen and/or air may be delivered via the LMA, although the option of adding inhalational agents, and thus limiting the amount of intravenous sedation, is available. An additional advantage of the LMA is the ability to provide full inhalational anesthesia in the event of a failed or inadequate block, without having to induce general endotracheal anesthesia. Finally, the patient may receive general endotracheal anesthesia as part of a combined technique.

TABLE 9. *Sedation scale*

Score	Degree of sedation
1	Fully awake and oriented
2	Drowsy
3	Eyes closed, rousable to command
4	Eyes closed, rousable to mild physical stimulation (shoulder shaking)
5	Unrousable to mild physical stimulation

Reprinted with permission from ref. 188.

TABLE 10. *Anesthesia options for shoulder surgery*

- Regional anesthesia
  - Minimal or no intraoperative intravenous sedation (patient awake)
  - Intraoperative intravenous sedation ("twilight sleep" to well sedated)
  - Combined with a laryngeal mask airway (LMA)
    - To secure a suspect airway (patient receives oxygen and/or air via LMA)
    - To augment intravenous sedation (oxygen + nitrous oxide)
    - To supplement an ISB with inhalational general anesthesia
- General anesthesia
  - Alone (intravenous muscle relaxants provide intraoperative motor block, intravenous narcotics provide intra- and postoperative analgesia)
  - Combined with an ISB
    - Inserted before the start of surgery (provides preemptive and intra- plus postoperative analgesia as well as muscle relaxation)
    - Inserted at the end of surgery (for postoperative analgesia)

Numerous intravenous agents have been used to provide pre- and intraoperative anxiolysis, sedation, and supplemental analgesia to improve patient comfort and satisfaction under regional anesthesia.[77,80,110,144,160,163,185,196] Propofol, supplemented by midazolam (anxiolysis and amnesia), and fentanyl (analgesia) are the agents of choice at the author's institution. Although the overall quality and ease of control of sedation is similar between midazolam and propofol, the former causes less pain on injection and provides better amnesia, whereas propofol causes less postoperative sedation and amnesia and results in a more rapid recovery of cognitive function. The discharge times appear to be similar.[14,125,168,193,196] Extreme caution needs to be observed if combinations of these drugs are used, because respiratory depression is an ever-present danger, particularly in the elderly.[2,63] The author favors a propofol infusion as the primary intraoperative sedative because of its ease of titration and rapid recovery. Its use may result in pain in the arm, particularly if a small vein on the dorsum of the hand is used.

This should be preempted with lidocaine 25 to 50 mg, fentanyl 50 g, or alfentanil 10 to 30 g/kg.[81,106,162] Supplementary analgesics or sedatives will decrease the requirements for propofol sedation.[129]

A final point in the care of the patient following an interscalene block relates to the presence of any of the harmless side effects that may be associated with the block (i.e., hoarseness and a Horner's syndrome). Although these side effects are temporary and harmless, they may be a cause for concern to the patient in the immediate postoperative period. Any patient suffering from these conditions should be reassured that these side effects are of a temporary nature.

The following step-by-step technique is used at the author's institution. The patient is placed on the operating room table, monitors are attached (EKG, noninvasive blood pressure cuff, pulse oximeter, and capnometer), and oxygen is administered via a nasal cannula at 3 to 5 L/min. Confirmation of the operative shoulder is obtained and an intravenous line inserted in the opposite arm. An attempt is made to avoid the antecubital fossa in inpatients to allow relative freedom of movement of the nonoperative arm. All patients are sedated to comfort prior to insertion of the block. The author favors fractionated doses of midazolam (0.5- to 1.0-mg boluses, usually limited to 2 to 3 mg) and fentanyl (25 to 50 μg boluses to a maximum of 100 μg) The objective is to maintain a calm and cooperative patient while avoiding oversedation. The patient should not be sedated to the point beyond which communication is lost, because this increases the risk of respiratory obstruction and/or depression; it also may mask the early warning symptoms and signs of an intravascular injection, as well as the symptom of an intraneural injection, i.e., severe pain on injection.[5]

The appropriate topographic landmarks are identified and the point of needle insertion determined. The skin over the area is sterilized with povidone-iodine or alcohol.[22] A skin wheal with a 26-gauge needle is raised at the planned point of insertion with 1% lidocaine.[33] The skin is punctured with an 18-gauge needle to avoid the use of significant force to penetrate the skin (the relative bluntness of the short-bevel needle makes penetration through intact skin difficult). Forceful penetration of the skin increases the risk of overshoot and direct damage to the underlying brachial plexus. The nerve block is performed using a peripheral nerve stimulator. Prior to performance of the block, confirmation that the positive lead is connected to the low-output (positive output) terminal of the nerve stimulator should be obtained. The distal end of the positive lead is connected to a ground electrode that is traditionally placed below (caudad to) the opposite clavicle. The negative lead of the nerve stimulator (from the negative output terminal) is attached to the needle (i.e., negative to needle to nerve).

The block needle is inserted through the skin puncture, with the bevel face angled down (rather than the customary bevel-up direction). This will increase the tactile sensation of "popping" through the interscalene sheath. The output of the nerve stimulator is gradually increased to 1.5 mAmps. The current should be increased slowly to avoid sudden, vigorous muscle contractions that may result from the tip of the needle being in close proximity to the nerve following initial insertion of the needle. With the current at 1.5 mAmps, the needle is advanced until a vigorous contraction of the appropriate muscle (biceps and/or deltoid) is obtained. The stimulating current is incrementally decreased and the needle position adjusted until an appropriate muscle twitch at or below 0.3 mAmps is obtained. Stimulation of the pectorals or triceps muscles is not regarded as an acceptable indication of correct needle placement. A diaphragmatic twitch is indicative of the needle being directed medial to the interscalene groove, because the phrenic nerve runs along the anterior surface of the scalenus anterior. The needle is withdrawn and redirected in a more lateral direction. A trapezius twitch (accessory nerve) indicates that the needle position is lateral to the interscalene groove and therefore should be redirected accordingly. An "immobile needle" technique allows administration of the local anesthetic while minimizing movement of the needle.[198] The patient is instructed not to move until completion of the injection. After gentle aspiration, 1 ml of local anesthetic is injected, after which gentle aspiration is repeated, because a plug of tissue may have obstructed the lumen of the needle during insertion. This would prevent the appearance of blood in the syringe during the initial aspiration. The following symptoms and signs are sought, particularly during the initial stages of the injection:

1. Aspiration of blood, indicating intravascular placement of the needle.
2. Complaint of pain or discomfort by the patient. A localized dull ache (pressure paresthesia) may be reported and is caused by pressure of the injected local anesthetic against the nerve.[202] This is distinct from severe pain on injection, which should be regarded as a sign of a potential intraneural injection. Should the patient complain of severe pain at any stage during the administration of the local anesthetic, the needle should be repositioned prior to completion of the block. If there is any suspicion that an intraneural injection may have occurred, a reasonable course of action would be to desist from further attempts at continuing or repeating the nerve block.
3. Disappearance of the muscle twitch after the injection of 1 to 2 ml of local anesthetic. This is indicative of the close proximity of the needle tip to the nerve. Injection of the local anesthetic increases the distance between the needle tip and the nerve, which, at the low currents used, results in the loss of muscle twitch.

The total dose of local anesthetic is injected in 3- to 5-ml aliquots, with gentle aspiration between each dose. During the entire procedure, the patient should be carefully observed for any symptoms and/or signs of an intravascular injection.

The final step is to confirm that the block is successful. The ability to accurately assess the onset and success of the block is as important as knowing how to perform the block. The time of development of the first signs of a successful block will vary with the test, as well as the local anesthetic agent used. In the author's experience, the sequence of onset of the money sign, the deltoid sign, or loss of sensation over C5–6 is variable, without one sign consistently appearing before another. However, with each specific local anesthetic agent, certain time limits are placed on at least one of the above indicators that the block is setting. This is important to avoid unnecessary operating room delays waiting for a potentially unsuccessful block to set. Although the first sign of a successful block may be almost immediate, this may not always be the case. The author uses the following cutoff times in determining whether an interscalene block is likely to be successful: 5 to 10 minutes for alkalinized mepivacaine 1.5% and 10 to 15 minutes for plain bupivacaine 0.5%.

The anesthesiologist should alert the surgeon to possible "gray areas" that might not be covered by an interscalene block. Supplementary skin infiltration to these areas is performed by the surgeon prior to skin incision.

Intraoperative sedation is provided by a continuous infusion of propofol that is started as soon as signs of a successful block are detected. The degree of sedation is tailored to the patient's needs, with an average infusion rate of 20 to 50 μg/kg/min. Midazolam and fentanyl are usually restricted to the preblock period, although small boluses (0.5 mg and 25 g, respectively) are occasionally administered intraoperatively to supplement the propofol infusion. These drugs should not be used in an attempt to save a failed interscalene block. The appropriate management of a failed block is to either repeat the block or convert to general anesthesia. The propofol infusion is often omitted in elderly and frail patients, because midazolam (with or without fentanyl) administered prior to the block may be adequate for the entire procedure.

Complications

Anesthetic complications of patients undergoing shoulder surgery can be subdivided into (a) complications directly associated with the use of an interscalene block and (b) complications unrelated to the use of the block.

Complications directly associated with the use of an interscalene block can be further subdivided into general complications, which can occur with the performance of any peripheral nerve block, e.g., pain and/or bruising at the injection site, hematoma formation, systemic toxicity, nerve damage, and sepsis.

Pain and/or bruising at the injection site, while not uncommon, is more of a minor annoyance than a complication and is related to the number of needle advances required to perform the block.[180] Hematoma formation and sepsis are exceedingly rare complications in which technique may play a major role.

Systemic toxicity following an interscalene block is uncommon and is usually the result of a direct intravascular injection rather than systemic absorption. Direct injection of minimal amounts of local anesthetics (e.g., bupivacaine 2.5 mg) into the vertebral artery can induce a grand mal seizure.[87] Brown et al.[20] reported a 0.7% (five of 659) incidence of seizures associated with the performance of interscalene blocks at a teaching institution. No adverse cardiovascular, pulmonary, or nervous system events were associated with any of the seizures. Urban and Urquhart[180] documented symptoms of an intravascular injection in two of 266 patients receiving an interscalene block, neither of whom went on to develop a seizure. The incidence of this complication can be minimized by fractionation of the local anesthetic injection into 3- to 5-ml boluses, with gentle aspiration between each bolus. Local anesthetic toxicity that is appropriately managed should not be regarded as a reason to cancel the surgery.

The relationship between peripheral nerve damage and regional anesthesia is controversial. Although there are many possible causes of nerve damage during the perioperative period (Table 11), in many cases, a definitive cause is impossible to establish.[24,167,190] In the American Society of Anesthesiology Closed-Claim Study, obtained from professional liability insurance company closed-claims data, Kroll et al. reported that nerve injury was responsible for 15% of the total number of claims (227 of 1,541).[88] The majority of these injuries occurred under general anesthesia (61%), rather than regional anesthesia (36%). The anesthetic technique in 3% was unrecorded. The most common nerve involved was the ulnar nerve (34%); the mechanisms responsible were recently reviewed.[119,166,190] The brachial plexus (23%) was the next group of nerves most frequently involved, followed by the lumbosacral nerve roots (16%) and spinal cord (6%). The remaining group was categorized as other/multiple nerves (21%). The investigators conclude that most anesthetic-related nerve injuries seem to occur without an identifiable mechanism.[88]

The overall incidence of nerve injury is in the region of 0.1% of all surgical cases.[47,112] In a study at the Virginia Mason Clinic in Seattle, Thompson and Liu report a 0.11% (30 of 26,167) incidence of postoperative nerve damage. Sixteen of these patients received regional anesthesia and, after careful evaluation, only three cases were suspect regarding the regional anesthetic. Because most resolve within days to weeks, the problem tends to escape our attention. Although these injuries are not always related to the regional anesthetic, historically regional anesthesia tends to be the scapegoat.[175]

Whether the incidence of nerve damage is influenced by use of a nerve stimulator or paresthesia technique in performing a peripheral nerve block is controversial. Some investigators have suggested that eliciting paresthesia results in nerve damage, whereas others have suggested that the use of a nerve stimulator and/or a short-bevel needle will reduce the incidence of postblock neuropathy. Moore et al.[104] contend that there are no statistically significant clinical data to support the suggestion that neuropathy results from any of these factors. They believe that the evidence to support the

TABLE 11. *Etiologic factors associated with perioperative nerve damage*

- Pre-existing (overt or latent) neurologic pathology
  - Metabolic conditions, e.g., diabetes, uremia, porphyria, amyloid
  - Nutritional, e.g., Beriberi, alcohol, pellagra
  - Infections, e.g., AIDS, acute inflammatory polyneuropathy (Guillain-Barré syndrome)
  - Obesity, cachexia
  - Preexisting but unidentified nerve tumors
- General anesthesia
  - Muscle relaxants may predispose to nerve damage
  - General anesthesia followed by performance of regional anesthesia
    - The mechanisms may involve direct trauma, pressure, ischemia, or any combination
    - Hypotension and hypothermia may potentiate the above
- Regional anesthesia
  - Excessive total dose
  - Excessively high concentration of local anesthetic agent
  - Pressure-related effects of high-volume injections
  - Vasoconstrictors
  - Needle injury
    - Direct trauma or hematoma formation resulting in nerve compression and/or ischemia
    - Intraneural injection
    - Paresthesia?
  - Injection of an incorrect (neurotoxic) solution
- Surgical causes
  - Malpositioning resulting in hyperextension or flexion of limbs
  - Prolonged operating time resulting in compression neuropathies
  - Direct nerve injury or interruption of nerve blood supply
  - Retractors
  - Tourniquet
  - Cold irrigating solutions (cardiac surgery → phrenic nerve/BP injuries)
  - Spinal cord ischemia → paraplegia (coarctation of aorta and dissecting aneurysms)
- Postoperative causes
  - Orthopedic splints and casts resulting in
    - Nerve compression or
    - Delayed swelling and edema (compartment syndrome)
  - Anticoagulation therapy may cause bleeding, resulting in direct compression of nerves and/or their blood supply

above arguments is based largely on extrapolation from animal data.

In 1977, Selander et al.[149] drew attention to the part played by the design of the needle tip in nerve injury. Based on their findings, they made the following observations: (a) nerve fascicles have a tendency to slide away from an advancing needle point, (b) short-bevel needles significantly reduce the risk of nerve injury compared with long-bevel needles, and (c) the degree of injury varies with the orientation of the long-bevel needle.

Selander et al.[150] attempted to ascertain whether paresthesia did indeed increase the risk of postanesthetic neurologic sequelae in a clinical setting. Patients undergoing hand surgery were prospectively observed. In one group the block was performed by eliciting paresthesia (290 patients), and in the other group (nonparesthesia group) pulsations of the axillary artery were regarded as being indicative of correct positioning of the needle (243 patients). Postoperatively, 18 (3.4%) of the patients had nerve lesions. In eight cases (1.5%), the nerve lesion was due to the effects of surgery, position, or plaster. Postanesthetic nerve lesions occurred in eight of 290 (2.8%) in the paresthesia group and two of 243 (0.8%) in the nonparesthesia group. In both of the latter cases unintentional paresthesias were elicited during the blocking procedure. Three patients complained of increased paresthesia on injection, whereas all complained of painful paresthesia. Their symptoms varied between light paresthesias lasting a few weeks to severe paresthesias with aching and paresis lasting more than 1 year. The earliest symptom appeared within 24 hours of the block and the latest not later than the third postoperative week. The investigators questioned whether the needle itself and/or a direct intraneural injection resulted in the postoperative neuropathies. They concluded that, whenever possible, nerve blocks should be performed without searching for paresthesias. Rough and repeated probing for paresthesia, especially with a thick sharp needle, can cause nerve damage, while "a gentle touch with the needle is probably harmless to the normal nerve."

Plevak et al.[123] reported a similar incidence of nerve damage following axillary brachial plexus block performed by either a transarterial (nonparesthesia) or paresthesia technique. In the transarterial group, the incidence of persistent paresthesias (lasting more than 48 hours) was 0.8% (2 of 239) versus 2.9% (14 of 477) in the paresthesia group. The success rate was similar (88% versus 85%).

In an attempt to further define the factors involved in nerve damage, Selander et al.[148] compared the effects of intrafascicular and topical application of bupivacaine on the rabbit sciatic nerve. They reported that topical application, in clinically recommended concentrations around the nerve, caused no detectable nerve injury. However, intrafascicular injections caused considerable axonal degeneration and damaged the blood–nerve barrier. The damage was the same when injecting physiologic saline solution (i.e., not due to the injected solution, but due to injection trauma alone), but it increased with increasing concentrations of bupivacaine, and especially with the addition of adrenaline (epinephrine). The increased axonal degeneration seen with adrenaline may be due to its pharmacologic effects on neural blood vessels, as well as toxic effects on the axons by preservatives added to prevent oxidation (sodium-pyrosulphite). Topical application of adrenaline did not cause any nerve damage. They commented that adrenaline increases the risk of neurologic sequelae once the nerve is injured (by needle trauma or intraneural injection), and concluded that intraneural injections should be avoided, and plain bupivacaine solutions should be routinely used. The possibility that epinephrine has a pathogenic role in the relatively rare reports of neurologic deficit following local anesthesia procedures has been raised by others.[108,113] Gentili et al. demonstrated the potential toxicity of local anesthetics in clinical concentrations when injected intraneurally and concurred that intraneural injections should be avoided.[60]

Operator experience plays an important role in the incidence of complications. Winchell et al.[197] reported a post-block neuropathy incidence of 0.36% (3 of 854), in which paresthesia was elicited by nine experienced anesthesiologists in private practice. Of these blocks, at least 1 paresthesia was elicited in 835. All operators made use of short-bevel needles.

Gentili and Wargnier[62] reported that a number of studies support the belief that paresthesia increases the risk of nerve trauma. The investigators concluded with their preferred axiom "no paresthesia no dysasthesia" to the "no paresthesia no anesthesia" axiom of Moore.

Moore et al. [104] counterargued that a more accurate statement by Gentili and Wargnier would be "no paresthesiae no dysasthesiae, but often failed anesthesia." They believe that the nerve stimulator has not been shown to be more reliable than using paresthesiae nor has it been demonstrated to be clinically safer. In addition, they stated that using the nerve stimulator while attempting to locate a nerve, particularly in unconscious patients, has not avoided neuropathy. These investigators have reviewed six medicolegal cases in which permanent brachial plexus neuropathy occurred when the nerve stimulator was used. None of these cases was reported in medical publications. Unfortunately, the details of the cases were not reported: Were the patients awake? Was unintentional paresthesia elicited? Was a definitive cause established? They concluded by suggesting that there are no statistically significant clinical data to demonstrate that eliciting paresthesia results in neuropathy. According to Moore et al., until a prospective blinded major clinical study provides us with statistically significant clinical information, investigators should not draw conclusions relating to clinical practice, which may have significant medicolegal connotations.

Some final comments on the subject by this author:

1. The incidence of nerve damage is probably influenced more by the skill and experience of the individual performing the block than whether a paresthesia or non-paresthesia technique is used.
2. The likelihood of an inadvertent intraneural injection occurring is significantly reduced by performing nerve blocks in patients who are not anesthetized or heavily sedated.
3. Although the success rate[4,65] and the complication rate might be similar (in experienced hands), a number of advantages are associated with the performance of a peripheral nerve block using a nerve stimulator: (a) less patient cooperation is required (i.e., an appropriate muscle twitch is an objective end point that is not dependent on the patient's interpretation of the site of paresthesia); (b) nerve blocks can be performed in patients in whom communication is difficult (e.g., language barrier, mentally challenged); (c) patients can be sedated to the point at which they are comfortable, but awake enough to report severe pain on injection (this level of sedation may interfere with the interpretation of a paresthesia); and (d) paresthesia can be an unpleasant experience, while the nerve stimulator is seldom (if ever) reported to be unpleasant.

Scrupulous documentation of paresthesias elicited (by design or inadvertently during a nonparesthesia technique), as well as the presence or absence of pain during the injection, is essential. Harmless side effects include a 10% to 17% incidence of hoarseness (ipsilateral recurrent laryngeal nerve block), 47% to 75% incidence of Horner's syndrome (stellate ganglion block),[152,186,189] and hemidiaphragmatic paresis (phrenic nerve block), the latter occurring in 100% of cases.[182–184]

Urmey et al.[183] demonstrated that ipsilateral diaphragmatic paralysis results in large decreases in a number of pulmonary function variables. This is not surprising, because the phrenic nerve is derived from the C3–5 nerve roots. Forced vital capacity and forced expiratory volume at 1 second were reduced by 27% ± 4.3% and 26.4% ± 6.8%, respectively. Peak expiratory and maximum mid-expiratory flow rates were also significantly reduced. The investigators suggest that an interscalene block should probably not be performed in patients who are dependent on intact diaphragmatic function and in those patients unable to tolerate a 25% reduction in pulmonary function. The situation may be aggravated when regional anesthesia is combined with general anesthesia, particularly with the patient in a lateral decubitus rather than the beach-chair position.[61]

Although this author regards these side effects as harmless, they may be of some concern to the patient. Should any of these side effects manifest themselves, the patient should be reassured of their harmless and temporary nature. A limited number of patients become acutely aware of a change in their breathing pattern, particularly an inability to inhale deeply and/or cough normally. This may create intense patient anxiety and should be treated with immediate reassurance and an increase in the depth of sedation. Occasionally, conversion to general anesthesia is required.

Specific complications are rare, but they can be severe and life threatening. They include direct injection into the vertebral artery or vein, pneumothorax,[3,186,189] high epidural,[32,89,143] total spinal[50,139] or subdural[173] injection, brainstem toxicity,[49] and bilateral plexus block.[72,94] The incidence of these complications can be significantly curtailed by using appropriate needles (short-beveled needles of limited length) and paying meticulous attention to detail during performance of the block.[5]

Although a pneumothorax may complicate any of the supraclavicular approaches to the brachial plexus, it is not commonly associated with the interscalene approach. In a closed claims analysis, Cheney et al. reported that adverse respiratory events infrequently lead to malpractice suits.[28] Pneumothorax was among the less common categories, accounting for 67 (3%) of the claims that were either needle related (nerve block or central venous catheter) or airway management related. Of the 27 cases that were related to nerve blocks, 11% were associated with interscalene blocks (Table 12). If a pneumothorax does occur, it is more than likely associated with poor technique, in which the point of needle insertion is lower than it should be (i.e., closer to the apex of the lung) or the caudad direction of the needle is overexaggerated.

A number of possible mechanisms have been described to explain the development of cervical epidural or spinal anesthesia. These include (a) advancement of the needle through an intervertebral foramen, followed by direct injection into the epidural, subdural, or subarachnoid space; (b) correct positioning of the needle outside the intervertebral foramen but with the needle tip within the dural cuff (which can extend as much as 8 cm beyond the intervertebral foramen); and (c) direct intraneural injection, followed by proximal spread of the local anesthetic solution. The avoidance of deep needle placement and maintenance of the caudal direction of the needle will decrease the likelihood of needle advancement between the transverse processes of the cervical spine directly into the epidural or subarachnoid space.[201]

Regional anesthesia is usually the anesthetic technique of choice in patients suffering from asthma or chronic obstructive airways disease, because airway manipulation under general anesthesia is avoided. However, bronchospasm associated with the use of this block has been reported.[93,174]

In addition to the above complications, a number of others may or may not be related to the use of an interscalene block.

A high incidence (17% to 24%) of potentially dangerous vasovagal events in patients undergoing arthroscopic shoulder surgery in the beach-chair position under an interscalene block have been reported.[36,134] These events were characterized by a sudden onset of severe hypotension and/or bradycardia, and were frequently associated with symptoms of lightheadedness or nausea. In one case, an asystolic cardiac arrest requiring resuscitation occurred.[36] The possibility of this occurring is particularly alarming, due to the limited access of the anesthesiologist to the patient in the beach-chair position.

These vasovagal responses have been attributed to activation of the Bezold-Jarisch reflex. Venous pooling secondary to the sitting position, coupled with a heightened cardiac contractile state, which has been compounded by the beta-adrenergic effects of epinephrine added to the local anesthetic, results in reflex arterial vasodilatation (activation of the parasympathetic nervous system) and a vagally mediated bradycardia.[35,64]

At the author's institution, the incidence of hypotension and bradycardia in patients undergoing shoulder surgery under an interscalene block in the beach-chair position is uncommon. Our technique differs from that described above, in that we do not add epinephrine to our local anesthetic solutions. Our findings may therefore support the mechanism proposed by D'Alessio et al. that epinephrine added to local anesthetics may aggravate the Bezold-Jarisch reflex. However, the degree of table tilt, as well as level of sedation, are not mentioned in the above reports. These factors may play a role in the incidence of vasovagal events. Because we tend to sedate our patients during surgery, this may decrease the possibility of a psychogenic cause for a vasovagal event. In addition, we favor a beach-chair position with an approximate 50 to 60 degree tilt, rather than the more extreme (greater than 60 degree) angle favored by some surgeons. As a result, the decrease in venous return may be less marked in our patients.

Hemodynamic and pulmonary changes have been documented in patients undergoing total hip arthroplasty. Proposed mechanisms include embolization of air, as well as systemic absorption of the monomeric liquid component of methylmethacrylate cement. Total shoulder arthroplasty performed in the beach-chair position results in the operative site being placed above the level of the patient's heart. As a result, open venous sinuses may entrain air, resulting in venous air embolism. Although air emboli have been documented during shoulder surgery, they have not proven to be of any clinical significance.

Methylmethacrylate cement may cause direct myocardial depression, peripheral vasodilatation, or direct lung injury.[13,76] Its use in total shoulder replacement has not been associated with adverse hemodynamic events or increased intrapulmonary shunting.[73]

TABLE 12. *Type and relative frequency of nerve blocks associated with claims for pneumothorax*

Type of block	% of total
Supraclavicular	37
Intercostal	33
Stellate ganglion	11
Interscalene	11
Suprascapular	7

POSTOPERATIVE PAIN MANAGEMENT

Shoulder surgery may be associated with severe postoperative pain. Prevention and control of postoperative pain are critical components of the perioperative management of patients undergoing shoulder surgery. Lack of pain at the end of the procedure, extending into the postoperative period, plays a particularly important role in situations in which early mobilization is encouraged. Additional benefits attributed to effective postoperative pain management include shorter recovery room (PACU) and hospital stay, as well as improved patient satisfaction. Regional anesthesia has been reported to be particularly successful in achieving these benefits.[19,30,34,82,169] Provision of preemptive and intense intraoperative analgesia that extends into the postoperative period results in lower overall pain scores and less use of parenteral narcotics with their attendant side effects. These side effects, together with inadequate pain control achieved with systemic opioid analgesics, result in delays in discharge, unplanned hospital admissions, and delays in postoperative passive joint motion exercises and recovery. Options available to optimize postoperative pain control following shoulder surgery include balanced analgesia (e.g., addition of ketorolac or NSAIDs to complement the primary anesthetic/analgesic technique); patient-controlled analgesia (PCA); cervical epidural anesthesia/analgesia; and interscalene block anesthesia/analgesia (e.g., single shot of a long-acting agent, or a continuous catheter technique).

The concept of balanced analgesia is based on the theory that the multimodal treatment of pain (in which drugs act by different mechanisms to produce additive or synergistic analgesia) is more effective than the use of any single analgesic drug or technique. In addition, the dose-related adverse effects of the individual drugs may be minimized.[38,79] The role played by the preemptive component of balanced analgesia is controversial.[16,27,37,78,84,204] Preoperative opiate medication[132] and local anesthetic blocks reduce postoperative orthopedic pain.[100] The addition of NSAIDs (e.g., ketorolac tromethamine) intra- and/or postoperatively provides safe and effective analgesia and decreases postoperative opioid analgesic requirements after surgery.[29,43,83,154,203] Side effects have been reported in less than 1% of patients following the use of ketorolac. Although rare, the most significant risks associated with its use are gastrointestinal (including ulceration, bleeding, and perforation), renal, bleeding (including postoperative wound bleeding), and hypersensitivity reactions. Patients should be carefully screened for anything in their histories that may predispose them to these complications. The drug should be used with caution if strict hemostasis is critical.[43]

The use of intravenous PCA offers several advantages over the use of intramuscular opioid analgesics. These include the ability of the patient to titrate their analgesia to their needs, resulting in superior analgesia with less total drug use, less sedation compared with intramuscular opioids, elimination of painful intramuscular injections, and a high degree of patient satisfaction.[53,130,154] However, its use may be associated with a number of opioid-related side effects, including nausea, sedation, and urinary retention. These side effects may slow down the patient's postoperative recovery and delay discharge from the hospital. The addition of NSAIDs to PCA may improve efficacy, decrease opioid usage, and decrease dose-dependent opioid-induced side effects, while maintaining and/or improving analgesia.[124,154]

The successful use of cervical epidural anesthesia in controlling postoperative pain following shoulder surgery has been reported.[205] This technique provides good surgical anesthesia and postoperative analgesia, with few complications and a high degree of patient acceptance. Postoperative analgesia may be provided by intermittent boluses or a continuous epidural infusion of local anesthetics with or without opioid analgesics. However, this technique provides unnecessary bilateral analgesia, may be more difficult to perform than an interscalene block, and may be associated with a higher incidence of severe complications in inexperienced hands.

The safety and efficacy of an interscalene block in providing intraoperative anesthesia and postoperative analgesia have been established.[19,30,34,82,169,170] Prolonged postoperative analgesia may be achieved with long-acting local anesthetic agents. Bupivacaine, tetracaine (supercaine), and etidocaine have resulted in 8 to 24 hours of postoperative analgesia.[82] As a result, the patient may remain pain free from the time of departure from the operating room, throughout his or her recovery room (PACU) stay, and for a variable duration on the floor. In the author's experience, lack of pain during the initial 12 hours following open shoulder surgery has a beneficial psychological impact on the overall pain reported by the patient. This benefit is even more impressive in ambulatory patients following arthroscopic shoulder procedures.[19] The awake, pain-free patient may in fact bypass phase I recovery and go directly to a reclining lounge chair in the phase II PACU.[111] If an extremity is still anesthetized at the time of discharge, care should be taken with positioning and padding of the affected limb. The patient should be given clear instructions on protection of the limb until the return of normal sensation. In addition, the patient should be instructed to take oral analgesics at the first sign of pain, because these blocks may rapidly recede. A delay in treating the pain may result in the development of severe pain that can become extremely difficult to control with oral analgesics. The patient should receive a follow-up call within 24 hours of discharge.

As with all joint surgery, movement of the shoulder joint in the early postoperative period is, in most cases, an important requirement following surgery. Although balanced analgesia is usually more effective than the use of opioids alone, this technique may still be inadequate in controlling pain with movement. The severity of the pain with movement causes the patient to use maximal doses of PCA, resulting in a high incidence of side effects. This limits the patient's use of PCA, resulting in an increase in the severity of the pain. Brachial plexus blocks utilizing long-acting local anesthetic agents are extremely effective for the duration of the block. However, complete anesthesia for a prolonged period of time is not always desirable, and the duration of these blocks is unpredictable. In addition, the block may recede rapidly, and, unless analgesics are administered early, the ensuing pain may be difficult to control.

The above problems have been overcome by utilizing continuous or intermittent infusions of local anesthetics and/or narcotics via catheters inserted within the brachial plexus sheath.[45,177] Low concentrations of local anesthetics provide postoperative analgesia, rather than complete anesthesia (accompanied by undesirable motor blockade) required for surgery. A number of advantages have been ascribed to the use of continuous perineural infusions of local anesthetics for postoperative pain control following upper limb surgery:

1. The ability to provide prolonged intraoperative anesthesia, as well as postoperative analgesia, to a specific and limited portion of the body. This allows the patient to remain ambulatory during the postoperative period.
2. The ability to provide extremely effective analgesia during the early, painful mobilization period following upper extremity joint surgery.
3. The ability to provide analgesia for repeated procedures of the upper extremity (manipulation under anesthesia) by simply injecting a bolus of local anesthetic via the catheter.

Insertion of an interscalene catheter using the classic approach is seldom successful in the short or long term. Insertion of the catheter/needle assembly at right angles to the sheath results in difficulty in advancing the catheter to an adequate depth and/or kinking of the catheter. The latter may result in difficulty in injecting through the catheter either immediately or by the following day. Anchoring the catheter is difficult, and dislodgment with neck movement is not uncommon.

A modified subclavian perivascular approach has become the technique of choice for interscalene catheter insertion. In this approach, the point of insertion is near the apex of the interscalene groove, and the needle is directed along the line of the interscalene groove in a caudad direction. Insertion of the catheter to an adequate depth is readily accomplished, resulting in stability with movement, as well as comfort to the patient. Correct positioning of the catheter needle assembly is confirmed with a nerve stimulator or paresthesia technique.

Potential complications associated with interscalene catheters are similar to those associated with a standard interscalene block. However, the incidence (particularly of local anesthesia toxicity, neurologic damage, and infection) is surprisingly small.

Tuominen et al.[178] reported a case of unintentional arterial catheterization resulting in acute bupivacaine toxicity. After the patient was successfully resuscitated, the catheter was left in place for further investigation. Contrast medium injected through the catheter indicated that the catheter was probably situated in the vertebral artery. This case was unusual, in that the patient had received four interscalene blocks within the previous 15 months. The investigators speculated that possible tissue damage from the needle, the catheter, or the local anesthetic[57,71] may have resulted in a weakened vessel wall, permitting penetration of the vessel by the catheter. It should be noted that repeated careful aspiration before and during the injection was negative for blood but did not prevent a serious toxic complication. Thus, patients receiving local anesthetics via interscalene catheters need to be carefully monitored, especially if a bolus is to be administered.

Concern regarding cumulative toxicity with continuous and/or intermittent infusions of bupivacaine has been expressed. However, supplementation of an axillary block with mepivacaine 30 minutes after the initial injection did not result in symptoms or signs of local anesthetic toxicity.[54] The safety of supplementing a bupivacaine axillary block, followed by a continuous infusion, has been established.[179] Despite the high doses and rather high peak venous concentration of bupivacaine, no toxic side effects were observed during the block or during the recovery period.

The pharmacokinetics of drugs used for brachial plexus infusions is similar to those seen with an epidural infusion. Once the steady state has been reached, the drugs infused do not accumulate if the rate of infusion remains unchanged.[128]

The use of a large initial bupivacaine dose injected into the interscalene sheath, followed by a continuous infusion for 48 hours, was shown to result in marked cumulation of bupivacaine and its metabolites (desbutylbupivacaine and 4-hydroxybupivacaine) in the plasma.[118] However, no toxic symptoms or potentially toxic concentrations were observed. The investigators concluded that a 48-hour continuous interscalene plexus infusion is safe, but prolonging the infusion beyond 48 hours may eventually give rise to bupivacaine toxicity.

Bupivacaine is bound to alpha-1 acid glycoprotein. The plasma concentration of alpha-1 acid glycoprotein increases as part of the stress response following surgery.[137] This increase continues for at least 5 days postoperatively, by which time its concentration has doubled.[68] Thus, a greater percentage of bupivacaine becomes bound to this acute-phase protein, with the result that the levels of free bupivacaine may remain unchanged or may even decrease as time goes by. The risk of systemic toxicity may therefore be reduced.[45,177]

Another potential complication associated with the use of brachial plexus catheters is the development of local or systemic infection. Gaumann et al.[59] cultured 11 catheter tips after removal following continuous axillary brachial plexus blocks. Eight cultures were negative (duration of placement was 3.6 ± 0.6 days), and three were positive (duration 8.6 ± 2.2 days). In none of the patients were there signs of local or systemic infection. The investigators concluded that the risk of infection was by far outweighed by the benefits. Lack of catheter-related infection is supported by a number of other studies.[1,142] Use of an aseptic technique, as well as the bacteriostatic properties of bupivacaine,[138,140] is probably responsible for this.

Minor (transient) complications have been reported with the use of continuous brachial plexus catheters. These include varying degrees of numbness of the upper limb, Horner's syndrome, hoarseness, and phrenic nerve paralysis.[117] Patients should be educated about the possibility of these side effects, to allay anxiety and improve patient satisfaction.

Occasional patient concern related to sensory and/or motor blockade associated with continuous infusions can be overcome by reducing the concentration of the infused drug, to achieve analgesia rather than anesthesia. In addition, the patient should be carefully monitored for signs of compartment syndrome, because pain may not be a reliable monitor for the development of this syndrome. The use of a continuous interscalene infusion may in fact be inappropriate in patients at high risk for compartment syndrome.[155]

A number of practical problems have been reported related to the use of interscalene catheters. These include difficulty in placing the catheter and catheter failure. The latter may be due to incorrect placement, kinking or curling of the catheter, as well as catheter migration, dislodgment, or leakage.[118,137,177] In the author's experience, a catheter-over-needle technique, although more difficult to initiate, is associated with fewer problems than a catheter-through-needle technique.

A few important precautions should be observed with the use of interscalene catheters. The catheter must be clearly labeled as a continuous brachial plexus catheter so as to avoid the mistaken administration of intravenous agents through the catheter.[115] In addition, the patient should be monitored for 30 to 60 minutes following a bolus dose of local anesthetic, because this is the time it takes for peak concentration to be achieved.[137]

The following technique of interscalene catheter insertion is practiced at the author's institution.

The patient is sedated to comfort with fractionated doses of midazolam and fentanyl. Following skin sterilization, a skin wheal is raised with local anesthetic at the apex of the interscalene groove. The skin is punctured with a sharp needle to avoid puckering of the catheter. An Arrow continuous brachial plexus catheter/needle assembly is then inserted in the direction of the interscalene groove at a 45-degree angle to the skin, and advanced until the needle pops through the brachial plexus sheath. A nerve stimulator is used to confirm the position of the needle within the sheath. Forty milliliters mepivacaine 1.5% (to which 4 ml 8.4% bicarbonate has been added) is injected via the needle. Expansion of the brachial plexus sheath with local anesthetic should facilitate insertion of the catheter. The catheter is inserted, an extension tube with a stop-cock is attached, and the patency of the system is tested with a few milliliters of local anesthetic before suturing in place. The catheter hub and proximal tubing are covered with a transparent impermeable dressing. The remainder of the tubing and stop-cock is securely taped and marked "interscalene catheter."

At the end of the surgical procedure, the patient remains in the PACU until the first sign of pain, at which time a bolus of 40 ml 0.25% bupivacaine is administered. The patient remains in the PACU for at least 45 minutes to assess the efficacy of the catheter and to monitor for signs of local anesthetic toxicity.

Once the position of the catheter has been confirmed, a continuous infusion of either 0.25% or 0.125% bupivacaine may be started at 3 to 10 ml per hour via an infusion pump. The infusion should be started within 2 hours of the bolus administration, because steady state is reached in approximately 18 hours (five half-lives). Because the bolus dose may last anywhere between 8 and 24 hours, in some patients the infusion may not have reached a level sufficient to provide adequate analgesia before the bolus dose wears off. Thus, an additional, albeit smaller, bolus (20 ml) of 0.5% bupivacaine may be required.[128] The patient should be monitored for 45 minutes as for the initial bolus. Bupivacaine 0.25% is usually adequate for postoperative analgesia, as well as control of pain associated with the use of continuous passive motion devices and exercises. Should breakthrough pain occur, the infusion may be increased to 0.375%, or a bolus of 0.375% or 0.5% may be administered. The aim, however, is to achieve adequate analgesia with minimum sensory and motor blockade.

Borgeat et al.[11] report the use of patient-controlled interscalene analgesia (PCIA) as a more refined method of controlling postoperative pain following major shoulder surgery. Patients received a continuous infusion of bupivacaine 0.15%, which might be supplemented with boluses as needed, i.e., PCIA. The rationale and technique is similar to PCA. Compared with PCA, the PCIA group experienced fewer side effects and greater patient satisfaction.

In the author's experience, a continuous interscalene block is a reliable, safe, and effective technique for producing prolonged postoperative analgesia following shoulder surgery.

CONCLUSION

Shoulder surgery may be safely performed under general or regional anesthesia. An interscalene brachial plexus block confers numerous advantages to the patient over general anesthesia. These include excellent intra- and postoperative analgesia, ideal operating conditions, and avoidance of side effects associated with general anesthesia. Prolonged postoperative analgesia can be achieved with an interscalene catheter.

REFERENCES

1. Ang E, Lassale B, Goldfarb G. Continuous axillary brachial plexus block—a clinical and anatomical study. *Anesth Analg* 1984;63:680–684.
2. Bailey P, Pace N, Ashburn M, Moll J, East K, Stanley T. Frequent hypoxemia and apnea after sedation with midazolam and fentanyl. *Anesthesiology* 1990;73:826–830.
3. Balas G. Regional anesthesia for surgery of the shoulder. *Anesth Analg* 1971;50:1036–1042.
4. Baranowski A, Pither C. A comparison of three methods of axillary brachial plexus anaesthesia. *Anaesthesia* 1990;45:362–365.
5. Barutell C, Vidal F, Raich M, Montero A. A neurological complication following interscalene brachial plexus block. *Anaesthesia* 1980;35:365–367.
6. Bashein G, Haschke R, Ready L. Electrical nerve location: numerical and electrophoretic comparison of insulated vs. uninsulated needles. *Anesth Analg* 1984;63:919–924.
7. Bedder M, Kozody R, Craig D. Comparison of bupivacaine and alkalinized bupivacaine in brachial plexus anesthesia. *Anesth Analg* 1988;67:48–52.
8. Benumof J. Laryngeal mask airway and the ASA difficult airway algorithm. *Anesthesiology* 1996;84:686–699.
9. Bernstein R, Rosenberg A. Ambulatory surgery. In: *Manual of orthopedic anesthesia and related pain syndromes*. New York: Churchill Livingstone, 1993:269–292.
10. Bernstein R, Rosenberg A. Regional anesthesia. In: *Manual of ortho-*

pedic anesthesia and related pain syndromes. New York: Churchill Livingstone, 1993:161–242.

11. Borgeat A, Schappi B, Biasca N, Gerber C. PCA versus PCIA after major shoulder surgery [Abstract]. *Anesth Analg* 1997;84(suppl):287.
12. Bourke D, Furman W. Improved postoperative analgesia with morphine added to axillary block solution. *J Clin Anesth* 1993;5:114–117.
13. Bouska G, Hecker R. The anesthetic implications of methylmethacrylate in prosthetic hip surgery. *Am J Anesthesiol* 1995;22:198–203.
14. Boyd O, Mackay C, Rushmer F, Bennett E, Grounds R. Propofol or midazolam for short-term alterations in sedation. *Can J Anaesth* 1993; 40:1142–1147.
15. Bridenbaugh L. The upper extremity: somatic blockade. In: Cousins M, Bridenbaugh P, eds. *Neural blockade*, 2nd ed. Philadelphia: JB Lippincott, 1988:387–416.
16. Bridenbaugh P. Preemptive analgesia—is it clinically relevant? *Anesth Analg* 1994;78:203–204.
17. Brown A. Early sign of successful bupivacaine interscalene block: the "money sign" [Letter]. *Reg Anesth* 1996;21:166–167.
18. Brown A, Broccoli E. An aid to the performance of interscalene blocks. *Anesthesiology* 1992;76:869–870.
19. Brown A, Weiss R, Greenberg C, Flatow E, Bigliani L. Interscalene block for shoulder arthroscopy: comparison with general anesthesia. *Arthroscopy* 1993;9:295–300.
20. Brown D, Ransom D, Hall J, Leicht C, Schroeder D, Offord K. Regional anesthesia and local anesthetic-induced systemic toxicity: seizure frequency and accompanying cardiovascular changes. *Anesth Analg* 1995;81:321–328.
21. Brull S, Lieponis J, Murphy M, Garcia R, Silverman D. Acute and long-term benefits of iliac crest donor site perfusion with local anesthetics. *Anesth Analg* 1992;74:145–147.
22. Burnett Y, Brennan M, Lubicky J, Kohli K. Efficacy of povidone-iodine, alcohol, and saline on the inhibition of bacterial growth from skin swabs in the caudal area. *Anesth Analg* 1995;80(suppl):62.
23. Buttner J, Ott B, Klose R. Effects of clonidine added to mepivacaine for brachial plexus block. *Anaesthetist* 1992;41:548–554.
24. Caplan R, Posner K, Cheney F. Perioperative ulnar neuropathy: are we ready for short cuts? *Anesthesiology* 1994;81:1321–1323.
25. Caplan R, Ward R, Posner K, Cheney F. Unexpected cardiac arrest during spinal anesthesia: a closed claims analysis of predisposing factors. *Anesthesiology* 1988;68:5–11.
26. Capogno G, Celleno D, Laudano D, Giunta F. Alkalinization of local anesthetics. *Reg Anesth* 1995;20:369–377.
27. Carpenter R. Clinicians remain hopeful about preemptive analgesia. *Anesth News* 1994;7:1.
28. Cheney F, Posner K, Caplan R. Adverse respiratory events infrequently leading to malpractice suits. *Anesthesiology* 1991;75: 932–939.
29. Code W. NSAIDs and balanced analgesia. *Can J Anaesth* 1993;40: 401–405.
30. Conn R, Cofield R, Byer D, Linstromberg J. Interscalene block anesthesia for shoulder surgery. *Clin Orthop Rel Res* 1987;216:94–98.
31. Conway J, Goldberg J, Chung F. Preadmission anaesthesia consultation clinic. *Can J Anaesth* 1992;39:1051–1057.
32. Cook L. Unsuspected extradural catheterization in an interscalene block. *Br J Anaesth* 1991;67:473–475.
33. Criswell J, Gauntlett I. Pain on intradermal injection with lidocaine. *Anaesthesia* 1991;46:691–692.
34. D'Alessio J, Rosenblum M, Shea K, Freitas D. A retrospective comparison of interscalene block and general anesthesia for ambulatory surgery shoulder arthroscopy. *Reg Anesth* 1995;20:62–68.
35. D'Alessio J, Rosenblum M, Weller R. Activation of the Bezold-Jarisch reflex in the sitting position for shoulder arthroscopy using interscalene block anesthesia. *Reg Anesth* 1994;19:75.
36. D'Alessio J, Weller R, Rosenblum M. Activation of the Bezold-Jarisch reflex in the sitting position for shoulder surgery using interscalene block. *Anesth Analg* 1995;80:1158–1162.
37. Dahl J, Kehlet H. The value of pre-emptive analgesia in the treatment of postoperative pain. *Br J Anaesth* 1993;70:434–439.
38. Dahl J, Rosenberg J, Dirkes W, Mogensen T, Kehlet H. Prevention of postoperative pain by balanced analgesia. *Br J Anaesth* 1990;64: 518–520.
39. De Andres J, Valia J, Gil A, Bolinches R. Predictors of patient satisfaction with regional anesthesia. *Reg Anesth* 1995;20:498–505.
40. de Jong R. Adverse effects and drug toxicity. In: *Local anesthetics*. St. Louis: Mosby, 1994:345–380.
41. de Jong R. Uptake, distribution, and elimination. In: de Jong R, ed. *Local anesthetics*. St. Louis: Mosby-Year Book, 1994:140–172.
42. de Jong R. Local anesthetic pharmacology. In: Brown D, ed. *Regional anesthesia and analgesia*. Philadelphia: WB Saunders, 1996: 124–142.
43. DeAndrade J, Maslanka M, Maneatis T, Bynum L, Burchmore M. The use of ketorolac in the management of postoperative pain. *Orthopedics* 1994;17:157–166.
44. DeKrey J, Balas G. Regional anesthesia for surgery of the shoulder. A review of 1500 cases. *Reg Anesth* 1981;4:46–48.
45. DeKrey J, Schroeder S, Buechel D. Continuous brachial plexus block. *Anesthesiology* 1969;30:332.
46. Dentz S, D'Ercole F, Edgar R, et al. Safety and efficacy of supplementing interscalene blocks [Abstract]. *Reg Anesth* 1996;21:22.
47. Dhuner K. Nerve injuries following operations: a surge of cases occurring during a 6 year period. *Anesthesiology* 1948;11:289.
48. DiFazio C. Toxicity of local anesthetics and dose selection. Presented at the XIIIth Annual ESRA, Barcelona, Spain, 1994:88–94.
49. Durrani Z, Winnie A. Brainstem toxicity with reversible locked-in syndrome after interscalene brachial plexus block. *Anesth Analg* 1991; 72:249–252.
50. Edde R, Deutsch S. Cardiac arrest after interscalene brachial-plexus block. *Anesth Analg* 1977;56:446–447.
51. Eledjam J, Deschodt J, Viel E, et al. Brachial plexus block with bupivacaine: effects of added alpha-adrenergic agonists: comparison between clonidine and epinephrine. *Can J Anaesth* 1991;38:870–875.
52. Elliott B. Positioning and monitoring. In: Wedel D, ed. *Orthopedic anesthesia*. New York: Churchill Livingstone, 1993:99–128.
53. Ferrante M, Rocco A, Gudman J, et al. A comparison of the efficacy of pain relief with PCA and standard intramuscular opioid therapy after total knee replacement. *Reg Anesth* 1987;12:94–95.
54. Finucane B, Yilling F. Safety of supplementing axillary brachial plexus blocks. *Anesthesiology* 1989;70:401–403.
55. Flory N, Van-Gessel E, Donald F, Hoffmeyer P, Gamulin Z. Does the addition of morphine to brachial plexus block improve analgesia after shoulder surgery? *Br J Anaesth* 1995;75:23–26.
56. Ford D, Pither C, Raj P. Comparison of insulated and uninsulated needles for locating peripheral nerves with a peripheral nerve stimulator. *Anesth Analg* 1984;63:925–928.
57. Foster A, Carlson B. Myotoxicity of local anesthetics and regeneration of the damaged muscle fibers. *Anesth Analg* 1980;58:727–736.
58. Gaumann D, Forster A, Griessen M, Habre W, Poinsot O, Della Santa D. Comparison between clonidine and epinephrine admixture to lidocaine in brachial plexus block. *Anesth Analg* 1992;75:69–74.
59. Gaumann D, Lennon R, Wedel D. Continuous axillary block for postoperative pain management. *Reg Anesth* 1988;13:77–82.
60. Gentili F, Hudson A, Hunter D, Kline D. Nerve injection injury with local anesthetic agents: a light and electron microscopic, fluorescent microscopic, and horseradish peroxide study. *Neurosurgery* 1980;6: 263–271.
61. Gentili M, Lefoulon-Gourves M, Mamelle J, Bonnet F. Acute respiratory failure following interscalene block: complications of combined general and regional anesthesia [Letter]. *Reg Anesth* 1994;19: 292–293.
62. Gentili M, Wargnier J. Peripheral nerve damage and regional anaesthesia [Letter]. *Br J Anaesth* 1993;70:594.
63. Gill S, Wright E, Reilly C. Pharmacokinetic interaction of propofol and fentanyl: single bolus injection study. *Br J Anaesth* 1990;65: 760–765.
64. Gold B, Weitz S, Lurie K. Intraoperative "syncope": evaluation with tilt-table testing. *Anesthesiology* 1992;76:635–637.
65. Goldberg M, Gregg C, Larijani G, Norris M, Marr A, Seltzer J. A comparison of three methods of axillary approach to brachial plexus blockade for upper extremity surgery. *Anesthesiology* 1987;66: 814–816.
66. Greenberg C, Brown A. Cost containment—utilization of techniques, personnel, equipment and supplies. In: White P, ed. *Ambulatory anesthesia and surgery*. London: WB Saunders, 1997:635–647.
67. Gross J, Bailey P, Caplan R, et al. Practice guidelines for sedation and analgesia by non-anesthesiologists: a report by the American Society of Anesthesiolgists task force on sedation and analgesia by non-anesthesiologists. *Anesthesiology* 1996;84:459–471.
68. Haasio J, Tuominen M, Rosenberg P. Continuous interscalene brachial plexus block during and after shoulder surgery. *Ann Chir Gynaecol* 1990;79:103–107.

69. Hartrick C, Raj P, Dirkes W Jr, Denson D. Compounding of bupivacaine and mepivacaine for regional anesthesia: a safe practice. *Reg Anesth* 1984;9:94–97.
70. Hilgier M. Alkalinization of bupivacaine for brachial plexus block. *Reg Anesth* 1985;8:59–61.
71. Hogan Q, Dotson R, Erickson S, Kettler R, Hogan K. Local anesthetic myotoxicity: a case and review. *Anesthesiology* 1994;80:942–947.
72. Huang K, Fitzgerald M, Tsueda K. Bilateral block of cervical and brachial plexuses following interscalene block. *Anaesth Intens Care* 1986;14:87–88.
73. Huffnagle S, Seltzer J, Torjman M, Marr A, Fenlin J. Does the use of methylmethacrylate cement in total shoulder replacement induce hemodynamic or pulmonary instability? *J Clin Anesth* 1993;5: 404–407.
74. Hynson J, Tung A, Guevara J, Katz J, Glick J, Shapiro W. Complete airway obstruction during arthroscopic shoulder surgery. *Anesth Analg* 1993;76:875–878.
75. Ichai C, Ciais J, Roussel L, et al. Intravascular absorption of glycine irrigating solution during shoulder arthroscopy: a case report and follow-up study. *Anesthesiology* 1996;85:1481–1485.
76. Johansen I, Benumof J. Methylmethacrylate: a myocardial depressant and peripheral dilator [Abstract]. *Anesthesiology* 1979;51:S77.
77. Johns F, Ziccardi V, Buckley M. Methohexital infusion technique for conscious sedation. *J Oral Maxillofac Surg* 1996;54:578–581.
78. Katz J, Kavanagh B, Sandler A, et al. Preemptive analgesia: clinical evidence of neuroplasticity contributing to postoperative pain. *Anesthesiology* 1992;77:439–446.
79. Kehlet H, Dahl J. The value of "multimodal" or "balanced analgesia" in postoperative pain treatment. *Anesth Analg* 1993;77:1048–1056.
80. Kestin I, Harvey P, Nixon C. Psychomotor recovery after three methods of sedation during spinal anaesthesia. *Br J Anaesth* 1990;64: 657–681.
81. King S, Davis F, Wells J, Murchison D, Pryor P. Lidocaine for the prevention of pain due to injection of propofol. *Anesth Analg* 1992;74: 246–249.
82. Kinnard P, Truchon R, St-Pierre A, Montreuil J. Interscalene block for pain relief after shoulder surgery: a prospective randomized study. *Clin Orthop Rel Res* 1994;304:22–24.
83. Kinsella J, Moffat A, Patrick J, Prentice J, McArdle C, Kenny G. Ketorolac trometamol for postoperative analgesia after orthopaedic surgery. *Br J Anaesth* 1992;69:19–22.
84. Kissin I. Preemptive analgesia. *Anesthesiology* 1996;84:1015–1019.
85. Klafta J, Roizen M. Current understanding of patients' attitudes toward and preparation for anesthesia: a review. *Anesth Analg* 1996;83: 1314–1321.
86. Kopacz D, Neal J, Pollock J. The regional anesthesia "learning curve." *Reg Anesth* 1996;21:182–190.
87. Kozody R, Ready L, Barsa J, Murphy T. Dose requirement of local anesthetic to produce grand mal seizure during stellate ganglion block. *Can Anaesth Soc J* 1982;29:489–491.
88. Kroll D, Caplan R, Posner K, Ward R, Cheney F. Nerve injury associated with anesthesia. *Anesthesiology* 1990;73:202–207.
89. Kumar A, Battit G, Froese A, Long M. Bilateral cervical and thoracic epidural blockade complicating interscalene brachial plexus block: report of two cases. *Anesthesiology* 1971;35:650–652.
90. Lanz E, Theiss D, Jankovic D. The extent of blockade following various techniques of brachial plexus block. *Anesth Analg* 1983;62: 55–58.
91. Lau K. Pneumomediastinum caused by subcutaneous emphysema in the shoulder. A rare complication of arthroscopy. *Chest* 1993;103: 1606–1607.
92. Lee H, Dewan N, Crosby N. Subcutaneous emphysema, pneumomediastinum, and potentially life-threatening tension pneumothorax. Pulmonary complications from arthroscopic shoulder decompression. *Chest* 1992;101:1265–1267.
93. Lim E. Inter-scalene brachial plexus block in the asthmatic patient. *Anaesthesia* 1979;34:370.
94. Lombard T, Couper J. Bilateral spread of analgesia following interscalene brachial plexus block. *Anesthesiology* 1983;58:472–473.
95. Macarthur A, Kleinman S. Rheumatoid cervical joint disease—a challenge to the anaesthetist. *Can J Anaesth* 1993;40:154–159.
96. Maurer P, Greek R, Torjman M, et al. Is regional anesthesia more time efficient than general anesthesia for shoulder surgery [Abstract]. *Anesthesiology* 1993;79:897.
97. McClain D, Finucane B. Interscalene approach to the brachial plexus: parasthesiae versus nerve stimulation. *Reg Anesth* 1987;12:80–83.
98. McClure J. Ropivacaine [Review]. *Br J Anaesth* 1996;76:300–307.
99. McKay W, Morris R, Mushlin P. Sodium bicarbonate attenuates pain on skin infiltration with lidocaine, with or without epinephrine. *Anesth Analg* 1987;66:572–574.
100. McQuay H, Carroll D, Moore R. Postoperative orthopaedic pain—the effect of opiate premedication and local anaesthetic blocks. *Pain* 1988;33:291–295.
101. Mitchell E, Murphy F, Wyche M, Torg J. Interscalene brachial plexus block anesthesia for the modified Bristow procedure. *Am J Sports Med* 1982;10:79–82.
102. Montgomery S, Raj P, Nettles D, Jenkins M. The use of the nerve stimulator with standard unsheathed needles in nerve blocks. *Anesth Analg* 1973;52:827–831.
103. Moore D, Bridenbaugh L, Thompson G, Balfour R, Horton W. Factors determining dosages of amide-type local anesthetic drugs. *Anesthesiology* 1977;47:263–268.
104. Moore D, Mulroy M, Thompson G. Peripheral nerve damage and regional anaesthesia [Editorial]. *Br J Anaesth* 1994;73:435–436.
105. Moran T, Little W, Mendez R, Trentalange M. Axillary blockade utilizing perineuronal meperidine a prospective, randomized, double-blind study. Orlando, FL: ASRA, 1995:33.
106. Morris R, McKay W, Mushlin P. Comparison of pain on skin infiltration of local anesthetics. *Reg Anesth* 1987;12:93.
107. Mulroy M. Complications of regional anesthesia. In: Mulroy M, ed. *Regional anesthesia: an illustrated procedural guide*. Boston: Little, Brown, 1989:31–43.
108. Myers R, Heckman H. Effects of local anesthesia on nerve blood flow: studies using lidocaine with and without epinephrine. *Anesthesiology* 1989;71:757–762.
109. Neal J, McMahon D. Induction of regional anesthesia: equipment. In: Brown D, ed. *Regional anesthesia and analgesia*. Philadelphia: WB Saunders, 1996:159–172.
110. Newson C, Joshi G, Victory R, White P. Comparison of propofol administration techniques for sedation during monitored anesthesia care. *Anesth Analg* 1995;81:486–491.
111. Pandit S, Pandit U. Phases of the recovery period. In: White P, ed. *Ambulatory anesthesia and surgery*. London: WB Saunders, 1997: 457–464.
112. Parks B. Postoperative peripheral neuropathies. *Surgery* 1973;74:348.
113. Partridge B. The effects of local anesthetics and epinephrine on rat sciatic nerve blood flow. *Anesthesiology* 1991;75:243–251.
114. Passannante A. Spinal anesthesia and permanent neurologic deficit after interscalene block. *Anesth Analg* 1996;82:873–874.
115. Patterson K, Scanlon P. An unusual complication of brachial plexus sheath cannulation. *Br J Anaesth* 1990;65:542–543.
116. Penning J. Pre-emptive analgesia: what does it mean to the clinical anaesthetist? *Can J Anaesth* 1996;43:97–101.
117. Pere P, Pitkanen M, Rosenberg P, et al. Effect of continuous interscalene brachial plexus block on diaphragm motion and on ventilatory function. *Acta Anaesthesiol Scand* 1992;36:53–57.
118. Pere P, Tuominen M, Rosenberg P. Cumulation of bupivacaine, desbutylbupivacaine and 4-hydroxybupivacaine during and after continuous interscalene brachial plexus block. *Acta Anaesthesiol Scand* 1991;35:647–650.
119. Perreault L, Drolet P, Farny J. Ulnar nerve palsy at the elbow after general anesthesia. *Can J Anaesth* 1992;39:499–503.
120. Peterson D. Shoulder block for anesthesia for shoulder reconstruction surgery. *Anesth Analg* 1985;64:373–375.
121. Pihlajamäki K, Lindberg R. Bupivacaine with and without adrenaline in interscalene brachial plexus blockade. Studies in patients with rheumatoid arthritis. *Br J Anaesth* 1987;59:1420–1424.
122. Pither C, Raj P, Ford D. The use of peripheral nerve stimulators for regional anesthesia: a review of experimental characteristics, technique, and clinical applications. *Reg Anesth* 1985;10:49–58.
123. Plevak D, Linstromberg J, Danielson D. Paresthesia vs nonparesthesia—the axillary block [Abstract]. *Anesthesiology* 1983;59:216.
124. Plummer J, Owen H, Ilsley A, Tordoff K. Sustained-release ibuprofen as an adjunct to morphine patient-controlled analgesia. *Anesth Analg* 1996;83:92–96.
125. Polster M, Gray P, O'Sullivan G, McCarthy R, Park G. Comparison of the sedative and amnesic effects of midazolam and propofol. *Brit J Anaesth* 1993;70:612–616.

126. Power I, Brown D, Wildsmith J. The effect of fentanyl, meperidine and diamorphine on nerve conduction in vitro. *Reg Anesth* 1991;16: 204–208.
127. Raj P. Ancillary measures to assure success (in peripheral nerve blocks). *Reg Anesth* 1980;5:9–12.
128. Raj P. Continuous brachial plexus analgesia. San Diego: ASRA, 1996: 499–502.
129. Ramirez-Ruiz M, Smith I, White P. Use of analgesics during propofol sedation: a comparison of ketorolac, dezocine, and fentanyl. *J Clin Anesth* 1995;7:481–485.
130. Ransom D, Leicht C. Postdelivery analgesia. In: Brown D, ed. *Regional anesthesia and analgesia*. Philadelphia: WB Saunders, 1996: 625–631.
131. Rice A, McMahon S. Peripheral nerve damage and regional anaesthesia [Letter]. *Br J Anaesth* 1993;70:527.
132. Richmond C, Bromley L, Woolf C. Preoperative morphine pre-empts postoperative pain. *Lancet* 1993;342:73–75.
133. Riegler F. Brachial plexus block with the nerve stimulator: motor response characteristics at three sites. *Reg Anesth* 1992;17:295–299.
134. Roch J, Sharrock N. Hypotension during shoulder arthroscopy in the sitting position under interscalene block. *Reg Anesth* 1991;15:64.
135. Roch J, Sharrock N, Neudachin L. Interscalene brachial plexus block for shoulder surgery: a proximal paresthesia is effective. *Anesth Analg* 1992;75:386–388.
136. Roizen M, Fischer S. Preoperative evaluation: adults and children. In: White P, ed. *Ambulatory anesthesia and surgery*. London: WB Saunders, 1997:155–172.
137. Rosenberg P, Pere P, Hekali R, Tuominen M. Plasma concentrations of bupivacaine and two of its metabolites during continuous interscalene brachial plexus block. *Br J Anaesth* 1991;66:25–30.
138. Rosenberg P, Renkonen O. Anti-microbial activity of bupivacaine and morphine. *Anesthesiology* 1985;62:178–179.
139. Ross S, Scarborough C. Total spinal anesthesia following brachial plexus block. *Anesthesiology* 1973;39:458.
140. Sakuragi T, Ishino H, Dan K. Bacteriacidal activity of clinically used local anesthetics on *Staphylococcus aureus*. *Reg Anesth* 1996;21: 239–242.
141. Salcedo E, Shay P, Berrigan M, et al. The pre-emptive analgesic effect of interscalene block prior to shoulder surgery. *Reg Anesth* 1996;21: 107.
142. Sarma V. Long-term continuous axillary plexus blockade using 0.25% bupivacaine—a study of three cases. *Acta Anaesthesiol Scand* 1990; 34:511–513.
143. Scammell S. Inadvertent epidural anaesthesia as a complication of interscalene brachial plexus block. *Anaesth Intens Care* 1979;7:56–57.
144. Schwieger I, Hall R, Szlam F, Hug C Jr. Anesthetic interactions of midazolam and fentanyl: is there acute tolerance to the opioid. *Anesthesiology* 1989;70:667–671.
145. Scott D. "Maximum recommended doses" of local anaesthetic drugs. *Br J Anaesth* 1989;63:373–374.
146. Selander D. Paresthesias or no parasthesias? Nerve complications after neural blockades. *Acta Anaesthesiol Belg* 1988;39:173–174.
147. Selander D. Peripheral nerve damage and regional anesthesia [Letter]. *Br J Anaesth* 1995;75:116–117.
148. Selander D, Brattsand R, Lundborg G, Nordborg C, Olsson Y. Local anesthetics: importance of mode of application, concentration and adrenaline for the appearance of nerve lesions. An experimental study of axonal degeneration and barrier damage after intrafascicular injection or topical application of bupivacaine (marcain). *Acta Anaesthesiol Scand* 1979;23:127–136.
149. Selander D, Dhunér K-G, Lundborg G. Peripheral nerve injury due to injection needles used for regional anesthesia: an experimental study of the acute effects of needle point trauma. *Acta Anaesthesiol Scand* 1977;21:182–188.
150. Selander D, Edshage S, Wolff T. Paresthesiae or no paresthesiae? Nerve lesions after axillary blocks. *Acta Anaesthesop; Scand* 1979;23: 27–33.
151. Selander D, Sjöstrand J. Longitudinal spread of intraneurally injected local anesthetics: an experimental study of the initial neural distribution following intraneural injections. *Acta Anaesthesiol Scand* 1978; 22:622–634.
152. Seltzer J. Hoarseness and Horner's syndrome after interscalene brachial plexus block. *Anesth Analg* 1977;56:585–586.
153. Seltzer J, Greek R, Maurer P, et al. The preemptive analgesic effect of regional anesthesia for shoulder surgery [Abstract]. *Anesthesiology* 1993;79:815.
154. Sevarino F, Sinatra R, Paige D, Ning T, Brull S, Silverman D. The efficacy of intramuscular ketorolac in combination with intravenous PCA morphine for postoperative pain relief. *J Clin Anesth* 1992;4: 285–288.
155. Sharrock N. Complications of orthopedic anesthesia. *Semin Anesth* 1996;15:288–294.
156. Sharrock N, Bruce G. An improved technique for locating the interscalene groove. *Anesthesiology* 1976;44:431–433.
157. Singelyn F, Gouverneur J, Robert A. A minimum dose of clonidine added to mepivacaine prolongs the duration of anesthesia and analgesia after axillary brachial plexus block. *Anesth Analg* 1996;83: 1046–1050.
158. Skues M, Welchew E. Anaesthesia and rheumatoid arthritis. *Anaesthesia* 1993;48:989–997.
159. Skyhar M, Altcheck D, Warren R, Wickiewicz T, O'Brien S. Shoulder arthroscopy with the patient in the beach-chair position. *Arthroscopy* 1988;4:256–259.
160. Smith I. Monitored anesthesia care: how much sedation, how much analgesia? *J Clin Anesth* 1996;8(suppl):76–80.
161. Smith I, White P. Use of the laryngeal mask airway as an alternative to a facemask during outpatient arthroscopy. *Anesthesiology* 1992;77: 850–855.
162. Smith I, White P, Nathanson M, Gouldson R. Propofol: an update on its clinical use. *Anesthesiology* 1994;81:1005–1043.
163. Sonne N, Clausen T, Valentin M, Halck S, Munksgaard A. Total intravenous anaesthesia for direct laryngoscopy: propofol infusion compared to thiopentone combined with midazolam and methohexitone infusion. *Acta Anaesthesiol Scand* 1992;36:250–254.
164. Sprung J, Distel D, Grass J, Bloomfield E, Lavery I. Cardiovascular collapse during anesthesia in a patient with preoperatively discontinued chronic MAO inhibitor therapy. *J Clin Anesth* 1996;8:662–665.
165. Stafford-Smith M. Impaired haemostasis and regional anaesthesia. *Can J Anaesth* 1996;43:R129–135.
166. Stoelting R. Postoperative ulnar nerve palsy—is it a preventable complication? *Anesth Analg* 1993;76:7–9.
167. Stoelting R. Nerve injury during anesthesia. *ASA Newsletter* 1994;58: 6–9.
168. Taylor E, Ghouri A, White P. Midazolam in combination with propofol for sedation during local anesthesia. *J Clin Anesth* 1992;4:213–216.
169. Tetzlaff J, Yoon H, Brems J. Patient acceptance of interscalene block for shoulder surgery. *Reg Anesth* 1993;18:30–33.
170. Tetzlaff J, Yoon H, Brems J. Interscalene brachial plexus block for shoulder surgery. *Reg Anesth* 1994;19:339–343.
171. Tetzlaff J, Yoon H, Brems J, Javorsky T. Alkalinization of mepivacaine improves the quality of motor block associated with interscalene brachial plexus anesthesia for shoulder surgery. *Reg Anesth* 1995;20: 128–132.
172. Tetzlaff J, Yoon H, O'Hara J, Reaney J, Stein D, Grimes-Rice M. Alkalinization of mepivacaine accelerates onset of interscalene block for shoulder surgery. *Reg Anesth* 1990;15:242–244.
173. Tetzlaff J, Yoon H, Dilger J, Brems J. Subdural anesthesia as a complication of an interscalene brachial plexus block. *Reg Anesth* 1994; 19:357–359.
174. Thiagarajah S, Lear E, Azar I, Salzer J, Zeiligsohn E. Bronchospasm following interscalene brachial plexus block. *Anesthesiology* 1984;61: 759–761.
175. Thompson G, Liu A. Perioperative nerve injury. In: Benumof JL, Saidman LJ (eds.) Anesthesia and Perioperative Complications. St. Louis: Mosby Year Book, Inc., 1992:160–172.
176. Tucker G, Mather L. Properties absorption, and disposition of local anaesthetic agents. In: Cousins M, Bridenbaugh, P, eds. *Neural blockade*. Philadelphia: JB Lippincott, 1988:47–110.
177. Tuominen M, Haasio J, Hekali R, Rosenberg P. Continuous interscalene brachial plexus block: clinical efficacy, technical problems and bupivacaine plasma concentrations. *Acta Anaesthesiol Scand* 1989; 33:84–88.
178. Tuominen M, Pere P, Rosenberg P. Unintentional arterial catheterization and bupivacaine toxicity associated with continuous interscalene brachial plexus block. *Anesthesiology* 1991;75:356–358.
179. Tuominen M, Rosenberg P, Kalso E. Blood levels of bupivacaine after single dose, supplementary dose and during continuous infusion in axillary plexus block. *Acta Anaesthesiol Scand* 1983;27:303–306.

180. Urban M, Urquhart B. Evaluation of brachial plexus anesthesia for upper extremity surgery. *Regional Anesth* 1994;19:175–182.
181. Urmey W. Upper extremity blocks. In: Brown D, ed. *Regional anesthesia and analgesia*. Philadelphia: WB Saunders, 1996:254–278.
182. Urmey W, Gloeggler P. Pulmonary function changes during interscalene brachial plexus block: effects of decreasing local anesthetic injection volume. *Reg Anesth* 1993;18:244–249.
183. Urmey W, McDonald M. Hemidiaphragmatic paresis during interscalene brachial plexus block: effects on pulmonary function and chest wall mechanics. *Anesth Analg* 1992;74:352–357.
184. Urmey W, Talts K, Sharrock N. One hundred percent incidence of hemidiaphragmatic paresis associated with interscalene brachial plexus anesthesia as diagnosed by ultrasonography. *Anesth Analg* 1991;72:498–503.
185. Urquhart M, White P. Comparison of sedative infusions during regional anesthesia: methohexital, etomidate, and midazolam. *Anesth Analg* 1989;68:249–254.
186. Vester-Andersen T, Christiansen C, Hansen A, Sorensen M, Meisler C. Interscalene brachial plexus block: area of analgesia, complications and blood concentrations of local anesthetics. *Acta Anaesth Scand* 1981;25:81–84.
187. Viel E, Eledjam J, DeLaCoussaye J, Athis F. Brachial plexus block with opioids for postoperative pain relief: comparison between buprenorphine and morphine. *Reg Anesth* 1989;14:274–278.
188. Wansbrough S, White P. Sedation scales: measures of calmness or somnolence? *Anesth Analg* 1993;76:219–221.
189. Ward M. The interscalene approach to the brachial plexus. *Anaesthesia* 1974;29:147–157.
190. Warner M, Warner M, Martin J. Ulnar neuropathy: incidence, outcome and risk factors in sedated or anesthetized patients. *Anesthesiology* 1994;81:1332–1340.
191. Wells D, Bjorksten A. Monoamine oxidase inhibitors revisited [Review]. *Can J Anaesth* 1989;36:64–74.
192. White P. Ambulatory anesthesia and surgery: past, present, and future. In: White P, ed. *Ambulatory anesthesia and surgery*. London: WB Saunders, 1997:3–34.
193. White P, Negus J. Sedative infusions during local and regional anesthesia: a comparison of midazolam and propofol. *J Clin Anesth* 1991; 3:32–39.
194. Wiener D, Speer K. The deltoid sign. *Anesth Analg* 1994;79:192.
195. Wildsmith J, Tucker G, Cooper S, Scott D, Covino B. Plasma concentrations of local anaesthetics after interscalene brachial plexus block. *Br J Anaesth* 1977;49:461–465.
196. Wilson E, David A, Mackenzie N, Grant I. Sedation during spinal anaesthesia: comparison of propofol and midazolam. *Br J Anaesth* 1990;64:48–52.
197. Winchell S, Wolfe R. The incidence of neuropathy following upper extremity nerve blocks. *Reg Anesth* 1985;10:12–15.
198. Winnie A. An "immobile needle" for nerve blocks. *Anesthesiology* 1969;31:577–578.
199. Winnie A. Interscalene brachial plexus block. *Anesth Analg* 1970;49: 455–466.
200. Winnie A. Clinical considerations: choice of local anesthetic agents. In: Winnie A, ed. *Plexus anesthesia*. Philadelphia: WB Saunders, 1990:197–202.
201. Winnie A. Considerations concerning complications, side effects, and untoward sequelae. In: *Plexus anesthesia*. Philadelphia: WB Saunders, 1990:221–266.
202. Winnie A. Perivascular techniques of brachial plexus block. In: Winnie A, ed. *Plexus anesthesia*. Philadelphia: WB Saunders, 1990:117–188.
203. Wong H, Carpenter R, Kopacz D, et al. A randomized, double-blind evaluation of ketorolac tromethamine for postoperative analgesia in ambulatory surgery patients. *Anesthesiology* 1993;78:6–14.
204. Woolf C, Chong M-S. Preemptive analgesia—treating postoperative pain by preventing the establishment of central sensitization. *Anesth Analg* 1993;77:362–379.
205. Zablocki A, Baysinger C, Epps J, Bucknell A. Cervical epidural anesthesia for surgery of the shoulder. *Orthop Rev* 1987;16:65–70.

Subject Index

Subject Index

M